Illana Rubenchik

Comprehensive Cytopathology

Marluce Bibbo, M.D., Sc.D., F.I.A.C.
Professor and Director,
Section of Cytopathology
The University of Chicago
Chicago, Illinois

Comprehensive Cytopathology

W.B. SAUNDERS COMPANY
A Division of Harcourt Brace & Company

Philadelphia   London   Toronto   Montreal   Sydney   Tokyo

W.B. SAUNDERS COMPANY
A Division of
Harcourt Brace & Company

The Curtis Center
Independence Square West
Philadelphia, PA 19106

Library of Congress Cataloging-in-Publication Data

Comprehensive cytopathology / [edited by] Marluce Bibbo.

    p.   cm.

ISBN 0–7216–2937–7

1. Cytodiagnosis.   I. Bibbo, Marluce.

RB43.C645

616.075′82–dc20   90–8535

Acquisitions Editor: Darlene Pedersen
Developmental Editor: Leslie Hoeltzel
Designer: Joan Wendt
Production Manager: Linda R. Turner
Manuscript Editor: Mary Anne Folcher
Illustration Coordinator: Walt Verbitski
Indexer: Ellen Murray

Comprehensive Cytopathology   ISBN 0–7216–2937–7

Printed in the United States of America

Last digit is the print number: 9   8   7   6   5   4

Dedication

To the memory of my father,
to my mother Yolanda
and to my siblings
Maria, Magda, Marley, Marcia, Mara and Marcos.

Contributors

George H. Anderson, M.B.B.S., F.R.C.P.(C.), F.I.A.C.
Clinical Professor of Pathology, Department of Pathology, University of British Columbia Faculty of Medicine; Director, Division of Cytology, Cancer Control Agency of British Columbia, Vancouver, British Columbia.
Chapter 3, Cytologic Screening Programs

Jan P. A. Baak, M.D., Ph.D.
Professor of Pathology and Head, Department of Quantitative Pathology, Free University Hospital, Amsterdam, The Netherlands.
Chapter 35, Morphometry

Gunter F. Bahr, M.D., F.I.A.C.
Professor and Chairman Emeritus, Department of Cellular Pathology, Armed Forces Institute of Pathology, Washington, D.C.; Professor, Cytology Laboratory, Beckenried, Switzerland.
Chapter 1, The Cell: Basic Structure and Function

Peter H. Bartels, Ph.D., F.I.A.C.
Professor of Optical Sciences and of Pathology, Optical Sciences Center, University of Arizona, Tucson, Arizona.
Chapter 33, Light Optical Microscopy, Chapter 36, Cell Image Analysis

Christine Bergeron, M.D., Ph.D.
Staff Pathologist, Institut de Pathologie et Cytologie Appliquées, Paris, France.
Chapter 39, In Situ Hybridization

Lisa M. Bibb, M.D.
Clinical Assistant Professor of Pathology, College of Medicine at Chicago, University of Illinois College of Medicine; Director, Section of Cytopathology, Illinois Masonic Medical Center, Chicago, Illinois.
Chapter 31, Effects of Therapy on Cytologic Specimens

Marluce Bibbo, M.D., Sc.D., F.I.A.C.
Professor and Director, Section of Cytopathology, The University of Chicago, Chicago, Illinois.
Chapter 4, Diagnostic Quality Assurance in Cytopathology, Chapter 7, Hormonal Cytology, Chapter 36, Cell Image Analysis

Sandra H. Bigner, M.D.
Professor of Pathology, Duke University Medical Center; Associate Chief, Division of Cytopathology and Cytogenetics, Duke University Medical Center, Durham, North Carolina.
Chapter 18, Central Nervous System

Ricardo Gonzalez Campora, M.D., M.I.A.C.
Associate Professor of Pathology, Faculty of Medicine; Jefe de Servicio de Anatomía Patológica, Hospital Universitario Virgen Macarena, Seville, Spain.
Chapter 25, Thyroid

Gordon Canti, M.B.B.S.(Lond), M.R.C.S., L.R.C.P., F.R.C.Path., M.I.A.C.
Consultant Cytopathologist (Retired), St. Bartholomew's Hospital, London, England.
Chapter 21, Skin

Cornelis J. Cornelisse, Ph.D.
Associate Professor of Analytical Cytology, Department of Pathology, State University of Leiden, Leiden, The Netherlands.
Chapter 37, Flow Cytometry

Dilip K. Das, M.D., Ph.D.
Deputy Director, Institute of Cytopathology and Preventive Oncology, New Delhi, India; Assistant Professor, Department of Pathology, Kuwait University, Safat, Kuwait.
Chapter 26, Lymph Nodes

Hugo Galera Davidson, M.D., F.I.A.C.
Professor of Pathology, Faculty of Medicine; Chairman of Pathology, Hospital Universitario *Virgen Macarena*, Seville, Spain.
Chapter 25, Thyroid

Wenancjusz M. Domagala, M.D., M.I.A.C.
Professor of Tumor Pathology, Medical Academy, Szczecin, Poland.
Chapter 38, Immunocytochemistry

Harvey E. Dytch, S.B., P.M.I.A.C.
Senior Scientific Analyst, Head, Artificial Intelligence/Adaptive Pattern Recognition Center, Section of Cytopathology, The University of Chicago, Chicago, Illinois.
Chapter 36, Cell Image Analysis

Stephen R. Ell, M.D., Ph.D.
Associate Professor of Radiology and Adjunct Associate Professor of History, University of Utah; Associate Professor and Chief of Chest Radiology, University of Utah School of Medicine; Chief, Radiology Service, Veterans Administration Medical Center, Salt Lake City, Utah.
Chapter 23, Imaging Techniques

Craig E. Elson, M.D.
Director of Cytopathology, Department of Pathology, Research Medical Center, Kansas City, Missouri.
Chapter 14, Respiratory Tract

Alex Ferenczy, M.D., M.I.A.C.
Professor of Pathology and Obstetrics and Gynecology, McGill University Faculty of Medicine; Department of Pathology, The Sir Mortimer B. Davis Jewish General Hospital, Montreal, Quebec, Canada.
Chapter 39, In Situ Hybridization

Denise Frias-Hidvegi, M.D., F.I.A.C.
Associate Professor of Pathology and Obstetrics and Gynecology, Northwestern University Medical School; Director of Cytology and Associate Pathologist, Northwestern Memorial Hospital and Veterans Administration Lakeside Medical Center, Chicago, Illinois.
Chapter 34, Electron Microscopy

John K. Frost, M.D., F.I.A.C.*
Professor of Pathology, Johns Hopkins University School of Medicine; Pathologist, Johns Hopkins Hospital, Baltimore, Maryland.
Chapter 6, Pathologic Processes Affecting Cells from Inflammation to Cancer

Ben J. Glasgow, M.D.
Resident in Ophthalmology, Jules Stein Institute, University of California, Los Angeles, UCLA Medical Center, Los Angeles, California.
Chapter 19, Eye

John R. Goellner, M.D., M.I.A.C.
Professor of Pathology, Mayo Medical School; Rochester Methodist Hospital and Saint Mary's Hospital, Rochester, Minnesota.
Chapter 5, Evaluation of the Cellular Sample

Prabodh K. Gupta, M.D., F.I.A.C.
Professor of Pathology and Laboratory Medicine and Director of Cytopathology and Cytometry Section, Division of Anatomic Pathology, University of

Pennsylvania Medical Center, Philadelphia, Pennsylvania.
Chapter 8, Microbiology, Inflammation and Viral Infections

A. Marion Gurley, M.B., Ch.B.
Senior Resident in Pathology, Northwestern University Medical School, Chicago, Illinois.
Chapter 34, Electron Microscopy

Steven I. Hajdu, M.D., F.I.A.C.
Professor of Pathology, Cornell University Medical College; Attending Pathologist and Chief, Cytology Service, Department of Pathology, Memorial Sloan-Kettering Cancer Center, New York, New York.
Chapter 20, Soft Tissue and Bone

Hi Young Hong, M.D.
Associate Pathologist, Riverview Hospital, Wisconsin Rapids, Wisconsin.
Chapter 31, Effects of Therapy on Cytologic Specimens

O. A. N. Husain, M.D., F.R.C.Path., F.R.C.O.G., F.I.A.C.
Consultant Pathologist and Director, Department of Cytopathology, Charing Cross Hospital (Medical School), London, England.
Chapter 16, Alimentary Tract (Esophagus, Stomach, Colon, Rectum)

Stanley L. Inhorn, M.D., F.I.A.C.
Professor of Pathology and Laboratory Medicine, University of Wisconsin Medical School; Medical Director, Wisconsin State Laboratory of Hygiene, Madison, Wisconsin.
Chapter 2, Basic and Clinical Cytogenetics

William W. Johnston, M.D., F.I.A.C.
Professor of Pathology, Duke University School of Medicine; Chief, Division of Cytopathology and Cytogenetics, Duke University Medical Center, Durham, North Carolina.
Chapter 14, Respiratory Tract

Ruth L. Katz, M.D., M.I.A.C.
Associate Professor of Pathology, Associate Pathologist and Chief, Section of Cytopathology, The University of Texas M. D. Anderson Cancer Center, Houston, Texas.
Chapter 28, Kidney, Adrenal and Retroperitoneum

Catherine M. Keebler, C.F.I.A.C.
Technical Director, Cytopathology Laboratory, University of Chicago Hospitals, Chicago, Illinois.
Chapter 4, Diagnostic Quality Assurance in Cytopathology, Chapter 32, Cytopreparatory Techniques

William H. Kern, M.D., F.I.A.C.
Clinical Professor of Pathology, University of Southern California School of Medicine; Medical Director, Department of Pathology, Hospital of the Good Samaritan, Los Angeles, California.
Chapter 17, Urinary Tract

*Deceased, 1990.

Torsten Löwhagen, M.D., F.I.A.C.
Consultant Cytopathologist, Division of Clinical Cytology, Department of Pathology, Karolinska Hospital, Stockholm, Sweden.
Chapter 24, Salivary Glands and Rare Head and Neck Lesions, Chapter 29, Prostate

Diane B. Mandell, C.T. (A.S.C.P.), C.M.I.A.C.
Supervisor, Cytology Service, University of California, Los Angeles, UCLA Medical Center, Los Angeles, California.
Chapter 19, Eye

Bernard Naylor, M.B., Ch.B., F.I.A.C.
Professor of Pathology, The University of Michigan; Director of Cytopathology, The University of Michigan Hospitals, Ann Arbor, Michigan.
Chapter 22, Pleural, Peritoneal and Pericardial Fluids

Alan B. P. Ng, M.D., F.I.A.C.
Professor of Pathology, University of Sydney, Sydney; Head, Department of Anatomic Pathology, Royal Prince Alfred Hospital, Camperdown, New South Wales, Australia.
Chapter 11, Endometrial Hyperplasia and Carcinoma and Extrauterine Cancer

Mary Osborn, Ph.D.
Honorary Professor, University of Göttingen; Scientific Staff Member, Max Planck Institute for Biophysical Chemistry, Göttingen, Federal Republic of Germany.
Chapter 38, Immunocytochemistry

Norman F. Pacey, M.D., F.I.A.C.
Head, Institute of Clinical Pathology and Medical Research, Cytology Department, Westmead Hospital, Westmead, New South Wales, Australia.
Chapter 10, Glandular Neoplasms of the Uterine Cervix

Dorothy L. Rosenthal, M.D., F.I.A.C.
Professor of Pathology, University of California, Los Angeles, UCLA School of Medicine; Head, Cytology Service, University of California, UCLA Medical Center, Los Angeles, California.
Chapter 19, Eye

Patricia E. Saigo, M.D., M.I.A.C.
Associate Professor, Cornell University Medical College; Associate Attending Pathologist, Memorial Sloan-Kettering Cancer Center, New York, New York.
Chapter 13, Unusual Tumors

Jan F. Silverman, M.D., M.I.A.C.
Professor, Department of Clinical Pathology and Diagnostic Medicine, East Carolina University School of Medicine; Director of Cytology, Pitt County Memorial Hospital, Greenville, North Carolina.
Chapter 27, Breast

Sol Silverman, Jr., D.D.S.
Professor and Chairman, School of Dentistry, University of California at San Francisco, San Francisco, California.
Chapter 15, Oral Cavity

Lambert Skoog, M.D., Ph.D.
Assistant Professor, Department of Pathology, Karolinska Institute; Consultant Cytopathologist, Division of Clinical Cytology, Department of Pathology, Karolinska Hospital, Stockholm, Sweden.
Chapter 24, Salivary Glands and Rare Head and Neck Lesions, Chapter 29, Prostate

Theresa M. Somrak, J.D., C.T.(A.S.C.P.), C.M.I.A.C.
Supervisor and Educational Coordinator, Cytopathology Laboratory, University Hospitals of Cleveland, Cleveland, Ohio.
Chapter 12, Vulva and Vagina

Kelly Sorensen, M.D.*
Assistant Professor of Pathology, Case Western Reserve University School of Medicine; Director of Cytopathology Laboratory, University Hospitals of Cleveland, Cleveland, Ohio.
Chapter 12, Vulva and Vagina

Edneia Miyki Tani, M.D., Ph.D.
Consultant Cytopathologist, Division of Clinical Cytology, Department of Pathology, Karolinska Hospital, Stockholm, Sweden.
Chapter 24, Salivary Glands and Rare Head and Neck Lesions, Chapter 29, Prostate

Hans J. Tanke, Ph.D.
Associate Professor of Cell Biology, Laboratory for Cytochemistry and Cytometry, State University of Leiden, Leiden, The Netherlands.
Chapter 37, Flow Cytometry

Liang-Che Tao, M.D., F.R.C.P.C.
Professor of Pathology, Indiana University School of Medicine; Director, Division of Cytopathology, Indiana University Hospital, Indianapolis, Indiana.
Chapter 30, Liver and Pancreas

Paul J. van Diest, M.D., Ph.D.
Staff Member, Department of Pathology, Free University Hospital, Amsterdam, The Netherlands.
Chapter 35, Morphometry

G. Peter Vooijs, M.D., Ph.D., F.I.A.C.
Professor of Pathology, Department of Pathology, University of Nijmegen; Chairman, Department of Pathology, St. Radboud Academic Hospital, The Netherlands.
Chapter 9, Benign Proliferative Reactions, Intraepithelial Neoplasia and Invasive Cancer of the Uterine Cervix

*Deceased, 1990.

Jami L. Walloch, M.D.
Clinical Assistant Professor, Loyola University Medical Center, Maywood; Associate Pathologist, Saint Therese Medical Center, Waukegan; Consultant Pathologist, Veterans Administration Hospital, Hines, Illinois.
Chapter 31, Effects of Therapy on Cytologic Specimens

George L. Wied, M.D., F.I.A.C.
Professor and Former Director, Section of Cytopathology, The University of Chicago, Chicago, Illinois.
Chapter 4, Diagnostic Quality Assurance in Cytopathology, Chapter 7, Hormonal Cytology, Chapter 36, Cell Image Analysis

Preface

As the body of knowledge in the field of cytopathology has increased dramatically over the past few years, especially with regard to applications of new technology, the need for a comprehensive textbook has become apparent. *Comprehensive Cytopathology* has been written to fill that void and to present in-depth coverage of the field. The goal has been to place within a single book discussions of general cytopathology (Part I in *Comprehensive Cytopathology*), diagnostic cytology (Part II) and special techniques (Part III). *Comprehensive Cytopathology* thus will serve as a reference for practicing cytopathologists, pathologists and cytotechnologists and as a valuable source for residents and cytotechnologists who are training in cytopathology.

Part I, General Cytology, consists of chapters on basic cell structure and function, basic and clinical cytogenetics, cytologic screening programs, diagnostic quality assurance in cytopathology, evaluation of the cellular sample and pathologic processes affecting cells from inflammation to cancer.

The chapters in Part II, Diagnostic Cytology, present information in a uniform format that includes sampling techniques, basic histology, cytologic features of the various lesions, correlation to clinical and histologic findings, differential diagnosis and diagnostic accuracy. Part II is organized into four sections. Section A contains seven chapters on diagnostic cytology of the female genital tract. Within Section B are nine chapters on cytology of various body sites, including the respiratory tract, oral cavity, alimentary tract, urinary tract, central nervous system, eye, soft tissue and bone, skin and pleural, peritoneal and pericardial fluids. Section C encompasses eight chapters on fine needle aspiration of various organs and body sites. Finally, Section D consists of one chapter that discusses the effects of therapy on cytologic specimens in all body sites.

A comprehensive book on cytopathology would be incomplete without chapters on special techniques, found in Part III. A chapter on cytopreparatory techniques is included and chapters describing the principles and applications of light optical microscopy, electron microscopy, morphometry, cell image analysis, flow cytometry, immunocytochemistry and *in situ* hybridization are also presented.

Among the unique features in *Comprehensive Cytopathology* are the emphasis on sampling methods to obtain cytologic specimens from all body sites, the relevant criteria for precise cytodiagnosis and the many existing pitfalls, the extensive number of illustrations depicting the main cytologic findings and the application of high technology to cytology.

As always in a comprehensive work, the reader may agree or disagree with inclusions or omissions of topics. It is no doubt true that as the field of cytopathology continues to progress, later editions of *Comprehensive Cytopathology* will reflect changes. In this first edition of *Comprehensive Cytopathology,* I have attempted, through an international group of experts, to present an up-to-date work that represents the state of the art, as the decade of the nineties continues to unfold.

Marluce Bibbo, M.D.

Acknowledgments

In the past 24 months I have worked with a group of internationally recognized experts in the field of cytopathology to produce this book, *Comprehensive Cytopathology*. My sincere thanks goes to them for their participation and patience with my criticisms. I hope that when they see the fruit of this "gestation" it will make it all worthwhile.

Many people have helped along the way. From the University of Chicago, I am grateful to my secretary and editorial assistants—Ms. Cheryl A. Harden, Ms. Wendy Hilgendorf and Ms. Joan Hives—for their help in communicating with the contributors and publisher, organizing and filing the manuscripts, checking the manuscripts for references, tables, and figures, and proofreading.

In addition, some junior colleagues were helpful with their critiques of the text, including Drs. Brendan Fitzpatrick, Kai Ni, Heidi Asbury and Shelly Underhill. All of my residents and cytotechnologists were a constant source of motivation throughout the editorial process.

I am immensely grateful to our publisher, W.B. Saunders, for all the support in the production of this book. In particular, I owe to Darlene Pedersen the encouragement to become the editor of a book of this magnitude. She not only convinced me that I could do it but also was there to assist me in all phases of the editorial process. Mr. Leslie Hoeltzel, Manager, Developmental Editors, was very helpful with the review of the manuscripts and communication with the contributors.

Many other individuals from the Saunders Company deserve recognition and thanks: Patricia A. Morrison, Chief of Design and Illustration Departments; Joan Wendt, Designer; Neil P. Litt, Desktop Publishing Manager; Linda R. Turner, Production Manager; Mary Anne Folcher, Senior Copy Editor; Jean Kenworthy, Marketing Manager; and others working in the various other departments.

Last, but not least, I wish to express my gratitude to my colleagues and friends for listening to my frustrations and helping me to survive this first edition of *Comprehensive Cytopathology*.

Contents

PART I

General Cytology

1

The Cell: Basic Structure and Function

Gunter F. Bahr

NUCLEUS

Eucaryotic cells, like those found in mammals and other higher organisms, are mainly characterized by the presence of a membrane-bound nucleus. Procaryotic cells, such as bacteria, lack a nucleus. Nucleated cells are generally 10 to 100 μm* in dimension, whereas non-nucleated procaryotic bacteria are about 1 to 10 μm in dimension.

The nucleus initiates and regulates most cellular activities. Of paramount importance for the cell are long molecules of deoxyribonucleic acid (DNA). DNA is a double helix composed of four deoxyribonucleotides (deoxyribonucleotide = base + sugar + phosphate) polymerized in an unbranched manner (Fig. 1–1). The DNA is packed into the nucleus in a specific fashion (Fig. 1–2). Histones, which are DNA-binding proteins, are necessary for this packing. The nucleus also contains a wide variety of other proteins employed in the replication and repair of DNA and its transcription into messenger ribonucleic acid (mRNA).

A gene is a sequence of deoxyribonucleotides that carry information that can be transcribed into RNA and translated for the synthesis of proteins. The human genome (the totality of all genes) is commonly assumed to contain 50,000 to 100,000 genes.

Before mitotic cell division can take place, the

genome has to be doubled by means of *DNA replication*. In DNA replication the molecule in Figure 1–1 splits along the middle and a new complementary strand is formed from each of the original parental strands, which serve as templates. Because each new DNA duplex contains half of the original parental DNA double strand, one says that DNA replication is *semiconservative*. A series of enzymes are involved in the process of DNA replication, which has several safeguard mechanisms to ensure that each new daughter cell contains an exact duplicate of the genome of the progenitor.

DNA AND CHROMATIN

The cell nucleus contains chromatin, the chromosomal material of the nonmitotic cell. It is readily stainable by the Papanicolaou procedure and consists of DNA, histones, nonhistone proteins, and a variable but generally small amount of RNA. Hematoxylin staining is in good proportion to cellular DNA content. Chromatin condenses to form chromosomes during cell division (see Fig. 1–2). As a teleologic argument, one may assume that chromatin condensation facilitates the logistics of properly distributing DNA between the two daughter cells and further making cell division possible (see Chapter 2, Basic and Clinical Cytogenetics).

As seen through the electron microscope, chromatin is visible as thin fibers (200 Å) arranged in a meshwork (Fig. 1–3). In healthy cells this meshwork appears to be evenly distributed throughout the nucleus. Whenever chemical or physical forces act on chromatin, it tends to clump, preferably towards the periphery of the nucleus, a situation referred to as *chromatin margination*. When cell degeneration occurs with partial loss of nuclear membrane integrity, smears tend to draw out the chromatin of polymorphonuclear leuko-

---

The nature of this chapter reflects the purpose of *Comprehensive Cytopathology*. It is restricted to mammalian, specifically human, cells and with respect to organs confines itself to those listed in the table of contents. An attempt is made to replace some older terminology with later terminology generally recognized in cell biology.

*1 mm = 10^3 μm = 10^7 Å (1 *Ångstrom* is nearly the distance between two carbon atoms in a molecule).

1 nm = 10 Å = 0.001 μm = (old term / millimicron) (nm = nanometer = 10^{-9} m).

The light microscope can resolve two particles 0.2 μm apart. The electron microscope can routinely resolve two particles 5 nm apart.

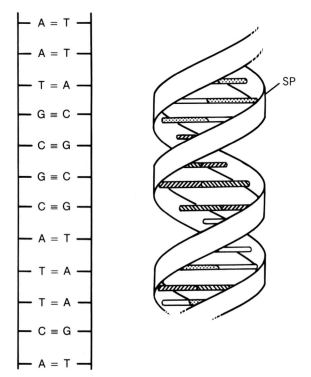

FIGURE 1–1. Schematic representation of the **DNA molecule**. On the left side, the complementary base pairing of adenine (A) with thymine (T) and cytosine (C) with guanine (G). The bases are held together with two (A=T) or three (G≡C) hydrogen bonds and are attached to a sugar phosphate (SP) backbone. On the right side, the DNA molecule is twisted to a double helix, yielding a schematic view of the actual DNA double helix.

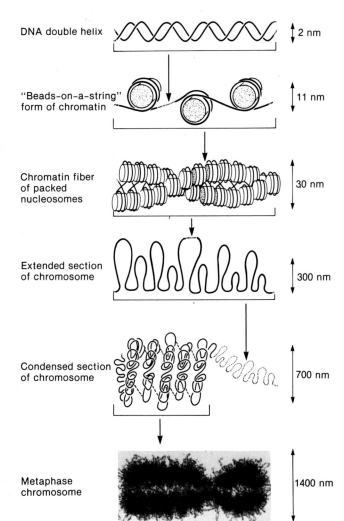

FIGURE 1–2. From the double helix of DNA to chromosomes. The DNA is wound around histone octamers giving the appearance of beads on a string. The beads, the histone octamer and two turns of double-stranded DNA, are called **nucleosomes** and are connected via linking DNA. A chromatin fiber of packed nucleosomes is but one of the versions proposed by which a chromatin fiber arises as seen in Figures 1–3 and 1–5. The micrograph of a metaphase chromosome demonstrates its fibrous nature. (Adapted with permission from The Molecular Biology of the Cell. Alberts B et al: New York, Garland Publishing, Inc., 1983.)

cytes and glandular cell nuclei, which can consequently be seen as long, blue-colored, hematoxylin-stained threads.

To understand the meshwork nature of chromatin (see Fig. 1–3) allows us to understand the morphologic events involved in its coarsening and clumping. Namely, when clumps appear, thinning or clearing must occur elsewhere. On the one hand, *hyper*chromasia means either more chromatin per volume of nucleus or decreased nuclear volume. *Hypo*chromasia, on the other hand, means either a volume increase (and thus thinning out or dilution of chromatin) or a loss of chromatin. In some cases, there may be as yet poorly understood chemical modifications involved in increased stain uptake.

PROTEIN SYNTHESIS

Protein synthesis is a complex, energy-consuming process. The initial step leading towards the synthesis of a functional protein involves *transcription* of the deoxyribonucleotide sequence of one gene into ribonucleic acid (RNA). Because this RNA carries the message needed to code for a specific protein, it is appropriately termed *mRNA*. The mRNA contains a sequence of ribonucleotides complementary to the

DNA sequence from which it was transcribed. During transcription, a DNA-dependent RNA-polymerase "fishes" ribonucleotides from the nucleoplasm and links them into a single strand of mRNA. The complementary base pairing of RNA to DNA follows the same rules as those in DNA replication, with the exception that the base uracil pairs with adenine instead of the base thymine. After a sequence of events collectively called RNA-processing, the mature mRNA passes through the nuclear envelope and complexes with cytoplasmic ribosomes containing *ribosomal RNA* (rRNA) and proteins (Fig. 1–4). The cytoplasm also contains *transfer RNAs* (tRNAs), so called because they carry amino acids, the building blocks of protein,

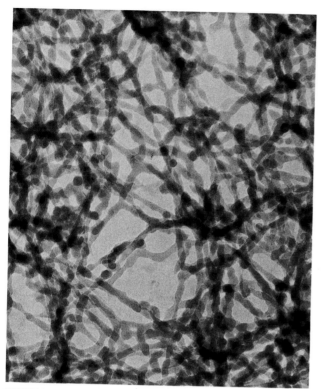

FIGURE 1–3. Electron micrograph of the **chromatin fiber meshwork** in a human lymphocyte interphase nucleus. Average fiber diameter is 20 nm. Final magnification ×100,000.

to the site of protein synthesis. As the ribosomes travel along the mRNA, the message is decoded, whereby three nucleotides in sequence *(codon)* code for one specific amino acid. Concurrently, the tRNA carrying the appropriate amino acid is called in and the amino acids are linked together with peptide bonds to form a protein (polypeptide).

NUCLEOLUS

Employing the Papanicolaou stain nucleoli appear as dark-red to cherry-red bodies within the nucleoplasm. Nucleoli are the sites of ribosome synthesis. The ribosomal DNA is transcribed into an rRNA precursor, which in turn is processed into ribosomal subunits before leaving the nucleolus. The ribosomal subunits do not function in protein synthesis until they have arrived in the cytoplasm.

Whenever cells are actively producing proteins, a prominent nucleolus is apparent. Such is continuously the case for liver cells (protein export) and intestinal epithelial cells (cell regeneration). In rapidly growing cancer cells large prominent nucleoli are a discriminating feature. When malignant cells cease to produce proteins for their own growth, as may be the case in a keratinizing squamous cell carcinoma, the nucleoli are reduced in size or disappear. Shrinking of the nucleolus can also be observed in starving cells. Cells of some other tissues neither produce much protein nor divide. Accordingly their nucleoli are very small or not visible

at all. An example are the cells of the prostate. Every healthy cell needs a nucleolus, however small, to regenerate the cell's own proteins.

Physiologically nucleoli undergo cyclic changes. They begin to disappear during prophase of cell division and reappear at the end of telophase (see Fig. 1–13, I and V).

Nucleoli are assembled from specific chromosomal regions, i.e., the stalks of so-called satellites, in the nucleolar context called *nucleolar organizer regions.* The human diploid chromosome complement contains ten chromosomes carrying satellites (Fig. 1–5). Evidence has accumulated suggesting that potentially all of them could produce nucleoli. Chromatin loops from each of the satellites participate in the formation of the final single nucleolus. The presence of ten nucleolar organizer regions of the human chromosome complement serves to explain multiple nucleoli in cells shortly after cell division. These gradually fuse.

An uneven rim of chromatin around the nucleolus is sometimes observable and is called *perinuclear chromatin.* It is now clear that this rim is composed of satellited chromosomes. Because this rim is more like a "peel" around the nucleolus, it may color the nucleolus as part of the chromatin, blue to dark blue-purple with hematoxylin in cytologic preparations.

Because order in the nucleus is disturbed in malignant cells, nucleolar organizer regions may be disjointed and give rise to multiple nucleoli. Moreover malignant cells often contain odd-shaped or spiculated nucleoli for the same reason. The usual two prominent nucleoli in liver nuclei, however, are the consequence of tetraploidy, i.e., a doubling of the diploid chromosome complement, frequently seen with age.

NUCLEAR ENVELOPE AND NUCLEAR SHAPE

The nucleus, as a defined cellular structure, disappears during cell division (see Fig. 1–13). Its limiting membrane, the nuclear envelope, can no longer be recognized with the light microscope. In most types of cells it is broken down into fragments to be reassembled during telophase, i.e., when the separated daughter chromatids arrive at the poles.

Two membranes of the lipid-bilayer type generally found in the cell constitute the nuclear envelope. The smooth, inner nuclear membrane envelops the nuclear content. During interphase, when the cell does not divide, the inner nuclear membrane is associated with chromatin fibers, which is the reason for the common observation that chromatin generally condenses onto the inner nuclear membrane. The outer nuclear membrane is part of the endoplasmic reticulum and when studded with ribosomes referred to as rough, hence, the term rough endoplasmic reticulum (rER) (see Fig. 1–4). Both membranes are bridged by special structures called *nuclear pores,* a misnomer as no pore-like openings are evident. Large quantities of vastly different-sized molecules are imported and exported by the nucleus through the nuclear envelope and its "pores."

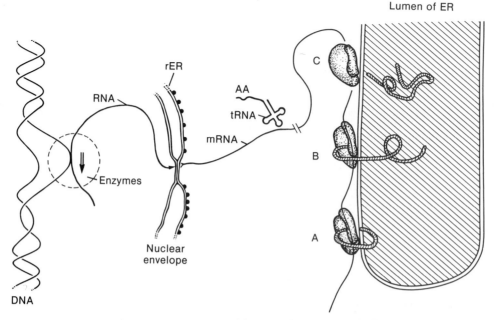

FIGURE 1–4. Protein and mRNA synthesis. DNA is unwound by special enzymes. Another enzyme transcribes the nucleotide sequence of one DNA strand into RNA. In RNA uridine is base paired to adenine instead of thymidine. The resulting RNA, or primary transcript, is further processed to become a messenger RNA (mRNA) that passes into the cytoplasm. The mature mRNA is then coupled to the 40S* and later to the 60S ribosomal subunits. Translation of the codon sequence (a sequence of three nucleotides) of single-stranded mRNA requires specific transfer RNAs (tRNAs) to bring in amino acids that are successively attached to the growing polypeptide chain. The newly synthesized protein is passed into the lumen of the endoplasmic reticulum (ER). (* S denotes the *Svedberg* constant, a measure of how fast a particle can be spun down in a centrifuge; it is therefore an indication of particle mass and shape.)

Situated immediately subjacent to the nuclear membrane one finds not only chromatin fibrils but a fibrous meshwork, the *nuclear lamina*. Inner and outer nuclear membranes together with the nuclear lamina and attached chromatin fibrils make the membrane visible to the light microscopist, an experience otherwise reserved for the electron microscopist. The visibility of the nuclear lamina alone varies greatly depending on its thickness.

The space between the two membranes of the nuclear envelope is called the perinuclear cisterna. When the cell is irradiated by x-rays the cisterna may enlarge focally in response to the injury. Such a vacuole so produced may become large enough to deform the nucleus into the shape of a bean.

To all light microscopic appearances a nucleus is a smooth sphere or spheroid. The forces involved in shaping the nucleus are not yet understood. The orderly arrangement of the chromosomes, as suggested in Figure 1–6, may help to maintain nuclear shape.

Unusual stress on the transcriptional and synthetic activities of the cell can affect the arrangement of interphase chromosomes. The stress of malignancy or viral assault can work havoc upon the nucleus. It loses its shape because additional chromosomes have to be accommodated. One of the earliest light microscopic signs of cytopathology is therefore nuclear enlargement. Sometimes clefts of varying depth and width become visible, and indentations and protrusions occur. All reflect ways in which rearrangements facilitate new metabolic requirements.

The average nucleus consists of about 25% dry substance, 18% of which is DNA and roughly the same percentage is histone. The rest are nonhistone proteins, the nucleolus and the nuclear membrane.

CYTOPLASM AND PLASMALEMMA

Most cells presented in this text appear to have homogeneous cytoplasm. Occasionally granules or inclusions can be observed when cells are routinely stained for light microscopy. Only with the aid of the electron microscope can a multitude of detail be resolved. By volume much of the cytoplasm is *cytosol*, a gel containing several billions of molecules of several thousand types. The cytoplasm contains many different organelles as well and is bounded by a lipid bilayer separating the cell from its environment. This barrier is the plasma membrane. To the clinical cytologist it is the cell membrane and by no means just a barrier. Rather it plays an active role as selective filter for nutrients to enter and waste products to leave the cell. The *plasma membrane* is vital for maintaining the proper concentration gradient between the inside of the cell and the cell's surroundings. This membrane is a lipid bilayer in which an assortment of proteins are embedded (Fig. 1–7).

Three types of lipids occur: phospholipids, cholesterol and glycolipids. They constitute the head of the lipid molecule with two fatty acids attached as the tail.

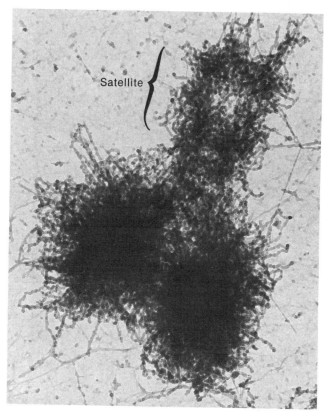

FIGURE 1–5. Satellite chromosome likely to belong to the G group. In this electron micrograph one of the ten human chromosomes potentially carrying satellites (marked by bracket) is depicted. The body of this chromosome—the two sister chromatids—is bent upwards from the object's plane towards the observer. It can be seen how, essentially, fiber loops constitute the chromosome. Average fiber diameter 20 nm. Magnification ×62,500.

One is a saturated, the other an unsaturated fatty acid. The double bond not only causes a bend in the molecule but accounts for the well-known osmiophilia of cell membranes in electron microscopic preparations. Without proteins a lipid bilayer is just a semipermeable membrane. Proteins are thought to float in the lipid bilayer, being laterally movable. Some of them are anchored to the fibrillar network or the cytoskeleton immediately subjacent to the plasma membrane. These proteins serve vital transport functions for ions such as sodium, potassium, calcium and magnesium. Recognition of a large number of external and internal molecules is another function, permitting or barring the passage through the plasma membrane. All cellular membranes are generally of the lipid bilayer type. There are, however, differences among them. The outer and inner layers of the plasma membrane differ with respect to their relative composition of phospholipids. The phospholipid heads face outwards to the exterior or to cytosol. Fatty acid tails are facing each other within the membrane. The exterior surface of the plasma membrane is covered by a carbohydrate cell coat, or *glycocalyx*, composed of oligosaccharides covalently bound to proteins in the plasma membrane and formstraight or branching chains. This coat is

thought to play an important role in recognizing "self" from "nonself." The glycocalyx may vary in thickness depending on the location of the cell. It may thus be thick on luminal faces of cells or barely detectable in tissues.

Especially in preparations of exfoliative cytology, a partition of the cytoplasm into *endoplasm* and *ectoplasm* can be noted, most perceivably in mesothelial cells. The ectoplasm is a thick gel with few cytoplasmic filaments, whereas the endoplasm accommodates all of the endoplasmic reticulum and all of the cellular organelles.

MITOCHONDRIA

Mitochondria are the purveyors of energy to most processes in the cell. They have therefore been called the powerhouses of the cell. In a liver cell about 1000 mitochondria can be found continuously powering the synthesis of, among others, blood proteins and lipids. An intermediate squamous cell has only a few mitochondria commensurable with low synthetic activity. By this reasoning the Hürthle cells and oncocytes possess considerable synthetic or energy-consuming activities.

Mitochondria produce energy by burning (oxidizing) carbohydrates and fatty acids to CO_2 and water. The

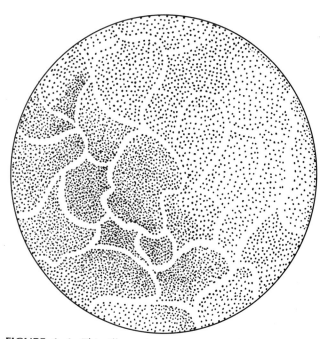

FIGURE 1–6. This illustration suggests how **chromosomes** may be distributed within the nucleus. Since it is known that chromatin is attached to the inner nuclear membrane, and since all chromatin is chromosomal, the attachment of chromosomes to areas at the inner nuclear membrane follows logically. Chromatin pattern is of interest to cytopathologists who frequently observe disturbances in this order. (Reproduced with permission from Compendium on Diagnostic Cytology, 6th ed. Wied GL, Keebler CM, Koss LG, Reagan JW (eds). Chicago, Tutorials of Cytology, 1988.)

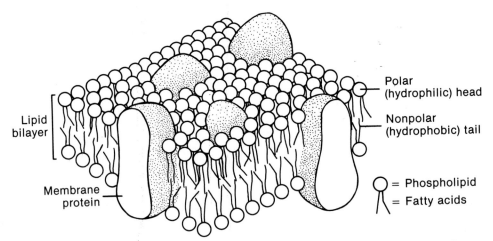

Lipid bilayer

Polar (hydrophilic) head

Nonpolar (hydrophobic) tail

Membrane protein

○ = Phospholipid

⚡ = Fatty acids

FIGURE 1–7. Schematic illustration of a piece of the plasma membrane modified after the **fluid-membrane model of Singer and Nicholson.** Lipid molecules are arranged in a bilayer: polar, hydrophilic heads (phospholipids) suggested by spheres, and their nonpolar, hydrophobic tails (fatty acids), by straight or bent tails. Embedded in the "sea" of lipid molecules, protein molecules appear to swim. Some protrude only to the cell exterior, and others reach through both layers. Among the latter are proteins involved in transmembrane transport, having valve-like channels. Both membrane proteins and lipids facing the cell exterior carry sugar residues with receptor properties.

product is energy-rich adenosine triphosphate, ATP. The ATP is consumed in synthesis, chemical additions and couplings; in active transport through membranes (ion pumps); in muscle contraction and movement of the cell (penetration of other tissues) and in cell division, just to mention some of the many energy-consuming cellular activities.

Although the covalent binding of hydrogen to oxygen is an explosive process, in mitochondria this energy can be transferred in increments and stored in ATP, a process that takes place in the respiratory chain of mitochondria. As the Papanicolaou stain does not enable one to visualize mitochondria, iron hematoxylin, according to Regaud, or acid fuchsin, according to Altmann, is generally used for this purpose. More specific histochemical stains are available, especially fluorescent ones, such as rhodamine 123. Mitochondria assume the shape of single spheres or long, often branching structures. Lengths of up to 7 μm and widths of 0.5 μm have been measured (Fig. 1–8).

Mitochondria are also divided during cell division. Much of the biosynthesis required for duplication is made on nuclear DNA–directed ribosomes in the cytoplasm. Mitochondria possess their own DNA that also plays roles in differentiation and inheritance, but it codes for only a few proteins. The complete base sequence of human mitochondrial DNA has been established. It is principally a closed molecular ring, about 5 to 6 μm in length.

LYSOSOMES

Another group of cytoplasmic organelles has been detected in presumably mitochondrial fractions of whole cells at centrifugation. This is a family of variously named organelles, all of which seem to stem from the Golgi apparatus. A lysosome is a membranous

bag containing up to 40 acid enzymes (hydrolases) with a pH of about 5, i.e., in the acid range. Many different types of lysosomes have been detected with histochemical probes. The various types of lysosomes are probably equipped for different tasks by various sets of hydrolases. On morphologic grounds, however, the types cannot be distinguished. An intact lysosome may enclose high concentrations of some or all of the following categories of enzymes: nucleases, proteases, glycosidases, lipases, phosphatases and sulfatases.

In one of several lysosomal diseases, the *Hunter-Hurler syndrome*, a hereditary disorder also called mucopolysaccharidosis, the absence of lysosomal enzyme leads to large lysosomal accumulations of incom-

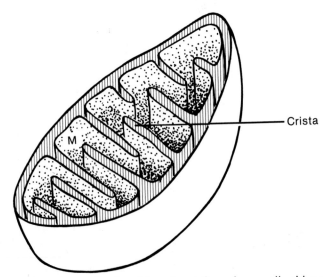

Crista

M

FIGURE 1–8. Mitochondrion. A cut through a small, oblong mitochondrion. Its compartmentalization is apparent. **Matrix space (M)** is filled with a concentrated suspension of different enzymes. The inner membrane is folded. These folds, termed **cristae,** increase the inner membrane's surface.

pletely degraded mucopolysaccharides (properly glycosaminoglycans) in the cell.

Among the normal functions of the lysosomes is the digestion of food particles, from the smallest grain via *pinocytosis* to entire bacteria and leukocytes via *phagocytosis*. Receptors at the plasma membrane react to small particles by invaginating it into the cytoplasm, eventually to be pinched off (Fig. 1–9). Smaller primary lysosomes join this food vacuole; its enzymes are thereby activated and digest the content. Usable molecules are selectively passed to the cytoplasm; indigestible molecules are secreted in a process reversing pinocytosis or phagocytosis (exocytosis), or they are stored, often permanently, in the cytoplasm. Examples are the deposition of anthracotic particles (black lung) in alveolar macrophages or the appearance of dustladen macrophages in sputum. In addition one may find a vacuole containing pieces of membranes and mitochondria being digested (autophagocytic vesicles) (see Fig. 1–9). Useful molecules are returned to the cytoplasm. The cytologist-pathologist encounters the effects of lysosomal enzymes in programmed cell death or autolysis of certain cells.

The *peroxisome* is another internal organelle enclosing enzymes. It contains chiefly catalase (40%) and other enzymes that use molecular oxygen to remove hydrogen from specific substrates. Catalase is an indispensable link in the oxidation of ethanol to acetaldehyde and in the detoxification of many drugs and other chemical compounds. Peroxisomes are believed to arise by budding from the endoplasmic reticulum.

ENDOPLASMIC RETICULUM

Diffusely distributed throughout the cytoplasm are fluid-filled sacs of the endoplasmic reticulum (ER). It is thought of as a continuous space, although it presents itself as an assembly of flat sacs and convoluted tubules. The ER is a single membrane totaling more than half of all internal membranes of the cell. One part of this membrane system facing the cytosol is studded with ribosomes. It is therefore called *rough* or *granular ER* (rER). The rER is continuous with the outer nuclear membrane (Fig. 1–10). The ER lacking ribosomes is termed *smooth endoplasmic reticulum* (sER).

Generally, the ER serves to separate newly synthesized molecules from the cytosol and to package and deliver these molecules to specific sites. Proteins, lipids and complex carbohydrates are synthesized with aid of the ER. The products are packaged in small transport vesicles and pinched off the ER to be transported to the nucleus, mitochondria, lysosomes or cell exterior as a process of secretion. A typical example of cells that manufacture and secrete proteins is that of the endocrine pancreas (see Fig. 1–10).

GOLGI APPARATUS

The Golgi apparatus, named after the Italian histologist *Camillo Golgi* who discovered it by means of silver stains, has most recently been considered part of the membrane system of which the ER is the main element (see Figs. 1–9 and 1–10). A Golgi apparatus is usually located in the vicinity of the nucleus close to the two centrioles that mark the cell's center. It is composed of stacks of flattened, smooth connected membrane sacs. Number and size of the Golgi apparatuses vary with cell type and cell function. It is particularly large in secretory cells such as goblet cells, in which it almost fills the cytoplasm. Small vesicles abound around the Golgi apparatus, apparently fulfill-

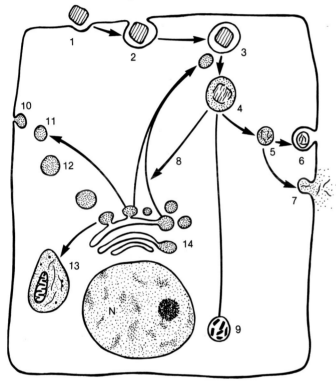

FIGURE 1–9. Lysosomal activities. Primary lysosomes filled with acid hydrolytic enzymes are budding on the Golgi membrane (14). When the cell phagocytizes a particle, its plasma membrane invaginates (1, 2) and releases the membrane-enclosed phagocytic vacuole into the cytoplasm. There, it is joined by a primary lysosome (3) with enzymes that immediately begin to break down the content of the vesicle (4). Usable molecules are transported within the cytoplasm (8). Indigestible or unwanted materials are excreted (5) in either a small vesicle (6) or suspension (7). Some indigestible materials are permanently stored by forming residual bodies (9). In endocytosis a small amount of suspended particles is enclosed in a vesicle (10). The vesicle is then digested by the contents of a primary lysosome (11, 12). Apparently wornout parts of the cytoplasm are enclosed in membranes to be digested for recycling of molecules. An autophagocytic vesicle results (13). Whenever primary lysosomes have joined material to be digested, the larger vesicle is referred to as a secondary lysosome. (N = nucleus.)

ing the task of transporting products to other cellular sites or the exterior (see Fig. 1–10). Although only a few functions of this organelle are fully understood, it can be said that it performs extremely complex biochemical operations. In the Golgi apparatus, generally, additions and deletions on proteins, lipids and carbohydrates are taking place, some of which have the nature of applying "addresses" to molecules and their packages to achieve correct distribution of products. Complexity of performance is expressed in a polarized structure. Golgi sacs are organized as crescents; the concave side seems to be the entrance to its chemical machinery, while products are leaving at the convex side (see Figs. 1–9 and 1–10). In addition to the previously mentioned goblet cells, further examples of its activities follow: in the pancreas it functions in the production of zymogen granules, in breast in the production of milk droplets and in bladder in the production of asymmetric membranes. One of several apparatuses is situated in glandular cells between the nucleus and the luminal surface. In parietal cells of the stomach and in a few other cell types an apparatus is situated between the nucleus and the basal surface of the plasma membrane. All cells have a Golgi apparatus.

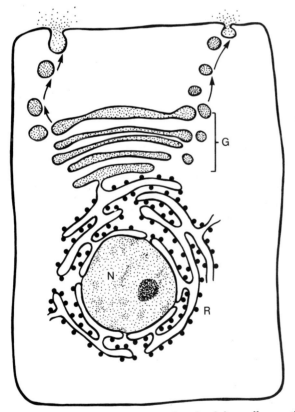

FIGURE 1–10. Schematic view of a **glandular cell secreting mucoproteins.** The protein part is synthesized on ribosomes and passed into the lumen of the endoplasmic reticulum (R) (see Fig. 1–4). From there it is transported to the Golgi sacs (G) to be joined with a mucopolysaccharide portion and packaged into vesicles to be secreted. Note the polarity of the cell: the nucleus (N) is situated in the basal half of the cell, and the Golgi apparatus is closer to the luminal surface.

CYTOSKELETON

Whenever cells move or change their shape a complex network of protein filaments is involved. Three major types of filaments are recognized: *microtubules, actin filaments* and *intermediate filaments* with widths of 25 nm, 6 nm and 7 to 11 nm, respectively. The last is a group to which keratin filaments (tonofilaments), neurofilaments and vimentin filaments belong. Numerous proteins are involved in the interaction of the filaments with their own kind and with other filaments in the cytoplasm.

Because pools of precursor molecules exist in the cytosol, microtubules and actin filaments can readily be assembled as well as broken down, which is a flexibility particularly useful in cell movement. The

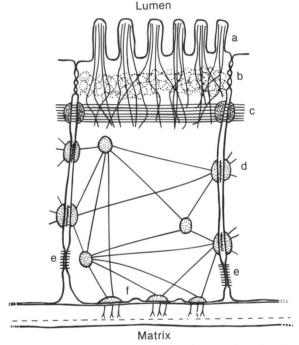

FIGURE 1–11. Schematic drawing that exaggerates the distribution of various **intercellular junctions** and the disposal of keratin and actin filaments in the cytoplasm. Microvilli (a) containing parallel arrays of actin filaments are held together by actin-bundling proteins (not shown here) and terminate in a dense meshwork called the **terminal web.** The membranes of neighboring cells seem to fuse in **tight junctions,** actually a system bonding one membrane to the other so that a type of barrier filter (b) is interposed in the intercellular space between luminal and matrix fluids. Tight junctions when seen en face present a delicate network of cell-to-cell contact. **Belt desmosomes** (c) are seen in cross section and as a belt girding the apical cytoplasm. A belt desmosome consists chiefly of actin filaments. **Spot desmosomes** (d) serve not only to anchor keratin filaments, crossing the cytoplasm, but to secure a hold onto the next cell. Two **gap junctions** (e) are illustrated. Small channels in gap junctions allow for the passage of small molecules and electrical signals. **Hemidesmosomes** (f) secure the cell base to the basal lamina. They too are anchoring points for the general keratin network.

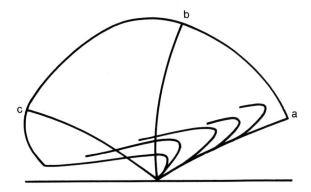

FIGURE 1–12. The beat of a cilium is schematically shown. Movement from **b** to **c** is called the effective stroke, whereas **a** depicts the cilium in the recovery stroke. Cilia beat in the respiratory tract, in the fallopian tubes and endometrium, in the endocervical canal, in the rete testis and on ependymal cells.

presence of so many filaments allows for order in the cytosol. Many organelles are believed to be attached to the cytoskeleton, thereby limiting their movement within preformed spaces. Microtubules originate at the cell center near the pair of centrioles. Three of the more outstanding functions of microtubules deal with the formation of the mitotic spindle (see Fig. 1–13), with the provision of stiffness but flexibility in cilia (Fig. 1–12) and with the anchoring of specific movable proteins in the plasma membrane.

Actin filaments have been found in all cells and in particularly high concentrations in fibroblasts. Of interest is also the presence of actin filaments in microvilli, finger-like protrusions from the plasmalemma that increase the absorptive area of many cells. About 25 actin filaments run from the apex of a microvillus into the cytoplasm and join a meshwork of other actin filaments subjacent to the plasma membrane (see Fig. 1–11). This meshwork is called the *terminal web*. With the help of actin fibers the body of a cell is tied in the middle (contractile ring) and thereby divided into two daughter cells during cytokinesis (see Fig. 1–13). Among several proteins frequently associated with actin is myosin, known also from striated muscle. In so-called *stress fibers*, 0.5 μm thick and up to 5 μm long, actin is associated with myosin in the cytoplasm. The exact function of this association is still unknown. The cytologist-pathologist will observe myoepithelial cells in both breast and prostate.

Of the intermediate filaments chiefly tonofilaments or keratin filaments are discussed because every epithelial cell contains keratin filaments. These run from one side of the cell to the other through the cytoplasm, not only forming a structural framework within the cell, but lending tensile strength to it as well (see Fig. 1–11).

In keratinizing epithelial cells keratin filaments accumulate and are crosslinked by other proteins and by disulfide bonds. The process usually starts at the periphery of the squamous cell and progresses towards the nuclear area where a narrow shell of organelle-filled cytoplasm persists until the nucleus becomes

pyknotic and dissolves. Keratin filaments are composed of one or several of the 19 cytokeratin molecules identified in tissues from which, by different polymerizations, appendices such as nails, hair, hoofs, beaks and feathers are produced.

The *cytosol*, or cell sap, a gel containing most of the free-floating molecules of the cell, surrounds all of the cytoplasmic organelles discussed so far. Evidence has been put forth stating how a meshwork of 1.5-nm fibers

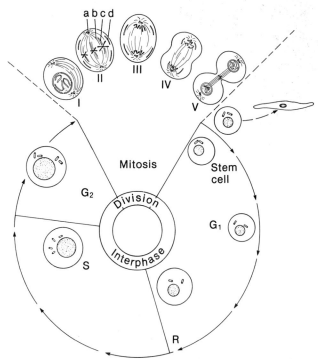

FIGURE 1–13. Cell cycle or generation cycle. The inner ring divides the life of the cell into periods of interphase and cell division. The majority of the cells discussed in this text are at interphase, most likely G1. When at G1, one of the daughter cells, a stem cell, may continue to point **R,** the **restriction point,** ready to begin the DNA synthesis necessary for subsequent cell division. The other daughter cell may be destined to differentiate, to mature and to die as a member in the protective shield of a squamous epithelium. A stem cell is said to be an "immortal cell." Some of the basal cells of squamous epithelium are stem cells as are the pluripotent cells of bone marrow from which blasts arise. In the S phase DNA is primarily synthesized. The products of this synthesis are sorted at G2 before mitosis begins. At the beginning of mitosis (schematically exaggerated), the nucleus begins division by condensing chromosomes at prophase to slender threads (I). The assembly of fully condensed chromosomes during metaphase follows (II). During anaphase (III) chromosome halves, the chromatids, are pulled apart by kinetochore microtubules (c), against bracing polar microtubules (b) to opposite ends of the cell. During telophase (IV) chromosomes are tightly gathered around the polar bodies and begin to decondense. During cytokinesis (V) the cytoplasm divides. At this point the nuclear envelope is reassembled from precursors (d). The behavior of the centrioles (a) at mitosis and at interphase is shown, as well as the disappearance of a nucleolus at I and reappearance at V.

accounts for the special properties of the cytosol, among them not to "run out" when the plasma membrane is cut. This is called the *microtrabecular meshwork*.

CELL JUNCTIONS

In the context of this text no free living cells are dealt with; rather, all cells considered are or have been members of an organ. All of them have experienced neighboring cells and have at some point "decided" whether they were at the right place, a process calling for complex biomolecular recognition mechanisms.

Three situations occur in which cell-to-cell contact is of special importance (see Fig. 1–11). Cells have to adhere to each other more or less firmly depending on the function of the organ. They must communicate with each other, e.g., to arrange for synchronous beating of the cilia. The epithelia lining small and large lumina act as barriers themselves and must tightly close intercellular spaces.

For cell-to-cell adherence, *spot desmosomes* have been deployed. These are rivet-like points where cells appear welded together. Keratin filaments end at spot desmosomes, and since this is the case for both cells so joined, the cytoskeleton of each is closely connected with that of the next cell. Spot desmosomes between neighboring cells are apparently distributed according to need.

A belt desmosome girds the apical portion of a columnar or cuboidal cell. It is called the *zonula adherences* and connects on the cytoplasmic side to a likewise circular bundle of actin filaments. In the intercellular space, the belt desmosomes of two cells are connected by short, poorly characterized filaments (see Fig. 1–11).

A third type of desmosome anchors the base of the cell to the basal lamina. Such fasteners are called *hemidesmosomes*, i.e., half desmosomes. Desmosomes of all types are dissolved when an aged or a dead cell leaves the organ but are rapidly reformed to fasten the new cells arising in cell division.

One finds the most prominent organelles for anchoring cells to each other and to their base in squamous epithelia, i.e., where physical and sometimes chemical wear is strongest, such as in the skin, in the oral cavity, in the vagina and in the cervix. Undissolved desmosomes bind immature metaplastic cells together, as well as sheets of repair cells. Increasingly malignancy means loss of cell-to-cell adherence. Strong hemidesmosomes fasten urothelial layers to the basal lamina.

In *tight junctions* a sheet of epithelial cells seals itself against the lumen as well as the tissue. The outer leaves of the two adjacent plasma membranes join so closely as to appear as one. Tight junctional proteins are localized in the space between the bilayered membranes in the form of beads on a string. Beaded strings, in turn, are connected to form a loose meshwork. Width and completeness of such meshworks vary with epithelial function.

Cells can communicate through narrow channels provided in *gap junctions* (see Fig. 1–11). Small molecules and electrical signals thus can pass from cell to cell. Gap junctions can be established between cells—even of another type—in minutes, probably from precursors floating in the plasma membrane. At the site where the gap junctions form, the two-cell membranes are separated by 2 to 4 nm, thus allowing for relatively large molecules to pass in between the two cells.

A *terminal bar* can sometimes be seen in cytologic preparations stained according to Papanicolaou. It appears that this light microscopic structure is the sum of belt desmosomes and actin filaments, as well as other protein filaments at the apical end of the cell. It is possible that the contractile belt desmosome plays a role in the sloughing off of the apical cell portion in ciliocytophoria. *Herxheimer's spiral* in the "tail" of some epithelial cells reflects cytoplasmic filaments of all types collected at the center of the cytoplasmic extension, probably more by mechanical effects than purposeful chemical binding.

EXTRACELLULAR MATRIX

In cytologic or pathologic studies the extracellular matrix (see Fig. 1–11) has oftentime played a subordinate role or none at all, unless such structures as cartilage, connective tissue or bone and teeth were considered. The histologist has usually separated the basement membrane, now *basal lamina*, from the rest of the intercellular cement or glue. In more recent years, however, the relevance of the matrix proteins and polysaccharides in regulating cell behavior and development has been further appreciated.

As it is now understood, polysaccharides are covalently linked to proteins yielding proteoglycans, also called mucoproteins. These and glucosaminoglycans form the highly hydrated ground substance in which all other elements are embedded. Such elements include collagen and elastin. Collagen, elastin and fibronectin are secreted by fibroblasts. Fibronectin is a protein facilitating adhesion of cells to substrates.

Another cell type, especially close to epithelia, is the macrophage, ready to migrate through the epithelial cell layer and appear on the luminal side. Nerve endings may do the same. Fibroblasts, however, are held back by the basal lamina.

Varying thickness reflects different filtering capacities in basal lamina. The membrane-like structure is a specialization of the general matrix. It contains a unique type of collagen, the proteins laminin and fibronectin. Each anatomic site places special demands on the basal lamina and are not yet fully understood.

CELL GROWTH AND DIVISION

Cytologists and pathologists frequently observe mitotic figures and conclude from a rough estimate of their proportion to nondividing cells whether a rapidly or slowly growing tissue is at hand. Since mitosis lasts approximately 2 hours, it is a handy marker for cell division. How much time a specific cell type needs to duplicate itself is difficult to derive from fixed tissue. Rather, the observation of live cells in tissue culture permits estimations of life cycle times. These vary from 8 hours to 4 days. Differences in division rates are predominately due to differences in the length of G1 (see Fig. 1–13).

The life of a cell begins with cell division (Fig. 1–13,V) and most often ends with a division; it is characterized by continuous synthesis and growth. Although this statement holds true for the synthesis of proteins, lipids and carbohydrates, DNA replicates only during a definable time of the cell cycle, the synthesis phase or S phase. In living cells, this phase can be marked by incorporation of radioactively labeled precursors, such as tritiated thymidine. Subsequent autoradiography reveals that thymidine is exclusively incorporated in the nuclei of cells that were in the S phase when tritiated thymidine was added to the culture.

A rapid means to estimate the numbers of cells in various phases of the cell cycle is to stain with DNA-specific fluorescent dyes followed by analysis in a flow-cytometer. This technique requires a suspension of single cells. For many cells of the human body it is not desirable to continue growing once the mature organ is established. Apparently, cells stop the cycle at the end of G1, i.e., before DNA replication is to commence. This point has been called the *restriction point*, R. It may be necessary at some point in time to start a cell into the cell cycle again. A hypothetic trigger protein has been suggested that should accomplish this reactivation. Normally the frequency of mitosis in liver is 1 or 2 in 10^4 cells. A classic example of reactivation can be seen among the remaining liver cells when some portion of the organ has been lost. Rapid cell division ensues. Liver regeneration serves to illustrate that some cells in organs divide only when needed and stop when the organ is regenerated. Those tissues having practically no mitotic frequency, such as the central nervous system, have great difficulty in regenerating.

Cells usually stop growing when they touch upon their own tissue or neighboring tissues. It is a characteristic feature of malignant cells not to cease cell division when the boundary of an adjacent organ has been reached.

Cells must maintain their structure and function by continuously renewing their wornout molecules and organelles. This process proceeds without visible indices, and neither light nor electron microscopist could detect such cell renewal processes without specific chemical markers. Some cells are destined to divide continuously and send one of the two daughter cells arising to programmed cell death. Well known is the "altruistic" death of basal cells in squamous epithelium. One of the daughters is an immortal cell and remains attached to the basal lamina, while its sister is differentiated to squamous superficial cells or mere squames, thus protecting the epithelium and the organism as well (Fig. 1–13, stem cell). Thus, the second type of cell renewal is cell division.

In Figure 1–13, cell division is depicted most schematically. Indicated are also the *centrioles*. Centrioles divide during the S phase of the cell cycle. During mitosis centriolar space acts as the attachment site for mitotic spindle fibers. In general, many microtubules end around the centrioles in an ill-defined mass. Stationary cells alter shape during cell division. At the end of G2 they round up and lose temporarily contact with their base and with their neighbors.

Acknowledgment. I wish to acknowledge the review and typing of the manuscript for this chapter by my daughter Nina I. Bahr, B.S., who is a student at the University of Zurich, Switzerland.

Recommended Related Literature

Alberts B, Bray D, Lewis J, Raff M, Roberts K, Watson JD: Molecular Biology of the Cell. New York, Garland Publishing, 1983.

Bloom W, Fawcett DW: A Textbook of Histology. Philadelphia, W. B. Saunders Co., 1975.

Karp G: Cell Biology. New York, McGraw-Hill, 1979.

Koss LG: Diagnostic Cytology, 3rd ed. Philadelphia, J. B. Lippincott Co., 1979.

Wied LG, Keebler CM, Koss LG, Reagan JW: Compendium on Diagnostic Cytology, 6th ed. Chicago, Tutorials of Cytology, 1988.

2

Basic and Clinical Cytogenetics

Stanley L. Inhorn

In many respects, the development of clinical cytogenetics has paralleled the emergence of clinical cytology as a major diagnostic laboratory specialty. The discipline of cytogenetics began over a century ago, when the merger of mendelian genetics and basic cytology led to the discovery of the law of constancy of chromosome number for each species.[31] Human cytogenetics developed a decade later than did clinical cytology, when in 1956 Tjio and Levan, using colchicine to arrest cells in metaphase and hypotonic solution to spread chromosomes on slides, determined that the diploid human chromosome number of man is 46.[132]

Many similarities exist between clinical cytology and human cytogenetics. In both disciplines, cellular features are examined through the microscope after appropriate cytopreparatory techniques. Both specialties require close working relationships between technologic and professional laboratory personnel in a setting that demands the utmost in quality assurance practices. In each field, there must be close cooperation and open communication between the laboratory and the clinician. Each specialty has inherent limitations.

Two major differences occur between clinical cytogenetics and clinical cytology. First, cytogenetic analyses are far more costly and demanding of personnel time. Second, in terms of medical applications, cytology has its greatest usefulness in the area of cancer screening and diagnosis. Although cytogenetics is used in the diagnostic workup of certain types of malignancies, its major role has been in the study of developmental and functional abnormalities. In conjunction with other genetic, laboratory, epidemiologic and clinical procedures, cytogenetics has helped to explain many aspects of abnormal development and problems of sex development. From a medical standpoint, there are six major areas of application for cytogenetic testing:

1. Patients with multiple congenital anomalies and their families
2. Prenatal diagnosis
3. Sex developmental abnormalities and infertility
4. Cancer diagnosis
5. Other specific uses (e.g., monitoring bone marrow transplants)
6. Research applications (e.g., mutagen testing).

Clinicians may request chromosome studies that are not warranted. Because of the high cost, limited laboratory resources and virtual absence of expected useful information, the cytogeneticist must counsel the physician to reconsider such a request. Examples of "nonindications" for chromosome studies are as follows:

1. An otherwise normal pubertal male with gynecomastia
2. A user of marijuana, LSD or other illicit drug
3. A patient with a history of exposure to Agent Orange
4. A patient with a known mendelian condition (e.g., osteogenesis imperfecta)
5. A phenotypically normal child with a learning disability, hyperactivity or other psychologic disorder
6. A patient with mild nonfamilial mental retardation without apparent malformations
7. A patient with a solitary congenital anomaly (e.g., cleft palate).

As in the case of clinical cytology, human cytogenetics has progressed and expanded scientifically as a result of technical improvements and discoveries made during the past three decades. Late developments in recombinant DNA technology have revolutionized cell biology, enabling investigators to create mutant genes and to perform genetic engineering of chromosomes. Furthermore, the new technology allows correlation of chromosomal morphology at the microscope level with molecular events at the gene level. Thus, the explosion of knowledge made possible by advances in molecular biology has brought the fields of cytogenetics and mendelian genetics together in a truly remarkable fashion. Another development that has benefited both cytogenetics and diagnostic cytology is the research on automated systems. Computerized chromosome analysis systems are available commercially for karyotyping and enhancing even poorly stained and overlapped chromosomes.

THE CELL CYCLE

Cytogenetics is the study of chromosome morphology and function. Because chromosomes are best visualized microscopically during certain phases of cell replication, dividing cell populations are required. If errors occur during the process of cell division, in either germ cells or somatic cells, numeric or structural chromosome abnormalities may result. Therefore, an understanding of the cell cycle is crucial to an appreciation of human cytogenetics.[8]

The cell cycle has been classically separated into a dividing phase (mitosis) and a resting stage (interphase). Resting phase is a misnomer, because this is the period in the cycle when the cell is most active metabolically. Chromosome replication actually occurs in a limited time period of interphase during which DNA synthesis takes place. This synthesis phase, called the *S phase,* lasts for about 8 hours and is initiated by the appearance of a diffusible S-phase activator in the cytoplasm. When completed, each chromosome has been duplicated. During the subsequent cell division (mitosis), each of the two daughter cells receives an identical set of chromosomes and enters the next interphase.

The first portion of interphase is designated as the *G1 phase*—G refers to the gap before the start of DNA synthesis. G1 is the most variable time period, depending on the cell type. In rapidly replicating tissues, G1 may last for only 10 to 12 hours. In tissues that have a low mitotic rate and in which only aged or damaged cells are replaced, G1 may last for weeks or months. G1 is the functional or differentiated stage of the cell cycle, in which the cell carries out its specific activity. The DNA content of the nucleus in G1 is species specific and is referred to as the diploid (2n) complement. At the termination of the S phase, replication of DNA in each chromosome results in the nucleus' containing the tetraploid amount (4n). Prior to the start of mitosis, there is a second gap (G2), lasting approximately 4 to 5 hours. During the *G2 phase,* no further DNA synthesis occurs. Thus, interphase is divided into three distinct periods—G1, S and G2—in terms of chromosome function. During G1, the nucleus is diploid and contains 46 chromosomes. During the S phase, the chromosomes are being replicated, and at its conclusion and for the relatively brief G2, the nucleus is tetraploid. Therefore, in a population of cells in which active replication is taking place,

a certain percent have the 4n DNA content. Measurements on such a population would show the average DNA content to be somewhere in the 2n to 4n range.

Mitosis and Meiosis

Mitosis is a process that permits the previously replicated chromosomes to be evenly divided into the two daughter cells. Mitosis (*M phase*) is thought to be initiated by one or more triggering factors that develop within the cytoplasm or are produced by specific cells and released into the circulation and the interstitial fluid. An internal stimulus has been named the M-phase promoting factor (MPF). A number of other mitotic stimulators have been identified, including the epidermal growth factor (EGF), fibroblast growth factor (FGF), interleukin-2 (IL-2) and platelet-derived growth factor (PDGF).

The changes that are seen in the nucleus during mitosis begin with the condensation of the chromosomes, which in interphase are positioned loosely in the nucleoplasm, each as a slender, long fiber consisting of DNA and associated proteins.[85] Because the individual chromosomes are several centimeters long in interphase, they must be folded extensively in order to fit into spheric nuclei with diameters in the μm range. Condensation and shortening of these fibers produce thicker chromosomes that become visible by light microscopy. This first phase of mitosis, resulting from biophysical changes induced by phosphorylation of associated histone molecules, is known as *prophase.* Further condensation of the chromosomes and disruption of the nuclear membrane signal the start of *prometaphase.* As the two centrosomes in the cytoplasm move to opposite poles of the nucleus, the microtubules extending from one to the other surround and permeate the nucleus. This structure is known as the *mitotic spindle apparatus.*

At this early stage of mitosis, each chromosome can be seen to have a *centromere* that binds two identical *chromatids.* The centromeres attach to the spindle fibers, and within a short time, all chromosomes migrate to the center of the spindle apparatus. During *metaphase,* the paired chromatids eventually form a so-called metaphase plate, with chromosomes positioned perpendicular to the spindle poles. The next event is *anaphase,* in which the centromeres split, and the chromatids of each chromosome are pulled to opposite poles by stretching of the spindle microtubules as the poles separate. This brief mitotic period is followed by *telophase,* in which the nuclear membrane reforms and the newly created chromosomes disperse into the nucleoplasm. As these last nuclear events occur, cytoplasmic organelles are roughly distributed to each daughter cell, and *cytokinesis* ends when the cleavage furrow becomes complete, thereby separating the two cells.

The human 46 chromosome complement consists of 22 pairs of *autosomes* plus the *sex chromosomes* (X and Y). In order to maintain the species number, the mature gametes can contain only 23 chromosomes when they fuse to form the diploid zygote. *Meiosis* is a specialized process whereby germ cells undergo two cell divisions: the first results in pairing of homologous chromosomes and the second results in reduction from 46 (the diploid number, 2n) to 23 chromosomes (the haploid number, n).

Prophase of the first meiotic division is a long and complex process in which the homologues pair and undergo changes, referred to as the leptotene, zygotene, pachytene, diplotene and diakinesis stages. By pachytene, synapsis (side-by-side pairing of homologues) is complete, providing an opportunity for *crossover* events to occur between the chromatids of the maternally derived member and those of the paternally derived homologue. Crossing-over between homologues refers to the exchange of chromatid segments following DNA breakage in each of two chromatids. Generally, two or more such genetic recombinations occur between each homologue. In diplotene, owing to progressive coiling and shortening, the bivalents dissociate and can be seen microscopically as duplicated homologues held together at the crossover sites, called *chiasmata*. The two X chromosomes in female cells behave like other homologues. The X and Y chromosomes in spermatogonia enter into end-to-end association, in which there may be pairing in a small region of their respective short arms, where crossing-over may occur in rare occasions.

When prophase I ends, the cell proceeds through stages that are comparable to mitosis, except that the centromere does not split. Chiasmata separate, and the centromere-spindle fiber mechanism pulls the paired chromosomes, with their recombinant segments, to opposite poles. Each daughter cell now contains 23 chromosomes, each with two sister chromatids. Meiosis II is a second cell division that occurs without prior DNA synthesis but otherwise proceeds as an ordinary mitosis. The second meiosis results in formation of four haploid nuclei, derived from a single germ cell.

Chromosome Structure

Each chromosome contains a single DNA molecule in the form of a double helix, with nucleotide base pairs on the inside of the helix and deoxyribose sugars and phosphates on the outside. Complexed to the DNA molecule are histones and nonhistone proteins. Pairs of four histones, known as the nucleosomal histones, are spaced regularly along the DNA molecule. The DNA wraps around these nucleosomes like beads on a string, as seen on electron microscopy. Nucleosomes are further packaged in groups to create a chromatin fiber that is 30 nm thick. This configuration is achieved through electrochemical forces induced by other proteins known as H1 histones.[19]

In addition to this basic 30-nm chromatin fiber structure, chromosomes are folded into looped domains that extend in various directions from the main axis of the chromosome. The loops vary in size and serve to further pack the long, slender chromatin fibers into the interphase nucleus. Despite the extensive looping, chromosomes are too thin to be seen by light microscopy except in certain cells. However, for many years, cytologists have noted areas of *heterochromatin* in interphase nuclei. Heterochromatin is now known to represent highly condensed chromatin in a helical configuration or supercoil, analogous to the loops of a telephone cord. From a functional standpoint, heterochromatin is transcriptionally inert and is composed of highly repetitive nucleotide sequences.[2] The less condensed chromatin is referred to as *euchromatin* and is transcriptionally active.

At the onset of mitosis, the entire chromosome undergoes a process of coiling and condensation, so that the euchromatic regions soon acquire the same configuration as the heterochromatic regions. Chromosomes thus become shorter and thicker, and by metaphase, each has a distinctive appearance that permits analysis by light microscopy.

CHROMOSOME ANALYSIS

As is true in all laboratory specialties, success depends on the integrity of each step in the diagnostic process. The six major steps in the total testing process are as follows:
1. Clinical question/test selection
2. Specimen collection/management
3. Technology/methodology selection
4. Laboratory analysis
5. Results validation/reporting
6. Application/interpretation of results.

These six sequential steps must be carried out in a fashion that incorporates quality assurance not only during each phase but more importantly at the interfaces between the steps in the diagnostic process.[62] The first step is important in assuring that the physician obtains appropriate specimens in clinical situations in which chromosome studies can be expected to yield useful information, of either a positive or negative nature. Because not all clinicians, whether they be specialists or primary care physicians, have extensive training in human genetics, it is essential that the physician and cytogeneticist's communications be open and functional. The physician must supply complete patient history and clinical information, which will vary depending on the medical problem. Results of previous studies on the patient or other family members should be documented.

Clinicians should be encouraged to telephone the laboratory with any questions regarding appropriateness of studies, sample collection and diagnostic protocols. To facilitate chromosome studies, descriptive brochures and instructional pamphlets produced by the laboratory can provide useful information, thereby decreasing the need for the physician to telephone the laboratory or vice versa.

Specimen Collection and Management

The main objective of specimen collection is to provide a sample of viable cells, taken aseptically, and to submit this sample to the laboratory in a fashion that permits growth and mitosis of selected cells. In most cases, these requirements are not difficult to fulfill. Peripheral blood provides a ready source of lymphocytes that can be stimulated to divide. Skin biopsy samples and specimens obtained at surgery or postmortem examination can be processed for cell/tissue culture. Amniotic fluid samples and chorionic villus biopsy specimens allow fetal diagnosis. Although time in transport is an important consideration regarding success in processing samples, many viable specimens will survive delays as long as a week. Most cytogenetics facilities are reference laboratories that accept specimens from physicians' offices and clinics. Thus, it is not unusual for specimens to take 1 or 2 days to reach a laboratory.

Blood samples in heparin anticoagulant and tissue samples in suitable balanced media will generally survive transport times of 48 to 72 hours if properly collected and prepared. Furthermore, biologic death is not the same as cell death, since postmortem specimens often yield satisfactory results. Even anecdotal reports of successful cultures from nonembalmed bodies that have been exhumed several days after death have been made. Specimens should be collected aseptically, using decontamination solutions, such as alcohol, that evaporate and are not toxic in residual amounts. Generally, antibiotics incorporated into culture media will eliminate any microorganisms that may be introduced into specimens. Even grossly contaminated specimens, such as aborted fetuses, may be salvaged with additional antibiotic treatment of cultures.

Three types of specimens are processed in the laboratory—direct preparations and short-term and long-term cultures.[139] Direct preparations may be made from sources that usually contain mitotic cells. These include bone marrow and fluids or washings from such sites as pleural and peritoneal cavities. Short-term blood cultures of 48 to 72 hours' duration depend on phytohemagglutinin or other substances that stimulate lymphocytes to dedifferentiate and begin mitotic activity. Long-term cultures can be started from various sources. Cells attach to culture flask surfaces and multiply as monolayer colonies. Once enough cells are present and dividing, they may be harvested for chromosome preparations.

Bone Marrow. Bone marrow was the tissue used by the English cytogeneticists in the late 1950s at the time of the rebirth of human cytogenetics. Squash preparation techniques, using Feulgen staining, were borrowed from plant and insect cytogeneticists. These methods have been replaced by more reliable techniques. For best results, 0.5 to 2 ml of marrow, collected in heparin, should be delivered within 1 hour after aspiration. Dilution with excess sinus blood should be avoided. The direct procedures place the aspirate into a solution such as a basic culture medium with heparin and colcemid (an analogue of colchicine). After 1 to 3 hours' incubation at room temperature, cells are centrifuged and resuspended in hypotonic (0.075 M) potassium chloride solution for 20 minutes at room temperature. Following centrifugation and

removal of supernatant, cells are fixed in cold glacial acetic-methanol fixative. A number of slide preparation techniques can be used to obtain maximum spreading of chromosomes, and various methods are available to obtain excellent staining results.

Although these direct procedures permit the examination of spontaneously dividing cells, results are not always successful. Mitotic rates may be low because of the disease process or the treatment modality. Chromosome morphology is frequently poor, especially in leukemia and preleukemia, and banding is often marginal. Cell synchronization techniques and short-term culture methods may help to correct these problems. To provide additional information in such cases, simultaneous examination of phytohemagglutinin-stimulated and unstimulated peripheral blood cultures may provide better material for chromosome analysis. Peripheral blood cultures also provide the cytogeneticist the opportunity to study spontaneously dividing cell populations as well as transformed lymphoblastoid cells.

Peripheral Blood. Peripheral blood is a convenient source of leukocytes. The discovery in 1960 that a bean extract, phytohemagglutinin, can transform small T lymphocytes into large lymphoblastoid cells opened a new era in clinical cytogenetics.[97] DNA synthesis begins after approximately 24 hours of incubation with phytohemagglutinin. Within 48 to 72 hours of incubation, cells enter mitosis. Other stimulants, such as pokeweed mitogen, can also be utilized for certain cases. Colchicine or an analogue is introduced into the culture for the last 3–4 hours of incubation to arrest the majority of cells in prometaphase or metaphase. Colchicine inhibits microtubule formation, thereby blocking development of the mitotic spindle apparatus. The convenience of peripheral blood cultures, made possible by the introduction of phytohemagglutinin and colchicine, has made it the most widely used source for chromosome analysis. Furthermore, it is possible to obtain excellent banding with cultured lymphocytes.

For most studies, 10 ml of blood is collected in heparin, and the leukocyte-rich plasma or buffy layer is separated for culture in appropriate media, supplemented with phytohemagglutinin. The most widely used culture media incorporate fetal bovine serum, glutamine and penicillin-streptomycin. Reduction in the supply of fetal bovine serum has led to the development of controlled process serum replacements to support the growth of cells in culture. If less than 10 ml is obtained, there may still be enough leukocytes to carry out the separation process. However, in infants, obtaining even a few milliliters of blood may be difficult. Volumes of less than 1 ml (5 to 10 drops in 5 ml of media) may be set up as whole blood cultures that usually yield enough dividing lymphocytes to provide satisfactory results. Failure of peripheral blood culture may be attributable to lymphocytopenia, poor response to phytohemagglutinin, excessive cellularity that causes depletion of culture media or other technical factors. Use of different stimulants, such as pokeweed mitogen, or adjustment of cell numbers may correct the problem. Blood collected in vacuum tubes or syringes can be conveniently shipped to the laboratory, and cultures can be set up several days after collection. However, extremes in ambient temperatures, freezing or exposure to excessive heat may destroy the viability of the cells for cytogenetic study. Depending on the leukocyte cellularity, different quantities of plasma or whole blood should be inoculated into culture tubes to obtain optimal results.

Tissue Culture. Tissue culture permits cytogenetic studies to be performed on cells from various organs of the body. Unless special techniques are used, however, most tissue cultures result in growth of stromal fibroblasts rather than parenchymal cells. This caveat applies to normal organs and to neoplasms alike. Skin samples, a common source, are obtained after decontamination of cosmetically remote sites. A tiny fragment (<3 mm) containing deep dermis is all that is required so that scar formation is avoided. From surgical specimens, aborted fetuses or autopsy cases, appropriate tiny samples are removed aseptically and placed in balanced salt solution or growth medium. Necrotic areas, fat or liver should not be selected. Fascia lata, lungs, areas close to large blood vessels and amniotic sacs are good sources from fetuses. To obtain cells other than fibroblasts, laboratories use soft agar methods, cloning techniques, washing methods, specialized growing surfaces and various cell identification markers.

In the laboratory, small biopsy samples are minced with scissors or scalpel blades into tiny fragments. These pieces are explanted onto surfaces of culture flasks and incubated in a 5% CO_2 atmosphere, using a suitable culture medium.[37] Several techniques can be used to promote attachment of the fragments and to encourage cell multiplication and migration onto the surface. Flasks are examined periodically, using an inverted microscope, and the medium is changed as required. Once sufficient monolayer growth is observed, usually in 7 days or more, cells are harvested for chromosome studies or subcultured.

An alternative procedure for handling tissue samples is to place the minced fragments in a trypsin-ethylene-diaminetetra-acetic acid (EDTA) or other enzyme solution, such as collagenase, and to agitate the mixture for 20 to 30 minutes. Once the tissues have dissociated, the solution is centrifuged and the cells are resuspended in growth medium for monolayer cultivation in a CO_2 incubator. Body fluids or body cavity washings can be handled like dissociated cells.

Amniotic Fluid. Amniotic fluid cultures permit the determination of the cytogenetic status of the fetus. Furthermore, amniotic fluid can be analyzed for its alpha-fetoprotein content, which is an indicator of neural tube defects and other congenital anomalies. Cells derived from the amnion can also be used to detect certain genetic conditions, including a number of inborn errors of metabolism.[111] Most amniocenteses are done between 13 and 20 weeks of gestation. With ultrasound guidance to locate the placenta, the safety of the technique is high. Compiled data from many studies have shown that amniocentesis increases the risk of spontaneous abortion by less than 1% above the natural risk. When 15 to 20 ml of amniotic fluid is collected, amniocyte cultures are almost always successful. Smaller volumes of fluid, with fewer cells, may delay growth so that results may not be obtained in a timely fashion.

A major consideration when examining amniotic fluid specimens is assuring that the cells analyzed are fetal and not maternal in origin. The quality of the specimen depends largely on the expertise of the obstetrician. The clinician should discard the first 1 to 2 ml of fluid and collect the sample itself in a different syringe to avoid maternal-cell contamination. The fluid should be transported to the laboratory in sterile nontoxic tubes. After centrifugation, the supernatant is withdrawn and saved for alpha-fetoprotein and other procedures, as indicated. The cells are resuspended in growth medium and distributed into multiple (at least two) culture flasks for incubation in a CO_2 atmosphere. Flasks should be placed in separate incubators to prevent possible loss of the specimen due to CO_2 or temperature (37°C) maintenance failure.[139]

Cytogenetic laboratories have tried various growth media and additives to improve success rates and to reduce the time from culture inoculation to reporting of results. A 10- to 14-day turnaround time is desired, especially in more advanced pregnancies. Different techniques and additives are employed to enhance cell attachment and to promote migration and cell division. Usually, flasks are left undisturbed for 4 to 5 days. At that time, in the case of a bloody specimen, the medium with any suspended cells is transferred to centrifuge tubes. After centrifugation, the pellet is resuspended in growth medium into a new culture flask. The original flasks are filled with fresh medium, and all flasks are incubated again in CO_2. When the rate of proliferation is judged to be adequate by microscopic examination, the flasks can be harvested for chromosome preparations.[139] The flasks are then replenished with fresh medium to be reincubated for later study if the original preparations yield too few satisfactory mitotic figures or yield ambiguous results.

Chorionic Villus Sampling. Chorionic villus sampling permits first-trimester diagnosis of genetic disorders. In large series, success rates of 98.7% have been achieved.[55] Chorionic villus sampling is generally performed 8 to 11 weeks following the last menstrual period, using a 16- to 18-gauge catheter under ultrasound guidance. The transcervical approach has been employed most widely, but starting in 1984, the transabdominal approach has gained broad acceptance.[122] Villus samples are obtained by placing the tip of the catheter into the chorion frondosum and exerting negative pressure with a 20-ml syringe.[55] Tissue samples of 15 to 30 mg are desirable, but even smaller samples can be grown successfully. Using a stereoscopic microscope, the villi are stripped free of decidual tissue. Cells from chorionic villi can be analyzed with either a direct technique or a culture method.

The direct technique developed by Simoni and associates[120] exposes the villi to a few hours of incubation with colcemid. Cells are then subjected to the usual hypotonic treatment and fixation. Various modifications of the direct technique include incubation times up to 48 hours, enzymatic treatment of villi to obtain cytotrophoblast cells and cell synchronization methods.[139]

Long-term cultures may also be obtained from chorionic villus sampling specimens following enzymatic treatment. Direct preparations seldom provide adequate information for a confident diagnosis to be made.[26] However, long-term culture has the disadvantages of possible maternal contamination and the greater time required for results to be obtained (usually 8 to 13 days). As to the question regarding safety of the chorionic villus sampling procedure, an ongoing study by the National Institute of Child Health and Human Development found that miscarriage occurred in 2% of the chorionic villus sampling patients, compared with 1.3% of the amniocentesis patients. Because chorionic villus sampling is performed earlier in pregnancy, some of the excess loss may be attributable to abortions that would have occurred naturally.[43]

Other Techniques. Other techniques have been developed to improve results from culture of clinical specimens.[139] These include culturing cells directly on cover glasses in petri dishes or in slide chambers and processing cultures *in situ*. A variety of media have been introduced to optimize growth from amniotic fluid, bone marrow and chorionic villus sampling. Stimulators, such as fibroblast growth factor, are commerically available. Alternative mitotic arresting agents (e.g., vinblastine), enzymes for harvesting (e.g., collagenase, pronase) and slide preparation techniques are employed. Cell synchronization can be achieved using methotrexate or fluorine-substituted uracil to inhibit DNA synthesis for a limited time period during incubation.[40]

Cell Storage. Cell storage can be achieved by cryopreservation. Low temperature freezers may be used, but liquid nitrogen provides more reliable preservation of cells for many years. Cells are stored in growth media containing glycerol or dimethyl sulfoxide (DMSO), and they can be readily recultured in order to carry out additional studies.[37] Cultures that might be preserved by a cytogenetics laboratory for future reference are tissues or prenatal specimens in which chromosomal abnormalities are shown or prenatal specimens in which metabolic diseases are suspected.

Banding Techniques

The rebirth of human cytogenetics in the late 1950s resulted in some confusion regarding the identification and classification of individual chromosomes. Dr. Charles E. Ford suggested convening a conference, by invitation, to decide on a standardized nomenclature. The report of this meeting, known as the 1960 Denver Conference, was entitled *A Proposed Standard System of Nomenclature of Human Mitotic Chromosomes.* In 1963, a second meeting, known as the London Conference, officially sanctioned the classification of the seven groups of chromosomes, A to G, as proposed

by Patau.[105] A third conference in Chicago in 1966 adopted a system for shorthand descriptions of the chromosome complement and its aberrations.

When analyzing nonbanded chromosomes, it is possible to reliably identify only chromosomes 1, 2, 3, 16 and Y. In exceptional karyotypes, pairs 17 and 18 and the largest and smallest C chromosomes, 6 and 12, may be distinguished.[63] The technique of labeling near the end of the S phase (late labeling) with tritiated thymidine, combined with autoradiography, enabled cytogeneticists to distinguish 4 from 5; 13, 14 and 15; 17 from 18; and 21 from 22.[116] This autoradiographic technique was too cumbersome for routine clinical use; however, it did distinguish one of the two X chromosomes in females on the basis of late labeling of its facultative heterochromatin. Thus, it was the first method that distinguished heterochromatin from euchromatin in metaphase chromosomes.

Q-Banding. Discovery by Caspersson's group that quinacrine mustard, a fluorochrome, produces differential staining of metaphase chromosomes ushered in a new era in cytogenetics in 1970.[17] This first banding procedure was the result of extensive studies of the chemistry of nuclei utilizing quantitative high-resolution microphotometric techniques.[16] It was soon found that the alkylating agent portion of the fluorochrome was not necessary to achieve banding because quinacrine dihydrochloride (Atebrine), Hoechst 33258, acridine orange and other fluorochromes also produce good banding. Depending on their affinities for adenine-thymine (AT) or cytosine-guanine (GC), the fluorochromes produce patterns similar to G-bands or R-bands, which are produced by nonfluorescent techniques.[139] The most intensely staining region, using quinacrine, is the terminal long arm of the Y chromosome. This method is, therefore, very useful in identifying the Y chromosome or Y translocations, especially in prenatal specimens. The bright Y long arm can also be seen in interphase cells of males. The so-called Y-chromatin body test on buccal smears is useful for rapid cellular sex determinations. The requirements for ultraviolet microscopy, special photographic methods and other technical problems such as fading of fluorescence on exposure to ultraviolet light, however, have limited the general utility of *Q (quinacrine)-banding.*

At the same time that Q-banding applications were being tried, apparently unrelated biochemical studies that were to provide more information on the functional correlates of chromosome structure were in progress. Using cesium chloride density gradients for DNA separation, Yunis and Yasmineh isolated a distinct fraction of DNA that differed from the main band DNA on the basis of its buoyant density.[155] This fraction, termed satellite DNA, is composed of short nucleotide sequences repeated in tandem thousands to millions of times per nucleus. Because of its repetitiveness, satellite DNA renatures rapidly after it denatures. Located primarily in heterochromatin, it is not involved in protein synthesis but serves a structural function. Satellite DNA has been localized to metaphase chromosomes on slides that have been subjected to NaOH plus heat pretreatment to denature the DNA. This *in situ* hybridization technique shows localization in the centromeres and secondary constriction regions of certain chromosomes.

C-Banding. In preparing slides for *in situ* hybridization, it was found that staining the treated (denatured) slides with Giemsa produced dark staining of the same regions that hybridize with satellite DNA.[154] The technique became known as *C-banding,* because of its selective staining of centromeres. It identifies heterochromatin, termed *constitutive heterochromatin,* in contrast to the heterochromatin of the inactive X, termed *facultative heterochromatin.* C-banding basically involves denaturing treatments using heat plus alkali, followed by reassociation under controlled conditions and staining with Giemsa.[4] C-banding produces prominent staining of the secondary constrictions of chromosomes 1, 9 and 16; the satellites on the D and G chromosomes and the distal portion of the Y long arm, in addition to less intense staining of all the centromeres. Variations in the length of heterochromatic regions, called *polymorphisms,* are commonly observed in the normal population. C-banding provides a means to demonstrate heritable variations in heterochromatin content: in this way, certain structural polymorphisms can be readily distinguished from significant chromosome alterations affecting euchromatin. A polymorphism present in one homologue of a chromosome pair can often change its appearance so extensively as to make matching difficult.

G-Banding. C-banding techniques have limited clinical usefulness other than that for demonstrating heterochromatin polymorphisms. However, as C-banding techniques were applied and modified in many laboratories, new methods that used Giemsa stain to produce banding patterns similar to those observed with quinacrine emerged. The methods are called *G-banding* because Giemsa staining is essential for band production. Giemsa dark bands correspond to quinacrine bright bands. G-banding can be produced by heat and saline pretreatment, Giemsa at pH 9, trypsin, potassium permanganate, urea, cesium chloride, detergents and other treatments.[63] G-banding can also be produced by treating living cells with such substances as actinomycin D, tetracycline or hydroxyurea for the last few hours of culture. One method, developed in 1971, yields bands that appear to be the reverse of G bands; thus, the technique is referred to as *R-banding.* R-banding is accomplished by immersing slides in a 10-mM phosphate buffer at 87°C, followed by Giemsa staining.[27]

The plethora of banding methods introduced in a short period of time created confusion regarding the proper terminology for bands and their usefulness in clinical cytogenetics. Consequently, at the Fourth International Congress of Human Genetics held in 1971 in Paris, a group of investigators developed a system for designating bands and regions of chromosomes. Certain changes were also made in the nomenclature developed at the three previous cytogenetics conferences. Two additional conferences resulted in a 1975 supplement to the Paris Conference. The supplement contains a three-letter code to describe banding techniques and a detailed system for designating polymorphisms. In 1976, at the Fifth International Congress, a standing committee on human chromosome nomenclature was elected. The committee produced a document called *An International System for Human Cytogenetic Nomenclature,* abbreviated ISCN (1978). Two updated versions have been published subsequently—ISCN (1981) and ISCN (1985).[65]

The most widely used banding technique in clinical practice is G-banding following trypsin pretreatment (GTG). The method is simple and reproducible and gives greater band resolution than do fluorescent methods. Slides can be retained permanently. A few laboratories prefer R-banding to G-banding for routine use. One major application of R-banding is to study possible aberrations of the light-staining terminal regions of some chromosomes.

The short-arm stalks of the five acrocentric chromosomes (D and G groups) are the sites of nucleolar RNA synthesis. These nucleolar organizing regions can be identified by a silver impregnation method.[139] *N-bands* appear as one or two dots of varying size.

Banding techniques permitted cytogeneticists to determine the approximate location of break points in cases of translocation and deletion. The limit of resolution was determined by the number of bands that could be distinguished—approximately 300 to 400 in the haploid karyotype—as noted in the report of the Paris Conference. In 1976, Jorge Yunis, of the University of Minnesota, introduced a technique that allowed discrimination of a larger number of bands by treating lymphocyte cultures with methotrexate.[149] By blocking the cell cycle at the beginning of the S phase, then adding thymidine to resume the cycle, a large population of cells is synchronized. In about 5 hours, many cells reach prometaphase, a stage in which chromosomes are more elongated. Between 800 and 1000 bands can be distinguished in prometaphase preparations. The ISCN (1985) report provided a diagram representing karyotypes at the 400, 550 and 850 band levels.[65] A convention was adopted for numbering and subdividing the bands in a consistent way. A variety of other specialized techniques have been developed for producing high resolution banding. Additional research methods are available for studying replication patterns and heterochromatin regions and for investigating inherent and acquired breakage and rearrangements.

Microscopy and Interpretation

Numeric Abnormalities. The analytic component of the cytogenetic testing process involves determining the *chromosome number* and detecting any structural abnormality. To determine the chromosome number in a cell culture preparation, the microscopist must examine prometaphase or metaphase spreads in which the complement appears to be intact and in which chromosomes are not too contracted or overlapping.

Mitotic plates can be examined under the microscope or in photographic enlargements. Each method has its advantages. Microscopic examination permits changing depth of focus to determine whether chromosomes are overlapped, touching or fused, broken, excessively stretched or condensed or otherwise problematic. With either method, the cytogeneticist must determine whether isolated chromosomes at some distance from the main aggregate are part of that cell. The slide-making process may cause disruption of nuclei so that one or more chromosomes may be located elsewhere. Another problem may arise when two mitotic plates are close together, and it may be difficult to determine whether certain chromosomes belong to one cell or the other. Usually, differences in the degree of contraction of chromosomes in the two cells allow the microscopist to assign the questionable chromosomes correctly.

Many clinical cytogenetics laboratories do their analyses from photographic enlargements. The cytogenetics technologist examines slides for suitable mitotic cells in which chromosomes are uniformly stretched and have minimal overlapping. The technologist photographs the cell and records its location on the slide by noting the readings of the coordinates on the stage micrometer. This permits the best of both techniques, because the cytogeneticist can then go back and examine the cell under the microscope if there are any questions. When overlaps occur, multiple photographic prints can be made, so that each individual chromosome can be cut out. Furthermore, photographs are needed for cutting out individual chromosomes and placing them according to size and appearance in a format known as a *karyotype* (Fig. 2–1).

The cytogeneticist must then determine the chromosome number of the cells and whether the complement appears to be normal. These are often accomplished by examining the photograph, counting the chromosomes and marking them with different colored wax crayons to designate their group or individual identity. Normal cells should contain 46 chromosomes. However, cells will be found that contain 45, 44 or fewer chromosomes and, occasionally, 47 or more. Variation from the modal number is referred to as *aneuploidy*. To determine whether aneuploidy represents a second cell line or is an artifact of preparation, it is necessary to count enough cells to rule out mosaicism. *Mosaicism* refers to the presence of two or more cell lines in one individual, such as the 45,X/46,XY mosaic, in which one population has 45 chromosomes with a single X and the other has 46 chromosomes with XY sex chromosomes. Significant mosaicism may arise as an error in meiosis, when nondisjunction or anaphase lag results in a gamete with an extra or missing chromosome. The first few postzygotic divisions also are highly susceptible to mitotic errors. In mosaic individuals, half the cells may have one complement and half another, or a second population of less than half may exist. Triple mosaicism can also occur.

To detect true mosaicism, various schemes have been designed. Patau devised a system in which 11 cells are analyzed. If only one cell is nonmodal, he calculated a 95% level of confidence that significant mosaicism does not exist. When two cells have the same chromosome extra or missing, additional cells have to be counted, according to the formula, in order to rule out significant mosaicism of greater than 25%, with a 95% level of confidence. In practice, most laboratories routinely examine, photograph or both between 15 and 20 cells and take additional photographs if needed. The finding of three cells with the same aneuploid complement in an analysis of 20 cells, for example, poses a diagnostic dilemma for the cytogeneticist. It is incumbent upon the examiner to study additional cells, or to study slides made from different culture flasks, to determine if the aneuploidy arose *in vitro* or is present in the subject. Reports should include the number of modal cells examined and the number of aneuploid or abnormal cells present, with each abnormality designated. Examples of numeric chromosome aberrations are as follows:

45,X	45 chromosomes, monosomy for X
47,XY,+13	47 chromosomes, XY sex chromosomes, trisomy for chromosome 13 (three 13s)
46,XX,+14,−18	46 chromosomes but aneuploid, XX sex chromosomes, with an extra 14 and missing an 18, also called pseudodiploid
69,XXY	triploid cell, with three haploid sets
92,XXXX	tetraploid cell (a type of polyploidy).

Structural Abnormalities. The more difficult aspect of cytogenetic analysis is determining the presence of *structural abnormalities*. This task has become even more formidable with the advent of extended banding and its capability of revealing tiny aberrations the size of one small band. To detect small structural changes, one must examine karyotypes carefully and compare homologous chromosomes. Larger aberrations can usually be identified on the metaphase or prometaphase spreads themselves. As will be explained in the next section, accurate results depend on high quality preparations and photographs, plus the expertise of the cytogeneticist.

Chromosomes are identified by their length, arm ratios, presence of secondary constrictions and presence of satellites. The centromere, which attaches the two chromatids, divides the chromosome into two parts or arms. If the arms are almost equal in length, the chromosome is called *metacentric;* if they are unequal, it is called *submetacentric.* The shorter arm is termed *p* and the longer arm is termed *q.* When the centromere is close to one end, the chromosome is designated *acrocentric.* All acrocentrics have stalks on their short arms, with attached satellites.

The karyotype is constructed by placing the cut-out chromosomes from the photograph on a karyotype form that lists them according to size and number (see Fig. 2–1). After the karyotype is made, each chromo-

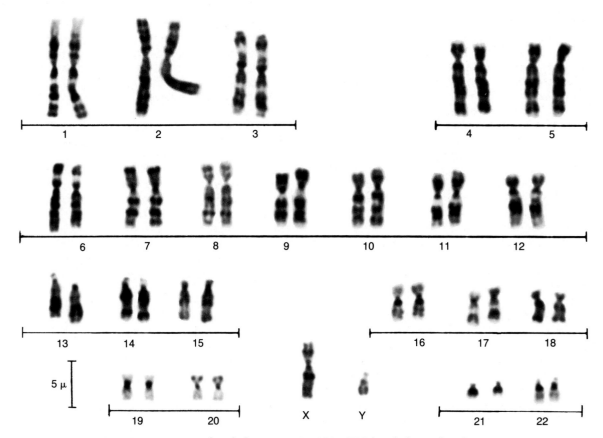

FIGURE 2–1. Normal male karyotype (46,XY), GTG banded, 400-band stage.

some is examined more closely for abnormalities. By placing the chromosome next to its homologue, it is possible to compare them and to note discrepancies. When banding techniques are used, each chromosome is considered to consist of a continuous series of bands.[65] *Bands* are distinguishable from adjacent segments by virtue of their lighter or darker staining intensity. Bands are located in *regions*, which are areas of chromosomes lying between two adjacent *landmarks*. Regions and bands are numbered consecutively from the centromere outwards on each chromosome arm. Bands are identified according to the chromosome number arm symbol, region number and band number. For example, 2p23 indicates chromosome 2, short arm, region 2, band 3. When extended banding techniques are used, existing bands may be subdivided into subbands, which are numbered sequentially from the centromere outward, e.g., 2p23.1, 2p23.2 and 2p23.3. Sub-bands may be further subdivided.

A standardized nomenclature, devised for describing the human chromosomes and their aberrations, is found in the latest ISCN (1985), along with accepted symbols and abbreviated terms.[65] Structural chromosome aberrations are designated by their breakpoints and band composition, using either a short system or a detailed system. The altered chromosome is placed within parentheses following the symbol identifying the type of aberration. When two or more chromosomes have been altered, the one with the lowest number is specified first followed by a semicolon, as is a sex chromosome if it is involved, e.g., t(4;10), t(X;15).

The types of aberrations include isochromosomes, deletions (terminal and interstitial), inversions (paracentric and pericentric), duplication of segments, rings, dicentrics, translocations (reciprocal, Robertsonian and whole-arm), insertions (direct and inverted), complex translocations and marker chromosomes. An example of a reciprocal translocation and its designation, using the short system as noted in ISCN (1985), is the following: 46,XY,t(2;5)(q21;q31). The same rearrangement as described by the long system follows: 46,XY,t(2;5)(2pter → 2q21::5q31 → 5qter;5pter → 5q31::2q21 → 2qter). Segments distal to bands 2q21 and 5q31 have been exchanged following breakage in the long arms of chromosomes 2 and 5.

Abnormalities such as those listed have to be distinguished from *variations in heteromorphic regions* in banded chromosomes. These heterochromatic regions are the centromeres (cen), the secondary constrictions (h) and satellites (s). Thus, 16qh+ designates a large secondary constriction region on the long arm of chromosome 16, and 15s+ indicates unusually large satellites on 15. A more complete description of polymorphisms can be used, by placing "var" for variable before the chromosome number.[65] A system for grading size of the variable region (1, very small to 5, very large) permits semiquantitation of the polymorphism, for example: 46,XX,var(4)(cen,G4). The centromeric region of chromosome 4 is large when stained with Giemsa.

Heterochromatin Polymorphisms. Heterochromatin polymorphisms are chromosome aberrations that result from changes in the amount or appearance of constitutive heterochromatin, causing the affected chromosome to have an unusual appearance (Fig. 2–2). For example, a number 16 with an elongated secondary constriction may be as large as a small C-group chromosome. Because heterochromatin is genetically inert, such polymorphisms should have no phenotypic expression. When the cytogeneticist examines a routine G-banded karyotype, a discrepancy in size and appearance between two homologues may intuitively be recognized as a polymorphism. To give credence to this diagnosis, C-banding should be performed. If the difference is due to a variation in constitutive heterochromatin, the C-banded karyotype will provide confirmation. If a child's specimen or a prenatal specimen is the subject, another level of confirmation is provided by studying the parents. If one or the other parent carries the same unusual chromosome, it would suggest that the variant is of no clinical significance. If the parents do not carry the variant, it must have arisen *de novo* and would have to be judged on its appearance alone. When heteromorphisms involve the short arms of the acrocentrics, the nucleolar organizing region technique may be helpful in diagnosis. For variations in the length of the Y long arm, both Q-banding and C-banding are useful.

In addition to heteromorphic variations, other polymorphisms are seen. One common polymorphism is pericentric inversion of chromosome 9 (Fig. 2–3). Pericentric inversions (involving the centromere and both arms) and paracentric inversions (involving either the short arm or the long arm) of other chromosomes are less common, and the majority are harmless. In one large study, 34 of 50 paracentric inversions were

familial.[80] The risk for paracentric inversion heterozygotes to have abnormal children is low, but it increases with the finding of recurrent abortion or abnormal children in other carriers in the family. There is need for caution in interpreting pericentric familial inversions in antenatal diagnosis, because a variety of unbalanced chromosomal abnormalities may result from crossing-over in the inverted segment. In addition, it may be difficult to recognize with confidence minute differences between apparently similar parental and fetal inversions.

The task confronting the cytogeneticst in determining whether the chromosome complement is normal or abnormal is indeed formidable. In most cases, the geneticist examines 15 to 20 G-banded metaphase plates and selects the best two or three for karyotyping. After determining the chromosome number and excluding mosaicism, the karyotypes are examined for structural aberrations. The cytogeneticist must decide whether the selected karyotypes are satisfactory for accurate evaluation or whether additional karyotypes will have to be prepared. In some cases, photography is unsatisfactory and should be repeated. When none of the metaphases or prometaphases are considered suitable for karyotyping, more cells may have to be photographed, or in some cases, new slides must be made from fixed cells in storage.

Most karyotypes are not perfect in every respect. There is often some degree of uneven condensation or extension that causes certain pairs to be unequal in length. Furthermore, chromosomes may be slightly curved, and it may be difficult to compare bands and regions. Overlaps can create major problems in analysis. To properly evaluate the complement, each pair

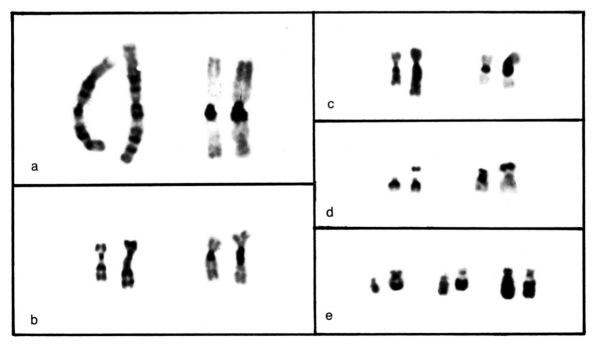

FIGURE 2–2. Common heterochromatin polymorphisms, with polymorphic chromosome placed to the right of its homologue. G-banded pair (left) and C-banded pair (right). *A,* Long arm of chromosome 1 (1qh+). *B,* Long arm of chromosome 9 (9qh+). *C,* Long arm of chromosome 16 (16qh+). *D,* Short arm satellite region of chromosome 21 (21ph+). *E,* Short (Y qh−), average and long (Yqh+) Y chromosomes resulting from differences in length of the heterochromatin.

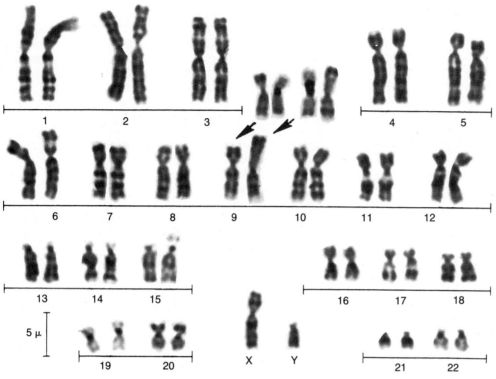

FIGURE 2–3. Male karyotype with pericentric inversion of chromosome 9. 46,XY,inv(9) (p11q12). The insert shows C-banding of the heterochromatic region. This cell also demonstrates prominent satellites on chromosome 15 (15ph+), a frequent polymorphism.

must be present in at least one of the karyotypes without major artifacts, as noted. Every chromosome must be examined closely and compared with its homologue, band-for-band, to determine whether it is normal or not. This decision relies on the knowledge, experience and skill of the cytogeneticist, who must be thoroughly familiar with the morphology and banding patterns of all chromosomes and must be able to detect any aberration. When certain chromosomes are problematic, for example a number 2, the observer may cut out additional number 2 pairs to compare them side-by-side. To assist, reference photographs of high-quality karyotypes at different banding levels should be available for comparison purposes. In addition, diagrams of chromosomes, known as *idiograms,* at the 400-band, 550-band and 850-band levels, reprinted in ISCN (1985), are helpful in evaluating possible deletions, insertions or other rearrangements.[65]

After examining the photographs and karyotypes, and checking any mitotic figures under the microscope if necessary, the cytogeneticist must write a report that states in clear terms whether the chromosome complement is normal or not. If it is abnormal, the nature of the chromosomal defect should be described, using both standardized nomenclature symbols and text that explains the findings in understandable language. If further studies on the subject or on family members are required, such recommendations should be made. In these cases, the subject should be referred to a clinical geneticist for counseling.

Quality Assurance

Reliability of cytogenetic analysis depends on the competence of all personnel in the laboratory and on the operation of the department. Many cytogenetics units started as research laboratories, and today many still combine research activities with diagnostic services. Some laboratories are located in clinical departments or genetics departments of universities. Others may be found in hospital clinical laboratories or in independent testing laboratories. Directors of such operations have come to realize that if reports that determine patient management are generated, the laboratory must be run with the same principles as other clinical laboratories. Systems must be in place to assure the highest quality performance and the most accurate results possible.

As noted in the section Chromosome Analysis, there are six major steps in the continuum of the total testing process. Controls must be in place at each step of the process as well as at the critical interfaces. In many respects, this evolution in cytogenetics regarding laboratory management parallels the changes seen in operation of clinical cytology laboratories. Quality assurance practices were introduced in earnest into diagnostic cytology in the 1970s, amidst increasing governmental and professional concerns about the reliability of cytology reporting. This concern led to more formal guidelines, standards setting and recommendations regarding the practice of cytology.[94] Quality specifications were spelled out for laboratory facilities and equipment, record keeping and reporting, specimen handling, diagnostic evaluation of slides, evaluation of screening accuracy, personnel qualifications and continuing education and automation.

In view of the many similarities between diagnostic cytology and clinical cytogenetics, professional societies, laboratory manufacturers, regulatory agencies, third party payers and practicing geneticists themselves began to recognize the need for establishing more consistent quality assurance practices for clinical cytogenetics. Another stimulant for standard setting was the concern over legal liability.

Federal Programs. The role of the federal government in laboratory regulation can be traced to two separate legislative acts that were passed in the 1960s. The 1965 amendments to the Social Security Act provided health insurance benefits for the aged. Standards were established by the federal government for accrediting independent laboratories under Medicare. In 1967, as part of the Partnerships in Health legislation, the Clinical Laboratories Improvement Act (CLIA), which provided for licensure of laboratories engaged in interstate commerce, was passed. Cytogenetics was not one of the disciplines identified separately in the regulations. In 1976, one of the federal agencies involved in these programs, namely, the Centers for Disease Control (CDC), convened an *ad hoc* meeting on genetic diseases. The meeting focused on newborn metabolic diseases, prenatal diagnosis for chromosomal disorders and alpha-fetoprotein testing. As a result of this meeting, CDC staff members proposed a number of standards, along with a laboratory examination checklist for CLIA regulation of cytogenetics laboratories. Many of the standards were general (e.g., that the cytogenetics section has a standard operating procedures manual), while others were specific (e.g., a minimum of 15 mitoses from two different containers are examined for amniotic fluid cultures). However, these guidelines were never incorporated into the CLIA regulations.

In 1978, CDC convened a conference for the development of methodology for cytogenetic proficiency testing. At that time, two programs were in existence— the New York State (NYS) program and the Province of Ontario Laboratory Proficiency Testing Program (LPTP). The NYS program requires that laboratories pass a proficiency test and have an on-site inspection. One part of the proficiency test is based on sets of banded slides sent to the laboratory. The laboratory photographs, karyotypes and analyzes these preparations and provides cytogenetic diagnoses. The second part of the examination requires the laboratory to submit banded karyotypes to the agency for evaluation by competent reviewers. The Ontario LPTP is a voluntary program of inspection and accreditation. Whole blood samples are sent to participants for culturing, slide preparation and analysis.

Professional Society Programs. Although CDC proposed to mount its own proficiency testing program based on elements of both the NYS and LPTP models, this activity was never approved. Other state health departments in the United States had neither the resources nor the expertise to follow the NYS lead, so further developments in the standards setting/regulatory arena in cytogenetics took place in the private sector. One major professional society that addressed the quality assurance issue in cytogenetics was the College of American Pathologists (CAP). The CAP has a long, distinguished history in the area of continuing education, laboratory management, performance

evaluation and voluntary regulation. The Laboratory Accreditation Program (LAP) is a rigorous one, based on inspection of a laboratory's operation and successful participation in proficiency testing. Approximately 4000 laboratories are accredited by the CAP. These include laboratories in acute-care hospitals, independent laboratories, limited-service general laboratories and specialty clinical laboratories dedicated to a single discipline.[54] The CAP's Interlaboratory Comparison Program offered 252 individual analytic challenges grouped into 51 surveys in 1986.

In 1986, the CAP introduced a proficiency testing program in cytogenetics. The survey consisted of 20 cytogenetics cases sent in quarterly shipments of five challenges.[53] Depending on the nature of the case, correct diagnoses were made in 60% to over 90% by the participants. The participants had the most difficulty with diagnoses that involved photographs of high-resolution chromosome banding. The CAP Survey CY (Cytogenetics) was designed with three primary objectives: (1) that all participants receive the same study materials; (2) that all responses be objective (preferably machine gradable); and (3) that consensus on any individual item be relatively high, to assure the fairness of the survey instrument. For the 1987 survey, in cases of rearrangements, breakpoints that were one or two bands on either side of the "correct" (refereed) response were considered to be acceptable. In 1988, a fresh blood sample from a woman having a benign chromosomal heteromorphism, a pericentric inversion of chromosome 2, was distributed as part of the survey.

Although the CY Surveys are available to any laboratory that wishes to participate, those laboratory directors who wish to receive CAP accreditation must enroll in the LAP program, which includes passing inspections, meeting rigorous standards of laboratory practice and successfully participating in the CY Surveys. Section IX of the Inspection Checklist deals exclusively with the operation of the cytogenetics unit. The laboratory must maintain a written program defining quality control procedures in use and a log of investigative efforts of failed cultures. There must be documentation of ongoing review of quality control activities, as well as corrective actions taken when controls exceed defined tolerance limits. Specimens and data must be handled in a fashion that minimizes the chance for errors. Reports must use the ISCN nomenclature correctly. Many other practice requirements are similar to those demanded for other sections of a clinical laboratory. Some specific standards include examining at least 100 cells for X and Y chromatin counts, at least 20 metaphases and two karyotypes for each case and average case banding at the 400-band level (or greater) of resolution.

One of the major scientific organizations in the field of genetics in the United States is the American Society of Human Genetics (ASHG). In the late 1970s, ASHG formed a Council on Accreditation and Certification and, in 1979, announced a program for certification of individuals in six categories, one being clinical cytogeneticist. A program for accrediting training programs was also proposed. Qualifications for certification and accreditation were developed, and an American Board of Medical Genetics was established to carry out these functions.

Paralleling the history of cytopathology and cytotechnology, a new organization, the Association of Cytogenetic Technologists (ACT), was founded in 1975. ACT joined the National Certifying Agency for Medical Laboratory Personnel to start a certification program for cytogenetics technologists. ACT holds national and regional meetings and publishes a journal, Karyogram. Several universities, including Thomas Jefferson University and the University of Iowa, have begun programs to train cytogenetic technologists.

Program Updates. In 1988, new rules for CLIA (known as CLIA–88) were proposed to go into effect on January 1, 1990. A set of regulations will be required to implement these rules. A major component will be new and enhanced proficiency testing requirements. For cytogenetics, regulations will be based on standards of the private sector and of New York State, which are the existing models for quality control standards. The New York State program has also served as a model for several voluntary regional programs that have developed in the United States as alliances of state genetics services programs.

In 1989, an ACT task force proposed chromosome analysis guidelines that would set minimum standards of performance. Minimum standards for amniotic fluid studies would require counting 15 to 20 cells from at least two independently established cultures, analyzing four to five cells and karyotyping two cells. *Analyzing* is defined as evaluating each chromosome and comparing the homologues band-for-band, from either the microscope or a photomicrograph. Karyotyping can be done from photographs or automated image analyzers. The ACT chromosome analysis guidelines suggest that each laboratory should establish protocols clearly defining standards for band resolution for its own cases and should address the consequences of an inadequate study. The 400-band level is suggested as a reasonable minimal goal for most specimens, particularly amniotic fluid. For children with multiple congenital anomalies and mental retardation (MCA-MR) or for couples with spontaneous abortions, the goal should be a band resolution of 550 or greater. A number of other guidelines and recommendations are made, including confirmation of abnormal cytogenetics results in prenatal diagnosis by cytogenetics studies of the newborn or abortus tissues. Turnaround time for prenatal diagnosis should be within 21 days for 90% of the specimens, preferably within 14 days.

Internal quality control methods and programs should be developed within the cytogenetics laboratory by the director and supervisor. Reagents and media must be carefully managed to assure success in cell culture and to avoid contamination problems. Depending on the specimen volume of the operation, cell culture reagents may be purchased in large volumes, frozen in smaller aliquots and thawed as needed. Lot numbers should be recorded for reference purposes, in cases of culture failure. Contamination should be minimized by using proper techniques and disposable labware. Biologic safety hoods must be properly maintained and monitored, and reagents should be purchased from sources that screen for mycoplasma, adventitious viral agents, endotoxin and bacteriophage. Manufacturers should certify that reagents will satisfactorily support cells in culture.

Another proposed guideline is that culture failure for blood samples (plasma separation technique) should be less than 2%; for whole blood samples (0.5 to 1 ml), it should be less than 5%. The rate of aneuploidy should be less than 20%. The average rate of single chromatid breaks should be 5 to 10%. Slides should be saved for 5 years. The fixed cells not made into slides should be kept until the case is thoroughly studied and the report submitted. In unusual or ambiguous cases, the fixed cells should be saved in a freezer indefinitely. A practice used in some laboratories is a grading system to measure the total number of mitotic spreads per slide and the percentage of mitoses with adequate morphology.[81]

Success in operating a clinical cytogenetics laboratory depends on implementation of a total quality assurance program. The laboratory director assumes responsibility for maintaining the quality of the testing process and ultimately the quality of the results. However, for the unit to function effectively, cytogenetics technologists and cytogeneticists must develop a close working relationship akin to that of cytotechnologists and cytopathologists in a diagnostic cytology laboratory. The ultimate objective is accuracy of results. The user of a laboratory has the right to assume that the information generated by the laboratory is correct.

CLINICAL CYTOGENETICS APPLICATIONS

When technologic improvements enabled investigators to study human chromosomes in the late 1950s, several research groups began to look at patients with well-recognized syndromes. In 1959, Lejeune and associates determined that Down syndrome was caused by an extra chromosome 21, thus establishing chromosomal aneuploidy as the cause of a common MCA-MR syndrome.[74] In the same year, two other research groups discovered that the Klinefelter syndrome was caused by an additional sex chromosome (47,XXY) and that the Turner syndrome was caused by monosomy of X (45,X). All three of these syndromes had been described many years previously, and their phenotypic expressions were thoroughly delineated. All three are common conditions. These startling discoveries stimulated a number of pediatricians, obstetricians, other clinicians and geneticists to examine patients and populations in whom new chromosomal abnormalities might be discovered.

Soon after clinical investigators began studying infants and children with multiple anomalies that did not fall within any of the recognized MCA-MR syndromes, two new syndromes were identified. Patau and colleagues described the trisomy 13 syndrome,[106] and

Edwards and colleagues described the trisomy 18 syndrome.[28] These findings, plus the description of a deleted chromosome 22 in cases of chronic myelogenous leukemia,[102] created an aura of intense interest in the potential insights that cytogenetics might offer in the fields of teratology, sex development and cancer biology.

Congenital Malformations

Early embryonic development is an extremely complex process, with the possibility of error occurring at any stage. Studies in laboratory animals have identified a number of agents, called *teratogens,* that can produce specific abnormalities in certain organs or regions of the body. Certain forms of radiation, a number of drugs and chemicals and several viruses are proven teratogens in one species or another. Epidemiologic and clinical investigations have identified a number of agents that are teratogenic for humans. These include such well-known agents as thalidomide, rubella virus and ionizing radiation. In addition to environmental factors, certain mendelian mutations are known to cause structural defects, such as the Marfan syndrome and achondroplasia. Other malformations may have multifactorial inheritance, the result of the joint action of genes at several loci. Many human conditions and traits are inherited in this manner. For example, cleft palate and neural tube defects are inherited multifactorially, but they may also be caused in some cases by environmental insults or by other etiologic mechanisms. The complexity of human development and the consequences of abnormal development have given rise to a subspecialty in pediatrics known as dysmorphology.[124]

Because chromosomal aneuploidies can cause MCA syndromes, clinicians must decide when to order chromosome studies in cases of congenital malformation. Indications for cytogenetic studies include the following:

1. Mental retardation with three or more dysmorphic features
2. Nonrecognizable or atypical congenital anomaly syndrome
3. Down syndrome for presence of translocation
4. Confirmation of presumed chromosomal syndrome (e.g., trisomy 13)
5. Parents of a child with a structural chromosome aberration
6. Offspring of a parent with a balanced chromosome rearrangement
7. Siblings of a positive parent and other relatives as indicated.

Grossly unbalanced structural autosomal syndromes are characterized by having multiple congenital anomalies in specific combinations, usually with impairment of growth, intellect and often gonadal function.[29] However, only about 6% of such individuals have a chromosome defect. If lymphocyte culture findings are negative and a patient is still suspected of having a structural chromosomal syndrome, fibroblast chromosome analysis should be considered because of the possibility of tissue mosaicism. In any given case, the malformations may be subtle, but the presence of a peculiar facial appearance, several minor anomalies, intrauterine and postnatal growth retardation and microcephaly should signal the possibility of a chromosome defect.

Down Syndrome. Down syndrome (mongolism), the most common cause of severe mental retardation, occurs in a frequency of 1:800 live births. Because many patients are available, studies of the Down syndrome (DS) have provided much information regarding the mechanisms causing aneuploidy and the inherent risks. Even before the trisomy 21 etiology was discovered, it was well known that the risk of having a DS offspring increases markedly with advanced maternal age. For maternal age 20, the risk is approximately 1:1900; for age 30, it is about 1:700; for age 40, it is approximately 1:100 and for age 45, it is almost 1:30.[56] Before the availability of chromosome studies, the woman who had one DS child could be told that her risk for a second DS child would be 1 to 2%, regardless of her age.

The mechanisms creating numeric chromosome abnormality include: (1) nondisjunction of chromosomes during meiosis or mitosis, (2) anaphase lag, in which one chromosome lags and is lost during mitosis, which can lead to mosaicism, and (3) polyploidization, in which various abnormal meiotic or mitotic events lead to triploidy (3n) or tetraploidy (4n).[140] Nondisjunction is considered to be the major cause of trisomy 21, and the maternal age effect indicates that the accident occurs most often during oogenesis. Studies of couples in whom the husbands were considerably younger than their wives have supported the observation that oogenesis is more susceptible to nondisjunction than is spermatogenesis. From a biologic standpoint, there is an obvious explanation for the sex difference. On the one hand, oogenesis is discontinuous, with all the oogonia entering meiosis during the embryonic period and coming to rest in prophase of the first meiotic division. Only at time of ovulation, some 14 to 50 years later, does meiosis resume. There is ample opportunity for errors to occur, perhaps as a result of exposure over a long time period to physical or chemical chromosomal mutagens.[42] Spermatogenesis, on the other hand, is continuous and may be active for the entire adult lifetime of the individual. Chromosomally abnormal spermatozoa presumably should not compete well against the millions of other normal sperm cells that are produced daily. Nonetheless, based on chromosomal markers, about 25% of trisomic DS has been attributed to paternal nondisjunction: the risk for fathers over age 55 is 1%.[49]

In addition to DS cases resulting from trisomy 21, other cases arise from translocation of the long arm of 21 to another chromosome. This results in a complement of 46 chromosomes but with three copies of 21q. Whereas the majority (95%) of DS cases are trisomy (47,+21), about 4 to 5% have a translocation, usually of a type called Robertsonian, involving fusion of long arms of two acrocentric chromosomes at their centromeres. The 21q is translocated to either the long arm of a G or to that of a D chromosome, usually a number 14. Translocations of D/G are about the same size and appearance as a C chromosome. For genetic counseling, it is important to know whether the child is a trisomic or translocation DS. In the trisomic case, especially if this is the second DS in the sibship, the question of parental predisposition must be raised. In the translocation circumstance, one must determine whether there is a balanced translocation in one of the parents or whether the translocation arose *de novo*.

Investigators have considered several mechanisms to explain nontranslocation recurrence of DS in a family. These include: (1) a parental mosaicism, (2) a structural rearrangement or heteromorphism distorting the meiotic process so that nondisjunction is more likely to occur, (3) a mendelian gene that increases the rate of nondisjunction, (4) a satellite association, (5) a reduced recombination on the nondisjoined chromosomes 21 and (6) environmental factors. From five surveys, it has been estimated that in 3% of couples producing a child with trisomy 21, one parent is a very low-order trisomy 21/normal mosaic.[50] Structural rearrangements that have been found in parents of two or more DS siblings include a D/D translocation carrier status in about 8% of couples (one of the parents). This translocation and other aberrations or polymorphisms may increase the risk of nondisjunction. Satellite association refers to the tendency of satellites on acrocentric chromosomes to adhere during mitosis or meiosis, with a presumed increased probability of nondisjunction. The evidence for this effect is limited. Studies of nucleolar organizing region variants in parents of DS children and controls do not show a demonstrable risk for nondisjunction in these variants.[126] Reduced recombination frequencies on nondisjoined chromosomes 21 in DS are consistent with the hypothesis that reduced chiasma formation predisposes an individual to nondisjunction.[143] Environmental agents that have shown an association with nondisjunction include radiation, thyroid disease and antithyroid antibodies. The data for oral contraceptives are inconclusive.[140]

Studies of DS patients and their families have provided much information regarding the inheritance of translocations. Most translocations resulting in DS arise *de novo*—55% of D/21 and 96% of G/21 translocations are new. When parents are found to be carriers of the D/21 translocation, it is important to know the risks for future pregnancies. If the father is a carrier, 2.4% of offspring will have DS, 58.8% will be balanced carriers and 38.8% will have normal chromosomes. For a mother, 11.0% of children will have DS, 40.0% will be carriers and 49.0% will have normal chromosomes.[47] When a parent carries a 21/21 translocation, it must have arisen in the affected parent because the carrier state cannot be inherited. Only affected offspring can result from a 21/21 carrier parent. When the parent has a 21/22 translocation, there is about a 10% chance of having a DS child.

The diagnosis of a DS infant or child should be readily apparent, based on manifestations specific to the condition and a number of other anomalies. Some of the defects are mild, while others, such as heart malformations, may be life-threatening. Many trisomy 21 conceptuses die *in utero*. A number die during the first few years of life, often as a result of defects in the immune system. Those that live to be adults continue to have severe mental retardation, hypotonia and short stature. Females may be fertile, but male DS patients are infertile, except in rare exceptions.[119]

Families in whom a DS infant has been born often seek genetic counseling to determine if there is a recurrence risk for future pregnancies and who in the family is at risk. Women in their late 30s and 40s who are contemplating pregnancy also want to know what their chances for having a DS child are. In the first instance, counselors can provide information, derived from risk tables compiled in the literature, depending on the chromosomal constitution of the proband, and other family studies as necessary. For older mothers, population-based risk tables can also be used for counseling. However, with the advent of amniocentesis, it is now possible to provide counseling based not only on prior cytogenetic studies, pedigree analysis, and risk tables, but on the chromosomal constitution of the fetus. Today, a large portion of the workload of many clinical cytogenetics laboratories is devoted to amniotic fluid studies to rule out trisomy 21. Of course, other trisomies and chromosomal aberrations can also be detected. Most of the patients are women over age 35 who have been counseled about the risk of trisomy.

The most frequent use of midtrimester amniocentesis is for ruling out DS and other chromosomal aneuploidies in older women. In the United States the cutoff age has been arbitrarily selected as 35 years, when the risk for DS is about 1:400. This guideline has been determined from cost-benefit analyses, availability of services and public policy issues. In the early 1980s, 25 to 26% of DS births were to women 35 years or older, who account for only 7% of births in the United States. Many women in the 30 to 34 age group are availing themselves of amniocentesis services, despite the age 35 guideline. Because 18% of DS births occurred in the 30 to 34 age group, which had 18.6% of all births, it has been recommended by some workers that amniocentesis be made available to women age 30 and older.[21]

A surge in the use of amniocentesis for the prenatal diagnosis of DS has occurred since a report in 1984 that second-trimester maternal serum alpha-fetoprotein (MSAFP) levels in DS pregnancies were lower, on the average, than in unaffected pregnancies. Further confirmation of this observation led to a suggestion that MSAFP measurement might serve as a screening test for DS, even though the two population levels overlap.[25] The background to this discovery lies in the wide application of MSAFP screening to detect open neural tube defects, ventral wall defects and certain other anomalies. MSAFP screening has maximal sensitivity at 16 to 18 weeks' gestation, when it will detect about 80% of open spina bifida cases and about 90% of anencephaly cases. Because this is a screening test, it must be confirmed by verification of fetal age by ultrasonography and a second blood sample. If the elevated MSAFP level is confirmed, then amniocentesis is recommended.[45] An amniotic fluid with elevated AFP is then tested for acetylcholinesterase (AChE), which is diagnostic for open neural tube defects.

MSAFP levels are influenced by maternal weight, race, gestational age, laboratory normative data and laboratory quality control. In the United States, use of different commercially available AFP reagents results in variable proportions of normal pregnancies with MSAFP levels falling below specific cutoffs, usually selected as 0.5 multiples of the median (MoM).[79] The screening efficacy of low MSAFP is not well defined. It is estimated that about 20% (with a range of 10 to 40%) of DS fetuses born to mothers under 35 could be identified by doing amniocenteses on women with "low" MSAFPs. This detection rate has to be measured against the cost, the diagnostic errors and the risk of unnecessary amniocenteses. Until the uncertainty about the reliability of risk tables of maternal age and gestational age–related MSAFP values is resolved, their use in making reproductive decisions remains controversial. First-trimester MSAFP screening[95] and effectiveness of amniotic fluid AFP in detecting chromosomal abnormalities other than DS[22] also require additional study.

Other Numeric Chromosome Abnormalities. When D and E trisomies (later identified as trisomy 13 and trisomy 18) were discovered in 1960, there were expectations that many other numeric aneuploidies would soon be found. Aside from a variety of sex chromosome aneuploidies, other trisomies and monosomies were not uncovered in patients or in surveys of various populations. It soon became apparent that autosomal trisomies other than 13, 18 and 21 are lethal except when mosaic, as is autosomal monosomy. Studies on spontaneous abortion specimens conducted in the 1960s and 1970s found that trisomy is the most common chromosomal finding, whereas autosomal monosomy is rare in this population, indicating probable early embryonic death.

Larger surveys of spontaneous abortion have shown that roughly 40 to 60% of cases are caused by abnormalities of chromosome number. Variations from series to series can be attributed to differences in length of gestation, preservation of specimens and selection criteria. In the chromosomally abnormal group, approximately 50% had trisomy; 15 to 20% were 45,X; 15 to 20% had triploidy; 6% were tetraploid and others had mosaicism or translocations and other structural defects. Sex chromosome aneuploidy other than 45,X is found infrequently in this population. In stillbirths and perinatal deaths, the incidence of chromosome abnormalities is 7 to 8%, and in livebirths it is approximately 0.5% (1 in 200). Those infants found to be chromosomally abnormal at birth have sex chromosome aneuploidy (37%), autosomal trisomy (23%) or structural aberrations (40%).[66]

Autosomal trisomy other than for chromosomes 13, 18 and 21, whether total or mosaic with a normal cell line, results in mental retardation, multiple anomalies and failure to thrive. The phenotypes for these chromosomal abnormalities have been defined, and the anomalies, with their frequency of occurrence, are summarized in several reference books.[115, 124]

Structural Chromosome Abnormalities. Structurally abnormal chromosomes result from breakage, which may be spontaneous or induced by a mutagenic agent. Breakage can occur in any stage of the cell cycle—during mitosis, meiosis or interphase (G1, S or G2). Breakage during G1, prior to DNA replication, will be present in both chromatids in the subsequent metaphase. When breaks are produced during G2, only one of the two chromatids is usually affected. Single breaks often rejoin or heal, and no visible effect may result. By comparison, breakage can lead to deletion of fragments or formation of balanced or unbalanced rearrangements, depending on the number of breaks and the nature of the rejoining process. Interchanges between two chromosomes can lead to formation of dicentric chromosomes (chromosomes with two centromeres) and other abnormal configurations that are unstable and are usually lost in subsequent mitoses. Acentric fragments will also be lost in later divisions. The mechanisms of chromosomal breakage and rearrangements are well described and illustrated in the textbook of Therman.[130]

Chromosomes can break at any site, and the variety of structurally abnormal chromosomes is therefore almost infinite.[130] The literature is replete with articles describing patients with various conditions caused by an unbalanced karyotype. With the advent of banding, it became possible to more precisely define the breakpoints and the exact nature of the defect. To assist clinicians and investigators alike, several catalogues of chromosomal variants have been published.[12, 115] Prior to banding, it was possible to detect aberrations if they were of sufficient size and in a location that permitted discrimination. Of course, with banding, such aberrations can be more definitively described (Fig. 2–4). Banding also permits detection of translocations, deletions and insertions as small as a single band (Fig. 2–5).

The catalogues of aberrations are useful in defining the syndromes or conditions that result from deletion or duplication of chromosomal segments. Deletion of a segment is called partial monosomy; duplication is called partial trisomy. These compiled data are useful for genetic counseling, for estimating the risk for transmission of rearrangements and for gene localization.[12] When compiling such catalogues, one must take into account the fact that determination of breakpoints is often not clear and depends on the quality of the preparations. Although prometaphase banding is ideal for determination of small aberrations, it is very time-consuming and requires much skill and experience.[115]

Analysis and comparison of published cases also permit identification of the critical segment in chromosomal syndromes. For example, the *cri du chat syndrome* was the first deletion syndrome described. The condition is caused by partial deletion of 5p, with the size of the deletion varying from small to about 60% of the length of the small arm.[130] By analyzing

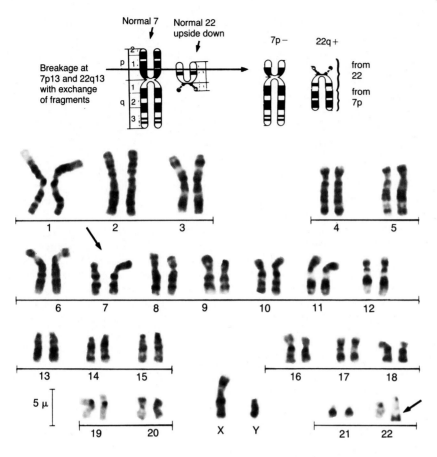

FIGURE 2–4. Karyotype with a balanced translocation between chromosomes 7 and 22, in a man whose wife has a history of spontaneous abortions: 46,XY,t(7;22)(p13.1;q13.3), GTG banded.

many cases, it has been possible to show that the critical segment is a small region in 5p15, probably 5p15.1.[99] Similarly, by reviewing 62 published cases of partial trisomy 13, investigators could localize certain features to the proximal long arm and others to the distal segment.[129]

When a newborn or child with an MCA-MR syndrome is studied, chromosome analysis may reveal an unbalanced structural defect (partial monosomy or partial trisomy). It then becomes necessary to examine the parents to determine if one or the other is a carrier of a balanced translocation or if the aberration arose *de novo*. If a parent is found to be a carrier of a balanced translocation, other children in the family plus parents or siblings of the affected parent will have to be studied to determine who else is a carrier and when the translocation arose. Locating and contacting all members of a large pedigree may become a monumental task. Often, family members do not have resources or insurance to pay for chromosomal analysis, so public health or research funding may be required. Translocation families are counseled regarding their risk of having: (1) offspring with balanced translocations, (2) spontaneous abortions due to lethal complements, especially deletions, and (3) children with the same MCA-MR syndrome as the proband, or a different abnormal phenotype, depending on which abnormal chromosome the child acquires during the segregation process. Although the overwhelming majority of persons with a balanced *de novo* reciprocal

translocation are phenotypically normal, there may be risk for mental retardation, male infertility or other adverse effects. Thus, the family histories accompanying the chromosomal studies in a pedigree analysis should be complete. It is always possible that a break involved an important gene locus or that a minute deletion occurred at the break site.[130]

Prenatal Diagnosis

Amniocentesis. Genetic amniotic fluid analysis is just one of a number of techniques available for prenatal diagnosis. These include ultrasonography, magnetic resonance imaging (MRI), fetoscopy and fetal blood sampling. For example, ultrasound is a very useful noninvasive technique that is often performed for uterine size incompatible with gestational age, polyhydramnios or oligohydramnios, suspected fetal death, bleeding or suspected twins. Ultrasound can detect a number of anomalies of the nervous system, internal organs, limbs, head and trunk.[58] The other techniques also have capabilities for diagnosing specific conditions and for ruling out at-risk disorders or malformations. The relief from anxiety that is provided a couple who have had a child with an inherited disorder or congenital anomaly is important in making reproductive decisions.[118] Amniocentesis has become a major diagnostic tool in the armamentarium of the obste-

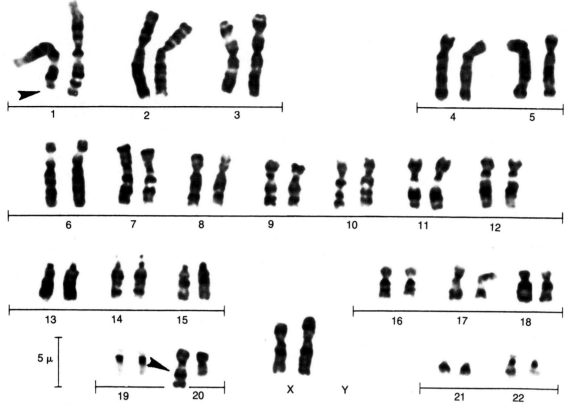

FIGURE 2–5. Female karyotype with a balanced translocation between chromosomes 1 and 20 in an amniotic fluid culture performed because of maternal age: 46,XX,t(1;20)(q32.1;q13.1), GTG banded.

trician. Of course, a normal infant cannot be guaranteed by any or all of these techniques.

The indications for amniocentesis are as follows:

1. Mother age ≥35 years or with increased risk for aneuploidy
2. Parental exposure to radiation or other mutagen
3. Parent is a known translocation carrier
4. Previous conceptus with aneuploidy or aberration
5. A pedigree with an X-linked disorder
6. Nonchromosomal indications—metabolic disorders, high MSAFP, and so forth.

Many of these indications relate to detection of a conceptus with chromosomal aneuploidy or aberration. In the case of X-linked disorders, a male fetus has a 50% chance of acquiring the disorder, so determining the sex provides important information to the family. A decision regarding continuation of pregnancy may now be made with additional input provided by recombinant DNA technology, which can diagnose hemophilia A and Duchenne muscular dystrophy in about 70% of cases.[118] A number of inborn errors of metabolism, mostly autosomal recessive disorders, can be diagnosed by using amniotic fluid or cells for biochemical or molecular biology studies. Thus, many disorders of amino acid, carbohydrate or mucopolysaccharide metabolism can be detected prenatally. The efficacy of MSAFP to detect DS and other aneuploidies has already been discussed in the section on DS. Although the screening test for DS is a low MSAFP, at least one chromosomal disorder, triploidy, has been associated with high MSAFP but normal amniotic fluid AFP.[35]

The use of amniocentesis for prenatal diagnosis introduced new clinical, diagnostic and ethical considerations, above and beyond those previously encountered by the cytogenetics laboratory. These include the following:

1. Potential damage to the placenta or fetus
2. Inadequate specimen, no growth, CO_2 or other technical failure
3. Specimen mix-up or contamination
4. Maternal cell contamination
5. Significance of 47,XXX; 47,XYY; "balanced" translocations; minute markers; low-order mosaicism
6. Interpretation of unusual chromosomal variants.

Amniocentesis is an invasive procedure, but with ultrasound guidance, puncture of the placenta or fetus should be averted. The risk of miscarriage is increased by less than 1%, as noted previously, and maternal complications such as amniotic fluid leakage, infection and vaginal bleeding are uncommon. Laboratory concerns include failure to grow or slow growth, sometimes related to paucity of amniocytes. If the growth rate appears to be unsatisfactory, or if an accident occurs in the laboratory, the obstetrician may have to be contacted for a second specimen. Obviously, the laboratory director tries to keep such occurrences to a minimum, by appropriate quality assurance practices described previously. Culture failure rate should be less than 1%. Maternal cell contamination can be avoided by proper collection techniques and clinician education.

As noted, amniocentesis introduces new diagnostic considerations. For example the 47,XXX and 47,XYY karyotypes are usually associated with no significant phenotypic changes. Women who are 47,XXX may be mentally retarded, but they are generally fertile. Males who are 47,XYY are fertile and usually of greater than average height, but some may have mental retardation or may develop psychosocial adjustment problems. Because the majority of these two sex chromosome aneuploidies will be phenotypically normal, counseling options are not as clear-cut as in other situations. If an apparently balanced translocation is detected, the parents must be studied to determine if either one has the same constitution. If one parent has the reciprocal translocation, one might counsel that the child will have no phenotypic abnormalities not present in the parent. However, one must issue the caveat that although the two translocations may be identical and may involve a minute deletion or gene mutation at a breakpoint, genes on the homologous chromosome may protect the parent, whereas the child may not inherit the same protection from genes on the other parental homologue.

From the standpoint of interpretation, the cytogeneticist must also deal with *de novo* Robertsonian translocations, which usually cause no mental or physical abnormalities.[13] An even more difficult problem is the presence of extra structurally abnormal chromosomes in amniotic fluid cultures. These marker chromosomes occur at the rate of 0.8 per 1000 cases.[57] They are often unidentified and simply called a marker, a minute or a fragment. Some are identified as an isochromosome of the short arms of one of the acrocentrics; others are designated as dicentric markers. Because their origin is often uncertain, it is difficult to provide meaningful information to the clinician. Another diagnostic dilemma is the presence of low order mosaicism for trisomy. Although true mosaicism occurs in only 0.25% of genetic amniocentesis, nearly 1.0 to 2.5% of amniotic fluid cell cultures contain a second cell line. The second cell line is considered to be an artifact of culture in most cases. Analytic methods to rule out true mosaicism and evaluation of cells from separate flasks or colonies will ordinarily be effective. Occasionally, however, these practices will result in diagnostic error.[18]

Unusual chromosomal variants present another challenge to the cytogeneticist. As discussed in the section on microscopy and interpretation, the cytogeneticist must be able to distinguish variations in the heterochromatic regions from significant structural aberrations. Use of special staining techniques is often helpful. Comparison with parental karyotypes may be necessary to determine the significance of a chromosomal variant.

Chorionic Villus Sampling. Chorionic villus sampling (CVS) presents many of the same problems and issues as amniotic fluid cell culture. In a collaborative study by seven different centers of transcervical CVS in first-trimester prenatal diagnosis, cytogenetic diagnoses were made in 97.8% of cases.[109] Only 17 of 2278 women (0.8%) required amniocentesis because the diagnosis was ambiguous. There were no errors in the determiion of sex or the identification of the major trisomies (21, 18 and 13). The investigators conclude that CVS is safe and effective, but it probably entails a slightly higher risk of procedure failure and of fetal loss than does amniocentesis. A unique problem that may occur in CVS cultures is mosaicism confined to the placenta as a result of viable mutations developing in trophoblast or extraembryonic mesoderm cells.[67] Such mosaicism has also been demonstrated in term placentas. The CVS discrepancies are usually designated as pseudomosaicism, but they actually represent constitutional mosaicism confined to the placenta. There is complete absence of mosaicism in the embryo in such cases, but some pregnancies result in unexplained fetal death, intrauterine growth retardation or perinatal morbidity—perhaps as a result of abnormal placental function.

Although short-term CVS culture may be more reliable in detecting mosaicism, with a lower risk of maternal contamination (from decidual cells), a decision to use direct, short-term or long-term CVS culture revolves around the quality of the chromosome preparations. A case has been made that subtle aberrations can be made using long-term culture only, which is more amenable to high quality banding procedures.[123]

Sex Developmental Abnormalities and Infertility

Chromosome studies have been instrumental in providing explanations to many puzzling questions regarding normal and abnormal sex development. The primary events in sex determinations are: (1) maternal and paternal meiosis, (2) gametogenesis, (3) fertilization, (4) postfertilization mitoses, (5) initiation of embryonic development, (6) initiation of gonadal ridge development, (7) differentiation of primordial germ cells and their migration to the gonadal ridges and (8) sex-specific gonadal differentiation.[64] The mechanism that determines whether the individual will be male or female is the combination of sex chromosomes at time of fertilization—an XY complement initiates testes and male development, whereas XX initiates ovaries and female development. The normal mature ovum always has an X, so it is the sperm, with either an X or a Y chromosome, that assigns genetic sex.

Role of the X Chromosome. The birth of individuals with abnormal sex chromosome complements (45,X; 47,XXX; 47,XXY; 48,XXXX and others); hermaphrodites, with both testicular and ovarian tissue; phenotypic females with a 46,XY constitution and phenotypic males with 46,XX karyotypes has provided insights into mechanisms of sex determination. From studies of Turner Syndrome patients, with 45,X or with a structurally abnormal second X, it would appear that two intact Xs are necessary for normal ovarian differentiation. Two Xs are required, even though one or the other X is randomly inactivated early in development in cells of the female embryo (the *Lyon hypothesis*). Random inactivation results in approximately half the cells of the mature female having a functioning, paternally derived X, and half having a functioning, maternally derived X. Inactivation of the second X produces facultative heterochromatin that can be seen in interphase nuclei of females as the *Barr body* (also called sex-chromatin or X-chromatin body). X inactivation occurs prior to the 5th week of development, before development of the gonads. That specific genes on the inactive X persist as female sex determiners seems unlikely. If such genes were present on the active X, they would have to be turned off by a gene or genes on the Y, since male cells also contain an active X.

Adults with monosomy X (45,X) or with additional Xs, such as tetrasomy X (48,XXXX), are phenotypic females, with ovaries and female genital sex development. The presence of a Y chromosome, no matter how many Xs may be present, usually guarantees that male gonadal and genital sex development will ensue. Therefore, the presence of a male sex determiner on Y is conclusive for man. In the latest edition of McKusick's catalogue, he notes that over 140 expressed genetic loci have been assigned to the X, with about an equal number suggested but not proved.[86] Although an X-inactivation center, a Y-regulator gene, an androgen-receptor protein gene (testicular feminization syndrome) and a gonadal dysgenesis locus (XY female type) have been identified, no specific ovarian-determining factor has been found on the X chromosome.

Role of the Y Chromosome. Despite its small size and the fact that approximately half its long arm is heterochromatic, the Y induces testicular and subsequent male development. Additional Ys, as in 47,XYY, provide no special advantage concerning male sex development. Variations in size of the Y chromosome in different males are due to differences in the relative length of the heterochromatic region. Even deletion of most or all of the quinacrine-fluorescent region results in no phenotypic effects or reduction in fertility.[89] Studies of patients with structural aberrations of the Y showed that the testis-determining factor (TDF) is located near the centromere, probably on the short arm. The distal end of Yp is the X-Y homologous, meiotic-pairing region. A male-specific transplantation antigen, the *H-Y antigen,* is considered by some investigators to be the same as the TDF.[142] *In vitro* laboratory experiments have shown that the presence of H-Y antigen on the cell surface induces testis development. A gene for H-Y, either structural or regulatory, is present near the Y centromere. However, a study of XX males and XY females suggests that the H-Y determinant and TDF are different entities and are spaced apart on the Y chromosome.[121] In addition to these loci, a stature or height-determining gene has been postulated on Yq as has a gene controlling tooth size.[3]

Despite existing uncertainties about mechanisms, it is clear that a testis-determining factor on the Y chromosome initiates testicular and subsequent male development. In addition, an X-linked gene, identified as the Y regulator locus, controls the expression of the TDF. Another regulator gene on the X governs the androgen responsiveness of target cells by production of androgen-receptor protein. In males, testicular development and subsequent production of testicular hormones result in differentiation of male internal and external genitalia. Normal development depends on the production of testosterone by Leydig cells and antimullerian hormone by Sertoli cells in the testis.

The presence of androgen-receptor protein and 5 α-reductase in certain target organs is also necessary. The 5 α-reductase converts testosterone to 5 α-dihydrotestosterone in the urogenital sinus, the prostate and the primordia of the external genitalia.[64] Thus, testes are required for wolffian duct differentiation and mullerian duct suppression. As in gonadogenesis, the inherent plan for genital development is female differentiation.

Indications for Chromosome Studies. Male development is clearly more complex than is normal female development, which requires only that there be two structurally intact X chromosomes, even though no ovarian-determining factor on the X is known and even though one X is inactivated early in development. Unlike male sex development, fetal hormones are not involved in female gonadal and genital differentiation. Thus, it is not surprising that there are many more types of male than female pseudohermaphroditism.[64] What then are the major indications for chromosome studies in the area of sex-related abnormalities?

1. Newborn with ambiguous genitalia
2. Female infant with lymphedema of extremities, coarctation of aorta or inguinal hernia
3. Prepubertal female with unexplained short stature
4. Individual with delayed puberty or incomplete sexual development (either sex)
5. Female with primary amenorrhea (>16 years) after other studies
6. Couples with unexplained infertility.

The majority of patients in all six of these categories will be found to have normal chromosome constitutions. However, when certain populations are studied, several sex chromosome abnormalities occur with regular frequencies. In spontaneous abortion, sex chromosome aneuploidy is rare, except for 45,X, which represents 15 to 20% of the chromosomally abnormal group. Because 15 to 20% of clinically recognizable pregnancies result in spontaneous abortion, of which about 50% are chromosomally abnormal, then about 4% of all conceptions that reach 12 to 20 weeks would be expected to have a 45,X complement. The incidence of 45,X in newborns is 1:10,000, indicating that over 95% of fetuses with this karyotype die *in utero*. This finding is not surprising in view of the fact that all other monosomies are lethal. In comparison, the presence of additional X or Y chromosomes is relatively common in newborns. Approximately one 47,XXX karyotype is found in 1000 live female newborns, whereas 1:1000 live male births has 47,XYY and 1:1000 has 47,XXY. Of the three, only 47,XXY, the Klinefelter karyotype, regularly results in gonadal dysgenesis. Although all three genotypes often occur in individuals who have normal appearance and normal intelligence and no external anomalies, these individuals, in aggregate, have an increased incidence of mental retardation, mental illness, such as schizophrenia, and difficulties in social adaptation.

Because all X chromosomes in excess of one are inactivated, an extra X would not be expected to have significant phenotypic effect in a female. Most 47,XXX females have normal female genitalia, feminine secondary sex development and average fertility. However, females with four or five X chromosomes have severe mental retardation and various physical anomalies. The initial publicity over reports that XYY males may be more aggressive and show criminal tendencies presented a biased picture, because it was based on a study of tall institutionalized criminals and psychopaths. Aside from a generally increased risk of behavioral disorder, the most obvious somatic effect of the extra Y is on height, because XYY men are on the average taller than XY men. There is normal male sex development and fertility.

The Klinefelter Syndrome. In contrast to the presence of an extra Y, which has no effect on male development, an additional X (47,XXY) leads to the Klinefelter syndrome, which is usually diagnosed after puberty on the basis of small testes, azoospermia and increased gonadotropins, with gynecomastia in about half the cases.[76] Almost half of the Klinefelter males are normal in appearance with average intelligence and come to medical attention only in the course of an infertility workup, or they may remain undetected. Small testes reflect atrophy and hyalinization of the seminiferous tubules, with few germinal cells present. Males with a 46,XY/47,XXY constitution may show less phenotypic effects than nonmosaic Klinefelter males. As in the case of females with extra Xs, the larger the number of additional X chromosomes in a male, the greater the severity of mental retardation and other somatic defects, especially skeletal malformations.

The Turner Syndrome. Most individuals with Turner syndrome die *in utero;* those who are liveborn have normal female external genitalia, so they do not present as an intersex problem. However, they often have lymphedema of the limbs and a redundancy of the skin of the neck with a low posterior hairline. In addition, a large number of major and minor anomalies are usually present, including serious cardiovascular defects, such as coarctation of the aorta. Another group of Turner syndrome cases is ascertained in children on the basis of marked shortness of stature. At puberty, the Turner syndrome genotype is suspected in females because of lack of secondary sex development and primary amenorrhea. Sex developmental failure results from the absence of follicles in the fibrous streak ovaries. Most 45,X individuals have normal intelligence, even though there is multiple system impairment. Importantly, the Turner syndrome is not associated with advanced maternal age as is observed in the XXX and XXY genotypes.

Patients with fewer dysmorphic features or taller stature may be suspected of being Turner syndrome mosaic, with a normal cell line (45,X/46,XX). Phenotypic variation with this mosaicism ranges widely, de-
pending on the percentage of normal cells and their tissue distribution. Patients may have a higher percentage of 45,X cells in tissues that are critical for sexual differentiation. In many cases, buccal smear and lymphocyte cultures will resolve the question of cryptic mosaicism in patients suspected of Turner syndrome; when results are conflicting, however, examination of skin biopsy or other tissues may yield a more accurate estimation of the extent of mosaicism.

Mixed Gonadal Dysgenesis. Another form of mosaicism that has even greater clinical significance is 45,X/46,XY, which is found in about 5% of patients with Turner syndrome. Depending on the proportion of each cell type, this mosaicism can give rise to a condition known as mixed gonadal dysgenesis. Most affected individuals are raised as girls because the external genitalia usually appear to be a clitoris and labia. The internal genitalia often show intersex features, and there may be a dysgenetic testis on one side and a streak gonad on the contralateral side.[64] Other cases have ovotestes or dysgenetic testes on both sides. Females with 45,X/46,XY show lack of feminine secondary sex development at puberty, plus they may have virilization. One third to one half of the cases appear clinically as the Turner syndrome phenotype with no virilization, despite the presence of testicular tissue.[1] In these individuals, the presence of dysgenetic testes is associated with a substantial risk of gonadal malignancy. The risk of gonadoblastoma and other tumors is 10% by age 15 and rises sharply to 73% by age 30.[83] Dysgenetic testes should be removed early to prevent the development of tumors and virilization. Therefore, all patients suspected of having Turner syndrome should be studied for possible mosaicism for XY. Those with no Y-bearing line have no increased risk of gonadal malignancy.

Structural Abnormalities of the Y. Structural abnormalities of the Y chromosome, including most deletions of the Y long arm, may have no phenotypic effects. However, an isochromosome of the Y long arm, 46,X,i(Yq), usually is found in an individual with a female phenotype and gonadal dysgenesis but no Turner syndrome stigmata, confirming the location of the TDF on the Y short arm. The absence of Turner syndrome features indicates the presence on the Y long arm of genes that prevent the physical stigmata of the syndrome, perhaps homologous to certain loci on the X short arm.

Structural Abnormalities of the X. Structural abnormalities of the X chromosome also provide insights into its functional anatomy. Isochromosome of the long arm, 46,X,i(Xq), occurs in some 20% of Turner syndrome patients and results in X-chromatin positive buccal smears. Even though the i(Xq) is invariably inactivated, patients have most features of Turner syndrome, including short stature, streak gonads and amenorrhea. They do, however, have a lower incidence of certain somatic abnormalities.[114] On the one hand, patients with short-arm deletions of the X are phenotypically similar to i(Xq) patients. On the other hand, long-arm deletion patients are usually of normal height and appearance, indicating that the genes that influence linear growth and prevent the Turner syndrome stigmata are located on the X short arm. Xq-patients do have gonadal dysgenesis, emphasizing the importance of two structurally normal X chromosomes for normal ovarian development.

Techniques of molecular biology have extended the gene map of the X chromosome.[30] Somatic cell *in situ* hybridization studies have located certain previously disputed traits to the X. The use of restriction enzymes to break the X into variable segments, known as restriction fragment length polymorphisms (RFLPs), have been used for mapping studies. Further sources of information have been the study of patients with X-autosome translocations and the localization of genes at the break sites. Over 200 DNA markers, located at specific regions on the X chromosome, can be used to study genetic linkages. Using the techniques of RFLPs and *in situ* DNA hybridization, for example, a deletion at Xq26-27 was associated with premature ovarian atrophy in a family.[73]

Sex Reversal. The finding of a male phenotype in individuals with XX sex chromosomes, male psychosexual identification, atrophic testes without evidence of ovarian tissue and absence of female genital organs has been termed *sex reversal*. Autosomal dominant inheritance, autosomal recessive inheritance and Y-autosomal and Y-X translocations have been postulated in the past to explain human XX maleness. Hybridization studies for the presence or absence of 23 Y-specific DNA restriction fragments identified Y-specific DNA in 12 of 19 XX males, suggesting that each of these individuals carries a single, contiguous portion of the Y chromosome in his genome.[138] Of practical importance is the ability of Y-specific DNA sequences to identify Y chromosome material in cases in which cytogenetic analysis alone led to misidentification in Turner syndrome mosaics.[38]

Infertility. Many couples seek medical attention because of reproductive dysfunction, infertility or recurrent spontaneous abortion. Male partner workups in infertility clinics include examination for developmental, endocrine or genetic defects. A number of studies of infertility show that 1 to 3% of male partners have Klinefelter syndrome. When examining men with azoospermia, 15 to 20% were found to be 47,XXY or variants.[104] In infertile males, 1% show X/XY mosaicism, and 1% have D-G or D-D Robertsonian translocations. The translocations may interfere with the processes of meiosis and spermatogenesis. Structural changes of the Y chromosome in 1 to 3% of infertile males are of unknown significance. A small number of female partners in infertility workups have chromosome abnormalities. These include the full gamut of sex chromosome aneuploidy plus other abnormalities.

Recurrent Abortions. Many studies have been made of recurrent spontaneous abortion (defined as two or more or three or more losses), with widely discrepant results. The results of these series depend on whether couples have exclusively experienced pregnancy loss or have had a mixed history of reproductive successes and failures. Conservatively, 2 to 6% of couples will be found to have a partner with a translocation (Rob-

ertsonian or balanced) or an occasional maternal X chromosomal aneuploidy or mosaicism. Qualitative or quantitative polymorphisms do not appear to play an important role in the etiology of multiple spontaneous abortions.[11]

Other Clinical Indications

Several clinical scenarios exist in which chromosome studies may provide useful information. These include the following:
1. Possible exposure to radiation or other mutagen
2. Bone marrow transplant for evidence of recolonization
3. Stillbirth where maternal factors have been ruled out
4. Genetic linkage study or genealogic study
5. Artificial insemination donor
6. X-linked mental retardation.

Ionizing radiation is a potent chromosome-damaging agent, causing breaks at any stage of the mitotic cycle or during meiosis. Many chemicals, called *clastogenic* agents, also break chromosomes, as do certain virus infections of cells. It is possible to determine extent of chromosome damage in persons who have been exposed to radiation because of medical reasons, occupation, or accident. The development of persistent clones of cells with dicentrics, reciprocal translocations, rings or other aberrations may indicate significant previous exposure. Therman proposed certain rules to help quantify chromosome-breakage studies.[130] Such studies have clinical relevance, because individuals with demonstrable chromosome damage may be at risk of developing neoplasms or of transmitting new mendelian mutations.

When a patient with leukemia receives a *marrow transplant* after measures to eradicate the recipient's own bone marrow, the physician is interested in knowing whether the cells that appear later in the circulation are from the donor or represent regrowth of residual leukemic recipient cells. This question is easily answered in male recipients from female donors, and vice versa, or when the leukemic cells are characterized by a consistent chromosomal rearrangement. In same-sex transplants, chromosome polymorphisms can be helpful in determining the identity of the cells.

Perhaps 1 to 2% of women who become pregnant will have a *stillbirth* (gestation greater than 20 weeks). About 5 to 10% of stillborns have chromosomal abnormalities, including lethal ones such as trisomy 18 and triploidy. The fact that reciprocal and Robertsonian translocations are also detected in this population may be a reason to suggest chromosome studies in such cases, even if no congenital malformations are apparent.

As more RFLP markers become available, analysis of linkage between two gene loci (e.g., one disease gene and one RFLP marker) and between a gene and a set of markers can be important, both for genetic counseling and for prenatal diagnosis. Progress in this field has been very rapid in recent years.[140] *Genetic linkage* studies can be used to determine if clinical conditions with similar characteristics occurring among members of unrelated families are identical in origin or have different etiologies. As far as study of prospective *artificial insemination donors* is concerned, it is necessary to assure that a donor does not carry a balanced translocation, since donors are customarily used for multiple inseminations.

In addition to chromosome breakage induced by radiation and other clastogens, spontaneous gaps and breaks can be observed in cell cultures from apparently healthy people. The frequency rates of gaps and breaks varies from laboratory to laboratory. In 1964, Schroeder and coworkers noted a high frequency of chromosomal breakage and rearrangements in blood of patients with Fanconi's anemia.[117] Subsequently, similar findings were observed in the Louis-Bar syndrome (ataxia telangectasia) and the Bloom syndrome. These rare autosomal recessive conditions are also associated with an increased risk of certain malignancies, such as leukemia. Soon after the discovery that the three hereditary syndromes show increased spontaneous *in vitro* chromosome instability, Lubs made the important observation of "satellites" on the end of the long arm of X in four males in a family with X-linked mental retardation.[78]

Mental retardation (MR), a major handicapping condition in our society, affects approximately 3% of the population. In cases of severe retardation or mild to moderate MR (IQ between 50 and 70), parents want to know whether the condition is heritable or not.[103] Evaluation includes a thorough three-generation pedigree; physicial, neurologic and sensory examination; and analysis of growth and development. Hundreds of different genetic causes (mendelian, chromosomal and multifactorial-genetic interaction) are known to produce or to be associated with MR. These include a large number of X-linked mutations.[136] In about 30% of families with multiple cases of MR, affected males have an X-chromosome structural fragile site marker, which corresponds to the satellites seen by Lubs.[135] Affected males often have macro-orchidism, which is detected after puberty. They may have no other characteristic physical findings, but some have minor anomalies such as prominent forehead, enlarged ears and long faces. Behavioral signs such as hand flapping and hyperactivity are also suggestive of fragile X.

Fragile X Syndrome. After 20 years of study, the fragile X syndrome is now recognized as the most common inherited cause of MR. To demonstrate the fragile site, designated fra(X)(q27), blood samples must be cultured in folate-deficient medium, or cells must be treated with fluorodeoxyuridine or methotrexate in culture. Protocols for testing specimens require rigid standardization and appropriate controls.[139] In affected males, from 10 to 50% of lymphocytes will show the aberration. Heterozygous females may be mildly retarded, but diagnosis of carrier status in female subjects is not as reliable because of variable expression of the fragile site. In a large Australian survey of intellectually handicapped persons, the prevalence of fragile X in males was 1:2610 and in females 1:4221.[137]

As a result of this survey, Turner and colleagues recommend screening for the fragile X in all mentally retarded people. If fra(X) is identified, females who are at risk of being carriers can be counseled and offered prenatal diagnosis. However, there are still many questions about the inheritance of fragile X, how it is inactivated and reactivated in females, penetrance and nonpenetrance of the mutant gene and the wide range of abnormalities in females who express the heterozygous state.[7] Over 100 other fragile sites have been reported using various culture conditions.[139] No pathologic role for other fragile sites has been shown, although they may predispose individuals to deletions and interchromosomal recombinations.[41]

Research and Public Health Applications

Techniques for analyzing chromosomes have opened new vistas in cellular biology, developmental biology and clinical medicine. Cytogenetics has been a vital factor in defining new entities, such as the fragile X syndrome, previously described. It continues to be an important tool for investigators in a variety of basic science and clinical disciplines. In the next section of this chapter, for example, the role of cytogenetics in cancer research is described. One practical application of chromosome technology, emanating from the research laboratory, is the use of cytogenetic methods as assays for environmental mutagens, a major public health concern.

Mutagenicity Testing. Mutagenicity testing raises many difficult questions because of the complexity of the genetic processes. Mutagens can cause gross chromosomal damage or gene mutations. They can affect germ cells or somatic cells. Some mutations may be eliminated; others may be transmitted to the next generations. Because humans cannot be used for mutagenicity testing, laboratory systems must be relied upon. The mouse has been used extensively for examining the effects of putative mutagenic agents at various levels of development. The most comprehensive data on this subject come from studies of radiation-induced mutation in mice.[140] Recognition of the potential genetic threat of radiation, resulting from this research, has led to worldwide efforts to control and monitor all radiation sources, to protect individuals and to prevent increase in background radiation levels. The public, their legislators and the scientific community alike have expressed similar concerns about the possible danger of chemical mutagens to the population.

Tens of thousands of chemicals are manufactured in quantity for use in industry, with large numbers of new compounds introduced every year. To determine potential mutagenic or carcinogenic activity of any one agent in animal studies is a difficult, time-consuming and expensive undertaking. Accordingly, investigators have explored the feasibility of short-term tests. The first short-term assay to provide useful information was the Ames test, which is based upon the responses of a mutant strain of *Salmonella typhimurium*. The success of the Ames test spurred the development of dozens of other short-term mutagen assays, which test for either gene mutations or chromosome aberrations.[77]

Cytogenetic assays may be performed on established cell lines, such as the Chinese hamster ovary line, or on human cells grown *in vitro*. Other systems can be used, including *in vivo* challenging of animals and subsequent study of their somatic cells and germ cells for chromosome damage. The most widely used end point in all such studies is the systematic analysis of metaphase cells for various types of chromosome and chromatid aberrations (breakage and rearrangements). As noted previously, such studies must be carried out by competent cytogeneticists, using well-defined diagnostic criteria and carefully controlled test conditions. Slides of treated and control cells, made and stained at the same time, should be coded and examined "blindly" by the microscopist.[130]

In systems that employ somatic cell cultures to evaluate chemical mutagenesis, the incidence of chromatid breakage has been used as an indicator of genetic damage following *in vivo* or *in vitro* exposure to a potential mutagen. In human lymphocyte cultures, spontaneous breakage may be found in upwards of 5% of untreated cells. Evaluation of a potential mutagenic effect must include statistically designed experiments that permit demonstration of a significantly higher incidence of chromatid breakage compared with the background level. Some studies have shown that short-term lymphocyte cultures may have an inherent limitation, in that they do not discriminate between lesions that affect DNA directly and those that result from damage to chromosomal proteins in G2, following DNA synthesis. The former result from true mutagenic exposure, whereas the latter can result from the stresses of fixation and slide making.[88] Thus, chromatid breakage alone is an unreliable indicator of mutagenic exposure, whereas quantification of chromosome-type rearrangements does reflect DNA damage. Experiments *in vivo* have shown that chromatid damage produced by nonmutagenic chemicals such as alcohol and cyclamate is not associated with chromosome-type rearrangements.[90]

Sister Chromatid Exchange. Another technique for detecting a mutagenic effect is analysis of sister chromatid exchange (SCE). The technique evolved from 1950s' research on chromosome replication, in which Taylor demonstrated the semiconservative segregation of DNA.[128] Autoradiography showed that, following replication, one chromatid is labeled and the other is not, so that any mitotic crossing-over between the sister chromatids can be visualized. The tritiated-thymidine method has been replaced by the less cumbersome bromodeoxyuridine (BrdU) technique, in which cells can be subsequently stained with Giemsa or with a fluorescent dye. As with chromosome breakage studies, SCE experiments must be designed with proper controls, since SCEs also occur spontaneously.

In addition to the background SCE rate, other factors must be considered in designing SCE studies. The question of localization of SCEs in certain regions of chromosomes has not been resolved. The results of chromosome breakage and SCE induction are not always in agreement. Nevertheless, SCEs are more numerous and simpler to score than chromosome breaks (Fig. 2–6). Although the biologic mechanisms responsible for SCE formations are not fully understood, scientists worldwide are increasingly using SCE in the evaluation of risk from exposure to chemical and biologic reagents.[146] In experimental studies using animals exposed *in vivo* and cells exposed *in vitro*, and in human case-control studies, assay techniques and study protocols can be adjusted to enhance study sensitivity and to minimize potential bias. In spite of their shortcomings, both chromosomal aberrations and SCE techniques may provide useful data when workers or other individuals are exposed to agents with known mutagenic effects.[127]

CHROMOSOMES AND CANCER

One of the primary criteria for cancer diagnosis in clinical cytology is hyperchromatic appearance of nuclei. This diagnostic hallmark, appreciated for years by pathologists, reflects the increased amount of nucleoprotein present in most malignant cells. Although other pathologists had described nuclear and mitotic abnormalities in tumor cells, Boveri in 1914 developed a somatic mutation theory of cancer based on his observations.[14] The theory proposed that malignant cells derive from normal cells as a result of alterations in the chromosome constitution. Unfortunately, the theory could not be tested until cytogenetic techniques improved in the 1950s. Squash techniques were then used to study the mouse Ehrlich ascites tumor, and soon thereafter investigators began examining human malignant exudates. A number of scientists, including Hauschka, Levan, Mitelman, Makino, Koller, Hsu and Sandberg, used newer cytogenetic methods to study the behavior of a variety of malignant cell populations and shifts in stemline karyotypes.[51] Because they were studying advanced or metastatic tumors, no insights were possible regarding the role of chromosome changes in early oncogenesis.

Hematologic Neoplasms

In 1960, Nowell and Hungerford detected a specific chromosome aberration in chronic myelogenous leukemia.[102] The so-called Philadelphia chromosome (Ph[1]) was later identified as a number 22, with deletion of the long arm. The excitement created by this discovery soon abated, however, as no additional specific markers were detected in other human neoplasms. Most solid tumors were found to have modal karyotype numbers in the near-triploid range, with a wide deviation in chromosome number from cell to cell. Even *clones,* cell populations derived from the same tumor

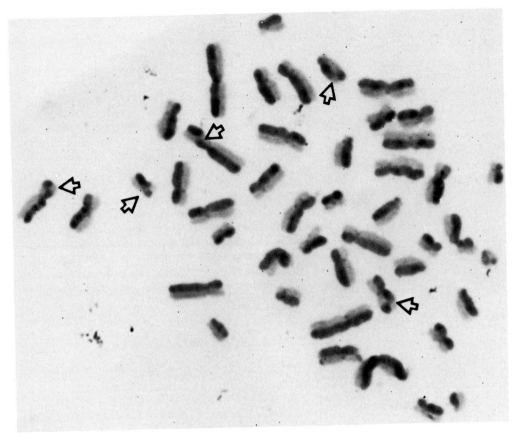

FIGURE 2–6. Sister chromatid exchanges (SCE) using bromodeoxyuridine technique. Arrows point to five exchanges in this male cell.

cell line, often had widely divergent modal numbers and inconsistent chromosome profiles. Some neoplasms, especially hematologic malignancies, were found to have modal numbers in the near-diploid range, but often these were pseudodiploid or had a marker chromosome, representing a stable rearrangement. As more solid neoplasms and leukemias were analyzed, however, the nonrandomness of karyotypic changes was noted in certain specific tumor types, but observations were limited by available methodology.[51] The advent of banding techniques and high resolution methods permitted more precise analysis of chromosome preparations from cancer cells and, thereby, greatly expanded research and clinical capabilities. Research horizons have been extended even further by the availability of molecular biology methods that permit greater understanding of chromosomal-genetic events in oncogenesis.

Although the mechanism of leukemogenesis is not clearly defined, certain etiologic agents have been identified such as ionizing radiation, oncogenic viruses and certain chemicals. One human type C retrovirus, human T cell leukemia virus (HTLV-1), has been isolated from lymphocytes of patients with adult T cell leukemia. Chemicals that have been determined to be leukemogenic include benzene and the alkylating agents.[148] A genetic component in leukemia has been inferred from the substantially increased risk of acute leukemia in the second twin if one of a set of monozygotic twins develops the disease in childhood. Other genetic associations include a predisposition to acute leukemia in three autosomal recessive chromosome breakage syndromes: Fanconi's anemia, Bloom's syndrome and ataxia telangiectasia. Furthermore, a striking increased risk of leukemia (10- to 20-fold) is present in children with DS.

Chronic Myelogenous Leukemia. The most thoroughly studied cancer, cytogenetically, is chronic myelogenous leukemia (CML), which evolves from a primitive myeloid stem cell in the bone marrow. The availability of the Ph[1] marker allowed investigators to study the natural history of CML and its evolution into acute leukemia. In most cases of newly diagnosed CML, the Ph[1] deletion is present in an otherwise apparently normal karyotype in all marrow-derived cells, indicating the clonal origin of the leukemia. Other somatic cells do not contain the Ph[1] deletion. The 10 to 15% of typical CML cases that do not display the Ph[1] deletion are referred to as Ph[1]-negative. Early studies showed that Ph[1]-positive cases occur in a younger population, who respond better to chemotherapy and have a longer life expectancy. Furthermore, the Ph[1] chromosome is consistently present in the erythroid and megakaryocytic precursor cells in the marrow, and the Ph[1]-positive stem line persists in the bone marrow of patients in complete clinical remission.

A second major discovery, made in 1973 by Janet Rowley, was that the Ph[1] chromosome develops not as a simple deletion of 22 but as a result of two breaks, the other involving the long arm of 9. Thus, in CML a reciprocal translocation occurs between 9 and 22, designated as t(9;22)(q34;q11) (Fig. 2–7). Because of

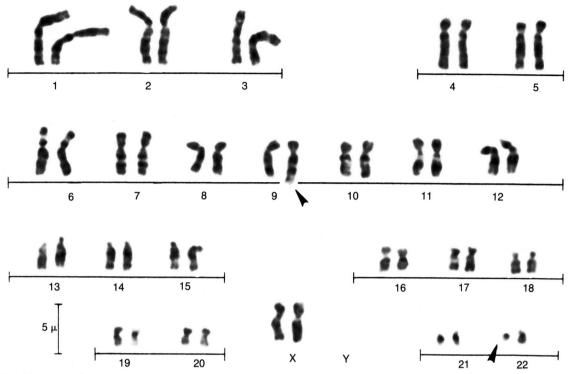

FIGURE 2–7. Leukemic cell from bone marrow of a female with **chronic myelogenous leukemia** showing the Ph¹ translocation between chromosomes 9 and 22: 46,XX,t(9;22)(q34;q11), GTG banded.

the greater length of the 9, the translocation to the end of its long arm is usually not as obvious as the aberration in 22. In high quality banded preparations, and especially in extended banding chromosomes, the t(9;22) can be readily seen.

During the course of Ph¹-positive CML, as the disease progresses, many patients develop additional chromosomal changes. In some cases, the more evolved Ph¹-positive line completely replaces the original Ph¹-positive line; in other cases, multiple clones with distinctive karyotypes coexist. Some clonal changes may be produced by therapy and do not necessarily signify a change in the clinical course of CML.[92] Studies of hundreds of cases of CML have shown that the major route for cytogenetic evolution involves the acquisition of an extra Ph¹, an extra chromosome 8 or the development of an isochromosome 17q, all three of which are associated with blastic crisis. Other less common changes are trisomy 19, trisomy 21 and the loss of a sex chromosome.[52] Another important finding is that translocations other than the t(9;22) occur in 5 to 10% of CML patients, and in some cases three or more chromosomes are involved in complex translocations.[51] Furthermore, as more Ph¹-negative CML patients were analyzed with improved banding and molecular techniques, it became apparent that many cases had cryptic rearrangements of chromosome 9 and 22. Other cases had been incorrectly classified as CML, but reevaluation showed that they were, in reality, chronic myeloproliferative disease, chronic myelomonocytic leukemia or other disorders. Travis and colleagues suggest that Ph¹-negative CML may be a nonentity.[133]

How the breakage and translocation between 22 and 9 are involved in leukemogenesis has been an enigma for hematologists. A possible answer has been provided by research involving *oncogenes*—genes that can transform cells to malignancy. Over 30 cellular oncogenes have been localized to individual bands or regions in the human genome.[51] Oncogenes are believed to exert their effects as a result of mutation or chromosomal breakage in a region adjacent to the oncogene, which activates the oncogene to increase the expression of its product. The coded oncogene products are considered to be involved in regulation of cell growth. Oncogenes belonging to the *ras*, *myc* and c-*abl* gene families have been identified in many common carcinomas, sarcomas, lymphomas and leukemias. In CML, two oncogenes are transferred as a result of the t(9;22) reciprocal translocation: c-*abl*, normally located in region q34 of chromosome 9, transfers to 22q, whereas c-*sis*, normally located in q11.2 of 22, moves to 9q. The c-*sis* does not appear to be altered or activated by this transfer, but c-*abl* is translocated adjacent to a site on 22, a 5.8-kbp DNA region, defined as the breakpoint cluster region (*bcr*).[6] The genetic alteration of c-*abl*, as a result of its fusion to the *bcr* locus on 22, creating a *bcr*-c-*abl* hybrid, directs the synthesis of a new 210,000-dalton, tyrosine-specific protein kinase. The aberrant protein is implicated in the pathogenesis of CML, perhaps as a cellular receptor for a growth factor. DNA probes in combination with other molecular techniques can be used to detect the altered *bcr* gene and to distinguish Ph¹-negative CML from other disorders.

Cytogenetic studies have become an important component in: (1) evaluating patients suspected of having leukemia, (2) functional classification of new cases, (3) predicting outcome of therapy, (4) monitoring the course of therapy, and (5) evaluating the results of bone marrow transplant. Many early leukemias are difficult to classify, so that cytogenetic analysis is often coupled with immunologic marker studies and morphologic examinations that incorporate cytochemical reactions to correctly identify leukemia cell types. Molecular probes are also becoming available for clinical application. Better culture techniques have improved the results of cytogenetic studies in recent years; however, marrow samples may yield chromosome preparations of poor quality or slides with few dividing cells. One practice that supplements the findings of bone marrow samples is the short-term culture of peripheral blood cells for the presence of spontaneously dividing cells. The finding of mitotic activity, chromosomal aberrations or both can correctly distinguish between leukemic and nonleukemic conditions in 97% of cases and may also predict those cases of myeloproliferative disorders that will progress to leukemia.[91] When peripheral blood is stimulated with phytohemagglutinin, malignant cells are sometimes identified dividing along with the normal lymphocytes.

Myelodysplastic and Myeloproliferative Disorders. Clearly, an important use of cytogenetics is in the investigation of patients with hematopoietic disorders that carry an increased risk for the development of leukemia. A number of conditions may be suspect, including myeloid metaplasia, polycythemia, myelofibrosis and myelodysplastic syndromes such as refractory anemia with excess of blasts. Because not all patients with one or another of these conditions progress to leukemia, the term "preleukemia" is not appropriate. The value of chromosome studies in the myelodysplastic syndromes (MDS) has been documented in numerous surveys. Approximately 80% of MDS patients with a cytogenetic abnormality develop leukemia.[100] The most common aberrations are 5q−, monosomy 7 and 7q−.[59] In chronic myeloproliferative disorders, such as idiopathic myelofibrosis and polycythemia vera, several specific numeric and structural chromosome changes have also been found, but a single karyotypic change is not as predictive of progression as is the presence of multiple cytogenetic abnormalities.

Acute Leukemias. The acute leukemias are a diverse group of hematopoietic malignancies in which early cytogenetic studies were not very informative or clinically useful. About 50% of patients had no demonstrable chromosomal findings. Before the use of banding techniques, the chromosomally abnormal cases were categorized as being hyperdiploid, hypodiploid or pseudodiploid.[134] In acute leukemia, in contrast to CML, both normal and malignant cells may coexist in the bone marrow. The most widely used morphologic classification, the French-American-British (FAB) system, divides acute lymphoblastic leukemia (ALL) into three categories, L1 to L3, and acute myelogenous leukemia (AML) into seven categories, M1 to M7.

Experience with AML has been similar to that with CML investigations. Whereas at first only about 50% of cases showed visible abnormalities, later studies have demonstrated karyotypic changes in over two thirds of patients.[96] In the last group, 55% show one specific chromosome rearrangement, and 45% show two or more.[51] More than 25 structural and numeric abnormalities have been reported in AML. Some have been associated primarily with specific leukemias, such as t(8;21) with FAB, M2 type, t(15;17) with M3 type, and inv(16) with M4 type. The t(8;21) and the inv(16) karyotypes have been associated with good prognoses.[36] Patients with normal karyotypes, with 45,X, missing the Y, and with t(15;17) have intermediate prognoses. Poor outcomes are generally seen in AML patients with t(9;22) translocation or with aneuploidy such as +8, −5 or −7. Interestingly, the t(9;22) appears to be identical to that seen in CML; however, the Ph[1] disappears during remission in AML but not in CML.[51]

Most cases of ALL occur in children between the ages of 2 and 4 years. AML is primarily a disease of adults, and the incidence rate increases sharply in the elderly. Analysis of marrow samples is successful in 70 to 80% of ALL cases.[112] Of patients with ALL, two thirds have characteristic acquired karyotypic changes in their leukemic cells, including more than 15 recurring types of rearrangements.[51] The more common types are t(1;19)(q23;p13); t(8;14)(q24;q32); t(9;22)(q34; q11); t(4;11)(q21;q23) and t(11;14)(p13;q13). The t(8;14) translocation is commonly diagnosed in L3, and the others in L1 or L2 leukemias.[9] In general, ALL patients with translocations do poorly and need aggressive therapy to prepare them for marrow transplant. Patients with hyperdiploidy (>50 chromosomes) have longest survival after chemotherapy, and patients with 40 to 45 or 47 to 49 chromosomes have intermediate prognoses.[151]

Chronic Lymphocytic Leukemia. The other major leukemia, chronic lymphocytic leukemia (CLL), is classified as a chronic lymphoproliferative disorder, along with hairy cell leukemia, multiple myeloma, adult T cell leukemia, mycosis fungoides and other entities. Most CLLs are B cell in origin and, as such, do not respond to phytohemagglutinin. Thus, this leukemia of middle-aged and elderly adults was difficult to study cytogenetically from blood cultures using standard methods.[51] The availability of B-cell mitogens, such as pokeweed mitogen, protein A, lipopolysaccharides from *Escherichia coli* and Epstein-Barr virus, permits study of lymphocytes in patients with CLL. About 40% of CLL cases have chromosome abnormalities, with trisomy 12 being the most common.[48] Patients with normal karyotypes generally have longer survival times than do patients with chromosomal changes. In a patient with a mixture of normal and abnormal karyotypes, the greater the percentage of abnormal cells, the worse the prognosis.[51]

Lymphomas. The majority of cytogenetic studies of the malignant lymphomas have been directed at the non-Hodgkin's lymphomas (NHL). Problems in clinical correlation are partially related to the lack of a uniform classification system for NHL. Nevertheless, as results from different cancer centers have been pooled and analyzed, at such conferences as the International Workshop on Chromosomes in Leukemia-Lymphoma in 1984, abnormal karyotypes have been found in 85% of cases.[51] Interest in the lymphomas began in 1972, when Manolov and Manolova described an abnormally long chromosome 14 (14q+) in tumor cells from a patient with Burkitt's lymphoma, a disease of B cells that predominantly affects children.[82] A few years later, it was shown that, as in the Ph[1] deletion in CML, the 14q+ in Burkitt's lymphoma was involved in a reciprocal translocation, in this case with chromosome 8, t(8;14)(q24;q32). Subsequently, two other translocations have been identified—t(8;22)(q24;q11) and t(2;8)(p11;q24). Because in Burkitt's lymphoma cases the break point on the long arm of chromosome 8 always involves band q24, its significance in the malignant transformation process is implied.

About 75% of Burkitt's lymphomas from all continents carry the t(8;14) translocation, whereas t(8;22) and t(2;8) are present in 16% and 9% of cases, respectively. The t(8;14) translocation is found in both the Epstein-Barr virus–positive and –negative types of Burkitt's lymphoma and in ALL-L3, a B cell–type leukemia.[151] Molecular studies have shown that the c-*myc* oncogene is located on band q24 of chromosome 8, and the human heavy chain immunoglobulin locus has been mapped to chromosome 14, the gamma chain locus to 22 and the kappa chain locus to 2. Subsequently, the c-*myc* oncogene has been shown to translocate from 8 to near the heavy chain locus on 14, whereas in the t(8;22) and t(2;8) translocations, the rearranged gamma and kappa chain immunoglobulin genes translocate from their respective positions on 22 and 2 to a chromosomal region distal to the c-*myc* oncogene on 8.[24] The effect of all three translocations is activation of the c-*myc* gene due to its positioning adjacent to long-range enhancers present in the three immunoglobulin loci. Although the precise function of the c-*myc* gene has not been determined, it is known to be associated with growth stimulation and is the cellular homologue of the transforming retroviral oncogene of avian myelocytomatosis virus, v-*myc*, which can induce B-cell lymphomas in chickens.[23]

In non-Burkitt's NHL, the most consistent finding has been the t(14;18)(q32;q21) translocation in *follicular lymphomas*, which constitute 40% of all NHL. In addition, a 6q− or an 18q+ has been found commonly in follicular large cell lymphoma, and trisomy 7 or 12, or both, has been found in most patients with follicular mixed small- and large-cell and follicular large-cell lymphomas.[151] In the nonfollicular lymphomas, the t(14;18) is rarely found. Increased clonal chromosomal variability in non-Burkitt's NHL usually indicates inability to sustain a prolonged remission. A molecular correlate for the t(14;18) translocation is the oncogene *bcl*-2 (B-cell leukemia-lymphoma), which maps to chromosome band 18q21, the site of the t(14;18) translocation.[98] Most studies have shown that t(14;18) results in the close apposition of the *bcl*-2 gene on chromosome 18 with the immunoglobulin heavy chain locus on 14. Regarding genomic alterations in patients

with *diffuse lymphomas,* translocations involving 14q are the most common finding. In large-cell or mixed-cell lymphoma, duplication of 3p is associated with a relatively good prognosis, whereas duplication of 2p or rearrangement of the *bcl*-2 oncogene indicates a poor prognosis.[152] The *bcl*-2 gene has been cloned, and its two protein products both appear to have growth regulatory function.[101]

Solid Tumors

Much of the early research in tumor cytogenetics focused on specific translocations in hematologic neoplasms. Undoubtedly, a factor in this selection process was the ease in obtaining suitable cell populations for study. Unlike bone marrow samples, preparations from solid tumors often yielded connective tissue cells rather than tumor cells. In addition, solid neoplasms, in contrast to leukemias, usually contain numerous karyotypic alterations, which make it difficult to establish the primary cytogenetic event. Determining the initial chromosomal change in sarcomas, which often have one or few karyotypic changes, is generally simpler than in carcinomas. Newer techniques, including exposure of cells to collagenase throughout the incubation period, methotrexate synchronization for better banding, modified hypotonic solution and frequent examination of incubating cells to assess mitotic activity, have improved results of cytogenetic studies of tumors.[113]

Despite improved methodology, cytogenetic studies of solid tumors are difficult. Many malignancies have chromosome numbers in the 60 to 90 range and have chromosomes that are so drastically changed that their origin can no longer be determined. Cytogeneticists refer to these as marker chromosomes. The difficulties in establishing cell lines from tumors and the changes that may occur *in vitro* make short-term culturing of tumor biopsy samples for chromosome analysis the preferred route. Short-term incubation (24 to 48 hours) can be coupled with the practice of sampling aliquots at 4-hour intervals to capture the mitotic wave.[107] A soft agar cloning procedure can be used to develop colonies of tumor cells in the agar matrix, while excluding fibroblasts and other cells that do not proliferate in this system.[20] Cells can be grown later on plastic surfaces for cytogenetic studies.

Childhood Cancers. The greatest insights into cancer initiation and progression as a result of cytogenetic studies have come from examination of several childhood cancers: retinoblastoma, Wilms' tumor and neuroblastoma. *Retinoblastoma* (Rb) is a common childhood tumor that occurs in both hereditary and nonhereditary forms. In 1963, a deletion in chromosome 13 was reported in a case of Rb,[75] but no further cytogenetic progress was made until prometaphase banding permitted Yunis and Ramsay to identify a deletion in the middle of band 13q14.[153] The significance of this finding was that the deletion is constitutional, that is, it is present in all cells of the patient.

Certain other unusual genetic features of Rb intrigued Alfred Knudson, a pediatrician-geneticist, who observed that 40% of children with retinoblastoma have inherited a genetic predisposition for Rb, which usually is bilateral. In the nonhereditary 60% group, the Rb generally affects one eye. Statistical analysis of data from unilateral and bilateral cases led Knudson to develop what is now called the *two-hit theory* of oncogenesis.[70] He proposed that both the hereditary and nonhereditary retinoblastomas are initiated by two mutations. In the inherited form, the first mutation is transmitted in germ cells. In nonhereditary cases, it occurs in somatic cells. For both types of tumors, a second mutation is necessary. However, genetic linkage studies have shown that even though most hereditary cases do not show the 13q14 deletion, there is a submicroscopic deletion in band 13q14 close to the esterase D locus.[125] Evidence exists that a retinoblastoma-susceptibility gene in band 13q14 operates in nonhereditary cases, perhaps as a result of chromosomal abnormalities that occur in retinal cells.[5]

Knudson theorized that the second event occurs at the same locus on the other homologous chromosome in one of four ways: submicroscopic mutation, chromosomal deletion, chromosomal loss, or genetic recombination.[72] The second hit can occur as a result of radiation, chemical exposure or other insult to a somatic target cell (in this case a retinoblast) that already carries a first hit, i.e., deletion of the Rb gene.

Although retinoblastoma was the prototype cancer for Knudson's research, he was also interested in using Wilms' tumor and neuroblastoma to test his model. Some cases of *Wilms' tumor* (nephroblastoma) are associated with aniridia, hemihypertrophy or other local hypertrophies, genitourinary and other abnormalities, and MR. The prediction that a deletion could account for this combination of Wilms' tumor and congenital abnormalities was confirmed with the detection of an 11p13 deletion.[34] A bank of 31 DNA probes, covering the area from proximal 11p14 to distal 11p12, and six reference loci have now been used to divide the 11p13 region into 16 intervals, and specific intervals have been correlated with phenotypic features such as aniridia and Wilms' tumor.[39] Patients with the constitutional predisposition to Wilms' tumor may have a visible deletion in one of the two chromosomes 11, but only 40% of patients with this deletion and aniridia actually develop the tumor. In identical twins with aniridia and the deletion, one twin may develop Wilms' tumor while the other does not.[32] These findings suggest that a deletion in band p13 in one chromosome 11 predisposes an individual to neoplasia but does not in itself induce the condition in the absence of a second mutation in the homologous chromosome.[151]

In cases of *neuroblastoma*, which can also be hereditary or nonhereditary, about 70% show a deletion of the terminal portion of chromosome 1 (1p32.2 → pter).[151] In many neuroblastomas, in addition, the presence of two types of structural abnormalities, *double minutes* (DMs) and *homogeneously staining regions* (HSRs), is noted. Both DMs and HSRs have been seen in direct preparations and cell lines from a wide variety of tumor types (e.g., breast carcinoma, small-cell lung carcinoma, colon carcinoid tumor).[60] They appear to be cytologic manifestations of specific gene amplification and may confer growth advantage to cells. The number of DMs per cell varies greatly because they do not have functioning centromeres. HSRs are pale regions in the chromosomes stained for G-banding. DMs and HSRs are rarely seen in the same cell.

From investigations of childhood cancers, the genes that have been identified as important for these tumors and at least some of their nonhereditary counterparts seem to cause cancer when both copies are defective or lost. The normal allele may be considered to be suppressing oncogenicity; accordingly, in 1983, Knudson coined the term *antioncogene*.[71] The tumor-promoting gene is different from the class of genes known as proto-oncogenes or oncogenes. The last class depends on gene expression of either an abnormal product or an increased amount of product. By comparison, the childhood cancer genes are regulatory genes and recessive in oncogenesis (both homologues must be affected), although predisposition is dominantly inherited.[72]

Solid Tumors of Adults. In solid tumors of adults, cytogenetic studies have not been as rewarding as has the research on childhood cancers. Nonetheless, certain specific neoplasms have been found to have consistent chromosomal abnormalities. In *meningioma*, monosomy 22 is found in 70% of tumors.[156] Many tumors show also loss of one or more other chromosomes. Yunis postulates that monosomy 22 and associated changes represent a secondary event because, in many cases, the majority of mitoses have normal chromosomes and only a subpopulation carries the alterations.[151] However, the loss of antioncogenes from 22q may be implicated in meningioma development.

A very common adult malignancy, *colorectal carcinoma*, has been studied extensively, but early results were difficult to interpret. For example, one study in 1979 reported analyzable results in 755 of tumors, and half of these permitted karyotyping with banding techniques. The cytogenetic data indicated only the nature of the hypodiploid, pseudodiploid and hyperdiploid patterns.[84] Using molecular techniques, two types of genetic alterations have been reported in colorectal tumors. Deletions of specific chromosomal regions can be detected by RFLP analysis of tumor DNA. The most frequent sites of allelic deletion are on 17p and 18q (75% of carcinomas).[69] The deleted sequences have been hypothesized to contain antioncogenes. The other genetic alteration involves mutations in *ras* proto-oncogenes, which convert these proto-oncogenes to oncogenic forms. *Ras*-gene mutations occurred in 58% of adenomas larger than 1 cm, in 47% of carcinomas, but in only 9% of adenomas under 1 cm, suggesting that they are not the first genetic alteration to occur during tumor development.[141]

Two other common tumors that have been studied extensively are carcinoma of the breast and small-cell lung cancer. Early *breast cancer* results were disappointing because of lack of mitotic activity and difficulty in analyzing metaphase cells. Effusions often yielded better results than did tumor biopsy samples.[51] From further studies, the most common finding has been structural changes in chromosome 1, especially involving 1q. Another aberration commonly found has been translocation or deletion of 16q. However, most primary breast carcinomas are chromosomally normal, and the aberrations found in effusions or metastases probably represent progression of disease. Genetic linkage studies of breast cancer susceptibility to nine oncogenes have not by themselves implicated oncogenes in initiation of breast cancer.[46] In one study of *small-cell carcinoma of the lung* (SCCL), a specific defect, deletion (3)(p14p23), was identified in all tumors.[145] This deletion has also been found in cases of renal cell carcinoma. Other investigators have not found the deletion to be universally present in SCCL; however, molecular analysis has shown that loss of alleles at 3p is consistently observed in SCCL and, occasionally, in nonsmall-cell lung cancer.[15]

Carcinogenesis and Tumor Progression

In the preceding sections, several genetic mechanisms involved in carcinogenesis have been described. Much of the work in this field is of recent vintage and involves newly applied molecular techniques. Since cancer biology is obviously a very complex subject, theories of carcinogenesis and their supporting data must be carefully scrutinized. Questions must be asked about the precise role of cytogenetic changes in the three classic stages of cancer development—*initiation*, *promotion* and *progression*. Initiation and promotion are involved in the transformation of normal cells to malignant ones. The existence of more than 40 *oncogenes* raises the following question: Do they represent as many as 40 distinct mechanisms of transformation, or can they be grouped into a small number of functional classes?[144] Are two or more oncogenes required to achieve full transformation, and at what steps in the process of multistep carcinogenesis *in vivo* do the oncogenes function?[10] How do other genes function in tumorigenesis?

The role of chromosomal aberrations in development of human neoplasia is inferred by the number of cancers that have nonrandom abnormalities, particularly deletions or translocations at a specific site. Thus, in CML, Burkitt's lymphoma, neuroblastoma and other malignancies, specific chromosome defects have been identified. In certain neoplasias, the rearrangement may activate an oncogene, such as c-*myc* in Burkitt's lymphoma. In the hereditary tumors such as retinoblastoma, the involved allelic site of the other homologue has to be affected by a second deletion or mutation, as proposed by Knudson. Another theory developed by Yunis is that certain chromosomes have constitutive *fragile sites* in homologous chromosomes. These sites are expressed as a chromosome break or gap when cells are cultured and receive special treat-

ment. Fragile sites in specific chromosome bands may predispose to chromosomal rearrangements, and some may represent oncogenic sites.[150] The example of Xq27 involved in X-linked MR illustrates that not all fragile sites are oncogenic.

Cell culture systems offer certain advantages for studying the different events in tumor development. Reznikoff and colleagues developed a model system using *human uroepithelial cells* (HUC) to study the genetic mechanisms of multistage carcinogenesis.[108] They began their investigations by growing HUC in cell culture and demonstrating a diploid karyotype. The cells were infected with SV40 virus which transformed the HUC into a cell line (SV-HUC–1) with an increased life span in culture. The transformed cells, however, were not capable of forming tumors when inoculated into athymic nude mice. Chromosome studies of four sample passages over a 19-month period showed pseudodiploidy, with extensive karyotypic changes due to formation, rearrangement and disappearance of different marker chromosomes.[93] The genetic instability led to continuous production of nonmodal cells with selection for the most balanced genome. All cells at a given passage contained at least five of seven characteristic marker chromosomes (Fig. 2–8).

SV-HUC-1 cells in early passages were exposed to 3-methylcholanthrene. After a 6-week post-treatment period of culture, cells inoculated into nude mice formed carcinomas.[108] All tumors retained some SV-HUC–1 chromosome markers, but each independent tumor was aneuploid and contained unique new marker chromosomes. Chromosomes usually altered in the malignant lines were numbers 3, 5, 6, 9, 11 and 13. When tumor cell lines were derived from carcinomas induced in nude mice, they retained the same distinctive chromosome markers. The stability of characteristic marker chromosomes distinguishes these malignant lines from the nonmalignant SV40-transformed parent line. Evolution of an adaptive neoplastic genome may select for cytogenetic stability.[147] A working hypothesis is that deleted chromosomal segments in transformed cells contained antioncogenes whose loss is required for expression of the tumorigenic phenotype, along with functional loss of the second allele. Mutational activation of the *ras* oncogene was apparently not involved in the tumorigenic transformation step in this HUC system.

CYTOGENETICS AND MOLECULAR BIOLOGY

The aim of traditional chromosome analysis is to characterize the entire chromosome complement of an individual, using the same level of resolution for all chromosome segments. With the advent of high-resolution techniques, it became obvious that technical problems such as overlaps and interhomologue variability are limiting factors.[110] A composite karyotype, in which chromosome arms were derived from many

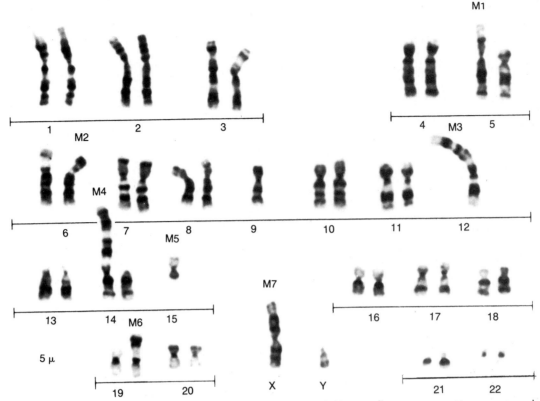

FIGURE 2–8. SV40 virus–transformed human uroepithelial cell with multiple rearrangements creating seven marker chromosomes, numbered consecutively and paired with the chromosome having the greatest homology, GTG banded.

different cells, was usually required. The time required for photography and analysis became prohibitive. The consensus from earlier studies was that high-resolution techniques are most efficiently used when there is some clue of where to focus attention. This consideration necessitates meaningful communication between the clinician and cytogeneticist.

Molecular techniques have further extended the horizons of the cytogeneticist. DNA probes, which are segments of DNA that have been radioactively labeled, can be used to bind (hybridize) to fragments of an individual's DNA complement that has been treated with restriction enzymes and separated by electrophoresis. By combining high-resolution microscopy, DNA probes and, in some cases, linkage studies, microdeletions of the X chromosome, such as glycerol-kinase deficiency mapped to band Xp21, have been identified.[33] This is an example of focused analysis, in which a genetic condition points to a particular chromosomal region that is not detected by ordinary karyotyping. The introduction of biotinylated gene probes now permits nucleic acid hybridization procedures to be performed without the use of radioisotopes. One practical use of a biotinylated gene probe is to detect the gene rearrangement of the breakpoint cluster region of chromosome 22 in CML in cases in which the qualilty or number of metaphase cells is suboptimal for detection of the Ph[1] deletion.[131]

A Y chromosome–specific DNA probe was used to correctly predict fetal sex in 51 of 54 cases.[44] In the later portion of this study, there were no diagnostic errors. As more probes are developed, opportunities for early diagnosis of chromosome abnormalities will increase. A powerful tool for linkage analysis is the use of RFLPs to detect differences in DNA strand sequences. Genotyping with DNA probes and RFLP analysis can be used to separate individuals who appear to be affected with the same disease from each other with respect to etiology and to identify carriers of a trait.[68]

The human DNA complement is believed to consist of 6 billion base pairs. A dream of many scientists has been to construct a map of the entire human genome by mapping all the genes and then determining the sequence of all the base pairs of nucleotides in the genes and in the remaining DNA. The National Research Council appointed a committee to study the possibility of mapping and sequencing the human genome.[87] Other federal agencies, including the National Institutes of Health, have also considered this enormous task. In 1988, an international organization, the Human Genome Organization, was formed and work is proceeding. Gene-mapping workshops are held periodically, and as new information becomes available, it can be applied to prenatal diagnosis, other patient diagnosis or carrier detection. *Genomics* will also be incorporated into tumor diagnosis, staging, prognosis and therapy. As McKusick states: The mapping and sequencing of the human genome constitute a new human anatomy.[87]

References

1. Adashi E, Farber M, Safaii HS, Mitchell GW: Mixed gonadal dysgenesis without virilization. Obstet Gynecol 50:397–400, 1977.

2. Adolph KW (Editor): Chromosomes and Chromatin. Boca Raton, FL, CRC Press, 1988.

3. Alvesalo L, Osborne RH, Kari M: The 47,XYY male, Y chromosomes, and tooth size. Am J Hum Genet 27:53–61, 1975.

4. Arrighi FE, Hsu TC: Localization of heterochromatin in human chromosomes. Cytogenetics 10:81–86, 1971.

5. Balaban G, Gilbert F, Nichols W, Meadows AT, Shields J: Abnormalities of chromosome 13 in retinoblastomas from individuals with normal constitutional karyotypes. Cancer Genet Cytogenet 6:213–221, 1982.

6. Barbacid M: Human oncogenes. *In* Important Advances in Oncology 1986. Edited by VT DeVita, S Hellman, SA Rosenberg. Philadelphia, JB Lippincott, 1986, pp 3–22.

7. Barnes DM: "Fragile X" syndrome and its puzzling genetics. Science 243:171–172, 1989.

8. Baserga R: The Biology of Cell Reproduction. Cambridge, MA, Harvard University Press, 1985.

9. Bennett JM, Catovsky D, Daniel MT, Flandrin G, Galton AG, Gralnick HR, Sultan C: Morphological classification of acute lymphoblastic leukemia: Concordance among observers and clinical correlations. Br J Haematol 47:551–561, 1981.

10. Bishop JM: Viruses, genes, and cancer: Retroviruses and cancer genes. Cancer 55:2329–2333, 1985.

11. Blumberg BD, Shulkin JD, Rotter JI, Mohandas T, Kaback MM: Minor chromosomal variants and major chromosomal anomalies in couples with recurrent abortion. Am J Hum Genet 34:948–960, 1982.

12. Borgaonkar DS: Chromosomal Variation in Man. A Catalog of Chromosomal Variants and Anomalies, 5th Edition. New York, Alan R Liss, 1989.

13. Boue J, Girard S, Thepot F, Choiset A, Boue A: Unexpected structural chromosome rearrangements in prenatal diagnosis. Prenat Diagn 2:163–168, 1982.

14. Boveri T: Zur Frage der Entwicklung maligner Tumoren. Jena, Gustav Fischer Verlag, 1914.

15. Brauch H, Johnson B, Hovis J, Yano T, Gazdar A, Pettengill OS, Graziano S, Sorenson GD, Poiesz BJ, Minna J, Linehan M, Zbar B: Molecular analysis of the short arm of chromosome 3 in small-cell and non-small-cell carcinoma of the lung. N Engl J Med 317:1109–1113, 1987.

16. Caspersson TO: The William Allan memorial award address: The background for the development of the chromosome banding techniques. Am J Hum Genet 44:441–451, 1989.

17. Caspersson T, Zech L, Johansson C, Modest E: Identification of human chromosomes by DNA-binding fluorescent agents. Chromosoma 30:215–227, 1970.

18. Cheung SW, Kolacki PL, Watson MS, Crane JP: Prenatal diagnosis, fetal pathology, and cytogenetic analysis of mosaic trisomy 14. Prenat Diagn 8:677–682, 1988.

19. Clark DJ, Thomas JO: Salt-dependent cooperative interaction of histone H1 with linear DNA. J Mol Biol 187:569–580, 1986.

20. Courtenay VD, Selby PJ, Smith IE, Mills J, Peckham MJ: Growth of human tumor cell colonies from biopsies using two soft-agar techniques. Br J Cancer 38:77–82, 1978.

21. Crandall BF, Lebherz TB, Tabsh K: Maternal age and amniocentesis: Should this be lowered to 30 years? Prenat Diagn 6:237–242, 1986.

22. Crandall BF, Matsumoto M, Perdue S: Amniotic fluid-AFP in Down syndrome and other chromosome abnormalities. Prenat Diag 8:255–262, 1988.

23. Croce CM: Chromosomal translocations, oncogenes, and B-cell tumors. Hosp Pract 20:41–48, 1985.

24. Croce CM, Tsujimoto Y, Erikson J, Nowell P: Chromosome translocations and B cell neoplasia. Lab Invest 51:258–267, 1984.

25. Cuckle HS, Wald NJ, Lindenbaum RH: Maternal serum alpha-fetoprotein measurement: A screening test for Down syndrome. Lancet I:926–929, 1984.

26. Czepulkowski BH, Heaton DE, Kearney LU, Rodeck CH, Coleman DV: Chorionic villus culture for first trimester diagnosis of chromosome defects: Evaluation by two London centers. Prenat Diagn 6:271–282, 1986.

27. Dutrillaux B, Lejeune J: Sur une nouvelle technique d'analyse du caryotype humain. CR Acad Sci (Paris) 272:2638–2640, 1971.

28. Edwards JH, Harnden DG, Cameron AH, Cross VM, Wolff OH: A new trisomic syndrome. Lancet I:787, 1960.

29. Elejalde BR, Opitz JM: Clinical cytogenetics. Postgrad Med 63:179–183, 207–214, 1978.

30. Federman DD: Mapping the X-chromosome. N Engl J Med 317:161–162, 1987.

31. Flemming W: Beitrage zur Kenntnis der Zelle und ihrer Lebenserscheinungen, III. Arch Mikrosk Anat 20:1–82, 1882.

32. Francke U: Specific chromosome changes in the human heritable tumors of retinoblastoma and nephroblastoma. *In* Chromosomes and Cancer from Molecules to Man. Edited by JD Rowley, JE Ultman. New York, Academic Press, 1983, pp 139–159.

33. Francke U: Elusive chromosome anomalies. Hosp Pract 21:175–193, 1986.

34. Francke U, Holmes LB, Atkins L, Riccardi VM: Aniridia-Wilms' tumor association: Evidence for specific deletion of 11p13. Cytogenet Cell Genet 24:185–192, 1979.

35. Freeman SB, Priest JH, MacMahon WC, Fernhoff PM, Elsas LJ: Prenatal ascertainment of triploidy by maternal serum alpha-fetoprotein screening. Prenat Diagn 9:339–347, 1989.

36. Freireich EJ: Hematologic malignancies: Adult acute leukemia. Hosp Pract 21:91–110, 1986.

37. Freshney RI: Culture of Animal Cells: A Manual of Basic Techniques. New York, Alan R Liss, 1987.

38. Gemmill RM, Pearce-Birge L, Bixenman H, Hecht BK, Allanson JE: Y chromosome–specific DNA sequences in Turner syndrome mosaicism. Am J Hum Genet 41:157–167, 1987.

39. Gessler M, Thomas GH, Couillin P, Junien C, McGilliwray BC, Hayden M, Jaschek G, Bruns GAP: A deletion map of the WAGR region on chromosome 11. Am J Hum Genet 44:486–495, 1989.

40. Gibas LM, Grujic S, Barr MA, Jackson LG: A simple technique for obtaining high quality chromosome preparations from chorionic villus samples using FdU synchronization. Prenat Diag 7:323–327, 1987.

41. Glover TW, Stein CK: Chromosome breakage and recombination at fragile sites. Am J Hum Genet 43:265–273, 1988.

42. Golbus MS: Oocyte sensitivity to induced meiotic nondisjunction and its relationship to advanced maternal age. Am J Obstet Gynecol 146:435–438, 1983.

43. Goldsmith MF: Trial appears to confirm safety of chorionic villus sampling procedure. JAMA 259:3521–3522, 1988.

44. Guyot B, Bazin A, Sole Y, Julien C, Daffos F, Forestier F: Prenatal diagnosis with biotinylated chromosome specific probes. Prenat Diagn 8:485–493, 1988.

45. Haddow JE, Knight GJ: Maternal serum alpha-fetoprotein screening: A test for the dedicated laboratory. J Med Technol 3:477–481, 1986.

46. Hall JM, Zuppan PJ, Anderson LA, Huey B, Carter C, King M-C: Oncogenes and human breast cancer. Am J Hum Genet 44:577–584, 1989.

47. Hamerton JL: Human Cytogenetics Vol 1: General Cytogenetics. New York, Academic Press, 1971.

48. Han T, Ozer H, Sadamori N: Prognostic importance of cytogenetic abnormalities in patients with chronic lymphocytic leukemia. N Engl J Med 310:288–292, 1984.

49. Hansson A, Mikkelsen M: The origin of the extra chromosome 21 in Down syndrome. Cytogen Cell Genet 28:107–122, 1976.

50. Harris DJ, Begleiter ML, Chamberlin J. Hankins L, Magenis RE: Parental trisomy 21 mosaicism. Am J Hum Genet 34:125–133, 1982.

51. Heim S, Mitelman F: Cancer Cytogenetics. New York, Alan R Liss, 1987.

52. Heim S, Mitelman F: Multistep cytogenetic scenario in chronic myeloid leukemia. *In* Advances in Viral Oncology, Vol 7. Edited by G Klein. New York, Raven Press, 1987, pp 53–76.

53. Hoeltge GA, Dewald G, Miles J, Palmer C: Proficiency testing in clinical genetics. Arch Pathol Lab Med 112:1085–1090, 1988.

54. Hoeltge GA, Duckworth JK: Review of proficiency testing performance of laboratories accredited by the College of American Pathologists. Arch Pathol Lab Med 111:1011–1014, 1987.

55. Hogge WA, Schonberg SA, Golbus MS: Prenatal diagnosis by chorionic villus sampling: Lessons of the first 600 cases. Prenat Diagn 5:393–400, 1985.

56. Hook EB: Rates of chromosome abnormalities at different maternal ages. Obstet Gynecol 58:282–285, 1981.

57. Hook EB, Cross PK: Extra structurally abnormal chromosomes (ESAC) detected at amniocentesis: Frequency in approximately 75,000 prenatal cytogenetic diagnoses and associations with maternal and paternal age. Am J Hum Genet 40:83–101, 1987.

58. Horger EO, Pai GS: Ultrasound in the diagnosis of fetal malformations. Am J Obstet Gynecol 147:163–170, 1983.

59. Horiike S, Taniwaki M, Misawa S, Abe T: Chromosome abnormalities and karyotypic evolution in 83 patients with myelodysplastic syndrome and predictive value for prognosis. Cancer 62:1129–1138, 1988.

60. Hubbell HR: Gene amplification in neoplasia and chemotherapy. Cancer Bull 35:132–137, 1983.

61. Inhorn SL: Chromosomal studies of spontaneous human abortions. In Advances in Teratology II. Edited by DHM Woollam. London, Logos Press, 1967, pp 37–99.

62. Inhorn SL, Addison BV (Editors): Proceedings of the 1986 Institute on Critical Issues in Health Laboratory Practice: Managing the Quality of Laboratory Test Results in a Changing Health Care Environment. Wilmington, DE, Du Pont, 1987.

63. Inhorn SL, Meisner LF: Mechanisms of chromosomal banding. In Pathology Annual 1975. Edited by SC Sommers. New York, Appleton-Century-Crofts, 1975, pp 145–176.

64. Inhorn SL, Meisner LF, Opitz JM: Abnormalities of sex development. In Endocrine Pathology, 2nd Edition. Edited by JMB Bloodworth. Baltimore, Williams & Wilkins, 1982, pp 375–418.

65. ISCN(1985): An International System for Human Cytogenetic Nomenclature. Edited by DG Harnden, HP Klinger, published in collaboration with Cytogen Cell Genet. Basel, Karger, 1985.

66. Jacobs PA: Epidemiology of chromosome abnormalities in man. Am J Epidemiol 105:180–191, 1977.

67. Kalousek DK: The role of confined chromosomal mosaicism in placental function and human development. Growth 4:1–3, 1988.

68. Kelly TE: Restriction fragment length polymorphism: Applications to linkage analysis. Growth 3:6–8, 1987.

69. Kern SE, Fearon ER, Tersmette KWF, Enterline JP, Leppert M, Nakamura Y, White R, Vogelstein B, Hamilton SR: Allelic loss in colorectal carcinoma. JAMA 261:3099–3103, 1989.

70. Knudson AG: Mutation and cancer: Statistical study of retinoblastoma. Proc Natl Acad Sci USA 68:820–823, 1971.

71. Knudson AG: Hereditary cancers of man. Cancer Invest 1:187–193, 1983.

72. Knudson AG: Hereditary cancers disclose a class of cancer genes. Cancer 63:1888–1891, 1989.

73. Krauss CM, Turksoy RN, Atkins L, McLaughlin C, Brown LG, Page DC: Familial premature ovarian failure due to an interstitial deletion of the long arm of the X chromosome. N Engl J Med 317:125–131, 1987.

74. Lejeune J, Gautier M, Turpin MR: Etude des chromosomes somatique de neuf enfants mongoliens. CR Acad Sci (Paris) 248:1721–1722, 1959.

75. Lele KP, Penrose LS, Stallard HB: Chromosome deletion in a case of retinoblastoma. Ann Hum Genet 27:171–174, 1963.

76. Leonard JM, Paulsen CA, Ospina LF, Burgess EC: The classification of Klinefelter's syndrome. In Genetic Mechanisms of Sexual Development. Edited by HL Vallet, IH Porter. New York, Academic Press, 1979, pp 407–419.

77. Liang JC: Cytogenetics and public health—Assays for environmental mutagens. Cancer Bull 35:138–143, 1983.

78. Lubs HA: A marker-X chromosome. Am J Hum Genet 21:231–244, 1969.

79. Macri JN: Critical issues in prenatal maternal serum alpha-fetoprotein screening for genetic anomalies. Am J Obstet Gynecol 155:240–246, 1986.

80. Madan K, Seabright M, Lindenbaum RH, Bobrow M: Paracentric inversions in man. J Med Genet 21:407–412, 1984.

81. Manhoff L, Clare N, Hunke M, Gonzalez L: A grading system for bone marrow cytogenetics and its use as a standard for quality control. Cancer Genet Cytogenet 9:167–171, 1983.

82. Manolov G, Manolova Y: Marker band on one chromosome 14 from Burkitt lymphoma. Nature 237:33–34, 1972.

83. Manuel M, Katayama KP, Jones HW: The age of occurrence of gonadal tumors in intersex patients with a Y chromosome. Am J Obstet Gynecol 124:293–300, 1976.

84. Martin P, Levin B, Golomb HM, Riddell RH: Chromosome analysis of primary large bowel tumors. Cancer 44:1656–1664, 1979.

85. McIntosh JR: Mechanisms of mitosis. Trends Biochem Sci 9:195–198, 1984.

86. McKusick VA: Mendelian Inheritance in Man, 8th Edition. Baltimore, Johns Hopkins University Press, 1988.

87. McKusick VA: Mapping and sequencing the human genome. N Engl J Med 320:910–915, 1989.

88. Meisner LF, Chuprevich TW, Inhorn SL: Mechanisms of chromatid breakage in human lymphocyte cultures. Acta Cytol 21:555–558, 1977.

89. Meisner LF, Inhorn SL: Normal male development with Y chromosome long arm deletion (Yq−). J Med Genet 9:373–377, 1972.

90. Meisner LF, Inhorn SL: Chemically induced chromosome changes in human cells in vivo. Acta Cytol 16:41–47, 1972.

91. Meisner LF, Inhorn SL, Chuprevich TW: Cytogenetic analysis as a diagnostic aid in leukemia. Am J Clin Pathol 60:435–444, 1973.

92. Meisner L, Inhorn SL, Nielsen P: Karyotype evolution of cells with the Philadelphia chromosome. Acta Cytol 14:192–199, 1970.

93. Meisner LF, Wu S-Q, Christian BJ, Reznikoff CA: Cytogenetic instability with balanced chromosome changes in an SV40 transformed human uroepithelial cell line. Cancer Res 48:3215–3220, 1988.

94. Melamed MR, Inhorn SL, Kachenmeister LA, Ng ABP, Rodner JH: Cytology. In Quality Assurance Practices for Health Laboratories. Edited by SL Inhorn. Washington, DC, American Public Health Association, 1978, pp 509–544.

95. Milunsky A, Wands J, Brambati B, Bonacchi I, Currie K: First-trimester maternal serum alpha-fetoprotein screening for chromosome defects. Am J Obstet Gynecol 159:1209–1213, 1988.

96. Misawa S, Hogge DE, Oguma N, Wiernik PH, Testa JR: Detection of clonal karyotypic abnormalities in most patients with acute nonlymphocytic leukemia examined using short-term culture techniques. Cancer Genet Cytogenet 22:239–251, 1986.

97. Moorhead PS, Nowell PC, Mellman WJ, Battips DM, Hungerford DA: Chromosome preparations of leukocytes cultured from human peripheral blood. Exp Cell Res 20:613–616, 1960.

98. Ngan B-Y, Chen-Levy Z, Weiss LM, Warnke RA, Cleary ML: Expression in non-Hodgkin's lymphoma of the bcl-2 protein associated with the t(14;18) chromosomal translocation. N Engl J Med 318:1638–1644, 1988.

99. Niebuhr E: Cytogenetic observations in 35 individuals with a 5p− karyotype. Hum Genet 42:143–156, 1978.

100. Nowell PC: Cytogenetics of preleukemia. Cancer Genet Cytogenet 5:265–278, 1982.

101. Nowell PC, Croce CM: Chromosomal approaches to oncogenes and oncogenesis. FASEB J 2:3054–3060, 1988.

102. Nowell PC, Hungerford DA: A minute chromosome in human chronic granulocytic leukemia. Science 132:1497, 1960.

103. Opitz JM: Diagnostic/genetic studies in mental retardation. Postgrad Med 66:205–214, 1979.

104. Opitz JM, Shapiro SS, Uehling DT: Genetic causes and workup of male and female infertility. Postgrad Med 65:247–254, 1979.

105. Patau K: The identification of individual chromosomes, especially in man. Am J Hum Genet 12:250–276, 1960.

106. Patau K, Smith DW, Therman E, Inhorn SL, Wagner HP: Multiple congenital anomaly caused by an extra chromosome. Lancet I:790–793, 1960.

107. Pathak S: Chromosome constitution of human solid tumors. Cancer Bull 35:126–131, 1983.

108. Reznikoff CA, Loretz LJ, Christian BJ, Wu S-Q, Meisner LF: Neoplastic transformation of SV40-immortalized human urinary tract epithelial cells by in vitro exposure to 3-methylcholanthrene. Carcinogenesis 9:1427–1436, 1988.

109. Rhoads GG, Jackson LG, Schlesselman SE, de la Cruz FF, Desnick RJ, Golbus MS, Ledbetter DH, Lubs HA, Mahoney MJ, Pergament E, Simpson JL, Carpenter RJ, Elias S, Ginsberg NA, Goldberg JD, Hobbins JC, Lynch L, Shiono PH, Wapner RJ, Zachary JM: The safety and efficacy of chorionic villus sampling for early prenatal diagnosis of cytogenetic abnormalities. N Engl J Med 320:609–617, 1989.

110. Riccardi VM: High-resolution karyotype-phenotype correlations and focused chromosome analysis. *In* Research Perspectives in Cytogenetics. Edited by RS Sparkes, FF de la Cruz. Baltimore, University Park Press, 1984, pp 53–62.

111. Rodeck CH, Nicolaides KH (Editors): Prenatal Diagnosis. New York, John Wiley & Sons, 1984.

112. Sandberg AA: The Chromosomes in Human Cancer and Leukemia. New York, Elsevier/North Holland, 1980.

113. Sandberg AA, Turc-Carel C: The cytogenetics of solid tumors: Relationship to diagnosis, classification and pathology. Cancer 59:387–395, 1987.

114. Santana JAM, Gardner LI, Neu RL: The X isochromosome-X syndrome (46,X,i(Xq)). Clin Pediatr 16:1021–1026, 1977.

115. Schinzel A: Catalogue of Unbalanced Chromosome Aberrations in Man. Berlin, de Gruyter, 1984.

116. Schmid W: DNA replication patterns of human chromosomes. Cytogenetics 2:175–193, 1963.

117. Schroeder TM, Anschutz F, Knopp A: Spontane Chromosomenaberrationen bei familiarer Panmyelopathie. Hum Genet 1:194–196, 1964.

118. Scott JA (Editor): Genetic Applications: A Health Perspective. Lawrence, KS, Learner Managed Designs, 1988, pp 208–230.

119. Sheridan R, Llerena J, Matkins S, Debenham P, Cawood A, Bobrow M: Fertility in a male with trisomy 21. J Med Genet 26:294–298, 1989.

120. Simoni G, Brambati B, Danesino C, Rossella F, Terzoli GL, Gerrari M, Fraccaro M: Efficient direct chromosome analyses and enzyme determinations from chorionic villi samples in the first trimester of pregnancy. Hum Genet 63:349–357, 1983.

121. Simpson E, Chandler P, Goulmy E, Disteche CM, Ferguson-Smith MA, Page DC: Separation of the genetic loci for the H-Y antigen and for testis determination on human Y chromosome. Nature 326:876–878, 1987.

121. Smidt-Jensen S, Hahnemann N: Transabdominal chorionic villus sampling for fetal genetic diagnosis. Technical and obstetrical evaluation of 100 cases. Prenat Diagn 8:7–17, 1988.

123. Smith A, Cohen M, den Dulk G, Guirguis A: Chorionic villus sampling—short-term versus long-term culture in a subtle 2;18 translocation. Prenat Diagn 9:217–220, 1989.

124. Smith DW: Recognizable Patterns of Human Malformation. Philadelphia, WB Saunders, 1982.

125. Sparkes RS, Murphree AL, Lingua RW, Sparkes M, Field LL, Funderburk SJ, Benedict WF: Gene for hereditary retinoblastoma assigned to human chromosome 13 by linkage to esterase D. Science 219:971–973, 1983.

126. Spinner NB, Eunpu DL, Schmickel RD, Zackai EH, McEldrew D, Bunin GR, McDermid H, Emanuel BS: The role of cytologic NOR variants in the etiology of trisomy 21. Am J Hum Genet 44:631–638, 1989.

127. Steenland K, Carrano A, Clapp D, Ratcliffe J, Ashworth L, Meinhardt T: Cytogenetic studies in humans after short-term exposure to ethylene dibromide. J Occup Med 27:729–732, 1985.

128. Taylor JH: A brief history of the discovery of sister chromatid exchanges. *In* Sister Chromatid Exchanges. Edited by RR Tice, A Hollaender. New York, Plenum Press, 1984, pp 1–10.

129. Tharapel SA, Lewandowski RC, Tharapel AT, Wilroy RS: Phenotype-karyotype correlation in patients trisomic for various segments of chromosome 13. J Med Genet 23:310–315, 1986.

130. Therman E: Human Chromosomes: Structure, Behavior, Effects, 2nd Edition. New York, Springer-Verlag, 1986.

131. Tilzer LL, Concepcion EG: Detection of the gene rearrangement in chronic myelogenous leukemia with biotinylated gene probes. Am J Clin Pathol 91:464–467, 1989.

132. Tjio JH, Levan A: The chromosome number of man. Hereditas 42:1–6, 1956.

133. Travis LB, Pierre RV, DeWald GW: Ph¹-negative chronic granulocytic leukemia: A nonentity. Am J Clin Pathol 85:186–193, 1986.

134. Trujillo JM: Chromosomal alterations in hematologic neoplastic disease. Cancer Bull 35:119–126, 1983.

135. Turner G, Brookwell R, Daniel A, Selikowitz M, Zilibowitz M: Heterozygous expression of X-linked mental retardation and X-chromosome marker fra(X)(q27). N Engl J Med 303:662–664, 1980.

136. Turner G, Opitz JM: Editorial comment: X-linked mental retardation. Am J Med Genet 7:407–415, 1980.

137. Turner G, Robinson H, Laing S, Purvis-Smith S: Preventive screening for the fragile X syndrome. N Engl J Med 315:607–609, 1986.

138. Vergnaud G, Page DC, Simmler M-C, Brown L, Rouyer F, Noel B, Botstein D, de la Chapelle A, Weissenbach J: A deletion map of the human Y chromosome based on DNA hybridization. Am J Hum Genet 38:109–124, 1986.

139. Verma RS, Babu A: Human Chromosomes: Manual of Basic Techniques. New York, Pergamon Press, 1989.

140. Vogel F, Motulsky AG: Human Genetics, 2nd Edition. Berlin, Springer-Verlag, 1986.

141. Vogelstein B, Fearon E, Hamilton SR: Genetic alterations during colorectal-tumor development. N Engl J Med 319:525–532, 1988.

142. Wachtel SS: H-Y Antigen and the Biology of Sex Determination. New York, Grune & Stratton, 1983.

143. Warren AC, Chakravarti A, Wong C, Slaugenhaupt SA, Halloran SL, Watkins PC, Metaxotou C, Antonarakis SE: Evidence for reduced recombination in the nondisjoined chromosomes 21 in Down syndrome. Science 237:652–654, 1987.

144. Weinberg RA: The action of oncogenes in the cytoplasm and nucleus. Science 230:770–776, 1985.

145. Whang-Peng J, Kao-Shan CS, Lee EC, Bunn PA, Carney DN, Gazdar AF, Minna JD: Specific chromosome defect associated with human small-cell lung cancer: Deletion 3p(14-23). Science 215:181–182, 1981.

146. Whorton EB, Tice RR, Stetka DG: Statistical design, analysis, and inference issues in studies using sister chromatid exchange. *In* Sister Chromatid Exchanges, Edited by RR Tice, A Hollaender. New York, Plenum Press, 1984, pp 431–440.

147. Wu S-Q, Christian BJ, Reznikoff CA, Meisner LF: Marker chromosome stability associated with neoplastic transformation of human uroepithelial cells. Cancer Genet Cytogenet 36:77–87, 1988.

148. Wyngaarden JB, Smith LH (Editors): Cecil Textbook of Medicine. Philadelphia, WB Saunders, 1988.

149. Yunis JJ: High resolution human chromosomes. Science 191:1268–1270, 1976.

150. Yunis JJ: The chromosomal basis of human neoplasia. Science 221:227–236, 1983.

151. Yunis JJ: Chromosomal rearrangements, genes, and fragile sites in cancer: Clinical and biologic implications. *In* Important Advances in Oncology 1986. Edited by VT DeVita, S Hellman, SA Rosenberg. Philadelphia, JB Lippincott, 1986, pp 93–128.

152. Yunis JJ, Mayer MG, Arnesen MA, Aeppli DP, Oken MM, Frizzera G: *bcl*-2 and other genomic alterations in the prognosis of large-cell lymphoma. N Engl J Med 320:1047–1054, 1989.

153. Yunis JJ, Ramsay N: Retinoblastoma and subband deletion of chromosome 13. Am J Dis Child 132:161–163, 1978.

154. Yunis JJ, Roldan L, Yasmineh WG, Lee JC: Staining of satellite DNA in metaphase chromosomes. Nature 231:532–533, 1971.

155. Yunis JJ, Yasmineh WG: Heterochromatin, satellite DNA, and cell function. Science 174:1200–1209, 1971.

156. Zang KD: Cytological and cytogenetic studies on human meningioma. Cancer Genet Cytogenet 6:249–274, 1982.

3

Cytologic Screening Programs

George H. Anderson

Screening for disease has played a significant role in medicine since the later part of the 19th century when public health authorities became aware that it was important to detect specific diseases in certain groups of the population. An obvious example of this type of screening is the requirement for radiologic examination of immigrants who might introduce infectious diseases, particularly tuberculosis, to their new country.

It is only in relatively recent years that the idea of screening for the early detection of cancer has gained widespread acceptance, particularly with the development of the techniques of exfoliative cytology initiated by the pioneer work of Dr. George Papanicolaou. With the publication of his paper in 1941,[43] it became apparent that this might be a test that could be of value in the early detection of cancer of the cervix. The widespread development of screening programs for the early detection of cancer of the cervix, particularly in North America and Europe, set the stage for the use of this technique in the examination of specimens from other organs. Over the past 40 years it has become apparent that cytology can be of assistance in the early detection of cancer occurring in many other sites.

Before discussing the use of cytology as a screening technique for cancer, it is necessary to establish the criteria that should be used to evaluate any screening tests for the early detection of disease. These criteria were outlined by Cochrane and Holland[10] in 1971 as follows:

1. *Simplicity*. The tests should be easy to administer by paramedical and other personnel.
2. *Acceptability*. Because screening is usually voluntary and a high rate of cooperation is necessary for an efficient screening program, the tests should be acceptable to the subjects involved.
3. *Accuracy*. The tests should give a true measurement of the attributes under investigation.
4. *Cost*. The expense of screening should be considered in relation to the benefits resulting from the early detection of disease.
5. *Precision*. The tests should give consistent results in repeated trials.
6. *Sensitivity*. The tests should have the ability to detect all members of the diseased population.
7. *Specificity*. The tests should have the ability to identify correctly all nondiseased people.

The last two criteria, sensitivity and specificity, are a measure of the validity of screening tests. To these can be added a third, the positive predictive value, which measures the probability of disease being present in patients whose findings are reported as positive.

In the context of cytologic screening *sensitivity* means the percentage of positive cases reported as being positive. It can be calculated using the following formula:

$$\text{Sensitivity} = \frac{\text{True positive}}{\text{True positive} + \text{False negative}} \times 100\%$$

In the context of cytologic screening *specificity* means the percentage of negative cases reported as being negative. It can be calculated using the following formula:

$$\text{Specificity} = \frac{\text{True negative}}{\text{True negative} + \text{False positive}} \times 100\%$$

Similarly, the positive predictive value can be calculated as follows:

$$\text{Positive predictive value} = \frac{\text{True positive}}{\text{True positive} + \text{False positive}} \times 100\%$$

When the value of a screening test for a potentially lethal disease such as cancer is assessed, one additional criterion becomes most important—the test should result in a reduction in the morbidity and mortality from the disease in question. At the present time, the only cytologic screening test that has been generally accepted as fulfilling this last criterion is the cervical smear, used for the detection of preinvasive lesions of the cervix. Nevertheless the value of cytologic techniques for the early detection of cancer in a number of other sites is well established and these will also be discussed in this chapter.

CERVIX

Requirements for a Cervical Smear Screening Program

The integration of a variety of procedures is essential for the successful development of a Papanicolaou smear screening program for preinvasive cancer of the cervix:
1. Collecting the smear
2. Processing the smear
3. Screening and interpreting the smear
4. Reporting the findings
5. Follow-up systems
6. Quality control.

If the performance in any one of these areas is less than optimal, this will reduce the efficiency and reliability of the whole system. The adequate performance of these elements will now be considered in some detail, with the exception of quality control, which is discussed in other chapters.

Collecting the Smear. The aim of collecting a cervical smear is to obtain a representative specimen from the squamocolumnar junction also known as the transformation zone or transitional zone of the uterine cervix, using an Ayre's spatula or a similar device. Because the majority of precursor lesions of invasive squamous carcinoma of the cervix arise in the region of the squamocolumnar junction, a smear cannot be considered adequate unless this area has been sampled. Having exposed the cervix using a bivalve speculum, a circumferential sample is obtained by turning the Ayre's spatula through 360 degrees, thus obtaining cells from the entire squamocolumnar junction. At times, difficulty may be experienced if the cervix is irregular in shape as may occur after childbirth, so that the collection technique may have to be modified to ensure that the entire area is sampled.

As a woman ages, usually starting at about 40 years, the squamocolumnar junction tends to migrate up the endocervical canal, making this area more difficult to sample with the Ayre's spatula. In older patients, with histories of negative smear finding, this is probably not important. However, even in younger women, experience has shown that as many as 20% of cervical smears do not contain endocervical cells. Their absence should be reported to the referring physician who may wish to repeat the smear or obtain an additional smear from the endocervical canal. This can be done either by using a cotton-tip applicator moistened with normal saline or by using an endocervical cytobrush. It is widely believed that an adequate cervical smear should always contain endocervical or squamous metaplastic cells, indicating that the upper margin of the squamocolumnar junction has been sampled.

Ideally the smear should be obtained at mid cycle, because cell morphology is most easily interpreted at this time, although this is not essential. The smear should not be obtained during active menstruation, because the presence of much fresh blood may make the smear impossible to interpret as may douching prior to the examination. Lubricant jelly should not be used on the vaginal speculum, although a small quantity of normal saline on the speculum will not affect cell detail. If a large amount of mucus or purulent exudate is on the surface of the cervix, this should be gently removed with a moistened cotton-wool swab prior to obtaining the sample.

Once the sample has been obtained, it should be placed on a glass slide, marked with the patient's name and spread smoothly down the length of the slide using the wooden spatula. Interpretation is greatly helped if the cells are spread over the surface of the slide in a uniform monolayer.

After spreading the cell sample it must be fixed immediately. Air drying, which starts to occur within 10 seconds of spreading the smear, may make the smear difficult or impossible to interpret. If an aerosol spray fixative is used it should be directed at the slide, which should be placed on a flat surface, from a distance of approximately 25 cm. If the aerosol nozzle is too close to the slide, it will tend to produce irregular ridging of the cellular material and may even blow it off the slide. The cells may also be fixed either by using 95% ethyl alcohol dropped onto the surface of the slide or by placing the slide into the alcohol for a minimum of 15 minutes. After fixation, the slide is allowed to air dry and is then sent to the cytology laboratory with a completed requisition.

Although fixation with an aerosol or alcohol fixative is the optimum method of cell preservation, it is also possible to air-dry smears without prior fixation; the smears are rehydrated in the laboratory using 50% glycerol and water.[1] This rehydration technique produces very acceptable results for squamous epithelial cells and has been employed by the British Columbia cytology laboratory for many years because of the inadequate fixation of many of the smears received by this large program. If this method is used glandular cells are often not well preserved.

When the smear is sent to the laboratory the accompanying requisition should contain some basic clinical information, necessary for adequate interpretation of the Papanicolaou smear. In addition to the patient's name and age and the date of the last menstrual period, any relevant clinical signs or symptoms and information relating to the use of birth control pills or an intrauterine contraceptive device should be provided. Any previous significant illness or surgery, particularly of a gynecologic nature, should also be included on the requisition. If the patient is being treated with estrogen compounds, steroids, digoxin, cytotoxic drugs or antiestrogens, this may affect the hormonal pattern and should be indicated on the requisition to avoid an incorrect interpretation.

Processing the Smear. Once received in the laboratory, the slide and requisition should be given a unique accession number. Appropriate information relating to the specimen is recorded, in a day book, card file or computerized file. It is essential that this accession process be performed accurately, with the correct accession number being placed on both the slide and the requisition, in order to avoid the potential risk of slides from different patients being mixed up.

Many variations of the original Papanicolaou staining technique have been published, and a detailed account of cytopreparatory techniques can be found in the chapter on cytopreparatory techniques.

Screening and Interpreting the Smear. Each smear must be screened in a systematic manner by a cyto-technologist who has received appropriate training and has successfully passed an examination certifying his or her competence. Examinations by the Canadian Society of Laboratory Technologists, the American Society of Cytology and the International Academy of Cytology may be considered examples of the level of proficiency that should be required of a competent screener. The number of smears that can be safely screened by cytotechnologists will vary according to the number of other duties they may be called upon to perform in the laboratory; for example, in a small laboratory, cytotechnologists may perform all of the tasks—accessioning the cases, staining and mounting the slides and screening the smears. In larger laboratories, clerical and laboratory aide staff may perform all of these duties except screening, leaving the cyto-technologists free to screen the smears. It has been recommended by the American Society of Cytology that "the average cytotechnologist should screen 20,000 gynecologic slides per year." This recommendation applies to cytoscreeners who perform no other duties in the laboratory and represents a maximum figure. In 1988 new legislation being introduced in the United States makes it likely that a figure of 80 to 100 slides will be considered the maximum number that can be screened during any 24-hour period by a cytotechnologist.

In a large laboratory that screens in excess of 50,000 to 100,000 smears per year, it is probably more efficient to establish a hierarchical system of screening in which the more junior, less experienced screeners pass on to the more experienced screeners those smears with abnormalities beyond a defined range. In the British Columbia Cytology Laboratory, with a workload in excess of 600,000 smears per year, the screening technologists examine a maximum of 85 to 90 slides per day. However, since the more senior technologists are responsible for reexamining smears with significant abnormalities and rescreening about 5% of the smears as part of the quality control program, the average productivity of this laboratory is about 65 slides per technologist per day.

The 1976 Canadian Task Force report on cervical cancer screening programs[4] recognized that patterns of practice could vary between laboratories. The report recommended that to perform at optimal efficiency, a cytology laboratory should examine a minimum of 25,000 cases per year. The 1982 update of this report[5] recommended that "to function most efficiently within a mass screening program a laboratory should process a sufficient number of cases annually to require staffing by a minimum of three qualified and experienced cytotechnologists, supervised by a cytopathologist and having an adequate clerical and technical support staff." Although this recommendation is aimed at achieving maximum efficiency, proficiency must also be considered. It is recognized that many laboratories with a smaller staff and fewer cases can perform reliably; however, it is unlikely that competence could be maintained if a laboratory were seeing fewer than 25 or 30 positive cases per year.

Reporting the Findings. The original numeric classification outlined by Papanicolaou is no longer considered adequate for reporting purposes both as a result of its lack of precision and as a result of variations in its use, introduced by a number of laboratories.

Current practice demands that cytologic reporting communicate the smear findings in descriptive terms, which may well include an anticipated histologic diagnosis if a biopsy is recommended. Although some disagreement still exists with regard to the final reporting responsibility for cervical smears, a well trained, experienced cytotechnologist can be expected to interpret negative smears and smears that show changes related to benign atypia. Smears that show abnormal cells consistent with dysplasia or worse should be referred for the interpretation and recommendations of a cytopathologist or other medically qualified person with appropriate training and experience in cytology.

Listed in the table is our reporting terminology for cervicovaginal cytology. This terminology is similar to that currently recommended in the Canadian Task Force Report[5] and the World Health Organization handbook on cytologic screening for cervical cancer.[14]

Follow-up System. An essential requirement of a cytology screening program is to provide adequate

---

Recommended Cervicovaginal Cytology Terminology for Reporting

Unsatisfactory (Reason to be Stated)

No Abnormal Cells
Metaplasia noted

Abnormal Cells Consistent with Benign Atypia (Nondysplastic)
Inflammatory effect
Trichomonas effect
Viral effect
Yeast effect
Irradiation effect
Keratinization
Atypical metaplasia
Condyloma effect
Other

Abnormal Cells Consistent with Dysplasia
Mild dysplasia (CIN I)*
Moderate dysplasia (CIN II)
Severe dysplasia (CIN III)

Abnormal Cells Consistent with Malignancy
Consistent with *in situ* squamous carcinoma (CIN III)
Consistent with invasive squamous carcinoma
Type unspecified

Abnormal Cells Not Specifically Classified
Comments to be attached

---

*CIN = cervical intraepithelial neoplasia.

follow-up and recall systems whether these are provided by the laboratory or by a centralized registry. The most important function of the follow-up system is to ensure that appropriate action has been taken once a cytologic abnormality has been reported. In addition, for those patients who have received treatment following the diagnosis of an abnormality at the level of severe dysplasia or carcinoma *in situ,* long-term follow-up is mandatory, since these patients have a significant risk of developing recurrent or new disease, sometimes many years after the treatment of the original lesion. Even those patients treated for carcinoma *in situ* by hysterectomy, with complete removal of the lesion, may develop new disease in the vagina, usually at the vault. This happens in about 1% of cases.

Over the past decade, the recommended method of investigation for patients with an abnormal Papanicolaou smear has become colposcopy. This technique, which was first described by Hinselman in the 1920s, involves the examination of the cervix by means of a magnifying instrument with a range of magnification from 5× to 20×. When the colposcopist identifies an area of abnormality, a small-bite biopsy sample is taken from a representative area of the lesion in order to confirm the colposcopic impression. If no lesion is identified, it is important to perform an endocervical curettage as well.

Screening Programs for Carcinoma of the Cervix

Screening programs for carcinoma of the cervix have a significant advantage in terms of their anticipated outcome because the natural history of the disease allows it to be detected at the preinvasive stage of dysplasia or carcinoma *in situ.* With appropriate treatment, progression to invasive cancer is prevented. This being so, screening programs can be expected to result in a reduced incidence and mortality from cancer of the cervix.

The report from the British Columbia Cytology Screening Program[2] covers the years from 1955 to 1985. Table 3–1 shows the increase in screening over this 30-year period. By 1965, roughly one third of the population of women at risk was being screened annually. Since the early 1970s, about 45% of the population has been screened each year. It was estimated that by 1970, 85% of the population at risk had been screened at least once and this coverage has been maintained.

Table 3–2 shows the pattern of screening during 1985, a pattern that has been consistent since about 1970. Of the screening effort annually, 85% is directed at women between the ages of 20 and 59 years. Approximately two thirds of the population between the ages of 20 and 34 are screened yearly, whereas the proportion in the population over age 60 is appropriately smaller.

Table 3–1 also shows the increasing number of cases of carcinoma *in situ* identified over 3 decades. By the end of 1988 over 30,000 cases of squamous carcinoma *in situ* have been detected and treated over a period of 33 years.

Table 3–3 demonstrates a significant increase in the detection rate of squamous carcinoma *in situ,* which occurred in British Columbia between 1972 and 1985. The rate of carcinoma *in situ* per 1000 women screened increased 4-fold between 1972 and 1980 for women between the ages of 20 and 24, nearly 3-fold for those between the ages of 25 and 29, with smaller increments for women up to the age of 45. The detection rate fell to somewhat lower levels for 1985 and by 1988 had fallen to 50% of the 1980 levels in women up to age 39.

Figure 3–1 shows that in British Columbia the incidence of clinically invasive squamous carcinoma of the cervix has fallen by 78% and mortality by 72% since the start of the program, reductions which the authors of the report believe are directly attributable to the cervical screening program.

Christopherson and coworkers,[7] in discussing the results of the Louisville screening program in Kentucky from 1953 to 1973, reported a reduction of 70% in mortality from cancer of the cervix in women between 30 and 59 years. They pointed out that the degree to which screening contributed to this observed reduction in mortality was difficult to assess because of the long time period involved and the improved socioeconomic factors during this same period. They concluded, however, that they were not aware of any evidence of a comparable drop in morbidity and mortality occurring in any population without mass cytologic screening.

Similarly, Dickinson, in describing the cervical cancer screening program in Olmstead County, Minnesota,[15] showed that the incidence of invasive cancer of

TABLE 3–1. Number of Women Screened and Number of Cases of Squamous Carcinoma *In Situ* of the Cervix in British Columbia

Year	Population Over Age 20 (× 1000)	Women Screened	Cases Detected	Rate Per 100,000
1955	422.9	11,707	52	12.3
1960	486.4	59,844	221	45.4
1965	543.2	161,556	504	92.8
1970	664.4	297,407	761	114.5
1975	805.5	355,917	1239	153.8
1980	926.2	433,329	1545	166.8
1985	1063.1	465,676	1420	133.6

Reproduced with permission from Anderson GH, et al: Organisation and results of the cervical cytology screening programme in British Columbia, 1955–1985. Br Med J 296:975–978, 1988.

TABLE 3–2. Number of Women Screened in British Columbia During 1985 by Age Group

Age Group	Female Population	Numbers Screened	% Age of Each Age Group Screened
15–18	103,000	25,571 (6%)	25%
20–34	380,800	224,970 (49%)	59%
35–59	415,800	168,186 (36%)	40%
60 and over	266,600	44,179 (9%)	16%
Total	1,166,200	462,906 (100%)	40%

Reproduced with permission from Anderson GH, et al: Organisation and results of the cervical cytology screening programme in British Columbia, 1955–1985. Br Med J 296:975–978, 1988.

the cervix fell by 46% between 1947 and 1967 and mortality for the disease by 48% during the same time period. He concluded that although it may take 10 years or more, cytologic screening will result in an improvement in both survival and mortality from cancer of the uterine cervix.

Macgregor and Teper[35] have reported a significant reduction in mortality from cancer of the cervix in the two regions in Scotland with comprehensive screening programs compared with the remainder of the United Kingdom. They also noted, as does Yule,[62] an increase in mortality from cancer of the cervix in women aged less than 35 in England and Wales where screening is less comprehensive in some areas. Laara and associates[34] in describing the results of screening programs in the Nordic countries stated that "organized screening programs have had a major impact on the reduction of mortality from cervical cancer in the Nordic countries."

Several case control studies have been reported in an attempt to estimate the relative risk of developing invasive cervical cancer in a woman with a prior negative screening history. The study by Clarke and Anderson[9] compared the Papanicolaou smear history of 212 patients with invasive cervical cancer with that of 1060 age-matched controls. In the 5 years before the year of diagnosis, 68% of these patients had a history of no cervical smears compared with 44% of the controls. These investigators concluded that the absence of cervical screening resulted in a significant relative risk of developing the disease and concluded

TABLE 3–3. Rates for Carcinoma *In Situ* Per 1000 Women Screened in British Columbia

Age Group	1972	1975	1980	1985
15–19	0.1	0.2	0.8	0.7
20–24	1.1	2.2	4.5	3.3
25–29	2.7	4.3	7.1	4.9
30–34	3.0	4.8	6.2	4.8
35–39	2.4	3.3	4.2	3.8
40–44	1.9	2.2	2.8	2.3
45–49	1.1	2.1	1.6	1.8
50–54	1.3	1.2	1.9	0.9
55–59	1.0	1.5	0.9	0.7
60–64	1.3	0.8	1.2	0.7
65–69	1.2	1.3	1.4	0.8
70–74	2.4	0.8	1.1	0.6
75 and over	1.0	0.8	1.2	0.9

Reproduced with permission from Anderson GH, et al: Organisation and results of the cervical cytology screening programme in British Columbia, 1955–1985. Br Med J 296:975–978, 1988.

that the Papanicolaou smear is an effective screening procedure for invasive cervical cancer.

A similar case control study reported by Macgregor and colleagues[36] from the northeast of Scotland showed a high relative protection, the inverse of the relative risk, for the first 2 or 3 years following a negative Papanicolaou smear and falling steadily with time after this.

Colposcopy has had a significant impact on the diagnosis and management of preinvasive lesions of the cervix. In British Columbia, for instance, in 1985 over 8000 new patients were referred for colposcopic examination, approximately 3000 of these patients having severe dysplasia or carcinoma *in situ*. This group represents over 1% of the women screened during that year. The introduction of colposcopy has resulted in the transfer of much of the responsibility for the diagnosis of preinvasive lesions of the cervix from the pathologist to the colposcopist and has introduced an additional potential source of diagnostic error, particularly in early invasive disease.

Prior to the advent of colposcopy, cone biopsy was the recommended diagnostic procedure for the evaluation of patients with persistently abnormal cervical smears. Townsend and colleagues [59, 60] have reported a number of instances of invasive cervical cancer developing in patients following colposcopic evaluation and treatment. In the majority of these patients the appropriate protocol was not followed at colposcopy, resulting in a misdiagnosis. Nevertheless, when properly performed by an experienced gynecologist, there is no doubt that colposcopy is very useful in the diagnosis and management of preinvasive lesions of the cervix, most notably in younger women. Many of these patients can be treated with cryotherapy or laser therapy, thus avoiding the potential complications of cone biopsy.

A word of caution is appropriate when studying incidence figures for cervical cancer. Most of this data is obtained from cancer registries that obtain their information from biopsy reports. Since the widespread utilization of colposcopy, which often results in the obtaining of a very small biopsy sample, the cancer registry may not always be able to distinguish reliably between carcinoma *in situ* and invasive cancer from a pathology report. In a report from British Columbia[23] involving a review of all new registrations of invasive cervical cancer diagnosed in the province between 1977 and 1979, of 521 new cases of invasive cervical cancer registered, 184 (35%) were subsequently found to be incorrectly registered. The majority of these incorrect

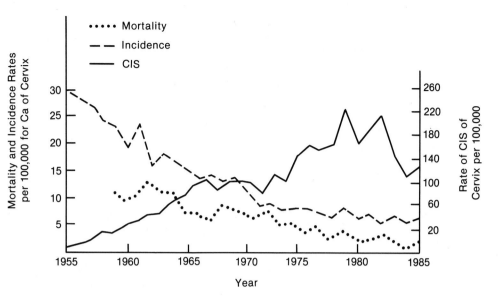

FIGURE 3–1. The incidence of **clinical invasive squamous (CIS) carcinoma** of the cervix and squamous carcinoma *in situ* 1955–85, and mortality from squamous carcinoma of the cervix, 1958–85, in British Columbia. (Age-standardized rates per 100,000 women over age 20.) (Reproduced with permission from Anderson GH, et al: Organisation and results of the cervical cytology screening programme in British Columbia, 1955–1985. Br Med J 296:975–978, 1988.) (Ca = cancer.)

registrations, 77%, proved on further study to be cases of preinvasive cervical cancer. This report also noted that 28 cases of invasive cervical cancer diagnosed in the province during the study period had not been reported to the registry, so that both over reporting and under reporting may occur.

Important factors in developing effective screening programs for cervical cancer are the age at which screening starts and the frequency with which it is performed. Considerable discussion has occurred in the development of appropriate recommendations in this regard, one of the most important factors in the decision being the estimated time taken for preinvasive lesions to develop into invasive carcinoma. Richart and Barron[49] calculated that of 1000 patients with undetected carcinoma *in situ*, about 25% will undergo transition to invasion within 5 years.

In British Columbia it is recommended that all women who are or who have ever been sexually active, have an annual Papanicolaou test and pelvic examination until the age of 35 years. After the age of 35, providing no significant abnormality has been detected on any of the previous examinations, the test may be performed less frequently at the discretion of the physician, after discussion with the patient. This recommendation is similar to the modified guidelines for Papanicolaou test frequency of the American Cancer Society,[18] which state "All women who are or have been sexually active, or have reached age 18 years, have an annual Pap test and pelvic examination. After a woman has had three or more consecutive satisfactory normal annual examinations, the Pap test may be performed less frequently at the discretion of her physician."

Unfortunately despite early hopes that screening for cervical cancer would eliminate this disease, it has become apparent that for a number of reasons this is not likely to occur in the near future. It is well recognized, for instance, that most of the women presenting with invasive cervical cancer have never had a Papanicolaou smear or have not had a smear for many years. Even if all of these noncompliant patients could be persuaded to participate in screening programs, the method itself is fraught with potential problems that result in a significant error rate in even the best programs. The reasons are discussed in the chapter on proliferative reactions, intra-epithelial neoplasm and invasive cancer of the uterine cervix. Nevertheless, although there is no reason for complacency, the accumulated experience of the past 40 years can leave no doubt of the vital role that carefully planned and efficiently run screening programs will continue to play in the early detection of preinvasive cancer of the cervix. Such programs clearly fulfill the criteria of Cochrane and Holland[10] outlined earlier in this chapter.

ENDOMETRIUM

The majority of patients presenting with endometrial carcinoma do so with Stage I disease,[11] which now has a 5-year survival rate of approximately 90% when patients are appropriately treated.[8] As yet no simple method provides a high degree of accuracy in the detection of carcinoma of the endometrium, although a number of devices are available for obtaining cells of endometrial origin. The routine cervical smear is an extremely inefficient method, depending on the chance of picking up endometrial cells from the region of the external os at the time the sample is collected.

In a review of 400 patients with carcinoma of the endometrium seen at the Cancer Control Agency of British Columbia, all of whom had routine cervical cytology prior to surgery, abnormal glandular cells were found in only 143 (36%). A more reliable source is a sample obtained from the vaginal vault, also known as a vaginal pool smear. Koss[27] reported the detection of 40 out of 63 cases (65%) of asymptomatic endometrial carcinoma using a vaginal smear but only 25% using a cervical smear. Reagan and Ng[47] reported an improved detection rate over the previous two methods using an endocervical aspiration smear. In four independent studies including 619 women with proven endometrial adenocarcinoma, 480 (77.5%) were detected by means of endocervical aspiration.

The most reliable method for the early detection of presymptomatic endometrial carcinoma is to obtain a sample directly from the endometrium. A number of reports in the literature have described a variety of endometrial cell sampling devices.[39] Cramer and Osborne[13] used the Milan-Markley Helix instrument in 170 patients at high risk for developing endometrial neoplasia—women with late menopause, obese women, hypertensive or diabetic women and women receiving estrogen medication. These investigators obtained cells adequate for diagnosis in 180 of 189 samples. They claimed that the sensitivity of the technique in their hands was 97%, specificity 96% and predictive value of a positive result 97%. They concluded that this technique is safe and dependable in assessing women at risk of developing endometrial hyperplasia and carcinoma. These investogators do not advocate this method as a general screening procedure for women at low risk.

Palermo and associates,[41] using the Endo-Pap sampler, obtained material from 153 patients who had a subsequent tissue diagnosis established by endometrial biopsy, curettage or hysterectomy. Adequate cytologic specimens were obtained in 93% of these patients. Of 32 patients with confirmed endometrial carcinoma, diagnostic material was obtained in 30 (94%). However, of 31 patients with hyperplasia only 10 (32%) were detected using this technique. Meisels and Jolicoeur[38] reported a similar experience using the Endo-Pap sampler in 1465 patients. Of 27 patients in this series with endometrial adenocarcinoma, 20 (74%) were correctly diagnosed and 7 (26%) were interpreted cytologically as having hyperplasia. However, of the 70 patients with endometrial hyperplasia, only 53% were correctly assessed using this endometrial sampler. Of the samples in this series, 8.7% were considered inadequate for interpretation.

Koss[30] has reported the results of screening a group of 2586 asymptomatic women for the detection of endometrial carcinoma and hyperplasia conducted between January 1979 and June 1982 utilizing the Milan-Markley Helix or the Isaacs cannula. The initial protocol for this study had also required a sample be obtained by endocervical aspiration and cotton swab-smear from the cervix in addition to the scrape smear.[29] Those two procedures were abandoned after the first 1000 or so cases had been examined as being noncontributory. In addition each woman had a scrape smear of the lateral vaginal wall to determine the maturation index and a vaginal pool smear. Of these women, 98% were past the age of 45 and 80% were postmenopausal. Of the initial cohort, 1567 were screened twice and 187 three times at annual intervals for a total of almost 4500 endometrial samplings. Sixteen occult carcinomas were detected on the first screening with an additional two patients presenting with symptoms within 12 months of the initial screening for a total of 18 carcinomas, a prevalence rate of 6.96 per 1000. A total of 21 patients were found to have hyperplasia, a prevalence rate of 8.1 per 1000. At the second screening

one additional case of occult carcinoma and three additional cases of endometrial hyperplasia were detected; two additional small carcinomas that were missed on screening were detected subsequently after vaginal spotting.

The investigators concluded that the currently available means of detection of occult endometrial carcinoma by direct sampling are only moderately reliable. Even more importantly, they emphasized that despite many years of experience in the interpretation of endometrial smears, the interpretation can be extremely difficult and "any thought that the endometrial smear is just another Papanicolaou smear is not based on realistic assessment of the level of diagnostic difficulty."

The sensitivity and specificity of the endometrial sampling techniques currently available for detecting asymptomatic endometrial carcinoma have not yet been clearly established. Koss and colleagues[29] suggested therefore that all women past the age of 50 should be screened at least once, because the majority of the occult lesions were discovered on the first screening. They also suggested that those women who are believed to be at high risk of developing endometrial carcinoma might possibly be screened more frequently, although concluding that the need for this is not yet clear.

Whatever the value of direct endometrial sampling may be, it should be remembered that any postmenopausal woman in whom endometrial cells are found on a Papanicolaou smear requires further investigation, because the presence of these cells after the menopause is always an abnormal finding even in the absence of cytologic abnormality. In addition, any woman over the age of 40 who is found to have endometrial cells after the mid cycle, unless she is wearing an intrauterine contraceptive device, requires similar investigation. The initial investigation may well be an endometrial aspiration smear which, in many instances, will yield diagnostic cells. However, negative findings on endometrial aspiration smear in a patient suspected of having endometrial carcinoma does not exclude this disease. An adequate investigation cannot be considered to have been completed until a fractional curettage of the endometrial cavity and endocervical canal have been performed.

LUNG

Over the past 25 years the incidence and mortality from cancer of the lung have increased steadily throughout the Western world. It is estimated that in the United States alone, there will be in 1990, 157,000 new cases and 142,000 deaths,[56] making carcinoma of the lung the commonest lethal malignant disease in this population. The majority of these cases are attributable to cigarette smoking, implying that it is a largely preventable disease. During recent years neither resectability (25%) nor 5-year survival rates (10%) have improved significantly.

It is generally believed that screening for cancer of the lung should be confined to high risk individuals: those who are middle aged or older with a long history of cigarette smoking, usually defined as a pack a day for 20 years or longer. At this time sputum cytology and chest radiography are the only two procedures considered to be reliable for the detection of early presymptomatic carcinoma of the lung, each being complementary to the other. Sputum cytology is most effective at detecting early stage squamous carcinoma, which is usually centrally located in major bronchi. Chest radiography is more effective in the detection of peripheral tumors, most commonly adenocarcinomas. Neither technique is particularly effective at detecting early stage small cell undifferentiated carcinoma largely because of the rapid growth of this tumor.

An adequate deep cough sputum sample must contain significant numbers of pulmonary macrophages indicating the origin of the specimen from the lower bronchial tree. Very few false positive results should occur if adequately trained and experienced personnel are used to screen the smears. Sputum cytology can also determine the tumor type with a high degree of accuracy as reported by Johnston and Frable.[26]

In the study published by Koss and associates[31] the accuracy of sputum examination was shown to be related to the number of specimens examined. In this study of 487 patients with bronchogenic carcinoma, 61% had the diagnosis established on the first specimen examined, this figure being increased to 89% after the examination of three specimens.

In 1971 the National Cancer Institute undertook the support of three long-term randomized control trials of screening for early lung cancer in large, high risk populations using chest films and sputum cytology.[40] The trials were completed in 1984 and were conducted at the Mayo Clinic, the Johns Hopkins Medical Institution and the Memorial Sloan-Kettering Cancer Center. The aim of the study was to determine whether the detection of lung cancer could be improved by adding modern cytologic screening techniques to either yearly chest films or chest films done every 4 months. In addition, the study was designed to determine whether mortality from lung cancer could be reduced significantly by this type of screening program combined with further sophisticated localizing methods and current treatment programs.

The three designated centers each initially screened approximately 10,000 asymptomatic cigarette smoking males. The results of these three trials suggested that sputum cytology alone will detect only about 20% of cancers of the lung, the majority of patients having early stage squamous carcinomas with favorable prognoses. All three groups reported a 5-year survival rate for these asymptomatic cytologically detected cases of approximately 80%.[19-21] This rate compares with a 5-year survival of only 10% for symptomatic patients. Unfortunately this apparent benefit may not be real, but may merely represent the earlier detection of a slowly growing lesion that results in prolonging the interval between diagnosis and death but does not prolong the individual's life span. Further studies are being done, and at this time screening for cancer of the lung is not recommended except as a part of a general health evaluation.

ESOPHAGUS

Cancer of the esophagus in the Western world is not a common disease, representing only 1% of the estimated new cancer cases for all sites in the United States for 1990.[57] For this reason it has not been considered an appropriate disease for early detection by screening in the Western world. However, cancer of the esophagus has been recognized as a relatively common disease in some areas of the world, particularly in northern Iran, parts of the African continent and in several areas of northern China, some of which have the highest rates of cancer of the esophagus in the world.

A detailed description of the epidemiologic characteristics of esophageal cancer in northern China has been provided by Shu[54] in his fascinating and detailed account of screening more than 500,000 patients for early esophageal cancer in these high risk areas of China between 1959 and 1979. In comparing the efficacy of cytology, endoscopy and radiography in the detection of early esophageal carcinoma Shu claims an accuracy as high as 94% for cytology, 75 to 92% for endoscopy and 67 to 82% for radiography.[55] He points out that in about 20% of these cases, the early lesions cannot be seen by either radiographic or endoscopic techniques. In this large series of patients, because 75% of the lesions detected by the massive screening program were either carcinoma *in situ* or minimally invasive, a surgical cure rate of 90% was achieved. This finding compares to a 5-year survival rate of only 5% in patients not detected by screening, who are first seen with symptoms of the disease, most commonly dysphagia.

Although the etiology of esophageal cancer in the Western world is strongly linked to the heavy use of alcohol and tobacco, the etiology of the disease in the high risk areas of China is still uncertain. Quite good evidence, exists, however, that it may be due to a combination of factors including fungi and their metabolites contaminating pickled vegetables and nitrosamine compounds present both in food and drinking water.

The method of collecting the cytologic samples from the esophagus in the Chinese studies utilizes an inflatable balloon covered by a silk mesh and attached to a rubber tube similar to a device originally described by Panico and Papanicolaou[42] and later improved by Brainsma.[3] Shen and associates[52] modified the balloon further, and even more modifications have resulted in the elimination of the outer silk mesh, the balloon being manufactured with a coarse granular outer surface. The latest balloon is also smaller than its predecessors, measuring only 2 cm in length with a maximum diameter of 1 cm and is designed to be partially filled with barium for localization by radiography.[54]

The technique involves the patient swallowing the device until it passes the gastric cardia. The balloon is then inflated with about 20 ml of air and is withdrawn slowly. After the balloon has traversed the esophagus, it is quickly withdrawn, the surface rinsed in normal saline and cytologic smears are prepared from these washings.

Because radiology and endoscopy will miss many early esophageal cancers, this cytologic technique may also be used to localize these early lesions. This localization is accomplished by obtaining successive samples in 5-cm steps down the esophagus from 20 cm to 38 cm. In a series of 129 patients with early esophageal cancer treated by surgery in the Peoples County Hospital at Linxian, this method of cytologic sampling accurately localized the lesion in 124 of 129 cases (97%).[54]

In addition to the early detection of cancer these studies have identified significant numbers of patients with squamous dysplasia and have defined the relationship between dysplasia and cancer of the esophagus. Shu,[54] reporting on the follow-up of 530 patients with severe dysplasia, for up to 12 years, found that nine of 17 patients (53%) in this group followed by repeated cytologic examination for 9 to 12 years developed carcinoma. These cytologic studies confirmed the assumed close relationship between dysplasia and cancer of the esophagus and found that severe dysplasia preceded early cancer by an average of 4 years. Shu also reported that regression may occur from severe to mild dysplasia.

STOMACH

The first description of the use of exfoliative cytology to detect carcinoma of the stomach was published by Marini from the University of Bologna in 1909.[37] Using gastric lavage he correctly diagnosed 32 of 37 cases of gastric and esophageal cancer. This degree of accuracy was particularly notable because unstained material was used to establish these diagnoses.

After Papanicolaou published his classic paper in 1941, exfoliative cytology was explored as a diagnostic tool for a number of other sites. During the 1950s the work of Rubin[50] and Raskin[46] at the University of Chicago was responsible for demonstrating the potential of the technique of gastric lavage in producing accurate and reproducible results for gastric cytology, detecting 288 of 379 (76.6%) cases of gastric carcinoma.[44] There were five false positive findings in this group, for a specificity of 98.2%. During this time Schade[51] in the United Kingdom, also published observations relating to the reliability of the technique in the diagnosis of early gastric cancer, concluding that "gastric cytology is a most useful addition to the diagnostic armamentarium in the fight against gastric cancer."

The development of direct vision fiber optic endoscopy in the 1960s resulted in a significant increase in the accuracy of gastric cytology. When cytology, in the form of gastric brushing, is combined with gastric biopsy the cumulative diagnostic accuracy of the two techniques can be as high as 98%.[58] Specificity using this technique is also high, Prolla and coworkers[45] reporting two false positive results (2.3%) in 85 cases with benign gastric ulcers.

With the exception of Japan, screening programs for gastric cancer have not been generally accepted, even in countries having a relatively high incidence of the disease, such as Iceland, Finland and Chile. In Japan, however, with the highest incidence of the disease in the world—three to four times that found in Western Europe and the United States—screening programs have been available for about 20 years.

Hirayama and associates[22] have reported a decrease in mortality from this disease in Japan since 1969, in both males and females between the ages of 40 and 69 years, of almost 50%. They attribute this decline in part to the mass screening program in Japan in which 3 to 4 million persons are examined annually. They pointed out a significant decrease in the reported incidence rates of gastric cancer in relatively recent years, the reasons for which are not known. The screening technique utilized in Japan is a sophisticated barium meal technique known as double contrast radiography, first developed by Shirakabe and colleagues.[53] In skilled hands this technique can detect carcinoma at the *in situ* stage as well as lesions with submucosal invasion only. This last patient group has a 20-year survival rate of 90%.[24] Fiber optic endoscopy, cytology and biopsy are used to confirm the presence of tumor in Japan, but are no longer used to screen.

BLADDER

Cancer of the bladder is one of the most common cancers in North America and Europe. The etiology of the majority of these tumors is not known, so that routine screening of the general population is not a practical measure. However, a number of well-recognized high risk groups are known; these classically have been industrial workers exposed to aromatic amines. The first of such groups was identified by Rehn[48], who in 1895 reported four cases of carcinoma of the bladder from a group of 500 workers in the German aniline dye industry. Cartwright[6] summarized the industrial and nonindustrial associations of bladder cancer including a number of new occupational risks recognized over the past 25 years. Crabbe[12] in the United Kingdom was the first to introduce a large cytology screening program aimed at detecting occupational cancer of the bladder in a group of 1000 male dyestuff workers. On the basis of voided urine cytology, 26 of these individuals were reported to have suspicious or positive smears, 15 being new patients and 11 being patients previously operated on for bladder tumors. Of these, 19 (73%) were confirmed by cystoscopy and 3 (12%) were considered to have suspicious findings on cystoscopy. Four (15%) were found to have false positive results. On the basis of these observations Crabbe recommended that regular cytologic screening should be widely utilized in factories where it is believed that workers may be exposed to bladder carcinogens.

Koss[28] reported on his observations of a group of workers exposed to paraaminodiphenyl; this is a potent bladder carcinogen that is inhaled, the products of its metabolism being excreted in the urine within 72 hours after exposure. He reported that carcinoma of the bladder developed in at least 10% of the exposed population. In following these patients over a period of years, Koss observed a progressive series of cytologic changes, some occurring as long as 10 to 15 years after exposure. He noted a gradual worsening of the cell changes from atypia or dysplasia to carcinoma *in situ,* comparing these changes to those observed in precancerous lesions of the uterine cervix. He also observed that progression from the stage of *in situ* carcinoma to invasive cancer appears to be significantly shorter in the urinary bladder than in the cervix.

The parasite *Schistosoma haematobium* has long been recognized as a significant cause of carcinoma of the bladder in many parts of the developing world, particularly Egypt. In this country a high risk population along the Nile delta is currently being screened using urine cytology.[16]

The screening of high risk patients for urinary cancer should be done by examining a sample of voided urine—samples obtained by means of catheterization may be difficult to interpret because of the presence of small papillary clusters of cells displaced by the catheter. Abnormal cells that provide a potential source of error may also be found in patients who have renal calculi and inflammatory disease and in patients who have undergone chemotherapy. The accuracy of urinary cytology is highly dependent on the degree of tumor differentiation. Farrow[17] correlated cytologic results with biopsy findings for 634 cases of carcinoma of the bladder. Cytology findings were positive or atypical in 94% of 245 high-grade tumors in this group, but abnormal in only 75% of 291 grade II tumors. The majority of grade I tumors were not detected by cytology. Farrow documented his experience with a large group of 10,338 patients examined both cystoscopically and cytologically. Of these patients, 1310 were found to have carcinoma of the bladder and 872 had positive or suspicious urine cytology, a sensitivity of 67%. Specificity in this series, however, was much greater: 95.4% of the patients with negative cytologic results having no bladder tumor. Farrow points out that if he had been examining a screening population, very few of whom would be expected to have positive cytologic results, the sensitivity of the test would almost certainly increase because of the reporting of more marginal abnormalities. This would be at the expense of specificity, because more false positive reports would result.

Koss and associates,[32] in discussing the diagnostic value of the cytologic examination of voided urine in 183 bladder tumors, reported an overall sensitivity of 82.5%. Of 103 high-grade tumors in this group, 94.2% were detected by cytology. This included 14 cases of flat carcinoma *in situ* all of which were detected by cytology. The method was much less effective for the low-grade tumors in this series, detecting 72% of the grade II tumors and only 17% of the grade I tumors. Figures such as these justify the use of screening programs for workers in high risk industries. The examination of a voided urine sample is a completely noninvasive procedure and when abnormal is a valuable indicator of the need for cystoscopy and other appropriate investigations.

Future Directions for Cytologic Screening

The development of a variety of automated techniques for examining cell structure and content has evolved steadily over the past 3 decades. These techniques, which include flow cytometry, cell image analysis and morphometry are described in detail in other chapters. The analysis of urothelial cells has proved to be particularly amenable to this type of examination. Koss and Sherman,[33] in reporting their experience with samples prepared from the sediment of voided urine demonstrated that computer image analysis can correctly discriminate between clearly benign and malignant urothelial cells with an error rate of about 5%. Tribukait,[61] using flow cytometry to measure DNA ploidy in 269 urothelial tumors, reported results very similar to those achieved by the cytologic examination of voided urine: 124 of 130 (95%) grade III tumors demonstrating aneuploidy as compared with 6 of 32 (19%) of grade I tumors in this series.

The rapidly increasing sophistication, speed and reliability of a number of the instruments used in analytic cytology suggest that some of these techniques may become the basis of fully automated systems for cytologic screening within the next decade.

References

1. Anderson GH: Cervical cytology. *In* Screening for Cancer. Edited by AB Miller. New York, Academic Press, p 91, 1985.
2. Anderson GH, Boyes DA, Benedet JL, Le Riche JC, Matisic JP, et al: Organisation and results of the cervical cytology screening programme in British Columbia, 1955-1985. Br Med J 296:975–978, 1988.
3. Brainsma AH: The value of cytology in the early diagnosis of carcinoma of the esophagus and stomach. Thesis, University of Utrecht, the Netherlands, 1957.
4. Canadian Task Force Report: Cervical cancer screening programmes. Can Med Assoc J 114:1003–1033, 1976.
5. Canadian Task Force Report: Cervical Cancer Screening Programs 1982. Health & Welfare Canada, Ottawa.
6. Cartwright RA: Screening for bladder cancer. *In* Screening for Cancer. Edited by AB Miller. New York, Academic Press, pp 399–402, 1985.
7. Christopherson WM, Lundin FE, Mendez WM, Parker JE: Cervical cancer control. Cancer 38:1357–1366, 1976.
8. Christopherson WM, Connelly PJ, Alberhaskey RC: Carcinoma of the endometrium. V. An analysis of prognosticators in patients with favorable subtypes and Stage I disease. Cancer 51:1705–1709, 1983.
9. Clarke AE, Anderson TW: Does screening by "Pap" smears help prevent cervical cancer. Lancet ii:1–4, 1979.

10. Cochrane AK, Holland WW: Validation of screening procedures. Br Med Bull 27:3–8, 1971.
11. Connelly PJ, Alberhaskey RC, Christopherson WM: Carcinoma of the endometrium. III. Analysis of 865 cases of adenocarcinoma and adenoacanthoma. Obstet Gynecol 59:569–574, 1982.
12. Crabbe JGS: Exfoliative cytological control in occupational cancer of the bladder. Br Med J 2:1072–1076, 1952.
13. Cramer JH, Osborne RJ: Endometrial neoplasia–screening the high risk patient. Am J Obstet Gyncol 139:285–288, 1981.
14. Cytological Screening in the Control of Cervical Cancer: Technical Guidelines. World Health Organization, Geneva, 1988.
15. Dickinson LE: Control of cancer of the uterine cervix. Gynecol Oncol 3:1–9, 1975.
16. El-Bolkainy MN: Cytology of bladder carcinoma. J Urol 124:20–22, 1980.
17. Farrow GM: Pathologist's role in bladder cancer. Semin Oncol 6:198–206, 1979.
18. Fink DJ: Change in American Cancer Society guidelines for detection of cervical cancer. Cancer 38:127–128, 1988.
19. Flehinger BJ, Melamed MR, Zaman MB et al: Early lung cancer detection: results of the initial (prevalence) radiologic and cytologic screening in the Memorial Sloan-Kettering study. Am Rev Respir Dis 130:555–560, 1984.
20. Fontana RS, Sanderson DR, Taylor WF, et al: Early lung cancer detection: results of the initial (prevalence) radiologic and cytologic screening in the Mayo Clinic study. Am Rev Respir Dis 130:561–565, 1984.
21. Frost JK, Ball WC, Levin ML, et al: Early lung cancer detection: results of the initial (prevalence) radiologic and cytologic screening in the Johns Hopkins study. Am Rev Respir Dis 130:549–554, 1984.
22. Hirayama T, Hisamichi S, Fujimoto I, Oshima A, Tominaga S: Screening for gastric cancer. In Screening for Cancer. Edited by AB Miller. New York, Academic Press, pp 367–376, 1985.
23. Husted JA, Anderson TW, Gallagher R: Accuracy of registration of invasive cervical cancer. Can Med Assoc J 129:1275–1277, 1983.
24. Ichikawa H, Yamada T: Double contrast radiography of the stomach. In Screening for Cancer. Edited by AB Miller. New York, Academic Press, pp 207–208, 1985.
25. Isaacs JH, Wilhoite RW: Aspiration cytology of the endometrium: office and hospital sampling procedures. Am J Obstet Gyncol 118:679–687, 1974.
26. Johnston WW, Frable WJ: The cytopathology of the respiratory tract. Am J Pathol 84:372–414, 1976.
27. Koss LG: Diagnostic Cytology and Its Histopathologic Bases, 3rd ed. Philadelphia, JB Lippincott, pp 427–429, 1979.
28. Koss LG: Diagnostic Cytology and Its Histopathologic Bases, 3rd ed. Philadelphia, JB Lippincott, pp 750–753, 1979.
29. Koss LG, Schreiber K, Oberlander SG, Moukhtar M, Levine HS: Screening of asymptomatic women for endometrial cancer. Obstet Gynecol 57:681–691, 1981.
30. Koss LG, Schreiber K, Oberlander SG, Moussouris HF, Lesser M: Detection of endometrial carcinoma and hyperplasia in asymptomatic women. Obstet Gynecol 64:1–11, 1984.
31. Koss LG, Melamed MR, Goodnes JT: Pulmonary cytology—a brief survey of diagnostic results from July 1st 1952 to December 31st 1960. Acta Cytol 8:104–113, 1964.
32. Koss LG, Deitch D, Ramanathan R, Sherman AB: Diagnostic value of cytology of voided urine. Acta Cytol 29:810–816, 1985.
33. Koss LG, Sherman AB: Image analysis of cells in the sediment of voided urine. In Computer Assisted Image Analysis Cytology. Edited by SD Greenberg. Monographs in Clinical Cytology. Edited by GL Wied, Vol. 9. Basel, S. Karger, pp 148–162, 1984.
34. Laara E, Day NE, Hakama M: Trends in mortality from cervical cancer in the Nordic countries: association with organised screening programmes. Lancet i:1247–1249, 1987.
35. Macgregor JE, Teper S: Mortality from carcinoma of cervix uteri in Britain. Lancet ii:774–776, 1978.
36. Macgregor JE, Moss SM, Parkin MD, Day NE: A case control study of cervical cancer screening in northeast Scotland. Br Med J 290:1543–1546, 1985.
37. Marini G: Uber die diagnose des Magenkarzinoms auf Grund der cytologischen des Spulwasser. Arch Verdawungskrankh 15:251–267, 1909.
38. Meisels A, Jolicoeur C: Criteria for the cytologic assessment of hyperplasias in endometrial samples obtained by the Endo-Pap endometrial sampler. Acta Cytol 29:297–302, 1985.
39. Milan AR, Markley RL, Fischer RS: Endometrial cytology using the Milan-Markley technique. Obstet Gynecol 48:111–116, 1976.
40. National Cancer Institute Cooperative Early Lung Cancer Group: NIH Publication no. 79-1972, 2nd ed. 2: Manual of Procedures. U.S. Government Printing Office, Washington, D.C., 1979.
41. Palermo VG, Blythe JG, Kaufman RH: Cytologic diagnosis of endometrial adenocarcinoma using the Endo-Pap sampler. Obstet Gyncol 65:271–275, 1985.
42. Panico FG, Papanicolaou GN, Cooper WA: Abrasive balloon for exfoliation of gastric cancer cells. JAMA 143:1308–1311, 1950.
43. Papanicolaou GM, Traut HF: The diagnostic value of vaginal smears in carcinoma of the uterus. Am J Obstet Gyncol 42:193–206, 1941.
44. Prolla JC, Kirsner JB: Handbook and Atlas of Gastrointestinal Exfoliative Cytology. Chicago, University of Chicago Press, p 3, 1972.
45. Prolla JC, Zavier RG, Kirsner JB: Exfoliative cytology in gastric ulcer. Its role in the differentiation of benign and malignant ulcers. Gastroenterology 16:33–37, 1972.
46. Raskin HF: Role of exfoliative cytology in the diagnosis of cancer of the digestive tract. JAMA 169:789–791, 1959.
47. Reagan JW, Ng ABP: The Cells of Uterine Adenocarcinoma, 2nd ed. In Monographs in Clinical Cytology. Edited by GL Wied, Vol. 1. Basel, S. Karger, pp 133–135, 1973.
48. Rehn L: Blasengeschwulste bei Fuchsinarbeitern. Arch Klin Chir 50:588–600,1895.
49. Richart RM, Barron BA: Screening strategies for cervical cancer and cervical intraepithelial neoplasia. Cancer 47:1176–1181, 1981.
50. Rubin CE, Massey BW, Kirsner JB et al: The clinical value of gastrointestinal cytologic diagnosis. Gastroenterology 25:119–138, 1953.
51. Schade ROK: A critical review of gastric cytology. Acta Cytol 3:7–14, 1959.
52. Shen C, Qiu SL: Exfoliative cytology of the esophagus: a preliminary report. Chin J Pathol 7:19–21, 1963.
53. Shirakabe H, Ichikawa H, Kumakura K, et al: Atlas of X-ray Diagnosis of Early Gastric Cancer. Philadelphia, JB Lippincott, 1966.
54. Shu YJ: In The Cytopathology of Esophageal Carcinoma: Precancerous Lesions and Early Cancer. Edited by LG Koss. Masson Publishing, New York, 1985.
55. Shu YJ: Cytopathology of the esophagus. Acta Cytol 27:7–16, 1983.
56. Silverberg E, Boring CC, Squires TS: Cancer Statistics, 1990. Cancer 40:20–21, 1990.
57. Silverberg E: Cancer Statistics, 1990. Cancer 40:18, 1990.
58. Thompson H: Screening for stomach cancer. In Screening and Monitoring of Cancer. Edited by BA Stoll. New York, John Wiley & Sons, p 178, 1985.
59. Townsend DE, Richart RM, Marks E, Nielsen J: Invasive cancer following outpatient evaluation and therapy for cervical disease. Obstet Gynecol 57:145–149, 1981.
60. Townsend DE, Richart RM: Diagnostic errors in colposcopy. Gynecol Oncol 12:5259–5264, 1981.
61. Tribukait B: Flow cytometry in surgical pathology and cytology of tumors of the genitourinary tract. In Advances in Clinical Cytology, Vol. 2. Edited by LG Koss, DV Coleman. New York, Masson Publishing, pp 165–189, 1984.
62. Yule R: Mortality from carcinoma of the cervix. Lancet i:1031–1032, 1978.

4

Diagnostic Quality Assurance in Cytopathology

George L. Wied
Marluce Bibbo
Catherine M. Keebler

Cytopathologists are concerned about and committed to quality assurance and quality control in their laboratories. These practices include, among others, the use of intralaboratory and extradepartmental consultations, case reviews, correlation of cytologic and histopathologic specimens, hierarchic review of cytopathology and review of completed diagnostic reports. Most of the quality assurance techniques are well described. [2, 4, 9, 11, 14, 15, 19, 20, 21, 34]

Until recently, however, formal organization and mandatory documentation of these quality assurance efforts may have been limited or deficient. Formal rules are often difficult to apply, because the types of programs vary depending on the volume and type of cytodiagnostic material and on the size and type of staff. Although the detailed design of the quality assurance program is up to the director of the cytopathology laboratory, basic quality control and quality assurance principles of structure, organization, documentation and systematic review apply.

The enactment of the Clinical Laboratory Improvement Amendment of 1988 by the United States Department of Health and Human Services, [32] the convening of two national conferences on cytologic quality assurance by the Centers for Disease Control, Atlanta, Georgia,[5, 24, 27] the publication of the Quality Assurance Manual by the College of American Pathologists (1988),[7] the American Medical Association Committee Report on the subject,[1] the proposal by the National Cancer Institute Workshop on *The Bethesda System* of reporting cytologic findings,[22] as well as editorials, letters to the editors[35] and general public interest in the assurance of high diagnostic standards fostered intense activities in the quality assurance and quality control sectors. [3, 4, 6, 10, 12, 13, 16–18, 23, 25, 26, 28–31]

QUALITY ASSURANCE MEASURES

Cytopathology is a practice of medicine and represents a medical consultation, about either gynecologic or nongynecologic anatomic sites. The basic principles of quality assurance apply to all types of cytologic specimens.

The following represents several *minimum* quality assurance stipulations to which probably most of us will agree at this time, without entering into details as to which specific quality assurance measures are currently proposed or enacted by governmental bodies or professional organizations.

Laboratory Directors. The laboratory should be directed by a legally qualified physician with a specialist qualification in Pathology, including special training and expertise in cytopathology. In a case in which the current laboratory director or codirector (associate cytopathologist) heads cytopathology without a board qualification in Pathology, but with special training in cytopathology, this condition may be approved under a "grandfather clause." The director or designated medical professional is responsible for proper performance and reporting of all tests done in the cytopathology laboratory. The director or designated cytopathologist should be physically present in the laboratory to direct the staff, be available for consultations, review all abnormal gynecologic cytology samples, review fine needle aspiration samples, review practically all nongynecologic samples and, preferably review a certain percentage of the "normal" gynecologic sample to assure continuing supervision of the staff.

Cytotechnologists. Cytotechnologists should meet one of the following requirements: Persons who have Cytotechnologist (American Society of Clinical Pa-

59

thologists)–registry certification or Health, Education and Welfare–registry certification and persons who have previously been admitted to the practice of cytotechnology by existing regulations under a grandfather clause.

Physical Laboratory Facilities. The laboratory should be clean, well lighted, adequately ventilated and functionally arranged so as to minimize problems in specimen handling, evaluation and reporting. The area for specimen preparation and handling should be separated from the area where specimens are interpreted (screening and reporting).

Safety Precautions. Laboratory personnel must be protected against hazards, be these chemical, biologic or others, by using well-ventilated hoods and biologic safety hoods for handling infectious material. Fire precautions should be posted and tested.

Equipment. An adequate number of binocular microscopes of good quality and proper working order must be available. The equipment should be under a service contract for periodic maintenance.

Specimen Collection. Cytologic specimens should be accepted and examined only if requested by a licensed medical practitioner and collected in accordance with instructions regarding recommended collection techniques. The cytopathology laboratory should inform the originator of the sample, if the specimens are "unsatisfactory" or "less than optimal" with a detailed identification as to which collection instructions resulted in the unsatisfactory or less than optimal sample.[22, 33]

Preparation, Fixation and Staining Procedures. The specimens must be identified with the patient's name and other criteria, such as unit number, and must be accompanied by a requisition form containing appropriate clinical information about the patient. The laboratory shall affix an accession number on each slide for further identification. Fixation while the specimen is still wet is recommended, and the Papanicolaou staining procedure is strongly suggested for most cytologic samples, unless additional staining procedures are warranted. Staining solutions and chemicals used in the cytopathology laboratory should be labeled as to the time of preparation, purchase, or both. Staining solutions should be filtered regularly to avoid contamination and should be covered when not in use.

Slide Screening Workload. Regulations as to the number of specimens a cytotechnologist may screen in a 24-hour period are currently under intensive review and may vary from state to state. Any regulation will have to set an arbitrary limit and may not do justice to the varying conditions that influence the quality of the screening performance. The percent of atypical cases screened versus the percent of negative cases in varying populations is a factor that should be considered when regulations are made. It is essentially a regulation that assures that the number and type of cytologic samples screened does not, through fatigue, adversely affect the cytotechnologist's performance. Some slides are easier and less fatiguing to screen, and some cytotechnologists tire earlier than others. As a general guideline, one may assume that an astute cytotechnologist may screen about 80 to 90 gynecologic cytology cases in a 24-hour period. Specimens from anatomic sites other than the female reproductive tract are more difficult to screen and should appropriately reduce the workload of the cytotechnologist. The interpretation of the cytotechnologist should become a permanent record and available for future review.

Cytologic Terminology. The vaginal/ectocervical/endocervical cytology sample should be preferably interpreted using *The Bethesda System.*[22] The nongynecologic material should be interpreted in medical terms, i.e., conform and correspond to diagnostic reporting systems in histopathology. Both the gynecologic and nongynecologic interpretations should avoid the Papanicolaou classifications or other similar numeric identifications or descriptive terms without clinical meaning.

Laboratory Records, Logs and Files. Each specimen should be recorded and a sequential accession number assigned together with the name of the patient and the originator of the sample. The cytologic samples should be retained on file for a minimum of 5 years or indefinitely if they exhibit abnormal features. The modern cytopathology laboratory should use a machine readable filing and data retrieval system. Such a system will permit the cytotechnologist to have information on all previous cytologic or histologic reports on a given patient on hand while he or she screens the material. Modern computerized data collection and retrieval systems are also essential for continuing quality control and assurance mechanisms. For performance evaluation of each cytotechnologist, a record of workload and diagnostic performance should be maintained as a part of the personnel data file.

INTERNAL QUALITY ASSURANCE MECHANISMS

Review. Specimens exhibiting significant cellular alterations should be reviewed by the cytopathologist. In the event that a particular patient exhibits abnormal or atypical cell findings while previous specimens were reported as "negative," all previous samples should be reviewed by the cytopathologist to ascertain that no "false negative" reporting has occurred. Specimens from a patient with atypical clinical findings should also be reviewed routinely by the cytopathologist. A certain percentage of "negative" samples should be routinely selected for review by the cytopathologist. At the discretion of the director, a certain percentage of "negative" samples may be submitted for rescreening by a senior cytotechnologist or by a cytopathologist.

Follow-up Procedures. Records of patients who had cytologic reports warranting repeated cell studies or biopsies or other follow-up procedures should be kept in an easily accessible file, preferably a computerized file, that permits rapid follow-up controls for quality assurance procedures.

EXTERNAL QUALITY ASSURANCE MECHANISMS

External quality assurance mechanisms with peer review by professional organizations or by state or federal governmental bodies are currently under review for possible implementation. Some states, e.g., New York, have a testing program for cytopathology laboratories enacted and operational for many years, [8] others have not even considered it. Any external program will be welcome by the high quality laboratory but may have problems in the funding and execution of an unbiased, objective and reproducible testing system. [15, 31]

CONTINUING EDUCATION PRACTICES

The laboratory director should conduct continuing educational procedures within the laboratory, provide up-to-date reading material, such as cytopathology textbooks, compendia on clinical cytology, cytologic journals and transparency teaching slide sets; and encourage participation of staff in ongoing educational events, such as local, regional, national and international cytology meetings or tutorials.

References

1. American Medical Association Committee Report of the Council on Scientific Affairs: Quality Control in Cervical Cytology: The Papanicolaou Smear, 1989.
2. Anderson GH, Flynn KJ, Hickey LA, Le Riche JC, Matisic JP, Suen KC: A comprehensive internal quality control system for a large cytology laboratory. Acta Cytol 31:895–910, 1987.
3. Ashton PR: American Society for Cytotechnology quality assurance survey data: Summary report. Acta Cytol 33:451–454, 1989.
4. Bonfiglio TA: Quality assurance in cytopathology: Recommendations and ongoing quality assurance activities of the American Society of Clinical Pathologists. Acta Cytol 33:431–433, 1989.
5. Centers for Disease Control. Proceedings of two conferences on the state of the art in quality control measures for diagnostic cytology laboratories. Atlanta, Georgia, March 12, 1988, September 1, 1988.
6. Clark AH: Current manpower pool in cytotechnology. Acta Cytol 33:455–459, 1989.
7. College of American Pathologists: Surgical Pathology/Cytopathology Quality Assurance Manual. Skokie, IL, 1988.
8. Collins DN, Kaufman W, Clinton W: Quality evaluation of cytology laboratories in New York State. Acta Cytol 18:404–413, 1974.
9. Erozan YS: Quality control in cytopathology. Clin Lab Med 6:707–713, 1986.
10. Gardner NM: In-house quality assurance program in a state cytology laboratory. Acta Cytol 33:487–488, 1989.
11. Gilbert FE, Hicklin MD, Inhorn SL, Koss LG, Naib ZM, Patten SF, Schwinn CP, Toll MW, Wied GL: Conclusions of a study group on standards of adequacy of cytologic examinations of the female genital tract. Acta Cytol 17:559–561, 1973.
12. Greenberg RS, Chow WH, Liff JM: Recent trends in the epidemiology of cervical neoplasia. Acta Cytol 33:463–470, 1989.
13. Gupta PK, Erozan YS: Cytopathology laboratory accreditation, with special reference to the American Society of Cytology programs. Acta Cytol 33:443–447, 1989.
14. Hindman WM: A proposal for quality control in gynecologic cytology. Acta Cytol 31:384–385, 1987.
15. Inhorn SL, Clarke E: A statewide proficiency testing program in cytology. Acta Cytol 15:351–356, 1971.
16. Kraemer BB: Quality assurance activities of the College of American Pathologists. Acta Cytol 33:434–435, 1989.
17. Lipa M, Fletcher A, Chen V, Nguyen GK, Colgan T, Magown J, Paraskevas M, Redburn J: Guidelines for Quality Assurance Programs in Cytopathology. Canadian Society of Cytology Bulletin, vol 5, no. 2, 1989.
18. Luff RD, Lobritz RW: Diagnostic performance of United States Air Force cytology laboratories: An eight-year experience in central monitoring. Acta Cytol 33:475–478, 1989.
19. Melamed MR: Quality control in cytology laboratories. Gynecol Oncol 12:206–211, 1981.
20. Melamed MR, Inhorn SL, Kachenmeister LA, Ng ABP, Rodner JH: Cytology. In Quality Assurance Practices for Health Laboratories. Edited by SL Inhorn. Washington, DC, Am Public Health Assoc, pp 509–544, 1978.
21. Mitchell H, Medley G, Drake M: Quality control measures for cervical cytology laboratories. Acta Cytol 32:288–292, 1988.
22. National Cancer Institute Workshop on Terminology: The Bethesda System. JAMA 262:931–934, 1989.
23. Parker JE: Education and training for cytopathologists: Its role in quality assurance. Acta Cytol 33:448–450, 1989.
24. Paris AL: Conference on the state of the art in quality control measures for diagnostic cytology laboratories: Background and introduction. Acta Cytol 33:423–426, 1989.
25. Penner DW: An overview of the College of American Pathologists' programs in surgical pathology and cytopathology: Data summary of diagnostic performance in cervical cytopathology. Acta Cytol 33:439–442, 1989.
26. Rube IF: Experience in managing a large-scale rescreening of Papanicolaou smears and the pros and cons of measuring proficiency with visual and written examinations. Acta Cytol 33:479–483, 1989.
27. Solomon D: Introduction to the proceedings of the conference on the state of the art in quality control measures for diagnostic cytology laboratories. Acta Cytol 33:427–430, 1989.
28. Steiner C: Cervical cancer screening from the public health perspective. Acta Cytol 33:471–474, 1989.
29. Taylor WR, Nadel MR, Smith RA, Hernandez C, Moser M, Friedell GH: Cervical cancer screening and demonstration projects to identify barriers to preventing cervical cancer mortality. Acta Cytol 33:460–462, 1989.
30. Taylor WR, Plott AE, Cheek SW, Martin FJ, Rothenberg RB: Epilogue: Establishment of the center for chronic disease prevention and health promotion. Acta Cytol 33:489–490, 1989.
31. Thompson DW: Canadian experience in cytology proficiency testing. Acta Cytol 33:484–486, 1989.
32. United States Department of Health and Human Services. Clinical Laboratory Improvement Amendment, 1988.
33. Vooijs GP, Elias A, van der Graaf Y, Poelen-van de Berg M: The influence of sample takers on the cellular composition of cervical smears. Acta Cytol 30:251–257, 1986.
34. Wied GL: Quality control standards for laboratories and cytotechnology registration. Acta Cytol 14:557, 1970.
35. Wied GL: Editorial and Letters to the Editor: Quality assurance measures in cytopathology. Acta Cytol 32:913–939, 1988.

5

Evaluation of the Cellular Sample

John R. Goellner

As in tissue pathology, in cytology the evaluation of the specimen involves a series of decisions and judgments, of which many are subconscious and made almost instantaneously. Cytologic specimens create a complication in that two types of laboratory personnel contribute to the evaluation—cytotechnologist and cytopathologist. These individuals are responsible together for the report as an end product. Evaluation of cellular samples is predicated on a number of factors. Didactic information that has been learned is certainly an important part of the background that the cytotechnologist and the cytopathologist bring to the examination of the specimen. However, the experience and the attitude of each are at least as important as knowledge. Experience allows the examiner to apply the appropriate aspects of didactic knowledge to a given case and to weigh the various factors that are involved. Attitude must always be one of alertness, care, caution and integration of what is known and what is observed about a given case.

SCREENING VERSUS DIAGNOSTIC CYTOLOGY

Basically, the first decision on a given cytologic specimen is, Is it within normal limits? If it is not, then, what is the cytologic abnormality and what does it indicate? Sometimes the cytologic findings are clear and unequivocal, and sometimes the prediction is an uncertain one, being suggestive rather than diagnostic. In relatively recent years, the development of fine needle aspiration has made cytologic study a more common procedure, and the cytology laboratory is expected to provide a definitive diagnosis, if possible. Aspiration cytology now is being used for diagnosis rather than for a screening procedure preliminary to open biopsy. This change places heavier responsibilities

on the cytology laboratory staff and makes the evaluation of the cellular sample a more difficult and exacting science.

The transition from screening, such as examining Papanicolaou smear material, to a more diagnostic mode, such as examining a fine needle aspirate from the pancreas, can be a difficult one. It entails a judgment as to whether or not the specimen is adequate to permit rendering a definitive diagnosis. In many cases the aspiration will be the final diagnostic effort and, if a positive diagnosis is made, treatment and prognostication will follow. It is important to remember the responsibility that this entails.

SPECIMEN ADEQUACY

The series of decisions made in evaluating a cytologic specimen probably are most frequently subconscious rather than conscious ones. Of course, as a specimen is being examined, the subconscious decisions often are raised to a conscious level; sometimes they are verbalized to oneself or to others. On a first quick examination of a slide, one may feel in a subconscious manner that very few cells are present. This feeling rapidly transforms itself into a more conscious question, Are there enough cells for a satisfactory specimen? The next question is again almost subconscious, What sort of specimen is this? This is because the numbers of cells expected and required vary depending on the type of specimen being examined. For example, one might compare cytologic study of spinal fluid, aspirate from the liver and a Papanicolaou smear.

On the one hand, with spinal fluid, one frequently encounters specimens that contain very few cells. The cell counts in normal spinal fluid may be very low and, depending on the volume of fluid obtained, there may be very few cells to examine. It would be reasonable to call such a specimen "negative," knowing that it is spinal fluid and that this situation is a normal occurrence.

On the other hand, aspiration from the liver ordinarily yields at least moderate numbers of cells, i.e., hundreds to thousands of cells. In addition, one expects to see liver cells in a liver aspirate. This finding is not necessarily always the case. Sometimes the needle aspirates only cells from a lesion, perhaps a metastatic carcinoma with only malignant cells present. Judgment must be exercised when one finds very few or no liver cells and no cells diagnostic of a pathologic abnormality—in fact, very few cells of any kind. If one sees muscle and fat or perhaps blood with inflammatory cells only, this finding would raise a question as to the adequacy of the sample. The exact point at which the sample is judged to be inadequate is difficult to define. Such a determination is best reached in concert with the physician who performed the aspiration, often the radiologist. It is ultimately the responsibility of that physician to judge whether or not the material obtained is representative. The decision is helped by the description of the aspirated material from the cytology laboratory. In some cases, the initial suspicion may be a metastatic tumor in the liver. However, after radiologic manipulation with various contrast studies, in addition to the attempted aspiration, the best judgment may be that this is not a metastatic lesion at all but perhaps a region of fatty metamorphosis in the liver, a cavernous hemangioma or some other benign condition. If this is the case, the fact that no tumor cells are present, and even the fact that no liver cells are present, would not necessarily make the specimen "unsatisfactory" or lead to a repeat aspiration (Fig. 5–1).

The cytologic findings must be integrated with the clinical situation and radiologic impression, and then a judgment is made as to whether or not the specimen is adequate. In some cases, very few cells are present but their nature or noncellular findings in the specimen may enable a diagnosis (Fig. 5–2). In other cases, large numbers of cells are present but they are irrelevant to the problem at hand and the specimen is "nondiagnostic" in this circumstance.

SPECIMEN ADEQUACY IN PAPANICOLAOU SMEAR CYTOLOGY

In regard to Papanicolaou smears, there is considerable debate about what constitutes an adequate specimen. Typically, the malignant and premalignant conditions of the cervix occur in the transition zone between squamous and glandular epithelium. This zone, therefore, is the area that needs to be sampled to detect the largest number of abnormalities. However, with advancing age, access to the transition zone becomes progressively more difficult as the process of squamous metaplasia moves the transition zone higher into the endocervical canal. The presence of endocervical cells or metaplastic squamous cells and a mucous

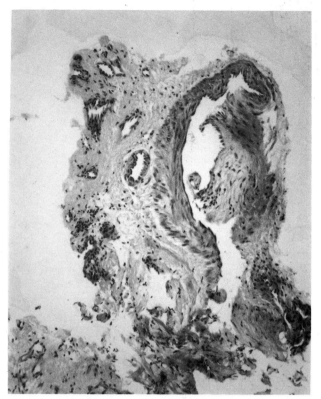

FIGURE 5–1. Fine needle aspirate from liver. Tissue fragments show benign hemangioma. No liver cells are present on tissue fragments or on smeared specimen that contained only blood, but the findings are diagnostic (hematoxylin and eosin; ×160).

endocervical component traditionally have been taken as evidence of sampling of the transition zone. The lack of these findings suggests that the transition zone has not been sampled and the specimen therefore is less than optimal.[5]

The debate centers on whether lack of cytologic evidence of transition zone sampling indicates that a specimen is completely inadequate and therefore repeat sampling is necessary.[8] This judgment should be made on the integrated information from the cytology laboratory and from the clinician caring for the patient. Consider the following two scenarios.

In one, the patient is 25 years old and is in a high-risk group for cervical disease by epidemiologic criteria. This is her first Papanicolaou smear, and she is unlikely to return for periodic Papanicolaou smears or follow-up care. A less-than-optimal specimen on this patient would be viewed with considerable concern because of her high-risk category and because she may not return for periodic care. In this case, the clinician might wish to recall the patient immediately for a repeat Pap smear.

In the second, the patient is 65 years old, is in a low-risk group for cervical disease by epidemiologic factors and returns yearly for a Papanicolaou smear and general physical examination. Knowing these facts about the patient and knowing that past smears have been negative over the years, the clinician might decide not to repeat the smear at this time.

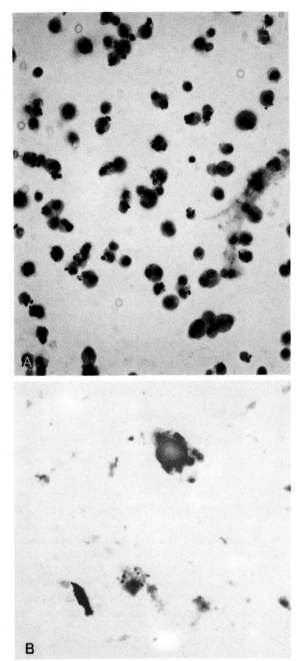

FIGURE 5–2. Aspirate from a cystic neck mass. The fluid contained degenerative foam cells (*A*) and psammoma bodies (*B*). These findings are highly suggestive of metastatic cystic papillary carcinoma of the thyroid, even though no viable thyroid cells are present (Papanicolaou smear; *A*, ×400, *B*, ×640).

Numerous other scenarios can be imagined and are encountered daily in clinical practice. In my opinion, dogmatic statements from the cytology laboratory as to what should be done next serve little useful function and only raise potential medicolegal complications. More desirable are a clear understanding between the laboratory and the clinician as to what the report indicates and trust in the clinician's ability to make a reasonable judgment as to the best course to pursue.

Because it is desirable to sample the squamocolumnar junction, consideration should be given to the collection techniques that facilitate this sampling. Current thinking is that a combination of the spatula and a technique for sampling the endocervical canal are more productive than using the spatula alone. The endocervical cytobrush and pipette sampling of the endocervix have been the two most successful methods. A number of reports have described increased detection of abnormalities with these techniques.[1, 10]

QUALITY VERSUS QUANTITY

Questions as to the adequacy of a specimen involve more than simply the numbers of cells. The presence of alveolar macrophages generally is considered to be crucial for a satisfactory sputum specimen in pulmonary cytology. The presence of these cells indicates sampling from the deeper portion of the respiratory tract, thus lending relative assurance that the specimen is representative and meaningful.[6] The quality of the cells present also is crucial. The judgment then becomes one of quality versus quantity. Cytologic material cannot be evaluated accurately without adequate fixation and staining. For this reason, emphasis traditionally has been placed on preparation techniques. This emphasis is appropriate because detailed observation of cellular features is crucial in arriving at the correct cytologic diagnosis. Common problems in proper visualization of a Papanicolaou smear include drying, excessive blood and inflammation. Common problems with aspirates include drying artifact as well as dilution by blood. It is important for those who prepare cytologic material to remember that, once a specimen is spread thinly onto a slide, drying commences immediately and can cause significant artifact within seconds. Unless it is intended that the material be read as an air-dried specimen, fixation should be accomplished within 1 or 2 seconds by immersion into alcohol or by spray fixation.

The cytologist or pathologist examining material that has been air dried will learn to look for thicker areas on the slide, which may have retained enough moisture to enable proper fixation. Diagnostic judgments based on artifactually air-dried cells are fraught with danger and may lead to untoward consequences (Fig. 5–3). Therefore, it is best to repeat the aspiration to obtain well-fixed material before a definitive diagnosis is rendered.

Another quality-versus-quantity judgment arises when there are a large number of slightly abnormal cells or a small number of very abnormal cells. The case in which there are large numbers of slightly abnormal cells must be judged as to whether or not the change is significant and should be investigated further. As the number of slightly abnormal cells decreases, one reaches a point where the decision is made not to pursue the problem, i.e., this mild change in a few cells is basically within normal limits. Each cytotechnologist and cytopathologist develops a per-

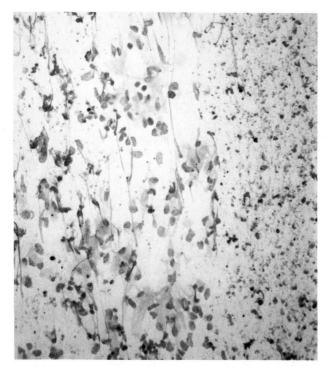

FIGURE 5–3. Aspirate from suspected colonic carcinoma metastatic to the liver. These cells were air dried and should not be used for diagnosis (Papanicolaou smear; ×160).

sonal "line" for the degree of change necessary to trigger a report of an abnormal finding. This line, one hopes, is relatively constant day after day and year after year and also relatively the same between cytotechnologists and cytopathologists. Lines may and should be moved in the light of subsequent feedback from tissue diagnosis; they should not be adhered to blindly or immutably.

A good deal of interobserver variation and even a surprising amount of intraobserver variation exist in diagnostic cytology and in histologic diagnosis as well. Various studies have documented these variations and they seem to be inevitable parts of the judgment process.[7, 9, 11] Cytotechnologists and cytopathologists are attempting to make themselves into reproducible diagnostic machines. They attempt to shut out extraneous influences, irritations, concerns and fatigue and to render reproducible and accurate diagnoses every hour of every day. This is an elusive goal. It certainly is clear that the desire for speed and efficiency begins to impact detrimentally on the decision-making process at some point. Currently there is much debate on this issue and the issue of whether quotas ought to be used by cytotechnologists, and perhaps cytopathologists, for daily workload levels.

In the absence of quotas, the temptation is to go through volumes of work so fast that cellular abnormalities either will not be noticed or will not be examined in enough detail and with enough care to render an accurate diagnostic impression. Current recommendations are in the range of approximately 80 to 100 cervical cytologic slides a day (an 8-hour work day without second jobs or overtime is assumed).[2,3] Comparable numbers are suggested for nongynecologic specimens although there is some debate as to whether exact numbers can be generated. The time needed to screen nongynecologic specimens varies greatly among different types of specimens (e.g., spinal fluid versus bronchial secretion), and it is difficult to average this out in a satisfactory manner. In addition, different individuals within the cytology laboratory screen and diagnose at different speeds. Therefore, a quota system is a rough approximation of average ability and may slow down those with an innate ability to go faster and, at the same time, place undue pressure on those who are naturally slower workers.

In general, the error a cytotechnologist makes is to miss abnormal cells entirely. In contrast, the error that the cytopathologist makes is to see abnormal cells and misjudge them. It is important for the cytotechnologist and for the cytopathologist to recognize where his or her problems will lie and to adjust his or her mental attitude to eliminate or minimize such problems.

CLINICAL INFORMATION

Another topic of importance in evaluation of the cytologic sample is the integration of clinical information with the cellular interpretation. Such information may range from practically none to a considerable amount. Some pathologists prefer to review the entire patient's history at the time they are asked to interpret an aspirated specimen. In cervical cytology, traditionally the minimum amount of information is given— usually age, often time of the last menstrual period, and, it is hoped, a modest amount of pertinent background information particularly related to neoplasia. Unfortunately, sometimes even this information is lacking and that may contribute to a less than optimal diagnosis. At the very least, the lack of such minimal information can lead to inefficiency in the laboratory because the cytologist and cytopathologist expend time to obtain the needed information.

A case in point would be the Papanicolaou smear that does not include the patient's age or menstrual status and that shows endometrial cells. The significance of these cells may vary from a normal finding to one suggestive of endometrial malignancy, depending on the two missing pieces of information.[4] If the clinician and his team understand this and provide such information routinely, the entire system works more smoothly and the patient is better served.

Another example would be the smear from a woman who has been treated for a neoplasm of the genital tract (adenocarcinoma of the endometrium). This history would alert the laboratory staff to the possibility of adenocarcinoma cells, which signals recurrent disease, or to the possibility of cellular changes, which is secondary to treatment (radiation effect on epithelial cells or reparative cells if surgery was fairly recent). Although one would hope that an accurate cytologic diagnosis could be established simply by observation of the cells, this background information makes framing of the question and reaching the conclusion easier and faster for the cytopathologist.

It is also possible to provide more information than the laboratory team wants or can use. For example, this overload of information is sometimes obtained with a thyroid aspirate—clinical thyroid status, findings on physical examination, thyroid scan results, and ^{131}I uptake as well as thyroid stimulating hormone and thyroxine values all are given to the cytopathologist. A simple note reading "cold nodule, ?malignancy" would be sufficient to state the question that the cytologic study is expected to answer.

The experience of the cytopathologist is important in properly weighing clinical information. The cells on the slide are still the crux of the matter. It is extremely important for the cytopathologist to be able to balance clinical bias with the microscopic examination. One mind set that may be useful in this regard is to remind oneself that any diagnosis that is made must be defensible to peer review, perhaps ultimately in a court of law. If the microscopic material does not justify a diagnosis, one should not make that diagnosis despite a heavy clinical bias. If the microscopic diagnosis is clear-cut and unarguable, heavy clinical bias to the contrary may not prevail: the cells are there and must be believed.

BACKGROUND KNOWLEDGE

It is very important for the cytopathologist and cytotechnologist to be aware of the relative probability of a given disease in a given organ in a given patient. This necessitates background knowledge of the various diseases that the cytology laboratory is expected to diagnose. Some situations are essentially inconceivable in a given situation and others are highly probable. In between, there are all degrees of probability and possibility. Endometrial carcinoma in a 30-year-old woman is extraordinarily rare but exceptions do occur (e.g., Stein-Leventhal syndrome). Papillary carcinoma of the thyroid occurs in young patients; anaplastic carcinoma does not. General knowledge such as this enables concentration first on the most likely diagnostic considerations.

CONTAMINATION PROBLEMS

Floaters or contaminants from accompanying cytologic material have always been a concern in cytology, as they have been in tissue diagnosis. Particularly with body fluid cytology, there is a considerable chance of cross-contamination, especially by a highly cellular positive specimen casting off malignant cells that contaminate a negative specimen. This problem has been recognized for years, and various laboratory techniques have been used in attempts to minimize it. It is always wise for the cytotechnologist and cytopathologist to keep the possibility of contamination in mind. More than one slide, in a multislide case, should contain the abnormal cells. If all the abnormal cells are on a filter

but not on accompanying sedimented material, there may have been an error in identification of the filter or the sedimented specimen. In addition, there generally should be more than one cell or one group of cells that establishes the diagnosis. The distribution of the abnormal cells should be logical and natural on body fluid specimens, not just along the cut edge of a filter preparation (perhaps from use of a contaminated pair of scissors) and not all along the edge of a filter preparation (perhaps from use of a contaminated filtering apparatus).

When the question of contamination arises, the cytopathologist must use his or her best judgment, often in concert with the clinician, to interpret the specimen properly. It often is very difficult to be completely sure that the problem really is contamination rather than actual abnormality. Further evaluation of the patient often is necessary. Repeat specimens may be needed. Additional laboratory examinations may need to be performed. Often, the problem is never resolved definitively and a "best guess" as to what happened is all that is possible. Thus, it is of extreme importance in the evaluation of the cytologic specimen to have accurate identification and careful handling to minimize the chance of error at every step from procurement to filing of the reports. Slip-ups in these areas are potentially tragic and often extremely difficult to rectify once they have occurred.

SUMMARY

A number of diverse factors play a role in the evaluation of a cellular sample. The quality of the preparation, the quality of the cell sample, the quality of the identification process, and the quality of the decision-making processes by the cytotechnologist and cytopathologist all play a part in this evaluation. It is a complicated process and one that is difficult to describe adequately to lay persons and even to medical persons from nonlaboratory disciplines. Much of what we do in cytology is recognition and, just as it is difficult to describe how one recognizes a familiar face on the street or a group of people on the street, so too it is difficult to explain how one recognizes subsets on the cellular level. I have attempted to discuss important conceptual areas in the recognition and diagnosis of cellular changes and to describe the decisions made in evaluating the cytologic sample.

References

1. Alons-van Kordelaar JJM, Boon ME: Diagnostic accuracy of squamous cervical lesions studied in spatula-Cytobrush smears. Acta Cytol 32:801–804, 1988.
2. American Medical Association. Report of the Council on Scientific Affairs. Quality Control in Cervical Cytology—The Papanicolaou Smear (Bohigian G, Chairman). Report: E (I–1988.)
3. Canadian Society of Cytology: Guidelines for Quality Assurance Programs in Cytopathology. (Lipa M, Chairman) vol 5, no 2, 1989.
4. Cherkis RC, Patten SF Jr, Dickinson JC, Dekanich AS: Signif-

icance of atypical endometrial cells detected by cervical cytology. Obstet Gynecol 69:786–789, 1987.

5. Elias A, Linthorst G, Bekker B, Vooijs PG: The significance of endocervical cells in the diagnosis of cervical epithelial changes. Acta Cytol 27:225–229, 1983.

6. Kato H, Konaka C, Ono J, Takahashi M, Hayata Y: Cytology of the Lung: Techniques and Interpretation. New York, Igaku-Shoin Medical Publishers, pp 38–39, 1983.

7. Koss LG: Dysplasia: A real concept or a misonmer? Obstet Gynecol 51:374–379, 1978.

8. Koss LG, Hicklin MD: Standards of adequacy of cytologic examination of the female genital tract: Conclusions of study group on cytology. Obstet Gynecol 43:792–793, 1974.

9. Robertson AJ, Anderson JM, Swanson Beck J, Burnett RA, Howatson SR, Lee FD, Lessells AM, McLaren KM, Moss SM, Simpson JG, Smith GD, Tavadia HB, Walker F: Observer variability in histopathological reporting of cervical biopsy specimens. J Clin Pathol 42:231–238, 1989.

10. Taylor PT Jr, Andersen WA, Barber SR, Covell JL, Smith EB, Underwood PB Jr: The screening Papanicolaou smear: Contribution of the endocervical brush. Obstet Gynecol 70:734–738, 1987.

11. Yobs AR, Plott AE, Hicklin MD, Coleman SA, Johnston WW, Ashton PR, Rube IF, Watts JC, Naib ZM, Wood RJ, Recalde AL, Ingram FR, Mangum CA: Retrospective evaluation of gynecologic cytodiagnosis. II. Interlaboratory reproducibility as shown in rescreening large consecutive samples of reported cases. Acta Cytol 31:900–910, 1987.

6

Pathologic Processes Affecting Cells from Inflammation to Cancer

John K. Frost

Cellular morphology bespeaks biologic activity. On the one hand, it reflects biologic behavior of the tissue and of the host; on the other hand, it reflects the genetic and molecular biology of the cells themselves. This intermediary position places examination of the cell in a key roll to our understanding of the myriad of normal and abnormal processes that affect this closely knit chain, from molecules to host.

Processes that affect cells are myriad, but cellular responses to them are limited. They fall into a few manageable categories, however, which can be characterized for better understanding. This allows for a better comprehension and more accurate diagnosis of the condition or conditions that are present and for the most prudent and efficacious therapy and management of the host.

CELLULAR STRUCTURES MOST KEY TO UNDERSTANDING BIOLOGIC BEHAVIOR

General biologic activity is reflected best in the cellular structures of the *nucleus*.[14] *Functional activity* is reflected mainly in the morphology of the *cytoplasm*, which displays the differentiation allowing a cell to perform its work (Fig. 6–1). In cells that are immediately wet fixed (e.g., 95% ethanol) and are properly prepared and stained by the Papanicolaou method,[20, 21] usual nuclear structures are either acidophilic or hematoxylinophilic.

Nucleoli

Nucleoli are the sites of production of proribosomes, consisting of RNA and RNA-associated protein. The latter is acidophilic when properly prepared, staining with the eosin and orange G of the Papanicolaou stain as a shade in the red-orange-yellow spectrum. This is a delicate balance, however, as nucleoli are also hematoxylinophilic if conditions are right to produce this artifact. Thus, if there is a general cellular overstaining with hematoxylin or an understaining with weak counterstains, nucleoli can stain with hematoxylin and be unable to take the acid counterstain. In this situation nucleoli are unable to be distinguished from chromocenters and thus cannot be definitely identified. This same inability to identify nucleoli is present in black and white photomicrography (see Fig. 6–1).

Rarely, nucleoli can incorrectly appear pale blue or green as a result of improper Papanicolaou staining techniques (e.g., contamination of counterstains by carryover from hematoxylin, acid wash, bluing reagent). In a Papanicolaou stain the outline of the acidophilic nucleolus is crisp and well defined, whereas in a Romanowsky stain (e.g., Wright, Giemsa, Diffquik) nucleoli stain pale blue and their borders usually are indistinct and poorly defined.

When nucleoli are definitely identified, the amount of their material that is present directly reflects the cell's degree of protein production. This can be either for building the cell's own substance (e.g., repair, replication, stimulation) or for making and secreting the extracellular material (e.g., mucus, ground substance). Nucleolar-associated chromatin is continuous with, and a part of, the chromatinic rim, the chroma-

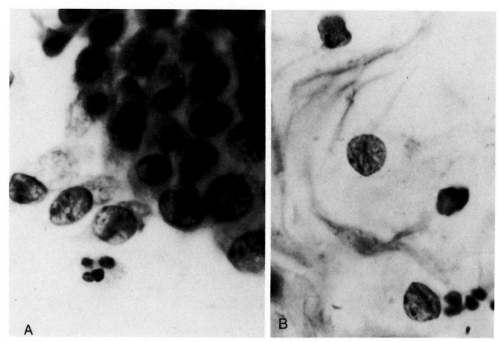

FIGURE 6–1. Euplasia—baseline normalcy. *A,* Normal euplastic columnar epithelial cells. Nuclei are round or rounded with a uniform chromatin-parachromatin pattern. The chromatinic rim is uniformly thick in each nucleus and is predictable from one nucleus to the next. The nuclear membrane is too thin to be visualized by light microscopy, but its shape determines the shape of the outer surface of the chromatinic rim. Each epithelial nucleus is approximately the same size as the entire nucleus and cytoplasm of the neutrophil, a good size and magnification indicator. The cytoplasm, in the shape of a column, determines the cell's function and, thus, its cell type. *B,* Normal euplastic keratinizing stratified squamous epithelial cells. The four epithelial nuclei show progressive stages of hypermaturation from the one rounded metabolic-type nucleus (center) about the size of the neutrophil (lower right), which has a uniform pattern of an intermediate cell, to the wrinkled and smudged karyopyknotic nucleus of a superficial cell (Papanicolaou stain (right center); fast vaginopancervical smear; × 1200). (Reproduced with permission from Frost JK: The Cell in Health and Disease, 2nd ed. Basel, S. Karger, 1986.)

tinic net or both, depending on the location of the nucleolus in the nucleus.

Chromatin

The chromatin, which is hematoxylinophilic, consists of DNA and DNA-associated protein. It is the DNA-associated protein that stains purple with hematoxylin not the DNA itself; however, the ratio of DNA to DNA-associated protein in a well-preserved cell is virtually constant, so that the degree of staining with hematoxylin reliably reflects the amount of DNA,[4] *if* the cell is well preserved. With degeneration, however, both the protein-staining characteristics (e.g., hypochromasia, normochromasia, hyperchromasia) and the DNA-protein ratio can be unpredictably altered, so that the degree of staining does not reflect the amount of DNA present.

The shade of purple, which a hematoxylinophilic structure exhibits, reflects its final pH after staining and mounting. It thus ranges from a red purple (low pH and most soluble) to a deep blue purple or "black" (high pH and most insoluble). The chromatin fibers during mitosis and meiosis are very tightly condensed and organized into chromosomes. During the intermitotic phase (i.e., metabolic phase) their structural

organization forms the *chromatinic rim, chromatinic net* and *parachromatin* (interchromatin).

Chromatinic Rim and Nuclear Membrane. The chromatinic rim is that structure of condensed biologically inactive chromatin (i.e., heterochromatin) that, under light microscopy, has been referred to in past years as the "nuclear membrane" (see Fig. 6–1). It is not the nuclear membrane, however, but consists of marginated, condensed heterochromatin that is attached to the inner surface of the true inner membrane of the nuclear envelope by the proteins of the nuclear lamina (Fig. 6–2).[9, 14] The thickness of this true inner nuclear membrane is so thin that it cannot be resolved by light microscopy, but its shape is accurately portrayed by the shape of the profile of the outer surface of the chromatinic rim. The thickness of the chromatinic rim, therefore, is not related to the thickness of the true nuclear membrane, but reflects the amount of condensed heterochromatin that is marginated against the true nuclear membrane.

Chromatinic Net. The chromatinic net is the network of condensed, biologically inactive heterochromatin that extends from the chromatinic rim throughout the nucleoplasm. Its degree and form of compaction depends on biologic activity and occurs in two major forms: *threads,* ranging from fine fibrils through coarser strands, and *granules* or chromocenters, ranging from

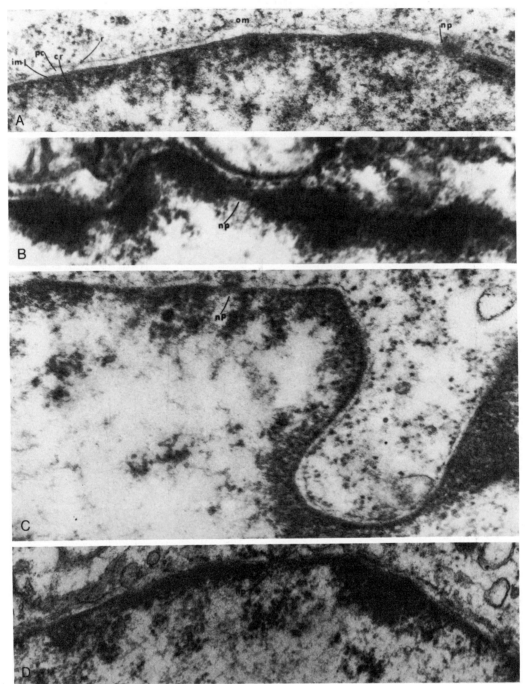

FIGURE 6–2. Nuclear Membrane. Electron micrographs of the region of the nuclear envelope of four separate nuclei. In each, the cytoplasm is above and the nucleoplasm is below. The nuclear envelope consists of the outer nuclear membrane *(om)* with occasional attached ribosomes *(r)*, the inner nuclear membrane and lamina *(im-1)* and the paranuclear cisterna *(pc)*. At least one nuclear pore *(np)* is depicted in each of the four nuclear views, with its protein complex projecting from nucleoplasm to cytoplasm. *A, Euplasia, columnar cell.* Smoothly rounded shape with a uniformly thin chromatinic rim of well-preserved condensed chromatin. *B, Retroplasia, columnar cell.* Wrinkled nuclear membranes with a smudged chromatinic rim and cleared parachromatin containing a few smudged granules of degenerated chromatin. *C, Proplasia, squamous metaplasia.* An undulated (wavy) nuclear membrane, with a chromatinic rim that is thicker than in euplasia *(A)* but is not degenerated or smudged as in retroplasia *(B)*. Parachromatin is cleared but contains a few threads and granules of well-preserved chromatin. *D, Malignant neoplasia, invasive lung carcinoma.* The inner nuclear membrane determines the shape of the outer surface of the chromatinic rim, even though the latter's thickness varies markedly from the chromatin condensing irregularly against the nuclear membrane. In this way, the inner surface of the chromatinic rim has an irregularity that is independent of the shape of its outer surface (Osmium/methacrylate; bronchial biopsy specimens; *A* and *D*, ×63,000; *B* and *C*, ×65,000). (Reproduced with permission from Frost JK: The Cell in Health and Disease, 2nd ed. Basel, S. Karger, 1986.)

fine granules ("ground glass"), to moderate granules, to coarse granules, to clumps.

Parachromatin. The parachromatin is the functional domain of the extremely small amount of biologically active euchromatin that is present in the nucleus at any given time—bathed in abundant nuclear sap (karyolymph) and supported by threads of biologically inactive heterochromatin. Parachromatin is very weakly hematoxylinophilic and is, thus, the pale region of the nucleus lying between the relatively enormous amount of biologically inactive heterochromatin compacted into the tightly condensed masses constituting the chromatinic net and chromatinic rim (see Fig. 6–1). Referred to in electron microscopy as the interchromatin areas, in light microscopy it is referred to as the parachromatin, principally by hematologists,[24] as it lies within or beside (L:para-) the condensed chromatin. It contains very little chromatin and, thus, is very palely hematoxylinophilic. The small bit of chromatin that it does contain, however, is rich in biologically active euchromatin with supporting threads of biologically inactive heterochromatin.[5, 14]

With increase of cellular activity, much of the heterochromatin in the parachromatin moves into the chromatinic net and rim, resulting in a higher proportion of euchromatin to heterochromatin and providing the euchromatin freer access to the substrates of the nuclear sap during its increased biologic synthetic activities. This movement of the heterochromatin out of the parachromatin produces increased pallor or "clearing" of the already pale parachromatin. Of great importance, this clearing of the parachromatin in increased activity is associated with crisp and distinctly defined chromatin-parachromatin interfaces, which indicates good preservation.

With decreased cellular activity of degeneration, however, both types of chromatin (heterochromatin and euchromatin) cohere and move out of the parachromatin to clump with the chromatinic net and chromatinic rim. Although this clearing of the parachromatin with degeneration can leave it as pale, as is the parachromatin with increased activity, the important discriminating difference between these two is that the chromatin-parachromatin interfaces are crisp and sharply defined in proplasia, and they become blurry and indistinct in degeneration.[14]

MORPHOLOGIC EFFECTS ON CELLS OF PROCESSES RESULTING IN BASELINE NORMAL ACTIVITY— EUPLASIA

Cells at their usual healthy state of being, living in "peace and harmony" with one another and their environment, and without pathologic processes affecting them, are generally referred to as "normal" and depicted as such in classic histology texts. Yet it is normal for cells to react to the host of pathologic processes to which they can be exposed, but by a limited number of mechanisms. In this way it is normal

for cells to be injured and to degenerate, to heal by repairing, to react to and compensate for stimulation and to adapt to chronic irritations. These are all normal reactions of the host to its environment; yet the reference morphology level of euplasia (*eu* = normal; *-plasia* = form, structure) is that form first referred to, which reflects activity of cells that are "living in peace and harmony," without stress from pathologic processes.

In euplasia (see Fig. 6–1), key nuclear structures appear in light microscopy to be as follows:

- *Round or rounded* (e.g., nucleus, nucleolus, chromocenter) (Figs. 6–1 and 6–3A)
- *Uniform or regular* (e.g., pattern of chromatin, parachromatin; thickness of chromatinic rim) (Figs. 6–1 and 6–2A)
- *Predictable* from one nucleus to another in a multinucleated cell (e.g., pattern of chromatin, parachromatin; numbers of nucleoli, chromocenters; degree of chromasia), or from one cell to another cell of the same type in a diagnostically true tissue fragment (Fig. 6–1A).

MORPHOLOGIC EFFECTS ON CELLS OF PROCESSES ASSOCIATED WITH CLASSIC INVASIVE CANCER— MALIGNANT CRITERIA

There is no perfect or absolute morphologic feature of cancer—or malignant criterion—that, when present, unequivocally means that this cell is from cancer or, when absent, means that there is no cancer. A few key morphologic changes occur, however, that signify a high likelihood of cancer being present. Careful evaluation of them can help lead a skilled diagnostician, experienced in this area, to a proper interpretation.[14] Most of these diagnostically valuable morphologic features, which are indicators of the effects of malignant neoplastic processes on cells, are present in the nucleus.

Nuclear Membrane Irregularities

Significant irregularities of shape are frequently present in the nuclear membrane of a cell from cancer, which are rarely present in other cells. As the nuclear membrane cannot be seen in light microscopy, its irregularities in shape are noted as irregularities in the shape of the profile of the outer surface of the chromatinic rim (Figs. 6–3D and 6–4). They are unpredictable and inexplicable, occurring for no reason that is explainable by normal, retrogressive or progressive processes. They have sharp characteristics in common, appearing as pointed spicules or razor-sharp angles projecting outwards into the cytoplasm or as sharply angled infoldings inward and toward the nucleoplasm.

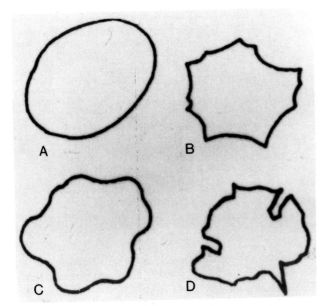

FIGURE 6–3. Nuclear membrane shape. This depicts the shape of the profile of the outer surface of the chromatinic rim. The nuclear membrane is too thin to be seen with the light microscope, but its shape determines the shape of the outer surface of the chromatinic rim. *A, Euplasia.* Normal baseline activity; rounded or oval. *B, Retroplasia.* Decreased activity; wrinkled concavities from water loss and shrinkage. *C, Proplasia.* Increased activity; undulated or wavy, in response to an increased need for transport activity across the membrane. *D, Malignant neoplasia.* Cancer; sharp and angled, unpredictable and inexplainable irregularities. (Reproduced with permission from Frost JK: The Cell in Health and Disease, 2nd ed. Basel, S. Karger, 1986.)

They cannot be explained away, such as being the sharp angles of nuclear molding caused by adjacent structures (e.g., nuclei, secretion, keratohyalin granules); the sharp angles between the concavities of a wrinkled, degenerated nucleus (Fig. 6–3B); or the sharp infoldings of nuclear lobulation or convolution that is associated with increased activity. Thus they are sharp, grotesque, unpredictable and inexplainable.

Chromatin

In cancer a general disarray occurs in the structural orderliness of the chromatin that is encountered in the normalcy of euplasia. Unpredictable and inexplainable sharp angles and pointed spicules replace the roundedness, so characteristic of euplasia, in certain key structures (e.g., large chromatin clumps of the chromatinic net (Fig. 6–5A) and along the inner aspect of the chromatinic rim).

The thickness of the chromatinic rim markedly varies from sharply irregular and massively thickened areas (clumped chromatin condensed against the lamina and true nuclear membrane) to extremely thinned segments (Fig. 6–2D). The last frequently are so thin that the chromatinic rim cannot be determined with the light microscope, other than as an invisible interface between nucleoplasm and cytoplasm (Figs. 6–4, 6–5A, 6–5F and 6–5H). Staining of chromatin is generally more darkly hematoxylinophilic in cancer (see Fig. 6–5). This hyperchromasia indicates increased DNA-associated protein and, thus, reflects a greater amount of DNA to be present.

Parachromatin

These pale areas of the nucleus, the parachromatin, can become even more cleared in two unpredictable ways: in the degree of clearing and in the size of the cleared areas (Figs. 6–4, 6–5A, 6–5C, 6–5G and 6–5H). In the first, the degree of clearing, one area can be clearer than the next area of the same size. In the second, the size of the cleared areas, regions of the nucleus that have the same degree of clearing can be of varying sizes and shapes. These are in striking contrast to the uniformity and regularity found in euplasia and proplasia. These differences can be present to an extreme degree, from slightly cleared areas to areas as clear as the perfectly clean portions of the

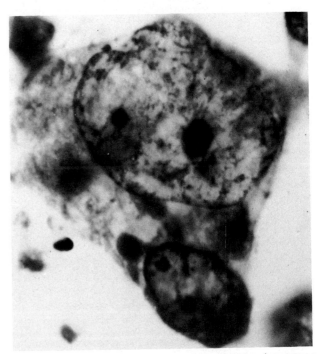

FIGURE 6–4. Nuclear membrane irregularities in cancer. Adenocarcinoma of the liver (hepatocellular carcinoma). Many small irregularities exist in the nuclear membrane (outer surface of the chromatinic rim) running along the upper right margin of the large nucleus (from 1 to 3 o'clock). At 11 o'clock, however, there is a large, deep irregularity with overhang and a sharp point. This macabre "bite" is unexpected and not explainable. Hazy secretion is in the opposite part of the cytoplasm, below the nucleus and away from the irregularity. Chromatin/parachromatin pattern is uneven, and the chromatinic rim varies markedly in thickness (Papanicolaou stain; fine-needle aspirate (FNA) of liver; ×1250). (Reproduced with permission from Frost JK: The Cell in Health and Disease, 2nd ed. Basel, S. Karger, 1986.)

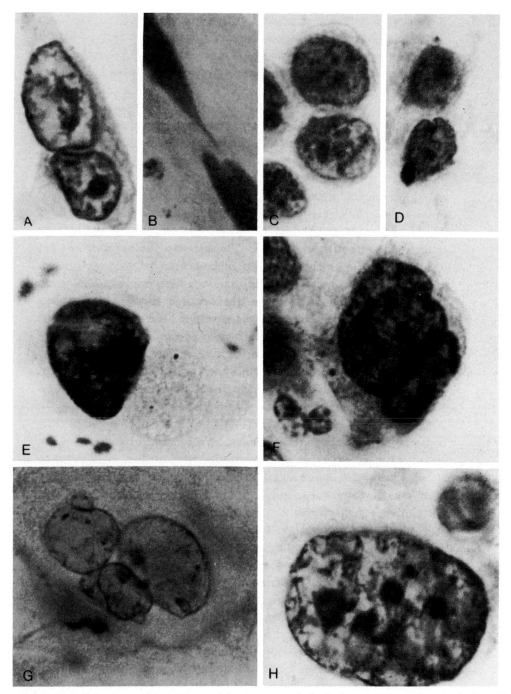

FIGURE 6–5. Criteria of malignant neoplasia. Many of the best morphologic features of cancer are depicted here; they are referred to and explained in the text by individual illustration (Papanicolaou stain; *A, B, C, D, F, G* and *H* ×2000; *E* and *H* ×1320). (Reproduced with permission from Frost JK: The Cell in Health and Disease, 2nd ed. Basel, S. Karger, 1986.)

slide. The hyperchromasia of the chromatinic rim and of the chromatinic net is in striking contrast to the hypochromasia, or clearing, of the parachromatin and accentuates the cellular pleomorphism. This pleomorphism and the irregularity of pattern become much more obvious if one mentally divides a nucleus into sections (e.g., quadrants) and compares them, to better perceive that each area has a different pattern than the other. This is in contrast to the structural uniformity encountered in euplasia.

Nucleolus

In response to the numerous pathologic processes present in malignant neoplasia, the nucleolus is frequently enlarged, irregular and sharply angled (Fig. 6–5H). The first two (nucleolar enlargement and irregularity) occur with increased protein production, such as in proplasia, and can be extreme in repair; thus, they do not discriminate between cancer and simple increased activity. In contrast the third (pointed spicules and sharp angles to the nucleolar outline), when present with the first two, constitutes a good indicator of malignant neoplasia.

Large nucleoli per se are generally not good indicators of malignancy because they are frequently present in simple protein production (e.g., cell stimulation, virus infection, repair). However, they can be helpful in differentiating leukemias and lymphomas, having conspicuous nucleoli in their malignant leukocytes, from benign leukocytes without prominent nucleoli. The presence of a nucleolus is also helpful in detecting invasive cancer, when nucleoli are present in apparently disarming dyskaryotic squamous cells that otherwise would be indicative only of squamous atypia, dysplasia or intraepithelial neoplasia.[14]

The number of nucleoli in a nucleus, per se, does not help discriminate cancer from noncancer, especially not from cell stimulation, which can have a large number of nucleoli in each cell.[2] However, an extreme variation in the numbers of nucleoli (i.e., of eight or more) between nuclei of either a multinucleated cell or a diagnostically true tissue fragment, is an increasingly significant indicator of a malignant process.

Mitosis

The presence of normal mitoses, per se, does not help in identifying cancer, as it is a common feature of proplasia in increased activity. However, the presence of abnormal mitoses (e.g., tripolar, tetrapolar and abnormally large numbers of chromosomes in a metaphase spread) is a valuable indicator of the probability of cancer.[14] The same can be said for aneuploidy. Either by determining the DNA ploidy by flow cytometry (low resolution) of a large number of cells,[15, 37, 38] by image analysis (high resolution) of fewer but individually identified cells[6, 16, 32, 40] or by karyotyping (individual chromosome identification and enumeration) of extremely few cells,[23] aneuploidy is a good indicator in favor of neoplasia, both malignant and premalignant (precursors). Like all malignant criteria, it is neither perfect nor absolute.

Multinucleation

It is not a malignant criterion to find multiple nuclei in a cell, as this is a frequent occurrence in proplasia (e.g., stimulation, repair). This finding does, however, afford valuable malignant criteria by descrying nuclear pleomorphism and nonpredictability of key nuclear features in comparing nucleus-to-nucleus of a multinucleated cell (Fig. 6–6). The key nuclear variations to evaluate include chromatin/parachromatin pattern, numbers and shape of chromatin aggregations and of nucleoli, parachromatin clearing, degree of nuclear chromasia, nuclear size and shape, thickness of chromatinic rims and nuclear membrane irregularities (Figs. 6–5D, 6–5E and 6–5F).

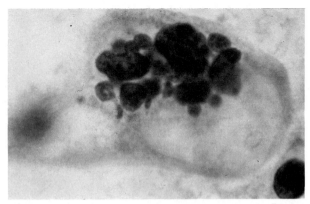

FIGURE 6–6. Cancer cell with multinucleation. Multinucleation is not a malignant criterion, as it is so much a part of increased activity (proplasia) that it, per se, does not help to distinguish the two. In a well-preserved cell with multinucleation, however, the opportunity arises to search for a loss of predictability in key features, when comparing nucleus to nucleus, which at times occurs in cancer. Note the marked variation in nuclear size and shape, nucleoli, chromocenters and chromasia (Papanicolaou stain; fast vaginopancervical smear; ×1250).

Relationships of Nucleus to Cytoplasm

An increased ratio of nuclear area to cytoplasmic area (N/C ratio) is frequently present in cancer. It is also found in precursor states (e.g., dysplasia, intraepithelial neoplasia), during increased activity and in normal small leukocytes. A large and well-preserved nucleus, of at least the size of an entire small macrophage, which has a scanty but well-preserved cytoplasm with an intact cell membrane, constitutes such a high N/C ratio favoring cancer.

Diagnostically True Tissue Fragment

The finding of a diagnostically true tissue fragment, per se, also is not a malignant criterion. However, in a well-preserved true tissue fragment, where the cells grew together and fragmented off as a unit (neither a secondary clustering together of primarily single cells nor a degenerated tissue fragment), one has another superb opportunity to evaluate for malignancy. As in a multinucleated cell, in a well-preserved and diagnostically true tissue fragment the same key nuclear features (plus N/C ratio) can be compared, cell-to-cell, for predictability in normalcy versus nonpredictability in cancer (Figs. 6–5D and 6–5E).

Good State of Preservation Essential for Diagnosis

Although cancer cells can and do degenerate (Figs. 6–5B and 6–5D), as do all cells, it is important that less than well-preserved cells *not* be the basis for the determination of the presence of cancer. Even "early" minimal degeneration of the nucleus can mimic many changes that, when present in a well-preserved cell, can represent valuable malignant criteria (e.g., hyperchromasia, parachromatin clearing, abnormal chromatin pattern, high N/C ratio). The error of using a less than well-preserved state has led to a number of false cancer diagnoses with unnecessary mental trauma, surgery, other therapy and even death.

In many instances the state of preservation can best be evaluated by determining the sharpness of the chromatin-parachromatin interfaces—those surfaces of condensed heterochromatin (chromatinic rim and chromatinic net) where they are bathed by the parachromatin. These interfaces are key to recognizing the well-preserved cell or to detecting the early stages of degeneration. With degeneration of the chromation thread, the denatured and dissolving DNA-associated protein "bleeds" into the surrounding parachromatin, producing a fuzziness or blurriness to the interfaces' surface.

Thus, the chromatin-parachromatin interfaces in well-preserved cells are crisp and well defined—as though the edges of the chromatin had just been cut by the sharp blade of a cookie cutter and had neither dissolved by degeneration nor bled into the parachromatin. In a well-preserved nucleus the surfaces of the interfaces match, in crispness, the well-defined outer surface of the chromatinic rim, which is held in sharp profile by the true inner nuclear membrane.

MORPHOLOGIC EFFECTS ON CELLS OF RETROGRESSIVE PROCESSES RESULTING IN DECREASED ACTIVITY—RETROPLASIA

Retrogressive or degradative processes which affect cells with decreased activity occur with such events as aging, injury, degeneration, death, necrosis and autolysis, resulting in the characteristic cellular structural changes of retroplasia (*retro* = backward; *-plasia* = form, structure). The inciting causes include external agents (e.g., trauma, heat, radiation, toxins), living organisms (e.g., viruses through helminths) and lack of blood supply (e.g., embolus, occlusion, hypoxia, anoxia, ischema, infarction).

Loss of a Cell's Control over its Water Content

A cell, unable to control its water content, can swell or shrink. Swelling produces hydropic degeneration with multiple vacuoles of varying sizes in the nucleus and, particularly, in the cytoplasm. The cell swells and, as the protein content is watered down, becomes proportionately less well stained or hypochromatic.

Eventually the cell membrane (plasma membrane, cytoplasmic membrane) ruptures with loss of some of the cytoplasm into the background. The result frequently appears to the unwary as a cell with a high N/C ratio (Fig. 6–7). Loss of all of the cytoplasm results in a truly bare nucleus of a degenerated cell. In order to avoid diagnostic error, this cell is to be recognized and clearly distinguished from a well-preserved cell with a high N/C ratio.

Cytoplasmic Staining

With degeneration, cytoplasmic proteins can appear blurry and lose their basophilia, becoming gray, yellow, orange or red. This resultant acidophilic cytoplasm should not be confused with cytoplasmic keratinization or with the presence of muscle or collagen, but should be recognized as degeneration. This form of degeneration is frequently a processing artifact from the use of improper fixative, or it occurs with air drying of the specimen before fixation, a part of the so-called air-drying artifact that plagues proper interpretation.

Nuclear Membrane Wrinkling

With loss of water and resultant shrinkage of nuclear volume, the nucleus collapses inwardly and the nuclear membrane wrinkles into a series of concavities (Figs. 6–2B and 6–3B). This finding must not be confused with the characteristic nuclear membrane irregularities of malignancy. Although cancer cells can degenerate, wrinkling of the nuclear membrane is not a feature of malignancy but of degeneration.

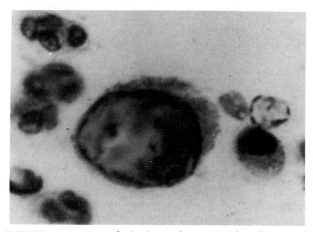

FIGURE 6–7. Retroplasia in a degenerated cell. Marked swelling of the nucleus has occurred either from residual proplasia or from water uptake. For size, compare with the well-preserved neutrophil at 11 o'clock. One-half of the nucleus (N) is bare with only a few whisps of cytoplasm (C), evidencing degenerative rupture of cell membrane and loss of cytoplasm, giving the false impression of an extremely high N/C ratio. The nucleus is hyperchromatic with large areas of clearing. The chromatin-parachromatin interfaces are extremely blurry as compared with the sharp outer profile of the chromatinic rim, especially from 12 to 3 o'clock (Papanicolaou stain; fast vaginopancervical smear; ×1500). (Reproduced with permission from Frost JK: The Cell in Health and Disease, 2nd ed. Basel, S. Karger, 1986.)

Chromatin Staining

The DNA-associated proteins of the chromatin (histone, nonhistone, enzymatic, structural), rather than the DNA itself, stain with hematoxylin. However, in the well-preserved nucleus the proportion of DNA to DNA-associated protein is so constant that the degree of hematoxylinophilia is a useful reflection of the quantity of DNA. With degeneration, by comparison, denaturation of nuclear protein affects its affinity for hematoxylin, resulting in either increase or decrease of hematoxylinophilia (see Fig. 6–7). The resulting hyperchromasia or hypochromasia, thus, has no dependable relationship to an increase or a decrease of DNA but is merely a result of degeneration, which cannot be read out accurately.

Chromatin-Parachromatin Interface Blurring

Protein solubility and binding are both altered by degeneration, so that bleeding of the chromatin occurs out into the parachromatin in the early stages of deterioration. This effect results in smudging or *blurring* of the normally crisply defined chromatin-parachromatin interfaces (Figs. 6–5D and 6–7).

Chromatin Coherence or Clumping

As the chromatin degenerates it becomes sticky, cohering together into larger aggregates of degenerated chromatinic clumps rather than the more orderly condensation and packing of well-preserved chromatin. This process leaves behind abnormally cleared areas of parachromatin virtually devoid of the finely divided chromatinic threads, which normally impart a faint hematoxylinophilia to the interchromatinic parachromatin. This degenerative clearing can be extreme. At times it mimics the clearing of increased activity in proplasia and cancer, except for the blurring of the chromatin-parachromatin interfaces (see Fig. 6–7). Fortunately, this blurring usually occurs early in degeneration and acts as an "early warning" that other morphologic changes that are present (e.g., hyperchromasia, parachromatin clearing, chromatin clumping, high N/C ratio) also may be due to degeneration rather than cancer. Thus, these changes lose value in that particular situation as possible criteria of malignancy, helping to avert a false cancer diagnosis.

Chromatin Gelatinization

As the masses of chromatin clumps further degenerate, they take on a blurred, gelatin-like appearance. This at times has been referred to incorrectly, as ground glass (e.g., in herpes). It is actually not finely granular, however, as is true glass ground by sandblasting and as is the ground glass finely granular chromatin

of mild proplasia in increased activity. It loses any particular pattern or form it may have had and degenerates into a truly formless mass of gelatinous denatured protein and admixed matter (Fig. 6–8).

MORPHOLOGIC EFFECTS ON CELLS OF PROGRESSIVE PROCESSES RESULTING IN INCREASED ACTIVITY—PROPLASIA

Innumerable processes, capable of causing progressive changes, can act upon cells with resultant increased general activity, but only a limited number of ways exist in which it is possible for the cells to react to them. Morphologic changes of proplasia reflect the multitude of progressive processes including stimulation, replication, reaction, repair from degeneration and, even, preinvasive neoplasia. Telltale minute differences evolve from intricate interplay among retroplasia, proplasia and the time sequence of interaction and progression of these features (see following discussion on mixed and changing processes), which may allow a differential to be noted and separate processes to be identified.

Proplasia, the morphologic changes of increased activity, continues to be characterized by the nonmalignant features of roundness of nuclear and cytoplasmic shapes, regularity of chromatin-parachromatin pattern and predictability of these structures from nucleus-to-nucleus in a multinucleated cell and from cell-to-cell in diagnostically true tissue fragments. It is identifiably discriminable from euplasia and retroplasia

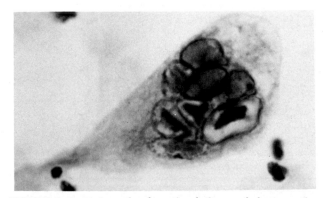

FIGURE 6–8. Herpes simplex stimulation and degeneration of an epithelial cell. This cell was first stimulated, with many features of proplasia still persisting (e.g., multinucleation and granular chromatin in the nucleus at 6 o'clock). The cell degenerated with many features of general retroplasia (e.g., blurring of chromatin-parachromatin interfaces, margination of chromatin, cytoplasm vacuolation and gelatinous degeneration of the upper four nuclei) and a few key features, which more specifically indicate herpetic infection (e.g., nuclear crowding and molding, similar to gallstones, and a central nuclear inclusion that is acidophilic with a peri-inclusion halo and transhalo bridges of blurry, degenerated chromatin strands) (Papanicolaou stain; fast vaginopancervical smear; ×600).

by a few key features, discussed subsequently. However, it shares these features with malignant neoplasia, from which it must be carefully and diagnostically differentiated by the absence of malignant criteria previously discussed.

Nuclear Membrane Undulation

With increased cellular activity the nuclear membrane is thrown into waves or undulations (Figs. 6–2C, 6–3C, 6–9 and 6–10). These facilitate the intensified transmembrane traffic necessitated by the increased metabolic activity.[39] It is neither the wrinkling of degeneration nor the unpredictable sharp irregularities of malignancy (Figs. 6–3B and 6–3C); from both of these, undulation is to be carefully differentiated.

Chromatin

The chromatin becomes more hyperchromatic with increased cellular activity. The chromatinic rim becomes somewhat granular and moderately thicker but maintains a uniform thickness within a given nucleus.

With mildly increased activity, the chromatinic net becomes more chromatic and finely granular (ground glass). As cellular activity increases, the amount of chromatin is greater and some of the fine granules coalesce into moderately sized granules and, with more heightened activity, into coarse granules. Overall nuclear hyperchromasia increases with cellular activity.

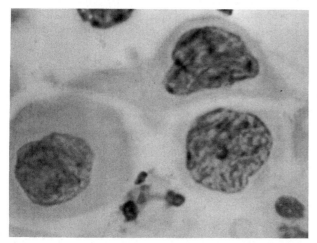

FIGURE 6–9. Proplasia, increased activity. These three epithelial nuclei demonstrate typical changes of increased activity including nuclear membrane undulation, uniformly thickened chromatinic rim, chromatin granulation, uniform parachromatic clearing and hyperchromasia. Because the cells are maturing towards squamous, there are no nucleoli. The cytoplasm is maturing poorly with a scanty moderately mature squame at 12 o'clock, a thick moderately mature cytoplasm at 9 o'clock and an immature cytoplasm at 3 o'clock (Papanicolaou stain; fast vaginopancervical smear; ×1500). (Reproduced with permission from Frost JK: The Cell in Health and Disease, 2nd ed. Basel, S. Karger, 1986.)

Parachromatin

In contradistinction to the chromatin, parachromatin becomes hypochromatic or cleared with increased activity, as biologically inactive heterochromatin moves out of the parachromatin and condenses into the chromatinic rim and net. This activity leaves a higher percentage of euchromatin in the small amount of chromatin remaining in the parachromatin. This parachromatin clearing is regularly distributed throughout the nucleus between the uniformly dispersed chromatin granules (see Figs. 6–9 and 6–10). This finding is in sharp contrast to the irregular parachromatin clearing, which can be encountered in cancer.

Nucleolus

Nucleoli can enlarge, multiply and become quite prominent in response to a great demand for heightened protein synthesis with increased activity. This finding is particularly true in columnar cells, where some of the largest, rounded nucleoli are found (see Fig. 6–10); however, other cell types can also produce prominent nucleoli with increased activity, particularly mesothelial cells, myocytes and fibroblasts. Even though they can be quite irregular, especially in radiation and repair (Fig. 6–11), these huge nucleoli of increased activity should not be confused with cancer. The corners of the nucleoli are rounded as are the ends of their spicules.[14, 18]

When cells with increased activity mature to stratified squamous epithelium, their nucleoli disappear as the cells mature near the surface, so that the cells exfoliate without nucleoli (see Fig. 6–9). Thus, squamous atypias, atypical metaplasias, dysplasias and intraepithelial neoplasias (e.g., cervical intraepithelial neoplasia or CIN) shed without nucleoli. Squamous cells under extreme repair (e.g., post radiation, estrogen-induced), however, can shed with prominent nucleoli (see Fig. 6–11). These can be large and irregular, but angles and spicules are rounded, not sharply pointed; the cells shed in tissue fragments.

Mitosis and Multinucleation

Rapidly growing cells exhibit many mitoses and considerable multinucleation (Figs. 6–8 and 6–10C). This finding is especially true in columnar epithelium (e.g., endocervix, bronchial tree) but can occur in virtually any tissue type. The mitoses are normal, however, and the occurrence of abnormal mitoses (e.g., tripolar, tetrapolar) makes one suspect the presence of a neoplasm. Multinucleation in simple proplasia is characterized by the predictability of one nucleus to another (see Fig. 6–10C) rather than the nonpredictability of cancer (see Fig. 6–6).

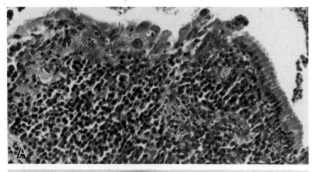

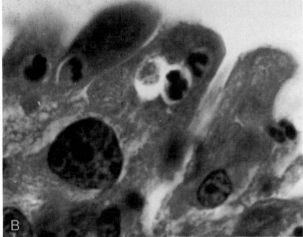

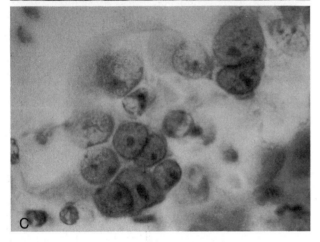

FIGURE 6–10. Chronic cervicitis with metaplasia, proplasia and retroplasia. *A,* The endocervical columnar epithelium (right) has given way to inflamed metaplasia (left) with a very active zone of transformation between, which exhibits extreme reaction, injury and repair (H&E stain; cervical biopsy; × 200). *B,* A higher power of this zone of transformation reveals greater detail of the extremely large columnar cell that is "fighting for its life." Two neutrophils have invaded its cytoplasm (as microphages, invading an injured secretory cell), as has one trichomonad that lies intracellularly and immediately to their left with its pale central nucleus and red cytoplasmic granules. The epithelial columnar cell's nucleus is large and hyperchromatic, with one prominent nucleolus. The parachromatin is cleared and uniformly distributed throughout the coarsely granular chromatinic net. The chromatinic rim is uniformly thickened, and the nuclear membrane is wavy. In addition to these changes of proplasia considerable blurring of the chromatin-parachromatin interfaces occurs, evidencing some retroplasia in this very "ill" cell. The cytoplasm is edematous with numerous small vacuoles (H&E stain; cervical biopsy; × 1200). (Reproduced with permission from Frost JK, et al: J Parasitol 47:302–303, 1961.) *C,* Extremely reactive endocervical columnar cells shed from another patient with the same condition. There are hyperchromasia, prominent nucleoli, high ratio of nucleus to cytoplasm and extensive multinucleation, but the nuclei are predictable, one-to-another, in key features (e.g., chromatin pattern, parachromatin clearing, chromasia, numbers of nucleoli, uniform thickness of the chromatinic rims, nuclear membrane undulation) demonstrating extreme proplasia in columnar cells (Papanicolaou stain; fast vaginopancervical smear; × 1000).

Relationships of Nucleus to Cytoplasm

As activity increases, two significant morphologic changes occur regarding the relationship of the nucleus to the cytoplasm. There is less ability for the cytoplasm to mature into its most mature cell type (e.g., stratified squamous, columnar) so that there is a greater immaturity to the cytoplasm of the cell with greatly increased activity (see Fig. 6–9). Additionally, the amount of cytoplasm the cell makes decreases relative to the amount of nucleoplasm, so that the N/C ratio increases, at times to an extreme degree.

MORPHOLOGIC EFFECTS ON CELLS OF MIXED AND CHANGING PROCESSES

Some of the most severe problems involving the diagnostic interpretation of morphologic changes in health and disease are caused by the presence of a confusing mixture of processes and their effects on cells. This problem figures significantly in a high percentage of legal proceedings held to settle alleged malpractice and constitutes one of the most serious pitfalls for the unwary—from the inexperienced through the highly accomplished.

Retroplastic changes in cells from degenerative proc-

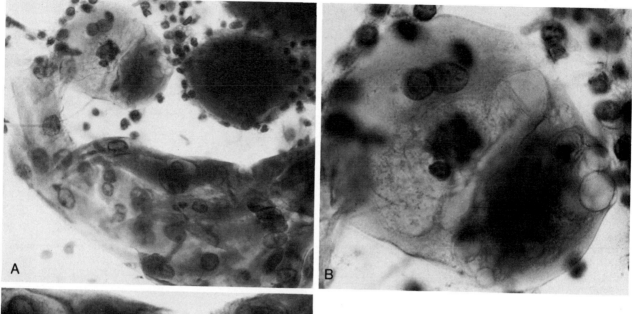

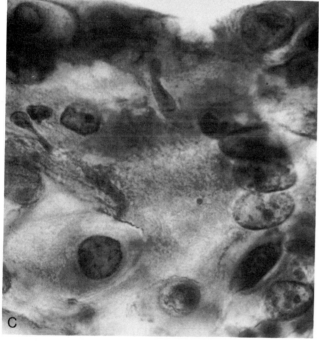

FIGURE 6–11. Radiation effect and extreme repair. Six weeks after the end of external irradiation for cervical cancer. *A*, A large tissue fragment of cells with radiation changes (left upper field), clusters of macrophages (right upper field) and extremely reactive, reparative epithelium (lower field) (×400). *B*, Marked radiation changes with cytoplasmic vacuoles, cytoplasmic enlargement without pallor, multinucleation and nuclear abnormalities (×1000). *C*, Marked reparative cellular changes. Prominent nucleoli that are rounded, multinucleation and large and hyperchromatic nuclei. Cytoplasm is abundant, however, and the cells hold together as a fragment of tissue, which is in favor of benignancy in extreme repair (×1000). (*A*, *B* and *C*, Papanicolaou stain; fast vaginopancervical smear.)

esses frequently mask the true nature of a more serious lesion present and, conversely, can make nonmalignant cells bear a close resemblance to cancer. Like tertiary syphilis in Oslerian medical history, degeneration can be the great mimic.

Unrecognized proplasia in reaction and healing can also lead to misdiagnoses. The two together in the same cell (retroplasia and proplasia), however, by far constitutes the most serious offender.

The finding of mixed processes usually results from evaluating, at a single point in time, a developing sequence of changing processes during a continuum of events.[12, 14] This evaluation is similar to taking a statement, or a thought, out of the context of the whole. An examination of a single, fixed specimen is comparable to viewing a single frame in a motion picture of a developing process, or in a series of interacting processes, and extreme care is needed in the interpretation of such evidence out of context.[14]

Injury and Repair

Following injury, the tissues mount an inflammatory response that is reflected in the leukoytes, blood and serum brought to the site. After the injurious event (e.g., trauma, infection, chemical, radiation), cells exhibit retroplastic changes of degeneration (see previous discussion), usually first including chromatin/parachromatin interface blurring in the nucleus and soon followed by either hydropic vacuoles in a swollen cytoplasm or wrinkling of the nuclear membrane. If the cell dies, these and other retroplastic features increase in severity as death and necrosis become morphologically more obvious.

If the cell survives, however, features of proplasia (see previous discussion) appear while retroplastic features are still present. Thus, during cellular repair and convalescence, nucleoli can become prominent (e.g., in columnar cells) (see Fig. 6–10); multinucleation and mitoses can occur; nucleoli enlarge and exhibit hyperchromasia of granular chromatin; cytoplasm becomes less mature (e.g., increased N/C ratio) and other proplastic reparative features appear. During this time features of retroplasia frequently continue for quite a while into convalescence (Fig. 6–10B), especially when inflammation continues in the surrounding tissues and proteolytic enzymes from degenerating granulocytes are discharged into the environment of cells, juices and background. In chronic inflammation and chronic irritation, with continuing injurious events, columnar epithelium changes to the more passively protective stratified squamous epithelium through the processes of squamous metaplasia.

Stimulation and Degeneration

Stimulatory events (e.g., chemicals, microorganisms, radiation) produce proplastic changes in the cells, which eventually return to normal after the stimulating effects wear off (see Fig. 6–11). Many processes that injure the cell, however, lead to death (see Fig. 6–8) or to convalescence with proplasia and eventual healing. Again, dependent upon the time of sacrifice of the cell (e.g., by exfoliation, brushing, needle aspiration), one will find features of pure proplasia (see Fig. 6–9), mixtures of proplasia and retroplasia (see Fig. 6–8) or pure retroplasia.

Chronic Irritation

Continuous stimulatory events, continuous degenerative events or a mixture of stimulatory and degenerative events—short of death to the cell—will lead to chronic irritation, exhibiting both proplastic and retroplastic changes. In this situation, columnar epithelium changes to the more protective stratified squamous epithelium through the process of squamous metaplasia.

Squamous Metaplasia

This benign, reversible and disarming process is a very important progression of events, particularly in the developmental spectrum in changes of neoplastic transformation, which lead to full-blown classic cancer (i.e., invasive malignant neoplasia). This process of squamous metaplasia—transformation from columnar epithelium through transformational epithelium to keratinizing stratified squamous epithelium—is covered in greater detail elsewhere.[14]

Under the influence of noxious agents or processes, columnar epithelium, which is very highly specialized for function (e.g., ciliary action, secretion, absorption) rather than protection, is transformed into another cell type. More precisely, the germinal cells change their maturational differentiation, as they mature toward the surface, from columnar epithelium to transformational epithelium to keratinizing stratified squamous epithelium.

Squamous metaplasia is most accurately recognized cytologically by the exfoliated mature squamous cells (intermediate and superficial cells), being smaller than normal squamous cells, and the less mature parabasal-like cells with or without keratinizing cytoplasm. Other features (e.g., columnar cells mixed with squamous cells) may provide the suspicion of metaplasia but are much less specific or diagnostic. The degree of activity or atypicality in the metaplasia is most accurately assessed by the degree of nuclear atypia or dyskaryosis.[14]

The earlier states in the process of squamous metaplasia (columnar, presquamous, transformational) are in transition to the final status of a more protective tissue (i.e., keratinized stratified squamous epithelium). Some reach the most protective state (e.g., highly keratinized stratified squamous epithelium) and remain there as long as the noxious processes are in effect. Others, upon reaching a given state and upon reduction or removal of the noxious processes, are transformed back toward the more healthy state of the original tissue (e.g., columnar epithelium).

A number of stages in this process of progression to squamous metaplasia, especially the transformational stage, are "restless," unstable and, apparently, more susceptible to neoplasic initiation and further mutational events in this highly promotional milieu. The most stable phase is referred to variously as "mature" metaplasia, "normal" metaplasia, "regular" metaplasia or "typical" metaplasia. This phase is recognized by normal appearing, euplastic nuclei.

Atypical Squamous Metaplasia, Dysplasia, *In Situ* Carcinoma and Intraepithelial Neoplasia

A more unstable phase of squamous metaplasia has been variously referred to as the presquamous phase and other terms (e.g., columnar phase, pink cell hyperplasia, subcolumnar atypia, reserve cell hyperplasia). Here the surface cells mature to columnar, but they frequently have nuclear atypia, secretion and other features of atypical functional differentiation.[14]

The most unstable phase of squamous metaplasia appears to be the transformational phase. Here the most mature surface cells show poorly directed orientation and functional differentiation. Some cells may have degrees of atypical columnar and secretory differentiation (Fig. 6–10), with atypical and unpredictable orientation, while other cells of the same lesion may show atypical tendencies to squamification and, yet, a large percentage are undifferentiated and immature. Their nuclei indicate an increased activity by being extremely proplasic with hyperchromatic granular chromatin, undulated nuclear membranes, cleared and uniformly distributed parachromatin and enlarged nuclei (see Fig. 6–9). No nucleoli are present in the cells exfoliated from these lesions.

With the continuous proplasia and resultant frequent mitoses, this is a more unsettled or "restless" epithelium. These cells are prime targets for mutational events, initiation and promotion through the course of neoplastic progression.

This atypical metaplasia[12, 33] has been called by various other names, including basal cell hyperactivity,[17] atypical hyperplasia,[29] dysplasia,[30] in situ carcinoma,[12, 14] and intraepithelial neoplasia.[31]

In using these terms, especially the last two, it is inferred that initiation has occurred, even though no diagnostic morphologic change is recognized to definitely note that event. It is also inferred that promotion is occurring, with continuing mutational changes bringing about neoplasic progression. In the cervix, CIN is currently being used more and more; while in the lung, bronchial intraepithelial neoplasia (BIN) is being suggested. As degenerative and inflammatory effects decrease and as the lesions increase in severity of morphologic atypia (e.g., CIN 1, 2, 3) (Figs. 6–9 and 6–12), there is a higher occurrence of cancer during the follow-up years.[1, 11, 16, 17, 26, 28–31, 33, 36]

Malignant Neoplasia, Invasive Cancer

In the cervix uteri and bronchus, the human sites chosen for the most intensive studies,[12, 14, 16, 28, 33, 35] and in in vitro and in vivo neoplastic transformation studies,[1, 3, 7, 19, 25, 34] the pattern of cellular morphology during this neoplastic progression, through in situ carcinoma, remains that of proplasia. Increasing nuclear atypia and cytoplasmic immaturity occur as the lesion becomes more severe (i.e., CIN 1, 2, 3).

As the processes associated with cancer continue and the neoplastic progression persists, the neoplasm develops the ability to invade and becomes an invasive malignant neoplasm, or cancer. At this stage of the progression, the cells change morphologically,[8, 10, 14, 27] including (1) prominent nucleoli appearing in their nuclei, (2) more abundant cytoplasm, (3) chromatin changing from coarse granules into larger and sharply angled clumps, (4) irregular clearing of the parachromatin and (5) nuclear membrane changing shapes from undulation to the unpredictable sharp and angled irregularities so characteristic of malignant neoplasia (see Fig. 6–5).

But even with this progression, the heterogeneity of cancer is evidenced by its retaining considerable cells from previous stages of its development, with many of the earlier clones still represented in the final lesion. This "rogues' gallery" of cells—cells shed from the lesser lesions along with the diagnostic cells of the most severe lesion present—is an interesting and a diagnostically important feature of this developing neoplasic progression. Especially in the cervix uteri and bronchus, this rogues' gallery of cells aids in the cytomorphologic recognition of the processes and the resultant cellular changes in the development of neoplasia.

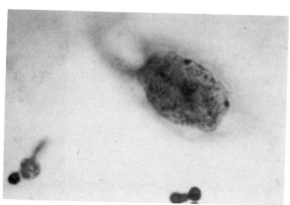

FIGURE 6–12. Proplasia with two sex chromatin bodies—trisomy X-sex chromosomes. This cell was shed from CIN 3. It has the proplastic features of increased activity (compare with Fig. 6–9) with undulation of the nuclear membrane, chromatin granules, hyperchromasia and uniform parachromatin clearing, but there are two Barr (sex chromatin) bodies, signifying at least three X-sex chromosomes. The intermediate cells of the patient's buccal smear and of this gynecologic smear revealed a normal XX (female) pattern (i.e., single Barr body). This X-trisomy in a proplastic cell strongly suggests aneuploidy; the latter can be detected in all of the three grades of dysplasia or CIN with cytogenetic studies[23] but usually is not detected by routine cytopathologic techniques (Papanicolaou stain; fast vaginopancervical smear; ×1200).

References

1. Albright CD, Frost JK, Pressman NJ: Cytologic preparations and objective morphologic analysis of cells from developing hamster squamous cell carcinomas. Anal Quant Cytol Histol 4:141, 1982.
2. Anastassova-Kristeva M: The nucleolar cycle in man. J Cell Sci 25:103–110, 1977.
3. Barker BE, Sanford KK: Cytologic manifestations of neoplastic transformation in vitro. J Natl Cancer Inst 44:39–63, 1970.
4. Bartels PH, Bahr GF, Bibbo M, Richards DL, Sonek MG, Wied GL: Analysis of variance of the Papanicolaou staining reaction. Acta Cytol 18:522–531, 1974.
5. Berezney R: The nuclear matrix: a structural milieu for the intranuclear attachment and replication of DNA. In International Cell Biology 1980-1981. Edited by HG Schweigher. Berlin, Springer-Verlag, pp 214–224, 1981.
6. Bibbo M, Bartels PH, Dytch HE, Wied GL: Computed cell image information. In Computer-Assisted Image Analysis Cytology. Monographs in Clinical Cytology. Edited by SD Greenberg. Basel, S Karger, vol. 9, pp 62–100, 1984.
7. Boone CW, Sanford KK, Frost JK, Mantel N, Gill GW, Jones GM: Cytomorphologic evaluation of the neoplastic potential of 28 cell culture lines by a panel of diagnostic cytopathologists. Int J Cancer 38:361–367, 1986.
8. Erozen YS, Pressman NJ, Donovan PA, Gupta PK, Frost JK: A comparative cytopathologic study of noninvasive and invasive squamous cell carcinoma of the lung. Anal Quant Cytol Histol 1:50–56, 1979.
9. Franke WW, Scheer U, Krohne G, Jarasch E-D: The nuclear envelope and the architecture of the nuclear periphery. J Cell Biol 91:39s–50s, 1981.

10. Frost JK: Concepts Basic to General Cytopathology, 4th ed. Baltimore, Johns Hopkins Press, 1972.
11. Frost JK, Ball WC Jr, Levin ML, Tockman MS, Erozan YS, Gupta PK, Eggleston JC, Pressman NJ, Donithan MP, Kimball AW, Jr: Sputum cytopathology: use and potential in monitoring the workplace environment by screening for biological effects of exposure. J Occup Med 28(8):692–703, 1986.
12. Frost JK, Erozan YS, Gupta PK: Cytopathology. *In* Atlas of Early Lung Cancer. Edited by National Cancer Institute Cooperative Early Lung Cancer Group. New York and Tokyo, Igaku-Shoin, 1983.
13. Frost JK, Petrakis NL, Wolde CE, Sanford KK, MacCardle RC, Stewart WE, Gey GO: Cell modulations, maturation and neoplastic transformation. Acta Cytol 6:399–402, 1962.
14. Frost JK: The Cell in Health and Disease, 2nd ed. Basel, S Karger, 1986.
15. Frost JK, Tyrer HW, Pressman NJ, Adams LA, Vansickel MH, Albright CD, Gill GW, Tiffany SM: Automatic cell identification and enrichment in lung cancer. III. Light scatter (size) and two fluorescent parameters (DNA, RNA) in squamous cell carcinoma. J Histochem Cytochem 27:557–559, 1979.
16. Fu YS, Reagan JW, Richart RM, Townsend EE: Nuclear DNA and histologic studies of genital lesions in diethylstilbesterol-exposed progeny. II. Intraepithelial glandular abnormalities. Am J Clin Pathol 72:515–520, 1979.
17. Galvin GA, Jones HW, TeLinde RW: The significance of basal-cell hyperactivity in cervical biopsies. Am J Obstet Gynecol 70:808–821, 1955.
18. Geirsson G, Woodworth FE, Patten SF, Bonfiglio TA: Epithelial repair and regeneration in the uterine cervix. I. An analysis of the cells. Acta Cytol 21:371–378, 1977.
19. Gey GO: Normal and malignant cells in tissue culture. Ann NY Acad Sci 76:547–549, 1958.
20. Gill GW, Frost JK, Miller KA: A new formula for a half-oxidized hematoxylin solution that neither overstains nor requires differentiation. Acta Cytol 18:300–311, 1974.
21. Gill GW, Plowden KM: Laboratory cytopathology techniques for specimen preparation. *In* Manual for the Thirty-first Postgraduate Institute for Pathologists in Clinical Cytopathology, 7th ed. Edited by JK Frost. Baltimore, The Johns Hopkins University School of Medicine and The Johns Hopkins Hospital, 1990.
22. Gupta PK, Frost JK: Cytologic changes associated with asbestos exposure. Semin Oncol 8:283–289, 1981.
23. Jones HW, Davis HJ, Frost JK, Park I, Salimi R, Tseng P, Woodruff JD: The value of the assay of chromosomes in the diagnosis of cervical neoplasia. Am J Obstet Gynecol 102:624–641, 1968.
24. Linman JW: Principles of Hematology. New York, MacMillan, 1966.
25. McDowell EM, Trump BF: Histogenesis of preneoplastic and neoplastic lesions in tracheobronchial epithelium. Surv Synth Path Res 2:235–279, 1983.
26. Nasiell M, Kato H, Auer G, Zetterberg A, Roger V, Karlen L: Cytomorphological grading and Feulgen DNA-analysis of metaplastic and neoplastic bronchial cells. Cancer 41:1511–1521, 1978.
27. Ng ABP, Reagan JW: Pathology and cytopathology of microinvasive squamous cell carcinoma of the uterine cervix. *In* Compendium of Diagnostic Cytology. Edited by GL Wied, LG Koss, JW Reagan. Chicago, Tutorials in Cytology, 1983.
28. Patton SF, Jr: Diagnostic Cytopathology of the Uterine Cervix, 2nd ed. Basel, S Karger, 1978.
29. Reagan JW, Hicks DJ, Scott RB: Atypical hyperplasia of the uterine cervix. Cancer 8:42–52, 1955.
30. Reagan JW, Patton SF, Jr: Dyplasia: A basic reaction to injury in the uterine cervix. Ann NY Acad Sci 97:662–682, 1962.
31. Richart RM: Natural history of cervical intraepithelial neoplasia. Clin Obstet Gynecol 10:748–784, 1967.
32. Rosenthal DL, Suffin SC: Predictive value of digitized cell images for the prognosis of cervical neoplasia. *In* Computer-Assisted Image Analysis Cytology. Monographs in Clinical Cytology. Edited by SD Greenberg. Basel, S Karger, vol. 9, pp 163–180, 1984.
33. Saccomanno G, Archer VE, Auerbach O, Saunders RP, Brennen LM: Development of carcinoma of the lung as reflected in exfoliated cells. Cancer 33:256–270, 1974.
34. Sanford KK, Parshad R, Stanbridge EJ, Frost JK, Jones GM, Wilkinson JE, Tarone RE: Analysis of chromosomal radiosensitivity during the G_2 cell cycle period and cytopathology of human normal X tumor cell hybrids. Cancer Res 46:2045–2049, 1986.
35. Saphir O, Leventhal ML, Kline TS: Podophyllin-induced dysplasia of the cervix uteri; its histological resemblance to carcinoma *in situ*. Am J Clin Pathol 32:446–456, 1959.
36. Tockman MS, Gupta PK, Meyers JD, Frost JK, Beglin SB, Gold EB, Chare AM, Wilkinson PH, Mulshine JL: Sensitive and specific monoclonal antibody recognition of human lung cancer antigen on preserved sputum cells: A new approach to early lung cancer detection. J Clin Oncol 6:1685–1693, 1988.
37. Tyrer HW, Frost JK, Pressman NJ, Adams LA, Albright CD, Vansickel MH, Tiffany SM: Automatic cell identification and enrichment in lung cancer. IV. Small cell carcinoma analysis by light scatter and two fluorescence parameters. Flow Cytometry 4: 462–472 (Universitetsforlaget), 1980.
38. Tyrer HW, Pressman NJ, Albright CD, Frost JK: Automatic cell identification and enrichment in lung cancer. V. Adenocarcinoma and large cell undifferentiated carcinoma. Cytometry 6:37–46, 1985.
39. Weiss P: The dynamics of the membrane-bound incompressible body: A mechanism of cellular and subcellular motility. Proc Natl Acad Sci (Washington) 52:1024–1029, 1964.
40. Wied GL, Bartels PH, Dytch HE, Bibbo M: Rapid DNA evaluation in clinical diagnosis. Acta Cytol 27:33–37, 1983.

PART **II**

Diagnostic Cytology

7

Hormonal Cytology

George L. Wied
Marluce Bibbo

The evaluation of the endocrinologic condition of the female patient by means of the study of vaginal cells is actually one of the earliest diagnostic applications of clinical cytology as we know it today. It dates back to 1847, when a Frenchman, Pouchet,[44] first published an atlas describing the vaginal epithelial cell changes that occur during the ovarian cycle. The early publications by Papanicolaou and his coworkers[36, 37, 39, 40, 58] also dealt with hormonal cell patterns. Papanicolaou[38] and, independently, the Rumanian investigator Babes[1] published the method of utilizing vaginal smears to detect cervical cancer. Hormonal cytology was, however, not widely applied until after the cytologic smear technique became an established method for detecting and diagnosing uterine lesions. This use of cytology occurred in the years following the publication of the monographs by Papanicolaou and his associates.[41, 42] The number of reports in the literature on methodology, results and efficiency of hormonal cytology has increased significantly since that time. Although excellent bioassays and correlative studies are now available,[4, 5, 17, 20, 22, 24, 31, 45, 53, 57, 77, 86, 87] it is still the consensus that, with certain limitations, the technique is an efficient, an inexpensive and a rapid method for establishing the hormonal condition of a patient as well as for assessing ovarian function from puberty throughout the reproductive years, menopause and senium.[50, 66] Hormonal cytology is also used to estimate time of ovulation, to determine ovarian dysfunction, to assess placental function or dysfunction in obstetrics, to assist in selecting hormonal therapy and to follow hormonal treatment results. The cytologic technique is also useful as an office method for the rapid classification of the hormonal stimulation of the vaginal epithelium.[8, 49, 50, 54, 64]

BASIC THEORY OF HORMONAL CYTOLOGIC CONSULTATION

The basic principle of hormonal evaluation of a patient by means of vaginal cytology is based on the assumption that the degree of cellular maturity or contextual morphology of the cell patterns is related—even quantitatively proportional—to the actual amount of sex steroids present. This assumption is only conditionally correct because (1) the estrogens, androgens and progestogens, which influence the appearance of vaginal epithelial cells, may act as synergists in some instances and as antagonists in other instances on the end organ (i.e., the vaginal epithelium) and (2) the degree of the end organ response, which generally remains constant in a given patient, varies from patient to patient. In certain conditions the degree of maturity of the vaginal epithelium may be proportional to the degree of the estrogenic effect. However, these ideal conditions are relatively rare and require detailed knowledge of endocrinology, cytophysiology and cytopathology for the interpreter to provide a clinically meaningful assessment of the hormonal condition of a particular patient. The cytologic screening for cervical cancer may be performed in most cases by a qualified cytotechnologist; a cytotechnologist may also count cytologic indices. However, meaningful cytodiagnostic hormonal consultations are assessments related to the history and age of the patient and to possible physiologic and pathologic changes and require, therefore, a medical and endocrinologic background.

SPECIMEN COLLECTION

Cytologic specimens for cancer diagnosis are usually taken from the vaginal fornix, the ectocervix and the endocervix.[55, 59, 70] For hormonal evaluation, the specimens should not exhibit inflammatory changes, glandular cells, "metaplastic cells" and anucleated squames. The specimens should consist of recently shed squamous cells that have exfoliated and have not been forcefully scraped from the vaginal epithelium (Fig. 7–1). The optimal site for obtaining a smear for hormonal evaluation is the lateral vaginal wall.[56, 75] Although in many cases it is possible to perform the hormonal evaluation on material obtained from the vaginal fornix, the quality of this sample is usually less than optimal. The material obtained from the posterior vaginal fornix usually contains cells that were exfoliated and accumulated over an extended period of time. Material from the vaginal fornix may also contain alone or in combination ectocervical, endocervical, or endometrial cells. This "pool effect" of the posterior fornix may be an advantage for cancer detection, but it is a disadvantage for assessing the hormonal status because it represents a contaminant in this situation. However, a specimen from the vaginal fornix may have to be used if a specimen from the lateral vaginal wall is unavailable.

Specimens should be taken either by lightly dipping an applicator into the secretion, without forceful scraping, or by aspiration. The specimen must be fixed immediately—while still wet—in 95% ethyl alcohol for at least 15 minutes or by a spray fixative if the routine Papanicolaou staining method is to be applied.[41] Alcohol fixation is also useful for other staining reactions, such as the Shorr method.[55]

A very rapid evaluation,[64] as proposed by Rakoff[49] and Rakoff and Takeda,[50] or phase-contrast microscopic evaluation,[23, 71] can be performed on a fresh drop of unfixed fluid. These techniques are particularly suitable as office procedures to be performed while the patient waits. However, part of the sample must be fixed and routinely stained for the cytologic diagnosis of possible atypia and for the medicolegal requirement of retaining cellular samples.

STAINING AND MICROSCOPIC TECHNIQUES

The following staining reactions and techniques are useful for hormonal evaluations.

The Papanicolaou Method

The Papanicolaou stain[41] provides the most satisfactory results and is probably the most universally applied cytologic technique. The various dyes (EA 36 and OG 6, Harris's and Gill's hematoxylins) are commercially available in ready-to-use form (from Ortho Corporation, Hartman-Leddon Company, and Ciba, Inc.). They may also be prepared from individual constituents of the dyes. The Papanicolaou staining procedure is described elsewhere in detail in this book.

The Shorr Method

The Shorr method[55] is a single differential stain and was designed specifically for hormonal assessment. The staining solution consists of the following:

Ethyl alcohol 50%	100	ml
Biebrich scarlet (water solution)	0.5	g
Orange G	0.25	g
Fast green FCF	0.075	g
Phosphotungstic acid c.p.	0.5	g
Phosphomolybdic acid c.p.	0.5	g
Glacial acetic acid	1.0	ml

The specimens are stained for 1 minute in the staining solution, carried through 70%, 80% and 95% absolute alcohols and xylol and mounted. The most mature cells stain orange-red; less mature cells deep green to pale green.

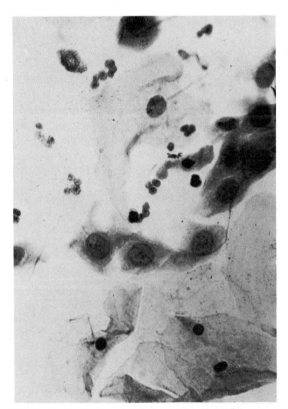

FIGURE 7–1. Cytologic sample from the vaginal wall containing **parabasal, intermediate and superficial cell types**. Specimens that are taken by forceful scraping of the wall with a wooden spatula can contain cells from the deep layers in addition to the freely exfoliating intermediate and superficial cells, as does this sample. Such samples cannot be used for hormonal interpretation (Papanicolaou stain; × 400).

Orcein Technique for Sex Chromatin

The demonstration of marginal nuclear chromatin bodies (sex chromatin)[62] can be accomplished using the Papanicolaou stain but may also be accomplished rather rapidly using the orcein stain, consisting of the following:

Orcein	1 g
Glacial acetic acid	45 ml
Distilled water	55 ml

The glacial acetic acid is heated in a flask on a hot plate to 80° to 85°C. Orcein is added while shaking both rapidly or stirring with a mechanical rod. This solution is gradually added to the distilled water at room temperature while stirring constantly. The flask is first stoppered and then bathed in cold running water, shaking the flask to cool the solution. The entire solution is filtered with No. 1 filter paper and stored in a brown bottle with a screw top. The stain improves with age. The technique also requires a fast green stock solution, consisting of the following:

Fast green	0.03 g
Ethyl alcohol 95%	100 ml

The fast green is added to the alcohol and stirred to dissolve.

For vaginal smears or buccal specimens, slight scrapings of the mucosa are fixed for 20 to 30 minutes in 95% ethyl alcohol. They are hydrated in 80%, 70% and 50% ethyl alcohols (five dips each), placed in distilled water (five dips) and stained in the orcein stock solution for 5 minutes. The specimen is then washed in distilled water for 10 to 15 seconds; dehydrated in 50%, 70%, 80% and 95% ethyl alcohols (five dips each); stained in a fast green stock solution for 1 minute, carried through 95% ethyl alcohol, absolute ethyl alcohol and xylene and then mounted.

Sex chromatin determinations should be made on all smears submitted with the diagnosis of primary amenorrhea. Atrophic smears that are negative for sex chromatin are found in cases of gonadal dysgenesis (XO or XY) and male pseudohermaphroditism (XY) (Fig. 7–2). Smears from cases of testicular feminization syndrome show good maturity, but the cells are negative for sex chromatin (Fig. 7–3).

The Rakoff Supravital Staining Technique

Rakoff[49] and Rakoff and Takeda[50] recommended a practical technique for immediate evaluation while the patient is in the office. The technique utilizes a supravital stain consisting of the following:

Aqueous solution of light green 10%	83 ml
Aqueous solution of eosin Y 1%	17 ml

Samples from the lateral vaginal wall are obtained with either a pipette or a cotton-tipped applicator. The secretions thus obtained are placed in 2 ml of physiologic saline solution, to which are added three drops

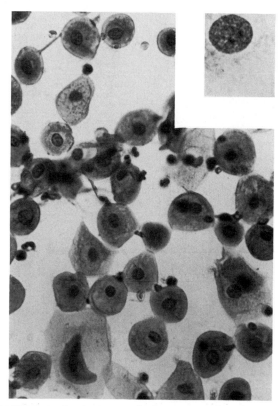

FIGURE 7–2. Cytologic sample from a patient with **Turner's syndrome**. The specimen consists of parabasal cells that are negative for sex chromatin (inset) (Papanicolaou stain; ×120). (Reproduced with permission from Rakoff AE, Takeda M: Gynecologic Endocrinopathies. *In* Teaching Slide Sets in Cytology, vol. 13. Wied GL (ed). Chicago, Tutorials of Cytology, 1979.)

of the staining solution. The solution is then gently agitated, and a drop or two of the stained sample is placed on a glass slide. A coverslip should be used so that individual cells are more easily visualized.

The staining reaction (Fig. 7–4) is roughly comparable to that obtained with the Papanicolaou technique. Superficial (karyopyknotic) squamous cells, which stain eosinophilic with the Papanicolaou technique, stain pink; intermediate cells stain blue-green. Nuclear detail is not visualized very satisfactorily with this stain. Subsequently, by adding a few drops of Lugol's solution to the test tube, glycogen-containing cells can also be distinguished. The advantages of the Rakoff stain are the rapidity and ease with which it can be used. Another major advantage is the rapid differentiation between intermediate and superficial cells. The main disadvantages are the instability of the stain (the solution must be prepared weekly), the lack of permanency of the preparation, the absence of definitive nuclear staining and the fact that the unfixed material is useful for only a relatively short period of time. However, for immediate assessments by the endocrinologically and cytologically trained clinician, supravital techniques are practical and useful.

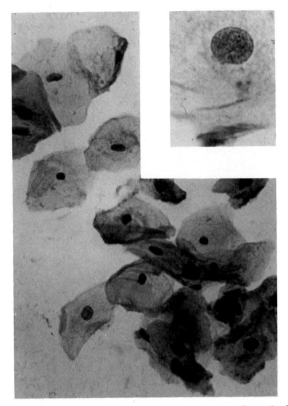

FIGURE 7–3. Cytologic sample from a patient with **testicular feminization syndrome**. The specimen consists of mature squamous cells that are negative for sex chromatin (inset) (Papanicolaou stain; ×120). (Reproduced with permission from Rakoff AE, Takeda M: Gynecologic Endocrinopathies. *In* Teaching Slide Sets in Cytology, vol. 13. Wied GL (ed). Chicago, Tutorials of Cytology, 1979.)

Phase-Contrast Microscopy Office Technique

The most rapid technique is one that does not require treatment of the specimen and that utilizes fresh and unfixed material. The phase-contrast microscope[56] provides these advantages. Most modern microscopes can be equipped with a phase condenser and phase objectives. Phase microscopes are also useful for the standardization of karyopyknosis on stained specimens.[71] The specimens should be thin and preferably contain few, if any, erythrocytes to guarantee good contrast patterns. The advantages of phase-contrast microscopy on fresh material are the immediate readability of the specimen, while the patient is still in the office, and the rapid determination of the microbiologic classification. The main diagnostic problem is that unfixed, unstained material often presents an unfamiliar cytomorphologic picture for those who have been trained to observe fixed, stained material. Unfixed, unstained cells are larger and exhibit more cytoplasmic details than do fixed, stained cells. Some of these details are lost when the cells are fixed and stained; such details have no diagnostic importance. Although it appears that phase-contrast microscopy is the most simple of

the aforementioned techniques, it suffers mostly from the fact that the specimen cannot be stored and reread and that inherent interpretative difficulties on fresh cell material restrict the technique to cytologists who are especially experienced in the analysis of fresh cell material samples (Figs. 7–5 to 7–9).

SQUAMOUS EPITHELIAL CELL TYPES FOR HORMONAL EVALUATION

Current terminology recognizes only three cell types (Fig. 7–10), compared with the great variety of cell types reported in older systems of terminology.[41, 46–49, 59–61, 73, 74] The vaginal epithelium normally exfoliates those cells that are on the surface of the epithelium. Theoretically, all normally exfoliated cells from healthy epithelial tissue could be considered "superficial," regardless of their degree of maturity, because they derive from the epithelial surface. The terminology currently in use does not refer to this actual superficiality in the epithelium when referring to "superficial," "intermediate" and "basal-parabasal" cells. To be technically correct, one would have to stipulate in each instance that one means superficial-type squamous epithelial cells, intermediate-type squamous epithelial

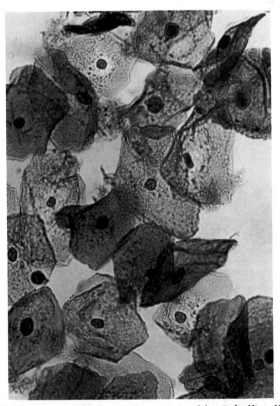

FIGURE 7–4. Cytologic specimen stained by **Rakoff's office procedure**. The squamous cells are sufficiently well stained to permit hormonal interpretation (×120). (Reproduced with permission from Rakoff AE, Takeda M: Gynecologic Endocrinopathies. *In* Teaching Slide Sets in Cytology, vol. 13. Wied GL (ed). Chicago, Tutorials of Cytology, 1979.)

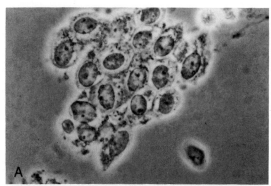

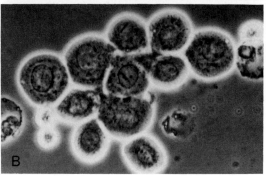

FIGURE 7–5. *A,* **Autolytic** and, *B,* **well-preserved parabasal cells** in a fresh (unfixed, unstained) cytologic sample (phase-contrast microscopy; ×120). (Reproduced with permission from Jenny JW: Phase Contrast Microscopic Cytologic Diagnosis: A Gynecologic Office Procedure. *In* Teaching Slide Sets in Cytology, vol. 27. Wied GL (ed). Chicago, Tutorials of Cytology, 1979.)

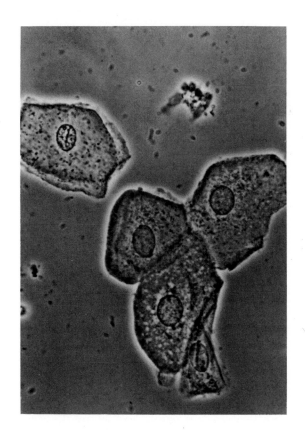

FIGURE 7–6. Fresh, unstained, **small intermediate cells** (phase-contrast microscopy; ×120). (Reproduced with permission from Jenny JW: Phase Contrast Microscopic Cytologic Diagnosis: A Gynecologic Office Procedure. *In* Teaching Slide Sets in Cytology, vol. 27. Wied GL (ed). Chicago, Tutorials of Cytology, 1979.)

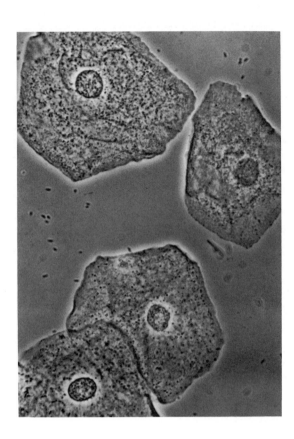

FIGURE 7–7. Fresh, unstained, **large intermediate cells** (phase-contrast microscopy; ×120). (Reproduced with permission from Jenny JW: Phase Contrast Microscopic Cytologic Diagnosis: A Gynecologic Office Procedure. *In* Teaching Slide Sets in Cytology, vol. 27. Wied GL (ed). Chicago, Tutorials of Cytology, 1979.)

FIGURE 7–8. Three large intermediate cells and one superficial cell that contains a brightly illuminated pyknotic nucleus, due to a deviation of the light over the dense corpora in the phase-contrast microscope (×120). (Reproduced with permission from Jenny JW: Phase Contrast Microscopic Cytologic Diagnosis: A Gynecologic Office Procedure. *In* Teaching Slide Sets in Cytology, vol. 27. Wied GL (ed). Chicago, Tutorials of Cytology, 1979.)

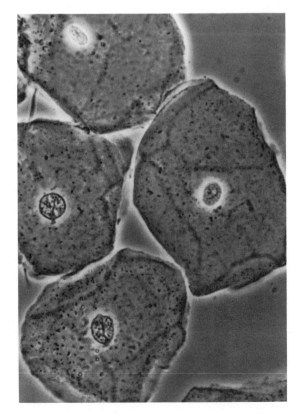

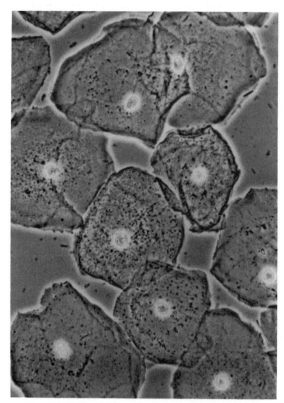

FIGURE 7–9. Flat superficial cells exhibiting pyknotic nuclei that show the light deviation under the phase-contrast microscope, which can be used to differentiate pyknotic from vesicular nuclei (×120). (Reproduced with permission from Jenny JW: Phase Contrast Microscopic Cytologic Diagnosis: A Gynecologic Office Procedure. *In* Teaching Slide Sets in Cytology, vol. 27. Wied GL (ed). Chicago, Tutorials of Cytology, 1979.)

cells and basal parabasal–type squamous epithelial cells. However, this distinction is generally understood by the users of the technique, and the terms are therefore abbreviated to superficial, intermediate and parabasal cells.[74]

Superficial Cells

Superficial cells are mature, usually polygonal, squamous epithelial cells. The cytoplasm stains either cyanophilic or eosinophilic, and the nucleus is pyknotic. The criterion for the superficial cell, in addition to the maturity of the cytoplasm, is the evidence of a pyknotic nucleus, regardless of the staining reaction of the cytoplasm. Superficial cells of the highest degree of maturity are flat and exhibit more or less prominent lines within the cytoplasm. These lines are apparently caused by the formation of prekeratin. Most superficial cells lie singly. Many exhibit an eosinophilic or orange-yellow staining reaction. The least mature superficial cells are folded, sometimes are crowded and exhibit a translucent cyanophilic cytoplasm. They may show a relatively prominent cellular outline, which is apparently a fixation artifact. Between the most mature superficial cells and the least mature superficial cells

are cells in transitional stages, which are identified by criteria indicative of degrees of maturity. A vast variety of combinations are seen, such as flat, cyanophilic, superficial cells with prekeratinization lines or folded, eosinophilic superficial cells with fine cellular borders and so forth. Another distinctive intracellular feature of certain mature, rapidly proliferating cells is the presence of intracellular granules.

The most important characteristic of superficial, as distinguished from intermediate, cells is the nuclear appearance.[72] The former have pyknotic nuclei (compressed, smaller nuclei with condensed chromatin), whereas the latter have vesicular nuclei (larger, oval or rounded nuclei). Several morphologic criteria have been offered for distinguishing the two types of nuclei. Pundel and Lichtfus[47] suggested a nucleometric criterion, i.e., all nuclei with diameters smaller than 6 μm should be called pyknotic. This procedure involves the use of some type of cytometric apparatus and is time consuming. The phase-contrast microscope may be employed on stained specimens.[71] In phase-contrast microscopy, an optical deviation of the light path causes the most dense corpora (pyknotic nuclei) to shine a brilliant red, whereas the vesicular nuclei (nonpyknotic nuclei) appear darker and more opaque than under the brightfield microscope.

Intermediate Cells

Intermediate cells are mature (i.e., usually polygonal) squamous epithelial cells, which may be either

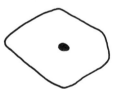

Superficial cell

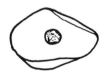

Intermediate cell

Parabasal cell

FIGURE 7–10. The three squamous cell types used for hormonal interpretation.

eosinophilic or cyanophilic, but which contain nonpyknotic vesicular nuclei, i.e., nuclei that exhibit structural details. The intermediate cell is a relatively large mature epithelial cell, usually as large as the superficial cell, that cannot be mistaken for a superficial cell because its nucleus is not pyknotic. It cannot possibly be mistaken for a basal-parabasal cell because the latter is usually a small, round or oval cell. Intermediate cells tend to exhibit cellular folding, and there is often crowding of the cells into small or large cell clusters. However, the most mature forms of intermediate cells may also be flat and lie singly. As mentioned in the section Superficial Cells, a variety of combinations of subcriteria are possible to help distinguish among the degrees of maturity (e.g., folded eosinophilic intermediate cells that lie singly or flat and cyanophilic intermediate cells that tend towards cluster formation). It becomes obvious that more than one criterion is required to describe the correct cellular pattern when one wishes to describe certain epithelial cells.

In the presence of *Bacillus vaginalis Doederlein,* intermediate cell patterns often exhibit cytolysis (Fig. 7–11). This lysis of the cytoplasm represents a peptolytic but normal process that is rarely encountered in superficial karyopyknotic cells and practically never in parabasal cells.

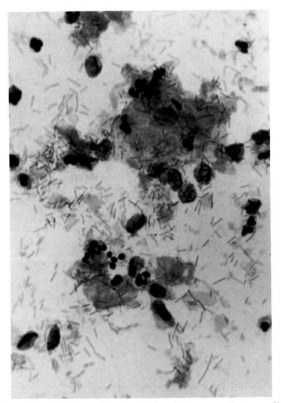

FIGURE 7–11. Extensive cytolytic changes on **intermediate squamous cells** due to the peptolytic influences of *Bacillus vaginalis*. The specimen exhibits free nuclei, cellular debris and abundant rod-like bacilli (Papanicolaou stain; ×400).

Basal-Parabasal Cells

Basal-parabasal cells often are not defined descriptively,[61] but are defined by stating that the group encompasses all normal cells, i.e., physiologically occurring squamous epithelial cells, that are neither superficial nor intermediate (Figs. 7–6 to 7–9). This group encompasses the small, oval or round, immature squamous epithelial cells. The cells usually contain relatively large structured, rarely degenerative pyknotic, nuclei (see Fig. 7–5). The staining reaction is generally cyanophilic or indistinct, rarely eosinophilic. The term *basal-parabasal* was selected because it actually represents a cell type and does not identify the actual epithelial layer from which the cells are derived. It seems highly unlikely that any cytopathologist would be able to identify a true basal cell (i.e., a cell from the *stratum germinativum*) by only observing its cytomorphology. It is quite conceivable that the exfoliated basal-parabasal cell may be derived from the surface layer of a quite highly developed epithelium that is immature and not clearly differentiated into the various cell layers of the epithelium. Basal-parabasal cell patterns do not exhibit bacterial (peptolytic) cytolysis, as observed on intermediate cells (see Fig. 7–11). Some show autolytic degeneration in the sense of a proteolytic, necrotic process.

CELL TYPES UNRELATED TO HORMONAL CONDITION

The interpreter of the specimen has to be aware of cell types that may occur in the female genital tract. These types are not necessarily atypical cells or cancer cells but include a variety of cells that occur as a result of benign changes, e.g., infections and metaplasia. These entities may alter the cell pattern significantly and often to such an extent that the hormonal evaluation is impaired.

Anucleated Squames

The vaginal epithelium does not normally exfoliate anucleate squamous cells as are found on the epidermis. If anucleated cells are found in the vaginal smear, the reason could be one of the following: (1) the smear was taken in the distal third of the vagina, in some instances contains anucleated squames that are similar to those from the labia and the external genitalia; (2) the specimen was taken from an ectocervix that contained an area of leukoplakia (hyperkeratosis); (3) the specimen was taken from a pregnant patient whose fetal membranes had ruptured, with the secretions containing anucleated squames from the epidermis of the infant; and (4) the smear was taken from a patient with an inflammatory reaction and in whom the occurrence of anucleated squames represents a protective mechanism of the epithelium against infection.

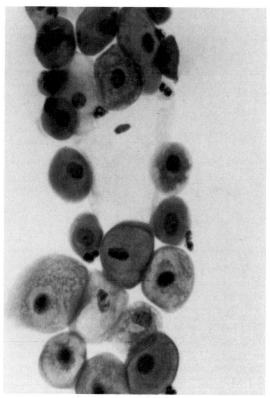

FIGURE 7–12. So-called metaplastic parabasal cells found in areas with **squamous metaplasia**. As a general rule, the presence of "metaplastic" cells in the cytologic sample indicates that the specimen was prepared on the ectocervix and cannot be used for hormonal interpretation (Papanicolaou stain; ×400).

Metaplastic Cells

Metaplastic cells are essentially small or large parabasal-type cells with prominent cellular borders, often exhibiting eccentric nuclei and sometimes containing a large intracellular vacuole. The staining in the center portion often differs from that in the marginal portion, i.e., the center is sometimes light brown. Also, there is essentially a darker-stained cytoplasm than that found in the parabasal cells. The presence of these cells is not diagnostic for squamous metaplasia per se, but the cells occur so frequently and almost exclusively in these conditions that the term *metaplastic cell* could be justified (Fig. 7–12). The presence of metaplastic cells eliminates the specimen from hormonal evaluation because it usually indicates that one is dealing with an ectocervical sample. Rarely, these cells occur in a vaginal smear in a patient with an epidermization border around a vaginal adenosis (e.g., the effect of exposure to diethylstilbestrol (DES) *in utero*).

Histiocytes

The presence of histiocytes, whether small-cell histiocytes, large-cell histiocytes or multinucleated foreign body giant cells, is usually indicative of a reactive condition that may preclude hormonal evaluation.

Paramenstrual debris and exodus of histiocytes are normal findings in smears prepared during the 6th to 10th days of the menstrual cycle.

Epithelial Cells Exhibiting Inflammatory Changes

Obviously benign epithelial cells may exhibit characteristic criteria of infection, which usually precludes hormonal interpretation. These changes are obvious in marked *Trichomonas* infections, in which the cells may exhibit prominent nucleoli, distorted staining reaction, perinuclear halo formation, increased activity of the nucleus, hyperchromatosis, macrokaryosis, and so forth. The presence of fungi, *Leptothrix*, coccoid bacteria, *Haemophilus vaginalis* (Fig. 7–13) and other specific or nonspecific criteria of infection belong in this group. Depending upon the degree of inflammatory or reparative changes present, such smears should not be used for hormonal evaluation.

Glandular Cells

Smears from the lateral vaginal wall should normally not contain endocervical or endometrial cells, unless the specimen was taken during the menstrual period. In some instances of extensive ectocervical ectopies, such as one encounters in pregnant patients, occasional

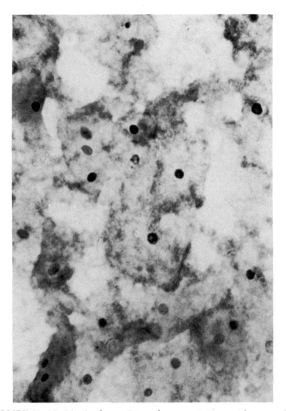

FIGURE 7–13. Vaginal specimen from a patient with **coccoid bacteria infection**. Pseudoeosinophilia and pseudopyknosis are due to the increased pH level. This specimen cannot be used for hormonal interpretation (Papanicolaou stain; ×400).

ectocervical cells may even be seen in specimens from the lateral vaginal walls. Generally, however, the presence of glandular cells of whatever cytomorphology is a sign for the cytopathologist to double check the area from which the specimen had in fact been obtained. In rare cases, vaginal adenosis may exfoliate glandular and metaplastic cells.

Precursor or Malignant Tumor Cells

The presence of atypical cells usually makes hormonal evaluation difficult or impossible. Some early cervical lesions, dysplasias, carcinomas *in situ,* early invasive lesions and endocervical and intrauterine lesions permit evaluation of the specimen from the lateral vaginal wall for hormonal assessment. As a matter of fact, the hormonal conditions in these cases are often of interest to cancer researchers and diagnosticians.

CELLULAR INDICES FOR HORMONAL ASSESSMENTS AND REPORTING PROCEDURE

Indices

Hormonal evaluations are sometimes expressed by means of indices (Fig. 7–14). The indices are assessments of the specimens as follows: (1) the karyopyknotic index (KPI = the ratio of superficial cells to intermediate cells); (2) the maturation index (MI = the percentage of superficial, intermediate and parabasal cells)[14, 35]; (3) the eosinophilic index (EI = the ratio of mature eosinophilic cells to mature cyanophilic cells); (4) the folded cell index (FCI = the ratio of folded mature cells to flat mature cells)[83, 84] and (5) the crowded cell index (CCI = the ratio of mature cells in clusters of four or more to cells in clusters of three or less).[83, 84] Other schemes and ratios have been proposed; most are now redundant inasmuch as the new terminology has eliminated all but the three types (superficial, intermediate and parabasal).[61, 74, 78a]

However, indices in exfoliative cytology are meaningful only when they relate to a previous index on the same patient. Under no circumstances can a cellular index assessed on patient A be an indication of the hormonal condition of patient B if both A and B exhibit an identical index—the response of the vaginal epithelium to hormonal stimuli differs from individual to individual. Prior to discussing the general problem of reporting the endocrinologic condition by means of indices, the various indices are discussed separately next.

Karyopyknotic Index

Assessment of the KPI is generally made on a minimum of 300 cells. The major problems of assessment of the KPI are as follows: (1) 300 cells is a relatively small sample, (2) the brightfield microscope does not permit a critical differentiation between pyknotic and vesicular nuclei and (3) differences of about ± 15% on the same case are possible between interpreters. Among the various indices, the KPI is most widely utilized.

Maturation Index

The MI[14, 35] is a count of the parabasal, intermediate and superficial cells (P:I:S). It is similar to the assessment of the KPI but with the additional evaluation of possible parabasal cells present. Because the MI seems to provide more data than the KPI, it is often considered a more informative index than the KPI. With rare exceptions, only one or two cell types occur in hormonal patterns: (1) parabasal cells alone, (2) parabasal and intermediate cells, (3) intermediate cells alone, (4) intermediate and superficial cells and (5) superficial cells alone. The occurrence of superficial cells alone is hypothetical—they practically never occur without an admixture of intermediate cells. The MI, like any index, is generally meaningless when the assessment is made on only one smear; a "shift to the left" or a "shift to the right" on repeated specimens from the same patient may have some clinical importance. If cell counts appear in all three bins of the MI, it is usually an indication that smears were taken by ectocervical scraping or that an inflammatory process is present.

Eosinophilic Index

The EI is not difficult to assess, but it is also the index that is most often altered by artifacts, such as pseudoeosinophilia due to poor fixation, poor staining technique or changes due to the influence of the vaginal pH. The EI, if determined without assessing the KPI or MI, is of limited value.

Folded Cell Index

The FCI[83, 84] assesses the tendency of the cells towards folding. A high FCI is usually found when the KPI is low and vice versa. This index is more simply assessed than is the KPI because cellular folding is clearly evident and not subject to the interpretative opinions that occur in determining nuclear pyknosis. Mature squamous cells that are folded are usually less mature than are flat cells that have lost the tendency to fold.

Crowded Cell Index

The CCI[73] assesses the tendency of the cell towards cluster formation. This is a relatively difficult index to

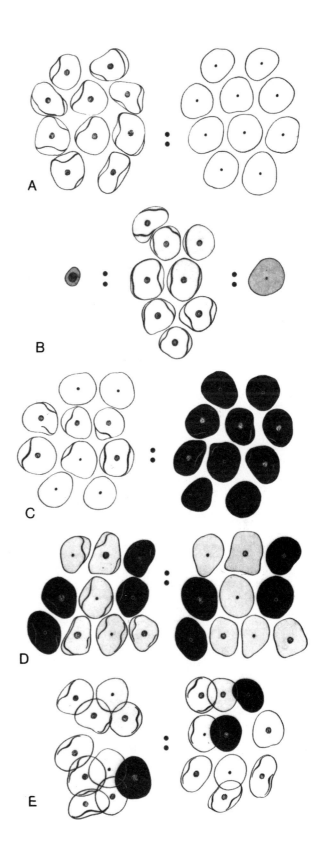

FIGURE 7–14. Schematic representations of the various **cytologic indices** used for the reporting of hormonal influences on the vaginal epithelium. *A,* Karyopyknotic index (KPI) = relation of mature superficial cells to mature intermediate cells, regardless of staining reaction. *B,* Maturation index (MI) = relation of superficial cells to intermediate cells to parabasal cells expressed in percentages and written as 10/80/10 for the example shown. *C,* Eosinophilic index (EI) = relation of mature eosinophilic squamous cells to mature cyanophilic squamous cells, regardless of nuclear appearance. *D,* Folded cell index (FCI) = relation of mature folded squamous cells to mature flat squamous cells, regardless of staining reaction and nuclear appearance. *E,* Crowded cell index (CCI) = relation of mature squamous cells in clusters of four or more cells to cells lying either singly or in clusters of less than four cells, regardless of staining reaction, nuclear appearance, cellular folding and flatness.

assess because cell clusters often contain so many cells that they do not lend themselves to accurate counting. Moreover, this index is usually parallel to the FCI.

Maturation Value

The maturation value (MV) introduced by Meisels[32] also utilizes the three main cell types (superficial, intermediate and parabasal cells), to which weights are assigned: superficial cells = 1.0, intermediate cells = 0.5 and parabasal cells = 0. The MV is not suggested as a means of reporting cytohormonal findings to the clinician. It is, however, a working mechanism useful for communication among cytologists.

Reporting Cytologic Findings

The clinician who requests a cytologic report on a patient's endocrinologic condition may receive differently worded versions of the same cellular findings.[69] One cytopathologist may state, for example, "only parabasal cells present" in a specimen from an atrophic epithelium or "no estrogen effect present." Another may say that the "KPI is zero." A third may report that "the MI is 100/0/0," while another may report "evidence of marked estrogenic deficiency or senile atrophy." Yet another may relate the age and menstrual history to the cytologic findings and so report that "the cytologic pattern is compatible with the age and menstrual history."

It would be ideal if the degree of maturity of the vaginal epithelium or any of the aforementioned indices would be directly related to the actual amount of estrogens present, thus permitting a diagnostic scale of marked estrogenic effect through moderate to slight effects, down to slight, moderate and marked estrogenic deficiencies. If this were true, a KPI of 60 would indicate an absolutely more marked estrogenic effect than would a KPI of 40, and an MI of 0/90/10 would mean a lesser hormonal stimulus than an MI of 0/75/25.

Unfortunately, this is not the case, as shown by the following example. The epithelial cell response to five daily administrations of 10 mg of estradiol benzoate in surgical castrate A is not necessarily the same as the response to five daily identical administrations to surgical castrate B or C, even when A, B and C exhibit the same initial patterns of epithelial atrophy. One patient might respond to a given dosage of estrogens with a KPI of 15, whereas another patient given the same dosage may respond with a KPI of 45. This dosage in a third patient might result in no karyopyknosis at all.

The presence of only intermediate cells is difficult to report in a clinically meaningful fashion by means of indices. In this case, an MI of 0/100/0 or a KPI of zero is of limited value to the clinician if not related to the clinical history, age and menstrual history of the particular patient. Intermediate cells occur when the patient is a normal newborn, an infant with luteoma, a normal child in the premenarche, a woman in the normal luteal phase, a normal pregnant patient, a secondary amenorrheic patient, a patient after hysterectomy and oophorectomy, a patient undergoing androgenic therapy or long-term estrogenic therapy, a patient receiving a combination therapy of estrogens and androgens or estrogens and progestogens, or, finally, a normal postmenopausal woman.

The hormonal interpretation of the cytologic specimen should be provided by an experienced cytopathologist with endocrinologic knowledge. The interpretation should be a meaningful and diagnostic communication and not merely an index. Cytopathologists should first indicate whether they were able to make a hormonal reading at all by asking the following questions: (1) Is the specimen taken from the vaginal wall or was it mistakenly taken from the ectocervix? (2) Is it free of anucleated squamous cells? (3) Is the specimen accompanied by an adequate clinical history, especially concerning hormonal therapy, if any? A negative reply to any of these three questions indicates that the report should read, "no hormonal evaluation possible."

For cases in which the hormonal evaluation can be performed, the clinician needs to know whether the cytologic pattern is compatible or incompatible with the age and menstrual history. The addition of indices is not needed. In the few cases in which the cytologic pattern is incompatible with the age and menstrual history, cytopathologists should provide further elucidation by stating why, in their opinion, the incompatibility exists, such as "too marked estrogenic effect for a patient 65 years of age" or "no cytologic evidence of corpus luteum hormone production, possibly anovulatory cycle, assuming this is a 28-day to 30-day cycle" or "postpartum cell type present, suggesting that the clinically existing pregnancy is already terminated (missed abortion)."

The clinician should request specific data in some cases. One may wish to know, for example, whether an existing infertility problem is due to deficient or no estrogenic or luteal hormone production. Cytologic smears on the 15th and 25th days of the cycle may result in a meaningful consultative statement from the cytopathologist, e.g., "The cytologic patterns indicate the presence of both normal estrogenic and luteal phases." For a posthysterectomy patient, the clinician may wish to know whether the ovaries are still functioning. These are only a few instances illustrating some of the cooperative efforts between clinician and cytopathologist—when questions are asked and are answered with clinically meaningful information.

Only in repeated or serial smears from the same patient would indices have some value, because one index could then be related to another. Indices are useful for assessing drug effects and their duration in experimental cases. However, for diagnostic evaluation of the individual case on a single specimen, the index is of no value to either the cytopathologist or the clinician. The indiscriminate issuance of indices rather than communicative reports may tend to become, for the cytopathologist or the cytotechnologist, a substitute for needed endocrinologic data. An index is given to the clinician, suggesting that the clinician be the one who finds the meaning for such an index rather than the cytopathologist or cytotechnologist.

Major Cell Patterns

In hormonal cytology there are actually only *two diagnostic* cell patterns:

1. The cell pattern exhibiting mature, flat, single-lying cells, most of which are superficial and some of which are intermediate. This cell pattern indicates unequivocally that the vaginal epithelium is stimulated by estrogens. No other hormone can induce this mature cell pattern.

2. The "atrophic" cell pattern consisting predominantly of parabasal cells, indicating lack of stimulation by estrogens.

Cell patterns between these two extremes are not per se diagnostic unless one knows the age of the patient, the menstrual history and other pertinent data, such as hormonal therapy, if any. These intermediate cell patterns consist predominantly of intermediate cells together with a few superficial or parabasal cells.

CYTOLOGIC PATTERNS

Infancy and Menarche

The cytologic patterns during the first days of the infant's life are similar to or identical with the cell patterns of the mother at the time of delivery—mostly intermediate cells, with a certain percentage of superficial cells (Fig. 7–15).[6] The cell patterns of the infant are characterized by the absence of leukocytes, erythrocytes and bacterial flora. However, this cell pattern changes rather rapidly, first by the influx of bacteria, then of leukocytes, and then by a steady, more or less rapid decrease of the proliferative index of the cell pattern. Using the MI to demonstrate the changes in a particular case, one may find at the time of birth an MI of 0/85/15, which decreases during the first 2 weeks to 20/80/0, and then in the next 3 to 4 weeks with atrophy, to an MI of 90/10/0 (Fig. 7–15). This is, however, only an example of a specific case and may vary from infant to infant. Erythrocytes may also be found in newborns' smears, especially around the 5th to 10th days.

The atrophic cell patterns (Fig. 7–16) are maintained throughout the early years of life and are gradually replaced by a noncyclic intermediate cell pattern, with an MI of 0/100/0 (Fig. 7–17) approximately 3 to 4 years prior to the onset of menstruation. The persistent intermediate cell pattern is accompanied by an absence of leukocytes, the presence of healthy vaginal flora (*Bacillus vaginalis Doederlein*) and sometimes the presence of bacterial cytolysis. This is a nondiagnostic cell pattern per se because identical patterns are found during the luteal phase of the normal cycle, during pregnancy, during secondary amenorrhea, during

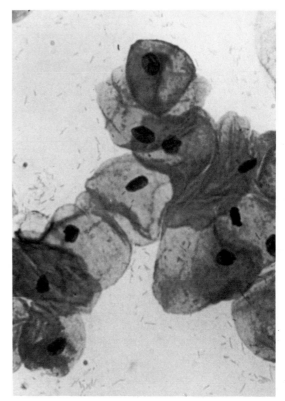

FIGURE 7–15. Cytologic sample from a newborn infant (4 days old) exhibiting **folded and crowded intermediate cells** similar to those in the mother's sample at the time of delivery. Note the first influx of microbiologic elements. The cell sample is generally sterile at the moment of birth (Papanicolaou stain; ×400).

menopause and after castration. However, one may give an occasional hormonal evaluation based on this cell pattern. In order to assess the cell patterns of the prepubertal patient, it is important to prepare repeated cell specimens, in weekly intervals throughout a 4- to 5-week period, to ascertain whether or not cyclic changes are already present.

Cyclic ovarian changes are usually found as long as 18 months prior to the actual onset of the menstrual cycle. One deals here with follicular growth and degeneration, without ovulation and corpus luteum formation. For the endometrium to respond to hormonal stimuli, a more prolonged and higher threshold dosage is required, as compared with the vaginal epithelial response.

Menstrual Cycle

During the menstrual cycle, characteristic alterations of the cytologic patterns occur. The main cell types during the menstrual cycle are (1) pattern of the menstrual period, (2) pattern of the proliferative (follicular) phase, (3) pattern at the time of ovulation, and (4) pattern of the secretory (luteal) phase.

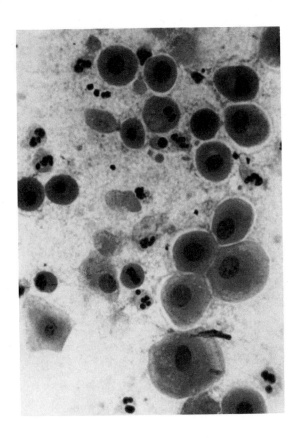

FIGURE 7–16. Cytologic sample from a 3.5-year-old child exhibiting **parabasal cell types, coccoid bacteria and leukocytes**. These changes occur several weeks after birth and persist until 2 to 4 years prior to the onset of menarche (Papanicolaou stain; ×400).

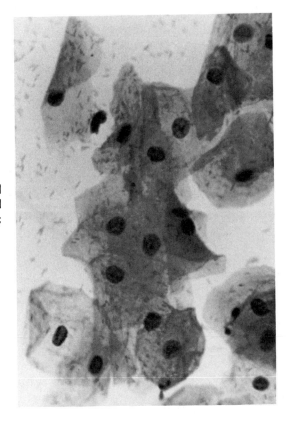

FIGURE 7–17. Cytologic sample (**vaginal smear**) from an 11-year-old child **prior to menarche**. There are small, folded intermediate cells and usually healthy vaginal flora, with no leukocytes (Papanicolaou stain; ×400).

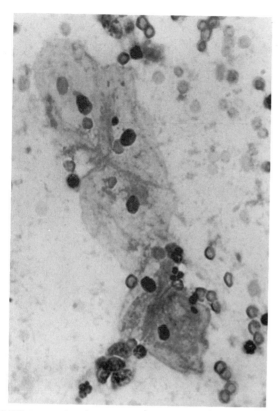

FIGURE 7–18. Cytologic sample **(vaginal smear)** taken **at the time of the menstrual period**. The specimen exhibits erythrocytes, leukocytes, intermediate cells, some endometrial cells and coccoid bacteria (Papanicolaou stain; × 400).

Menstrual Period

During the menstrual period, the cellular pattern is not always typical for a particular diagnostic hormonal pattern. It consists mainly of erythrocytes, leukocytes, coccoid bacteria and some endometrial, intermediate and superficial cells (Fig. 7–18).

Proliferative Phase

After the cessation of the menstrual period, there are only occasional erythrocytes along with a decrease in the number of leukocytes and an increase in the number of superficial cells versus intermediate cells. The cells have a tendency to flatten out and lie singly as the proliferative phase progresses (Fig. 7–19). During the 6th to 10th days of the cycle, an exodus of histiocytes and paramenstrual debris are normal findings.

Ovulatory Pattern

The ovulatory pattern represents the maximal height of cellular maturity for a given patient (Fig. 7–20). The KPI has no set number for determining the time when ovulation usually occurs. One patient may ovu-

late with a KPI of 35, whereas another may ovulate with a KPI as high as 85. For the individual patient, however, the KPI level recurs at ovulation with only minor deviations. At the time of ovulation, the cells are mostly flat and lie singly. Many of the cells are eosinophilic and contain pyknotic nuclei. The cells exhibit very fine, indistinct, sometimes barely visible cellular borders.

Postovulatory and Secretory Phases

The first apparent cellular change after ovulation has occurred is that the cellular border becomes more prominent, with the beginning of cellular folding (Fig. 7–21). The relative number of superficial cells decreases rather rapidly within the next 7 days, thus reducing the KPI. Shortly before the onset of menstruation, the cell pattern consists predominantly of folded and crowded intermediate, often cytolytic, cells. In the late luteal or premenstrual phase, the smear is usually free of leukocytes and coccoid bacteria (Figs. 7–22 and 7–23).

Patients with primary amenorrhea and in whom hormonal therapy has never been initiated usually exhibit only atrophic cell types (see Fig. 7–4) or an intermixture of parabasal-basal cell types with a few

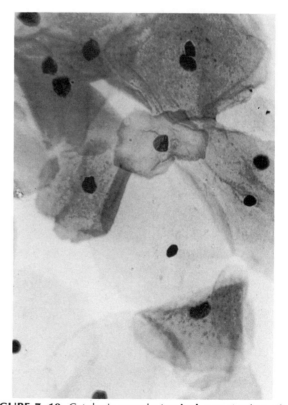

FIGURE 7–19. Cytologic sample **(vaginal smear)** taken **after the menstrual period and prior to ovulation** (proliferative phase). Intermediate and superficial cells are present, the background is free of leukocytes and the previously present coccoid bacteria are largely replaced by healthy vaginal flora (Papanicolaou stain; × 400).

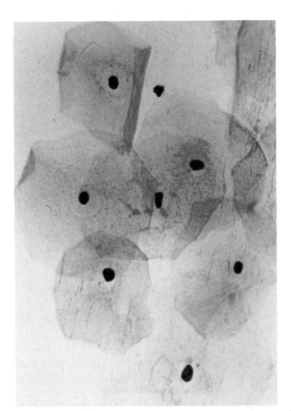

FIGURE 7–20. Cytologic sample **(vaginal smear)** taken **at the time of ovulation**. The cells are mostly flat superficial-type squamous epithelial cells, with healthy vaginal flora and practically no leukocytes (Papanicolaou stain; ×400).

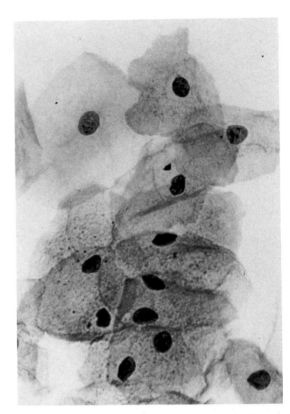

FIGURE 7–22. Cytologic sample **(vaginal smear)** taken **during the luteal (secretory) phase** of the cycle. The cells are practically all intermediate-type squamous epithelial cells; they are folded and show a tendency towards crowding (Papanicolaou stain; ×400).

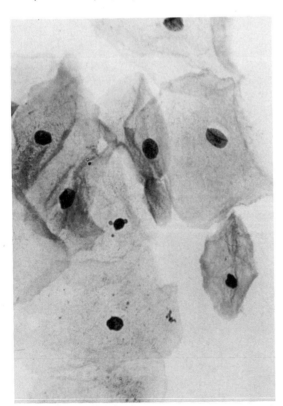

FIGURE 7–21. Cytologic sample **(vaginal smear)** taken **during the postovulatory days**. As the first indication of incurred ovulation, the cells exhibit increased folding and relatively sharp cellular outlines, which are fixation artifacts (Papanicolaou stain; ×400).

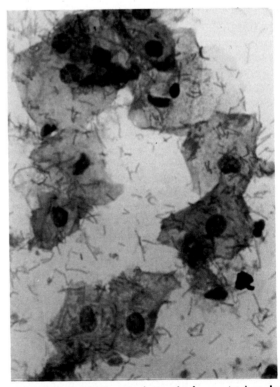

FIGURE 7–23. Cytologic sample **(vaginal smear)** taken **during the last days of the luteal phase**. The cells exhibit bacterial cytolysis. Although there are practically no leukocytes, abundant, relatively long *Bacillus vaginalis* organisms are present (Papanicolaou stain; ×400).

more mature cell types (see Fig. 7–5). The cell pattern is that normally found during infancy (see Fig. 7–16). A patient with primary amenorrhea who exhibits an intermediate cell type is usually more amenable to hormonal therapy as compared with a patient who exhibits an atrophic epithelium. In patients with primary amenorrhea, one will always determine the presence of "sex chromatin bodies" (the marginal chromatin bodies on the nuclear envelope).[49, 50] An absence of marginal chromatin bodies in parabasal cells suggests Turner's syndrome (see Fig. 7–1) or the testicular feminization syndrome (see Fig. 7–2) if the cells are mature.

Nonpregnant patients whose normal menstrual cycle ceased prior to physiologic menopause (secondary amenorrhea) usually exhibit the intermediate cell type (an MI of 0/100/0). The same intermediate pattern may be found also after surgical removal of the ovaries or during the luteal phase of the normal menstrual cycle or during normal pregnancy. Therefore, assessment of the hormonal condition in the secondary amenorrheic patient requires comprehensive information on the patient's age, menstrual history and possible medication.

To predict the day of ovulation, e.g., for successful artificial insemination, daily smears should be obtained during three complete menstrual cycles, plus preparation of temperature curves. These will help predict, with some degree of accuracy, when ovulation will occur during the upcoming fourth cycle. The patient may prepare her own specimens by inserting an empty container of a Tampax tampon in the vagina, thus avoiding contamination of the specimen with vulvar cells. Then, with a premoistened cotton-tipped applicator inserted diagonally inside the container, the vaginal wall can be slightly scraped, the material put on a glass slide and immediately fixed. The specimens should be examined at one diagnostic session. This procedure is relatively simple because the interpreter is required only to obtain an impression of which specimen exhibits the highest proliferative cell pattern. No counts of cellular indices are necessary. Approximately 80 slides of the three monthly cycles may be examined in less than 20 minutes. The slides from the days of highest cellular maturity during each of the 3 months are identified, and a comparison is made with the temperature curves. If the results coincide, it is relatively certain that ovulation has been determined accurately and that the anticipated date of ovulation for the forthcoming cycle may be predicted rather confidently.

Pregnancy and Postpartum

Pregnancy

The normal cell patterns during pregnancy occur in a similar sequence but are slower than those observed in the normal menstrual cycle between the time of ovulation and the late luteal phase (Figs. 7–24 to 7–26).[3, 14, 18, 19, 27, 30, 31, 37, 48, 65, 80] The changes of the cell

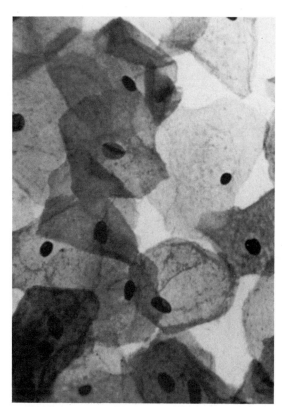

FIGURE 7–24. Cytologic specimen taken **during pregnancy (at 3.5 months).** The material exhibits predominantly intermediate cells and a few superficial cells (Papanicolaou stain; ×400).

patterns described in the section Menstrual Cycle are similar to those expected to occur in early pregnancy. However, in some cases it may take 3 to 5 months to achieve the complete intermediate cell type (an MI of 0/100/0), which is the normal cell pattern during pregnancy.

The presence of extremely marked cellular maturity in pregnancy usually indicates the presence of progesterone deficiency. During normal pregnancy, parenteral or oral administration of estrogen (not local application) does not induce increased cellular maturity. Therefore, if proliferation during pregnancy occurs as a result of estrogen administration, it may be concluded that a hormonal disturbance exists.

One of the significant cytologic criteria of a poor prognosis during pregnancy is the sudden shift, not influenced by exogenous hormones, from the intermediate cell type to either (a) the considerably higher mature type or to (b) the considerably lower mature type. In the case of a, this shift usually indicates progesterone deficiency; in case of b, it usually indicates a discontinuance of the pregnancy, regardless of whether the fetus is still *in utero*. Cellular changes due to infection have to be excluded. These inflammatory changes—resulting from infection, regeneration or metaplasia—also induce a pseudoatrophic cell pattern mimicking the postpartum cell type. In order to differentiate these cell types, parenteral estrogen administration is suggested. Resulting marked maturation up to superficial cell layers usually indicates that the

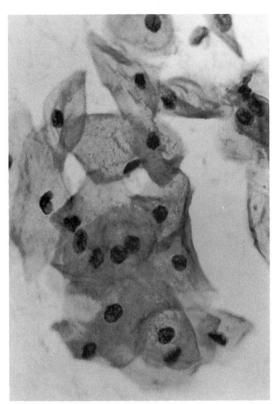

FIGURE 7–25. Cytologic specimen taken **during pregnancy (at 5 months).** The sample contains mostly small folded and crowded intermediate cells (Papanicolaou stain; ×400).

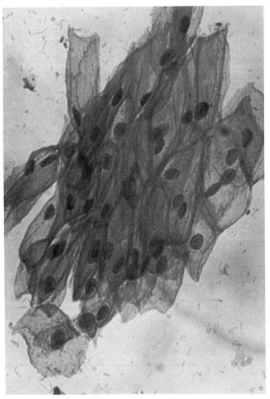

FIGURE 7–26. Cytologic specimen taken **late in the pregnancy** exhibits abundant folded and crowed intermediate cells (Papanicolaou stain; ×400).

previously low proliferative pattern was due to a hormonal deficiency and not to infection, regeneration or metaplasia.

Many causes exist for abortions other than endocrinologic causes. Therefore, clinically threatened abortions may or may not be accompanied by an abnormal hormonal cell pattern. However, cell patterns are known that indicate "inevitability of abortion" and are cytodiagnostically useful. Inevitable abortion may be predicted when the cytologic specimen exhibits endometrial cells.

Differences in the cytomorphology of postmature abortions have been described by some workers.[34, 37] However, other investigators' examinations[18, 19, 66] and our own examinations could not duplicate these findings. Further studies on this topic are needed.

The presence of *vernix caseosa* cells (anucleated squames that usually stain yellowish with the Papanicolaou technique) is evident and may indicate rupture of fetal membranes. Kittrich[26] recommended the following staining technique to differentiate fetal from maternal cells: several drops of a 0.05% aqueous solution of Nile blue sulfate added to a fresh smear on a glass slide, then covered with a coverslip, will color the fat-containing fetal cells orange and the maternal cells, which contain little, if any, lipid, blue.

Postpartum

Postpartum vaginal smears show predominantly atrophic patterns for 5 to 6 weeks after delivery in lactating women (Figs. 7–27 and 7–28). Varying degrees of atrophy may persist for as long as several months. However, Danos[7] seldom encountered the cytohormonal pattern expected for this period and implied that atrophic smears rarely are observed 6 weeks after delivery. Likewise, Butler and Taylor[6] stated that smears from postnatal clinics in Manchester, England, did not support generally accepted views. They found the classic postpartum smear in only 28% of 84 patients. Whereas atrophic smears were seen in almost 30% of 27 samples taken on the 6th postpartum day, the incidence of atrophy fell to a mere 5.3% of 75 samples taken 6 weeks after delivery.

A study by McLennan and McLennan[30] showed that atrophic smears predominate 3 to 6 weeks after delivery in women who are lactating. Only a third of the nonlactating patients have atrophic patterns. In addition, these investigators showed a progressive increase occurs in the incidence of estrogenic patterns observed beyond the 6th postpartum week, irrespective of the persistence of lactation. The incidence of mixed patterns was constant (about 5%), regardless of lactation or time beyond delivery. This study confirms the traditional view of hormonally related puerperal vaginal cytology patterns and is at variance with claims that vaginal atrophy is unusual in the puerperium.

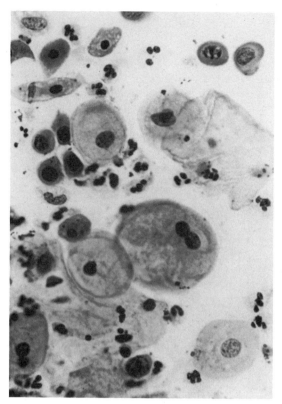

FIGURE 7–27. Cytologic specimen taken **during the postpartum period (6th week postpartum)**. This sample from a **lactating patient** shows an "atrophic"-type patten, with an inflammatory reaction and, usually, coccoid bacteria (Papanicolaou stain; ×400).

Postmenopause, Senium and Status Postcastration

The cytologic patterns of the postmenopausal years are mirror images of patterns observed during premenarche and menarche.[9, 11, 17, 20, 33, 36, 43, 67] A period of cyclic changes is evidenced on the vaginal epithelium that is no longer manifested on the endometrium. These cyclic changes are followed by a noncyclic intermediate cell pattern and, in many instances, but not inevitably, by complete epithelial atrophy (Fig. 7–29 to 7–35).

A variety of reactions deviate from this general pattern. In some instances, atrophy may occur a few months after cessation of menstruation; in other instances, atrophy may never occur, and the intermediate cell pattern (with an MI of 0/100/0) persists throughout the life of the woman.[66, 67] The same is true for surgical castrates. Young individuals who undergo surgical castration while still menstruating retain an intermediate pattern and may never exhibit atrophy. Most probably, adrenal hormones are responsible for maintaining the intermediate type of proliferation in these cases.

The fact that the presence of atrophic or intermediate cell patterns may indicate inactivity or absence of ovarian function should also be taken into consideration when reporting hormonal patterns on patients with breast carcinoma. This finding is especially important when the surgeon is seeking an indication as to the best course of therapy on the basis of the hormonal report.

Administered Sex Steroid Hormones

Cytologic Effects of Administered Estrogens

The parenteral or oral administration of estrogens induces epithelial proliferation in practically all physiologic conditions (Fig. 7–36),[10, 20, 21, 25, 35, 59, 63, 68, 76, 77] with the exception of normal pregnancy. It should be noted, however, that *local* estrogen administration also induces cellular maturity during normal pregnancy.

In an attempt to inhibit some facets of the aging process in postmenopausal women, long-term estrogenic therapy has been in vogue (see Fig. 7–35). The cytologic follow-up of these patients allows the assessment of the hormonal status prior to hormone administration and the determination of the duration of effectiveness of a particular estrogenic substance.

Cytologic Effects of Administered Progestogens

The cytologic effects of progestogens depend on the initial cell type existing prior to the time of initial

Text continued on page 108

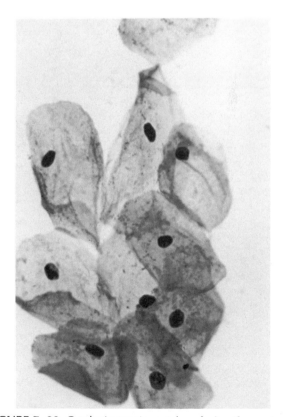

FIGURE 7–28. Cytologic specimen taken **during the postpartum period (6th week postpartum)**. This particular sample was taken from a **nonlactating woman** and exhibits intermediate and superficial cells (Papanicolaou stain; ×400).

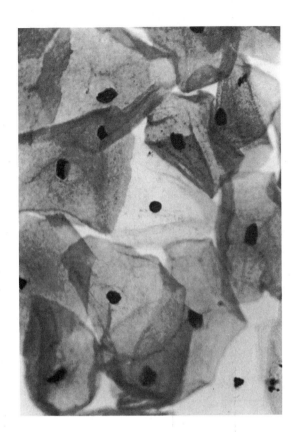

FIGURE 7–29. Cytologic specimen from a **menopausal patient 8 months after the cessation of menstruation**. The sample exhibits large intermediate and superficial cells. In some cases, discernible cyclic changes may still be present. In others, this type of pattern is static and noncyclic (Papanicolaou stain; × 400).

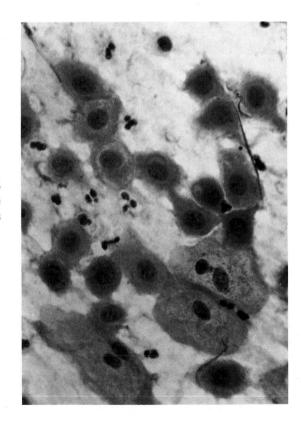

FIGURE 7–30. Cytologic specimen from a **postmenopausal patient (4 years postmenopausal)** exhibits intermediate and parabasal cells in various degrees of degeneration, leukocytes and coccoid bacteria (Papanicolaou stain; × 400).

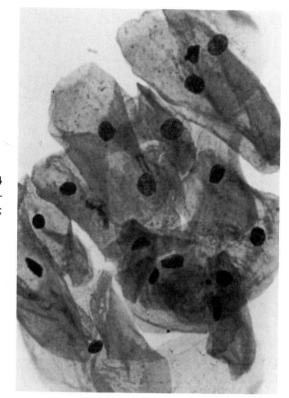

FIGURE 7–31. Cytologic specimen from a **postmenopausal patient (4 years postmenopausal)** exhibits well-preserved intermediate and superficial cells, *Bacillus vaginalis* and no leukocytes (Papanicolaou stain; ×400).

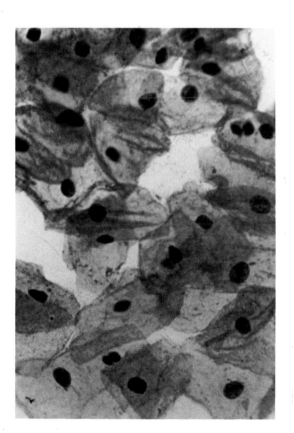

FIGURE 7–32. Cytologic specimen from a **surgical castrate (8 years after surgery)** exhibits well-preserved folded and crowded small intermediate cells, a few superficial cells, *Bacillus vaginalis* and no leukocytes (Papanicolaou stain; ×400).

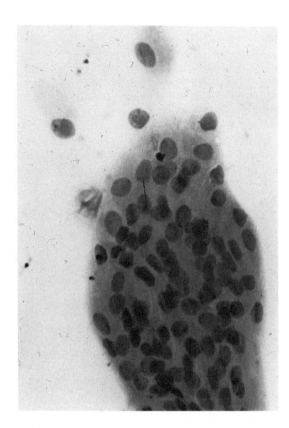

FIGURE 7–33. Cytologic specimen from a **postmenopausal patient (10 years postmenopausal)** exhibits autolytic parabasal cells in clusters (Papanicolaou stain; ×400).

FIGURE 7–34. Cytologic specimen from a **postmenopausal patient (15 years postmenopausal)** exhibits anisocytotic parabasal cells in various degrees of degeneration, leukocytes and coccoid bacteria (Papanicolaou stain; ×400).

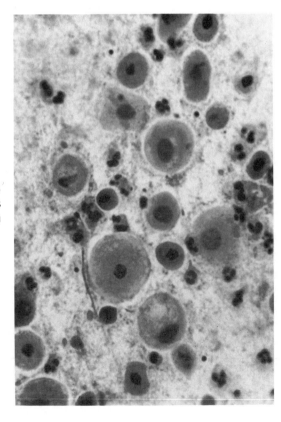

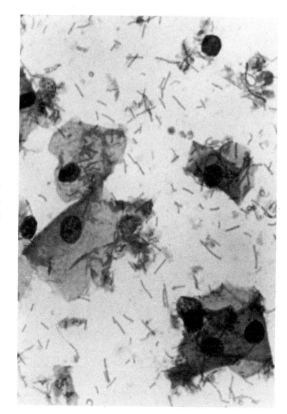

FIGURE 7–35. Cytologic specimen from a **postmenopausal patient who had a long-term administration of estrogens**. The slide contains intermediate cells in different stages of bacterial cytolysis, a peptolytic process caused by *Bacillus vaginalis* (Papanicolaou stain; ×400).

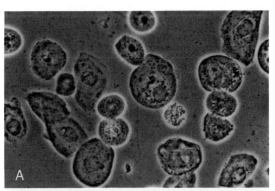

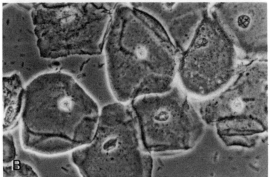

FIGURE 7–36. Cytologic samples showing *(A)* **an atrophic pattern** (parabasal cells) and *(B)* **the resulting cell pattern** (superficial cells) after estrogen administration (phase-contrast microscopy; ×120). (Reproduced with permission from Jenny JW: Phase Contrast Microscopic Cytologic Diagnosis: A Gynecologic Office Procedure. *In* Teaching Slide Sets in Cytology, vol. 27. Wied GL (ed). Chicago, Tutorials of Cytology, 1979.)

administration.[16, 28, 29, 51, 52, 79, 81, 82] If, on the one hand, the proliferative condition at that time was one stimulated by estrogens (e.g., an MI of 0/40/60), the result of administering progestogens is a decrease in the cellular maturity (e.g., an MI of 0/95/5) (Fig. 7–37). If, on the other hand, the initial pattern was one of atrophy (an MI of 100/0/0), progestogen administration may in some cases induce epithelial growth of an irregular and a mixed type (e.g., an MI of 20/80/0), or in some cases no proliferative effect is seen (e.g., an MI of 100/0/0). If the initial cell type was an intermediate cell pattern (an MI of 0/100/0), no changes are generally induced by administering progestogens.

Cytologic Effects of Administered Androgens

The cytologic effects of administered androgens also depend on the cell type existing prior to the initial hormone administration.[40, 49, 50, 60] The results are very similar to those described for administered progestogens. Sex steroids may act as antagonists when androgens (or progestogens) are added to existing estrogen administration. They act to some extent as synergists when the initial cell type is one of atrophy.[78]

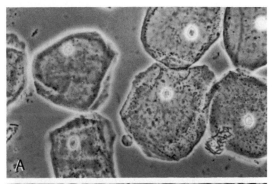
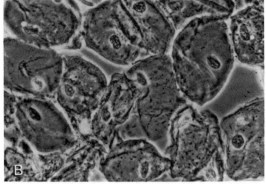

FIGURE 7–37. Cytologic samples showing *(A)* **an estrogen-stimulated pattern** (flat and single superficial cells) and *(B)* **the resulting cell pattern** (folded and crowded intermediate cells) after administration of progestogenic substances (phase-contrast microscopy; ×120). (Reproduced with permission from Jenny JW: Phase Contrast Microscopic Cytologic Diagnosis: A Gynecologic Office Procedure. *In* Teaching Slide Sets in Cytology, vol. 27. Wied GL (ed). Chicago, Tutorials of Cytology, 1979.)

Gynecologic Endocrinopathies

The cytologic patterns in gynecologic endocrinopathies were well described by Rakoff[49] and Rakoff and Takeda.[50]

Turner's Syndrome

In most cases of Turner's syndrome, the vaginal smear exhibits predominantly or only parabasal cells (see Fig. 7–2), which are almost always sex-chromatin negative. Patients with primary amenorrhea should undergo sex chromatin examinations. Atrophic cell patterns with sex chromatin–negative nuclei are encountered in gonadal dysgenesis (XO or XY) and in male pseudohermaphrodites (XY).

Testicular Feminization Syndrome

The vaginal smear of a patient with testicular feminization syndrome usually exhibits a mature cell pattern with superficial and intermediate squamous cells (Fig. 7–3). However, the cells are sex chromatin-negative. Negative findings for sex chromatin in mature squamous cell patterns are practically diagnostic for testicular feminization syndrome.

Stein-Leventhal Syndrome

The cytologic patterns in cases of Stein-Leventhal syndrome are uncharacteristic—different stages of cellular maturity may be in evidence. Some cases show well-matured cells (superficial and large intermediate cells), others show only intermediate cells and yet others show predominantly parabasal cells.

Virilizing Adrenal Tumor and Androgenic Syndrome

In virilizing adrenal tumor and androgenic syndrome, the cell pattern often demonstrates predominantly intermediate cells and some parabasal cells, along with rare superficial cells (Fig. 7–38). It may be one of the rare exceptions that the MI shows numbers in the three bins, such as MI = 20:77:3. However, no diagnostic decision as to presence of a virilizing tumor can be made on the basis of such cellular pattern.

Secondary Amenorrhea in Patients with Anorexia Nervosa

The cell pattern in extreme cases of anorexia nervosa shows complete atrophy (parabasal cells only), often accompanied by atrophic vaginitis (Fig. 7–39). This pattern is due to a decrease in pituitary gonadotropins, with secondary ovarian failure.

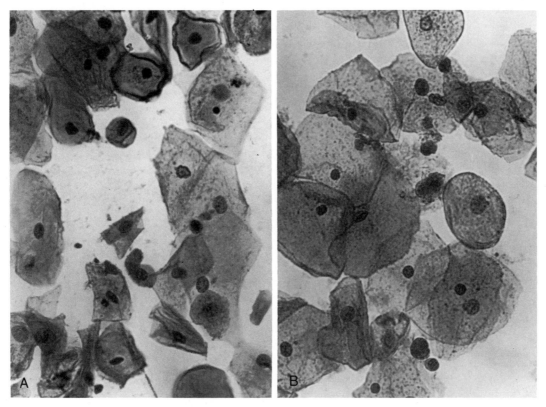

FIGURE 7–38. Cytologic samples from *(A)* a patient with **a virilizing adrenal tumor** and *(B)* a patient with **an androgenic syndrome**. In both instances, a rare admixture of intermediate and superficial cells is seen with a very few parabasal cells (Papanicolaou stain; ×120). (Reproduced with permission from Rakoff AE, Takeda M: Gynecologic Endocrinopathies. *In* Teaching Slide Sets in Cytology, vol. 13. Wied GL (ed). Chicago, Tutorials of Cytology, 1979.)

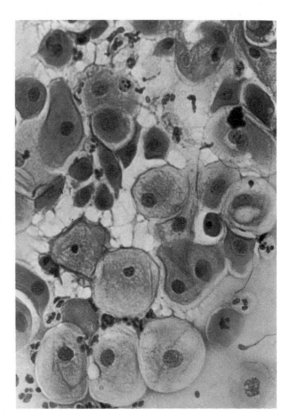

FIGURE 7–39. Cytologic sample from a patient with **anorexia nervosa and secondary amenorrhea**. The specimen exhibits an anisocytotic atrophic cell type (Papanicolaou stain; ×120.) (Reproduced with permission from Rakoff AE, Takeda M: Gynecologic Endocrinopathies. *In* Teaching Slide Sets in Cytology, vol. 13. Wied GL (ed). Chicago, Tutorials of Cytology, 1979.)

Granulosa Cell Tumor

A persistent highly mature cell pattern may be caused by exogenous estrogen administration, which may be contained in cosmetic substances or may be caused by steroid hormones taken without medical supervision. Only after any possible exogenous cause is excluded should one consider the presence of a granulosa-cell tumor. Figure 7–40 shows the very mature cell pattern in a case of granulosa-cell tumor and the resulting decrease of cellular maturity after the tumor was surgically removed.

Precocious Puberty

The cytologic evaluation of children suspected of precocious puberty can only effectively be done in those age groups in which one would expect normally to find an atrophic cell pattern: from 1 to maximally 5 years of age. After the age of 5 years, intermediate cells are already in the vaginal smears of some healthy children; this factor makes the identification of precocious puberty based on cell maturity rather difficult. The typical cell pattern of precocious puberty, in an infant, exhibits intermediate and superficial cells where one would normally expect to find only parabasal cells.

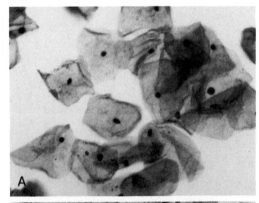
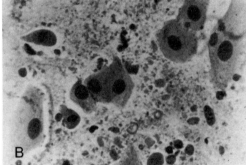

FIGURE 7–40. Cytologic samples from a patient with a granulosa cell tumor, (A) before and (B) after surgical removal of the tumor. The preoperative sample shows a marked estrogen stimulation, whereas the postoperative sample shows an atrophic cell pattern (phase-contrast microscopy; ×120). (Reproduced with permission from Rakoff AE, Takeda M: Gynecologic Endocrinopathies. In Teaching Slide Sets in Cytology, vol. 13. Wied GL (ed). Chicago, Tutorials of Cytology, 1979.)

THE ESTROGEN PROLIFERATION TEST: AN AID IN DIFFERENTIAL CYTODIAGNOSIS

Papanicolaou[41] first suggested the administration of estrogen in patients whose vaginal smears exhibited equivocal cellular criteria. His recommendation for a short-term, low-dosage estrogen administration was to induce growth and maturation of the normal squamous epithelium without affecting the morphology of malignant tumor cells. Boschann[5] later called this phenomenon a "hormonal deafness" of malignant tumor cells to the administration of estrogen. Thus, if malignant tumor cells are present in the cell sample, the repeat cell sample should reveal clearly defined malignant tumor cells amidst abundant mature squamous epithelial cells and an essentially clean background.[25, 41, 85]

The majority of atrophic cell patterns (see Figs. 7–5, 7–16, 7–30, 7–33 and 7–34) may be unequivocally identified as such, i.e., as normal, immature epithelial cells whose presence is due to deficient steroid hormonal stimulation of the vaginal epithelium. Occasional difficulties in interpreting atrophic cell patterns may sometimes be due to the inexperience of the individual evaluating the cell sample.[2, 12, 13, 15] However, certain cell patterns exist that may, even in retrospect, present diagnostic problems even for the experienced interpreter. In fact, atrophic cell patterns remain a challenge and provide some of the most interesting but difficult case studies.

Epithelial atrophy accompanied by inflammatory cell changes may be misinterpreted as malignant because of certain similarities between cells deriving from reparative and inflammatory processes and those deriving from malignant lesions (Figs. 7–41 to 7–43). Parabasal cells from the patient with epithelial atrophy tend to degenerate proteolytically and result in an autolytic cell pattern that may bear certain similarities to highly degenerated tumor cells from the necrotic surface of a squamous cancer (Figs. 7–44 and 7–45).

The estrogen test is performed in our institution either by the local administration of an estrogenic substance daily through 3 days (vaginal cream) with repeat smears on the 5th day or by the intramuscular injection of 20 mg of long-acting estrogenic substance with repeat smears on the 7th day. The reappearance of the atrophic cell pattern occurs as early as 15 days and as late as 6 months after cessation of the administration of estrogens. The proliferative test may be suggested (1) when it is doubtful whether one is dealing with benign immature cells or with a malignant condition and (2) when it is doubtful whether one is dealing with a recurrent lesion or with radiation cell changes.

Response to the Estrogen Proliferation Test

The results of short-term administration of estrogens in patients with epithelial atrophic cell changes were

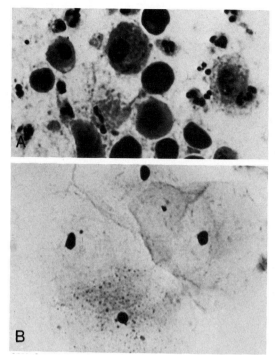

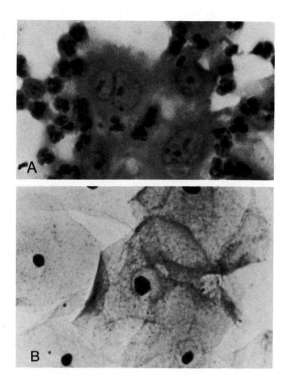

FIGURE 7–41. Cytologic patterns of *(A)* **an atrophic cell type** in a postmenpausal patient and *(B)* **a marked estrogenic effect** after estrogen administration (Papanicolaou stain; ×400).

FIGURE 7–42. Cytologic samples showing *(A)* **the regenerative changes** (tissue repair) and *(B)* the **disappearance of the reparative changes** and then the replacement with mature squamous cells after estrogen administration (Papanicolaou stain; ×400).

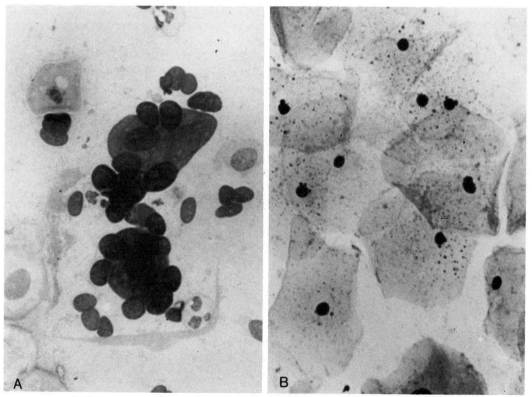

FIGURE 7–43. *A,* **Bare nuclei** in an atrophic cell pattern may be difficult to interpret. *B,* After estrogen administration, only **normal, mature squamous cells** are present (Papanicolaou stain; ×400).

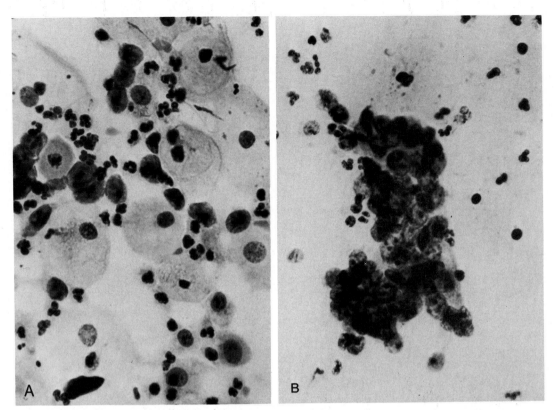

FIGURE 7–44. *A*, **Bare nuclei and immature cells**. Some of the bare nuclei could be misinterpreted as darkly stained trichomonads surrounded by parabasal cells. *B*, After estrogen administration, the slide contains well-preserved cells from a poorly differentiated malignant tumor, along with leukocytes and mature normal cells (Papanicolaou stain; ×400).

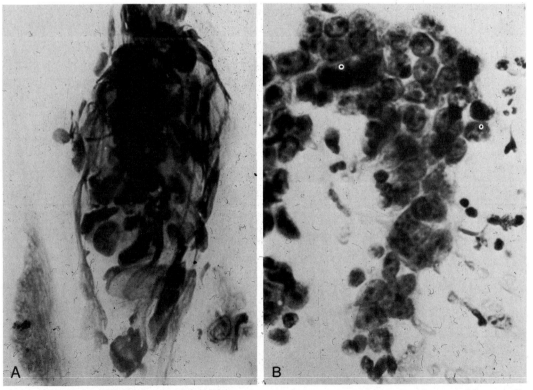

FIGURE 7–45. *A*, **Highly degenerated nuclear material** from a postmenopausal patient previously treated for a malignant lesion. *B*, After estrogen administration, the **degenerative changes disappeared** and the malignant tumor cells are now clearly identifiable as such (Papanicolaou stain; ×400).

shown to induce the following changes in the cell sample: (1) the background becomes "clean"; (2) the superficial and intermediate cells become the predominant cell types in the sample; (3) the previously present parabasal cells do not appear in the repeat smears or, if present, are few in number; (4) the cells characteristic of squamous metaplasia increase in number, in both endocervical and ectocervical samples, and (5) the degree of epithelial response varies from patient to patient.

After the estrogen test administration, the cell sample may appear deceptively normal at first glance because of the abundance of normal squamous epithelial cells and the significant decrease of tumor diathesis. These cell samples require diligent screening on the part of the cytotechnologist, more so than samples in which the tumor diathesis may provide a clue.

Although the estrogen proliferation test is not considered useful in the presence of lesions deriving from glandular epithelium, it is helpful in ruling out the presence of a squamous cell carcinoma or dysplasia of the uterine cervix or vagina in patients with questionable atrophic cell patterns. With increasing experience, the cytologist will need to request fewer estrogen proliferation tests. But even for the experienced, the test administrations may be useful in equivocal cases and may help to avoid unnecessary biopsies.

References

1. Babes AA: Diagnostic du cancer du col uterin par les frottis. Presse Med 36:451–454, 1928.
2. Bibbo M, Keebler CM, Wied GL: The cytologic diagnosis of tissue repair in the female genital tract. Acta Cytol 15:133–137, 1971.
3. Birtch PK: Hormonal cytology of pregnancy. Clin Obstet Gynecol 4:1062–1074, 1961.
4. Boquoi E, Hammerstein J: Discrepancies between colpocytology and urinary steroid hormone excretion in women treated with clomiphene citrate or gonadotropins for anovulatory sterility. Acta Cytol 13:332–346, 1969.
5. Boschann H: Personal communication.
6. Butler EB, Taylor DS: The postnatal smear. Acta Cytol 17:237–240, 1973.
7. Danos ML: Postpartum cytology: Observations over a four year period. Acta Cytol 12:309–312, 1968.
8. Dart LH, Turner TR: Fluorescence microscopy in exfoliative cytology. Lab Invest 8:1513–1522, 1959.
9. Davidson HB, Hecht EL, Winston RL: The significance of abnormal menopausal vaginal smears. Am J Obstet Gynecol 57:370–375, 1949.
10. Diczfalusy E: Mode of action of contraceptive drugs. Am J Obstet Gynecol 100:136–163, 1968.
11. Dove GA, Morley F, Batchelor A, Lun SF: Oestrogenic function in postmenopausal women. J Reprod Fertil 24:1–8, 1971.
12. Ehrmann RL, Younge PA, Lerch MA: The exfoliative cytology and histogenesis of an early primary malignant melanoma of the vagina. Acta Cytol 6:245–254, 1962.
13. Frable WJ, Smith JH, Perkins J, Foley C: Vaginal cuff cytology: Some difficult diagnostic problems. Acta Cytol 17:135–140, 1973.
14. Frost KJ: Gynecologic and obstetric cytopathology. In Novak's Gynecologic and Obstetric Pathology: With Clinical and Endocrine Relations, 7th ed. Edited by ER Novak, JD Woodruff. Philadelphia, WB Saunders, 1973.
15. Gard PD, Fields MJ, Noble EJ, Tweeddale DN: Comparative cytopathology of squamous carcinoma in situ of the cervix in the aged. Acta Cytol 13:27–35, 1969.
16. Greenblatt RB: One-pill-a-month contraceptive. Fertil Steril 18:207–211, 1967.
17. Gronroos M: Vaginal smear in postmenopause and its correlation with the urinary excretion of estrogens, 17-ketosteroids and gonadotrophins. Acta Obstet Gynecol Scand [Suppl] 5:117, 1965.
18. Hammond DO: A critical evaluation of the value of vaginal cytology for determination of "biologic term." Acta Cytol 9:340–343, 1965.
19. Hammond DO: Vaginal cytology at the end of pregnancy. Acta Cytol 10:230–231, 1966.
20. Hustin J, Van den Eynde JP: Cytologic evaluation of the effect of various estrogens given in postmenopause. Acta Cytol 21:225–228, 1977.
21. Jackson MCN: Oral contraception in practice. J Reprod Fertil 6:153–173, 1963.
22. Jayle MF, Genet P, Pujol J, Veyrin-Forrer F: The relationship between the appearance of vaginal smears and the rate of excretion of urinary steroids. Acta Cytol 4:16–25, 1960.
23. Jenny JW: Phase Contrast Microscopic Cytologic Diagnosis: A Gynecologic Office Procedure. In Teaching Slide Sets in Cytology, vol. 27. Edited by GL Wied. Chicago, Tutorials of Cytology, 1979.
24. Joensson G, Diczfalusy E, Plantin LO, Roenl L, Birke G: Estradurin (polyestradiol phosphate) in the treatment of prostatic carcinoma: A clinical and steroid metabolic study. Acta Endocrinol [Suppl] 83:3–41, 1963.
25. Keebler CM, Wied GL: Use of the estrogen test as an aid in differential diagnostic problems related to screening the cell sample from the postmenopausal patient. Acta Cytol 18:482–493, 1974.
26. Kittrich M: Zytodiagnostik des Fruchtwasserabflusses mit Hilfe von Nilblau. Geburtshilfe Frauenheilkd 23:156–163, 1963.
27. Lichtfus CJP: Vaginal cytology at the end of pregnancy. Acta Cytol 3:247–251, 1959.
28. Martinez-Manatou J, Giner-Velasquez J, Cortes-Gallegos V, Aznar R, Brdjas B, Guitterez-Najara Rudel NW: Daily progestogen for contraception: A clinical study. Br Med J 2:730–732, 1967.
29. Martinez-Manatou J, Giner-Velasquez J, Rudel H: Continuous progestogen contraception: A dose relationship study with chlormadinone acetate. Fertil Steril 18:57–62, 1967.
30. McLennan MT, McLennan CE: Hormonal patterns in vaginal smears from puerperal women. Acta Cytol 19:431–433, 1975.
31. McRae DJ: Correlation between vaginal cytology and urinary hormone assays in pregnancy. Acta Cytol 11:45–50, 1967.
32. Meisels A: The maturation value. Acta Cytol 11:249, 1967.
33. Montanari GD, Marconato A, Montanari GR, Grismondi GL: Granulation tissue on the vault of the vagina after hysterectomy for cancer: Diagnostic problems. Acta Cytol 12:25–29, 1968.
34. Morris JMcL, van Wagenen G: Compounds interfering with ovum implantation and development. Am J Obstet Gynecol 96:804–823, 1966.
35. Nyklicek O: Importance of vaginal cytogram for diagnosis and therapy in the deficiency of estrogenic hormones. Gynecol Invest 131:173, 1951.
36. Papanicolaou GN: On the continuation of sexual rhythm in a woman after menopause. Anat Rec 64:37, 1936.
37. Papanicolaou GN: The diagnosis of early human pregnancy by the vaginal smear method. Proc Soc Exp Biol Med 22:436–437, 1925.
38. Papanicolaou GN: New cancer diagnosis. In Proceedings of the Third Race Betterment Conference, New York, 1928.
39. Papanicolaou GN: The sexual cycle in the human female as revealed by vaginal smear. Am J Anat 52:519–637, 1933.
40. Papanicolaou GN, Ripley HS, Shorr E: Suppressive action of testosterone propionate on menstruation and its effects on vaginal smears. Endocrinology 24:339–346, 1939.
41. Papanicolaou GN, Traut HF: Diagnosis of Uterine Cancer by the Vaginal Smear. New York, Commonwealth Fund, 1943.
42. Papanicolaou GN, Traut HF, Marchetti AA: The Epithelia of Woman's Reproductive Organs. New York, Commonwealth Fund, 1948.
43. Patten SF Jr: Diagnostic Cytology of the Uterine Cervix. In Monographs in Clinical Cytology, vol 3. Edited by GL Wied. Basel, S Karger, 1969.

44. Pouchet FA: Theorie Positive de l'Ovulation Spontanee et de la Fecondation des Mammiferes et de l'Espece Humaine, Basee sur l'Observation de Tante la Serie Animale. Paris, Bailliere, 1847.

45. Puittarajurs BV, Taylor W: The relationship between urinary excretion of ovarian hormone metabolites and cornification of the vaginal epithelium during the menstrual cycle. J Endocrinol 18:67–76, 1959.

46. Pundel JP: Vaginal cytology at the end of pregnancy. Acta Cytol 3:253–263, 1959.

47. Pundel JP, Lichtfus C: La pycnose nucleire des cellules vaginales. Bull Soc R Belge Gynecol Obstet 26:630, 1956.

48. Pundel JP, Van Meensel F: Gestation et Cytologie Vaginale. Paris, Masson & Cie, 1951.

49. Rakoff AE: Gynecologic endocrinology. In Progress in Gynecology, vol, 2. Edited by JV Meigs, S Sturgis. New York, Grune & Stratton, 1950.

50. Rakoff AE, Takeda M: Gynecologic Endocrinopathies. In Teaching Slide Sets in Cytology, vol, 13. Edited by GL Wied. Chicago, Tutorials of Cytology, 1979.

51. Reyniak JV, Sedlis A, Stone D, Connell E: Cytohormonal findings in patients using various forms of contraception. Acta Cytol 13:315–322, 1969.

52. Rudel HW, Martinez-Manatou J, Maqueo-Topete M: The role of progestogens in the hormonal control of fertility. Fertil Steril 16:158–169, 1965.

53. Schneider V, Friedrich E, Schindler AE: Hormonal cytology: A correlation with plasma estradiol, measured by radioimmunoassay. Acta Cytol 21:37–39, 1977.

54. Shorr E: New technic for staining vaginal smears. III. A single differential stain. Science 94:545–546, 1941.

55. Shorr E, Papanicolaou GN: Action of gonadotropic hormones in amenorrhea as evaluated by vaginal smears. Proc Soc Exp Biol Med 41:629–636, 1939.

56. Soost HJ: Comparative studies on the degree of proliferation of the vaginal and ectocervical epithelium in the hormonal evaluation of a patient by means of exfoliative cytology. Acta Cytol 4:199–209, 1960.

57. Stern E, Crowley LG, Weiner JM, Hopkins CE, Marmoston J: Correlation of vaginal smear patterns with urinary hormone excretion. Acta Cytol 10:110–118, 1966.

58. Stockard CR, Papanicolaou GN: A rhythmical "heat period" in the guinea pig. Science 46:1176–1182, 1917.

59. Symposium on administered estrogens. Acta Cytol 2:331–337, 1958.

60. Symposium on androgenic effects. Acta Cytol 1:70–71, 1957.

61. Symposium on cytological terminology. Acta Cytol 2:26–27, 1958.

62. Symposium on sex chromatin. Acta Cytol 6:1–12, 1962.

63. Teter J: The use of selected cytologic indices for evaluation of estrogenicity of synthetic compounds. Acta Cytol 16:366–375, 1972.

64. von Bertalanffy L, Masin F, Masin M: Use of acridine orange fluorescence technique in exfoliative cytology. Science 124:1024–1025, 1956.

65. von Haam E: The cytology of pregnancy. Acta Cytol 5:320–329, 1961.

66. Wachtel E: Exfoliative Cytology in Gynaecological Practice. Washington, DC, Butterworth, 1964.

67. Wied GL: Climacteric amenorrhea: A cytohormonal test for differential diagnosis. Obstet Gynecol 9:646–649, 1957.

68. Wied GL: The cytologic changes of vaginal epithelial cells and the leukorrhea following estrogenic therapy. Am J Obstet Gynecol 70:51–59, 1955.

69. Wied GL: Hormonal evaluation of a patient through cytologic interpretation. Acta Union Int Cancer 14:277–285, 1958.

70. Wied GL: Importance of the site from which vaginal smears are taken. Am J Clin Pathol 25:742–750, 1955.

71. Wied GL: Phase contrast microscopy in office technique for prescreening of cytologic vaginal smears. Am J Obstet Gynecol 71:806–818, 1956.

72. Wied GL: Suggested standard for karyopyknosis: Use in hormonal reading of vaginal smears. Fertil Steril 6:61–65, 1955.

73. Wied GL (moderator): Symposium on hormonal cytology. Acta Cytol 12:87–92, 1968.

74. Wied GL: Terminology of cytologic reporting of endocrinologic conditions. Acta Cytol 8:383–384, 1964.

75. Wied GL, Bahr GF: Vaginal, cervical and endocervical smears on a single slide. Obstet Gynecol 14:362–367, 1959.

76. Wied GL, Bibbo M: The effects of sex steroids on the vaginal epithelium. In Advances in Steroid Biochemistry and Pharmacology. Edited by MH Briggs. New York, Academic Press, 1970.

77. Wied GL, Bibbo M: Evaluation of the endocrinologic condition of the patient by means of vaginal cytology. In Compendium on Diagnostic Cytology, 4th ed. Edited by GL Wied, LG Koss, JW Reagan. Chicago, Tutorials of Cytology, 1976.

78. Wied GL, Bibbo M: Hormonal cytology of the female genital tract. In Pathways to Conception. Springfield, IL, Charles C Thomas, 1971.

78a. Wied GL, Bibbo M: Evaluation of endocrinologic condition by exfoliative cytology. In Gynecologic Endocrinology, 3rd ed. Edited by JJ Gold, JB Josimovich. New York, Harper and Row, 1980.

79. Wied GL, Davis ME: Comparative activity of progestational agents on the human endometrium and vaginal epithelium of surgical castrates. Ann NY Acad Sci 71:599–616, 1958.

80. Wied GL, Davis ME: Cytologic screening during pregnancy. Clin Obstet Gynecol 6:573–603, 1963.

81. Wied GL, Davis ME: Synergism and antagonism of sex steroids as determined on the vaginal epithelial cells. Ann NY Acad Sci 83:207–216, 1959.

82. Wied GL, Davis ME, Frank R, Segal PB, Meier P, Rosenthal E: Statistical evaluation of the effect of hormonal contraceptives cytological smear pattern. Obstet Gynecol 27:327–334, 1966.

83. Wied GL, del Sol JR, Dargan AM: Progestational and androgenic substances tested on the highly proliferated vaginal epithelium of surgical castrates. I. Progestational substances. Am J Obstet Gynecol 75:98–111, 1958.

84. Wied GL, del Sol JR, Dargan AM: Progestational and androgenic substances tested on the highly proliferated vaginal epithelium of surgical castrates. II. Androgenic substances. Am J Obstet Gynecol 75:289–300, 1958.

85. Wied GL, Keebler CM: Hormonal cytology. In Teaching Slide Sets in Cytology, vol. 8. Edited by GL Wied. Chicago, Tutorials of Cytology, 1973.

86. Wied GL, Manglano JI: A comparative study of the Papanicolaou technic and the acridine-orange fluorescence method. Acta Cytol 6:554–568, 1962.

87. Young S, Bulbrook RD, Greenwood FC: The correlation between urinary estrogen and vaginal cytology. Lancet 1:350–353, 1957.

8

Microbiology, Inflammation and Viral Infections

Prabodh K. Gupta

The lower female genital tract, the vulva, the vagina, the cervix and the uterine cavity, is in direct communication with the external environment and so is prone to the various noninfectious and infectious inflammatory reactions. Although most of these remain confined locally, sometimes the infectious processes can be progressive and the organisms may ascend to the fallopian tubes and the ovaries. Occasionally, microbial infections can disseminate via the peritoneal space or the hematogenous or lymphatic routes.

It must be appreciated that although a large number of women harboring genital infections may remain asymptomatic, vaginal infection may produce a number of clinical symptoms. Increased vaginal secretions, along with sloughed vaginal epithelial cells, bacteria and inflammatory cells, constitute the symptomatic *leukorrhea*. Vulvovaginal irritation, itching, pain, ulceration with bleeding and warty growths are some of the other common presenting features of vaginal infections.

VAGINAL MICROBIOLOGY

In healthy women, the vaginal milieu is polymicrobial and contains a large number and variety of aerobic as well as obligate and facultative anaerobic organisms.[91] The most frequently recovered bacteria include *lactobacilli, Streptococcus viridans* and *Staphylococcus*

epidermidis; all of these women are asymptomatic. *Bacteroides* and *Gardnerella vaginalis* may be culturable from 20% and 30 to 50% of the asymptomatic women, respectively. *Staphylococcus* occurs infrequently in the healthy vaginal flora. Table 8–1 depicts the microorganisms that can be commonly recovered from vaginal specimens.

Pregnancy does not appear to affect the microbial composition of the vagina significantly. Estrogen hormones and similar substances help in the epithelial maturation of the vagina and support the growth of an extraordinary number of microbes. Transplacental hormonal exchanges influence the vaginal epithelium of the newborn infant. Bacterial composition and an adult type of microenvironment may occur in a newborn female infant. Menarchal and menopausal changes also affect the bacterial make-up of the vagina. Hormone or hormone-like medications, oral contraceptives, intrauterine contraceptive devices (IUDs), barrier diaphragms, pessaries and other similar substances and contraptions may directly or indirectly influence the microbial balance of the lower genital tract.[58] Common factors influencing the vaginal microbial flora are presented in Table 8–2. It must be appreciated that the vaginal flora is dynamic in health. It contains a large

TABLE 8–1. Common Microbial Organisms in the Vaginal Flora

Lactobacilli	*Bacteroides* species
Diphtheroids	*Peptococcus* species
Staphylococcus species	*Peptostreptococcus* species
Streptococcus species	*Fusobacterium* species
Enterobacter (not group A)	*Clostridium* species
Gardnerella vaginalis	*Bifidobacterium*

TABLE 8–2. Common Factors Influencing Vaginal Microbial Flora

Physiologic	Diseases and Drugs	Local Factors
Parturition	Hepatic disorders	Infections
Pregnancy	Hormonal imbalance	IUD
Menstruation	Metabolic diseases	Pessary
Menopause	Erosion and infections	Diaphragm
	Oral contraceptives	Vaginal douche
	Hormonal mimic drugs	Surgery
	Antibodies	Trauma
		Abortion
		Sexual exposure

115

TABLE 8–3. Cytologic Features of Vaginopancervical Smears in Infective Processes

General	Cellular Degenerative Changes	Cellular Reactive Changes
Background changes	Nuclear	Hyperplasia and repair
Acute and chronic inflammation and cellular obscuring	Cytoplasmic	Metaplasia
		Parakeratosis
Fresh and old blood		Hyperkeratosis
Cytolysis		Pseudoparakeratosis
Cell distribution changes		Multinucleation
		Histiocytic proliferation
		Dysplasia

number of organisms that, under not too well understood circumstances, may become pathogenic and cause disease.

General Features

There are a number of general cytologic features that represent the effects of infective processes. These include the changes listed in Table 8–3. Specific cytologic alterations frequently are associated with certain infections; they are described in their respective areas. Only some of these may occur in specific inflammatory conditions.

Background

Inflammation and Morphologic Obscuring. Overgrowth of microbes in the vaginal milieu may result in obscuring of the morphologic details in the smear (Figs. 8–1 and 8–2). In such smears, numerous polymorphonuclear leukocytes are present, often interspersed with a large number of histiocytes. Excessive bacterial growth may also contribute to cellular obscuring. It must be realized that no meaningful evaluation of

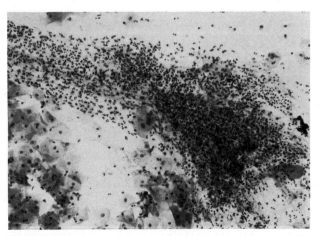

FIGURE 8–1. Heavy, acute inflammatory reaction to **polymicrobial infection** (Papanicolaou stain; vaginopancervical smear; ×273.5).

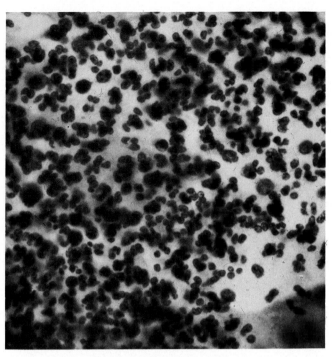

FIGURE 8–2. Polymicrobial infection. High-power view of the same specimen as in Figure 8–1. Notice the overwhelming, acute inflammatory response intermixed with numerous macrophages. In this particular case, recurrent cervical carcinoma cells were embedded in the inflammatory exudate (Papanicolaou stain; vaginopancervical smear; ×700).

cellular change may be possible on such smears. In all such cases, it is almost mandatory that appropriate therapy be initiated and a repeat smear examined before an opinion is rendered. Atrophic epithelium of the vagina is particularly prone to inflammatory changes. In cases with overwhelming inflammatory exudate it may not be possible to differentiate vaginitis from cervicitis and endocervicitis.

Cellular specimens from specific areas, e.g., the vaginal, cervical, and endocervical smear,[99] or vulvar or lateral vaginal wall scrapings, may reveal inflammatory response in one or more preparations that can help localize the infective process within the lower genital tract. A specific cervical inflammation with predominant lymphohistiocytic reaction is observed in follicular cervicitis. Granulomatous reaction may occur with foreign bodies (suture, IUD and so forth) or specific infections such as tuberculosis.

Bleeding. Both fresh and old bleeding may be observed in infectious processes. Postmenopausal women with atrophic, thin vaginal mucosa may bleed more easily. Similar changes may occur in *Trichomonas vaginalis* infection, which produces the typical "strawberry lesion."[35] Capillaries at the tips of papillae can readily bleed. Whereas the fresh bleeding is recognizable without much difficulty, old bleeding observed as fibrin should be differentiated from mucus. Fibrin threads are uniformly thick and reveal nodal formations at the points of intersections of interlacing threads. Sometimes, hemosiderin pigment may be observed. It is generally seen within the macrophages,

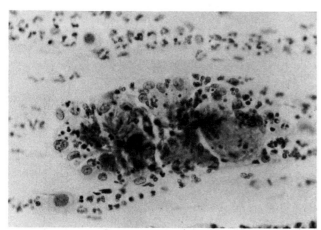

FIGURE 8–3. Hematoidin crystals, also known as cockleburs, seen in this specimen. These orangeophilic, amorphous structures are often associated with old bleeding, as in abortion, or with major blood group incompatibility between husband and wife during pregnancy (Papanicolaou stain; vaginopancervical smear; ×875).

but can occur extracellularly. Sometimes, old hemorrhage may contain hematoidin crystals that appear as cockleburs, as described by Hollander and Gupta (Fig. 8–3).[45]

Cytolysis. Cytolysis commonly affects the intermediate squamous epithelial cells. The process is believed to be glycogen dependent. Late menstrual cycle and pregnancy often reveal lactobacilli overgrowth. Pale staining, vesicular nuclei with little or no cytoplasm of the intermediate cells predominate in such smears. Numerous lactobacilli may occur interspersed with the cellular remnants (Fig. 8–4).

Cellular Changes. In the healthy state, normal women almost always have only two cell types, i.e., intermediate and superficial cells in their vaginopancervical smears. Heavy inflammation frequently causes an exfoliation of parabasal cells in the vaginal smear.

Although often present in postmenopausal women and in the immediate postpartum period, occurrence of three types of cells in the premenopausal age group should be carefully evaluated. Also, caution should be exercised in rendering hormonal evaluation in smears with excessive inflammation. The parabasal cells may exfoliate from ulceration of the squamous epithelium of the vagina and the ectocervix.

Under the persistent effect of various microbial infections and inflammatory reactions, both squamous and columnar epithelial cells may undergo degenerative changes. Almost all of these changes are nonspecific, but their identification helps in the proper interpretation of more serious cellular features. This is critical because most degenerative changes are accompanied by concurrent regenerative and reactive changes.

Cellular Degeneration. The cytoplasm of the squamous and columnar cells may be completely or partially dissolved in inflammatory states. However, the major changes are observed within the nuclei. These have been detailed by Frost.[23] Briefly, the nuclei may become compact, dense and pyknotic with loss of all chromatinic details (Fig. 8–5). Such nuclei may have a distinct clearing or hollow all around them, giving the perinuclear "halo" (Fig. 8–6) that is often seen in association with *Trichomonas* and other infections. Nuclei that are undergoing degenerative changes frequently lose the sharp details of their nuclear envelope, the chromatin and the interphase. The nuclear chromatin may clump irregularly or appear beaded along the nuclear margins. They become blurry and opaque. Other changes include nuclear swelling, with partial or total disintegration of the nuclear envelope, karyorrhexis and karyopyknosis (Fig. 8–7).

Cellular Regenerative (Repair) Changes in Inflammatory Reactions. The epithelial cells of the lower genital tract (ectocervix, endocervix and transforma-

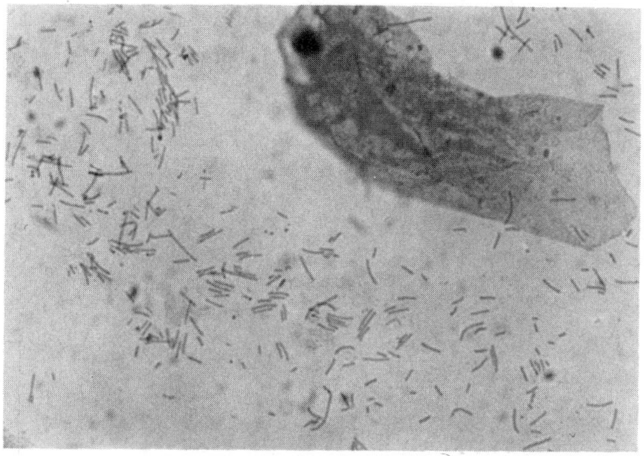

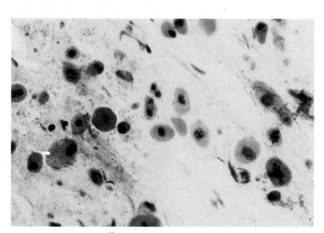

FIGURE 8–5. Nuclear degeneration. Notice the pyknotic and degenerating nuclei that show nuclear fragmentation and lack of detail (Papanicolaou stain; vaginopancervical smear; ×875). (Reproduced with permission from Gupta PK, Heustis DG, Bonfiglio TA, Neiberg RK, Lin F: Cytology of the female genital tract. *In* Practical Cytopathology. Astairita RW (ed). New York, Churchill Livingstone, 1990.)

FIGURE 8–4. *Lactobacillus.* Notice the numerous elongated bacillary structures. These appear predominantly under the effect of progesterones and can be overwhelming, causing extensive cytolysis as during pregnancy (Papanicolaou stain; vaginopancervical smear; ×1378).

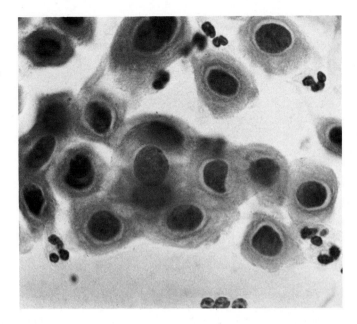

FIGURE 8–6. Perinuclear clearing or halos. This kind of degenerative change is often seen in inflammatory conditions like trichomoniasis. The nuclei of such cells may show varying degrees of degeneration (Papanicolaou stain; vaginopancervical smear; ×1378).

tion zone), under the influence of persistent irritation (infections and noninfections) and repair, undergo morphologic changes commonly referred to as metaplasia. This essentially reflects a benign process of tissue repair. Geirsson and coworkers[26] referred to these as atypical reparative changes (ARC). The majority of these changes are believed to be derived from the columnar and squamous epithelia, but reserve or pleopotential cells may also partake in the genesis of the metaplasia. It must be appreciated that there is a continuum of changes observed in the healing phase and the changes, for convenience, are grouped under the term metaplasia.

The earliest discernible changes are referred to as presquamous metaplasia: columnar differentiation phase, or type I ARC of the cervical columnar epithelium. Under the effect of chronic irritations and repair processes, the surface cells of the columnar epithelium continue to mature, and there is a proliferation of the basal or reserve cells. These small, undifferentiated cells commonly occur in small tissue fragments. They have high nucleocytoplasmic ratios and prominent nucleoli (Fig. 8–8). The nuclear chromatin is fine and uniformly distributed, and the nuclear membrane is well delineated and thin. These may have an inflammatory background. The cells of subluminal origin can often be mistaken for undifferentiated neoplasia.

As the changes evolve, the subluminal cells differentiate from the germinal layers upwards. These changes reflect the immature squamous metaplastic epithelium and have been referred to as ARC type II.

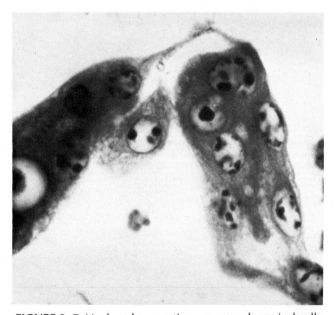

FIGURE 8–7. Nuclear degeneration among endocervical cells infected with **adenovirus infection.** The infected cells show disintegration of the nuclear envelope, karyorrhexis and karyopyknosis (Papanicolaou stain; vaginopancervical smear; ×1378).

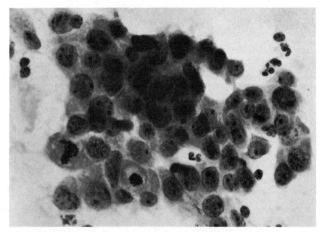

FIGURE 8–8. Columnar phase of **squamous metaplasia.** Numerous columnar metaplastic cells with prominent nuclei and coarse chromatin pattern are seen. Notice the mitotic figures and the inflammatory background (Papanicolaou stain; vaginopancervical smear; ×875).

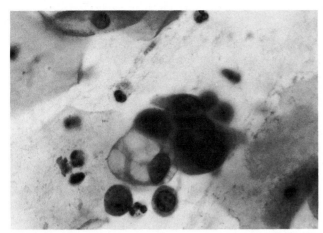

FIGURE 8–9. Squamous metaplastic changes with **columnar cell hyperplasia.** Notice the excessive mucus production and goblet cell formation in these columnar cells. An occasional cell has dense cytoplasm revealing a squamoid differentiation. The background is acute inflammatory (Papanicolaou stain; vaginopancervical smear; × 1378).

The cells may appear to be columnar and have excessive goblet proliferation and mucus production. Signet-ring forms may be recognized. These cells can have numerous macronucleoli, coarse chromatin and modest but pale cytoplasm. If not carefully examined, the changes can be mistaken for adenocarcinoma of the endocervix (Fig. 8–9).

Keratinizing Stratified Squamous Metaplasia. As the changes progress from the subluminal via the presquamous to the keratinizing stratified squamous phase, the cells become oval or polygonal with sharp borders and dense cytoplasm. They lie in sheets and reveal no obvious cilia and mucus. Intercellular bridges may be seen at times. These cells with their metaplastic changes have been called ARC type III. The nuclear changes may be reactive or degenerative with pyknosis. These cells may be mistaken for squamous cell carcinoma (Fig. 8–10).

Squamous Epithelium

When stressed, as by a chronic infective injury, squamous epithelium responds in a number of ways. These changes essentially represent alteration of functional differentiation of the affected cells and are mostly cytoplasmic in nature. Proper identification of these cytoplasmic features is necessary, as they may mask a more serious underlying disease process. These changes are hyperkeratosis, parakeratosis, basal cell hyperplasia, pseudoparakeratosis and dyskeratosis, and have been discussed elsewhere in this book. These changes reflect abnormalities of maturation with normal keratin formation in cells that normally do not reveal these changes.

Dyskeratosis is mentioned here for its relationship with viral infections and developing cancer. This represents an abnormality of the squamous cells in which the cytoplasmic maturation is altered. The affected

cells reveal premature, hypermature or atypical keratinization. It is a common occurrence in the presence of chronic infections, such as human papilloma virus (HPV). The cytomorphologic features are further detailed in the appropriate sections.

Endocervical Columnar Epithelium

Under the effect of chronic infection, stimulation and irritation, columnar epithelial cells undergo certain changes. These include squamous metaplasia (discussed earlier) and columnar cell hyperplasia and hyperplastic polyps.

Columnar Cell Hyperplasia. Columnar cells of the endocervix frequently enlarge and produce excessive mucus. Such changes occur in chronic irritation of the endocervical canal, such as among women using IUDs[34] and are discussed separately.

The Hyperplastic Polyp. Hyperplastic endocervical columnar cells may proliferate to produce finger-like epithelial processes—polyps. As described by Ramzy[78] and Frost,[22] these polyps are three-dimensional structures with three distinct planes—a floor or base composed of a sheet of polygonal cells, a middle plane that makes the sides of the polyp and a top or surface layer that, like the base, is also a sheet of polygonal cells. In the center of the polyp a connective tissue core that contains fibroblasts, collagen and capillary vessels may be recognizable.

INFECTIONS OF THE FEMALE GENITAL TRACT

Bacterial Infections

Bacterial Vaginitis. One of the most common causes of vaginal discharge is *nonspecific vaginitis*, as de-

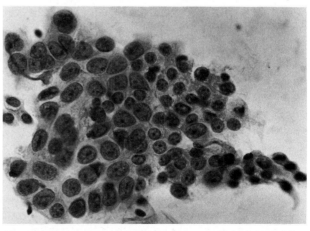

FIGURE 8–10. Metaplastic changes revealing **keratinizing stratified squamous metaplasia.** These cells are polygonal and appear as immature squamoid in configuration. Occasionally, intercellular bridges may be observed in such cell groups (Papanicolaou stain; vaginopancervical smear; × 875).

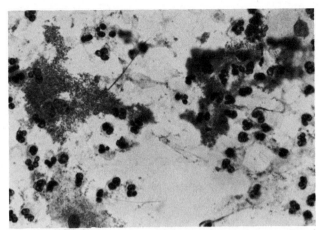

FIGURE 8–11. **Mixed coccobacillary organisms** in the background. Notice the acute inflammatory reaction and pronounced epithelial cell degeneration (Papanicolaou stain; vaginopancervical smear; ×875).

scribed by Gardner and Dukes.[25] It is also known as *nonspecific vaginosis,* so named by Blackwell and Barlow,[11] or *bacterial vaginosis,* a term used by Spiegel and associates.[92] Schnadig and coworkers[83] have suggested the term *bacterial bacteriosis* for the entity.

Bacteria most commonly infect the female genital tract. Nonspecific organisms including mixed bacteria and coccobacilli were reported to occur in nearly 20% of patients seen by Bibbo and Wied[10] at the University of Chicago. These infections are frequently seen in children and may be hormonally dependent. Vaginal or vaginopancervical smears often reveal a number of bacilli and cocci organisms (mixed infections) as detailed by Wied and Bibbo (Fig. 8–11).[100] These organisms, although diffusely scattered, may occur in clumps and as microcolonies. Specific species identification can only be made by appropriate microbiologic isolation techniques but is generally not considered necessary for clinical management of the disease.

Lactobacillus Vaginitis. Lactobacilli are a heterogenous group of organisms that are normally present in the vaginal flora. They occur in abundance in the late luteal phase and in pregnancy, prefer an acid environment and are common among women on hormonal medications and in the premenarchal and menopausal age groups. They are gram-positive, immobile, non-spore-forming anaerobes or faculative anaerobes. Certain species may be aerobic in their growth characteristics. The glycogen-rich intermediate cells are often lysed in the presence of lactobacilli. Smears in such cases show cellular crowding, cytolysis with cytoplasmic debris and numerous bare nuclei occurring in a predominantly bacillary background.

Depending upon the day of the menstrual cycle, lactobacilli may be observed in up to 50% of healthy women. In the symptomatic population, the observed figure may be lower, about 20%. It is debatable if pure lactobacilli (an unlikely occurrence) produce vaginitis, although vaginal discharge and leukorrhea may occur as a result of excessive cytolysis.

Gardnerella Vaginitis. *G. vaginalis* is the current

term used to describe the organism variously named as *Haemophilus vaginalis* and *Corynebacterium vaginalis.* The organisms were first described by Gardner and Dukes.[24] They stated, "Any woman whose ovarian activity is normal and who has a gray, homogenous, malodorous vaginal discharge with a pH of 5.0 to 5.5 that yields no trichomonads is likely to have *Haemophilus vaginalis* vaginitis."

Morphologically, the organisms are gram-negative or gram-variable, 0.1 to 0.8 nm in diameter and appear bacillary or coccobacillary. The microbe, although it shares many characteristics with *Corynebacterium,* is catalase-negative and now classified separately. Petersdorf and colleagues[74] and Ledger and associates[60] found that as many as 40 to 50% of women may have vaginal infection with *G. vaginalis* and be asymptomatic. Leukorrhea and pruritus with inflamed vaginal mucosa and occasional punctate hemorrhages are commonly observed among symptomatic women. It is believed that patients with pure *G. vaginalis* infection are asymptomatic when the vaginal pH is less than 4.5. The synergistic relationship is altered when secondary organisms interplay with *G. vaginalis.* A raised pH over 4.5 (5.0 to 6.5) and an interaction with various bacteroides and peptococci may produce the clinical disease.

Patients with a high pH of the vagina have a vaginal discharge with a distinct fishy odor. This odor is more manifest when the pH is further raised by potassium hydroxide (KOH) in the *whiff test.*[102] Such preparations of vaginal reactions and KOH, when examined microscopically, have the diagnostic *clue cells* (Fig. 8–12). Normal polygonal squamous cells have thin, transparent cytoplasm that is covered over by tiny coccobacillary forms of *G. vaginalis.* Changes are best seen at the edge of the "infected" cells. The cell borders may be indistinct and on a different plane of focus. Similar "clue cells" are observed in the fixed and stained Papanicolaou preparations (Fig. 8–13). A variable

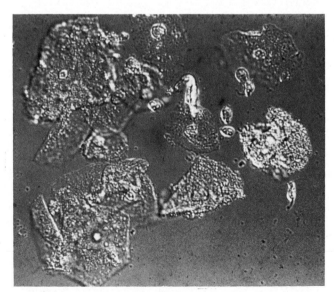

FIGURE 8–12. **"Clue cells."** This photomicrograph was taken under phase contrast. (Unstained; vaginopancervical smear; ×546). (Courtesy of Dr. Belur Bhagavan.)

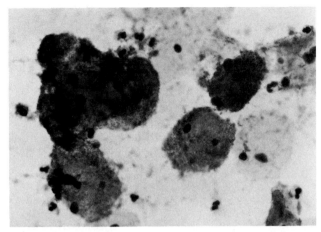

FIGURE 8–13. *Gardnerella vaginalis* infection. Notice the presence of numerous "clue cells." The background is relatively clean. The organisms are not only covering the surface of the epithelial cells but are stretching beyond the outlines of such cells (Papanicolaou stain; vaginopancervical smear; ×700).

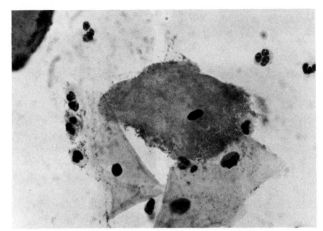

FIGURE 8–15. The single epithelial cell in the center reveals the sticking of the **coccobacillary organisms** gathered at the edges. The cytoplasm appears devoid of any microbial organisms. Such cells should not be considered diagnostic for *Gardnerella vaginalis* infection (Papanicolaou stain; vaginopancervical smear; ×1102).

amount of acute inflammation may be present in the background. Mere complete or partial covering of the squamous epithelial cells by the organisms (Fig. 8–14), or their sticking to the cellular margins (Fig. 8–15) per se should not be considered diagnostic for *G. vaginalis*. To be diagnostic, clue cells should have bacterial organisms not only covering the surfaces of the affected cells but also spreading beyond the margins of the squamous cells.

A high degree of diagnostic accuracy exists in cytologic detection of clue cells and culture confirmation for *G. vaginalis*. Schnadig and coworkers[83] cultured *G. vaginalis* in nearly 90% of the cases that contained clue cells. This infection is believed to be sexually transmissible, and an accurate diagnosis is necessary.

Micrococcus Vaginitis (Toxic Shock). This group of microbes includes a large number of gram-positive coccoid organisms commonly observed in female genital tract smears, and gram-negative diplococci. *Staphylococcus aureus* may be recovered from the vagina in about 5% of normal women. These organisms frequently cause vaginitis and vaginal discharge, and may produce toxic shock syndrome. This association was documented by Shands and coworkers in 1980.[86] The organisms characteristically occur singly and can be seen within the polymorphonuclear leukocytes or other infected epithelial cells. Occasionally fragments of tampon fibers may be observed in vaginal smears (Fig. 8–16). The finding of coccoid organisms or tampon fibers in the vaginal smears does not have any correlation with the clinical occurrence of toxic shock syndrome.

Gonococcus Vaginitis. This gram-negative diplococcus causes abundant, purulent vaginal exudate. The infection affects the urethra and the perivaginal glands.

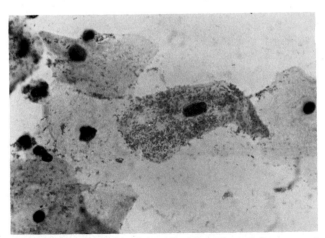

FIGURE 8–14. Total and partial obliteration of the two epithelial cells by the **coccobacillary organisms.** Cells that are covered only on the surface should per se not be considered diagnostic for *Gardnerella vaginalis* infection (Papanicolaou stain; vaginopancervical smear; ×1102).

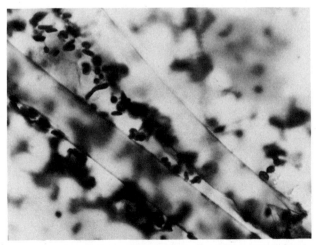

FIGURE 8–16. Tampon fibers. The two splinter-like objects are cellulose fibers from a tampon. Occasionally, these may have a capillary in the center, which may contain red blood cells (Papanicolaou stain; vaginopancervical smear; ×551).

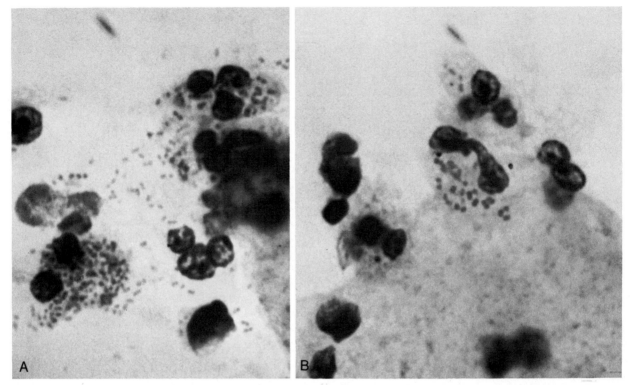

FIGURE 8–17. Gonococcal organisms. These two fields of the same slide reveal diploid structures within the polymorphonuclear leukocytes, on the surface of the epithelial cells and outside the cells. Although these organisms can be conveniently detected in Papanicolaou-stained preparations, such a diagnosis should not be rendered based on these preparations alone (Papanicolaou stain; vaginopancervical smear; ×1722).

The organism occurs as bean-shaped diplococci that are often seen on the surface of squamous cells. The gonococci are better observed in the air-dried areas of the smears, such as the edges. Within the swollen polymorphonuclear leukocytes, diplococci may be present in large numbers (Fig. 8–17). Gonococcus vaginitis is a venereal infection with important social and medical implications. Although detectable cytologically, we do not advise rendition of such a diagnosis on cytologic examination of Papanicolaou stained smears alone; they may be indistinguishable from other cocci organisms, phagocytosed debris or chlamydial organisms.

Curved Anaerobic Bacterial Vaginitis. These motile, anaerobic, rod-shaped organisms resemble *Wolinella* and have been recognized as a cause of nonspecific vaginitis by Hjelm and colleagues.[43] Although these bacteria cannot be easily diagnosed in Papanicolaou stained smears, they can be detected in wet mount preparations. Clinically, the presentation is of nonspecific vaginitis.

Foreign Body Vaginitis. A forgotten tampon is the most common cause of this type of vaginitis, in which there is a secondary overgrowth of anaerobic organisms. The tampons may irritate and ulcerate the vaginal wall and ectocervix. Occasionally, fragments of tampons can be observed in vaginal smears. Their presence is not diagnostic of vaginitis. Heavy acute inflammation, mucus and foreign body giant cells may be observed.

Granuloma Inguinale. This venereally transmitted infection is caused by gram-negative, encapsulated coccobacillary organisms called *Calymmatobacterium Donovani*. The infection produces large, ulcerated lesions that histologically reveal inflammatory granulation tissue and numerous macrophages. These macrophages are easily identifiable in ethanol-fixed Papanicolaou stained smears. They are plump and swollen and have a lobulated cytoplasm (Fig. 8–18). Within the cytoplasm a large number of coccobacillary (1 to 2μ) structures (Donovan bodies) are seen. These are

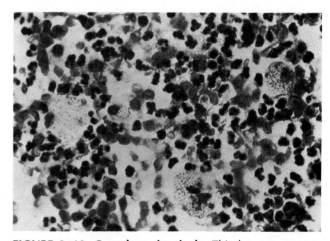

FIGURE 8–18. Granuloma inguinale. This low-power magnification reveals an acute inflammatory background with numerous pale, lobulated macrophages that contain the diagnostic organisms (Papanicolaou stain; vaginopancervical smear; ×875).

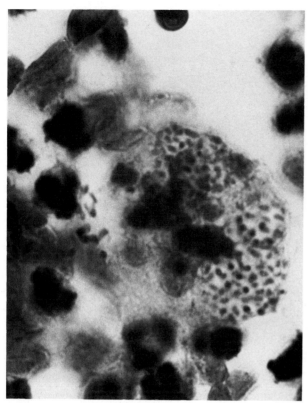

FIGURE 8–19. Donovan bodies. A higher magnification of the photomicrograph seen in Figure 8–18 reveals the detail of a single macrophage. Within the lobulated structures numerous safety pin–shaped bacillary structures are seen (Papanicolaou stain; vaginopancervical smear; ×1378).

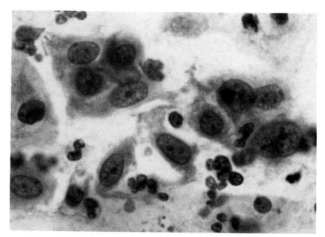

FIGURE 8–20. Detail of **epithelioid cells.** These cells from a case of tuberculosis of the cervix appear in syncytial formation. They have "soft" cytoplasm and irregular nuclear forms. Notice also the lymphoid cells present in the background (Papanicolaou stain; vaginopancervical smear; ×1102). (Case courtesy of Dr. S. Bhambhani.)

safety-pin shaped with terminal or polar thickening of the cell walls (Fig. 8–19). The organisms stain faintly with hematoxylin and eosin (H + E) dyes. They can be stained with Romanowsky or silver stains. Varying degrees of acute inflammation are commonly observed in the smears. The infection is more common in the tropics, and the incidence is high in India and New Guinea. Although reported, an association of granuloma inguinale and squamous cell carcinoma is controversial. It is true that the infection may cause extremely bizarre pseudoepitheliomatous hyperplasia of the squamous epithelium that can mimic neoplasm.

Tuberculosis. This is a disease of the tropics and is almost always secondary to extragenital, most often pulmonary, tubercular infection. The involvement is more common in the fallopian tubes and the endometrium and is thus difficult to detect cytologically. Angrish and Verma[1] reported a number of cases of cervical tuberculosis that were detected cytologically. The cervical smears reveal large aggregates of epithelioid cells. These appear as pale, cyanophilic cells in a syncytial formation with indistinct and arborizing borders and vesicular, oval nuclei (Fig. 8–20). Intermixed with these one may occasionally observe Langhans' type multinucleated giant cells (Fig. 8–21). These cells may contain as many as 20 to 30 peripherally arranged vesicular nuclei. A variable number of lymphocytes may be present in the background. Secondary infection is common in these ulcerated lesions, and heavy, acute

inflammatory exudate may be present. A cytologic diagnosis of granulomatous disease, probably tuberculosis, can be suggested under appropriate clinical and cytologic settings and situations in which a complete granuloma may be observed under low power microscopy (Fig. 8–22).

Malacoplakia. Malacoplakia is a rare disorder that may infect the cervix. We have observed two cases occurring in postmenopausal women with atrophic smears and persistent vaginal discharge.[50] Numerous macrophages with the characteristic intracytoplasmic, laminated inclusions (Michaelis-Gutmann bodies) may be observed (Fig. 8–23). They can be stained for calcium by appropriate histochemical techniques.[76]

Actinomyces. These organisms belong to the order of higher bacteria that also include Mycobacteriaceae and Streptomycetaceae. There are three common spe-

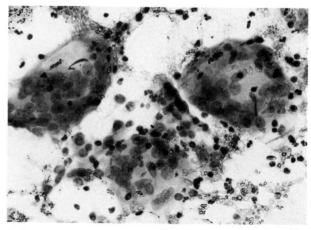

FIGURE 8–21. Langhans' type multinucleated giant cells. These cells are from a case of tuberculosis of the cervix. Notice the numerous lymphocytes in the background in a relatively clean preparation (Papanicolaou stain; vaginopancervical smear; ×700). (Case courtesy of Dr. S. Bhambhani.)

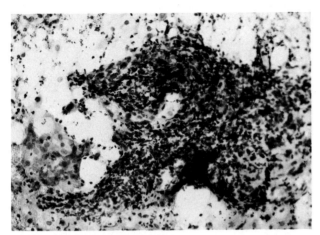

FIGURE 8–22. Tuberculous granuloma. This low-power view reveals a sampling of a total granuloma in the smear. Notice the multinucleated giant cells on the left side, the acute and chronic lymphocytic infiltration in the center and the necrotic element on the right side (Papanicolaou stain; vaginopancervical smear; ×218). (Specimen courtesy of Dr. S. Bhambhani.)

cies of *Actinomyces*—*A. israelii*, *A. bovis*, and *A. naeslundii*. These bacteria are nonmotile, nonspore-forming and anaerobic or facultative anaerobes. They are gram-positive and occur in filamentous and diphtheroid forms.

Although a common occurrence in the tonsilar crypts, tartar of teeth and the alimentary tract, *Actinomyces* do not occur as commensals in the vaginal flora. In the female genital tract, ascending infection is the most common mode of occurrence of the clinical disease; however, rarely, hematogenous, lymphatic or dissemination of infection from the alimentary tract or other distant sources may occur. Ascending infection occurs in the presence of intrauterine or intravaginal contraptions, IUDs of various types being the most common. Vaginal pessaries, surgical clamps and foreign bodies, including forgotten tampons, have all been

associated with vaginal *Actinomyces*. The clinical disease may manifest as much as 12 months after the retrieval of the *Actinomyces*-associated IUD.

Gupta has reviewed the subject and the relationship of *Actinomyces* with the clinical female genital tract disease.[32] It is appropriate to say that nearly 10% of women using an IUD may develop vaginal *Actinomyces* infection at some stage. If such users have symptoms of lower genital tract infection such as pelvic pain, vaginal discharge, bleeding, fever or lower abdominal tenderness, approximately one quarter of these women may have genital *Actinomyces* infection. Of the women using an IUD and being admitted to the hospital for clinically suspected pelvic inflammatory disease, about 40% may harbor the organism in the lower genital tract.[14, 62] Dissemination of the infection to distant sites has been documented by de la Monte and coworkers[19] and Hager and Majmudar.[40]

Cytomorphology of Actinomyces. In close proximity generally of the calcified and mineralized fragments of a disintegrating IUD, the *Actinomyces* organism can be detected in Papanicolaou stained vaginal smears. Typically, the organisms appear as spidery, amorphous clumps that are darker in the center (Fig. 8–24). These aggregates of *Actinomyces* in the cervicovaginal smears have been referred to as Gupta bodies by Hager and Majmudar. Upon careful examination, numerous filamentous organisms with acute angle branching patterns are recognizable in these clumps (Fig. 8–25). They appear uniformly thick and may be beaded. The filaments generally extend to the outer limits of the dark clumps. Occasionally only a few delicate, branching filamentous forms may occur scattered randomly in the

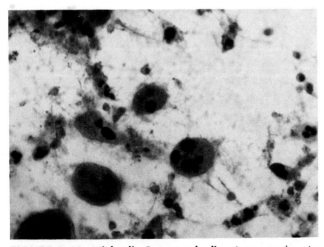

FIGURE 8–23. Michaelis-Gutmann bodies. Intracytoplasmic laminated structures from a case of malacoplakia of the cervix (Papanicolaou stain; vaginopancervical smear; ×875). (Case courtesy of Drs. K. Kapila and K. Verma.)

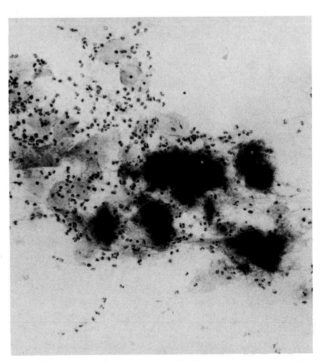

FIGURE 8–24. *Actinomyces.* In this low-power view, notice the distribution of dark, spidery structures along the endocervical component in the smear (Papanicolaou stain; vagino-pancervical smear; ×273).

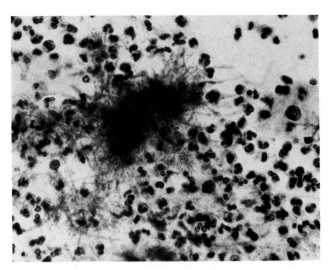

FIGURE 8–25. A higher magnification than that of Figure 8–24 of one of the colonies of **Actinomyces.** Notice the numerous filamentous structures radiating from the center. If carefully examined, such filaments often reveal acute-angle branching. A heavy, acute inflammatory reaction is present in the background (Papanicolaou stain; vaginopancervical smear; ×868).

smear. Calcified filamentous forms that may not be stainable by antigen antibody techniques, club forms or the Splendore Hoeppli phenomenon may be identified in Papanicolaou stained smears. Typical sulphur granules may be observed in smears obtained from symptomatic patients (Fig. 8–26). These per se are not diagnostic of *Actinomyces,* and proper morphologic identification of the filamentous forms is necessary in all cases. Various other morphologic forms have been detailed by Gupta and coworkers[36] and Gupta.[32]

Actinomyces organisms can be stained with modified Gram, periodic acid-Schiff (PAS) and silver stain. A definitive species diagnosis can be made by specific antigen antibody reaction using an immunoenzymatic or immunofluorescence technique or bacterial culture procedures.[89]

Actinomyces can be diagnosed with a high degree of accuracy in properly prepared Papanicolaou stained smears. Immunodiagnostic and culture techniques may be used to further confirm the species of the organisms. A number of organisms, including *Candida,* dermatophytes, *Nocardia* and bacterial aggregates, foreign substances such as sulfa drug crystals and contraceptive creams, among others, may resemble *Actinomyces* organisms. Hematoidin crystals described by Hollander and Gupta[44] have a resemblance to sulfur granules. The differential diagnosis of *Actinomyces* as seen in the vaginopancervical smears is given in Table 8–4.

We believe vaginal *Actinomyces* infections are acquired most commonly from exterior sources. Orogenital contact may be an important mode of acquiring the genital *Actinomyces* infection. It is believed that the "tail" of the IUD acts as a carrier for the ascent of the vaginal organisms. The tissue damage produced by the body and edges of the IUD causes a change in the oxygen reduction potential and alteration in the microbial milieu of the vagina. The changed environment is conducive to the growth of *Actinomyces.* Infection has been observed with all types of IUDs, although it is more common with devices with polyfilamentous thread and angular forms.

Occasionally, *Actinomyces* may occur with "black yeast," a fungus commonly found in unclean bathtubs and fixtures. It has large, dark-fruiting bodies, *Aureobasidium pullulans* (Fig. 8–27). As reported by de Moraes-Ruehsen and associates,[20] *Entamoeba gingivalis,* a protozoa of the oral cavity, may be found in association with *Actinomyces* in vaginal specimens (Fig. 8–28). An orogenital route of *Actinomyces* infection is a distinct possibility. These nonpathogenic protozoa should be distinguished from *Entamoeba histolytica* that occur in the alimentary tract and may cause lower genital tract infection and have been discussed separately.

IUD-Associated Cellular Changes. In addition to the alterations in the microbial environment and *Actinomyces* infection, usage of the IUD is associated with cellular changes. These occur in women who have used an IUD for 10 to 12 weeks or for a longer duration and as a result of chronic irritation by the IUD thread; they involve the endocervical cells and the endometrial

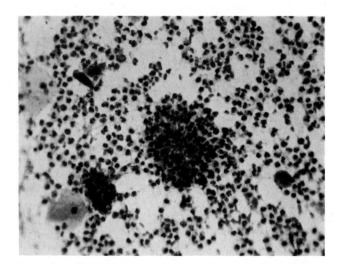

FIGURE 8–26. "Sulfur granule." In the center are radiating filamentous structures of *Actinomyces* organisms. "Sulfur granules," per se, are not specific for *Actinomyces.* When present with *Actinomyces* infections, however, patients generally are found to be symptomatic (Papanicolaou stain; vaginopancervical smear; ×636).

TABLE 8–4. Differential Diagnosis of Actinomyces in Vaginal Smears

	Filamentous Structures
Other Organisms	*Candida, Aspergillus, Nocardia, Penicillium, Trichophyton, Leptotrichia, Lactobacilli*
Miscellaneous Structures	Fibrin threads, mucus threads, sulfa crystals, cotton and synthetic fibers
	Nonfilamentous Structures
	Contraceptive cream, bacterial clumps, hematoxylin pigment, spermatozoa, hematoidin, foreign material (spores, pollen, douche ingredients)

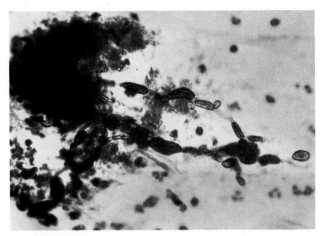

FIGURE 8–27. *Aureobasidium pullulans.* A smear from a patient with an IUD and *Actinomyces* reveals numerous large, budding yeast-like structures. These black organisms can vary in color from light yellow, to gold-brown, to black (Papanicolaou stain; vaginopancervical smear; ×551). (Reproduced with permission from Gupta PK: Intrauterine contraceptive device: vaginal cytology, pathologic changes and their clinical implications. Acta Cytol 26:571–613, 1982.)

cells located by the body of the IUD. It is important to properly recognize these morphologic features, since they can mimic and be confused with dysplastic and neoplastic cellular changes. There is no conclusive evidence for the association of squamous dysplastic changes and IUD usage. Squamous cell changes are essentially reactive and reparative in nature. These occur in about 40% of women using IUDs. DNA analysis of IUD-associated cellular changes does not reveal any aneuploidy.

The picture is further complicated by an interplay among the reactive-proplastic and degenerative-retroplastic changes occurring over a prolonged period of time and affected by polymicrobial and physiologic factors.

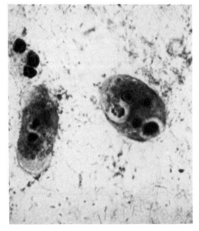

FIGURE 8–28. *Entamoeba gingivalis.* These irregular histiocyte-like structures have nuclei with central karyosomes and ingested leukocytic material within the cytoplasm (Papanicolaou stain; vaginopancervical smear; ×1378).

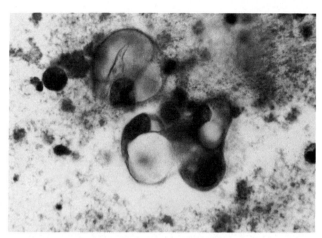

FIGURE 8–29. Extremely bizarre **glandular cells** occurring in an inflammatory background in a patient with IUD usage. Such cells, if not carefully examined, can be mistaken to represent a neoplastic process (Papanicolaou stain; vaginopancervical smear; ×1378).

Endocervical columnar cells may become hyperplastic with large papillary tissue fragments. Bibbo and coworkers[9] and Gupta and colleagues[34] have systematically reviewed these changes. Columnar cell hyperplastic changes should be distinguished from adenocarcinoma (Fig. 8–29). They may mimic papillary tumors of ovarian or endometrial origin. Single cells can be extremely bizarre and resemble neoplasia. The presence of heavy inflammation and degenerative changes helps diagnostically. The salient features of these cellular changes are summarized in Table 8–5. The presence of psammoma or calcified bodies among IUD users is not an indication of neoplasm.

Another cell type, best described as indeterminate cell changes or "IUD cells," probably arises from the endometrial surface. Such conclusions are supported by the work of Gupta and coworkers.[34] These high nucleocytoplasmic ratio cells should be distinguished from the third type of cell described by Graham[28] and *in situ* carcinoma cells. Nuclear degeneration, the presence of nucleoli and a hiatus between normal and abnormal cells help differentiate these cells from true neoplastic cells (Fig. 8–30). The salient features are summarized in Table 8–6. Occasionally, the endometrial-type reactive cells and the IUD cells may occur together.

TABLE 8–5. Comparison of IUD-Associated Columnar-Type Cells and Adenocarcinoma Cells

Feature	IUD Columnar Cells	Tumor Cells
Tumor diathesis	Absent	Present
Distribution	Endocervical component	Random
Inflammation	Present	Variable
Cellular degeneration	Present	Absent
"Bubble gum" cytoplasm	Present	Absent
Bare nuclei	Absent	Present
Cellular preservation	Poor	Good
Atypical histiocytic cells	Absent	Present

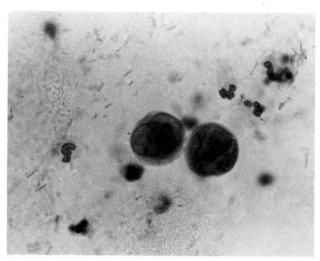

FIGURE 8–30. "IUD cells" from a patient wearing an IUD. These high nucleocytoplasmic (N/C) ratio cells appear to be of endometrial origin. They frequently show multinucleation, nuclear degeneration and nucleoli. If not carefully examined, these can be easily mistaken to represent cervical intraepithelial neoplasm (Papanicolaou stain; vaginopancervical smear; ×1378). (Reproduced with permission from Gupta PK: Intrauterine contraceptive device: vaginal cytology, pathologic changes and their clinical implications. Acta Cytol 26:571–613, 1982.)

Bi- and multinucleated giant forms and psammoma body formation are other findings that may be observed in the presence of the IUD and *Actinomyces*. These develop from the endometrial surface changes. Extensive squamous metaplasia of the endometrial surface may occur in some cases as the result of prolonged endometritis accompanying the IUD.

Leptotrichia buccalis. These microbes, also known as just *Leptotrichia*, are gram-negative, nonspore-forming anaerobic organisms. They occur in the oral and vaginal cavities as very thin, segmented, large, filamentous structures. Occasionally, branching may be observed (Fig. 8–31). Morphologically they may be indistinguishable from certain forms of Doederlein's bacillus. Most frequently (75 to 80%), cases of *Leptotrichia* have concomitant *T. vaginalis* infection. Numerous other infective organisms, including *Candida* and *G. vaginalis* may occur in the presence of *L. buccalis* infection.

An investigative study on the prevalence of *Lepto-*

TABLE 8–6. Comparison of IUD Cells and Cervical Intraepithelial Neoplasia (CIN) Cells

Feature	IUD Cell	CIN Cell
Distribution	Endocervical	Endocervical
Tissue fragments	Frequent	Uncommon
Inflammation	Present	Absent
Cellular degeneration	Present	Absent
Preservation	Poor	Good
Cellular hiatus	Present	Absent
Nucleoli	Present	Absent
Multinucleation	Present	Absent
IUD columnar cells	Present	Absent

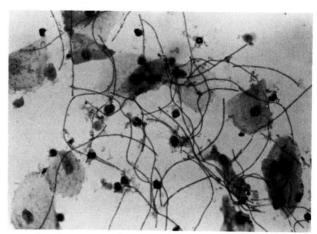

FIGURE 8–31. *Leptotrichia buccalis.* These elongated bacilary structures are commonly found in association with trichomoniasis. Occasionally, acute-angle branching may also be observed in these structures (Papanicolaou stain; vaginopancervical smear; ×875).

trichia in cervicovaginal smears was made by Bibbo and Wied.[10] They observed an associating *Leptotrichia* organism in 75% with trichomonads, 1.5% with Doederlein's bacillus, and about 1% among patients with fungal or *G. vaginalis* infection. The vast majority (47%) of the 1000 patients were oral contraceptive users. Pregnancy and menopause were other physiologic features, followed by the postpartum state, that were often associated with the presence of *L. buccalis* in cervical smears. Sometimes acute inflammatory changes may be observed in the presence of *Leptotrichia*.

Mycoplasma. These are the smallest known organisms capable of growing in cell-free media. A correlation between the occurrence of a "dirty" smear and mycoplasma was documented by Jones and Davson.[48] Mardh and coworkers[63] confirmed these findings and reported the occurrence of coccoid organisms both on the surface and in between the squamous epithelial

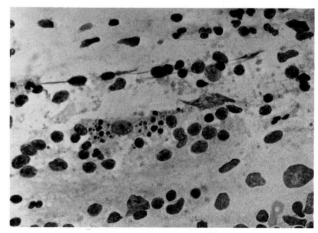

FIGURE 8–32. Follicular cervicitis. Notice the tingible body macrophages in the center surrounded by mature reactive lymphoid cells (Papanicolaou stain; vaginopancervical smear; ×1102).

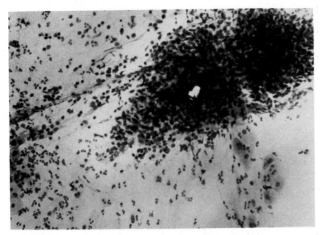

FIGURE 8–33. Follicular cervicitis. Notice the occurrence of a germinal follicle capillary in this particular smear (Papanicolaou stain; vaginopancervical smear; ×551).

cells in dirty smears in cases of *Mycoplasma*. Such features appear to have limited practical value.

Follicular Cervicitis. Also referred to as lymphocytic cervicitis, this is a specific type of cervical and sometimes vaginal infection in which the predominant feature is the occurrence of lymphoid follicles in the subepithelial areas. When examined cytologically, numerous mature and reactive lymphoid cells and germinal macrophages (tingible bodies) are seen (Fig. 8–32). At times a capillary from the germinal center of the lymphoid follicle may be scraped and observed in the smear (Fig. 8–33).[80] There is evidence that nearly 50% of the cases of follicular cervicitis are associated with *Chlamydia* infection.[37, 73] Follicular cervicitis is not uncommonly seen in postmenopausal atrophic smears. Precise pathogenesis of this condition is not well understood.

Viral Infections

Diseases caused by these intracellular organisms are among the most common in the human body and include a most heterogeneous group of clinical conditions. Although some of the viral infections have been affecting humanity for thousands of years, changes in society, social habits, medical practice and advances in diagnostic capabilities have resulted in a great many new viral diseases. Even though smallpox has been eradicated from the world, through the use of antibiotics and immunosuppressive therapies numerous dormant viral infections have become manifest.

Being intracellular by nature, viruses co-opt cellular metabolic processes in their replication. In addition to the nature of the affected tissues, the virus, general and local immune responses and the particular enzymatic derangements are important in determining the cytomorphologic changes and the nature of the tissue injury or injuries. In some common viral infections, these cellular changes may be quite typical and considered of diagnostic significance.

General Features of Viral Infection

Inclusion Formation. These are discrete, dense, homogeneous, round or oval intracellular structures consisting of viral particles in a matrix and generally represent a stage in the replication of the virus. These do not occur in all viral infections; their formation depends upon a particular agent and upon the affected tissue. Certain inclusions are typical and diagnostic. Inclusions may be observed within the nuclei, the cytoplasm or both together.

Hydropic or Ballooning Degeneration. This is often an effect of organelle membrane damage caused by the virus. Certain degenerative changes precede or accompany the development of inclusion bodies and are often used in the diagnostic evaluation of cellular changes (Fig. 8–34).

Necrosis. Viruses may cause coagulative necrosis and characteristic cytoplasmic changes. Most often the cytoplasm becomes opaque and thickened and loses its transparency and crispness. Nuclear degenerative changes with karyolysis and karyorrhexis may occur (Fig. 8–35). Only ghost forms of the infected cells may remain.

Giant Cell Formation. Alterations in the membrane composition of the infected cells contribute to the fusion of cells to produce syncytial and giant forms.

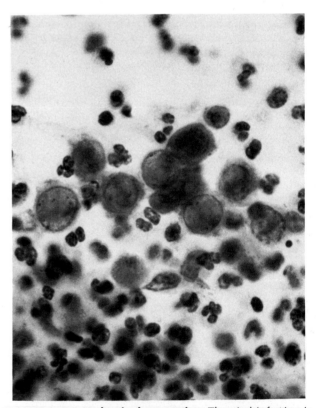

FIGURE 8–34. Hydropic degeneration. The viral infection in this specimen is causing this change in the infected cells. The cells have a clearing of the chromatin pattern, a migration of the chromatin to the nuclear margins and an obliteration of the nuclear detail. (Papanicolaou stain; vaginopancervical smear; ×818).

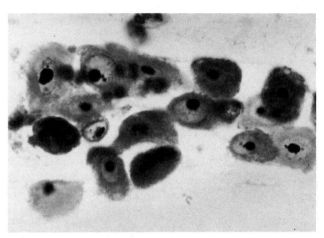

FIGURE 8–35. Nuclear degeneration with fragmentation and lysis of the chromatin pattern. This case represents the adenovirus infection in Figure 8–7 (Papanicolaou stain; vaginopancervical smear; ×700).

Sometimes nuclear inclusions may occur within the multinucleated forms.

Cellular Proliferation. Transient cellular proliferation is commonly seen in viral infections. These changes may be extreme and mimic dyskaryosis and neoplastic forms (Fig. 8–36).

Cellular Cohesion. In certain viral infections, the initial step is attachment to the host cell; viral proteins (antireceptors) adsorb to the cell surface furnished with appropriate receptors. The interaction may alter not only the surface of the infected cell but also the structure of the virion. Although not fully understood, viral detachment and readsorption perhaps contribute to cell clumps or plaque formation.

Cytoskeletal Changes. Cytoplasmic and nuclear changes frequently occur not as a result of the damage caused by the virus, but rather as a result of specific reorganization of the cellular or skeletal elements necessary for its growth. Alteration in intermediate keratin filaments and microtubules and cellular metabolism contribute to the formation of ciliocytophthoria

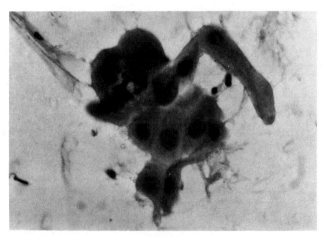

FIGURE 8–36. Atypical cellular proliferation in a case of **human papilloma virus (HPV) infection** (Papanicolaou stain; vaginopancervical smear; ×1102).

seen in certain viral infections. It should be distinguished for detached ciliary tufts (DCT) described by Hollander and Gupta,[44, 46] which may be observed in lower genital tract smears in the absence of any viral infection. *In vivo* hemadsorption observed occasionally may be a related phenomenon (Fig. 8–37).

Oncogenesis. Both *in vitro* and *in vivo* neoplastic transformation of the viral-infected cells may occur. Numerous DNA viruses and a group of retroviruses are capable of neoplastic transformation in the infected cells. These commonly manifest as dyskaryosis and atypical nuclear changes.

No Change. Quite often, in the presence of florid viral infection, no discernible morphologic changes may occur in the infected cells and tissues.

The previously mentioned cellular manifestations may or may not be reflected in all cytologic preparations and in the presence of all viral infections.

Specific Infections

Specific viral infections commonly observed in the female genital tract include herpes. *Herpes* is a Greek word meaning "to creep." It is believed that this word was used in relation to certain clinical features of an infection that eventually was found to be related to the particular DNA virus. Presently, there are at least six different diseases that occur in human beings from this group of viruses. These are

- Herpes simplex virus, Type 1 (HSV 1)
- Herpes simplex virus, Type 2 (HSV 2)
- Cytomegalovirus (CMV)
- Varicella zoster
- Epstein-Barr (EB) virus
- Human B-cell lymphoma virus or HSV 4

The first four infections may affect the female genital tract and are detectable cytologically.

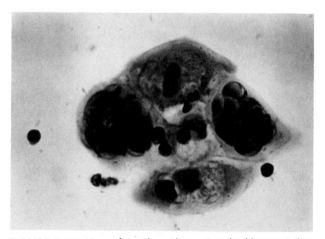

FIGURE 8–37. Hemadsorption. This patient had herpes infection at the time these and many other similar cells were seen. This phenomenon has been observed by us on numerous other occasions, and in every case the patient has had a concomitant viral infection. The significance of such a change is not well known (Papanicolaou stain; vaginopancervical smear; ×700).

Herpes Simplex Virus. Distinction between HSV 1 and HSV 2 was made based upon serologic studies by Schneweis.[85] Most people acquire antibodies to HSV 1 during the first 2 years of their life. Herpetic vulvovaginitis or stomatitis due to HSV 1 may occur at the time of initial infection, generally in infancy or early adolescence. Infection is mostly asymptomatic, or it may be accompanied by upper respiratory tract or ocular symptoms. Morphologically, HSV 1 and HSV 2 cellular changes appear identical.

Although congenital or neonatal transmission may occur, HSV 2 generally occurs after puberty and the onset of sexual activity. Cutaneous lesions, commonly vesicles, tend to occur in the same area repeatedly; the interval between successive eruptions varies considerably even in the same individual. Stress, menses and other unrelated ailments may precipitate an eruption in an otherwise healthy person. Following the initial infection, the virus remains dormant in the sacral (S2 through S4) dorsal root ganglia in the spinal cord. Its presence in the cord has been documented by McDougall.[64]

In more recent years there has been an increase in the occurrence of HSV 2 cases; it is generally attributed to changed sexual and social habits. Using seroepidemiologic data, an association of HSV 2 and cervical cancer has been established by Kessler[53] and others. Aurelian and coworkers,[3] Gilman and colleagues,[27] and Anthony and coworkers,[2] among others, have reported specific proteins to be associated with cervical cancer. Gupta and associates[33] reported HSV antigens in dysplastic and cervical carcinoma cells. Studies using radiolabeled probes have demonstrated HSV messenger RNA in carcinoma *in situ* cells by Jones.[49] Recent experimental studies support the etiologic role of HSV in the causation of human cervical cancer. Obviously, the precise nature of HSV 2 in the development of human cervical cancer is far from resolved at this point. Current interests and investigations point to a probably more prominent role of HPV infection in such proliferative processes.

Herpes Simplex Genitalis Virus, Type 2. For nearly 2500 years, people have used the word herpes in medical literature. Lawrence Corey[17] has briefly discussed the history of genital herpes. It was first described by John Astrue in 1736 in the French literature. Over 100 cases of "herpes progenitalis" were reported in the late 19th century.

Experimental transmission of herpes in human beings was established by Lipshutz[61] in 1921. He concluded that there were differences between oral (HSV 1) and genital herpes (HSV 2) infections. The work of Nahmias and coworkers[66] in the 1960s demonstrated two separate antigens that occur among HSV 1 and HSV 2 cases.

HSV 2 is one of the most common sexually transmitted genital infections; over 300,000 new cases are recorded in the United States annually. The prevalence of infection varies in the various groups. Although in general populations the incidence of infection is not well established, genital HSV infection was diagnosed among 4.2% of those attending the Sexually Transmitted Disease Clinic in Seattle, Washington, in 1980. Women presenting at the student health services have been found to have HSV 2 about seven to ten times more commonly than gonorrhea. Data from the Centers for Disease Control (CDC) suggest that the prevalence of HSV 2 is increasing and that the infection is occurring in social groups that previously did not have the disease.

Primary infection may be asymptomatic or accompanied by severe constitutional symptoms. Commonly, fever, headache and myalgia occur before the appearance of mucocutaneous lesions. Visible lesions appear between 2 and 7 days following exposure to the virus. Local pain and itching, dysuria, vaginal discharge and inguinal lymphadenopathy may be present. The lesions are painful and often multiple. Large ulcerations that start as papules or vesiculae spread rapidly. They form pustules that coalesce and break down. Unless complicated by secondary infection, these ulcers heal in 5 to 10 days with re-epithelization. Residual scarring is uncommon. Systemic symptoms and inguinal lymphadenopathy occur mainly in primary HSV 2 infection.

The cytologic diagnosis of HSV infection is important and must be made on well-preserved cells that have typical diagnostic features and have not been altered by air-drying, fixation or inflammation. Such a diagnosis may determine proper management of patients, especially pregnant women with genital ulcerations. An HSV diagnosis, with its social and medical implications, should only be rendered when unequivocal evidence is present.

The smears should be prepared from the edge and bed of the ulceration, not from the contents of the vesiculae. The latter generally contain serosanguinous material with acute inflammatory cells, eosinophils and some macrophages. Although use of air-dried smears and their examination after Romanowsky stain (Tzanck preparation)[94] have been advocated, we do not recommend this for genital lesion diagnoses. Heavy inflammation, cellular obscuring and degeneration often make interpretation difficult and may severely compromise the diagnostic value of air-dried smears. Cellular samples obtained from the cleared ulcer beds should be immediately fixed in 95% ethanol and examined after Papanicolaou staining.

The virus may infect the immature squamous, metaplastic and endocervical columnar cells. Initially, the changes are proplastic and somewhat nonspecific. The infected cells may occur singly, in groups and in tissue fragments. There is cyto- and karyomegaly, and the nucleocytoplasmic ratio is not much altered. These cells demonstrate a combination of reactive (proplastic) and degenerative (retroplastic) changes. The nuclei of the infected cells show changes in the chromatin structure of hydropic or ballooning degeneration. The chromatinic material becomes extremely finely divided and is uniformly dispersed in the nuclear sap. The chromatin-parachromatin interphase is obliterated, and nuclei assume a faintly hematoxylinophilic, homogenized appearance. Some chromatinic material may be matted against the inner leaf of the nuclear envelope, which may appear uniformly thick and conspicuous. The altered nuclear morphology is commonly referred to as ground glass, bland, gelatinous, glassy or opaque. In some cases the redistribution of chromatin may result in a beaded appearance of the nuclear margins.

Nucleoli may be present and conspicuous, may have associated chromatin, and may not appear typically bright acidophilic. Although the nucleoli generally remain round or oval, sometimes irregular shapes may be observed.

In the later stages of HSV infection, the cells undergo the effects of viral replication and DNA integration. The cells may assume multinucleation. Multinucleation is observed in nearly 80% of the smears from cases of genital HSV infection. The infected nuclei may have the same homogenous chromatin pattern described previously. The nuclei appear tightly packed within the cells and reveal distinct internuclear molding (Fig. 8–38). At times they may be overlapping and not molding. Large and single intranuclear inclusions appear within these nuclei. The nuclear inclusions are generally round or oval in shape. They can be angulated and sharp (Fig. 8–39). They lack structure and are densely eosinophilic. Depending upon the staining procedure employed, they may appear cherry red. The intranuclear inclusion is often surrounded by a clear zone, or halo, which separates it from the nuclear membrane. Most often the halo is as clear as the background of the slide. Sometimes it may retain delicate, homogenous, diffuse hematoxylinophilia. Small, inconspicuous chromatin granules can occur in the peri-inclusion halo. Inclusions may occur in infected single cells that are observed in nearly one third of the cases of HSV 2 infection. Intranuclear inclusions may not be present in all of the nuclei within the multinucleated giant cells.

The cytoplasm in the infected cells at this early stage of HSV infection is dense. It may lose its transparent appearance and become opaque. Often it stains bright cyanophilic.

HSV-infected cells can become atypical; the enlarged

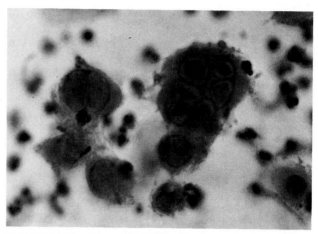

FIGURE 8–39. Herpes genitalis infection. Notice the multinucleated cells containing intranuclear inclusions (Papanicolaou stain; vaginopancervical smear; ×700).

cells may assume bizarre shapes (Fig. 8–40). They may be hyperchromatic, degenerated and misinterpreted as tumor cells. The cytoplasm may show changes of the cytoskeletal structure and become dense or opaque uniformly or focally. The latter may represent keratohyaline material. Degenerative vacuoles, the ectoplasmic-endoplasmic differentiation with spiral fibrils of Erbeth, as described by Patten,[72] may be present between the two zones. The fibrillary apparatus of Herxheimer appears as delicate, uniformly thin spirals that originate at the nucleus and travel down the cytoplasm and may be observed in cells with squamous differentiation features.

Multinucleated giant cells per se do not establish the diagnosis of HSV infection. Proper nuclear features and inclusions must be identified for such diagnosis. Virus-infected cells or virocytes should be distinguished from other giant cells such as trophoblasts, foreign body giant cells following extraneous intervention with foreign bodies or surgery, nonspecific giant cells seen in postmenopausal smears and reactive multinucleated cells found in cases of cervicitis.

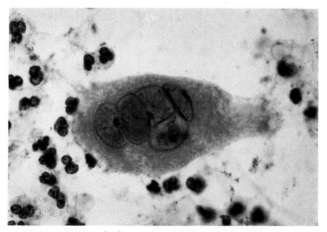

FIGURE 8–38. Early herpes genitalis infection. The multinucleation shows a homogeneous chromatin pattern and molding of the nuclei within the giant cell. The internuclear inclusions are not conspicuous (Papanicolaou stain; vaginopancervical smear; ×700).

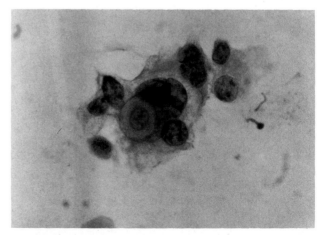

FIGURE 8–40. Bizarre columnar cells in a smear with **herpes genitalis infection** (Papanicolaou stain; vaginopancervical smear; ×875).

Ng and coworkers[70] described the morphologic differences between primary and recurrent herpes. Paucity of intranuclear inclusions and occurrence of chromatinic homogeneity and "ground glass" changes were often reported in primary herpes, whereas inclusions were predominant among cases with postprimary infection. This observation has not been confirmed by the studies of Vesterinen and associates[98] and other workers, although these have been adapted by the World Health Organization. Morphologically, HSV 2 and HSV 1 cannot be differentiated. Such a diagnosis can only be rendered either by appropriate serologic reactions or viral cultures.

Cytomegalovirus. These large (1800 to 2000 Å) DNA viruses belong to the herpes group that includes HSV 1, HSV 2, varicella zoster and EB virus. CMV is ubiquitous and circulates commonly in the general population. As with herpesviruses, CMV establishes itself in the host and causes persistent infection and recurrent disease. In the genital tract, reinfection may occasionally occur. Unlike other herpesviruses, however, clinically overt manifestations of viral replication are seen only rarely. The infection spreads by intimate contact through body secretions, including saliva, tears, urine, endocervical mucus, semen and transplanted organs.

Nearly 50 to 60% of adult women have circulating antibodies to CMV. Serologic evidence of infection is more common in low socioeconomic groups. Cervical shedding of CMV occurs in nearly 10% of the female population.[79] These figures vary in different populations; e.g., the recovery rate for CMV in the cervical specimens has been reported to be 28% in Japan. In a number of studies summarized by Kumar and coworkers[57] the incidence of primary genital CMV infection has been reported between 0.2 and 2.2%. Most primary genital CMV infection cases are clinically asymptomatic. Stagno and colleagues[93] reported symptomatic episodes in only one out of 21 cases, and Griffiths and associates[29] in only one out of 14 pregnant women with primary CMV infection. Almost always these symptoms are infectious mononucleosis–like and include lethargy, malaise and fever.

Characteristically, epithelial tissues, including salivary gland, alimentary tract, bronchial and alveolar lining cells, hepatocytes, renal tubule cells, hematopoietic cells and endocervical and endothelial cells, are targeted by CMV infection. Cytologically, the infected cells, endocervical columnar, perhaps, occur more commonly in the cervical smears than are recognized. According to Naib,[68] the CMV-bearing cells occur within the endocervical glands, and not many cells may be observed in the epithelium of the endocervical canal. Proper cellular specimens, as can be obtainable with a cytobrush or similar technique, may be more rewarding. Also, since almost all women are asymptomatic, very little effort may be made to screen these smears critically for CMV-associated changes. In a certain number of patients, concomitant CMV and HSV infections may occur. It is not infrequent to overlook the not-so-obvious CMV-infected cells in such cases. At times, the cytomorphologic identification of CMV and its differentiation from HSV may be extremely difficult.

The CMV-infected cells may be multinucleated and somewhat enlarged (Fig. 8–41). The nuclear degenerative changes may be similar to those in HSV. We have observed that the internuclear molding tends to be less obvious in CMV-infected cells, as compared with HSV. Infected endocervical cells are anisocytic. They contain round intranuclear inclusions, generally acidophilic, which are disproportionately large when compared with the total size of the nuclei. These inclusions have a clear zone of halo around them, and frequently threads of chromatinic material may stretch between the inclusion and the inner leaf of the nuclear membrane, which may be considerably thickened with the chromatinic material in apposition against it (Fig. 8–42), giving a wheel spoke appearance. The infected cells may have an intracytoplasmic, irregular inclusion.

Endocervical cells may be buried among inflammatory or other epithelial cells and may be hard to screen in routine fashion. In selected cases, CMV-specific monoclonal antibodies can be used to establish the presence of infected cells.

Herpes Zoster. Varicella zoster is related to varicella (chickenpox) that is so common in childhood and infancy. Herpes zoster (shingles) infection may involve the vulva and vagina. Lesions often appear in patients who were exposed to the Varicella virus in childhood. They occur in older individuals along the distribution of sensory nerves as extremely painful vesiculae or blisters and tend to be unilateral.

A smear from the base of the lesion often reveals numerous multinucleated giant cells with little intercellular molding. Numerous infected single cells may occur. Intranuclear inclusions may be basophilic, large

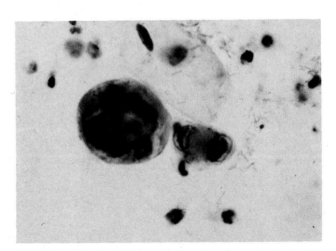

FIGURE 8–41. The degenerated multinucleated cells in this case represent **viral infection.** The accompanying cell has distinctly large intranuclear inclusions. The inclusion-bearing cells are not enlarged. This case represents a cytomegalovirus infection of the cervix (Papanicolaou stain; vaginopancervical smear; ×700). (Reproduced with permission from Gupta PK, Heustis DG, Bonfiglio TA, Neiberg RK, Lin F: Cytology of the female genital tract. In Astairita RW (ed): Practical Cytopathology, pp. 23–140. New York, Churchill-Livingstone, 1990.)

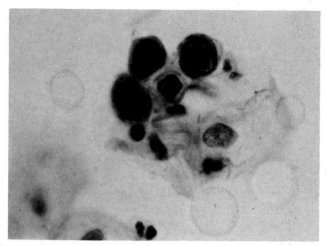

FIGURE 8–42. Cytomegalovirus infection. Notice the infected columnar-type cells with disproportionately large but distinct intranuclear inclusions (Papanicolaou stain; vaginopancervical smear; ×700). (Reproduced with permission from Gupta PK, Heustis DG, Bonfiglio TA, Neiberg RK, Lin F: Cytology of the female genital tract. In Astairita RW (ed): Practical Cytopathology, pp. 23–140. New York, Churchill-Livingstone, 1990.)

and inseparable from the markedly thickened inner nuclear membrane. Infected parabasal-type cells may show some cytoplasmic degenerative changes. Intracytoplasmic vacuolation and hyalinization may be present.

Human Papilloma Virus (HPV). HPVs belong to the family *Papovaviridae*, which includes double-stranded DNA members, papilloma viruses and polyomaviruses.

The papilloma virus genome is approximately 8000 basepairs in length. It has three functioning areas including genes for early viral function, the late region containing genes for viral structural proteins and a noncoding regulatory region. The viral capsid has two proteins and polypeptides.

Papilloma virus has been isolated from over 60 animal species including mammals, reptiles and amphibians. The vast majority of these viruses infect epithelial surfaces of either the skin or mucosa and cause self-limiting warty growth. The papilloma viruses are species-specific and do not cross-infect.

In humans, utilizing molecular hybridization and restriction enzyme analyses, so far 60 distinct HPV types have been identified. These different HPV types tend to be site-specific. Some of the common HPV types and the specific lesions they commonly are associated with are given in Table 8–7. It can be appreciated that HPV types 6 and 11 are commonly associated with warty condyloma, flat condyloma and low-grade dysplasia (cervical intraepithelial neoplasia [CIN] grade I), whereas HPV types 16, 18, 31 and 35 are often found in high-grade cervical dysplastic (CIN grades II and III) lesions and cervical carcinoma *in situ*.

HPV has a predilection for mature keratinocytes in the superficial squamous epithelial cells. The presence

TABLE 8–7. Common Human Papilloma Virus Lesions (At Least 60 Types)

HPV Type	Lesion
1, 2, 3, 4, 10, 28	Common warts
6, 11, 31, 42, 45	Anogenital condyloma, low-risk (CIN grade I) lesions
16, 18, 31, 33, 35, 39	High-Risk (CIN grade II and III) lesions—anogenital, laryngeal, esophageal, lung cancer (possibly)
26, 27	Warts, immune deficiency, renal transplant

of HPV antigen in squamous cells can be demonstrated by using polyclonal rabbit antihuman wart virus antibodies or exploiting the cross-reactivity feature of the bovine papilloma virus antibodies with HPV antigens. In conditions in which the HPV DNA is integrated with the infected cell DNA, as in high-grade dysplasia (CIN grades II and III), carcinoma *in situ* or squamous cell carcinoma, molecular techniques are necessary to detect the viral genome.

Papilloma Virus and Cancer. The virus is believed to enter the body through small, inconspicuous cuts or abrasions on the skin or mucous membrane. It stimulates the growth of the prickle cell layer. The growth is by clonal expansion and, as suggested by Broker and Butcher,[13] it pushes aside the normal epithelium to form warts. Virus replication occurs in the nucleus.

In addition to the numerous benign, self-limiting warty growths, papilloma viruses are associated with a number of neoplasms occurring in animals, such as rabbits and cattle. The most convincing evidence for an association of HPV with human genital warts is in the demonstration of HPV DNA and RNA in at least 80% of all cervical, vulvar and penile squamous cell carcinomas, in a similar proportion of premalignant CIN lesions and in 95% of genital condylomas.[103] HPV types 6 and 11 predominate in benign warty lesions, whereas 16 and 18 occur in 60 to 70% of all cervical tumors investigated. Other HPV types (31, 33, 35 and 45) and some uncharacterized HPV types are detectable in the additional 20% of cervical neoplastic tissues. HPV types 16 and 18 have also been found in several human cervical cancer cell lines, including the famous HeLa cell. Limited success has been achieved in transformation experiments conducted using HPV subgenomic particles and human epidermoid cell lines.

Historic Perspective. The typical cytomorphologic changes now associated with HPV infection were first documented by Ayre in 1949.[4] Papanicolaou in his *Atlas of Exfoliative Cytology*[71] published in 1954 presented magnificent illustrations depicting cellular changes presently recognized as HPV-associated. Koss and Durfee[56] in 1956 used the term *koilocytic atypia* to describe the surface epithelial changes of the cervix and its relationship with cancer. Naib and Masukawa[69] in 1961 published a paper entitled, "Identification of Condyloma Acuminata Cells in Routine Vaginal Smears." Additional papers on the same topic were published by Ayre,[5] Sagiroglu[81] and De Girolami.[18] Ayre[5] for the first time suggested a possible viral etiology of cervical dysplastic lesions. In the mid-70s,

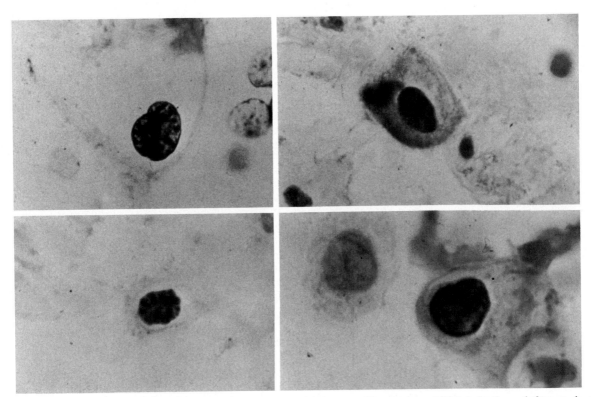

FIGURE 8–43. This composite represents four different cases of **human papilloma virus (HPV) infection of the cervix.** These smears have been stained with rabbit anti-HPV antibodies using immunoenzymatic reaction. In addition to the typical koilocytotic cell, the other, atypical, metaplastic and parabasal type cells also contain the viral antigens (immunoenzymatic stain with chromogen dimethylaminoazobenzene (DAB); ×868).

Meisels and Fortin[65] and Purola and Savia[75] independently defined a set of cellular changes that are associated with cervical condylomatous lesions and HPV infection. Also, *flat condyloma,* indistinguishable from cervical dysplasia, was recognized as a separate viral-related entity. The presence of virus particles within the koilocytes in cervical tissues was demonstrated by Laverty and coworkers[59] ultrastructurally. In 1980, Woodruff and colleagues[101] demonstrated the presence of HPV capsid antigen in genital condylomas using polyclonal rabbit antihuman wart virus antibodies. Gupta and associates[30] employed Papanicolaou and immunoenzymatic stained cells in cervical smears and demonstrated viral particles in cervical dysplastic cells identified by the viral antigen detection system.

Immunoenzymatic studies may reveal the presence of HPV antigens in 0.5 to 5% of the cells in the smears. Abundance of HPV infection, accompanying inflammatory reaction *(G. vaginalis)* and the degree of dysplastic changes determine the proportion of the antigen-positive cells. In up to 80% of these cases, corresponding cervical biopsy tissue may reveal identical results. Antigenically stained cells may include parabasal, intermediate and metaplastic types (Fig. 8–43). Antigen positivity has no relationship to the age, but is instead dependent upon the degree and depth of condylomatous change in the squamous epithelium. Nearly 90% of the cases with two-thirds thickness involvement may reveal the HPV antigen. Condylomatous and low-grade lesions (CIN grade I) reveal HPV antigens more commonly.

Nucleic acid hybridization was described in 1975 by Southern.[90] It has been used extensively for study of HPV DNA in vaginal secretions and infected cells, both in the smears and tissues. *In situ* hybridization, which permits localization of labeled DNA or RNA probes within the cellular preparations and tissue sections, was developed by Brahic and Haase[12] in 1978. Gupta and coworkers[31] used radiolabeled HPV DNA probes and established the presence of viral genomes in infected dysplastic cells in cervical smears (Fig. 8–44). RNA probes have been developed and used by Stroler and Broker[95] among others. Radiolabeled probes have more recently been replaced by immunoenzymatic techniques. Filter dot and more recently polymerase chain reaction (PCR) techniques have been utilized to investigate the presence of extremely small quantities of the viral genome in infected specimens. It must be realized that most of the sophisticated techniques presently have limited practical value. Biotin-labeled DNA probes may help identify high-risk (HPV types 16 and 18) versus low-risk (HPV types 6 and 11) infections in clinical samples. Its relevance to the clinical and therapeutic management of patients with cervical dysplasia and HPV infections is presently controversial.

Cytomorphology. Cytomorphologic identification of cellular changes is presently the most convenient, rapid, economical and sensitive available procedure for detection of HPV infection in the genital tract. As discussed previously, HPV infection generally manifests as verrucous or flat-surface epithelial lesions. Both

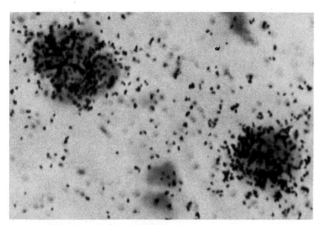

FIGURE 8–44. Human papilloma virus (HPV) infection. This slide has been processed for *in situ* hybridization using an S³⁵-labeled HPV-16 probe. The radiolabeled granules are distinctly seen on the surface of the infected nuclei (Autoradiograph with hematoxylin; vaginopancervical smear; ×1102).

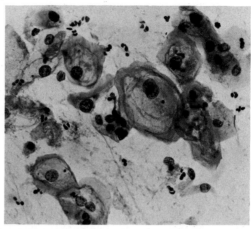

FIGURE 8–45. Typical koilocytotic cells. The smear reveals one normal intermediate squamous cell in the left upper corner. Notice the peripheral condensation of the cytoplasm of these cells, giving a "wire-loop" appearance. Also, the sharp margins and the angulations of these infected cells are lost, and they have become rounded and translucent (Papanicolaou stain; vaginopancervical smear; ×700).

lesions have the same basic pathognomonic features; additionally, the papilliferous lesions reveal surface hyper- and parakeratosis and papillomatosis.

HPV, being a DNA virus, affects both the nucleus and cytoplasm of the infected cells. It is generally believed that the virus gains entrance into the susceptible cell through the plasma membrane. The cytoplasmic changes of the infected cells—dyskeratosis—is a prominent feature of HPV infection. HPV DNA may occur within the epithelial cell nucleus either as unintegrated or integrated forms. Consequently, nuclear changes are commonly seen with HPV infection. These, however, tend to be more pronounced in cases of HPV DNA integration with the epithelial cell nuclear DNA. Such lesions typically appear as dysplastic and atypical. Chromosome and ploidy alteration, a hallmark of CIN or dysplastic change, may occur in these cases.

The classic manifestation of HPV infection is the presence of the koilocyte, so named by Koss and Durfee.[56] The cell has also been called nearo-carcinoma by Ayre,[5] and balloon cells by Meisels and Fortin.[65]

A typical koilocyte is a squamous epithelial cell (Fig. 8–45). Most commonly intermediate cells and sometimes metaplastic-type koilocytic cells may occur. The latter may be indistinguishable from parabasal cells.

The HPV-infected cells show blunting of the sharp angles of the squamous cells. The squamous angular forms tend to become rounded, and the cell assumes a softer, rounded or ovoid appearance. Typically, the cytoplasm shows a peripheral condensation and produces a "wire looping" effect, in which the cytoproteins gel at the margins, leaving an almost empty shell. This cytoplasm generally appears structureless and opaque, or waxy. It may be acidophilic and appear as a brighter reddish-orange, resembling a deep pumpkin red or a shade thereof. The typical koilocytotic cell has a large cavity or halo intracytoplasmic space. This space has a sharp peripheral margin, and the nucleus contained within this most often is eccentrically located; that is,

this is a large *paranuclear*, and not a *perinuclear*, halo. The latter is generally small with soft margins and is seen in the infectious process, such as in trichomoniasis. It may also have a variable pale or faint cytoplasm within it. Occasionally, phagocytosed material may be observed within the koilocytic space (Fig. 8–46).

Ultrastructurally, viral particles can be more easily detected in warty lesions occurring in the skin than in those in the genital tract and airways. Intranuclear icosahedral nonenveloped virions of 40 to 50 nm can be observed. At times, some particles may also be seen within the cytoplasm. Such findings are believed to be artifactual.

Immunocytologic investigations may reveal high-molecular-weight cytokeratin within the koilocytic space. No viral antigens can be demonstrated with the paranuclear halo of koilocytes by immunoenzymatic techniques.

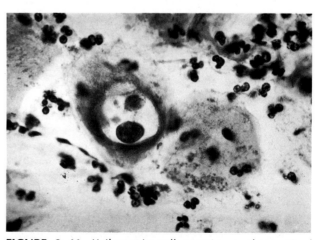

FIGURE 8–46. Koilocytotic cell contains a phagocytized trichomonad in the center from a case with **human papilloma virus (HPV) infection** (Papanicolaou stain; vaginopancervical smear; ×1378).

Diagnostically, the koilocyte is an excellent indicator of HPV infection. It has a high degree of specificity. Properly selected and evaluated, nearly 90% of the cases of condyloma with koilocytic change were found to have demonstrable HPV antigen by immunoenzymatic techniques. Although highly specific, the koilocyte alone has low sensitivity for detection of HPV infection. Based upon examination of routine vaginopancervical smears, in our experience nearly 60% of the cases of condyloma reveal obvious koilocytes; an additional 20% of the smears will reveal the diagnostic cell if carefully screened. About one third of the cases of HPV infection may be missed cytologically if the diagnosis is made solely on the basis of koilocytic changes. Schneider and colleagues[84] have reported that only 20% cases of HPV infection may be detected cytologically. We feel this is too low and probably not correct. It is obvious that the conflicting reports in the literature about the diagnostic value of vaginopancervical smears for HPV infection are based upon excessive reliance on the koilocyte as the sole diagnostic feature.

It is well known[55] that the most vulnerable area of the ectocervical-endocervical interface is the transformation zone, an area situated between the squamous-lined ectocervix and the columnar-lined endocervix. HPV infection is believed also to originate in this region. Once established, the infection may move proximally or distally and affect the adjacent epithelial cells. The ectocervical squamous epithelial changes that manifest as koilocytes and other dyskeratotic forms are more obvious and more common, but the proper recognition of these nonclassic changes can improve the diagnostic value of routine vaginopancervical smears.

Quite often, a diagnosis of HPV infection or condylomatous changes can be *suspected* with the lower magnification ($\times$ 100 to $\times$ 200) examination of the vaginopancervical smear. The infected cells may occur with or without inflammation, concomitant infection or endocervical component. It is not uncommon to be able to suggest a diagnosis of HPV infection in an otherwise less-than-satisfactory smear that is rich in vaginal components and has minimal endocervical representation.

The HPV-infected cells tend to stick together. The presence of groups or clumps of deeply acidophilic, opaque squamous cells in an otherwise well-fixed (no air-drying artifacts) and -stained smear may be telltale evidence of HPV infection (Fig. 8–47). A careful evaluation of such groups may reveal a number of squamous cells that have lost their sharp, polygonal shapes; they have become rounded and blunt. The cells may be overlapping, as commonly seen in pregnancy and late postovulatory smears, but they do not remain transparent and thin. They become dense, and may be opaque. The normal gradual centrifugal thinning of the intermediate and superficial cell cytoplasm is lost. Any degree of change between a normal-appearing squamous cell and the typical koilocyte may be present in these cells. Besides the HPV-infected cells occurring as aggregates, syncytial or pseudoepithelial formation may be observed.

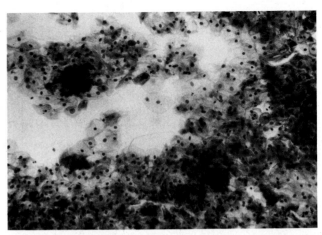

FIGURE 8–47. Human papilloma virus infection (HPV). This low-power view demonstrates the cellular clumping or plaque formation so commonly observed in this infection (Papanicolaou stain; $\times$172).

Ectocervical involvement by HPV may result in infected cells with dyskeratosis. Although frequently observed in cases of squamous cell carcinoma, some of the abnormal cytoplasmic features, especially changes in tinctorial character, occur commonly in HPV-infected cells. Abnormal shape is another feature affecting the squamous epithelial cells. Frayed edges (Fig. 8–48), fiber and tadpole formations are some of the features observed in HPV-infected squamous cells. Nuclear changes must be evaluated in these cases for proper interpretation of cytomorphology.

Parakeratosis (Fig. 8–49) is another feature that sometimes is seen in association with HPV infections. This finding is important in cases that may not have an inflammatory background. The parakeratotic cells can reveal abnormal keratinization or dyskeratosis. Hyperkeratosis may be seen as anucleated squames. This per se is not considered suggestive of HPV infection, but a better cellular sample should be examined in such cases.

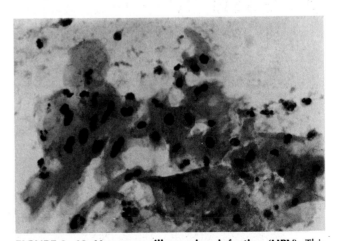

FIGURE 8–48. Human papilloma virus infection (HPV). This photomicrograph reveals the dyskeratosis that frequently accompanies the viral infection. Some of the cells are elongated, fiber-shaped and bizarre. These keratinized cells, if not carefully examined, can be mistaken for evidence of invasive cancer (Papanicolaou stain; vaginopancervical smear; $\times$875).

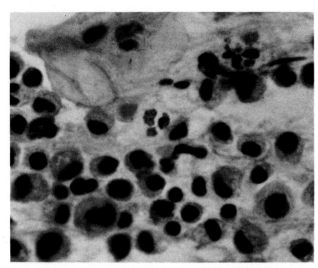

FIGURE 8–49. Human papilloma virus (HPV) infection. Notice the numerous parakeratotic cells. These keratinized orangeophilic cells have nuclear pleomorphism and hyperchromasia. They should be differentiated from pseudoparakeratosis commonly seen among oral contraceptive users (Papanicolaou stain; vaginopancervical smear; ×551).

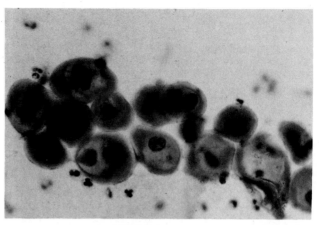

FIGURE 8–50. Human papilloma virus (HPV) infection. These cyanophilic metaplastic-type cells reveal evidence of HPV infection. Notice the nuclear variation in shape and size, the eccentric location of the nuclei and the peripheral condensation of the cytoplasm (Papanicolaou stain; vaginopancervical smear; ×1102). (Reproduced with permission from Gupta PK, Heustis DG, Bonfiglio TA, Neiberg RK, Lin F: Cytology of the female genital tract. In Astairita RW (ed): Practical Cytopathology, pp 23–140. New York, Churchill Livingstone, 1990.)

In cases in which the HPV infection may dominate the transformation zone or involve the endocervical canal, the infected cells as observed in vaginopancervical smears appear cyanophilic and may not be the keratinized squamous type. Atypical repair-type cells discussed elsewhere may dominate the smear. Very commonly these cases have immature, metaplastic-type cells infected with HPV in the smear (Fig. 8–50). They appear as single and basophilic with dense cytoplasm and round or oval shapes. They may be as small as parabasal or appear as big as intermediate cells. Some anisocytosis is common in these cells. The cytoplasm may show peripheral condensation similar to that seen in typical koilocytes. The nuclei may be eccentrically located, reveal size variation and show features of increased activity such as enlargement, chromatin granularity and bi- or multinucleation. The nucleoli are inconspicuous. When the infection is nested in the transformation zone, parakeratotic and metaplastic-type cells may predominate. Small tissue fragments can be seen sometimes. In cases with infection involving the ecto- and endocervical regions, a mixture of mature, parakeratotic squamous cells and metaplastic-type cells with evidence of HPV infection may all appear together (Fig. 8–51).

Using the diagnostic criteria mentioned previously and as summarized in Table 8–8 and Figure 8–52, we have nearly 100% correlation between the cytodiagnosis of HPV, its histology and detection of HPV by molecular techniques. The sampling procedures and the interval between the cytosmear and appropriate tissue studies are important. Changes observed in the endocervical cells in HPV infection, in our experience, have not been sufficiently specific to be useful diagnostically.

Nuclear changes, although not specific, are commonly observed among HPV-infected cells. The nuclei

may not show any changes; they may degenerate and appear hyperchromatic and pyknotic or reveal chromatin margination and abnormal clearing. Bi- and multinucleated forms in the squamous cells occur often. The nuclei may be enlarged, but changes most often are proplastic with pale, finely divided chromatin gran-

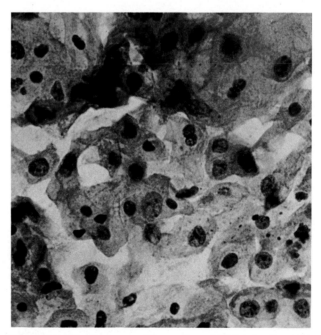

FIGURE 8–51. Human papilloma virus (HPV) infection. This infection appears to involve the ectocervix and the transformation zone simultaneously. Both mature squamous cells and immature metaplastic-type cells are observed in this smear. Some of the cells show small tissue fragment formation. Multinucleation and keratinization are also observed. (Papanicolaou stain; vaginopancervical smear; ×172).

TABLE 8–8. Cytomorphologic Features of Human Papilloma Virus Infection

Affected Cell
Keratinized, mature squame
Keratinized, immature squame
Undifferentiated transformation zone
Cellular Configuration
Clumps
Single
Tissue fragments
Cellular Shape
Loss of polygonal form, blunt or rounded corners
Cellular Margin
Thickened, wire loop appearance
Cell Size
Iso- and anisocytosis
Cytoplasm
Variable translucency and condensation
Koilocytosis
Nucleus
Karyomegaly
Bi- and Multinucleation
Minimal dyskaryosis
Associated Changes
Parakeratosis
Hyperkeratosis

ules distributed uniformly within the enlarged nucleus. The nucleoli are absent or inconspicuous in these cells. The nuclear membrane may be loose and wavy. It may be degenerated and appear folded and somewhat wrinkled, giving the typical raisin-like appearance so often observed in HPV infections (Fig. 8–53).

HPV and Cervical Dysplasia. The more recently established Bethesda system of gynecologic cytology reporting recognizes condyloma and varying degrees of dysplasia. The same terminology is being used to describe the HPV-related lesions.

Morphologically, it can be difficult to distinguish a condyloma from mild dysplasia or a CIN grade I lesion, both cytologically and histologically. An awareness of this difficulty has led to the two lesions being grouped together as low-grade dysplastic lesions. In our and some other laboratories, most of the time CIN grade I is identified and reported separately from condyloma. In contrast to condyloma, CIN grade I lesions have enlarged nuclei and hyperchromasia. Chromatin granules are uniformly distributed, and they tend to be isodiametric in size, moderately coarse and appear identical. No parachromatin clearing and abnormal clumping is observed (Fig. 8–54). At times the nuclear membrane may be undulating and appear folded and wrinkled. Most affected cells are intermediate squames.

According to the Bethesda system[6] for reporting gynecologic cytodiagnoses, CIN grades II and III are grouped together as "high-grade" cervical dysplastic lesions. CIN grade II or moderate dysplasia has distinct nuclear chromatin granularity, which is uniform and coarse and may be unevenly distributed within the affected intermediate and parabasal-type cells. Parachromatin clearing is inconspicuous (Fig. 8–55). This is essentially a state of further exaggeration of the changes seen in CIN grade I. Whereas all condylomas and three quarters of CIN grade I may reveal HPV antigen-positive cells, only two thirds of CIN grade II smears may manifest such findings. CIN grade III, or

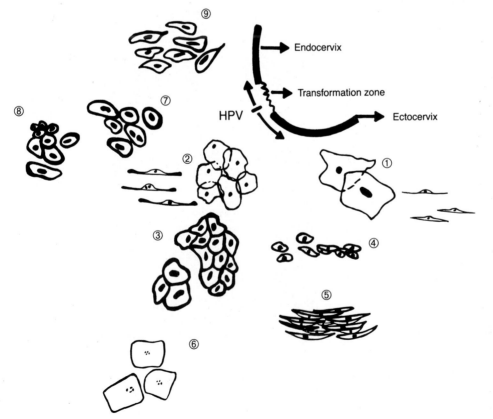

FIGURE 8–52. A diagrammatic representation of cellular changes in the cervix following **human papilloma virus (HPV) infection** (see text).
1. Normal squamous cells.
2. Koilocytotic cells.
3. Plaques of HPV-infected cells.
4. Parakeratotic cells.
5. Dyskaryosis with atypical forms.
6. Hyperkeratosis with anucleate squames.
7. Metaplastic-type HPV-infected cells. These cyanophilic cells have eccentric nuclei and peripheral cytoplasmic condensation.
8. HPV-infected cells from the transformation zone. These appear undifferentiated.
9. HPV-infected cells from the transformation zone. These cells are of an unclassified type.

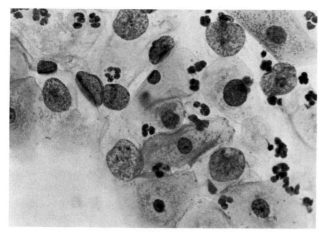

FIGURE 8–53. Human papilloma virus (HPV) infection. Notice the uniformly distributed chromatin pattern in these infected cells with pure condylomatous changes. Some of the nuclei have a folded, irregular nuclear membrane that corresponds to the "raisinoid" change seen in the tissue sections (low-grade dysplasia) (Papanicolaou stain; vaginopancervical smear; ×868).

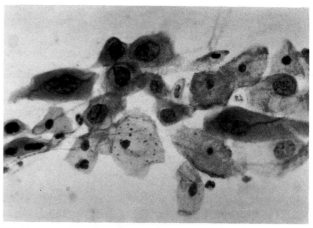

FIGURE 8–55. Human papilloma virus (HPV) infection with cervical intraepithelial neoplasm (CIN II) changes. In comparison to Figure 8–54, the nuclear chromatin pattern is more irregular, coarser and hyperchromatic. In the new terminology, such a pattern will be grouped as high-grade dysplastic change (Papanicolaou stain; vaginopancervical smear; ×700.)

severe or marked dysplasia, may be indistinguishable from carcinoma *in situ*. The biologic behavior and management of these lesions is essentially identical.

The affected cells tend to appear mostly singly and are more immature. They have distinct hyperchromasia with coarse but uniform chromatin granularity, nuclear membrane undulation and uniformity. No nucleoli or parachromatin clearing is generally seen. At times, the affected cells may be in small groups and fragments. Atypical, keratinized and bizarre dyskeratotic forms may appear in some cases.

Rarely (less than 5%), CIN grade III cells may be antigen-positive. The integrated HPV genome, however, can be detected within the infected cells by molecular hybridization techniques. A comparison of the two commonly used hybridization techniques is given in Table 8–9. In a given specimen, when only a few HPV infected cells are present, they may be more easily visualized by the *in situ* technique and radiolabeled probes than by the Southern blot hybridization. In the presence of widespread infection, with low copy numbers, although no diagnostic cellular changes may be present, the Southern blot or PCR techniques can be more rewarding. An excellent correlation between the cytomorphologic and molecular detection of HPV has been documented by Katz and associates.[51]

Recently introduced immunoenzymatic (biotin) and radiolabeled probes are useful in separating the low-risk (HPV types 6 and 11) infections from the high-risk (HPV types 16, 18, 31, 35 and others) ones, and may be important in the clinical management of cases. It must be appreciated that a small proportion of low-risk infection (HPV types 6 and 11) may progress to cancer. The American College of Obstetrics and Gynecology recommends "that all cases of dysplasia be

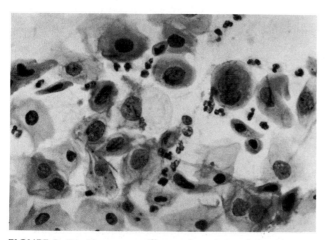

FIGURE 8–54. Human papilloma virus (HPV) infection with cervical intraepithelial neoplasm (CIN I) changes. Notice that the nuclei in the upper portion are more hyperchromatic and have coarser nuclear granularity as compared with the nuclei in the lower portion which have a uniformly distributed chromatin pattern and are considered to represent a condyloma (low-grade dysplasia) (Papanicolaou stain; vaginopancervical smear; ×700).

TABLE 8–9. Comparison of Hybridization Techniques for Detection of Human Papilloma Virus Infection

	In Situ	Southern Transfer
Cellular localization	Possible	Not possible
Morphologic identification of infected cells	Possible	Not possible
Retrospective studies	Possible	Not possible
Tissue for study	Fresh or fixed	Fresh only
Sensitivity[51]	Moderate	High
Diagnosis of genotype	Possible	Possible
Diagnosis of subtype	Not possible	Possible
Multiple testings of single specimen	Not possible	Possible

clinically managed irrespective of the type of HPV found within them."

Using more sensitive techniques such as the PCR, HPV genomes have been detected in a large number of tumors, including endocervical and ovarian adenocarcinoma and vulvar, vaginal, cervical and anal carcinoma. Obviously, the last word on the relationship of HPV and human cervical and other cancer is not written as yet. The interrelationship of immunologic, cellular and mutagenic events and the role of other genital infections such as HSV and CMV may all be important in understanding the biology of this common genital infection.

It is not uncommon for HPV to manifest clinically in the condition of altered immune response. Pregnancy and physical and emotional stress may precipitate clinical HPV disease. Similarly, prolonged immunosuppression, as after a kidney transplant, and chemotherapy may cause clinical HPV disease. In fact, the first case reported by Gupta and coworkers[38] of dysplasia after azathioprine (Imuran) therapy is now believed to represent a case with condylomatous changes in the cervical epithelium. Increased incidence of condyloma in patients with acquired immunodeficiency syndrome (AIDS) is also well documented.

Polyomavirus. In addition to HPV, another member of the papovavirus family—BK virus—may occasionally be observed in the vaginopancervical smear. BK virus is seen frequently as a urothelial infection following renal transplantation and immunotherapy and immunosuppression. Rarely, intranuclear large basophilic inclusions may be seen in the vaginal smear. One case (Fig. 8–56) depicts a typical BK virus inclusion observed in a kidney transplant recipient. It is also possible that the affected cell is a parabasal type with BK virus infection. Cross-contamination of the vaginal

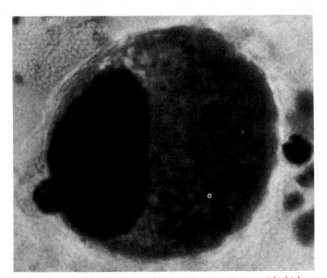

FIGURE 8–56. BK virus infection in a patient with kidney transplant and immunosuppression. This cell represents the intranuclear basophilic inclusion. This patient had concomitant BK virus infection in the urothelium. The contamination of vaginal contents from the urothelial cells cannot be entirely excluded in this one instance (Papanicolaou stain; vaginopancervical smear; ×1378).

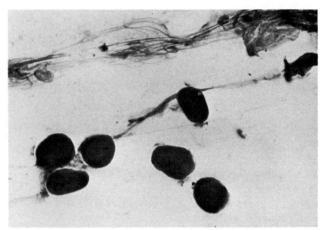

FIGURE 8–57. Molluscum bodies. Notice the dark, large intercytoplasmic inclusions (Papanicolaou stain; vulvar smear; ×875).

contents from the urinary tract, however, is a distinct possibility.

Molluscum Contagiosum. This was first described by Thomas Bateman in 1814. Like other pox viruses, the genome is a single, linear molecule of double-stranded DNA. The virus contains a virus-specified, DNA-dependent RNA polymerase and has not been cultured in in vitro systems.

A typical molluscum contagiosum lesion consists of a localized mass of hypertrophic, hyperplastic epidermal cells that push the basement membrane down and produce on the epidermal surface a pearl-white, somewhat umbilicated tumor. The germinal cells in the lesion multiply rapidly. Each cell enlarges and is filled with dense acidophilic intracytoplasmic inclusion called molluscum body (Fig. 8–57). To be diagnostic, each molluscum body must be intracytoplasmic and should have a compressed hematoxylinophilic nucleus on the outside. The tinctorial character of the inclusion may change with the age of the lesion.

Chlamydial Infection

Chlamydia trachomatis is one of the most common sexually transmitted diseases. Although documented perhaps earlier, C. trachomatis was first visualized by Halberstaeder and von Prowazek[41] in 1907 in a conjunctival scraping. The growth cycle of C. trachomatis was described back in the early 1930s.[97] The first isolation of C. trachomatis from a nonlymphogranuloma venereum case was done in 1959 by Jones and coworkers.[47] The patient was the mother of a newborn infant with ophthalmia neonatorum. In addition to the well-known culture techniques,[82] immunodiagnostic techniques, including immunofluorescence and immunoenzymatic techniques, radioimmunoassays and more recently molecular hybridization techniques, have been introduced in the diagnostic armamentarium for C. trachomatis.

Nearly 50% of women with C. trachomatis infection may be asymptomatic. Genitourinary disease, including urethritis, vaginitis, cervicitis, endometritis, salpingitis and pelvic inflammatory disease (PID) may occur in women infected with *C. trachomatis* organisms. The infection can also affect the neonate during passage through the birth canal and cause neonatal pneumonia or may be transmitted to the sexual partner, causing urethritis, prostatitis and epididymitis. Systemic disease may be associated with *C. trachomatis* infection; perihepatitis, endocarditis and gastroenteritis have been associated with *C. trachomatis* infection. The cases are few and precise data is lacking. The clinical chlamydial diseases are summarized in Table 8–10. The precise role of *C. trachomatis* infection in all of the clinical diseases mentioned in Table 8–10 is variable. Taylor-Robinson and Thomas[96] summarized the data that are presented in Table 8–11.

C. trachomatis is an obligate intracellular organism. It shares certain both bacterial and viral characteristics. The organism does not stain with a Gram stain. It contains both RNA and DNA, is susceptible to antibodies, divides by binary fusion and has a rigid cell wall.

A comparison of some of the common characteristics of *Chlamydia*, bacteria and viruses is given in Table 8–12.

Chlamydia organisms occur in two major forms: the infective, extracellular elementary body and the intracellular initial and intermediate forms or bodies, also referred to as reticulate particles. Elementary bodies measure about 300 nm. These are liberated from the infected cells and are phagocytosed by the susceptible cells, which most frequently are squamous metaplastic or endocervical columnar cells. There is some evidence of *Chlamydia* organisms infecting the parabasal cells of the lower genital tract. Shurbaji and associates[88] have documented the occurrence of chlamydial organisms within the prostatic epithelium and urothelium. As seen by life cycle studies, once within the infected cells the elementary bodies reorganize and enlarge. They repeatedly replicate by binary fission and, after undergoing the intermediate stages of development, produce intracytoplasmic inclusions that are large pockets of numerous elementary bodies. The infected cell finally lyses, liberating numerous elementary bodies to restart the cycle. This life cycle in a cell culture, e.g., McCoy cell line, is completed within 48 to 60 hours.

The infected epithelial cell can undergo a number of

proplastic and retroplastic changes. These include enlargement of the nuclei and cytomegaly, hyperchromasia and nucleolar prominence. Multinucleation may occur. The retroplastic changes commonly include cytoplasmic vacuolation and protein precipitation that may appear as nonspecific inclusions. Some serologic evidence exists for the possible association of *Chlamydia* infection and cervical dysplasia, but it is not well accepted.

In a symptomatic patient the body will react to chlamydial infection, and the occurrence of intense polymorphonuclear leukocytic response in the vaginopancervical smears is the most common single feature of symptomatic chlamydial infection. This was one of the major features observed among chlamydial cases by Kiviat and associates.[54] Quinn and coworkers[77] found the presence of intense polymorphonuclear leukocytic exudation as the single most common feature among cases of genital *Chlamydia* infection.

Although direct detection of *Chlamydia* in appropriately stained representative smears has been practiced for the longest period of time, the diagnostic value of direct smear examination in specimens other than conjunctival smears has been questioned repeatedly. A number of advances in the *Chlamydia* diagnosis have been made in more recent years. Improved culture techniques, direct immunofluorescence antigen detection and enzyme-linked immunosorbent assay (ELISA)-based tests have been introduced with a high degree of specificity and sensitivity. In a recent summary statement, the CDC, however, enumerated the

TABLE 8–11. Relationship of *Chlamydia Trachomatis* and Various Associated Diseases

Disease	Relationship
Acute and chronic cervicitis	Established
Follicular cervicitis	Established
Salpingitis	Established
Lymphogranuloma venereum	Established
Nongonoccal urethritis	Established
Postgonococcal urethritis	Established
Reiter's syndrome	Established
Neonatal pneumonia	Established
Conjuncivitis	Established
Epididymitis	Questionable
Cervical atypia	Questionable
Abortion	Questionable

TABLE 8–10. Chlamydial Diseases

Infections in Men	Infections in Women	Infections in Infants
Nongonoccal urethritis	Cervicitis	Conjunctivitis
Postgonococcal urethritis	Conjunctivitis	Pneumonia
Conjunctivitis	Subclinical genital infection	Gastroenteritis (possibly)
Subclinical genital infection	Salpingitis	
Epididymitis	Dysplasia (possibly)	
Reiter's syndrome	Infertility	
Systemic disease	Systemic disease	

TABLE 8–12. Common Characteristics of *Chlamydia*, Bacteria and Viruses

Feature	*Chlamydia*	Bacteria	Viruses
Ubiquitous nature	Yes	Yes	Yes
Multiplication in cell-free medium	No	Yes	No
Multiplication dependent on host-cell nucleic acid	No	No	Yes
Smallest reproductive forms—less than 350 nm	Yes	No	Yes
Cell wall or peptidoglycan present	Yes	Yes	No
DNA and RNA present	Yes	Yes	No
Various metabolic systems present	Yes	Yes	No
Multiplication inhibited by:			
Antibodies alone	Yes	No	Yes
Antibiotics	Yes	Yes	No

state of *Chlamydia* diagnosis. It stated, "Despite the encouraging improvement in diagnostic capability, current tests are not ideal. They are relatively difficult to perform, require considerable experience and have limited application."[15]

Although tissue cell culture is used as a "gold standard" for the diagnosis, more recently Kellogg[52] critically reviewed the various diagnostic methods and their limitations. Briefly stated, the number of swabs cultured, site of epithelial sampling, type of collection device, storage, evaluation of symptoms, serum immunoglobulin levels and antibodies, any treatment to stabilize the cellular membranes including antibodies and steroid preparations and other drugs, micturation and various inhibiting substances in the vaginal secretions can have a bearing on the diagnostic value of *Chlamydia* cultures. Also, selection of container, cell line and pretreatment, inoculation technique and culture duration, concomitant infections and contamination and type of stain used to detect growth of the organism in the cell line all have a bearing on the performance of the culture techniques. Cultures for *Chlamydia* are generally more valuable in younger patients with primary first-time infection. Antigen assays, on the other hand, are dependent upon the population make-up. These results tend to be less positive in asymptomatic and older patients. The size of the population, clinical disease, quality of the specimen and reading threshold also determine the results of direct *Chlamydia* diagnostic procedures.

The cytologic detection of *Chlamydia* has been documented by Naib,[67] Gupta and coworkers[37] and Bibbo and Wied.[10] Elementary bodies that are abundant in symptomatic individuals and may be easily cultured cannot be detected in Papanicolaou stained specimens. Romanowsky-stained specimens can be helpful for such identification, especially when the sample is examined under darkfield illumination. A golden-yellow discoloration is observed within the *Chlamydia* organisms. Also, the presence of heavy, acute inflammation may

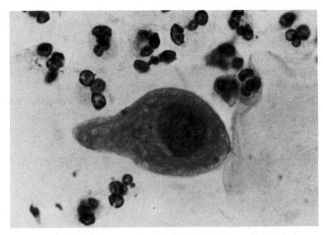

FIGURE 8–59. *Chlamydia* **infection.** In addition to the "moth-eaten," rarefied appearance seen in the cells in Figure 8–58, numerous fine-walled vacuolated structures are also seen in these cells. The structures represent the intermediate forms in the development of *Chlamydia* infection (Papanicolaou stain; vaginopancervical smear; × 868).

cause cellular obscuring and degeneration, rendering the fine cytoplasmic details incomprehensible. Cellular degenerative changes, on the other hand, can cause intracytoplasmic structures that may mimic chlamydial inclusions. It must be appreciated that cytoplasmic degenerative changes may occur in the presence of *Chlamydia* infection also, but they per se are not sufficient for a diagnosis.

Intracytoplasmic aggregates of minute elementary bodies occurring within the metaplastic cells is the earliest discernible feature of *Chlamydia* infection (Fig. 8–58). These may undergo degeneration with small, pinhead structures surrounded by a halo that is thin-walled (Fig. 8–59). These intermediate forms may be prominent and give the infected cell a "moth-eaten" appearance. A careful study of such cells often shows clumps of elementary bodies, also.[39] At times the intracytoplasmic aggregates of elementary bodies can condense and produce distinctly identifiable intracytoplasmic nebular inclusions.[87] These are large, homogeneous or finely granular structures with ill-defined

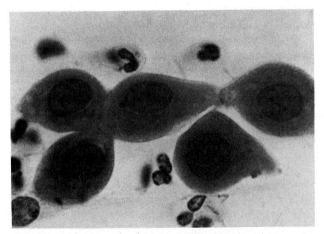

FIGURE 8–58. Changes of *Chlamydia* **infection.** Notice the "moth-eaten" rarefied appearance with minute dot-like structures within the cytoplasm. The larger vacuolated areas represent cytoplasmic degeneration (Papanicolaou stain; vaginopancervical smear; × 1102).

TABLE 8–13. Cytologic Features of *Chlamydia* Infection

Background:	Acute inflammation with numerous polymorphonuclear leukocytes and macrophages
Infected cells:	Metaplastic columnar cells, and possibly parabasal cells either singly or in tissue fragments
Morphology:	Intracytoplasmic elementary bodies; faint, acidophilic coccoid structures occurring diffusely or focally; moth-eaten appearance; reticulate and intermediate bodies occurring intracellularly as thin-walled target forms
	Nebular forms occurring as dense intracytoplasmic structures; multinucleation and cellular reactive changes.

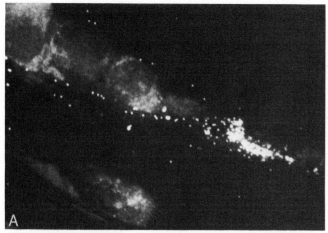

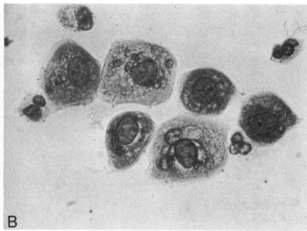

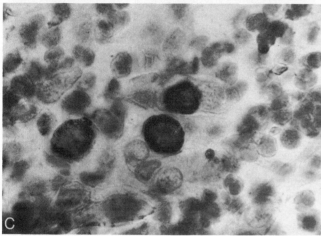

FIGURE 8–60. *Chlamydia* **infection.** Intracytoplasmic organisms are detectable using antichlamydial monoclonal antibodies (vaginopancervical smear). *A*, Elementary bodies (immunofluorescence with FITC; ×1378). *B*, Intermediate forms (immunoperoxidase with AEC chromogen; ×868). (Reproduced with permission from Gupta PK, Heustis DG, Bonfiglio TA, Neiberg RK, Lin F: Cytology of the female genital tract. In Astairita RW (ed). Practical Cytopathology, pp. 23–140. New York, Churchill Livingstone, 1990.) *C*, Nebular forms (immunoperoxidase with AEC chromogen; ×868). (FITC = fluorescein isothiocyanate; AEC = amino-ethyl carbazole.)

and indistinct walls. Ultrastructurally, nebular inclusions contain the chlamydial organisms. The *Chlamydia* organisms can be identified using appropriate antigen detection techniques in most of the infected cells (Fig. 8–60). When properly done, the cytodiagnosis of *Chlamydia* has a high degree of specificity and sensitivity. The cytomorphologic features are summarized in Table 8–13.

Cellular degeneration with intracytoplasmic inclusion formation as commonly observed after radiation and chemotherapy, secretions and coccoid organisms can all be mistaken for *Chlamydia*. The value of proper history and a high-quality representative smear and staining cannot be overemphasized.

Fungal Infections

Candida albicans and *Torulopsis glabrata* are now grouped together, the latter being called *Candida glabrata*. *Candida* infection generally involves the vulva, the vagina and sometimes the cervix. A large proportion (about 40%) of women with detectable *Candida* organisms may be asymptomatic. Clinically, the infection produces a white, cheesy, thick discharge with a burning sensation and intense itching. Pruritus is a common symptom of *Candida* infection involving the vulvar region. Sometimes there may be minimal vaginal discharge. In Papanicolaou stained smears, numerous filamentous organisms may occur, revealing pseudo and true hyphal forms (Fig. 8–61). Yeast-budding forms may be common (Fig. 8–62). Sometimes the organisms cause a peculiar fern-like arrangement of epithelial cells. Fungal organisms can be suspected in such cases also when the background contains numer-

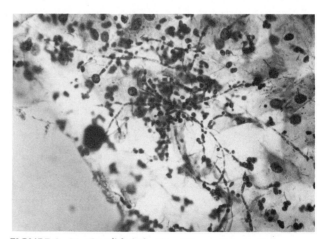

FIGURE 8–61. *Candida* **infection.** The numerous filamentous structures with the septate and pseudoseptate branching pattern and budding yeast forms are clearly seen (Papanicolaou stain; vaginopancervical smear; ×875).

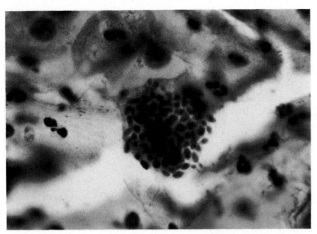

FIGURE 8–62. Budding yeast forms in *Candida* infection. The precise significance of the pure yeast form in vaginal smears is not well understood (Papanicolaou stain; vaginopancervical smear; ×1378).

ous fragmented leukocytic nuclei. Although the organisms can be conveniently seen in KOH preparations, a high degree of correlation exists between the Papanicolaou detection of *Candida* and fungal cultures.

Rare cases of blastomycosis have been observed in vaginal smears. *Alternaria, Aspergillus* and other fungi seen in the vaginal specimens are most often contaminants and nonpathogens.

Parasitic Infections

Trichomonas vaginalis. *T. vaginalis* is a protozoan and the most common parasitic organism. It is one of the four species *(T. tenax, T. hominis, T. fecalis* and *T. vaginalis)* and is the only pathogen to human beings. The most frequent infection occurs in the lower female genital tract, although nongenital infections including neonatal pneumonia, perinephric abscess, cutaneous lesion and alimentary tract infection have all been documented, as has been human prostatic disease. Host factors such as endocervical glands and mucus, various immunoglobulins, the complement system and leukocytes, macrophages and the polymicrobial vaginal environment are some of the important contributing factors for clinical symptoms.

The clinical disease is often described as occurring in acute, chronic and latent phases. Nearly 50% of the women who have this infection harbor this parasite in the latent phase and are asymptomatic. During the symptomatic phase, the organisms occur in the vagina, and occasionally in the secretions of the Skene and Bartholin glands. In approximately 10 to 20% of the women, lower urinary tract infection may occur and present as dysuria and urethral discharge. The organism may be recovered from clean catch urine specimens. It has also been recovered from purulent tubal material. The precise role, if any, of *T. vaginalis* infection in the development of PID, although documented, is controversial.

The incubation period of *T. vaginalis* infection is between 4 and 28 days. A foamy vaginal discharge occurs in 10 to 25% of patients. It may be malodorous, copious and frothy and greenish-yellow. Vulvar vaginitis and symptoms of PID including inguinal lymphadenopathy may occur. "Strawberry vagina" with reddening of the mucosa and small, punctate hemorrhagic spots is typical. The strawberry cervix, although classic, is seen in less than 5% of infected patients.

The disease may exacerbate in the latent phase during or immediately following the menstrual period. The clinical disease is more common during pregnancy. Frost[21] observed *Trichomonas* in 19% of pregnant women. The affect of *Trichomonas* infection on the newborn infant and postpartum endometrial infection is documented but not universally accepted.

Cytopathologic Features. Although the organism can be observed by a number of techniques such as darkfield, hanging drop and wet mount preparations, and PAS, Romanowsky and immunoenzymatic staining methods, excellent morphologic details are seen using wet fixation and Papanicolaou stained vaginal smears. "Routine" vaginopancervical smears are most valuable diagnostically. Since the organisms occur in the vagina, vaginal pool material or secretions from the posterior fornix are more sensitive. Vaginal douching in the preceding 24 hours, dilution of the secretions by menstrual blood, inflammation with cellular obscuring, marked cytolytic changes as in pregnancy or late luteal phase and atrophic cellular changes may all make the detection of *T. vaginalis* difficult. In asymptomatic women the organisms are best detected by examining cervical material obtained by endocervical canal scraping or aspiration.

In well-stained and representative vaginopancervical smears, *T. vaginalis* can be suspected by a number of features. These include the occurrence of aggregates of leukocytes covering the surfaces of the isolated, mature squamous epithelial cells (Fig. 8–63). These leukocytic agglomerations have been called "BB shots"

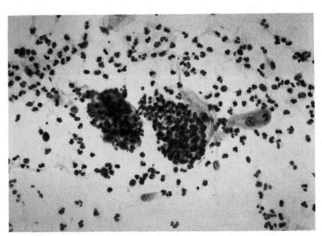

FIGURE 8–63. *Trichomonas vaginalis* infection revealing the aggregations of leukocytes on the surface of squamous epithelial cells, also called "BB shot" or "cannonball" appearance. Such leukocytic aggregations, per se, should not be considered diagnostic for *Trichomonas* infection (Papanicolaou stain; vaginopancervical smear; ×437).

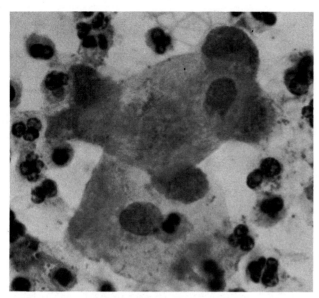

FIGURE 8–64. *Trichomonas vaginalis* infection. Notice the attachment of a number of trichomonads at the edges of the squamous epithelial cell in the center of the field. Numerous polymorphonuclear leukocytes are also observed at the periphery of such cells (Papanicolaou stain; vaginopancervical smear; ×1102).

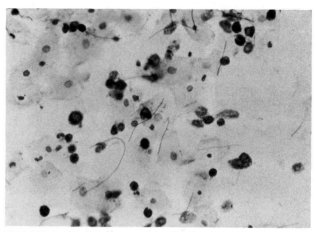

FIGURE 8–65. *Trichomonas vaginalis* organisms have been stained with mouse antitrichomonad vaginalis monoclonal antibody and immunoenzymatic technique. Notice the varied forms of the organisms in this smear (Immunoenzymatic stain with DAB chromogen; vaginopancervical smear; ×1093). (DAB = dimethylaminoazobenzene.)

and "cannonballs," and represent a number of *T. vaginalis* feeding on the squamous epithelial cell that, in turn, is phagocytosed by the leukocytes and macrophages. The attachment of *T. vaginalis* to the margins of the squamous epithelial cells can be easily studied by appropriate immunoenzymatic techniques (Fig. 8–64).

Sometimes, *T. vaginalis* may be suspected by observing *Leptotrichia* in the vaginal smears. These are large, generally nonbranching, curved bacillary structures distinct from lactobacilli and are described in detail previously. Bibbo and Wied[10] observed *Leptotrichia* and *Trichomonas* together in 95% of over 1000 cases examined.

In posthysterectomized women *T. vaginalis* occurs most often without the accompaning inflammatory reaction. In such smears, numerous mature squamous cells and *T. vaginalis* organisms occur with minimal changes, and only some bacteria may occur as accompaniments.

Cytopathologically, *T. vaginalis* frequently appears as small, round or oval structures. Their size may vary from that of the nucleus of a leukocyte to that of the parabasal cell. Extremely large, giant forms of *Trichomonas*, 150 to 200 μ in size, have been observed. The organisms stain a cytoplasmic color that may vary according to the pH of the vagina, staining quality and fixation. Generally, they are cyanophilic or delicate lavender in color. Bizarre, elongated or tadpole forms may occur (Fig. 8–65). Although frequently occurring singly, in cases of severe infection and immunosuppression, large microcolonies of the organisms may appear in the smear. The organisms always have a distinct, faint, vesicular nucleus (Fig. 8–66). Most often it is eccentric. Sometimes a number of acidophilic, uni-

formly sized granules may be observed within the organisms. *T. vaginalis* multiplies by binary fission and the organisms may be observed in mitosis. Some correlation has been observed between the size of the *T. vaginalis* and their pathogenicity. It is believed that the smaller organisms cause more fulminant and symptomatic infection.

Histologically, the organisms, although inconspicuous in routine H + E stained cervical tissues, may be detected by PAS, Masson's trichrome and appropriate immunodiagnostic techniques. They often occur on the surface of both squamous and endocervical epithelial cells, but may be seen within the epithelium. Pericellular ("chicken wire") edema may occur among the squamous epithelial cells. Reserve cell hyperplasia, squamous metaplasia and epithelial papillomatosis with capillary proliferation may occur. Some of these

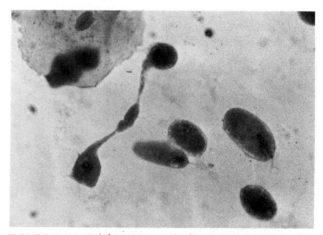

FIGURE 8–66. *Trichomonas vaginalis* organisms. Notice the round and oval-shaped organisms. To be diagnostic, they must contain a hematoxylinophilic faint, definite, vesicular nucleus. Intracytoplasmic acidophilic granules may also be present (Papanicolaou stain; vaginopancervical smear; ×1102).

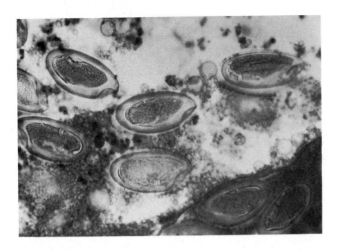

FIGURE 8–67. *Enterobius vermicularis.* These ovoid eggs of the organisms most commonly are considered contaminants. Occasional cases of lower genital tract infection and disease caused by *Enterobius* have been recorded (Papanicolaou stain; vaginopancervical smear; ×875).

changes may be nonspecific in nature but are often seen in cases of trichomoniasis.

Although reactive and atypical epithelial cellular changes may occur with *Trichomonas,* there is no convincing evidence of pure *T. vaginalis* infection causing nuclear chromosomal changes or aneuploidy, and thus dysplasia or preneoplastic epithelial changes. Concomitant infection with *Chlamydia,* herpes and HPV, among others, may occur in cases with *T. vaginalis* infection. There is some evidence of suspecting the presence of *Chlamydia* within *T. vaginalis* organisms. Bare nuclei and mucus must be distinguished from trichomonads.

Enterobius Vermicularis. *E. vermicularis* is a nematode that is commonly found in the tropics. Although alimentary tract infection is common, an occasional report exists of its occurrence in the endometrium, fallopian tubes and other sites.

Most often the eggs of *E. vermicularis* occur as a contaminant in vaginal pool material, especially among women with poor personal hygiene. These eggs are 50 to 60 μ by 20 to 25 μ. They are flattened on one side (Fig. 8–67). The shell is double-walled and smooth. Within the egg, an embryo can often be recognized. Only rarely the larvae may be seen in the vaginal smear (Fig. 8–68).

Trichuriasis. This is a nematode infection caused by

Trichuris trichiura. The eggs of this alimentary tract parasite may occur in the vaginal smear as a contaminant. The eggs are barrel shaped and 50 to 55 μ by 20 to 25 μ in size. They have a thick shell with a brownish discoloration. Bipolar colorless prominence is typical and diagnostic (Fig. 8–69). The infection is seen in tropical countries.

Entamoeba Histolytica. *E. histolytica* is a protozoa that may infect the lower genital tract. Clinically, the affected area is ulcerated and fungating and can be misdiagnosed clinically as neoplasm. Intermixed with necrotic material, numerous trophozoite forms can be seen (Fig. 8–70). These histiocytic-type organisms have biphasic cytoplasm with vesicular nuclei containing a central karyosome. Ingested red blood cells are often seen within the cytoplasm. Only rarely a cyst form may be observed in the vaginal smear (Fig. 8–71). This most likely represents a contaminant from the alimentary tract.

Entamoeba Gingivalis. These protozoa may be seen in vaginopancervical smears in association with *Actinomyces.* Such a relationship was documented by Ruehsen and associates.[20] These histiocytic-type organisms have numerous ingested fragments of leukocytic nuclei and cellular debris in the cytoplasm. They do not contain intracytoplasmic red blood cells that are commonly observed in *E. histolytica* infection.

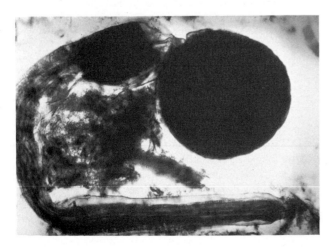

FIGURE 8–68. *Enterobius vermicularis* infection. This smear reveals a larva. The presence of such an organism in a smear is rare (Papanicolaou stain; vaginopancervical smear; ×136).

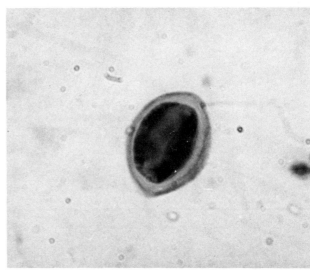

FIGURE 8–69. *Trichuris trichiura.* These eggs contain clear polar structures. The infection most often is considered contamination from the alimentary tract (Papanicolaou stain; vaginopancervical smear; ×700). (Case courtesy of Dr. S. Bhambhani.)

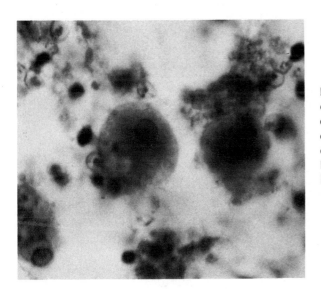

FIGURE 8–70. *Entamoeba histolytica* infection. This infection, common in tropical countries, clinically occurs as a fungating exophytic lesion that can be mistaken for invasive neoplasm. The organisms are generally round to oval in shape with nuclei and a central karyosome. In contrast to the *Entamoeba histolytica* seen in Figure 8–28, the cytoplasm contains red blood cells and not leukocytic debris (Papanicolaou stain; vaginopancervical smear; ×1102).

FIGURE 8–71. A cyst of ***Entamoeba histolytica.*** Finding of such cysts in a vaginal smear is considered extremely rare and a contamination from the alimentary tract (Papanicolaou stain; vaginopancervical smear; ×1102). (Case courtesy of Dr. S. Bhambhani.)

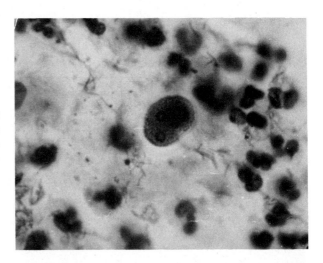

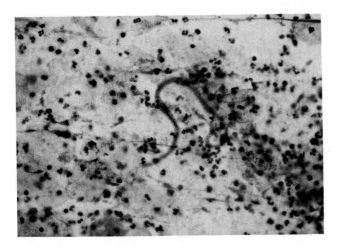

FIGURE 8–72. Microfilariae. These organisms are frequently observed in tropical countries where filariasis is common. The various kinds of organisms can be distinguished by the features of the mouth and the caudal end (Papanicolaou stain; vaginopancervical smear; ×136). (Case courtesy of Dr. S. Bhambhani.)

FIGURE 8–73. An ovum of *Ascaris lumbricoides*. Both fertilized and unfertilized ova can be seen in this vaginal smear (Papanicolaou stain; vaginopancervical smear; ×700). (Case courtesy of Dr. S. Bhambhani.)

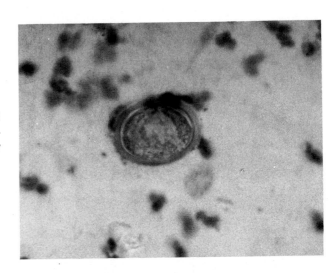

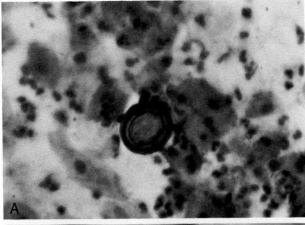

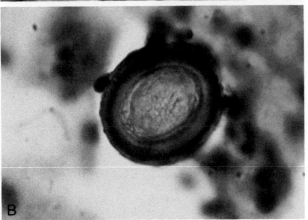

FIGURE 8–74. An egg of *Hymenolepis nana*. This tapeworm infection is seen in the tropics, and the eggs are generally seen as a contamination from the alimentary tract (Papanicolaou stain; vaginopancervical smear). (Case courtesy of Dr. S. Bhambhani.) *A*, Lower power, an oval egg (×700). *B*, Higher power, details of the egg (×1102).

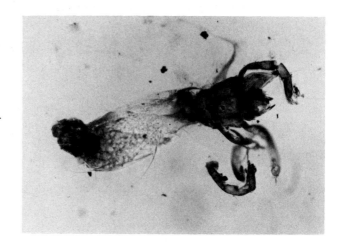

FIGURE 8–75. Human body louse, ***Pediculus humanus*** (Papanicolaou stain; vaginopancervical smear; ×273).

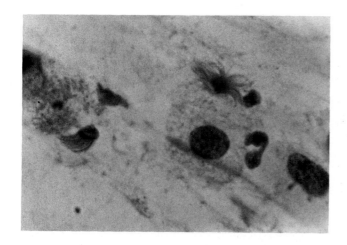

FIGURE 8–76. Detached ciliary tuft. These ciliated structures have, in the past, been reported as ciliated parasites (Papanicolaou stain; vaginopancervical smear; ×1722).

Filariasis. The most common nematode causing vascular space infection is *Wuchereria bancrofti*. Microfilariae may sometimes be seen in vaginal smears in endemic areas (Fig. 8–72).[16] The microfilariae are generally 200 to 200 μ in length. They have a pointed tail with an elongated terminal nucleus. A 5 to 15 μ caudal space is present beyond the nucleus terminally.

Ascariasis. This nematode infection is caused by *Ascaris lumbricoides*. Although alimentary in habitat, the organism may migrate to various parts of the body and be seen in pulmonary and vaginal specimens. In vaginal smears, both unfertilized and fertilized ova may be observed (Fig. 8–73).[7]

Cysticercosis. *Hymenolepis nana* is a cestode that causes alimentary tract symptoms. The eggs may occur in the vaginal smear as a contaminant from the feces (Fig. 8–74).[8] Eggs of the various tapeworms can be distinguished by detailed morphologic examination.

Arthropods. Water fleas or mites, but more commonly human body louse *Pediculus humanus* or human pubic louse *Phthirus pubis* may be seen as contaminants in the vaginal smear (Fig. 8–75).

The DCT (Fig. 8–76) can masquerade as parasites and have been reported as "ciliated protozoa." The appearance of DCT is a physiologic occurrence when ciliated tufts are shed in the vaginal smear.

Other organisms including *Schistosoma*, *Toxoplasma*, varicella, *Balantidium coli* and *Trubatrix aceti* (vinegar eels) have been observed in vaginal smears.

AIDS. Most of the parasitic infections, although uncommon in Western populations, are being observed with increased frequency among patients with AIDS. Single and multiple infections occur in women who are human immunodeficiency virus (HIV) positive with a history of intravenous drug abuse or heterosexual relationships. An association of HIV-induced immunosuppression with HPV infections and CIN has more recently been reported.[42]

References

1. Angrish K, Verma K: Cytologic detection of tuberculosis of the uterine cervix. Acta Cytol 25:160–162, 1981.
2. Anthony DD, Wentz WB, Reagan JW, Heggie AD: Induction of cervical neoplasia in the mouse by herpes simplex virus type 2 DNA. Proc Natl Acad Sci USA 86:4520–4524, 1989.
3. Aurelian L, Gupta PK, Frost JK, Rosenshein NB, Smith CC, Tyrer HW, Mantione JM, Albright CD: Fluorescence activated separation of cervical abnormal cells using herpesvirus antigenic markers. Anal Quant Cytol 1:89–102, 1979.
4. Ayre JE: The vaginal smear: "Precancer" cell studies using a modified technique. Am J Obstet Gynecol 58:1205–1219, 1949.
5. Ayre JE: Role of the halo cell in cervical carcinogenesis: A virus manifestation in premalignancy? Obstet Gynecol 15:481–491, 1960.
6. The 1988 Bethesda system for reporting cervical/vaginal cytological diagnoses. NCI workshop. JAMA 262:931–934, 1989.
7. Bhambhani S: Egg of *Ascaris lumbricoides* in cervicovaginal smear. Acta Cytol 28:92, 1984.
8. Bhambhani S, Milner A, Pant J, Luthra UK: Ova of *Taenia* and *Enterobius vermicularis* in cervicovaginal smears. Acta Cytol 29:913–914, 1985.
9. Bibbo M, Harris MJ, Wied GL: Microbiology and inflammation of the female genital tract. *In* Compendium on Diagnostic Cytology. Edited by GL Wied, LG Koss, JW Reagan. Chicago, Tutorials of Cytology, pp 61–75, 1976.
10. Bibbo M, Wied GL: Cytology of Inflammatory Reactions, Tissue Repair, Effects of IUD, Contaminants and Microbiologic Classification Including Chlamydial Organisms, vol 30, 3rd ed. Chicago, Tutorials of Cytology, 1982.
11. Blackwell A, Barlow D: Clinical diagnosis of anaerobic vaginosis (nonspecific vaginitis). A practical guide. Br J Vener Dis 58:387–393, 1982.
12. Brahic M, Haase AT: Detection of viral sequences of low reiteration frequency by *in situ* hybridization. Proc Natl Acad Sci USA 75:6125–6129, 1978.
13. Broker TR, Butcher M: Papillomaviruses: Retrospective and prospective. *In* Cancer Cell 41 DNA Tumors, Venise. Cold Spring Harbor, New York, Cold Spring Harbor Publications, 1986.
14. Burkman RT, Schlesselman S, McCaffrey L, Gupta PK, Spence MR: The relationship of genital tract *Actinomyces* and the development of pelvic inflammatory disease. Am J Obstet Gynecol 143:585–589, 1982.
15. Centers for Disease Control: *Chlamydia trachomatis* infection: Policy guidelines for prevention and control. MWR 34:53–74, 1985.
16. Chandra K, Annousamy R: An unusual finding in the vaginal smear. Acta Cytol 19:403, 1975.
17. Corey L: Genital herpes. *In* Sexually Transmitted Diseases. Edited by KK Holmes, P-A Mardh, PF Sparling, PJ Wiesner. New York, McGraw-Hill, pp 449–473, 1984.
18. De Girolami E: Perinuclear halo versus koilocytotic atypia. Obstet Gynecol 29:479–487, 1967.
19. de la Monte SM, Gupta PK, White CL III: Systemic *Actinomyces* infection. A potential complication of intrauterine contraceptive devices. JAMA 248:1876–1877, 1982.
20. de Moraes-Ruehsen M, McNeill RE, Frost JK, Gupta PK, Diamond LS, Honigberg BM: Amebae resembling *Entamoeba gingivalis* in the genital tracts of IUD users. Acta Cytol 24:413–420, 1980.
21. Frost JK: *Trichomonas vaginalis* and cervical epithelial changes. Ann NY Acad Sci 97:792–799, 1962.
22. Frost JK: Concepts Basic to General Cytopathology, 4th ed. Baltimore, Johns Hopkins Press, pp 23–25, 1972.
23. Frost JK: The Cell in Health and Disease, 2nd ed. Basel, S Karger AG, pp 97–109, 1986.
24. Gardner HL, Dukes CD: *Haemophilus vaginalis* vaginitis: A newly defined specific infection previously classified as "nonspecific" vaginitis. Am J Obstet Gynecol 69:962–976, 1955.
25. Gardner HL, Dukes CD: *Hemophilus vaginalis* vaginitis. Ann NY Acad Sci 83:280–289, 1959.
26. Geirsson G, Woodworth FE, Patten SF, Bonfiglio TA: Epithelial repair and regeneration in the uterine cervix. 1. Analysis of the cells. Acta Cytol 21:371–378, 1977.
27. Gilman SC, Docherty JJ, Clarke A, Rawls WE: Reaction patterns of herpes simplex virus type 1 and type 2 proteins with sera of patients with uterine cervical carcinoma and matched controls. Cancer Res 40:4640–4647, 1980.
28. Graham RM. The Cytologic Diagnosis of Cancer, 3rd edition. Philadelphia, WB Saunders, pp 79–92, 1972.
29. Griffiths PD, Campbell-Benzie A, Heath RB: A prospective study of primary cytomegalovirus infection in pregnant women. Br J Obstet Gynaecol 87:308–314, 1980.
30. Gupta JW, Gupta PK, Shah KV, Kelly DP: Distribution of human papillomavirus antigen in cervicovaginal smears and cervical tissues. Int J Gynaecol Obstet 2:160–170, 1983.
31. Gupta JW, Gupta PK, Rosenshein NB, Shah KV: Human papillomavirus detection in cervical smears: A comparison of *in situ* hybridization, immunochemistry and cytopathology. Acta Cytol 31:387–396, 1987.
32. Gupta PK: Intrauterine contraceptive device: Vaginal cytology, pathologic changes and their clinical implications: Review and lead article. Acta Cytol 26:571–613, 1982.
33. Gupta PK, Aurelian L, Frost JK, Carpenter MM, Klacsmann KT, Rosenshein NB, Tyrer HW: Herpesvirus antigens as markers for cervical cancer. Gynecol Oncol 12:S232–S258, 1981.
34. Gupta PK, Burroughs F, Luff RD, Frost JK, Erozan YS: Epithelial atypias associated with intrauterine contraceptive devices (IUD). Acta Cytol 22:286–291, 1978.

35. Gupta PK, Frost JK: Human urogenital trichomoniasis epidemiology, clinical and pathological manifestations. *In* Proceedings of the Symposium on Trichomonads and Trichomoniasis. Edited by J Kulda, J Cerkasov. Acta Univ Carol 30:399–410, 1988.

36. Gupta PK, Hollander DH, Frost JK: Actinomycetes in cervicovaginal smears: An association with IUD usage. Acta Cytol 20:295–297, 1976.

37. Gupta PK, Lee EF, Erozan YS, Frost JK, Geddes ST, Donovan PA: Cytologic investigations in *Chlamydia* infection. Acta Cytol 23:315–320, 1979.

38. Gupta PK, Pinn VM, Taft PD: Cervical dysplasia associated with azathioprine (Imuran). Acta Cytol 13:373–376, 1969.

39. Gupta PK, Shurbaji MS, Mintor LJ, Ermatinger SV, Myers J, Quinn TC: Cytopathologic detection of *Chlamydia trachomatis* in vaginopancervical (Fast) smears. Diagn Cytopathol 4:224–229, 1988.

40. Hager WD, Majmudar B: Pelvic actinomycosis in women using intrauterine contraceptive devices. Am J Obstet Gynecol 133:60–63, 1979.

41. Halberstaedter L, von Prowazek S: Uber z elleinschlüsse parasitarer natur. beim Trachom Arb Gesundheista 26:44–47, 1907.

42. Henry MJ, Stanley MW, Cruikshank S, Carson L: Association of human immunodeficiency virus—induced immunosuppression with human papilloma virus infection and cervical intraepithelial neoplasia. Am J Obstet Gynecol 160:352–353, 1989.

43. Hjelm E, Hallen A, Forsum U: Motile anaerobic curved rods in nonspecific vaginitis. Eur J Sex Transmit Dis 1:9, 1982.

44. Hollander DH, Gupta PK: Detached ciliary tufts in cervicovaginal smears. Acta Cytol 18:367–369, 1974.

45. Hollander DH, Gupta PK: Hematoidin cockleburs in cervicovaginal smears. Acta Cytol 18:268–269, 1974.

46. Hollander DH, Gupta PK: DCT, CCP and pseudo-protozoa. Acta Cytol 23:258–259, 1979.

47. Jones BR, Collier LH, Smith CH: Isolation of virus from inclusion blennorrhoea. Lancet 1:902–905, 1959.

48. Jones DM, Davson J: *Mycoplasma hominis* in Ayre's smears. Nature 213:828–829, 1967.

49. Jones KW: Detection of herpes simplex virus type 2 in RNA in human cervical biopsies by *in situ* cytological hybridization. *In* Oncogenesis and Herpes Viruses, vol 3, II, 24(2). Edited by G de-Thbe, W Henle, F Rapp, W Davis. Lyon, France, International Agency for Research on Cancer, p 917, 1978.

50. Kapila K, Verma K: Intracellular bacilli in vaginal smears in a case of malacoplakia of the uterine cervix: Letter to the editor. Acta Cytol 33:410–411, 1989.

51. Katz RL, Ferre F, Sneige N, Bruner J, Silva EG, Panish M, Payne LG, Pyle P, Follen-Mitchell M: Comparison of the sensitivity of cytomorphology, slot-blot hybridization and polymerase chain reaction for the detection of human papillomavirus in cervical brushings. Acta Cytol 33:696, 1989.

52. Kellogg JA: Clinical and laboratory considerations of culture *vs.* antigen assays for detection of *Chlamydia trachomatis* from genital specimens. Arch Pathol Lab Med 113:453–460, 1989.

53. Kessler II: Venereal factors in human cervical cancer: Evidence from marital clusters. Cancer 39[Suppl 4]:1912–1919, 1977.

54. Kiviat NB, Paavonen JA, Brockway J: Cytologic manifestations of cervical and vaginal infections. I. Epithelial and inflammatory cellular changes. JAMA 253:989–996, 1985.

55. Koss LG: Diagnostic Cytology and Its Histopathologic Bases, 3rd ed. Philadelphia, JB Lippincott, pp 288–289, 1979.

56. Koss LG, Durfee GR: Unusual patterns of squamous epithelium of the uterine cervix: Cytologic and pathologic study of koilocytotic atypia. Ann NY Acad Sci 63:1245–1261, 1956.

57. Kumar ML, Gold E, Jacob IB, Ernhant CB, Nankervis GA: Primary cytomegalovirus infection in adolescent pregnancy. Pediatrics 74:493–500, 1984.

58. Larsen B, Galask RP: Vaginal microbial flora: Composition and influences of host physiology. Ann Intern Med 96[Suppl 6, pt 2]:926–930, 1982.

59. Laverty CR, Russell P, Hills E, Booth N: The significance of noncondylomatous wart virus infection of the cervical transformation zone. A review with discussion of two illustrative cases. Acta Cytol 22:195–201, 1978.

60. Ledger WJ, Campbell C, Wilson JR: Postoperative adnexal infection. Obstet Gynecol 31:83–89, 1968.

61. Lipschutz B: Untersuchungen uber die aetiologic der krankheiten der herpesgruppe. Arch Derm Syph (Berlin) 136:428, 1921.

62. Luff RD, Gupta PK: Actinomyces-like organisms in wearers of intrauterine contraceptive devices. Am J Obstet Gynecol 129:476–477, 1977.

63. Mardh P-A, Stromby N, Westrom L: *Mycoplasma* and vaginal cytology. Acta Cytol 15:310–315, 1971.

64. McDougall JK: *In situ* cytological hybridization to detect herpes simplex virus RNA in human tissue. *In* Antiviral Mechanism in the Control of Neoplasia. Edited by P Chandra. New York, Plenum, p 233, 1979.

65. Meisels A, Fortin R: Condylomatous lesions of the cervix and vagina. I. Cytologic patterns. Acta Cytol 20:505–509, 1976.

66. Nahmias AJ, Dowdle WR, Naib ZM, Highsmith A, Harwell RW, Josey WE: Relation of pock size on chorioallantoic membrane to antigenic type of herpesvirus hominis. Proc Soc Exp Biol Med 127:1022–1028, 1968.

67. Naib ZM: Cytology of TRIC agent infection of the eye of newborn infants and their mothers' genital tracts. Acta Cytol 14:390–395, 1970.

68. Naib ZM: Exfoliative Cytopathology, 3rd ed. Boston, Little, Brown, pp 104–113, 1985.

69. Naib ZM, Masukawa N: Identification of condyloma acuminata cells in routine vaginal smears. Obstet Gynecol 18:735–738, 1961.

70. Ng ABP, Reagan JW, Lindner E: The cellular manifestations of primary and recurrent herpes genitalis. Acta Cytol 14:124–129, 1970.

71. Papanicolaou GN: Atlas of Exfoliative Cytology. Cambridge, Massachusetts, Harvard University Press, color plate A-IV, 1954.

72. Patten SF Jr: Diagnostic Cytopathology of the Uterine Cervix, 2nd ed, revised. Basel, S Karger AG, p 64, 1978.

73. Paavonen J, Brunham R, Kiviat N, Stevens C, Kuo C, Stamm WE, Holmes, KK: Cervicitis—etiologic, clinical and histopathologic findings in chlamydial infections. *In* Proceedings of the 5th International Symposium on Human Chlamydial Infections, Lund, Sweden, June 15–19. Edited by P-A Mardh, KK Holmes, JD Oriel, P Piot, J Schacter. New York, Elsevier, p 141, 1982.

74. Petersdorf RG, Curtin JA, Hoeprich PD, Peeler RN, Bennett IL Jr: A study of antibiotic prophylaxis in unconscious patients. N Engl J Med 257:1001–1009, 1957.

75. Purola E, Savia E: Cytology of gynecologic *Condyloma acuminatum*. Acta Cytol 21:26–31, 1977.

76. Qualman SJ, Gupta PK, Mendelsohn G: Intracellular *E. coli* in urinary malakoplakia: A reservoir of infection and its therapeutic implications. Am J Clin Pathol 81:35–42, 1984.

77. Quinn TC, Gupta PK, Burkman RT, Kappus EW, Barbacci M, Spence MR: Detection of *Chlamydia trachomatis* cervical infection: A comparison of Papanicolaou and immunofluorescent staining with cell culture. Am J Obstet Gynecol 157:394–399, 1987.

78. Ramzy I: Clinical Cytopathology and Aspiration Biopsy. Fundamental Principles and Practice. Norwalk, Connecticut, Appleton and Lange, p 9, 1989.

79. Reynolds DW, Stagno S, Hosty TS, Tiller M, Alford CA Jr: Maternal cytomegalovirus excretion and perinatal infection. N Engl J Med 289:1–5, 1973.

80. Roberts TH, Ng ABP: Chronic lymphocytic cervicitis: Cytologic and histopathologic manifestations. Acta Cytol 19:235–243, 1975.

81. Sagiroglu N: Progression and regression studies of precancer (anaplastic or dysplastic) cells, and the halo test. Am J Obstet Gynecol 85:454–469, 1963.

82. Schachter J, Dawson CR: Human Chlamydial Infections. Littleton, Massachusetts, PSG Publishing, pp 181–219, 1978.

83. Schnadig VJ, Davie KD, Shafer SK, Yandell RB, Islam MZ, Hannigan EV: The cytologist and bacterioses of the vaginalectocervical area: Clues, commas and confusion. Acta Cytol 33:287–297, 1988.

84. Schneider A, Meinhardt G, De-Villiers E-M, Gissmann L:

Sensitivity of cytologic diagnosis of cervical condyloma in comparison with HPV-DNA hybridization studies. Diagn Cytopathol 3:250–255, 1987.

85. Schneweis KE: 2μm Antigenen aufbau des herpes simplex virus. Zeitschrift fur Immunitaetisforschung 124:173–196, 1962.

86. Shands KN, Schmid GP, Dan BB, Blum D, Guidotti RJ, Hargett NT, Anderson RL, Hill DL, Broome CV, Band JD, Fraser DW: Toxic-shock syndrome in menstruating women: Association with tampon use and *Staphylococcus aureus* and clinical features in 52 cases. N Engl J Med 303:1436–1442, 1980.

87. Shiina Y: Cytomorphologic and immunocytochemical studies of chlamydial infections in cervical smears. Acta Cytol 29:683–691, 1985.

88. Shurbaji MS, Gupta PK, Myers JD: Immunohistochemical demonstrations of chlamydial antigens in association with prostatitis. Mod Pathol 1:348–351, 1988.

89. Shurbaji MS, Gupta PK, Newman MM: Hepatic actinomycosis diagnosed by fine needle aspiration: A case report. Acta Cytol 31:751–755, 1987.

90. Southern EM: Detection of specific sequences among DNA fragments separated by gel electrophoresis. J Mole Biol 98:503–517, 1975.

91. Spiegel CA, Amsel R, Eschenbach D, Schoenknecht F, Holmes KK: Anaerobic bacteria in nonspecific vaginitis. N Engl J Med 303:601–607, 1980.

92. Spiegel CA, Eschenbach DA, Amsel R, Holmes KK: Curved anaerobic bacteria in bacterial (nonspecific) vaginosis and their response to antimicrobial therapy. J Infec Dis 148:817–822, 1983.

93. Stagno S, Pass RF, Dworsky ME, Henderson RE, Moore EG, Walton PD, Alford CA: Congenital cytomegalovirus infection: The relative importance of primary and recurrent maternal infection. N Engl J Med 306:945–949, 1982.

94. U.S. Department of Health and Human Services, Public Health Service: Sexually transmitted disease fact sheet, 39th ed. Atlanta, Centers for Disease Control, 1981.

95. Stroler MH, Broker TR: *In situ* hybridization detection of human papillomavirus DNAs and messenger RNAs in genital condylomas and a cervical carcinoma. Hum Pathol 17:1250–1258, 1986.

96. Taylor-Robinson D, Thomas BJ: The role of *Chlamydia trachomatis* in genital tract and associated diseases. J Clin Pathol 33:205–233, 1980.

97. Thygeson P: The etiology of inclusion blennorrhea. Am J Ophthalmol 17:1019–1035, 1934.

98. Vesterinen E, Purola E, Saksela E, Leinikki P: Clinical and virological findings in patients with cytologically diagnosed gynecologic herpes simplex infections. Acta Cytol 21:199–205, 1977.

99. Wied GL, Bahr GF. Vaginal, cervical and endocervical cytologic smears on a single slide. Obstet Gynecol 14:362–367, 1959.

100. Wied GL, Bibbo M: Question 6: Microbiologic classification of the cellular sample. *In* Management of Patients with Vaginal Infection: An Invitational Symposium. FP Zuspan (Coordinator), M Bibbo, HL Gardner, HC Hesseltine, WC Keettel, WR Lang, GL Wied. J Reprod Med 9:1–16, 1972.

101. Woodruff JD, Braun L, Cavalieri R, Gupta PK, Pass F, and Shah KV: Immunological identification of papillomavirus antigen in condyloma tissues from the femal genital tract. Obstet Gynecol 56:727–732, 1980.

102. Wynn RM: Vaginitis and Related Problems. Proceedings of a Symposium sponsored by the Department of Obstetrics and Gynecology, University of Arkansas for Medical Science. Norwalk, Connecticut, The Purdue Frederick Company, 1980.

103. zur Hausen H: Papillomaviruses in human cancer. Cancer 59:1692–1696, 1987.

9

Benign Proliferative Reactions, Intraepithelial Neoplasia and Invasive Cancer of the Uterine Cervix

G. Peter Vooijs

Diagnostic cytology of the uterine cervix was not the first application of cytology in clinical diagnosis of diseases, but it is definitely the most widespread and best known. In its early days vaginal cytology was primarily directed at the diagnosis of invasive cancer of the uterine cervix and of the endometrium, but later cytologists began to realize that cervical lesions were best recognized in direct scrapes of the cervical mucosa. The concept that invasive carcinoma of the cervix is antedated by an intraepithelial neoplastic change—carcinoma *in situ*—was postulated at the beginning of this century.[161] These intraepithelial changes were believed to be potentially progressive precursors of invasive cancer. Subsequently it became known that the spectrum of abnormal changes of the epithelial lining of the uterine cervix was much wider than previously known. Cytologists soon became aware that these noninvasive epithelial abnormalities of the uterine cervix could also be diagnosed in the direct scrapes. With meticulous comparison between the characteristics of the cells in cytologic smears and the histologic changes found in the same patients, the cytologic characteristic of intraepithelial lesions of the cervix became better defined and the accuracy of cervical cytology in predicting the histopathologic change improved.

All epithelial abnormalities of squamous character derive from ectocervical squamous basal cells and endocervical reserve cells. Depending on the strength of the negative stimulus on the differentiating and maturing basal cells and endocervical reserve cells and, in a later stage, immature metaplastic cells, the ultimately resulting cells will have a more or less differ-

entiated aspect. This explains not only common morphologic features in the different variants of dysplasia and ultimately in the most dedifferentiated intraepithelial variant, carcinoma *in situ*, but also the extremely common co-occurrence of carcinoma *in situ* and dysplastic changes of different severity.

Despite a relatively high proportion of incorrect diagnoses, in large-scale population-screening programs, cervical cytology has proved to be the most effective tool for the diagnosis of cervical cancer. After an initial increase in the number of severe epithelial lesions diagnosed in the population the majority of lesions diagnosed are of slight to moderate severity. It is well known that the majority of these lesions will regress to a less abnormal change after a variable time. In this respect it is justified to follow these changes cytologically, when the cytodiagnostic service is of high quality.

For a correct interpretation of abnormalities a thorough knowledge of the cytologic and histologic characteristics of cervical cancer and its potential precursor lesions is necessary.

THE NORMAL UTERINE CERVIX

Histology and Cytology

Ectocervix

The vagina and the outer portion of the uterine cervix—the ectocervix—are lined with nonkeratinizing

153

squamous epithelium. Embryologically this epithelium is derived from a solid epithelial plate growing inwards from the urogenital sinus up to the level of the later endocervical canal. This solid plate replaces, at the level of the vagina and the ectocervix, the primitive cuboidal epithelium from the fused müllerian ducts from which also the columnar epithelium, lining the fallopian ducts, the uterine corpus and the endocervical part of the cervix, originates. The fusion site of these two types of epithelium is called the *squamocolumnar junction* (Fig. 9–1). The location of this fusion site varies considerably, depending on physiologic and pathologic conditions. During reproductive years the squamocolumnar junction is located at the entrance of the endocervical canal, the *external os,* but owing to hormonal influences or as a result of stromal edema that has changed the configuration of the cervix, it may be located inside the endocervical canal or on the surface of the cervix. When located on the external surface of the cervix, part of the columnar cell lining of the endocervical canal is present on the ectocervical face. This causes a usually well-demarcated reddening of the surface that is easily recognizable at inspection. This outward bulging of the endocervical mucosa, referred to as *ectropion, eversion* or *false erosion,* should be differentiated from a *true erosion* of the epithelium, which by definition is a loss of the lining mucosa, leaving the underlying cervical stroma barren. During childhood and after menopause the squamocolumnar junction is located inside the canal.

During reproductive years the morphology of the stratified squamous epithelium, the function of which is primarily a protective one, is cyclically changing under the influence of ovarian hormones. In its fully matured stage the epithelium of vagina and ectocervix can be subdivided into several layers (Fig. 9–2). For correlation with the different cell types present in cervical cytologic specimens, a subdivision into three layers is most practical. Beginning with the deepest layer, these are (1) basal cell and parabasal cell layer,

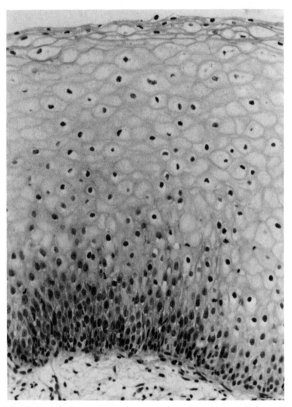

FIGURE 9–2. Normal mature stratified nonkeratinizing squamous epithelium, covering the ectocervical surface (hematoxylin and eosin; ×165).

(2) intermediate cell layer and (3) superficial cell layer. Under physiologic circumstances epithelial regeneration takes place in the basal layer, usually composed of a single layer of relatively primitive cells with scarce cytoplasm and large oval to round nuclei with prominent nucleoli. Under normal circumstances true basal cells are not present in cervical smears unless, at the taking of the smear, the entire epithelial layer has been removed, leaving the underlying stroma denuded. Parabasal cells are unusual in smears from women in reproductive years, unless certain pathologic processes occur, particularly a reduced or absent estrogenic hormonal stimulation. They are the predominant cell type in smears from women in postmenopause and from children.

Parabasal cells are round to oval in shape, have a small cytoplasmic body and relatively large oval to round nuclei (Fig. 9–3; see also Fig. 9–16). The cytoplasm is relatively dense, has distinct borders, may contain vacuoles and commonly stains cyanophilic. After drying of the vaginal or cervical surface, due to absence of estrogenic stimulation or after exposure to air, the cytoplasm stains eosinophilic.

The major part of the thickness of the epithelium is formed by the intermediate cell layer. With maturation of the cells towards the surface, the cells become better differentiated, reflected by an increase of the cytoplasmic volume and signs of specific functional qualities of the cytoplasm, such as storage of glycogen or secretory products. Cells are bound to each other by

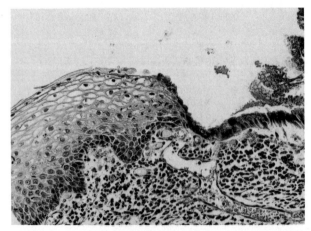

FIGURE 9–1. Squamocolumnar junction. Fusion site of the stratified nonkeratinizing squamous epithelium of the ectocervix and the mucus-producing columnar epithelium lining the endocervical canal (hematoxylin and eosin; ×100).

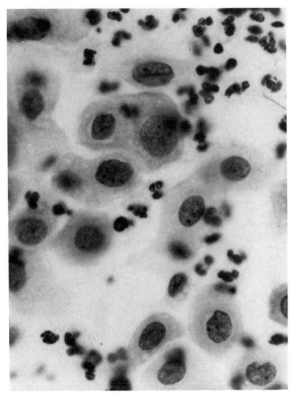

FIGURE 9–3. **Parabasal cells.** Round to oval cells with relatively large nuclei and scant dense, cyanophilic cytoplasm. Admixture of leukocytes is due to inflammation (Papanicolaou stain; ×625).

ess can be accelerated significantly under estrogenic stimulation. Although the influence of estrogenic hormones is predominantly evident on the vaginal epithelium, the ectocervical squamous and endocervical columnar epithelium, contrary to what is often stated, also show a cellular reaction to ovarian hormones. During reproductive years a reduced maturation of the cervical squamous epithelium may be found as the result of the action of oral hormonal contraceptives. Prior to reproductive age, the start of which is marked by the first menstrual period, or menarche, the epithelial lining of the vagina and ectocervix is relatively thin and composed of less mature cells of a parabasal type (Fig. 9–5). Cells do not contain glycogen. Also, during pregnancy, as a result of the relative predominance of progesterone, maturation of the epithelium becomes reduced. The epithelial lining is then composed of intermediate-type cells, with cyanophilic staining cytoplasm, often with a pronounced outer zone. These rather characteristic cells are also called *navicular cells.* Sometimes the underlying stroma shows a large-cell—decidual—reaction, as is physiologic in the endometrial stroma (Fig. 9–6). (See also Chapter 7 on hormonal cytology.) These large stromal cells, when present in smears, may cause differential diagnostic problems with cells from invasive processes, particularly adenocarcinomas, because of large prominent nucleoli (Fig. 9–7). Their occurrence in sheets and as single cells, not in clusters, together with the evenly distributed, finely granular nuclear chromatin, against the back-

intracellular bridges called desmosomes. Cytoplasm of intermediate squamous cells is cyanophilic in staining. Nuclei become only slightly reduced in size during the passage of the cells through the intermediate cell layers. The round to oval nuclei have a diameter of about 8 to 10 μm, have a clearly defined nuclear membrane (Fig. 9–4; see also Fig. 9–18) and contain an evenly distributed, finely granular chromatin.

The most superficial layers are composed of fairly large polygonal cells that are loosely attached to each other. These cells do not proliferate and represent an end stage in the maturation process of nonkeratinizing stratified squamous epithelium. Intercellular attachments—desmosomes—become loose, and cells constantly exfoliate from the surface. Cells are polygonal and have a clear, translucent, usually pink-staining, occasionally cyanophilic cytoplasm, sharply defined boundaries and a small, often pyknotic central nucleus. Superficial cells have a diameter of approximately 40 μm. The nuclear diameter is 3 to 5 μm. The eosinophilic staining of the cytoplasm is caused by the presence of prekeratin proteins. Sometimes fibrillary strands of keratin can be recognized in the cytoplasm of the most superficial eosinophilic staining cells. Rarely superficial cells may contain keratohyalin granules in the cytoplasm, which are supposed to be derived from the granular cell layer of an altered—keratinized—stratified squamous epithelium.

The entire maturation cycle of the normal squamous cell takes approximately 4 days. The maturation proc-

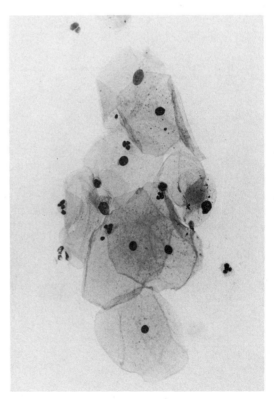

FIGURE 9–4. **Normal superficial and intermediate squamous cells** desquamated from normal nonkeratinizing squamous epithelium (Papanicolaou stain; ×400).

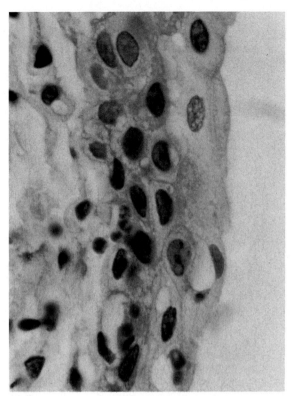

FIGURE 9–5. Atrophy of **ectocervical squamous epithelium**. Epithelial layer is reduced in thickness and almost entirely composed of immature parabasal type cells (hematoxylin and eosin; ×625).

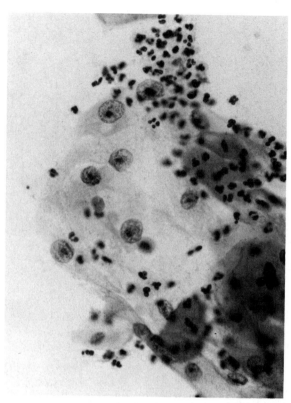

FIGURE 9–7. Large stromal cells in cervical smear during pregnancy show large nuclei with prominent nucleoli and an evenly distributed finely granular chromatin (Papanicolaou stain; ×275).

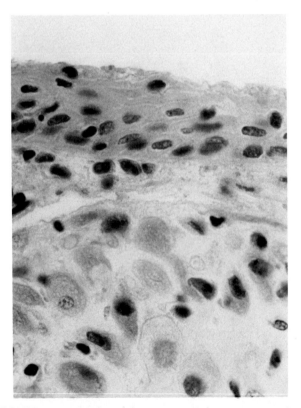

FIGURE 9–6. Atrophy of the **ectocervical squamous epithelium** during pregnancy. Decidual change of cervical stromal cells (hematoxylin and eosin; ×250).

ground of the pregnancy, should provide the correct diagnosis.

Also after the last menstrual period—menopause—the epithelium reduces in thickness and again becomes atrophic. The epithelial cells do not contain glycogen and the epithelium in its atrophic state becomes highly vulnerable to even small traumata and often shows signs of inflammation (see Figs. 9–3, 9–16 and 9–17). An absolute or relative reduction in the level of circulating estrogenic hormones leads to lysis of the cytoplasm of vaginal and cervical squamous cells, as is evident during the second, or luteal, phase of the menstrual cycle, during pregnancy, during lactation and after menopause. Cytolysis may be conspicuous, resulting in a large number of bare nuclei throughout the smear (Fig. 9–8).

Continuous stimulation by estrogenic hormones causes hypertrophy of the superficial layers of the ectocervical squamous epithelium and induces hypersecretion of the endocervical columnar epithelium. The superficial squamous layers are composed of large polygonal cells with clear, slightly eosinophilic staining cytoplasm and very small, almost completely pyknotic nuclei. The presence of these cells in smears from women in postmenopause, particularly when endometrial cells are also found, should be a warning signal of an endometrial abnormality induced by the continuous estrogenic growth stimulus and requires additional diagnostic evaluation.

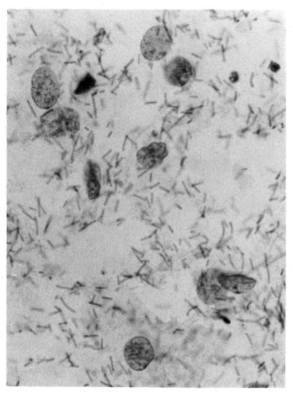

FIGURE 9–8. Cytolysis. Bare nuclei are due to lysis of the cytoplasm. Doederlein bacilli are conspicuous (Papanicolaou stain; ×625).

Endocervix

The epithelial lining of the endocervical canal is formed by a single layer of tall columnar cells (Fig. 9–9). Owing to an arrangement of the nuclei on different levels and variability in size of the columnar cells this epithelial lining often has a pseudostratified appearance. The surface of the endocervical canal is irregularly shaped, with invaginations extending up to 8 mm deep into the cervical stroma (Fig. 9–10). In tissue sections these invaginations are often tangentionally cut and appear as round or oval epithelial stromal inclusions and then are often referred to as *endocervical glands,* even though the uterine cervix does not contain glands in the strict sense. The lining columnar epithelial cells are the source of the mucus that covers the epithelium and composes the mucus plug that fills the endocervical canal. The configuration of the epithelium, the amount of mucus produced and the consistency of the mucus vary with the hormonal status.

In the normal cervical smear endocervical columnar cells appear as tall columnar cells with a large body of clear, finely or coarsely vacuolated, faintly cyanophilic, clear cytoplasm (Fig. 9–11). Ciliated cells may be present. Endocervical cells usually are arranged in strips of parallel arranged cells or in tight sheets. When present in sheet-like arrangements, cell boundaries may create a honeycomb pattern (Fig. 9–12). It is not unusual to find stripped, bare nuclei due to lysis of the fragile cytoplasm. Basally located nuclei are round to

oval and often rather variable in size, with a finely granular, evenly distributed chromatin. In most nuclei one or two small nucleoli can be observed. In cases of increased proliferative activity of the endocervical epithelium the cells and their nuclei show a rather wide variation in size and shape and nucleoli may become prominent and variable in size. Multinucleation of cells is not uncommon. In well-preserved cytologic specimens ciliated columnar cells may be recognized. The morphologic variants of ciliated and mucus-producing cells refer to the müllerian origin of the endocervical epithelium. The presence of ciliated cells has no special significance. It is therefore no sign of an epithelial abnormality.

In tissue sections often a single layer of primitive cells can be observed beneath the columnar cell layer. These cells, also called *reserve cells,* are thought to be multipotential germinative cells, which under physiologic conditions produce normal endocervical columnar cells (Fig. 9–13). In pathologic states reserve cells may proliferate and, depending on the severity of the stimulus, produce abnormal, less well differentiated columnar cells or, through the process of metaplasia, squamous metaplastic cells.

Immunocytochemistry of Normal Cervical Epithelium. The structure and shape of the cell are maintained by an internal cytoplasmic structure, the cytoskeleton. In this cytoskeleton on the basis of their ultrastructural appearance and biochemical composition, three different types of filaments can be distinguished. Next to microtubules and microfilaments,

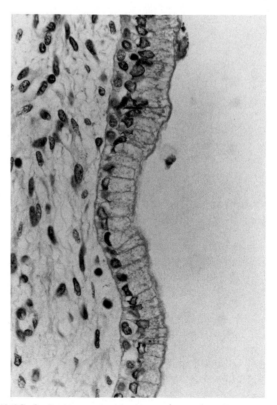

FIGURE 9–9. Mucus-producing **columnar cells** lining the endocervical canal (hematoxylin and eosin; ×425).

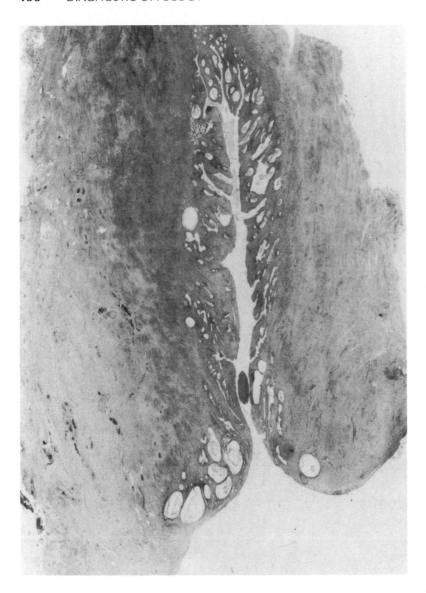

FIGURE 9–10. Low-power view of **uterine cervix**. Deep stromal invaginations of endocervical mucosa greatly increase the surface of the mucus-producing columnar epithelium (hematoxylin and eosin; ×15).

filaments measuring 8 to 11 nm in diameter are commonly seen in mammalian cells. These so-called *intermediate-sized filaments*, which are extremely insoluble and have an entirely different biochemical composition from that of microtubules and microfilaments, often constitute a considerable part of the intracellular matrix. There are five types of intermediate filament, and they occur in tissue-specific combinations.[108, 141]

Keratins have been recognized as epithelium-specific intermediate filament proteins and as comprising a family of at least 19 different polypeptides (not including the hair keratins). The tissue-specific intermediate filament proteins are retained during malignant transformation. Tumors of epithelial origin thus retain cytokeratins as the structural protein for the intermediate filaments.[141] Keratin immunocytochemistry has proved to be a valuable additional technique in the routine diagnosis of cancers that pose problems upon morphologic examination. Broad-spectrum monoclonal antibodies can be used to separate epithelial tissues from nonepithelial tissues. Combinations of the 19 different

keratin proteins are distributed in a more or less tissue-specific fashion as initially detected by two-dimensional gel electrophoresis.[108]

Mainly based on gel electrophoretic studies normal ectocervical epithelium was found to contain keratins 1, 4, 5, 6, 13, 14, 15 and 19, with some variability in the expression of keratins 2, 8, 10, 11, 16 and 17. Endocervical cells contain keratins 7, 8, 18 and 19, with variability in the expression of keratin 4.[35] Reserve cells contain keratins 5, 17, 19 and varying amounts of keratin 4.[203] Reserve cells show an unequivocal distribution of keratin 18 and contain keratins 5, 7, 8, 18 and 19. Immature squamous metaplasia has a keratin expression pattern that on the one hand is characteristic of endocervical columnar cells and on the other hand characteristic of an epithelium that has undergone squamous differentiation. This change becomes emphasized when we compare immature squamous metaplasia with mature squamous metaplasia. The pattern of keratin expression in immature squamous metaplasia was shown to differ from that in normal squamous

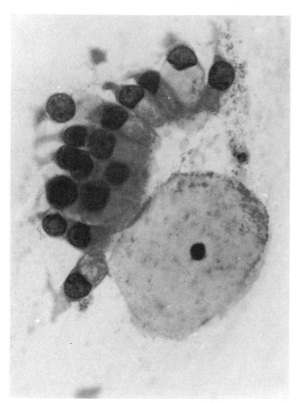

FIGURE 9–11. Superficial squamous cell and tall columnar cells with eccentrically located nuclei and abundant vacuolated cytoplasm. Ciliated cells may be present (Papanicolaou stain; ×500).

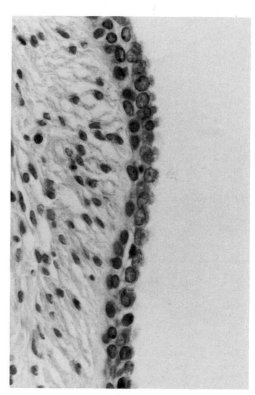

FIGURE 9–13. Single layer of **reserve cells** beneath endocervical columnar cells (hematoxylin and eosin; ×425).

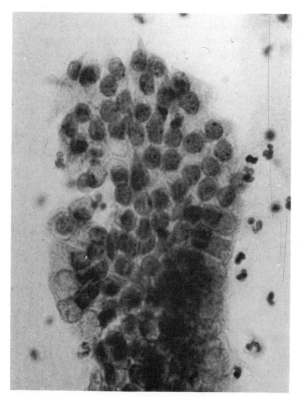

FIGURE 9–12. Sheet of **columnar cells**. Sharply outlined cytoplasmic boundaries create a honeycomb pattern (Papanicolaou stain; ×400).

epithelium. Keratin 19 is present in the full thickness of immature squamous metaplastic epithelium, as opposed to normal squamous epithelium, in which only the basal cell component reacts positively. Keratins 8 and 18, indicative of a columnar differentiation of the cells, become absent. The expression of keratins 4, 10, 13 and 14 increases with squamous differentiation (Figs. 9–14 and 9–15).[117]

Puts and coworkers[138] studied the presence of vimentin-positive cells present in normal ecto- and endocervical epithelium, subcolumnar reserve cell hyperplasia and squamous metaplastic and dysplastic epithelium of the uterine cervix. They demonstrated a relatively large number of vimentin-positive and Langerhans cells in normal ectocervical stratified squamous metaplastic epithelium, a small number in endocervical columnar epithelium and a larger number in subcolumnar reserve cell hyperplasia and in immature squamous metaplasia. Mature squamous metaplastic epithelium showed a great resemblance to normal ectocervical stratified squamous epithelium, both in numbers and distribution of Langerhans cells.

Atrophy

Usually a smear from an atrophic epithelium does not cause diagnostic problems. Cells are of the basal-parabasal cell type, with a high nucleocytoplasmic ratio. Cells are often arranged in syncytia with indistinct cell borders. Usually nucleoli are absent.

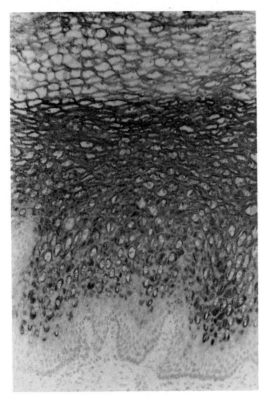

FIGURE 9–14. Expression of **keratin 4** in intermediate and superficial cell layers of mature stratified nonkeratinizing squamous epithelium. Basal cell layers do not stain (Immunoperoxidase method; ×110).

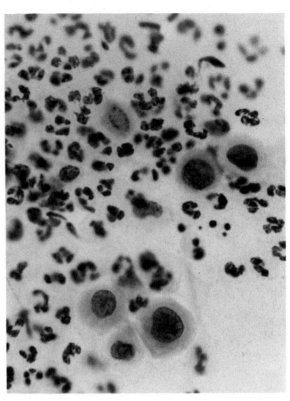

FIGURE 9–16. Parabasal type cells and leukocytes in a cervical smear taken postmenopause (Papanicolaou stain; ×625).

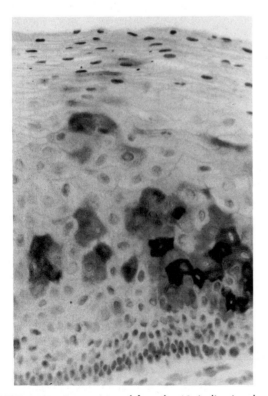

FIGURE 9–15. Expression of **keratin 10** indicating keratin production in the intermediate cell layer of stratified nonkeratinizing squamous epithelium (Immunoperoxidase method; ×250).

In cases of inflammation and atrophy (senile vaginitis) cell changes due to infection and degeneration may cause diagnostic problems (Figs. 9–16 and 9–17). Nuclear chromatin becomes coarsely granular and hyperchromatic. Owing to erosion or ulceration of the superficial stromal layers regeneration of the epithelium is induced. From these parabasal-type cells with relatively large nuclei, prominent nucleoli may appear.[21] In these cases differential diagnosis with an epithelial abnormality may become difficult and at times virtually impossible. However a short course of locally applied or oral estrogenic hormones will induce maturation (Fig. 9–18). Since epithelial abnormalities do not react to the estrogenic stimulus, or at least not into the same degree as normal epithelia do, abnormal cells will stand out clearly and diagnosis can be readily made. In our material after a short course of oral estrogenic hormones, the number of smears with significant drying artifacts was reduced from 66% to 32% and the percentage of smears with a marked to moderate inflammatory exudate from 73% to 55%.

BENIGN PROLIFERATIVE REACTIONS

Hyperkeratosis

The covering epithelium of the vagina and ectocervix apparently still has the potential for further "differen-

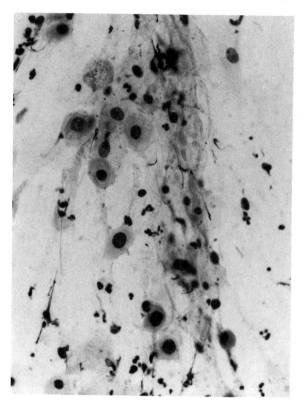

FIGURE 9–17. Cervical smear taken postmenopause with evidence of **inflammation, degenerative nuclear changes and drying artifacts** (Papanicolaou stain; ×250).

tiation," as is demonstrated when this epithelium comes under the influence of chronic, rather severe stimulation. An example of such a chronic stimulation is descensus uteri (prolapse of the uterus), but it may also occur with inflammatory processes or as a reaction to hyperestrinism of long duration. The epithelium increases its protective role by increasing the overall thickness of the epithelium (acanthosis). In addition a granular layer and the development of several layers of keratinized cells—hyperkeratosis—may occur (Fig. 9–19). Hyperkeratosis implies an excessive formation of keratin over the surface of the stratified squamous epithelium. It should be stressed that keratinization of the stratified squamous epithelium of the vagina and cervix represents an abnormal differentiation. At clinical examination this area may appear as a white patch, a sign of leukoplakia. In the cytologic smear leukoplakia can be recognized by the presence of numerous anucleated squames[130] lying as single squames or in sheets (Fig. 9–20). These are often folded and have a pale yellowish-pink color. Remnants of nuclei may be visible as a central clear zone, so-called nuclear ghosts. Cells from the granular cell layer may be encountered in the smear, resembling intermediate or superficial squamous cells, containing eosinophilic or cyanophilic keratohyalin cytoplasmic granules.

Parakeratosis

Parakeratosis is another protective reaction of the nonkeratinizing squamous epithelium of the genital

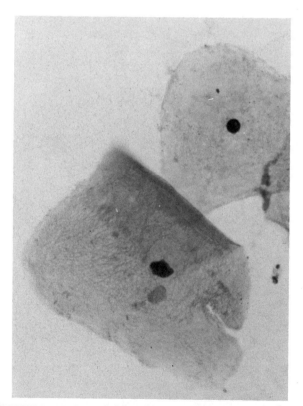

FIGURE 9–18. Superficial and intermediate squamous cell in cervical smear after short course of estrogenic hormones because of epithelial atrophy postmenopause (Papanicolaou stain; ×550). (Same case as in Figures 9–16 and 9–17.)

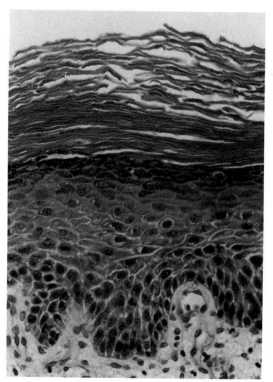

FIGURE 9–19. Hyperkeratosis. Multiple layers of keratin composing the surface of the squamous epithelium. A granular cell layer has been formed beneath the keratin layers (hematoxylin and eosin; ×300).

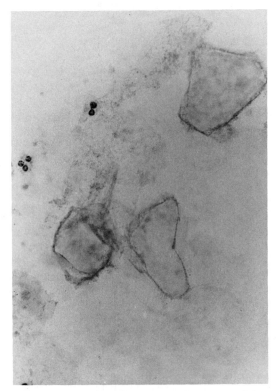

FIGURE 9–20. Anucleated squames desquamated from the superficial layers of keratinized—hyperkeratotic—squamous epithelium (Papanicolaou stain; ×500).

mous metaplasia. The term metaplasia implies the transformation of one cell type into another type of cell, the latter being of a lower organizational order. As applied to the uterine cervix the term refers to the process of replacement of simple columnar epithelial lining the endocervical canal and glands by a stratified squamous epithelium.

Squamous metaplasia may be arbitrarily subdivided into:

- Reserve cell hyperplasia
- Immature squamous metaplasia
- Mature squamous metaplasia.

Reserve cell hyperplasia is transformed in immature squamous metaplasia, which with increasing differentiation gradually turns into mature squamous metaplasia. The maturation of immature squamous metaplasia tends to be more pronounced in the distal part of the endocervical canal.

Factors in the initiation and promotion of squamous metaplasia are chronic irritation of a physical nature such as that caused by an intrauterine contraceptive device (IUD), chemical irritants, inflammation with cell destruction and endocrine changes at the beginning of, during and after reproductive age. Some of the chemical stimuli that induce squamous metaplasia in subcolumnar reserve cells are also capable of inducing cancer in the uterine cervix of the experimental animal.

Squamous metaplasia as such should not be regarded as a change that necessarily and inevitably precedes

tract, characterized by the presence of varying numbers of layers of small squamous cells, sharply demarcated from the underlying superficial zone. The nuclei are small, frequently pyknotic and hyperchromatic.

In cytologic specimens cells from parakeratosis appear as relatively small, superficial squamous cells, lying isolated or in sheets (Fig. 9–21). Shapes vary from round or oval to polygonal or spindle shaped. Cytoplasmic staining usually is dark or light eosinophilic, rarely cyanophilic.

Nuclei are small and often hyperchromatic owing to pyknosis. Although hyperkeratosis and parakeratosis are usually associated with a relatively mature squamous epithelium, a counterpart may overlay an abnormal change such as dysplasia or squamous cell carcinoma. The patient with cellular evidence of hyperkeratosis or parakeratosis should be re-examined to exclude a more serious lesion, camouflaged by the overlying hyperkeratotic or parakeratotic epithelial layer. The physician should be advised to take two smears in succession. The first scrape is intended to remove the superficial abnormally keratinized layers. In the material obtained with the second scrape, the true nature of the underlying epithelium will become apparent.

Squamous Metaplasia

The most common protective mechanism of the endocervical epithelium of the uterine cervix is squa-

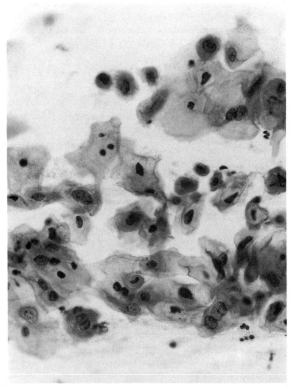

FIGURE 9–21. Parakeratosis. Small superficial squamous cells with sharply outlined cytoplasmic borders and small often pyknotic nuclei (Papanicolaou stain; ×260).

the development of cancer, but the concept of squamous metaplasia is of great importance in the understanding of carcinogenesis in the uterine cervix.

Basal Cell Hyperplasia—Reserve Cell Hyperplasia

Reserve cell hyperplasia is defined as the appearance of one or more layers of primitive, undifferentiated cells in a subcolumnar position between an overlying endocervical lining epithelium and an underlying basement membrane. The earliest form of reserve cell hyperplasia is a single layer of subcolumnar cells[127] (Fig. 9–22). A proliferation of the subcolumnar reserve cells may involve only one or two layers of cells beneath columnar epithelium or may attain a considerable thickness.

There is much controversy as to the origin of these reserve cells. Hypotheses concerning their origin include:[178]

1. Ingrowth of basal cells from the stratum germinativum of adjacent normal stratified squamous epithelium

2. Origin from fetal squamous basal cells in the preexisting stratified squamous epithelial lining of the urogenital sinus

3. Origin from undifferentiated fetal rests

4. Origin from endocervical columnar cells

5. Origin from cervical stromal cells

Fluhmann[47] arbitrarily states that the primitive subcolumnar cells are of epithelial origin and arise above the basement membrane directly from the columnar cells by a process termed *prosoplasia*. The evidence is lacking to definitely exclude their origin from stromal cells.

The epithelium lining the endocervical canal is derived embryologically from the coelomic epithelium lateral to the urogenital ridge and the subsequently developed müllerian system. The stroma of the uterine cervix, derived from the primitive mesoderm at the site of the urogenital ridge, may regain certain of its embryologic potentialities to supply replacement cells through a poorly defined basement membrane. However, the most logical derivation is from the same coelomic epithelium as that from which the columnar cells are derived.

Contrary to what is often stated these reserve cells are not comparable with the basal cells of the original stratified squamous epithelium, since these cells are already dedicated to the formation of squamous cells, whatever the degree of final differentiation (maturation) may be.

Reserve cell hyperplasia per se is not a significant reaction biologically, but it is a frequently occurring nonspecific reaction of the endocervical mucosa.[128, 129]

Cytology. Cells are usually arranged in the form of a sheet. Cell borders are usually poorly defined, which often gives the cell aggregates the appearance of a syncytium, lacking the loss of polarity and the disorganization usually observed in a carcinoma *in situ*.

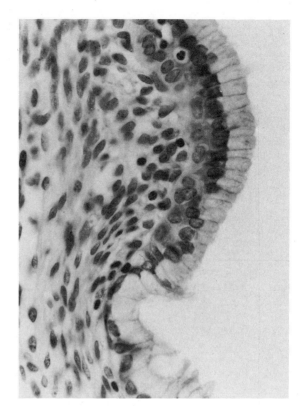

FIGURE 9–22. Reserve cell hyperplasia. The earliest form of reserve cell hyperplasia is the appearance of a single layer of primitive cells beneath the endocervical columnar lining epithelium (hematoxylin and eosin; ×425).

In cervical smears it is not unusual to find a single layer of columnar endocervical cells tightly attached to the margin of a sheet of reserve cells. Pure reserve cells are infrequently identifiable in cervical smears. Presence of reserve cells in cervical smears probably implies that the overlying columnar layer has been dislodged. When present these reserve cells are usually arranged in larger syncytial aggregates called microbiopsies. Cells are relatively small and irregular and polygonal in shape. The small amount of cytoplasm, which is ill defined, is cyanophilic and may be finely vacuolated. Nuclei are small, relatively uniform in size and shape and bean shaped, round or oval and may show longitudinal grooves. Nuclear chromatin is finely granular and is comparable with the nuclear chromatin of the normal interphase nucleus of the columnar cell. Hyperchromasia is uncommon, but in marked proliferation nuclear chromatin may be arranged in coarser chromatin masses.[144] Nucleoli are not identifiable.[128, 130]

The cells arising in reserve cell hyperplasia are noteworthy, since in some instances they are reminiscent of those seen in carcinoma *in situ*. A proliferation of the subcolumnar reserve cells may involve only one or two layers of cells beneath columnar epithelium or may attain a considerable thickness. The proliferation not only simulates carcinoma *in situ* but actually may represent a developmental stage of this process.[144] In the cytologic specimen cells are usually arranged in the form of a sheet. Cell borders are often poorly defined, giving the cell aggregates the appearance of a syncytium but lacking the loss of polarity and the disorganization usually observed in a carcinoma *in situ*.

Reserve cell hyperplasia represents theoretically the earliest stage in immature squamous metaplasia in the uterine cervix. The concept of reserve cell hyperplasia as a stage in squamous metaplasia based on the embryonic rest hypothesis was initially proposed by Eichholz.[39]

Reserve cell hyperplasia is in all instances related to the endocervical canal.[128] The predominant site of pure reserve cell hyperplasia is in the proximal part of the endocervical canal, somewhat more proximal than the site of maximal involvement of immature squamous metaplasia.

A surface reaction with any degree of differentiation towards a squamous cell type is more logically placed within the category of immature squamous metaplasia in spite of the persistence of an overlying endocervical columnar epithelium.

Immature Squamous Metaplasia

Immature squamous metaplasia represents the morphologic spectrum of epithelial changes from a single

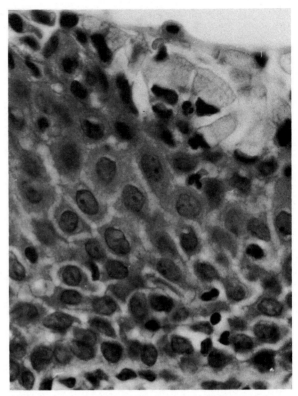

FIGURE 9–24. Immature squamous metaplasia. Layers of relatively immature squamous cells beneath endocervical columnar cells (hematoxylin and eosin; ×500).

or multiple layers of reserve cells to an epithelium composed of three or more layers of cells with features of mature nonkeratinizing squamous epithelial cells (Figs. 9–23 to 9–25; see also Fig. 9–30). Unlike reserve cells, cells derived from areas of immature squamous metaplasia are more often isolated (Figs. 9–26 to 9–28). Their tendency to occur as single cells is correlated with the degree of maturation of the parent epithelium. The majority of cells are round to oval, with the number of polygonal cells increasing with maturation. The cytoplasm of immature squamous metaplastic cells is dense, homogeneous but sometimes vacuolated and cyanophilic in staining reaction (Fig. 9–29). Cells from immature squamous metaplasia vary from round to oval to polygonal. The cytoplasm is homogeneous, relatively dense and predominantly cyanophilic. Cytoplasmic vacuolization is frequently observed in the presence of inflammation or as a consequence of degeneration. Nuclei, particularly in the more immature cells, are large, creating a high nucleocytoplasmic ratio (see Fig. 9–28). Often in cervical smears cells from immature squamous metaplastic changes demonstrate some degree of atypia. Cells and nuclei show a slight irregularity in size and shape, which is understandable because most metaplastic changes occur under the influence of some irritating factor (Fig. 9–30; see also Fig. 9–29). Differential diagnosis with dysplastic changes should be made on the basis of the evenly distributed, finely granular nonhyperchromatic chromatin and the presence of nucleoli.

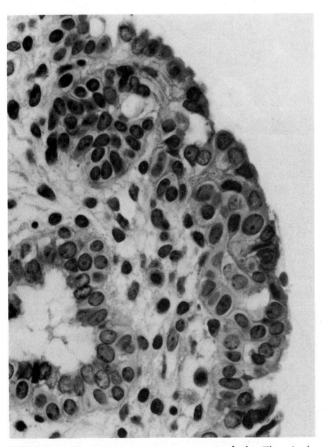

FIGURE 9–23. Immature squamous metaplasia. The single layer of endocervical columnar cells has been replaced by immature squamous metaplastic cells showing slight irregularity in size and shape. In the vesicular nuclei are finely granular nonhyperchromatic chromatin and prominent nucleoli (hematoxylin and eosin; ×400).

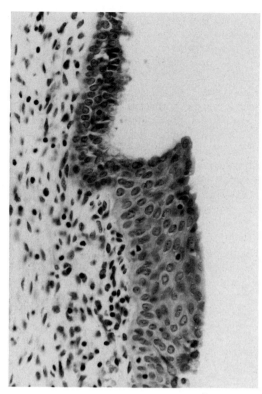

FIGURE 9–25. Immature squamous metaplasia. Multiple layers of relatively mature squamous metaplastic cells have replaced the endocervical columnar lining (hematoxylin and eosin; ×200).

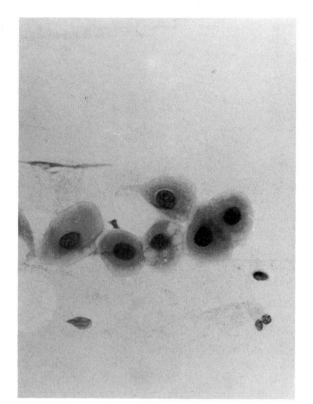

FIGURE 9–27. Immature squamous metaplasia. Singly lying cells with relatively dense homogeneous or vacuolated cytoplasm (Papanicolaou stain; ×400).

Mature Squamous Metaplasia

Squamous metaplasia is represented by a spectrum of epithelial changes resulting in an admixture of cells of varying maturity in the cellular sample.

The *squamocolumnar junction* bears no constant relationship to the anatomic external os, and the external os has no histologic landmarks to delineate it.

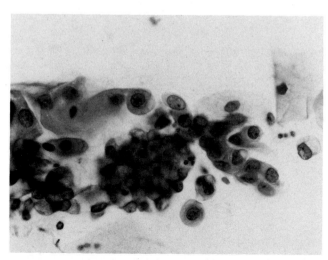

FIGURE 9–26. Immature squamous metaplasia. Immature squamous metaplastic cells lying singly and in a sheet next to endocervical columnar cells (Papanicolaou stain; ×625).

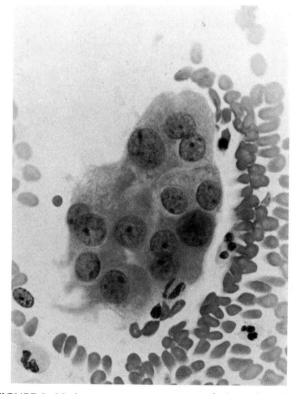

FIGURE 9–28. Immature squamous metaplasia. Cells with a high nucleocytoplasmic (N/C) ratio. Large nuclei with prominent nucleoli and a finely granular chromatin (Papanicolaou stain; ×410).

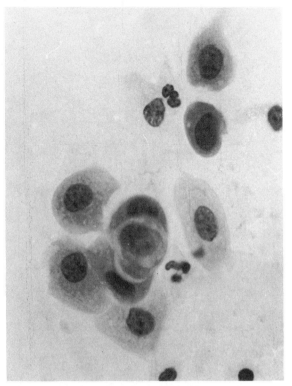

FIGURE 9–29. Slightly atypical **immature squamous metaplastic cells**. Finely granular nuclear chromatin and small multiple nucleoli (Papanicolaou stain; ×625).

The increase in linear extent of squamous metaplasia in the endocervical canal and the region of the transformation zone with increasing age is inversely related to the reduction of the linear extent of reserve cell hyperplasia.

Mature squamous epithelium encompasses the classic three layers of nonkeratinizing squamous epithelium, making mature squamous metaplastic epithelium virtually indistinguishable from the original ectocervical squamous epithelium. Foci of mature squamous metaplasia may be indistinguishable from the normal ectocervical mucosa. The only clue to its metaplastic origin are underlying endocervical glands (Fig. 9–31).

Presence of squamous metaplasia in cervical smears was reported by von Haam and Old[191] to be 41.5%. Howard and coworkers[68] reported an 83% incidence, and Carmichael and Jeaffreson[26] found it to be present in 41% of cervices examined histologically.

The relationship of age to prevalence of squamous metaplasia was found by von Haam and Old[191] to be 86.2% in the 3rd decade and 69.2% in women over 60 years of age. In 101,000 first cervical smears from women 35 to 54 years of age, 62.5% contained squamous metaplastic cells. The prevalence of squamous metaplasia rises significantly from the 3rd to the 5th decade.[6]

Cytology. Cells originating from squamous metaplasia tend to be isolated, less frequently occurring in loose sheets. The number of cells will vary with the extent of the epithelial change, the localization of the

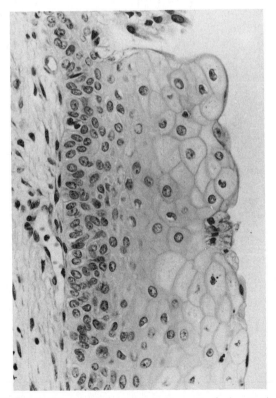

FIGURE 9–30. Immature squamous metaplasia. Epithelial lining composed of relatively mature squamous metaplastic cells. In the superficial layers maturation is still incomplete resulting in cells with relatively high nucleocytoplasmic (N/C) ratios. Cytoplasmic borders are distinct. A small island of columnar cells is recognizable in the superficial layer (hematoxylin and eosin; ×310).

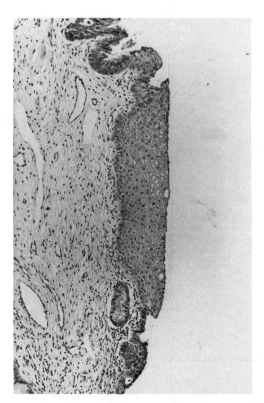

FIGURE 9–31. Mature squamous metaplasia. An island of mature squamous metaplastic epithelium bordered by endocervical columnar epithelium. Mature squamous metaplastic epithelium has great resemblance to stratified squamous epithelium of the ectocervix (hematoxylin and eosin; ×130).

lesion and the method of sampling.[128, 129] Cells from squamous metaplasia characteristically have distinct borders and are predominantly round, oval or polyhedral. In immature squamous metaplasia the cytoplasm is homogeneous and cyanophilic, whereas in a more mature type of metaplasia, it is characterized by a more densely staining outer zone or ectoplasm and a clear central perinuclear zone or endoplasm (Fig. 9–32). At the periphery of the cells, remnants of the fibrillar apparatus, observed in normal squamous cells, may be demonstrated. The nuclei are relatively small, round or oval, usually centrally located and uniform in size and have a basically finely granular chromatin in which there are small aggregates or chromocenters.[144] Sometimes mature squamous metaplastic cells can be differentiated from cells derived from the original ectocervical squamous epithelium by their slightly denser staining cytoplasm.

Cells from a slightly to moderately atypical squamous metaplastic change may pose major problems to the inexperienced cytologist (Figs. 9–33 to 9–35). Within this group of diagnostically difficult lesions, there is a subset that is associated with abnormal cytologic smears, that are colposcopically abnormal and that have the histologic and cytologic features of atypical immature squamous metaplasia (AIM).[34]

The cytoplasm gives information related to the maturity and specific tasks of the cell, whereas the nucleus reflects not only maturity but also the degree of dedifferentiation of a cell (malignant potential). Nuclei in

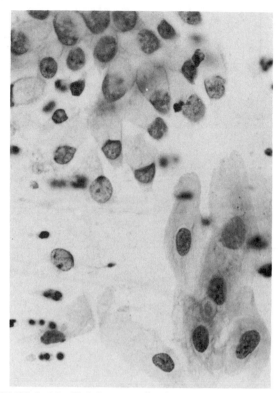

FIGURE 9–33. Slightly atypical relatively **mature squamous metaplastic cells.** Cells resembling ectocervical squamous cells with slightly irregular somewhat enlarged nuclei next to endocervical mucus-producing columnar cells (Papanicolaou stain; ×625).

atypical squamous metaplasia appear to be large but only relative to the size of the cytoplasm. Absolutely, the nuclei in atypical squamous metaplasia are much smaller than nuclei in dysplastic changes. In squamous metaplasia, hyperchromasia is generally absent. Hy-

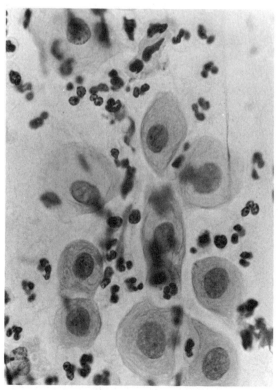

FIGURE 9–32. Mature squamous metaplasia. Round to oval cells with relatively large nuclei. Cytoplasm showing dense outer zone, "ectoplasm," and lighter inner zone "endoplasm" (Papanicolaou stain; ×625).

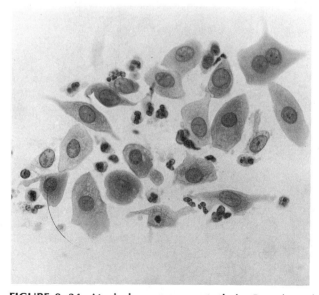

FIGURE 9–34. Atypical squamous metaplasia. Round, oval and polygonal cells with slightly enlarged, slightly irregular nuclei. Nuclear chromatin is finely granular and evenly distributed (Papanicolaou stain; ×425).

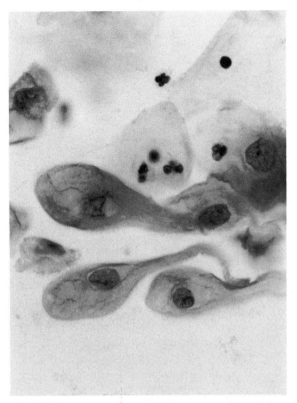

FIGURE 9–35. Cells from **atypical squamous metaplasia** simulating a dysplasia because of abnormal size and shape of the cells. Nuclei are enlarged but relatively small in comparison with the size of the cytoplasmic body (Papanicolaou stain; ×550).

perchromasia in nuclei of dysplastic cells reflects an abnormality in DNA synthesis, e.g., an abnormal number of chromosomes in that particular nucleus.

Mature squamous metaplasia is also referred to as

- Epidermization (Fig. 9–36)
- Complete squamous metaplasia
- Squamous prosoplasia, Stage V (Fluhmann[47]).

Atypia

The word *atypia* means not normal, or not typical for a normal cell of this particular tissue. The term atypia is a minimally defined descriptor in diagnostic cytopathology. The term atypia should not be used as a noun but only as a descriptor of an observation with additional specification of the severity of the atypia. When the word atypia is used in a descriptive diagnosis, the degree of aberration from the normal should be further specified, as should what specific type of cells the observer has referred to. The use of the word atypia without further specification should be avoided, since it then can be used too often as a substitute for a careful description and definition. Commonly the word atypia is used as a descriptive diagnosis when indicating minimal to slight aberrations from the normal. Features most frequently causing such a diagnosis of slight to minimal atypia are nuclear enlargement

and aberrations from the normal configuration of the cells (Fig. 9–37). Most often causative processes are inflammation, regenerative reactions, certain deficiency states such as folic acid deficiency and the earliest changes in an epithelium that is in neoplastic transformation.

In 70,625 first smears, minimally atypical squamous cells and squamous metaplastic cells were diagnosed in 16.8% of smears. When related to the mode of contraception these diagnoses of minimal atypia were made in 14.1% of smears from women using oral contraceptives and in 24.3% of smears from women using IUDs. Diagnoses of minimal to slight atypical changes such as "some abnormal squamous cells present" and "atypical squamous metaplastic cells present" should be followed by a repeat smear after 12 months.[194] Patten[130] advises maintaining patients with evidence of cytologic atypia under surveillance at yearly intervals. Moderate atypia, frequently observed in reparative reactions, should be followed by a repeat smear after 3 months.[194]

Reactive and Regenerative Changes

A reactive change is an epithelial reaction to injury characterized by the presence of sometimes highly atypical cells of endocervical and squamous metaplastic origin.

The epithelia covering the uterine ectocervix and endocervical canal are under the constant influence of physiologic stimuli but also of ever-changing external stimuli.[130]

Regenerative epithelial reactions are commonly found in patients after

- Radiotherapy
- Recent hysterectomy
- Cautery or biopsy
- Cryocoagulation diathermy
- Past history of severe cervicitis
- Partial or complete destruction of the epithelium by infection and inflammation.

These environmental changes result in a variety of morphologic responses, which may be classified as destructive, protective or reparative. All of these reactive changes may result in some form of epithelial atypia in that certain morphologic features are present that represent a departure of the normal.

Repair epithelium in experimental animals has been found to be more susceptible to the action of carcinogenic agents than nontraumatized tissue.[151]

Regeneration of cells as a manifestation of a reparative change can occur in squamous epithelium, in squamous metaplastic epithelium and in columnar epithelium.[15] Geirsson and colleagues[56] found 51.3% of the cells in tissue repair to be of glandular origin, 38.7% of squamous metaplastic origin and 10% of squamous origin.

Reparative reactions are frequent in patients who have had severe recurrent cervicitis and in patients who have had recent treatment, such as punch biopsies, conization, cryosurgery, laser therapy and endocervical

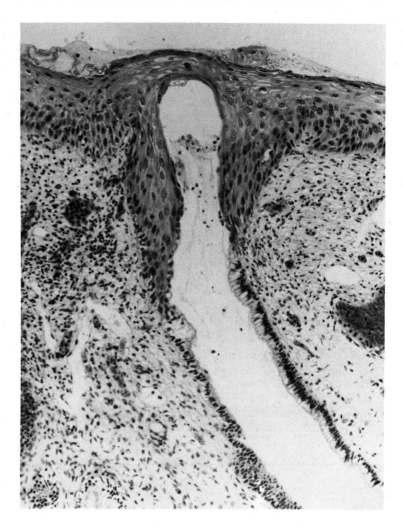

FIGURE 9–36. Epidermization. Relatively mature squamous metaplastic epithelium bridging an invagination of the endocervical mucosa into the stroma. Complete blocking of the invagination may lead to large mucus-filled cysts, Naboth's ovula in the cervix (hematoxylin and eosin; ×101).

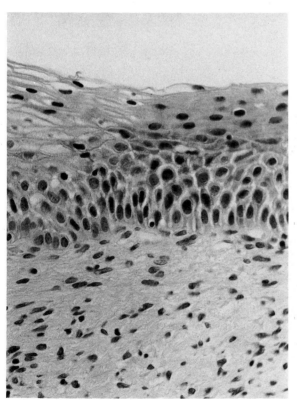

FIGURE 9–37. Minimally atypical **squamous epithelium.** Irregular arrangement of cells and slightly abnormal nuclei in the basal and parabasal layers. Reduced maturation of cells and slight nuclear enlargement in more superficial layers (hematoxylin and eosin; ×250).

curettage. This type of reaction is also found after hysterectomy, together with evidence of granulation tissue, in the postirradiation stage and in cases of true erosion or ulceration of the cervical stroma, which may be caused by a prolapsed uterus, by pressure necrosis from a ring or a shield pessary or by an IUD.

Cytology. Reparative changes are characterized morphologically by significant nuclear enlargement and usually the presence of large, prominent nuclei as a sign of an active protein synthesis in the fast-growing cells, which try to replace the damaged epithelial cells (Fig. 9–38).

Cells from reparative epithelium usually desquamate as large, sheet-like aggregates with indistinct cytoplasmic boundaries. In these aggregates mitoses may be present (Fig. 9–39). It is not unusual to find that leukocytes have infiltrated the larger aggregates of epithelial cells. Rarely abnormal singly lying cells are found. The cells have a wide variation in size and shape. The cytoplasm is usually cyanophilic and sometimes is finely vacuolated or may contain large vacuoles. Nuclei mostly are round to oval with some nuclear enlargement and variation in nuclear size. Nucleoli are prominent, and sometimes multiple macronucleoli are present. As a rule the nuclear chromatin is finely granular, almost always evenly distributed and not hyperchromatic. Essentially cells have the characteristics of immature columnar cells (Fig. 9–40), immature

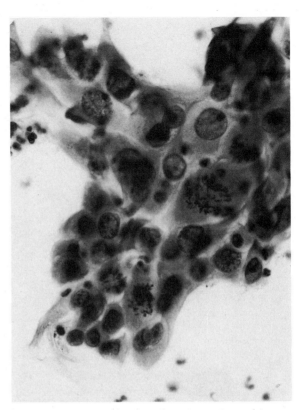

FIGURE 9–39. Reparative reaction. Syncytium of immature cells with multiple mitoses (Papanicolaou stain; ×325).

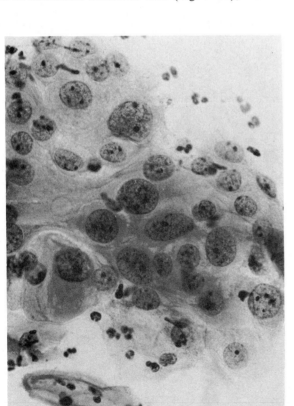

FIGURE 9–38. Reparative reaction. Syncytial arrangement of immature cells with relatively large, round to oval nuclei, prominent nucleoli and a finely granular evenly distributed nuclear chromatin. Conspicuous variation in nuclear size (Papanicolaou stain; ×350).

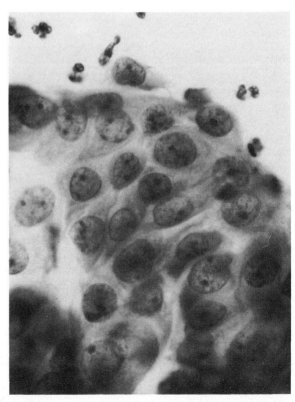

FIGURE 9–40. Reparative reaction. Aggregate of immature cells with features of columnar cells. Round to oval, eccentrically located nuclei, finely granular nuclear chromatin and one to two prominent nucleoli (Papanicolaou stain; ×625).

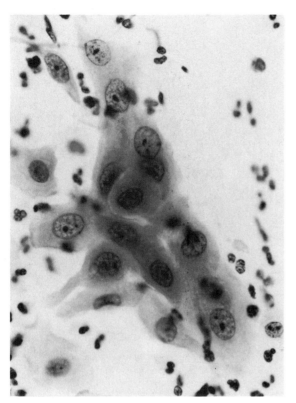

FIGURE 9–41. Atypical reparative reaction. Sheet-like aggregate of immature cells with variation in cellular size and shape, together with a somewhat coarse, slightly hyperchromatic nuclear chromatin and very prominent nucleoli (Papanicolaou stain; ×550).

squamous cells or immature squamous metaplastic cells.[152] Depending on the severity of the stimulus causing the epithelial damage, the replacing epithelium—regeneration and repair—will be blocked in its maturation and show a degree of abnormal configuration or hyperchromasia (Figs. 9–41 and 9–42).

The *differential diagnosis* between cells from reparative changes and cells from invasive neoplastic processes may be difficult. The predominant arrangement of cells in sheet-like aggregates, even though the cytoplasmic boundaries may be indistinct, together with the normochromatic, finely granular, evenly distributed chromatin, and the presence of macronucleoli usually can provide the correct diagnosis. In no other epithelial abnormality and particularly in no invasive process do these three characteristics occur simultaneously.

Inflammation-Associated Cellular Changes

Inflammation alone causes minor cytologic abnormalities, such as a dual staining reaction, lysis or vacuolization of the cytoplasm, slightly disproportionate nuclear enlargement and an increase of the nucleocytoplasmic ratio (Fig. 9–43). Nuclear chromatin is more often hypochromatic than hyperchromatic. (See Chapter 8 on Microbiology, Inflammation and Viral Infections for additional information.)

Degenerative Changes. Degenerative changes of nuclei such as folding of the nuclear membrane, karyorrhexis, karyolysis and pyknosis in cases of inflammation must be differentiated from abnormal nuclear changes in premalignant or malignant epithelial lesions.

Cytomorphologic alterations caused by inflammation or physical or chemical trauma usually are nonspecific. Changes are cell destruction, cytolysis, karyorrhexis (Fig. 9–44) and karyolysis. In cases of nuclear alterations, such as nuclear enlargement, binucleation and multinucleation, as well as coarse clumping and irregular distribution or a complete loss of structure of the chromatinic material, the differential diagnosis with true atypical changes, such as dysplastic reactions or even invasive carcinoma, becomes relevant (Fig. 9–45). Usually the correct diagnosis can be made on the basis of the cytoplasmic vacuolization due to hydropic degeneration and the fading of nuclear contours due to autolysis.

Unsatisfactory Quality. Occasionally extreme admixture of inflammatory cells can obscure epithelial cells or dilute the number of diagnostic cells in a specimen, thus reducing the chance of detection of abnormal cells. In women participating in a large population-screening program, the number of smears unsatisfactory for cytologic diagnosis was 6.8%.[97] Poor quality of the smears was caused by too few epithelial cells

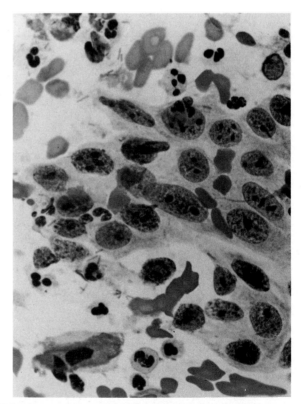

FIGURE 9–42. Atypical reparative reaction. Sheet-like aggregate of immature cells with indistinct cytoplasmic borders, round to oval nuclei, coarse, somewhat hyperchromatic nuclear chromatin and very prominent, often pleomorphic macronucleoli. In the left lower corner, a moderately atypical squamous metaplastic cell (Papanicolaou stain; ×450).

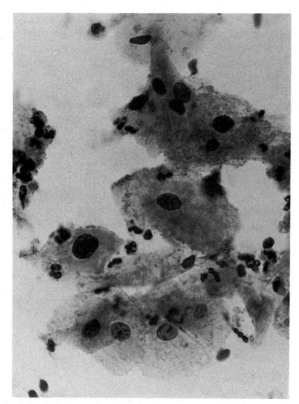

FIGURE 9–43. Slight **atypia** of squamous cells in a cervical smear with evidence of a bacterial infection (Papanicolaou stain; ×350).

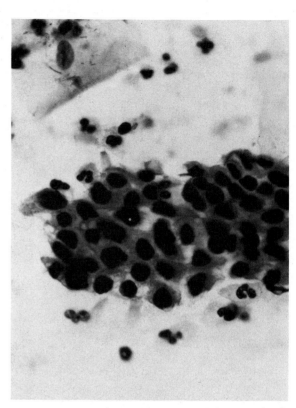

FIGURE 9–45. Degenerative changes in endocervical columnar cells. Hyperchromasia due to condensation of the chromatinic material. Loss of nuclear structure. Differential diagnosis with a severe epithelial lesion on the basis of sharply outlined cytoplasmic borders. Honeycomb pattern (Papanicolaou stain; ×500).

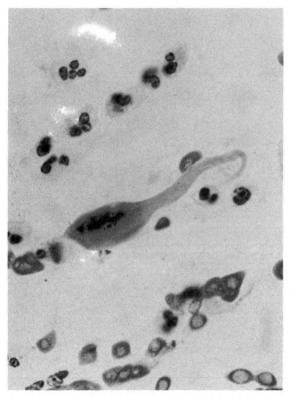

FIGURE 9–44. Karyorrhexis. Loss of nuclear structure, dissolved nuclear membrane, irregular clumping of chromatinic material. On the basis of the shape, this cell must be considered to be derived from an epithelial abnormality (Papanicolaou stain; ×625).

present or because of a strong admixture of erythrocytes or inflammatory cells. Of the smears that were considered evaluable, endocervical columnar cells and squamous metaplastic cells were found significantly more frequently in smears showing signs of bacterial inflammatory reaction or the presence of *Trichomonas vaginalis*. A significant proportion of smears without signs of inflammation were less reliable for cytologic diagnosis.

An inflammatory exudate has been reported to be associated with approximately 32% of dysplastic reactions.[143] In a large population study, a significantly higher percentage of smears without signs of epithelial abnormalities were found in the absence of signs of inflammation.[97] In these smears the occurrence of minimal epithelial atypia was even significantly lower than expected. The prevalence of mild and moderate dysplasia was also lower than expected but not significantly so. The percentage of smears without any sign of inflammation rose significantly with age. The distribution of epithelial changes in the group of smears with signs of bacterial infection did not differ significantly from the expected numbers. In contrast, epithelial abnormalities were significantly more common in smears showing evidence of *T. vaginalis* (Fig. 9–46), as were changes consistent with severe dysplasia and carcinoma *in situ*. In smears with evidence of *Candida albicans* (moniliasis) significantly more minimally atyp-

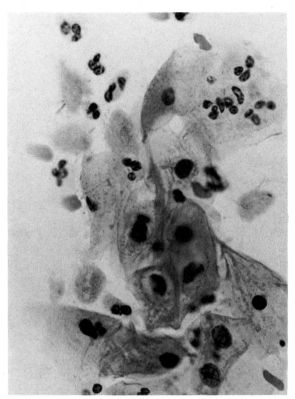

FIGURE 9–46. Evidence of ***Trichomonas vaginalis* infection**. Trichomonads can be recognized between slightly atypical squamous cells. In the center is a cell with a clear perinuclear halo (Papanicolaou stain; × 450).

ical epithelial changes were found, which seemed more a reaction of the epithelium to the inflammatory stimulus than a dysplastic change. This was not paralleled by a higher proportion of smears with squamous metaplastic cells present, nor was there evidence of a higher proportion of mild to moderate dysplastic changes.

Epithelial Abnormalities. The finding that the presence of inflammatory signs or microorganisms is more common in smears consistent with dysplasia or carcinoma, and the lack thereof to be suggestive for atypia or dysplasia,[51, 52] was not confirmed. The exception to that finding was *T. vaginalis*; this parasite was found four times more frequently than expected in smears consistent with severe dysplasia and carcinoma *in situ*.

La Vecchia and coworkers[91] also found significant associations of a history of *T. vaginalis* and *C. albicans* with cervical intraepithelial neoplasia (CIN) lesions, but not with invasive cancer. Frisch[51] found 4% of smears originally diagnosed as inflammatory atypia to be underreported, since in subsequent smears these atypias had "progressed" to CIN.

Schachter and colleagues[163] reported a significantly increased risk for cervical neoplasia in women with antibodies to *Chlamydia trachomatis*, and Hanekar and associates[67] found in patients with *Chlamydia*-associated epithelial abnormalities that the progression rate to CIN grade III after 2 years' follow-up was significantly higher than in a control group with comparable epithelial changes but without evidence of *Chlamydia* infections. They suggest that *Chlamydia* may be a

cocarcinogen or a potentiating agent in the progression of cervical intraepithelial lesions. In patients with persistent inflammatory atypia Noumoff[122] found in colposcopically directed biopsies in about one third of the patients underlying CIN, of which, again, about one third was of greater severity than CIN grade I. On the basis of these data he advises that all patients with persistent inflammatory atypia should undergo colposcopic evaluation.

It may be difficult to decide whether the epithelial abnormality is a nonspecific response to the inflammatory stimulus or a true preneoplastic intraepithelial lesion. The cytologic report should clearly state the diagnostic dilemma, and recommendation for a repeat examination after a follow-up interval should be part of the report.

This minimal to mild atypia may eventually be followed by the appearance of cellular changes consistent with a mild dysplasia. Smears with signs of atypia related to inflammation should therefore be repeated after 1 year.[194]

Immunosuppression

Immunosuppression either due to immunodeficiencies or caused by medication conveys a significant risk for infections with herpes simplex virus Type 2 and human papilloma virus (HPV) and for developing neoplastic conditions (Fig. 9–47).[98, 99] Patients at risk

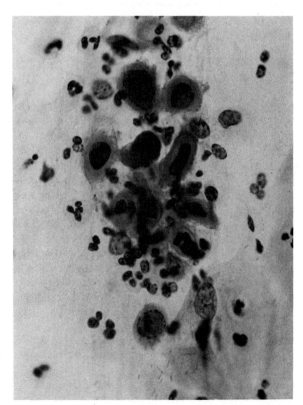

FIGURE 9–47. Changes consistent with a **herpes simplex Type 2 virus**. Nuclear enlargement and dense opaque nuclear chromatin. At the left of the cell group is a singly lying cell with an enlarged nucleus and a "ground-glass" nucleus (Papanicolaou stain; × 450).

are those receiving immunosuppressive drugs because of transplants or for various other conditions, patients with Hodgkin disease and patients with cancer following treatment with cytostatics.[66, 134, 165] The reported significantly increased risk for cervical cancer with the number of pregnancies is an interesting association in view of the fact that pregnancy is considered a transient state of immunodepression.[18, 91]

Intrauterine Contraceptive Devices

The most severe reactive changes, those that most closely mimic intraepithelial neoplasia, both of squamous as well as of glandular type, are associated with the presence of an IUD.[59, 159] Composing cells may show severe cellular and nuclear polymorphism, an increased nucleocytoplasmic ratio, prominent nucleoli and cytoplasmic vacuolization. Often severely atypical cells arranged in clusters are present. There is usually a marked inflammatory reaction. The differential diagnosis with cells derived from an adenocarcinoma may be extremely difficult, but the cytopathologist can avoid this erroneous diagnosis, since these IUD-related changes usually are found in relatively young women and in the presence of an IUD. This, however, stresses the importance of correct and complete clinical information, accompanying the request for a cytologic examination. Sometimes it may be necessary to remove the device and to repeat the cytologic examination after an interval of 4 to 6 weeks. Usually the epithelial abnormalities will have disappeared by then.

Condylomatous Lesions and Epithelial Abnormalities

It has been recognized that certain intraepithelial neoplastic lesions of the human cervix, first defined as koilocytotic warty atypia by Koss and Durfee,[87] would now be diagnosed as condylomatous lesions, caused by an infection with HPV. HPV, in particular the subspecies 6, 11, 16, 18 and 31, known as causative agents in warty condyloma acuminatum of the vulva and vagina, were thought to be important sexually transmitted etiologic factors in the genesis of cervical cancer.[69, 124] These subtypes were reported to play an important role in the development of progressive intraepithelial precancerous changes of the squamous epithelium, but also in those of the endocervical epithelium of the cervix. Condyloma acuminatum is found in younger age groups than is dysplasia and is quite frequent in the sexually active teenager.[104]

Types 6 and 11 are most commonly associated with condyloma acuminatum of the cervix and with cervical intraepithelial neoplastic lesions of mild to moderate severity. Types 16 and 18 are usually associated with more severe epithelial abnormalities and with invasive cancer.

This has resulted in reports stating that presence of types 16 and 18 in preinvasive lesions might be an indicator of a progressive behavior of such a particular lesion. However, only a long prospective study could support evidence for such an association. Present epidemiologic evidence implicating HPV as a cause of cervical neoplasia is still rather limited. Most of the present evidence comes from studies that do not satisfy basic epidemiologic requirements. Most significant methodologic shortcomings are with the usually small number of subjects studied, the potentially biased selection of individuals and the low accuracy of differential cytologic diagnosis between papilloma virus infections and preneoplastic lesions.[16, 112] With the increased sensitivity of molecular biologic methods HPV subtypes, often more than one type, have been demonstrated in a very high percentage of apparently healthy individuals without any evidence of a cervical epithelial abnormality.[96, 166] Koilocytosis and multinucleation were found to have predictive value for mild and moderate dysplasias with a relatively low risk of progression. Positivity to HPV was twice as frequent in the group of lesions that were regressive.[164]

For a more detailed overview of the relation between HPV and epithelial abnormalities of the cervix see Chapter 8 on Microbiology, Inflammation and Viral Infections.

Dysplasia of the cervical and vaginal epithelium is frequently associated with condyloma. Condyloma acuminatum is usually detected by cytologic screening because of the characteristic morphology of cells exfoliating from its surface. These lesions were previously often misdiagnosed as dysplasias.

In the differential diagnosis with CIN it is relevant that condylomata occur at a younger mean age, are found in the transformation zone and the cervical portio, are polyploid, often regress and contain HPV antigens in the majority of cases. Koss,[84] contrary to what most authors favor, prefers to use the term CIN grade I with features of condyloma.

Histology. Cervical lesions are of three types. The most frequent form is a flat, acanthotic epithelial change with well-preserved basal layers and marked nuclear degeneration with perinuclear halos towards the surface that also shows dyskeratotic changes (Fig. 9–48). The classic proliferative, papillomatous condyloma is found much less frequently and the third type, even rarer, is an endophytic "inverted" condyloma. The flat and endophytic condylomata represent new lesions that were previously not described on the cervix. Many of the condylomatous lesions were described as dysplasias. This led Meisels and coworkers[103] to believe that this sexually transmitted viral lesion represented a precursor of cervical neoplasia in view of the fact that condyloma acuminata has been proved to undergo malignant transformation in a few cases and that it behaves epidemiologically in a way similar to carcinoma of the cervix.

Cytology. Even though there are certain features that are characteristic of condyloma and CIN, these two lesions cannot always be distinguished clearly by morphologic means. Some features may help in differentiating between them.

The koilocytes are the predominant cellular features of infection with HPV.[102] Koilocytes must be differen-

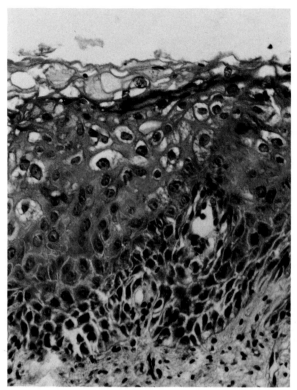

FIGURE 9–48. Condylomatous change with **slight nuclear atypia** and irregular arrangement of the cells in the squamous cell layer (hematoxylin and eosin; ×155).

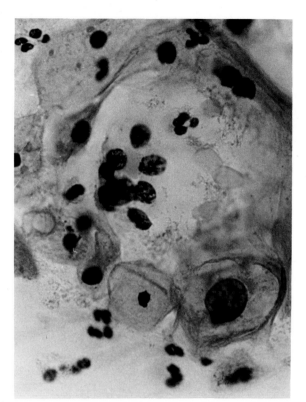

FIGURE 9–49. Koilocytotic cell. Large perinuclear halo. Dense outer zone of the cytoplasm and an enlarged nucleus with finely granular nuclear chromatin (Papanicolaou stain; ×500).

tiated from cells with perinuclear halos occurring with other types of infection, such as trichomoniasis. In these cells however nuclear abnormalities are not as outspoken and halos tend to be smaller and less well demarcated. Once the cellular pattern is recognized condyloma acuminatum becomes the most frequent epithelial lesion diagnosed in a mass screening program.[104]

The pathognomonic change is the koilocytotic cell: This is a superficial or intermediate squamous cell, which displays a large perinuclear halo with irregular, clear-cut edges and a dense, often amphophilic, sometimes almost hyaline cytoplasm in the area surrounding the perinuclear cavity (Fig. 9–49). In condyloma cells are generally mature and often display an ample amphophilic cytoplasm, the chromatin is usually poorly defined and the nuclei may show various stages of degeneration. The nuclear membrane is not distinct and nucleoli usually are absent. In intraepithelial abnormalities, cells are mostly immature with scant cyanophilic cytoplasm, the chromatin details are distinct, the nuclear membrane is clearly visible and somewhat irregular and small nucleoli can be recognized.[101, 102] Abnormal differentiation becomes evident by an underdeveloped, cytoplasmic body and a relatively enlarged nucleus, leading to an increased nucleocytoplasmic ratio (Fig. 9–50). Nuclear shapes are round to oval and often irregular. Particularly in the more severe abnormalities the nuclear chromatin is increased and often irregularly distributed. Cellular changes originate in pre-existent squamous epithelium or more often in squamous metaplastic epithelium.

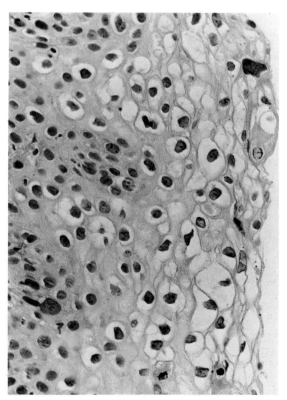

FIGURE 9–50. Condylomatous change in **mature squamous epithelium**. Irregularity in nuclear size and shape and conspicuous nuclear halos (hematoxylin and eosin; ×250).

Structural features typical of the condylomatous epithelium are common in dysplastic changes. Dysplastic changes are often (25% of the time) accompanied by a micropapillary change of the surface. These lesions are probably also due to infection by the papilloma virus, yet their significance is unknown and the possibility of a precancerous lesion cannot be ruled out except by a very long term follow-up study. It may be assumed that this virus may affect the cervical and vaginal epithelium without any typical papillary condylomatous lesion resulting.[137]

Sensitivity. Cytology may detect the majority of lesions with koilocytotic features but may not detect focal CIN grades I, II and III lesions associated with these condylomatous changes.[171]

Cellular changes due to HPV infection may mimic the changes found in cases of well-differentiated squamous cell carcinoma. Usually the right diagnosis may be made on the basis of the less outspoken nuclear abnormalities in HPV-induced epithelial lesions.

Neither cytology nor histology can detect the asymptomatic, colposcopically negative, latent HPV infection, which can be detected by hybridization tests only. The great intra- and interobserver variability in the cytologic and histologic diagnosis of condyloma and CIN indicates that there is a great amount of subjectivity in evaluating the morphologic characteristics of a lesion. The correlation between morphologic signs of HPV infection and the results of HPV-DNA hybridization indicates that the sensitivity of the cytologic and histologic features of HPV infection are in the range of 15 to 36%.[111] Future diagnosis of HPV should include hybridization.[101]

SQUAMOUS INTRAEPITHELIAL NEOPLASIA

Terminology. "The primary function of a diagnostic terminology is to communicate to the referring physician the interpretation of a specimen in descriptive terms that will have clear implications for appropriate patient management. Many practicing physicians do not have detailed knowledge of cytopathology. Thus the cytologic report should not only be scientifically accurate but also easily understood."[42] The terminology currently used in cytopathology is variable, inconsistent and sometimes ambiguous, which has made many cytopathologists and clinicians confused and uncertain about the meaning of some terms. Failure to understand the clinical meaning of a cytopathologic evaluation may lead to inappropriate patient management.

The cytology report should consist of a concise description of abnormal cellular findings in well-defined and generally accepted terms, followed, if appropriate, by a prediction of the histologic condition, and should also include a recommendation for the further management of the patient.[40, 42, 194, 198, 199]

In pathology, the basis for any system of classification is morphologic. However, where possible, the classification should relate to the biologic significance or potential of the process.[131]

Papanicolaou Classification. The Papanicolaou classification of cytologic findings in epithelial lesions has led to different interpretations. Also, the Papanicolaou system does not provide for the diagnosis of noncancerous lesions.

"The groups of the Papanicolaou system do not reflect the current understanding of cervical neoplasia and the Papanicolaou classes do not have an equivalent in tissue diagnostic terminology."[116] Epithelial abnormalities of the uterine cervix form a morphologic and most likely also a biologic continuum.

The rationale for distinguishing between dysplasia and carcinoma *in situ* on a cytomorphologic basis is to permit the best possible correlation between the cellular and tissue sample and with the final clinical outcome of the epithelial change.

Years of experience have demonstrated the difficulty of splitting dysplastic cervical lesions into the diagnostic triad of mild, moderate and severe dysplasia. In our own experience cytologic diagnoses of mild or severe dysplasia and carcinoma *in situ* proved to be fairly accurate. The cytologic diagnoses of moderate dysplasia were less accurate. A large proportion (57%) of moderate dysplasias were absent or had regressed to a less severe lesion at follow-up 6 months after primary diagnosis. On the other hand in about 20% of cases during follow-up a more severe lesion was found.[186, 200]

A National Cancer Institute (NCI) working group recommended discontinuing the use of the Papanicolaou classification as a means for reporting. The Papanicolaou classification is deficient in advising about the true nature of abnormalities unless it is accompanied by a verbal description of the cytologic findings.

In order to establish some order, all lesions that are known to be reactions to infections, inflammation or reparative reactions (regeneration) should be excluded, as well as benign proliferative reactions in the endocervical canal such as reserve cell hyperplasia and squamous metaplasia, since these in themselves are not considered to be stages in the process of carcinogenesis.[116]

The NCI working group adopted a new classification based on only two categories:

Low-grade squamous intraepithelial lesions
● Changes consistent with HPV infection
● Mild dysplasia (CIN grade I)

High-grade squamous intraepithelial lesion
● Moderate dysplasia (CIN grade II)
● Severe dysplasia (CIN grade III)
● Carcinoma *in situ* (CIN grade III)

It was thought that using only two categories would reduce the present inconsistencies in terminology. The proposed terminology is related to the expected clinical behavior of the epithelial abnormalities and is management-oriented in that it includes a recommendation for the preferred follow-up procedure in an individual case. The new classification is thought to provide a basis for communicating the diagnostic interpretation of a specimen in unambiguous descriptive or diagnostic terms that will have clear implications for proper patient management.[116]

The expectations from the working group about the impact of the new terminology and classification are quite high. It is, however, unlikely that our understanding of the clinical behavior of intraepithelial lesions of moderate to severe grade will improve with the proposed system.

Dysplasia

The term *dysplasia* means disordered form (disordered differentiation). Reagan and associates[149] introduced the term dysplasia to describe these disordered growth patterns and reported that the majority of these intraepithelial changes would regress spontaneously or persist unchanged if left untreated.

"In the uterine cervix, the term dysplasia is applied to a spectrum of heteroplastic reactions involving stratified squamous or squamous-like (metaplastic) epithelium. As the term implies, this group of reactions is characterized by malformation or disordered development, manifested morphologically by variations in cytoplasmic maturation in association with certain nuclear abnormalities."[127, 128]

The definition of dysplasia is derived from the definition of carcinoma *in situ*, which is defined as "an intraepithelial abnormality in which throughout its whole thickness, no differentiation takes place." "All other disturbances of differentiation in the squamous epithelial lining, the glands, or covering of the surface are to be classified as dysplasia. They may be characterized as a high or a low degree, terms that are preferable to suspicious and nonsuspicious, as the proposed terms describe the histologic appearance and do not express an opinion."[207]

In the definition of the World Health Organization dysplasia is "a lesion in which part of the thickness of the epithelium is replaced by cells showing varying degrees of atypia." The lesions were further graded as mild, moderate and severe.[135] Most pathologists determine these grades of dysplasia on the basis of the proportion of the epithelial thickness occupied by the abnormal cells, taking into account the degree of atypia of these cells. The latter grading has raised much discussion, since a number of authors do not believe that this grading is sufficiently correlated to biologic behavior. The dual terminology has led gynecologists to assume that dysplasia and *in situ* carcinoma are two biologically distinct entities with different progressive potential and that dysplastic lesions may not require treatment.[30] Some studies have shown that the behavior of these intraepithelial lesions cannot be predicted with accuracy and that even mildly abnormal changes, when left untreated, may progress to carcinoma *in situ* and invasive cancer.[45, 90] Burghardt[23] reported on the direct development of invasive cancer from dysplasia without an interphase of *in situ* carcinoma.

The marked variation in morphology, even from one site to another within the same cervix, is undoubtedly the cause for the confusion in terminology and the difficulties in evaluating the biologic significance of these reactions.

Fundamentally dysplasia represents a reaction to injury in the sense that a stimulus acting upon a normal epithelium results in some morphologic alteration of that epithelium.

It is unpredictable where (or when) the stimulus will initiate an abnormal reaction, i.e., in mature stratified squamous epithelium, mature squamous metaplasia or immature squamous metaplasia. The form of dysplasia that results may then depend on the maturity of the epithelium that reacts. The morphologic features of a dysplastic reaction involving an immature squamous metaplastic epithelium are relatively uniform and will differ from a similar reaction involving mature stratified squamous epithelium.

The stimulus exerts its effect on the cells of the basal layer of mature ectocervical stratified epithelium or on the reserve cells or immature squamous metaplastic cells in the endocervical canal. Initially this would be demonstrated by a defect in the mitotic mechanism of the cell, resulting in scattered cells with an abnormal DNA content, demonstrated by the appearance of enlarged nuclei with an abnormally distributed hyperchromatic chromatinic material. Differentiation of the cytoplasm is disturbed owing to an abnormal stimulus from the nucleus.

With a continuing stimulus persistence of some of the abnormal cells capable of complete division and survival might lead to an increase of the number of abnormal cells. Continued selection and persistence of the abnormal cells will increasingly involve multiple layers of the lining epithelium, thus increasing the severity of the lesion.

Cervical Intraepithelial Neoplasia

Because of a great deal of confusion about the clinical significance of the terms dysplasia and carcinoma *in situ*, the term cervical intraepithelial neoplasia, or CIN, was introduced in an effort to bring a more active approach to the evaluation and treatment of noninvasive epithelial abnormalities of the cervix.[152]

The concept of CIN reflects the basic unity of precancerous changes, regardless of the phenotype of such epithelial abnormalities.[152–155] It was meant to replace the prior system of nomenclature, such as dysplasia and carcinoma *in situ*.

Data on the progression rate of dysplasias of different grades of severity and carcinoma *in situ* stress the continuous nature of the epithelial alterations ultimately leading to invasive squamous cell cancer. On this basis it seemed advisable to abandon the artificial distinction between dysplasia and carcinoma *in situ*.[155]

The terminology of CIN subclassified into grades of dedifferentiation essentially has not provided an advantage over the former subclassification of dysplasias. It has always been recognized that within the group of dysplasias a proportion of the lesions may progress to a more severe abnormality, eventually even to an invasive process. Many cases of CIN are not truly neoplastic in nature but represent a nonspecific response to injury from chronic irritation or inflammation. Although the presence of an inflammatory process does not exclude the possibility that the epithelial abnormality is not truly neoplastic in nature, it remains true that a residue of cases will remain in which nonspecific reactive changes mimic very closely those of true CIN.[21] Richart and Barron[155] apply strict criteria to lesions before they can be included in the group of CIN. However these are only applicable in retrospect when epithelial changes have proved to persist during a certain period of time. As stated by the authors the progressive or indolent nature of dysplastic lesions cannot be judged on the basis of mere light microscopic examination. This, however, is equally impossible in grading intraepithelial neoplasias. A relatively large percentage of the lesions do not progress during long-term follow-up. Within the morphologic spectrum of CIN one must include lesions known as koilocytotic atypia, recognized as due to papilloma virus infection. CIN can be graded from I to III to reflect the degree of epithelial abnormality, provided that no prognostic significance is attached to this classification. The implication of the CIN concept is that all patients with abnormalities, whatever their grade, must be referred to colposcopic examination to be evaluated further.[84] Koss[84] advises following CIN grade I (mild dysplasia) with cytology or destroying the lesion. In daily practice the subclassification into CIN grades I through III has not reduced the number of women referred for colposcopic evaluation or biopsies, and the diagnoses CIN grades I through III still include a large number of lesions that will spontaneously regress, since they were of a reparative or a reactive nature.

Electron Microscopy. Although it is possible to subclassify CIN into mild, moderate and severe dysplasia and carcinoma in situ by light microscopy, such a subclassification is difficult at the subcellular level.

The nuclear enlargement may reflect the increase in DNA synthesis that accompanies the decreased generation time in dysplasia and carcinoma in situ. Mitotic figures are rarely observed in normal epithelium but are frequently seen in dysplasia and carcinoma in situ, in keeping with the more rapid growth rate. The mitotic figures in dysplasias do not generally differ from those in normal epithelium, but rare mitotic figures are observed in which the number of chromosomes in nuclei appear to be increased.[173]

In a comparative study between normal and dysplastic cells using scanning electron microscopy Kenemans and coworkers[76, 77] demonstrated differences in surface architecture between the basal and luminal side of normal intermediate squamous cells and between normal and abnormal cells, both in exfoliated cells and in cells from tissue specimens. The luminal side of epithelial cells bears microridges and the basal side contains microvilli. In all cases of histologically established (moderate or severe) dysplasia there was a remarkable increase in the number of microvilli and a decrease in the number of desmosomes. Abnormal configuration of microvilli was also observed in epithelial abnormalities. These changes have also been documented in cells from invasive carcinoma. The decrease in number of desmosomes is in accord with the finding that neoplastic cells are more loosely attached to one another than are normal cells.

The lack of adhesiveness between the epithelial cells in dysplasia and carcinoma in situ could also account for the increased number of leukocytes in the altered epithelium, since it would facilitate the penetration of the epithelium by inflammatory cells.

Surface cells in dysplasia, although they may appear flattened under the light microscope, have cytoplasm containing large numbers of ribosomes, numerous mitochondria and decreased or absent storage of glycogen, which is in keeping with their less-differentiated state. Increased numbers of ribosomes and polyribosomes have also been reported in cervical squamous cell carcinoma.[173, 174]

Cervical Intraepithelial Abnormalities

Origin and Localization. Dysplastic reactions occur significantly more frequently on the anterior as opposed to the posterior lip of the uterine cervix[151] and are usually localized in the endocervical mucosa at the transformation zone in the region of the cervical os or in the epithelium covering the ectocervix or portio vaginalis.

The majority of abnormal surface reactions begin within the area of the endocervical-lining epithelium and mimic in an abnormal fashion various stages in the process of squamous metaplasia.[131] There is some confusion about the exact site and cells of origin of cervical intraepithelial abnormalities. Koss[83] indicates as the site of origin of over 90% of the intraepithelial abnormalities the area of squamous epithelium bordering the columnar epithelium, known as the squamocolumnar junction or transformation zone (Fig. 9–51). The remaining less than 10% of lesions are then thought to originate in the area of the columnar epithelium. This would mean that the cell of origin of most of the intraepithelial lesions would be the basal cell of the original ectocervical squamous epithelium overlying an area without gland-bearing stroma. This is in conflict with the observation by Reagan and Patten[148] that only 11.1% of a series of dysplasias were located in an area of the cervix without underlying glands. In 48.9% of specimens, the site of involvement was partially related to gland-bearing stroma, and the remaining 40% of the lesions were confined to a site with underlying glands.[130] From these data it appears that in 88.9% of their specimens there had been at least partial involvement of the area in which squamous metaplasia occurs as the basic reaction to injury of the columnar epithelium. The latter distribution is more in line with the experience from routine clinical practice that the majority of intraepithelial changes, and virtually all of the severe intraepithelial abnormalities, extend into the invaginations of the columnar epithelium. It is a common observation that the severity of the change in the invaginations is less than the surface change.

Morphology Related to Origin. From the spectrum

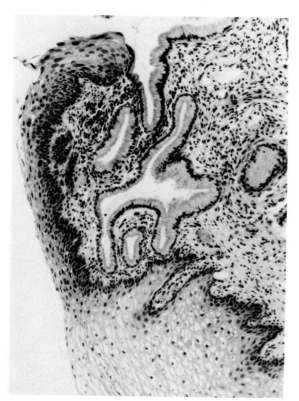

FIGURE 9–51. Transformation zone. The most distal part of the endocervical columnar epithelial lining bordering the original stratified squamous nonkeratinizing epithelium has been replaced by mildly atypical squamous metaplastic epithelium (hematoxylin and eosin; ×123).

of morphologic patterns of intraepithelial abnormalities occurring on the ectocervix and in the epithelial lining of the endocervical canal it is evident that the potential of reserve cells to differentiate into squamous epithelium through an intermediate stage of immature squamous metaplasia gradually diminishes in the proximal direction along the canal. This is reflected in the epithelial abnormalities originating at different sites. The dysplastic reactions occurring close to the squamocolumnar junction usually still demonstrate some maturation into squamous-like epithelium in the superficial layers, whereas abnormalities occurring proximally in the canal lack this squamous differentiation completely and seem to be composed entirely of undifferentiated primitive cells (atypical reserve cells). The resemblance to squamous epithelium of the more distal lesions does not necessarily mean that these, although often erroneously named "better differentiated" when compared with classic carcinoma *in situ*, would have a less malignant potential. In this respect the relatively large-cell severe dysplasia should be considered of comparable severity as the more classic carcinoma *in situ* and treated accordingly.

Grading. The current concept of dysplasia and *in situ* carcinoma is that these form a continuous spectrum of a developing intraepithelial abnormality. Many have felt such a continuum to be in conflict with a subdivision into grades. However, on the basis of histologic crite-

ria, it is not only possible to grade the severity of the change, but it is also clinically relevant, since grading provides a basis for the mode of treatment. Grading lesions also makes these lesions accessible for retrospective and prospective studies, which are the only available means to get more insight in the true nature of these changes. The fact that it has been proved to be very difficult to diagnose these lesions accurately and reproducibly can never be the reason to refrain from categorizing these lesions.

Grading of dysplastic reactions may give more insight into the morphologically different types of dysplasia as well as into the biologic potential of these types.

The more closely the lesion resembles normal epithelium, the less severe that lesion is thought to be. The more primitive cell types predominate that lack signs of differentiation, the more severe a lesion is considered to be. Thus it is possible to apply the terms minimal, slight, moderate and severe to differentiate on a morphologic basis—phenotypically—one lesion from another.

Unfortunately the degree of morphologic abnormality does not necessarily correlate with the biologic potential of the epithelial change.[128] Because of this frequent lack of correlation Friedell[50] recommended a morphologic classification incorporating both qualitative and quantitative information.

Fundamentally the intraepithelial neoplastic—dysplastic—reaction is characterized by premature keratinization of component cells and abnormal differentiation of a variable number of cell layers that, in the most severe forms, encompasses all cell layers throughout the whole thickness of the mucosal lining.

In all dysplastic changes, by definition, in the uppermost layers of the epithelium, cells remain that have features of normal epithelial cells. This is usually more apparent in dysplasias originating in the original squamous epithelium than in changes involving the squamous metaplastic epithelium.

Cells in the upper layers of dysplasia have features indicating differentiation. However, the nuclei are usually enlarged and more hyperchromatic in comparison with normal squamous epithelial cells, and there is a remarkable variation of the nuclei of the cells, in contrast to the rather uniform size and shape of nuclei in normal epithelial cells at a comparable level.

In lesions involving mature squamous epithelium individual cell keratinization and keratohyalin pearl formation are not uncommon.

Mitoses are usually found. In less severe lesions, mitoses, both normal and abnormal forms, are confined to the lower half of the epithelium. In more severe changes mitoses can also be found in the upper third of the mucosal lining.

Occurrence. More recently the mean age at which cervical intraepithelial lesions are diagnosed seems to be gradually decreasing. This might be related to changes in sexual behavior within Western countries and a lowering of the age of first sexual activity. Although several observers have reported that invasive cancers are also diagnosed with greater frequency in younger women,[111] this has so far not resulted in a

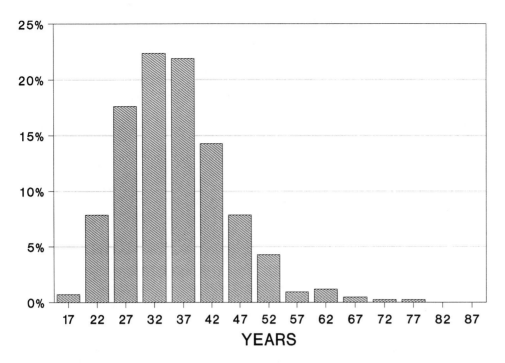

FIGURE 9–52. Moderate dysplasia. Histologic diagnoses. Age distribution—average age is 36.8 years (SD-9.1) and N = 420. (Data from the Nijmegen Registry of Cervical Cytology, 1978-1987.)

greater mortality from cervical cancer in women in younger age groups. The reported increased frequency of intraepithelial lesions in younger women may in part be due to an increased frequency of cytologic testing and not be a true increase in the number of intraepithelial abnormalities.

On the basis of cellular evidence of dysplasia Patten [129] reported a prevalence of 0.98% in 57,469 nongravid women. Regan and coworkers [147] reported a prevalence of 0.77% in a study of 10,533 women. On the basis of histologic evidence the prevalence has been reported to vary between 1.2% [100] and 3.2%. [147] In our own material in women 35 through 55 years of age mild and moderate dysplasia was found in 1.6% and severe dysplasia and *in situ* carcinoma in 0.3% of women at first screening. [186]

Age at Detection. The stages of evolution of the dysplastic process might be reflected in the age at detection. Based on cellular evidence of dysplasia, the mean age at detection was 34.7 years. [127] Patients with slight dysplasia were found to have a mean age of 32.0 years, with moderate dysplasia the mean age was 35.7 years and in patients with severe dysplasia the mean age was 38.4 years. [127]

Reagan and associates [147] reported a mean age of 34.2 plus or minus 1.6 years in women having only minimal to slight dysplastic lesions and of 41.4 plus or minus 3.0 years in reactions classified as severe dyspla-

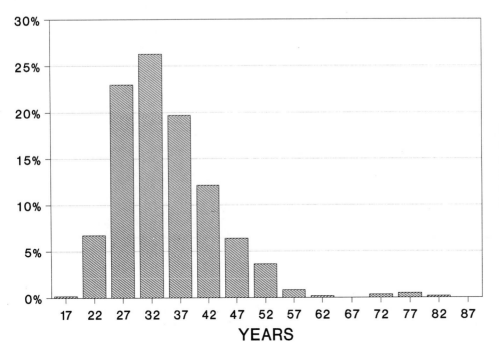

FIGURE 9–53. Severe dysplasia. Histologic diagnoses. Age distribution—average age is 35.7 years (SD-8.7) and N = 609. (Data from the Nijmegen Registry of Cervical Cytology, 1970–1987).

sia. In our own series the average age of detection of moderate dysplasia was 36.8 years and of severe dysplasia 35.7 years (Figs. 9–52 and 9–53).

Histology. In the dysplastic reaction abnormal cells are present throughout all layers of the epithelium. Inversely related to the severity of the lesion going from the basal layers to the surface, signs of differentiation will occur. The morphology of cells composing the superficial layers of a dysplastic reaction is related to the severity of the dysplastic reaction. This is evidenced by a relative increase in the cytoplasmic volume, well-defined cell boundaries and a reduction in the size of the nucleus and thus a lower nucleocytoplasmic ratio. The dysplastic reaction is characterized by premature keratinization of component cells, abnormal differentiation of the cells composing the epithelial lining and abnormally large nuclei in association with varying degrees of cytoplasmic maturation (usually varying degrees of abnormal maturation of the cytoplasm).

Cells present in the upper layers of the mucosa reflect in their morphology the entire cascade of maturation steps throughout the epithelium. The more dedifferentiated the cell in the most basal layers, the less influence maturation stimuli will have during this cell's passage through the layers of the epithelium, and the greater the remaining abnormality of the cell that finally reaches the superficial layers will be. From the morphology of these superficial cells, which are mechanically removed from the superficial layers of the mucosa, the experienced cytopathologist can rebuild an image of the histopathologic appearance of the mucosal lining at the site of the scrape and thus give an impression of the severity of the abnormality at that site.

Cytology. Shortly after the introduction by Ayre[7, 8] of the spatula for making cervical smears, it was reported that precancerous and cancerous changes still confined to the mucosa of the cervix could be detected in these cytologic samples.[8, 9, 48, 136] The number of abnormal cells in a cell preparation taken from epithelial lesions of comparable severity may differ from one case to the other, depending on the method of collection and the skill of the person who has taken the sample.[198] In general the number of abnormal cells is related to the severity (and the extent) of the lesion. The lesser the abnormality, the fewer abnormal cells are found in the specimen. The more severe the lesion, the higher the number of abnormal cells. On the basis of cell population evaluation, one can obtain rather specific information on differentiation characteristics of the parent lesion.[131] With experience a more definitive interpretation can be made on the basis of cellular specimens, since both cancerous and noncancerous changes in the surface mucosa of the uterine cervix are reflected in the desquamated cells.[144]

Abnormal cells originating from the surface of epithelial abnormalities may be subdivided morphologically into two groups. Those showing signs of differentiation of squamous type have, depending on the degree of maturation, features reminiscent of superficial, intermediate or parabasal squamous cells (Figs. 9–54 and 9–55). When signs of differentiation are

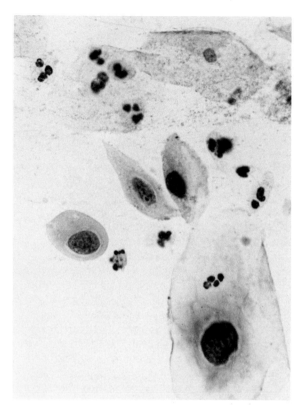

FIGURE 9–54. Slight dysplasia. Cells of squamous type with slightly enlarged nuclei and some hyperchromasia. Compare with squamous metaplastic cell and normal superficial squamous cell (Papanicolaou stain; ×425).

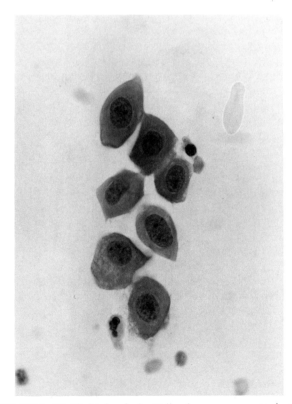

FIGURE 9–55. Slight dysplasia. Cells of squamous metaplastic type with slightly enlarged nuclei. The nuclear chromatin is finely granular and very slightly hyperchromatic (Papanicolaou stain; ×625).

almost completely absent, cells bear a resemblance to reserve cells.

Patten,[128] in an attempt to provide a morphologic terminology for dysplasia that might be applicable to both histologic and cellular material and might provide evidence for biologic potential, introduced a subclassification of dysplasia for routine use. The major subdivisions were (1) keratinizing (ectocervical) dysplasia, (2) nonkeratinizing dysplasia and (3) metaplastic dysplasia.

In a series of 2453 cases the nonkeratinizing variant was observed approximately seven times more frequently than the metaplastic type and 25 times more frequently than the keratinizing variant. Admixtures of these different types are most often represented by the simultaneous occurrence of cells consistent with the nonkeratinizing and metaplastic variants. Of this series about 85% of dysplasias in a 5-year period progressed to *in situ* carcinoma. The reactions are further classified as to severity by adding the terms minimal, slight, moderate and marked (severe).[131]

Arrangement of Cells. Abnormal cells from dysplastic lesions usually lie singly and have well-defined cell borders. In the majority of specimens atypical cells are also found in sheets. Usually cell borders are still recognizable. The presence of cell aggregates with indistinct cell borders in a cellular specimen indicates a reduced tendency to maturation in the mucosal lining. This reduced maturation is a reflection of the dedifferentiation of the component epithelial cells that lack the stimulus to mature. In such an aggregate the component cells are regularly arranged with relation to one another. Less frequently cells may be arranged in syncytial masses. Here the component cells are irregularly arranged with relation to one another and have indistinct cell borders. A syncytial arrangement is more commonly associated with carcinoma *in situ* and invasive cancer.

In almost all cases of dysplasia sheetlike arrangements are found. Syncytial masses are found in only 10% of specimens and are always associated with a severe epithelial abnormality.[128, 130]

Cell Size. The volume and the condition of the cytoplasm is a reflection of the state of maturation and differentiation of the cells. Usually there is an admixture of cells of varying maturity. In view of the site of origin of dysplasias and the preceding metaplastic process in the endocervical canal, the size of cells involved in dysplastic changes may vary from almost the size of a normal superficial squamous cell in minimal abnormalities to the size of an immature basal cell or a very immature squamous metaplastic cell in more severely abnormal changes.

Relating cell size to the severity of the histopathologic change in dysplasias, those samples containing dysplastic cells with cell areas predominantly in the range of normal squamous cells tend to originate from a less atypical (less severe) dysplastic reaction. These reactions are more frequently located on the portio vaginalis or in relation to the external cervical os. Those samples with dysplastic cells possessing cell characteristics more reminiscent of squamous metaplastic cells are more likely to have arisen in the area

of the distal portion of the endocervical canal (transformation zone).

Most of the abnormal cells observed in the presence of dysplasia, carcinoma *in situ* and invasive cancer will possess cell sizes as observed in cells from immature squamous metaplasia and reserve cell hyperplasia. The relative nuclear area, nuclear shape and particularly intranuclear chromatin architecture should then provide the basis for the right diagnosis.[130]

Cell Configuration. The shape of an abnormal cell in a sample may also reflect the maturity of the parent tissue reaction. In dysplasia there is a predominance of polygonal cells, comprising about 55% of the abnormal cell population (52.7%[143] and 56%[209]). Round or oval forms, indicative of a less mature reaction, represented about 40% of the abnormal cells in samples studied (41.6%[143] and 40%[209]).

A predominance of polygonal forms, often found together with eosinophilic staining of the cytoplasm, suggests an origin from a dysplastic reaction, originating in original squamous stratified epithelium, and a predominance of oval forms is suggestive of a dysplastic reaction in an area of squamous metaplasia, most likely the transformation zone of the endocervical canal. The presence of spindle-shaped or elongated cells may indicate the presence of (abnormal) keratinization at the surface of the epithelium. The elongated cells often show fibrillary structures in the cytoplasm. The presence of these fibrils is indicative of keratinization in the dysplastic process. Keratinization overlying a dysplastic reaction most often occurs in the ectocervical epithelium, but occasionally a keratinizing dysplasia may be found in the endocervical canal in a metaplastic epithelium.

Anucleated squames, sometimes with pale yellow cytoplasm, may also be found. When contamination from the vulvar mucosa can be excluded, the presence of these squames should always lead to an extra awareness on the part of the cytopathologist. Sometimes severe dysplastic reactions or even keratinizing squamous cancer may be covered by a thick layer of hyperkeratosis.

When making a scrape from this area the cellular material obtained may be restricted to keratinized squames. Owing to the resistant cover, deeper layers have not been sampled and the true lesion remains obscure.

When anucleated squames are diagnosed in a cell sample, even without atypical cells being observed, a repeat smear should be advised and the physician should be specifically instructed to sample any area of leukoplakia (literally *white patch*) very carefully, preferably by taking successive smears from the same area, thus gradually uncovering the nonkeratinized part of the lesion.

Nuclear Morphology. Nuclear characteristics are the main determinants for the grading of an epithelial abnormality. Although cytoplasmic features may provide additional information as to the origin and degree of maturation of a cell, the main important denominator of the severity of an epithelial abnormality remains nuclear changes.

Nuclear atypia should be classified as mild, moderate

or severe. Cytoplasmic changes should be classified according to quantity, density, staining quality and shape.

The morphology of the cell nuclei in cases of epithelial changes comprises a combination of any number of the following:[42]

- Disproportionate nuclear enlargement
- Irregularity in form and outline
- Hyperchromasia
- Irregular chromatin condensation
- Abnormalities of the number, size and form of the nucleoli
- Multinucleation.

Papanicolaou[125, 126] introduced the term *dyskaryosis* to designate certain cytologic patterns observed in vaginal and cervical smears from cases of early carcinoma and some other pathologic lesions of the uterine cervix in which the exfoliated cells are characterized by marked nuclear abnormalities consistent with the generally accepted criteria of malignancy, although the cells as a whole may show no significant deviation from their standard normal type. He described the morphology of dyskaryotic cells as follows: "The nuclei show distinct abnormal features such as enlargement, hyperchromasia, anisokaryosis, bi- or multinucleation et cetera." Patten[128] strongly advocates avoiding the use of subjective terminology to describe morphologic changes and thus rejects the use of the term dyskaryosis "which although useful during the developmental stages of applied cytology, presently has no place in the vocabulary of the diagnostic cytologist except for historical reflection."[128] The working party of the British Society of Cytology,[42] however, endorsed the recommendation made by Spriggs and associates[179] to use the terms dyskaryosis and dyskaryotic in the description of nuclear abnormalities in both squamous and endocervical cells in intraepithelial lesions as well as in invasive carcinoma.

Relative Nuclear Area. The relative nuclear area is an expression of nuclear area in relation to cytoplasmic area. The relative nuclear area increases with the severity of the lesion from minimal dysplasia to carcinoma *in situ*.

Nuclei of dysplastic cells are relatively large when compared with their normal counterparts. The greater size of the nuclei is a reflection of the reduced maturation of the cell, indicated by a relatively large nucleus and a relatively small amount of cytoplasm.

Actual nuclear area is of less practical importance in routine diagnostic cytology because of the lack of a possibility for an accurate comparison with an object of known size.

Mild Dysplasia (CIN Grade I)

Histology. In mild dysplasia there is a slight disturbance of the regular arrangement of cells. The upper two thirds of the epithelium usually show a relatively regular arrangement of cells with preserved stratification. These layers are composed of cells, recognizable as intermediate-type and superficial squamous–type

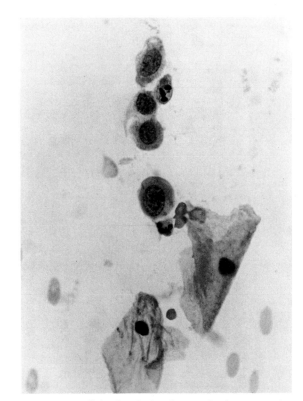

FIGURE 9–56. Slight dysplasia of metaplastic type. Enlarged nuclei and increased nucleocytoplasmic (N/C) ratio. Compare cell size with the superficial squamous cells and the two leukocytes (Papanicolaou stain; ×600).

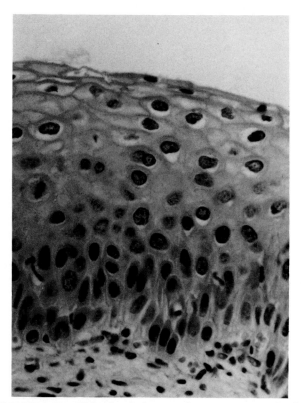

FIGURE 9–57. Slight dysplasia. Irregular arrangement of cells in the basal and parabasal layers. Reduced maturation and slightly enlarged, somewhat hyperchromatic nuclei in the most superficial layers (hematoxylin and eosin; ×250).

cells, with slightly reduced cytoplasmic volume and slightly increased nuclear size. Nuclei are usually of normal round to oval shape and have a minimally hyperchromatic nuclear chromatin. Aberrations of the nuclear morphology are predominantly limited to the most basal layers of the epithelium.

Cytology. Cells from mildly atypical lesions such as mild dysplasia (CIN grade I) usually have plentiful clear, translucent cytoplasm with well-defined angular borders. Cells resemble intermediate- and superficial-type squamous cells with a somewhat reduced cytoplasmic body and a slightly enlarged nucleus, occupying less than one third of the total area of the cell (Fig. 9–56; see also Figs. 9–54 and 9–55). Nuclear chromatin is finely granular, evenly distributed and only slightly hyperchromatic (Fig. 9–57).

Moderate Dysplasia (CIN Grade II)

Histology. In moderate dysplasia there is a moderate disturbance of stratification. Usually only the upper one third of the epithelium still shows evidence of stratification of cells of superficial and intermediate cell size. The uppermost layers are still composed of flat squamous cells, although nuclei may be enlarged and slightly hyperchromatic. Occasionally the surface layers are keratinized, with loss of nuclei and the formation of a granular layer (Fig. 9–58). Nuclear

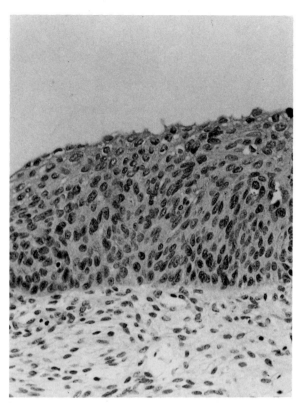

FIGURE 9–59. Moderate dysplasia. Disturbed maturation in all cell layers. In the uppermost layers stratification is still recognizable. Moderate increase of nuclear size. Irregular nuclear shapes and some hyperchromasia (hematoxylin and eosin; ×130).

abnormalities may be seen throughout the epithelium, particularly in the more basal layers. Cell arrangement is disturbed in up to two thirds of the thickness of the epithelium (Figs. 9–59 and 9–60). In these disturbed layers mitoses, sometimes abnormal, are present in increased numbers.

Cytology. The size of abnormal cells is more variable. Next to some abnormal cells of the superficial squamous cell type, smaller cells of the intermediate and parabasal cell type are usually found (Fig. 9–61). Most cells are round to oval, but occasionally spindle cells and elongated and bizarre shapes may be found. Cytoplasmic staining is cyanophilic, but a relatively high number of cells may show eosinophilia of the cytoplasm. Nuclei are enlarged and round to oval, sometimes elongated or irregularly shaped (Fig. 9–62). Nuclear chromatin is evenly distributed and slightly to moderately hyperchromatic (Fig. 9–63). Nucleoli are usually absent. The nucleocytoplasmic ratio is increased, both by nuclear enlargement and by reduction of the cytoplasmic volume (Figs. 9–64 and 9–65). The nucleus generally occupies less than half of the total area of the cell.

According to Koss[84] virtually all lesions classified as moderate dysplasia (CIN grade II) must be considered as neoplastic events in the squamous epithelium. Some of the abnormalities may resemble flat condylomas, and in a proportion of these moderately abnormal lesions HPV may be documented, particularly with the

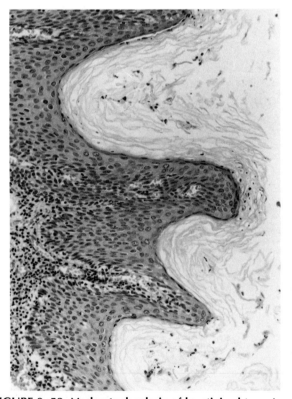

FIGURE 9–58. Moderate dysplasia of keratinized type. Irregular arrangement of cells in basal and intermediate cell layers. Reduced maturation, nuclear enlargement and irregularities in nuclear size and shape still appear in the more superficial layers. Abnormal keratin formation (hematoxylin and eosin; ×260).

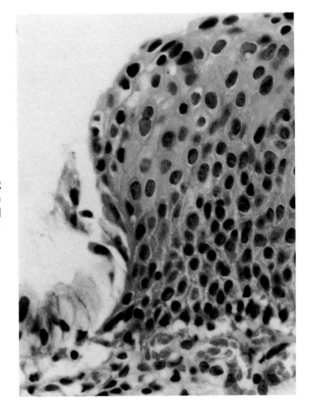

FIGURE 9–60. Moderate dysplasia of metaplastic type bordering endocervical mucus-producing columnar cells. Disturbed maturation of superficial layers. Nuclei show irregular sizes and shapes. Increased hyperchromasia of nuclear chromatin (hematoxylin and eosin; ×310).

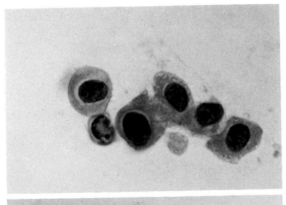

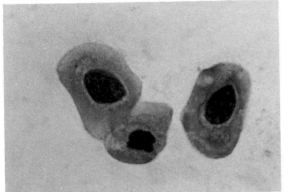

FIGURE 9–61. Moderate dysplasia. Cells of squamous and squamous metaplastic type. Nuclear enlargement, moderate hyperchromasia of the finely granular chromatin. Increased nucleocytoplasmic (N/C) ratio (Papanicolaou stain; ×625).

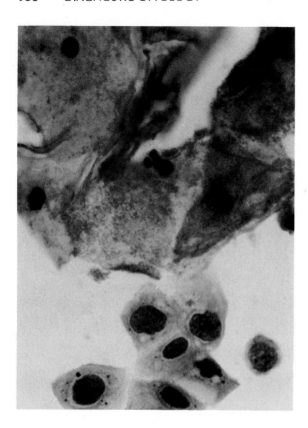

FIGURE 9–62. Moderate dysplasia. Nuclei are enlarged and show irregularities in shape. Nuclear chromatin is evenly distributed and finely granular (Papanicolaou stain; ×625).

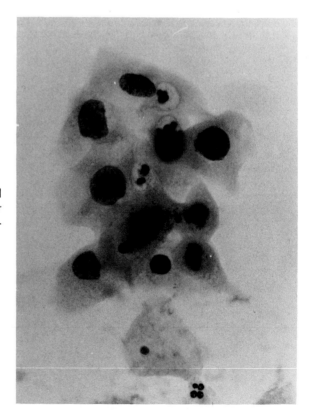

FIGURE 9–63. Moderate dysplasia. Irregularly shaped cells and enlarged nuclei. Moderate hyperchromasia of finely granular nuclear chromatin. Compare size of cells and nuclei with superficial squamous cell (Papanicolaou stain; ×400).

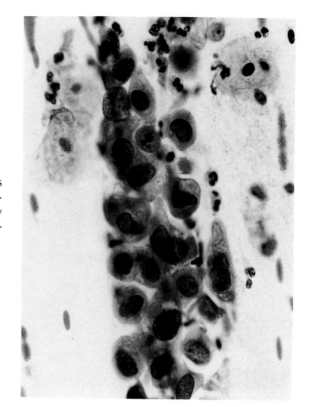

FIGURE 9–64. Moderate dysplasia. Round, oval and elongated cells with enlarged, somewhat irregularly shaped nuclei. Increased nucleo-cytoplasmic (N/C) ratio. Finely granular, slightly and moderately hyperchromatic nuclear chromatin. Compare with intermediate squamous cells (Papanicolaou stain; ×500).

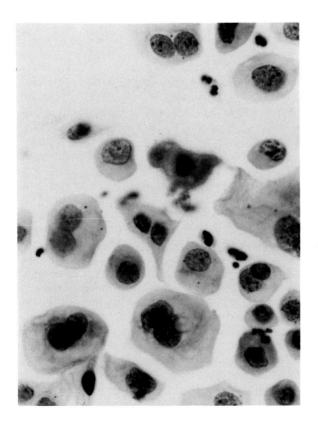

FIGURE 9–65. Moderate to severe dysplasia. Cells vary in size and shape. Nuclei are round to oval and irregular in shape. Nuclear chromatin is in part finely, in part coarsely, granular and moderately hyperchromatic. Increased nucleocytoplasmic (N/C) ratio (Papanicolaou stain; ×450).

application of recent highly sensitive *in situ* hybridization techniques. Meisels and associates[105] proposed the term *atypical condylomas* for these lesions. Because of their progressive potential, Koss[84] advises eradicating all moderately abnormal lesions under colposcopic control. This also applies to the atypical condylomas that are associated with other forms of CIN.

Severe Dysplasia and Carcinoma In Situ (CIN Grade III)

Histology. In severe dysplasia cells show a greatly disturbed arrangement in all three layers of the epithelium (Fig. 9–66). Stratification is only present in the most superficial layers (Fig. 9–67). Throughout the entire epithelium cells show a reduced maturation with loss of cytoplasmic volume and an increased nuclear size. Cells and nuclei vary in size and shape and often have irregular forms. Differentiation in intermediate-type and superficial squamous–type cells may be lost (Fig. 9–68). Nuclei have a hyperchromatic, irregularly distributed, coarsely granular chromatin. Mitoses may be found throughout all epithelial layers. The abnormal changes often extend into the stromal invaginations of the endocervical epithelium (Fig. 9–69).

Cytology. The size of the cells in severely abnormal

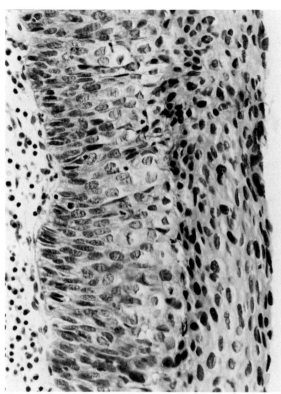

FIGURE 9–67. Severe dysplasia. Palisade arrangement of cells in lower half of the epithelium. Upper half of the epithelium is composed of abnormal cells with irregular nuclei and hyperchromatic nuclear chromatin lying parallel to the surface. The sudden change in the polarity of the cells in this abnormal epithelium may reflect a sudden change in the environment during the development of the lesion (hematoxylin and eosin; ×250).

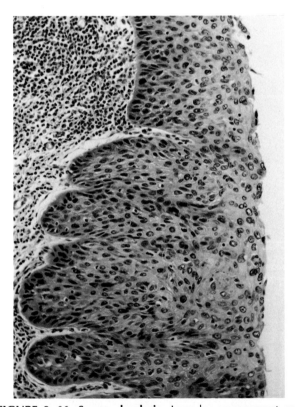

FIGURE 9–66. Severe dysplasia. Irregular arrangement and disturbed maturation of cells involving almost the entire thickness of the epithelium. Only in the most superficial layers do cells show an increased cytoplasmic volume resulting in a lower nucleocytoplasmic (N/C) ratio (hematoxylin and eosin; ×128).

intraepithelial changes is comparable with the parabasal cell type. Cytoplasm is usually sparse, typically forming a small rim around the nucleus (Fig. 9–70). Cells are round to oval and often irregular or elongated (Figs. 9–71 and 9–72). In the keratinizing squamous lesions there are sometimes large cells with plentiful, often eosinophilic, cytoplasm. Cells occur lying singly as well as in aggregates. In the most severe intraepithelial lesions aggregates have a syncytial composition, with indistinct cell borders and irregularly arranged nuclei (Fig. 9–73). The morphology of these aggregates is consistent with the histologic evidence of the lack of cell maturation and the irregular arrangement of nuclei in the most superficial layers of severely abnormal epithelium (Figs. 9–74 and 9–75). The nucleus occupies usually at least two thirds of the total area of the cell. Nuclei have a hyperchromatic, irregularly distributed, coarsely granular chromatin (Fig. 9–76). In actively proliferating lesions eosinophilic-staining nucleoli may be observed, but more often these are obscured by the dense hyperchromatic chromatin. Some severe dysplasias show an extreme irregularity in shape and size of the composing cells. In cervical smears these lesions may present with large, bizarre-shaped cells with highly abnormal hyperchromatic nuclei. Differential diagnosis

Text continued on page 193

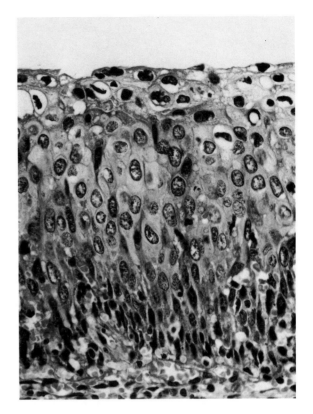

FIGURE 9–68. Severe dysplasia. Only in the most superficial layers are signs of maturation identifiable, by a change in polarity and a somewhat increased cytoplasmic volume of the cells. Vacuolation of the cytoplasm of the superficial cells (koilocytosis) may be caused by infection with human papilloma virus (HPV) but is more often a sign of degeneration (hematoxylin and eosin; ×250).

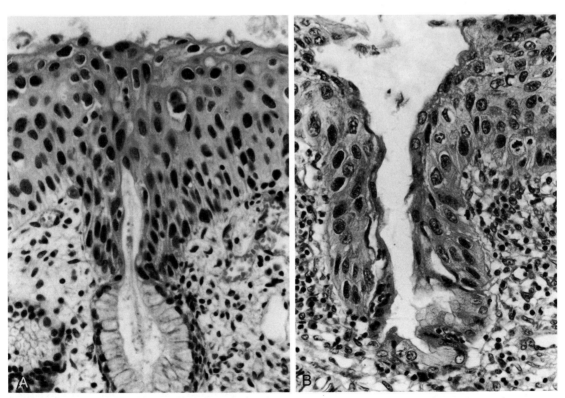

FIGURE 9–69. *A* and *B*, **Severe dysplasia of metaplastic type.** Extension of the epithelial abnormality into the stromal invagination, with *(B)* replacement of the lining columnar epithelium (hematoxylin and eosin; *A* ×150 and *B* ×280).

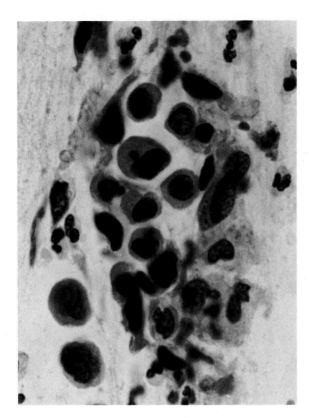

FIGURE 9–70. Severe dysplasia. Cells of parabasal cell type with a small rim of cytoplasm around a large, often irregularly shaped, hyperchromatic nucleus. High nucleocytoplasmic (N/C) ratio (Papanicolaou stain; ×625).

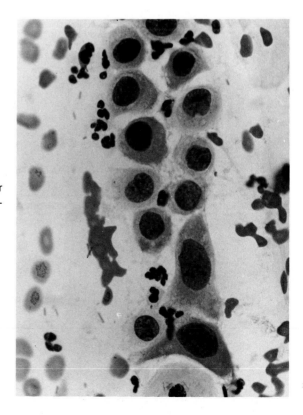

FIGURE 9–71. Severe dysplasia. Cells and nuclei are round to oval or irregularly shaped. Finely granular and coarse, moderately hyperchromatic nuclear chromatin (Papanicolaou stain; ×625).

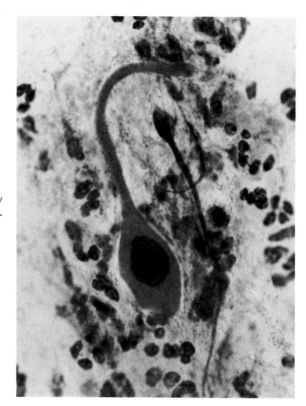

FIGURE 9–72. Severe dysplasia. Large elongated cell with relatively large nucleus and dense, hyperchromatic nuclear chromatin (Papanicolaou stain; ×625).

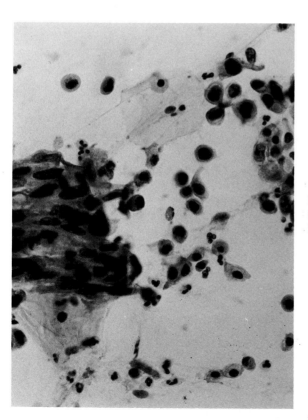

FIGURE 9–73. Severe dysplasia. Singly lying cells and cells in a syncytial aggregate with indistinct cell borders and irregularly shaped hyperchromatic nuclei (Papanicolaou stain; ×250).

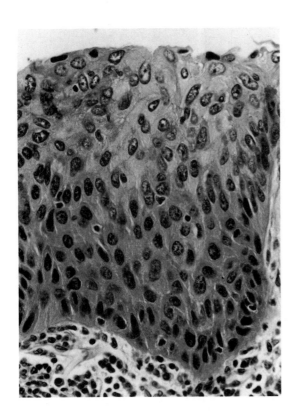

FIGURE 9–74. Severe dysplasia. Irregular arrangement of immature abnormal squamous cells in the most superficial layers (hematoxylin and eosin; ×315).

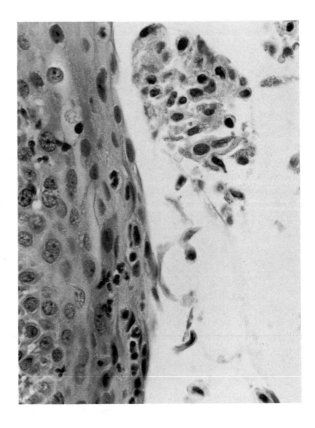

FIGURE 9–75. Dysplasia. Cells desquamating from the superficial layers reflect the lack of maturation and the grade of abnormality of the epithelial lesion (hematoxylin and eosin; ×250).

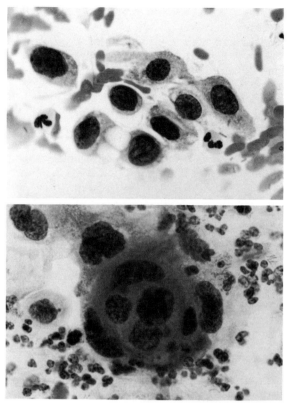

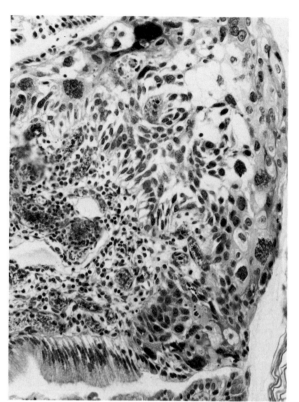

FIGURE 9–76. **Severe dysplasia.** Cells in a syncytial aggregate and singly lying with relatively large irregular nuclei and a dense, coarsely granular irregularly distributed hyperchromatic nuclear chromatin (Papanicolaou stain; ×400).

FIGURE 9–77. **Dysplasia of metaplastic type.** Irregular arrangement of sometimes bizarre-shaped abnormal cells (hematoxylin and eosin; ×125).

with an invasive squamous cell cancer may at times be extremely difficult (Figs. 9–77 and 9–78).

Biologic Significance Follow-up

The evolution of invasive squamous cell cancer involves a number of stages with increasing intraepithelial abnormality designated as dysplasia, carcinoma *in situ* and microinvasive carcinoma. Although it is not usually possible to predict the malignant potential of an epithelial abnormality (premalignant lesion), there is evidence to indicate that mild dysplasias are more prone to spontaneously regress, and conversely, severe dysplasia and carcinoma *in situ* are more apt to persist or progress.

Dysplasia may follow a variable course.

Regression. The dysplastic reaction may undergo spontaneous regression. The lesion may disappear in a matter of weeks and become undetectable at a short-term follow-up screening, or it may take a much longer time, the lesion becoming gradually less abnormal in a matter of months or even years. In some cases the disappearance may be caused by a desquamation of the abnormal epithelium due to minimal trauma.

A dysplastic epithelium tends to separate more easily from the supporting stroma than the normal epithelium does. This may account in part for the disappearance of dysplastic reactions after initial cytologic diagnosis

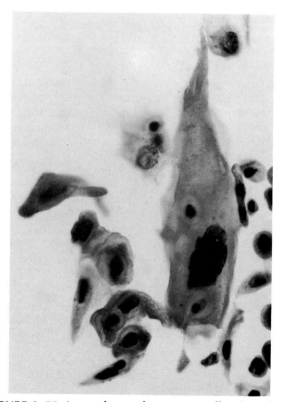

FIGURE 9–78. **Large abnormal squamous cell** with multiple irregular, hyperchromatic nuclei. Compare the size of this cell with the other abnormal squamous cells (Papanicolaou stain; ×625).

in women during cytologic follow-up. In these instances the diagnostic test essentially becomes a cure for the lesion.

In studies reporting on regression or progression after confirmation of the cytologic diagnosis by histology, part of the observed regression during follow-up must be ascribed to the surgical procedure, as may be the case in studies reporting on follow-up of dysplasias diagnosed during pregnancy, due to the traumatic effects to the cervix during childbirth.[176] Spontaneous regression may therefore be lower than cited in these studies, whereas progression may be higher in cases without bioptic intervention or that are diagnosed during pregnancy.

Even if a regression does not follow the biopsy, however, it is entirely possible that the biology of the lesion is altered in a variety of ways. If the smear is positive following a biopsy and later becomes negative the assumption that the lesion regressed spontaneously may be invalid.[152]

Koss and colleagues,[89] in a long-term follow-up study of individual patients with carcinoma *in situ* and related lesions, noted that a single biopsy could eradicate an area of intraepithelial neoplasia. There can be no doubt that punch biopsies can eradicate areas of CIN completely, either directly by complete removal or indirectly by altering the balance between the host and the neoplasm so that areas of residual CIN regress, thus producing an immediate cure, a delayed cure or a change in the distribution of an area of CIN.[152] In follow-up studies after biopsies no valid figure for the regression rate can be derived, since the proportion of cures that are inadvertently produced by the diagnostic procedures rather than occurring spontaneously cannot be determined.

Persistence. Dysplasia may also persist during a variable period of time before regressing or progressing to a more severe lesion, such as marked dysplasia, carcinoma *in situ* or invasive cancer. Documented cases of marked dysplasia have persisted for as much as 20 years without showing a malignant progression. There is unanimity among authors that dysplasia in certain circumstances can progress to carcinoma *in situ* and finally to invasive cancer.

Progression. Slight dysplasias may also antedate the appearance of a severe intraepithelial lesion or an invasive cancer by many years. Most prospective studies, when carried out without intercurrent intervention through biopsies or frequent repeat smears, indicate that less than 15% of dysplasias will progress.[131]

The fact that the presence of HPV infection was proved to be associated with the presence of premalignant lesions of mild to marked severity had given hope to the idea that the identification of the virus and its different species would have value in the identification of progressive intraepithelial abnormalities. However, it has been shown that with more sensitive techniques the virus can be identified in the large majority of women during reproductive years, which makes the presence of this virus useless in determining progressive potential.

Follow-up Studies: Literature Review. Christopherson[28] followed more than 200 patients with dysplasia from 1 to 13 years. Patients were admitted on the basis of a biopsy diagnosis of dysplasia that later was cytologically confirmed. During the observation period 30% of the lesions regressed to normality, 49% of lesions persisted, 20% showed progression to carcinoma *in situ* and 1.3% progressed to invasive cervical cancer.

In a study of 120 women with cytologic evidence of dysplasia, during long-term follow-up for up to 9 years, Scott and Ballard[167] found a regression or complete involution in 60% of women; progression to carcinoma *in situ* in this series was 4.1%. In 223 women followed for an average of 3.8 years progression to carcinoma *in situ* was 5.8%.[168] In a retrospective study of 364 women with dysplastic reactions of varying severity that were initially detected and followed closely by cytology alone for a minimum of 9 months and a maximum of 24 months, Patten[127] found the reaction to regress or disappear in 71.9% with slight dysplasia, 44.2% with moderate dysplasia and 16.3% with marked dysplasia. Furthermore, during this period of observation, only those cases that were initially classified as marked dysplasia progressed to *in situ* carcinoma. Of cases initially diagnosed as marked dysplasia, 6.8% (3) developed carcinoma *in situ* from 10 to 17 months later. None of these cases were seen to develop invasive cancer. In a retrospective study of 102 women with moderate dysplasia Patten noted regression in 44.2%, persistence in 42.2% and progression in 13.6% during follow-up from 9 to 23 months.

Progression occurred on the average 3 years after initial diagnosis of dysplasia. Patten[128] stated that on the basis of data available it could be expected that 5 to 10% of dysplastic reactions could be expected to antedate the subsequent appearance of *in situ* cancer. From reported series it seems likely that in less than 1.5% of patients with evidence of dysplasia will an invasive cancer subsequently develop.[28, 100, 167]

Nasiell and associates[114] followed 894 women with cytologically diagnosed moderate dysplasia by cytology without major treatment. During a follow-up period of 78 months they observed regression of the moderate dysplasia in 54%. Average follow-up time for patients with continuous normal cytology after disappearance of dysplasia was 53 months. During follow-up for 51 months progression was observed in 30% and persistence in 16%. In 54% of patients biopsies were performed. In patients without biopsies regression was 50%, progression 35% and persistence 15%, which implies a statistically significant difference between biopsied and nonbiopsied patients. In patients over 51 years of age fewer lesions progressed than in younger patients and the progression time was also significantly longer.

In 3.8% of patients with persistent moderate dysplasia followed for an average of 50 months, cytology periodically gave no evidence of an abnormality. The risk of progression of moderate dysplasia was 5 to 9 cases per 100 women per year. When related to an incidence of carcinoma *in situ* of 4 in 100,000 women per year, the yearly progression risk of moderate dysplasia can be calculated to be 2000 times greater than for a woman without cervical dysplasia. Regression showed only slight variation between different age groups.

Tanaka and coworkers[182] followed 230 cases with an initial diagnosis of mild dysplasia cytologically and colposcopically for from 2 to 10 years. Regression of the epithelial abnormality was observed in 73.5% of cases, persistence in 20% and progression in 6.5% of cases. Out of 15 cases that showed progression, 10 cases of *in situ* carcinoma or microinvasive carcinoma developed. The average period after which progression was diagnosed was 54.8 months.

An important factor in explaining the wide variation between the results obtained in different follow-up series is the highly subjective character of the histologic diagnosis of intraepithelial neoplasia. Various pathologists will return a diagnosis on the same lesion varying from mild dysplasia to carcinoma *in situ*.[49]

Clinical management of intraepithelial lesions of the cervix depends greatly on the cytologic and histologic definitions of dysplasia. The diagnosis of dysplasia is often considered inconsequential by uninformed physicians, who fail to take appropriate action.[162]

Rate of Progression: Transit Time. On the basis of all available evidence it may be concluded that the rate of progression of dysplastic lesions is strongly related to the severity of the lesion as evaluable by cytologic analysis.

Data from long-term population studies in a population that has been screened intensively allow true incidence figures to be measured and can provide evidence from the ratios between mild and severe intraepithelial lesions that the majority of mild and moderate intraepithelial changes eventually regress or persist for a prolonged period.

In the Nijmegen screening program the ratio between mild and moderate dysplasias on the one hand and severe dysplasias and *in situ* carcinomas on the other hand was 4:1 at second screening. It is often not understood that the ratio of precancerous lesions to invasive cancer is probably on the order of 10 to 1, possibly even higher.[86]

A suggestion of a fast transition time between normal epithelium and severe dysplasia should only be made after the more likely possibility of false-negative cytology because of poor sampling has been excluded. In cases of severe epithelial abnormalities the number of unsatisfactory or less reliable smears is much increased, owing to admixture of inflammatory cells, cell debris or blood.

The results of these studies strongly support a conservative approach in the clinical management of patients diagnosed with mild to moderately atypical epithelial abnormalities.

Rate of Progression: Review of the Literature. Richart and Barron[155] followed 557 patients with cervical dysplasia detected by cytologic and colposcopic examinations without interference of punch biopsies or other treatment. They estimated the time spent in each stage of dysplasia prior to its progression to carcinoma *in situ*.

At the end of the follow-up period transition probabilities were calculated and transit times of mild, moderate and severe dysplasia to carcinoma *in situ*

were computed. The transit times ranged from a median of 86 months for patients with very mild dysplasia, 58 months for mild dysplasia and 38 months for moderate dysplasia to 12 months for severe dysplasia. The median transit time to carcinoma *in situ* for all dysplasias was 44 months. In a 10-year period moderate dysplasia was calculated to progress to a more severe lesion in about 90% of the cases. They reported the progression rates to be relatively stable, and they concluded that in time almost all cases of dysplasia would develop into carcinoma *in situ* if left untreated. Although progression from one smear class to another might be an age-related phenomenon, there was no obvious gradient in the ages. Similarly there was no evidence that progression from one class to another was solely time-dependent. During long-term follow-up a substantial proportion of patients remained in the stage in which they were detected and did not progress to a higher-stage disease over a definite period of time. These data cannot be considered as representative for true regression and persistence rates because patients entered in the study were highly selected, since one of the criteria for acceptance was a persistence of the lesion over at least a three-smear interval. This eliminated many lesions due to repair and other processes that cytomorphologically cannot be discriminated from dysplasia and that had regressed during the interval.

Bamford and coworkers[10] reviewed the smears preceding the histologic diagnosis in 100 cases of CIN grade III, diagnosed in an intensively screened population. These suggest that the transition time from normality to CIN grade III may be shorter than has generally been assumed. However, they provide no information about the quality and cellular composition of the smears that were reviewed.

Cytologic Follow-up. Given a correct cytologic diagnosis we do not consider it necessary to immediately biopsy lesions of minimal or moderate severity, since only a small proportion of these lesions will progress to a more marked abnormality, whereas the time it takes a lesion to progress provides ample time to detect a lesion at successive cytologic examinations. In view of the relatively large proportion of lesions that will regress spontaneously and the median duration of progression time to a more severe lesion, patients with initial diagnoses of mild and moderate dysplasias should be followed by regular cytologic smears for varying periods of time before further therapy is recommended. Only after persistence of the lesion has been confirmed are further follow-up procedures, including colposcopy, warranted.

A cytologic diagnosis of severe dysplasia or *in situ* carcinoma is usually followed by colposcopy and biopsy, which at confirmation of the process are followed by cryocautery, laser treatment, conization or hysterectomy.

Follow-up Interval. There is no unanimity about when and to what extent follow-up examinations of cytologically diagnosed cervical abnormalities should be carried out.[71, 193, 194] In cases of minimal epithelial abnormalities a repeat smear should be advised after 12 months. In cases consistent with mild to moderate dysplasia a repeat smear after 3 months should be recommended. When the abnormality is also diagnosed in the repeat smear the patient should be referred for further evaluation including colposcopy. This should also be the procedure when a more severe lesion is diagnosed in the repeat smear. When the lesion is not confirmed in the repeat smear a second repeat smear should be made again after 3 months. If the lesion remains absent or appears to be of less severity, the follow-up interval can be doubled to 6 months and later to 12 months.

It is well known that sometimes initial findings of mild to moderately atypia at follow-up prove to be of a more serious kind.[115, 184, 185, 200] With a follow-up procedure as described, it is therefore mandatory that the execution of repeat examinations is well supervised by the laboratory. Only when this condition is fulfilled is an initial cytologic follow-up of mild to moderate abnormalities warranted.[194]

The procedure described is presently adopted for the nationwide screening program in the Netherlands.[193, 194, 197] In cases of cytologic diagnoses consistent with mild dysplasia or a more severe lesion detected outside the screening program, an immediate referral for colposcopic evaluation is agreed upon by all parties involved.

Colposcopy

The colposcope is well suited for follow-up studies of cervical intraepithelial neoplasia because of its lack of influence on the natural history of the disease.[151] An optimal cancer detection system for preclinical asymptomatic cervical lesions should combine a cytologic examination with a colposcopic follow-up examination. The principal goal of cervical cytology is to detect precancerous lesions and asymptomatic, preclinical cancer. The purpose of cytologic screening is to signal these abnormalities and to induce further evaluation of lesions that have proved to be persistent or that may progress. Colposcopy could have an important place in the evaluation of these patients. Colposcopically guided biopsies may clarify inconclusive cytologic findings and give an assessment of the location, size and extent of a lesion. There is a good correlation between the presence of abnormalities detected by colposcopy and histologically, but little correlation between colposcopic categories and histologic grades of intraepithelial lesions.[111]

Cellular Reactions Simulating Dysplasia

Certain stimuli may cause reactions in the cervical mucosa that may stimulate dysplasia. Chronic inflammatory processes and instrumental treatment for erosion or other surface abnormalities of the cervix (electrocautery, cryotherapy, laser treatment) may induce changes that may be confused with dysplastic changes when relevant clinical information is lacking. Certain medications, particularly those used in the systemic treatment of malignancies or in the course of immunosuppression in patients with organ transplants, may also induce cellular changes of a dysplastic nature. In rare instances folic acid deficiency may cause an increase of both cytoplasm and nucleus. Even though extremely large nuclei may occur, the nucleocytoplasmic ratio remains within the limits of a minimal abnormality because of a correlated increase of the cytoplasmic body, often creating rather characteristic giant cells. In contrast with dysplastic changes nuclei are hypochromatic.[189] Similar changes may be found as an effect of radiotherapy or treatment with alkylating drugs.[84]

Prognosis of Dysplasia and DNA Cytophotometry

Light microscopically observed severely abnormal epithelial lesions cannot be subdivided into regressive, persistent or progressive subtypes. An alternative for visual light microscopic evaluation of these lesions is the study of DNA ploidy.[210] In one study the DNA content in dysplasia proved to be higher than normal, but the mode of the DNA index distribution fell entirely within the diploid range. Some cells had DNA values in the tetraploid and the hyperdiploid range, but a significant relationship between aberrant DNA values in dysplasia and DNA profiles of carcinoma in situ and invasive carcinoma could not be established.[211]

The wide range of DNA values found in dysplasia and carcinoma in situ indicates that dysplasia and carcinoma in situ contain a highly variable population of cells whose range of DNA content is similar to that found in invasive cancer. A high proportion of cells in these lesions have abnormal chromosome numbers, but no chromosomal feature is distinctive of dysplasia, carcinoma in situ or microcarcinoma, nor is any marker chromosome characteristic for early cervical neoplasia.[179] In some studies DNA ploidy analyses indicated a high percentage of aneuploidy in CIN grade III lesions. On this basis DNA aneuploidy was considered to be a marker for progression.[53, 73] In dysplasia and carcinoma in situ clonal proliferation may already be occurring. However, there is also much evidence of the opposite kind: wide scatter of chromosome counts without a recognizable similarity from cell to cell. DNA estimations usually do not indicate a dominant aneuploid stem line. By the time microinvasion is identifiable there is evidence that a new clone has overgrown the rest of the epithelium. Most cases have one distinct stem line but sometimes can have several.[4, 5]

According to some investigators quantitative DNA determinations in cytomorphologically equivalent dysplastic cervical cells do not offer additional means of predicting the outcome of the epithelial change. In patients with moderate cervical dysplasia, there were no significant differences between cell populations from moderate dysplasias that subsequently progressed to carcinoma in situ and from lesions that regressed to normality. The DNA distribution pattern of both groups was different from that of normal cells.[113]

A striking association was found between DNA ploidy and age. In women under 35 years with CIN grade III lesions aneuploidy was present in 27% and the majority of the lesions showed a polyploid pattern, whereas in women over 50 years of age aneuploidy was found in 88%. These findings suggest that processes finally progressing to invasive cancer may have different biologic characteristics in these two age groups. A diploid DNA pattern does not necessarily imply a regressive or persistent behavior of intraepithelial abnormalities.[4, 5, 61]

Postradiation Dysplasia

After successful radiotherapy for a malignancy of the cervix, a small percentage of patients, following a latent period varying from 6 months to more than 20 years, will develop an abnormality of the cervical or vaginal mucosa that has the characteristics of dysplasia. Essentially the characteristics of a postradiation dysplasia are those of classic dysplasia. Accompanying the cellular evidence of dysplasia is the evidence of increased maturation of squamous cells, comparable with estrogen-induced maturation and the characteristics of radiation changes such as multinucleation, dual staining reaction and vacuolization of the cytoplasm. The appearance of superficial squamous cells may antedate the appearance of a cellular abnormality.[132] The biologic significance of a postradiation dysplasia remains uncertain.

Accuracy

With the exception of invasion the basic changes of importance in the recognition of primary cancer are apparent both in tissues and cells.[144] Since there is no single distinguishing feature that is in itself invariably pathognomonic of cancer in the cell or the epithelial lesion of origin, more than one fundamental change must be present in order to warrant an interpretation of cancer. Usually cell samples show dysplastic cells with a variable degree of atypia.

A prerequisite for the study of cellular pathology is an intimate knowledge of the component cells in the parent tissues in order to learn the origin of various cells identified in cellular preparations. Since the cellular sample represents a very comprehensive sample of the surface changes, there are many instances in which cellular evidence of a change is not apparent on so-called punch biopsies. For this reason the presence of a lesion can only be excluded when the pathologic study is comprehensive. This is an important consideration when dealing with evidence gained by cell studies.[144]

Clinicians increasingly show an inclination to reduce the amount of tissue removed for diagnostic or even therapeutic purposes. For diagnostic purposes multiple biopsies preferably taken under colposcopic control or a very shallow conus are most often used. Thus a severe lesion of limited extent bordered by less severe changes may not be present in the histologic material. When comparing cytologic and histologic findings, this may lead to the conclusion that a severe lesion diagnosed cytologically apparently was overestimated: a *false-positive diagnosis.*

With the use of collection techniques that provide comprehensive samples of the uterine cervix, most reactions occurring in the cervix can be recognized on the basis of the cellular changes alone.[128] The number of cells diagnostic for a specific, benign proliferative reaction depends on the extent of the epithelial change and the method used for collecting the cells. In a well-sampled specimen, cells from these multiple atypical mucosal changes may be found next to another. In a less adequate sample in which only part of the circumference of the ectocervix and the endocervical canal is represented by the cells in the sample, only part of the abnormal changes may be recognizable. This may lead to an underestimation of the severity of the lesion or, when the sample is highly inadequate, to a *false-negative diagnosis.*

Moreover in cases in which sampling of the cervix has been done less expertly the number of abnormal cells may be relatively low. In routine screening situations this low number of cells may remain unobserved or, because of the paucity of abnormal cells, erroneously lead to an underestimation of the severity of the lesion.

The initial cellular sample collected from the cervix usually contains the greatest number of abnormal cells. Subsequent samples may contain few abnormal cells even after an interval of 2 to 3 weeks. Since after only a short interval samples are taken from less-matured lesions, diagnoses on repeat studies made after too short an interval are likely to overestimate the severity of the lesion. Therefore, when follow-up of the lesion is done cytologically or when confirmation of the lesion is required prior to biopsy the repeat study should not be performed within 4 weeks.

In cases of discrepancies between cytologic and histologic diagnoses in all cases, both the cytologic and the histologic specimens have to be reviewed. When at review the original cytologic diagnosis is confirmed a repeat histologic examination may be requested.

Carcinoma *In Situ*

Broders[20] introduced the term carcinoma *in situ* to describe epithelial lesions entirely composed of cells that have all the features of malignant cells but that do not exhibit invasive growth. This term has become widely used since. Other terminologies that have been in use are incipient cancer, surface cancer, Bowen's disease of the cervix, intraepithelial cancer, carcinomatoid change and preinvasive or noninvasive cancer.[128, 149, 150]

Carcinoma *in situ* is now generally accepted as a precursor of invasive squamous cell carcinoma.

Origin, Localization and Extent. The morphologic variations that can be observed when studying the spectrum of lesions directly associated with carcinoma *in situ* suggest a common pathway in the development of dysplasia and carcinoma *in situ*. The basic factor in the mechanism of the genesis of carcinoma *in situ* is reserve cell hyperplasia. The cells arising in reserve cell hyperplasia are noteworthy, since in some instances they are reminiscent of those seen in carcinoma *in situ*. A proliferation of the subcolumnar reserve cells may involve only one or two layers of cells beneath columnar epithelium or may attain a considerable thickness. The latter not only simulates carcinoma *in situ* but actually may represent a developmental stage of this process.[144]

The stimulus that has induced a proliferation of reserve cells as such also blocks the differentiation of these reserve cells into immature and then mature squamous metaplastic cells. Thus, by proliferation primitive undifferentiated cells finally compose the entire lesion. Each pathway in the development of carcinoma *in situ*, localized in the endocervical canal, begins with or mimics reserve cell hyperplasia. If some differentiation occurs in the epithelial substrate prior to conversion to carcinoma *in situ*, such as occurs in squamous metaplasia or dysplasia of metaplastic type, the ensuing lesion is of large-cell type. A lack of differentiation of the epithelial substrate would result in an *in situ* lesion composed entirely of small primitive cells.[128]

The majority of cases of carcinoma *in situ* originate in the area of the transformation zone, bordering the original anatomic separation between stratified squamous epithelium and columnar epithelium. The farthest limit of CIN is determined by the farthest limit of reserve cell hyperplasia (squamous metaplasia, repair epithelium).[151] In the most distal part of this area the stimulus for a metaplastic change of the columnar epithelium is apparently the strongest. This may also be the reason why distally in the canal large-cell carcinomas *in situ* are much more frequent than proximally, where small-cell variants are more often seen.

It may well be that the potential for metaplastic change in the more proximal parts of the canal is lower, resulting in a lower frequency of mature squamous metaplastic changes and also a higher frequency of poorly differentiated epithelial abnormalities.

Epithelial changes preceding a small-cell carcinoma *in situ* likely do not develop through precursor lesions showing some squamous differentiation. It is probably very difficult to differentiate between early small-cell intraepithelial changes and the finally resulting small-cell carcinoma *in situ*. In a small number of women participating in the Nijmegen population-screening program a small-cell lesion was identified that was composed of rather immature small cells, which histologically showed a pseudostratified, somewhat columnar arrangement. In a few women who had no intercurrent smears or biopsies taken for various reasons, classic small-cell *in situ* carcinomas were found at repeat examination 3 to 4 years later.

The biologic significance of these pseudostratified small-cell precursor lesions, which biologically may be comparable with the more distally located severe dysplasias, needs further clarification. On a cytomorphologic as well as on a histologic basis it is possible to subclassify abnormal intraepithelial lesions quite specifically into categories that can be arbitrarily labeled dysplasia and carcinoma *in situ*.

Age at Detection. Most authors report an average age at detection of about 40 years (41.6 years[29, 149, 150, 181] and 42.5 years with a range of 22 to 91 years).[128] In our own material average age at first histologic diagnosis of *in situ* carcinoma was 39.4 years with a range of 17 to 82 years (Fig. 9–79). More recently the mean age at detection is reported to be lower. This reduction in average age has been related to an earlier onset of sexual activity but may at least in part be attributed to a more intense cytologic screening.

In our own registry the age-distribution curve showed a bimodal pattern, with peak incidences at 35

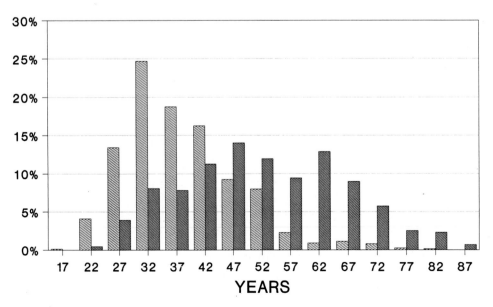

FIGURE 9–79. Carcinoma *in situ* (CIS) and invasive cancer (INV CA). Histologic diagnoses. Age distribution—average age of patients with carcinoma *in situ* was 39.2 years (SD-9.8) and N = 879. Average age of patients with invasive cancer was 53.0 years (SD-13.9) and N = 435. (Data from the Nijmegen Registry of Cervical Cytology, 1970–1987.)

and 50 years.[61, 186] These peaks were correlated with peak incidences of invasive squamous cancer at about 48 years and over 60 years of age.

Histology. The subjective nature of morphologic classification criteria initially caused a wide variation in the spectrum of histologic substrates diagnosed as carcinoma *in situ*. However, experience in the classification of carcinoma *in situ* combined with clinically correlated studies has increasingly narrowed the histologic spectrum to a point of relatively uniform agreement on certain morphologic patterns.[128]

The best description of the characteristic cytomorphologic and architectural changes of carcinoma *in situ* is given in the definition adopted by the International Committee on Histological Terminology for Lesions of the Uterine Cervix in Vienna in 1961.[207]

"Only those cases should be classified as carcinoma *in situ*" that, in the absence of invasion, show a surface epithelium in which, throughout its whole thickness, no differentiation takes place (Fig. 9–80). The process may involve the cervical glands without hereby creating a new group.

"It is recognized that the cells of the uppermost layers may show some flattening (Fig. 9–81). The very rare case of an otherwise characteristic carcinoma *in situ* that shows a greater degree of differentiation belongs to the exception for which no classification can provide."[207] The World Health Organization definition

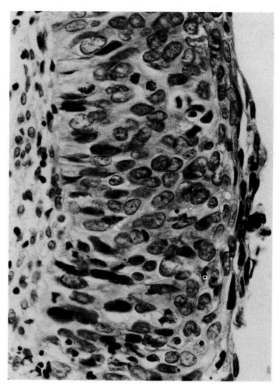

FIGURE 9–81. Carcinoma *in situ*. Irregular arrangement of cells and almost complete lack of maturation. Parallel arrangement of cells only in the most superficial layers. Mitoses can be recognized at all levels (hematoxylin and eosin; ×450).

of a carcinoma *in situ* is "a lesion in which all or most of the epithelium shows the cellular features of carcinoma."[135] This definition also includes an epithelial abnormality with some evidence of maturation in the most superficial layers and thus also encompasses a lesion that many pathologists would regard as a severe dysplasia.

In general the term carcinoma *in situ* is employed to describe a reaction replacing the normal surface epithelium or the epithelium of the invaginations of the surface epithelium or both, in which all the layers of the epithelium are composed of abnormal poorly differentiated or largely undifferentiated cells.[128]

The lesion may be composed of large or small cells, but essential in the classification of a lesion as carcinoma *in situ* is that the entire thickness of the epithelium is composed of poorly differentiated cells virtually without signs of maturation (differentiation) towards the surface (see Fig. 9–81). It is not unusual to find continuous with the surface lesion in the invaginations an epithelial change that shows a better maturation with the more superficial layers composed of cells recognizable as squamous (metaplastic).

Thus, together with a characteristic carcinoma *in situ* on the surface of the endocervical canal, it is not unusual to find a moderate to severe dysplasia (of squamous metaplastic type) in the invaginations of the endocervical canal.[128] Both normal and atypical mitoses are present at all levels of the epithelial reaction (see Fig. 9–81). This contrasts with moderate and severe

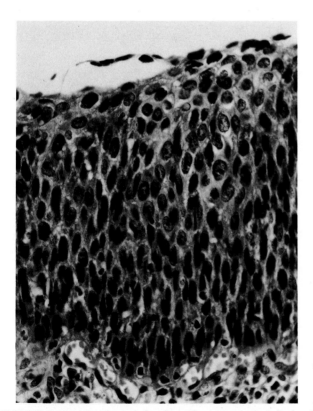

FIGURE 9–80. Carcinoma *in situ*. Almost complete lack of maturation and parallel arrangement of cells throughout the entire epithelium. Disturbed palisade arrangement of cells in the most basal layers (hematoxylin and eosin; ×250).

dysplastic lesions, in which mitoses usually are absent in the most superficial layers. On a histologic and cytologic basis Reagan and coworkers[144] proposed a subclassification of carcinoma *in situ* into small-cell carcinoma *in situ* and large-cell carcinoma *in situ*. Although useful in recognizing morphologic variations and studying the morphogenesis of these lesions, this classification has not provided significant information on the biologic potential of these lesions.[128] Patten[131] subdivides *in situ* carcinomas into large-cell type, intermediate type and small-cell type. The intermediate type seems to be the dominant morphologic variant in his material. The large-cell type, although relatively rare, appeared to be increasing in frequency. The once-dominant cell type of small-cell *in situ* carcinoma was observed with decreasing frequency.

At the time of his reporting it was not yet evident whether this change in the distribution of morphologic variants of *in situ* carcinoma was paralleled by a change in the distribution of morphologic variants of invasive cancer. The lesion is characteristically located in the area of the transformation zone. The overall extent and distribution of carcinoma *in situ* is comparable with that observed for reserve cell hyperplasia and immature squamous metaplasia. Extension of the surface change into the invaginations occurs in over 90% of cases.[146] Richart[151] observed that extension into the portio vaginalis occurred in about 55% of cases and that 3% of *in situ* cancers had an extension into the vaginal fornix.

Cytology. The number of abnormal cells in cellular samples is usually greater in cases of carcinoma *in situ* than with dysplasias. The cellular changes of importance in the recognition of *in situ* cancer are those exhibited by cells desquamated or forcibly scraped from the epithelial surface.

Arrangement of Cells. In situ carcinoma, because of the undifferentiated nature of the component cells, lacks the characteristic cytoplasmic changes of differentiation (maturation). The cells are either isolated or, because of a disturbance in cytoplasmic division during cell division, cells adhere together and are arranged as syncytial aggregates (Figs. 9–82 and 9–83). Most samples do contain isolated cells, but aggregates of abnormal cells predominate. A scraping of the cervix forcibly removes cells from the surface. In view of the high number of cells arranged in syncytial masses, in these situations taking a smear is essentially performing multiple microbiopsies. In a syncytial group cells are arranged irregularly and have indistinct cell borders and overlapping nuclei (Fig. 9–84). The latter two features differentiate these syncytial aggregates from sheets that are found in the presence of dysplasias and in which the more distinct cell borders and the more regular arrangement of the cells are a reflection of the relatively higher differentiation (maturation) of the dysplastic epithelium, in comparison with the epithelium composing the *in situ* carcinoma.

Cell Size and Shape. Cells from a carcinoma *in situ* lesion are relatively small compared with cells from normal stratified squamous epithelium or dysplastic cells. Cells from the histologically large-cell variant of carcinoma *in situ* are predominantly in the range of

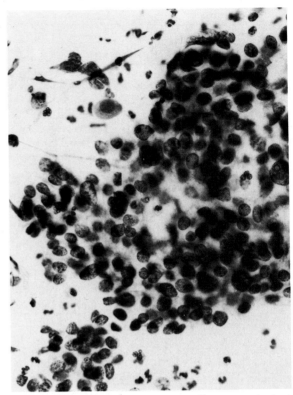

FIGURE 9–82. Carcinoma *in situ*. Cells occur singly but predominantly in syncytial aggregates with indistinct cell borders. Cells have only a minimal amount of cytoplasm. Nuclei, although relatively small, vary greatly in size (Papanicolaou stain; ×250).

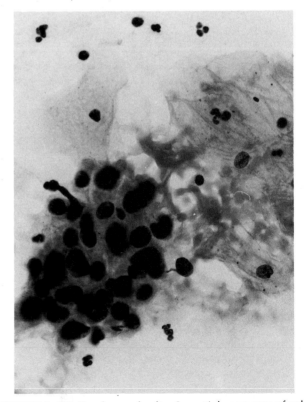

FIGURE 9–83. Carcinoma *in situ*. Syncytial aggregate of cells with indistinct cytoplasmic borders. Nuclei vary in size and shape and are frequently overlapping. Nuclear chromatin is dense and hyperchromatic (Papanicolaou stain; ×250).

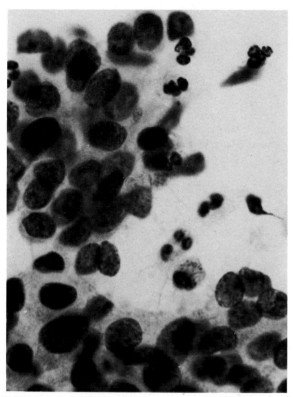

FIGURE 9–84. Carcinoma *in situ*. Syncytial aggregate of cells. Nuclei vary in size and shape and frequently overlap. Nuclear chromatin is irregularly distributed and coarsely granular (Papanicolaou stain; ×625).

small immature squamous metaplastic cells. Similarly, cells from a histologically small–type carcinoma *in situ* are in the range of reserve cells. From a series of cytologic specimens in cases of histologically proven *in situ* carcinomas, Patten[128] computed a mean cell area of 238 μm. The cells are predominantly round to oval in shape, reflecting the immature character of these cells. Irregular or elongated cell forms are related to a specific superficial change of the lesion. The sparse cytoplasm stains predominantly basophilic, a cytoplasmic staining reaction that reflects the lack of keratinization in these undifferentiated cells. The few cells showing an eosinophilic staining reaction are most likely derived from a coexisting dysplasia. Owing to the highly vulnerable cytoplasm in cases of carcinoma *in situ*, the finding of cells with damaged cytoplasm or with bare nuclei is frequent (Fig. 9–85).

Nuclear Morphology. The lack of a differentiation stimulus, usually associated with a relatively rapid cell growth, becomes apparent from the round to oval shape of the nuclei. On the average nuclei of cells derived from *in situ* carcinoma are usually somewhat smaller than nuclei derived from dysplastic cells. Patten[128] computed a mean nuclear area of 125 μm. The nuclear membrane in isolated cells is usually well defined; at higher magnification nuclear grooves may be seen that are rather characteristic of these undifferentiated cells, even though they are most likely artifacts due to fixation (Fig. 9–86; see also Fig. 9–85). The

chromatin varies from finely granular and unevenly distributed to coarsely granular and hyperchromatic (see Fig. 9–86). The number of small nuclei with coarse hyperchromatic chromatin is correlated with the degree of dedifferentiation of the cells from the carcinoma *in situ*. Another characteristic of *in situ* carcinoma cells, recognizable at high magnification, is the interrupted nuclear membrane due to irregular sedimentation on the membrane of the coarsely granular chromatin. It is rare to find eosinophilic staining nucleoli, but chromocenters or "false" nucleoli are rather common (see Fig. 9–86). "True" nucleoli may be obscured by the coarse hyperchromatic chromatin but are definitely present, as they are related to the high proliferation rate of the lesion. The absence of nucleoli would be in contradiction to the relatively high proliferative activity, which is evident from the presence of mitoses even in the uppermost layers of the epithelium. Macronucleoli, which are usually present in nuclei from invasive cancer cells, are only rarely seen in *in situ* carcinomas.

Relative Nuclear Area. The relative nuclear area (nuclear area in relation to cytoplasmic area) with an average value of 50% better reflects the primitive character of these cells from *in situ* carcinomas than just the size of the cell or the nucleus.

Reagan and Hamonic[144] reported the presence of

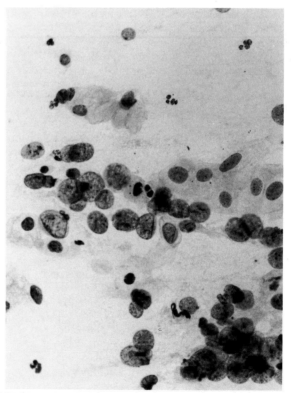

FIGURE 9–85. Carcinoma *in situ*. Syncytial aggregate with indistinct cell borders and multiple isolated bare nuclei. Compare size with intermediate squamous cells and columnar cells in upper half of this field. Nuclei have sharply outlined membranes, an irregular distribution of finely granular chromatin and conspicuous nuclear grooves (Papanicolaou stain; ×250).

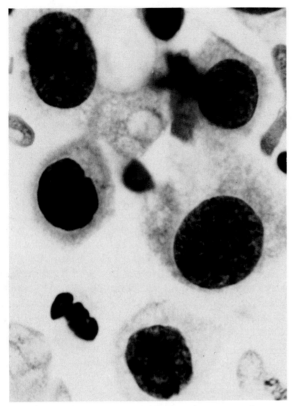

FIGURE 9–86. Carcinoma *in situ*. Coarsely granular irregularly distributed nuclear chromatin. Large irregular condensations of chromatin—chromocenters—should be differentiated from nucleoli. Deep nuclear groove in nucleus at the lower margin (Papanicolaou stain; ×1250).

inflammatory exudate in specimens from *in situ* cancers in 68% of cases compared with 32% in specimens from dysplasias. In our own material from a population-screening program the percentage of smears showing an inflammatory exudate in cases of carcinoma *in situ* and severe dysplasia (85.1%) was not significantly different from the percentages of smears found with less severe changes or without signs of epithelial abnormalities.[97]

Biologic Significance

It is generally agreed that the majority of lesions classified as carcinoma *in situ* are actively proliferating lesions that, if left alone, will finally turn into an invasive cancer. However, with presently available knowledge and techniques, it is virtually impossible from cytologic, histologic or clinical data to predict which reaction will regress and which will progress to a more severe lesion.

It is generally accepted that all invasive cancers of the uterine cervix develop from a carcinoma *in situ* or from a severe dysplasia. However, there is massive evidence that not all *in situ* carcinomas or severe dysplasias progress into an invasive process; many regress into a lesion of less severity or disappear completely. This means that these lesions diagnosed as intraepithelial cancer are essentially not malignant in nature.

Many studies have tried to uncover the characteristics of those *in situ* carcinomas that progress into an invasive process, to discriminate these from the lesions that show regression but that appear light-microscopically identical. Data on the follow-up of severe dysplasias and *in situ* carcinomas are not abundant, since most lesions are immediately treated when diagnosed. Available data indicate that only a relatively small number of lesions will eventually progress to an invasive squamous cell carcinoma.[49, 58, 65, 80, 89]

Prospective studies designed to follow the course of *in situ* carcinoma suggest a relatively slow evolution to invasive carcinoma. Analyses of incidence rates and mortality indicate that the length of the preinvasive stage is on the order of 12 to 15 years. Reports of so-called fast-growing cancers, which are claimed to have passed very quickly through a premalignant preinvasive phase as should be evidenced by a negative cytologic examination shortly prior to the diagnosis of the invasive process, appear with some periodicity in the literature. However, on careful analysis of available evidence, the accuracy of the preceding cytologic diagnosis usually does not stand, since false-negative diagnoses due to sampling errors cannot be excluded. In our own registry of premalignant and malignant lesions of the uterine cervix, encompassing 17 years prior to and during a population-screening program, difference in mean age between *in situ* cancer and invasive cancer was 13.7 years (carcinoma *in situ*: mean age 39.2 years; invasive cancer: mean age 52.9 years).

Developmental Carcinoma *In Situ*. Reagan and colleagues[149] described the morphologic characteristics of a group of epithelial lesions that they considered to be developmental carcinoma *in situ*. Comparable cytologic features in women who ultimately were proved to have carcinoma *in situ* were described by Koss and Durfee.[87] Compared with classic carcinoma *in situ*, cells more frequently lie singly than in arranged syncytial masses. When present in aggregates, cells more often had a sheet-like rather than a syncytial arrangement. In almost all instances there was a significant admixture of dysplastic cells in the smears. Average cell size was between the mean sizes for dysplastic cells and *in situ* carcinoma cells. Also, for the distribution of cell shapes values proved to be between the values found for dysplasias and *in situ* carcinomas. Nuclear chromatin was predominantly finely granular and unevenly distributed. The lesions usually showed a more orderly growth pattern and a relatively low mitotic activity.

Cytology. The cellular characteristics of this so-called developmental carcinoma *in situ* were reminiscent of cells found in proliferating reserve cells. The mean age at which this developmental *in situ* cancer was found antedated the mean age of classic *in situ* carcinoma by 5 years.

Fawdry[43] found "early recurrences" of carcinoma *in situ* within a year after hysterectomy in 0.9% of women who had a hysterectomy after a diagnosis of carcinoma *in situ*. During subsequent long-term follow-up invasive squamous cell carcinomas of the vaginal vault were found in 0.3% of patients. These figures stress the importance of cytologic follow-up by vaginal vault smears in women who have had a hysterectomy for a severe epithelial abnormality of the cervix.

Co-Occurrence of Dysplasia and Carcinoma In Situ

An area in which discrepancies in the grading of lesions still occurs is the discrimination between severe dysplasia and carcinoma *in situ*. Although for the sake of a better understanding of the biologic behavior of intraepithelial lesions it is still advocated to differentiate as much as possible between severe dysplasia and carcinoma *in situ*, in routine diagnosis such a strict separation is not very relevant. Both changes are considered to be of a high potential for progression to an invasive lesion, and clinical management is usually identical. In view of the influence from local environmental factors and because of the origin from different stem cells, the markedly dysplastic change, which usually still shows some maturation of the most superficial layers into squamous cells, originating in the original ectocervical squamous epithelium, is likely to be fully comparable with the characteristic carcinoma *in situ*, originating in the endocervical canal through a squamous metaplastic interphase and in which characteristically any sign of maturation, even in the most superficial layers, is absent.

Approximately 80% of *in situ* carcinomas coexist with dysplasia. Graphic distribution of these lesions suggests that when coexistence occurs, dysplasia lies distal from carcinoma *in situ*.[128] Both dysplasia and carcinoma *in situ* occur more frequently on the anterior lip of the cervix.

A possible explanation is that the anterior lip is more frequently traumatized. The radial extent of cervical intraepithelial neoplasia on the portio epithelium is greatest in the carcinoma *in situ* population. Also, the size and distribution of carcinoma *in situ* on the exposed portion of the cervix is more constant than in dysplasia.

Of patients with carcinoma *in situ* 45% had only dysplasia on the exposed portion of the cervix. The difference in the distribution of carcinoma *in situ* and dysplasia may be accounted for by the increased size of the lesion in patients with carcinoma *in situ*[151] and also by the age-related size differences between dysplasia and carcinoma *in situ*.[148]

The hypothesis that dysplasia represents a younger (smaller and less extensive) precursor of carcinoma *in situ* is supported by the colposcopic and cytologic observation in the individual case. The lesions are not biologically different, but the patient with a carcinoma *in situ* has a lesion that has been present for a longer time and involves a larger area of the cervix. Our knowledge of the biologic behavior of carcinoma *in situ* is still incomplete; an untreated lesion may develop into an invasive cancer, regress to a less severe lesion, completely disappear or persist for an indeterminate period of time.[149] Dysplasia and carcinoma *in situ* both occur in the area of the transformation zone.

Co-occurrence of Carcinoma In Situ and Adenocarcinoma In Situ

Carcinogenic changes in the uterine cervix can be considered to be part of a field carcinogenic process. This means that the carcinogenic stimulus does not exert its action on an isolated cell that becomes the stem cell of a malignant proliferation, but on a larger area of the epithelium. This may be the explanation for the common observation that next to a severe lesion changes of different, often lesser severity are found. It also explains the common multifocal occurrence of epithelial abnormalities.

This field stimulus apparently not only influences squamous and squamous metaplastic epithelium but also the columnar epithelium of the endocervical canal. The co-occurrence of abnormal columnar cell changes together with abnormalities of the squamous and squamous metaplastic epithelium is becoming increasingly frequent.

In a series of 42,863 first cervical smears, minimally to severely atypical columnar cell changes were observed in 69% of cases of severe dysplasia, carcinoma *in situ* and microinvasive and invasive cancer (Figs. 9–87 and 9–88). In 13% of cases this atypia was diagnosed as an adenocarcinoma *in situ* (Figs. 9–89 and 9–90).

The increased prevalence of these atypical columnar

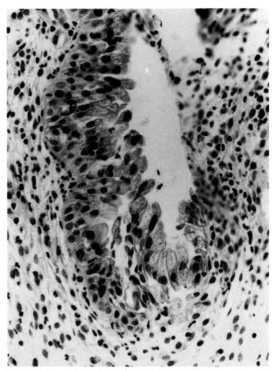

FIGURE 9–87. Mild atypia of endocervical columnar epithelium. Pseudostratified columnar epithelium with irregular arrangement of nuclei, variation in nuclear size and scattered nuclear hyperchromasia (hematoxylin and eosin; ×250).

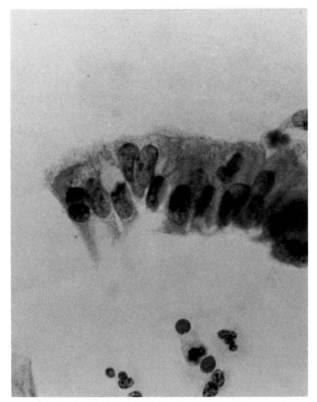

FIGURE 9–88. Mildly atypical columnar cells. Irregular arrangement of nuclei and variation in nuclear size and shape. Slight hyperchromasia of regularly distributed nuclear chromatin. Usually one to two nucleoli present (Papanicolaou stain; ×625).

cell changes may be due to a new factor that also causes columnar cell abnormalities but is more likely caused by an increased sensitivity of screeners to columnar cell changes, correlated with an increased awareness of the significance of endocervical columnar cells as a quality parameter for cervical smears.[196, 199] For a detailed description of the cytomorphologic characteristics of adenocarcinoma *in situ* see Chapter 10 on cytology of Glandular Neoplasms of the Uterine Cervix.

Dysplasia and Carcinoma In Situ During Pregnancy

In general the cellular features of dysplastic changes in pregnant women are identical to the changes observed in nongravid women. Often dysplastic changes remain undetected in view of the significantly larger number of smears of unsatisfactory quality. Particularly during the first trimester of pregnancy smears may contain a large number of relatively small, immature atypical cells. In general, dysplastic reactions during the first months of pregnancy tend to be composed of relatively small cells, thus suggesting a severe abnormality. These relatively immature dysplastic changes may lead to a dilemma: whether the patient should undergo histologic evaluation or not. In most instances,

with progression of pregnancy a reduction of the severity of a dysplastic reaction occurs. In a study of 87 women with dysplasia during pregnancy Slate and Merritt[176] found 45% of lesions to regress, 29% to persist and 25% to progress to a more severe abnormality after a variable period of time.

As a general rule, unless clinical symptoms suggest a severe lesion, routine cytologic diagnosis should be avoided during the first trimester. Contrary to widespread belief there is no evidence that dysplastic lesions and carcinoma *in situ* behave differently during pregnancy. The morphologic features of *in situ* carcinoma do not differ from those presented for the nongravid patient. The growth rate of preinvasive epithelial changes is not greater during pregnancy.

Surgical procedures may induce overstimulation or may damage the cervix and thus may interfere with the pregnancy. In general it is fully warranted to carefully follow the abnormality during pregnancy, even in cases of carcinoma *in situ*, and to postpone treatment of the epithelial change till after childbirth. It is advocated that surgical treatment be instituted only after cytologic reconfirmation of the lesion, when normal menstrual cycling has resumed and epithelial atrophy has been reversed. In some of the cases the epithelial abnormality will disappear after childbirth, possibly owing to the passage of the newborn through the cervical canal or because of a change in hormonal influence on the cervical epithelium, potentially changing the balance (or imbalance) between the host tissue and the abnormal epithelium.

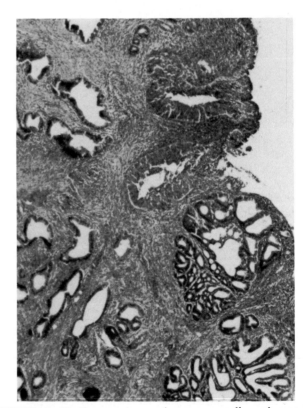

FIGURE 9–89. Co-occurrence of **squamous cell carcinoma *in situ*** and **adenocarcinoma *in situ*** (hematoxylin and eosin; ×130).

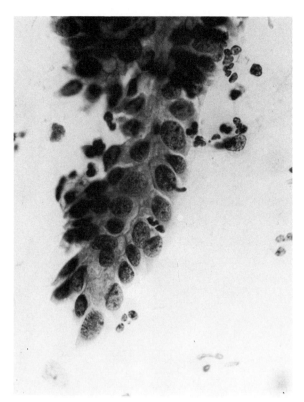

FIGURE 9–90. Adenocarcinoma *in situ.* Papillary aggregate of cells with partly overlapping nuclei. Variation in size of predominantly round to oval nuclei. Moderate hyperchromasia of predominantly finely granular and regularly distributed nuclear chromatin. One to multiple nucleoli present (Papanicolaou stain; ×350).

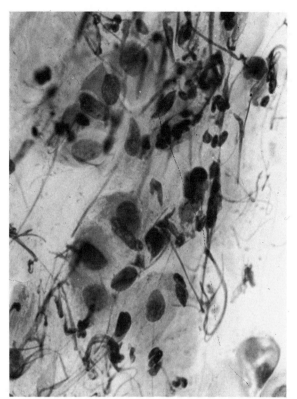

FIGURE 9–91. Atrophy in postmenopause. Cells with an increased nucleocytoplasmic (N/C) ratio against a background of cellular debris and inflammatory cells (Papanicolaou stain; ×500).

Dysplasia and Carcinoma In Situ *in the Postmenopausal Patient*

Dysplasia and carcinoma *in situ* occurring during postmenopause are often difficult to diagnose because of the lack of mature squamous and columnar cells in the smears. Owing to the lack of estrogenic stimulation cells remain rather small, often the size of parabasal cells or relatively immature squamous metaplastic cells. Aggregates of small cells with densely staining nuclei are a common finding in smears from women in postmenopause. Relative nuclear enlargement due to a reduced development of the cytoplasm, which is in turn caused by a low estrogenic stimulus, may mimic the nucleocytoplasmic ratio found in epithelial lesions (Figs. 9–91 and 9–92). These cells are often erroneously diagnosed as dysplastic cells or cells consistent with *in situ* carcinoma.

To avoid unnecessary biopsies it is advisable to repeat the cytologic examination after a short course of oral or local hormonal estrogenic medication. In the majority of cases the supposedly dysplastic change will have disappeared through maturation of the epithelium under the estrogenic stimulus (Fig. 9–93; see also Fig. 9–18). Since abnormal epithelial cells are less sensitive to the maturation stimulus from the estrogenic hormones, true abnormal cells can be recognized much more easily between the now-matured surrounding

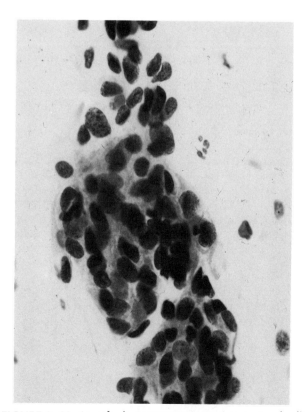

FIGURE 9–92. Atrophy in postmenopause. Aggregate of cells with indistinct cell borders, increased nucleocytoplasmic (N/C) ratio, variation in nuclear size and shape and hyperchromasia (Papanicolaou stain; ×400).

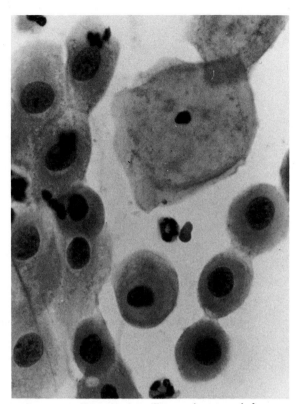

FIGURE 9–93. Effect of a short course of **estrogenic hormones.** Maturation of squamous cells. Some minimal atypia of parabasal cell type remaining. No evidence of an epithelial abnormality (Papanicolaou stain; ×500). (Same case as in Figure 9–91.)

epithelial cells (Fig. 9–94). With this relatively simple procedure in cases of epithelial atrophy with pseudoabnormalities, unnecessary biopsies can be avoided. In view of the higher rate of complications in cases of surgical interventions involving atrophic tissues this must be considered an important benefit to these women. Kaminski and coworkers[75] reviewed 115 consecutive patients over 50 years of age with known abnormal cytologic findings, diagnosed at routine cervical screening. There was a strong association between epithelial abnormalities and atrophy. After correction of the estrogen deficiency, the epithelial abnormality reverted to normal in a statistically significant percentage of patients. Findings were epithelial atrophy in 58% of patients and no epithelial abnormalities in 37%. Two patients had CIN grade I and two patients CIN grade II. One patient showed evidence of HPV infection. In our own material the lesion disappeared completely in 18% of cases, and moderate to severe atypia was reduced to slight atypia in 55% of cases. The estrogenic stimulus induced a marked increase in maturation in 68% of smears. The smears were easier to read because of a reduction in the admixture of inflammatory cells and the degree of cytolysis of the cytoplasm of atrophic cells, resulting in a clear background against which truly abnormal cells usually stand out clearly.

INVASIVE CANCER OF THE UTERINE CERVIX

Epidemiology. Worldwide, cancer of the cervix is the second most common cancer in women. In developing countries this type of cancer even ranks first, whereas in developed countries it ranks tenth. In most developed countries the frequency of cervical cancer and the mortality rate for cervical cancer have dropped since the 1950s. Cervical smears are important in the prevention of cancer of the cervix.[62, 64, 70, 86] The first priority is to screen the group that has never been examined. An increase in the number of screenings by reducing the interval between screenings is reported to have only a marginal benefit.

Olesen[123] analyzed the number of previous smears in 428 women who developed invasive cancer of the cervix and compared these with previous screenings in age- and area-matched controls. He reported that 55% of the cancer patients and 33% of the controls had never been screened before. This was a highly significant difference. Regular screening reduced the relative risk for invasive cancer in the screened population to about 0.25. When only symptomless patients were analyzed the relative risk was reduced to 0.15. Even the group

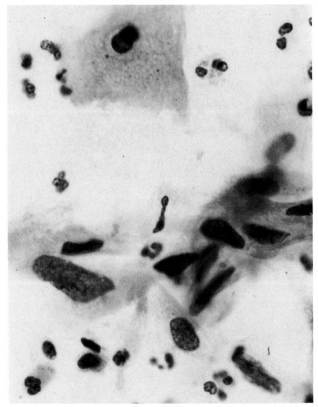

FIGURE 9–94. Effect of a short course of **estrogenic hormones.** Maturation of squamous cells and some highly atypical squamous cells with increased nucleocytoplasmic (N/C) ratio, irregular nuclei and dense hyperchromatic nuclei. Abnormal cells are consistent with severe dysplasia. (Papanicolaou stain; ×625). (Same case as in Figure 9–92.)

of patients that was screened more than 5 years previously had a reduction in relative risk for developing invasive cancer to 0.67. The incidence rate of invasive cancer in the age group participating in the Nijmegen screening program dropped significantly 3 years after the start of the program. After two negative smears, in only 0.01% of the screened women was a severe epithelial abnormality detected.[186]

In recent years an increase in the incidence rate of cervical cancer in younger women has been suggested. This may well be an effect of more frequent screening and screening in younger age groups, since mortality rates have not (yet) shown an increase in these age groups.[187] In some countries, however, an increase in mortality rates for cervical cancer in young women has been reported since the late 1960s,[3, 31, 57] suggesting the effect of the introduction of some new risk factors in recent years, particularly among young women.[111] Independently of her age, a woman's risk of cervical cancer is strongly associated with sexual activity, more specifically with the number of partners and with age at first intercourse.[17] The epidemiologic pattern strongly suggests the role of a sexually transmitted agent because of the striking associations between the temporal, socioeconomic and geographic distributions of mortality rates of cervical cancer and incidence rates of sexually transmitted diseases.[12] Although other factors such as long-term use of oral contraceptives, smoking, specific dietary factors and immunosuppression may also be important, the exact role and the relative contribution of each of these factors can only be determined after the sexually transmitted agent that may be the main cause of cervical cancer has been identified with certainty.[111]

For over 20 years much attention has been given to herpes simplex virus Type 2 as an etiologic agent of cervical neoplasia, but conclusive evidence of a causal role has never been obtained.[16, 110] According to current hypothesis, HPV is etiologically involved. Even though there is evidence for this from laboratory studies, it will be very difficult to prove this hypothesis epidemiologically.[16, 111, 180]

Microinvasive Carcinoma

Microinvasive carcinoma is the earliest stage in the genesis of an invasive cancer that can be recognized histologically.

With the implementation of large-scale population-screening program, an increasing number of these preclinical, nonsymptomatic processes are being detected. Over a 30-year period the percentage of microinvasive cancers diagnosed at the University Hospitals of Cleveland increased from 1.2% of the squamous cancers seen in the period ending in 1947 to 23.5% of the cervical cancers detected in a comparable period ending in 1972. Of the women with microinvasive cancer, 62.1% were asymptomatic and 56.1% had normal-appearing cervices at the time of diagnosis.[118] These cancers with limited extent have a very good prognosis. Since these cancers occur several years prior

to the average age of detection of frankly invasive cancers, the patient is often still under 40 years of age and requests, if in anyway possible, to have as conservative a treatment as possible. Microinvasive carcinoma in its early stages is often found originating from an overlying severe epithelial abnormality (CIN grade III: severe dysplasia and carcinoma in situ), but occasionally, particularly in more extensive lesions, invasion seems to arise from a lesion of lesser severity. This, however, may be a pseudodifferentiation in an originally severe lesion. This phenomenon may have caused the confusion about the potential for progression of mild to moderately atypical epithelial lesions.

The concept of microinvasive carcinoma was introduced by Mestwerdt[106] for invasive processes with a maximum depth of invasion of 5 mm. Microinvasive carcinomas were made into a subgroup of Stage I invasive cancers because of the much better survival in this group of lesions. The depth of invasion has since been the crucial parameter for the choice between a relatively conservative approach and radical treatment. The subject of microinvasion has been associated with 2 decades of confusion. Investigators have reported conflicting results in what appears to be the same subset of patients.[38] The volume of the tumor, histologically determined by depth of stromal invasion and linear extension along the surface and semiquantitated from multiple parallel sections, is the real denominator of the stage of the disease. There has been much confusion about the exact definition of microinvasive carcinoma. In the literature the maximum depth of invasion is given as 1 mm, 3 mm, 5 mm, 7 mm and 9 mm. The ideal definition of microinvasive carcinoma should enable a clear decision between a conservative approach and radical treatment, but unfortunately there is still no internationally accepted definition of microinvasive carcinoma. Also the original definition adopted by the International Federation of Gynecology and Obstetrics (FIGO) did not fulfill this requirement. In 1985 the oncology committee of the Federation changed the definition of limited-stage cervical cancer and better defined microinvasive carcinoma.[46] It is now widely accepted that to be considered as a microinvasive cancer the depth of invasion, measured from the base of the epithelium from which it develops, should not exceed 5 mm and the largest diameter (lateral extent) should not exceed 7 mm. Vascular involvement should not alter the staging but should be specifically recorded, as it may affect treatment decisions in the future.[46] The depth of invasion should be measured from the basement membrane of the neighboring noninvasive epithelium. Preclinical carcinoma of the cervix should include minimal microscopically evident stromal invasion as well as small cancers of measurable size. Based on the histologic evaluation of the tissue removed, which should include the entire lesion, Stage IA tumors are further subdivided into Stage IA1 tumors, which include lesions with minute foci of invasion visible only microscopically, and Stage IA2 tumors, which are macroscopically measurable. Lesions of greater size should be staged as IB. Since as a rule it is impossible to estimate clinically whether a cancer of the cervix has extended to the corpus, extension to the corpus should be disregarded.[46]

Histology. The diagnosis of microinvasive carcinoma should only be made on a histologic specimen that contains the entire lesion. Punch biopsy taken under colposcopic control and endocervical curettage specimens are inadequate to provide a reliable diagnosis of microinvasion.

Histologically two separate entities may be recognized.[92–94]

- Early stromal invasion
- Microinvasive carcinoma.

Early Stromal Invasion. In early stromal invasion cell nests protrude from the basal layer of the overlying epithelium into the surrounding stroma or singly lying nests are located within 1 mm of the overlying epithelium (Fig. 9–95). These changes are usually too small to be measured accurately and reproducibly. The earliest sign of invasive growth is a usually rather well circumscribed small nest of cells "dropping" from the severely abnormal, essentially noninvasive surface epithelium into the stroma. The cells composing this protruding peg seem better differentiated owing to a relatively large body of eosinophilic staining cytoplasm, which is the basis of a lower nucleocytoplasmic ratio in the invading cells than in the cells of the epithelium of origin (Fig. 9–96).[22] The invading body of cells is well demarcated and surrounded by a dense infiltrate

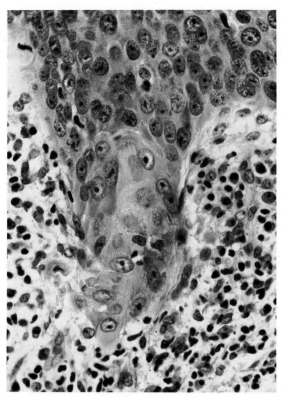

FIGURE 9–96. Microinvasive cancer. Early stromal invasion. Cells protruding into the surrounding stroma, showing an increased cytoplasmic volume and a decreased nucleocytoplasmic (N/C) ratio (hematoxylin and eosin; × 400).

of lymphocytes and plasma cells, which characteristically leave a loose, somewhat edematous clear zone, free of inflammatory cells around the invading cell groups.[24, 25, 92, 93] The increased amount of eosinophilic cytoplasm is probably not a sign of improved differentiation, but on the contrary a reflection of dedifferentiation enabling the cell to break through the basement membrane and to proliferate despite the host's immune response in the surrounding stroma.

This rather characteristic histologic picture usually enables the pathologist to differentiate between extensions of the abnormal epithelium into invaginations, noninvasive nests of abnormal surface epithelium due to tangential sectioning and truly invasive cells in an early stromal invasion.

Microinvasive Carcinoma. The depth of invasion in microinvasive carcinoma originally was determined to be less than 5 mm.[1, 2] The prognosis of the disease is most clearly determined by the volume of the tumor. Thus the extent of invasion in microinvasive carcinoma should not be measured in one direction only. Measurements should also encompass the spread of the lesion parallel to the surface epithelium, analyzed in multiple parallel sections (Fig. 9–97). This enables the pathologist to get a fairly accurate impression of the volume of the tumor, which is directly related to the chance of vascular invasion and thus with prognosis. Measurements should be made with an ocular micrometer that is calibrated for each objective. A practical

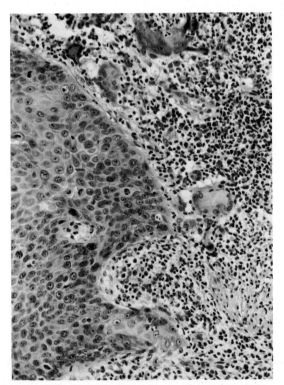

FIGURE 9–95. Microinvasive cancer. Early stromal invasion. Nests of tumor cells lying within 1 mm from the basal layer of the overlying epithelium. Dense infiltrate of lymphocytes and plasma cells in the surrounding stroma (hematoxylin and eosin; × 128).

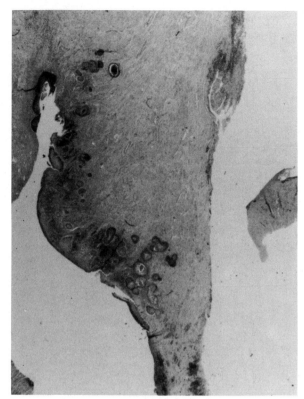

FIGURE 9–97. Microinvasive cancer. Multiple nests of invasive cancer within 5 mm from the basal layers of the ectocervical and endocervical epithelium (hematoxylin and eosin; ×15).

into such a space (Fig. 9–98). In many specimens tumor cell nests are found in tissue spaces. These, however, lack an endothelial lining; there is no evidence of a continuous growth from the tumor into these spaces. They are the result of shrinkage of the stroma during fixation. Ferenczy[44] feels that true involvement of capillary-like spaces should exclude the tumor from the category of microinvasive cancers, irrespective of the depth of invasion. Ng and Reagan[117, 118] reviewed the frequency of lymph node metastasis of 96 women who had had hysterectomy and radical lymph node resection. With a depth of infiltration under 1 mm no lymph node metastases were found. With a depth of infiltration of from 1 to 5 mm the frequency of lymph node involvement increased from 3.2% to 11.1%. In the total group metastatic spread to lymph nodes was found in 4% of cases. Burghardt[22] found no recurrent cancers after 3 to 11 years' follow-up in 9 cases with early stromal invasion or microinvasion up to 5 mm and in all cases with involvement of capillary spaces. Roche and Norris[160] found no spread to lymph nodes in 30 cases with microinvasion of 2 to 5 mm (average 3.2 mm) in depth. In 57% of these women capillary-like space involvement was found. Seski and colleagues[172] reported on lymph node involvement in one out of four women with microinvasion up to 3 mm and capillary-like space involvement, whereas in a group of 37 women with comparable depth of invasion but without capillary-like space involvement, lymphatic spread could not be

approach is to measure the diameter of field of vision for each objective once with a stage micrometer and to relate these measurements to a specimen under study.[30] A diagnosis of a microinvasive cancer should not be made unless the entire histologic specimen has been carefully examined. Presence of tumor tissue in the resection margins of the specimen should be excluded in view of the high risk of residual cancer in patients with conization specimens with tumor tissue present in the resection margins of the cone. Sedlis and colleagues[169] found residual cancer in 12 out of 15 patients with tumor presence in the resection margins of the conization specimen. In about half of these patients residual tumor growth in the uterus was more extensive than in the cone.

The risk of distant spread of a microinvasive carcinoma is related to the depth of invasion, the lateral extent of the lesion and the lymphatic channel involvement. The single most important histologic parameter for the determination of prognosis in microinvasive cancer is the extension of tumor growth into capillary-like spaces (lymphatic channels or microarterioles).[160] Of less importance in the determination of prognosis are the growth pattern of the lesion and the host's immune response to the tumor. Confluence of invading foci seems to be of relevance only for prognosis, where it contributes to the overall extent of the tumor.[30] A diagnosis of invasion of capillary-like spaces should be supported by the presence of an endothelial lining of these spaces[22] and a continuous growth from the tumor

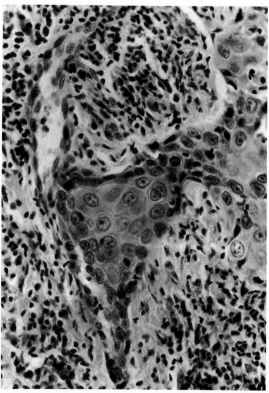

FIGURE 9–98. Microinvasive cancer. Invasion of capillary-like space. Tumor cells invading luminal space lined in part by endothelial cells and in part by tumor cells (hematoxylin and eosin; ×310).

demonstrated. Although the results of these studies are conflicting, capillary-like space involvement should be considered an important risk factor and warrants the choice of more radical treatment.[30, 38]

Cytology. Cytologic features consistent with microinvasive cancer are still very difficult to interpret. Many authors stress the fact that a diagnosis of microinvasive carcinoma cannot be reliably made from a cytologic specimen. However, some cytologic features are strongly associated with a more-advanced epithelial abnormality than that of a CIN grade III type of lesion.

Arrangement of Cells. Cells are often arranged in syncytial aggregates (Fig. 9–99). In microinvasive carcinoma the number of abnormal cells on the average is lower than in outright invasive cancer.

Nuclear Morphology. Nuclear chromatin is more often uniformly finely or coarsely granular and less often irregularly distributed or opaque than in outright invasive cancer (Fig. 9–100). Nucleoli are usually found, but macronucleoli are infrequent (Fig. 9–101). The most consistent nuclear feature associated with invasive growth is the appearance of irregularly shaped nucleoli, together with a relative increase in the amount of cytoplasm.

Evidence of Tissue Destruction. Obviously related to the depth of invasion, evidence of tissue destruction was considerably less frequently found than in overt invasive cancer.[118, 120] Related to the depth of invasion and the amount of tissue destruction by the invading process, cellular features are more reminiscent of either carcinoma *in situ* or frankly invasive cancer. In a series

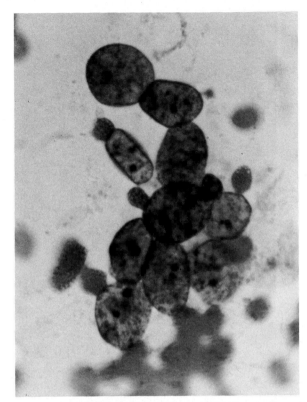

FIGURE 9–100. Microinvasive cancer. Round to oval nuclei with irregular distribution of coarsely granular hyperchromatic nuclear chromatin and pleomorphic nucleoli (Papanicolaou stain; ×850).

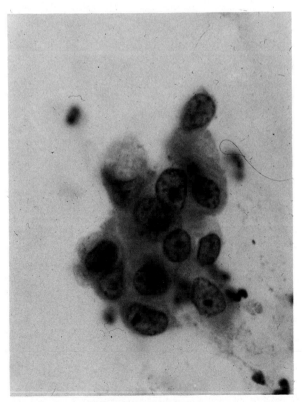

FIGURE 9–99. Microinvasive cancer. Syncytial aggregate of epithelial cells with indistinct cell borders. Irregular distribution of nuclear chromatin and nucleoli varying in size and shape (Papanicolaou stain; ×625).

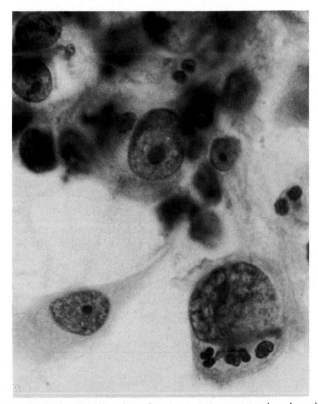

FIGURE 9–101. Microinvasive cancer. Large round and oval nuclei with coarsely granular irregularly distributed nuclear chromatin and irregular macronucleoli (Papanicolaou stain; ×650).

of 52 cases of proven microinvasive cancer, Ng and colleagues[120] found cellular characteristics of microinvasive cancers with an epithelial infiltration of 0.1 to 2.0 mm to resemble those of *in situ* carcinoma and dysplasia, whereas those in cases of microinvasion of 3.1 to 5.0 mm were more reminiscent of frankly invasive cancer. Cellular features consistent with microinvasive cancer were found to be most distinctive with a depth of invasion between 2 and 3 mm.

Accuracy. Ng and coworkers[117] and Ng and Reagan[118] state that on the basis of cellular characteristics the diagnosis of microinvasive cancer can be made accurately and reproducibly in a high proportion of cases. From 56 cases of proven microinvasive cancer 80% were correctly recognized as microinvasive in the cellular samples. In a review study of 100 cases obtained from patients with lesions associated with cancer of the cervix, correct interpretation was made in 97% of cases of *in situ* carcinoma, in 87% of cases of microinvasive cancer and in 97% of cases of outspoken cancer. Nguyen[121] reviewed 42 cases of histologically proven microinvasive squamous cell carcinomas with invasion of less than 3 mm. At review microinvasion could be suggested on the basis of cellular features in approximately 60% of cases. Cytologic prediction was 14% in cases with stromal invasion less than 1 mm; it increased to 73% and 88% when stromal invasions were up to 2 and 3 mm, respectively, in depth.

These figures demonstrate that in selected series the cytologic diagnosis of microinvasive carcinoma can be made with high accuracy. A review situation, however, is essentially different from a screening situation, in which the incidence of severe abnormalities is usually very low. In those routine screening situations the primary diagnosis of "changes consistent with microinvasive cancer" is made less frequently and with less accuracy. The effort to cytologically diagnose epithelial abnormalities as accurately as possible is encouraged. It is, however, advisable to mention the possibility of a microinvasive cancer rather than give such a diagnosis with certainty. In general in routine cytodiagnosis making a firm diagnosis of a microinvasive carcinoma should be avoided. In addition to a diagnosis of an invasive cancer the possibility of the process being microinvasive may be mentioned. Such a diagnosis is based on very delicate differences between the characteristics of *in situ* carcinomas and invasive cancers. A suggestion of too high a precision would be misunderstood against the background of the relatively high rate of false diagnoses, which unfortunately are still being made and may potentially reduce clinical acceptance of diagnostic cytopathology.

Invasive Cervical Cancer

Invasive cancer was defined by the International Committee on Histological Terminology for Lesions of the Uterine Cervix as "any lesion in which epithelial formations invade the underlying stroma by infiltration or destruction is to be classified as invasive carcinoma."[207]

TABLE 9–1. Distribution of Histologic Types in Primary Invasive Cancers of the Cervix

Squamous cell cancer	
Nonkeratinizing	43.3%
Keratinizing	29.1%
Small cell cancer	10.9%
Adenosquamous carcinoma	7.0%
Adenocarcinoma	6.2%
Clear cell carcinoma	1.5%
Adenocanthoma	0.8%
Adenoid cystic carcinoma	0.2%

In a large series of primary invasive cancers of the cervix Ng and Reagan[119] found the distribution of histologic types shown in Table 9–1.

Keratinizing and nonkeratinizing squamous cell cancer may originate from the original nonkeratinizing stratified ectocervical squamous epithelium and from metaplastic epithelium in the endocervical canal.

Small-cell carcinoma originates in undifferentiated precursor cells of the endocervical columnar epithelium, which lack every differentiation into columnar or squamous epithelium. The group of small-cell cancers is probably not a homogeneous group. Jones and associates,[74] based on the ultrastructural demonstration of neurosecretory granules in the cytoplasm of these cells, suggested that part of these tumors were of neuroendocrine origin and probably originated from amine precursor uptake and decarboxylation (APUD) cells in the cervix. This finding is supported by the demonstration of argentafin (Kultchitsky) cells in small-cell cancers of the cervix, which suggests a relationship with small-cell cancers of the bronchus (extrapulmonary small-cell cancer).[183] Adenocarcinomas with the subtype of clear cell carcinoma originate from the endocervical columnar epithelium, derived from the embryologic müllerian epithelium. Adenocarcinomas are also found that originate from mesonephric duct remnants, known as mesonephric carcinomas. Adenocarcinomas with an admixture of a benign or a malignant squamous component—adenoacanthoma and adenosquamous carcinoma—most likely originate from undifferentiated precursor cells of the endocervical columnar epithelium, with a dual development into columnar epithelium and squamous epithelium. For a detailed description of adenocarcinomas and precursor lesions see Chapter 10 on Cytology of Glandular Neoplasms of the Uterine Cervix.

Age at Detection. Patten[127] in a series of 61 cases found a mean age at detection of 53.4 years. Reagan and Hicks[146] found a mean age of 48.2 years. In our own series of 435 cases of squamous cell cancer of the cervix, the mean age was 53.0 years (standard deviation of 13.9 years) (see Fig. 9–79).

Clinical Considerations. In its earliest stages invasive cancer may not disturb the configuration of the cervix and may remain undetected during palpation or even at colposcopic inspection. MacLean and coworkers[95] found in a series of women diagnosed with invasive cancer that the majority had never had a cytologic smear taken or had not had smears taken frequently enough. Of 122 women diagnosed with invasive cancer only 12 women (10%) had ever before been examined cytologically.

In our experience, in women 55 years and older, invasive cervical cancer is almost always diagnosed in a more advanced clinical stage. Only two out of 47 women with invasive cancer diagnosed in this age group had a cytologic cervical smear taken at any time in their life. Since 39% of invasive cancers were diagnosed in this age group, a considerable reduction in mortality could be realized if these women were screened periodically.[13]

Macroscopically malignant cervical tumors can be divided into two categories. Exophytic growth, consisting of papillary excrescences or warty-like masses, protrudes above the surface. This kind of tumor most often originates in the epithelium of the ectocervix or the portio vaginalis. Endophytic growth is a growth pattern most commonly found in tumors originating proximally from the external os.

In squamous cell carcinoma the most important prognostic factors are the extent of the tumor, differentiation grade and histologic type or subtype. The extent of the neoplasm at the time of diagnosis is still the most important factor in prognosis. Women with lymph node involvement have only half the life expectancy of women without distant spreading of the tumor.[133] This makes an accurate determination of the extent of the tumor at the time of diagnosis of utmost importance. The type of the tumor, the degree of differentiation and the host's immune response are only of secondary importance for the final outcome of the disease. Cervical carcinoma may spread along the mucosal surface and by direct growth into adjacent structures and along tissue spaces. Distant spread occurs via the lymphatic system and less frequently via blood vessels.

Local growth of the tumor is upwards into the body of the uterus or downwards into the vagina. In a horizontal plane the tumor may grow into the wall of the bladder and the rectum as well as laterally, eventually reaching the wall of the pelvis. The extent (stage) of the disease is determined according to the FIGO staging system, based on findings from physical examination (Table 9–2).[46]

The involvement of vascular structures by the primary tumor is related to the frequency of lymph node involvement. Van Nagell and coworkers[188] reported lymph node metastases in 6% of patients without vascular involvement and in 34% in patients with invasion in lymphatics and small blood vessels. Barber and associates[11] found 5-year survival in patients with IB carcinomas without vascular involvement (90%) to be significantly better than in patients who showed vascular involvement (59.4%). In Stage IB and IIA carcinomas lymph nodes were found in 20 to 45% of patients.[133] Most frequently involved are the external iliac, obturator and hypogastric nodes, followed in order of frequency by the common iliac, parametrial and paracervical nodes.

Histology. The classification of types and subtypes of a malignant tumor should reflect a correlation between the specific morphology and the biologic behav-

TABLE 9–2. 1985 Modification of FIGO Staging of Carcinoma of the Cervix Uteri

Stage	Description
0	Preinvasive carcinoma (CIN grade III [carcinoma *in situ*]).
I	Carcinoma strictly confined to the cervix (extension to the corpus should be disregarded).
IA	Preclinical carcinomas of the cervix, i.e., those diagnosed only by microscopy.
IA1	Minimally microscopically evident stromal invasion.
IA2	Lesions detected microscopically that can be measured. The upper limit of the measurement should not show a depth of invasion of more than 5 mm taken from the base of the epithelium, either surface or glandular, from which it originates, and a second dimension, the horizontal spread, must not exceed 7 mm; larger lesions should be staged as IB.
IB	Lesions of greater dimensions than stage IA2, whether seen clinically or not. Preformed space involvement should not alter the staging but should be specifically recorded so as to determine whether it should affect treatment decisions in the future.
II	Invasive carcinoma that extends beyond the cervix but has not reached either lateral pelvic wall; involvement of the vagina is limited to the upper two thirds.
III	Invasive cervical carcinoma that extends to either lateral pelvic wall, or the lower third of the vagina or both.
IV	Invasive carcinoma that involves the urinary bladder or rectum or both, or extends beyond the true pelvis.

ior of the tumor variant, and it should enable universal recognition and classification of morphologic characteristics to ensure uniform reporting and registration. Tumors composed of poorly differentiated cells in general are more aggressive than tumors composed of well-differentiated cells.[190, 204] The most widely used grading system was proposed by Broders.[19] This grading system was based on the proportion of well-differentiated cells in the total cell population composing a tumor (Table 9–3).

Broders later recognized that in tumors of the uterine cervix there was no counterpart for the grade I epidermoid cancer of the skin and recommended using three grades with keratinization as the decisive parameter for differentiation. Broders' grading system has had a very positive influence on the reproducibility of grading of malignant tumors.

However, in squamous cell carcinomas of the cervix signs of keratinization were interpreted as a characteristic of differentiation. This may be correct in cases of carcinomas originating in keratinizing epithelium. In the uterine cervix, with its nonkeratinizing stratified squamous epithelium, keratinization should be regarded as a sign of abnormal differentiation. Keratinized cells are not sensitive to radiation. This is the

TABLE 9–3. Grading System For Malignant Tumors

Percentage of Differentiated Cells	Grade
75–100%	Grade I
50–75%	Grade II
25–50%	Grade III
0–25%	Grade IV

underlying cause for the discrepancy between histologic grade of differentiation, which suggests a relatively good prognosis for the patient, and the poor reaction of the tumor to radiotherapy, or as Patten stated, "When keratinization is used as an index of differentiation for the classification of invasive carcinoma of the uterine cervix, there is relatively little correlation between differentiation and biologic behavior and/or radiocurability."[128] Reagan and coworkers[145] and Sidhu and colleagues[175] found no correlation between histologic grade and survival.

In view of the poor correlation between differentiation grade and biologic behavior, Wentz and Reagan[205] proposed a classification of squamous cell cancers of the cervix based on histologic characteristics. Subclassification of the tumors was based on growth pattern, cellular characteristics and stromal reaction at the site of infiltration. One of the major advantages of this grading system is that it permits a morphologic correlation between cytologic and tissue specimens and it refers to the cells from which the malignant tumor was derived. Based on the reaction to radiotherapy this classification correlates better with the biologic behavior of the neoplasms. Wentz and Reagan's classification of squamous cell cancers of the cervix included large-cell nonkeratinizing cancers, keratinizing cancers and small-cell cancers. Wentz and Lewis[204] found 5-year survival in large-cell nonkeratinizing cancers to be 78.6%, in keratinizing cancers to be 47.8% and in small-cell cancer to be 20%. Survival was best in large-cell nonkeratinizing tumors and poorest in small-cell cancers. Later, in view of the wide variation in cell sizes present in large-cell nonkeratinizing squamous cell cancers, the prefix large-cell was dropped.[128] In 1973 this classification was adopted by the World Health Organization.[158]

Cytology

Cell Size and Shape. The cells originating in squamous cell carcinoma are smaller than normal squamous cells. Round and oval forms are more numerous than in dysplasia. Elongated cells are common in invasive cancer, many of them containing intracytoplasmic fibrils. The configuration of a cell depends in part on surface tension, viscosity of cytoplasm, the mechanical action exerted by adjoining cells, the rigidity of the cell membrane and the functional adaptation.

Arrangement of Cells. Cells are often arranged in syncytial masses in which cells have indistinct boundaries. This aggregation form is also a "microbiopsy" demonstrating altered cellular polarity. Cytoplasmic eosinophilia is more often observed in the cells of invasive cancer.

Nuclear Morphology. The nuclear configuration is in part related to the shape of the cell. Invasive cancer has the largest proportion of nonisodiametric nuclear forms.[145] Cytologic specimens do not always reflect underlying disease. This is particularly important in regard to invasive cancer. In improperly made smears the sampled material may be composed almost exclusively of the debris covering the invasive lesion due to necrosis of the most superficial layer and thus fail to reflect the true nature of the disease. Scattered abnor-

mal cells may remain undetected during routine screening, leading to a false-negative diagnosis. This is still not very well recognized. Specimens of unsatisfactory quality because of admixture of debris, blood and leukocytes should be carefully rescreened by a second observer and the cytologic examination should be repeated shortly.

Relative Nuclear Area. The mean nuclear area of tumor cells is more than twice the mean area of normal squamous cells. This is significantly different from the larger mean nuclear area of cells in dysplasia and carcinoma *in situ*.

Cells in dysplasia have the highest absolute nuclear size, but their relative nuclear area is relatively low. In general, the relative nuclear area is larger in more primitive cells and smaller in mature cells.

Nonkeratinizing Cancer

This tumor characteristically invades with large masses that have round, well-demarcated, blunt borders and that are separated by thick bands of stromal cells (Fig. 9–102). The surrounding stroma usually contains a moderately cellular mononuclear infiltrate. Epithelial pearl formation by definition is absent. In-

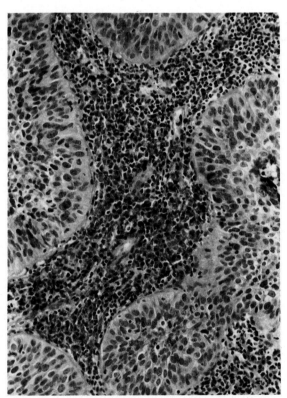

FIGURE 9–102. Nonkeratinizing squamous cell cancer. Tumor nests invade with blunt edges. The stroma contains a dense inflammatory infiltrate. Tumor cells are relatively rich in cytoplasm. Mitoses are frequently seen. No evidence of keratinization. Nuclei vary greatly in size. Nucleoli are conspicuous even with this magnification (hematoxylin and eosin; ×163).

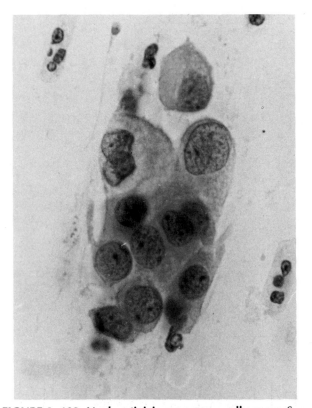

FIGURE 9–103. Nonkeratinizing squamous cell cancer. Syncytial aggregate of tumor cells with indistinct cell borders. Moderate amount of cytoplasm causing an intermediate nucleocytoplasmic (N/C) ratio. Nuclei are round to oval or irregularly shaped. Nuclear chromatin is moderately hyperchromatic, coarsely granular and irregularly distributed. Nucleoli are conspicuous (Papanicolaou stain; ×625).

dividual cell keratinization may occur. Light microscopically it may be difficult to classify these tumor as squamous in origin. In those cases the immunocytochemical demonstration of keratin 14 may be of assistance. Keratin 14 can only be demonstrated in keratinizing cells. In nonkeratinizing cancers positivity in scattered cells can often be demonstrated, even when light-microscopically individual cell keratinization is not recognizable. Usually a moderate number of mitoses can be observed. In cytologic specimens cells most often occur in syncytial aggregates with usually ill-defined cytoplasmic borders (Fig. 9–103). Owing to the often extensive necrosis of these neoplasms, cellular debris, blood cells and proteinaceous material cause a dirty background in the smear, which even in the absence of diagnostic tumor cells should raise suspicion of a malignant process being present (Fig. 9–104). The majority of cells are round to oval, sometimes polygonal. Moderate variation in size and shape is usually present. Tumor cells having phagocytosed inflammatory cells or epithelial cells are relatively frequent. The cells have a relatively large body of cyanophilic cytoplasm and have large round to oval nuclei (Fig. 9–105). Nuclei are relatively large and mostly round to oval. The nuclear chromatin is hyperchromatic, irregularly distributed and usually coarsely

granular (Fig. 9–106). Nucleoli are frequently observed. Macronucleoli are found in less-differentiated tumors and can be considered an expression of the high proliferative activity of the tumor cells.

Particularly in cases of moderately to poorly differentiated nonkeratinizing squamous cell carcinomas the cytologic differential diagnosis with a poorly differentiated adenocarcinoma may be difficult. In cases of adenocarcinomas the cells are often aggregated as clusters with overlapping nuclei. The nuclei are eccentrically located and nuclear chromatin is only slightly to moderately hyperchromatic and very irregularly distributed, leaving intranuclear clear spaces (Fig. 9–107). Often nuclear chromatin is sedimented against the nuclear membrane, which then becomes sharply outlined.

Keratinizing Cancer

The tumors are composed of irregular masses of cells that are usually sharply demarcated against the surrounding stroma (Fig. 9–108). Characteristically, infiltrating nests are irregular in shape and often elongated (Fig. 9–109). Blunt borders of infiltrating masses are less frequently seen. Cytoplasmic keratinization of

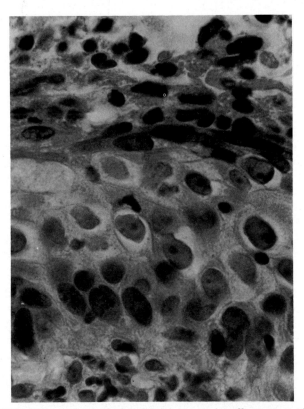

FIGURE 9–104. Nonkeratinizing squamous cell cancer with a layer of cellular debris, proteinaceous material and cells with degenerated hyperchromatic nuclei on the surface. In less adequately prepared cytologic smears often only this degenerated material is present. Compare lack of cellular detail with sharply outlined detail of underlying vital tumor cells (hematoxylin and eosin; ×275).

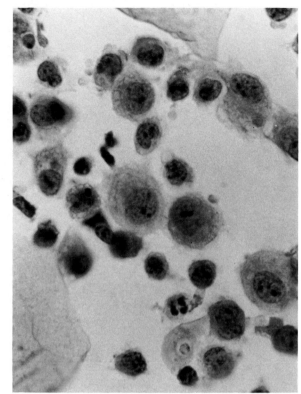

FIGURE 9–105. Nonkeratinizing squamous cell cancer. Singly lying tumor cells with a relatively large cytoplasmic body causing an intermediate nucleocytoplasmic (N/C) ratio. Coarsely granular unevenly distributed nuclear chromatin and conspicuous nucleoli that vary in size and shape (Papanicolaou stain; ×625).

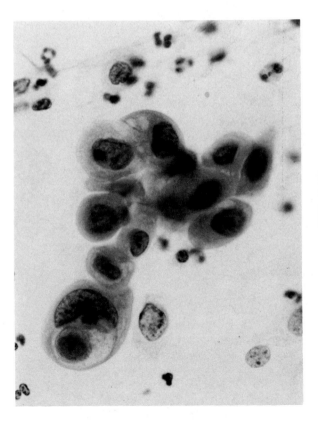

FIGURE 9–106. Nonkeratinizing squamous cell cancer. Tumor cells with variable amount of cytoplasm and irregular nuclei. Coarsely granular irregularly distributed hyperchromatic nuclear chromatin. Phagocytosis of tumor cell (Papanicolaou stain; ×500).

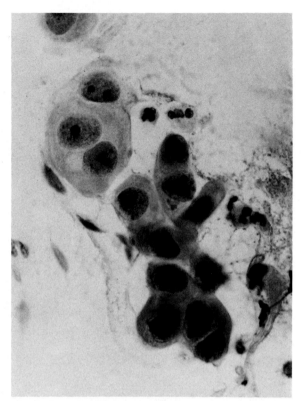

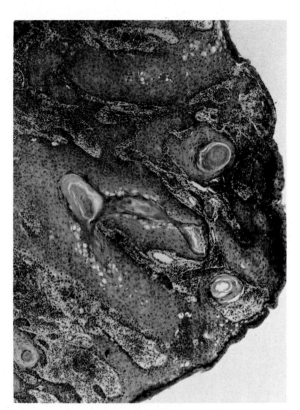

FIGURE 9–107. Cells from **adenocarcinoma** in a sheet-like arrangement. These cells have to be differentiated from cells derived from nonkeratinizing squamous cell carcinoma. Differentiation is possible on the basis of cells in cluster-like aggregates with eccentrically located nuclei. Usually cells from adenocarcinomas have a slightly to moderately hyperchromatic irregularly distributed nuclear chromatin and large very prominent nucleoli (Papanicolaou stain; × 400).

FIGURE 9–108. Keratinizing squamous cell cancer at low-power magnification showing infiltration of stroma by large masses of tumor cells. Keratin "pearl" formation is conspicuous (hematoxylin and eosin; × 36).

individual cells and formation of epithelial pearls are characteristic features. From a practical standpoint a single, well-formed epithelial pearl includes a neoplasm in the category of a keratinizing carcinoma.[128]

Superficial hyperkeratosis and atypical parakeratosis may be present. The surrounding stroma usually shows a mononuclear infiltrate of moderate density. Typically a small rim around the infiltrating nests is free of inflammatory cells. Squamous cell differentiation is conspicuous. Mitotic activity may be variable and is low in those parts of the tumor with a relatively large number of cells showing signs of cytoplasmic keratinization. Necrosis is often conspicuous.

In cytologic specimens tumor cells frequently lie singly. Elongated, caudate or bizarre cell forms are often present (Fig. 9–110). Admixture with cellular debris and blood cells in these tumors, due to their often exophytic growth, is less frequently seen than with large-cell nonkeratinizing cancers.

Cells usually have a relatively large amount of cytoplasm, which often is abundant in the large bizarre cells (Figs. 9–111 and 9–112). The cytoplasm commonly stains eosinophilic. Together with the presence of numerous large irregular cells, cytoplasmic eosinophilia is characteristic of keratinizing cancer. Nuclei

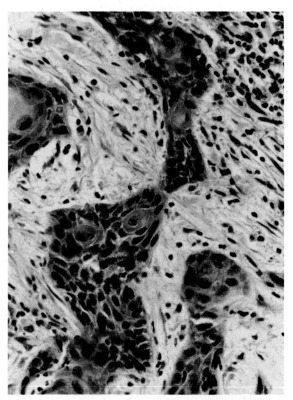

FIGURE 9–109. Keratinizing squamous cell cancer. Characteristic pattern of infiltration by tumor-elongated nests with sharp edges (hematoxylin and eosin; × 260).

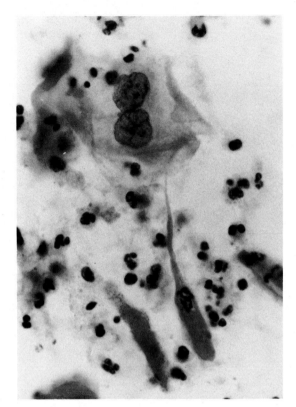

FIGURE 9–110. Keratinizing squamous cell cancer. Binucleated tumor cell. Nuclei have irregular shape and irregular distribution of coarsely granular chromatin. Elongated cell with degenerated nucleus (Papanicolaou stain; ×625).

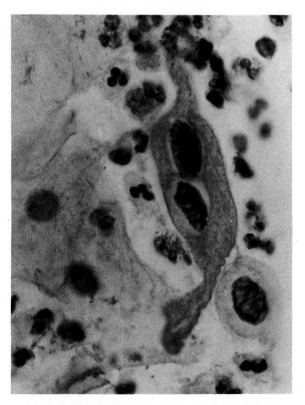

FIGURE 9–111. Keratinizing squamous cell cancer. Large binucleated cell. Cytoplasm showing fibrillary keratin structures. Nuclei are irregularly shaped and have a coarsely granular hyperchromatic chromatin (Papanicolaou stain; ×625).

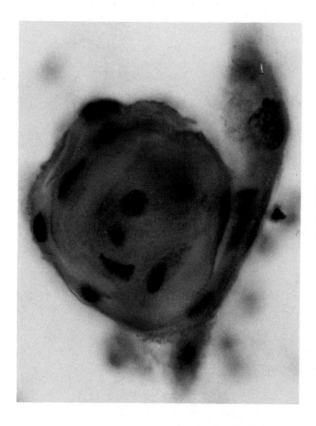

FIGURE 9–112. Keratinizing squamous cell cancer. Keratin "pearl" in cytologic specimen. Nuclei vary in size and shape. Irregularly distributed nuclear chromatin. Some nucleoli can be recognized (Papanicolaou stain; ×625).

may be round to oval but more frequently are elongated or irregular in shape. Bizarre nuclear forms may be present. Nuclear chromatin is hyperchromatic and coarsely granular. Nuclei with a very dense hyperchromatic—opaque—chromatin are especially frequent in highly keratinized cancers.

Verrucous Carcinoma

Verrucous carcinoma is an uncommon variant of keratinizing squamous cell carcinoma.[72] This unusual, locally invasive, slow-growing tumor is characterized by its warty appearance.

Histologically the tumor is composed of papillary excrescences of well-differentiated, only minimally atypical squamous cells, often with surface keratinization (Fig. 9–113). Invasive parts of the tumor lack the atypia characteristic of keratinizing squamous cell carcinoma, and it may be difficult to prove frank invasion.[44]

In view of the very high recurrence rate of verrucous carcinoma wide excision is necessary. The reaction of the tumor to radiotherapy is doubtful.[37]

Cytologically the cells from a verrucous carcinoma may not be indicative of a severe epithelial abnormality, and cytologic diagnosis of the clinically overt lesion is often negative for malignancy.

Adenosquamous Carcinoma

In adenosquamous cancer there is a malignant squamous component and a malignant adenomatous component (Fig. 9–114). The squamous component usually is of the nonkeratinizing or small-cell type. Rarely a keratinizing squamous component may be found. The cytologic features of cells from the squamous cancer component and cells from the adenocarcinomatous

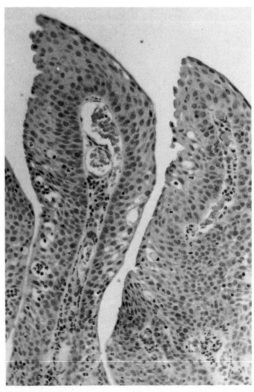

FIGURE 9–113. Verrucous carcinoma. Papillary excrescences composed of only minimally atypical squamous cells (hematoxylin and eosin; ×138).

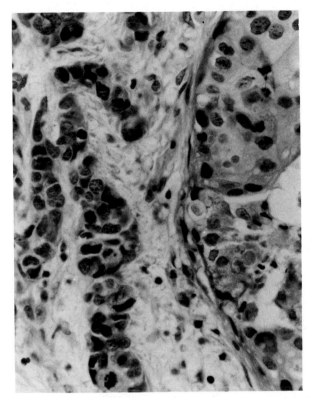

FIGURE 9–114. **Adenosquamous cancer** showing poorly differentiated adenocarcinoma and nonkeratinizing squamous cancer components (hematoxylin and eosin; ×250).

imens the tumor cells are relatively small with large nuclei and scanty cyanophilic cytoplasm, causing a high nucleocytoplasmic ratio (Fig. 9–117). Nuclei may be round to oval but more often are irregular and have a hyperchromatic, coarsely granular chromatin. Nucleoli are usually present but may be obscured by the dense chromatinic material.

Immunocytochemistry in Intraepithelial Neoplasia and Invasive Cancer

The development of chain-specific monoclonal antibodies (mAbs) to individual keratins allows the immunocytochemical distinction between reserve cells, immature and mature squamous metaplasia and normal ectocervical squamous and endocervical columnar epithelium as well as between different types of epithelial abnormalities (CIN grades I, II and III).

By using several monoclonal antibodies directed against different epitopes of the same keratin polypeptide (for instance, different mAbs against keratin 18), it is possible to detect structural alterations resulting from biologic activity or neoplastic transformation. The degree of differentiation in a squamous cell cancer can be determined by the use of keratin 10 or 13 antibodies. Keratin 10 is a marker of keratinization. It may be

component are similar to those described for these respective cancer types (Fig. 9–115). In the cytologic specimen both cell types can be found within the same cell cluster. This in contrast to the rare situation in the cervix of both a squamous cell carcinoma and a separate adenocarcinoma occuring.

Small-Cell Cancer

Small-cell cancer used to be categorized as a subtype of squamous cell cancer. More recently, however, on the basis of immunocytochemical and electron-microscopic evidence these tumors are considered to be of neuroendocrine derivation. They should therefore be grouped together with the carcinoid tumors. In view of the differential diagnostic problems these tumors may present in cytologic specimens, they are discussed here in more detail. In comparison with keratinizing and nonkeratinizing squamous cell cancer, small-cell cancer usually has a more proximal localization in the cervical canal.

Small-cell cancer grows rather diffusely in large masses separated by thin strands of stromal cells (Fig. 9–116). Boundaries with the surrounding stroma are often ill defined. Cells show a relatively high variation in size. There is no evidence of individual cell keratinization or epithelial pearl formation. Mitoses usually are numerous. In some tumors, cells show a positive reaction to neuroendocrine markers. In cytologic spec-

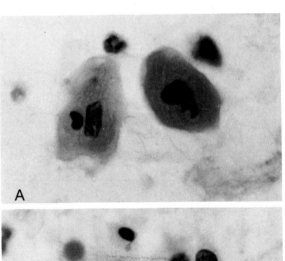

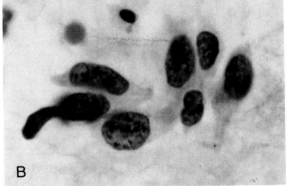

FIGURE 9–115. **Adenosquamous cancer.** Cells with characteristics of squamous cell cancer (A) occurring together with cells consistent with poorly differentiated adenocarcinoma (B) (Papanicolaou stain; ×625).

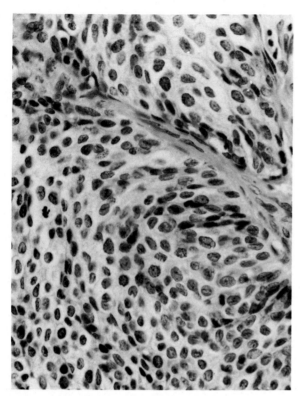

FIGURE 9–116. Small cell cancer. Large masses of tumor cells with minimal cytoplasm separated by small strands of stromal cells (hematoxylin and eosin; ×250).

of the lesion morphologically described as CIN grade III. CIN grade II lesions in invaginations of the endocervical canal had an identical pattern to lesions on the surface of the canal. The staining pattern in CIN grade III was comparable with that found in invasive squamous cell carcinoma. Puts and associates[139] used anti-cytokeratin antibodies to keratins and found no qualitative differences in staining reactions between epithelial lesions of varying degrees of severity. They did find a variable number of Langerhans cells in 32 dysplastic lesions but no specific pattern in distribution between lesions of different severity.[138] They speculated that differences in the number of Langerhans cells might be correlated to differences in the dysplastic processes, as well as to differences in host response and thus could potentially be an indicator of a tendency to regression or progression.

Smedts and coworkers[177] investigated the expression of keratins in normal cervical epithelia, metaplastic epithelium and cervical intraepithelial neoplasia grades I, II and III with a panel of chain-specific mAbs. This allowed the detection of individual keratins 4, 5, 7, 8, 10, 13, 14, 18 and 19 at the single-cell level. The results showed that, during the transformation of reserve cells into immature squamous metaplasia, this epithelium acquired keratins typical of the ectocervical squamous epithelium, whereas keratins typical of reserve cells expressed in cells of the more superficial layers of squamous epithelium, even when light microscopically no signs of keratinization are detectable.

Broadly cross-reacting mAbs give positive reactions in virtually all epithelial tissues and primary and metastatic epithelial cancers, including squamous cell carcinomas of different differentiation grades and small-cell anaplastic carcinomas. Antibodies to keratins 7 and 18 have proved useful to distinguish between different subgroups of carcinomas. The antibodies to keratin 18 can among others recognize adenocarcinomas but do not normally react with squamous cell carcinomas.[140] Keratin 7 mAbs in general gave no staining reaction with (keratinizing) squamous epithelia. This antibody reacts with columnar cells in the cervix.[142]

Moll and coworkers[109] showed the presence of cytokeratins 5, 7, 8, 17, 18 and 19 in immature squamous metaplasia and a changed pattern of keratin expression in mature squamous epithelium and mild dysplasia (Fig. 9–118). In invasive carcinoma they found a similar pattern as in mature squamous epithelium.

Whittaker and colleagues[206] in abnormal cervical epithelium found cytokeratins 10, 11, 13 and 16 to be irregularly distributed in CIN grade III. There was a patchy pattern distribution of positivity. Areas of positivity alternated with negative areas. They could not demonstrate a consistent and progressive change in cytokeratin content from normal epithelium through CIN grades I and II. Their observations suggest that an abrupt change occurred at the time of development

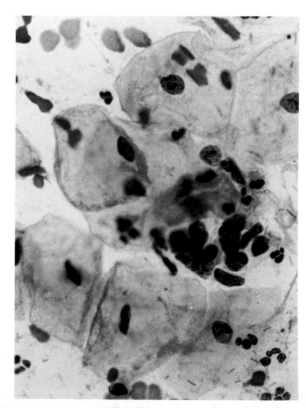

FIGURE 9–117. Small cell cancer. Small tumor cells with scanty cytoplasm and large irregularly shaped nuclei. Compare with superficial and intermediate squamous cells. Nuclei show large variation in size and shape. Nuclear chromatin is coarsely granular and hyperchromatic (Papanicolaou stain; ×400).

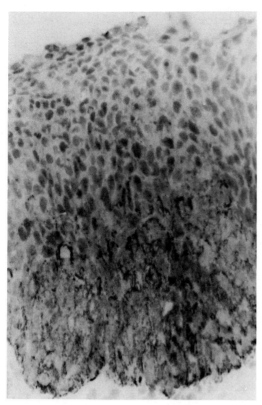

FIGURE 9–118. Severe dysplasia of metaplastic type. Positive-staining reaction for keratin 8 in basal and parabasal cell layers indicating an increase in cytoplasmic characteristics of simple epithelium in this abnormal originally squamous metaplastic epithelium (immunoperoxidase method; ×250).

keratins 13 and 14 decreased, in some areas becoming completely absent. This emphasized the increased expression of a keratin pattern characteristic of simple epithelium with increasing dysplastic change.

Keratins 8, 18 and 19 have been found in cervical squamous cell carcinomas as well as in adenocarcinoma. The expression of these keratins in reserve cells might indicate that these cells are the common progenitor cells with a dual differentiation potential on the one hand through a phase of metaplasia into squamous epithelial abnormalities and on the other hand through differentiation into a columnar cell–type abnormality. The dual expression of squamous cell–type and columnar cell–type keratins in immature squamous metaplasia seems to support this hypothesis.

EFFICACY OF CERVICAL CYTOLOGY IN THE DETECTION OF SQUAMOUS LESIONS

Mortality from cervical cancer has dropped significantly during the last decades, which can be attributed to the widespread use of preventive cervical cytologic screening. The reader is referred to Chapter 3 on Cytologic Screening Programs for additional information.

and columnar cells were lost. This change continued during further differentiation into mature squamous metaplasia. Premalignant transformation resulted in a partial loss of the keratins typical of squamous epithelium and acquisition of keratins typical of simple epithelia.

In the course of increasing epithelial atypia through grades I to III of intraepithelial neoplasia, keratins characteristic of simple epithelia appear in dysplastic lesions (Fig. 9–119). In CIN grade I approximately half and in CIN grade II (moderate dysplasia) a third of cases show some dispersed positivity for keratins 8 and 18, whereas keratin 19, which in mature squamous epithelium stains basal layers, now shows loss of polarity and stains an increasing part of the entire thickness of the dysplastic epithelium, often in an irregular fashion.

Compared with mature squamous epithelium the expression of keratins 4, 5, 13 and 14 decreased and the staining pattern became variable (Figs. 9–120 and 9–121). This indicated that dysplastic epithelium related to the progression of the severity of the abnormality progressively lost its squamous keratin phenotype and acquired keratin characteristics of simple epithelium.

These changes were even more evident in cases of CIN grade III, in which in all cases the expression of keratins 8 and 18 was abundant and expression of

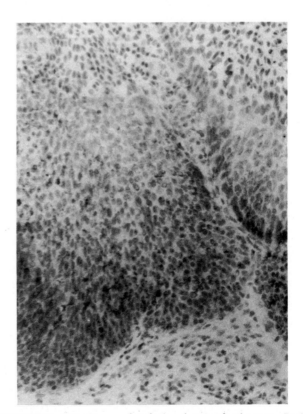

FIGURE 9–119. Severe dysplasia of metaplastic type. Positive-staining reaction for keratin 18 in basal and parabasal cell layers indicating an increase in cytoplasmic characteristics of simple (glandular) epithelium in this abnormal originally squamous metaplastic epithelium (immunoperoxidase method; ×100).

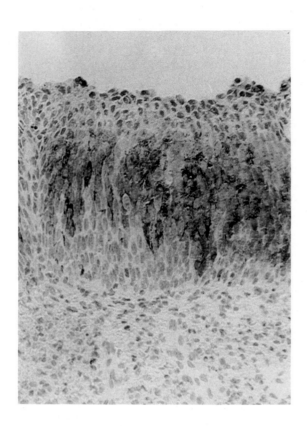

FIGURE 9–120. Severe dysplasia. Positive-staining reaction for keratin 4 in intermediate cell layers. No staining reaction in basal, parabasal and superficial cell layers (immunoperoxidase method; ×100).

FIGURE 9–121. Severe dysplasia. Scattered areas of positive staining for keratin 14 in basal and parabasal cell layers. No positivity in intermediate and superficial cell layers (immunoperoxidase method; ×250).

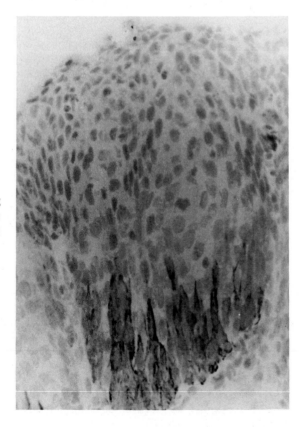

For the detection of cervical cancer, cytologic testing is most appropriate. Squamous cell carcinoma is highly vulnerable to detection technology and therefore secondary prevention. High-risk groups have been defined and cancer precursors, i.e., dysplasia of the cervix and carcinoma *in situ*, have been described.[60] Criteria that are essential in the suitability of cervical cancer for routine screening are an easy to perform, reliable test, acceptability to patients, a prolonged preclinical phase and the availability of effective therapy that is more efficient and less of a burden to patients than treatment for clinical cancer.

The purpose of screening cytologic samples is to identify amidst a multitude of normal cells those cells that are consistent with a premalignant or malignant change. The samples may also disclose functional characteristics of the cells or important findings such as infections and infestations.

The detection system of a cytologic cervical smear examination leading to the discovery and treatment of precancerous lesions and early cancer of the cervix has been shown to be effective in reducing the rate of morbidity and mortality from high-stage invasive cervical cancer in appropriately screened populations.[185] There is ample evidence that the cervical smear has contributed in a remarkable fashion to the prevention of invasive carcinomas of the uterine cervix.[86]

After the implementation of well-organized screening programs remarkable drops in the incidence and mortality rates have been documented.[55, 63, 64, 107, 186, 187] However, there is no evidence that the Papanicolaou test has succeeded anywhere in the complete eradication of this theoretically preventable disease, which emphasizes the importance of identifying the potential failures of this detection system and of analyzing the reasons for them.[86] Cytologic case finding may fail because of inadequate sampling, insufficient training, insufficient time devoted to screening (excessive work load), inadequate clinical information, inadequate supervision of laboratory procedures, relatively high intra- and interobserver variability of cytologic diagnoses and inadequate follow-up procedures.

The cervical smear is a safe, easy and inexpensive method for the screening of large numbers of sexually active women. When a cervical cytologic report states the presence of an epithelial abnormality it has a high rate of accuracy. "The cytologic screening of cervical specimens is a complex matter and, regardless of its problems, has contributed in a tangible and statistically significant way to the reduction of morbidity and mortality from carcinoma of the uterine cervix."[85] It can be stated without any restriction that the cervical smear test is perhaps the only effective screening test known today. Nevertheless systematic screening has nowhere been able to eradicate the disease completely. This failure of the screening system is due to multiple causes.[86] The complex cancer detection system is prone to errors at all levels, such as the initial clinical examination, the taking of the smear and screening and interpretation of the abnormalities in the cytologic specimen. Finally the report from the pathologist may be misinterpreted by the clinician who requested the test to be made.[86] To reduce the problem of false-negative diagnoses quality control of the taking of the cytologic sample and the cytologic diagnostic procedure is important. To reduce the consequences of false-negative results it may be advisable to make a repeat smear 1 year after the initial smear. After two negative smears a longer interval of 3 years or even 5 years seems justified.[64, 187] The number of preclinical asymptomatic invasive cancers and of preinvasive cancers diagnosed depends largely on the prevalence of these abnormalities in the population under study, the sensitivity and specificity of the cytologic test and the efficacy of follow-up procedures.

Sensitivity, Specificity and Predictive Value. The reader is referred to Chapter 3 on Cytologic Screening Programs for definitions of sensitivity, specificity and predictive value.

A detection program for cervical cancer should not only be directed towards the detection of invasive cancer but should also include the detection of severe epithelial abnormalities that can be considered potential precursors of invasive cancer. Sensitivity figures should therefore not only encompass invasive cancer, as in most reports on the accuracy of screening, but should also be calculated for a spectrum of severe epithelial abnormalities considered as potential precursors. In most studies only the screening history of women with invasive cancer is reviewed.

To determine with maximum possible accuracy the sensitivity of the cytologic diagnosis, however, the total number of women from the same population and in the same time period who were cytologically tested and found to have severe epithelial abnormalities (severe intraepithelial neoplasia and invasive cancer), or "true positives," should be known as well. Since it is clearly impossible to histologically examine each cervix from women who have been screened, sensitivity has to be calculated in an indirect way. All women with negative smears have to be followed for a sufficiently long time. The longer the follow-up, the more cases will be detected that were in an undetectable, asymptomatic, preclinical phase at the time of the test and that otherwise cannot be distinguished from the truly missed cases that become evident during the follow-up period.

Day[36] suggested avoiding the most common inaccuracies in calculating sensitivity by using only incidence rates. Inaccuracies result from the inclusion of cases that become apparent during follow-up but that were still in an undetectable preclinical stage at the time of the negative cervical screening test; cases can be missed at the time of screening and not become evident during the time of follow-up, and in some of the women the lesion may have regressed during follow-up. For cervical cancer Day's method unfortunately is of limited value, since incidence rates in the absence of screening must also be known. The latter situation is, however, fortunately becoming increasingly rare. Cervical cytodiagnosis has been the subject of many investigations evaluating the quality of this method as a diagnostic test.[70] In the literature cytologic false-negative rates in cervical cytology vary widely. A number of studies have shown rates varying from 15 to 55% in the presence of invasive cervical cancer[14, 32] and from 6 to 45% in the presence of squamous cell carcinoma *in situ*.[32, 33, 157, 169]

Cecchini and coworkers[27] calculated the protective interval for CIN grade III to be 3 years. No differences in the risk for developing CIN grade III were observed between women with only one initial screening and women rescreened within the 3-year interval. The sensitivity of screening was calculated with and without colposcopy. When screening sensitivity was assumed to be a constant, the sensitivity of the cytology-colposcopy combination was 0.71, with 0.64 for cytology alone. When sensitivity was assumed to decrease in subsequent screening rounds, the complex sensitivity was calculated to be 0.60, with 0.50 in subsequent rounds and 0.52 for cytology alone. We calculated sensitivity of screening for the detection of severe dysplasia, carcinoma *in situ* and invasive cancer both separately and as a group.[184] For those women with a tissue diagnosis of severe dysplasia, carcinoma *in situ* and invasive cancer who had participated in the screening program the cytologic diagnosis of the smear, taken up to 48 months before the tissue diagnosis was made, was recorded. When severe dysplasia, carcinoma *in situ* and invasive cancer were considered together in the evaluation of false-negative diagnoses after 24 and 36 months, sensitivity figures were 94% and 89% respectively. When only carcinoma *in situ* and invasive cancers were considered sensitivity figures after 24, 36 and 48 months were 95%, 92% and 89% respectively. Sensitivity was relatively high, being 99%, 98% and 97% respectively, when only invasive cancers were considered to be falsely negative in the analysis of diagnoses after 24, 36 and 48 months. If an epithelial abnormality is diagnosed in a woman who previously had a negative test result there are two possibilities: (a) The epithelial abnormality did not exist when the former negative smear was taken, or (b) the epithelial abnormality did exist but was not recognized (screening or interpretation error), or was not present in the cell sample (sampling error). To calculate the sensitivity of cervical cytology, information has to be obtained on the number of false-positive results and false-negative diagnoses. Almost all of these studies evaluated sensitivity and specificity, e.g., the validity of the test.[54, 185, 199] Much less research has been done on the reproducibility of the light microscopic diagnosis.[81]

Observer Variability. Observer variability is the variation in scoring by observers. It can be divided into intraobserver variability, interobserver variability and the variability due to inaccuracy of the assessment system, such as changes within the microscope or fading of staining.

Intraobserver variability is defined as the difference in scoring by the same observer when evaluating the same specimen on two separate occasions, correcting for the inaccuracy of the system. Interobserver variability is defined as the difference in scoring between observers.[82] The observer variability in cervical cytology has only rarely been evaluated.[41, 79, 81, 82, 184, 193] Intraobserver variability proved to be an important factor in incorrect diagnoses. Intraobserver variability was found to be rather inconsistent. Overdiagnoses as well as underdiagnoses were made by all observers without evidence of a consistent pattern when reviewing previously screened cases. Inconsistency was not significantly reduced with longer experience in cytodiagnostics.[81, 82] It was found that 9.1% of smears with false-negative and 52.9% of smears with false-positive diagnoses were correctly diagnosed at a second rescreening by the same observer. Intraobserver variability was less than 17% when the same observer screened the same smear twice. However, average intraobserver variability differed considerably for individual observers. The intraobserver variability seemed only slightly influenced by the years of experience in cytopathology. Interobserver variability also showed considerable differences between observers. There was a strong influence of the years of full-time experience in cytopathology of the observer on the grading of squamous and squamous metaplastic abnormalities. Evans and coworkers,[41] in one of the few studies on observer variability, suggested that cytodiagnosis in itself was not an appropriate field for quality control because it is essentially an expression of opinion. From our studies we have deduced that intraobserver variability is the main cause of false diagnoses.[81, 82] When wrongly diagnosed, severe epithelial abnormalities are more often underestimated than completely overlooked. Apart from training in cytopathology, the establishment of laboratory protocols for multiple screening of even minor abnormalities and the institution of a well-supervised protocol for repeat examinations after cytologic diagnoses of epithelial abnormalities of mild and moderate severity seem to be the most effective means of reducing the number of severe epithelial abnormalities that remain undetected at cervical cytologic screening.

Quality Control. The cytologic report should encompass the following items:

- A statement about the adequacy of the specimen, including an explanation of the problems encountered for less than fully satisfactory specimens and a determination of whether a repeat specimen is necessary.
- A descriptive diagnosis, comprising the presence and character of any inflammatory changes, the expected histopathologic change in the squamous or squamous metaplastic cervical mucosa and changes in columnar cells from the endocervical mucosa or an abnormality related to the endometrium. A recommendation for further action to be taken on the basis of the cytologic diagnosis should be given, when indicated.[40, 116, 193, 194, 198, 199, 208]

Quality control by the laboratory seems the best way to reduce sampling and screening errors.[193] Gay and associates[54] found that for all types of malignancy the majority of errors were due to poor sampling. They found an overall false-negative rate of 20% for invasive processes. They further stated that if all the errors made by laboratory personnel could be eliminated, in their material the false-negative rate in the presence of malignancy could have been reduced from 20% to 12%, the latter value simply due to inadequate cell samples. Reporting inadequate smears is an important step in ensuring the quality of laboratory performance. An adequate cytologic sample is a smear that discloses abnormalities of epithelial cells from the uterine sample and thus triggers further action.[85] Such a sample includes a sufficient number of cells representative of the area sampled, fixed and stained in a manner that allows interpretation.[78]

In an adequate cervical smear endocervical columnar cells, squamous metaplastic cells and squamous cells should be present. The cytopathologist should evaluate whether a specimen submitted is of sufficient quality to enable an adequate diagnosis. This evaluation encompasses the cellular composition of the sample, the quality of the cellular material and technical aspects of the smear, such as staining, cellularity, admixture of blood and inflammatory cells and adequacy of the specimen in relation to the clinical information. If the specimen is less than optimal, the consulting cytopathologist has an obligation to inform the referring physician of such a conclusion and the reasons for it. A significantly lower number of epithelial abnormalities were diagnosed in smears without endocervical cells present than in smears that did show endocervical cells.[40, 199]

In a cohort study we showed that the absence of endocervical cells could not be ascribed to a physiologic phenomenon but was the result of inadequate sampling of the uterine cervix.[199] It is generally assumed that obtaining a cervical smear is an easily executed, clinically simple procedure. This is not true. In our experience well-trained paramedical sample takers perform far better than most physicians who are relatively untrained.[198] Taking duplicate smears could possibly reduce the error, but this is a very costly procedure when routinely practiced in large-scale screening programs.[170]

Many variables influence the detection rate of abnormalities in cervical smears, including the sampling technique used, the preparation of the patient, the fixation and staining of the smears, the accuracy of the screening, the daily work load and the interpretation of morphologic changes. All smears should be screened according to a strict laboratory protocol. We have adopted the procedure that smears with diagnoses of even minor abnormalities made by a cytotechnologist with short-term experience are always checked by a cytotechnologist with long-term experience. Also a protocol for multiple screening by more than one observer of specimens at high risk for a false diagnosis should be instituted. Included in this high-risk category are smears from women in postmenopause, with clinical symptoms of irregular bleeding and with a previous history of cancer.

Smears of unsatisfactory quality for cytologic diagnosis should also be screened by more than one observer, since in cases of severe epithelial lesions the proportion of unsatisfactory smears is significantly higher.

As a procedure for quality control it is often advocated that 10% of smears initially diagnosed as negative should be rescreened. Considering that at most 10% of smears show an abnormality, rescreening normal specimens is a very unrewarding and time-consuming procedure. It may take several years before an unreliable observer is detected.[70, 81, 82, 86, 212] Much more effective in reducing the number of screening errors are quality-promoting procedures such as good supervision of daily work load to avoid too large a volume to be screened per working day, a screening protocol for multiple screening of selected specimens, which because of anamnestic, clinical or cytomorphologic reasons are thought to be at high risk for a false diagnosis and good supervision and training of both cytotechnologists and cytopathologists.[193, 208]

The cytologic report should contain properly worded recommendations for further patient evaluation.[116, 194] To be able to provide proper recommendations all clinical information is essential to the cytopathologist. The clinician should take the advice of the cytopathologist as a strong recommendation but should institute a different treatment strategy when intercurrent clinical information or special circumstances warrant this.

Review. A good procedure for quality control is the review of previous cytologic and histologic material. The degree of abnormality may differ between the cytologic sample and the subsequently taken biopsy. Nevertheless it is usually very possible to determine the causes for discrepancies. Since cytologic diagnosis is highly dependent on the ability of the observer to refer the cellular and nuclear changes to a complex histologic architecture of the lesion, cytologic and histologic characteristics are very instructive. According to Koss and Hicklin[88] one of the best methods of quality control is the comparison of cytologic findings with histologic findings and *vice versa* and by long-term follow-up of patients.

Inadequate sampling of the cervix can account for about half of the false-negative cytologic diagnoses. Taking smears should be avoided during the first 4 days of the menstrual cycle. In women using oral contraceptives the number of inadequate or less reliable smears is significantly increased. In all instances the best collection time is from day 5 through day 14 of the menstrual cycle.[198, 201, 202] The best smears submitted to our laboratory were taken with a relatively recently developed ectocervical brush. The percentage of smears containing endocervical columnar cells was higher and the number of unsatisfactory smears was significantly lower when compared with spatula-made smears[192, 196] and with combined spatula and endocervical brush smears.[195]

REFERENCES

1. Anderson MC: The pathology of cervical cancer. Clin Obstet Gynecol 12:87–119, 1985.

2. Anderson MC, Burghardt E, Coppleson JWM, Kolstadt P, Richart RM, Wade-Evans T: *In* Pre-clinical Neoplasia of the Cervix. Edited by JA Jordan, F Sharp, A Singer. London, Royal College of Obstetricians and Gynaecologists, 1982.

3. Armstrong B, Holman D: Increasing mortality from cancer of the cervix in young Australian women. Med J Aust 1:460–462, 1981.

4. Atkin NB: Prognostic value of cytogenetic studies of tumors of the female genital tract. *In* Advances in Clinical Cytology vol 2. Edited by LG Koss, DC Coleman. New York, Masson, pp 103–121, 1984.

5. Atkin NB, Kay R: Prognostic significance of modal DNA value and other factors in malignant tumours, based on 1465 cases. Br J Cancer 40:210–221, 1979.

6. Auerbach SH, Pund ER: Squamous metaplasia of the cervix uteri. Am J Obstet Gynecol 49:207–213, 1945.

7. Ayre JE: A simple office test for uterine cancer diagnosis. Can Med Assoc J 51:17–22, 1944.

8. Ayre JE: Selective cytology smear for diagnosis of cancer. Am J Obstet Gynecol 53:609–617, 1947.

9. Ayre JE: Cervical cytology in diagnosis of early cancer. JAMA 136:513–517, 1948.

10. Bamford PN, Beilby JOW, Steele SJ, Vlies R: The natural history of cervical intraepithelial neoplasia as determined by cytology and colposcopic biopsy. Acta Cytol 27:482–484, 1983.

11. Barber HRK, Sommers SC, Rotterdam H, Kwa T: Vascular invasion as a prognostic factor in stage Ib cancer of the cervix. Obstet Gynecol 52:343–348, 1978.

12. Beral V: Cancer of the cervix: A sexually transmitted infection? Lancet i:1037–1040, 1974.

13. Berkhout FJ, Vooijs GP, van't Hof-Grootenboer B, Kaiser M, van der Graaf Y: Prevalence of invasive cervical cancer and *in situ* carcinoma in the city of Nijmegen, the Netherlands. Results of twelve years of screening. Submitted.

14. Berkowitz RS, Ehrmann RL, Lavizzo-Mourey R, Knapp RC: Invasive cervical carcinoma in young women. Gynecol Oncol 8:311–316, 1979.

15. Bibbo M, Keebler CM, Wied GL: The cytologic diagnosis of tissue repair in the female genital tract. Acta Cytol 15:133–37, 1971.

16. Bosch FX, Munoz N: Human papillomavirus and cervical neoplasia: A critical review of the epidemiological evidence. *In* Human Papillomavirus and Cervical Cancer. Edited by N Munoz, FX Bosch, OM Jensen. Lyon, France, IARC Scientific Publications No. 94, pp 135–151, 1989.

17. Brinton LA, Fraumeni JF Jr: Epidemiology of uterine cervical cancer. J Chronic Dis 39:1051–105, 1986.

18. Brinton LA, Hamman RF, Huggins GR, Lehman HF, Levine RS, Mallin K, Fraumeni JF: Sexual and reproductive risk factors for invasive squamous cell cervical cancer. J Natl Cancer Inst 79:23–30, 1987.

19. Broders AC: Carcinoma: Grading and practical application. Arch Pathol Lab Med 2:376–381, 1926.

20. Broders AC: Carcinoma *in situ* contrasting with benign penetrating epithelium. JAMA 99:1670–1674, 1932.

21. Buckley CH, Butler EB, Fox H: Cervical intraepithelial neoplasia. J Clin Pathol 35:1–13, 1982.

22. Burghardt E: Early Histological Diagnosis of Cervical Cancer. Philadelphia, WB Saunders, pp 319–362, 1973.

23. Burghardt E: Premalignant conditions of the cervix. Clin Obstet Gynecol 3:257–295, 1976.

24. Burghardt E: Diagnostic and prognostic criteria in cervical microcarcinoma. Clin Oncol 1:323–333, 1982.

25. Burghardt E, Holzer E: Diagnosis and treatment of microinvasive carcinoma of the uterine cervix. Obstet Gynecol 49:641, 1977.

26. Carmichael R, Jeaffreson BL: Squamous metaplasia of the columnar epithelium in the human cervix. J Pathol 52:173–186, 1941.

27. Cecchini S, Palli D, Casini A: Cervical intraepithelial neoplasia. III. An estimate of screening error rates and optimal screening interval. Acta Cytol 29:329–333, 1985.

28. Christopherson WM: Concepts of genesis and development in early cervical neoplasia. Obstet Gynecol Surv 24:842–850, 1969.

29. Christopherson WM, Parker JE: Carcinoma *in situ*. *In* Dysplasia, Carcinoma *in Situ* and Micro-invasive Carcinoma of the Cervix Uteri. Edited by LA Gray. Springfield, Illinois, Charles C Thomas, 1964.

30. Coleman DV, Evans DMD: Biopsy Pathology and Cytology of the Cervix. London, Chapman and Hall, pp 240–259, 1988.

31. Cook GA, Draper GJ: Trends in cervical cancer and carcinoma *in situ* in Great Britain. Brit J Cancer, 50:367–375, 1984.

32. Coppleson LW, Brown B: Estimation of the screening error rate from the observed detection rates in repeated cervical cytology. Am J Obstet Gynecol 119:953–958, 1974.

33. Creasman WT, Rutledge F: Carcinoma *in situ* of the cervix. An analysis of 861 patients. Obstet Gynecol 39:373–380, 1972.

34. Crum CP, Egawa K, Fu YS, Lancaster WD, Barron B, Levine RU, Fenoglio CM, Richart RM: Atypical immature metaplasia (AIM): A subset of human papilloma virus infection of the cervix. Cancer, 51:2214–2219, 1983.

35. Czernobilsky B, Moll R, Franke WW: Intermediate filaments of normal and neoplastic tissues of the female genital tract with emphasis on problems of differential tumor diagnosis. Pathol Res Pract 179:31–37, 1984.

36. Day NE: Estimating the sensitivity of a screening test. J Epidemiol Community Health 39:364–366, 1985.

37. Demian SDE, Bushkin FL, Echevarria RA: Perineural invasion and anaplastic transformation of verrucous carcinoma. Cancer, 32:395–401, 1973.

38. DiSaia PJ: Conservative management of the patient with early gynecologic cancer. CA 39:135–154, 1989.

39. Eichholz K: *In* Basal Cells in the Epithelium of the Human Cervical Canal. Edited by R Carmichael, BL Jeaffreson. J Pathol Bacteriol 49:63–68, 1939.

40. Elias A, Linthorst G, Bekker B, Vooijs GP: The significance of endocervical cells in the diagnosis of cervical epithelial changes. Acta Cytol 27:225–229, 1983.

41. Evans DMD, Shelley G, Cleary B, Baldwin Y: Observer variation and quality control of cytodiagnosis. J Clin Pathol 27:945–950, 1974.

42. Evans DMD, Hudson EA, Brown CL, Boddington MM, Hughes HC, Mackenzie EFD, Marshall T: Terminology in gynaecological cytopathology: Report of the working party of the British Society for Clinical Cytology. J Clin Pathol 39:933–944, 1986.

43. Fawdry RD: Carcinoma *in situ* of the cervix: Is posthysterectomy cytology worthwhile? Br J Obstet Gynecol 91:67–72, 1984.

44. Ferenczy A: Carcinoma and other malignant tumors of the cervix. *In* Pathology of the Female Genital Tract, 2nd ed. Edited by A Blaustein. New York, Heidelberg, Berlin, Springer Verlag, 1982.

45. Fidler HK, Boyes DA, Worth AJ: Cervical cancer detection in British Columbia. Br J Obstet Gynecol 75:392–404, 1968.

46. International Federation of Gynecology and Obstetrics: Changes in definitions for clinical staging for carcinoma of the cervix and ovary. Am J Obstet Gynecol 156:263–264, 1987.

47. Fluhmann CF: Comprehensive Review of "Squamous Metaplasia." The Cervix Uteri and Its Diseases. Philadelphia, WB Saunders, 1961.

48. Foote JW Jr, Li KYY: Smear diagnosis of *in situ* carcinoma of the cervix. Am J Obstet Gynecol 56:335–339, 1948.

49. Fox CH: Biologic behaviour of dysplasia and carcinoma *in situ*. Am J Obstet Gynecol 99:960–972, 1967.

50. Friedell GH: Terminology for epithelial abnormalities of the uterine cervix. Am J Clin Pathol 44:280–282, 1965.

51. Frisch LE: Inflammatory atypia: An apparent link with subsequent cervical intraepithelial neoplasia explained by cytologic underreading. Acta Cytol 31:869–872, 1987.

52. Frisch LE: Inflammatory atypia and the false-negative smear in cervical intraepithelial neoplasia. Acta Cytol 31:873–877, 1987.

53. Fu YS, Reagan JW, Richart RM: Definition of precursors. Gynecol Oncol 12:220–231, 1981.

54. Gay JD, Donaldson LD, Goellner JP: False-negative results in cervical cytologic studies. Acta Cytol 29:1043–1046, 1985.

55. Geirsson G: Organization of screening in technically advanced countries: Ireland. *In* Screening for Cancer of the Uterine

Cervix. Edited by M Hakama, AB Miller, NE Day. Lyon, France, International Agency for Research on Cancer, pp 239–250, 1986.

56. Geirsson G, Woodworth FE, Patten SF, Bonfiglio TA: Epithelial repair and regeneration in the uterine cervix. I. An analysis of the cells. Acta Cytol 21:371–378, 1977.

57. Green GH: Rising cervical cancer mortality in young New Zealand women. NZ Med J 89:89–91, 1979.

58. Green GH, Donovan JW: The natural history of cervical carcinoma in situ. Br J Obstet Gynecol 77:1–9, 1970.

59. Gupta PF, Burroughs F, Luff RD, Frost JK, Erozan YS: Epithelial atypias associated with intrauterine contraceptive devices (IUD). Acta Cytol 22:286–291, 1978.

60. Gusberg SB: Detection and prevention of uterine cancer. Cancer 62:1784–1786, 1988.

61. Hanselaar AGJM, Vooijs GP, Oud PS, Pahlplatz MMM, Beck JLM: DNA ploidy patterns in cervical epithelial neoplasia grade III, with and without synchronous invasive squamous cell carcinoma: Measurements in nuclei isolated from paraffin embedded tissue. Cancer 62:2537–2545, 1988.

62. Hajdu SI: American Cancer Society report on the cancer related health checkup. Acta Cytol 24:369–370, 1980.

63. Hakama M: Trends in the incidence of cervical cancer in the Nordic countries. In Trends in Cancer Incidence, Causes and Practical Implications. Edited by K Magnus. Washington, DC, Hemisphere Publishing Corp, pp 279–292, 1988.

64. Hakama M, Chamberlain J, Day NE, Miller AB, Prorok PC: Evaluation of screening programmes for gynecological cancer. Br J Cancer 52:669–673, 1985.

65. Hall JE, Walton L: Dysplasia of the cervix. Am J Obstet Gynecol 100:662–671, 1968.

66. Halpert R, Fruchter RG, Sedlis A, Butt K, Boyce JG, Sillman FH: Human papillomavirus and lower genital neoplasia in renal transplant patients. Obstet Gynecol 68:251–258, 1986.

67. Hanekar AB, Leiman G, Markowitz S: Cytologically detected chlamydial changes and progression of cervical intraepithelial neoplasias. A retrospective case-control study. Acta Cytol 29:661–664, 1985.

68. Howard L Jr, Erickson CC, Stoddard LD: A study of the incidence and histogenesis of endocervical metaplasia and intraepithelial carcinoma: Observations on 400 uteri removed for noncervical disease. Cancer 4:1210–1233, 1951.

69. Howley PM: On human papillomaviruses. N Engl J Med 315:1089–1090, 1986.

70. Husain OAN: Diagnostic errors in cytology in "preclinical" neoplasia of the cervix. In Proceedings of the Ninth Study Group of the Royal College of Obstetricians and Gynecologists, London, pp 111–132, 1982.

71. International Academy of Cytology: Policy statement on the frequency of gynecologic screening. Acta Cytol 24:371–372, 1980.

72. Isaacs JH: Verrucous carcinoma of the female genital tract. Gynecol Oncol 4:259–269, 1976.

73. Jakobsen A, Baek Kristensen P, Kvist Poulsen H: Flow cytometric classification of biopsy specimens from cervical intraepithelial neoplasia. Cytometry 4:166–169, 1983.

74. Jones HW, Plymate S, Gluck FB, Miles PA, Greene JF: Small cell nonkeratinizing carcinoma of the cervix associated with ACTH production. Cancer 38:526–533, 1976.

75. Kaminski PF, Sorosky JI, Wheelock JB, Stevens CW Jr: The significance of atypical cervical cytology in an older population. Obstet Gynecol 73:13–15, 1989.

76. Kenemans P, Davina JHM, de Haan RW, van der Zanden P, Vooijs GP, Stolk JG, Stadhouders AM: Cell surface morphology in epithelial malignancy and its precursor lesions. In Scanning Electron Microscopy III. Chicago; SEM, Inc, 1981.

77. Kenemans P, van der Zanden PHT, Stolk JG, Vooijs GP, Stadhouders AM: Cell surface ultrastructure in neoplasia of the uterine cervix. Biology of the cancer cell. In Proceedings of the fifth meeting of the European Association for Cancer Research. Edited by P Kenemans. Vienna, September 1979. Amsterdam, Kugler, 1980.

78. Kern WH: Replies to questions on quality assurance measures in cytopathology: In Quality Assurance Measures in Cytopathology. Edited by GL Wied. Acta Cytol 32:922–923, 1988.

79. Kern WH, Zivolich MR: The accuracy and consistency of the cytologic classification of squamous lesions of the uterine cervix. Acta Cytol 21:519–523, 1977.

80. Kinlen LJ, Spriggs AI: Women with positive cervical smears but without surgical intervention. A follow-up study. Lancet ii:463–465, 1978.

81. Klinkhamer PJJM, Vooijs GP, de Haan AFJ: Intraobserver and interobserver variability in the diagnosis of epithelial abnormalities in cervical smears. Acta Cytol 32:794–800, 1988.

82. Klinkhamer PJJM, Vooijs GP, de Haan AFJ: Intraobserver and interobserver variability in the quality assessment of cervical smears. Acta Cytol 33:215–218, 1989.

83. Koss LG: Diagnostic Cytology and Its Histopathologic Bases, 3rd ed. Philadelphia, JB Lippincott, pp 285–393, 1979.

84. Koss LG: Precancerous lesions of the epithelia of the uterine cervix. In Compendium on Diagnostic Cytology, 6th ed. Edited by GL Wied, CM Keebler, LG Koss, JW Reagan. Chicago, Tutorials of Cytology, pp 96–104, 1988.

85. Koss LG: Replies to questions on quality assurance measures in cytopathology: In Quality Assurance Measures in Cytopathology. Edited by GL Wied. Acta Cytol 32:923–924, 1988.

86. Koss LG: The Papanicolaou test for cervical cancer detection. A triumph and a tragedy. JAMA 261:737–743, 1989.

87. Koss JL, Durfee GR: Unusual patterns of squamous epithelium of uterine cervix: Cytologic and pathologic study of koilocytotic atypia. Ann NY Acad Sci 63:1245–1261, 1956.

88. Koss LG, Hicklin MD: Standards of adequacy of cytologic screening of the female genital tract. Conclusions of study group on cytology. Obstet Gynecol 43:792–793, 1974.

89. Koss LG, Stewart FW, Foote FW, Jordan MJ, Bader GM, Day E: Some histologic aspects of behavior of epidermoid carcinoma in situ and related lesions of the uterine cervix. A long term prospective study. Cancer 16:1160–1211, 1963.

90. Kottmeier HL: Evolution et traitement des epitheliomas. Rev Franc Gynaecol Obstet 56:821–825, 1961.

91. La Vecchia C, Franceschi S, Decarli A, Fasoli M, Gentile A, Parazzini F, Regallo M: Sexual factors, venereal disease, and the risk of intraepithelial and invasive neoplasia. Cancer 58:935–941, 1986.

92. Lohe KJ: Early squamous cell carcinoma of the uterine cervix. I. Definition and histology. Gynecol Oncol 6:10–30, 1978.

93. Lohe KJ: Early squamous cell carcinoma of the uterine cervix. III. Frequency of lymph node metastases. Gynecol Oncol 6:51–59, 1978.

94. Lohe KJ, Burghardt E, Hillemans HG, Kaufmann C, Ober KG, Zander J: Early squamous cell carcinoma of the uterine cervix. II. Clinical results of a cooperative study in the management of 419 patients with early stromal invasion and microcarcinoma. Gynecol Oncol 6:31–50, 1978.

95. MacLean AB, Lay MP, Kelleher PR, Carnielo RJ: Cytology, colposcopy and cervical neoplasia. NZ Med J 98:756–758, 1985.

96. Macnab JCM, Stephen A, Walkinshaw MB, Cordiner JW, Clements JB: Human papillomavirus in clinically and histologically normal tissue of patients with genital cancer. N Engl J Med 315:1052–1058, 1986.

97. Makkus L, Vooijs GP, van't Hof-Grootenboer B: Inflammatory signs in cervical smears. Submitted, 1990.

98. Matas AJ, Simmons RL, Kjellstrand CM, Buselmeier TJ, Najarian JS: Increased incidence of malignancy during chronic renal failure. Lancet i:883–885, 1975.

99. Matas AJ, Simmons RL, Najarian JS: Chronic antigenic stimulation, herpesvirus infection, and cancer in transplant recipients. Lancet i:1277–1279, 1975.

100. McKay DG, Terjanian B, Paschiachioda D, Younge PA, Hertig AT: Clinical and pathologic significance of anaplasia (atypical hyperplasia) of the cervix uteri. Obstet Gynecol 14:2–21, 1959.

101. Meisels A, Alonso de Ruiz P: Human papillomavirus—Related changes in the genital tract. In Human Papillomavirus and Cervical Cancer. Edited by N Munoz, FX Bosch, OM Jensen. Lyon, France, IARC Scientific Publications No. 94, pp 67–85, 1989.

102. Meisels A, Fortin R: Condylomatous lesions of the cervix and vagina. I. Cytologic patterns. Acta Cytol 20:505–509, 1976.

103. Meisels A, Fortin R, Roy M: Condylomatous lesions of the cervix. II. Cytologic, colposcopic and histopathologic study. Acta Cytol 21:379–390, 1977.

104. Meisels A, Roy M, Fortier M, Morin C: Condylomatous lesions of the cervix. Morphologic and colposcopic diagnosis. Am J Diagn Gynecol Obstet 1:109–116, 1979.

105. Meisels A, Roy M, Fortier M, Morin C, Casas-Cordero M, Shah KV, Turgeon H: Human papillomavirus infection of the cervix: The atypical condyloma. Acta Cytol 25:7–16, 1981.

106. Mestwerdt G: Probeexzision und Kolposkopie in de Fruehdiagnose des Portiokarzinoms. Zentralbl Gynakol 4:326–332, 1947.

107. Miller AB: Evaluation of the impact of screening for cancer of the cervix. *In* Screening for Cancer of the Uterine Cervix. Edited by M Hakama, AB Miller, NE Day. Lyon, France, International Agency for Research on Cancer, pp 149–160, 1986.

108. Moll R, Franke WW, Schiller DL, Geiger B, Krepler B: The catalog of human cytokeratins: Patterns of expression in normal epithelia, tumors, and cultured cells. Cell 31:11–24, 1982.

109. Moll R, Levy R, Czernobilsky B, Holweg-Majert P, Dallenbach-Hellweg G, Franke WW: Cytokeratins of normal epithelia and some neoplasm of the female genital tract. Lab Invest 49:599–609, 1983.

110. Morse AR, Coleman DV, Gardner SD: An evaluation of cytology in the diagnosis of herpes simplex virus infection and cytomegalovirus infection of the cervix uteri. Br J Obstet Gynaecol 81:393–398, 1974.

111. Munoz N, Bosch FX: Epidemiology of cervical cancer. *In* Human Papillomavirus and Cervical Cancer. Edited by N Munoz, FX Bosch, OM Jensen. Lyon, France, IARC Scientific Publications No. 94, pp 9–39, 1989.

112. Munoz N, Bosch X, Kaldor JM: Does human papillomavirus cause cervical cancer? The state of the epidemiological evidence. Br J Cancer 57:1–5, 1988.

113. Nasiell K, Auer G, Nasiell M, Zetterberg A: Retrospective DNA analyses in cervical dysplasia as related to neoplastic progression or regression. Anal Quant Cytol 1:103–106, 1979.

114. Nasiell K, Nasiell M, Vaklavinkova V: Behavior of moderate cervical dysplasia during long term follow up. Obstet Gynecol 61:609–614, 1983.

115. Nasiell K, Roger V, Nasiell M: Behavior of mild cervical dysplasia during long term follow up. Obstet Gynecol 67:665–669, 1986.

116. National Cancer Institute Terminology and classification: Report of a workshop on the terminology for cervical and vaginal cytology. *In* Bethesda, Maryland, Working Group on Terminology and Classification, 1989.

117. Ng ABP, Reagan JW: Microinvasive carcinoma of the uterine cervix. Am J Clin Pathol 52:511–529, 1969.

118. Ng ABP, Reagan JW: Pathology and cytopathology of microinvasive squamous cell carcinoma of the uterine cervix. *In* Compendium on Diagnostic Cytology, 6th ed. Edited by GL Wied, CM Keebler, LG Koss, JW Reagan. Chicago, Tutorials of Cytology, pp 114–122, 1988.

119. Ng ABP, Reagan JW: The pathology and cytopathology of squamous cell carcinoma of the uterine cervix. *In* Compendium on Diagnostic Cytology, 6th ed. Edited by GL Wied, CM Keebler, LG Koss, JW Reagan. Chicago, Tutorials of Cytology, pp 123–131, 1988.

120. Ng ABP, Reagan JW, Lindner EA: The cellular manifestations of microinvasive squamous cell carcinoma of the uterine cervix. Acta Cytol 16:5–13, 1972.

121. Nguyen GK: Exfoliative cytology of microinvasive squamous-cell carcinoma of the uterine cervix. A retrospective study of 42 cases. Acta Cytol 28:457–460, 1984.

122. Noumoff JS: Atypia in cervical cytology as a risk factor for intraepithelial neoplasia. Am J Obstet Gynecol 156:628–631, 1987.

123. Olesen F: A case control study of cervical cytology before diagnosis of cervical cancer in Denmark. I. J Epidemiol 17:501–508, 1988.

124. Oriel JD: A natural history of genital warts. Br J Vener Dis 47:1–13, 1971.

125. Papanicolaou GN: Atlas of Exfoliative Cytology. Cambridge, The Commonwealth Fund, 1954.

126. Papanicolaou GN, Traut HF: Diagnosis of Uterine Cancer by the Vaginal Smear. New York, The Commonwealth Fund, 1943.

127. Patten SF: Dysplasia of the uterine cervix. *In* New Concepts in Gynecologic Oncology. Edited by GC Lewis, WB Wentz, RC Jaffe. Philadelphia, FA Davis, pp 33–44, 1966.

128. Patten SF: Diagnostic cytology of the uterine cervix. *In* Monographs in Clinical Cytology, vol 3. Edited by GL Wied. Baltimore, Williams and Wilkins, pp 52–181, 1969.

129. Patten SF: Diagnostic cytology of the uterine cervix. *In* Monographs in Clinical Cytology, 2nd ed, vol 3. Edited by GL Wied. Baltimore, Williams and Wilkins pp 42–261, 1978.

130. Patten SF: Benign proliferative reactions of the uterine cervix. *In* Compendium on Diagnostic Cytology, 6th ed. Edited by GL Wied, CM Keebler, LG Koss, JW Reagan. Chicago, Tutorials of Cytology, pp 83–87, 1988.

131. Patten SF: Morphologic subclassification of preinvasive cervical neoplasia. *In* Compendium on Diagnostic Cytology, 6th ed. Edited by GL Wied, CM Keebler, LG Koss, JW Reagan. Chicago, Tutorials of Cytology, pp 105–113, 1988.

132. Patten SF, Reagan JW, Obenauf M, Ballard L: Post-irradiation dysplasia of the uterine cervix and vagina. An analytical study of cells. Cancer 16:173–182, 1963.

133. Piver MS, Chung WS: Prognostic significance of cervical lesion size and pelvic node metastases in cervical carcinoma. Obstet Gynecol 46:507–510, 1976.

134. Porreco R, Penn I, Droegemueller W, Greer B, Makowski E: Gynecologic malignancies in immunosuppressed organ homograft recipients. Obstet Gynecol 45:359–364, 1975.

135. Poulsen ME, Taylor CW, Sobin LM: Histological Typing of Female Genital Tract Tumours. Geneva, World Health Organization, pp 15–18, 55–62, 1975.

136. Pund ER, Nettles JB, Caldwell JD, Nieburgs H: Preinvasive and invasive carcinoma of the cervix uteri: Pathogenesis, detection, differential diagnosis and pathologic basis for management. Am J Obstet Gynecol, 55:831–837, 1948.

137. Purola E, Savia E: Cytology of gynecologic condyloma acuminatum. Acta Cytol 21:26–31, 1977.

138. Puts JJG, Moesker O, de Waal RMW, Kenemans P, Vooijs GP, Ramaekers FCS: Immunohistochemical identification of Langerhans' cells in normal epithelium and in epithelial lesions of the uterine cervix. Int J Gynecol Pathol 5:151–162, 1986.

139. Puts JJG, Moesker O, Kenemans P, Vooijs GP, Ramaekers FCS: Expression of cytokeratins in early neoplastic epithelial lesions of the uterine cervix. Int J Gynecol Pathol 4:300–313, 1985.

140. Ramaekers FCS, Huysmans A, Moesker O, Kant A, Jap PHK, Herman CJ, Vooijs GP: Monoclonal antibodies in keratin filaments specific for glandular epithelia and their tumors: Use in surgical pathology. Lab Invest 49:353–361, 1983.

141. Ramaekers FCS, Puts JJG, Moesker O, Kant A, Huysmans A, Haag D, Jap PHK, Herman CJ, Vooijs GP: Antibodies to intermediate filament proteins in the immunohistochemical identification of tumours: An overview. Histochem J 15:691–713, 1983.

142. Ramaekers F, Huysmans A, Schaart G, Moesker O, Vooijs P: Tissue distribution of keratin 7 as monitored by a monoclonal antibody. Exp Cell Res 170:235–249, 1987.

143. Reagan JW, Hamonic MJ: Dysplasia of the uterine cervix. Ann NY Acad Sci 63:1236–1244, 1956.

144. Reagan JW, Hamonic MJ: The cellular pathology in carcinoma *in situ*: A cytohistopathological correlation. Cancer 9:385–402, 1956.

145. Reagan JW, Hamonic MJ, Wentz WB: Analytical study of the cells in cervical squamous cell cancer. Lab Invest 6:241–250, 1957.

146. Reagan JW, Hicks DJ: A study of *in situ* and squamous cell cancer of the uterine cervix. Cancer 6:1200–1214, 1953.

147. Reagan JW, Hicks DJ, Scott RB: Atypical hyperplasia of the uterine cervix. Cancer 8:42–45, 1955.

148. Reagan JW, Patten SF: Dysplasia: A basic reaction to injury in the uterine cervix. Ann NY Acad Sci 97:662–682, 1962.

149. Reagan JW, Seidemann IL, Patten SF: Developmental stages of *in situ* carcinoma in uterine cervix: An analytical study of cells. Acta Cytol 6:538–546, 1953.

150. Reagan JW, Seideman IL, Saracusa Y: The cellular morphology of carcinoma *in situ* and dysplasia or atypical hyperplasia of the uterine cervix. Cancer 6:224–235, 1953.

151. Richart RM: Colpomicroscopic studies of the distribution of dysplasia and carcinoma *in situ* on the exposed portion of the human uterine cervix. Cancer 18:950–954, 1965.

152. Richart RM: The influence of diagnostic and therapeutic procedures on the distribution of cervical intraepithelial neoplasia. Cancer 19:1635–1638, 1966.

153. Richart RM: Natural history of cervical intraepithelial neoplasia. Clin Obstet Gynecol 10:748–784, 1967.

154. Richart RM: Cervical intraepithelial neoplasia: A review. *In* Pathology Annual. Edited by SC Sommers. New York, Appleton-Century-Crofts, pp 301–328, 1973.

155. Richart RM, Barron BA: A follow-up study of patients with cervical dysplasia. Am J Obstet Gynecol 105:386–393, 1969.

156. Richart RM, Barron BA: Screening strategies for cervical cancer and cervical intraepithelial neoplasia. Cancer 47:1176–1181, 1981.

157. Richart RM, Vaillant HW: Influence of cell collection techniques upon cytological diagnosis. Cancer 18:1474–1478, 1965.

158. Riotton G, Christopherson WM: Cytology of the female genital tract. *In* International Histological Classification of Tumours, No. 8. Geneva, World Health Organization, 1973.

159. Risse EKJ, Beerthuizen RJCM, Vooijs GP: Cytologic and histologic findings in women using an IUD. Obstet Gynecol 58:569–573, 1981.

160. Roche WD, Norris HJ: Microinvasive carcinoma of the cervix: The significance of lymphatic invasion and confluent patterns of stromal growth. Cancer 36:180–186, 1975.

161. Rubin IC: The pathological diagnosis of incipient carcinoma of the uterus. Am J Obstet Gynecol 62:668–676, 1910.

162. Rylander E: Cervical cancer in women belonging to a cytologically screened population. Acta Obstet Gynecol Scand 55:361–366, 1976.

163. Schachter J, Hill EC, King EB, Heilbron DC, Ray RM, Margolis AJ, Greenwood SA: *Chlamydia trachomatis* and cervical neoplasia. JAMA 248:2134–2138, 1982.

164. Schlaen I, Gonzalez-Garcia MR, Weismann EA: Predictive value of phenotypic cytologic characteristics in early dysplastic cervical lesions. Acta Cytol 32:298–302, 1988.

165. Schneider A, Kay S, Lee HM: Immunosuppression as a high risk factor in the development of condyloma acuminatum and squamous neoplasia of the cervix. Acta Cytol 27:220–224, 1983.

166. Schneider A, Sawada E, Gissmann L, Shah K: Human papillomaviruses in women with a history of abnormal Papanicolaou smears and in their male partners. Obstet Gynecol 69:554–562, 1987.

167. Scott RB, Ballard LA: Problems of cervical biopsy. Ann NY Acad Sci, 97:767–781, 1962.

168. Scott RB, Ballard LA: Cytology and its office application as viewed by the clinician. Clin Obstet Gynecol 5:179–195, 1962.

169. Sedlis A, Sall S, Tsukuda Y, Park R, Manham C, Shingleton HM, Blessing JA: Microinvasive carcinoma of the uterine cervix: A clinical pathologic study. Am J Obstet Gynecol 133:64–74, 1979.

170. Sedlis A, Walters AT, Balin H, Hontz A, Lo Scuito L: Evaluation of two simultaneously obtained cervical cytological smears: A comparison study. Acta Cytol 18:291–296, 1974.

171. Selvaggi SM: Cytologic detection of condylomas and cervical intraepithelial neoplasia of the uterine cervix with histologic correlation. Cancer 58:2076–2081, 1986.

172. Seski JC, Abell MR, Morley GW: Microinvasive squamous carcinoma of the cervix: Definition, histologic analysis, late results of treatment. Obstet Gynecol 50:410–414, 1977.

173. Shingleton HM, Richart RM, Wiener J, Spiro D: Human cervical intraepithelial neoplasia. Fine structure of dysplasia and carcinoma *in situ*. Cancer Res 28:695–706, 1968.

174. Shingleton HM, Wilbanks GD: Fine structure of human cervical intraepithelial neoplasia *in vivo* and *in vitro*. Cancer 33:981–989, 1974.

175. Sidhu GS, Koss LG, Barber HRK: Relation of Histologic factors to the response of Stage I epidermoid carcinoma of the cervix to surgical treatment. Obstet Gynecol 35:329–388, 1970.

176. Slate TA, Merritt JW: The behavior of cervical atypias and carcinoma *in situ* during pregnancy: A study of 120 patients. *In* Proceedings of the First International Congress on Exfoliative Cytology. Philadelphia, JB Lippincott, pp 128–132, 1961.

177. Smedts F, Ramaekers FCS, Robben H, Pruszczynski M, van Muijen G, Lane B, Leigh I, Vooijs GP: Changing patterns of keratin expression during progression of cervical intraepithelial neoplasia. Submitted.

178. Song J: The human uterus: Morphogenesis and embryological basis for cancer. Springfield, Illinois, Charles C Thomas, pp 12–35, 1964.

179. Spriggs AJ, Butler EB, Evans DMD, Grubb C, Husain OAN, Wachtel GE: Problems of cell nomenclature in cervical cytology smears. J Clin Pathol 31:1226–1227, 1978.

180. Summary Report. *In* Human Papillomavirus and Cervical Cancer. Edited by N Munoz, FX Bosch, OM Jensen. Lyon, France, IARC Scientific Publications No. 94, pp 1–8, 1989.

181. Sullivan JJ: Symposium on probable or possible malignant cervical lesions: Carcinoma *in situ*. Acta Cytol 6:183–184, 1962.

182. Tanaka H, Kimura E, Onda T, Ishida N, Tenjin Y: Establishing guidelines for dealing with mild dysplasia through cytology and colposcopy (follow-up study). Nippon Sanka Fujinka Gakkai Zasshi 37:2681–2690, 1985.

183. Tataeishi R, Wade A, Hayakawa K, Hongo J, Ishii S, Terekawa N: Argyrophil cell carcinomas (apudomas) of the uterine cervix. Virchows Arch [A] 366:260–274, 1975.

184. Van der Graaf Y, Vooijs GP: False negative rate in cervical cytology. J Clin Pathol 40:438–442, 1987.

185. Van der Graaf Y, Vooijs GP, Gaillard HLJ, Go DMDS: Screening errors in cervical cytologic screening. Acta Cytol 31:434–438, 1987.

186. Van der Graaf Y, Vooijs GP, Zielhuis GA: Population screening for cervical cancer in the region of Nijmegen, the Netherlands, 1976–1985. Gynecol Oncol 30:388–397, 1988.

187. Van der Graaf Y, Zielhuis GA, Vooijs GP: Cervical screening revisited. Acta Cytol 34:366–372, 1990.

188. Van Nagell JR, Donaldson ES, Wood EG, Parker JC: The significance of vascular invasion and lymphocyte infiltration in invasive cervical cancer. Cancer 49:379–383, 1978.

189. van Niekerk WA: Cervical cytological abnormalities caused by folic acid deficiency. Acta Cytol 10:67–73, 1966.

190. von Hansemann D: Ueber asymmetrische zellteilung in Epithelkrebsen und deren biologische Bedeutung. Virchows Arch [A] 119:229–326, 1890.

191. von Haam E, Old JW: Reserve cell hyperplasia, squamous metaplasia and epidermization: *In* Dysplasia, Carcinoma *in situ* and Micro-invasive Carcinoma of the Cervix Uteri. Edited by LA Gray, Springfield, Illinois, Charles C Thomas, pp 41–82, 1964.

192. Vooijs GP: Biometrically designed spatula for cervical scraping. Acta Cytol 31:82, 1987.

193. Vooijs GP: Replies to questions on quality assurance measures in cytopathology: *In* Quality Assurance Measures in Cytopathology. Edited by GL Wied. Acta Cytol 32:936–938, 1988.

194. Vooijs GP: Guidelines in abnormal findings in cytological studies of the cervix uteri (Dutch). Ned Tijdschr Geneeskd 132:640–641, 1988.

195. Vooijs GP: Significance of cellular composition of smears for the reliability of cytological diagnoses. *In* New Frontiers in Cytology. Modern Aspects of Research and Practice. Edited by K Goertler, GE Feichter, S Witte. Berlin, Heidelberg, New York, London, Paris, Tokyo, Springer-Verlag, pp 412–420, 1988.

196. Vooijs GP: Endocervical brush device. Lancet, i:784, 1989.

197. Vooijs GP, Casparie van Velsen JAGM, Peters FATM, Beck JLM: National registry of cervical cytologic diagnoses in the Netherlands. Acta Cytol 33:825–830, 1989.

198. Vooijs GP, Elias A, van der Graaf Y, Poelen van de Berg M: Samplers' influence on the cellular composition of cervical smears. Acta Cytol 30:251–257, 1986.

199. Vooijs GP, Elias A, van der Graaf Y, Veling S: Relationship between the diagnosis of epithelial abnormalities and the composition of cervical smears. Acta Cytol 29:323–328, 1985.

200. Vooijs GP, Van der Graaf Y, de Schipper F: PAP class IIIA:

A "proliferating" problem in cervical cytology. Eur J Obstet Gynecol Reprod Biol 29:219–226, 1988.

201. Vooijs GP, van der Graaf Y, Elias AG: Cellular composition of cervical smears in relation to the day of the menstrual cycle and the method of contraception. Acta Cytol 31:417–426, 1987.

202. Vooijs GP, Van der Graaf Y, Vooijs MA: The presence of endometrial cells in cervical smears in relation to the day of the menstrual cycle and the method of contraception. Acta Cytol 31:427–433, 1987.

203. Weikel W, Wagner R, Moll R: Characterization of subcolumnar reserve cells and other epithelia of human uterine cervix. Virchows Arch [Cell Pathol] 54:98–110, 1987.

204. Wentz WB, Lewis GC: Correlation of histologic morphology and survival in cervical cancer following radiation therapy. Obstet Gynecol 26:228–232, 1965.

205. Wentz WB, Reagan JW: Survival in cervical cancer with respect to cell type. Cancer 12:384–388, 1959.

206. Whittaker JR, Samy AMJ, Sunter JP, Sinha DP, Monaghan JM: Cytokeratin expression in cervical epithelium: An immunohistological study of normal, wart virus-infected and neoplastic tissue. Histopathology 14:151–160, 1989.

207. Wied GL: Editorial: An international agreement on histological terminology for lesions of the uterine cervix. Acta Cytol 6:235–236, 1962.

208. Wied GL, Bonfiglio TA, Cardin V, Drake M, Gupta PK, Holzner JH, Kern WH, Koss LG, Masubuchi K, Meisels A, Pfitzer P, Proctor DT, Richart RM, Rilke F, Rosenthal DR, Saigo PE, Stormby N, Suprun HZ, Vooijs GP, Wikely GW, Winkler BA: Replies to questions on quality assurance measures in cytopathology. Acta Cytol 32:913–939, 1988.

209. Wied GL, Legoretta G, Mohr D, Rauzy A: Cytology of invasive cervical carcinoma and carcinoma *in situ*. Ann NY Acad Sci 97:759–766, 1962.

210. Wied GL, Messina AM, Rosenthal E: Comparative quantitative DNA measurements of Feulgen-stained cervical epithelial cells. Acta Cytol 10:31–37, 1966.

211. Wilbanks GD, Richart RM, Terner JY: DNA contents of cervical intraepithelial neoplasia studied by two wavelength Feulgen cytophotometry. Am J Obstet Gynecol 98:792–799, 1967.

212. Wood RJ, Hicklin MD: Rescreening as a quality control procedure in cytopathology. Acta Cytol 21:240–246, 1977.

10

Glandular Neoplasms of the Uterine Cervix

Norman F. Pacey

Glandular neoplasms of the cervix uteri are assuming an increased importance to the cytopathologist.

It is claimed that adenocarcinoma and adenosquamous carcinoma of the cervix uteri have been changing their frequency in recent years. Reporting from the University Hospitals of Cleveland, Reagan and Ng[38] found that in the 5-year period ending in 1946, adenocarcinoma and adenosquamous carcinoma accounted for 5% of cervical cancers, whereas in the 5-year period ending in 1971, they accounted for 16% of cervical cancers. Tasker and Collins[48] were also early in noting the increasing incidence of adenocarcinoma, representing 5.9% of all cervical malignancies from 1953 to 1967 and 9.5% in the period from 1967 to 1972 in Ontario, Canada. Similarly, at the University of California, Brand and coworkers[13] found that the relative incidence of cervical adenocarcinomas from 1959 to 1979 was 5%, but between 1979 and 1982, this relative incidence of adenocarcinomas rose to 11%, and to 18% if adenosquamous carcinomas were included.

Adenocarcinoma and adenosquamous carcinoma now constitute a significant proportion of all invasive cancers of the cervix uteri in many recent reports (Table 10–1).

Data from two of the major oncology centers in Sydney, Australia—the Royal Hospital for Women, Paddington, and the Westmead Hospital—support this contention that adenocarcinoma has increased in relative incidence.[33] These data show that adenocarcinoma and adenosquamous carcinoma of the cervix have more than doubled in relative incidence in the 1970s and 1980s at these two institutions.

These cancer types now total 21.5% and 24% respectively of all cancers of the cervix presenting to these hospitals, and data from the third major oncology center in Sydney (King George V Hospital, Camperdown) show a similar figure of 22.3% for 1980 to 1982.[43]

A number of factors could be contributing to this trend. There is definitely a relative decrease in squamous carcinomas, as the result of screening activity. In some parts of the world, there could be an increase in absolute numbers of adenocarcinomas and adenosquamous carcinomas. Better cytologic criteria for identifying cases and improved recognition of mixed patterns by the histopathologists could also have contributed to this change.

The only answer lies in improved cytodiagnosis of adenocarcinoma and its precursors. Improved cytodiagnosis and treatment of the precursor lesions could decrease the incidence and mortality rates of invasive adenocarcinomas just as screening has done for squamous cancer.

TABLE 10–1. Proportion of Adenocarcinomas and Adenosquamous Carcinomas in Total Series of Invasive Carcinomas of Cervix Uteri

Gallup and Abell[19]	9.5%
Weiss and Lucas[50]	12.8%
Tamimi and Figge[46]	15.5%
Reagan and Ng[37]	16%
Horowitz and coworkers[24]	16%
Berek and coworkers[7]	18.2%
Shingleton and coworkers[41]	18.5%
Mayer and coworkers[32]	20% (adenocarcinoma only)
Julian and coworkers[27]	28%
Davis and Moon[14]	34%

TABLE 10–2. Age Incidence

	Mean Age (Years)	Range (Years)
Endocervical dysplasia	36	33–38
Adenocarcinoma *in situ*	37	22–70
Early or microinvasive adenocarcinoma	41	28–66
Invasive adenocarcinoma and adenosquamous carcinoma	49	26–85

Reproduced with permission from Bousfield L, et al: Acta Cytol 24:283–296, 1980.

INVASIVE ADENOCARCINOMA

Age Incidence

The age incidence of the range of glandular neoplasia of the cervix at our institution is summarized in Table 10–2.

For invasive adenocarcinoma, there is a wide age scatter. Most cases occur in the 4th, 5th and 6th decades, but according to some, it is also the usual form of cervical malignancy in the first 2 decades of life. Pollack and Taylor[36] reported that 78% of cervical cancers in their series that were seen in the first 2 decades of life were adenocarcinomas. We have not seen any cases in that age group.

Etiologic Factors

Horowitz and coworkers[24] have suggested that patients with squamous carcinoma and adenocarcinoma could represent two distinct populations with different risk factors. In their series, patients with adenocarcinoma appeared to be from a more affluent socioeconomic background with significantly more education, greater income and less risk of unemployment. They found less of a linkage with early first intercourse and smoking. Brand and colleagues[13] confirmed that there are as yet no recognized etiologic factors for cervical adenocarcinoma, and no relationship has been established with age at first intercourse, sexual activity or smoking.

Schwartz and Weiss[40] claim indirect evidence of a relationship with oral contraceptive use, but no studies have demonstrated a causal link. Any such study would, in fact, need to be controlled for all the confounding variables, especially the presence or absence of genital wart virus infection.

Our own studies on the histologic features of adenocarcinoma *in situ* (AIS) show that this precursor lesion will involve some or all of the transformation zone if there is an associated squamous abnormality.[26] Otherwise, without exception, the lesion arose contiguous to the squamocolumnar junction.

There was also a high incidence of associated squamous abnormalities (cervical intraepithelial neoplasia or worse, with or without wart virus infection in 60% of cases) and of wart virus infection alone recognized by histologic or cytologic criteria in an additional 7% of cases. These observations have led us to believe that the etiologic factors for the later invasive stages of adenocarcinoma and squamous carcinoma should have an identical etiology.

Smotkin and associates[42] have identified human papilloma virus type 16 or type 18 DNA in a small number of adenocarcinomas and adenosquamous carcinomas, and they have also suggested that there may be a common etiologic link between squamous carcinomas and adenocarcinomas.

Histology

The histologic classification of invasive adenocarcinoma used in our department is that of Tock and Shilkin,[49] slightly modified. It is logical and can accommodate the various alternative classifications summarized by Korhonen[28] and Anderson.[2]

1. Pure adenocarcinoma
   a. Adeniform
   b. Papillary
   c. Trabecular (and scirrhous)
   d. Mucoid
   e. Medullary
   f. Anaplastic
   g. Mixed
2. Combined glandular and squamous cell carcinoma
   a. Mixed (collision)
   b. Adenosquamous (blended)
   c. Mucoepidermoid
3. Adenoma malignum or minimal deviation adenocarcinoma
4. Clear cell carcinoma
5. Adenoid cystic carcinoma and adenoid basal carcinoma.

Tock and Shilkin[49] described the common subtypes succinctly as follows:

1. Pure adenocarcinoma
   a. The adeniform pattern is the most common, in which a pattern of endocervical gland structures are reproduced.
   b. The papillary pattern is an extension of the former pattern with formation of intraluminal papillary processes.
   c. The trabecular pattern shows solid cords of cells infiltrating the stroma. We have seen one example with a scirrhous pattern mimicking that of primary breast cancer but in which the tumor clearly arose from carcinoma *in situ*.
   d. Mucoid tumors show malignant glandular cells in pools of mucin.
   e. Medullary tumors occur in solid sheets with negligible glandular formation, although cellular mucin production is evident.
   f. Anaplastic tumors are not readily distinguishable from anaplastic squamous cancer, except for foci of abortive glandular formation and minimal evidence of mucin production seen with special stains.
   g. Mixed patterns are most commonly a combination of adeniform and papillary subtypes.
2. Combined glandular and squamous cell carcinoma
   a. Mixed (collision) tumors occur when the adenocarcinoma and the squamous cell carcinoma

have demonstrably separate origins and infiltrate each other.

b. The group with blended elements is referred to as adenosquamous carcinoma. Glassy cell carcinoma is now regarded as an undifferentiated form of adenosquamous carcinoma.[17, 47]

c. Those tumors having mainly squamous cell characteristics but containing scattered or clumped cells with intracytoplasmic mucin are labeled mucoepidermoid carcinomas.[17]

Cytology

Our cytologic classification of invasive adenocarcinoma of the cervix is simple. Primary adenocarcinoma is divided into (1) *well-differentiated adenocarcinoma* and (2) *poorly differentiated adenocarcinoma.* Mixtures of both well-differentiated adenocarcinoma and poorly differentiated adenocarcinoma may also occur.

The degree of differentiation is graded on the basis of nuclear appearance; cellular features are of secondary importance.[17, 28, 37]

This simple cytologic classification aids us in the better recognition of the abnormal material in the smear. It is also completely compatible with any histologic classification.

Fu and colleagues[17] also found a good correlation with survival when the degree of differentiation is determined solely on the basis of nuclear morphology rather than the more traditional histologic and architectural features. In their studies, the well-differentiated tumors had slightly enlarged, hyperchromatic, relatively uniform round to elongated nuclei. The nucleoli were small and inconspicuous. Mitoses were fewer than 10 per 10 high power fields. In poorly differentiated tumors, the nuclei were large and irregular in size and shape. Nucleoli were large and multiple, and mitotic figures were frequent. The 5-year survival rates for well-differentiated and poorly differentiated adenocarcinomas were 67% and 19% respectively; for mixed carcinomas the 5-year survival rates were poor regardless of the degree of differentiation of the glandular component.[17]

In a further elegant refinement, Fu and associates[18] added nuclear DNA quantitation. They found that well-differentiated tumors were more likely to have low-ploidy (<3N) stem cells, whereas poorly differentiated tumors usually had high-ploidy (>3N) stem cells. Tumors with low-ploidy stem cells were found to have a significantly better prognosis than high-ploidy tumors with a comparable degree of nuclear differentiation. Patients with advanced clinical Stage III and IV tumors were found to have a poor outlook regardless of ploidy.[18]

This additional study explained the occasional discrepancies found in clinical behavior when using this simple classification based upon nuclear appearances.

The more unusual histologic subtypes such as clear cell carcinoma, adenoid basal carcinoma and adenoma malignum have individual features that will be discussed separately.

Background

We have found that fresh blood or a dense inflammatory exudate is much more commonly found in the general background of smears than is indicated in published reports.[37] This finding raised practical difficulties in diagnosis in two ways. First, screening is very much more difficult because of the increased cellular content. Second, cellular changes can occur that raise difficulties in diagnosis. Heavy bloodstaining of a smear can cause delay in fixation and later difficulty in staining. Delayed fixation produces nuclear swelling and alteration in the nucleocytoplasmic ratio in both normal and malignant cells so that malignant cells may be overlooked (Fig. 10–1). The difficulty in staining manifests as apparent hypochromasia, probably due to failure of the hematoxylin stain to penetrate the fatty film arising from the blood. Infection, and particularly trichomonal infection, also produces changes in both malignant and benign cells that reduce the contrast between benign and malignant cells, so that the latter can be overlooked (Fig. 10–2).

Where it is present, tumor diathesis is, of course, a very valuable feature, but we have found tumor diathesis in only one quarter of cases. Some care is also necessary in interpretation.

A false or apparent tumor diathesis can occur in two situations. Many postmenopausal women can have a background to their smears similar to tumor diathesis. Occasionally, a similar background is apparent in trichomonal infections. Both situations require careful screening to eliminate the presence of cancer in any account, and diagnostic difficulty can be reduced in the first instance by resmearing after a course of estrogen therapy and in the latter, after treatment for trichomoniasis. Finally, the background may be perfectly clean in a small percentage of cases.

The second feature to note is the number of atypical

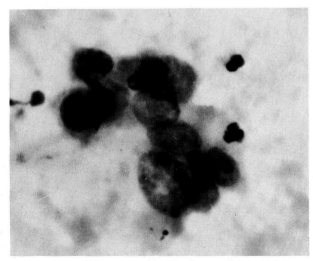

FIGURE 10–1. A strip of **abnormal endocervical cells** with enlarged hypochromatic nuclei caused by heavy blood staining in the smear (Papanicolaou stain; ×600).

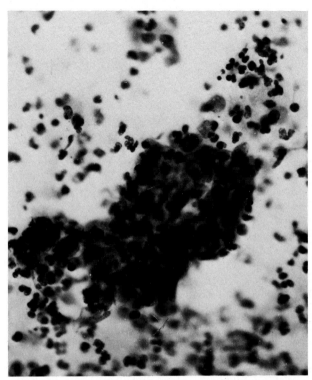

FIGURE 10–2. A group of **well-differentiated adenocarcinoma cells** in a background of inflammatory cells and trichomonads (Papanicolaou stain; ×400).

TABLE 10–3. Architectural Features in Invasive Adenocarcinoma

Exfoliative Features	Well-differentiated Adenocarcinoma	Poorly Differentiated Adenocarcinoma
Sheets		
Crowded	+ + +	+ +
Disoriented	+	+ +
Supercrowded	+ +	0
Papillary groupings	+ + +	+ +
Rosettes	+ + + +	+
Strips	+ + + +	+ +
Clusters and balls	+ +	+ +
Acinar or gland formation	+ + + +	+ + + +
Syncytia	+	+
Single malignant	+	+ +

+ = 5–25%; + + = 26–50%; + + + = 51–75%; + + + + = 76–100%.

or malignant cells. There is a wide variation depending upon (1) the type of sampling technique utilized, (2) the anatomic location of the lesion, (3) the histologic pattern and (4) surface necrosis and inflammation. We are used to seeing very few cells diagnostic of squamous invasive cancer on a smear, but it is apparent from our series that we still usually require abundant malignant material in glandular neoplasms to make the diagnosis with any degree of confidence.

Architecture

The arrangement of the malignant cells is of paramount importance in the diagnosis of adenocarcinomas (Table 10–3).

Adenocarcinomas, particularly well-differentiated adenocarcinomas and AIS, tend to shed cells in sheets and in tissue fragments (Fig. 10–3). These have to be studied closely to identify diagnostic features. Sheets may rarely retain the honeycomb formation seen in normal endocervical material, but more commonly crowding and overlapping of nuclei mask individual cell outlines. In such cases, cellular detail must be sought from gland openings within sheets or torn-open glands around sheet edges. Supercrowding of nuclei is a feature particularly diagnostic of invasion (Figs. 10–4 and 10–5) and is seen in almost half of our well-differentiated adenocarcinomas. Small sheets or

"strips," which may be fragments avulsed from gland edges, may occur. Palisading (or side-by-side arrangement) and pseudostratification of nuclei may be seen in suitable fragments, corresponding with the appearance in histologic sections.

Circular groups of cells with peripheral nuclei and cytoplasm directed towards the center are termed *rosettes*. These may be seen in AIS or in invasive well-differentiated adenocarcinomas (Fig. 10–6).

Papillary grouping may also be recognized in well-differentiated adenocarcinomas of papillary type (see Fig. 10–3).

Especially in poorly differentiated adenocarcinomas, one may see compact cellular "balls and clusters" (Fig. 10–7) with excentric nuclei, pleomorphism and three-dimensional piling (Fig. 10–8). These cellular arrangements may be particularly important in cytodiagnosis because individual cellular criteria of malignancy, especially nuclear criteria, may not be striking in poorly differentiated adenocarcinomas. Degenerative changes do not obscure this diagnostic arrangement of cells (Fig. 10–9).

Isolated cells are not so common in adenocarcinomas in our experience, contradicting textbook descriptions. They usually contribute little to the diagnostic process.

Syncytia (Figs. 10–10 and 10–11) are small, destratified sheets in which the cytoplasm is bubbly and pale staining with ill defined edges and no cell borders evident within the sheet. The nuclei usually show significant variation in size compared with the more uniform nuclear size of crowded sheets. The nuclei are round. At least some of the nuclei show prominent nucleoli with irregularly distributed chromatin (clumping and clearing).

Squamoid or nonstratified sheets are occasionally present. These squamoid sheets are difficult to evaluate because it is sometimes difficult to distinguish them from degenerated or atypical squamous cells seen in inflammatory conditions. It is of more diagnostic value when these squamoid cells are still attached to abnormal endocervical sheets (Figs. 10–12 to 10–14).

Text continued on page 241

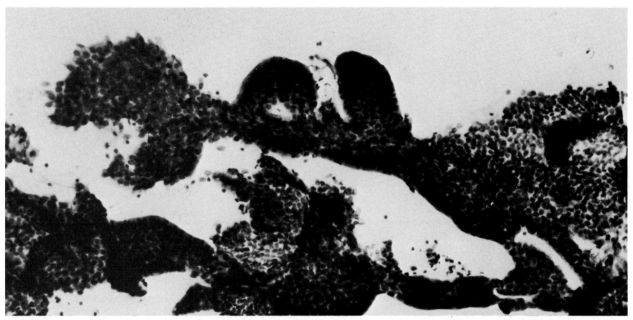

FIGURE 10–3. Well-differentiated adenocarcinoma. Malignant cells are shed in sheets and tissue fragments. Note the gland openings and the papillary projections. The background is clean (Papanicolaou stain; ×100).

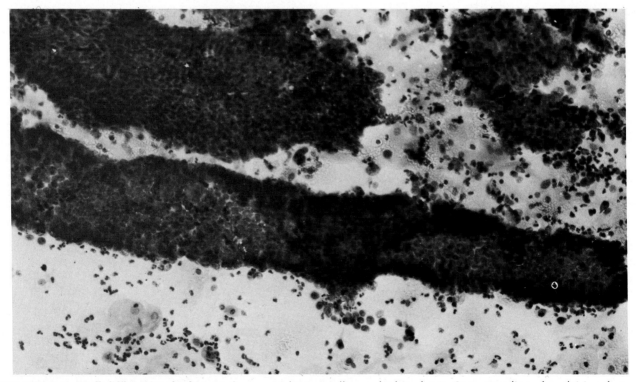

FIGURE 10–4. Well-differentiated adenocarcinoma. Malignant cells are shed in sheets. Supercrowding of nuclei is a feature strongly favoring the presence of invasion. The background is inflammatory (Papanicolaou stain; ×200).

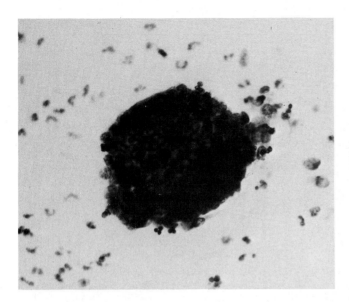

FIGURE 10–5. Well-differentiated adenocarcinoma. In this tissue fragment, the malignant nuclei show supercrowding (Papanicolaou stain; ×400). (Reproduced with permission from Ayer B, Pacey F and Greenberg M: The cytologic diagnosis of adenocarcinoma *in situ* of the cervix uteri and related lesions. II. Microinvasive adenocarcinoma. Acta Cytol 32:318–324, 1988.)

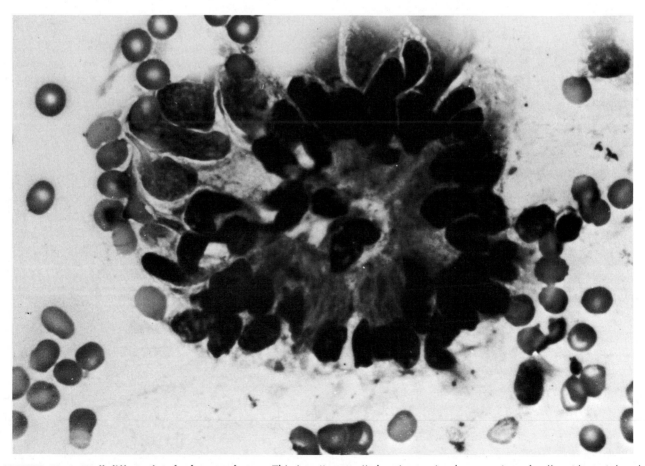

FIGURE 10–6. Well-differentiated adenocarcinoma. This is a "rosette," showing a circular grouping of cells with peripheral, pseudostratified nuclei. Nuclei are oval and hyperchromatic with coarse granularity and inconspicuous or absent nucleoli (Papanicolaou stain; ×600).

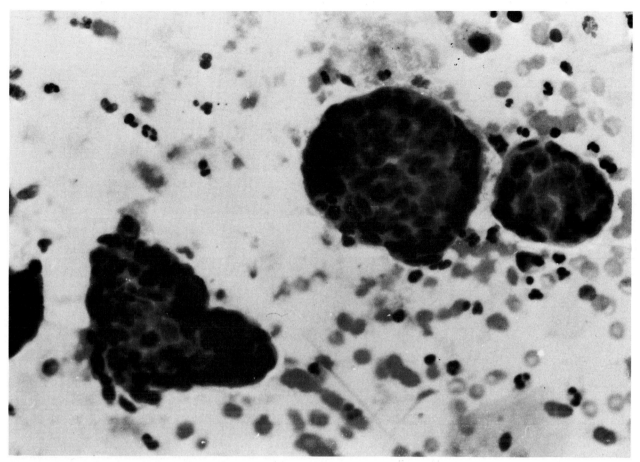

FIGURE 10–7. Poorly differentiated adenocarcinoma. Compact "balls and clusters" of malignant cells have well-defined structures. The background shows fresh blood (Papanicolaou stain; ×400).

FIGURE 10–8. Poorly differentiated adenocarcinoma. The clusters are much less obvious in this example. The nuclei are eccentric and show three-dimensional piling. Chromatin is finely granular and evenly distributed. Hyperchromasia is absent. Round disproportionate nucleoli are prominent in some cells. The background shows fresh blood (Papanicolaou stain; ×400).

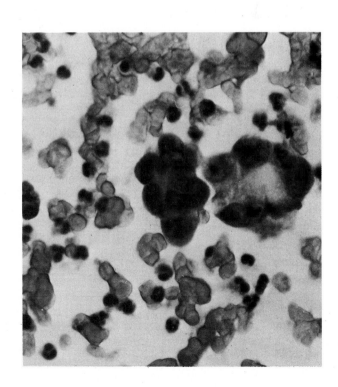

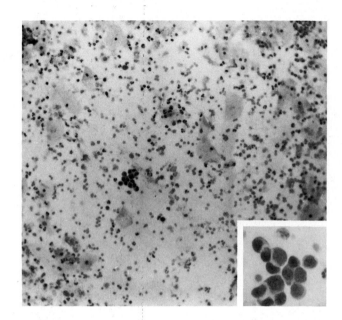

FIGURE 10–9. Poorly differentiated adenocarcinoma. Infrequent groupings of small degenerate cells are easily dismissed in screening. Note the inflammatory background (Papanicolaou stain; ×100). The inset shows the characteristic glandular groupings at a higher power (Papanicolaou stain; ×400).

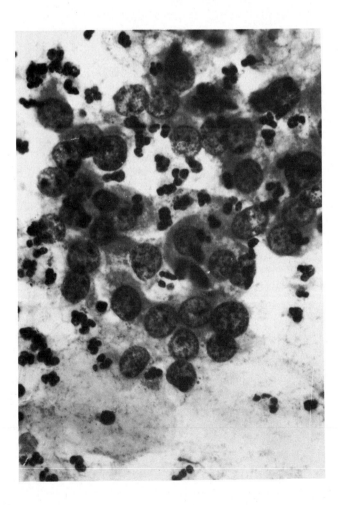

FIGURE 10–10. Poorly differentiated adenocarcinoma. This loose syncytial arrangement shows round variably sized nuclei, moderate hyperchromasia and moderate granularity irregularly distributed. Nucleoli are indistinct (Papanicolaou stain; ×400).

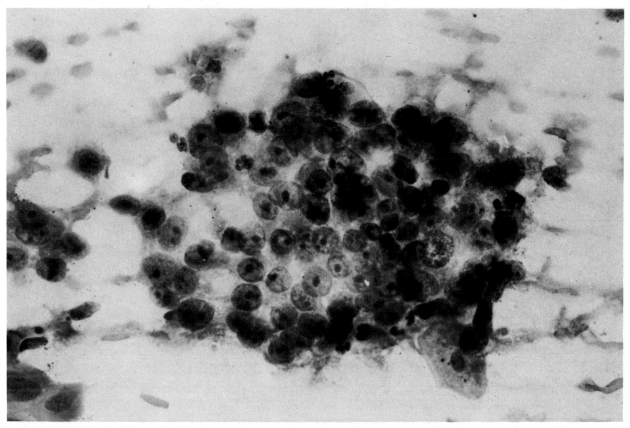

FIGURE 10–11. Poorly differentiated adenocarcinoma. The cells are dissociating in this sheet. Nuclei show prominent single round nucleoli, disproportionately enlarged in some nuclei. Slight hyperchromasia and variable granularity are shown (Papanicolaou stain; ×400).

FIGURE 10–12. "Microinvasive adenocarcinoma." Squamoid cells are seen as a part of an endocervical sheet of adenocarcinoma *in situ* and exhibit markedly contrasting cytoplasmic and nuclear features (Papanicolaou stain; ×400). (Reproduced with permission from Ayer B, Pacey F and Greenberg M: The cytologic diagnosis of adenocarcinoma *in situ* of the cervix uteri and related lesions. II. Microinvasive adenocarcinoma. Acta Cytol 32:318–324, 1988.)

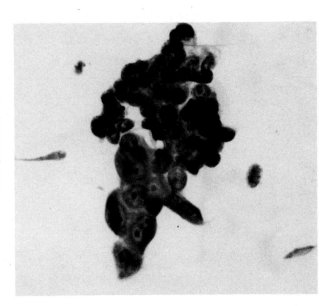

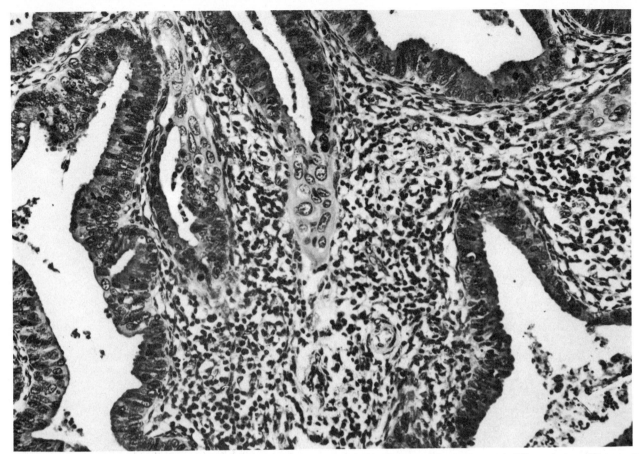

FIGURE 10–13. "Microinvasive adenocarcinoma." Foci of early stromal invasion show squamoid differentiation. The nuclei are enlarged, round, variable in size with "salt-and-pepper" distribution of chromatin (hematoxylin and eosin; ×250).

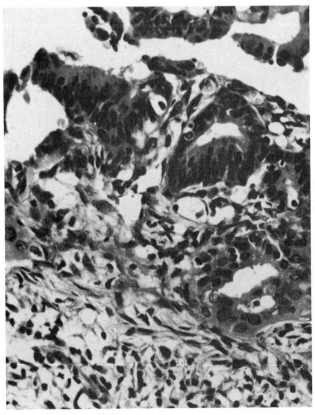

FIGURE 10–14. "Microinvasive adenocarcinoma." Foci of early stromal invasion, showing squamoid differentiation, arise from the tips of "exophytic" outgrowths of a gland with adenocarcinoma *in situ* (hematoxylin and eosin; ×250).

Nuclear Features

Well-Differentiated Adenocarcinomas

Nuclear Size. One quarter of cases have very small nuclei less than the size of normal endocervical nuclei. When this criterion is present, it is one of the most diagnostic features of well-differentiated adenocarcinoma (see Figs. 10–4 and 10–5). Of our cases, 40% have nuclei in the normal to 1½ times normal endocervical nuclear size. The remaining cases may reveal marked enlargement or marked variation in nuclear size.

Nuclear Shape. Almost half have round nuclei, one third have oval nuclei and the remaining one sixth show irregularly shaped nuclei.

Degree of Chromasia. One third show only normal chromasia or slight hyperchromasia, 50% show moderate hyperchromasia and surprisingly few (16%) reveal marked hyperchromasia.

Chromatin Pattern. Most have a finely or moderately granular pattern, whereas only 15% have a coarsely granular pattern. In 60% of cases, the distribution is even, and in the remaining 40% it is irregular.

Nucleoli. Nucleoli are usually absent or small, but in a quarter of cases, prominent nucleoli are to be expected in at least some of the nuclei. Marked variation in nucleolar size is very rare. Nucleoli may be single but are multiple in most cases. It is unusual for nucleoli to be other than round. These nuclear features are illustrated in Figures 10–3 through 10–6.

Poorly Differentiated Adenocarcinoma

Nuclear Size. This must be studied in cells free from degenerative changes and free from the secondary effects of inflammation. There is a substantial deviation from the mean nuclear size for normal endocervical cells, which is 8 μ.

Marked variation in nuclear size, ranging from 8 to 25 μ or more within the same group, is very frequent, and most of the other cases also show nuclear enlargement, marked in some.

Nuclear Shape. Round (62%) or irregular (34%) shapes are to be expected. Oval shapes are rare.

Degree of Chromasia. Slight or absent hyperchromasia may be seen in 50% of cases; 40% and 10% show moderate and marked hyperchromasia, respectively.

Chromatin Pattern. In contrast to well-differentiated adenocarcinoma, two thirds show irregular distribution of chromatin, and only one third show even distribution. Three quarters of cases show finely granular chromatin, and the remainder show moderately granular chromatin. Coarse granularity of chromatin is rare in our experience.

Nucleoli. One can expect tremendous variation in findings here. Nucleoli may be absent altogether, even in poorly differentiated adenocarcinomas. Nucleoli may range from small to large. Multiple nucleoli are more common, but one has to be particularly careful in the presence of single nucleoli. Nucleoli are much more likely to be round in shape than irregular.

These nuclear features are illustrated in Figures 10–8, 10–10 and 10–11.

Early invasive adenocarcinoma or adenocarcinoma invading to less than 5 mm in depth from the surface has also been termed *microinvasive adenocarcinoma* by some (see Figs. 10–13 and 10–14). The cytologic criteria are identical to those of frank invasive adenocarcinoma (Table 10–4) and so are included in the previous description. The fact that such cases are now regularly identified by cytologic means is encouraging, but long-term follow-up will be necessary to establish whether there is a more favorable prognosis for such cases to warrant a separate entity.

The more unusual subtypes of adenocarcinoma need special mention.

Adenoma Malignum. This rare type of adenocarcinoma has the nuclear features of poorly differentiated

TABLE 10–4. Comparison of Adenocarcinoma *In Situ*, Microinvasive and Invasive Adenocarcinoma

Features	Adenocarcinoma *In Situ*	Microinvasive Adenocarcinoma	Invasive Adenocarcinoma
Average age	37	41	49
Number of abnormal cells	Abundant	Abundant	Abundant
Cell sheets	Always present	Always present	Always present
Rosettes, strips	Present	Present	Present
Supercrowding of cells	Absent	Present	Present
Syncytia	Absent	Present	Present
Papillary formations	Not frequent	Common	Often seen
Dissociation of cells	Rare	Often seen	Common
Nuclear shape	Oval and round	Oval, round or bizarre	Round or bizarre
Nuclear size	Variable	Variable, but more pleomorphism seen	Marked pleomorphism
Nucleoli	Absent to prominent; occasionally multiple	Small to prominent; can be multiple	Small; often multiple
Background	Tumor diathesis absent	Tumor diathesis in some cases	Tumor diathesis in approximately one third of cases
Associated squamous atypia	Present in 50% of cases	Present in about 50% of cases	Present in 20% of cases

(Reproduced with permission from Ayer B, et al: Acta Cytol 31:397–411, 1987.)

adenocarcinoma but may retain a deceptively normal columnar configuration.

Szyfelbein and coworkers[45] reported that numerous endocervical cells were present in flat, coherent, monolayered sheets, multilayered sheets and three-dimensional clusters. Gland openings within sheets (acinus formation) are illustrated and described as typically crowded and overlapping. They also illustrate a cellular strip (ribbon) showing loose pseudostratification. All of these are architectural features of great diagnostic significance.

The neoplastic cells vary from small and cuboidal to large and columnar. They range from subtle abnormalities that are easily overlooked to frankly malignant changes. The nuclei are round or oval and vesicular, with fine to more coarsely dispersed chromatin. Chromatin margination was seen in two of three cases. Nucleoli are occasionally prominent. From the illustrations, they are seen to be occasionally multiple and irregular; they also can be single and disproportionately enlarged.

Clear Cell Adenocarcinoma. This subtype generated considerable interest previously with the fear that maternal exposure to diethylstilbestrol during pregnancy could predispose the female fetus to later development of clear cell adenocarcinoma of the vagina and cervix.[22, 23]

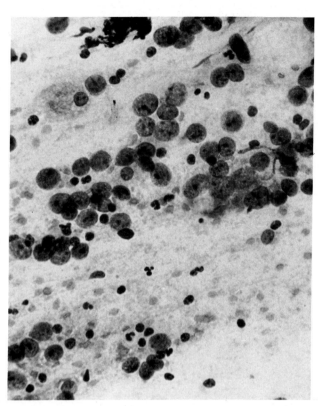

FIGURE 10–16. Clear cell carcinoma. Many bare nuclei are a frequent feature in this type of cancer. The nuclei are large and round and show moderately granular and even chromatin. Nucleoli are occasionally multiple but, in the nuclei towards the upper edge, single and enlarged. The background shows diathesis and blood (Papanicolaou stain; ×400).

In our experience, more-advanced cases of the disease have been indistinguishable cytologically from other forms of poorly differentiated adenocarcinoma.[51] However, there has been diagnostic difficulty in the literature in regard to the cytologic findings in early stage clear cell carcinoma.

Our experience has been as follows. The nuclear characteristics are those of poorly differentiated adenocarcinoma with nuclear size enlargement and prominent, round, disproportionate nucleoli as the most important criteria, and other criteria, such as hyperchromasia, are not constant and just as likely to be absent (Fig. 10–15). Bare nuclei in large numbers characterize our cases, but, of course, are not of diagnostic significance in themselves (Fig. 10–16).

It is cellular pattern that may lead to these cases being dismissed too lightly. In our cases, the cervical smears all contained numerous abnormal cells that occurred singly and in loose sheets. The abnormal cells were large. In those cells in which the cytoplasm was well preserved, it was abundant, pale staining and cyanophilic (Fig. 10–17). This cellular configuration has led to difficulty in our laboratory in distinguishing the lesion from squamous atypia and, in particular, from repair (regeneration) occurring in squamous dysplasia.

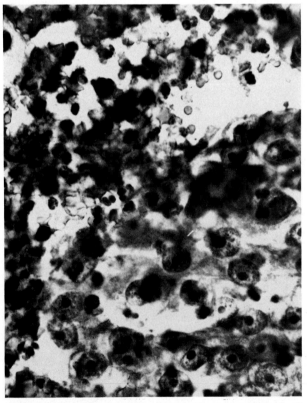

FIGURE 10–15. Clear cell carcinoma. These dissociated cells show delicate, lacy, indistinct cytoplasm. The nuclei are enlarged and round with finely granular, dispersed chromatin. The most striking feature is the single, round, disproportionately enlarged nucleoli (Papanicolaou stain; ×600).

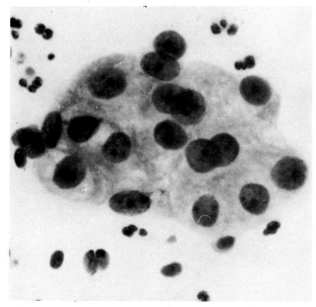

FIGURE 10–17. Clear cell carcinoma. Well-preserved adenocarcinoma grouping with large round or oval nuclei and occasionally prominent nucleoli. The cytoplasm is abundant and finely vacuolated, and the cytoplasmic borders are ill defined (Papanicolaou stain; ×600).

Thus, these two subtypes have characteristic nuclear features of poorly differentiated adenocarcinoma but may have deceptively bland cytoplasmic features, such as normal columnar shape in the case of adenoma malignum and abundant cytoplasm, that mislead one into thinking of a squamous origin in the case of clear cell adenocarcinoma.

Adenoid Basal Carcinoma and Adenoid Cystic Carcinoma. These as yet have no defined cytologic criteria of recognition.

ADENOCARCINOMA *IN SITU*

Friedell and McKay[16] were the first to recognize AIS of the cervix as a histologic entity. They defined several criteria supporting the concept of AIS. Their own article illustrates the first two of these. The remaining criteria have all been well established in further studies.
1. This lesion histologically resembles carcinoma but without demonstrable invasion of the stroma (their Case 1).
2. Similar morphologic changes occur at the periphery of unquestionably invasive adenocarcinoma (their Case 2).
3. An *in situ* lesion can be followed through to its development into an invasive adenocarcinoma. This criterion has now been met, using both the review of previous cytologic smears[8, 11, 29] and by retrospective histologic study of biopsy material.[10]
4. The similarity of the cytologic features of exfoliated cells from histologically proven *in situ* lesions to those found in smears from patients with microin-

vasive and invasive carcinoma of the same type is demonstrable.[5]
5. The average age of patients with AIS is several years younger than that of patients with invasive cancer, suggesting that the *in situ* form precedes the development of the invasive form of cancer.[11]

Histology

AIS has recently been classified on histologic grounds[1, 26] as follows:
1. Endocervical type, characterized by luminal accumulations of mucin-containing cytoplasm in at least some cells in a gland.
2. Endometrioid type, characterized by features similar to those of endocervical AIS but with intracellular mucin being entirely absent. The presence of a small amount of mucin along the luminal border is permitted.
3. Intestinal type, containing areas of AIS in which there are prominent collections of neoplastic goblet cells. The presence of argentaffin or Paneth cells is not a prerequisite for the designation of intestinal type.
4. Mixtures of these patterns.
5. Mucoepidermoid carcinoma *in situ*.[44]
6. Clear cell AIS.[21]

This classification is based upon the World Health Organization classification for invasive adenocarcinoma. It suffers from the disadvantage of the endocervical type being overwhelmingly predominant. Endocervical-type pattern is present in 96% of cases (either alone (57%), with associated intestinal-type pattern (29%) or mixed with endometrioid pattern (13%)) and the endometrioid pattern is in 4% of cases. This classification also does little to assist in cytologic detection.

Again, our cytologic classification of AIS of the cervix is simple. AIS is divided into (1) *well-differentiated AIS* and (2) *poorly differentiated AIS*. The basis for this cytologic classification is to aid in identification from cytologic material.

Cytology

We have found a clear background in one third of cases. An inflammatory background is the most com-

TABLE 10–5. Architectural Features in Adenocarcinoma *In Situ*

Exfoliation Features	Well-differentiated AIS	Poorly Differentiated AIS
Tightly crowded sheets	+ + + +	+ + +
Loosely crowded sheets	0	+ +
Strips off sheets	+ + + +	+ + + +
Isolated strips	+ + + +	+ + + +
Rosettes	+ + + +	+ + + +
Gland openings	+ + + +	+ + + +
Feathering	+ + + +	+ + +

+ + = 26–50%; + + + = 51–75%; + + + + = 76–100%.

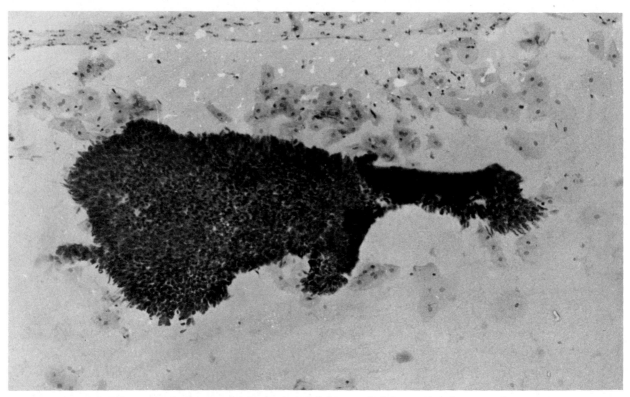

FIGURE 10–18. Well-differentiated adenocarcinoma *in situ*. Tightly crowded sheets of malignant cells occasionally show short strips of cells with pseudostratified nuclei extending off the edge (left side) or feathering (right side) (Papanicolaou stain; ×100).

mon, occurring in almost two thirds of cases. A blood-stained background is present in half, with or without accompanying inflammation. Degenerative changes in the smears, usually in association with inflammatory changes, appear in 20% of the cases.

The architectural features are of primary diagnostic importance (Table 10–5).

Tightly crowded sheets of malignant glandular cells are present in all cases of well-differentiated AIS and in 60% of cases of poorly differentiated AIS (Figs. 10–18 and 10–19). In the remaining cases of poorly differentiated AIS, loosely crowded sheets are present in which pseudostratification is minimal.

A particular diagnostic feature in both types of AIS is the presence of short strips of cells with pseudostratified nuclei extending off the edges of the crowded sheets, as seen in Figures 10–18 and 10–19.

Other highly significant features included isolated strips of varying lengths (Figs. 10–20 and 10–21) with palisading and pseudostratified nuclei, and the small circular groups of cells known as rosettes, with peripheral pseudostratified nuclei and cytoplasm oriented towards the central lumen (Figs. 10–22 to 10–24). Not only do these features aid especially the beginner in the accurate identification of AIS, but they also make possible accurate classification into well-differentiated and poorly differentiated types, as well as classification into endocervical, endometrioid and intestinal histologic subtypes.

Gland openings within crowded sheets are present in most cases of AIS (see Fig. 10–19), but the charac-

teristic palisading and pseudostratification are seen at a diagnostic level in only a quarter of cases of well-differentiated AIS and only rarely in poorly differentiated AIS.

Feathering is a feature that is occasionally useful in diagnosis (see Fig. 10–18). Nuclei denuded of columnar cytoplasm retain their polarity and pseudostratification, giving a frayed or feathered appearance. Occasional sheets with an otherwise undifferentiated appearance can be identified as AIS by observing even small foci of feathered edging.

Isolated cell distribution is rare and is of little diagnostic value.

Small three-dimensional balls of glandular cells are sometimes seen in the endometrioid pattern of AIS. These are always seen as a feature in addition to the other characteristic architectural features seen in AIS (Fig. 10–25).

Nuclear Features

Well-Differentiated Adenocarcinoma In Situ

Nuclear Size. The usual size is 8 to 15 μ, but larger sizes (15 to 20 μ) are noted in about 15% of cases. The small-cell variant, with nuclei smaller than the 8 μ length of normal endocervical cells, is rare but important because it is likely to be dismissed in screening (Fig. 10–26).

Text continued on page 249

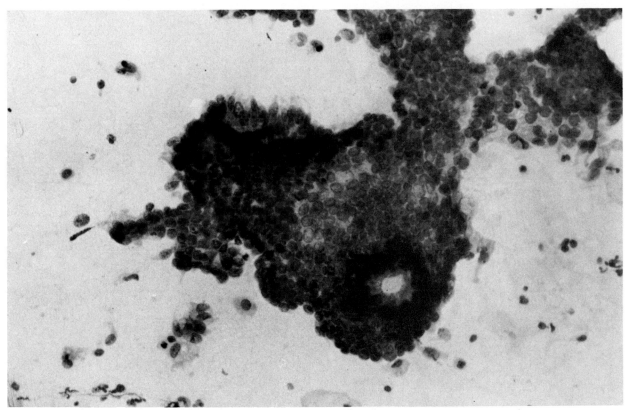

FIGURE 10–19. **Well-differentiated adenocarcinoma** *in situ.* Crowded sheet with a gland opening around which the centrifugal-like distribution of nuclei and the pseudostratified arrangement of nuclei aid in characterization (Papanicolaou stain; ×200). (Reproduced with permission from Ayer B, Pacey F, Greenberg M and Bousfield L: The cytologic diagnosis of adenocarcinoma *in situ* of the cervix uteri and related lesions. I. Adenocarcinoma *in situ.* Acta Cytol 31:397–411, 1987.)

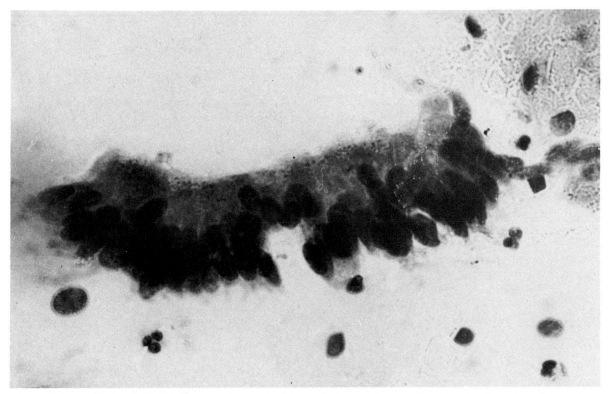

FIGURE 10–20. **Well-differentiated adenocarcinoma** *in situ* **(endocervical type).** This strip of cells shows diagnostic nuclear pseudostratification. The nuclei are oval and hyperchromatic with moderately coarse even chromatin. Abundant cytoplasm and a glandular edge are seen (Papanicolaou stain; ×600). (Reproduced with permission from Ayer B, Pacey F, Greenberg M and Bousfield L: The cytologic diagnosis of adenocarcinoma *in situ* of the cervix uteri and related lesions. I. Adenocarcinoma *in situ.* Acta Cytol 31:397–411, 1987.)

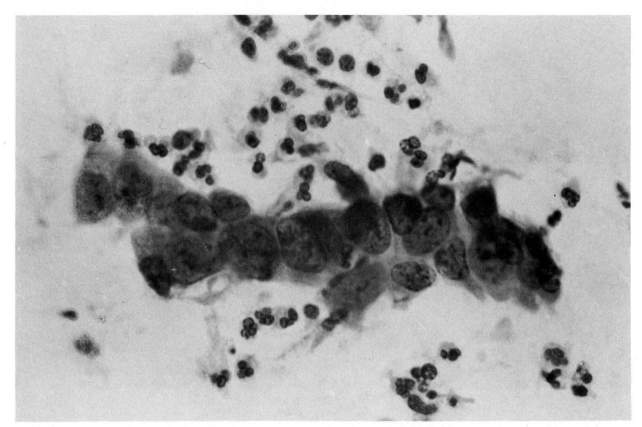

FIGURE 10–21. Poorly differentiated adenocarcinoma *in situ* (endocervical type). This strip of cells shows less nuclear pseudostratification. The nuclei are round or irregular in shape and very greatly enlarged. Chromasia is much less than that in Figure 10–20. Chromatin is finely granular and usually distributed evenly. Multiple small nucleoli are seen (Papanicolaou stain; ×600). (Reproduced with permission from Ayer B, Pacey F, Greenberg M and Bousfield L: The cytologic diagnosis of adenocarcinoma *in situ* of the cervix uteri and related lesions. I. Adenocarcinoma *in situ*. Acta Cytol 31:397–411, 1987.)

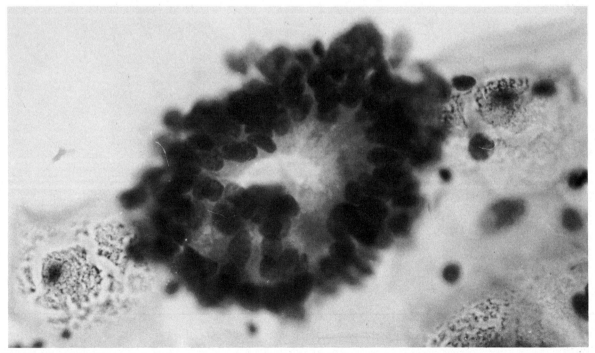

FIGURE 10–22. Well-differentiated adenocarcinoma *in situ* (endocervical type). A circular group of cells, known as a "rosette." Nuclear pseudostratification and nuclear criteria establish the diagnosis. The abundant cytoplasm characterizes the histologic type (Papanicolaou stain; ×600). (Reproduced with permission from Ayer B, Pacey F, Greenberg M and Bousfield L: The cytologic diagnosis of adenocarcinoma *in situ* of the cervix uteri and related lesions. I. Adenocarcinoma *in situ*. Acta Cytol 31:397–411, 1987.)

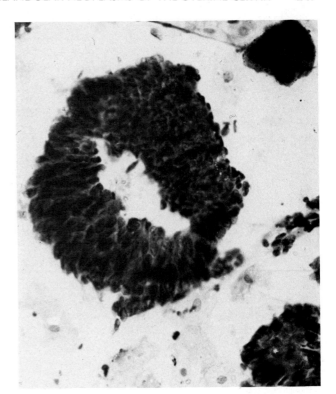

FIGURE 10–23. Well-differentiated adenocarcinoma *in situ* (endometrioid type). This "rosette" is more chunky and shows much less free cytoplasm along the glandular edge, characterizing it as the endometrioid type (Papanicolaou stain; ×200). (Reproduced with permission from Ayer B, Pacey F, Greenberg M and Bousfield L: The cytologic diagnosis of adenocarcinoma *in situ* of the cervix uteri and related lesions. I. Adenocarcinoma *in situ*. Acta Cytol 31:397–411, 1987.)

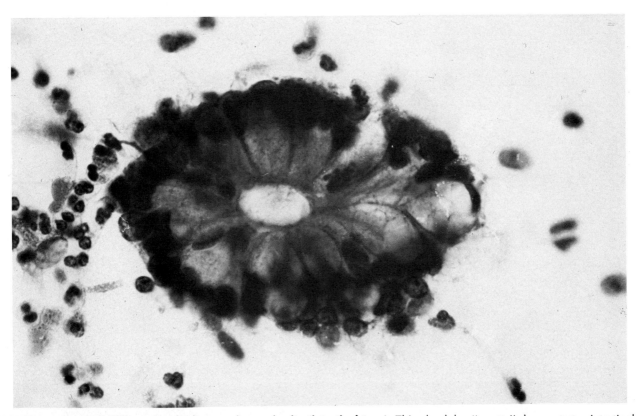

FIGURE 10–24. Well-differentiated adenocarcinoma *in situ* (intestinal type). This glandular "rosette" demonstrates intestinal-pattern adenocarcinoma *in situ* with goblet cells (Papanicolaou stain; ×600). (Reproduced with permission from Ayer B, Pacey F, Greenberg M and Bousfield L: The cytologic diagnosis of adenocarcinoma *in situ* of the cervix uteri and related lesions. I. Adenocarcinoma *in situ*. Acta Cytol 31:397–411, 1987.)

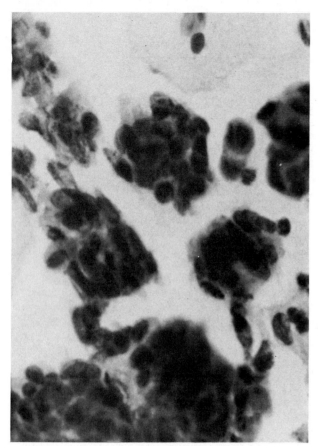

FIGURE 10–25. Well-differentiated adenocarcinoma *in situ* (endometrioid type). The glandular groupings on the right are three-dimensional balls, contrasting in arrangement with the other short strips of cells in which stratified nuclei completely obliterate the cytoplasm (Papanicolaou stain; ×400).

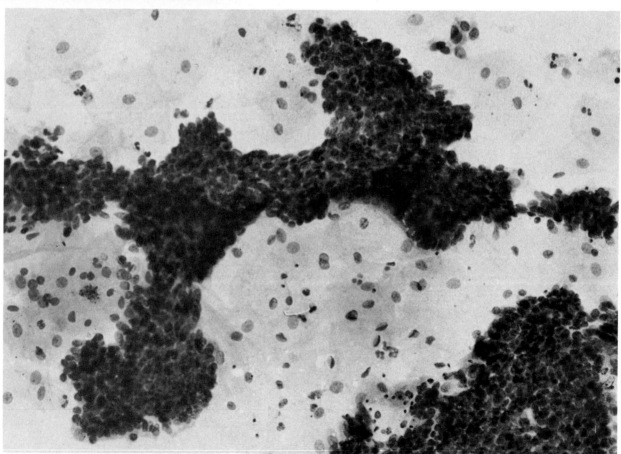

FIGURE 10–26. Well-differentiated adenocarcinoma *in situ*. The small cell variant, with nuclei smaller than the usual normal endocervical cell nuclei or normal intermediate cell nuclei, is easily dismissed during screening (Papanicolaou stain; ×200). (Reproduced with permission from Ayer B, Pacey F, Greenberg M and Bousfield L: The cytologic diagnosis of adenocarcinoma *in situ* of the cervix uteri and related lesions. I. Adenocarcinoma *in situ*. Acta Cytol 31:397–411, 1987.)

Nuclear Shape. The shape of the nucleus is oval.

Degree of Chromasia. Moderate hyperchromasia is present in 90% of cases and marked hyperchromasia in 10%.

Chromatin Pattern. Finely granular chromatin is present in one quarter of cases and moderately granular chromatin in three quarters. Coarse chromatin is rare. An even distribution of chromatin is to be expected.

Nucleoli. Nucleoli are absent in half the cases and present in at least some cells in the sample in half the cases. Of those cases with nucleoli, the nucleoli are usually small and round but may be medium-sized.

Poorly Differentiated Adenocarcinoma In Situ (Figs. 10–27 to 10–29)

Nuclear Size. Nuclei are 8 to 15 μ in about half of the cases and larger than 15 μ in length in the other half; they are greatly enlarged (up to 25 μ) in a small number.

Nuclear Shape. Oval nuclei predominate in half the cases and round nuclei in the other half. Bizarre shapes are unusual.

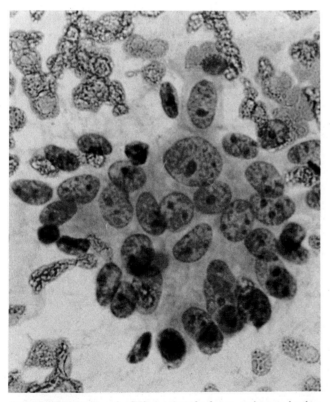

FIGURE 10–27. Poorly differentiated adenocarcinoma *in situ*. This glandular "rosette" shows little nuclear stratification. The nuclei are round but variable in size. Chromatin is finely granular and evenly distributed. Nucleoli are very prominent features (Papanicolaou stain; ×400). (Reproduced with permission from Ayer B, Pacey F, Greenberg M and Bousfield L: The cytologic diagnosis of adenocarcinoma *in situ* of the cervix uteri and related lesions. I. Adenocarcinoma *in situ*. Acta Cytol 31:397–411, 1987.)

Degree of Chromasia. Hyperchromasia is absent or slight in nearly half the cases, and just show over half the cases show moderate hyperchromasia.

Chromatin Pattern. Half the cases have finely granular chromatin, and half have moderately granular chromatin. An even distribution of chromatin is almost universal.

The most important feature is the variation from the normal vesicular pattern; this is quite distinctive even when the nuclei are only mildly hyperchromatic and the chromatin is only finely granular.

Nucleoli. Nucleoli are present in all our identified cases of poorly differentiated AIS. They are small, medium-sized and prominent in increasing order of likelihood. Multiple nucleoli are most unusual.

Differential Diagnosis

It should now be apparent that the cells of cervical adenocarcinoma precursors and most of their variants are shed in cohesive sheets, just as are normal endocervical cells. Sheets of normal endocervical cells may contain gland openings, and there may be short strips of columnar epithelium coming off the edges of the sheets. Isolated strips of normal columnar epithelium are a frequent finding in smears, and even occasional rosettes can be found. The differences are twofold. First, normal columnar cells do not show pseudostratification and they maintain the normal honeycomb architecture and picket fence arrangement.

Second, the normal nuclear structure is retained; nuclei are round or oval with evenly dispersed vesicular chromatin and often one or two tiny but distinctive nucleoli. The cytoplasm is abundant, lacy and vacuolated.

Endocervical cells are particularly prone to inflammatory changes from a large variety of causes. The tendency to shed in sheets, strips and even rosettes remains, but small balls and clusters of inflammatory endocervical cells are not unusual. The endocervical cells show dedifferentiation, with nuclear enlargement, granularity of chromatin even up to coarse, irregular distribution of chromatin and the presence of nucleoli (Fig. 10–30). Such inflammatory changes frequently coexist with squamous metaplasia, again tending to shed in sheets and monolayers. These cells also show nuclear enlargement, chromatin irregularities, multiple irregular nucleoli and occasional and unpredictable hyperchromasia due to tetraploidy.

Degenerative changes frequently coexist, especially if the original cause of the inflammatory reaction is an agent such as *Trichomonas*, which actively damages the cells. This damage is then followed by repair, again causing specific abnormalities in endocervical cells, some of which mimic malignant criteria.

The conclusion from all of this is that the cytologist faced with interpreting cellular changes in situations in which the cytodiagnosis of adenocarcinoma and its precursors is being considered must have a good working knowledge of the appearance of normal endocervical cells under a wide range of conditions, especially

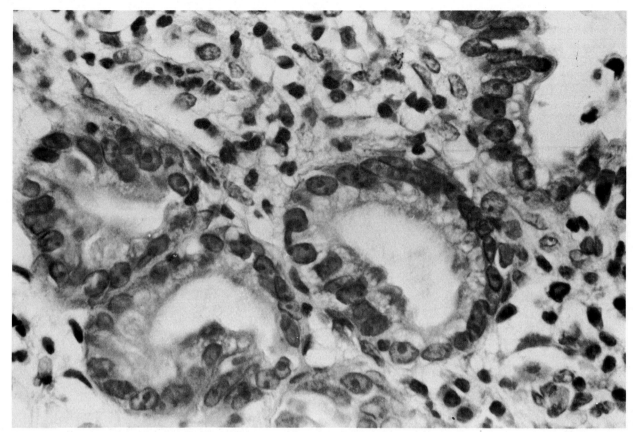

FIGURE 10–28. Poorly differentiated adenocarcinoma *in situ.* Histologic section that corresponds very closely to the previous cytologic patterns (Fig. 10–27). No pseudostratification is seen, but the nuclei are enlarged and round, though irregular, with enormous single round nucleoli in some of them. Cellular shape remains columnar (hematoxylin and eosin stain; ×400).

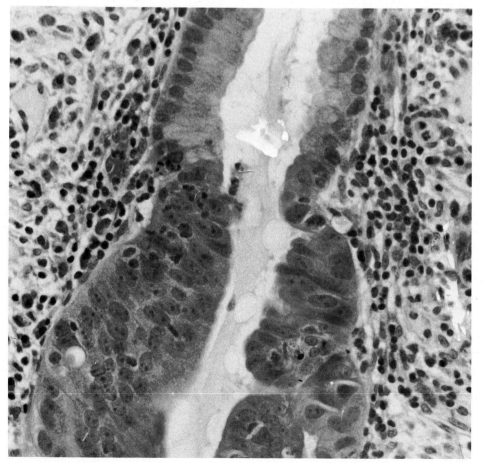

FIGURE 10–29. Poorly differentiated adenocarcinoma *in situ.* This histologic section shows a different pattern with much more obvious pseudostratification. The nuclei tend to be oval in shape and greatly enlarged. Chromasia is identical to the adjacent normal endocervical cells at the top of the section, but prominent nucleoli are evident (hematoxylin and eosin stain; ×400).

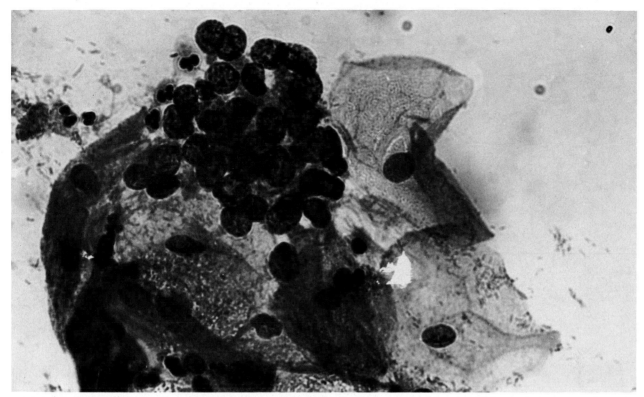

FIGURE 10–30. Groups of **reactive endocervical cells** resemble adenocarcinoma with enlarged hyperchromatic nuclei, coarse chromatin and occasional nucleoli (Papanicolaou stain; ×400).

when inflammatory changes, degenerative changes, necrosis or repair may be present alone or in combination.

Endometrial cells are usually shed from the endometrium and are found in Papanicolaou smears in degenerate form. Differential diagnosis from malignancy is usually easy, especially if one has a good history including date of last menstrual period and if the smear taker avoids the menstrual period.

Under certain circumstances, endometrial cells are exfoliated by direct action of the spatula, and in this situation there are some traps to avoid. Endometrial cells collected in this way will appear in the smear as sheets with gland openings and as strips showing pseudostratified nuclei. Furthermore, normal endometrial cells have a higher nucleocytoplasmic ratio, appear hyperchromatic and have a coarser chromatin and larger and more prominent nucleoli. Unless the cells are recognized as of endometrial origin, they are easily mistaken for AIS or for invasive adenocarcinoma of the cervix.

Such situations could arise in the following circumstances.

1. *Cervical endometriosis.* We have seen two examples, the second predicted in advance. Large sheets and strips presented on the smears in a well-preserved state and on a number of occasions, irrespective of the time of the cycle. The cells were recognized as of endometrial origin, considerably aided in the second case by the coexistence of large numbers of endometrial stromal cells of typical appearance. The colposcopic appearance of cervical endometriosis has now been defined, and it is not unreasonable to request help from the colposcopist if this diagnosis is seriously entertained in the future.

2. *Postcone biopsy smears.* Cone biopsy results in considerable shortening of the cervical canal and sometimes complete removal of endocervical epithelium so that endometrial tissue is now brought within direct reach of the spatula. Postcone biopsy smears are screened with a high index of suspicion, so the unwary can overreact to the presence of high endocervical cells or debrided endometrial cells in the smears (Fig. 10–31). In such circumstances, it is advisable to review the smear with the histology of the cone biopsy and with the previous abnormal Papanicolaou smear that led to the cone biopsy. However, it is as well to note that occasionally one could see AIS or invasive adenocarcinoma after a cone biopsy or after conservative management such as cryotherapy for a squamous abnormality thought originally to exist alone.

3. *Sampling with an endocervical brush.* This sampling technique is very effective in obtaining thicker sheets, strips and rosettes of normal endocervical epithelium than can be found with the usual modified Ayre spatula. Such thick sheets can appear to show prominent pseudostratification of nuclei at times. The nuclei are, however, all completely normal and this, plus the history of sampling with the endocervical brush, should alert one to what is happening.

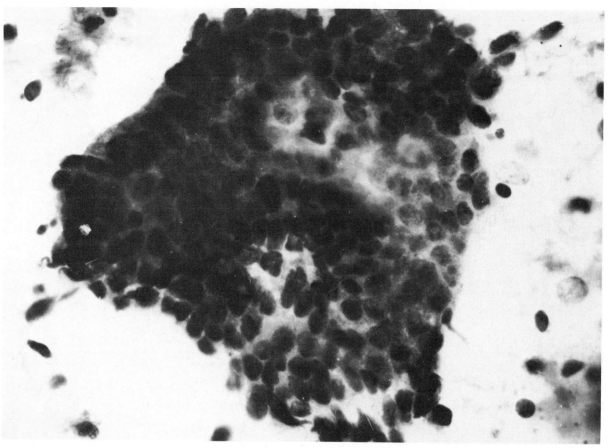

FIGURE 10–31. Sheet of **endocervical cells** after cone biopsy. These cells from the high endocervical canal reveal crowding with hyperchromatic and pseudostratified nuclei and mimic adenocarcinoma *in situ* (Papanicolaou stain; ×400).

The endocervical brush is also likely to drag down a sample from the endometrial cavity, with the attendant difficulties already discussed.

Another common finding generally not appreciated by either the cytopathologist or the histopathologist is tubular metaplasia of the endocervical epithelium.[35] The cervical epithelium is composed of ciliated columnar secretory cells interspersed with smaller, dark, intercalated cells. In Papanicolaou smears, one sees ciliated columnar cells, which should alert one to the possibility of the diagnosis, and a loose, slight pseudostratification. Nuclear appearances show larger nuclei, up to twice the size of normal endocervical cell nuclei, that are moderately hyperchromatic, granular and evenly distributed.

In the presence of an endocervical polyp, endocervical cells may exhibit changes such as marked nuclear enlargement, nuclear hyperchromasia, prominent nucleoli and even variation in nuclear size, all criteria that can be seen in the presence of malignant lesions. One has to exercise a certain degree of caution when a woman has a history of cervical polyps, and one may occasionally have to ask the clinician if clinical examination showed evidence of a polyp. However, in our series, a 28-year-old woman with a cervical polyp also had a coexistent adenocarcinoma.

Not surprisingly, it can occasionally be extremely difficult to differentiate AIS from squamous carcinoma *in situ* on cytologic criteria alone.

AIS may be predicted on cytologic criteria, demanding a diagnostic cone biopsy, with only squamous carcinoma *in situ* later confirmed by histology. Some appearances traditionally reported by histopathologists as squamous carcinoma *in situ* may represent mixed *in situ* lesions. Rosenthal and coworkers[39] observed dyskaryotic glandular cells compatible both visually and by digital image analysis with a diagnosis of AIS; yet, on later histopathologic examination, these cells were seen in cases reported as showing only squamous carcinoma *in situ*. Others have also noted this practical difficulty in accurate diagnosis.[30] Special stains for mucin secretion are certainly indicated in histologic sections in such cases.

Another area of difficulty occurs when squamous carcinoma *in situ* is present, with extension downwards into the endocervical glands. In these cases, the malignant squamous cells are inclined to be shed in sheets rather than individually, as we have observed over many years of experience (Fig. 10–32).

In some cases, normal or slightly atypical endocervical cells may persist along one edge of these sheets of malignant cells, leading the observer to assume the sheets of malignant cells are all glandular in origin. Neither of these two misdiagnoses should be regarded as a false-positive.

Finally, the presence of mesonephric remnants in histologic sections is characterized by small, cleftlike acini lined by a single layer of cuboidal epithelium.

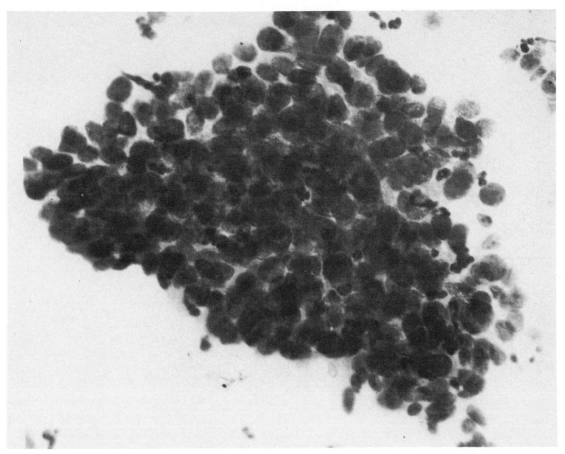

FIGURE 10–32. Sheet of **malignant cells** with apparent pseudostratification and a gland opening, from a case of cervical intraepithelial neoplasia III with glandular extension (Papanicolaou stain; ×400).

The cells and nuclei are bland with scanty cytoplasm.[34] We have never seen this condition directly involve the surface epithelium, so the exfoliation of these cells onto smears is unlikely.

Cells from malignancy other than that arising primarily from the female genital tract are occasionally observed in cervical smears. Possible origins of such cells in these smears are as follows:

1. Malignant cells traverse a route similar to that of an ovum.
   a. Peritoneal or pelvic involvement from any primary site, plus ascites as part of a carcinomatosis
   b. From ovary (Fig. 10–33)
   c. From fallopian tube
2. Malignancy can spread directly to the cervix or vagina from either rectum or bladder.
3. Cells can metastasize to uterus or vagina (as part of a generalized carcinomatosis). Usual origins have been ovary or breast, but stomach, lung and a host of other sites have been described as primary sites of origin.
4. Extrauterine cancer plus a second primary tumor can appear within the genital tract.

Examples of all of these have been identified in our laboratory. They are largely of academic interest and usually signify a poor prognosis. One exception to this gloomy prognosis can be the fallopian tube carcinoma. This is usually originally thought to be an endometrial cancer, because the cytologic findings are identical. Dilatation and curettage (D & C) fails to confirm the diagnosis, and repeat D & C also fails. In such cases, it is important to further investigate and to exclude fallopian tube cancer, since early diagnosis can significantly alter the prognosis towards a favorable outcome.

Diagnostic Accuracy

Our approach to the cytologic diagnosis of adenocarcinoma and its precursors is based on the following premises:

1. AIS cannot yet be recognized or localized by colposcopic means and so accurate prediction from the Papanicolaou smear is essential.
2. Squamous carcinoma *in situ* can be identified and localized accurately by colposcopy and yet coexistent AIS would be completely overlooked.
3. The further investigation and treatment of squamous carcinoma *in situ* alone is very different from the treatment of AIS alone or coexistent with squamous carcinoma *in situ*.

However, it is as well to realize that within the range

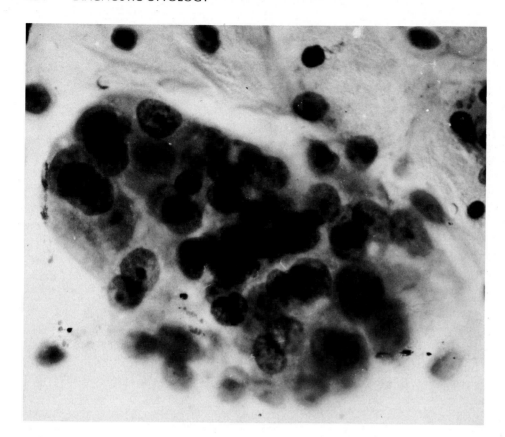

FIGURE 10–33. Ball of **malignant glandular cells** shown in cervical smear, of extrauterine origin from ovary (Papanicolaou stain; ×600).

of adenocarcinoma and its precursors, an invariably accurate prediction is not always possible on cytologic grounds. Further investigation after a cytologic prediction of a glandular lesion certainly includes colposcopy and target biopsy to exclude overt invasive cancer. Accurate diagnosis will then usually depend upon a diagnostic cone biopsy, whereas this investigatory procedure is now rarely performed for squamous abnormalities.

The accuracy of cytologic prediction has been reported from our department in previous publications.[3–5, 11]

The prospective diagnostic accuracy for AIS was 78.5%, and on review, this could be increased to 98.5%. This rate varies between well-differentiated AIS and poorly differentiated AIS. For well-differentiated AIS the criteria are now well established and, hence, the diagnostic accuracy is higher.

An accurate diagnosis of poorly differentiated AIS is much more difficult, with a tendency to overdiagnose such cases as invasive. Smears from poorly differentiated cases of AIS show large nuclei with prominent nucleoli that are occasionally multiple, and the nuclei may not show pseudostratification; hence, the possibility of invasion cannot always be ruled out by cytologic criteria alone.

Furthermore, in very inflammatory smears, the distinction between reactive and neoplastic cells is always difficult. Such cells share so many common criteria that they have sometimes been overidentified as invasive adenocarcinomas. Even on review, this distinction can be extremely difficult. We have found false-nega-

tive diagnosis and false underdiagnosis to be an occasionally problem in the cytodiagnosis of AIS of the cervix uteri.

On several occasions, indicated in our previous publications, review of Papanicolaou smears reported as negative in years when AIS was not so well known has revealed unreported AIS. In some cases, this review has even established the diagnosis when the findings in the current smear have been obscured by inflammatory changes or degeneration.

False underdiagnosis resulted when AIS was missed initially owing to the abundance of atypical squamous cells in four cases of coexisting squamous carcinoma *in situ* and in one case of coexisting invasive squamous cell carcinoma.

There are some reports in the literature concerning the accuracy of diagnosis of invasive adenocarcinoma. Korhonen[28] reported a diagnostic accuracy of cytology of 86% with 14% false-negative results. Reagan and Ng[37] found the diagnostic accuracy of cytology to be 97.4%. Predictive accuracy for invasive adenocarcinoma in our latest series was 95.7%; a few cases were thought to be AIS in the initial smears.[5]

However, a more realistic picture of diagnostic accuracy of cytology smears is revealed in large review series of cases and when the history of previous smears is taken into account. Thus, Littman and colleagues[31] found that cytologic evaluation was not responsible for the detection of any one of 13 mixed adenosquamous carcinomas of the cervix uteri. In eight cases, pretreatment cytologic smears had been reported as negative and yet all contained malignant cells on review.

Hurt and coworkers[25] confirmed that in their series no less than 42% of those cases in which cytology had been performed had a negative result reported.

Benoit and associates[6] found that patients with adenocarcinoma or adenosquamous carcinoma were much more likely to have negative screenings prior to diagnosis than patients with squamous carcinoma. Of 84 patients with Stage I cancers of the cervix, 25 had negative screening within 3 years prior to diagnosis, and in no less than 12 of those (48%), adenocarcinoma or adenosquamous carcinoma developed. The smears were not reviewed to see if sampling error or laboratory error contributed to this, although the discussion covered both possibilities.

Gallup and coworkers[20] reviewed the previous smear histories of 20 patients with adenosquamous carcinoma of the cervix. Of these patients, 55% had had negative smears within the last year. Five of six patients with lesions greater than 2 cm had negative smears.

Boddington and associates[8] actually reviewed the smears of 13 women who had previously had a total of 25 smears from 2 to 8 years before diagnosis. In six patients (eight smears) this review "showed cells which, with hindsight, could be called either clearly malignant, or else suspicious of adenocarcinoma."

The authors also noted that no less than five of these 13 patients had negative or inadequate cervical smears at the time of clinical diagnosis. In fact, in their whole series, the overall false-negative rate for invasive adenocarcinomas was 26.7%.

In light of this discussion, it would be well to remember that cytology should not be recommended as the definitive diagnostic investigation for invasive adenocarcinoma of the cervix uteri. If the clinician is suspicious of invasive cancer at clinical examination, then he or she should proceed to colposcopy and biopsy regardless of the cytologic findings.

References

1. Akahori T, Hasegawa K, Ohtsu F, Kinugasa M, Takeuchi K: Cytologic studies of cervical adenocarcinoma. Acta Obstet Gynecol Jpn 39:70–78, 1987.
2. Anderson MC: In Obstetrical and Gynaecological Pathology, 3rd ed. Edited by Haines and Taylor. Edinburgh, Churchill Livingston, pp 288–296, 1987.
3. Ayer B, Pacey F, Greenberg M, Bousfield L: The cytologic diagnosis of adenocarcinoma in situ of the cervix uteri and related lesions. I. Adenocarcinoma in situ. Acta Cytol 31:397–411, 1987.
4. Ayer B, Pacey F, Greenberg M: The cytologic diagnosis of adenocarcinoma in situ of the cervix uteri and related lesions. II. Microinvasive adenocarcinoma. Acta Cytol 32:318–324, 1988.
5. Ayer B, Pacey F, Greenberg M: The cytologic diagnosis of invasive adenocarcinoma of the cervix uteri. Cytopathology. (accepted for publication).
6. Benoit AG, Krepart GV, Lotocki RJ: Results of prior cytologic screening in patients with a diagnosis of Stage I carcinoma of the cervix. Am J Obstet Gynecol 148:690–694, 1984.
7. Berek JS, Hacker NF, Fu YS, Sokale JR, Leuchter RC, Lagasse LD: Adenocarcinoma of the uterine cervix: Histologic variables associated with lymph node metastasis and survival. Obstet Gynecol 65:46–52, 1985.
8. Boddington MM, Spriggs AI, Cowdrell RH: Adenocarcinoma of the uterine cervix: Cytological evidence of a long preclinical evolution. Br J Obstet Gynaecol 83:900–903, 1976.
9. Boon ME, Alons-van Kordelaar JJ, Rietveld-Scheffers PE: Consequences of the introduction of combined spatula and cytobrush sampling for cervical cytology: Improvements in smear quality and detection rates. Acta Cytol 30:264–270, 1986.
10. Boon ME, Baak JPA, Kurver JPH, Overdiep SH, Verdonk GW: Adenocarcinoma in situ of the cervix: An underdiagnosed lesion. Cancer 48:768–773, 1981.
11. Bousfield L, Pacey F, Young Q, Krumins I, Osborn R: Expanded cytologic criteria for the diagnosis of adenocarcinoma in situ of the cervix and related lesions. Acta Cytol 24:283–296, 1980.
12. Boyes DA: The value of a Pap smear program and suggestions for its implementation. Cancer 48:613–621, 1981.
13. Brand E, Berek JS, Hacker NF: Review: Controversies in the management of cervical adenocarcinoma. Obstet Gynecol 71:261–269, 1988.
14. Davis JR, Moon LB: Increased incidence of adenocarcinoma of the uterine cervix. Obstet Gynecol 45:79–83, 1975.
15. Ferry J, Scully R: Adenoid cystic carcinoma and adenoid basal carcinoma of the uterine cervix. Am J Surg Pathol 12:134–144, 1988.
16. Friedell GH, McKay DG: Adenocarcinoma in situ of the endocervix. Cancer 6:887–897, 1953.
17. Fu YS, Reagan JW, Hsiu JG, Storaasli JP, Wentz WB: Adenocarcinoma and mixed carcinoma of the uterine cervix. I. A clinicopathologic study. Cancer 49:2560–2570, 1982.
18. Fu YS, Reagan JW, Fu AS, Janiga KE: Adenocarcinoma and mixed carcinoma of the uterine cervix. II. Prognostic value of nuclear DNA analysis. Cancer 49:2571–2577, 1982.
19. Gallup DG, Abell MR: Invasive adenocarcinoma of the uterine cervix. Obstet Gynecol 49:596–603, 1977.
20. Gallup DG, Harper RH, Stock RJ: Poor prognosis in patients with adenosquamous cell carcinoma of the cervix. Obstet Gynecol 65:416–422, 1985.
21. Hasumi K, Ehrmann RL: Clear cell carcinoma of the uterine endocervix with an in situ component. Cancer 42:2435–2438, 1978.
22. Herbst AL, Robboy SJ, Scully RE, Poskanzer DC: Clear cell carcinoma of the vagina and cervix in girls: Analysis of 170 registry cases. Am J Obstet Gynecol 119:713–724, 1974.
23. Herbst AL, Ulfelder H, Poskanzer DC: Adenocarcinoma of the vagina: Association of maternal stilbestrol therapy with tumor appearance in young women. N Engl J Med 284:878–881, 1971.
24. Horowitz IR, Jacobson LP, Zucker PK, Currie JL, Rosenshein NB: Epidemiology of adenocarcinoma of the cervix. Gynecol Oncol 31:25–31, 1988.
25. Hurt GW, Silverberg SG, Fable WJ, Belgrad R, Crooks LD: Adenocarcinoma of the cervix: Histopathologic and clinical features. Am J Obstet Gynecol 129:304–315, 1977.
26. Jaworski R, Pacey F, Greenberg M, Osborn R: The histologic diagnosis of adenocarcinoma in situ and related lesions of the cervix uteri: Adenocarcinoma in situ. Cancer 61:1171–1181, 1987.
27. Julian CG, Diakoku NH, Gillespie A: Adenoepidermoid and adenosquamous carcinoma of the uterus: A clinical pathological study of 118 patients. Am J Obstet Gynecol 128:106–115, 1977.
28. Korhonen MO: Adenocarcinoma of the uterine cervix. Acta Pathol Microbiol Immunol Scand [Suppl] 264:1–51, 1978.
29. Krumins I, Young Q, Pacey F, Bousfield L, Mulhearn L: The cytologic diagnosis of adenocarcinoma in situ of the cervix uteri. Acta Cytol 21:320–329, 1977.
30. Laverty CR, Farnsworth A, Thurloe J, Bowditch R: The reliability of cytological prediction of cervical adenocarcinoma in situ. Aust NZ J Obstet Gynaecol 28:307–312, 1988.
31. Littman P, Clement PB, Henriksen B, Wang CC, Robboy SJ, Taft PD, Ulfelder H, Scully RE: Glassy cell carcinoma of the cervix. Cancer 37:2238–2246, 1976.
32. Mayer EG, Galindi J, Davis J, Wurzel J, Aristizabal S: Adenocarcinoma of the uterine cervix: Incidence and role of radiation therapy. Radiology 121:725–727, 1976.
33. Osborn RA: Personal communication, 1989.
34. Ostor AG, Pagan R, Davoren RAM, Fortune DW, Chanen W, Rome R: Adenocarcinoma in situ of the cervix. Int J Gynecol Pathol 3:179–190, 1984.

35. Pacey F, Ayer B, Greenberg M: The cytologic diagnosis of adenocarcinoma *in situ* of the cervix uteri and related lesions. III. Pitfalls in diagnosis. Acta Cytol 32:325–330, 1988.

36. Pollack RS, Taylor HC: Carcinoma of the cervix during the first two decades of life. Am J Obstet Gynecol. 53:135–141, 1947.

37. Reagan JW, Ng ABP: The Cells of Uterine Adenocarcinoma. *In* Monographs in Clinical Cytology, Vol 1, 2nd ed. Edited by GL Wied. Basel, S Karger, pp 88–113, 1973.

38. Reagan JW, Ng ABP: Cellular detection of glandular neoplasms of the uterine cervix. *In* Compendium on Diagnostic Cytology, 6th ed. Edited by GL Wied. Chicago, Tutorials of Cytology, pp 146–153, 1988.

39. Rosenthal DL, McLatchie C, Stern E, White BS, Castleman KR: Endocervical columnar cell atypia coincident with cervical neoplasia characterized by digital image analysis. Acta Cytol 26:115–120, 1982.

40. Schwartz SM, Weiss NS: Increased incidence of adenocarcinoma of the cervix in young women in the United States. Am J Epidemiol 124:1045–1047, 1986.

41. Shingleton HM, Gore H, Bradley DH, Soong SJ: Adenocarcinoma of the cervix. I. Clinical evaluation and pathologic features. Am J Obstet Gynecol 139:799–814, 1981.

42. Smotkin D, Berek JS, Fu YS: Human papillomavirus DNA in adenocarcinoma and adenosquamous carcinoma of the uterine cervix. Obstet Gynecol 68:241–244, 1986.

43. Spurrett BS. Personal communication regarding records of Royal Prince Alfred Hospital, Camperdown, Australia, 1988.

44. Steiner G, Friedell GH: Adenosquamous carcinoma *in situ* of the cervix. Cancer 18:807–810, 1965.

45. Szyfelbein WM, Young RH, Scully RE: Adenoma malignum of the cervix: Cytologic findings. Acta Cytol 28:691–698, 1984.

46. Tamimi HK, Figge DC: Adenocarcinoma of the uterine cervix. Gynecol Oncol 13:335–344, 1982.

47. Tamimi HK, Marit EK, Hesla J, Cain JM, Figge DC, Greer BE: Glassy cell carcinoma of the cervix redefined. Obstet Gynecol 71:837–841, 1988.

48. Tasker JT, Collins JA: Adenocarcinoma of the uterine cervix. Am J Obstet Gynecol 118:344–358, 1974.

49. Tock E, Shilkin K: Pathological studies on adenocarcinoma of the uterine cervix in Singapore. Pathology 6:275–286, 1974.

50. Weiss RJ, Lucas WE: Adenocarcinoma of the uterine cervix. Cancer 57:1996–2001, 1986.

51. Young QA, Pacey NF: The cytologic diagnosis of clear cell adenocarcinoma of the cervix uteri. Acta Cytol 22:3–6, 1978.

11

Endometrial Hyperplasia and Carcinoma and Extrauterine Cancer

Alan B. P. Ng

Over the past 3 decades, the frequency of endometrial carcinoma has been progressively rising while that of cervical squamous cell cancer has been declining. The increase in the number of endocervical adenocarcinoma cases is less conspicuous. As early as 1965, the frequency of endometrial carcinoma surpassed that of cervical squamous cancer in many countries, including the United States.[15] This increase is in part due to the rising age of the population, the changing social conditions, the greater use of unopposed estrogen and the relative lack of good screening programs for the detection of endometrial carcinoma and its precursors. Preliminary evidence indicates that with the decreased use of unopposed estrogen, there has been some parallel decline in the frequency of endometrial cancer.[25] However, today, it is still the most common cancer of the female genital tract in many countries.

This chapter dicusses cytologic techniques pertinent to the detection of endometrial disease and extrauterine cancer. Discussion of endometrial cells is divided into those forcibly removed by direct endometrial sampling and those spontaneously desquamated as are seen in endocervical and vaginal samples, because the method of cellular preparation, approach and criteria

TABLE 11–1. Cervical Scrape and Aspiration Samples— 270,000 Samples Over 9 Years

Nature of Endometrial Cells	Cases	Percent (%)
Normal endometrial cells		
First half of cycle	1688	0.6
Second half of cycle or postmenopause	3024	1.2
Hyperplastic endometrial cells	594	0.2
Malignant endometrial cells	121	0.04
Total	5427	2.0

utilized and the differences in morphologic changes vary in these two procedures. Basic histology and histopathology, normal and abnormal endometrial cells, malignant cells derived from extrauterine origin and their differential diagnosis are discussed. Accuracy based on various cellular techniques in the detection of endometrial cancer and precursor changes as well as extrauterine cancer is presented.

SAMPLING TECHNIQUES

Cytology can contribute to the detection of endometrial carcinoma, including early lesions, and its precursors, if increased awareness by laboratory staff in the search for endometrial cells, improved education in the recognition of normal and abnormal endometrial cells and improved cellular sampling techniques and quality of sample are in evidence. Endometrial cytology probably represents the most difficult area in gynecologic cytology. Endometrial cells are not frequently present in routine cellular samples; however, when present, they may be significant and are not often recognized. Furthermore, cell samples that are optimal for the detection of cervical squamous cell cancer and its precursors are not optimal for the detection of endometrial carcinoma.

Based on 5427 consecutive cases of 270,000 cytologic samples over a 9-year period, when each case consisted of a cervical scrape and endocervical aspiration, 2% of cases contained normal or abnormal endometrial cells (Table 11–1). Most of the endometrial cells were seen in the endocervical aspirate sample. Normal-appearing endometrial cells were seen in 1.8% of the cases, 0.6% were seen when the specimens were collected during the first half of the menstrual cycle and 1.2% during the second half of the cycle or the postmenopausal period. Hyperplastic endometrial cells were reported in 594 or 0.2% of cases. Malignant endometrial cells were recorded in 121 or 0.04% of cases. Of the 5427 cases that contained normal or abnormal endometrial cells, endometrial cells were seen in 5415 or 99.8% from the endocervical aspirate sample and only 1109 or 24% from the cervical scrape sample. The frequency of endometrial cells seen in women of reproductive age depends on the day of the cycle that the cell sample is obtained.[24, 31]

An optimal sample should consistently provide a large concentration of well-preserved representative cells and be readily obtained.[16] *Direct endometrial sampling* is optimal and provides an adequate amount of well-preserved material for the study of endometrial pathology. It can be performed in the physician's office or in outpatient clinics and does not require a general anesthetic. Major complications, such as uterine perforation, in competent hands are rare. However, the procedure has to be performed under sterile conditions by a physician; it is relatively expensive and time consuming and creates more discomfort when compared with routine Papanicolaou smears. The endometrial sample is also more difficult to interpret, requiring more experience and practice. Currently, a lack of consistency and sufficient data on differentiating normal from pathologic hyperplasia, and pathologic hyperplasia from well-differentiated carcinoma on a cellular basis, exists. This procedure will not be cost-effective for mass screening and should probably be applied to those women who are at high risk for the development of endometrial cancer and to those in whom endometrial disease is suspected, such as in the presence of endometrial cells in cervical samples of older or postmenopausal patients. Periodic endometrial sampling of postmenopausal women, for example every 3 years, may increase the detection rate of endometrial cancer and its precursors.

Techniques that may obtain endometrial cells based on spontaneous desquamation from the endometrium include *endocervical, cervical* and *vaginal sampling.* These procedures are inexpensive and simple to perform. The ectocervical scrape and contents from the posterior vaginal fornix are not ideally suited for the detection of endometrial carcinoma and, especially, endometrial hyperplasia. Endometrial cells when seen in the vaginal samples are usually few in number and tend to show degenerate changes making accurate evaluation difficult. Short of direct endometrial sampling, the endocervical sample is the next most valuable cytologic technique in detecting endometrial cancer and, to a lesser extent, endometrial hyperplasia. As the endocervical canal is in close proximity to the endometrial cavity, endometrial cells collected from this location tend to be better preserved and are relatively more abundant when compared with vaginal and ectocervical samples. Thus, the endocervical sample together with the ectocervical sample is not only ideal in the evaluation of cervical squamous and endocervical lesions but is also suitable for the detection of endometrial cancer and often its precursors, short of applying the more complex endometrial sampling procedure.

These two sampling procedures—cervical scrape and endocervical sampling—should be employed for all cases, especially if endocervical, endometrial, or both lesions are suspected. Numerous types of endocervical and endometrial samplers are now commercially available; however, some of them become expensive when large numbers are used. Often, a modified Ayre spatula with an extended, elongated tip is adequate for sampling the endocervix and secretions in the canal. This technique is much more economical than many endocervical samples. The use of a glass endocervical aspirator with a rubber bulb, if properly carried out, is also more economical.

The utilization of a nonabsorbable cotton swab to collect material from the endocervical canal is generally inferior, as the sample usually contains a limited number of representative cells and the cells tend to be distorted making accurate evaluation difficult or impossible. Irrespective of the type of sampler, the person performing the procedure must be familiar and comfortable when using the instrument. It should not cause too much discomfort to the patient, and the technique should provide an adequate amount of material for evaluation. Furthermore, the cost of the sampler should be taken into consideration.

CLINICAL INFORMATION

Another important prerequisite in the evaluation of the endometrium by the cytologic approach is the provision of pertinent clinical information if optimal benefit is to be obtained in the detection of endometrial pathology. The nature of the sample should be indicated in the requisition form, as it may assist in the preparation and approach to the evaluation of the cell sample. The patient's age, the date of onset of the last menstrual period and the date the cellular sample was obtained, permitting calculation of the exact day of the cycle, and the menopausal status should be provided. For example, the presence of normal-appearing endometrial cells in an endocervical sample seen in the second half of the menstrual cycle in a woman of 20 may not be as important, as the cause is usually not related to neoplasia, whereas the presence of normal-appearing endometrial cells in the second half of the cycle in a woman of 48 or in a postmenopausal woman is more likely to be associated with endometrial neoplasia. The use of any exogenous hormones, intrauterine devices or recent intrauterine instrumentation may cause shedding of endometrial cells at a time that is not normally expected. Relevant clinical diagnosis and the existing complaint should also be noted in the requisition form. Sometimes, on the basis of the cellular evidence, it may be possible to resolve the clinical problem or complaint. Although some of this information will not be applicable in every case, the contribution of the cellular evaluation is directly related to the amount of pertinent clinical information provided.

HISTOLOGY OF NORMAL ENDOMETRIUM

The endometrium is a modified mucosa lining the uterine cavity. During the reproductive years, the endometrium undergoes regular cyclic changes as a result of ovarian hormonal influence. Depending on the stage of the menstrual cycle, the endometrium varies in thickness from 1 mm to 8 mm and consists of the thin basal layer, which abuts the myometrium, and the functional layer lying superficial to the basal layer. The functional layer can be divided into the superficial or compacta layer, consisting of relatively few glands and abundant stroma, and the deep or spongiosa layer containing an abundance of glands and relatively less stroma. The functional layer is extremely sensitive to ovarian hormonal influence, whereas the basal layer is not. The epithelial cells lining the surface and glands of the functional layer consist predominantly of secretory cells, whereas ciliated and intercalated cells are less frequently encountered. The intercalated cell type is considered to be degenerative or nonactive secretory cell. The epithelial cells in the basal layer are low columnar with basal nuclei. They are nonsecretory and nonciliated. The cells in the endometrial stroma are called endometrial stromal cells, which may be divided into superficial stromal cells located in the superficial portion of the functional layer and deep stromal cells located in the spongiosa portion and basal layer.

Based on a 28-day menstrual cycle, the changes of the endometrium may be divided into menstrual phase day 1 to 4; proliferative phase day 5 to 14, also known as follicular or preovulatory phase; and the secretory phase day 15 to 28, also known as postovulatory or luteal phase. The day of onset of menstrual bleeding is considered to be day 1 of the cycle, and the bleeding lasts for about 4 days when most of the functional layer of the endometrium is desquamated in minute fragments, cell clusters and single cells. The basal layer remains intact with some residual functional layer, which then begins to regenerate and proliferate from day 5 to day 14 owing to stimulation by estrogen from the ovary. This stimulation results in a rapid increase in the thickness of the endometrium with the formation of new endometrial glands and stroma.

At the beginning of the proliferative phase, the surface and glandular epithelia are composed of relatively small cuboidal cells. The glands are straight and narrow. Towards the end of the proliferative phase, the cells assume a pseudostratified columnar form and are attached to the basement membrane, but not all cells reach the surface of the glandular lumen. The nuclei are basal or intermediate in location. The glands increase in size and appear tortuous. The stromal cells are small, spindle-shaped or stellate with scanty cytoplasm and indistinct cell borders. The nuclei are round, oval or reniform. A longitudinal groove may be seen in the nuclei of deep stromal cells.

Ovulation usually occurs in the middle of a 28-day cycle heralding in the secretory phase from day 15 to day 28. Under the influence of progesterone and estrogen from the ovary, glycogen appears as subnuclear vacuoles in the cytoplasm beneath the nucleus and displaces the nucleus from the basal position of the cell. The vacuoles migrate around the nucleus to lie in the apical portion and then discharge into the glandular lumen as secretions. The endometrial glands become plumper and more tortuous. The stromal cells, especially from the superficial layer, accumulate cytoplasmic volume, become larger and appear polyhedral, resulting in an epithelioid-appearance with more distinct cell borders. These cells are known as predecidual or pseudodecidual cells or if pregnancy occurs decidual cells. Ciliated cells are most numerous during the middle and late proliferative phase and the early secretory phase. If pregnancy does not occur, with the cessation of hormones from the ovary, desquamation of the endometrium occurs, resulting in menstrual flow, marking the beginning of a new cycle.

In postmenopausal women, the endometrium eventually becomes thin and atrophic and the epithelial cells become smaller, low columnar or cuboidal. The stromal cells also become smaller with inconspicuous cytoplasm.

NORMAL ENDOMETRIAL CELLS

Considerable experience is required to master the identification of the normal features of endometrial cells, partly because these cells are small and minor structural changes may be significant. Their cellular appearance changes in response to hormonal and other stimulation, and several types of endometrial cells are known. The appearance of the endometrial cells is related to many factors, most important of which are the site of origin of the several different cell types of the endometrium, the stage of the menstrual cycle, the menopausal status, the perspective from which the cells are viewed, the state of preservation of the cells, the method used to collect the sample and the processing and staining technique.

Normal Cells Removed by Direct Sampling

The number of cells and their distribution in a sample depend in large part on the technique of endometrial sampling. Thus, the Vakutage or Vabra device samples often contain fragments of macroscopic tissue as well as single cells and groups of cells, whereas an endometrial sampler contains a sample that can be smeared on a glass slide and fixed in the same manner as a routine Papanicolaou smear. Macroscopic tissue fragments are also less likely to be obtained. Grossly recognizable tissue fragments are best embedded in paraffin for sectioning and interpreted as in routine surgical specimens (Fig. 11–1). Often endocervical cells are seen in endometrial samples and should be differentiated from endometrial cells. The appearance of endocervical cells is similar to that of endocervical or

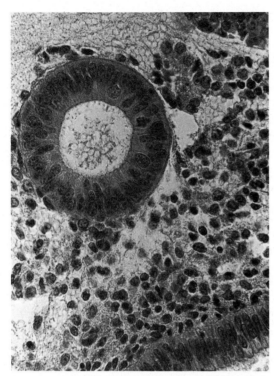

FIGURE 11–1. Proliferative endometrium. Microfragment showing endometrial gland and stroma. Cell block preparation from a direct endometrial sample (hematoxylin and eosin; ×400).

The secretory or nonciliated cell is the most common of the cells found. During the proliferative phase, the cell area varies from 60 μ to 80 μ², about half to two-thirds the size of normal endocervical cells. The cytoplasmic border is ill-defined, making accurate evaluation of cell size difficult. The scanty cytoplasm is cyanophilic and finely vacuolated. The nucleus is round or oval and is approximately the same size as the nucleus of a normal intermediate squamous cell (40 μ²). The chromatin is uniformly powdery and finely granular with one or two chromocenters. Micronucleoli are infrequently seen.

In the secretory phase, the epithelial cells in sheets are more spaced apart owing to an increased cytoplasmic volume, and the cytoplasmic border is more distinct. Depending on the perspective from which the cells are viewed, subnuclear vacuolization may be seen during the early secretory phase. Later, vacuolization becomes more diffuse to see. The cytoplasmic stain changes from cyanophilia to an intermediate or slight eosinophilia, as secretion accumulates. The nucleus becomes displaced to the base or periphery of the cell and may be indented. The discharge of secretion from the cell is followed by a reduction in cytoplasmic volume and cell size. Late in the secretory phase, associated shrinkage of the nucleus and variable evidence of degeneration occur. The intercalated cells probably represent compressed, nonfunctioning secre-

cervical scrape samples.[23] Normal endometrial cells are observed at any time during the menstrual cycle and postmenopausal period. The three types of epithelial cells are the secretory cell, ciliated cell and intercalated cell. In addition, superficial and deep stromal cells are present. The relative frequency of these cells is related to the stage of the menstrual cycle and the functional state of the epithelium.[24]

Normal endometrial cells are seen in aggregates and, less frequently, singly. The aggregates occur in sheets of various sizes and shapes with or without glandular openings, smaller groupings and strips (Fig. 11–2). Epithelial, stromal or both cell types may be seen in the same sheet. The aggregates have uniform cell and nuclear size and normal polarity and architectural arrangement. The sheets are usually monolayer and are more frequently encountered during the secretory phase. Mitotic figures may be seen, especially during the proliferative phase. Occasionally blood vessels may be seen. Stomas of glands when identified are usually uniform in size and are more closely approximated and smaller in the proliferative phase and more widely separated and larger in the secretory phase. When viewed in proper perspective, the stomas are lined by a single layer of cells that is relatively uniform. The cells are regularly arranged in relationship to one another.

Depending on the perspective from which the epithelial cells are viewed, they may appear columnar, cuboidal, round or oval. The appearance of the stromal cells is dictated by the cell type and phase of the cycle.

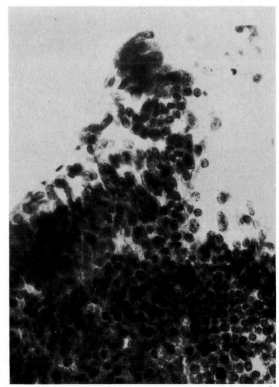

FIGURE 11–2. Proliferative endometrium. Sheets of endometrium where the cells are regularly arranged in relationship to one another and uniform in size and shape. Smear preparation from a direct endometrial sample (Papanicolaou stain; ×400).

tory cells. They are long, thin, prismatic forms with distention in the vicinity of the oval or slightly elongated nucleus. Ciliated cells are prismatic in form and when viewed in the proper perspective, cilia may be identified. A distinct row of anchoring granules may be present beneath the fine border of the cell, occurring alone or with cilia.

During the early proliferative phase, endometrial stromal cells have a mean area of 45 μ^2. They become progressively larger and reach a size of 100 μ^2 in the late secretory phase. This increase in size and the following changes are seen mainly in superficial stromal cells. The cells are round or oval with an ill-defined cytoplasmic outline and scanty cytoplasm with an amphophilic stain. Unless associated with degenerative changes, large cytoplasmic vacuolization is inconspicuous in stromal cells. The nuclear size progressively increases during the menstrual cycle from 35 to 50 μ^2. The nucleus is round, oval or reniform. The nuclear chromatin is finely granular, becoming more granular as the proliferative phase progresses. Small nucleoli may be seen in some cells. Mitoses may occur in the stromal cells. During the secretory phase, especially at the late stage, a conspicuous increase of cytoplasmic volume occurs owing to glycogen accumulation with peripheral condensation of the cytoplasmic matrix, giving the round, oval or polygonal cell an epithelioid appearance. The cytoplasm remains weakly staining and appears foamy. The fully developed stromal cells are characteristic of decidual cells.

The deep stromal cells, especially those originating from the basal layer, tend to remain unchanged throughout the menstrual cycle or under hormonal influence. They remain small, spindle shaped, and sometimes stellate in form. Another type of endometrial stromal cell is the granular or "K" cell, which is relatively inconspicuous. The cytoplasm is scanty, finely vacuolated and contains small acidophilic granules. The nucleus is oval or reniform and usually excentric. The nucleus has finely granular chromatin and small chromatocenters. They are seen more frequently during the late secretory phase.

During the menstrual phase, the sheets and cell clusters are fragmented and single normal cells are more frequently encountered. They appear necrotic or degenerate. Cellular aggregates consisting of a peripheral rim of epithelial cells and a central core of stromal cells, similar to those seen in "exodus" in endocervical or vaginal samples, are present. Associated blood, inflammatory cells and cellular debris are present in the specimen. Few inflammatory cells, especially lymphocytes and neutrophils, are seen in endometrial cell samples, and they may be derived from the cervix or from the endometrium and do not usually indicate infection.

Endometrial samples obtained from postmenopausal women usually contain fewer fragments and glandular stomas are inconspicuous. The cellular features are similar to those seen in early proliferative phase or appear atrophic; however, mitoses are absent. Thus, the cells are small and appear normal.

When macroscopic fragments are obtained by the endometrial sampling technique, they are processed by the cell block technique as for surgical specimens. These fragments, although relatively small, permit histologic interpretation as for tissue changes described employing criteria similar to those applied to histologic specimens.

Endometrial samples often contain varying numbers of endocervical columnar cells and sometimes squamous and squamous metaplastic cells from the cervix.

Spontaneously Desquamated Normal Cells

Cells that are spontaneously desquamated from the endometrium and found in the cervical or vaginal secretions are quite different in appearance than those forcibly removed from the endometrium.[24] In obeying the law of surface tension, the desquamated endometrial cells tend to round up to look like soap bubbles in many instances. Consequently, endometrial cells with columnar configurations and in sheets are inconspicuous in the cervical or vaginal aspirates. Singly, they appear round, oval or low cuboidal. In aggregate, they approach a cell-ball pattern with molding of the peripheral margin or closely approximated groupings of varying shapes and sizes. The conditions at the time of desquamation, the environment into which they are shed and the interval that has elapsed since the cells were shed further modify the appearance of the desquamated cells. If these factors are unfavorable, the endometrial cells may be so degenerate and few in number that detailed study and accurate evaluation become difficult or impossible. The cervical mucus is usually a good environment for the preservation of desquamated endometrial cells when compared with material in the posterior vaginal fornix. For this reason, samples obtained from the cervical canal are more apt to be satisfactory for cell evaluation than those obtained from the vagina.

Endometrial cells that are spontaneously desquamated may be of epithelial or stromal origin. Often, it is not possible to distinguish betwen endometrial epithelial and stromal cells. Epithelial cells are seen singly and in aggregates. Aggregates may be small or large and appear as tight compact cell balls. A loose or tight monolayer of cells of varying sizes and shapes is seen where the cells and nuclei have a comparable size with a normal polarity (Fig. 11–3). Sometimes, poorly formed or part of acinous groupings are identified; however, the cells are regularly arranged and singly layered.

In single cells and cell aggregates, the endometrial cells appear small, slightly larger than large lymphocytes and neutrophils, with a round, an oval or a low cuboidal configuration (Fig. 11–4). The cytoplasmic border is poorly defined, and the scanty cytoplasm appears foamy or finely vacuolated and stains weakly cyanophilic or indeterminate and, less often, eosinophilic. Large distinct cytoplasmic vacuoles are less frequently present. Neutrophils in cytoplasmic vacuoles, a sign of degenerative or reactive change, are

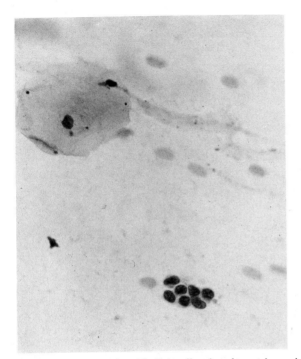

FIGURE 11–3. Normal epithelial cells of endometrium, day 6 of menstrual cycle. The nuclear size is comparable to that of the intermediate squamous cell. Endocervical aspirate (Papanicolaou stain; ×480). (Reproduced with permission from Ng ABP, Reagan JW, Cechner RL: The precursors of endometrial cancer: A study of their cellular manifestation. Acta Cytol 17:439–448, 1973.)

infrequently seen in endometrial cells. This is a non-characteristic feature that can be seen in other cell types, especially endocervical columnar and squamous metaplastic cells.

Degenerate single cells and cell aggregates of endometrial cells often have a eosinophilic cast over them, a feature also seen in poorly fixed or air-dried cells stained with the Papanicolaou stain. The nucleus measures about 35 to 40 μ^2, approximately the size of the nucleus of a normal intermediate squamous cell. It is round or oval and usually excentric in location. In viable and well-preserved cells, the chromatinic material is finely granular and evenly distributed. One or two distinct small chromocenters are observed. Micronucleoli are rarely encountered in normal endometrial cells. Sometimes, the nuclear membrane may appear to be irregularly or regularly thickened due to deposition of chromatinic material beneath the nuclear membrane, known as "chromatinic membrane," a manifestation of early cell death. Pyknotic dark nuclei are also encountered.

The superficial stromal cells also occur singly and in loose aggregates (Fig. 11–5). They are generally bigger than epithelial cells with some variation in size. The cell size, distinction of cytoplasmic border and cytoplasmic volume depend on stage of menstrual cycle and hormonal influence. The cytoplasm can be scanty or moderately abundant with inconspicuous cell borders. It stains weakly cyanophilic or amphophilic with

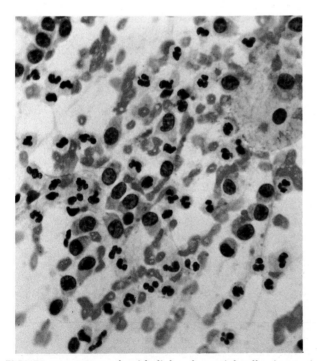

FIGURE 11–4. Normal epithelial endometrial cells, day 3 of menstrual cycle. Most of the cells occur singly and appear round or cuboidal in form. Endocervical aspirate (Papanicolaou stain; ×520).

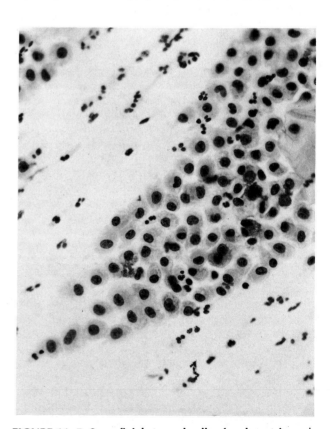

FIGURE 11–5. Superficial stromal cells of endometrium, day 6 of menstrual cycle. The cells are most readily recognized when in groups. Endocervical aspirate (Papanicolaou stain; ×360).

fine small vacuoles. Larger vacuoles are less frequently encountered.

The nucleus is round, oval or reniform and may be centrally or excentrically located. The nuclear size may vary from 35 to 50 μ^2. Large stromal cells with a round or polygonal appearance that contain a moderate amount of cytoplasm, giving them an epithelioid appearance, are known as decidual cells. Decidual cells may be seen in late secretory phase, during pregnancy and with exogenous progestational effect. In contrast, deep stromal cells, occurring singly or in aggregates, are no larger than endometrial epithelial cells, and they are oval or spindle shaped with ill-defined cell borders and scanty weakly staining cyanophilic or amphophilic cytoplasm (Fig. 11–6). The nuclei are oval or spindle shaped and more hyperchromatic, but the chromatin remains uniformly granular. Infolding of the nuclear envelope, producing a longitudinal nuclear groove, is sometimes seen. Stromal cells, especially deep stromal cells, are prone to be desquamated together with double-contoured masses made up of an inner core of stromal cells and an outer rim of epithelial cells on days 6 to 10 in the normal cycle, referred to as exodus (Fig. 11–7). These double-contoured masses are accompanied by a moderate number of stromal cells and neutrophils with a clean background. During the first few days of the menstrual cycle, excessive blood and degenerate material with endometrial cells are often seen in cervical or vaginal samples.

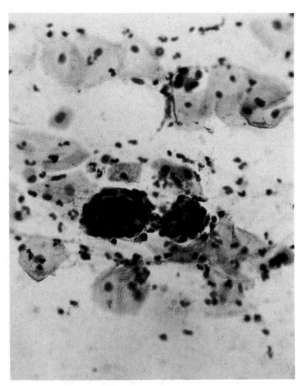

FIGURE 11–7. Normal endometrial cells in characteristic cell balls observed at "exodus," day 9 of menstrual cycle. Endocervical aspirate (Papanicolaou stain; ×320).

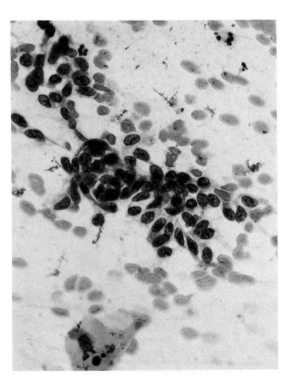

FIGURE 11–6. Deep stromal cells of endometrium, day 7 of menstrual cycle. Endocervical aspirate (Papanicolaou stain; ×480).

Frequency and Significance of Spontaneous Desquamation

During menstruation, as a result of ischemia, a large portion of the functional layer of the endometrium is shed. Thus, it might be anticipated, in samples collected from the cervical canal or the posterior vaginal fornix, that endometrial cells are observed frequently on days 1 to 5 of the menstrual cycle and progressively less frequently on days 6 to 14. Endometrial cells are identified in about 50% of the samples on day 1 of the cycle, 80 to 90% on days 2 to 5, 50% on days 6 to 7, 10 to 20% on days 7 to 10 and 5% on days 11 to 14. Spontaneously desquamated endometrial cells are rarely seen in healthy women from samples collected during the secretory phase, being observed in about 1% of cases. Endometrial cells are rarely seen in samples from healthy postmenopausal women.[24]

During the first few days of the cycle, not only are endometrial cells frequently seen, they are seen in large numbers, consisting of small and large aggregates as well as single cells with a bloody background and inflammatory cells. The number of endometrial cells is in the thousands. In contrast, the number of abnormal cells spontaneously desquamated from hyperplastic and malignant endometrial lesions are relatively few, usually varying from a few cells in hyperplasia to a few hundred cells in carcinoma. During the later part of the first half of the cycle, the number of endometrial cells present progressively decreases. When endometrial cells are shed during the secretory phase or postmenopausal period, they are usually relatively few in number.

For practical purposes, the presence of endometrial cells during the first half of the cycle is due to physiologic shedding, and when seen in the second half of the cycle and in the postmenopausal period, it is related to abnormal shedding and must be explained. The number of endometrial cells due to abnormal shedding are usually less than 100 cells per sample in the majority of cases. Many benign endometrial lesions may cause abnormal shedding of normal-appearing endometrial cells. The frequency of the abnormal changes and the nature of the changes are dependent on the age and menopausal status of the woman. Endometrial epithelial cells, stromal cells, or both may be shed during the immediate postpartum period, during pregnancy and during impending abortion or immediate postabortion period. Other benign conditions that may cause abnormal shedding of endometrial cells include dysfunctional uterine bleeding, contraceptive hormonal therapy, estrogen therapy, intrauterine devices, anovulatory changes, recent endometrial instrumentation, endometritis, pyometra, benign endometrial polyp, submucous myoma and endometriosis especially of the cervix and vagina. Based on the review of the clinical data of 2238 consecutive cases in which normal-appearing endometrial cells were observed during the second half of the cycle or postmenopausal period, associated benign processes are shown (Table 11–2).[16] A large percentage apparently have no associated clinical findings; however, many on subsequent investigation, including endometrial curettage, showed endometrial polyps or benign endometrial changes such as anovulation and endometritis. The benign conditions are most frequently encountered in women 40 years and younger. Estrogen use is the most frequently recorded finding among postmenopausal women.

In a small percentage of women with pathologic endometrial hyperplasia and invasive adenocarcinoma, endometrial cells are shed that appear within normal limits and do not have cytologic features of pathologic hyperplasia or malignancy. This finding is rarely associated with women under 40 years of age as shown in a study in Table 11–3 in which tissue diagnosis was available for evaluation with cytologic findings.[16] Association with endometrial cancer and its precursors increases with the greater age of the patient after 40

TABLE 11–2. Abnormal Shedding of Endometrial Cells in Benign Conditions

Clinical Information	Number	Percent (%)
Dysfunctional bleeding	401	17.2
Contraceptive hormone	255	11.0
Intrauterine device	26	5.4
Estrogen therapy	56	2.4
Myomas	42	1.8
Others*	26	1.1
Negative history	1422	61.1
Total	2328	100.0

*Endometritis, endometriosis, pregnancy, post-partum, recent endometrial instrumentation. (Reproduced with permission from Ng ABP, Reagan JW: Normal endometrial cells and their significance in the detection of benign and malignant endometrial lesions. *In* Compendium on Diagnostic Cytology, 6th ed. Edited by GL Weid, CM Keebler, LG Koss, JW Reagan. Chicago, Tutorials of Cytology, p 162, 1988.)

years of age, and this finding is particularly significant in postmenopausal women. Furthermore, the frequency and nature of endometrial changes were not significantly different in asymptomatic and symptomatic women.[20]

Some 57% of the women with associated carcinoma and 70% with pathologic hyperplasia were asymptomatic at the time of cellular study. The cancer was usually well-differentiated, focal and confined to the endometrium. Of the cases with normal or benign endometrial lesions, two thirds were asymptomatic at the time of cellular study. As shown in Table 11–4, different types of endometrial cells were identified irrespective of the nature of the endometrial disease. Normal epithelial endometrial cells were most frequently identified alone. Both epithelial and stromal cells were frequently encountered, and endometrial stromal cells were infrequently encountered alone in cellular samples.

A number of healthy women having no endometrial or benign endometrial diseases, endometrial polyps or pathologic endometrial hyperplasia shed a comparable number of normal-appearing endometrial cells, averaging about 60 cells per slide. In contrast, an average of 110 normal-appearing endometrial cells per slide were seen in women with endometrial cancer. However, in samples that contain abnormal endometrial cells, an average of 160 hyperplastic and 430 malignant endometrial cells per sample were observed in patients with endometrial hyperplasia and endometrial carcinoma, respectively.[19, 24]

TABLE 11–3. Abnormal Shedding of Normal-Appearing Endometrial Cells in Relation to Age

Tissue Diagnosis	<40 Years	40 to 49 Years	50 to 59 Years	>60 Years
Normal/benign endometrium (%)	90	63	44	40
Endometrial polyp (%)	9	28	41	29
Endometrial hyperplasia (%)	1	7	11	18
Adenocarcinoma (%)	0	2	4	13
Total cases	195	237	188	76

Modified after Ng ABP, Reagan JW, Hawkiczek S, Wentz BW: Significance of endometrial cells in the detection of endometrial carcinoma and its precursors. Acta Cytol 18:356–361, 1974.

TABLE 11–4. Types of Normal-Appearing Endometrial Cells in Relation to Endometrial Disease

Endometrial Cell Type in Samples	Endometrial Tissue Diagnosis			
	Normal/Benign	*Polyp*	*Hyperplasia*	*Carcinoma*
Epithelial (%)	52	52	59	65
Epithelial & Stromal (%)	34	40	32	31
Stromal (%)	14	8	9	4

Modified after Ng ABP, Reagan JW, Hawkiczek S, Wentz BW: Significance of endometrial cells in the detection of endometrial carcinoma and its precursors. Acta Cytol 18:356–361, 1974.

CYTOLOGY OF BENIGN ENDOMETRIAL LESIONS

Benign endometrial changes commonly seen include the various causes of dysfunctional bleeding secondary to hormonal imbalance, exogenous hormonal effects, pregnancy changes, intrauterine-device effects, endometritis, polyps and benign tumors such as a submucous leiomyoma. Cytologic specimens from direct endometrial samples or cervical or vaginal aspirates are not usually used and are not optimal specimens in the diagnosis of benign endometrial conditions. They are utilized primarily for the detection of endometrial cancer and its precursors. With few exceptions, the characteristic cytologic features of benign endometrial lesions appear within normal limits, slightly atypical or reactive and may be confused with and must be differentiated from malignant or premalignant changes. Sometimes, benign endometrial lesions shed normal-appearing endometrial cells at a time they are not normally expected to in vaginal or cervical aspirates. Any abnormal shedding of endometrial cells or any cytologic atypia of endometrial cells should be investigated. Although most are due to benign lesions, some may be associated with cancer and its precursors.[20] Unless such changes are investigated, usually by evaluating a tissue sample, it is not possible to accurately delineate most of the benign endometrial entities from neoplastic causes by cytology alone. This factor is particularly important in perimenopausal and postmenopausal women.

Direct Endometrial Sample

Not many characteristic diagnostic cytologic changes in cellular samples are associated with benign endometrial lesions except when tissue fragments are present, which are then best processed and interpreted as histologic tissue specimens. Sometimes, in cell samples, some cytologic changes may indicate benign endometrial lesions. In samples from patients on exogenous progesterone therapy or oral contraceptives, decidual changes of stromal cells with small narrow openings of glands, widely spaced and indicating atrophy, may be seen in fragments of endometrial tissues as is seen in tissue preparations.

In pregnancy, multinucleated syncytial trophoblastic cells may be seen in cell samples. Cytotrophoblasts are less characteristic. Arias-Stella reaction changes are seldom recognized in cytologic specimens except in tissue fragments. The cellular diagnosis of acute or chronic endometritis is difficult, as the presence of inflammatory cells in cell samples does not imply infection of the endometrium. If inflammatory cells such as plasma cells are seen in the stroma of tissue fragments, a diagnosis of chronic endometritis can be made. However, plasma cells seen free in a cell sample may or may not represent chronic endometritis, as they are more likely to originate from the endocervical canal. Occasionally, in suppurative inflammation or pyometra, the cell sample contains pus consisting of many neutrophils with necrotic material. Usually such a diagnosis is made on clinical evaluation. Rarely are characteristic changes of specific infections of endometrium seen in endometrial samples such as tuberculosis, cytomegalic inclusion disease, herpes simplex and chlamydial infection. The diagnosis of endometrial polyp in cellular samples is difficult unless tissue fragments are obtained, processed and interpreted as tissue specimens.

Sometimes, a reactive change, involving the surface epithelium and within glands, is seen and consists of enlarged cuboidal or columnar cells with increased cytoplasmic volumes that stain more densely eosinophilic, giving a metaplastic oncocytic appearance. The cytoplasm may show vacuolization and neutrophils within it, a sign of degeneration. The nuclei are slightly enlarged, round or oval, often excentric and may contain small nucleoli. However, the chromatin is uniformly distributed. The changes are nonspecific and are seen in association with many benign endometrial lesions. When desquamated they appear as small clusters or singly, resembling immature metaplastic cells of the endocervix except that the cytoplasm tends to be eosinophilic.

Cervical or Vaginal Sample

As discussed, sometimes benign endometrial lesions shed endometrial cells that may be identified in vaginal or cervical aspirates. They may be epithelial or stromal in origin. Usually, the number of cells are few in the sample and vary from a few cells per sample to about a 100 cells per sample. They do not appear to be significantly different from normal endometrial cells except that they are seen in the second half of the cycle or during the postmenopausal period. Occasionally, decidual cells or trophoblastic cells are seen.

ENDOMETRIAL CARCINOGENESIS

The development of endometrial carcinoma may follow two major pathways, both originating from primitive multipotential endometrial cells from the basal layer.

1. The most common and well-known pathway follows a series of developments of abnormal proliferative changes of increasing severity (pathologic hyperplasia). They culminate in invasive cancer over a period of time in a large percentage of cases, if left untreated, and influencing factors persist to act on the affected endometrium. Endometrial carcinoma occurring by this pathway is known as the "good prognostic group," as the tumor is of low-grade malignancy or better differentiated with precursor changes. It is less invasive, estrogen related and tends to be positive for estrogen and progesterone receptors. These types of tumors occur in a slightly younger age group, after the fifth or early sixth decade of life. This group constitutes about 70 to 80% of endometrial cancer. Most are well-differentiated adenocarcinomas, adenoacanthomas and mucinous and secretory carcinomas.

2. The secondary pathway is less common and appears to be associated with an apparent spontaneous development of cancer from the primitive endometrial cells without, it seems, going through the morphologic precursor phases, or it goes through a short imperceptible noninvasive phase before invasion. This is known as the "poor prognostic group," as the tumors tend to be poorly differentiated and more invasive with poorer prognoses. The tumors appear to be unrelated to estrogen and less likely to be positive for estrogen and progesterone receptors. They occur in an older age group, after the sixth or seventh decade of life. This group constitutes about 20 to 30% of endometrial cancers. Most are poorly differentiated adenocarcinomas, adenosquamous carcinomas, clear cell carcinomas and poorly differentiated papillary serous adenocarcinomas.

The proposed pathways of endometrial carcinogenesis have important implications in early detection, investigation, management and prognosis. The good prognostic group permits a morphologic precursor detection before cancer develops and is more likely to be symptomatic during precursor changes. The occurrences are less likely in the poor prognostic group, which also is less likely to produce symptoms until the disease is advanced.

PATHOLOGIC ENDOMETRIAL HYPERPLASIA—PRECURSORS OF ENDOMETRIAL CANCER

Histology

In the endometrial cancers that appear to have morphologic precursor changes, the changes are known as pathologic hyperplasia, denoting an abnormal proliferation of the endometrium in contrast to the normal physiologic hyperplasia during the menstrual cycle. In general, the hyperplasia becomes progressively more severe as carcinogenesis progresses. Certain arbitrary subdivisions can be made that relate to biologic behavior. Diverse names have been given to these lesions. The terminology used, although not ideal, is probably best known to both pathologists and clinicians. The biologic behavior of these lesions has been better documented. The terms used are as follows: adenomatous hyperplasia (later known as simple hyperplasia without atypia) and atypical hyperplasia and adenocarcinoma in situ, which can be grouped together as atypical adenomatous hyperplasia or adenomatous hyperplasia with atypia. Cystic hyperplasia has also been included in the terminology and is now considered to be relatively unimportant in endometrial carcinogenesis but is part of a change due to unopposed estrogenic effect. Pathologic endometrial hyperplasia is usually associated with a state including unopposed endogenous or exogenous estrogenic stimulation. The definitive diagnosis is made on microscopic examination of the endometrial tissue.[18]

Cystic Hyperplasia. Usually, there is an abundance of endometrial tissue with an increased number of normal and enlarged glands, irregularly distributed and separated by hyperplastic stroma, giving it a Swiss cheese–like appearance. The glands are usually lined by a single layer of slightly enlarged tall columnar cells similar to those seen in the physiologic proliferative phase and some cells are ciliated. The oval or elongated nuclei are normal in size and slightly enlarged, usually basal and infrequently intermediate in location. Micronucleoli are infrequently evident.

Adenomatous Hyperplasia. The number of endometrial glands are increased and crowded and irregularly located in the stroma. The glands are normal or smaller than normal in size and are characterized by outpouchings of the proliferating glands, forming bud-like projections, which may become pinched off to form small nests of closely packed, round daughter glands. The epithelial cells in the glands resemble those of physiologic proliferative endometrium, having a single layer of slightly enlarged oval or elongated nuclei. Stratification of the cells is inconspicuous. Micronucleoli are infrequent.

Atypical Hyperplasia. In adenocarcinoma in situ (adenomatous hyperplasia with atypia), the number of abnormal glands are increased, sometimes markedly, and are irregularly located in the stroma. The glandular pattern becomes more complex, and abnormal cellular changes are obvious and more severe. The glands may appear moderately enlarged, normal or smaller in size and sometimes are closely related to one another but separated by definite bands of stroma. Combined papillary infoldings, sometimes resulting in bridging of the glands, and outpouchings may be evident, and in advanced disease these can be conspicuous. Focally, back-to-back glands may be seen but are not conspicuous. The presence of extensive back-to-back formation of glands may suggest early invasive cancer.

Stratification of the abnormal enlarged epithelial cells is evident with varying degrees of altered cellular polarity. The enlarged columnar cells appear wider and have a relatively more conspicuous cyanophilic and sometimes slightly eosinophilic cytoplasm. The cells are obviously larger than cells of adenomatous hyperplasia without atypia. The nuclei are more hyperchromatic, enlarged and tend to appear more rounded rather than elongated. They are either basal or intermediate in location. Granularity of the chromatin is increased, and nuclear clearing is inconspicuous. Micronucleoli are encountered in some of the cells, and macronucleoli are uncommon. Necrosis and inflammation are usually absent. In advanced disease, especially with conspicuous back-to-back glands or bridging of the glands, it is not possible to differentiate these changes from early invasive carcinoma.

It is not unusual to see the various stages of carcinogenesis of the endometrium in the same specimen. The various types of epithelial variations or metaplasia seen in normal endometrium, such as tubal, eosinophilic, clear-cell and mucinous changes, and squamous metaplasia, can be observed in pathologic hyperplasia. The most common is squamous metaplasia, which can be seen in up to 10% of cases.[18]

Cytology from Direct Endometrial Sample

Although interest in this has increased, the cellular characteristics and microhistology of pathologic hyperplasia in cell samples prepared from direct endometrial samples are not adequately documented and evaluation requires more experience. Differentiation of normal endometrial cells from reactive and hyperplastic endometrial cells, and of hyperplasia from well-differentiated malignant endometrial cells, requires further detailed characterization. However, certain general features of hyperplastic endometrial cells are known that are similar to those described for endocervical aspirates.[2, 12, 13, 18] When tissue fragments, small or large, consisting of glands and stroma are present, the diagnosis of endometrial hyperplasia can be made on the basis of histopathologic criteria.

Optimal sampling and cellular preparations made from direct endometrial sampling contain an abundance of normal and hyperplastic endometrial fragments and cells, occurring in aggregates and less frequently singly. Depending on the technique, the aggregates may appear as tissue fragments; sheets containing epithelia; stromal or both stromal and epithelial cells; small loose aggregates of epithelial, stromal, or both cell types and whole or part of the glandular structures and strips of epithelial cells (Fig. 11–8). Depending on the type of hyperplasia, the glandular stomas in endometrial sheets are variable in size and shape and tend to be more crowded and irregularly spaced. In cystic hyperplasia, glandular stomas are enlarged, and crowding is not conspicuous. In

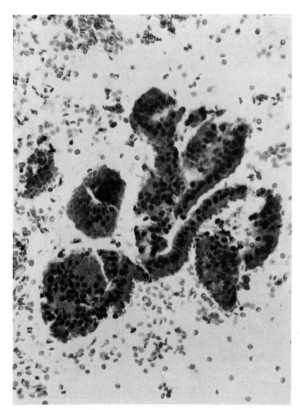

FIGURE 11–8. Strips and loose aggregates of **hyperplastic endometrial epithelium** with no significant cytologic atypia obtained from a postmenopausal woman with adenomatous hyperplasia. Smear preparation from a direct endometrial sample (Papanicolaou stain; ×250).

adenomatous hyperplasia without atypia, glandular stomas are smaller and crowded but separated. In adenomatous hyperplasia with atypia (atypical hyperplasia and adenocarcinoma *in situ*), glandular stomas appear more crowded but separated, and they are smaller, normal or slightly larger than normal in size. Marked crowding of glands with a back-to-back pattern is uncommon. Papillary infoldings may be appreciated within glands. In cystic and adenomatous hyperplasia without atypia, the epithelial cells and nuclei are slightly enlarged and are regularly arranged in the glands and in tighter cell aggregates (Fig. 11–9). The nuclei are uniform throughout with finely granular chromatin. Micronucleoli are not conspicuous. Tight three-dimensional groups are rare. In adenomatous hyperplasia with atypia, the atypical endometrial cells are arranged around glands and are more crowded and stratified, with slight pleomorphism in size. The cells are obviously enlarged, with moderate amounts of cytoplasm, and stain cyanophilic, amphophilic or slightly eosinophilic. The nuclei are also enlarged and crowded around glands with no significant alteration of nuclear polarity. The slightly hyperchromatic nuclei are round with uniform granular chromatin in most cells, and some may show irregular distribution of chromatin. Nucleoli are seen in some of the cells and are small or intermediate in size. Loose and tight groupings may also be observed and single cells are not conspicuous. Tissue necrosis is not evident; however, the cell sampling may contain red blood cells and a few inflammatory cells. Occasionally, within endometrial glands or contiguous to them, clusters of squamous metaplastic cells at various stages of maturation may be identified.

Cytology from Endometrial Aspirate or Vaginal Sample

The spontaneous desquamation of hyperplastic endometrial cells is inconsistent and the endometrial cells when present are few in number. Samples from the posterior vaginal fornix are less likely to contain endometrial cells and when present are fewer in number and in a poorer state of preservation than those seen in endocervical aspirates. Some endometrial cells may appear within normal limits, whereas others appear hyperplastic and abnormal. They are usually seen in women who are over 40 years of age during the second half of the cycle or during postmenopause. When endometrial cells are seen in these phases of life, the possibility of pathologic hyperplasia or even carcinoma of the endometrium should be considered.[19]

Changes in endometrial cells associated with pathologic hyperplasia include cellular and nuclear enlargement, slight nuclear hyperchromasia, alterations in nuclear chromatin and frequency of nucleoli. The degree of cellular abnormality is related to the severity of the endometrial hyperplasia.[7, 18] The altered cells are often accompanied by erythrocytes and evidence of an estrogenic effect, whereas the milieu associated with invasive endometrial carcinoma is not evident. Although the cytologic features of cystic hyperplasia, adenomatous hyperplasia, atypical hyperplasia and

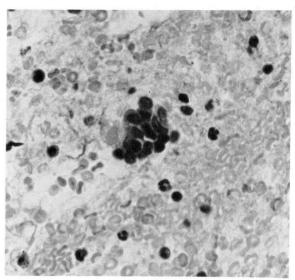

FIGURE 11–9. An aggregate of **hyperplastic endometrial cells** without atypia from a postmenopausal woman with **adenomatous hyperplasia.** Smear preparation from a direct endometrial sample (Papanicolaou stain; ×480).

adenocarcinoma *in situ* have been characterized, from the practical and biologic behavior points of view, they can be grouped into adenomatous hyperplasia with no atypia (cystic and adenomatous hyperplasia) and those with atypia (atypical hyperplasia and adenocarcinoma *in situ*). Table 11–5 shows a comparative study of the two groups of pathologic hyperplasia and grade I endometrial carcinoma.[18, 24] The findings are based on endocervical aspirate samples.

In endometrial hyperplasia without atypia, the number of endometrial cells encountered averages 100 cells and six aggregates per smear. Up to a fourth of the cells appear within normal limits and the rest appear hyperplastic. Some are normal endometrial stromal cells and most are of the epithelial type. The endometrial cells appear in loose two-dimensional or flat small aggregates, usually from five to 15 cells per aggregate, forming a modified part or whole acini pattern in some of the aggregates (Fig. 11–10). Tight groupings or three-dimensional cell balls with overlapping of the nuclei are not usually seen. The cells and nuclei appear similar within each group and are regularly related to each other. Single cells, especially endometrial stromal cells, are less frequently encountered and are more difficult to recognize. The hyperplastic endometrial cells are only slightly larger than their normal counterparts, and this characteristic is often difficult to appreciate as the cell borders are usually indistinct. The cells are round or oval and sometimes low cuboidal in form. The cytoplasm is scanty, weakly staining, appears cyanophilic or amphophilic and is finely vacuolated. Large vacuoles with or without leukocytes are infrequently encountered. They usually represent degenerate changes and may be seen more frequently in vaginal samples.

TABLE 11–5. A Comparative Study of Pathologic Hyperplasia and Grade I Carcinoma

Cellular Features	Hyperplasia		Adenocarcinoma Grade I
	No Atypia	Atypia	
Abnormal cells/slide	50	100	200
Groupings/slide	1	8	18
Cell area (μ²)	95	120	130
Number area (μ²)	45	55	60
Nuclear hyperchromasia	+ +	+ +	+
Uniformly granular chromatin (%)	95	70	20
Irregularly granular chromatin (%)	5	30	80
Total nucleoli (%)	4	25	73
Micronucleoli (%)	4	23	70
Macronucleoli (%)	0	2	3
Tumor diathesis (% of cases)	0	0	90

Modified after Ng ABP, Reagan JW: The pathology and cytopathology of microinvasive adenocarcinoma and precursors of endometrial carcinoma. *In* Compendium on Diagnostic Cytology, 6th ed. Edited by GL Weid, CM Keebler, LG Koss, JW Reagan. Chicago, Tutorials of Cytology, p. 180, 1988.

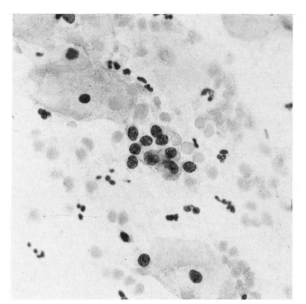

FIGURE 11–10. Cystic hyperplasia of endometrium. Minimal increase of nuclear size with uniform granular chromatin and slight hyperchromasia. Two larger cells with more conspicuous cytoplasm are endometrial stromal cells. This specimen was taken from a 48-year-old woman on day 22 of the menstrual cycle. Endocervical aspirate (Papanicolaou stain; ×480). (Reproduced with permission from Ng ABP, Reagan JW, Cechner RL: The precursors of endometrial cancer: A study of their cellular manifestation. Acta Cytol 17:439–448, 1973.)

Similarly, the nuclei are only slightly larger than normal and are centrally or excentrically located within the cells. They are round or oval and less frequently reniform. Unless degenerate, the nuclear membrane is not prominent and the nucleus is slightly hyperchromatic. The chromatinic material appears slightly more granular than normal and is uniformly distributed. Two to three chromocenters are seen, and micronucleoli are rarely encountered. The nucleus appears similar from cell to cell, and nuclear clearing is usually absent. The background of the smear is clean with no tumor diathesis. Estrogenic effect may be evident in the smears from postmenopausal women.

In pathologic hyperplasia with atypia (atypia hyperplasia and adenocarcinoma *in situ*), the endometrial cells encountered average 250 cells and 12 aggregates per smear; however, most of the cells appear hyperplastic and less than 5% appear within normal limits. Most are hyperplastic epithelial cells and a small proportion are endometrial stromal cells. The number of cells per group usually vary from 5 to 25 cells. The aggregates appear as loose two-dimensional groupings, having modified part or whole acini patterns with moderate variations in size of the cells and nucleus. The cellular and nuclear polarity are not significantly altered. Tight groupings and cell balls are infrequently encountered. Single cells are encountered but infrequently. The hyperplastic endometrial cells appear to be obviously larger than normal, round or oval in form, and low cuboidal cells are infrequently seen (Fig.

11–11). The cytoplasmic border is indistinct. The cytoplasm is scanty, weakly staining, appears cyanophilic or amphophilic and is finely vacuolated. Large distinct vacuoles with or without leukocytes are uncommon.

The nuclear size may vary from within normal limits to obviously enlarged; however, most are larger than normal. The nuclei are centrally or excentrically located and appear round or oval, rarely reniform. The nuclear membrane is not conspicuous. The nucleus is slightly hyperchromatic with more granular chromatinic material. Most nuclei are uniformly distributed with two to three chromocenters. Up to 30% of the nuclei show obvious or early nuclear clearing where the chromatinic particles are not evenly distributed within the nucleus. Nucleoli are seen in up to 25% of the cells, and they are usually single. They are usually micronucleoli, and macronucleoli are rarely seen. The background of the smear lacks tumor diathesis. Estrogenic effect is often present in the smears from postmenopausal women.

Certain differences are evident between the cytologic features of adenomatous hyperplasia without atypia and that with atypia and between adenomatous hyperplasia with atypia and grade I endometrial adenocarcinoma, as shown in Table 11–5.[18] The number of endometrial cells and cell aggregates are generally higher for endometrial hyperplasia with atypia than that without atypia. Up to 25% of the endometrial cells appear within normal limits in hyperplasia without atypia, and almost all endometrial cells are hyperplastic with atypia. The cell and nuclear sizes of hyperplasia

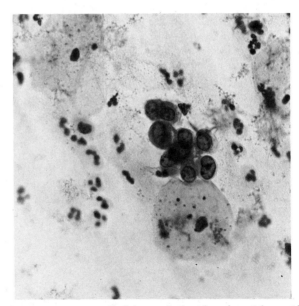

FIGURE 11–11. Atypical hyperplasia of endometrium. Although the endometrial cells are still regularly related to one another, note the definite increase in cellular and nuclear size and the presence of micronucleoli in some cells but no significant nuclear clearing. Endocervical aspirate (Papanicolaou stain; ×520). (Reproduced with permission from Ng ABP, Reagan JW, Cechner RL: The precursors of endometrial cancer: A study of their cellular manifestation. Acta Cytol 17:439–448, 1973.)

with atypia are obviously larger than their normal counterparts, whereas those without atypia show only slightly or minimal enlargement. Up to 30% of the nuclei have an early or obvious irregular distribution of a chromatinic nature within the nucleus. About 70% have uniform distribution of chromatin, and up to 25% of the cells have a single micronucleolus in hyperplasia with atypia. In contrast, in hyperplasia with no atypia, the chromatin material is invariably uniformly distributed and micronucleoli are rare.

When compared with pathologic hyperplasia with atypia, cell samples containing grade I endometrial adenocarcinoma have significantly more abnormal endometrial cells and greater numbers of aggregates. The cells and nuclei are also larger. The aggregates may be loose and form modified whole or part acini. Tight groups or cell balls are evident with overlapping or crowding of the nuclei and loss of cellular and nuclear polarity. In contrast, in hyperplasia with atypia, the cell aggregates are loose with no cell ball formation, no overlapping of nuclei and no loss of cellular and nuclei polarity. The nuclei of viable malignant endometrial cells are usually slightly less hyperchromatic than those of pathologic hyperplasia. Over 80% of malignant cells have an irregular distribution of the chromatinic material, and up to 75% have micronucleoli. About 30% of hyperplasia with atypia cells have an early or obvious irregular distribution of the chromatinic material, and only up to 25% have micronucleoli. A tumor diathesis, consisting of a watery granular background, cellular detritus with few inflammatory cells and red blood cells, is seen in 90% of grade I adenocarcinomas and is absent in pathologic hyperplasia. Thus, cells derived from pathologic hyperplasia without atypia more closely resemble those of normal endometrial cells. Conversely, to some degree, the cellular abnormalities of hyperplasia with atypia approach those associated with grade I endometrial adenocarcinoma.

The cytologic features of early focal or microinvasive adenocarcinoma are not well documented and appear to be more similar to those observed in pathologic hyperplasia with atypia. Less frequently, the features are similar to those observed in grade I endometrial carcinoma, in which both hyperplastic and malignant cells are seen. A tumor diathesis is usually absent.

ENDOMETRIAL CARCINOMA

Histology

In many Western countries, endometrial cancer is the most frequent malignant tumor encountered in the female genital tract. The most common malignant tumor of the endometrium is of epithelial origin, and endometrial stromal cell tumor and malignant mixed müllerian tumor (epithelial and sarcoma components) are much less frequently encountered.

Carcinoma may originate from any site of the endometrium and infrequently from a preexisting benign polyp. Carcinoma is rarely seen primarily in adeno-

myosis. It is usually of multicentric origin and less frequently unicentric. In early cancer, the affected endometrium may appear slightly thickened and granular and, later, becomes polypoid or papillary and infiltrating. Ultimately, hemorrhage and necrosis may occur. Diffuse involvement of the endometrium may occur. In some poorly differentiated cancers and certain histologic cell types, such as adenosquamous carcinoma, direct invasion in the endocervix occurs more frequently. Extension of cancer is by direct invasion to involve myometrium and pelvic tissues and organs, with lymphatic spread to regional lymph nodes. Hematogenous spread to distant sites usually occurs later in the disease process.

Microscopically, most carcinomas of the endometrium are of columnar or glandular epithelial cell origin and are known as adenocarcinomas. Normal endometrial pattern is lost with disorganization of the glandular structures. The abnormal glands are increased in number, back to back, with little or no discernible stroma, are variable in size and shape and are usually similar to or smaller than their normal counterparts. A papillary pattern may be seen and is dominant in some tumor types. The glandular pattern becomes less conspicuous or absent in more anaplastic neoplasms and is replaced by sheets of tumor cells. The malignant cells are larger than normal and may appear columnar, cuboidal, polygonal or round. The cells lining the glands may be single layered or stratified with altered polarity. The cytoplasm is scanty or moderate in amount and stains weakly cyanophilic. The nuclei are enlarged, round or oval with an abnormal chromatin pattern. Nucleoli of varying size and number are seen in many of the cells. Mitotic activity is evident. Hemorrhage, necrosis and clusters of foam-cell histocytes may be seen. Psammoma bodies are infrequently identified. The histologic features are modified by the degree of differentiation and histologic subtypes of the tumor.

Some pathologic factors that are important in influencing the histopathologic and cytologic features and in the management and prognosis of endometrial carcinoma include the histologic type, the degree of differentiation of the glandular component and the extent of the neoplasm.[14]

Of the histologic types of carcinoma, the typical (endometrioid) adenocarcinoma constitutes about 60% of cases; adenocarcinoma with a benign-appearing squamous component (adenoacanthoma) 20%; adenocarcinoma with a malignant squamous component (adenosquamous carcinoma) 10%; papillary serous adenocarcinoma 7% and clear cell carcinoma 1%. The other 2% of cases represent secretory carcinoma, pure mucinous carcinoma, undifferentiated carcinoma and, rarely, spindle cell carcinoma, neuroendocrine tumor and ciliated cell carcinoma.[14] Sometimes, various components are seen in the same tumor. In adenoacanthoma, the glandular component is usually well differentiated. In adenosquamous carcinoma, the glandular component is usually moderately differentiated.

Papillary serous adenocarcinoma is characterized by the presence of papillary fronds of tumor cells with a distinct central stalk consisting of connective tissue stroma and blood vessels. The tumors are usually moderately to poorly differentiated. Clear cell carcinoma of the endometrium is morphologically, ultrastructurally, histochemically and biologically comparable to its counterpart in the vagina, cervix and ovary, and they share a common müllerian cell origin. The malignant cells are characterized by a moderate amount of clear cytoplasm. The tumor is usually poorly differentiated. Secretory adenocarcinoma is a well differentiated adenocarcinoma in which the cytoplasm shows secretory activity similar to that in physiologic secretory cells of the endometrium. Pure mucinous carcinoma of the endometrium is uncommon and appears morphologically similar to mucinous carcinoma elsewhere, such as the ovary, endocervix and colon. The tumor is usually relatively well differentiated with varying amounts of mucin intra- and extracellularly.[14, 24, 25]

Malignant tumors having cells that resemble those of the normal parent tissue are said to be differentiated whereas those composed predominantly of primitive cells are said to be undifferentiated. In general, differentiated neoplasms are usually less malignant, giving a better prognosis than poorly differentiated neoplasms. The most widely used method for evaluating the differentiation of a malignant tumor is that described by Broders in which grade I represents the most well-differentiated and grade IV the least differentiated. Modifications of Broders's grades include well-, moderately and poorly differentiated, reducing the four grades into three, grade I to grade III. For practical purposes in cytology, endometrial adenocarcinoma can be grouped into well-differentiated (Broders's grades I and II) and poorly differentiated (Broders's III and IV). Approximately 80% of typical endometrial adenocarcinomas of the endometrium represent grades I and II, and 20% are grades III and IV. Most adenoacanthomas and secretory and mucinous carcinomas are well differentiated and less aggressive, whereas most adenosquamous cancers, serous papillary adenocarcinomas and clear cell cancers are poorly differentiated and more aggressive.

The degree of differentiation is manifested by microscopic features including growth pattern and the appearance of tumor cells. In well-differentiated tumors, a glandular pattern with varying degrees of papillary proliferation predominates and solid sheets of tumor cells are not evident. With increasing dedifferentiation, solid sheets of tumor cells and papillary patterns become increasingly conspicuous and acini structures become increasingly infrequent. In the least differentiated tumor, the tumor is composed predominantly of sheets of tumor cells and malignant glands are rarely encountered. With increasing lack of differentiation, the shape of the cells changes from columnar to cuboidal, round or polygonal. Focally, pleomorphism is evident in the less differentiated tumors. The cellular and nuclear size increase progressively as the tumor becomes less differentiated, nucleoli are more frequently encountered and become larger, mitotic activity increases and necrosis and hemorrhage become

more conspicuous. Foam-cell histiocytes in the stroma are observed more frequently in well-differentiated tumors. These histologic changes of differentiation are reflected in the cytologic features seen in cellular samples.

The extent of endometrial involvement by tumor and the aggressive infiltrating growth pattern influence cellular desquamation. Extensive involvement of the endometrium; increasing dedifferentiation of the tumor cell with increasing hemorrhage and necrosis; certain tumor types, such as adenosquamous carcinoma and papillary carcinomas, are features making the endometrium more prone to shed cells and in greater numbers, as a result of the decreased mutual adhesiveness of the tumor cells.

Cytology from Direct Endometrial Samples

Direct endometrial samples obtained from women with endometrial carcinomas usually contain an abundance of cellular material.[2, 13, 22, 24] Depending on the technique used, the specimens may contain all or some single cells, cell aggregates, microtissue fragments and large fragments of tumor tissue. When macroscopically recognizable fragments are obtained, they are processed by the cell block technique and are evaluated with the same criteria as the histologic study of surgical specimens, which are well documented (Fig. 11–12).

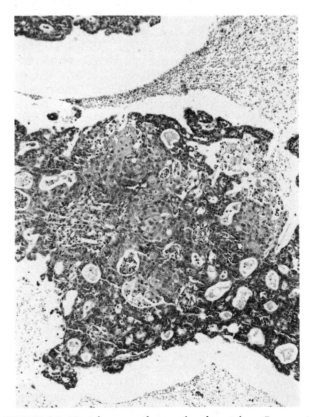

FIGURE 11–12. Adenoacanthoma of endometrium. Fragment of malignant endometrial adenocarcinoma with clusters of benign-appearing squamous cells. Cell block preparation from Vabra sampler (hematoxylin and eosin; ×100).

This type of sample is more readily interpretable and provides more specific information as to the histologic type and degree of differentiation of the endometrial carcinoma. Differentiation from other types of nonmalignant tissue is facilitated. If no gross fragments are present, the specimen is smeared or concentrated in a glass slide and stained with the Papanicolaou stain, evaluated as a cytologic specimen.

The specimens obtained may contain malignant cells occurring singly, in aggregates or microfragments; hyperplastic endometrial cells in aggregates or microfragments and, less frequently, singly, and even benign endometrial cells occurring singly, in aggregates or microfragments. Often, benign endometrial cells and sometimes squamous or squamous metaplastic cells are present, usually representing contaminants from the cervix and, less frequently, from a squamous metaplasia from the endometrium. Depending on the extent of cancer, cell type and degree of differentiation, the background or diathesis of the specimen in cellular samples may not show a tumor diathesis and appears clear if the tumor is focal with minimal or no necrosis and hemorrhage. In contrast, a tumor diathesis is usually present if cancer is extensive and aggressive with hemorrhage and necrosis.

When single cells or cell groups are present, the criteria are similar to those described for malignant cells that spontaneously desquamate into the endocervical canal or vagina fornix (refer to this section for criteria). However, the malignant cells from direct endometrial samples are abundant, cell aggregates are larger and the cellular details are better preserved facilitating interpretation (Fig. 11–13). Microfragments are of sizes varying from single abnormal whole or partial glands to large sheets or fragments of tumor cells of different sizes and shapes. The gland openings are crowded or compressed and are of varying sizes and shapes.

Papillary folds or diffuse sheets of tumor cells with no glandular stomas may be evident, especially in undifferentiated tumors. The malignant cells in the glands, papillae or sheets are crowded with overlapping cells or cell stratification. The cellular and nuclear polarity are altered and irregularly arranged in relationship to one another. The shape of the cells, especially when viewed within glands, is low columnar or cuboidal; however, most cells appear round or oval. Strips of abnormal cells are also encountered; however, this pattern is seen more frequently in normal and abnormal endocervical columnar cells.

The cells and nuclei are enlarged, and the cellular and nuclear sizes increase with further lack of differentiation. Variation occurs in the size of cells and nuclei. Because of the crowding of the cells, the cytoplasm is often inconspicuous. Overlapping and crowding of the enlarged nuclei with the long axis irregularly arranged are evident. The chromatinic material is slightly more granular and irregularly distributed. Nucleoli are seen and their frequency, size and number increase with greater dedifferentiation of the tumor. Mitotic activity may be seen in some of the cells. Many of the larger cell aggregates tend to have

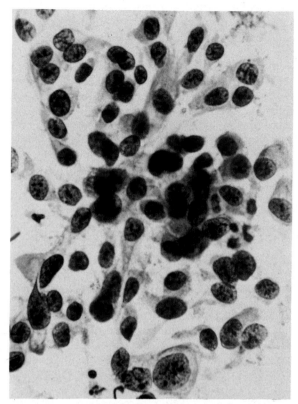

FIGURE 11–13. Poorly differentiated adenocarcinoma of endometrium. Monolayer of cell aggregates and single cells that are large with malignant features. Smear preparation from an endometrial sample (Papanicolaou stain; ×500).

a sheet-like appearance and are less likely to be large three-dimensional cell balls. Sometimes, a benign or hyperplastic endometrial fragment or cell cluster is seen contiguous to the malignant fragments or cells. They may occur separately in the specimen. Clusters of foam-cell histiocytes are often observed, and psammoma bodies are rarely identified.

Sometimes, morulae and, less frequently, sheets of benign-appearing squamous metaplastic cells are seen within abnormal glands or contiguous to them, representing an adenoacanthoma. Sheets of malignant squamous cells may be seen contiguous to or separate from malignant glandular cells, representing an adenosquamous carcinoma. The squamous carcinomas are usually of the large-cell nonkeratinizing type and, less frequently, they are of the keratinizing type. Small-cell cancer component is rare. The cytologic criteria for recognizing benign squamous metaplastic cells and malignant squamous cells are similar to those described for the cervix. In serous papillary carcinoma, papillary cell groupings and papillary tissue fragments are seen in the specimen.

The cytoplasm of clear cell carcinoma may be moderately abundant with clear or foamy cytoplasm; however, its recognition as a clear cell type of cancer cytologically is not often possible. Hobnail-shaped cells may be seen within glands. Mucinous carcinomas may not be recognized cytologically because not all large cytoplasmic vacuoles are mucin producing. In fact, most are degenerative and a mucin stain may be needed for a definitive diagnosis. The cytoplasmic vacuoles of mucin-secreting cells often have pale eosinophilic coloration. Secretory carcinoma is difficult to recognize in cell groups or single cells, and they appear as well-differentiated adenocarcinomas with more conspicuous small vacuoles in some of the cells. If large fragments are present, a diagnosis of the various subtypes may be facilitated using histologic features.

Cytology from Endocervical Aspirate or Vaginal Sample

General Characteristics of Endometrial Adenocarcinoma

Cellular samples that depend solely on spontaneous desquamation contain far fewer cells derived from endometrial carcinoma. The cytologic features are modified and appear different when compared with samples obtained by direct sampling of the endometrium. The cytologic features described for endometrial carcinoma are based primarily on endocervical aspirate samples. Although the criteria utilized are also similar in samples obtained from the vaginal fornix, vaginal samples when compared with endocervical samples are more likely not to contain abnormal endometrial cells. When present, they are fewer in number and are more likely to show degenerate changes. In a poorer state of preservation detailed evaluation is more difficult, resulting in decreased detection rate.

Of all the features that have been attributed to the cells of endometrial carcinoma, the most important are the distribution and interrelationship of the cells; the cell and nuclear size; the changes in the nuclear structure; the appearance of the nucleolus and the milieu in which they exist.[24, 25] Not all cell samples that depend on spontaneous desquamation of cells from the endometrium of patients with endometrial carcinoma contain endometrial cells. Their presence and the number of cells depend on many factors, including the person collecting the sample; the technique and nature of equipment utilized; the anatomic variations, such as a narrowed cervical canal and the intrinsic nature of the tumor extent, degree of differentiation and histologic cell type of cancer.

When abnormal endometrial cells are present in samples collected by spontaneous desquamation, they are usually much less conspicuous than abnormal cells derived from primary cervical cancers. The number of abnormal endometrial cells vary from case to case. In some cases, especially those of early endometrial cancer, the endometrial cells present are few in number consisting of no more than 50 to 100 per sample. It may contain in addition to malignant cells, normal-appearing and hyperplastic endometrial cells. In cell samples containing abnormal endometrial cells, approximately one-third each of the samples contains less than 250 abnormal endometrial cells per sample, 250 to 500 abnormal cells per sample and over 500 abnormal cells per sample. The abnormal cells occur singly

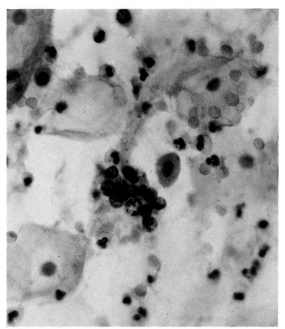

FIGURE 11–14. Well-differentiated adenocarcinoma of endometrium. Abnormal acinus structure with irregular cellular arrangement and loss of cellular polarity. Note the irregular distribution of chromatin and chromatin pattern are different from cell to cell. Endocervical aspirate (Papanicolaou stain; ×480). (Reproduced with permission from Ng ABP, Reagan JW, Cechner RL: The precursors of endometrial cancer: A study of their cellular manifestation. Acta Cytol 17:439–448, 1973.)

and in aggregates. Single malignant endometrial cells are difficult to identify, particularly when the tumor is well differentiated. The number of cells per aggregate is variable; however, the majority consists of a few cells to 30 cells per group. Larger aggregates are less frequently encountered. Cell aggregates usually have a peripheral smooth molded or rounded appearance. Depending on the grade, tumor pattern and histologic cell type, the aggregates may appear as modified whole or part acinar; loose or tight clusters with no specific pattern; cell balls; papillary and sheet like. Strips and fully formed rosettes, often seen in normal and abnormal endocervical lesions, are rare. When the cells occur in aggregates, the relationship of malignant cells is lost. A loss of nuclear polarity occurs where the nuclei are irregularly arranged in relationship to one another. Nuclear overlapping and crowding may be evident (Figs. 11–14 to 11–18).

Although the appearance of the malignant cells is dependent in part on the degree of differentiation and histologic cell type of the tumor, the cells and nuclei are larger than their normal counterparts and hyperplastic cells. The mean cell area is about 150 μ^2 with a variation of 100 to 200 μ^2. Variations in size and shape of cells in each sample are not usually conspicuous. The configuration of the cells is not always discernible because of indistinct cytoplasmic borders of the cells, particularly in dense groups. The malignant cells are usually round, oval or low cuboidal. A columnar form is seen in less than 5% of the cells. Bizarre malignant

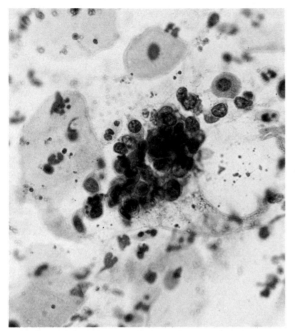

FIGURE 11–15. Adenocarcinoma of endometrium. Broders's grade II. Tight cell cluster and few single malignant cells. Note the mild tumor diathesis. Endocervical aspirate (Papanicolaou stain; ×480).

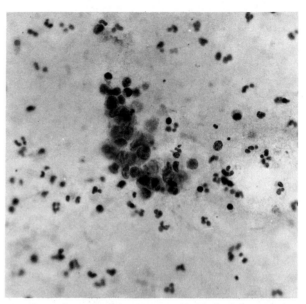

FIGURE 11–17. Adenocarcinoma of endometrium. Broders's grade II. Note many pyknotic nuclei and degenerate malignant cells. Watery granular background, cellular detritus and few inflammatory cells constitute a tumor diathesis. Vaginal sample (Papanicolaou stain; ×500).

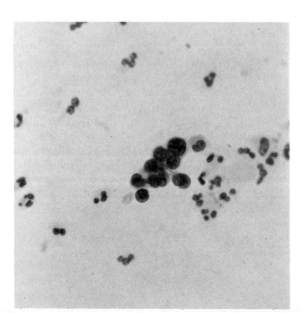

FIGURE 11–16. Adenocarcinoma of endometrium. Broders's grade II. Loose cluster of malignant cells and a single stromal cell with a reniform nucleus. Endocervical aspirate (Papanicolaou stain; ×480).

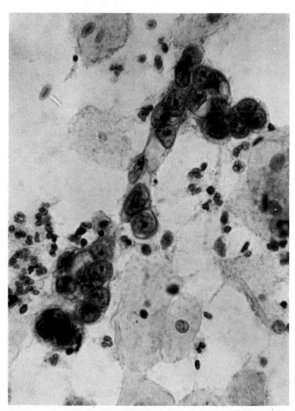

FIGURE 11–18. Poorly differentiated adenocarcinoma of endometrium. Broders's grade IV. There is marked cellular and nuclear enlargement. Macronucleoli are evident. Endocervical aspirate (Papanicolaou stain; ×500).

cells are rarely identified. The malignant cells usually have indistinct cell borders with scanty cytoplasm.

Moderate to abundant cytoplasm is seen in about 10% of cells. Using the EA65 modification of the Papanicolaou staining method, the cytoplasm appears cyanophilic in about two thirds of the cells, and the remaining one third stain weakly eosinophilic or indeterminate. Dense staining of the cytoplasm and strong cytoplasmic eosinophilia are uncommon. The cytoplasmic matrix is characteristically diffusely and finely vacuolated in over two thirds of the cells and homogeneous in less than one third of the cells. A granular cytoplasm is seen in less than 5% of the cells. Large discrete cytoplasmic vacuoles, single or multiple, are not seen in every sample and are present in about 5% of cells in some samples. They may or may not contain neutrophils within the vacuoles.

The vacuoles may distort the cellular configuration and compress the nucleus, producing a signet-ring appearance. With few exceptions, these large vacuoles are secondary to degenerative changes and do not represent true secretions of the cells. They are also seen frequently in degenerative endocervical columnar and squamous metaplastic cells of the cervix.

The mean nuclear area of malignant endometrial cells is about 70 μ^2 with a variation of 50 to 90 μ^2, depending on the degree of differentiation of the tumor. However, variation in size and shape of the nucleus is usually not conspicuous within each cell sample. The nucleocytoplasmic ratio is high, and the nuclear area usually represents over 50% of the cellular area. The nucleus is mononucleated, and multinucleation is rare. Depending on the perspective, they are mixed; the nucleus is often excentrically located in the cell and less frequently is it centrally located. The nucleus is usually round or oval in shape, infrequently indented or reniform, and rarely is it bizarre in configuration. The nuclear membrane is usually distinct, and deposition of chromatin beneath the nuclear membrane known as chromatininc membrane, a sign of cell death, represents about 5% of the cells. The nucleus is usually normochromic or slightly hyperchromatic. Marked hyperchromasia is seen in less than 10% of cells.

The nature of the chromatinic material and its distribution within the nucleus are characteristic for malignant cells. The chromatic material shows clumping and irregular distribution within the nucleus, resulting in areas of nuclear clearing. Furthermore, the resulting abnormal chromatin pattern varies from cell to cell. In about 90% of the malignant cells, there is an irregularly distributed finely clumped chromatin, and the remaining 10% have an irregularly clumped, coarsely granular chromatin or pyknosis.

The frequency, size and number of nucleoli are dependent on the degree of differentiation and the histologic cell type of the tumor. Generally over 75% of malignant endometrial cells contain one or more discernible nucleoli. Of those with nucleoli, over two thirds of the cells have a single nucleolus and less than one third have multiple nucleoli. Over 80% of the nucleoli are small (micronucleoli) and less than 20% are large (macronucleoli). The nucleoli are usually

round, and irregular forms are seen in only about 2% of cells. Discrete inclusions within the nucleus of uncertain nature are rarely seen, being present in less than 0.5% of malignant cells. Mitoses are infrequently seen and are observed in less than 10% of cell samples. It is not always possible to determine whether the dividing cell is of epithelial or histiocytic origin.

Along with the malignant endometrial cells, other changes in cell samples may be observed. An obvious tumor diathesis is seen in many of the samples. This consists of a watery granular transudate or, less frequently, an exudate in which inflammatory cells are more conspicuous; erythrocytes both recent and old; fibrin and cellular detritus. The degree of changes may vary, and evidence of a tumor diathesis may also vary from minimal to obvious changes. Generally 90% of cell samples show tumor diathesis. Early invasive cancers that are well differentiated may have an inconspicuous or absent diathesis, whereas extensive poorly differentiated cancers are more likely to be associated with an apparent diathesis. The changes of a tumor diathesis are the result of tissue destruction by tumor and tumor necrosis. Large foam-cell histiocytes, occurring singly or in loose clusters, are frequently seen.[4, 24] Occasionally, psammoma bodies are identified.[6, 24] An associated estrogenic effect may be seen in cell samples; however, cell samples that show an atrophic cell pattern may equally be likely to show malignant endometrial cells. An estrogenic effect is more likely to be seen in samples from women with a well-differentiated adenocarcinoma and is more likely to be absent with a tumor that is undifferentiated or aggressive in growth. The features described for endometrial adenocarcinoma in endocervical samples are based on optimal quality of the samples and some of these features may at times be difficult to evaluate.

Pathologic Factors Influencing Cellular Features

The distribution and appearance of malignant endometrial cells and the background of the cell samples are influenced by the differentiation of the glandular component, histologic cell type and extent of disease.[8–11, 24, 25, 27]

Tumor Differentiation. The evaluation of the degree of differentiation of adenocarcinoma is based on Broders's grades.[24] For practical purposes, the cytologic evaulation may be grouped into well differentiated (Broders's grades I and II) and poorly differentiated (Broders's grades III and IV). As shown in Table 11–6, significant differences are seen in the cytologic characteristics of well-differentiated and poorly differentiated adenocarcinoma. In addition to the features of malignancy, the major differences between well-differentiated and poorly differentiated adenocarcinoma reside in the number of abnormal cells, growth pattern of tumor, cellular and nuclear size, nature of the nucleolus and tumor diathesis (see Figs. 11–14, 11–15, and 11–18). Furthermore, not all cell samples from women with endometrial adenocarcinoma contain ma-

TABLE 11–6. Cytologic Features of Endometrial Adenocarcinoma When Related to Tumor Differentiation

Cellular Features	Broders's Grade			
	I	II	III	IV
No. of cells/slide	200	400	600	600
No. of groups/slide	18	20	30	30
Cell area (μ^2)	132	150	176	198
Nuclear area (μ^2)	60	67	85	92
Nucleoli (cell %)	73	97	100	100
Single (cell %)	65	63	52	40
Multiple (cell %)	8	34	48	60
Micronucleoli (cell %)	70	86	64	55
Macronucleoli (cell %)	3	11	36	45
Round nucleoli (cell %)	73	97	99	85
Irregular nucleoli (cell %)	0	0	1	15
Tumor diathesis (% of cases)	90	93	100	100
Histiocytes (% of cases)	34	33	18	5

Modified after Reagan JW, Ng ABP: The cells of uterine adenocarcinoma, 2nd ed. Basel, S Karger, 1973.

lignant endometrial cells. In patients with grade I endometrial cancer, only 64% of the samples contained malignant cells, whereas 83% of samples from women with grade IV cancer contained endometrial cells. With increasing lack of differentiation, there are increasing numbers of cells and cell aggregates, increasing cellular and nuclear size and increasing numbers and size of the nucleolus.

In undifferentiated cancer, irregular configuration is seen in some of the macronucleoli. The shape of the endometrial cells changes from round-oval or cuboidal in well-differentiated cancers to a rounder or polygonal configuration with a centrally placed nucleus and slightly more conspicuous cytoplasmic volume in undifferentiated cancers.

In well-differentiated adenocarcinomas, most of the cell aggregates are small and are composed of a modified acinar. A lumen may be evident that is surrounded by low cuboidal or round cells, which are irregularly arranged in relationship to one another. The malignant cells are loosely clustered together. Tight compact, papillary or sheet-like aggregates are infrequently encountered.

In poorly differentiated adenocarcinoma, the cell aggregates tend to be relatively larger, tight and compact or cell balls. Papillary structures are of different sizes and shapes, and sheet-like structures are more frequently encountered. However, a modified acinar pattern and loose small aggregates are inconspicuous or absent.

Not all cell samples from well-differentiated adenocarcinomas reveal an apparent diathesis and, when present, tend to be less conspicuous and focal in the smear. In contrast, a diathesis is usually evident in cell samples from undifferentiated cancers and tends to be more conspicuous. Sometimes evidence of hemorrhage or necrosis, or both, is pronounced, which may interfere with detailed evaluation of the tumor cells. Foam-cell histiocytes are more frequently encountered in well-differentiated than in poorly differentiated tumors. Most undifferentiated carcinomas of the endo-

metrium in which cell type is unclear show cellular features of poorly differentiated adenocarcinoma. These differences seen in cellular samples correlate with the histologic features of well-differentiated and poorly differentiated carcinoma of the endometrium.

Histologic Cell Types. With few exceptions, it is difficult to diagnose cytologically specific cell types of adenocarcinoma of the endometrium. Usually the cellular features reflect the endometrial origin of the tumor and the changes of differentiation of the tumor but not the specific histologic subtypes of the carcinoma.[1, 9, 10, 13, 24, 25]

Secretory Adenocarcinoma. The cellular features of secretory adenocarcinoma are basically those of a typical grade I endometrial adenocarcinoma and are not distinctive of a secreting cancer. Because much of the cytoplasm of the malignant cell is cytolysed during passage to the cervical canal, evaluation of secreting activity is not possible. Some of the better-preserved cells may show more distinguished cytoplasmic vacuoles, which may or may not represent secretion and may be due to degenerative changes (Fig. 11–19). A tumor diathesis is often absent or inconspicuous.

Clear Cell Adenocarcinoma. This is usually a poorly differentiated adenocarcinoma representing grade III and less frequently grade IV neoplasms. Thus, the cellular changes are those of a grade III to IV adenocarcinoma and are often not distinctive. The tumor cells occur singly, in compact masses or in a sheet-like arrangement. They are large, round or polygonal, and some of the cells have a moderate amount of cytoplasm that appears diffusely vacuolated or granular and is fragile (Fig. 11–20). A clear cytoplasm seen in a tissue specimen is seldom seen in a cellular sample. The enlarged nuclei often contain multiple nucleoli, and macronucleoli are common. A tumor diathesis is usually evident. The cellular changes resemble those de-

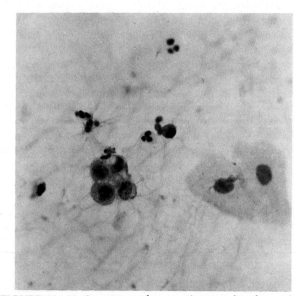

FIGURE 11–19. Secretory adenocarcinoma of endometrium. Broders's grade I. The cytoplasm is more conspicuous and vacuolated. Endocervical aspirate (Papanicolaou stain; ×500).

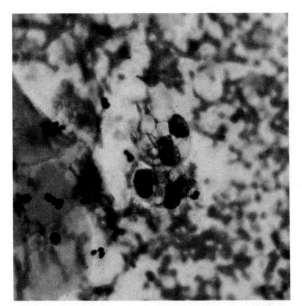

FIGURE 11–20. Clear cell adenocarcinoma of endometrium. Broders's grade IV. The malignant cells are poorly differentiated with prominent clear cytoplasm and indistinct cell borders. Endocervical aspirate (Papanicolaou stain; ×480).

rived from their counterparts in the cervix, vagina and ovary.

Mucinous Adenocarcinoma. Most mucinous carcinomas of the endometrium are relatively well differentiated, representing grade II tumors. Thus, the cellular changes are basically those of a grade II adenocarcinoma and may be indistinguishable from a typical endometrial grade II adenocarcinoma. Special stains for the presence of mucin are usually necessary to confirm a mucin-secreting adenocarcinoma. In some cell samples, the malignant cells contain more conspicuous cytoplasm with large distinct vacuoles that contain a homogeneous pale, slightly eosinophilic fluid representing that mucin secretion is present.

Although these vacuoles may be difficult or impossible to differentiate from degenerative changes, the vacuoles of degenerative changes are clear and often contain neutrophils. Often the vacuoles of mucinous carcinoma are so large that they distend the cell borders, and occasionally signet-ring cells are seen. When mucin is extensive, the smear during preparation is sticky and the cell samples have a pale homogeneous streaky background that represents extracellular mucin. The last is indistinguishable from mucin production by endocervical cells.

Serous Papillary Adenocarcinoma. Most tumors of this type are grade III adenocarcinomas and less frequently grade II or IV neoplasms. The basic cellular changes are those described for these grades. However, the characteristic feature of this tumor is that the cell aggregates appear predominantly papillary in form and in different sizes and shapes (Fig. 11–21). The papillary groupings may appear as small compact cell balls, elongated sausage-like tight groups with peripheral molding of the cellular border and irregular tight

clusters of cells with radiating papillary fronds. Occasionally, when viewed at its proper perspective, a central core of connective tissue with or without capillaries, representing the stalk of the papilla, may be identified in some cell aggregates. Psammoma bodies are also more likely to be encountered. Papillary forms may be seen in other histologic types of adenocarcinoma but are usually not conspicuous. For comparable grades, tumors that are predominantly papillary in type shed more cells than nonpapillary tumors.

Undifferentiated Carcinoma. The cytologic features of these tumors are those described for grade IV adenocarcinoma.

Adenocarcinoma with a Squamous Component. This may be divided into those adenocarcinomas with a benign-appearing squamous component (adenoacanthoma) and those with a malignant squamous component (adenosquamous carcinoma). In both types, the endometrial origin of the tumor is based on the cytologic features of the malignant glandular component described for endometrial adenocarcinoma. The glandular component of an adenoacanthoma is usually well differentiated (grade I or II) and is cytologically of the endometrial type.

Because the morphologic features of squamous metaplasia or mature squamous cells derived from endometrial carcinoma are similar to their counterparts

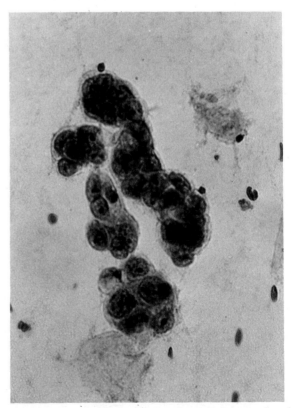

FIGURE 11–21. Papillary serous adenocarcinoma of endometrium. Tight, elongated and small cell-ball papillary pattern. The malignant cells and nuclei are markedly enlarged with macronucleoli representing a poorly differentiated adenocarcinoma. Endocervical aspirate (Papanicolaou stain; ×480).

in the cervix, it is often not possible to make a diagnosis of adenoacanthoma of the endometrium from endocervical or vaginal samples that contain separate groups or single malignant glandular endometrial cells and separate squamous cells. Usually the separate squamous metaplastic cells are derived from the cervix.

In some cases in which the squamous metaplastic cells form part of an aggregate with malignant glandular cells, the cellular diagnosis of adenoacanthoma can be considered. This is more likely to occur if the squamous component in the tumor is conspicuous. The squamoid component may show immature metaplastic cells comparable to the morulae of Dutra in tissue specimens, mature squamous metaplastic cells and mature squamous cells, which may be nonkeratinizing or keratinizing with pearl formation. Sometimes the squamous cells may demonstrate dysplastic or *in situ* carcinoma changes.

In adenosquamous carcinoma of the endometrium, both a malignant glandular component with features of endometrial adenocarcinoma and a malignant squamous component are evident in the cellular samples (Figs. 11–22 and 11–23). The proportion of each cell type in the parent tumor will influence the frequency of the cell types seen in the cell sample. Usually, the glandular component of endometrial type predominates or both components are equally conspicuous. A predominant squamous component is less frequently encountered. The glandular component is usually of grade II or III endometrial adenocarcinoma, and grade I or IV component is less frequently present. As in the cervix, the squamous component may be of keratinizing, nonkeratinizing or small-cell type. The most frequent cell type is the large-cell nonkeratinizing, and the least frequent is the small-cell type. Sometimes it is difficult to differentiate sheets of grade IV adeno-

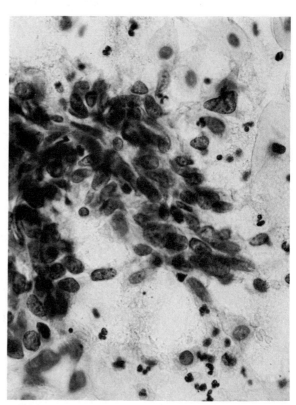

FIGURE 11–23. Malignant squamous component of **adenosquamous carcinoma of endometrium.** The squamous component is of the large cell nonkeratinizing type. Endocervical aspirate (Papanicolaou stain; × 480).

carcinoma from a squamous large-cell nonkeratinizing carcinoma component. The last cells have a more homogeneous cytoplasm, the chromatin is more granular and the macronucleoli are less conspicuous. The two components are usually identified as separate groups or single cells. Less frequently, the two cell types are identified in the same aggregate.

Adenosquamous carcinoma of the endometrium is a more aggressive cancer than adenoacanthoma and is more likely to shed cells and in greater numbers. It is thus more likely to be detected in cellular samples. As adenosquamous carcinoma of the endometrium tends to involve the endocervix in a large percentage of cases, it is not always possible to distinguish it from its cervical counterpart on the basis of the cellular evidence. Its differentiation is based primarily on the cellular differences between the malignant glandular component originating in the cervix and endometrium. It is rare to encounter cervical samples that contain both a malignant glandular and a malignant squamous component that are due to primary cervical squamous carcinoma and primary endometrial adenocarcinoma. In these cases the squamous cell component predominates and the malignant glandular component is less conspicuous and shows features of endometrial adenocarcinoma. Because primary squamous cell carcinoma of the endometrium is rare, it is also extremely rare to encounter such a tumor coexisting with an endocervical adenocarcinoma or cervical squamous cell cancer.

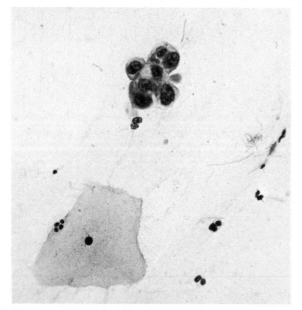

FIGURE 11–22. Adenosquamous carcinoma of endometrium. Malignant glandular component, Broders's grade II. The malignant squamous component is shown in Figure 11–23. Endocervical aspirate (Papanicolaou stain; × 480).

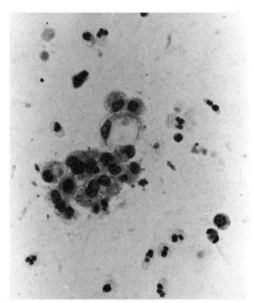

FIGURE 11–24. Malignant glandular component in **malignant müllerian tumor of uterus.** Endocervical aspirate (Papanicolaou stain; × 480).

Malignant Mixed Müllerian Tumor. This tumor consists of an admixture of malignant epithelial and malignant mesenchymal components in which the sarcoma often predominates (Figs. 11–24 and 11–25). The most common epithelial component is of a glandular type and is often associated with a malignant squamous component. The most common sarcoma component is stromal sarcoma or fibrosarcoma (homologous type or

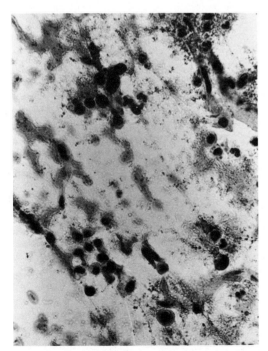

FIGURE 11–25. Stromal cell sarcoma component in **malignant müllerian tumor of uterus.** The sarcoma cells tend to occur singly with some variation in size and shape. Note tumor diathesis. Endocervical aspirate (Papanicolaou stain; × 480).

carcinosarcoma). Rhabdomyosarcoma, bone, cartilage and glial tissue are less frequently present (heterologous type). Cell samples may contain a malignant glandular component of an endometrial type with or without squamous component and may or may not contain sarcoma cells of stromal, striated muscle or other sarcoma cell types.

Extent of Carcinoma

Cellular changes in relation to the extent of endometrial carcinoma depend on the extent of endometrial mucosa involvement by cancer and the extent of invasiveness of the cancer into the myometrium, pelvis, cervix and elsewhere. Focal involvement of the endometrial mucosa by cancer usually representing early disease is much less likely to shed cells, and if cells are shed they are usually limited in number. Most focal cancers are well differentiated and are often associated with precursor changes or normal endometrium. Cell samples obtained from focal cancers that contain endometrial cells have few cells and may show a combination of normal, hyperplastic and malignant well-differentiated adenocarcinoma cells. A tumor diathesis is more likely to be absent and if present is inconspicuous. In some cases, evidence is found of precipitated protein with a watery background. Focal poorly differentiated adenocarcinoma is less frequently encountered and tends to shed less cells, showing features of this adenocarcinoma. These lesions are less likely to be associated with precursor changes, and hence hyperplastic cells are infrequently encountered with the malignant cells.

In contrast, tumors with extensive involvement of the endometrial mucosa and invasion into the myometrium are more prone to shed cells in greater numbers, and a tumor diathesis is more frequently encountered and more pronounced. A relationship exists between the invasiveness of an endometrial cancer and the differentiation of the neoplasm. Poorly differentiated cancers are usually more invasive. As a result it is difficult to determine whether any given manifestation is a reflection of differentiation or extent or both. With involvement of the endocervix by endometrial carcinoma, it may sometimes be difficult to differentiate it from a primary endocervical adenocarcinoma in cellular samples. Usually the cellular characteristics of the parent tissue of origin assist in differentiation.

MALIGNANT CELLS OF EXTRAUTERINE ORIGIN

The ability to recognize malignant cells of extrauterine origin from those of primary uterine origin in cellular samples is of importance, as it will determine the nature of the investigation. Furthermore, the presence of malignant cells in uterine samples in patients with known extrauterine cancer provides information about the extent of the neoplasm. Infrequently, evidence of extrauterine neoplasm is first appreciated in a routine cellular sample. Malignant tumor cells identified in cellular samples of the uterus and vagina are, in the majority of cases, from primary uterine neoplasms and, less frequently, of extrauterine origin. The latter are usually of the glandular type and only rarely of the squamous, sarcoma, lymphoid or leukemic cell type.[5, 21, 24, 29, 30]

Factors that are considered to be of importance in influencing the shedding of malignant cells of extrauterine origin into the uterus or vagina include the site of primary tumor, extent and location of the neoplastic spread, ascites and patency of the uterine tubes. In cellular samples that contain malignant cells of extrauterine origin, the predominant primary site of the tumor will be located in the pelvis or abdominal cavity. The most common sites are the ovary and gastrointestinal tract; primary tumor from the uterine tube, pancreas, urethra, breast and abdominal mesothelium and malignant melanoma are less frequently encountered. Other rare primary neoplasms include lung, urinary bladder, gall bladder, and appendix. At the time of cellular detection, metastasis to the pelvis and peritoneum, often associated with ascites, will be appreciated in the majority of cases. Only about a fourth of cases will show metastasis to the mucosa of the uterus or vagina or both. The patency of the uterine tubes also facilitates the passage of malignant cells from the abdomen to the uterine and vaginal cavities for cellular detection.[21]

The source of the malignant cells will determine the appearance of the cellular samples. The tumor cells observed in endometrial, endocervical or vaginal sam-

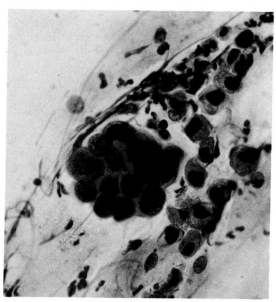

FIGURE 11–27. Mammary ductal carcinoma. Malignant tumor cells as an aggregate and single cells. Although leukocytes are evident, a tumor diathesis is absent in the sample. Endocervical aspirate (Papanicolaou stain; ×480). (Reproduced with permission from Ng ABP, Teeple D, Lindner E, Reagan JW: The cellular manifestations of extrauterine cancer. Acta Cytol 18:108–117, 1974.)

ples may originate directly from the primary tumor or its metastasis in the pelvis or abdominal cavity, passing through the lumens of the uterine tubes. Under these conditions, evidence of an adverse host response is usually absent in the cellular sample. A lack of tumor diathesis is seen in 80% of cell samples containing malignant cells of extrauterine origin (Figs. 11–26 and 11–27). Less than 20% have a diathesis, and in these cases vaginal or uterine metastasis, or both, with mucosa involvement and ulceration are seen. Furthermore, in many cases, the diathesis is not conspicuous in the presence of poorly differentiated malignant cells. In contrast, less than 10% of cell samples obtained from women with primary endometrial carcinoma and less than 15% of cell samples obtained from women with primary endocervical adenocarcinoma lack a tumor diathesis. In endometrial samples, the presence of glandular cells, especially when poorly differentiated with benign endometrial cells or fragments, may suggest an extrauterine cancer. A diathesis is usually lacking. The number of abnormal cells seen are variable, and these cells are usually less conspicuous than those of primary uterine tumors.

The cellular features of malignant cells of extrauterine origin are usually poorly differentiated. In the majority of cases, it is not possible to determine the primary site or histologic subtype of the tumor (see Fig. 11–27). However, infrequently, the arrangement and morphology of the cell aggregates may reflect the tissue of origin and differentiation of the parent tumor. When malignant cells with a papillary pattern of extrauterine origin are identified, the most common primary site is from the ovary (see Fig. 11–26) and very

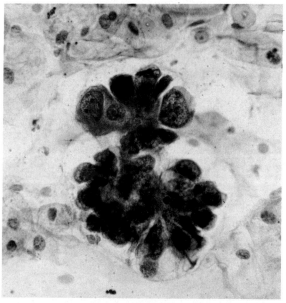

FIGURE 11–26. Serous papillary adenocarcinoma of ovary. Papillary grouping of poorly differentiated malignant tumor cells. Note absence of tumor diathesis. Endocervical aspirate. (Papanicolaou stain; ×480). (Reproduced with permission from Ng ABP, Teeple D, Lindner E, Reagan JW: The cellular manifestations of extrauterine cancer. Acta Cytol 18:108–117, 1974.)

infrequently the pancreas, mesothelium or thyroid. Similarly, psammoma bodies with malignant cells should suggest an ovarian origin; however, they have been observed in the presence of benign and malignant lesions of the endometrium, mesothelium, pancreas, lung, thyroid and kidney.[6, 21]

Except for a lack of a tumor diathesis, the cellular characteristics of extrauterine neoplasms, originating in the uterine tube, have many of the features of endometrial adenocarcinoma. Evidence of a watery transudate may be associated with uterine tube or endometrial cancer. When malignant cells of extrauterine origin are organized in a linear arrangement, a primary mammary or a specific type of gastric cancer should be considered. In some cases of well-differentiated adenocarcinoma of the colon, the cell samples may contain tall columnar cells with elongated nuclei arranged in a palisading pattern. The cellular features of lymphoma or leukemia are characterized by single abnormal cells of lymphoid origin. Sarcoma cells, primary or secondary, are rarely seen.

Thus, when malignant cells especially of a poorly differentiated adenocarcinoma are observed without an associated tumor diathesis, the presence of an extrauterine origin should be considered.[21]

DIFFERENTIAL DIAGNOSIS OF NORMAL AND ABNORMAL ENDOMETRIAL CELLS

Endometrial Compared with Endocervical Adenocarcinoma

In cell samples collected from the endocervical canal, significant differences are noted between endometrial and endocervical adenocarcinoma as shown in Table 11–7.[24, 25] Although the number of abnormal cells are related to the degree of differentiation, generally the number of cells of endocervical adenocarcinoma are much higher than endometrial carcinoma (Figs. 11–14 and 11–28). This finding is due to the location of the sampling. The arrangement of malignant cells of endocervical origin tends to occur in strips, sheets, rosettes and irregular masses, whereas malignant endometrial cells occur in small loose clusters of modified acinous structures; tight cells balls and sheets are seen only in undifferentiated adenocarcinoma. For comparable grades of differentiation, malignant endocervical cells and nuclei are larger and have more nucleoli and macronucleoli. The chromatin is more granular and hyperchromatic than malignant endometrial cells. Malignant cells of columnar form are more frequently seen in endocervical adenocarconoma, whereas the cells are round or oval in endometrial adenocarcinoma.

Using the EA65 stain, cells derived from endocervical adenocarcinoma tend to have a granular eosinophilic cytoplasm and less often cyanophilic. Malignant endometrial cells tend to have finely vacuolated cyanophilic or indeterminate-staining cytoplasm. In vaginal samples, columnar form is inconspicuous in both endo-

TABLE 11–7. Differences Between Endometrial and Endocervical Adenocarcinoma

Cellular Characteristics	Endometrial Adenocarcinoma	Endocervical Adenocarcinoma
No of cells/cm²	50	1300
Cell area (μ²)	140	190
Nuclear area (μ²)	60	90
Columnar forms (%)	5	60
Eosinophilic cytoplasm (%)	30	80
Cyanophilic cytoplasm (%)	55	10
Granular cytoplasm (%)	5	75
Vacuolated cytoplasm (%)	65	25
Nuclear hyperchromasia	+	+ +
Multiple nucleoli (%)	25	75
Macronucleoli (%)	15	40
Chromatin	Irregular finely granular	Irregularly finely or coarsely granular
Cellular arrangement	Loose cell clusters Modified acini Tight cell balls Sheets (undifferentiated)	Strips, sheets, rosettes, masses

Modified after Reagan JW, Ng ABP: The cells of uterine adenocarcinoma, 2nd ed. Basel, S Karger, 1973.

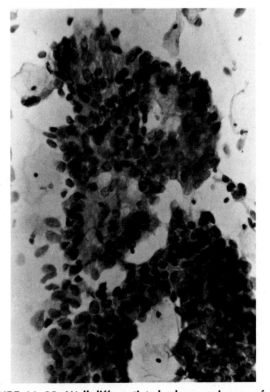

FIGURE 11–28. Well-differentiated adenocarcinoma of endocervix. Malignant cells are abundant. When viewed in proper perspective, the malignant cells are columnar in form. The cells tend to occur in a sheet-like arrangement. Compare with Figures 11–14 and 11–15. Endocervical aspirate (Papanicolaou stain; × 300).

metrial and endocervical adenocarcinoma. The differentiation of adenosquamous carcinoma from the endometrium and cervix is based on the characteristics of the malignant glandular component.

Endometrial Compared with Extrauterine Adenocarcinoma. Most extrauterine adenocarcinomas are poorly differentiated and are usually not associated with a tumor diathesis in vaginal and uterine samples (endocervical and endometrial), whereas a tumor diathesis is usually associated with a poorly differentiated endometrial or endocervical adenocarcinoma. Although other differences may be present as described, the presence or absence of a tumor diathesis in the presence of a poorly differentiated adenocarcinoma is the most important reliable variable.[21, 24]

Endometrial Adenocarcinoma Compared with Cervical Squamous Carcinoma. Small-cell cancer of the cervix and its precursors may be confused with well-differentiated adenocarcinoma of the endometrium. In well-differentiated adenocarcinoma of the endometrium, the samples contain relatively few cell aggregates and appear as loose altered acinar or tight clusters with molded peripheral border. The cells may be cuboidal with an excentric nucleus. The chromatin is irregular and finely granular with micronucleoli. The tumor diathesis is watery with granular material and few inflammatory cells and cellular detritus. The cytoplasm is finely vacuolated. When compared with endometrial carcinoma, in small-cell carcinoma, the cell sample contains many cells occurring singly and in aggregates. The aggregates are in syncytial form with no altered acinar pattern or tight clusters with molded peripheral border. The nuclei are more hyperchromatic with more granular chromatin. Nucleoli are less conspicuous. The tumor diathesis is more prominent with more conspicuous degree of cellular detritus, inflammatory cells and hemorrhage. The cytoplasm is scanty and granular. Nucleoli and diathesis are absent in small-cell carcinoma *in situ*.

Large-cell type of squamous carcinoma may be confused with poorly differentiated adenocarcinoma. Although cell samples from poorly differentiated adenocarcinomas may contain sheet-like or syncytical cell aggregates, papillary groups and tight cell ball clusters may be present as well. The cytoplasm remains finely vacuolated; the chromatinic material remains relatively and finely granular; the macronucleoli are conspicuous and diathesis is watery and granular, with some cellular detritus and inflammatory cells. In contrast, cell samples from large-cell nonkeratinizing squamous cell carcinoma contain many more abnormal cells, occurring singly or syncytially with no papillary or tight cell ball pattern. The cytoplasm stains more densely and homogeneously, the nuclei are more hyperchromatic and the chromatin is more granular, with more conspicuous nuclear clearing. Macronucleoli are less conspicuous, and tumor diathesis with more conspicuous cellular detritus and inflammatory cells is evident.[23, 24]

Irradiated malignant cells in cell samples may sometimes be difficult to evaluate as to cell type and origin of tumor. Malignant glandular cells may lose their characteristic features and mimic cells of squamous type. Malignant squamous cells may take on some characteristics of a glandular component.

Benign Lesions Simulating Adenocarcinoma. The most common entity that is often confused with adenocarcinoma is reactive endocervical, parabasal or immature squamous metaplastic cell aggregates of the cervix.[3, 17] When compared with endometrial adenocarcinoma, reactive cervical cells are relatively large with few single cells and most tend to occur in aggregates, which are sheet-like and often show irregular cytoplasmic processes (Fig. 11–29). Mitotic figures and inflammatory cell infiltrate are often seen in the sheets of cells. When in a monolayer, the cytoplasm is moderately abundant and may appear vacuolated, and the nucleocytoplasmic ratio is variable but usually low. Often some cells in the sheets appear relatively normal, whereas others appear atypical. The nuclei are enlarged, and often macronucleoli are evident. However, irregular distribution of chromatinic material is inconspicuous or absent. Although there may be a hemorrhagic inflammatory background in the cell sample, a tumor diathesis is usually absent. These reactive cells usually disappear when inflammation subsides on repeat cell studies.

Degenerative changes, especially in immature metaplastic cells of the cervix, may be confused with adenocarcinoma (Figs. 11–30 and 11–31). The most common degenerative change is the presence of cytoplasmic vacuoles. These vacuoles in small metaplastic cells may push the nucleus to one side and when seen in aggregates may be mistaken for adenocarcinoma. The cytoplasm of metaplastic cells has a densely staining homogeneous cyanophilic cytoplasm. Even in the presence of degenerative cytoplasmic vacuoles, usually

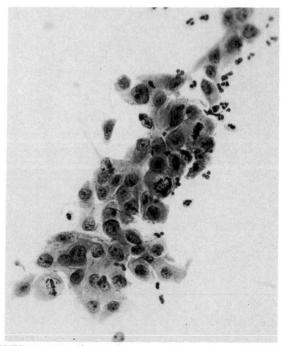

FIGURE 11–29. Sheet of **regenerative endocervical cells.** Note mitotic structures. Compare with Figures 11–15 and 11–28. Endocervical aspirate (Papanicolaou stain; ×320).

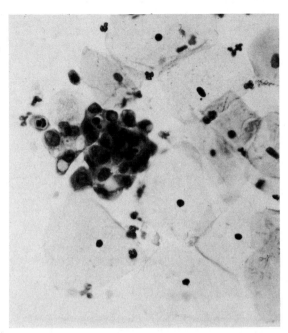

FIGURE 11–30. Vacuolated immature metaplastic cells simulating adenocarcinoma. Endocervical aspirate (Papanicolaou stain; × 400).

a thin rim of dense-staining cytoplasm is still recognizable. The nuclei of metaplastic cells are uniformly granular with no nuclear clearing or nucleoli.[17]

Arias-Stella cells have been rarely described and are difficult to differentiate from other cell types in cervical and endometrial samples. They are relatively simple to appreciate in endometrial samples that contain tissue fragments. In cellular aggregates they lack the cytologic features of malignancy. Syncytial trophoblasts are multinucleated in cervical and endometrial samples. Cytotrophoblasts are more difficult to identify except when tissue fragments are present.[26, 28]

The presence of bare nuclei of endocervical origin, especially in cell samples from postmenopausal women, occurring singly and in aggregates, has been mistaken for adenocarcinoma. The bare nuclei are relatively uniform in size and shape, and the nuclei appear bland with no nucleoli. An interpretation of adenocarcinoma or other cellular abnormality should not be made primarily on bare or free nuclei.

Artificial changes in endocervical columnar cells and in cells derived from benign proceses induced by improper collection, fixation or staining may produce changes simulating adenocarcinoma. These include cellular and nuclear enlargement; cytoplasmic vacuolization; chromatin alterations, such as irregular clumping of chromatin material and nuclear clearing, and nuclear inclusions. Great caution should be taken in interpreting cells in poorly prepared specimens. When detailed study is difficult or impossible, it is advisable to report such a specimen as "unsatisfactory for proper evaluation" and repeat the cell study.[17]

DIAGNOSTIC ACCURACY

Many factors contribute to the ultimate accuracy achieved in diagnostic cytopathology of the female genital tract. Clinical and pathologic aspects of the patient influence the optimal evaluation of a cell sample. These include configuration and abnormalities, particularly of the cervix and body of uterus; age of patient; presence or absence of infection; menses or abnormal uterine bleeding; type, severity, anatomic location and distribution of one or more disease processes to be detected by evaluating the cellular samples; biologic aspects of the tumor in relation to extent of disease; degree of differentiation of tumor; histologic cell type of tumor and extent of necrosis and inflammation.

The qualitative and quantitative superiority of cellular material collected in a cell sample is influenced by the motivation and ability of the individual who is collecting the specimen, the type and method of collection, the method of cell film preparation, the fixation and staining procedures as well as the time interval between cytologic studies.

Particularly pertinent to the evaluation of endometrial cells, the laboratory staff (cytotechnologists and cytopathologists) must be intimately familiar with the recognition of endometrial cells and their changes, as these probably represent the most difficult area in gynecologic cytology. Because of the plethora of influencing factors, it is practically impossible to achieve 100% accuracy in diagnostic cytopathology, especially endometrial cytology.

Using direct endometrial sampling, accuracy for the detection of endometrial hyperplasia when tissue

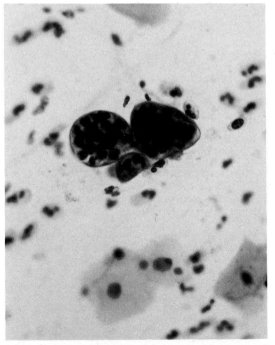

FIGURE 11–31. Vacuolated immature squamous metaplastic cells with intracytoplasmic leukocytes simulating adenocarcinoma from a woman who is wearing an intrauterine device. Endocervical aspirate (Papanicolaou stain; × 480).

fragments are obtained is over 90% and for the detection of adenocarcinoma it is over 95%. If no tissue fragments are present and diagnosis is based on cellular changes, the accuracy is about 50% for endometrial hyperplasia and 90% for endometrial carcinoma.[2, 8, 12, 13, 24, 25]

The sensitivity for detection of endometrial hyperplasia based on spontaneous desquamation of endometrial cells (endocervical or vaginal sample) is very low and is not optimal for a screening program. It is, however, a simple method for detecting some endometrial conditions when endometrial cells are identified in routine samples. In our experience, endometrial cells are seen in about 25% of cases in patients with adenomatous hyperplasia with atypia (atypical hyperplasia and adenocarcinoma *in situ*) and about 10% of cases in patients with adenomatous hyperplasia without atypia (adenomatous and cystic hyperplasia) in endocervical aspirate samples. Endometrial cells are seen in vaginal samples in about 5% for cell hyperplasias. However, when endometrial cells are present, the diagnosis of endometrial hyperplasia in these cases is relatively high, up to 75% specificity in endocervical aspirates.[7, 19, 24]

The overall accuracy for the diagnosis of endometrial adenocarcinoma by vaginal samples is less than 50%. In contrast, the overall accuracy rate for the detection of endometrial carcinoma by the endocervical samples is about 70%. In some cases, up to 15%, only normal-appearing endometrial and hyperplastic endometrial cells are seen in the endocervical sample from patients with endometrial cancer. Furthermore, the detection rate for well-differentiated adenocarcinomas is less than 60% and about 80% for poorly differentiated adenocarcinomas and adenosquamous cancers.[24, 25, 27]

References

1. An-Foraker SH, Kawada CY: Cytodiagnosis of endometrial malignant mixed mesodermal tumor. Acta Cytol 29:137–141, 1985.
2. Bibbo M: The Vakutage method in the detection of endometrial cancer and its precursors: *In* Compendium on Diagnostic Cytology, 6th ed. Edited by GL Wied, CM Keebler, LG Koss, JW Reagan. Chicago, Tutorials of Cytology, p 213, 1988.
3. Bibbo M: "Look-alikes" in cytology of the female genital tract. *In* Compendium on Diagnostic Cytology, 6th ed. Edited by GL Wied, CM Keebler, LG Koss, JW Reagan. Chicago, Tutorials of Cytology, p 236, 1988.
4. Blumenfeld W, Holly EA, Mansur DL, King EB: Histiocytes and the detection of endometrial carcinoma. Acta Cytol 29:317–322, 1985.
5. Boken R, Perkovic M, Bakotin J, Milasinovic D, Mojsovic D: Cytology and histopathology of metastatic malignant melanoma involving a polyp on the uterine cervix. A case report. Acta Cytol 29:612–615, 1985.
6. Fujimoto I, Masubuchi S, Miwa H, Fukuda K, Yamaguchi S, Masbuchi K: Psammoma bodies found in cervicovaginal and/or endometrial smears. Acta Cytol 26:317–322, 1982.
7. Kashimura M, Baba S, Shinohara M, Kashimura Y, Saito T, Hachisuga T: Cytologic findings in endometrial hyperplasia. Acta Cytol 32:335–340, 1988.
8. Koss, LG, Schreiber K, Oberlander SG, Moussouris HF, Lesser M: Detection of endometrial carcinoma and hyperplasia in asymptomatic women. Obstet Gynecol 64:1–11, 1984.
9. Kuebler DL, Nikrui N, Bell DA: Cytologic features of endometrial papillary serous carcinoma. Acta Cytol 33:120–126, 1989.
10. Kusuyama Y, Yoshida M, Imai H, Kosomichi T, Mabuchi Y, Yokota H: Secreting carcinoma of the endometrium. Acta Cytol 33:127–130, 1989.
11. Lozowski MS, Mishriki Y, Solitare GB: Factors determining the degree of endometrial exfoliation and their diagnostic implications in endometrial adenocarcinoma. Acta Cytol 30:623–627, 1986.
12. Meisels A, Jolicoeur C: Criteria for the cytologic assessment of hyperplasias in endometrial samples obtained by the Endopap endometrial sampler. Acta Cytol 29:297–302, 1985.
13. Milan AR, Markley RL: Endometrial cytology by a new technic. Obstet Gynecol 42:469–475, 1973.
14. Ng ABP: Some pathologic factors significant in management and prognosis of endometrial carcinoma. *In* Compendium on Diagnostic Cytology, 6th ed. Edited by GL Wied, CM Keebler, LG Koss, JW Reagan. Chicago, Tutorials of Cytology, p 208, 1988.
15. Ng ABP, Reagan JW: The pathology and cytopathology of squamous cell carcinoma of the uterine cervix. *In* Compendium on Diagnostic Cytology, 6th ed. Edited by GL Wied, CM Keebler, LG Koss, JW Reagan. Chicago, Tutorials of Cytology, p 123, 1988.
16. Ng ABP, Reagan JW: Normal endometrial cells and their significance in the detection of benign and malignant endometrial lesions. *In* Compendium on Diagnostic Cytology, 6th ed. Edited by GL Wied, CM Keebler, LG Koss, JW Reagan. Chicago, Tutorials of Cytology, p 162, 1988.
17. Ng ABP, Reagan JW: Normal, benign and neoplastic processes simulating adenocarcinoma of uterus. *In* Compendium on Diagnostic Cytology, 6th ed. Edited by GL Wied, CM Keebler, LG Koss, JW Reagan. Chicago, Tutorials of Cytology, p 176, 1988.
18. Ng ABP, Reagan JW: The pathology and cytopathology of microinvasive adenocarcinoma and precursors of endometrial carcinoma. *In* Compendium on Diagnostic Cytology, 6th ed. Edited by GL Wied, CM Keebler, LG Koss, JW Reagan. Chicago, Tutorials of Cytology, p 180, 1988.
19. Ng ABP, Reagan JW, Cechner RL: The precursors of endometrial cancer: A study of their cellular manifestations. Acta Cytol 17:439–448, 1973.
20. Ng ABP, Reagan JW, Hawkiczek S, Wentz BW: Significance of endometrial cells in the detection of endometrial carcinoma and its precursors. Acta Cytol 18:356–361, 1974.
21. Ng ABP, Teeple D, Lindner EA, Reagan JW: The cellular manifestations of extrauterine cancer. Acta Cytol 18:108–117, 1974.
22. Palermo VG: Interpretation of endometrium obtained by the endo-Pap sampler and a clinical study of its use. Diag Cytopathol 1:5–12, 1985.
23. Patten SF Jr: Diagnostic cytology of the uterine cervix, 2nd ed. Basel, S Karger, 1978.
24. Reagan JW, Ng ABP: The cells of uterine adenocarcinoma, 2nd ed. Basel, S Karger, 1973.
25. Reagan JW, Ng ABP: The cells of endometrial cancer. *In* Compendium on Diagnostic Cytology, 6th ed. Edited by GL Wied, CM Keebler, LG Koss, JW Reagan. Chicago, Tutorials of Cytology, p 194, 1988.
26. Schneider V: Cytology in pregnancy. *In* Compendium on Diagnostic Cytology, 6th ed. Edited by GL Wied, CM Keebler, LG Koss, JW Reagan. Chicago, Tutorials of Cytology, p 51, 1988.
27. Schneider ML, Wortmann M, Weigel A: Influence of the histologic and cytologic grade and the clinical and postsurgical stage on the rate of endometrial carcinoma detection by cervical cytology. Acta Cytol 30:616–622, 1986.
28. Shrago SS: The Arias-Stella reaction: A case report of a cytologic presentation. Acta Cytol 21:310–313, 1977.
29. Takashina T, Ito E, Kudo R: Cytologic diagnosis of primary tubal cancer. Acta Cytol 29:367–372, 1985.
30. Takashina T, Ono M, Kanda Y, Sagae S, Hayakawa O, Ito E: Cervicovaginal and endometrial cytology in ovarian cancer. Acta Cytol 32:159–162, 1988.
31. Vooijs GP, Van der Graaf Y, Yooijs MA: The presence of endometrial cells in cervical smears in relation to the day of the menstrual cycle and the method of contraception. Acta Cytol 31:427–433, 1987.

12

Vulva and Vagina

Kelly Sorensen
Theresa M. Somrak

Vulvar and vaginal exfoliative cytology, although not a substitute for biopsy, may provide valuable information about the nature of a lesion with little discomfort to the patient. Although unsuspected cancer is rarely identified by this approach, a wide variety of infectious and inflammatory diseases, dermatologic diseases and benign and malignant tumors have characteristic cytologic features.

VULVA

Technique

Technical success in procuring an optimal specimen from the vulva depends on the method utilized. Scrapings are best obtained through the use of physical force using a variety of instruments, i.e., the edge of a glass slide, scalpel blade or other instrument. A warm, moist saline towel or cloth placed over the lesion to be sampled softens the superficial keratinized layer, resulting in a more cellular specimen with a reduction in the amount of drying artifact. Vigorous scraping may be required to dislodge cellular material covered by a thick layer of keratin, which should be discarded for a more cellular second scrape. Moist or ulcerated lesions may be sampled by touching a glass slide directly against the lesion or by swabbing the edge of the ulcer and spreading the material on a slide. All slides should be immediately fixed with spray fixative or 95% ethanol for optimal preservation. Pigmented lesions are perhaps best biopsied unless the surface is ulcerated or the specimen can be easily obtained through nonaggressive methods. Cysts of the vulva are best aspirated via the fine needle aspiration biopsy technique.

Histology

The vulva is composed of the mons pubis, the labia majora, the labia minora, the clitoris, the vestibule and the Bartholin glands. Except for the Bartholin glands these structures are covered by stratified squamous epithelium. The Bartholin glands are paired, mucus-secreting glands lying in the posterior aspect of the labia majora. Their main excretory ducts are lined by stratified squamous epithelium, as are the ducts of the minor vestibular gland.

Infectious and Inflammatory Diseases

A number of infectious and inflammatory diseases may involve the vulva. Proper specimen collection and culturing is often necessary for the complete identification of a causative agent. Many venereal and nonvenereal processes have characteristic morphologic appearances on Papanicolaou smears that suggest the causative agent. Common viral infections such as herpes simplex (a common cause of vulvar ulcers) and the human papilloma virus (condyloma acuminatum) have readily identifiable cytopathic effects. The use of podophyllin in the treatment of genital warts results in nuclear alterations, which can result in the diagnosis of squamous dysplasia or squamous carcinoma *in situ*.[7] Podophyllin is believed to have a direct cytotoxic effect resulting in enhancement of the nuclei with increased hyperchromasia of the nuclear chromatin. The cytoplasm is often vacuolated and stains eosinophilic. The effects of trichloroacetic acid and salicylic acid also used in the treatment of condyloma is keratolysis without discernible cytopathic effects. Uncommon viral infections such as molluscum contagiosum (Fig. 12–1), cytomegalovirus, varicella, herpes zoster, variola, Epstein-Barr virus and vaccinia may rarely involve the vulva as a part of a systemic infection. Mycotic vulvar infections are usually secondary to *Candida albicans* or *Candida tropicalis*. Unusual fungal organisms include *Torulopsis glabrata* and the superficial dermatophytic mycoses, including tinea cruris, tinea versicolor and tinea circinata. Deep mycotic infections of the

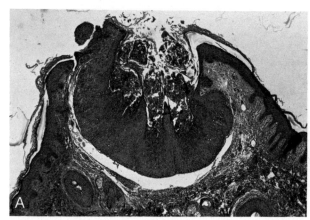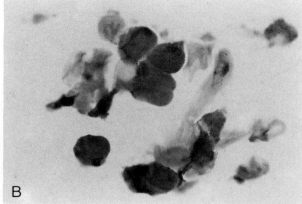

FIGURE 12–1. Molluscum contagiosum, vulva. *A,* Umbilicated lesion with central corps ronds (hematoxylin and eosin; ×20). *B,* Molluscum bodies with dense eosinophilic cytoplasm (Papanicolaou stain; ×500).

vulva (blastomycosis, sporotrichosis, coccidioidomycosis and actinomycosis) are rare. Parasitic infections such as trichomoniasis, amebiasis and schistosomiasis usually involve the vagina as well as the vulva. The diagnosis can easily be made by identifying the organism on a cytologic preparation or in a biopsy specimen.

Bartholin gland infections are caused by a variety of anaerobic and aerobic organisms. Both ductal and acinar elements may be infected, resulting in a blockage of secretion and causing the formation of an abscess that may be diagnosed by fine needle aspiration.

Inflammatory and dermatologic diseases of the vulva include vulvar vestibulitis syndrome, Behçet syndrome, Crohn's disease, malakoplakia, contact dermatitis, psoriasis, pemphigus vulgaris (Fig. 12–2), bullous pemphigoid, lichen planus, erythema multiforme, vulvar dystrophy and a variety of dermatologic tumors such as seborrheic keratosis, syringomas and hidradenoma papilliferum (Fig. 12–3). Such lesions are most frequently diagnosed clinically or by biopsy rather than by a cytologic sample. Pemphigus may be suggested by the presence of isolated or loose aggregates of acantholytic cells taken from the base of the ulcer.

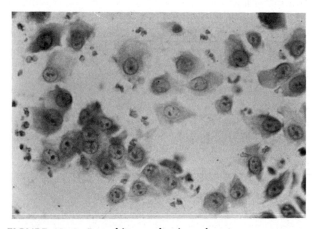

FIGURE 12–2. Pemphigus vulgaris, vulva. Loose aggregates of acantholytic cells with prominent nucleoli (Papanicolaou stain; ×500).

Vulvar Dystrophy

Vulvar dystrophies are divided histopathologically into three major categories: (1) hyperplastic, (2) atrophic and (3) mixed dystrophies.[20] The degree of hyperkeratosis determines its clinical appearance. The variable clinical appearances with regard to color of the lesion, degree of hyperplasia or extent of disease process offer little indication as to whether or not an underlying dysplasia is present signifying possible malignant potential. Clinically all of the external structures of the vulva including the skin of the perianal region and thigh may be involved.

Histologically hyperkeratosis and acanthosis are usually present. Parakeratosis may be noted. Cytologically an increased number of anucleate squames are generally present. Because of the presence of anucleate squames from normal skin, caution should be exercised in coming to a conclusion about the pathologic significance of anucleate squames. The squamous cells retaining their nuclei may demonstrate reactive changes such as slight nuclear enlargement; however, significant degrees of nuclear atypia and pleomorphism are not observed unless an underlying dysplasia is present (Fig. 12–4).

Lichen sclerosis most frequently occurs in the postmenopausal period; however, women of any age may be affected. Histologically the epidermis may be of normal thickness, hyperplastic in the early stages or atrophic in the advanced stages. A hyalinized zone of collagen is noted beneath the epidermis, below which are plasma cells and lymphocytes. Separation of the basal layer from the basement membrane may result in the formation of bullae. Cytologic features similar to those of the hyperplastic dystrophies are noted in lichen sclerosis, including varying degrees of anucleate squames or parakeratotic cells. Many of the dystrophies are clinically mixed dystrophies. Therefore, distinction of the type of dystrophy based on the cytologic appearances is impossible. Significant cytologic atypia is not present.

Epithelial dysplasias are noted in approximately 16%

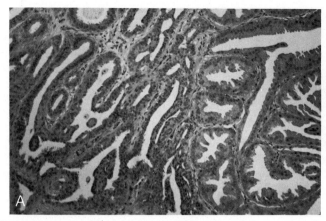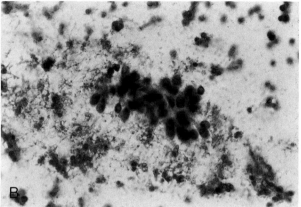

FIGURE 12–3. Hidradenoma papilliferum, vulva. *A,* Complex glandular and tubular structure with papillary projections supported by delicate fibrovascular core (hematoxylin and eosin; ×80). *B,* Columnar cells showing little pleormorphism or atypia resembling breast ductal cells (Papanicolaou stain; ×500).

of the mixed dystrophies, 10% of the hyperplastic dystrophies and rarely in lichen sclerosis alone.[20, 22, 28] The risk of dystrophy developing into invasive squamous carcinoma is between 1 and 10%.[15] If cellular atypia is absent, the risk of developing a squamous carcinoma is minimal.

The potential for a dysplastic dystrophy to develop into a malignant process is related to the severity of the dysplasia. In mild and moderate dysplasia, the epithelium histologically contains cells with enlarged nuclei and abundant cytoplasm. The upper level will show considerable cytoplasmic differentiation. The nuclei are slightly enlarged and hyperchromatic. Mitoses may be observed above the basilar layer. Hyperkeratosis or parakeratosis may be noted. In severe dysplasia the cells are smaller and have an increased nucleocytoplasmic ratio. The nuclei are hyperchromatic and coarsely granular. At the surface, cytoplasmic differentiation may occur with increasing amounts of cytoplasm. Nuclear pyknosis may occur in the upper levels, as may isolated cell keratinization. Mitoses are seen from the basilar level to the surface. Cytologically the dysplastic cells are usually polygonal in form with varying amounts of eosinophilic cytoplasm.

In the more advanced dysplasias, the cells have a round or oval configuration. Variable nuclear enlargement is noted together with some variability in nuclear size. Marked variability in size is uncommon. Hyperkeratosis or parakeratosis is usually present. In most cases, one can separate severe dysplasia and carcinoma *in situ* from the mild to moderate dysplasias based on the number of dysplastic cells and the extent of the cytologic abnormality. The cellular changes with mild dysplasia are subtle and often overlooked. Frequently the area containing the mild dysplasia is not sampled owing to lack of clinical distinction from areas of dystrophy without atypia.

Malignant Vulvar Neoplasms

Malignant tumors of the vulva make up approximately 5% of all gynecologic malignancies.[15] The frequency with which each type occurs is as follows: 51% squamous carcinoma, 25% squamous carcinoma *in situ,* 8% metastatic tumor, 8% Paget's disease, 5% malignant melanoma, 2% adenocarcinoma, 2% basal cell

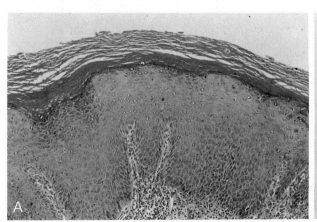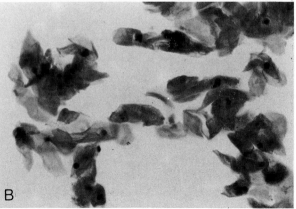

FIGURE 12–4. Hyperplastic dystrophy, vulva. *A,* Skin with acanthosis, hyperkeratosis and chronic dermal infiltrate (hematoxylin and eosin; ×20). *B,* Hyperkeratosis (Papanicolaou stain; ×500).

carcinoma and 1% sarcoma.[10] Most vulvar carcinomas occur in an older population.

Squamous Cell Carcinoma *in Situ.* This condition of the vulva has been noted in women of all ages. Data suggest that squamous cell carcinoma *in situ* is increasing in frequency and is occurring in a younger age group.[14] Approximately 40% of the cases occur in women younger than 40 years of age.[14] Studies have linked both the herpes simplex virus and the human papilloma virus to the development of vulvar malignancies.[21, 27] Other factors that have also been implicated include physical and chemical agents such as ionizing irradiation, arsenicals and immunosuppression.

Pruritus is the most common symptom. Genital warts are present in 15 to 30% of the patients.[4, 28] Multifocality on the vulva or prior cervical dysplasia is present in approximately one fourth of patients.[4, 14] Clinically, lesions of squamous cell carcinoma are generally slightly raised, usually with a sharply defined border. The surface may be erythematous, hyperkeratotic or scaly. Hyperpigmentation may be noted. Ulceration is unusual. Colposcopic examination or a magnifying lens may be helpful to delineate the borders of the lesion. The use of toluidine blue O is not effective because of the variability of toluidine blue O in staining lesions with hyperkeratosis, resulting in high numbers of false-positives and false-negatives.[14]

Histologically squamous cell carcinoma *in situ* demonstrates a proliferation of immature epithelial cells with an increased nucleocytoplasmic ratio, nuclear hyperchromasia and multinucleation. Hyperkeratosis or parakeratosis is usually present. Maturation disturbances are frequently noted along the surface. Koilocytotic changes are noted frequently within and adjacent to the lesion (Fig. 12–5A). Cytologic scraping of the lesion reveals abnormal cells occurring singly or in loose aggregates. The cells are polygonal with well-defined cytoplasmic borders. Variation in size and shape of the cells is usually noted; however, lesions may mimic either a basal cell carcinoma having small uniform cells or a large-cell squamous carcinoma having marked variability. The nuclei are enlarged and hyperchromatic with granular chromatin. Anucleate squames and parakeratotic cells are usually observed (Fig. 12–5B).

The clinical presentation is of marked importance before establishing a diagnosis of bowenoid papulosis because there are no well-accepted histologic criteria that separate bowenoid papulosis from squamous carcinoma *in situ.* Bowenoid papulosis occurs in a somewhat younger age group. The lesions appear slightly elevated and are small in size. Many of the lesions show varying amounts of pigmentation. Spontaneous regression occurs commonly. The histologic findings are those of dysplasia, ranging from moderate dysplasia to carcinoma *in situ.* Human papilloma virus antigens have been identified in several of the lesions.[3, 21]

Squamous Cell Carcinoma. The majority of all malignant vulvar tumors are invasive squamous cell carcinomas. Squamous cell carcinoma of the vulva usually affects elderly women, with a mean age of 63 to 67 years.[1, 13] Clinically most patients present with a tumor mass with or without pruritus, pain or perineal bleeding. The most frequent sites of involvement are the labia majora or labia minora or the clitoris. Tumor size correlates with lymph node metastases and prognosis.

Histologically, vulvar squamous carcinoma can be subdivided into a keratinizing type, a large-cell nonkeratinizing type and a small-cell type. The majority are of the keratinizing type, with differentiation showing prominent intercellular bridges, cytoplasmic keratinization and the formation of keratin pearls. Large-cell nonkeratinizing carcinoma by definition lacks keratin pearls. Small-cell carcinoma and spindle cell lesions may occasionally occur. No correlation has been noted between the histologic type, degree of differentiation and lymph node metastases when considered independently.[15]

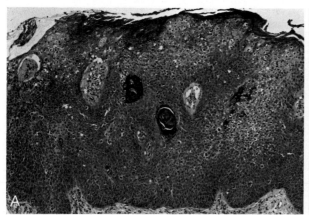 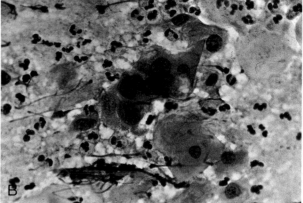

FIGURE 12–5. Squamous cell carcinoma *in situ* **of vulva.** *A,* The entire thickness of the epithelium is composed of small atypical immature cells. Dyskeratotic cells and mitoses are noted throughout the epithelium (hematoxylin and eosin; ×20). *B,* Loose aggregates of atypical cells having hyperchromasia, increased nucleocytoplasmic (N/C) ratio. Nuclear pleomorphism is noted (Papanicolaou stain; ×500).

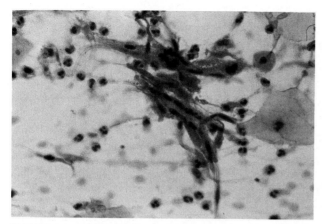

FIGURE 12–6. Keratinizing squamous carcinoma, vulva. Aggregates of spindle-shaped squamous cells showing little atypia or nuclear pleomorphism typical of well-differentiated carcinomas (Papanicolaou stain; ×500).

The cytologic characteristics resemble for the most part their cervical counterparts. The abnormal cells may occur in aggregates or singly depending on the tumor type and method of preparation. Owing to the presence of increased numbers of desmosomal junctions, those tumors showing evidence of keratinization are more frequently found in aggregates. The cells are polygonal, with well-defined cell borders and eosinophilic cytoplasm. Variation in the size and shape may be noted, with occasional bizarre forms having cytoplasmic processes that create elongated or tadpole forms. The nuclei are relatively uniform, although usually enlarged and hyperchromatic. Anucleate squames or parakeratotic cells are frequently noted (Fig. 12–6).

Verrucous Carcinomas. These are large, cauliflowerlike tumors that have a well-demarcated base. Histologically the tumors are composed of exophytic papillary fronds with hyperkeratosis or parakeratosis on the surface. The tumor is well demarcated from the underlying stroma, with the rete pegs having blunt pushing borders. Nuclear pleomorphism is mild. Keratin pearls are usually present. In cytologic smears from verrucous carcinomas, the cells usually occur in aggregates that retain their cytoplasmic processes. Sheets of hyperkeratotic and parakeratotic cells are usually present. Little cellular or nuclear pleomorphism is present. Owing to marked histologic and cytologic similarity to pseudoepitheliomatous hyperplasia and condyloma acuminatum, verrucous carcinomas are difficult to diagnosis, and a biopsy that includes the base of the lesion is often necessary.

Basal Cell Carcinoma. This is a disease predominately of postmenopausal women having an average age of 65 years and constituting 2 to 3% of all vulvar malignancies. It most frequently involves the labia majora.[39] Grossly, the lesion can show marked variability in appearance and size. Histologically, these basal cell carcinomas are similar in appearance to basal cell carcinomas from other sites. The tumor is composed of nests of uniform cells with scanty cytoplasm. A characteristic feature is the peripheral palisading observed in the outermost layer of epithelial cells. The nuclei are small and round or oval in shape (Fig. 12–7A). Morphologic variants having both the cystic features and sclerotic stroma have been described. Metastases to lymph nodes are rare, with two cases having been reported.[26, 51] Care should be observed with perirectal lesions to distinguish basal cell carcinomas of the skin from the basaloid cloacogenic carcinoma of the rectum. Cytologically few cases of basal cell have been described. The cells are small and uniform in size with a scant amount of poorly defined cytoplasm. The nuclei are enlarged and uniform in size with hyperchromatic chromatin. Nucleoli may be observed (Fig. 12–7B).

Paget's Disease. This disease of the vulva affects predominately white postmenopausal women having an average age of 67 years.[12, 31] Although Paget's disease histologically is similar in all sites at which it occurs, the natural history and morphogenesis differ. Clinically, the lesions appear as irregular, generally well-demarcated erythematous or eczematous islands that frequently ulcerate. The labia majora are the most

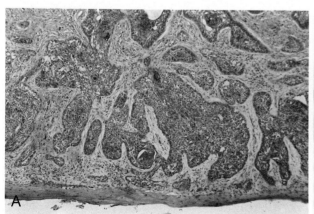
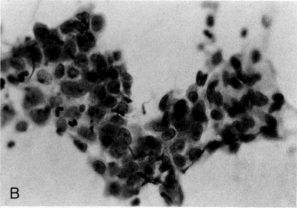

FIGURE 12–7. Basal cell carcinoma, vulva. A, Infiltrating nests of basaloid cells with peripheral palisading that originates from the basal epidermis (hematoxylin and eosin; ×20). B, Aggregates of small uniform cells having scanty cytoplasm and prominent nucleoli (Papanicolaou stain; ×500).

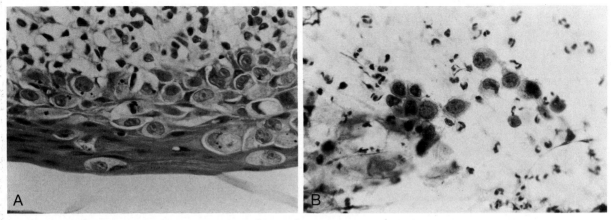

FIGURE 12–8. Paget's disease, vulva. *A*, Clusters of mucin-positive cells at the base of the epidermis showing migration to the surface (hematoxylin and eosin; ×20). *B*, Loose aggregates of atypical glandular cells with moderate amounts of cytoplasm. Nuclear chromatin is variable with occasional nucleoli (Papanicolaou stain; ×500).

frequently involved site. The theories about vulvar Paget's disease state that its morphogenesis differs from that of mammary Paget's disease, which invariably has an associated intraductal or invasive ductal carcinoma of the breast. Current theories suggest an origin from the basal layer of the epidermis and its appendages or from cells derived from the sweat glands or the Bartholin gland. Only 30% of the patients with vulvar Paget's disease will have demonstrable invasive carcinoma.[15] Progression to an invasive carcinoma only rarely occurs. Prognosis depends upon whether an invasive carcinoma is present and the extent of the disease. Recurrences due to inapparent histologic involvement of the margins of resection are frequent. The prognosis of patients with underlying invasive carcinoma and lymph node metastases is poor.

Paget's disease histologically is characterized by the presence of large, pale cells with mucicarmine-positive cytoplasm that are isolated or occur in aggregates in the epidermis. Occasional signet-ring forms are noted. Involvement of the hair follicles, pilosebaceous units, sweat ducts and less frequently sweat glands may be observed. Invasion of the dermis may be in the form of sheets, glands or cords. Rarely invasive carcinoma may occur directly from the epidermis. Melanin granules within Paget's cells have been observed (Fig. 12–8*A*). Cytologically, Paget's cells are isolated or occur in groups. The cells are large, with variable amounts of cytoplasm that stains indeterminately. The nuclei are enlarged and usually eccentrically placed with occasional signet-ring forms. One or more nucleoli are generally present. "Cell within cell" groupings are said to be characteristic (Fig. 12–8*B*).[32] Distinction of the cytologic characteristics of Paget's disease lesions from those having underlying invasive adenocarcinoma has not been possible (Fig. 12–9).

Carcinoma of the Bartholin Glands. This is rare; patients have an average age of 49.5 years.[53, 54] A number of histologic variants have been noted, including squamous cell carcinoma, adenocarcinoma, undifferentiated carcinoma, transitional cell carcinoma, adenoid cystic carcinoma, adenoacanthoma and adenosquamous carcinoma. Because none of the cell types are unique for Bartholin gland carcinoma, the cytologic patterns correlate with the histologic pattern. Involvement of the superficial portion of the skin overlying the gland may make distinction from a primary vulvar neoplasm difficult.

Melanomas. These are uncommon malignant tumors of the vulva.[6] The most frequent sites of involvement include the labia majora and labia minora. The peak incidence is the 6th through 8th decades.[37] The most frequent complaint is that of a mass in the vulvar region accompanied by bleeding or pruritus. Two thirds of the lesions are pigmented. The superficial spreading form is the most frequently noted histologic type, with nodular melanoma being the least common variant. Prognosis correlates with Clark's level and Breslow's depth of invasion.[42] Histologically atypical melanocytes are noted migrating through the squamous epithelium or into the dermis. The cells occur in loose aggregates that have a nevoid or epithelioid appearance. Nuclear

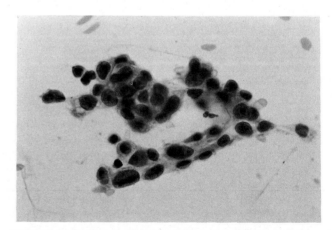

FIGURE 12–9. Paget's disease with invasive adenocarcinoma. Aggregate of malignant cells with ill-defined cytoplasmic borders, pleomorphic nuclei with variable chromatin and occasional nucleoli (Papanicolaou stain; ×500).

pleomorphism is prominent with prominent macronuclei. Variable amounts of melanin pigment may be noted. The cytologic appearance of melanoma reveals large pleomorphic cells with varying amounts of cytoplasm that are isolated or occur in loose aggregates. The nuclei are enlarged and round or oval. Binucleation and multinucleation are frequently noted. Macronucleoli are frequent. Intracytoplasmic melanin may be noted in the pigmented lesions.

VAGINA

Technique

Most cytology samples from the vagina should be obtained prior to manipulation of the cervix in order to avoid contamination. Excess mucus secretion should be removed with cotton balls. In sampling for adenosis, some authors recommend a circumvaginal scraping of the upper vagina. An alternative method is a four-quadrant scrape of the anterior, posterior and lateral walls using a downwards motion to avoid cervical contamination.

Histology

The vagina extends from the ectocervix to the vestibule or introitus. Recesses are noted in the upper portion of vagina between the cervix and vagina that are known as the vaginal fornices. The vagina is lined with a stratified squamous mucosa that is hormonally sensitive.

Infectious and Inflammatory Diseases

A number of infections and inflammatory disease processes may involve the vagina; these have been covered elsewhere in detail. Atrophic vaginitis occurs as a result of loss of estrogenic stimulation, resulting in thinning and shrinkage of the tissue. Cell scrapings usually reveal intermediate or atrophic cells. Trauma may result in infections with inflammatory reactions and repair. Vaginitis emphysematosa is a self-limited disease characterized by multiple cystic cavities in the lamina propria that may extend into the mucosa. It is believed to be related to infections by *Trichomonas vaginalis* and *Haemophilus vaginalis*.[19] The cavities usually have no discernible cell lining, although multinucleated giant cells or inflammatory cells may be found. Cytologic scrapes usually reveal inflammatory cells with occasional giant cells and reparative changes. Figure 12–10 depicts a case of malakoplakia in the vagina.

Vaginal Cysts

The majority of vaginal cysts are inclusion cysts lined with squamous mucosa and contain keratinous debris.

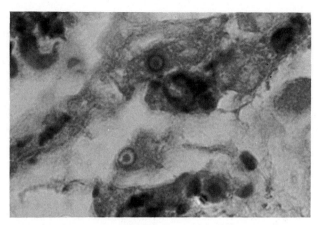

FIGURE 12–10. Malakoplakia, vagina. Michaelis-Gutmann bodies within histiocytes (Papanicolaou stain; ×500).

They are usually traumatic in origin. The remainder of vaginal cysts are usually of müllerian origin and are lined with columnar or cuboidal mucus-secreting cells. They are usually located along the anterolateral vaginal wall. Cysts of mesonephric origin are believed to be rare. Scrapes of such lesion usually result in only normal-appearing squamous epithelial cells. Needle aspiration may provide a worthwhile clue about the origin and nature of the lesion. Endometriosis of the vagina is uncommon.[18] Endometriosis is usually thought to be secondary to implantation at the time of surgery, but even this is thought to be a rare event.

Vaginal Adenosis

Vaginal adenosis is defined as the presence of glandular epithelium or the mucinous products in the vagina.[50] The incidence of adenosis in women not exposed to diethylstilbestrol (DES) varies markedly, ranging from 0 to 40.8%.[44, 48] The change is most frequently observed in the upper one third of the vagina, with the anterior vaginal wall being more commonly involved than the posterior or lateral walls. The gross appearance of the lesion depends upon the age of the patient, with early lesions appearing as grapelike clusters or as white areas. Adenosis in younger women may be confined to the surface. Involvement of the lamina propria is usually noted. With time glands may be noted only in the lamina propria. Evidence obtained via visual and colposcopic studies as well as cellular findings suggest that adenosis undergoes spontaneous involution in the majority of cases. With the passage of time squamous metaplasia occurs on the surface and ultimately replaces the glandular epithelium in the lamina propria. Microglandular hyperplasia of vaginal adenosis has been observed.

Histologically the columnar epithelium may resemble that of the endocervix, the endometrium or the uterine tube, with the majority of adenosis being of endocervical type (Fig. 12–11*A*). In cellular samples of adenosis obtained by scraping the vagina, columnar epithelial cells resembling endocervical cells can be identified. These may be seen alone or in combination

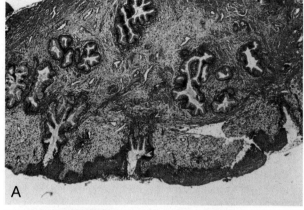

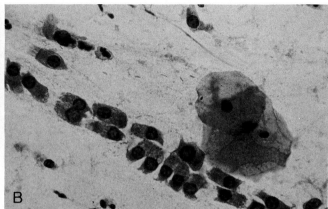

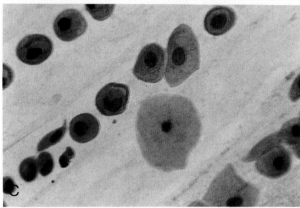

FIGURE 12–11. Adenosis, vagina. *A*, Numerous glands are noted in the lamina propria, which extend to the surface mucosa lined by squamous epithelium (hematoxylin and eosin; ×20). *B*, Tall columnar cells (Papanicolaou stain; ×500). *C*, Metaplastic squamous cells (Papanicolaou stain; ×500).

with immature or mature squamous metaplastic cells. With involution only squamous metaplastic cells may be noted. Occasionally anucleate squamous cells indicative of hyperkeratosis are seen (Fig. 12–11*B* and *C*).

Diethylstilbestrol Offspring

A variety of changes have been reported in women exposed to DES *in utero*. Changes attributed to DES have included malignant neoplasms (clear cell carcinoma), cervical erosions, genital ridges, cervical hoods, adenosis and varying abnormalities of the uterus.[48]

The least common change is the development of clear cell carcinoma. The risk of developing clear cell carcinoma in DES-exposed women from birth to age 34 years is estimated at 0.1%.[34] The risk of development increases from age 15, plateauing from 17 to 22 years of age and declining afterwards. The neoplasm most frequently originates from the anterior vaginal wall, less frequently from the posterior or lateral aspects. Although the majority (55%) of the clear cell carcinomas were of vaginal origin, 42% were of cervical origin.[24]

Three histopathologic patterns have been noted, including a tubulocystic, a solid and a papillary pattern. The cells have abundant clear cytoplasm with demonstrable glycogen on periodic acid-Schiff stains. Bulging of the nuclei towards the glandular lumen occurs, prompting the designation of hobnail cells (Fig. 12–

12*A*). Cytologically the cells derived from clear cell carcinoma may be isolated or occur in aggregates. The cells are usually uniform in size. The cytoplasm is often poorly stained and finely vacuolated. The nucleus is enlarged and hyperchromatic and may range from coarsely clumped to finely granular. Macronucleoli are frequently observed (Fig. 12–12*B*).

One of the most common changes observed in women exposed to DES *in utero* is adenosis. Its frequency has been reported to occur in from 35% to over 90% of the female offspring in exposed women.[24, 49] Adenosis has been noted to coexist with clear cell carcinoma in 95% of the cases studied.[46] However, at present no proof exists that significant epithelial abnormalities are more common in DES-exposed women than in unexposed women. Atypical variants of adenosis have been described as having nuclear and cytoplasmic abnormalities.[47]

Additional described abnormalities have included uterine abnormalities as documented by hysterosalpingography and abnormalities in the male offspring, including hypotrophic testicles and microphallus.[2]

Benign Neoplasms and Tumor-like Conditions

Fibroepithelial polyps of the vagina are uncommon neoplasms that clinically are commonly mistaken for a malignancy. The polyps are covered by stratified squa-

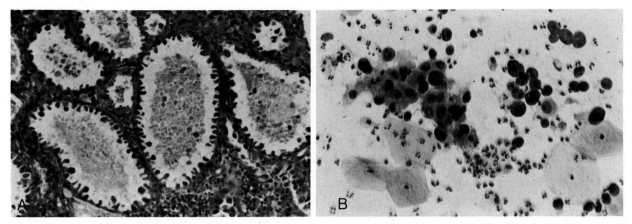

FIGURE 12–12. Clear cell carcinoma, vagina. *A,* Tubulocystic pattern with intraluminal "hobnail" cells (hematoxylin and eosin; ×80). *B,* Loose aggregates of relatively uniform cells with pleomorphic nuclei and occasional macronucleoli (Papanicolaou stain; ×500).

mous epithelium, which overlies loose to dense connective tissue that has large pleomorphic nuclei. Cytologic scrapes reveal normal squamous cells without atypia.

Malignant Neoplasms

Primary malignant neoplasms of the vagina are extremely uncommon, representing only 1 to 2% of all malignant tumors of the female genital tract.[15] Because of the close relationships of the vagina to other anatomic sites, it is estimated that 80 to 90% of the neoplasms are secondary, originating from adjacent sites.

Age-specific incidence rates for intraepithelial and infiltrative cancers are quite different from those observed for cervical cancer. The peak incidence rates for both intraepithelial and infiltrating cancers occur later, suggesting either a longer latency period or that different stimuli may be involved.

Abnormalities confined to the epithelium of the vagina are less common than their counterparts in the cervix. They may be confined to the vagina or coexist with changes in the cervix, either concurrent or arising at varying intervals following detection and treatment of the cervical lesion. Such intraepithelial changes most frequently involve the upper vagina or apex. Multicentricity may be observed in some cases. Histopathologically the changes are similar to those observed in the cervix. Varying degrees of cellular differentiation, mitotic activity and nuclear atypia are noted in the abnormal cells, which are indistinguishable from their counterparts in the cervix. Because the majority of preinvasive vaginal neoplasms are clinically silent, cytology remains the most effective way of detecting these changes. Cytology was positive in 80 to 88% of the patients with vaginal carcinoma *in situ.*[17, 25]

In women treated by radiotherapy, abnormalities have been identified in the vaginal and cervical specimens. Early radiation changes include cellular and

nuclear enlargement, cytoplasmic polychromasia, multinucleation and vacuolation of the cytoplasm. With time, atrophic cells become the dominant population. Development of dysplastic changes after a latency period of several months to years is termed postirradiation dysplasia. The cells are enlarged and irregular in shape with cytoplasmic polychromasia. The nuclei are enlarged and hyperchromatic.[40] The change is frequently associated with a resistance or recurrence of the cervical cancer depending upon the time at which the postirradiation dysplasia was detected.[52]

Squamous cell cancer is the most common primary malignant neoplasm of the vagina. According to the International Federation of Gynecology and Obstetrics definition, primary vaginal tumors must occur in the vagina without involvement of the cervix or vulva.[29] Patients with prior cervical or vulvar cancer should have a disease-free interval of 5 years from invasive cervical carcinoma.[41] Most patients with primary vaginal carcinoma are postmenopausal. Bleeding and discharge are the most common symptoms. Histologically most vaginal cancers are of the large-cell type; keratinizing carcinomas are less common and small-cell neoplasms are rare. Prognosis depends upon the stage of the disease.

Cytologic preparations reveal features analogous to that of cervical carcinoma with varying degrees of differentiation observed (Fig. 12–13).[35]

Verrucous carcinomas are well-differentiated variants of squamous carcinoma, consisting of an exophytic growth pattern that clinically is usually well demarcated. Verrucous carcinoma generally grows by direct extension. Metastasis to the lymph nodes is rare. Histologically, the epithelium is quite mature. Dyskeratosis and epithelial pearls are often noted. Parakeratosis and hyperkeratosis are noted at the surface.

Scrapes of verrucous carcinomas reveal abundant hyperkeratotic or parakeratotic cells.[43] The cells occur predominantly in aggregates with little pleomorphism. The nuclei show little variation or increase in size. Hyperchromasia is usually not marked. A biopsy that

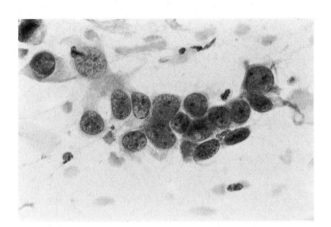

FIGURE 12–13. Squamous cell carcinoma, large-cell type, vagina. Large, pleomorphic cells with coarsely granular hyperchromatic nuclei and scanty delicate cytoplasm (Papanicolaou stain; ×500).

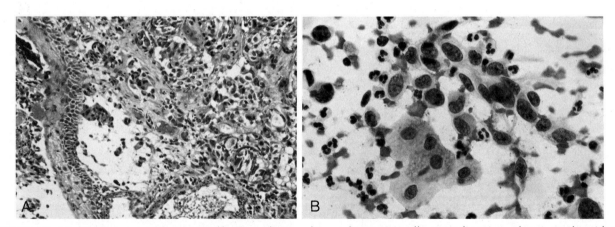

FIGURE 12–14. Melanoma, vagina. *A,* Infiltrating pleomorphic melanocytic cells extending into dermis and epidermis (hematoxylin and eosin; ×80). *B,* Loose aggregates of large pleomorphic cells having granular hyperchromatic nuclei and an occasional macronucleolus (Papanicolaou stain; ×500).

includes the base of the lesion is often necessary to establish the correct surgical diagnosis.

Primary adenocarcinoma of the vagina excluding clear cell carcinomas are rare. Numerous variants have been described, including those having adenoid cystic, mucinous[38] and mixed adenocarcinoma and argentaffin carcinomas.[16]

Sarcoma botryoides, stromal sarcomas, leiomyosarcomas and malignant melanomas (Fig. 12–14) are rare primary neoplasms of the vagina. Other benign and malignant mesodermal tumors that have been noted include lipoma, hemangioma, lymphangioma, fibrous histiocytoma and lymphoma.[15]

Metastatic Tumors

Metastatic neoplasms to the vulva and vagina occur either through direct extension or hematogenous or lymphatic spread within neoplasms of the female genital tract. The vagina is most commonly involved, followed by the ovaries and vulva.[33] Extragenital neoplasms are more likely first to involve the ovary. In the vulva, cervical cancers are the most frequent site of the primary tumor, followed by the endometrium, the urethra and the kidneys.[8] Metastatic diseases make up 84% of all neoplasms of the vagina. In the vagina the cervix was the most common primary site followed by the endometrium, the colon, the rectum and the ovaries.[15] Histologically and cytologically most metastatic diseases show the same degree of differentiation as the primary tumor.

References

1. Benedet JL, Turko M, Fairey RN: Squamous carcinoma of the vulva: Results of treatment, 1938 to 1976. Am J Obstet Gynecol 134:201, 1979.
2. Bibbo M, Gill WR, Azizi F: Follow-up study of male and female offspring of DES exposed mothers. Obstet Gynecol 49:1, 1977.
3. Braun L, Farmer ER, Shah KV: Immunoperoxidase localization of papilloma virus antigen in cutaneous warts and bowenoid papulosis. J Med Urol 12:187, 1983.
4. Buscema J, Woodruff JD, Parmly TH: Carcinoma *in situ* of the vulva. Obstet Gynecol 55:225, 1980.
5. Cagler H, Tamer S, Hreshshysmon MM: Vulvar intraepithelial neoplasia. Obstet Gynecol 60:346, 1982.
6. Ching PF, Woodruff JM, Lewis JL: Malignant melanoma of the vulva: A report of 44 cases. Obstet Gynecol 45:638, 1975.
7. Connors RC, Ackerman AB: Histological pseudomalignancies of skin. Arch Dermatol 112:1767, 1976.
8. Covington EE, Brendle WK: Breast carcinoma with vulvar metastases. Obstet Gynecol 23:910, 1964.
9. Cruz-Jimenez PR, Abell MR: Cutaneous basal cell carcinoma of vulva. Cancer 54:1860, 1975.
10. Dehner LP: Metastatic and secondary tumors of the vulva. Obstet Gynecol 42:47, 1973.
11. Dodson MG, O'Leary JA, Averette HE: Primary carcinoma of Bartholin's gland. Obstet Gynecol 35:578, 1970.
12. Fenn ME, Morley GW, Abell MR: Paget's disease of vulva. Obstet Gynecol 38:660, 1971.
13. Figge DI, Gaudenz R: Invasive carcinoma of the vulva. Am J Obstet Gynecol 119:382, 1974.
14. Friedrich EG, Wilkenson EF, Fu YS: Carcinoma *in situ* of the vulva: A continuing challenge. Am J Obstet Gynecol 136:830, 1980.
15. Fu YS, Reagan JW: Pathology of the Uterine Cervix, Vagina and Vulva, 1st ed. Philadelphia, WB Saunders, 1989.
16. Fukushima M, Twiggs LB, Okagaki T: Mixed intestinal adeno-carcinoma–argentaffin carcinoma of the vagina. Gynecol Oncol 23:387, 1986.
17. Gallup DG, Morley GW: Carcinoma *in situ* of the vagina. A study and review. Obstet Gynecol 46:334, 1975.
18. Gardner HL: Cervical and vaginal endometriosis. Clin Obstet Gynecol 9:90, 1966.
19. Gardner HL, Feret P: Etiology of vaginitis emphysematosa. Am J Obstet Gynecol 88:680, 1964.
20. Gardner HL, Kaufman RH: Benign disease of the vulva and vagina, 2nd ed. Boston, GK Hall, 1981.
21. Gross G, Hagedvin M, Ikenberg H: Bowenoid papulosis: Presence of human papilloma virus (HPV) structural antigens and of HPV 16 related DNA sequences. Arch Dermatol 121:858, 1985.
22. Hart WR, Norris HJ, Helwig EB: Relation of lichen sclerosis et atrophicus of the vulva to the development of carcinoma. Obstet Gynecol 45:369, 1975.
23. Herbst AL, Norusis MJ, Rosenow PJ: An analysis of 346 cases of clear cell adenocarcinoma of the vagina and cervix with emphases on recurrence and survival. Gynecol Oncol 7:111, 1979.
24. Herbst AL, Robboy SJ, Scully RE: Clear cell adenocarcinoma of the vagina and cervix in young females. An analysis of 170 registry cases. Am J Obstet Gynecol 119:713, 1974.
25. Hernandez-Linares W, Puthawala A, Nolan JF: Carcinoma *in situ* of the vagina: Past and present management. Obstet Gynecol 56:356, 1980.
26. Jimenez HT, Fenoglis CM, Richart RM: Vulva basal cell carcinoma with metastasis. A case report. Am J Obstet Gynecol 121:285, 1975.
27. Kaufman RH, Dressman GR, Burke J: Herpes virus–induced antigens in squamous cell carcinoma *in situ* of the vulva. N Engl J Med 305:483, 1981.
28. Kaufman RH, Garner HL, Brown DJ: Vulvar dystrophies: An evaluation. Am J Obstet Gynecol 120:363, 1974.
29. Kottmeier HL: The classification and clinical staging of carcinoma of the uterus and vagina: A report by the Cancer Committee of the International Federation of Gynecology and Obstetrics. J Int Fed Gynecol Obstet 1:83, 1963.
30. Krain LS, Rosenthal L, Newcomer VP: Pemphigus vulgaris involving the cervix associated with endometrial carcinoma of the uterus. A case report with immunofluorescent findings. Int J Dermatol 12:220, 1973.
31. Lee SC, Roth LM, Erlich CE: Extramammary Paget's disease of the vulva. A clinicopathologic study of 13 cases. Cancer 39:2540, 1977.
32. Masukawa T, Friedrich EG: Cytopathology of Paget's disease of the vulva. Diagnostic abrasive cytology. Acta Cytol 22:476, 1978.
33. Mazur MT, Hsueh W, Gersell DJ: Metastases to the female genital tract. Analysis of 325 cases. Cancer 93:1978, 1984.
34. Melnick S, Cole P, Anderson D: Rates and risks of diethylstilbestrol-related clear cell adenocarcinoma of the vagina and cervix: An update. N Engl J Med 316:914, 1987.
35. Merchant S, Murad TM, Dowling EA: Diagnosis of vaginal carcinoma from cytologic material. Acta Cytol 18:494, 1974.
36. Merino MJ, Livols VA, Schwartz PE: Adenoid basal cell carcinoma of the vulva. Int J Gynecol Pathol 1:299, 1982.
37. Morrow CP, Rutledge F: Melanoma of the vulva. Obstet Gynecol 39:745, 1972.
38. Naves AE, Monti JA, Chechoni E: Basal-like carcinoma in the upper third of the vagina. Am J Obstet Gynecol 137:136, 1980.
39. Palladino VS, Duffy JL, Bures GL: Basal cell carcinoma of the vulva. Cancer 24:460, 1969.
40. Patten SF, Reagan JW, Obenauf M: Post irradiation dysplasia of uterine cervix and vagina: An analytical study of the cells. Cancer 16:173, 1963.
41. Peters WA, Kumar NB, Morley GW: Carcinoma of the vagina: Factors influencing treatment outcome. Cancer 55:892, 1985.
42. Phillips GL, Twiggs LB, Okagaki T: Vulva melanoma: A micro staging study. Gynecol Oncol 14:80, 1982.
43. Ramzy I, Smart MS, Collins JA: Verrucous carcinoma of the vagina. Am J Clin Path 65:644, 1976.

44. Ricci JU, Lisa JR, Thom CH Jr: The vagina in reconstructive surgery: A histological study of its structural components. Am J Surg 77:542, 1949.

45. Robboy SJ, Kaufman RH, Prat J: Pathologic findings in young women enrolled in the National Cooperative Diethylstilbestrol Adenosis (DESAD) Project. Obstet Gynecol 51:528, 1978.

46. Robboy SJ, Welch WR, Young RH: Topographic relation of cervical ectropion and vaginal adenosis to clear cell adenocarcinoma. Obstet Gynecol 60:546, 1982.

47. Robboy SJ, Young RH, Welch WR: Atypical vaginal adenosis and cervical ectropion: Association with clear cell adenocarcinoma in diethylstilbestrol-exposed offspring. Cancer 54:869, 1984.

48. Sandburg EC: Benign cervical and vaginal changes associated with exposure to stilbestrol *in utero*. Am J Obstet Gynecol 125:777, 1976.

49. Sherman AI, Goldrath M, Berlin A: Cervical-vaginal adenosis after *in utero* exposure to synthetic estrogens. Obstet Gynecol 44:531, 1974.

50. Skully RE: Pathology and Pathogenesis of Diethylstilbestrol Related Disorders of the Female Genital Tract. Symposium on DES. Edited by AL Herbst. Am College of Obstetrics and Gynecology, 1977.

51. Sworn MJ, Hammond GT: Metastatic basal cell carcinoma. Case report. Br J Obstet Gynaecol 86:332, 1979.

52. Wentz WB, Reagan JW: Clinical significance of post irradiation dysplasia of uterine cervix. Am J Obstet Gynecol 106:812, 1970.

53. Wharton LR Jr, Everett HS: Primary malignant Bartholin's gland tumors. Obstet Gynecol Surv 6:1, 1951.

54. Wheelock JB, Goplaerud OR, Dunn LJ: Primary carcinoma of the Bartholin's gland: A report of ten cases. Obstet Gynecol 63:820, 1984.

13

Unusual Tumors

Patricia E. Saigo

There are so many unusual and rare tumors of the female genital tract that the scope of this unit had to be limited. It focuses, therefore, upon those tumors likely to be encountered in cervicovaginal smears.

NEUROENDOCRINE CARCINOMA OF THE UTERINE CERVIX

Neuroendocrine carcinoma of the uterine cervix is a type of rare malignant tumor first described by Albores-Saavedra in 1972.[2] The incidence based on data from several retrospective series varies from 0.6%[87] to 5%.[136] The patients, all adults, range in age from 26 to 83 years, with mean ranges of 42 to 58 years.[2, 10, 87, 123, 136, 143] No epidemiologic profile or particular risk factors have been identified.

Most of the women are symptomatic, with bleeding as the most common complaint. An occasional tumor has been discovered during treatment for some other condition.[143] There have been only a few patients presenting with symptoms referable to a functioning endocrine tumor.[82, 119, 129, 136, 139]

Histology

The neuroendocrine component has several patterns. One is the well-differentiated pattern with rosettes, not often seen in cervical tumors. Another pattern is the trabecular or ribbon arrangement (Fig. 13–1). Still another is the solid streaming pattern, which may include the spindly type of cytologic change.

Although these tumors may be composed solely of neuroendocrine carcinoma, many also have components of adenocarcinoma or epidermoid carcinoma in greater or lesser proportions.[51, 123, 143]

All of these tumors have evidence of neuroendocrine differentiation documented by electron microscopy or by histochemical and immunologic methods. Argyro-phil granules (Fig. 13–2), but no argentaffin granules, have been identified. A variety of polypeptides (see Fig. 13–2) have been detected in these tumors, including serotonin, adrenocorticotropic hormone (ACTH), beta human chorionic gonadotrophin, calcitonin and human growth factor. Although polyamines can be demonstrated immunologically, rarely do the patients have symptoms referable to their peripheral effects.[123, 129]

Cytology

The results of the evaluation of gynecologic smears have not been routinely included in the reported studies. Very few tumors were initially discovered by cytology,[51, 53, 123, 128] and all six patients reported by Walker and coworkers[143] had no tumor cells detected

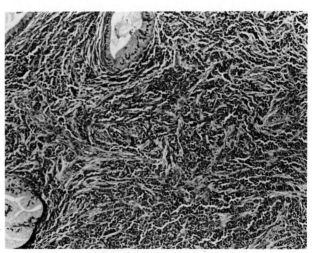

FIGURE 13–1. The histopathology of the case illustrated in Figure 13–4 shows the **trabecular arrangement of infiltration** (hematoxylin and eosin; × 50).

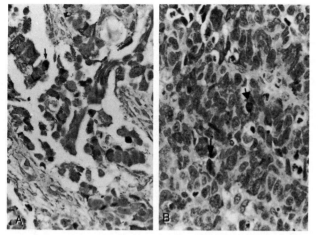

FIGURE 13–2. Special stains document the **neurosecretory granules.** *A,* The arrow points to a cell containing the dark granules in the Grimelius reaction (×100). *B,* Chromogranin (arrows) is demonstrated using an immunologic reaction (×200).

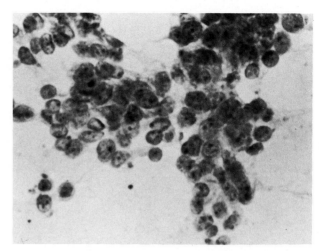

FIGURE 13–3. The cells of this **neuroendocrine carcinoma** are small with scant cytoplasm. Their nuclei contain finely granular chromatin and small, punctate nucleoli (Papanicolaou stain; ×300).

in their smears. Because most of the tumors are large and obvious by visual inspection, biopsy is the most common method of establishing the diagnosis. Even in those reports in which cytology was done, except for the case report by Miles and coworkers,[95] no description of the cytopathologic findings are included. No specific characteristics for the diagnosis of neuroendocrine carcinoma were found in their case, which displayed cytologic evidence of both squamous and glandular differentiation as well as features suggesting neuroendocrine differentiation. The cytologic description of this type of tumor in cervicovaginal smears is scant,[83, 95, 118] compared with the numerous reports referable to the carcinoid–oat-cell carcinoma spectrum of the pulmonary[66, 147, 150] and pancreatic[9] neuroendocrine tumors.

The four cases of cervical neuroendocrine carcinoma in our laboratory showed a spectrum of cytologic variability. In the well-differentiated neuroendocrine carcinomas, the cells were small with scant basophilic cytoplasm and round to oval nuclei containing small, punctate nucleoli (Fig. 13–3), resembling the cells of bronchial carcinoid tumors. In other cases, the small cells were present either as the sole component of the smear or as a component of a smear containing cells clearly recognizable as adenocarcinoma. When the cells of neuroendocrine carcinoma were admixed with those of adenocarcinoma, they were not as apparent and were easily overlooked.[118] In other cases, the cells from the neuroendocrine carcinoma were not well preserved and resembled those of oat-cell carcinoma. The chromatin was smudged or coarsely granular (Fig. 13–4).

Summary of Cytologic Findings

- Small cells with scant basophilic cytoplasm
- Often small, punctate nucleoli in oval nuclei
- Smudged chromatin in poorly differentiated cancers.

Pathogenesis

Neuroendocrine cells have been demonstrated in the normal cervical epithelium with histochemical and immunologic techniques. Fox and associates[47] reported an argyrophil cell in each of two cases of 120 normal cervices examined using Bodian's protargol method; no argentaffin-positive cells were noted using the diazo method. In an investigation of 97 cases of cervical cancers to identify those of neuroendocrine carcinoma, Tateishi and coworkers[136] found 19 out of 54 cases with normal cervical mucosa to be reactive with the Grimelius reaction. Six of the cases contained argyrophilic

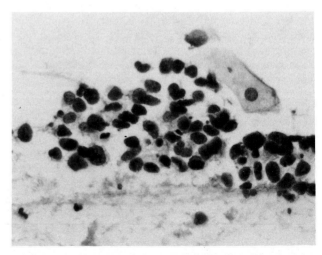

FIGURE 13–4. In this case of **neuroendocrine carcinoma,** the chromatin of the tumor cells is coarse and smudged, obscuring the nucleoli in many cells, although they are evident in an occasional cell (Papanicolaou stain; ×300).

TABLE 13–1. Clinical Outcome of Neuroendocrine Carcinoma

Author	Stage of Disease				Outcome			
	I	II	III	IV	NED	AWD	DOD	DOC
Walker and coworkers[143]	4	5	2	3	1	1	11	1
Barrett and coworkers[10]	5	0	1	1	1	0	5	1
Silva and coworkers[123]	5	2	1	1	2	0	7	0
Gersell and coworkers[51]	9	3	2	1	3	2	10	0

NED = No evidence of disease; AWD = alive with disease; DOD = died of disease; DOC = died of other causes.

cells in the endocervical glands, eight in the squamous epithelium and five in both. Other investigators[45] identified argyrophilia in 11 out of 210 cases (5%) and using immunologic reactions found that all 11 contained serotonin and six contained calcitonin as well. No other polypeptides (ACTH, bombesin, gastrin, glucagon, motilin, neurotensin, pancreatic polypeptide, somatostatin, insulin and alpha human chorionic gonadotrophin) were identified.

Scully and colleagues[119] investigating carcinomas lacking the histologic appearance of neuroendocrine differentiation found argyrophilia in six of ten cases of minimal deviation adenocarcinoma and in three of 21 adenocarcinomas of the cervix. Of these nine tumors four contained serotonin and two neurotensin; none contained calcitonin, gastrin, ACTH, glucagon or insulin.

Because nearly half of the tumors in large series contain other types of carcinoma,[51] it is likely that these tumors originate from a stem cell capable of focal or total histologic and biochemical neuroendocrine differentiation. Tumors with the histologic pattern of a neuroendocrine carcinoma that have electron-dense organelles or the appropriate biochemical products or both are classified as a neuroendocrine carcinoma. When only the morphologic or the biochemical expression is present, it is no longer included in this category.

Clinical Course

The prognosis is poorer for these tumors than for squamous or epidermoid carcinoma or adenocarcinoma

(Table 13–1). Of the 22 patients with Stage I tumors, six (27%) were alive with no evidence of disease in follow-ups ranging from 16 months to 12 years. In contrast, a 76% 5-year survival is anticipated for those with adenocarcinoma.[117] A comparison of short-term survival of those with undifferentiated carcinomas of the cervix with neurosecretory granules with those without showed 25% and 67% survival, respectively.[10] Even when the carcinoma was an incidental discovery, the prognosis was not favorable; the patient was alive with disease at 12 months.[143] Metastases to lungs, lymph nodes and liver offer an opportunity to follow and confirm dissemination of the disease by aspiration cytology. In another series reported by Albores-Saavedra and associates,[3] those with better-differentiated tumors survived longer than those with poorly differentiated tumors. This has not been consistently reported.

CARCINOMA OF THE FALLOPIAN TUBE

Adenocarcinoma of the fallopian tube is the rarest of all gynecologic cancers, with an incidence ranging from 0.13 to 1.6%.[4, 61] The women, all adults, range in age from 21 to 84 years, with mean ages of 55 to 57 years (Table 13–2). Most are postmenopausal. About 20 to 40% are nulliparous,[91, 110, 148] although a rate as high as 71% has been reported.[18]

The symptom complexes of pain-menorrhagia or abnormal bleeding–leukorrhea and pain-vaginal discharge or bleeding–pelvic mass have been described as the classic symptoms of carcinoma of the fallopian tube. Sedlis[121] reported that 5% have the first set of symptoms and 20% the second, which is less than the 57% found by others.[18] However, in most other series, the patients present with one complaint, abnormal bleeding, described by at least half the patients, followed by abdominal discomfort or pain and finally an abdominal mass. The abdominal pain or discomfort is thought to be due to the distention of the fallopian tube by the carcinoma. Even patients with Stage I disease are symptomatic, with abnormal bleeding reported in six of seven such patients.[62] In patients with a pelvic mass, the mass may be unrelated to the fallopian tube carcinoma and is often leiomyomata.

The syndrome of crampy lower abdominal pain followed by profuse watery discharge (hydrops tubae

TABLE 13–2. Clinical Data of Patients with Adenocarcinoma of the Fallopian Tube

Author	Average Age			Clinical Stage			
	Number of Patients	Years	(Range)	I	II	III	IV
Yoonessi[148]	47	53	(21–78)	4	26	17	0
Raju and Wiltshaw[111]	22	54	(39–70)	6	12	4	0
Amendola and coworkers[4]	34	57	(21–81)	16	4	12	2
Murray and coworkers[91]	30	55	(33–82)	9	11	7	3
Podratz and coworkers[110]	47	57	(46–84)	12	14	17	4
Hirai and coworkers[62]	15	56	(42–73)	7	3	3	2
King and coworkers[73]	17	60	(44–83)	6	5	6	0

profluens) has been emphasized by some[120] and found in as many as 15% of some series,[38, 111] but not in others. This symptom complex is indicative of tubal disease, but it is not specific for carcinoma of that organ. Because of discharge into the vagina of fluid bathing the tumor, the likelihood of detecting malignant cells in this setting should be great. In the analysis by Hirai and colleagues,[61] two of ten patients described a watery discharge, but the cytology samples failed to contain tumor cells. They ascribed the absence of tumor cells to the expulsion of copious amounts of fluid, which removed the diagnostic cells with its flow. Brewer and Guderian[20] had two patients presenting with watery discharge; the diagnosis of an adenocarcinoma was made on cervicovaginal smear in one and suspected in the other.

Despite the presence of symptoms, 19 to 35% have no detectable abnormality on physical examination.[41, 109] Ultrasonography was used to detect the tumor in six patients with normal pelvic examinations.[73]

Asymptomatic patients are reported in nearly every series, with rates varying between 6 and 14%.[41, 109] Yoonesi[148] reported four patients in whom the tubal carcinoma was an incidental finding: One was discovered during herniorrhaphy, two in the abdominal hysterectomy specimen removed for cervical epidermoid carcinoma *in situ* and one at autopsy. One of the patients with cervical carcinoma *in situ* had a cervical smear that was suggestive of carcinoma *in situ* but not of the tubal carcinoma.

Patients at risk for carcinoma of the fallopian tube are reputedly those with tubal infections, particularly tuberculous salpingitis, although the number of patients with this risk factor is small in most series, ranging from 6 to 19%.[4, 38, 41, 59, 110] In the combined series of 115 patients reported by Peters and colleagues,[109] 37% had evidence of pelvic inflammatory disease based on the gross or histologic examination; among patients with Stage I disease, the association was 54%. One of two patients with tuberculosis had a uterine infection in Yoonesi's[148] study, and three patients in the series reported by Tamimi and Figge[135] had documented extrasalpingeal tuberculosis with no evidence of salpingeal infection.

Regardless of which one of the several staging systems is applied, only a fourth to a third of the patients have tumors limited to the tube (see Table 13–2). Attempts at earlier detection have included the use of radiologic techniques such as ultrasonography, contrast medium studies and hysterosalpingography. Routine cervicovaginal cytology has not been a sensitive method for screening, with detection rates ranging from 0 to 20% in large series; the highest rate, 60%, has not been duplicated (Table 13–3). Therefore, Hirai and associates[61] advocated aspiration of the endometrial cavity, which successfully detected abnormal cells in 50% in their population compared with the 20% in routine cervicovaginal smears. Although this technique was sensitive in their study group, it was not in the series reported by King and coworkers,[73] in which all eight patients in whom endometrial aspiration was performed failed to disclose any tumor cells.

TABLE 13–3. Results of Cervicovaginal Smears in Women with Carcinoma of the Fallopian Tube

Author	Number of Patients	Cytologic Results	
		Negative	Positive
Sedlis[121]	40	16	24 (60%)
Boutselis and Thompson[18]	14	12	2 (14%)
Benedet and coworkers[14]	NS	NS	4
Yoonesi[148]	47	43	4 (9%)
Roberts and Lifshitz[112]	28	28	0
Amendola and coworkers[4]	34	30	4 (12%)
Eddy and coworkers[41]	23	16	7 (30%)
Podratz and coworkers[110]	31	29	2 (6%)
Hirai and coworkers[61]			
VCE	15	12	3 (20%)
Endom Asp	12	6	6 (50%)
Cul de sac Asp	12	5	7 (58%)
King and coworkers[73]			
VC	11	9	2 (18%)
Endom Asp	8	8	0

Negative = Negative for malignant cells; Positive = positive for malignant cells; NS = not stated; VCE = vaginocervical-endocervical smear; Endom Asp = endometrial aspirate; VC = vaginocervical smear; Cul de sac Asp = Cul de sac aspiration.

In some reports, the abnormality detected in the routine cervicovaginal smear did not indicate a fallopian tube carcinoma, but another process. It was during the work-up and treatment for the other condition that the fallopian tube carcinoma was discovered.

Histology

Most of the malignant tumors are adenocarcinomas (Fig. 13–5), often papillary and with psammoma bodies. These carcinomas resemble ovarian carcinomas, and criteria elaborated to establish the carcinoma as primary in the fallopian tube has been described by Hu and coworkers.[68] No predilection exists for one or the other tube, and bilateral carcinomas have been

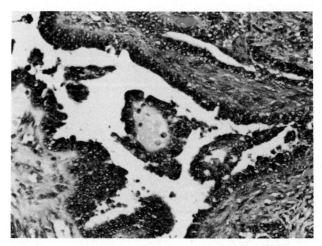

FIGURE 13–5. The histopathology of the **adenocarcinoma** identified in the smear in Figure 13–6 is shown here. The cells form small clusters present in the lumen of the fallopian tube (hematoxylin and eosin; ×100).

found in about 5 to 26%.[38, 62, 91, 120] The most common location is the region of the ampulla and fimbria; rarest is the interstitial portion of the tube.[61, 110] Because most patients present with abnormal bleeding, endometrial curettage is performed. Even in these specimens, the appearance of adenocarcinoma is not sufficiently distinctive.[14] Only in retrospect is the diagnosis of fallopian tube carcinoma made.

Less common are the mesodermal mixed tumors of the fallopian tube, which accounted for 4% (2 out of 47) to 12% (2 out of 17).[73, 110] The cytologic appearance of this type of tumor in cervicovaginal smears has not been described, although one patient had had four abnormal smears.[75] In another study, all three patients with smears had no evidence of tumor in them; the one patient who had had an endocervical curettage for vaginal spotting had fragments of tumor in that specimen.[103] Histologically, these tumors resemble their ovarian and endometrial counterparts with the admixture of adenocarcinoma and sarcoma that may be myosarcoma or undifferentiated sarcoma.[85]

Squamous carcinoma was found in two of 47 patients.[110]

A rare occurrence is carcinoma originating in the prolapsed portion of the fallopian tube retained after a vaginal hysterectomy.[42] Ehlen and coworkers reported on a 68-year-old woman who, 25 years following a vaginal hysterectomy for fibroids, complained of vaginal bleeding.[42] A 0.5-cm nodule noted at the vaginal apex was biopsied, revealing a moderately differentiated infiltrating adenocarcinoma of the left fallopian tube. Tumor cells were not noted in the vaginal smear.

Prolapse of the fallopian tube following hysterectomy is a common clinical occurrence, but the cytologist is only rarely challenged by this problem. In a report of four patients with cytologic specimens from the vaginal apex following vaginal hysterectomy without salpingo-oophorectomy, one patient had small cells suggestive of endometrial cells.[124] In the absence of the uterus, they concluded that these cells represented benign tubal epithelial cells. The other smears contained cells consistent with the healing process. Biopsy of the prolapsed tubes may reveal very atypical cells arranged in a cribriform pattern, and the authors advise caution in making the diagnosis of an adenocarcinoma in this clinical setting.

Cytology

Although abnormal smears are reported in many series, few detail the characteristics of the tumor cells. Benson[15] recognized two types of cells: One group consisted of moderate-sized cells containing round to oval nuclei with coarse chromatin, nucleoli and vacuolated cytoplasm; the other consisted of small cells with pyknotic nuclei and scant cytoplasm. The tumor cells resemble those of an endometrial or ovarian carcinoma (Fig. 13–6). Because of the rarity of tubal carcinomas, the cytologist is more likely to suggest an origin in the endometrium or the ovary.[15, 50] Hirai and

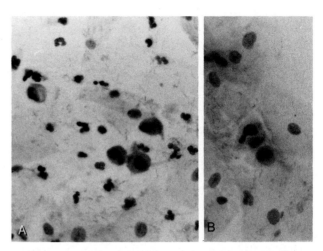

FIGURE 13–6. This **composite of two groups of cells** was found in the vaginal smear. Very few cells were observed, some were poorly preserved (A), whereas others were arranged in small clusters (B). The background was free of blood and necrotic debris (Papanicolaou stain; × 300).

colleagues[61] illustrate cell clusters in endometrial aspirates in which about half have "clean" backgrounds. The lack of a tumor diathesis has also been noted in the cervicovaginal smears, similar to the smear pattern associated with malignant cells of other extrauterine tumors.

As is evident in the descriptions of the exfoliated cells, there is nothing distinctive or unique about the cells from an adenocarcinoma of the fallopian tube apart from their classification as malignant cells of glandular origin. As part of the müllerian-derived epithelium, the normal and neoplastic cells share characteristics common to the tumors of the ovaries, the endometrium and the endocervix.

Tumor cells in other types of cytologic specimens, ascitic fluids (Fig. 13–7) and peritoneal wash speci-

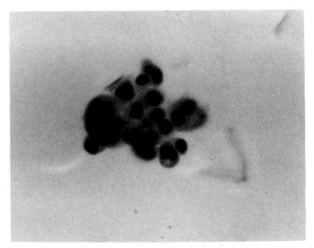

FIGURE 13–7. Many clusters of cells were present in the ascites from a woman with **widely disseminated tubal carcinoma.** The cytologic features were those of adenocarcinoma, but there were no characteristics that indicated a particular source of the carcinoma (Papanicolaou stain; × 300).

mens, were found to be important in the prognosis of the patients by some, but not by others. Because a third of the patients will have extratubal spread, ascites is common and the detection of tumor cells in those specimens likely. Podratz and coworkers[110] found a significant difference in survival for those patients whose wash specimen or peritoneal fluid specimen did contain malignant cells compared with those in whose specimens tumor cells were absent. The former had a 5-year survival of 20% compared with the latter's 67%. However, this was not found in another review of 31 patients with these examinations in whom the mean survival was 24 months regardless of the cytologic findings.[41]

An interesting observation in the review of patients with abnormal cytologic findings in cervicovaginal smears is that conditions other than that of fallopian tube carcinoma are likely to be identified. In the treatment for the condition identified in the smear, a fallopian tube carcinoma is present simultaneously. The most common type of abnormal cells are those of dysplasia, carcinoma *in situ* or invasive carcinoma of the uterine cervix.[41, 148] Less common are findings indicating an adenocarcinoma or hyperplasia of the endometrium or the endocervix.[41] In some cases, two independent carcinomas, one in the endometrium and the other in the fallopian tube, are found. In only one of the seven patients in one study[41] and one of four in another[14] could the abnormal smears be attributed to the fallopian tube cancer.

The differential diagnoses include adenocarcinomas of the endometrium or of the ovary. The smear pattern from the former is more likely to contain a tumor diathesis, but fallopian tube carcinomas are also associated with bleeding. The cells from an endometrioid-type ovarian adenocarcinoma would be similar to those of a tubal carcinoma. A fallopian tube carcinoma is highly probable when these malignant cells are present in a patient with an unremarkable pelvic examination and no detectable abnormality in endometrial curettings.

Summary of Cytologic Findings

- Small cells with eccentric oval nuclei
- Cell clusters
- Small nucleoli
- Few tumor cells
- "Clean" background.

Clinical Course

At the time of initial exploration, about half to three fourths of the patients have spread of disease to other organs, usually intraperitoneal. The most common sites of metastases are in the omentum and peritoneum, the ovaries and the uterus.[4] Transcoelomic spread is the major cause of treatment failure, occurring in 35% of patients with Stage I disease.[38] Intra-abdominal recurrences were the most common, present in 21%.[110] Extraperitoneal recurrences were associated with intra-

peritoneal disease; the sites of metastases include the lymph nodes, the liver, the lungs, the pleura, the vagina and the brain.[91, 110]

The 5-year survival for those with Stage I disease ranges from 25 to 77%.[4, 41, 112] The 5-year survival rates for Stage II disease vary from 27 to 58%.[91, 111] Few patients with Stage III and IV disease survive for 5 years.

An interesting phenomenon is the high rate of synchronous or metachronous malignant tumors occurring in other organs of the female genital tract as well as in other organs. One series found synchronous tumors in eight of 34 (24%) patients: two in the ovary, five in the endometrium and two in the cervix; one patient had an independent tumor in the ovary and in the endometrium.[4] Others have reported that 18 to 21% have had another primary tumor preceding the fallopian tube cancer in the breast, the ovary or the colon; two cutaneous melanomas have also been reported.[91, 110] A primary tubal carcinoma cannot always be differentiated from a metastasis from the prior cancer, and four patients were excluded from one series for this reason.[91]

SARCOMAS OF THE FEMALE GENITAL TRACT

Sarcomas constitute about 5% of the primary malignant tumors of the female genital tract. They can be divided into two large categories: the mixed tumors and the monomorphic sarcomas. The following discussion is limited to those in which cytology is most likely to have a role.

Müllerian Mixed Tumors

Müllerian mixed tumors are composed of two kinds of tissue: one epithelial and the other mesenchymal. Although this type of malignant neoplasm may be found in the ovary, the fallopian tube or the cervix, the most common site is the uterine corpus, where it makes up about 1 to 2% of all malignant uterine cancers. Nearly all of the women are postmenopausal, although there are rare instances of females under the age of 40 years.[69, 86] While the risk factors associated with endometrial carcinoma may be present, there is a stronger association with a history of irradiation in the distant past. An average of 11 to 17% of patients have this history,[11, 69] although a rate of 53% (10 out of 19) has been reported.[102] Of interest is one report of 30 women who had had prior pelvic irradiation for benign (22 patients) and malignant (8 patients) conditions.[93] In this study, half of the women in the latter group had mesodermal mixed tumors (Stages III and IV), whereas only one of the former group did (Stage I). Another study found that the mean age of the postirradiation group was younger, 62 years compared with 69 years for the nonirradiated group.[142]

The chief complaint from women with uterine tumors is abnormal bleeding. About a fourth of the patients have the tumor protruding through cervical os,[11] and origin from the cervix, although rare, should be considered.[57] A third of the patients have extra-uterine spread and may also have symptoms and findings consistent with involvement of the adnexal and intra-abdominal organs.

Primary ovarian mesodermal mixed tumors make up less than 1% of primary ovarian cancers and have clinical presentations similar to those of the other epithelial cancers with spreading to pelvic and abdominal organs: pelvic pain, abdominal enlargement and weight loss.[39, 98] Bilateral involvement is frequent.[98, 137] Ascites is frequently noted because only rarely is the disease confined to the ovary.[137] The history of prior pelvic irradiation is not an associated precondition.[102]

Mesodermal mixed tumors also occur in the fallopian tubes.

Histology

The tumor is often polypoid, filling the entire endometrial cavity and protruding through the external os (Fig. 13–8). The tumor may be seen invading the underlying myometrium or extending into the endocervix.

Histologically, these tumors contain adenocarcinoma and less frequently squamous carcinoma or a mixture of both types. The adenocarcinomatous component is often papillary. The sarcomatous portion of the tumor can be represented by leiomyosarcoma, stromal sarcoma or anaplastic sarcoma; this type is referred to as the homologous type. When the sarcomatous element is composed of malignant mesenchymal elements foreign to the uterus such as rhabdomyosarcoma (Fig. 13–9), osteosarcoma or chondrosarcoma, the tumor is referred to as heterologous. Some feel that there is a difference in prognosis, whereas others do not.[11, 30] King and Kramer[74] suggest that the identification of

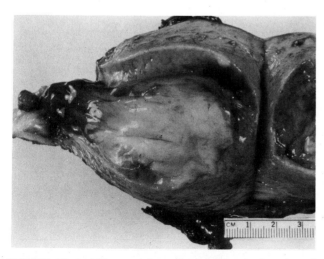

FIGURE 13–8. This **mesodermal mixed tumor** is a broad-based polypoid mass filling the entire endometrial cavity and protruding through the cervix, which has been partially removed.

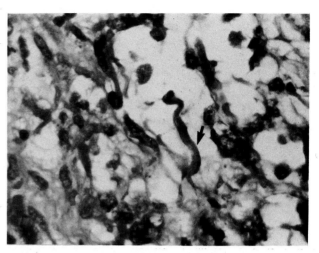

FIGURE 13–9. Rhabdomyosarcoma may form the predominant component of the mesodermal mixed tumor as it did here. Note the cross striations (arrow) in one cell (hematoxylin and eosin; ×200).

heterologous elements depends upon the diligence of the observer and that the separation of these two types is arbitrary.

Cytology

The role of cytology as a screening mechanism for this type of endometrial cancer is limited. Of the 11 patients from whom cervicovaginal cytology was obtained, only three were diagnosed with a malignant tumor based on their smears.[11] A slightly higher yield was reported by Massoni and Hajdu.[86] The five patients reported by An-Foraker and Kawada[5] all had malignant or suspicious glandular cells noted on their cervicovaginal specimens; however, the specimens collected by the Isaacs cell sampler provided evidence of the sarcomatous elements in addition to the carcinoma in the routine smears.

Tumors cells were more often present in the vaginal specimen than in the cervical one.[63] The carcinomatous element was present in 38%, of which adenocarcinoma was more common than was squamous carcinoma.[86] Sarcomatous elements were noted in 29%.[86] In a detailed tabulation, all five cases contained malignant glandular cells and two also contained malignant squamous cells; a variety of malignant mesenchymal elements were represented in greater and lesser numbers.[5] The type most consistently represented was the spindly, malignant stromal cell.

The tumor cells lie in a bloody background. The cells of adenocarcinoma may resemble those of ordinary endometrial adenocarcinoma or those of clear cell carcinoma (Fig. 13–10), with round nuclei containing prominent nucleoli. The arrangement is often papillary. The sarcomatous elements (Fig. 13–11) are more difficult to discern because they may have lost their spindle or elongated shape and may not exfoliate in a manner permitting ready identification and classification. They are often single, with lacier, ill-defined

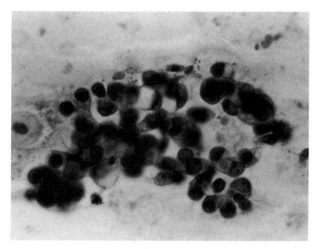

FIGURE 13–10. The **adenocarcinoma** exfoliated from a mesodermal mixed tumor is of the clear cell type with round nuclei containing prominent nucleoli (Papanicolaou stain; ×300).

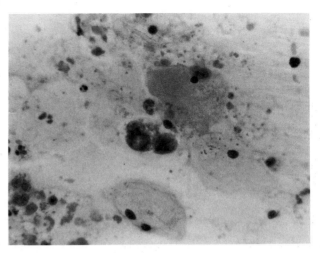

FIGURE 13–12. These **large tumor cells,** one of which is multinucleated, have ill-defined cytoplasmic borders suggesting that they are from the sarcomatous component of the tumor (Papanicolaou stain; ×300).

cytoplasmic borders and a finer but still hyperchromatic chromatin arrangement. Multinucleation and cellular gigantism are frequent (Fig. 13–12). Of the heterologous elements, rhabdomyosarcoma may be seen, but the characteristic cross-striations may not be sufficiently preserved in cytologic material to make a specific diagnosis. The cells of chondrosarcoma are round with blue-gray cytoplasm and round nuclei containing red nucleoli. Those of osteosarcoma are large with dusty brown-pink cytoplasm; they may be multinucleated. Limited representation of the sarcomatous portion of this malignant tumor may be due to the covering of the carcinoma, which prohibits these cells from exfoliating (Fig. 13–13).

Gynecologic cytology for ovarian tumors has not been helpful, and in none of the smears from the 11 patients with mesodermal mixed tumors of the ovary were malignant cells detected.[39] However, nine patients (81%) had ascites.

The cytology of ascites and peritoneal washings will be discussed together. The most prevalent cell type represented is adenocarcinoma; the least common occurrence is the presence of sarcomatous cells exclusively.[52, 69, 101] The cells of adenocarcinoma form clusters of cells with thin, lacy cytoplasm and round or oval, slightly hyperchromatic nuclei with prominent nucleoli. Sarcomatous cells may resemble the cells of adenocarcinoma because they may become round, their cytoplasm may become lacy and they may even form cell clusters. They are recognizable as sarcomatous when they are single, have caudate or elongated shapes and have ill-defined cytoplasmic borders (Fig. 13–14); multinucleation may be present, and the nuclear chromatin is finer with prominent nucleoli.

Because recurrent and metastatic disease is common, aspiration cytology may be helpful in confirming the diagnosis (Fig. 13–15).[106]

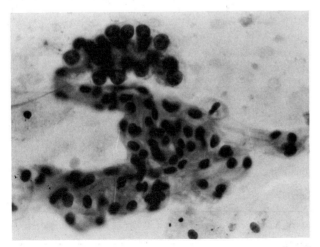

FIGURE 13–11. In this field, a papillary group of cells represents the **adenocarcinoma** adjacent to the spindly, sarcomatous cells that have retained their elongated shape (Papanicolaou stain; ×300).

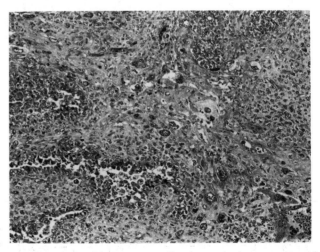

FIGURE 13–13. The **sarcoma** lies beneath the covering of adenocarcinoma and is composed of leiomyosarcoma (hematoxylin and eosin; ×200).

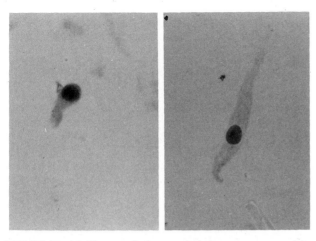

FIGURE 13–14. These cells from a **rhabdomyosarcoma** of the uterus were noted in the ascites. Note the preservation of the elongated shape, the thin cytoplasm and the ill-defined borders (Papanicolaou stain; × 300).

Summary of Cytologic Findings

- Cells of adenocarcinoma, often papillary
- Squamous carcinoma
- Elongated malignant cells (sarcoma)
- Bloody background (gynecologic specimens).

Clinical Course

These uterine tumors are very aggressive, with an overall 5-year survival of 38%. The survival for patients with disease limited to the uterus was 52%, compared with 28% for those with spread beyond the uterus.[127] Even among the group with limited disease, those whose pelvic washings contained tumor cells in the absence of visible extrauterine spread had a worse prognosis (0 out of 3 survived) than those without this finding (9 out of 15 survived).[52]

Most recurrences—95% of locoregional and 85% of distant metastases—are noted within 3 years.[126] Intrapelvic and intra-abdominal metastases are the most common, although metastases to more distant sites such as the lungs, bones and the brain have been reported.[73]

Survival for those with ovarian mesodermal mixed tumor is dismal. None of the 12 patients reported in one study survived 5 years, except for one patient with Stage I disease who had been followed for 2.5 years.[12]

Monomorphic Sarcomas of the Uterus

Monomorphic sarcomas of the uterus are uncommon, composing no more than 2% of the malignant tumors of the uterus. Of these, the most common are endometrial stromal sarcoma and leiomyosarcoma.

Stromal Sarcoma

Endometrial stromal sarcoma is a disease found in young as well as old women, with mean ages ranging from 42 to 53 years.[151] About half are premenopausal. The most common complaint is abnormal bleeding. Less commonly, the patients present with abdominal pain. Upon examination, there may be a tumor protruding through the external cervical os, but the most common finding is an enlarged uterus.

Histology

Histologically, the tumor shows a monomorphic pattern of infiltration by small, uniform cells resembling the stromal cells of proliferative endometrium (Fig. 13–16). The tumor may form a discrete mass, infiltrate diffusely into the endometrium and myometrium or extend into the lymphatic channels (endolymphatic

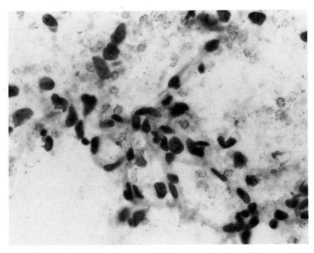

FIGURE 13–15. The lung aspirate contained malignant spindle cells, consistent with metastasis from a known **mesodermal mixed tumor** (Papanicolaou stain; × 300).

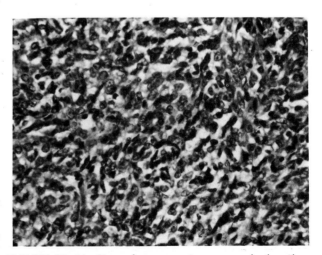

FIGURE 13–16. Stromal sarcoma is composed of uniform small spindly cells with scant cytoplasm. They may form small glands as in the center of the field (hematoxylin and eosin; × 200).

stromal miosis). The mitotic rate is low (below 10 per 10 high power field [hpf]) in low-grade tumors, whereas it is much higher in high-grade tumors. Grading should be performed when the entire specimen is available, rather than on small fragments or on the cytology, although the latter has been suggested.[97] The application of flow cytometry may change the grading criteria currently applied, which is based solely on histopathology.[7]

About 20% of the low-grade tumors are Stage I tumors, but about half will recur in the pelvis within 3 years.[72] The indolent nature is reflected in the high 10-year survival for both Stage I (88%) and Stage IV (75%) patients.[72] High-grade sarcomas are more aggressive, with recurrences in the pelvis within 2 years.[151] Tumor cells may exfoliate into the ascitic fluid, where they are present singly and in small, loose clusters; molding may also be present.[65] The most common site of distant metastases is in the lungs.[113]

Cytology

Cytology as a screening procedure has not been effective; in only about half of these patients have malignant cells been identified in their smears, even after retrospective review.[13] Exfoliation of cells requires involvement of the endometrium and ulceration of the surface to release tumor cells. It may also depend on the grade of the tumor; one group found that their case with the high-grade stromal sarcoma had cells in the vaginal smear, whereas the other, who had a low-grade sarcoma, did not.[97]

The cellular patterns noted in the smears vary from the single cell arrangement to the formation of loosely cohesive clusters (Fig. 13–17). The cytoplasm is wispy, with ill-defined borders, and comet cells have been described as cells whose cytoplasm seems to merge with the nucleus and extend excentrically as a trailing tail.[67] The nuclei are round or oval with irregular

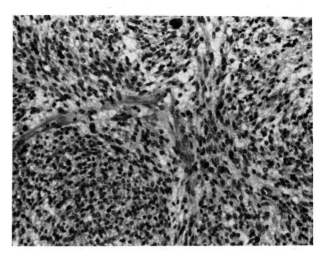

FIGURE 13–18. The interlacing muscle group pattern is a feature of the histologic appearance of **leiomyosarcoma** (hematoxylin and eosin; ×100).

borders. Most of the cells are uniform, although giant tumor cells have been reported.[67]

The differential diagnoses of these small uniform cells presenting in a bloody smear with necrotic debris are endometrial carcinoma, anaplastic small-cell carcinoma and anaplastic sarcoma.

Summary of Cytologic Findings

- Small spindle-shaped cells
- Single cells or small loose clusters
- Wispy ill-defined cytoplasm
- Little pleomorphism.

Leiomyosarcoma

Although leiomyomata uteri are present in an estimated 20% of women, leiomyosarcoma accounts for about 1.5% of the malignant tumors of the uterus. The mean age is in the 6th decade. The patient presents with abnormal bleeding or pelvic pain or discomfort. On examination the uterus is enlarged.

Because most leiomyosarcomas are intramural, tumor cells are rarely present in cervicovaginal smears. Hajdu and Hajdu[55] found only six of their 38 patients had malignant cells in their cervicovaginal smears. Vaginal smears were more likely to contain the malignant cells.

Histology

Histologically, leiomyosarcoma is composed of bundles of spindle cells occurring in a whorled or storiform arrangement (Fig. 13–18). The less-differentiated tumors are more cellular and show much more pleomorphism. Mitotic counts are important in establishing the grade of the smooth muscle tumor. Those with 10 or more mitoses per 10/hpf are likely to be aggressive tumors with spread to the pelvis and peritoneum and

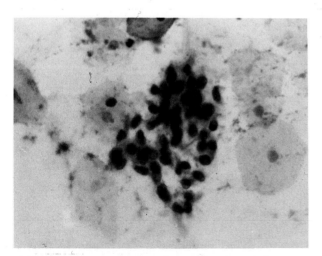

FIGURE 13–17. The small uniform cells of **stromal sarcoma** have formed a loose group. The arrangement of the wispy cytoplasm is "comet"-like in a few cells (Papanicolaou stain; ×300).

to metastasize to the lungs.[113] Pulmonary metastases may occur in the absence of local recurrence and may be the initial site of recurrence.[16] Transthoracic aspiration of these masses can establish the diagnosis of recurrence (Fig. 13–19).

Currently available methods cannot always differentiate between these two types of sarcoma because some tumors have features of both[72] and have been referred to as stromomyoma.

Other monomorphic sarcomas are rare. They include chondrosarcoma,[29] osteosarcoma[33] (Fig. 13–20) and rhabdomyosarcoma.[36]

Cytology

In cytologic preparations these tumor cells are elongated spindly cells with nuclei located about midway between the pointed ends (Fig. 13–21). The cytoplasm is thin with ill-defined borders. The cells may be single or they may be arranged in a whorl (Fig. 13–22), the so-called storiform or pinwheel arrangement. When the cells have rounded up, the cytoplasm is denser and more eosinophilic, although the periphery is still ill defined. Giant tumor cells and multinucleation may be seen. The nuclei, which can be convoluted, have coarse, hyperchromatic chromatin and single or multiple nucleoli. Exfoliated cells from the epithelioid variant have more abundant eosinophilic cytoplasm and excentrically placed nuclei (Fig. 13–23), mimicking an adenocarcinoma.

The differential diagnoses for the spindly tumor cells include other types of spindle cell sarcomas such as fibrosarcoma, malignant fibrous histiocytoma and malignant peripheral nerve sheath tumors. Because these are rare in the female genital tract, it is unlikely that they would be considered in the absence of prior knowledge of such a tumor in a given patient. More likely is the interpretation of these cells as the cytologic representatives of a poorly differentiated carcinoma that has undergone spindly metaplasia or the sarcomatous component of mesodermal mixed tumor.

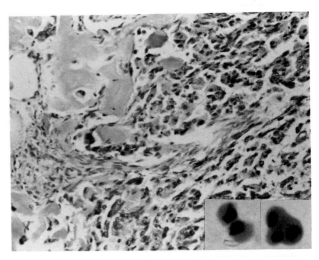

FIGURE 13–20. This **osteogenic sarcoma** was present in the uterus of a 31-year-old woman (hematoxylin and eosin; ×200). Two years later, the pleural fluid contained the malignant cells (inset) consistent with metastases (Papanicolaou stain; ×300).

Summary of Cytologic Findings

- Elongated spindly cells
- Ill-defined cytoplasmic borders
- Coarse chromatin in oval, convoluted nuclei
- Single or multiple nucleoli
- Multinucleation common
- Occasional giant tumor cells.

LYMPHOMA AND LEUKEMIA

In 1989, the American Cancer Society estimated that, in that year, 20,000 women would be diagnosed with lymphoma and Hodgkin's disease and another 12,000 with leukemia.[22] Although a fourth of all lymphomas originate in extranodal sites, the female genital tract is rarely the site of primary lymphomas, with only 1% considered to have originated there, most com-

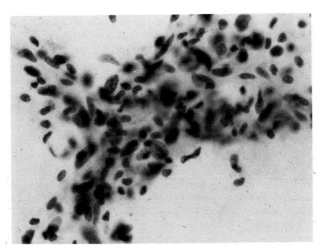

FIGURE 13–19. In a lung aspirate, **metastatic leiomyosarcoma** has a cytologic appearance similar to that in a vaginal smear (Papanicolaou stain; ×300).

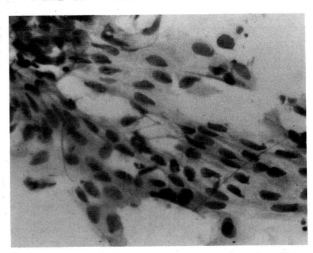

FIGURE 13–21. Long spindly cells with oval nuclei characterize the cells of **leiomyosarcoma** (Papanicolaou stain; ×300).

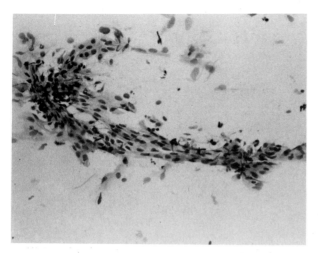

FIGURE 13–22. At lower magnification, the arrangement of **interlacing muscle groups** is evident (Papanicolaou stain; ×100).

monly in the ovary.[48] Secondary spread of lymphoma and leukemia to the female genital tract occurs in up to 40% of cases.[25, 78, 114] Because the lymphoma may be widely disseminated at the time of diagnosis, it is difficult to determine whether the disease presented in the female genital tract as part of generalized disease or whether the lymphoma began in the genital organs. Crisp and coworkers[32] emphasize the importance of proper staging to evaluate the extent of disease and, thereby, to properly stage and treat the patient. When symptoms are referable to the cervix, colposcopy may assist in visualizing an abnormal pattern, unlike those associated with intraepithelial squamous neoplasms.[94]

In two large series of lymphoma and granulocytic sarcoma involving the uterus and the vagina, the cervix was most commonly involved, in 69% of cases (29 out of 42), followed by the vagina in 19% (8 out of 42) and finally the corpus in 12% (5 out of 42).[26, 58] The

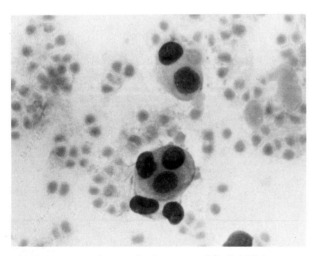

FIGURE 13–23. These cells from an **epithelioid leiomyosarcoma** may be confused with carcinoma because of the clustering pattern. In other areas the cells were less cohesive (hematoxylin and eosin; ×300).

patients ranged in age from 20 to 80 years with a median in the 5th decade.

The symptoms resemble those of other gynecologic neoplasms. Abnormal bleeding is associated with tumor involvement of the vagina, the cervix and the endometrium.[23, 24, 26] The chief complaint of pelvic mass or abdominal discomfort has also been reported in patients with tumors in the vagina, the uterus and the ovary.[24, 54] A few patients are asymptomatic despite having a tumor detectable on physical examination in the ovary, the cervix, the vagina and the pelvis.[24, 54, 58] Cervical lymphoma was an incidental finding in three women in whom hysterectomies were performed for leiomyoma.[58]

Two patients in each of two series presented with granulocytic sarcoma of the cervix.[26, 58] Granulocytic sarcoma is rare, occurring as the initial presentation in 0.6% of patients with granulocytic leukemia.[81] Therefore, it is noteworthy that Lucia and associates[84] found leukemic infiltrates in 41% of uteri at autopsy of which 33% were granulocytic leukemias.

The most common gross appearance of the cervix was that of generalized enlargement; other findings were a polypoid mass protruding through the external cervical os and multinodular masses.[58, 88] Vaginal involvement presented as diffuse thickening. Endometrial tumors were apparent when they formed polypoid tumors, as did one of the two tumors in Harris and Scully's[58] series; however, most had no visible tumor masses.

Histology

Lymphomas are divided into two large groups: Hodgkin's disease and non-Hodgkin's lymphoma. The involvement of the female genitalia in Hodgkin's disease is uncommon (12%) compared with involvement by non-Hodgkin's lymphoma (35%).[78] In one series, only one of 15 patients had Hodgkin's disease.[26] Hahn[54] included two cases: one had primary involvement of the vulva and the other had secondary involvement of the parametrium in a generalized process.

Terminology for the non-Hodgkin's lymphomas is based on several schemata. Using the Working Formulation, the distribution in one series showed that about half of the cervical lymphomas (Fig. 13–24), all but one vaginal and both endometrial ones, were diffuse large-cell lymphomas.[58] Another notable finding in this series was that a third of the cervical tumors and one of the vaginal ones were follicular lymphomas, an observation also made by Chorlton and colleagues.[26] Harris and Scully[58] found sclerosis a prominent feature. The collagenous tissue compresses the tumor cells, introducing an artifact that creates an impression of a nonlymphomatous malignant process.

Granulocytic sarcoma, although uncommon, has been reported as presenting in the cervix prior to the development of leukemia.[24, 58, 122] The diagnosis can be confirmed by a positive chloracetate esterase stain, but this stain can be misleading; one of two cases reported by Harris and Scully[58] gave a negative reaction.

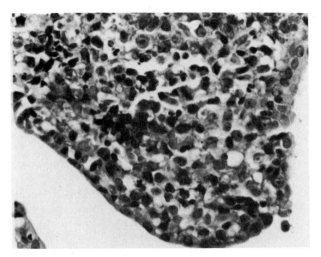

FIGURE 13–24. A **large cell lymphoma** is present beneath the endocervical epithelium (hematoxylin and eosin; ×300).

Lymphoma should be suspected when the tumor under scrutiny does not resemble the common carcinomas and sarcomas of this location. The same caveat applies to "inflammatory" lesions with an unfamiliar appearance. Because lymphomas rarely present in the female genital tract, misinterpretations of histologic material have included small-cell carcinoma, sarcoma and inflammatory processes.[24, 58, 122] Despite this, these patients have done well, and a review of the prior material is prompted by recurrence of the tumor.

Cytology

The role of cytology is limited in those patients with primary as well as secondary involvement of the genital organs, because the disease is most likely subepithelial in the cervix or vagina and is more likely to involve the ovary, in which case exfoliation into cervicovaginal smears is serendipitous. Because ulceration of the mucosal surface is rare, the opportunity to sample the tumor cells even in accessible locations such as the cervix and vagina is limited. The cervicovaginal smears were diagnostic in four of seven patients in one review.[78] In the report of a case and a review of the literature, Whitaker[145] found a third of the cases of lymphoma of the cervix had positive smears, two cases of Hodgkin's disease and three cases of reticulum cell sarcoma (large-cell lymphoma). However, in another report, the tumor cells were identified in only two of ten cases with cervicovaginal cytology.[58] The researchers attributed the lack of success to the protective epithelial covering. This is illustrated in a report in which the patient with the positive smear had an ulcerated lesion, whereas the other patient whose epithelium was intact had a negative one.[23] Even in patients with tumor cells in the smear, the diagnosis of lymphoma or leukemia has been missed or misinterpreted in both the cytologic and histologic material, probably because of the rarity of this type of tumor in gynecologic material. The small cells have been interpreted as small-cell carcinoma, endometrial carcinoma and sarcoma, and the patients were treated accordingly.[24, 58, 88]

The apparently more common involvement of the female genital organs, particularly the uterus, by leukemic infiltrates suggests that the likelihood of identifying leukemic cells in cervicovaginal smears is greater than the likelihood of identifying lymphoma. In a study of 61 cases with 68 smears available for review, leukemic cells were found in 17 (28%) cases: seven cases of myelogenous leukemia, five of monocytic leukemia and five of lymphocytic leukemia.[25] The researchers attributed the high rate of abnormal smears to the loss of integrity of the overlying epithelial surface and to bleeding, which would permit circulating leukemic cells in the blood to appear in the smear.

The smear pattern in the non-Hodgkin's lymphomas and in the leukemias is one of a monomorphic population of tumor cells. In the small-cell or lymphocytic lymphomas, the tumor cells are small, slightly larger than the red blood cells, with scant basophilic cytoplasm and excentric nuclei (Fig. 13–25). The nuclei are bean shaped or oval with coarse granular cytoplasm and prominent nucleoli. Others, large-cell or histiocytic lymphomas, are composed of larger cells. Some cells have nuclear protrusions (Fig. 13–26), as have been described for those cells in body cavity fluids,[71, 92] whereas others do not, despite a search for them.[134]

The cytology of Hodgkin's disease has been described.[104] The smears contain large tumor cells, often binucleated—the Reed-Sternberg cells—in a background of lymphocytes, plasma cells and eosinophils.

The differential diagnoses include follicular cervicitis or chronic cervicitis, small-cell anaplastic carcinoma and sarcoma. In follicular cervicitis, there is a pleomorphic infiltrate of immature and mature lymphocytes. The nuclei of the immature lymphocytes contain small punctate nucleoli and evenly dispersed chromatin

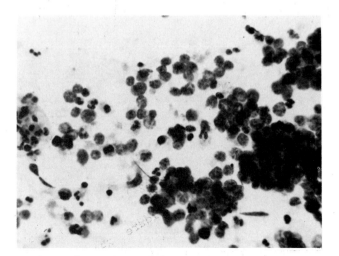

FIGURE 13–25. These malignant cells from a **small cell lymphoma** are diagnostic for that disease when they are scattered singly. The large masses of cells may be misinterpreted as representing a carcinoma (Papanicolaou stain; ×300).

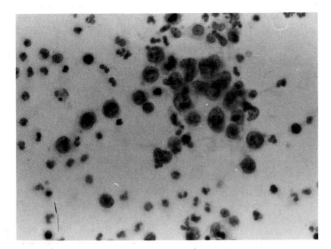

FIGURE 13–26. Other **lymphomas** are composed of larger cells with lobulated nuclei containing prominent nucleoli (Papanicolaou stain; × 300).

without coarse condensation around the nuclear envelope. Nipplelike nuclear protrusions are absent. The cellular pattern of chronic cervicitis includes a mixture of many mature lymphocytes (Fig. 13–27) and scattered plasma cells. The lymphocytes have small, pyknotic nuclei and no nucleoli. In the smears of anaplastic carcinoma, the cells are small with deeply hyperchromatic, irregularly shaped, pleomorphic nuclei. Nucleoli are not prominent and may not be present at all; cytoplasm is more abundant. Although the cells of lymphoma are arranged singly, those of anaplastic carcinoma show occasional intercellular associations and may even mold. One pitfall differentiating small-cell lymphomas from carcinomas is that the lymphoid cells may touch one another, giving the illusion of cell clusters (see Fig. 13–25) rather than the diagnostic single isolated cell pattern associated with nonepithelial tumors. Small-cell sarcomas may resemble the cells of a carcinoma in smears rather than lymphoma because they may form cell groups that resemble clusters.

The smears from Hodgkin's disease contain a variety of cell types, lymphocytes, plasma cells and eosinophils. Even in a patient with Hodgkin's disease with all the other attendant cells in the smear, Reed-Sternberg cells are required for the diagnosis of Hodgkin's disease.

The malignant leukemic cells depend upon the type of leukemia. The commonest type of leukemia that involves the uterus is granulocytic or myelocytic. These cells resemble granulocytes, but their nuclei are less pyknotic and immature band forms and misshapen multilobated forms are present (Fig. 13–28). Cursory examination of these smears may lead one to the conclusion that there is acute inflammation rather than a leukemic infiltrate. The other types of leukemia, monocytic and lymphocytic, both chronic and acute, have cells that resemble those of the lymphomas, small and large cell. It may not be possible to separate these types of lymphomas using the Papanicolaou stained preparation; however, a diagnosis of leukemia or lymphoma can be rendered.

Summary of Cytologic Findings

- Small cells arranged singly
- Scant cytoplasm
- Convoluted nuclei often with prominent nucleoli
- Large binucleated cells in Hodgkin's disease
- Monomorphic cell population except for Hodgkin's disease
- Pleomorphic population of plasma cells, eosinophils and lymphocytes in Hodgkin's disease.

MALIGNANT MELANOMA

Malignant melanoma of the female genital tract accounts for 3 to 5% of all melanomas.[35] In this organ system, the most common site is the vulva, where it is the second most common malignant tumor, accounting for 2 to 11% of the malignant tumors,[99, 146] or one

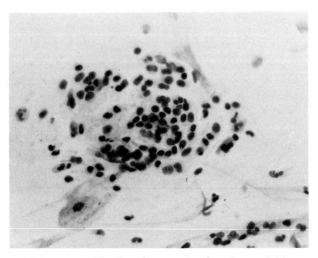

FIGURE 13–27. The lymphocytes in **chronic cervicitis** are small and uniform (Papanicolaou stain; × 300).

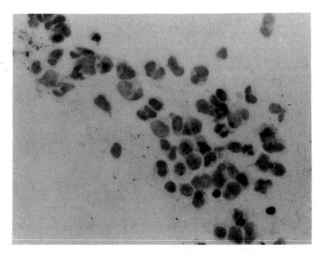

FIGURE 13–28. The cells of **acute myelogenous leukemia** are in immature blast forms as well as a few band shapes (Papanicolaou stain; × 300).

melanoma for every 27 epidermoid carcinomas.[99] About 3% of the vaginal malignant tumors are malignant melanomas.[27]

The mean age of patients with vulvar melanoma is 55 years, with a range of 15 to 84 years. The most common complaints are an enlarging mole or tumor, itching or bleeding.[146] Rarely, such melanomas are identified during a routine gynecologic examination. The most common locations are the labia minora and the clitoris. Vulvar melanomas are rarely evaluated by exfoliative cytology and are most often biopsied.

Cytology is more likely to be useful in the detection and follow-up of patients with vaginal melanomas. In a review of the literature, Levitan and coworkers[80] found 129 cases of vaginal melanomas. The mean age was 57 years and the range from 22 to 83 years; three fourths of the patients were older than 50 years. The most common presenting symptom was abnormal bleeding, followed by vaginal discharge; least common was the presence of a mass. Tumors, ranging in size from 0.5 cm to larger than 5 cm,[27] were often located in the distal vagina.

Treatment of both vaginal and vulvar melanomas is surgical. Local recurrences in the vagina and vaginal metastases from vulvar melanomas may occur several years after primary excision.[19, 27] Follow-up by periodic cytologic examination was found useful in a case of vaginal melanoma with repeated vaginal recurrences and excisions over a 3-year period.[115]

Primary cervical melanoma is even rarer, with only a few cases reported. In a review of the literature, Mordel and colleagues[96] summarized the 20 cases acceptable as primary cervical melanomas. The average age was 55 years, with a range of 26 to 74 years; the peak age group was in the 7th decade. Patients most commonly presented with abnormal vaginal bleeding. On physical examination, the commonest finding was a polypoid mass. In a case report, a 51-year-old woman presented with brain metastases and had a cervical melanoma detected in her cervical smear.[149]

Cutaneous melanomas are commoner, with an incidence of 2.7% and an estimated increasing incidence rate of 3.4% per year.[22] Metastatic spread from the skin tumors is usually to the lungs, the lymph nodes, the liver and the brain, but in autopsy series 23 of 85 (27%) women had metastases to the uterus including the uterine cervix.[96, 108] About 4% of patients with melanoma present with metastases, most commonly in the lungs, and no identifiable primary source.[8] A report documented a case in which the cytologic diagnosis of malignant melanoma was the first indication of metastasis to the endometrium from a cutaneous primary source subsequently located in the back.[132] The patient had no other evident sites of metastatic spread and died 5 months later of myocardial infarction.

Histology

The histology of primary melanomas shows an intraepithelial proliferation of abnormal melanocytes. In the epidermis the tumor cells may form small clusters or disseminate throughout the epithelium as single cells. The infiltrating tumor may be composed of eosinophilic round or spindly cells with central nuclei containing prominent nucleoli. Multinucleation is often present. The cells may be deeply pigmented (Fig. 13–29) or amelanotic. In the latter, histochemical or immunologic stains or electron microscopy or both may be required to determine the precise nature of the malignant neoplasm.

Metastatic melanoma lies beneath the mucosa and will not have the intraepithelial changes associated with melanoma originating at this site.

Cytology

Ehrman and associates[43] reported the first cases of the cytology of primary melanoma of the vagina. This report is of special significance because the cytologic report of malignant cells was the first indication of a malignant tumor in the vagina in one case, a 60-year-old woman whose complaint was slight vaginal bleeding without any provoking factor and whose physical examination revealed marked senile vaginitis. No clinical indication of a malignant process was apparent. In the other cases of primary cervical, vaginal and vulvar melanomas reported since then, tumors were visible. In a review of 722 specimens representing a variety of specimen types from 79 patients with melanoma, including two with primary vaginal melanoma, only 3% of the smears containing malignant cells were of cervicovaginal origin.[56]

The cytology of both primary and metastatic melanoma to the cervix and vagina shows marked cellular pleomorphism. Single cell arrangement is a consistent feature of this tumor,[43, 56] although sheets of tumor cells have also been reported.[17] The cells may be round or oval, or in some instances more polygonal, with amphophilic or basophilic cytoplasm and ill-defined, occasionally lacy, cell borders (Fig. 13–30). The pres-

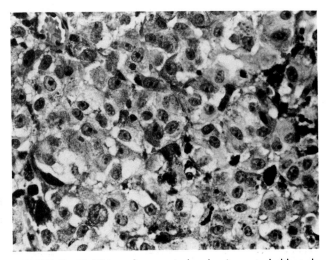

FIGURE 13–29. This **melanoma** is deeply pigmented although the cells in the smear (Fig. 13–30) are not (hematoxylin and eosin; ×200).

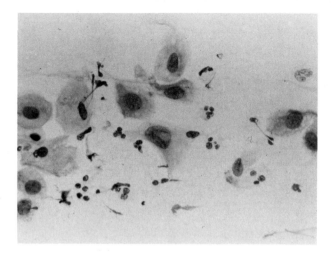

FIGURE 13–30. Melanoma may mimic many different kinds of cells. In this field, the tumor cells are polygonal with ill-defined, lacy cytoplasmic borders. The nucleus of the cell in the center has an intranuclear cytoplasmic inclusion. Compare the tumor cells with the intermediate cells to the left (Papanicolaou stain; ×300).

ence of pigment (Fig. 13–31) has been noted by some,[49, 132] but has not been found consistently.[17, 43, 149] Pigment in gynecologic smears is not readily apparent and is often inconspicuous despite deep pigmentation of the tumor from which it came. A diligent search is often necessary.

Prominent nucleoli are often present[132] in excentric hypochromatic or hyperchromatic nuclei.[17] Multinucleated and binucleated cells, both large and small, are generally present. Spindle cells have been reported.[64] Invagination of the cytoplasm into the nucleus resulting in an intranuclear vacuole has been reported[56] but has not been a consistent feature.[115, 132, 149]

The differential diagnoses include epidermoid carcinoma, adenocarcinoma and spindle cell sarcoma. The cells of epidermoid carcinoma are also generally arranged singly. The nuclei tend to have coarse, more hyperchromatic chromatin and do not tend to have nucleoli. Keratinized cells with large, black, opaque nuclei in pearl formation may be found as well. Orangeophilic cytoplasm may be factitiously produced by degeneration of the cytoplasm, so all aspects of the cytomorphology and smear pattern must be considered. The cells from an adenocarcinoma have prominent nucleoli and excentrically placed nuclei, but their cytoplasm is translucent and has well-defined cell borders. The tumor cells often form cell balls or clusters and may phagocytize other tumor cells. Of the genital adenocarcinomas, the ones that exfoliate cells that could mimic melanoma are the serous-type adenocarcinomas of the ovary and endometrium. The associated pigment from bleeding may further confuse the observer.

Melanin in histiocytes (Fig. 13–32) may suggest the presence of melanoma, but melanin must be found within malignant cells to establish the diagnosis of melanoma.

Adjunctive histochemical stains may be helpful. Among these are the Fontana-Masson and the potassium ferricyanide stains. Investigation of cytologic preparations with regard to the reactivity of these cells to specific antibodies has been reported. Ordóñez and coworkers[107] studied 11 fluid and 21 fine needle aspiration specimens containing tumor cells from 32 patients with melanoma and 15 fluid and 21 fine needle aspiration specimens containing malignant cells from patients with a variety of other tumors. Their results indicated that 24 of the 32 (75%) specimens containing the cells of malignant melanoma reacted positively to mouse monoclonal antibody HMB-45; none of the other tumors tested reacted to this antibody. All but one melanoma stained positively for S-100 protein; that one reacted with that to HMB-45. Four specimens, one each from metastatic ovarian, mammary and pros-

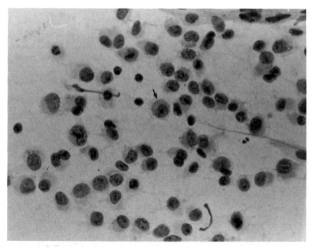

FIGURE 13–31. These cells from **melanoma** metastatic in the endocervix are small and could be overlooked in the atrophic smear. The nuclei contain small prominent nucleoli. The cell in the center (arrow) has melanin pigment around its periphery (Papanicolaou stain; ×300).

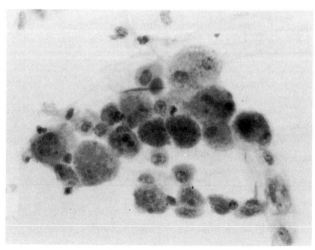

FIGURE 13–32. Histiocytes have phagocytized melanin that obscures the nuclei of some cells (Papanicolaou stain; ×300).

tate carcinoma and a neurogenic sarcoma, showed reactivity to S-100 protein. Another study[6] showed that all but one of 20 specimens was negative for keratin; all were positive for vimentin. Another study on histologic material indicates that the staining reaction differs for cutaneous and mucosal melanomas.[46] Caution should be exercised in interpreting cells reacting with HMB-45 because it has been found in two of 100 cases of breast cancer and in six of 100 samples of benign breast tissue.[17a] It now is evident that a variety of tumors contain a number of antigens, some of which are more common to a particular group of tumors. Therefore, the results of a panel of antibodies, rather than the reaction of a single antibody, should be considered in evaluating the cytology and the pattern of reactivity before drawing a conclusion.

Summary of Cytologic Findings

- Pleomorphism with binucleated or multinucleated cells
- Single cell arrangement
- Ill-defined, lacy cytoplasmic borders
- Prominent nucleoli
- Melanin pigment in tumor cells.

Clinical Course

The prognosis of vulvar melanoma is related to the thickness of the tumor. Chung and colleagues[28] established that patients with tumors greater than 2 mm thick had an unfavorable prognosis. A compilation of several studies showed an overall 5-year survival rate of 36%.[99] Similar results were found in their evaluation of the 19 patients with vaginal melanomas.[27] The 5-year survival based on data from several series was 5%.[99]

TROPHOBLASTIC TUMORS

Trophoblastic tumors of the uterus are associated with gestation, which may either be concurrent with the discovery of the neoplasm or have preceded the discovery of the tumor. Classification of this broad, all-inclusive group is intricate, and the reader is directed to several excellent discussions.[37, 90] This discussion is limited to hydatidiform mole and choriocarcinoma.

The incidence of gestational trophoblastic disease in the United States is low, estimated at one in 2000 to 2500 pregnancies,[37] compared with that in some other countries, where the incidence is as high as 9.9 in 1000 pregnancies.[90] Women at greatest risk are those at the ends of the reproductive spectrum, those under 20 and over 40 years, although this disease has been found in women throughout their reproductive years and several years following menopause. The uterus is the most commonly affected site, although trophoblastic disease has been found in the fallopian tubes and in the ovaries.

Patients present with bleeding and rarely with the expulsion of vesicles of molar tissue. There may be asymptomatic patients; a study of elective abortions found one molar pregnancy in 600 consecutive specimens.[31]

The most common trophoblastic tumor is hydatidiform mole. These are further subdivided into complete and partial moles. The former have a diploid chromosomal complement, of which about 90% have the chromosomal complement of 46,XX and, far less often, 46,XY. Both sets of chromosomes are paternally derived.[37, 90] About 3 to 16% of complete molar pregnancies are associated with an invasive mole, and 2.5% go on to choriocarcinoma.[34, 40, 90] Follow-up is accomplished by monitoring the serum levels of the beta subunit of human chorionic gonadotropin (hCG) levels.

In the partial mole, a conceptus is identified, and the pregnancy may even go to term. The chromosomal complement is triploid, 69,XXY in 70%, 69,XX in 27% and 69,XYY in 3%.[131] The extra set of chromosomes is paternal. Most tumors are confined to the uterus, and evacuation of the tumor may be curative. The outcome for partial moles is favorable and unassociated with the development of choriocarcinoma.[34] Caution in making the diagnosis of partial mole based on the use of DNA flow cytometry should be exercised; triploidy was found in six of 59 (10%) abortion specimens, but only three were found to correlate with the histologic criteria for partial moles.[140]

Choriocarcinoma is found in one in 20,000 to 40,000 pregnancies in the United States. About 33 to 50% follow a molar pregnancy, 25 to 33% a spontaneous abortion and 25 to 33% a normal gestation.[40] In a small proportion of cases the tumor is found after a long interval following the gestation,[34] but this may be the result of choriocarcinoma originating in the placenta during gestation that is undetected by gross and microscopic examination.[21] The most common sign of uterine choriocarcinoma is bleeding. Because of the highly vascular nature of the tumor, patients may also present with metastases to the lungs, the brain or the vagina.[21]

Choriocarcinoma, when unassociated with gestation, is more often found in the ovaries as a part of or composing the entirety of a germ cell tumor.[77, 141] This is very rare; the few acceptable cases have been reported in premenarchal girls. The nature of gestational trophoblastic disease precludes ready acceptance of ovarian nongestational choriocarcinoma in women of reproductive age or in recently postmenopausal women.[77]

Extragenital choriocarcinoma has been reported in which the tumor is in part or *in toto* represented by neoplastic tissue that appears histologically identical to gestational trophoblastic tissue and produces the same biochemical product, hCG. The gastrointestinal tract is the most common site for the origin of these tumors.[116, 138]

Histology

Molar tissue is composed of thin-walled, discrete vesicles that on histologic examination are large edem-

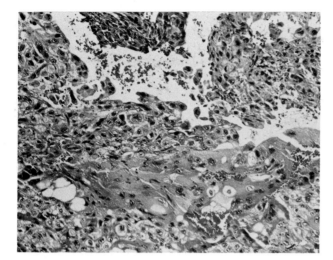

FIGURE 13–33. Choriocarcinoma is composed of cytotrophoblasts and syncytiotrophoblasts (hematoxylin and eosin; ×200).

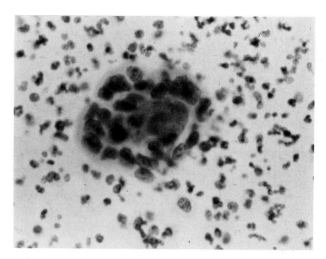

FIGURE 13–35. Cytotrophoblasts are arranged in a cluster found in ascites (Papanicolaou stain; ×300).

atous chorionic villi with central cisterns and proliferation of trophoblastic tissue. The trophoblasts may show much atypia. In partial moles, evidence of fetal tissue may also be present.

Choriocarcinoma is composed solely of trophoblastic tissue without any chorionic villi (Fig. 13–33). The tumor is often quite hemorrhagic, infiltrating deeply into the myometrium (Fig. 13–34) or located only in the myometrium. Exfoliation of material from this type of tumor results in a bloody smear, with few, if any, recognizable tumor cells.

Cytology

There is little in the literature about the cytology of trophoblastic cells, probably because the contribution by cytology is limited in making the initial diagnosis

and in the follow-up, which is accomplished almost exclusively by monitoring serum beta hCG levels.

The tumor cells are of two kinds. One is the cytotrophoblast, which is a polygonal cell with a single nucleus containing a prominent nucleolus (Fig. 13–35). It is about the size of decidual cells,[133] which have more distinct cellular membranes. The cytoplasm is translucent and cyanophilic or eosinophilic. The other cell is the syncytiotrophoblast (Fig. 13–36), a large, bizarre, multinucleated cell. The cytoplasm is dense, eosinophilic and occasionally vacuolated.

These cells are found in bloody smears and may form large aggregates (Fig. 13–37). It may not be possible to differentiate hydatidiform mole from choriocarcinoma.[44]

Summary of Cytologic Findings

- Polygonal mononucleated cells
- Prominent nucleoli

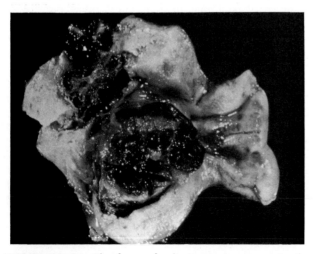

FIGURE 13–34. The **hemorrhagic tumor** is present in the endometrial cavity as well as infiltrating deeply into the myometrium.

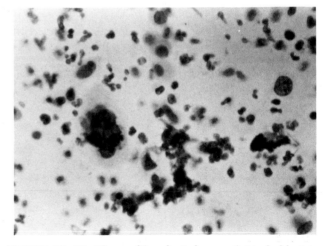

FIGURE 13–36. The **multinucleated syncytiotrophoblast** is present in the left side with a cytotrophoblast at the right (Papanicolaou stain; ×300).

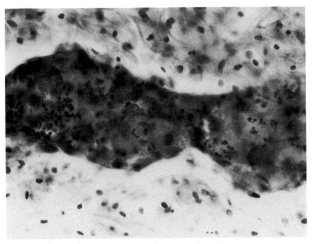

FIGURE 13–37. This large aggregate of cells was found in the smear of a young patient with **hydatidiform mole** and represents molar tissue (Papanicolaou stain; ×300).

- Multinucleated cells
- Mixture of these cells around an edematous core (hydatidiform mole) or in sheets (choriocarcinoma).

Clinical Course

Gestational trophoblastic disease has an excellent prognosis.[34, 37] About 4 to 10% of patients with partial moles have persistent disease requiring treatment.[100, 130] In patients with choriocarcinoma, cytotoxic agents are highly effective, even when there are metastases. The most common sites of metastases are the lungs (Fig. 13–38), the liver, the brain and the vagina.[21, 44, 60]

EXTRAUTERINE TUMORS

Metastatic extragenital carcinomas rarely involve the uterine cervix. Only five cervical metastases were iden-

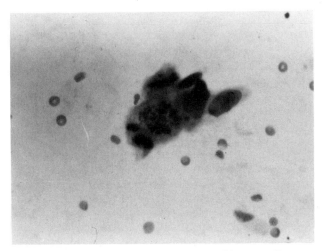

FIGURE 13–38. These malignant trophoblastic cells were found in the bronchial wash of a patient with **metastatic choriocarcinoma** (Papanicolaou stain; ×300).

tified in 149 women with extragenital cancers; most of these were adenocarcinomas.[89] Analyzing the situation from a different perspective, about half of the adenocarcinomas in the uterine cervix involve that organ secondarily.[1] Most common is direct extension by endometrial carcinomas. Less common are metastases from tumors originating in the adjacent organs such as colorectal carcinoma and transitional cell carcinoma. The most common distant tumors are from the ovary, the breast and the stomach.[70, 79, 144]

Metastases to the uterine corpus are also uncommon. Only seven of the 149 extragenital cancers involved the endometrium.[89] Of these, the most common were colorectal, breast and gastric carcinoma.[76, 89]

The tumors metastatic to the vagina were most commonly colorectal carcinomas, followed by breast carcinoma and transitional cell carcinoma. Metastases from breast cancer particularly may occur many years after removal of the primary tumor and a long disease-free interval.[89]

Cytology

Cytologic examination of cervicovaginal smears as a method of identifying metastases may be useful because 6% are asymptomatic, and the abnormal cervicovaginal smear is the first indication of distant disease.[105] Unfortunately, most of the patients are symptomatic with complaints of abnormal bleeding or have evidence of disseminated disease. The proportion of abnormal smears as a result of extrauterine disease is low, 1% of all abnormal smears or one in 10,000 cases.[105]

The tumor cells are most commonly found in the vaginal pool samples. A tumor need not involve the uterus at all; the tumor cells gain passage through the fallopian tubes, thence through the endometrial cavity and endocervical canal into the vaginal pool smear.[125] The number of cells is relatively small and the background is more likely to be clean rather than to contain blood and cellular debris.[70, 105] In those instances in which the surface is ulcerated, necrosis will accompany the tumor cells. This is particularly true for those tumors that invade by direct extension, as from the rectum.

Cytology will reflect the type of adenocarcinoma seen in the primary site. The most common type of malignant cell is that of adenocarcinoma originating from the ovary.[105] Ovarian adenocarcinomas will most likely be of the serous subtype and will be present as papillary clusters displaying marked pleomorphism. Psammoma bodies may accompany the cells, but this is not a common finding. The key to making an accurate assessment is to discern that these cells do not resemble the tumor cells associated with endometrial or endocervical adenocarcinoma. The exception is the unusual papillary serous-type adenocarcinoma of the endometrium. Other types of ovarian carcinoma, endometrioid and clear cell subtypes, resemble their uterine counterparts. In the absence of blood and necrosis, dissemination from the ovary is likely; however, concurrent endometrial cancers are found in

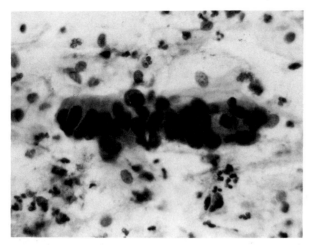

FIGURE 13–39. Metastatic colonic carcinoma forms groups of tall columnar cells with basally placed nuclei (Papanicolaou stain; × 300).

about a third of the women with endometrioid-type ovarian carcinoma.

Adenocarcinoma of colorectal origin is composed of tall columnar cells (Fig. 13–39). The basally placed nuclei are very hyperchromatic, often with coarse chromatin and prominent nucleoli. These cells may be interpreted as those of an endocervical adenocarcinoma. However, the nuclei of the cells from colorectal carcinomas contain much coarser chromatin granules.

The cells of metastatic mammary carcinomas are usually very uniform and may resemble the cells of carcinoma *in situ* (Fig. 13–40). They may be inapparent because their chromatin may be rather hypochromatic and may also resemble histiocytes or even endometrial cells.

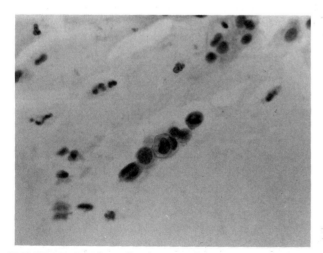

FIGURE 13–40. The cells of **metastatic mammary carcinoma** are arranged in a single file in this field, but they are not always arranged so. This arrangement in cervicovaginal material is more often associated with epidermoid carcinoma *in situ*. The small cluster of cells in the middle of the group identifies these cells as glandular in nature (Papanicolaou stain; × 300).

Gastric adenocarcinomas are characterized by small cells with excentric nuclei and large cytoplasmic mucin vacuoles. There are often few cells in the smear, especially if there is no direct involvement of the uterus. Even in the presence of cervical metastases, only four of six smears contained tumor cells.[70]

It behooves the cytologist to be familiar with the cells of the tumors of the uterus and the vagina so that, when confronted with the unfamiliar, the proposal of an extrauterine cancer can be offered confidently.

References

1. Abell MR, Gosling JRG: Gland cell carcinoma (adenocarcinoma) of the uterine cervix. Am J Obstet Gynecol 83:729–755, 1962.
2. Albores-Saavedra J, Poucell S, Rodriquez-Martinez HA: Primary carcinoid of the uterine cervix. Pathologia 10:185–193, 1972.
3. Albores-Saavedra J, Rodriquez-Martinez HA, Larraza-Hernandez O: Carcinoid tumors of the cervix. Pathol Annu, 14:273–291, 1979.
4. Amendola BE, LaRouere J, Amendola MA, McClatchey KD, Han IH, Morley GW: Adenocarcinoma of the fallopian tube. Surg Gynecol Obstet 157:223–227, 1983.
5. An-Foraker SH, Kawada CY: Cytodiagnosis of endometrial malignant mixed mesodermal tumor. Acta Cytol 29:137–141, 1985.
6. Angeli S, Koelma IA, Fleuren GJ, Van Steenis GJ: Malignant melanoma in the fine needle aspirates and effusions. An immunocytochemical study using monoclonal antibodies. Acta Cytol 32:707–712, 1988.
7. August CZ, Bauer KD, Lurain J, Murad T: Neoplasms of endometrial stroma: Histopathologic and flow cytometric analysis with clinical correlation. Hum Pathol 20:232–237, 1989.
8. Baab GH, McBride CM: Malignant melanoma. The patient with an unknown site of primary origin. Arch Surg 110:896–900, 1975.
9. Banner BF, Myrent KL, Memoli VA, Gould VE: Neuroendocrine carcinoma of the pancreas diagnosed by aspiration cytology. A case report. Acta Cytol 29:442–448, 1985.
10. Barrett RJ III, Davos I, Leuchter RS, Lagasse LD: Neuroendocrine features in poorly differentiated and undifferentiated carcinomas of the cervix. Cancer 60:2325–2330, 1987.
11. Barwick KW, LiVolsi VA: Malignant mixed müllerian tumors of the uterus. A clinicopathologic assessment of 34 cases. Am J Surg Pathol 3:125–135, 1979.
12. Barwick KW, LiVolsi VA: Malignant mixed mesodermal tumors of the ovary. A clinicopathologic assessment of 12 cases. Am J Surg Pathol 4:37–42, 1980.
13. Becker SN, Wong JY: Detection of endometrial stromal sarcoma in cervicovaginal smears. Report of three cases. Acta Cytol 25:272–276, 1980.
14. Benedet JL, White GW, Fairey RN, Boyes DA: Adenocarcinoma of the fallopian tubes. Experience with 41 patients. Obstet Gynecol 50:654–657, 1977.
15. Benson PA: Cytologic diagnosis in primary carcinoma of fallopian tube. Case report and review. Acta Cytol 18:429–434, 1974.
16. Berchuck A, Rubin SC, Hoskins WJ, Saigo PE, Pierce VK, Lewis JL Jr: Treatment of uterine leiomyosarcoma. Obstet Gynecol 71:845–850, 1988.
17. Bokun R, Perkovic M, Bakotin J, Milasinovic D, Mojsovic D: Cytology and histopathology of metastatic melanoma involving a polyp on the uterine cervix. A case report. Acta Cytol 29:612–615, 1985.
17a. Bonetti F, Colombari R, Manfrin E, Zamboni G, Martignoni G, Mombello A, Chilosi M: Breast carcinoma with positive results for melanoma marker (HMB-45). Am J Clin Pathol 92:491–495, 1989.
18. Boutselis JG, Thompson JN: Clinical aspects of primary car-

cinoma of the fallopian tube. Am J Obstet Gynecol 111:98–101, 1971.

19. Brand E, Fu Y, Lagasse L, Berek J: Vulvovaginal melanoma: Report of seven cases and literature review. Gynecol Oncol 33:54–60, 1989.

20. Brewer JI, Guderian AM: Diagnosis of uterine-tube carcinoma by vaginal cytology. Obstet Gynecol 8:664–672, 1956.

21. Brewer JI, Mazur MT: Gestational choriocarcinoma. Its origin in the placenta during seemingly normal pregnancy. Am J Surg Pathol 5:267–277, 1981.

22. Cancer Facts and Figures. New York, American Cancer Society, pp 8–13, 1969.

23. Carr I, Hill AS, Hancock B, Neal FE: Malignant lymphoma of the cervix uteri: Histology and ultrastructure. J Clin Pathol 29:680–686, 1976.

24. Castaldo TW, Ballon SC, Lagasse LD, Petrill ES: Reticuloendothelial neoplasia in the female genital tract. Obstet Gynecol 54:167–170, 1979.

25. Ceelen GH, Sakurai M: Vaginal cytology in leukemia. Acta Cytol 62370–62372, 1962.

26. Chorlton I, Karnei RF, King FM, Norris HJ: Primary malignant reticuloendothelial disease involving the vagina, cervix and corpus uteri. Obstet Gynecol 5:735–748, 1974.

27. Chung AF, Casey MJ, Flanner JT, Woodruff JM, Lewis JL Jr: Malignant melanoma of the vagina—Report of 19 cases. Obstet Gynecol 55:720–727, 1980.

28. Chung AF, Woodruff JM, Lewis JL Jr: Malignant melanoma of the vulva: A report of 44 cases. Obstet Gynecol 45:638–646, 1975.

29. Clement PB: Chondrosarcoma of the uterus: Report of a case and review of the literature. Hum Pathol 9:726–732, 1978.

30. Clement PB, Scully RE: Uterine tumors with mixed epithelial and mesenchymal elements. Semin Diag Pathol 5:199–222, 1988.

31. Cohen BA, Burkman RT, Rosenshein NB, Antienza MF, King TM, Parmley TH: Gestational trophoblastic disease within an elective abortion population. Am J Obstet Gynecol 135:452–454, 1979.

32. Crisp WE, Surwit EA, Grogan TM, Freedman MF: Malignant pelvic lymphoma. Am J Obstet Gynecol 143:69–74, 1982.

33. Crum CP, Rogers BH, Andersen W: Osteosarcoma of the uterus: Case report and review of the literature. Gynecol Oncol 9:256–268, 1980.

34. Czernobilsky B, Barash A, Lancet M: Partial moles: A clinicopathologic study of 25 cases. Obstet Gynecol 59:75–77, 1982.

35. Das Gupta F, D'Urso J: Melanoma of female genitalia. Surg Gynecol Obstet 119:1074–1078, 1964.

36. Daya DA, Scully RE: Sarcoma botryoides of the uterine cervix in young women: A clinicopathologic study of 13 cases. Gynecol Oncol 29:290–304, 1988.

37. Dehner LP: Gestational and nongestational trophoblastic neoplasia. A historic and pathobiologic survey. Am J Surg Pathol 4:43–58, 1980.

38. Denham, JW, Maclennan KA: The management of primary carcinoma of the fallopian tube. Cancer 53:166–172, 1984.

39. Dinh TV, Slavin RE, Bhagavan BS, Hannigan EV, Tiamson EM, Yandell RB: Mixed mesodermal tumors of the ovary: A clinicopathologic study of 14 cases. Obstet Gynecol 72:409–412, 1988.

40. Driscoll SG: Gestational trophoblastic neoplasms: Morphologic considerations. Hum Pathol 8:529–538, 1977.

41. Eddy GL, Copeland LJ, Gershenson DM, Atkinson EN, Wharton JT, Rutledge FN: Fallopian tube carcinoma. Obstet Gynecol 64:546–552, 1984.

42. Ehlen T, Randhawa G, Turko M, Clement PB: Post-hysterectomy carcinoma of the fallopian tube presenting as vaginal adenocarcinoma. A case report. Gynecol Oncol 33:382–385, 1989.

43. Ehrmann RL, Younge PA, Lerch VL: The exfoliative cytology and histogenesis of an early primary malignant melanoma of the vagina. Acta Cytol 6:245–254, 1962.

44. Elston CW: Trophoblastic tumours. The histopathology of trophoblastic tumours. J Clin Pathol 10:111–131, 1976.

45. Fetissof F, Arbeille B, Boivin F, Sam-Giao M, Henrion C,

Lansac J: Endocrine cells in ectocervical epithelium. An immunohistochemical and ultrastructural analysis. Virchows Arch [A] 411:293–298, 1987.

46. Fitzgibbons PL, Chaurushiya PS, Nichols PW, Chandrasoma PT, Martin SE: Primary mucosal malignant melanoma: An immunohistochemical study of 12 cases with comparison to cutaneous and metastatic melanomas. Hum Pathol 20:269–272, 1989.

47. Fox H, Kazzaz B, Langley FA: Argyrophil and argentaffin cells in the female genital tract and in ovarian mucinous cysts. J Pathol Bacteriol 88:479–487, 1964.

48. Freeman C, Berg JW, Cutler SJ: Occurrence and prognosis of extranodal lymphomas. Cancer 29:252–260, 1972.

49. Garcia-Valdecasas R, Rodriguez-Rico L, Linares J, Galera H, Salcattierre V: Malignant melanoma of the vagina. A case diagnosed cytologically. Acta Cytol 18:535–537, 1974.

50. Garret R: Extrauterine tumor cells in vaginal and cervical smears. Obstet Gynecol 14:21–27, 1959.

51. Gersell DJ, Mazoujian G, Mutch DG, Rudloff MA: Small-cell undifferentiated carcinoma of the cervix. A clinicopathologic, ultrastructural, and immunocytochemical study of 25 cases. Am J Surg Pathol 12:684–698, 1988.

52. Geszler G, Szpak CA, Harris RE, Creasman WT, Barter JF, Johnston WW: Prognostic value of peritoneal washings in patients with malignant mixed müllerian tumors of the uterus. Am J Obstet Gynecol 155:83–89, 1986.

53. Habib A, Kaneko M, Cohen C: Carcinoid of the uterine cervix. A case report with light and electron microscopic studies. Cancer 43:535–538, 1979.

54. Hahn GA: Gynecologic consideration in malignant lymphomas. Am J Obstet Gynecol 75:673–683, 1958.

55. Hajdu SI, Hajdu EO: Cytopathology of Sarcomas and Other Nonepithelial Malignant Tumors. Philadelphia, WB Saunders, pp 183–212, 1976.

56. Hajdu SI, Savino A: Cytologic diagnosis of malignant melanoma. Acta Cytol 17:320–327, 1973.

57. Hall-Craggs M, Toker C, Nedwich A: Carcinosarcoma of the uterine cervix: A light and electron microscopic study. Cancer 48:161–169, 1981.

58. Harris NL, Scully RE: Malignant lymphoma and granulocytic sarcoma of the uterus and vagina. A clinicopathologic analysis of 27 cases. Cancer 53:2530–2545, 1984.

59. Harrison CR, Averette HE, Jarrell MA, Penalver MA, Donato D, Sevin B-U: Carcinoma of the fallopian tube: Clinical management. Gynecol Oncol 32:357–359, 1989.

60. Heaton GE, Matthews TH, Christopherson WM: Malignant trophoblastic tumors with massive hemorrhage presenting as liver primary. A report of two cases. Am J Surg Pathol 10:342–347, 1986.

61. Hirai Y, Chen J-T, Hamada T, Fujimoto I, Yamauchi D, Hasumi K, Masubuchi K, Sakamoto A: Clinical and cytologic aspects of primary fallopian tube carcinoma. A report of ten cases. Acta Cytol 31:834–840, 1987.

62. Hirai Y, Kaku S, Teshima H, Shimizu Y, Chen J-T, Hamada T, Fujimoto I, Yamauchi K, Sakamoto A, Hasumi K, Masubuchi K: Clinical study of primary carcinoma of the fallopian tube: Experience with 15 cases. Gynecol Oncol 34:20–26, 1989.

63. Holmquist ND: The exfoliative cytology of mixed mesodermal tumors of the uterus. Acta Cytol 6:373–375, 1962.

64. Holmquist ND, Torres J: Malignant melanoma of the cervix. Report of a case. Acta Cytol 32:252–256, 1988.

65. Hong IS: The exfoliative cytology of endometrial stromal sarcoma in peritoneal fluid. Acta Cytol 25:277–281, 1981.

66. Horan DC, Bonfiglio TA, Patten SF Jr: Fine needle aspiration cytopathology of bronchial carcinoid tumors. An analytical study of the cells. Acta Cytol 26:105–109, 1982.

67. Hsiu J-G, Stawicki ME: The cytologic findings in two cases of stromal sarcoma of the uterus. Acta Cytol 23:487–489, 1979.

68. Hu CY, Taylor ML, Hertig AT: Primary carcinoma of the fallopian tube. Am J Obstet Gynecol 59:58–67, 1950.

69. Kanbour AI, Buchsbaum HJ, Hall A, Kanbour AI: Peritoneal cytology in malignant mixed müllerian tumors of the uterus. Gynecol Oncol 33:91–95, 1989.

70. Kashimura M, Kashimura Y, Matsuyama T, Tsukamoto N,

Sugimori H, Taki I: Adenocarcinoma of the uterine cervix metastatic from primary stomach cancer. Cytologic findings in six cases. Acta Cytol 27:54–58, 1983.

71. Katayama I, Hajian G, Evjy JT: Cytologic diagnosis of reticulum cell sarcoma of the uterine cervix. Acta Cytol 17:498–501, 1973.

72. Kempson RL, Hendrickson MR: Pure mesenchymal neoplasms of the uterine corpus: Selected problems. Semin Diag Pathol 5:172–198, 1988.

73. King A, Seraj IM, Thrasher T, Slater J, Wagner RJ: Fallopian tube carcinoma: A clinicopathological study of 17 cases. Gynecol Oncol 33:351–355, 1989.

74. King ME, Kramer EE: Malignant müllerian mixed tumors of the uterus. A study of 21 cases. Cancer 45:188–190, 1980.

75. Kinoshita M, Asano S, Yamashita M, Matsuda T: Mesodermal mixed tumor primary in the fallopian tube. Gynecol Oncol 32:331–335, 1989.

76. Kumar NB, Hart WR: Metastases to the uterine corpus from extragenital cancer. A clinicopathologic study of 63 cases. Cancer 50:2163–2169, 1982.

77. Kurman RJ, Norris HJ: Malignant germ cell tumors of the ovary. Hum Pathol 7:551–564, 1977.

78. Lathrop JC: Views and reviews: Malignant pelvic lymphomas. Obstet Gynecol 30:137–145, 1967.

79. Lemoine NR, Hall PA: Epithelial tumors metastatic to the uterine cervix. A study of 33 cases and review of the literature. Cancer 57:2002–2005, 1986.

80. Levitan Z, Gordon A, Kaplan A, Kaufman R: Primary malignant melanoma of the vagina: Report of four cases and review of the literature. Gynecol Oncol 33:85–90, 1989.

81. Liu PI, Ishimaru T, McGregor DH, Okada H, Steer A: Autopsy study of granulocytic sarcoma (chloroma) in patients with myelogenous leukemia, Hiroshima-Nagasaki 1949–1969. Cancer 31:948–955, 1973.

82. Lojek MA, Fer MF, Kasselberg AG, Glick AD, Burnett LS, Julian CG, Greco FA, Oldham RK: Cushing's syndrome with small cell carcinoma of the uterine cervix. Am J Med 69:140–144, 1980.

83. Lozowski W, Hajdu SI, Melamed MR: Cytomorphology of carcinoid tumors. Acta Cytol 23:360–365, 1979.

84. Lucia SP, Mills H, Lowenhaupt E, Hunt ML: Visceral involvement in primary neoplastic diseases of the reticulo-endothelial system. Cancer 5:1193–1200, 1952.

85. Manes JL, Taylor HB: Carcinosarcoma and mixed müllerian tumors of the fallopian tube. Report of four cases. Cancer 28:1687–1693, 1976.

86. Massoni EA, Hajdu SI: Cytology of primary and metastatic uterine sarcomas. Acta Cytol 28:93–100, 1984.

87. Matsuyama M, Inoue T, Ariyoshi Y, Doi M, Suchi T, Sato T, Tashito K, Chihara T: Argyrophil cell carcinoma of the uterine cervix with ectopic production of ACTH, beta-MSH, serotonin, histamine and amylase. Cancer 44:1813–1823, 1979.

88. Matsuyama T, Tsukamoto N, Kaku T, Matsukuma K, Hirakawa T: Primary malignant lymphoma of the uterine corpus and cervix. Report of a case with immunocytochemical analysis. Acta Cytol 23:228–232, 1989.

89. Mazur MT, Hsueh S, Gersell DJ: Metastases to the female genital tract. Analysis of 325 cases. Cancer 53:1978–1984, 1984.

90. Mazur MT, Kurman RJ: Gestational trophoblastic disease. *In* Blaustein's Pathology of the Female Genital Tract, 3rd ed. Edited by RJ Kurman. New York, Springer-Verlag, pp 835–875, 1987.

91. McMurray EH, Jacobs AJ, Perez CA, Camel HM, Kao M-S, Galakatos A: Carcinoma of the fallopian tube. Management and sites of failure. Cancer 58:2070–2075, 1986.

92. Melamed M: The cytological presentation of malignant lymphomas and related diseases in effusions. Cancer 16:413–431, 1963.

93. Meredith RF, Eiser DR, Kaka Z, Hodgson SE, Johnston GA Jr, Boutselis JG: An excess of uterine sarcomas after pelvic irradiation. Cancer 58:2003–2007, 1986.

94. Mikhail MS, Runowicz CD, Kadish AS, Romney SI: Colposcopic and cytologic detection of chronic lymphocytic leukemia. Gynecol Oncol 34:106–108, 1989.

95. Miles PA, Herrara GA, Mena H, Trujillo I: Cytologic findings in primary malignant carcinoid tumor of the cervix. Acta Cytol 29:1002–1008, 1985.

96. Mordel N, Mor-Yosef S, Ben-Baruch N, Anteby S: Case report: Malignant melanoma of the uterine cervix: Case report and review of the literature. Gynecol Oncol 32:375–380, 1989.

97. Morimoto N, Ozawa M, Kato Y, Kuramoto H: Diagnostic value of mitotic activity in endometrial stromal sarcoma. Report of two cases. Acta Cytol 26:695–698, 1982.

98. Morrow CP, d'Ablaing G, Brady LW, Blessing JA, Hreshchyshyn MM: A clinical and pathological study of 30 cases of malignant mixed müllerian epithelial and mesenchymal ovarian tumors: A Gynecologic Oncology Group study. Gynecol Oncol 18:278–292, 1984.

99. Morrow C, DiSaia P: Review. Malignant melanoma of the female genitalia: A clinical analysis. Obstet Gynecol Surv 31:233–271, 1976.

100. Mostoufi-Zadeh M, Berkowitz RS, Driscoll SG: Persistence of partial mole. Am J Clin Pathol 87:377–380, 1987.

101. Motoyama T, Watanabe H: Ascitic fluid cytologic features of malignant mixed mesodermal tumor of the ovary. Acta Cytol 31:63–67, 1987.

102. Mukai K, Varela-Duran J, Nochomovitz LE: The rhabdomyoblast in mixed müllerian tumors of the uterus and ovary. Am J Clin Pathol 5:101–104, 1980.

103. Muntz HG, Rutgers JL, Tanaza HM, Fuller AF Jr: Carcinosarcomas and mesodermal mixed tumors of the fallopian tube. Gynecol Oncol 34:109–115, 1989.

104. Nasiell M: Hodgkin's disease limited to the uterine cervix. A case report including cytological findings in the cervical and vaginal smears. Acta Cytol 8:16–18, 1964.

105. Ng ABP, Teeple D, Lindner EA, Reagan JW: The cellular manifestations of extrauterine cancer. Acta Cytol 18:108–117, 1974.

106. Nguyen G-K: Cytopathologic aspects of a metastatic malignant mixed müllerian tumor of the uterus. Report of a case with transabdominal fine needle aspiration biopsy. Acta Cytol 26:521–526, 1982.

107. Ordóñez NG, Sneige N, Hickey RC, Brooks TE: Use of monoclonal antibody HMB-45 in the cytologic diagnosis of melanoma. Acta Cytol 32:684–688, 1988.

108. Patel JK, Kidolkar MS, Picren JW, Moore RH: Metastatic pattern of malignant melanoma. A study of 216 autopsy cases. Am J Surg, 135:807–810, 1978.

109. Peters WA III, Andersen WA, Hopkins MP, Kumar NB, Morley GW: Prognostic features of carcinoma of the fallopian tube. Obstet Gynecol 71:757–762, 1987.

110. Podratz KC, Podczaski ES, Gaffey T, O'Brien PC, Schray MF, Malkasian GD Jr: Primary carcinoma of the fallopian tube. Am J Obstet Gynecol 154:1319–1326, 1986.

111. Raju KS, Wiltshaw E: Primary carcinoma of the fallopian tube. Report of 22 cases. Brit J Obstet Gynaecol 88:1124–1129, 1981.

112. Roberts JA, Lifshitz S: Primary adenocarcinoma of the fallopian tube. Gynecol Oncol 13:301–308, 1982.

113. Rose PG, Piver MS, Tsukada Y, Lau T: Patterns of metastasis in uterine sarcoma. An autopsy study. Cancer 63:935–938, 1989.

114. Rosenberg SA, Diamond HD, Jaslowitz B, Craver LF: Lymphosarcoma: A review of 1269 cases. Medicine 40:31–84, 1961.

115. Sagebiel RW, Gates EZ, Hill LC: Cytologic detection of recurrent vaginal melanoma. Acta Cytol 22:353–357, 1978.

116. Saigo PE, Brigati DJ, Sternberg SS, Rosen PP, Turnbull AD: Primary gastric choriocarcinoma. An immunohistological study. Am J Surg Pathol 5:333–342, 1981.

117. Saigo PE, Cain JM, Kim WS, Gaynor JJ, Johnson K, Lewis JL Jr: Prognostic factors in adenocarcinoma of the uterine cervix. Cancer 57:1584–1593, 1986.

118. Saigo PE, Wolinska WH, Kim WS, Hajdu SI: The role of cytology in the diagnosis and follow-up of patients with cervical adenocarcinoma. Acta Cytol 29:785–794, 1985.

119. Scully RE, Aguirre P, DeLellis RA: Argyrophilia, serotonin and peptide hormones in the female genital tract and its tumors. Review. Int J Gynecol Pathol 3:51–70, 1984.

120. Sedlis A: Primary carcinoma of the fallopian tube. Obstet Gynecol Surv 16:209–226, 1961.

121. Sedlis A: Carcinoma of the fallopian tube. Surg Clin North Am 58:121–129, 1978.

122. Seo IS, Hull MT, Pak HY: Granulocytic sarcoma of the cervix as a primary manifestation. Cancer without overt leukemic features for 26 months. Cancer 40:3030–3037, 1977.

123. Silva EG, Kott MM, Ordóñez NG: Endocrine carcinoma intermediate cell type of the uterine cervix. Cancer 54:1705–1713, 1984.

124. Silverberg SG, Frable WJ: Prolapse of fallopian tube into vaginal vault after hysterectomy. Arch Pathol Lab Med 97:100–103, 1974.

125. Song YS: The significance of positive vaginal smears in extra-uterine carcinomas. Am J Obstet Gynecol 73:341–348, 1957.

126. Spanos WJ Jr, Peters LJ, Oswald MJ: Patterns of recurrence in malignant mixed müllerian tumor of the uterus. Cancer 57:155–159, 1986.

127. Spanos WJ Jr, Wharton JT, Gomez L, Fletcher GH, Oswald MJ: Malignant mixed müllerian tumors of the uterus. Cancer 53:311–316, 1984.

128. Stahl R, Demopoulos RI, Bigelow B: Carcinoid tumor with a squamous cell carcinoma of the cervix. Gynecol Oncol 11:387–392, 1981.

129. Stockdale AD, Leader M, Phillips RH, Henry K: The carcinoid syndrome and multiple hormone secretion associated with a carcinoid tumour of the uterine cervix. Case report. Br J Obstet Gynaecol 93:397–401, 1986.

130. Szulman AE, Philippe E, Boué JG, Boué A: Human triploidy: Association with partial hydatidiform moles and nonmolar conceptuses. Hum Pathol 12:1016–1021, 1981.

131. Szulman AE, Surti U: The syndromes of hydatidiform mole. I. Cytogenetic and morphologic correlations. Am J Obstet Gynecol 131:665–671, 1978.

132. Takeda M, Diamond SM, DeMarco M, Quinn DM: Cytologic diagnosis of malignant melanoma metastatic to the endometrium. Acta Cytol 22:503–506, 1978.

133. Taki I: Cytology of hydatidiform mole, invasive mole, and choriocarcinoma. Compendium of Diagnostic Cytology, 6th ed. Edited by GL Wied, CM Keebler, LG Koss, JW Reagan. Chicago, Tutorials of Cytology, pp 232–235, 1988.

134. Taki I, Aozasa K, Kurokawa K: Malignant lymphoma of the uterine cervix. Cytologic diagnosis of a case with immunocytochemical corroboration. Acta Cytol 29:607–611, 1985.

135. Tamimi HK, Figge, DC: Adenocarcinoma of the uterine tube: Potential for lymph node metastases. Am J Obstet Gynecol 141:132–137, 1981.

136. Tateishi R, Wada A, Hayakawa K, Hongo J, Ishii S, Terakawa N: Argyrophil cell carcinomas (apudomas) of the uterine cervix. Virchows Arch [A] 366:257–274, 1975.

137. Terada KY, Johnson TL, Hopkins M, Roberts JA: Clinicopathologic features of ovarian mixed mesodermal tumors and carcinosarcomas. Gynecol Oncol 32:228–232, 1989.

138. Trillo AA, Accettullo LM, Yeiter TL: Choriocarcinoma of the esophagus: Histologic and cytologic findings. A case report. Acta Cytol 23:69–74, 1979.

139. Tsukamoto N, Hirakawa T, Matsukuma K, Kaku T, Matsuyama T, Kamura T, Saito T: Carcinoma of the uterine cervix with variegated histological patterns and calcitonin production. Gynecol Oncol 33:395–399, 1989.

140. Van Oven MW, Schoots CJF, Oosterhuis JW, Keij JF, Dam-Meiring A, Huisjes HJ: The use of DNA flow cytometry in the diagnosis of triploidy in human abortions. Hum Pathol 20:238–242, 1989.

141. Vance RP, Geisinger KR: Pure nongestational choriocarcinoma of the ovary. Report of a case. Cancer 56:2321–2325, 1985.

142. Varela-Duran J, Nochomovitz LE, Prem KA, Dehner LP: Postirradiation mixed müllerian tumors of the uterus. A comparative clinicopathologic study. Cancer 45:1635–1631, 1980.

143. Walker AN, Mills SE, Taylor PT: Cervical neuroendocrine carcinoma: A clinical and light microscopic study of 14 cases. Int J Gynecol Pathol 7:64–74, 1988.

144. Way S: Carcinoma metastatic in the cervix. Gynecol Oncol 9:298–302, 1980.

145. Whitaker D: The role of cytology in the detection of malignant lymphoma of the uterine cervix. Acta Cytol 20:510–513, 1976.

146. Wilkinson EJ, Friedrich EG Jr: Diseases of the vulva. In Blaustein's Pathology of the Female Genital Tract, 3rd ed. Edited by RJ Kurman. New York, Springer-Verlag, pp 83–84, 1987.

147. Wilson RA: An unusual second primary tumor. Report of a case of atypical carcinoid of the lung. Acta Cytol 22:362–365, 1978.

148. Yoonesi M: Carcinoma of the fallopian tube. Obstet Gynecol Surv 34:257–270, 1979.

149. Yu HC, Ketabchi M: Detection of malignant melanoma of the uterine cervix from Papanicolaou smears. A case report. Acta Cytol 31:73–76, 1987.

150. Zaharopoulos P, Wong JY, Stewart GD: Cytomorphology of the variants of small-cell carcinoma of the lung. Acta Cytol 26:800–808, 1982.

151. Zaloudek C, Norris HJ: Mesenchymal tumors of the uterus. In Blaustein's Pathology of the Female Genital Tract, 3rd ed. Edited by RJ Kurman. New York, Springer-Verlag, pp 2384–2393, 1987.

14

Respiratory Tract

William W. Johnston
Craig E. Elson

In the introduction to his famous 1954 *Atlas of Exfoliative Cytology*, George N. Papanicolaou comments, "During the past decade much progress has been made in the adaptation of the cytologic method to the diagnosis of cancer. This is attested by the expanding use of the method to cover a greater number of organs and by its rapidly increasing utilization in diagnostic laboratories in this country and abroad." Later in his chapter on the respiratory system he notes further, "The use of the cytologic method in the diagnosis of malignant lesions of the respiratory tract has been generally acclaimed as one of its most successful applications. Statistics show that its diagnostic accuracy is higher than that of bronchoscopy. The cytologic method may indeed provide not only an accurate diagnosis of a malignant neoplasm but often a recognition of its type."[402]

These highly prophetic words were reflected in the studies published during the 1950s and 1960s, a remarkably fertile period of development for respiratory cytology. Multiple publications reported new techniques, detection of neoplastic cells, and cytohistologic correlations. The studies of Archer,[9] Wandall,[567] Bamforth,[24-25] Grunze,[196] Russell,[472] Woolner,[588-597] McDonald,[347, 348, 360] Papanicolaou,[402-405, 574] Farber,[130-136] Clerf,[86-88] Herbut,[222-225] Foot,[155, 156] Umiker,[547-553] Richardson,[444, 445] Koss,[288-293] and Spjut[509] were significant contributions among these early investigations.

During the same period of time, significant developments were also occurring in transthoracic needle biopsy studies, although studies were not quite as profuse as those involving sputum and bronchial material. The Dahlgren and Nordenstrom[102] monograph on transthoracic needle biopsy published in 1966 stimulated widespread interest. They concluded that their 87% rate of diagnostic accuracy was due to improve-

ments in fluoroscopic monitoring, newly developed thin-walled needles and refinements in cytologic methods of diagnosis.

Now, more than 3 decades after the publication of the Papanicolaou atlas, the study of cellular specimens from the respiratory tract is established in major hospitals and clinics throughout the world as a vital diagnostic procedure in the evaluation of any patient with suspected primary or secondary lung cancer, a prior established history of lung cancer or any suspected lung lesion in which morphologic confirmation is indicated. The emergence of fine needle aspiration (FNA) has enhanced further the diagnostic usefulness of clinical cytology in lung cancer diagnosis. The numerous and excellent reviews, atlases and monographs embracing all aspects of respiratory cytology are an eloquent testimony to this prominence.[138, 160, 161, 168, 220, 247, 251, 253, 254, 260, 261, 266, 289, 290, 293, 316, 469, 473, 528, 605] This chapter explores the contributions made to pulmonary pathology by morphologic study of sputum, bronchial washings, bronchial aspirates, bronchial brushings, bronchoalveolar lavage specimens (BAL) and transthoracic FNA from the lung.

SAMPLING AND CYTOPREPARATORY TECHNIQUES

The purpose of this section is to review the major types of cytologic preparations that are now used in most laboratories. The specimens discussed here include sputum, bronchial washings, bronchial brushings, BALs and FNAs.

The diagnostic accuracy of cytology begins with a foundation of excellence in cytopreparation of these specimens. A specimen from the respiratory tract that has been prepared for cytologic examination should exhibit an abundance of well-preserved and stained diagnostic cellular material, should have been prepared rapidly and with relative ease and should survive permanent slide storage. Many laboratories have studied techniques for the best realization of these objectives. Paraffin embedding and section of sputum[1, 332, 579] is not a productive technical approach to respiratory cytology, but it is of use in FNA as well as any other specimen in which visible chunks of tissue are removed along with cells. Various techniques for freeing tumor cells from mucus by lysis were interesting in theory but were frequently too laborious and time consuming to be practical.[52, 124, 219, 284, 318, 346, 413, 529, 530] Several major techniques have stood the test of time and are the most widely utilized today. They are the wet-film preparation[116] and fixation from fresh or prefixed respiratory material,[589] the Saccomanno blender technique,[203, 476] as modified from the carbowax method of Sims, membrane filtration,[76, 147, 207, 519] cytocentrifugation,[153] and Wright-stained, air-dried smears. These methods are used for spontaneously produced sputum, induced sputum, bronchial washings and brushings, BALs and FNAs. The Papanicolaou method of staining is the most generally accepted one and, in the United States in particular, it has gained widespread popularity. In many European laboratories, air-dried smears stained by a Romanowsky stain are preferred; however, this technique for FNAs is gaining acceptance in laboratories in the United States.

The following types of cellular specimens and techniques for cellular preparation are those currently most commonly utilized in the contemporary clinical cytology laboratory. The cytologic pattern may vary depending upon the type of preparation and knowledge of these variations is essential for accurate cytologic diagnosis.

Sputum

Sputum, a highly specialized product of the respiratory tract, is the result of the interaction between the mucociliary apparatus and immune system of the host and between the animate and inanimate invaders from the environment. Composed predominantly of mucus, it also contains a large variety of cellular and noncellular materials produced by the host and substances that have been inhaled. It is the most frequently examined specimen obtained from the respiratory tract. A number of cytopreparatory techniques are utilized in preparing it for examination.

Fresh and Unfixed Sputum

The simplest sputum specimen is one in which a fresh, early morning specimen, produced by a deep cough, is collected and brought immediately to the laboratory without any fixation. It is examined grossly for tissue fragments and blood-tinged areas. Smears from these areas and other randomly sampled areas are prepared and fixed immediately in 95% ethyl alcohol. Staining of these smears is by the traditional Papanicolaou method. Sputum prepared in this manner has the advantage of displaying cells and other components that exhibit excellent preservation and staining. It is the method preferred by us and has been in use in our laboratory for nearly 30 years. Risse and associates[446, 447] in a 1987 study emphasized the importance of blood in sputum. They found that in patients with primary lung cancer, the presence of blood in the sputum was highly significant from the point of view of its association with a correct positive cytologic diagnosis in sputum.

Prefixed Sputum

If it is not possible to transmit unfixed material to the laboratory, prefixed sputum may be obtained by instructing the patient to expectorate into a wide-mouthed small jar, half filled with 70% ethyl alcohol. Preservation of cells trapped in mucus may be only fair because of failure of the alcohol to penetrate into the cell. The mucus may also become rubbery producing greater difficulties in getting a good smear.

Sputum Prefixed With Alcohol and Carbowax (Saccomanno)

Saccomanno has described a method of cytopreparation of sputum that has gained wide popularity. It involves the collection of sputum in a mixture of 50% ethyl alcohol and 2% polyethylene glycol (Carbowax). In the laboratory, the specimen is broken up in a Waring-type blender, and smears are prepared from the centrifuged cell button. This technique has several major advantages, including concentration of cells and the possibility of preparing teaching slides from interesting cases.[476] It is used in our institution for the collection of sputum from outpatients. This method produces a number of artifacts in tumor cells, which are different from those found in smears prepared from fresh sputum. For example, tissue fragments and fungal fragments may be disrupted. Secretory vacuoles in tumor cells may be exploded, and cells from small-cell undifferentiated carcinoma may be dispersed.

In a reported study, Perlman and associates[410] reviewed 204 sputum samples that had been made using both slide preparations directly from fresh, unfixed sputum and the Saccomanno technique. The diagnostic accuracy for 55 squamous carcinomas was similar (fresh 95%, Saccomanno 86%) but significantly less in the Saccomanno preparations of 22 small-cell carcinomas (fresh 100%, Saccomanno 24%) and 26 adenocarcinomas (fresh 96%, Saccomanno 52%). Four cases negative on fresh smears were suspicious or diagnostic of cancer on the Saccomanno slides. No cases of small-cell undifferentiated carcinoma were observed in which the Saccomanno preparation added information not available on the fresh smears.

Induced Sputum

In those patients who cannot produce sputum spontaneously by deep coughing, a specimen of sputum may be induced.[26, 41, 47, 55, 173, 394, 408, 450, 458–461, 510, 541] The basic principle involves the inhalation of some appropriate solution that has been aerosolized. The inspired vapor stimulates mucus production. One popular method employs a heated (37°C) solution of 15% sodium chloride and 20% propylene glycol. After inhaling these vapors for approximately 20 minutes, the patient will usually produce copious satisfactory sputum.[127]

Bronchoscopy

The development of the rigid bronchoscope in the late 19th century by Gustav Killian formed the foundation of a technology by which the mucosal surfaces of the bronchi could be directly visualized and sampled for both tissue and cellular evaluation. In later years this technology has been furthered by the introduction of flexible catheters advanced into the bronchi under fluoroscopic control and perhaps even more importantly by the development of the flexible fiberoptic bronchoscope. These developments have been summarized by Walloch.[566]

Bronchial Aspirates and Washings

Introduction of the bronchoscope into the lower respiratory tract enables the examiner to obtain specimens by means of a suction apparatus that aspirates secretion. Washings from the visualized areas may also be collected by the instilling of 3 to 5 ml of a balanced salt solution through the bronchoscope and reaspiration of the resulting material. Once the bronchoscope is removed, direct smears may be made with immediate fixation in 95% ethyl alcohol. The aspirates and washings may be treated in several different ways. They may be centrifuged and smears prepared from the cell buttons, they may be subjected to membrane filter preparation or they may be centrifuged and the resulting buttons embedded in paraffin for histologic sectioning. In our experience, a judicious combination of direct smears and membrane filter preparations of the aspirates and washings yields the best diagnostic results.

Bronchial Brushings

The development of the flexible fiberoptic bronchoscope has made it possible for the operator to view much smaller bronchi of the lung than was formerly possible with the rigid tube bronchoscope alone.[123–126] With this apparatus the examiner may both visualize and brush a suspected lesion and submit the resulting cytologic material for laboratory examination. The techniques for preparation of cellular specimens from the bronchial brush are similar to those utilized for bronchial aspirates and washings.

Bronchoalveolar Lavage

Bronchoalveolar lavage (BAL) involves the infusion and reaspiration of a sterile saline solution in distal segments of the lung via a fiberoptic bronchoscope.[72, 315, 316, 513, 514] This technique has been utilized in the therapy of such diseases as pulmonary alveolar proteinosis, cystic fibrosis, pulmonary alveolar microlithiasis and asthma but has proved later to be of value in the diagnosis of pulmonary disease.[105, 316] Although it has been employed in the detection of lung cancer[315] and the evaluation of interstitial lung disease,[105] perhaps the most important diagnostic application of BAL is the detection of opportunistic infections in immunocompromised hosts.[108, 392, 513, 514] The use of this technique is discussed in detail by Linder and coworkers[315] and Linder and Renard.[316]

Fine Needle Aspiration

The cytology of the respiratory tract has been revolutionized by a combination of two factors: evolution of highly sophisticated radiologic imaging techniques, making possible the precise visualization and localization of masses in the lungs, and the reintroduction of a technique of sampling of such visualized lesions by the insertion into them of a fine bore needle.[250, 331, 358, 389, 417, 418, 438, 488, 517] In this procedure a fine needle attached to a syringe is passed through the chest wall or bronchial wall into the pulmonary mass visualized by fluoroscopy, computed tomography or bronchoscopy. The aspirated cellular specimen is examined by conventional cellular techniques. The importance and usefulness of the techniques are rapidly gaining wide recognition throughout the world, and they have the potential of becoming the premiere tools for the evaluation of pulmonary lesions.

Indications and Contraindications

Although some variation occurs among institutions in their policies on indications for the performance of FNA, the following ones are those most generally used and have been summarized by Stitik[512] and by Heaston and associates:[220] (1) suspected lung cancer that is inoperable; (2) a solitary pulmonary mass suspected of being the source of probable metastatic disease; (3) a solitary pulmonary nodule and known primary malignancy outside the lung; (4) a patient who refuses exploratory thoracotomy for suspected lung cancer; (5) multiple pulmonary masses; (6) an undiagnosed pulmonary mass; (7) a suspected superior sulcus tumor; (8) a patient who fails to respond to appropriate antituberculosis therapy; (9) a suspected infectious process particularly in the immunocompromised patient and (10) a patient with suspected lung cancer on whom five consecutive early morning deep-cough specimens of sputum and one bronchial brushing or washing have been negative for malignant tumor cells. The last indication should be one on which all of the others are dependent.

The contraindications for FNA include (1) patients who are debilitated or uncooperative or who have an uncontrollable cough; (2) patients who have hemorrhagic diathesis, who are undergoing anticoagulation therapy or who have suspected vascular lesion or pulmonary hypertension and (3) patients who have echinococcus cyst. Complications have included pneumothorax, hemoptysis and hemothorax.

The general technique of FNA came into use at our institution in the early 1970s. Among the total number of aspirates examined from all body sites, 30% have been from the lung. In the medical center's most current procedure, any patient found to have a demonstrable radiographic abnormality in the lung fields is a potential candidate for FNA. The decision on whether or not to proceed with the aspiration is based upon the level of suspicion that the visualized nodule or density represents a cancer or an infectious process and on the morphologic evidence provided by prior cytologic and histologic specimens obtained from the respiratory tract. All aspirations are performed by a radiologist using fluoroscopy or computed tomography.

Transbronchial Fine Needle Aspiration

Transbronchial FNA as described by Tsuboi and associates,[545] Hayata,[217] Rosenthal and Wallace,[470] and Horsley and associates[231] is a special modification of needle aspiration for those cases in which the lung neoplasm has not invaded through the mucosa into the bronchial lumen and thus is not accessible through sputum or bronchial brushing. This procedure involves the insertion of a flexible needle through the fiberoptic bronchoscope, penetration of the bronchial wall and aspiration of cytologic material lying beyond.

In a reported study, Wagner and associates[563] found an accuracy rate of 56% for transbronchial aspiration as compared with 48% for wash, 56% for brush, 35% for sputum and 71% for forceps biopsy all in the same patients.

Preparation

In the preparation of the cellular specimen from a fine needle aspirate, the most important principle is that the diagnostic cellular material should be within the barrel of the needle and not within the barrel of the syringe. To ensure that this relationship remains undisturbed, the needle should be disconnected from the syringe, the syringe refilled with air and the syringe and needle reconnected. One now is in a position to expel the contents of the needle onto a slide or into a small amount of any solution desired. Excellent smears are simply prepared by gently laying one slide over the slide holding the drops of expelled material, permitting the weight of the upper slide to spread the material, pulling the slides apart horizontally and quickly dropping them into 95% ethyl alcohol.

At our institution, the following procedure is followed. A 22-gauge Chiba needle with a 20-ml syringe is inserted percutaneously into the lung mass. From the aspirate two direct smears are prepared for immediate wet fixation in 95% ethyl alcohol and staining with the Papanicolaou method. The remaining aspirate is then mixed with 10 ml of a balanced salt solution and brought to the laboratory for further procedures. The cellular suspension is centrifuged, and aliquots are processed for membrane filters, direct smears, cytocentrifuge specimens and cell blocks. For immediate consultation, a drop of concentrated suspension is mixed on a glass slide with a 0.4% aqueous solution of toluidine blue and a cover slip is placed.

This simple preparation provides excellent nuclear detail, but like other aqueous stains, it does not lend itself to permanent storage. By this procedure the radiologist can be given an immediate assessment of the cellular content of the aspirate and therefore an implied assessment of whether or not it is satisfactory for diagnosis.[401] If it is determined to be hypocellular, the aspiration can be repeated immediately. When extensive necrosis is observed, the radiologist is advised to obtain additional material from the periphery of the nodule, where well-preserved tumor cells are more likely to be found. The presence of bacteria, fungi or inflammation are reported immediately to the radiologist so that appropriate cultures may be obtained. Based upon the findings in the wet preparation the specimen can be evaluated for additional cytochemical or immunocytochemical stains or for electron microscopic evaluation.

ANATOMY AND HISTOLOGY

The respiratory system has a number of known functions that include cleansing and warming of inspired air, gaseous exchange between the alveoli and capillaries, immunologic and cellular host protection mechanisms, voice production and olfaction. As with other organ systems, it probably has a number of additional important functions yet to be discovered. The gross and microscopic anatomy of the respiratory system is a remarkable example of a structure designed for maximum efficiency in carrying out a series of complex functions. The anatomy relevant to clinical cytology is discussed here. This has been well reviewed by Murray[363] and Wang.[568]

A pair of lungs composed of many microscopic air sacs, the alveoli, promotes the exchange of oxygen and carbon dioxide with the capillary blood. A series of tubes, first bronchioles and then bronchi, converging to form the trachea, connect the alveoli to the upper respiratory tract and, ultimately, through the nose and oral cavity to the external environment. Each lung is enclosed in a sealed expansile cavity surrounded by bone and muscle. Through the action of these diaphragmatic and intercostal muscles, those cavities or cages expand and contract so as to suck air into the alveolar spaces and to expel its altered contents back out to the exterior of the body.

The oral cavity and portions of the pharynx and nose are lined by a nonkeratinizing stratified squamous epithelium. A less thick squamous epithelium covers the vocal cords. Although the morphologic examination of specimens from these areas does not constitute a component of the discipline of respiratory cytology, superficial and intermediate squamous cells are constantly exfoliating and consequently are commonly present in sputum and bronchial specimens.

The major portions of the upper and lower respiratory tracts are lined by a pseudostratified and ciliated columnar epithelium (Figs. 14–1 and 14–2). This mucosa covers the surfaces of portions of the nasal cavities, the sinuses and portions of the larynx and the tracheobronchial tree. In histologic sections, this epithelium may show two or three layers of nuclei, but each cell is anchored into the basement membrane. Nestled between these cells and adjacent to the basement membrane are small round-to-polygonal cells believed to represent basal or reserve cells. Mucus-producing goblet cells may be seen between the ciliated cells (Figs. 14–3 and 14–4). Their number is variable and dependent on absence or presence of environmental irritants and certain diseases. Two rare cell types include brush cells of unknown function and argyrophil or Kulchitsky-like cells.

As the terminal bronchioles are approached, the lining epithelial cells begin to change. Ciliated cells,

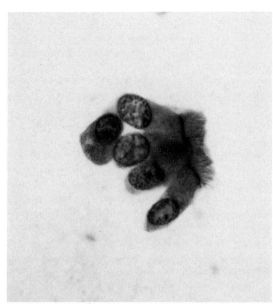

FIGURE 14–2. Ciliated bronchial epithelium. Bronchial brushing (Papanicolaou stain; ×1000).

although still present, are less numerous (Figs. 14–5 and 14–6). Nonciliated Clara cells become numerous with some projecting plump protoplasmic protrusions into the lumen. These cells are believed to have a number of important functions, including the secretion of the hypophase material of surfactant, detoxification of inhaled toxic substances and cellular reparative functions. Goblet cells, normally not present, may be found in the bronchiolar epithelium of smokers.

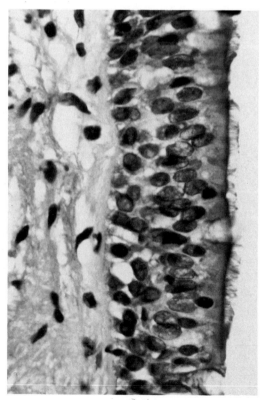

FIGURE 14–1. Normal bronchial mucosa. Note cilia, terminal bars, several rows of nuclei and scattered goblet cells. Bronchial biopsy (hematoxylin and eosin; ×680).

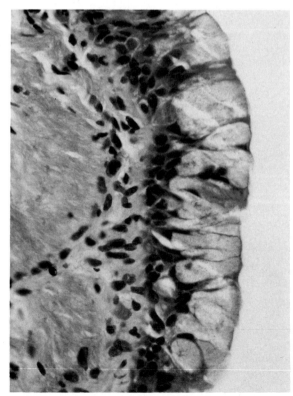

FIGURE 14–3. Goblet cell hyperplasia in bronchial epithelium. Bronchial biopsy (hematoxylin and eosin; ×400).

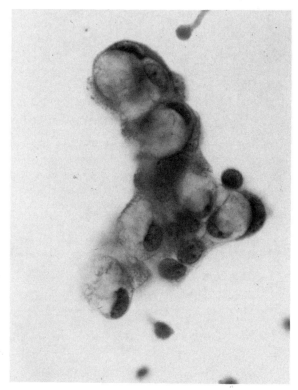

FIGURE 14–4. Goblet cell hyperplasia. Nuclei of the goblet cells are flattened and displaced to the periphery of the cells. Cilia can be observed at the edge of this cell cluster. Bronchial washing (Papanicolaou stain; ×1000).

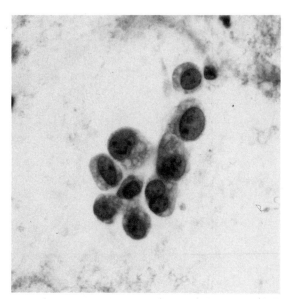

FIGURE 14–6. Reactive bronchiolar and alveolar epithelium. Sputum (Papanicolaou stain; ×680).

The alveoli are lined by an epithelium composed of two cell types (Fig. 14–7). The type I cells or pneumocytes are long and flattened and line more than 90% of the alveolar surface. The type II cells or pneumocytes are cuboidal with prominent nucleoli. They are characterized ultrastructurally by prominent microvilli and osmophilic lamellated inclusion bodies. These cells are the source of surfactant, the chemical

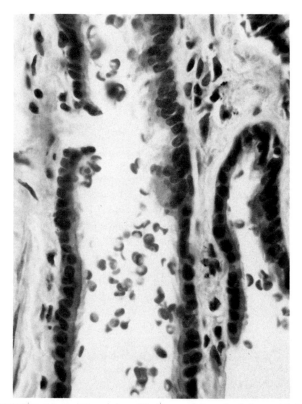

FIGURE 14–5. Normal epithelium of terminal bronchiole. Pulmonary resection (hematoxylin and eosin; ×520).

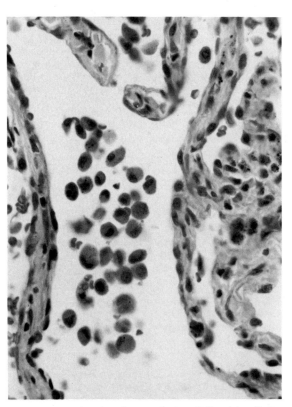

FIGURE 14–7. Alveolar duct and alveoli lined by flattened pneumocytes. Carbon-laden macrophages are also present. Pulmonary resection (hematoxylin and eosin; ×400).

substance that coats the lining of the alveoli and prevents their collapse on expiration. They also have been shown to be the chief cell types involved in repair of the alveolar epithelium. Also of significance in cytologic evaluations are the alveolar macrophages found both within the alveolar air spaces and within the extracellular lining of the alveolar surface. These macrophages are discussed in more detail in a further section of this chapter.

CYTOLOGY OF NORMAL AND BENIGN COMPONENTS

The morphology of benign cellular components of respiratory cellular material has been well-described in the literature by Farber and associates,[136] Woolner and McDonald,[597] Koss,[288, 290, 292] and Frost and associates.[168, 169] Electron microscopy of sputum has been studied by Kory.[287]

The components of respiratory specimens (sputum, bronchial aspirates or brushings, BALs and FNAs), in the absence of neoplasm, may be divided into epithelial cells, macrophages, leukocytes, intrinsic noncellular inanimate components, extrinsic noncellular inanimate components and living organisms.

Cytology of Normal Epithelial Cells

The normal epithelial components of sputum consist of squamous epithelial cells exfoliating from the oral cavity and pharynx, columnar cells exfoliating most frequently from the tracheobronchial tree and occasionally from the upper respiratory tract, bronchiolar cells, and alveolar pneumocytes. Squamous cells are present most commonly in sputum. Ciliated columnar cells and goblet cells are most common in bronchial specimens and BALs. Lesser numbers may be seen in FNAs. Bronchiolar cells and alveolar pneumocytes probably will not be recognized, unless they are hyperplastic or atypical.

Squamous Cells

Squamous cells, usually of oral origin, are commonly seen in specimens of sputum and bronchial material. A mixture of intermediate and superficial squamous cells is most frequent. The intermediate cells are characterized by a round-to-oval vesicular nucleus embedded in a uniformly thin, cyanophilic cytoplasm. The superficial cells have pyknotic nuclei and orangeophilic cytoplasm. Occasionally, anucleate squames and parabasal cells may also be present.

Ciliated Bronchial Columnar Cells

The individual bronchial cell is characterized in profile by a columnar or prismatic shape ending in a tail. The nucleus is oriented towards this tail and shows a finely granular chromatin pattern with one or more small nucleoli (Fig. 14–2). In longitudinal profile the nucleus may appear to be wider in diameter than the cell itself, but more careful examination will reveal a thin margin of cytoplasm between nuclear membrane and cytoplasmic membrane. Cilia with a terminal plate are present. Ciliated columnar cells are characteristically seen in bronchial washings, aspirates or brushings, in BALs and FNAs. They should not be present in large number in sputum, except in postbronchoscopy specimens, or in cases in which extensive damage to the respiratory epithelium has occurred. Scattered single cells and small cell clusters of bronchial epithelium are commonly found in BALs and in FNAs.

Goblet Cells

A less commonly encountered epithelial cell present in the bronchial epithelium lining is the mucus-producing bronchial cell, or goblet cell. Such cells are readily recognized by the presence of either single or multiple vacuoles filled with mucus. These goblet cells are more common in patients with chronic tracheobronchial disease, such as asthmatic bronchitis, chronic bronchitis and bronchiectasis. Occasionally, they are present in bronchial brushings and FNAs in such great numbers that a mucus-producing adenocarcinoma may be suggested. Examples of goblet cells are shown in Figure 14–4.

Epithelial Cells from Bronchioles and Alveoli

Although the utilization of a number of modern laboratory techniques has enabled one to differentiate a variety of subtypes of terminal bronchiolar and alveolar cells, conventional light microscopic examination of cytologic specimens in the absence of disease does not permit the observer to appreciate these various cell types. Indeed, the terminal bronchiolar and alveolar cells in their normal forms are probably not present in cytologic material very often. These cells are relatively small, and when present in cytologic material appear as rounded single cells with finely vacuolated cytoplasm and centrally placed nuclei with one to two small nucleoli (see Fig. 14–6). Some may bear cilia. With such morphology they are usually interpreted as alveolar macrophages. Among various specimen types, these cells are likely to be most commonly encountered in BALs and FNAs, and if they are reactive, they may be a diagnostic pitfall in such specimens.

Cytology of Abnormal Epithelial Cells

Squamous Cells

Abnormal but benign squamous cells may be exfoliated in the presence of a number of diseases of the mouth. Infection, inflammation and ulceration may release parabasal cells. These may be confused with metaplasia. Chronic mucosal irritation with leukoplakia may produce masses of anucleate squames. The rare disease pemphigus may result in the exfoliation of extremely abnormal-appearing immature squamous cells with enlarged nuclei and centrally placed macronucleoli. These cells are easily mistaken for cancer cells.

Bronchial Cells

So-called irritation forms of bronchial epithelium may occur in response to a wide variety of insults varying from microorganisms to environmental toxins. These altered cells are characterized by marked nuclear enlargement, coarsening of the chromatin pattern and one or more enlarged nucleoli.[423–428, 477] Nuclear enlargement may be at a magnitude of 10 to 20 times the diameter of a normal bronchial cell nucleus (Figs. 14–8 to 14–11). Saito and associates[479] have described in some detail the atypical reparative changes in bronchial cells following brushing.

Another extremely common response to irritation is the presence of multinucleation; however, the nuclei are small and mirror images of one of another (Fig. 14–12).[70–71, 229] These cells have been studied extensively by Chalon and associates.[70–71] Although such cells may be seen after a wide variety of insults, they are most commonly seen following instrumentation.

Hyperplasia of Bronchial Epithelium. Koss[288] and Koss and Richardson[292] were among the first investigators to note the diagnostic pitfall posed by hyperplasia of bronchial epithelial cells. These changes may occur in association with a number of chronic diseases of the lung, including tuberculosis,[180, 334, 399] bronchiectasis,[272] chronic bronchitis and asthma.[373, 378, 477, 480] Nay-

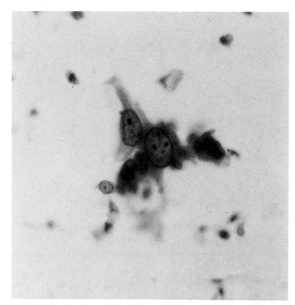

FIGURE 14–9. Reactive bronchial epithelium. Bronchial brushing (Papanicolaou stain; × 400).

lor and Railey[378] described a patient with chronic asthmatic bronchitis in whom papillary tissue fragments exfoliating from hyperplastic bronchial epithelium were noted and incorrectly diagnosed as adenocarcinoma. These tissue fragments have come to bear the name "Creola bodies" after the patient in whom they were

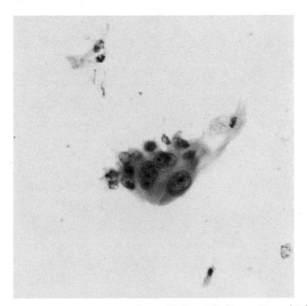

FIGURE 14–8. Reactive bronchial epithelium. Bronchial brushing (Papanicolaou stain; × 400).

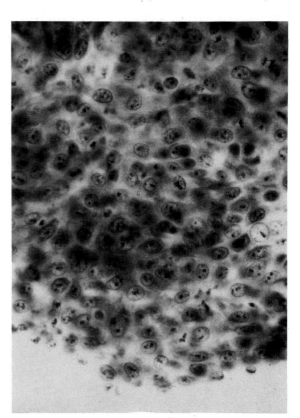

FIGURE 14–10. Reparative epithelium from a patient exposed to malathion. These cells form a cohesive sheet and exhibit abundant cytoplasm, prominent nucleoli and nuclear enlargement. Bronchial brushing (Papanicolaou stain; × 400).

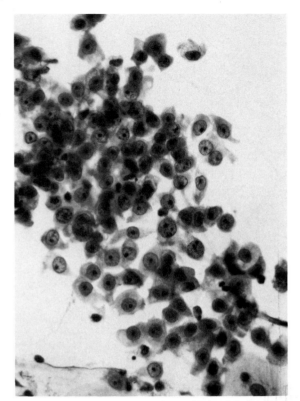

FIGURE 14–11. Highly reactive bronchial epithelium from a patient with adult respiratory distress syndrome. Although the cells show some variation in nuclear size and prominent nucleoli, the cytoplasm maintains a distinct cuboidal to columnar shape. An extensive search revealed a few ciliated cells with identical nuclear features. Sputum (Papanicolaou stain; ×400).

seen. The fragments may be seen in the sputum and bronchial brushings from 42% of cases of asthmatic bronchitis. The cytologic presentation is that of papillary clusters of cells partially covered on the surface by well-differentiated, ciliated respiratory epithelium. Some nuclear molding is seen between individual cells, although chromatin and nucleolar structures remain relatively unremarkable. At times nuclear detail may be obscured because of the thickness of the tissue fragment. A varying number of vacuolated mucus cells may also be present in these fragments. The key to their benignity is to be found in the finely granular chromatin pattern, regular uniform nucleoli and the presence of cilia (Fig. 14–13).

Hyperplasia of Type II Pneumocytes. In the presence of insult, type II pneumocytes may enlarge, proliferate and produce differential diagnostic problems. In such circumstances they may be present either as single cells or as small papillary tissue fragments composed of enlarged cells with prominent nucleoli. Hyperdistended vacuoles may be present in the cytoplasm. Differential diagnosis of such cells becomes a rather formidable problem of determining whether these cells are coming from one of the benign disease processes, such as tuberculosis, pulmonary fibrosis, thermal injury, thromboembolism with or without pulmonary infarction, anthracosis, interstitial pneumonia, systemic lupus erythematosus, acute toxic alveolar damage, oxygen toxicity and organizing pneumonia, or whether they are actually derived from bronchioloalveolar carcinoma.[39, 40, 80, 93, 272, 273, 340, 354, 555, 556, 582]

Pulmonary infarcts are cited in the literature as being particularly prone to give rise to such cells in sputum[42]; however, in my experience, they are most frequently encountered in association with pneumonias of various

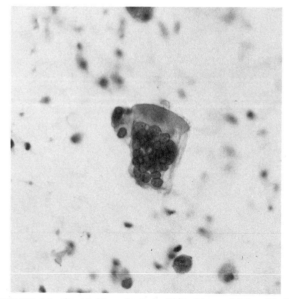

FIGURE 14–12. Multinucleated ciliated bronchial epithelial cell. Bronchial brushing (Papanicolaou stain; ×400).

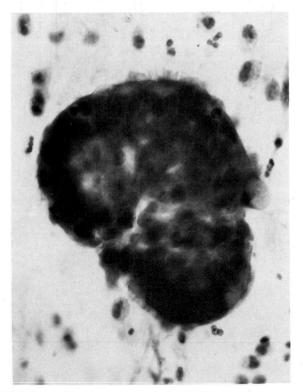

FIGURE 14–13. Hyperplastic bronchial epithelium from a patient with asthma. Note uniformity of nuclei, cilia and terminal bars. Sputum (Papanicolaou stain; ×520).

TABLE 14–1. A Profile of Signs and Diseases in 43 Patients Without Cancer But With Cytologic Diagnoses Suspicious For Malignancy

Disease Category	Number Patients	Percent Patients
Pneumonia	17	39.5
Smoking history	9	20.9
Hemoptysis	7	16.3
Chronic obstructive pulmonary disease	7	16.3
Granulomatous disease	7	16.3
Chronic bronchitis	6	14.0
Abscess	4	9.3
Mass	4	9.3
Infarct	2	4.6
Other	8	18.6

Reproduced with permission from Johnston, WW: Cytologic correlations. *In* Pulmonary Pathology. Edited by DH Dail, SP Hammar. New York, Springer-Verlag, 1987.

forms and etiologies (see Table 14–1). Frable and associates,[161] and Johnston and Frable[260, 261] have stressed a diagnostic distinction between the poorly preserved cell clusters associated with infarcts and the well-preserved cells forming ball-like clusters without molding but with deep depth of focus, which are originating in bronchioloalveolar carcinoma.[161, 260, 261] Silverman and associates[500] have reported one case in which a pulmonary infarct was diagnosed by FNA. Hyperplastic type II pneumocytes in FNAs can constitute one of the most dangerous of diagnostic pitfalls. Insistence upon a specimen of high cellularity for positive cancer diagnosis will be a major factor in avoiding such an error. Figures 14–14 and 14–15 illustrate the atypical cell clusters from two separate pa-

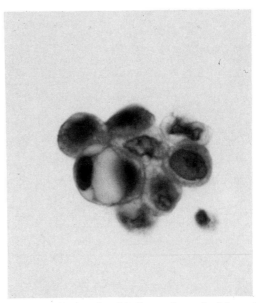

FIGURE 14–15. Normal epithelium of terminal bronchiole. Pulmonary resection (hematoxylin and eosin; ×520).

tients who were suspected, from cytology, of having bronchioloalveolar carcinoma. Findings, at autopsy, in the second case revealed chronic organizing pneumonia with hyperplasia of type II pneumocytes (Fig. 14–16). Other examples of hyperplasia of type II pneumocytes are depicted in Figures 14–17 through 14–20. A special

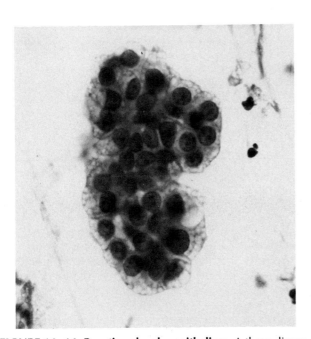

FIGURE 14–14. Reactive alveolar epithelium. A three-dimensional papillary fragment of type II pneumocytes from a patient with organizing pneumonia. Such fragments may be virtually indistinguishable from those exfoliated from bronchioloalveolar carcinoma. Sputum (Papanicolaou stain; ×680).

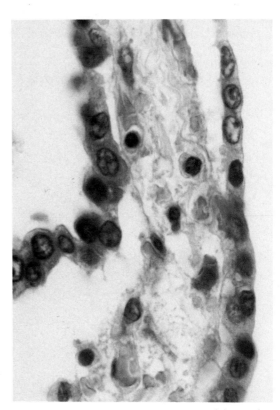

FIGURE 14–16. Organizing pneumonia and hyperplasia of **type II alveolar pneumocytes.** The cells depicted in Figure 14–15 are from the same case. Section of lung at autopsy (hematoxylin and eosin; ×400).

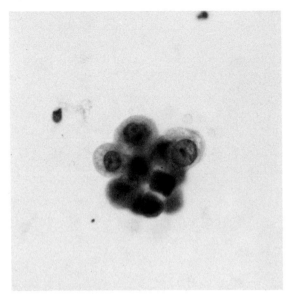

FIGURE 14–17. Reactive alveolar epithelium. A three-dimensional radiating "flower petal" group of type II pneumocytes from a patient with organizing pneumonia. Similar groups may be observed in bronchioloalveolar carcinomas. Bronchial washing (Papanicolaou stain; ×680).

situation of hyperplasia of type II pneumocytes in response to chemotherapy is discussed in the section under that title.

Squamous Metaplasia and Reserve Cell Hyperplasia

The term metaplasia is used to define a morphologic entity in which one differentiated cell type ordinarily

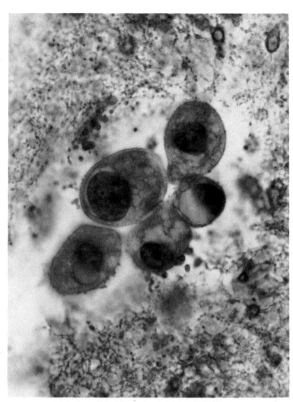

FIGURE 14–19. Hyperplastic type II pneumocytes. Sputum (Papanicolaou stain; ×1000).

composing a part, covering or lining of a tissue is replaced by a differentiated cell of another type.[312, 329] Squamous metaplasia, when employed in reference to the lung, describes the replacement of the ciliated pseudostratified bronchial epithelium normally lining the trachea and bronchi by a truly stratified and flattened epithelium that resembles squamous epithelium.

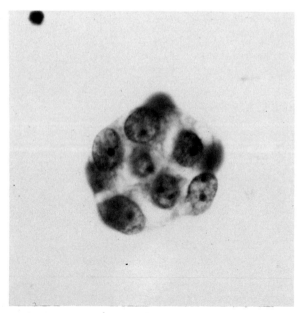

FIGURE 14–18. Reactive alveolar epithelium. A three-dimensional ball-like cluster of type II pneumocytes mimicking the configuration that may be seen in bronchioloalveolar carcinoma. Sputum (Papanicolaou stain; ×400).

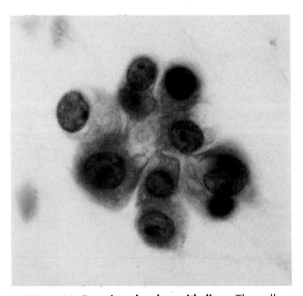

FIGURE 14–20. Reactive alveolar epithelium. The cells possess moderate to abundant vacuolated cytoplasm and are arranged in a radiating "flower petal" pattern. Sputum (Papanicolaou stain; ×1000).

Although squamous metaplasia probably represents an attempt of the host to repair an epithelial surface that has been damaged by varying environmental living and nonliving toxic agents,[474, 475, 477, 478, 485, 555] the attempted repair in itself inflicts additional damage to the lung, replacing the highly functional and protective ciliated bronchial epithelium with a nonfunctional and nonprotective squamous-like epithelium. Cigarette smoke appears to be the most common environmental toxin associated with the development of squamous metaplasia.[15, 17-21] Chronic bronchitis and bronchiectasis will frequently show foci of this epithelial change.

The development of squamous metaplasia is antedated by a proliferation of reserve or basal cells. As this proliferation continues, it begins to form a multilayered epithelium that intervenes between the columnar epithelial cells and the basement membrane (Figs. 14–21 and 14–22). As these reserve cells gradually mature, an epithelium is produced that more and more resembles a stratified squamous epithelium (Fig. 14–23).

Cytology

In cytologic materials, reserve cell hyperplasia is recognized by the presence of tissue fragments composed of small, uniform, tightly cohesive cells possessing darkly stained nuclei and a thin rim of cyanophilic cytoplasm. Nuclear molding is present, but uniformity is also present throughout the fragment. No tendency towards fragmentation of the cluster is seen (Fig. 14–24). Necrosis does not occur. At times reserve cell hyperplasia may be very alarming in appearance and

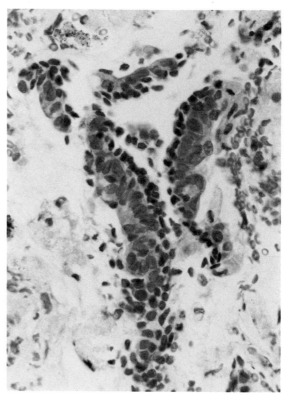

FIGURE 14–22. Bronchial epithelium with early hyperplasia of reserve cells. Bronchial washing. Cell block preparation (hematoxylin and eosin; ×400).

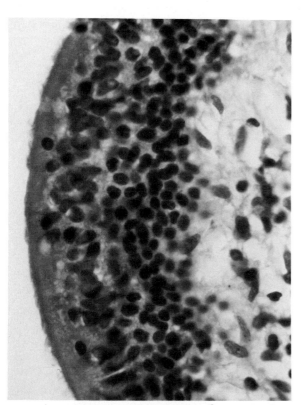

FIGURE 14–21. Reserve cell hyperplasia in bronchial epithelium. Bronchial biopsy (hematoxylin and eosin; ×680).

must be distinguished from small-cell undifferentiated carcinoma. Other small-cell neoplasms, such as leukemias and lymphomas, should not be confused with reserve cell hyperplasia, as they characteristically exfoliate into the respiratory material as single cells. Reserve cell hyperplasia may be present in all types of respiratory specimens but is most frequent in bronchial brushings.

Cells from squamous metaplasia may occur as single cells or as small tissue fragments (Figs. 14–25 and 14–26).[475] As fragments, they are grouped in a uniform, monolayered cobblestone-like arrangement with striking uniformity between the cells. Some fragments may exhibit flattening of one surface, presumably that which was adjacent to the lumen of the bronchus. Although they resemble maturing squamous cells, they are smaller and possess a higher nucleocytoplasmic ratio. As squamous metaplasia mimics maturing squamous epithelium, metaplastic cells of varying degrees of maturity may be present. The nuclei may be intensely karyopyknotic. Squamous metaplasias are capable of undergoing changes characterized by increasing degrees of nuclear abnormality. These metaplasias exhibit an increase in nucleocytoplasmic ratio, a thickening of the nuclear membrane, an increase in granularity and hyperchromasia of the chromatin and the appearance of nucleoli (Fig. 14–27). These abnormalities have been called by various names, including atypical squamous metaplasia and squamous metaplasia with dys-

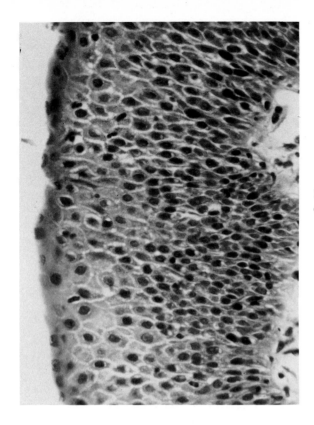

FIGURE 14–23. Squamous metaplasia in bronchial epithelium. Bronchial biopsy (hematoxylin and eosin; ×400).

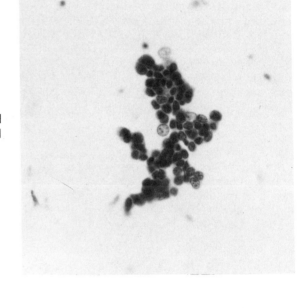

FIGURE 14–24. Reserve cell hyperplasia. The nuclei are small and hyperchromatic with areas of striking nuclear molding. Bronchial brushing (Papanicolaou stain; ×400).

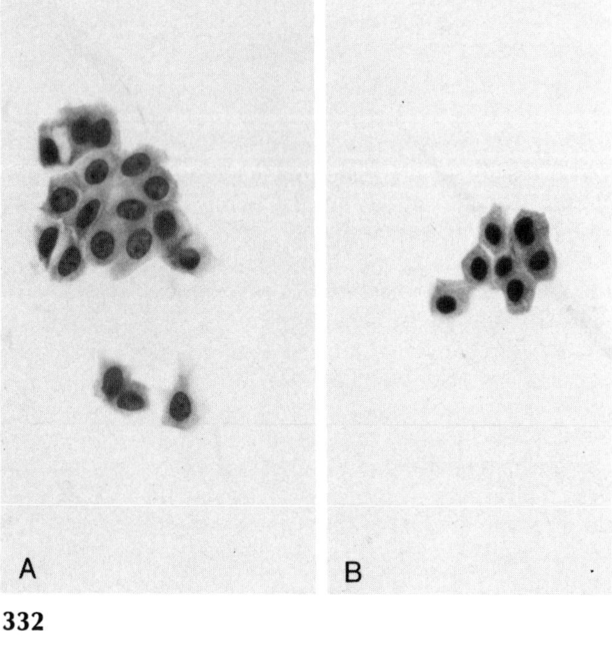

FIGURE 14–25. *A* and *B*, **Squamous metaplasia.** Sputum (Papanicolaou stain; ×400).

A

B

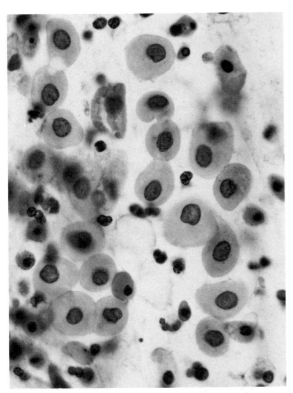

FIGURE 14–26. Squamous metaplasia. The cells have sharp cytoplasmic borders and nuclei that are not enlarged and that show uniformity of size and fine chromatin. Sputum (Papanicolaou stain; × 680).

plasia.[157, 174, 194, 277, 281, 371–373, 375, 377, 387, 522] They have been observed in the presence of longstanding chronic irritation of the tracheobronchial tree, particularly cigarette smoking, and they are believed by many investigators to antedate the appearance of carcinoma of the lung. In about 60% of patients, however, these atypical metaplastic cells are associated with non-neoplastic

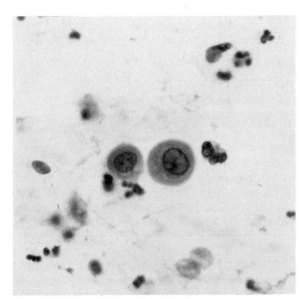

FIGURE 14–27. Squamous metaplasia with mild dysplasia. Sputum (Papanicolaou stain; × 680).

TABLE 14–2. Cancer Types Present in 28 Patients With Cytologic Diagnosis of Atypical Squamous Metaplasia

Cancer Primary in the Lung	Number Patients	Percent Patients
Squamous cell carcinoma	9	32.2
Adenocarcinoma	5	17.8
Large-cell undifferentiated carcinoma	5	17.8
Small-cell undifferentiated carcinoma	5	17.8
Cancer Metastatic to the Lung		
Mammary carcinoma	2	7.2
Squamous cell carcinoma	1	3.6
Chondrosarcoma	1	3.6
Total	28	100

Reproduced with permission from Johnston WW: Cytologic correlations. *In* Pulmonary Pathology. Edited by DH Dail, SP Hammar. New York, Springer-Verlag, 1987.

conditions of the lung, most notably pneumonia (Tables 14–2 and 14–3).[249] Figures 14–28 to 14–30 illustrate a particularly severe atypical metaplasia and hyperplasia of type II pneumocytes occurring in a young adult. Atypical metaplasia is discussed further in the section The Inconclusive Cytologic Specimen.

A special morphologic type of cell probably originating in atypical squamous metaplasia is the so-called "Pap" cell, originally seen by Dr. Papanicolaou in a specimen of his own sputum. He described these cells as follows: "Cells with atypical features, which in some instances may cause a suspicion of malignancy, are often seen in cases of chronic inflammatory conditions including pneumonia, tuberculosis and bronchiectasis. Some of these cells have a distinctive form and therefore a diagnostic value, such as the cell known in our laboratory as the 'Pap' cell because it was first noted 7 years ago in the author's sputum during an exacerbation of a chronic inflammatory condition of the upper respiratory tract. It is a relatively small acidophilic cell with an elliptic form and an ovoid pyknotic nucleus. Dense clusters of cells of this type have been seen in many cases of chronic respiratory infections. In such cases a characteristic fading of the nucleus is often noted, particularly in the later resolving stages of the inflammatory process.

TABLE 14–3. A Profile of Signs and Diseases in 42 Patients Without Cancer But With Cytologic Diagnosis of Atypical Squamous Metaplasia

Disease Category	Number Patients	Percent Patients
Pneumonia	12	28.6
Chronic obstructive pulmonary disease	10	23.8
Granulomatous disease	10	23.8
Chronic bronchitis	9	21.4
Smoking history	8	19.0
Hemoptysis	3	7.1
Abscess	3	7.1
Thromboemboli	3	7.1
Other	5	11.9

Reproduced with permission from Johnston, WW: Cytologic correlations. *In* Pulmonary Pathology. Edited by DH Dail, SP Hammar. New York, Springer-Verlag, 1987.

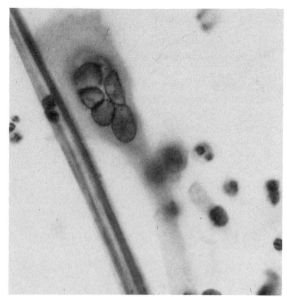

FIGURE 14–28. Atypical squamous metaplasia from a young adult quadraplegic with pneumonia and oxygen toxicity. Sputum (Papanicolaou stain; ×400).

"The exact nature, origin and diagnostic and prognostic significance of the 'Pap' cells has not as yet been established. According to one view they are small squamous cells from the upper portion of the respiratory tract. Another view supported by good evidence is that they represent a squamous metaplastic change of epithelial cells of the ciliated type."[402]

Bronchopulmonary Dysplasia

A special incidence in the occurrence of atypical squamous metaplasia was described in neonates with

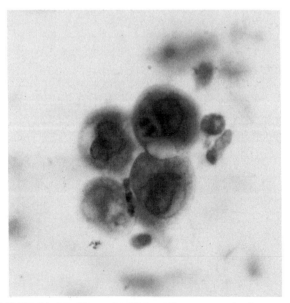

FIGURE 14–29. Hyperplastic type II pneumocytes in sputum from the same case as in Figure 14–28 (Papanicolaou stain; ×1000).

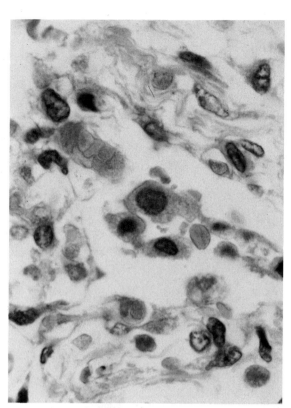

FIGURE 14–30. Autopsy lung from case described in Figures 14–28 and 14–29. Cells similar to those shown in sputum line the **alveolar apaces** (hematoxylin and eosin; ×400).

respiratory distress syndrome by Northway and associates[390] in 1967 and was termed bronchopulmonary dysplasia. Additional studies have been reported by D'Ablang and associates[99] and by Kanbour, Doshi and associates.[114, 267] In the early stages, the cellular findings in tracheal aspirates include bronchial cells and metaplastic cells. As the disease progresses the metaplastic cells become more atypical. Bronchopulmonary dysplasia is a well-known complication in babies with hyaline membrane disease who have received intensive care with oxygen and respirators.

Epithelial Cellular Changes Following Radiation Therapy, Chemotherapy and Toxic Chemicals

Severe morphologic changes in benign cells of the lung and upper respiratory tract may occur at varying intervals following treatment with ionizing radiation or with a variety of drugs. These cells may be so severely altered that they may be mistaken for cancer cells. Knowledge of a history of prior therapy with such agents is the best safeguard against an erroneous cancer diagnosis.

Cellular alterations in response to radiation therapy may involve both squamous cells and columnar cells and are characterized by cytomegaly with both cytoplasmic and nuclear enlargement, multinucleation, macronucleoli and cytoplasmic vacuolization (Fig. 14–31).

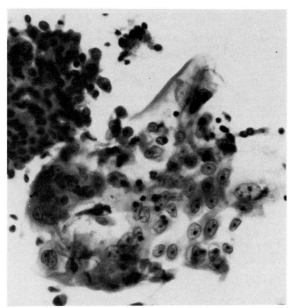

FIGURE 14–31. Radiation changes. Compared with the adjacent bronchial epithelium, the cells in the center of the field exhibit nuclear enlargement with a concomitant increase in the amount of cytoplasm, prominent nucleoli and multinucleation. Bronchial brushing (Papanicolaou stain; × 325).

An acute radiation response can stimulate such cellular changes within the area that had been irradiated or at a remote site. For example, a patient who had received radiation treatment to the neck could exhibit changes in bronchial epithelium; a patient who had received radiation treatment to the left lung could exhibit changes in the right lung. As the radiation response in the lung becomes more chronic, a diffuse interstitial fibrosis ensues. Epithelial abnormalities may persist and run the gamut from focal areas of squamous metaplasia of the lining bronchial cells to severe squamous atypia. A false-positive diagnosis of squamous cell carcinoma on specimens of sputum and bronchial material is a potential dangerous pitfall in such a patient.

A number of drugs used for anticancer chemotherapy may be associated with the production of severe changes in the lung parenchyma.[221] These drugs include the alkylating agents busulfan, cyclophosphamide, chlorambucil, melphalan, bleomycin,[32] bis-chlorethyl-nitrosurea (BCNU) and the antimetabolites methotrexate and azathioprine.[31] The toxic injury to the lung is that of diffuse alveolar damage. The initial phase of this damage consists of pulmonary edema and hemorrhage. The striking feature of this phase that permits this type of alveolar damage to be differentiated from that resulting from causes other than from these drugs is the presence of atypical epithelial cells in great abundance. It has been shown by Bedrossian and associates[31] that these atypical cells are in fact abnormal type II pneumocytes that have undergone degranulation and loss of lamellar bodies. These atypical pneumocytes may shed into sputum or be harvested in brushings, BALs or FNAs. These pneumocytes are

most likely to be seen, however, in BALs.[236] Bedrossian has emphasized the significance of the presence of these cells in sputum and BALs. They may herald the progression of the drug-induced lung damage to diffuse fibrosis.[31]

Cells resulting from chemotherapy are prone to occur singly and to show cytomegaly, hyperchromasia and macronucleoli (Fig. 14–32 A and B). In addition to type II pneumocytes, cells of the tracheobronchial epithelium and the terminal bronchiolar epithelium may be involved. A major key to the correct recognition of these cells lies in the tendency of many of them to be roughly rectangular in shape, to occur singly, to be sparse and to exhibit nuclear degeneration. Some may show remnants of cilia.

We have observed extremely atypical changes in the bronchial epithelium of a farmer who inhaled the insecticide parathion. Stein and associates[511] have reported macrophage abnormalities in patients on amiodarone, an antiarrhythmatic drug.

Other Cellular Components

A variety of cells of nonepithelial origin may appear in various types of cytologic specimens from the lungs. The type and frequency of these cells will be dependent on the type of specimen and the disease process in the patient. Perhaps the most frequent cell encountered is

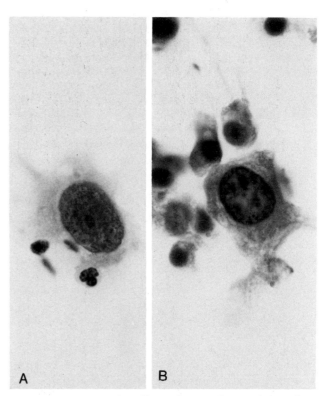

A   B

FIGURE 14–32. A and B, **Chemotherapy changes** in a patient being treated for **acute leukemia.** The cells show nuclear enlargement, hyperchromasia and abnormal chromatin distribution, but the cytoplasm maintains a columnar or "boxcar" shape. Bronchial brushing (Papanicolaou stain; × 1000).

the pulmonary alveolar macrophage. Although it was once believed that the macrophage originated from the alveolar lining epithelium, it is now established that the pulmonary alveolar macrophage originates in the bone marrow.[290] The presence of this characteristic cell most frequently laden with particles of carbon helps to establish that a specimen of sputum is satisfactory. Risse and associates, in 1987 reports,[446, 447] noted that in patients with primary lung cancer, sputum samples with true-positive cytologic diagnoses contained significantly more cells from the lower respiratory tract, such as alveolar macrophages and bronchial columnar cells, than did sputum samples with false-negative cytologic diagnoses. The macrophages are recognized by the excentric position of the nucleus, abundant foamy cytoplasm and the phagocytosed material, usually carbon. On occasion the nuclei may assume a bean shape and show one or more nucleoli and cytoplasmic processes.[565] A study by Mylius and Gullvag[364] has shown an increase in the alveolar macrophage count with a higher level of particulate pollution in the workplace.

Binucleated and multinucleated giant cell macrophages are not infrequently encountered. These cells may be seen in association with chronic lung disease of many varieties, including sarcoidosis (Fig. 14–33),[4, 558] tuberculosis,[22, 376, 452, 535] infections with nontuberculous mycobacteria,[497] giant cell interstitial pneumonia[557] and other inflammatory diseases,[430] but they are not diagnostic and may be seen in respiratory

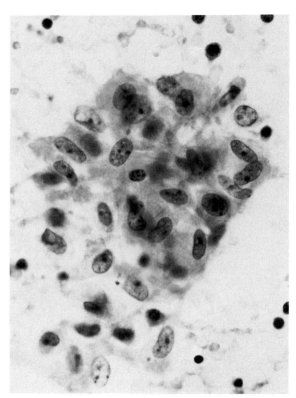

FIGURE 14–34. Epithelioid macrophages from a patient with **sarcoidosis.** Note the abundant cytoplasm and bland nuclear appearance. Fine needle aspiration (FNA) of lung (Papanicolaou stain; ×680).

material in the absence of clinical disease. With granulomatous disease, characteristic epithelioid cells may be shed (Fig. 14–34). Large vacuoles containing lipid have been reported in pulmonary macrophages in the presence of lipoid pneumonia (Fig. 14–35).[322, 498] Multinucleated cells laden with lipid may be numerous, and they may mimic adenocarcinoma or liposarcoma. Tabatowski and associates[525] have reported the finding of nonpigmented alveolar macrophages and phagocytic multinucleated giant cells in the bronchial washings from a hard-metal worker with giant cell interstitial pneumonia.[525] In the presence of intra-alveolar hemorrhage, macrophages laden with hemosiderin may appear in the cellular specimen (Fig. 14–36).

Other cells originating from circulating blood, which may be seen in respiratory cellular samples, include lymphocytes,[539] eosinophils, neutrophils and plasma cells. Lymphocytes may be associated with a chronic inflammatory process or with a rupture of a lymphoid follicle in the wall of a bronchus (Fig. 14–37). These cells may stream out in the mucus strands mimicking the exfoliation pattern of small-cell undifferentiated carcinoma. Absence of necrosis, molding and nuclear abnormalities help to rule out carcinoma. Eosinophils may be seen most frequently in association with asthmatic bronchitis but also with any disease in which there is a component of allergy. Charcot-Leyden crystals may accompany the eosinophils (Fig. 14–38). Plasma cells are commonly encountered in chronic inflammatory exudates.

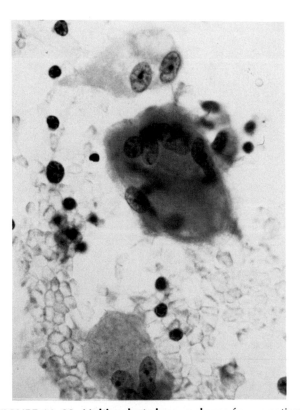

FIGURE 14–33. Multinucleated macrophages from a patient with sarcoidosis. Fine needle aspiration (FNA) of lung (Papanicolaou stain; ×680).

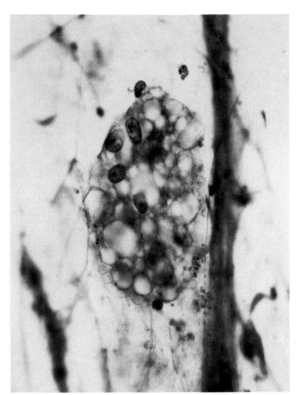

FIGURE 14–35. Multinucleated macrophage with numerous cytoplasmic vacuoles from a patient with **lipoid pneumonia.** Sputum (Papanicolaou stain; ×520).

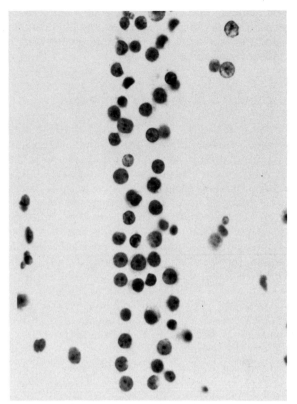

FIGURE 14–37. Follicular bronchitis. Small lymphocytes presumably arising in a ruptured lymphoid follicle. Sputum (Papanicolaou stain; ×680).

Cellular specimens obtained by FNA may contain a variety of cells unique to them because of the anatomic route followed by the needle as it is inserted percutaneously into the lung. Thus, such a specimen may contain squamous epithelial cells, cells from various skin appendages, fibrofatty connective tissue, striated muscle, capillaries and mesothelium. The last occurs in monolayered sheets and may be a diagnostic pitfall

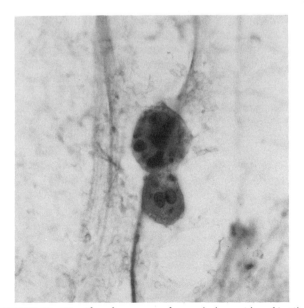

FIGURE 14–36. Alveolar macrophages laden with refractile granules of hemosiderin. Sputum (Papanicolaou stain; ×400).

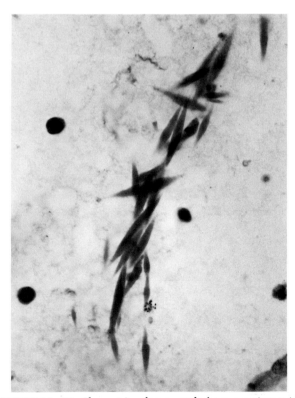

FIGURE 14–38. Charcot-Leyden crystals from a patient with **asthma.** Bronchial washing (Papanicolaou stain; ×680).

if it is reactive and hyperplastic. Rarely fragments of liver tissue may be present when the physician performing the aspiration had tried to enter the lung too far inferiorly on the chest wall.

Noncellular Inanimate Components

In addition to cells from the host and living microorganisms, many different nonliving structures and substances may be present in specimens from the lower respiratory tract. The presence of some may indicate specific problems. Others may serve only to confuse and to produce incorrect diagnoses. Some may be derived from the patient, may have been inhaled or may have contaminated the specimen after it has been taken from the patient.[484] Structures and substances produced by the host include Curschmann's spirals, inspissated mucus spheres, amyloid, alveolar proteinosis, ferruginous bodies, psammoma bodies and corpora amylacea. Inhaled or contaminating structures include food, pollen granules and any materials floating around in the laboratory's environment during the cytopreparation procedure.

Curschmann's spirals are casts of small bronchioles formed from inspissated mucus (Fig. 14–39). They are seen in any condition characterized by the chronic and excessive production of mucus. Asthmatic bronchitis is a classic example. Occasionally, small inspissated masses of mucus will round up and adhere to one another so as to suggest nuclei. In extreme situations

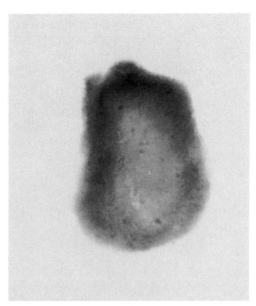

FIGURE 14–40. Pulmonary alveolar proteinosis. Specimens typically contain numerous rounded fragments of amorphous material, such as the one shown. Bronchoalveolar lavage (Papanicolaou stain; ×1000).

the nuclear hyperchromasia and molding of small-cell undifferentiated carcinoma may be suggested.

The cytology of bronchial amyloidosis has been reported by Chen.[79] Hsiu and associates[234] have reported the diagnosis of primary amyloidosis by FNA of a hilar mass. Both reports described the amyloid as presenting as amorphous eosinophilic masses, some having scalloped edges. These masses showed a green birefringence under polarized light with Congo red staining.

Koss has discussed the cytology and histochemistry of acellular masses derived from patients with alveolar proteinosis.[290] In a study performed in his laboratory no histochemical differences could be found between the eosinophilic amorphous masses of this protein and those in the sputum of patients without the disorder. Electron microscopy has now confirmed that the lamellar bodies visible by light microscopy in the proteinaceous material are surfactant (Figs. 14–40 and 14–41). The pathogenesis of this disease is still under debate but may be related to underlying defects in macrophage function.[103]

Ferruginous bodies have been noted in tissues and cellular specimens from the lungs for many years. They all were formerly called asbestos bodies reflecting the belief that all were formed as a reaction to inhaled fibers of asbestos. Now it is recognized that a number of different inhaled mineral fibers may result in quite similar structures.[191] These bodies are composed of various substances, including iron, which are encrusted upon a thin needle-like fiber (Fig. 14–42). Increasing attention is being focused upon their relationship to bronchogenic carcinoma.[7, 453, 454] Leiman and Markowitz[308] have recommended further evaluation of a pulmonary mass when the FNA shows only asbestos bodies. Roggli and associates[453–455] have stressed that

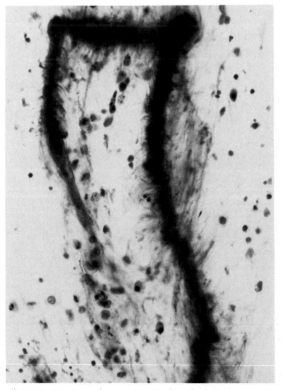

FIGURE 14–39. Curschmann's spiral with dense central core of inspissated mucus. Sputum (Papanicolaou stain; ×325).

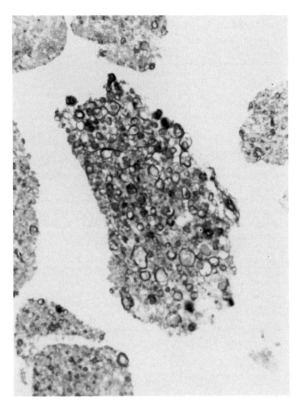

FIGURE 14–41. Pulmonary alveolar proteinosis. The amorphous material observed in cytologic preparations is found to contain numerous whorls of lipid when evaluated by semithin sections. Bronchoalveolar lavage, semithin Epon section (toluidine blue stain; × 1000).

the finding of even one ferruginous body in respiratory material or a FNA is indicative of large numbers of these in the lung. Roggli and associates have also evaluated the asbestos body content of broncholavage

fluid from 20 patients with a history of occupational asbestos exposure. Large numbers of asbestos bodies in the broncholavage fluid were indicative of considerable occupational exposure, whereas occasional bodies were a nonspecific finding.[454]

In a 1988 report, Wheeler and associates found bronchial washing specimens stained with Prussian blue to be more sensitive than sputum for the identification of asbestos bodies.[578]

Psammoma bodies (calcospherites) and corpora amylacea are the names given to several varieties of dark-staining, rounded bodies with concentric rings and radial striations, which may appear in respiratory material. Corpora amylacea are composed of glycoproteins and do not calcify. Psammoma bodies are calcified and contain phosphates, iron, magnesium and sudanophilic material. Corpora amylacea are seen under circumstances of heart failure, pulmonary infarction and chronic bronchitis. Psammoma bodies have been associated with the rare disease pulmonary microlithiasis and with malignant neoplasms, including bronchioloalveolar carcinoma and small-cell undifferentiated carcinoma (see Fig. 14–97).[29, 202, 494]

Any structure that can be breathed into the respiratory passages or any particle of masticated food is capable of appearing in the respiratory specimen and of producing great confusion to the examiner if its identity is not recognized. Plant cells may be confused with cancer cells, and structures such as pollen and starch granules may be confused with infectious organisms (Fig. 14–43). Plant cells and other food particles have also been reported in FNAs from aspiration pneumonia.[94]

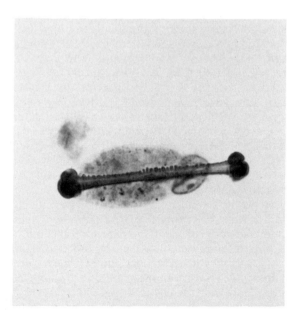

FIGURE 14–42. Ferruginous body partially engulfed by a macrophage, from a patient with **asbestosis.** Sputum (Papanicolaou stain; × 1000).

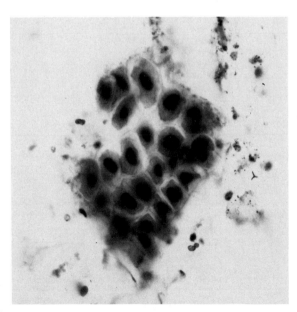

FIGURE 14–43. Vegetable cells. Such cells may mimic atypical squamous cells because of their orangeophilia, nuclear hyperchromasia and sharp cytoplasmic borders. Careful examination, however, reveals the presence of cell walls. Sputum (Papanicolaou stain; × 400).

CYTOLOGY OF RESPIRATORY INFECTIONS

This section describes observations and experiences in the cytologic detection of the most important and common pulmonary infections. It is not intended to be an exhaustive review of pulmonary infectious disease. Rather it is limited to a presentation of those organisms that the cytologist is most likely to encounter (Table 14–4). The major emphasis is on cytologic detection of some mycoses and several miscellaneous parasitic organisms that are frequently associated with opportunistic infection. The necessity for close cooperation among the cytology laboratory, the clinical microbiology laboratory and the patient's physician is implicit in this discussion. Special stains for bacteria, acid-fast bacteria, fungi and parasites should be obtained when appropriate (Table 14–5). Viral infections may produce changes of diagnostic significance in squamous, bronchial, bronchiolar and alveolar epithelial cells.

Among those patients with suspected respiratory infections, a new and unique group has emerged consisting of those with preexisting diseases of various etiologies who have developed new respiratory signs and symptoms demanding evaluation and therapy.

TABLE 14–4. Infectious Organisms Detectable in Cytologic Specimens From the Lung

Viruses
 Herpes simplex
 Herpes zoster
 Cytomegalovirus
 Adenovirus
 Measles virus
 Parainfluenza virus
 Respiratory syncytial virus
Bacteria
Gram-positive and gram-negative
 Staphylococcus aureus
 Pseudomonas aeruginosa
 Legionella sp.
Acid-fast
 Mycobacterium tuberculosis
 Mycobacterium avium and *M. intracellulare*
Fungi
 Actinomyces bovis
 Nocardia asteroides
 Blastomyces dermatitidis
 Cryptococcus neoformans
 Histoplasma capsulatum
 Candida albicans
 Paracoccidioides brasiliensis
 Coccidioides immitis
 Aspergillus fumigatus
 Aspergillus niger
 Phycomycetes
Parasites
 Pneumocystis carinii
 Toxoplasma gondii
 Strongyloides stercoralis
 Dirofilaria immitis
 Echinococcus
 Paragonimus kellicotti
 Paragonimus westermani
 Cryptosporidium

TABLE 14–5. Staining Characteristics of Infectious Organisms Commonly Seen in Cytologic Specimens From the Lung

Organism	Papanicolaou Stain	Special Stain
Mycobacterium tuberculosis	–	Acid-fast, auramine-O
Mycobacterium avium and *M. intracellulare*	–	Acid-fast, auramine-O
Staphylococcus aureus	±	Gram
Pseudomonas aeruginosa	±	Gram
Legionella sp.	–	Dieterle, fluorescence with antisera
Nocardia asteroides	±	Gram, acid-fast
Blastomyces dermatitidis	+	PAS, Meth.-Ag.
Cryptococcus neoformans	+	PAS, alcian blue
Coccidioides immitis	+	PAS, Meth.-Ag.
Histoplasma capsulatum	±	Meth.-Ag.
Geotrichum candidum	+	Meth.-Ag.
Candida albicans	+	PAS, Meth.-Ag.
Aspergillus fumigatus	+	PAS, Gram
Phycomycetes sp.	+	PAS, Meth.-Ag.
Strongyloides stercoralis	+	Meth-Ag, Giemsa
Pneumocystis carinii	±	Toluidine blue, Meth.-Ag, Wright

PAS = periodic acid–Schiff; Meth.-Ag = methenamine silver.

These patients have histories involving many disease backgrounds, but frequently encountered are those patients with established pulmonary or extrapulmonary cancer, who are under various programs of radiation therapy and chemotherapy; patients who have primary immune deficiencies and patients who have immune responses suppressed by drugs.[238] In the last two groups are renal allograft recipients and the alarmingly increasing population of patients with acquired immune deficiency syndrome (AIDS).[204, 205] When a patient with one of these histories develops a problem in the lungs, it can be related to any one of the following factors: recurrence of neoplasm, a new disease unrelated to the preexisting one, lung changes induced by the chemotherapeutic agents or opportunistic lung infection. Any one of these disease states can be life-threatening to the patient and must be immediately diagnosed correctly and treated. The role of the cytology laboratory in the diagnosis of opportunistic infections of the lower respiratory tract merits major consideration, because a number of these infectious agents lend themselves readily to detection and correct diagnosis by cytologic methods and principles.[245–248, 252, 257, 263, 366]

Viral Infections

In a review, Rosenthal[468] placed the role of cytology in the diagnosis of viral infections of the lung into appropriate perspective when she noted: "Definite viral diagnosis is made by viral culture, DNA probes, immunocytochemistry or other specific diagnostic techniques. However, the changes appreciated in the specimens stained by the Papanicolaou technique can provide a rapid preliminary diagnosis, which will enable the clinicians to begin therapy on an informed basis, before the definitive diagnosis is provided by more sophisticated methods. Avoiding a delay in treatment, albeit currently experimental, may be lifesaving to a patient who is threatened by an overwhelming viral infection. Cytologic diagnosis can provide this critical information."[468]

Many reports describe cellular changes in cells from the respiratory tract in association with a number of different viral infections,[585] including adenovirus,[290] herpes simplex,[162, 370] herpes zoster,[468] measles,[30] cytomegalovirus,[242, 285, 572] and parainfluenza and respiratory syncytial virus.[368, 531] The cellular changes occurring in these patients can be divided into three general categories. First is a cellular alteration observed and named ciliocytophthoria by Papanicolaou in 1956.[403] This is a peculiar degeneration of the ciliated respiratory epithelium in which a pinching off occurs between the cilia-bearing cytoplasm and the nucleated cytoplasm, resulting is an anucleated mass of cytoplasm-bearing cilia and a degenerating nucleus with cytoplasm (Fig. 14–44).[403, 415, 416] A second type of cellular alteration most frequently associated with viral pneumonia may occur and produce diagnostic problems in differentiation from cancer. This alteration is a form of regeneration and atypia of the respiratory epithelium appearing in sputum and bronchial material as tissue fragments composed of cells bearing enlarged hyperchromatic nuclei with prominent nucleoli. The tightly cohesive features of the cells in the tissue fragments and the absence of atypical cells lying singly help in avoiding the incorrect diagnosis of cancer. The third type of cellular alteration is much more specific and may be diagnostic for certain viral infections. Most frequently observed are the changes seen in association with infection with herpes simplex virus. The hallmark of cellular alteration produced by herpes is that of cells with multiple molded nuclei, which may contain eosinophilic irregular inclusion bodies or exhibit a peculiar type of nuclear degeneration that appears as slate gray,

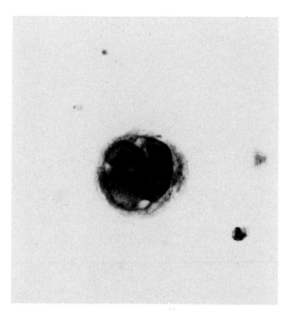

FIGURE 14–45. *Herpes simplex.* This cell shows the characteristic multinucleation, nuclear molding, "ground-glass" appearance of the nuclei and peripheral margination of the chromatin. Sputum (Papanicolaou stain; × 1000).

homogenized contents (Fig. 14–45). Alveolar lining cells infected by herpes zoster are indistinguishable from those infected by herpes simplex.

Cells infected by the cytomegalovirus are larger and may show some multinucleation, but they have fewer nuclei and none of the molding as seen in herpes simplex. Large amphophilic, smooth, intranuclear inclusions, surrounded by very prominent halos and marked margination of chromatin on the inner surface of the nuclear membrane, are present. Within the nucleus, cytomegalovirus particles take on a protein envelope and migrate out into the cytoplasm where they appear as cytoplasmic inclusions that are manifested as a textured appearance to the cytoplasm. An example of a cell infected with the cytomegalovirus is shown in Figure 14–46.

Infection with adenovirus produces two types of intranuclear inclusions in bronchiolar and alveolar lining cells. The first type consists of a small red body surrounded by a well-circumscribed clear halo. The second is a homogeneous basophilic mass almost completely replacing the nucleus. Ciliocytophthoria may be quite pronounced. The most characteristic cytologic finding in measles pneumonia is the presence of multinucleated giant cells containing eosinophilic inclusions that are present both within the nucleus and cytoplasm. The respiratory syncytial virus also stimulates a proliferation of multinucleated giant cells with cytoplasmic basophilic inclusions surrounded by halos.

Bacterial Infections

Although the majority of lung infections produced by bacteria do not lend themselves to primary diagnosis by conventional cytologic methods, a few instances

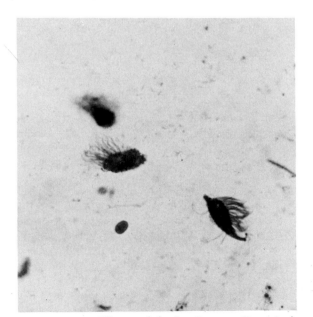

FIGURE 14–44. Ciliocytophthoria. Sputum (Papanicolaou stain; × 1000).

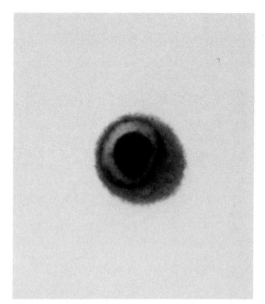

FIGURE 14–46. Cell showing changes of **cytomegalovirus infection,** including an intranuclear inclusion with surrounding halo and peripheral margination of the chromatin. Bronchial washing (Papanicolaou stain; ×1700).

occur in which the cytologic specimen may be extremely helpful.

Gram-positive and Gram-negative Bacteria

It is not at all uncommon for specimens of sputum to show bacillary and coccal forms of bacteria. These rarely indicate pulmonary infection but rather are the result of bacterial overgrowth. Actinomyces may be seen as contaminants from the tonsillar crypts. Similar observations are also usually true for bronchial material. In contrast, the presence of bacteria in a cytologic specimen from an FNA may be of extreme importance. A striking example is to be found in a 45-year-old physician-patient with pyoderma gangrenosum and hypogammaglobulinemia who developed several cavitary lesions in his left lower lobe. An FNA specimen revealed the presence of many bacilli that were gram-negative and found on culture to be *Pseudomonas aeruginosa*. We have also seen *Staphylococcus aureus* in the form of botryomycosis diagnosed by FNA. In evaluating such specimens, it is important to remember that although the Papanicolaou stain will render bacteria visible, their red or blue staining has no connection to true gram-negative or gram-positive findings.

Opportunistic infections with *Legionella pneumophila* and *L. micdadei* are worthy of note as they appear to be increasing in frequency.[565] *Legionella* is an extremely small gram-negative rod. Specimens of sputum, bronchial material and particularly FNAs stained by the Dieterle method of silver impregnation may reveal the organisms. Much greater sensitivity in detection of this organism is being achieved by immunofluorescence microscopy, however, utilizing anti-*Legionella* antisera, which are now commercially available.

Acid-fast Bacteria

The search for acid-fast organisms in a cytologic specimen is likely to be most useful for a patient with suggestive morphologic evidence of granulomatous inflammation and necrosis or an extremely suggestive clinical history. Patients infected with *Mycobacterium avium-M. intracellulare* complex may show large alveolar macrophages, which on acid-fast stain, reveal large numbers of branching acid-fast bacilli. Cell blocks prepared from FNA are useful for acid-fast staining when it is suspected that a tuberculous lesion has been aspirated. Fluorescence microscopy with auramine-O may also reveal the organisms. Maygarden and Flanders[344] reported the cytologic findings from three patients with AIDS in which mycobacteria were seen on the routine modified Wright-stained slides without special stains. The organisms appeared as negative images—unstained rod-shaped structures against the deep blue background of the stain. Nocardiosis should be suspected when an FNA reveals the presence of delicate branching filamentous rods with an inflammatory reaction consisting mainly of neutrophils. Positive acid-fast stains further enforce this diagnosis.

Fungal Infections

Many of the respiratory fungal infections are readily detectable by cytologic methods. In these diseases the etiologic agent is visible and in some cases has a morphology on which a specific diagnosis may be based. The detection of these fungi in a stained cytologic specimen may be the first clue to the nature of the patient's problem. The accuracy of observation is dependent on the ability of the cytologist to appreciate the various forms that the fungi may assume.

Pulmonary Blastomycosis

Blastomycosis (North American blastomycosis, Gilchrist's disease) is a chronic infectious disease of both granulomatous and suppurative types that may involve lungs, skin, bones and genitourinary tract. It is caused by infection with the dimorphic fungus *Blastomyces dermatitidis*. The disease is endemic in many parts of the United States, including the Ohio, St. Lawrence and Mississippi River Valleys and the southeastern United States. It has also been found in southern Manitoba, Mexico and parts of South America and Africa. The natural habitat of *B. dermatitidis* is believed to be the soil from which infectious conidia are inhaled.[38] The symptoms, signs and changes seen radiologically may closely resemble the appearance and progression of lung cancer. Symptoms may consist of cough, dyspnea, chest pain, low-grade fever, weight loss and weakness. The sputum may become purulent or blood streaked. In well-developed cases, the radiologic findings may include unilateral, dense, irregular shadows, which may be produced by lung cancer, hilar adenopathy, consolidation or cavitation.[74, 92] Sputum production may be present in 50 to 80% of patients and is usually found to contain organisms.

In cytologic materials that have been fixed in 95% alcohol and stained by the Papanicolaou technique, *B. dermatitidis* appears as single or budding spheric cells 8 to 15 μ in diameter with thick refractile walls. The thickness of the walls may impart to these forms a "double-contoured" appearance. No hyphae are seen. An important criterion for morphologic confirmation of blastomyces is the nature of the budding. Single budding is characteristic. The bud has a tendency to remain in close apposition to the mother cell such that a flattening of the two surfaces occurs. Staining is of little help as an aid in identifying this organism. The wall is highly refractile and may stain cyanophilically. The cytoplasm stains variably. In some cells scattered brownish-red granules are seen embedded in an otherwise nonstaining cytoplasmic mass. In other cells the entire cytoplasmic mass may shrink within the cell wall and may show cyanophilic staining. The unwary may mistake these yeast cells for those of human origin. The cell wall is mistaken for cytoplasm and the cytoplasmic mass is mistaken for a nucleus (Fig. 14–47).[104, 257, 302] The Splendore-Hoeppli phenomenon around these organisms in cytologic preparations has been reported by Subramony and colleagues.[518]

The inflammatory reaction induced by infection with *B. dermatitidis* may vary from that of the production of classic tuberculoid granulomata to the production of microabscesses with a predominance of neutrophils. The cytologic examination of respiratory cellular material from such cases reflects this spectrum of inflammatory reactivity. Occasionally, one may also see multinucleated giant cells with the organism within; however, more frequently giant cells without apparent organisms are seen. The cellular picture has nothing specific to suggest that infection with blastomyces has occurred.

The presence in itself of these organisms is diagnostic for infection. All varieties of respiratory and FNA specimens may reveal the organisms. The following cases are fairly typical of patients with pulmonary blastomycosis whose disease has been diagnosed in our laboratory.

A 62-year-old man with diabetes mellitus was transferred from another hospital. A chest radiograph at that time had revealed fluffy white infiltrates in both lungs. He had been treated with large doses of penicillin and corticosteroids. Cytologic examination of a specimen of sputum revealed the characteristic budding yeast-like forms of *Blastomyces dermatitidi*. He died several days later. An autopsy revealed systemic blastomycosis. In this case the possibility of carcinoma of the lung was considered in the differential diagnostic interpretation of the radiologic findings. Had these organisms not been identified, the patient most likely would have received an exploratory thoracotomy.

In another case, a 9-year-old girl presented with a cavitary lesion in the left lower lobe. An FNA was performed and revealed the budding yeasts of *Blastomyces dermatitidi*. The child lived in a part of North Carolina where this disease is endemic.

Pulmonary Cryptococcosis

Cryptococcosis is a systemic infectious disease that is caused by the yeast-like fungus, *Cryptococcus neoformans*. Although infection most often involves the central nervous system, it may also involve lung, skin, bones, liver, adrenal, kidney, prostate, endocardium and pericardium. The causative agent is an encapsulated organism that reproduces by budding. It has a worldwide distribution; is found in the soil and is most frequent in soil contaminated with bird droppings, particularly those of pigeons. Primary portal of entry into the human host is through the respiratory tract. Prevalence of human disease is highest in the United States and Australia. Although the organism is classified as a primary pathogen, it is more often encountered as a cause of an opportunistic infection.[74]

Pulmonary cryptococcosis may encompass a spectrum of disease that ranges from that with no symptoms to that with a chronic course and associated with extrapulmonary infection. Patients with the disease may present with chronic cough, fever, chest pain, blood-streaked sputum or mucoid sputum and weight loss. Radiologic findings may include simple or multiple nodules that resemble primary lung cancer or metastatic cancer, consolidation and pleural effusion.

The budding yeast of *C. neoformans* has been reported in cytologic preparations of sputum, bronchial material, BALs and FNAs.[200, 431, 464, 496] Like blastomyces, single budding is characteristic of this yeast; however, in contrast to blastomyces, the single bud of cryptococcus pinches off leaving a markedly attenuated

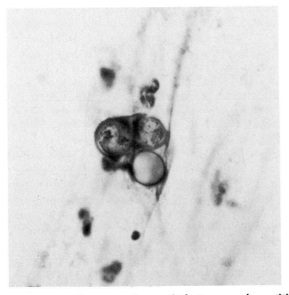

FIGURE 14–47. Three yeast forms of *Blastomyces dermatitidis* exhibiting well-defined cell walls. Typically, internal structure can be discerned, although this is absent in one of the cells shown. Sputum (Papanicolaou stain; ×1000).

isthmus of attachment to the mother yeast cell and thus assuming a tear-drop shape. The cell is ovoid to spheric, thick-walled and 5 to 20 μ in diameter (Fig. 14–48). It is usually surrounded by a gelatinous capsule, which may require special stains for visualization (periodic acid–Schiff, mucicarmine or Alcian blue) (Fig. 14–49). Occasionally, however, even with Papanicolaou staining alone, the capsule can be visualized. It may stain faintly cyanophilically, or it may be seen as a nonstaining space between cell body and displaced mucus. The visual effect is similar in principle to an India ink preparation.

Of additional significance in the correct identification of these organisms in respiratory specimens is the frequency with which they may be at the small end of the size spectrum. Because of this small size, they may be easily overlooked. Additionally, the cryptococci are much more variable in their internal morphology than the blastomyces. A rather vague, empty appearance to the internal structure of the organism may be encountered. A dark area within the organism possessing a refractile appearance is frequently observed and is similar to that of the internal structure of a starch granule. We believe that this appearance is due to the presence of trapped air within a depression in the wall of the organism beneath the coverslip. It is well known from preparing specimens of the female genital tract that if one does not exclude all air as the coverslip is lowered onto the mounting medium, bubbles of trapped air will give a dark refractile appearance.

The inflammatory reaction provoked by *Cryptococcus* may be extremely slight, completely absent or granulomatous. The following case history is a fairly characteristic profile of patients in whom *Cryptococcus* is diagnosed.

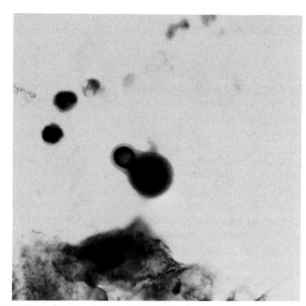

FIGURE 14–49. *Cryptococcus neoformans.* This field illustrates the typical narrow-based budding and variation in cell size as well as prominent staining of the capsule (periodic acid–Schiff stain; ×1000).

A 57-year-old man had been receiving large doses of steroid medication for regional enteritis. Gradually he had developed increasing shortness of breath and cough. Radiographs of the lung showed multiple pulmonary nodular densities. Metastatic carcinoma was suspected. An FNA showed the presence of typical budding yeast forms of *Cryptococcus neoformans*. These cytologic observations were confirmed by positive culture findings.

Pulmonary Coccidioidomycosis

Coccidioidomycosis is a chronic granulomatous infection most frequently involving the lungs but rarely also spreading to other organs in the body. The causative agent is the dimorphic fungus *Coccidioides immitis.* Infection is by inhalation of the highly infectious arthroconidia (arthrospores) formed by disarticulation of mycelia in the soil. In the United States, coccidioides is endemic in a number of southwestern states including California, Arizona, New Mexico, Nevada, Utah and Texas. It is also endemic in certain parts of Central and South America.

Primary infection for the otherwise healthy individual may be without symptoms, or the individual may present with an upper respiratory infection or a lower respiratory infection with cough, chest pain, fever, chills, night sweats, weakness and sputum production. Radiologic studies are usually nonspecific showing infiltrates, consolidation or pleural effusion. The majority of these pulmonary infections resolve spontaneously; however, a small number of patients will experience residual disease, including a pulmonary nodule, cavity, progressive pneumonia and chronic pulmonary disease. Immunocompromised patients and those with diabetes mellitus are particularly prone to develop chronic disease.

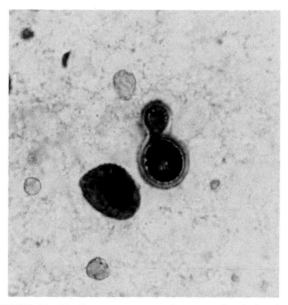

FIGURE 14–48. *Cryptococcus neoformans.* The dark refractile appearance of the larger yeast cell results from the trapping of air under the organism. Bronchial washing (Papanicolaou stain; ×1300).

The gross and histopathologic changes of pulmonary coccidioidomycosis are characterized by granulomatous inflammation, caseous necrosis, cavition and fibrosis. Thus, this disease bears striking resemblance to pulmonary tuberculosis. Histologic examination of tissues reveals the large spherules containing endospores. Occasional hyphal forms may also be present.[74]

Spherules and endospores of *C. immitis* have been reported in cytologic preparations of sputum, bronchial washings and FNAs.[197] In Papanicolaou-stained material the spherule appears as a nonbudding spheric, thick-walled structure, measuring 20 to 60 μ in diameter. Staining characteristics are variable and of little aid in identification. The spherules may be empty or may contain endospores. These are round, nonbudding structures measuring 1 to 5 μ in diameter (Fig. 14–50). It is not difficult to confuse the empty spherules with nonbudding forms of *B. dermatitidis*. Occasionally, arthrospores may be present in sputum. The following case histories are illustrative.

A 55-year-old woman with fever, cough and bloody sputum production was admitted to the hospital. Radiographs of the chest revealed bilateral pulmonary infiltrates. Significant in the history of the patient was the presence of diabetes mellitus that had been difficult to control. Characteristic spherules of coccidioides were present in a Papanicolaou-

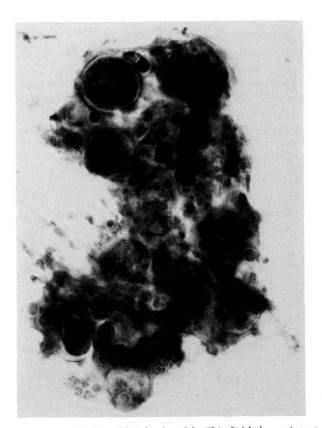

FIGURE 14–50. *Coccidioides immitis.* This field shows intact spherules containing endospores, ruptured spherules and free endospores. Note the resemblance of the enlarging endospores to *Blastomyces dermititidis.* Sputum (Papanicolaou stain; ×400).

stained specimen of sputum. Culture results were confirmatory.

Another characteristic case is that of a 45-year-old resident from Southern California who presented with a 2-cm nodule in the periphery of the left lower lobe. An FNA was obtained and revealed the classic spherules of coccidioides. A confirmatory thoracotomy was performed.

In a 1986 study Freedman and associates demonstrated the utility of FNA in the diagnosis of pulmonary coccidioidomycosis. In a series of 112 FNAs performed on solitary pulmonary nodules, eight cases were identified as coccidioidomycosis by the presence of spherules in the aspirated material.[166]

Pulmonary Histoplasmosis

The term histoplasmosis actually refers to two different and clinically distinct entities. The more common use of the term is applied to a systemic disease produced by the dimorphic fungus *Histoplasma capsulatum* var. *capsulatum*. A second disease, endemic to Africa and called African histoplasmosis, is produced by infection with *Histoplasma capsulatum* var. *duboisii*. Pulmonary involvement with this disease is much less common than that with *H. capsulatum* var. *capsulatum*. The mycelial phase of the latter organism is found in soil and other areas heavily contaminated with bird droppings. Although it is worldwide in distribution, some highly endemic areas include the Mississippi and Ohio River valleys in the United States, Mexico, Guatemala, Peru and Venezuela. Respiratory infection occurs by inhalation of the highly infectious conidia. Rapid systemic dissemination though infected macrophages may occur. The majority of pulmonary infections are asymptomatic and resolve spontaneously. A minority of patients may develop acute pulmonary disease, systemic disease or chronic pulmonary disease. Disseminated disease has been reported as a complication of lymphoproliferative disease, anticancer chemotherapy, organ transplantation in association with immunosuppressive drugs and AIDS. Young children are more susceptible to disseminated disease. Chronic pulmonary disease mimics tuberculosis with granulomatous inflammation, caseous necrosis, cavitation and fibrosis. A special form of the disease of particular interest to the cytologist is the peripheral "coin" lesion also referred to as histoplasmoma. These lesions are always suspicious signs of carcinomas and must be evaluated. An FNA is an appropriate technique for initial evaluation.

H. capsulatum has been reported in sputum, bronchial washings, FNAs and gastric washings from patients with symptoms. The organism is so small as to make recognition on Papanicolaou-stained specimens difficult. With special staining, particularly methenamine silver, it may be visualized as a 2- to 4-μ round-to-oval, single budding yeast-like organism (Fig. 14–51). For diagnostic purposes it should be intracellular in macrophages or neutrophils. A number of small budding yeasts present as contaminants are remarkable

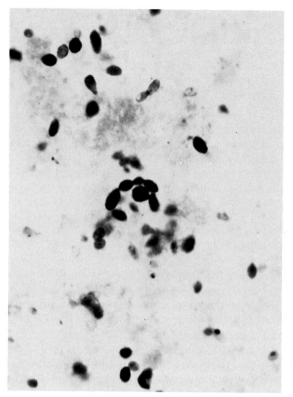

FIGURE 14–51. *Histoplasma capsulatum.* Fine needle aspiration (FNA) of lung (methenamine silver stain; ×1000).

in their resemblance to *Histoplasma;* however, they are usually found extracellularly.[248]

We have seen histoplasmosis in such diverse cytologic specimens as touch preparations from mediastinal lymph nodes, tracheal aspirates from an infant and an FNA from a peripheral subpleural nodule.

Pulmonary Candidiasis

Various species of the genus *Candida,* but most frequently *Candida albicans,* are capable of producing superficial, mucocutaneous and systemic fungal infections in humans. As noted by Chandler and Watts,[74] candidiasis is the most frequently encountered opportunistic fungal infection and accounts for approximately 50% of such infections among immunocompromised patients. In the healthy human, *C. albicans* makes up a part of the flora of the oral cavity, upper respiratory tract, digestive tract and vagina.

Pulmonary candidiasis is almost exclusively a fungal infection that occurs in patients who have underlying disease or who are immunocompromised. The symptoms and signs consist of fever, cough, dyspnea and pulmonary infiltrates on radiography. Because of the frequent presence of *Candida* species in the absence of disease, laboratory confirmation of pulmonary candidiasis is difficult. Positive findings in cultures of sputum and bronchial material may be ambiguous. Conclusive diagnosis of pulmonary infection should be provided either by open biopsy in which microscopic examination provides evidence of parenchymal inva-

sion by organisms or by transthoracic FNA in which organisms are demonstrated and confirmed by cultural identification.

Species of *Candida* are the most frequently encountered fungi in cytologic specimens. Because of this frequency, their clinical significance may be discounted. All *Candida* species may appear as small, oval, 2- to 4-μ budding yeasts. Occasionally, they may elongate into pseudohyphal forms with additional budding at the points of constriction (Fig. 14–52). Although their presence in pulmonary material is not usually significant, it may reflect an overwhelming candidiasis in the compromised host.[248] We have experienced such a situation in an immunocompromised patient in whom the finding of candidal pseudohyphae in a bronchial brushing correlated with a blood culture positive for *Candida albicans.* This patient died 2 days later. Ness and associates[379] have recommended testing bronchoalveolar lavage fluids for *Candida* antigen to distinguish between *Candida* pneumonia and *Candida* colonization of the respiratory tract or oral contamination.

Pulmonary Paracoccidioidomycosis

Paracoccidioidomycosis (South American blastomycosis) is a chronic systemic fungal infection that is caused by the dimorphic pathogen *Paracoccidioides brasiliensis.* The disease is largely confined to Central and South America and has been reported in Mexico,

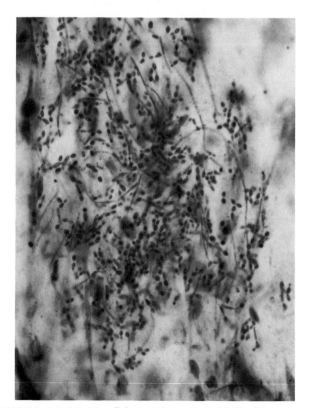

FIGURE 14–52. *Candida sp.* Sputum (Papanicolaou stain; ×400).

Brazil, Colombia and Venezuela. Infection is believed to occur through inhalation of fragments from the mycelial phase. Pulmonary symptoms include cough, hemoptysis, dyspnea, fever, malaise and weight loss. Radiographic changes are nonspecific and may include infiltrates, nodular densities, consolidation and cavitation.[74] The yeast-like phase of the organism is present in the infected tissue and may be seen in cytologic specimens of sputum, bronchial material, BALs and FNAs. The organisms of paracoccidioides are highly characteristic and virtually diagnostic. In alcohol-fixed, Papanicolaou-stained cytologic specimens, the fungus appears as an oval-to-round yeast, measuring 6 to 40 μ in diameter. Multiple budding is characteristic and manifested by many buds attached by their necks to the parent yeast. This appearance has been compared with that of the pilot's wheel of a ship, with the tiny buds corresponding to the handles of the wheel.

In a 1984 study, Tani and Franco,[534] on review of respiratory cytologic material from 45 patients with paracoccidioidomycosis, were able to identify the organisms in more than 95% of the patients.

Pulmonary Aspergillosis

Pulmonary aspergillosis has been defined by Chandler and Watts[74] as a spectrum of pulmonary infections that includes allergic reactions, fungal growth in a preexisting lung cavity, tracheobronchitis, chronic destructive infection of the lung parenchyma and rapidly progressive fungal invasion of the parenchyma and pulmonary vessels. The last is most likely in severely immunocompromised patients.[74]

The causative organisms, members of *Aspergillus* species, are found throughout the world. In descending order of frequency, organisms responsible for infection are *Aspergillus fumigatus*, *A. flavus* and *A. niger*. Pulmonary aspergillosis is acquired through the inhalation of the organism's airborne spores. These spores are quite small, measuring less than 4 μ in diameter, and are capable of reaching the most peripheral parts of the lungs. Because exposure to *Aspergillus* spores is a very common event for all humans and aspergillosis is uncommon, the immune state of the patient is probably the most significant determining factor. The presenting signs and symptoms of a patient with pulmonary aspergillosis will be dependent on the underlying disease and the type of *Aspergillus* infection.

We have observed *Aspergillus* sp. in cytologic specimens of sputum (50% of cases), bronchial washings (23% of cases), bronchial brushings (3% of cases) and FNAs (20% of cases). In Table 14–6 is summarized a sampling of the varieties of aspergillosis as seen in our institution over the past 25 years.

The most characteristic presentation of the organism is that of thick, uniform, septate hyphae 3 to 6 μ in width with 45 degree-angle, brush-like branching (Fig. 14–53). The mycelial growth in pulmonary aspergillosis is only rarely associated with the presence of conidiophores or fruiting heads, so that confusion with phycomycosis may occur. However, fungi producing the

last disease are only rarely septate. The presence of septate, branching hyphae in cytologic material is strong morphologic evidence of infection. Culture findings alone may be positive in the absence of true infection. Occasionally conidiophores may be seen. The morphology of these structures gives *Aspergillus* its name (i.e., aspergillum—a brush or perforated globe for sprinkling holy water). They expand into large vesicles at the end, the surfaces of which are covered with sterigmata bearing long chains of spores (Fig. 14–54). Their presence confirms *Aspergillus* sp. Intracavitary fungus balls of the lung produced by *Aspergillus* as well as other fungi may produce marked cellular atypias easily mistaken for squamous cell carcinoma.[290, 323] Occasionally their presence may be associated with the production of crystals of calcium oxalate.[137, 442] Identification of oxalate crystals in the cytologic specimen may be the first clue to the presence of *Aspergillus*. These crystals are particularly striking in infections with *A. niger*. The following observed case is typical of the many examples of pulmonary aspergillosis that are seen in our laboratory.

A 59-year-old man with a long history of rheumatoid arthritis treated with steroids was admitted with *Salmonella* pneumonia. Specimens obtained from bronchial brushing revealed many branching septate hyphae characteristic for species of *Aspergillus*. Culture findings were positive for *A. fumigatus*.

Pulmonary Mucormycosis

Pulmonary mucormycosis is an opportunistic infection produced by a variety of fungi in the order Mucorales. It has also been referred to as phycomycosis and zygomycosis. The most frequent pathogen cultured from infected patients is *Rhizopus* sp.; however, a number of other organisms have been reported. These include *Mucor*, *Absidia*, *Rhizomucor*, *Cunninghamella*, *Mortierella*, *Saksenaea*, *Syncephalastrum* and *Apophysomyces*. All of these organisms are ubiquitous in nature and some are commonly seen as molds growing on bread, fruit and other foods. Infection may occur when a severely immunocompromised or debilitated patient inhales the sporangiospores. Pulmonary mucormycosis is most commonly observed in patients with acute leukemia or lymphoma. It also occurs in the presence of diabetes mellitus, anticancer chemotherapy, renal failure and severe burns. Infected patients present with fever and pulmonary infiltrates that may progress to infarction and occasionally cavitation. Infarction results because of the propensity of the organism to invade through the walls of the pulmonary vessels and thrombose their lumens.[74]

The cytologic diagnosis of mucormycosis is dependent on the correct recognition of hyphal fragments. Regardless of which organism is producing the infection, the infecting hyphal fragments are quite similar. The hyphae may exhibit considerable variation in size and shape. They may be quite large, varying from 6 to 50 μ in diameter. Branching is at irregular intervals and is usually at right angles. The hyphae are usually

TABLE 14–6. Presentation of Pulmonary Aspergillosis in Cytology

Patient	Underlying Disease	Clinical Presentation	Type of Cytologic Specimen Positive for Organisms	Comments
66 male	Acute myelogenous leukemia	Pulmonary infiltrates	FNA	Chemotherapy
3 female	Immunodeficiency disease	Mass in right upper lobe	FNA	
69 male	Asbestosis	Areas of lung consolidation	FNA	Many ferruginous bodies also present
71 male	Acute myelogenous leukemia	Bilateral pulmonary infiltrates	Sputum	Chemotherapy and steroids
58 male	Malignant lymphoma	Mass in left upper lobe	Bronchial brushings	
20-month old female	Immunodeficiency disease	Bilateral pneumonia	Bronchial washings	
48 female	Adult respiratory distress syndrome	Bilateral air space disease	Sputum	
15 male	Aplastic anemia	Pulmonary infiltrates	Bronchial washings	
31 male	Sarcoidosis	Pulmonary infiltrates	Bronchial brushings	Steroids
59 male	Acute myelogenous leukemia	Pulmonary infiltrates	Bronchial washings	Chemotherapy
75 male	Chronic obstructive pulmonary disease	Pulmonary infiltrates	Sputum	Steroids and oxygen
67 female	Chronic obstructive pulmonary disease	Bronchitis	Sputum	
53 male	Emphysema	Cavity right upper lobe	Sputum	Fruiting heads and oxylate crystals present
62 male	Chronic alcoholism	Mass in right upper lobe	Sputum	
15 female	Löeffler's syndrome	Pneumonia	Sputum	
55 female	Chronic bronchitis	Bronchitis	Sputum	
44 male	Chronic obstructive pulmonary disease	Mass in right upper lobe	Sputum	
64 male	Chronic obstructive pulmonary disease	Multiple lung cavities		Treated with steroids for *Pseudomonas* sepsis
70 male	Small-cell undifferentiated carcinoma	Pneumonia	Bronchial washings	Chemotherapy
59 male	Rheumatoid arthritis and diabetes mellitus	Pneumonia	Sputum	Steroids
60 male	Large-cell undifferentiated carcinoma		Sputum	Fungus growing on surface of tumor

FNA = Fine needle aspiration.

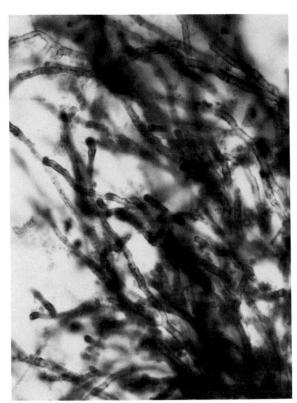

FIGURE 14–53. *Aspergillus.* Typical branching, septate hyphal fragments with parallel cell walls. Sputum (Papanicolaou stain; ×680).

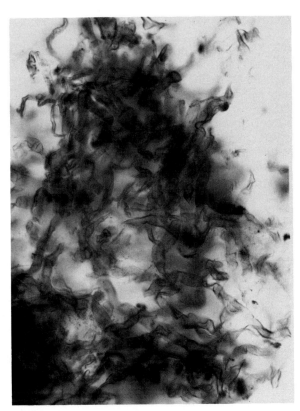

FIGURE 14–55. Mucormycosis. Characteristic branching, ribbon-like hyphal fragments without obvious septa. Bronchial brushing (Papanicolaou stain; ×400).

nonseptate and coenocytic. The tendency of the hyphal fragments to fold and wrinkle gives them a ribbon-like appearance. Because of this as well as their hyaline nature, they may be easily misinterpreted as fragments of plant fibers or other foreign material (Fig. 14–55).

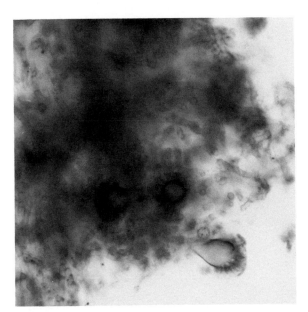

FIGURE 14–54. Fruiting heads of **aspergillus** from a patient with a cavitary squamous cell carcinoma colonized by *Aspergillus fumigatus.* Bronchial washing (Papanicolaou stain; ×520).

Other Fungi

Other fungi that have been implicated in lung infections include *Torulopsis glabrata,* a small yeast-like fungus: *Fusarium spp.* with hyphae resembling those of *Aspergillus; Trichosporon spp.* with small yeast-like cells, septate hyphae and arthrospores; *Geotrichum candidum* with septate hyphae, spheric cells and rectangular arthrospores; *Penicillium sp.* with small round, nonbudding yeast-like cells with transverse septa; *Chrysosporium parvum* var. *crescens* with its very large spheric adiaconidia, etiologic agent of the pulmonary mycosis adiaspiromycosis; *Curvularia sp.* with pigmented hyphae; *Sporothrix schenkii,* with its small ovoid-to-cigar-shaped yeast-like cells, *Petriellidium bovdii,* with septate branching hyphae;[74] *Fonsecaea pedrosoi* cultured from an FNA of pulmonary phaeohyphomycosis;[603] *Penicillium marneffei* in a BAL;[73] *Actinomyces sp.*;[305] and *Alternaria sp.*[434]

Parasitic Infections

A growing number of parasites are being diagnosed in respiratory material. The two most frequent ones, *Pneumocystis carinii* and *Strongyloides stercoralis* are emphasized in this section.[23, 264, 335]

Pneumocystis carinii *Pneumonia*

Prior to 1960, the organism *Pneumocystis carinii* was little more than an academic curiosity. It was rarely diagnosed clinically, and when seen at autopsy, was found to be present almost exclusively in debilitated premature infants. However, in recent years, the incidence of *P. carinii* pneumonia has been increasing and is now recognized as occurring potentially in any situation of impaired immune response.[201] More particularly, it is observed in infants who are premature or debilitated and in patients who have immunologic disorders and immunoglobulin defects and in those who are undergoing therapy with corticosteroids and chemotherapy. The infection has been found with high frequency in patients who have received renal allografts. The infection has also been described as a complication in AIDS.[152, 158, 184, 190, 278, 320, 395, 422, 441, 463] The introduction of effective therapeutic drugs has markedly increased the clinical importance of a diagnosis.[506]

Cytology

On Papanicolaou-stained material, the organisms may be difficult to identify, because their staining may be quite variable and faint. A most typical presentation on the smear is a mass of partially eosinophilic amorphous material. Within this mass may be a suggestion of small superimposed circlets. Although this presentation may or may not be diagnostic for pneumocystis, such material should raise an immediate suspicion of its presence, and the material should be further evaluated by special stains. In such a situation, one would decolorize this slide and restain with methenamine silver. This procedure immediately brings out the diagnostic features of these organisms. On methenamine silver stains the organism is seen mainly as a spheric cyst measuring 6 to 8 μ in diameter or approximately the diameter of an erythrocyte (Fig. 14–56). Certain variations of this form can be seen: the organism can be cup shaped, crescent shaped or crinkled. Depending on the surface of the organism which is exposed to view, small interior structures can be seen that take the forms of rings, dots or commas. Some laboratories prefer to use a Giemsa stain or toluidine blue for identification of this organism. With these stains, one is able to identify up to eight trophozoites occurring within the cyst. These structures are about 0.5 to 1.0 μ in diameter and easily overlooked and may be confused with granules or cell fragments.

A renewed interest has taken place in the initial recognition of *P. carinii* in smears stained by the Papanicolaou method. Greaves and Strigle[190] have described these organisms in such smears as appearing in the form of casts of alveoli. These casts are composed of masses of organisms packed together with a smooth border around the periphery of the masses, representing the molding induced by the alveolar walls. Tinctorial characteristics of these masses vary from eosinophilic to cyanophilic. In our experience, casts may be seen in sputum, bronchial material, BALs and FNAs. They may be extremely numerous in the presence of massive infection such as that seen in patients with

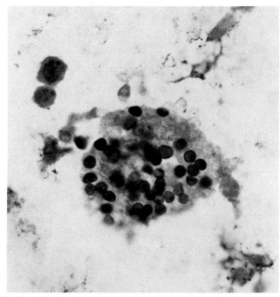

FIGURE 14–56. *Pneumocystis carinii.* Alveolar cast stained with methenamine silver, showing the typical appearance of the cyst form of the organism. Bronchial washing (methenamine silver stain; ×680).

AIDS and are conclusively diagnostic for *P. carinii* (Fig. 14–56 to 14–58). Ghali and associates[184] have reported apple-green fluorescence of these masses in Papanicolaou-stained smears when exposed to ultraviolet light. Chandra and associates[75] have reported the Diff-quik stain to be positive in 76% of cases.[75]

In the literature, one can find reports of success in diagnosing this organism in sputum,[159] tracheal aspirates,[278] washings from the hypopharynx and bronchus, bronchial brushings,[441] BAL[152, 395] and FNA.[261] Among these, BAL has clearly emerged as the one most likely

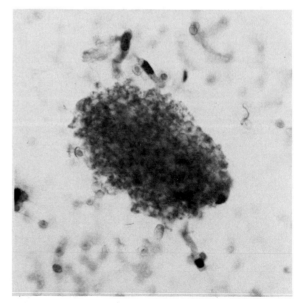

FIGURE 14–57. *Pneumocystis carinii.* A three-dimensional alveolar cast exhibiting the characteristic honeycomb appearance. Bronchial washing (Papanicolaou stain; ×520).

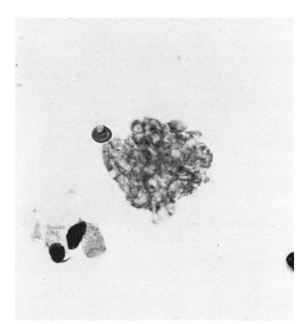

FIGURE 14–58. *Pneumocystis carinii.* Alveolar cast with honeycomb pattern. Bronchial washing (Papanicolaou stain; ×1000).

to yield organisms.[392] Organisms easily confused with pneumocystis are the small budding yeasts, notably *Histoplasma capsulatum*, *Candida sp.* and *Saccharomyces*. The most reliable distinguishing characteristic is the presence of budding. The bronchial brushing illustrated in Figure 14–57 is from a 27-year-old man who was admitted for evaluation of high fever and bilateral pulmonary infiltrates. A typical alveolar cast composed of *Pneumocystis* organisms is depicted. The patient was diagnosed as having AIDS and died 2 weeks later. Figure 14–58 shows a similar cast at higher magnification. The cysts are clearly visible.

Pulmonary Strongyloidiasis

Respiratory infection with *Strongyloides stercoralis*[573] has been found mostly in patients who are receiving very heavy steroid therapy for such conditions as rheumatoid arthritis, renal transplantation and severe asthmatic bronchitis. Pulmonary infection is produced when the filariform larvae migrate through the intestinal wall into the blood stream and finally penetrate into the alveolar spaces. A hemorrhagic pneumonia is produced there. The organisms are readily identified in the bloody sputum expectorated by these patients.[77, 186, 237, 271, 571] The filariform larvae observed measure 400 to 500 μ in length and exhibit a closed gullet and slightly notched tail. In extreme cases, filariform larvae, rhabditiform larvae and ova may all be observed in the alveoli.

Our laboratory has observed five examples of infection of the lower respiratory tract by the filariform larval stage of *Strongyloides stercoralis*. One patient was a 45-year-old man who had received a cadaveric kidney transplantation and because of increasing evidence of renal failure on the third

postoperative day, had been given high-dose steroids. He was readmitted 3 weeks later with cough, dyspnea, abdominal pain and bloody diarrhea. He developed pulmonary edema and transtracheal aspirates revealed filariform larval forms of *S. stercoralis*.

In another case, a 77-year-old man had been treated with 40 mg/day of prednisone for asthma. Sputum cytologic examination revealed both rhabditiform and filariform larvae of *S. stercoralis*. The patient died 2 weeks later and was found at autopsy to have had widely disseminated strongyloidiasis.

In Figure 14–59 is shown the filariform larval stage of *S. stercoralis* from a nematodal infection, which was involving the intestine and lungs of the first patient described. The primary diagnosis was established by cytologic examination of the tracheal aspirates. The organism is identified as being in the filariform larval stage because of its length of 400 to 500 μ and closed gullet. To be considered in the differential diagnosis are *Ascaris lumbricoides* and hookworms, both *Necator americanus* and *Ancylostoma duodenale*. An important criterion in this differential diagnosis is a blunt and slightly notched tail. This is in contrast to the tails of the filariform larvae in both hookworm and *Ascaris*, which are sharply pointed.

Evidence exists that infection of the respiratory tract with *S. stercoralis* was rare prior to the introduction of steroid therapy. Although migration through the respiratory tract is a part of the life cycle of *Strongyloides*, the larvae ordinarily do not linger in the lungs and produce, at most, minor irritation. In the immunosuppressed patient hyperinfection in the gastrointestinal tract occurs, and the organism apparently is capable of mounting a respiratory infection. In autopsies performed at our institution between 1930 and 1975, there

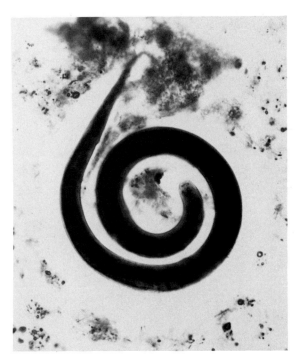

FIGURE 14–59. Filariform larva of ***Strongyloides stercoralis.*** Sputum (methenamine silver stain; ×680).

were only two instances of respiratory infection with *S. stercoralis*. One was in a premature, debilitated infant. The second was in a patient with leukemia who had been treated with steroid therapy. Gocek and associates[186] have reported one case of unsuspected pulmonary strongyloidiasis coexisting with adenocarcinoma of the lung. Vieyra-Herrera and associates[559] from Mexico have reported a fatal pulmonary infection from the parasite in a patient with AIDS.

Pulmonary Dirofilariasis

Dirofilaria immitis is the dog heart worm. Mosquitoes feeding upon the blood of infected dogs ingest the infectious microfilariae. If a human is bitten by such a mosquito, the infective larvae will migrate to the heart and die and will then be carried into pulmonary arteries. There they produce luminal obstruction and infarction. The lesion produced appears on a radiograph as a 2- to 3-cm peripheral nodule. An FNA may show the worm with granulomatous reaction. Seven cases (one diagnosed by FNA) were reported by Ro and associates.[449] Hawkins and associates have also reported one case diagnosed by FNA.[218]

Other Parasites

Also described in the respiratory cytologic literature are diagnoses of pulmonary echinococcosis,[6, 53, 179, 181, 542] *Paragonimus kellicotti*,[345] trichomoniasis,[396] *Entamoeba gingivalis*,[107] *P. westermanii*,[583] microfilaria,[362] *Toxoplasma gondii* and *Cryptosporidium*.[516]

INCONCLUSIVE CYTOLOGIC SPECIMEN

In prior sections of this chapter emphasis has been placed upon those cytologic changes likely to become pitfalls for false-positive cancer diagnoses. Another major issue that must be addressed in the laboratory control of diagnostic accuracy is that regarding the significance of inconclusive cytologic diagnoses, or those diagnoses in which the cytologic study is unable to confirm conclusively the presence of cancer or to rule it out in the specimen.

The scientific literature on cytology of the respiratory tract is ambiguous on this subject. Some investigators in the past have chosen either to ignore these inconclusive diagnoses in their studies or to group them together with positive cancer diagnoses. Others have recorded them but did not evaluate them. One of us (WWJ) has studied 205 patients in whose cytologic specimens of sputum or bronchial material some variety of an inconclusive diagnosis had been made.[249] These data are summarized in Tables 14–4 through 14–6. The most frequent inconclusive diagnoses made were either "atypical squamous metaplasia" or "atypical cells suspicious for malignancy." In 70 patients, a cytologic diagnosis of atypical metaplasia was made. In 28 of these patients, or 40% of the group, this diagnosis was followed by a tissue confirmation of cancer (see Table 14–4). In nearly one third of these, the cancer was a squamous cell carcinoma with the other neoplasms scattered through a variety of other tumor types. In the remaining 42 patients, the follow-up studies revealed the presence of some variety of non-neoplastic disease, usually inflammatory in origin (see Table 14–5). In these patients various types of pneumonias comprised the most frequently associated category of disease. Some 135 patients had originally been given a cytologic diagnosis of "atypical cells suspicious for malignancy." In 92, or approximately 68% of these patients, this suspicion of cancer was confirmed by tissue examination. In 43 patients, or approximately 32%, no cancer was found. In this last group of patients, the most common underlying disease process was pneumonia (see Table 14–6).

Risse and associates[448] evaluated the significance of severe dysplasia in sputum samples. They defined dysplasia as the presence of atypical squamous metaplastic cells with an increased nucleocytoplasmic ratio, hyperchromasia and irregular nuclear shape. In a group of 46 patients with diagnoses of severe dysplasia on sputum, follow-up showed a malignant process in 21 patients (46%).[448]

In 1964 Koss and associates[291] reported cytologic results obtained on 1886 patients for two 1-month periods. Of these, 362 patients were proved to have cancer. A total of 63 diagnoses of "suspicious" (for cancer) were rendered. Of these, 38 or 60.3% were among the proven cancer group. Among the possible sources for diagnostic error, these investigators noted viral pneumonitis, prior radiation, hyperplasia of bronchial lining, aspergilloma and human error or judgment based upon insufficient evidence.[291]

PATHOLOGY OF LUNG CANCER

The major focus of respiratory cytology is the diagnosis of lung cancer. Thus, a chapter of this type would not be complete without a discussion of this all too common disease. Although the information provided in this section is but a brief overview of the vast literature on carcinoma of the lung, the clinical, epidemiologic and morphologic features discussed here should provide a useful context, within which the cytologic diagnosis of lung cancer may be considered.

Carcinoma of the lung is now reported to be the most commonly diagnosed noncutaneous malignancy in the world.[209, 297] In the United States, it has long been recognized as the leading cause of death from cancer in males.[598] According to relatively recent estimates, it is now emerging as the most common cause of death from malignancy in females.[493] The overall incidence of carcinoma of the lung continues to increase, and it is estimated that for the next year, more than 155,000 new cases will be diagnosed in this country and over 142,000 patients will die of the disease.[493]

Overwhelming clinical, epidemiologic and experimental evidence exists implicating cigarette smoking in the etiology of lung cancer.[18, 21, 165, 602] Approximately 80 to 85% of lung cancer deaths are attributed to smoking.[148] Although the association is strongest for squamous cell carcinomas and small-cell undifferentiated carcinomas, even in the case of adenocarcinoma, most patients are cigarette smokers.[11] Other factors, which have been implicated in the development of lung cancer, include asbestos exposure, for which a synergistic effect with cigarette smoking has been described,[507] radon exposure,[188, 432] nickel,[27] arsenic,[397] beryllium[564] and vinyl chloride.[575]

Although all major types of lung carcinoma are believed to arise within the epithelium that lines the respiratory tract, the *in situ* carcinomas that have been identified are largely those of the squamous type.[18, 64] They are thought to arise in a progressive epithelial dysplasia occurring in metaplastic squamous epithelium.[18] Areas of atypical epithelial proliferation occurring in association with adenocarcinomas have been observed,[354] suggesting that such areas may give rise to adenocarcinoma. Attempts to identify an *in situ* lesion of small-cell undifferentiated carcinoma, however, have been unsuccessful.[473] The not uncommon occurrence of heterogeneity in lung cancer,[3, 440, 455] as evidenced by the existence of adenosquamous carcinomas and combined small-cell/large-cell carcinomas, would lend support to the theory that lung carcinomas arise from precursor cells of endodermal origin, capable of expressing one or more patterns of cellular differentiation.[3, 599] The previous claims of a separate neural crest origin[407] for small-cell carcinoma would appear unfounded, in view of the occurrence of mixed small-cell/large-cell carcinomas and in light of the observation by Yesner[600] that small-cell undifferentiated carcinomas may convert, over a period of time, to large-cell carcinomas.

Table 14–7 shows a classification, modified from that of the World Health Organization (WHO)[294] and the

TABLE 14–7. Histologic Classification of Major Neoplasms of the Lung

Squamous cell carcinoma
Well-differentiated
Moderately differentiated
Poorly differentiated
Adenocarcinoma
Acinar
Papillary
Bronchioloalveolar
Large-cell undifferentiated carcinoma
Giant cell
Small-cell undifferentiated carcinoma
Oat cell
Intermediate
Combined
Adenosquamous carcinoma
Bronchial gland carcinoma
Adenoid cystic
Mucoepidermoid
Carcinoid
Metastatic tumors

Armed Forces Institute of Pathology Fasicle[69] on malignant epithelial tumors of the lung. Squamous cell carcinomas are characterized by histologic findings that mimic, to a greater or lesser degree, the features of normal squamous epithelium (Figs. 14–60 and 14–61). These include keratinization, which is manifested by the presence of either keratin pearls or individually keratinized cells, and so-called intercellular bridges, which are spicules of cytoplasm observed at the sites of desmosomal junctions. In well-differentiated neoplasms, these features are identified without difficulty, whereas in poorly differentiated tumors, they are much less common, with the predominant histologic pattern consisting of nests and sheets of undifferentiated cells. (Fig. 14–62). Areas of squamous dysplasia or carcinoma *in situ* may be observed in the adjacent bronchial epithelium (Fig. 14–63). Electron microscopy of these tumors reveals, in addition to desmosomes, variable numbers of cytoplasmic tonofilament bundles.[112]

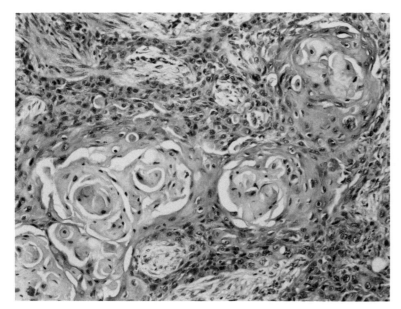

FIGURE 14–60. Keratinizing squamous cell carcinoma with keratin pearl formation. Pulmonary resection (hematoxylin and eosin; ×130).

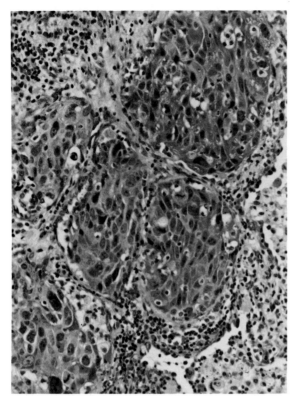

FIGURE 14–61. Moderately differentiated squamous cell carcinoma. Pulmonary resection (hematoxylin and eosin; ×170).

Although primary peripheral squamous cell carcinomas have been described,[60] the majority occur centrally,[11] arising in the segmental, lobar or main stem bronchi. These neoplasms frequently attain a large size[28, 60] and tend to occur with pneumonia due to bronchial obstruction. They are much more likely to undergo central necrosis with cavitation than are the other types of lung cancer.[78, 515] The prognosis for squamous cell carcinoma, although poor, is nevertheless somewhat better than that for other lung carcino-

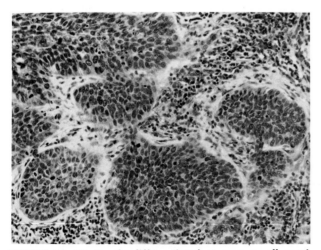

FIGURE 14–62. Poorly differentiated squamous cell carcinoma. Pulmonary resection (hematoxylin and eosin; ×170).

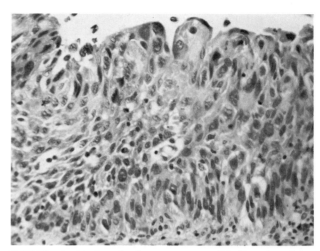

FIGURE 14–63. Dysplastic squamous epithelium in a bronchus. This field was adjacent to an area of invasive squamous cell carcinoma. Pulmonary resection (hematoxylin and eosin; ×250).

mas,[177] in part because of its tendency to metastasize later than other types.[577] Patients with well-differentiated keratinizing squamous cell carcinomas tend to fare better than those with poorly differentiated tumors.

Adenocarcinomas have been recognized for many years as the most common type of lung cancer occurring in females.[561] In later years, these tumors have been diagnosed with increasing frequency, to the point that in some series, they are the most commonly diagnosed type of lung carcinoma.[95, 554, 560] Although part of this increase may result from the broadened WHO definition of adenocarcinomas[294] and the relative increase in the number of women with lung cancer, as some have suggested,[560] other workers have demonstrated an increased incidence independent of these factors.[95]

Histologically, adenocarcinomas may be characterized by the presence of glandular structures (Fig. 14–64), papillary structures, a bronchioloalveolar pattern, or histochemically documented mucin production in tumors with a solid pattern.[294] A bronchioloalveolar pattern is defined as growth of cuboidal or columnar tumor cells along alveolar or fibrovascular septa (Figs. 14–65 to 14–68).[333] Distinction of this pattern from a papillary pattern is frequently arbitrary. Although adenocarcinoma may be divided into acinar, papillary and bronchioloalveolar subtypes, based upon the predominant pattern, mixed acinar and papillary (or bronchioloalveolar) areas frequently occur within the same tumor.[294, 601] Ultrastructurally, all types of pulmonary adenocarcinomas can exhibit a variety of features, including those reminiscent of goblet cells, bronchiolar (Clara) cells or type II pneumocytes.[280]

The majority of adenocarcinomas occur in the periphery of the lung[36] and frequently involve the overlying pleura. Scarring is a common finding in adenocarcinomas[36] and has led some to suggest that it represents a predisposing factor for the development of malignancy.[16] In some circumstances, such as diffuse

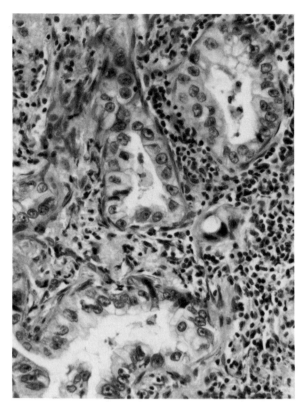

FIGURE 14–64. Acinar adenocarcinoma. Lung biopsy (hematoxylin and eosin; ×250).

interstitial fibrosis, it is apparent that scarring predates the neoplasm.[354] However, the bulk of the literature would indicate that in most cases, the scarring occurs as a response to the tumor.[61, 330, 490]

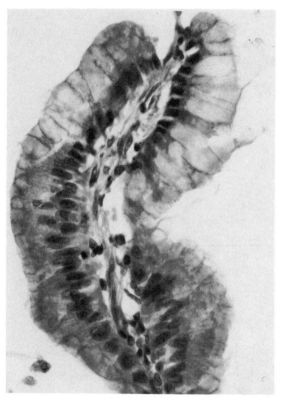

FIGURE 14–66. Bronchioloalveolar carcinoma, mucinous (type I). Lung resection (hematoxylin and eosin; ×400).

Bronchioloalveolar carcinoma (BAC) is a heterogeneous group of neoplasms[37, 85, 113, 118, 125, 313, 333, 356] characterized by a predominant pattern of growth of cylindric tumor cells along alveolar or fibrovascular septa.[294]

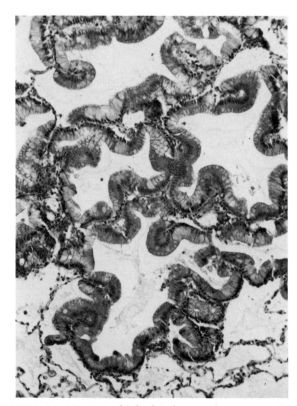

FIGURE 14–65. Bronchioloalveolar carcinoma, mucinous (type I). Lung resection (hematoxylin and eosin; ×100).

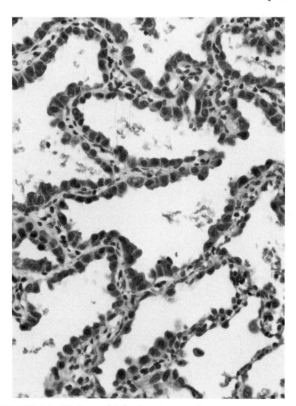

FIGURE 14–67. Bronchioloalveolar carcinoma, nonmucinous (type II). Lung resection (hematoxylin and eosin; ×250).

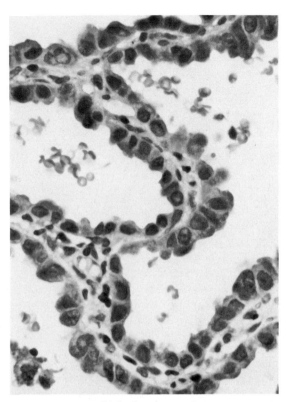

FIGURE 14–68. Bronchioloalveolar carcinoma, nonmucinous (type II). Lung resection (hematoxylin and eosin; ×520).

A similar histologic pattern may be produced by adenocarcinomas metastatic from the stomach, pancreas, colon and kidney, and consequently one must exclude such tumors before an unequivocal diagnosis of BAC can be rendered.[467] The radiographic appearance of BAC may be that of a solitary nodule; multiple, often bilateral nodules or a diffuse infiltrate, so that except for the solitary nodule it may radiographically mimic metastatic cancer in bilateral nodules and pneumonitis a in diffuse infiltrate.[356] The multinodular pattern has been attributed to aerogenous spread of tumor cells within the lung.[313] Two histologic types of bronchioloalveolar carcinoma have been described: a mucinous variety, characterized by tall columnar cells with abundant intracellular and extracellular mucin (type I) (see Figs. 14–65 and 14–66) and a nonmucinous type, which lacks obvious mucin production and instead is characterized by cuboidal or columnar cells, typically arranged along the septa in a hobnail-like fashion (type II) (see Figs. 14–67 and 14–68).[118, 333] By electron microscopy, the former exhibit features of goblet cells,[34, 193, 280] whereas the latter show similarities to Clara cells and type II pneumocytes.[2, 89, 193, 241, 262, 280, 296, 492]

The prognosis of adenocarcinomas overall is somewhat worse than that of squamous cell carcinomas,[177] despite the higher rate of resectability of the former.[11,36] This is in part due to the tendency of adenocarcinomas to metastasize earlier in their course.[577] As a group, bronchioloalveolar carcinomas do not differ significantly in prognosis from other adenocarcinomas.[37] However, those patients presenting with bronchioloalveolar carcinomas occurring as solitary nodules have a

considerably better prognoses,[333, 356] with a reported 5-year survival of approximately 60%.[85] It has been suggested that nonmucinous (type II) differentiation may be a useful predictor of improved survival,[333] although it would appear that the presence or absence of aerogenous spread is more important than cell type in this regard.[85]

The term large-cell undifferentiated carcinoma encompasses those primary nonsmall-cell carcinomas, which lack histologic evidence of either adenomatous or squamous differentiation (Fig. 14–69).[294] When examined by electron microscopy, most cases show evidence of differentiation, more commonly adenomatous (i.e., junctional complexes and intercellular or intracellular lumens lined by microvilli) than squamous;[5, 82, 110, 230] a few show neuroendocrine features[110] and the remainder lack specific findings. Such ultrastructural evidence of differentiation, however, appears to have no bearing on survival.[5] Large-cell undifferentiated carcinoma, in general, has a poorer prognosis for the patient than either adenocarcinoma or squamous cell carcinoma.[5, 391]

Giant cell carcinoma (Fig. 14–70), a variant of large-cell undifferentiated carcinoma, is characterized by the presence of pleomorphic multinucleated giant tumor cells.[369] Neutrophils are often observed within the cytoplasm of these cells. A similar histologic appearance may result when neoplasms of other types are treated by radiation. Giant cell carcinomas arising in the pancreas, liver, thyroid and other organs may metastasize to the lung. The prognosis for the patient

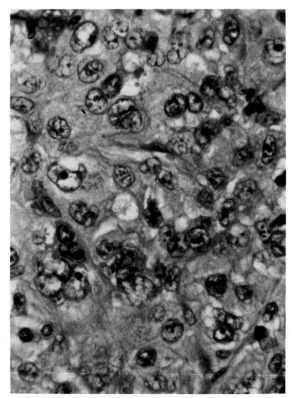

FIGURE 14–69. Large-cell undifferentiated carcinoma. Lobectomy specimen (hematoxylin and eosin; ×520).

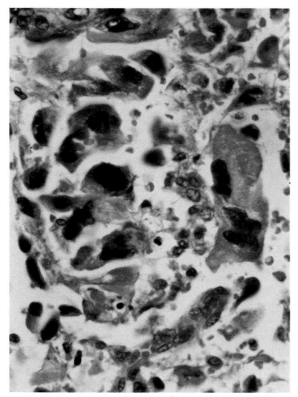

FIGURE 14–70. Giant cell carcinoma. Pulmonary resection (hematoxylin and eosin; ×680).

with giant cell carcinoma is extremely poor.[369, 569] Lipford and associates[317] have suggested that the presence of tumor giant cells in limited stage lung cancer is predictive of an unfavorable outcome, regardless of the differentiation of the rest of the tumor, although this observation has not been confirmed by others.[126] Adenosquamous carcinomas contain, by definition, significant areas of both glandular and squamous differentiation.[294] Although in several studies they compose less than 5% of lung carcinomas,[12, 149, 275] they are diagnosed with greater frequency when tumors are extensively sampled.[455] Adenosquamous carcinomas tend to occur more peripherally than do squamous cell carcinomas[149] and their behavior is reportedly similar to that of adenocarcinomas.[68] If ultrastructural criteria are used, many squamous cell carcinomas, adenocarcinomas and large-cell undifferentiated carcinomas would be reclassified as adenosquamous carcinomas.[14]

Small-cell undifferentiated carcinoma of the lung has been subdivided into three types, based upon cytologic features: the oat-cell type, intermediate cell type and combined small-cell/large-cell type.[294] Cells of oat-cell carcinoma are approximately twice the size of lymphocytes and possess scanty cytoplasm, a high nuclear to cytoplasmic ratio, nuclear hyperchromasia with finely dispersed granular chromatin and absent or inconspicuous nucleoli (Fig. 14–71). Mitotic figures and necrosis are usually present. In areas of cell degeneration, the nuclei appear pyknotic and exhibit a characteristic molding against each other. In bronchial biopsies, crush artifact is frequently present and is sometimes so pronounced as to render the biopsy uninterpretable.

Better-preserved areas will reveal sheets of cells with occasional perivascular pseudorosettes.[600]

The cells of the intermediate cell variant show a chromatin pattern similar to that of the oat-cell type but have larger nuclei with more abundant cytoplasm (Fig. 14–72) and not infrequently exhibit distinct nucleoli.[63] In some cases, spindle-shaped cells may predominate.[63] Combined small-cell undifferentiated carcinomas include those cases that contain components of both small-cell undifferentiated carcinoma and large-cell carcinoma (squamous, large-cell undifferentiated or adenocarcinoma).[56, 294] By electron microscopy, a few dense core neurosecretory granules may be demonstrated in most cases of small-cell undifferentiated carcinoma[122] and some may show ultrastructural evidence of squamous or glandular differentiation.[83] The latter findings, however, should not alter the histologic diagnosis.

Most patients with small-cell undifferentiated carcinoma present with disseminated disease and consequently are not considered surgical candidates.[63] Combination chemotherapy has brought about some prolongation of life, but the overall 2-year survival is only about 5%.[63] Although some have suggested otherwise,[106, 388] it would appear that the intermediate cell variant does not differ significantly in behavior from the oat-cell type.[211, 228, 343] The prognosis of the combined small-cell undifferentiated carcinomas is said to be similar to,[211] or worse than,[228, 433] that of the other

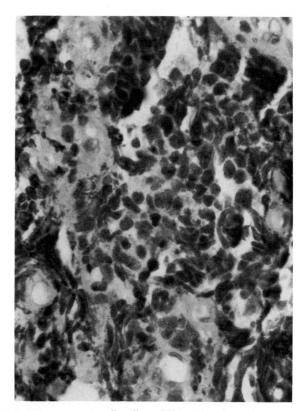

FIGURE 14–71. Small-cell undifferentiated carcinoma, oat cell type. Note the prominent nuclear molding and areas of crush artifact. Bronchial biopsy (hematoxylin and eosin; ×680).

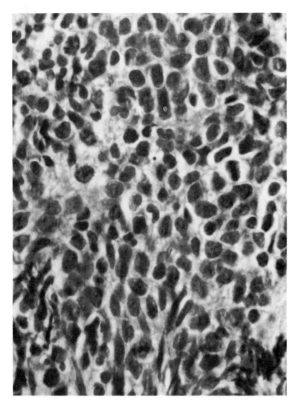

FIGURE 14–72. Small-cell undifferentiated carcinoma, intermediate cell type. The cytoplasm is more abundant than in the oat cell variety. Some nuclei have a fusiform shape. These are visible nucleoli. Bronchial biopsy (hematoxylin and eosin; ×680).

types. Because the therapeutic approach to small-cell undifferentiated carcinoma may differ significantly from that of the nonsmall-cell carcinoma, accurate histologic and cytologic distinction between these two groups is of paramount importance.

Lung cancer may come to clinical presentation by a variety of signs and symptoms, the most common of which are weight loss, cough, dyspnea, weakness, chest pain and hemoptysis.[11, 84] In other situations, an opacity on a chest radiograph may be the first clue to the presence of a neoplasm. In one series of 955 cases, nearly half of all "coin lesions" observed by radiography were malignant and most of these (78%) were primary lung cancers.[543] Some patients may present with symptoms related to ectopic hormone production. The syndromes of inappropriate antidiuretic hormone production and Cushing's syndrome are most closely associated with small-cell undifferentiated carcinoma, whereas hypercalcemia due to production of a parathyroid-like hormone has been described with squamous cell carcinoma.[599]

Carcinoma of the lung tends to spread initially via lymphatics to regional lymph nodes and hematogenously to distant organs, most commonly the liver, adrenals, bone and brain.[601] By far the most important factor for predicting prognosis of these tumors is stage,[192] as determined by tumor size, lymph node involvement and presence or absence of distant metastases.[361] Histologic features reported to be associated

with survival include cell type, as previously discussed, vascular invasion,[90] presence or absence of a plasmacytic infiltrate[317] and extent of tumor necrosis.[126]

CYTOLOGY OF LUNG CANCER

At the present time, most of the major medical institutions throughout the world utilize some variety or combination of different cytologic specimens in the diagnostic workup of a patient with suspected lung cancer. Sputum continues to be the most frequently examined specimen, but bronchial washings and brushings, BALs and FNAs are gaining positions in the use of cytology. These procedures used appropriately in concert have the capability of both diagnosing and classifying correctly the vast majority of the common lung neoplasms. Sputum examined as multiple specimens will detect the more central tumors, whereas bronchial brushings and FNAs will detect the remaining ones, usually occurring as the more peripheral or even subpleural lesions. Recalling the histogenesis of primary lung cancers is very persuasive as an aid in comprehending exactly why it is that cytologic diagnosis of the respiratory tract has been so successful. It is mainly because most primary lung cancers arise from the epithelium lining the respiratory passages and have the potential of shedding cancer cells into specimens of sputum or of having their cells harvested for cytologic diagnosis by methods of fiberoptic bronchoscopy, BAL or FNA.[72, 111, 161, 294]

As an example of the distribution of lung tumors likely to be encountered in a large laboratory of cytology and surgical pathology, a summary of several large series including the experience of our laboratory is presented in Table 14–8. Our experience includes the major types of lung cancer and their relative frequencies based on a combination of cytologic and histologic diagnoses. The relative incidence of adenocarcinoma was noted to increase, and the absolute incidence of lung cancer in women also increased, corresponding to trends observed elsewhere.

Squamous Cell Carcinoma

Squamous Cell Carcinoma In Situ

Squamous cell carcinoma of the lung is the only malignant tumor of the lung for which a preinvasive or *in situ* phase has been well documented.[48] Although our knowledge of the histogenesis of this tumor is still quite rudimentary, some basis exists for the belief that squamous cell carcinoma of the lung shares with its counterpart in the uterine cervix a demonstrable preinvasive stage of development in which the epithelium of the tracheobronchial tree undergoes a series of alterations, which can be morphologically classified as atypical metaplasia or dysplasia and carcinoma *in situ*.

A number of reports in the literature have documented the cytologic manifestations of these biologic events.[352, 355] Saccomanno,[473–477] in his cytologic studies

TABLE 14–8. Histologic Classification and Relative Incidence of Lung Cancer

Histologic Type	Percent Distribution				
	Armed Forces Institute of Pathology[69]	*Roswell Park*[560]	*Mayo Clinic*[591]	*Memorial-Sloan Kettering*[150, 351]	*Duke University*
Squamous cell carcinoma	40	38	30	33	39
Adenocarcinoma	(20)	(27)	24	45	(27)
Acinar	17	24			22
Bronchioloalveolar	3	3			5
Large-cell undifferentiated carcinoma	20	9	19	6	17
Small-cell undifferentiated carcinoma	20	19	26	16	16
Adenosquamous carcinoma	1	1			1

on cigarette-smoking uranium miners, has reported the progression of dysplastic changes in metaplastic epithelium to carcinoma *in situ* and invasive carcinoma. He divided the observed cellular changes into the categories of regular metaplasia, mildly atypical metaplasia, moderately atypical metaplasia, markedly atypical metaplasia, carcinoma *in situ* and invasive carcinoma. Using similar criteria, Nasiell and associates[375] have described increasing degrees of aneuploidy that suggest progression toward neoplasia.[375] Unfortunately little published data are available that give information on progression and regression rates between these atypias and invasive cancer.

The extent to which cytologic techniques are capable of contributing to the detection of these preinvasive lesions is being evaluated most effectively in three major screening projects for the early detection of lung cancer in high risk populations. Under the sponsorship of the National Cancer Institute, a Cooperative Early Lung Cancer Group (Memorial Sloan-Kettering, Johns Hopkins and Mayo Clinic) has been examining the usefulness of prolonged surveillance of persons without clinical or radiographic evidence of lung cancer but with increased risk for developing the disease.[127, 150, 154, 351, 588] For example, the participants admitted to the Mayo Clinic Lung Project were enrolled from a group of asymptomatic men of 45 years of age or older at increased risk of lung cancer because of their smoking histories. The project design called for an initial chest radiograph and sputum cytology (3-day pooled sputum) three times per year. To date these studies have led to the detection of 58 *in situ* or early invasive carcinomas. The investigators conclude from such studies that cytologic techniques are of proven value in screening programs for the detection of *in situ* squamous cell carcinomas and that conservative surgical resection of such cases is associated with a remarkably high cure rate for the disease.[588]

In specimens of sputum the cells shed from *in situ* squamous cell carcinoma appear as single small cells of round-to-oval shape. The cytoplasm frequently is densely keratinized, and the nuclei show obvious malignant features including nuclear enlargement with increased nucleocytoplasmic ratios, irregularity of the nuclear membranes and dense hyperchromasia. Nucleoli may be present. Although some variation in cell size and shape occurs, it is much less striking than the

bizarre extremes in pleomorphism seen in invasive squamous cell carcinoma. Most cases will also fail to show the necrosis and inflammatory exudate more frequently observed in advanced invasive lesions (Fig. 14–73). Occasionally one may encounter a population of uniform cells possessing a densely granular chromatin and thin rim of cytoplasm virtually indistinguishable from those cells shedding from a carcinoma *in situ* of the uterine cervix. It is agreed by most investigators, however, that *in situ* squamous cancers of the lung do not shed a population of cells that would permit an accurate distinction from invasive cancer. Bronchial brushings may yield small tissue fragments or microbiopsies of carcinoma *in situ*. The cytology of squamous cell carcinoma *in situ* has been described in detail by Woolner,[588] Erozan and Frost,[127–129] Koss,[290] Kato and associates,[269] Hayata[217] and Koprowska and associates.[286]

Invasive Squamous Cell Carcinoma

Invasive squamous cell carcinomas usually exfoliate large numbers of diagnostic neoplastic cells into the

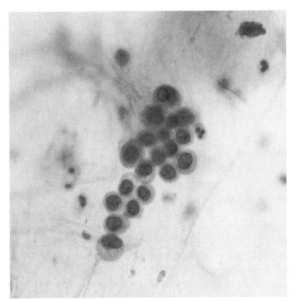

FIGURE 14–73. Squamous cell carcinoma *in situ*. Sputum (Papanicolaou stain; × 400).

sputum, washings or brushings. In sputum the neo-plastic cells occur singly and in loose clusters (Fig. 14–74). Tissue fragments are rare. Intact keratin pearls and intercellular bridges, although important in the histologic diagnosis of squamous cell carcinoma, are uncommonly observed. Marked cellular pleomorphism is characteristic of these tumors. Bizarre cytoplasmic shapes of almost infinite variety may occur. Classic forms such as the caudate or "tadpole" cell (Fig. 14–75), the fiber or spindle cell (Fig. 14–76) and the "third-type" cell similar in morphology to that seen in squamous cell carcinoma of the cervix are present (Fig. 14–77). The nuclei exhibit enlargement and marked hyperchromasia with a tendency toward pyknosis. When the chromatin pattern is preserved, it is arranged into irregular, sharp-bordered clumps with abnormal clearing of the parachromatin. As a result of the densely staining chromatin, nucleoli are observed less frequently than in other types of malignant neoplasms. They may, however, be conspicuously large in some cells. Their presence is more frequently associated with squamous cell carcinomas of a lesser degree of differ-entiation. Nucleocytoplasmic ratios may range from extremely high to very low owing to the marked variability in the amount of cytoplasm produced by these neoplastic cells. Keratinization of the cytoplasm is indicated by an intense hyaline appearance with either a bright orangeophilic staining or a deep cyano-

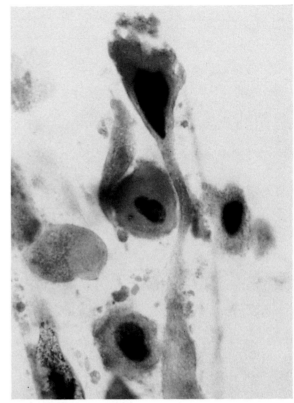

FIGURE 14–75. Keratinizing squamous cell carcinoma. Tad-pole cell (caudate cell). Sputum (Papanicolaou stain; ×1000).

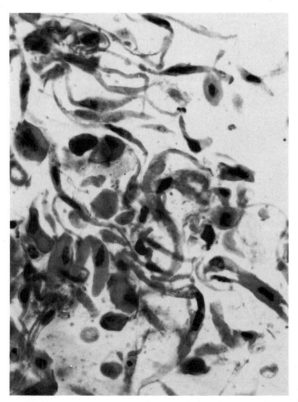

FIGURE 14–74. Keratinizing squamous cell carcinoma. At low magnification, numerous spindle cells and other cells with bizarre shapes are seen. Note the striking hyperchromasia of the nuclei, the dyscohesion and the hard-appearing cyto-plasm. Sputum (Papanicolaou stain; ×400).

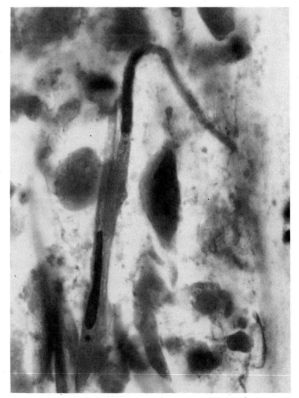

FIGURE 14–76. Keratinizing squamous cell carcinoma. Fiber cells. Sputum (Papanicolaou stain; ×1000).

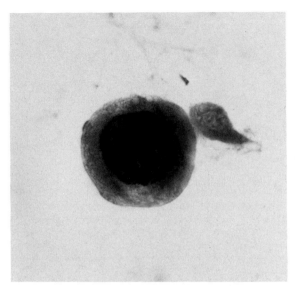

FIGURE 14–77. Keratinizing squamous cell carcinoma. "Third" type cell. Saccomanno sputum (Papanicolaou stain; ×1000).

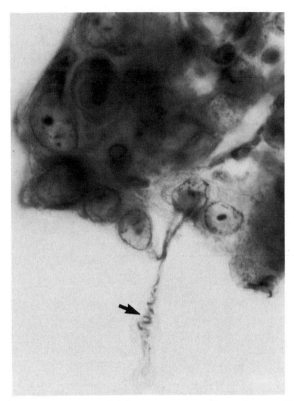

FIGURE 14–78. Keratinizing squamous cell carcinoma. Depicted is a twisting (arrow) between the keratinized and nonkeratinized cytoplasmic interface (Herxheimer's spiral). Sputum (Papanicolaou stain; ×400).

philia. Ectoendoplasmic ringing or the Herxheimer spirals (Fig. 14–78), as described by Frost,[168] is another striking feature of abnormal keratinization in the cytoplasm. These cytologic features are summarized in Table 14–9. In bronchial specimens and FNAs, keratinizing squamous cell carcinomas exhibit findings similar to those observed in sputum, although tissue fragments are more common.

As the differentiation of the squamous cell carcinoma decreases, nuclear and cytoplasmic features of squamous differentiation are less apparent (Figs. 14–79 to 14–81). In sputum, poorly differentiated squamous cell carcinomas appear as single cells and cell clusters, whereas in bronchial brushing specimens and FNAs, there is a noticeable tendency towards formation of large irregular sheets of cells.[45a] The only cytologic evidence of squamous differentiation may lie

TABLE 14–9. Well-Differentiated Squamous Cell Carcinoma

Cytology Feature	Sputum	Bronchial Wash	Bronchial Brush	BAL	FNA
1. Single cells	+	+	+	+	+
2. Striking pleomorphism of cell outline	+	+	+	+	+
3. Chromatin irregularly dispersed and densely hyperchromatic	+	+	+	+	+
4. Karyopyknosis	+	−	−	−	−
5. Nucleoli inconspicuous or absent	+	−	−	−	−
6. Nucleoli obscured by dense chromatin	+	−	−	−	−
7. Cytoplasm intensely orangeophilic and hyaline	+	+	−	+	−
8. Aberrant shapes	+	+	+	+	+
9. Ecto endoplasm, refractile ringing and sharp cytoplasmic outlines	+	−	−	−	−
10. Irregular cytoplasmic thinning manifested as caudate cells and spindle cells	+	+	+	+	+
11. Keratinized squamous ghosts	+	+	+	+	+
12. Keratin pearls	±	−	−	−	±
13. Small tissue fragments	−	−	+	−	+
14. Large irregular sheets	−	−	+	−	+
15. Inflammation and necrosis	+	−	−	−	+
16. Herxheimer spirals	+	+	+	+	+

BAL = bronchoalveolar lavage; FNA = fine needle aspiration.

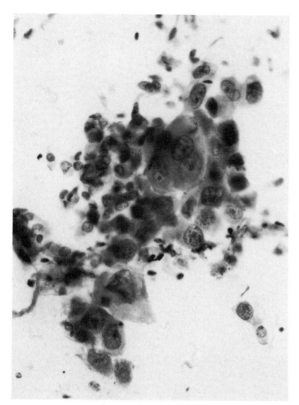

FIGURE 14–79. Moderately differentiated squamous cell carcinoma. Note the sharply defined cytoplasmic borders of many of the tumor cells and the large size of the nuclei in comparison to those of the bronchial epithelial cells. Bronchial brushing (Papanicolaou stain; ×400).

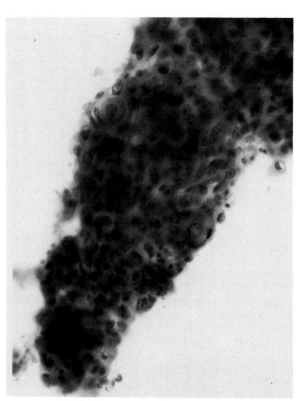

FIGURE 14–81. Poorly differentiated squamous cell carcinoma. Within this sheet of cells, small squamous pearls can be observed. Fine needle aspiration (FNA) of lung (Papanicolaou stain; ×325).

in the sharp appearance of the cytoplasmic borders and in the tendency of the cells to form a monolayer. The cytoplasm of these cells is generally cyanophilic. Because of sampling, cells of squamous cell carcinoma

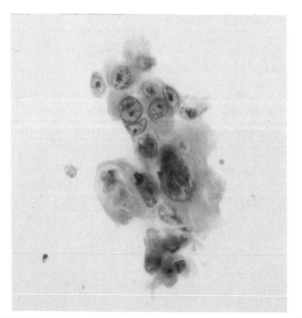

FIGURE 14–80. Moderately differentiated squamous cell carcinoma. Sputum (Papanicolaou stain; ×400).

obtained by bronchial brushing or fine needle aspiration may exhibit less differentiation than those observed in sputum from the same patient. Cytologic features of poorly differentiated squamous cell carcinoma are listed in Table 14–10.

In FNAs from squamous cell carcinomas, the specimen will reflect the degree of differentiation and tissue preservation present at the site of the needle tip. When necrotic tumor with large masses of keratinized squamous ghosts dominate the cytologic picture, aspiration of a more peripheral portion of the tumor will increase the chance of obtaining diagnostic tumor cells.

A unique cytologic picture may be produced in sputum when a keratinizing squamous cell carcinoma cavitates by extruding its necrotic core into the bronchial lumen.[78] This picture has been described in detail by Lavoie and associates.[303] The background is extremely necrotic with keratinized ghosts and an intense inflammatory reaction. Markedly pleomorphic degenerating tumor cells with karyopyknosis is abundant. Cavitary squamous cell carcinoma must be differentiated from a cavitary fungus ball as discussed in the infectious disease section of this chapter. In the fungus ball, the specimen will reveal atypical metaplastic cells, some severely atypical, rather than truly malignant cells. Careful search of the specimen may reveal the causative organism. It must be remembered, however, that fungus balls may also arise in cavitary squamous carcinomas.

TABLE 14–10. Poorly Differentiated Squamous Cell Carcinoma

Cytologic Feature	Sputum	Bronchial Wash	Bronchial Brush	BAL	FNA
1. Mixture of single pleomorphic cells and tissue fragments	+	+	+	+	+
2. Chromatin irregularly dispersed and hyperchromatic	+	+	+	+	+
3. Prominent nucleoli	+	+	+	+	
4. Cytoplasm hyaline but cyanophilic	+	+	+	+	+
5. Some tendency of cytoplasm to form refractile ringing	+	+	+	+	+
6. Large irregular sheets	−	−	+	±	
7. Occasional cell may show orangeophilia	+	+	+	+	+

BAL = bronchoalveolar lavage; FNA = fine needle aspiration.

Squamous metaplasia with dysplasia is distinguished from keratinizing squamous cell carcinoma by the lesser degree of atypia in the former. In sputum, plant cells (see Fig. 14–43) may occasionally mimic keratinizing squamous cell carcinoma. Sheets of reactive or reparative epithelium exhibiting prominent nucleoli and variation in nuclear size can be distinguished from poorly differentiated squamous cell carcinoma by the more uniform chromatin and nuclear membranes, the maintenance of cell polarity within groups and the paucity or absence of single cells in the reactive cases.[45]

Adenocarcinoma

Depending on their location and size, adenocarcinomas may exfoliate large numbers of diagnostic cells, few cells or no cells at all. Small peripheral tumors are least likely to provide diagnostic material in sputum or bronchial specimens. Although the cellular pattern reflective of the adenocarcinoma group is readily identified in specimens of respiratory material, attempts to further classify the adenocarcinoma into acinar, papillary or bronchioloalveolar cell types are less successful. The reader may consult further the work of Roger, Nasiell and associates,[451] Smith and Frable[504] and Gupta[198] who have studied the differences in cytologic presentation among the various adenocarcinomas. Cytologic features of these neoplasms are summarized in Tables 14–11 and 14–12. Papillary adenocarcinomas have not been separately tabulated, because their cytomorphology, similar to their histomorphology, shows considerable overlap with bronchioloalveolar carcinoma.

Adenocarcinomas appear in cytologic material with both single cells and cell clusters (Figs. 14–82 to 14–88). The chromatin in well-differentiated tumors is typically finely granular to powdery in appearance. The nuclei are enlarged and round to oval with varying degrees of nuclear membrane abnormalities. They may, however, be so bland in appearance that one must rely on other features, such as variation of cell size and shape, cell crowding, disorganization within groups and lack of cohesion, to establish a diagnosis of malignancy. In many adenocarcinomas of the acinar type, the presence of centrally placed macronucleoli is a prominent feature. The cytoplasm may vary in appearance from homogeneous to extremely vacuolated. The vacuoles may be multiple and small, imparting a delicate foamy appearance to the cytoplasm, or may be large, causing indentation and margination of the nucleus. Expression of vacuoles in adenocarcinoma is, in the experience of our laboratory, less common in specimens prepared by the Saccomanno blender technique.[261] In well-differentiated neoplasms, the cells may assume a columnar shape, whereas in other cases, many cells will exhibit extremely high nucleocytoplasmic ratios and will be recognized only as undifferentiated malignant tumor cells.

Cell groups in specimens of adenocarcinoma may consist of ball-like clusters (see Fig. 14–85), papillary fragments (see Fig. 14–87), loose clusters or true acini

TABLE 14–11. Acinar Adenocarcinoma

Cytologic Feature	Sputum	Bronchial Wash	Bronchial Brush	BAL	FNA
1. Mixture of cell clusters, tissue fragments and single cells	+	+	+	+	+
2. Vesicular, lobulated and eccentrically placed nuclei	+	+	+	+	+
3. Chromatin extremely finely dispersed and powdery	+	+	+	+	+
4. Macronucleoli centrally placed	+	+	+	+	+
5. Cytoplasm foamy and cyanophilic, finely vacuolated or showing hyperdistended secretory vacuoles	+	+	+	+	+
6. Tissue fragments may show only clusters of tumor cells arranged in syncytial groupings or true acini, tubules and papillary structures.	+	+	+	+	+
Large irregular sheets	−	−	+	−	−
Small irregular sheets	+	+	+	+	+

BAL = bronchoalveolar lavage; FNA = fine needle aspiration.

TABLE 14–12. Bronchioloalveolar Carcinoma

Cytologic Feature	Sputum	Bronchial Wash	Bronchial Brush	BAL	FNA
1. Ball-like cell clusters	+	–	–	–	–
2. Papillary fronds	+	+	+	+	+
3. Nuclei round to oval with bland, finely granular chromatin	+	+	+	+	+
4. Nucleoli but inconspicuous	+	+	+	+	+
5. Single cells may bear a strong resemblance to alveolar macrophages, which may also be present in large numbers.	+	–	–	+	+
6. Cytoplasmic villi may mimic cilia.	+	+	+	+	+
7. Cells may or may not exhibit secretory vacuoles.	+	+	+	+	+

BAL = bronchoalveolar lavage; FNA = fine needle aspiration.

with central lumens (see Fig. 14–88). With decreasing differentiation of the neoplasm, one sees increasing nuclear hyperchromasia, coarsening of chromatin, more irregular nuclear contours and greater cellular pleomorphism, such that the cytomorphology begins to merge with that of large-cell undifferentiated carcinoma.

Bronchioloalveolar Carcinoma

The histologic diagnosis of bronchioloalveolar carcinoma is based on a predominant pattern of growth of cuboidal or columnar cells along alveolar or fibrovascular septa.[333] Although this pattern may sometimes be appreciated in FNAs,[495] one obviously does not have benefit of this architectural feature in sputum or bronchial specimens. However, a number of cytologic features are seen (Table 14–12), which are typical of bronchioloalveolar carcinomas and may allow one to suggest this diagnosis in cytologic material. Like other adenocarcinomas, bronchioloalveolar carcinoma tends to exfoliate both as single cells and cell groups. The nuclei are characteristically round to oval and uniform in size, with finely granular or powdery chromatin and small inconspicuous nucleoli (Fig. 14–89).[125, 198, 324, 451, 495, 504, 538] A minority of cases, however, show prominent nucleoli.[198, 451, 495, 536, 538] Nuclear folds are commonly present (Fig. 14–90),[198, 324, 451] and in some cases nuclear pseudoinclusions (invaginations of cytoplasm into the

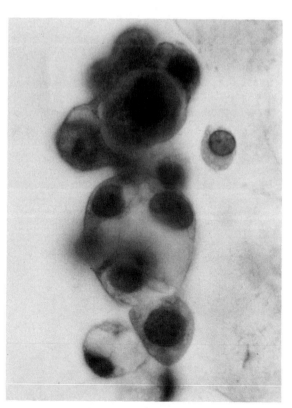

FIGURE 14–82. Acinar adenocarcinoma. Sputum (Papanicolaou stain; ×1000).

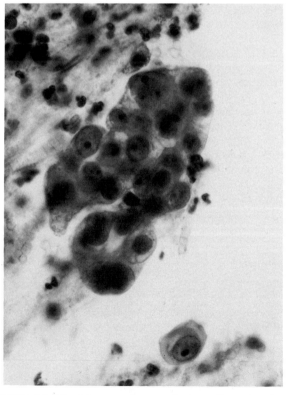

FIGURE 14–83. Adenocarcinoma. A three-dimensional cell cluster showing variation in nuclear size, powdery chromatin, prominent nucleoli and delicate finely vacuolated cytoplasm. Sputum (Papanicolaou stain; ×520).

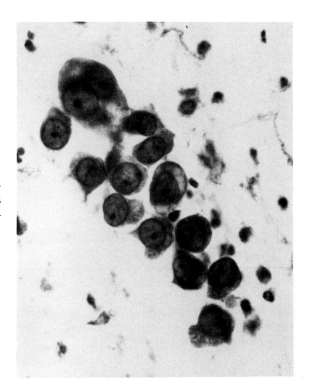

FIGURE 14–84. Adenocarcinoma. Saccomanno sputum. Some cytoplasmic vacuoles can be observed, although expression of vacuoles tends to be less prominent than in freshly prepared sputum (Papanicolaou stain; ×680).

nucleus) are observed (Fig. 14–91).[125, 494] The cytoplasm varies in amount from modest to abundant and, like that of other adenocarcinomas, may be homogeneous, granular, finely vacuolated or distended by single or multiple large vacuoles (Fig. 14–92 and 14–93).

Smith and Frable,[504] Elson and associates[125] and Silverman and associates[495] have emphasized the extreme depth of focus in the three-dimensional cell clusters of bronchioloalveolar carcinoma. Frequently, the cell groups exhibit a radiating "flower-petal" or "cartwheel" pattern (Fig. 14–94).[125] Papillary-shaped fragments lacking fibrovascular cores are also common (Fig. 14–95).[198, 251, 324, 451] In some cytologic preparations

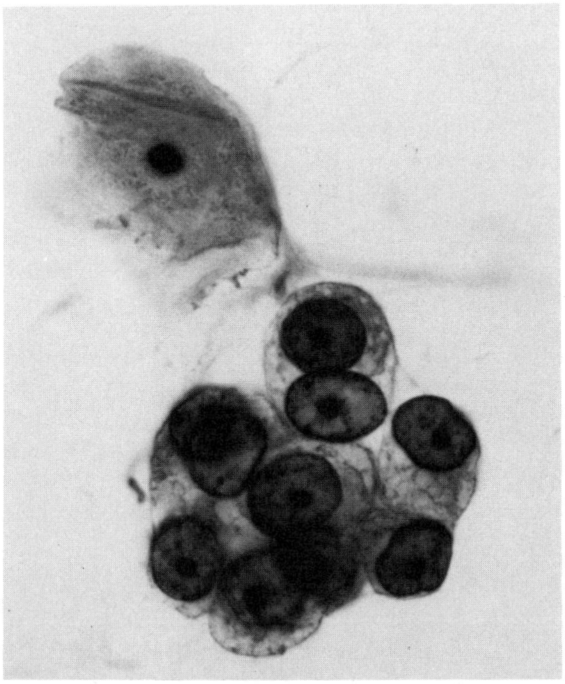

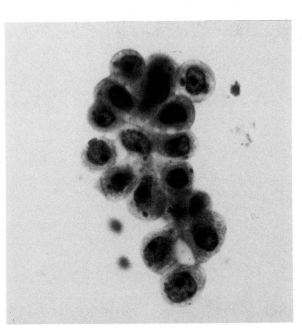

FIGURE 14–85. Adenocarcinoma. This cell cluster shows some depth of focus, and the cells exhibit central macronucleoli and vacuolated cytoplasm. Sputum (Papanicolaou stain; ×1000).

FIGURE 14–86. Adenocarcinoma with erythrophagocytosis. Erythrocytes and fragments of erythrocytes are seen within the cytoplasm of the tumor cells. Sputum (Papanicolaou stain; ×680).

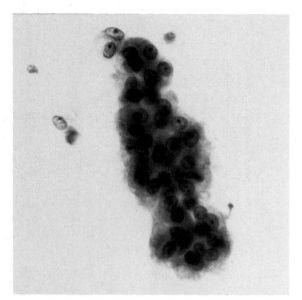

FIGURE 14–87. Papillary cell cluster. Histologically, this tumor showed areas of bronchioloalveolar differentiation. Sputum (Papanicolaou stain; ×520).

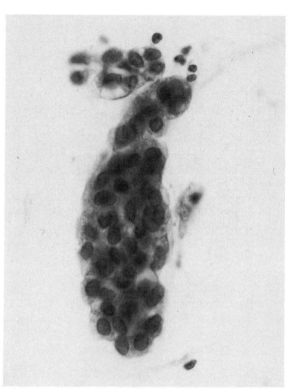

FIGURE 14–89. Papillary cell cluster from a patient with **bronchioloalveolar carcinoma.** Note the bland appearance of the nuclei. A nuclear pseudoinclusion is present at one tip of the cluster. Sputum (Papanicolaou stain; ×520).

numerous nonpigmented macrophage-like cells will be present (Fig. 14–96).[125, 324, 451, 495] It may be extremely difficult or impossible to determine in individual cases, whether these cells represent tumor cells or macrophages.[451] Their presence, however, should prompt a search for three-dimensional, diagnostic clusters of similar cells. In a small number of cases, psammoma bodies may be encountered (Fig. 14–97),[202, 324, 494, 538] and exceptionally they may be the only cytologic clue to the presence of carcinoma.[125] Some tumor cells with features of type II pneumocytes may possess numerous distended microvilli, which may be mistaken for cilia in cytologic preparations.[262, 307]

The cytologic appearance of bronchioloalveolar car-

cinoma in FNAs is similar to that described, except that sheets of tumor cells may be prominent[495, 538] and, as mentioned, tissue fragments containing alveolar septa may be present.

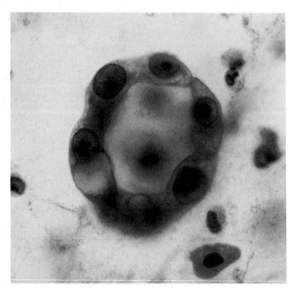

FIGURE 14–88. Adenocarcinoma. This three-dimensional cell cluster is a true acinus with a central lumen, visualized here by focusing the microscope at the midpoint of the cell cluster. Sputum (Papanicolaou stain; ×680).

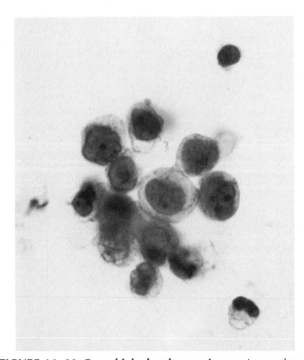

FIGURE 14–90. Bronchioloalveolar carcinoma. Loose three-dimensional cell cluster exhibiting prominent nuclear folds in some of the cells. Sputum (Papanicolaou stain; ×1300).

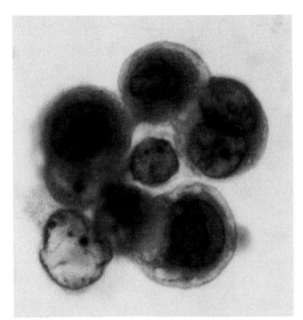

FIGURE 14–91. Bronchioloalveolar carcinoma. Cell cluster showing a nuclear pseudoinclusion. Bronchial brushing (Papanicolaou stain; ×1700).

Tao and coworkers[536] have observed that diffuse and multifocal bronchioloalveolar carcinomas are far more likely to exfoliate tumor cells in sputum and bronchial specimens than is the solitary nodular form of the

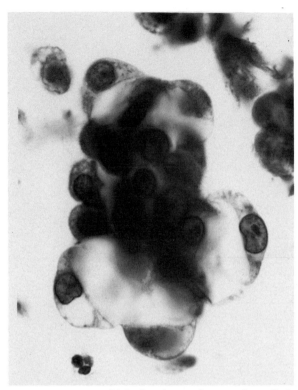

FIGURE 14–93. Bronchioloalveolar carcinoma. This cell cluster shows distended cytoplasmic vacuoles, variation in nuclear size and a few prominent nucleoli. Sputum (Papanicolaou stain; ×1000).

disease. For the latter, FNA is a much more effective means of obtaining tumor cells.[536]

Overall, the mucinous (type I) tumors possess more abundant cytoplasm and more innocuous nuclear features than do the nonmucinous tumors and therefore

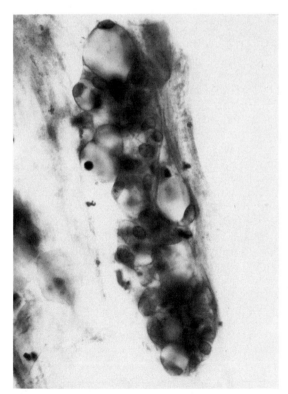

FIGURE 14–92. Bronchioloalveolar carcinoma. The tumor cells show small nuclei with powdery chromatin, occasional nuclear folds and large secretory vacuoles. Sputum (Papanicolaou stain; ×400).

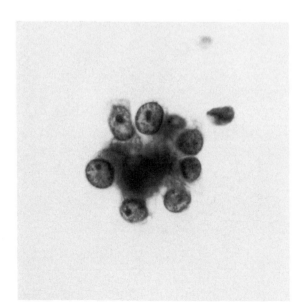

FIGURE 14–94. Bronchioloalveolar carcinoma. This three-dimensional cell cluster shows a radiating "flower petal" or "cartwheel" pattern. Prominent nucleoli are present in some of the cells. Sputum (Papanicolaou stain; ×1300).

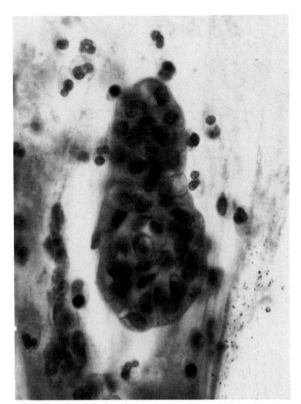

FIGURE 14–95. Papillary cell cluster from a patient with **bronchioloalveolar carcinoma**. Sputum (Papanicolaou stain; ×680).

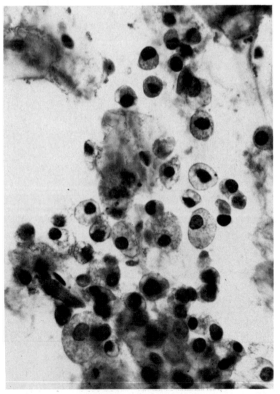

FIGURE 14–96. Bronchioloalveolar carcinoma. Single cells with abundant vacuolated cytoplasm. Distinguishing between single tumor cells and macrophages may be very difficult. Sputum (Papanicolaou stain; ×520).

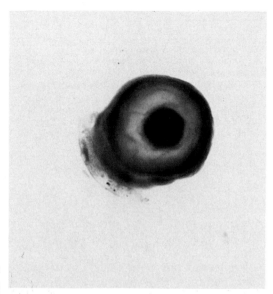

FIGURE 14–97. Psammoma body from a patient with **bronchioloalveolar carcinoma**. For this patient, psammoma bodies were the only cytologic clue to the presence of the neoplasm. Sputum (Papanicolaou stain; ×1000).

the former are more likely to be overlooked during routine cytologic screening.[125] However, so much overlap exists between the cytologic features of the type I and type II tumors in exfoliated material that the investigators would consider such specimens unreliable for distinguishing between the two patterns.[125]

The possible confusion of bronchioloalveolar carcinoma with reactive alveolar epithelium has been discussed. As mentioned, bronchial goblet cell hyperplasia may occasionally be confused with this neoplasm. Some metastatic adenocarcinomas with bland nuclear features, particularly carcinoma of the breast, may closely resemble bronchioloalveolar carcinoma in cytologic preparations. Wang and Nieberg[570] have reported a case of so-called sclerosing hemangioma, a tumor of presumed type II pneumocyte origin, which was erroneously diagnosed as bronchioloalveolar carcinoma by FNA.

A small percentage of bronchioloalveolar carcinomas are poorly differentiated and exhibit pronounced nuclear atypia, similar to that observed in other poorly differentiated adenocarcinomas.[125, 198, 261, 495, 536, 538] In view of this and the fact that pulmonary adenocarcinomas not infrequently exhibit mixed acinar and bronchioloalveolar patterns, it is unreasonable to expect that cytologic preparations will consistently permit the distinction of bronchioloalveolar carcinomas from other adenocarcinomas[125] just as it is unreasonable to expect this from a transbronchial biopsy specimen.[66] Such a distinction, from a practical standpoint, is far less important than is the recognition that cells exhibiting the bland features described here may indeed be derived from a malignant neoplasm.

Large-cell Undifferentiated Carcinoma

The cytologic characteristics of large-cell undifferentiated carcinoma are shown in Table 14–13. These

TABLE 14–13. Large-Cell Undifferentiated Carcinoma

Cytologic Feature	Sputum	Bronchial Wash	Bronchial Brush	BAL	FNA
1. Mixture of large single cells and syncytial groups	+	+	+	+	+
2. Nuclei round to lobulated with irregularly dispersed, intensely staining chromatin	+	+	+	+	+
3. Nucleoli may be large and vary in number from cell to cell.	+	+	+	+	+
4. Cytoplasm usually cyanophilic and varies from granular to foamy; cytoplasmic outline frequently ill defined.	+	+	+	+	+
5. Cells may shed in syncytial groupings with randomly oriented overlapping nuclei.	+	+	+	+	+

BAL = bronchoalveolar lavage; FNA = fine needle aspiration.

neoplasms exfoliate large numbers of diagnostic cells and appear in respiratory specimens both as single cells and as tissue fragments. The single cells are large and possess multiple criteria for malignancy, including high nucleocytoplasmic ratios; marked aberrations in the chromatin patterns; abnormal nuclear contours and multiple, enlarged, irregular nucleoli. Cytoplasm may be wispy or homogeneous with a tendency towards cyanophilia. No evidence of keratinization is seen, and insufficient cytoplasmic differentiation is seen to warrant a diagnosis of adenocarcinoma (Fig. 14–98). The large tissue fragments, which may be present, lack any recognizable architectural pattern such as squamous pearls, acini or papillary structures. Occasionally seen is the giant cell carcinoma variant of large-cell undifferentiated carcinoma, so named because of the presence of many multinucleated tumor giant cells (Fig. 14–99).[57, 58, 96, 365, 369, 412, 532, 569] Differential diagnostic considerations for large-cell undifferentiated carcinoma include metastatic undifferentiated carcinomas, amelanotic malignant melanomas, sarcomas, chemotherapy changes and radiation changes. Benign irradiated epithelial cells may possess very large nuclei but their equally abundant cytoplasm should help to differentiate them from tumor cells. Previously irradiated neoplasms may exhibit bizarre giant cells indistinguishable from those observed in giant cell carcinoma.

All of the nonsmall-cell carcinomas of the lung may exfoliate only large anaplastic malignant tumor cells into the cytologic specimens, so that the cytologic diagnosis of large-cell undifferentiated carcinoma is made. Furthermore, sampling methods such as bronchial brushings or FNA may reach only undifferentiated portions of squamous or adenocarcinomas. FNAs obtained from poorly differentiated adenocarcinomas have, in the experience of our laboratory, been particularly difficult to classify correctly.

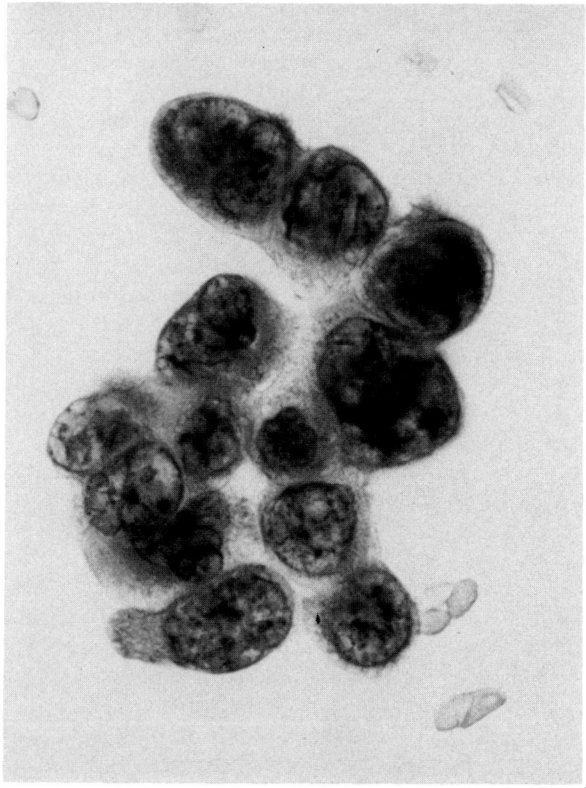

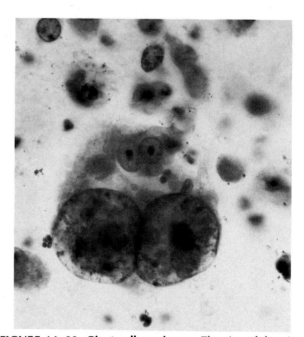

FIGURE 14–98. Large-cell undifferentiated carcinoma. The cells possess high nuclear to cytoplasmic ratios, abnormal chromatin distribution and marked nuclear membrane abnormalities. Bronchial brushing (Papanicolaou stain; ×1000).

FIGURE 14–99. Giant cell carcinoma. The size of the giant tumor cell can be appreciated by comparing it with the neutrophils in the field. Fine needle aspiration (FNA) of lung (Papanicolaou stain; ×680).

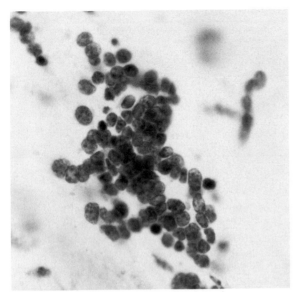

FIGURE 14–100. Small-cell undifferentiated carcinoma, oat cell type. The characteristic features of oat cell carcinoma, including nuclear molding, hyperchromatic granular chromatin and high nuclear to cytoplasmic ratios are seen. Sputum (Papanicolaou stain; ×680).

Small-cell Undifferentiated Carcinoma

As mentioned, small-cell undifferentiated carcinoma of the lung may be subclassified into oat-cell carcinoma, intermediate cell carcinoma and a combined cell type (small-cell carcinoma in combination with squamous

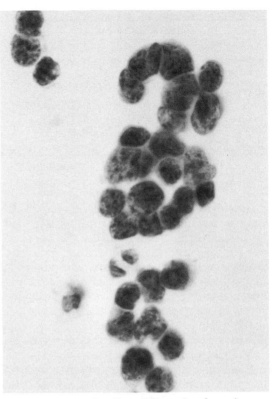

FIGURE 14–102. Small-cell undifferentiated carcinoma, oat cell type. Sputum (Papanicolaou stain; ×1000).

cell carcinoma, large-cell undifferentiated carcinoma or adenocarcinoma).[69, 239, 294] The relative frequencies of these histologically confirmed subtypes as encountered in our laboratory during a 5-year period are shown in Table 14–14. Cytologic characteristics are

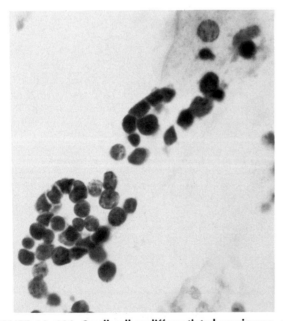

FIGURE 14–101. Small-cell undifferentiated carcinoma, oat cell type. Note the presence of nuclear pyknosis, hyperchromasia and nuclear molding. Sputum (Papanicolaou stain; ×680).

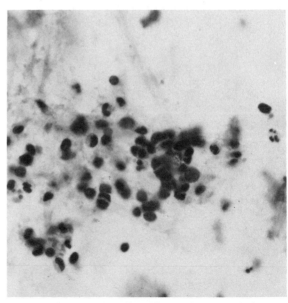

FIGURE 14–103. Small-cell undifferentiated carcinoma. Note nuclear pyknosis, intense molding and necrotic tumor. Sputum (Papanicolaou stain; ×400).

TABLE 14–14. Classification of Small-Cell Undifferentiated Carcinoma

	Cases	Percent
Oat cell carcinoma	179	88.6
Intermediate cell carcinoma	10	5.0
Combined*	13	6.4
	202	100.0

*Small-cell carcinoma with foci of squamous cell carcinoma or adenocarcinoma.

Reproduced with permission from Johnston WW: Cytologic correlations, *In* Pulmonary Pathology. Edited by DH Dail, SP Hammar. New York, Springer-Verlag, 1987.

summarized in Table 14–15. The individual cell from oat-cell carcinoma varies from approximately 1½ times to 2 times the size of a lymphocyte. It is round to oval in shape possessing a centrally placed nucleus with a uniform but deeply staining chromatin pattern and a very high nucleocytoplasmic ratio. Nucleoli are occasionally visible but are generally inconspicuous.

The exfoliation pattern into sputum for this neoplasm may vary from large numbers of cells and tissue fragments to several cells present on only one slide out of many examined. In specimens of freshly prepared sputum, large numbers of tumor cells may be found entrapped in strands of mucus. A most characteristic presentation results when clusters of these small tumor cells exhibit extreme molding and are superimposed upon irregular nuclear outlines (Figs. 14–100 to 14–102). As this tumor is highly prone to necrosis, the cellular specimen will frequently reflect this, with cells exhibiting karyopyknosis, disintegration of the cytoplasm and formation of cyanophilic masses of necrotic debris (Figs. 14–103 and 14–104).[367, 604] In specimens of sputum prepared by the Saccomanno technique, nuclear molding may be much less evident because of greater dispersion of the cells from the mechanical process. Individual nuclei also tend towards more opaqueness. Cells of the intermediate cell subtype of small-cell undifferentiated carcinoma possess slightly larger nuclei with a larger rim of cytoplasm and, on occasion, conspicuous nucleoli.

In the combined type of small-cell undifferentiated carcinoma, the cellular specimen may reveal several

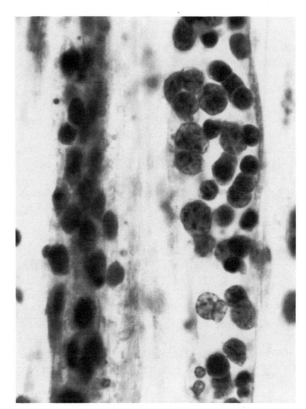

FIGURE 14–104. Cells derived from **small-cell undifferentiated carcinoma** exhibiting nuclear molding. An adjacent mucus streak contains necrotic tumor cells. Sputum (Papanicolaou stain; ×1000).

morphologic possibilities: it may show a combination of malignant cells diagnostic for small-cell undifferentiated carcinoma and malignant cells diagnostic for either squamous cell carcinoma or adenocarcinoma;[457] it may reveal malignant cells from small-cell undifferentiated carcinoma only or it may reveal malignant cells from squamous cell carcinoma or adenocarcinoma only.

The cytologic presentation of small-cell undifferentiated carcinoma in bronchial brushings and FNAs can vary from one that is characteristic to one that produces a significant problem in differential diagnosis.[35] In most

TABLE 14–15. Small-Cell Undifferentiated Carcinoma

Cytologic Feature	Sputum	Bronchial Wash	Bronchial Brush	BAL	FNA
1. Very small cells arranged in loose clusters with some single cells.	+	+	+	+	+
2. Cells arranged along mucus threads.	+	−	−	−	−
3. Individual cell is about 1½ times the size of a lymphocyte.	+	+	+	+	+
4. Nuclei may vary from round to very irregular. Chromatin is uniformly dispersed but hyperchromatic to pyknotic.	+	+	+	+	+
5. Nucleoli may be present but are usually inconspicuous or absent.	+	+	+	+	+
6. Cytoplasm is extremely scanty, presenting only as a thin cyanophilic rim.	+	+	+	+	+
7. Intercellular molding is striking and an important diagnostic feature.	+	−	−	−	−
8. A tumor diathesis may be present.	+	+	+	+	+

BAL = bronchoalveolar lavage; FNA = fine needle aspiration.

cases, large numbers of tumor cells may be present. The finding of tissue fragments is of diagnostic importance to exclude lymphoma, but this differential may be more difficult to determine than that in sputum. Most cells are well-preserved with discernible nuclear chromatin pattern and occasional nucleoli. They usually appear larger and with less molding than when seen in sputum. A tumor diathesis is helpful in excluding carcinoid tumors, although the rarely encountered atypical carcinoids may cause exceptional difficulty in the differential diagnosis (Fig. 14–105). The intermediate cell carcinomas in the experience of our laboratory have caused the greatest interpretative difficulty, being at times suggestive of poorly differentiated squamous cell carcinomas (Fig. 14–106).

The ability of cytology to correctly predict the histology of small-cell undifferentiated carcinoma is summarized in Table 14–16 in a review of histologically confirmed small-cell undifferentiated carcinoma in our laboratory. In no case did the cytology incorrectly predict that a small-cell undifferentiated carcinoma would be found; however, there were five cases in which the cytology revealed only squamous cell carcinoma components of tumors that were later shown by histologic examination to be combined types of small-cell carcinoma.

Adenosquamous Carcinoma

As discussed, the reported incidence of adenosquamous carcinoma is related to the diligence with which histologic sections, cytologic specimens and electron microscopic preparations are examined. The duality of differentiation of these neoplasms may be reflected in the cytologic specimens. A diagnosis of adenosqua-

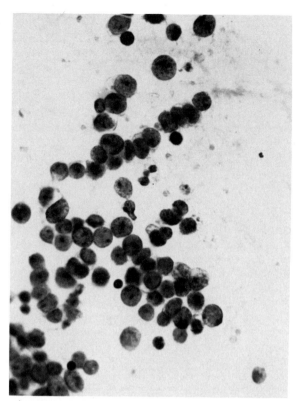

FIGURE 14–106. Small-cell undifferentiated carcinoma intermediate cell type. The nuclei, on average, are somewhat larger than those of the oat cell type and some exhibit distinct nucleoli. Sputum (Papanicolaou stain; ×680).

mous carcinoma should be entertained when a single cytologic specimen of sputum, a bronchial brushing or an FNA exhibits malignant tumor cells in which there is evidence for both keratin production and secretory activity.

Carcinoid

The majority of primary carcinoid tumors of the lung occur within the walls of larger bronchi and probably originate in bronchial submucosal glands.[67] Although carcinoids typically appear as exophytic endobronchial lesions, tumor cells are rarely observed in

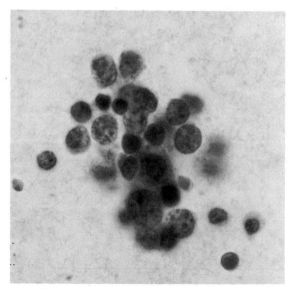

FIGURE 14–105. Small-cell undifferentiated carcinoma in fine needle aspiration (FNA). Note the dual cell population produced by a mixture of well-preserved and necrotic tumor cells. This is a helpful feature in differentiating this lesion from atypical carcinoid. FNA (Papanicolaou stain; ×1000).

TABLE 14–16. Predictability of Cytologic Diagnosis of Small-Cell Undifferentiated Carcinoma in Histologically Confirmed Cases

Cytologic Diagnosis	Number Patients	Percent Patients
Small-cell undifferentiated carcinoma	78	81.3
Combined	5	5.2
Undifferentiated malignant neoplasm	8*	8.3
Squamous cell carcinoma	5	5.2
Total	96	100.0

*Two cases intermediate cell carcinoma histologically; two cases possible atypical carcinoid histologically.

Reproduced from Johnston WW: Cytologic correlations. *In* Pulmonary Pathology. Edited by KH Dail, SP Hammar. Springer-Verlag, New York, 1987.

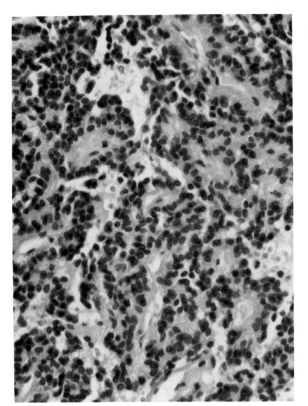

FIGURE 14–107. **Carcinoid tumor,** composed of small uniform cells, which form rosettes separated by vascular connective tissue. No nuclear atypia, necrosis or mitotic figures are evident. Lung biopsy (hematoxylin and eosin; ×325).

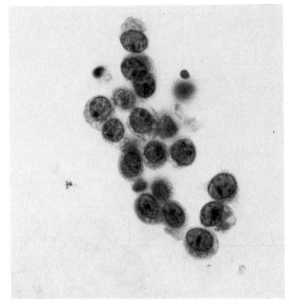

FIGURE 14–108. **Carcinoid tumor.** Bronchial brushing (Papanicolaou stain; ×1000).

totic figures, necrosis and even nuclear molding, so that the cytologic features begin to merge imperceptibly with those of small-cell undifferentiated carcinoma (Fig. 14–110).[10, 398, 523, 584] In general, atypical carcinoids exhibit more cytoplasm and less nuclear atypia than

sputum,[325, 393] because of the intact bronchial mucosa overlying the tumor. In tissue sections, the tumor cells may be arranged in ribbons, trabeculae, rosettes, acini[67] or papillary structures[336] separated by highly vascular connective tissue septa (Fig. 14–107). When observed in bronchial brushing specimens and FNAs, the tumor cells occur singly as well as in sheets and three-dimensional ball-like clusters.[183] The cells are characterized by small, round-to-oval, uniform nuclei with a stippled, granular chromatin pattern and small nucleoli (Fig. 14–108). Cytoplasm is scant to moderate in amount and may vary from homogeneous to lace-like in appearance. Necrosis is absent unless the lesion has been traumatized or secondarily infected. Peripheral carcinoids in FNA specimens may show the typical morphology described but on occasion may exhibit a spindle cell pattern.[51, 97, 115, 437] When there is any question as to the tumor type in routine cytologic preparations, additional studies, such as immunoperoxidase stains for chromogranin or electron microscopy for documenting neurosecretory granules, may be extremely helpful.

Atypical carcinoids constitute only about 10% of all carcinoid tumors.[580] They may occur centrally, but more commonly they arise in the periphery of the lung. Histologically, these carcinoids maintain the overall architecture of carcinoid tumors (Fig. 14–109),[195, 357] but cytologically they are characterized by greater cellular pleomorphism, nuclear hyperchromasia, mi-

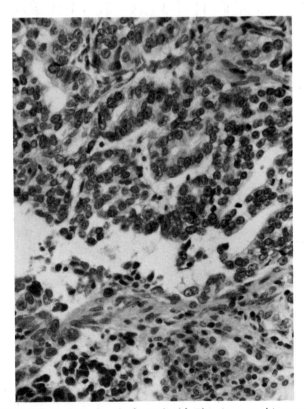

FIGURE 14–109. **Atypical carcinoid.** The tissue architecture of a carcinoid tumor is maintained but mitotic figures, nuclear hyperchromasia and focal nuclear molding are present. Pulmonary resection (hematoxylin and eosin; ×250).

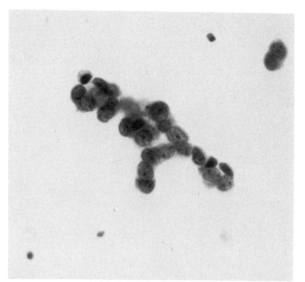

FIGURE 14–110. Cells derived from an **atypical carcinoid.** The high nuclear to cytoplasmic ratios and focal nuclear molding in this field call to mind features of small-cell undifferentiated carcinoma. Bronchial brushing (Papanicolaou stain; ×680).

small-cell undifferentiated carcinoma. Nevertheless, this differential diagnosis may be exceedingly difficult or impossible in cytologic material, just as it is in transbronchial biopsy material.[357] In view of this and the fact that atypical carcinoids are frequently resectable[580] and associated with a 2-year survival of greater than 50%,[63] it has been suggested that stage I small-cell tumors of the lung diagnosed by cytology or small biopsy should be considered for resection.[357] It has also been proposed that the term well-differentiated neuroendocrine carcinoma should be substituted for atypical carcinoid.[265]

Adenoid Cystic Carcinoma

The trachea[232] and, less commonly, the large bronchi may give rise to adenoid cystic carcinomas, which are identical in appearance to those occurring in the salivary glands.[65, 337] These tumors may appear as an endobronchial mass or as a circumferential area of bronchial constriction.[406] Because these neoplasms are covered by intact mucosa, sputum specimen findings are usually negative. In bronchial brushings and needle aspirates, adenoid cystic carcinoma occurs as three-dimensional clusters of small uniform cells, which surround spheric or cylindric cores of homogeneous, hyaline, basal lamina material (Fig. 14–111). The tumor cells, which have round-to-oval, hyperchromatic nuclei and small nucleoli, are also found singly and in small clusters in cytologic preparations. Patients with these neoplasms may survive for many years, but because of the high frequency of recurrence of this lesion, the ultimate prognosis is poor.[91, 206]

Other Primary Neoplasms of the Lung

In addition to the lung cancers discussed, less frequently other primary neoplasms of the lung may exfoliate diagnostic cells into cellular specimens from the respiratory tract or be diagnosed by FNA. These neoplasms include mucoepidermoid tumor,[537] leiomyosarcoma,[151, 295, 483] pulmonary blastoma,[164, 508] Hodgkin's[120, 172, 274, 310, 439, 520, 586] and non-Hodgkin's lymphomas,[328, 443, 465, 487, 489] endobronchial granular cell tumor,[171, 185] solitary papilloma of the bronchus,[456, 471] angiosarcoma,[382] carcinosarcoma,[240] chondrosarcoma,[342] malignant fibrous histiocytoma,[270, 299] bronchial gland carcinoma[383] and clear cell tumor.[384] Occasionally, two or more synchronous neoplasms of lung or of an adjacent site, such as larynx, may be diagnosed in one or more specimens of sputum and bronchial material.[581]

Mucoepidermoid carcinomas of the large bronchi, like adenoid cystic carcinomas, tend to occur with symptoms related to bronchial irritation or obstruction. The cytologic features have been described by Tao and Robertson[537] and are similar to those of mucoepidermoid tumors of the salivary glands.

On rare occasions pulmonary blastomas may be sampled in specimens of respiratory cytology. One such case has been observed in our laboratory, in

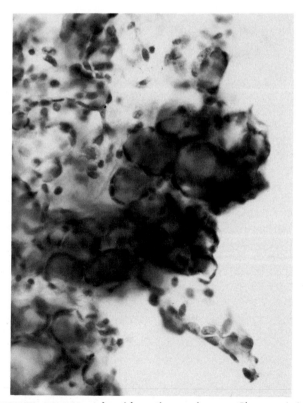

FIGURE 14–111. Adenoid cystic carcinoma. Characteristic three-dimensional clusters of small cells surrounding cores of hyaline material. Bronchial brushing (Papanicolaou stain; ×400).

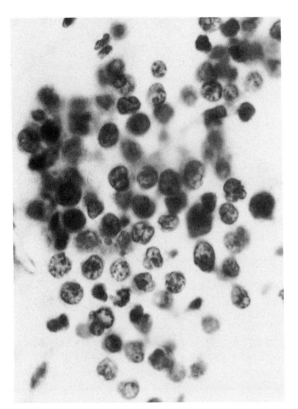

FIGURE 14–112. Large-cell lymphoma. Sputum (Papanicolaou stain; ×1000).

which sputum contained cells that were interpreted as adenocarcinoma. A thoracotomy was performed and a pulmonary blastoma removed. Review of the cytologic specimen revealed tiny fragments of small malignant cells adherent to the differentiated glandular component. These undoubtedly represented the mesenchymal component of the tumor.[508]

Non-Hodgkin's lymphomas may be encountered in all types of respiratory cytologic specimens. Characteristic findings include the presence of small, single, malignant cells, some having sharp indentations or bulbous protrusions of the nuclear membranes and prominent nucleoli (Fig. 14–112). Diagnosis of Hodgkin's disease (Fig. 14–113) is absolutely dependent on the finding of Reed-Sternberg cells: malignant tumor cells with two mirror-image nuclei, each possessing a macronucleolus. Just as in surgical pathology, Reed-Sternberg cells must be considered necessary but not sufficient for a diagnosis of Hodgkin's disease. In our experience, most cells in respiratory specimens that exhibit the features described for Reed-Sternberg cells are derived from carcinomas or malignant melanomas.

Neoplasms Metastatic to the Lung

Although cancer metastatic to the lung is more common than primary lung cancer, cytologic evidence of its presence in specimens of sputum and bronchial material is not reported as frequently as that of the primary tumors.[54, 59, 123, 276, 466] There are several reasons

for this. First, exfoliative cytologic techniques are not called upon as frequently for suspected metastatic cancer to the lung as they are for suspected primary cancer. Second, unless the tumor has metastasized to the alveolar space, it must ulcerate through the bronchial mucosa to produce exfoliation of cells. The studies of Koss,[290] and Kern and Schweizer[276] have shown that cells from metastatic tumors to the lung may be seen in respiratory material in 50 to 70% of cases. Patterns of malignant cells that deviate from those recognized for the primary lung tumors are strongly suggestive of the presence of cancer metastatic to the lung. Metastatic tumors to the lung occurring as diffuse nodules or as single tumors involving a major bronchus have different cytologic patterns.[54] In cases of diffuse metastases, tumor cells may occur in clusters simulating a pattern of bronchioloalveolar carcinoma but with far fewer cells. Occasionally, a cell cluster may actually represent the cast of an alveolar space. The background of the smear is unusually clean with virtually no macrophages. At times it is possible to recognize the primary site of the neoplasm by noting cell characteristics and spatial arrangement. When large, single metastases have produced exfoliation through an ulcerated bronchus, a primary lung carcinoma may be mimicked. All available surgical tissue should be compared with the cytology, as it may be possible to say whether or not the tumor cells are consistent with the previous primary cancer. Differences noted between the cytologic specimen and the original tissue specimen may signal the presence of a second cancer that is either metastatic to the lung or a new primary cancer of the lung.

Tables 14–17 and 14–18 depict the pattern and frequency of cancers of nonpulmonary origin manifested in specimens of sputum, bronchial washings,

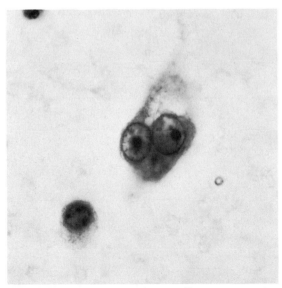

FIGURE 14–113. Reed-Sternberg cells in sputum from a patient with pulmonary involvement with **Hodgkin's disease.** Note the mirror-image nuclei with prominent nucleoli. Sputum (Papanicolaou stain; ×1000).

TABLE 14–17. Malignant Neoplasms Metastatic to Lung or Arising in Adjacent Sites with Malignant Cells in Sputum or Bronchial Material

Squamous cell carcinoma		40%
Adenocarcinoma		34%
Breast	15%	
Kidney	6%	
Colon	5%	
Lymphoma/leukemia		8%
Other		18%

Reproduced with permission from Johnston WW: Cytologic correlations. *In* Pulmonary Pathology. Edited by KH Dail, SP Hammar. Springer-Verlag, New York, 1987.

bronchial brushings and FNAs seen in our laboratory during a 10-year period. Although squamous cell carcinomas appear to be the most common, the appearance of their cells in respiratory material is most frequently secondary to the presence of the primary neoplasm in an anatomic site adjacent to the respiratory tract, e.g., larynx, pharynx, oral mucosa, tonsil, tongue and esophagus.

Adenocarcinomas are by far the most common true metastatic neoplasms detected in sputum and bronchial material. Among these, adenocarcinomas from the breast, kidney and colon are the most often seen. Each one of these may, on occasion, have a cytologic appearance that is so characteristic as to permit a cytologic diagnosis strongly suggestive of that particular neoplasm. Ductal carcinoma of the breast that has metastasized to the lung may show scattered tumor cells occurring singly and as small clusters. The cells are large and polygonal in shape with macronucleoli (Fig. 14–114). One tumor cell may mold the nucleus of an adjacent cell into an "owl-eyed" configuration.[13] Tumor cells from renal cell carcinoma will occur singly and in flat tissue fragments. Depending on the differentiation of the tumor, nucleoli may be small or extremely large. The cytoplasm is characteristically

TABLE 14–18. Neoplasms Metastatic to the Lung Diagnosed by Fine Needle Aspiration

Type of Neoplasm or Tissue of Origin	Number Patients	Percent Patients
Malignant melanoma	70	26.8
Urinary and male genital tract	45	17.2
Breast	39	14.9
Female genital tract	33	12.6
Gastrointestinal tract	26	10.0
Bone and soft tissues	22	8.4
Lymphoma	10	3.8
Mediastinum	3	1.2
Unclassified	9	3.5
Adrenal	1	0.4
Salivary glands	1	0.4
Thyroid	1	0.4
Neuroblastoma	1	0.4
	261	100.0

Reproduced with permission from Johnston WW: Cytologic correlations. *In* Pulmonary Pathology. Edited by KH Dail, SP Hammar. New York, Springer-Verlag, 1987.

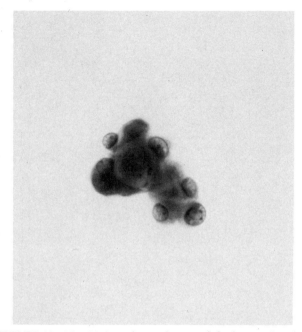

FIGURE 14–114. Metastatic carcinoma of the breast showing the so-called owl's eye pattern of cell wrapping. Fine needle aspiration (FNA) of lung (Papanicolaou stain; ×680).

granular or cleared. Stains for mucin will be negative (Fig. 14–115).

In some adenocarcinomas metastatic from the colon, patterns suggestive of the colonic origin of the neoplasm may be manifested in cytologic material. The first pattern is that of tissue fragments of tumor with columnar differentiation and elongated nuclei forming a palisade-like arrangement. The nuclei are very hyperchromatic with macronucleoli. Extensive tumor ne-

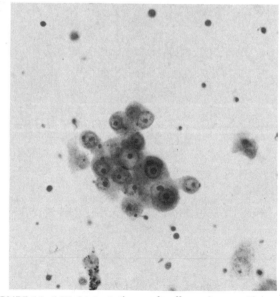

FIGURE 14–115. Metastatic renal cell carcinoma. The tumor cells exhibit abundant granular cytoplasm and macronucleoli. Fine needle aspiration (FNA) of lung (Papanicolaou stain; ×520).

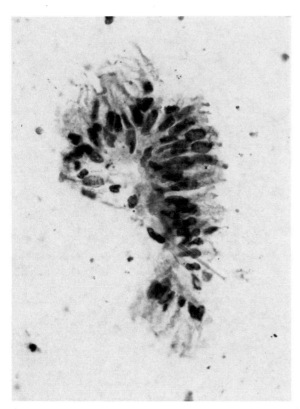

FIGURE 14–116. Metastatic colon carcinoma showing the characteristic palisading of columnar tumor cells and elongated nuclei. Fine needle aspiration (FNA) of lung (Papanicolaou stain; ×520).

crosis is a frequent and very characteristic finding (Fig. 14–116). The second pattern is that of clusters of malignant signet ring–type cells with striking peripheral displacement of the nucleus by a secretory vacuole (Fig. 14–117). Stains for mucin will be positive. Two

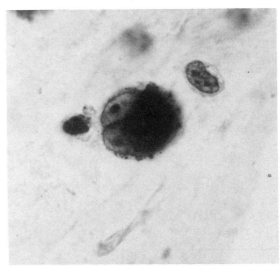

FIGURE 14–118. Metastatic malignant melanoma. The cytoplasm is heavily pigmented with melanin. Bronchial brushing (Papanicolaou stain; ×1000).

examples of metastatic malignant melanoma with and without pigment are shown in Figures 14–118 and 14–119. Although the intranuclear cytoplasmic invagination in the cell in Figure 14–119 is frequently seen in melanoma, it is not diagnostic and its presence does not rule out other lesions including benign ones. Other neoplasms metastatic to the lung reported in sputum or bronchial material have included choriocarcinoma,[98] giant cell tumor of bone,[121, 524] medullary carcinoma of the thyroid,[208] melanoma,[306] mesothelioma,[119] immunoblastic lymphadenopathy[187] and adamantinoma of the tibia.[526]

The opportunity to study the cytology of tumors metastatic to the lungs has been markedly increased by the use of FNA to sample the pulmonary nodules

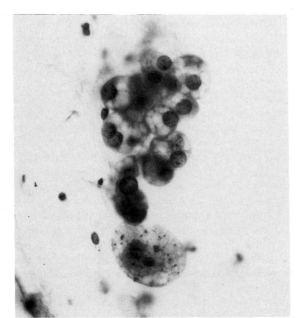

FIGURE 14–117. Metastatic adenocarcinoma from colon showing signet-ring tumor cells. Sputum (Papanicolaou stain; ×400).

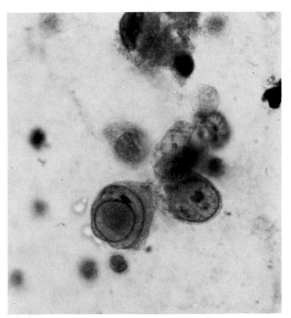

FIGURE 14–119. Cell from **metastatic malignant melanoma** showing an intranuclear cytoplasmic invagination. Fine needle aspiration (FNA) of lung (Papanicolaou stain; ×1000).

of metastatic disease. This aspect of the development of FNA of the lung has been unusually innovative in that it has resulted in a major modification of the diagnostic approach to the patient with suspected metastatic tumor. Before the advent of FNA, such patients would have been subjected to thoracotomy or treated on the bases of radiologic and clinical findings. In these patients the aspirates usually reveal the answers to the critical questions of malignancy, differentiation and organ of origin. In patients with multiple primary cancers, additional information may be provided about which primary has metastasized.

In the diagnostic assessment with FNA of a patient with suspected cancer metastatic to the lung, the case should be approached in the same manner as evaluation of tissue from open biopsy. The patient's clinical history must be reviewed for either documentation or prior suspicion of a preexisting neoplasm. All prior histologic and cytologic specimens should be reviewed and the cellular changes in the FNA compared with the preexisting diagnostic material. In the absence of known prior cancer, immunocytochemical techniques may be of some help.

Table 14–18 summarizes our experience with such patients. Metastatic neoplasms have represented 15% of the total patient population examined by FNA of the lung in our laboratory. With reference to the type of neoplasm, tissue or organ system of origin, malignant melanoma was seen in 26.8%; neoplasms from the urinary and male genital tract in 17.2%; adenocarcinoma from the breast in 14.9%; neoplasms, usually squamous cell carcinomas, from the female genital tract in 12.6%; adenocarcinomas from the gastrointestinal tract in 10.0% and neoplasms from the bones and soft tissues in 8.4%. In terms of histologic type, the six most common metastatic neoplasms were malignant melanoma, adenocarcinoma of the breast, adenocarcinoma of the colon, transitional cell carcinoma of the bladder, squamous cell carcinoma of the cervix and adenocarcinoma of the kidney. The large number of melanomas in this series is a specific example of the significant role that needle aspiration may play in the therapeutic management of patients with cancer metastatic to the lung. An example of metastatic transitional carcinoma as seen in an FNA of the lung is depicted in Figure 14–120.

A marked difference occurs between the cytologic presentation of neoplasms metastatic to the lung in FNAs and in specimens of sputum and bronchial material. This difference lies mainly in the amount of cellular material available for study. Most metastatic masses when aspirated yield large numbers of tumor cells and tissue fragments. Extensive necrosis and inflammation may also be present and partially obscure the tumor. Once a cancer diagnosis is established the major diagnostic decision will be the determination of metastatic cancer versus primary lung cancer. Paraffin sections of cell blocks become useful when special stains and immunocytochemistry are needed for differential studies. Tissue fragments fixed in glutaraldehyde are extremely valuable for electron microscopy.

Other metastases reported in the literature as diagnosed by FNA have included lymphoma,[50] malignant

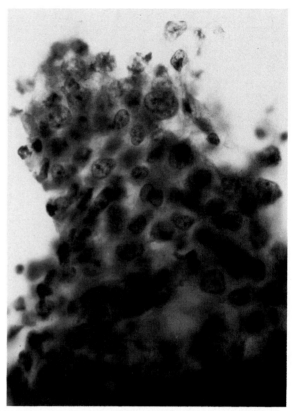

FIGURE 14–120. Metastatic transitional cell carcinoma. Fine needle aspiration (FNA) (Papanicolaou stain; ×680).

schwannoma,[499] adenoid cystic carcinoma,[8] ameloblastoma,[311] malignant fibrous histiocytoma,[233, 325, 385] thymoma[400] and dermatofibrosarcoma protuberans.[409]

In a 1986 study, Kim and associates[279] reported the morphologic features of cells aspirated from 17 sarcomas metastatic to the lung. The group included five malignant fibrous histiocytomas, three fibrosarcomas, three leiomyosarcomas, three endometrial stromal sarcomas, one osteosarcoma and two poorly differentiated sarcomas.

DIAGNOSTIC ACCURACY

In the writing on clinical laboratory tests, when expressing predictive accuracy, it has become fashionable to use the terms "sensitivity" and "specificity" as introduced by Galen and Gambino.[178] Sensitivity is the mathematic expression of the ability of a clinical test to detect disease in a diseased population. Specificity is the mathematic expression for the ability of a test to refrain from falsely diagnosing disease in a nondiseased population.[109] Sensitivity is a measure of the percentage of known diseased patients with positive test results among all the diseased patients evaluated. The specificity is the percentage of patients with negative test results among all known patients without disease tested. Expressed mathematically

$$\text{Sensitivity} = TP/(TP + FN)$$
$$\text{Specificity} = TN/(TN + FP).$$

TABLE 14-19. Diagnostic Accuracy of Sputum and Bronchial Material

Investigator	Year	Specimen Type	Sensitivity (%)	Specificity (%)
Koss et al.	1964	Sputum ×3	89	99.8
		Sputum ×5	96.1	
Erozan and Frost	1970	Bronchial washings ×1	61	NS
		Sputum ×1	42	
		Sputum ×3	82	
		Sputum ×5	91	
Bibbo et al.	1973	Bronchial brushings	70	98
Bedrossian et al.	1976	Sputum ×3	57	NS
		Bronchial washings	76	
		Bronchial brushings	76	
Johnston and Bossen	1981	Sputum ×1	27	99.9
		Bronchial washings/brushings ×1	22	
		Sputum/bronchial brushings ×5	87	
Pilotti et al.	1982	Sputum ×3	57	NS
		Bronchial brushings	67	
Ng and Horak	1983	Sputum ×3	83	NS
		Bronchial washings	74	
Truong et al.	1985	Sputum	60	99.9
		Bronchial washings	66	
		Bronchial brushings	77	
Tanaka	1985	Sputum ×1	27	NS

NS = not supplied.

TP = true positives; FN = false negatives; TN = true negatives and FP = false positives.

In diagnostic cytology these equations become one means of expressing the false negative and false positive rates. Although useful, they are only a partial expression of the more broad concept of diagnostic accuracy in cytology. Such accuracy embraces not only the assessment of presence or absence of cancer in a given specimen but also prediction of cancer differentiation and identification of benign disease states. This section of the chapter discusses these various facets of accuracy when applied to sputum, bronchial material and FNA. The complicated and difficult "gray" area where cancer can neither be diagnosed conclusively nor excluded has been discussed in a preceding section.

Sensitivity and Specificity of Specimens of Sputum and Bronchial Material

Studies in the literature document the level of accuracy that may be achieved in the detection and classification of lung neoplasms through the use of sputum, bronchial washings and bronchial brushings.* Some of these are summarized in Table 14–19. In 1964 Koss and his associates[291] reported on their study of 149 patients with histologically proven lung cancer and on whom three or more satisfactory sputum specimens had been examined, the largest series that had been published up until that time. The overall accuracy (sensitivity) of cytology in detecting the presence of the tumor was 89% when three or more cytologic specimens of sputum were examined. Their specificity

*See references 81, 159, 175, 176, 182, 199, 210, 212–216, 235, 243, 244, 256, 258–261, 268, 282, 283, 301, 304, 314, 319, 321, 338, 339, 341, 350, 380, 381, 414, 419, 420, 440, 462, 481, 482, 491, 503, 521, 533, 544, 562, 587, 606.

was 99.8%. Two false-positive diagnoses were recorded.[291]

The importance of multiplicity of specimen examination was also studied by Erozan and Frost in 1970.[128] Among their patients with lung cancer, one bronchoscopic examination yielded diagnostic cytology in 61%, whereas one sputum specimen yielded diagnostic cytology in only 42%. Diagnostic yield, however, increased to 82% with three sputum examinations and to 91% with five.[128] Bedrossan and his associates[33] in 1976 reported a sensitivity of 56% in cancer detection when three sputum samples were examined. This rate increased to 76% when either bronchial brushings or bronchial washings were utilized.[33] In 1982 Pilotti and colleagues[419, 420] reported for sputum an overall sensitivity of 58% and for bronchial brushings a 67% rate. Ng and Horak[380, 381] reported in 1983 an overall sensitivity of 74% for bronchial washings and 83% for three sputum samples. Truong and associates[544] in their 1985 study determined that the overall sensitivities of sputum, bronchial washings and bronchial brushings were 60%, 66% and 77% respectively. Their false positive rate was 2.8%.[544] Tanaka and associates[533] examined the accuracy of cytologic diagnosis and typing in 154 patients. Central lesions were detected in 57 to 64% of the cases by either 3-day pooled sputum or aerosol-induced specimens.[533]

Sputum has shown the highest levels of sensitivity in the detection of the more centrally located tumors, but this sensitivity has also declined drastically for the peripheral cancers. Bronchial brushing techniques for these peripheral lesions have improved diagnostic accuracy in cancer detection up to the levels of 70 to 88% of cases.[44, 46, 139–146, 170, 212, 216, 341, 587]

In 1973 Bibbo and associates[46] reported 693 specimens obtained by a fluoroscopically controlled bronchial brushing technique. The series included 224 confirmed primary tumors and 30 metastatic tumors. For primary tumors the average diagnostic yield (sensitiv-

TABLE 14–20. Total Respiratory Cytopathologic Specimens on Which the Study Was Based

	Number
Respiratory specimens	9,892
Patients diagnosed as having cancer by cytopathology	363
Patients diagnosed as having cancer by cytopathology also diagnosed from tissue	232
Patients treated on the basis of a cytopathologic diagnosis	125
False-positive cytopathologic diagnoses	6

From Johnston WW: Ten years of respiratory cytopathology at DUMC. I. The cytopathologic diagnosis of lung cancer during the years 1970 to 1974 noting the significance of specimen number and type. Acta Cytol 25:103–107, 1981.

ity) was 70% and 53% for metastatic lesions. In 160 cases, sputum samples taken before brushings showed tumor cells in only 7% of cases; however, sputum samples after brushing showed an increase to 66% tumor detection rate. Nine false-positive diagnoses were recorded and reported as a 2% rate.[46] Bibbo has emphasized the excellence of cellular preservation and the increased amounts of tumor cells arranged in irregular sheets as compared with sputum and bronchial washings.[44, 45a]

In 1975 Johnston and Bossen[258] reported on the results of the examination of 9892 consecutive specimens of sputum samples, bronchial washings and bronchial brushings. The patient groups on which these studies are based are shown in Tables 14–20 and 14–21. Specimens from 363 patients were interpreted as diagnostic of cancer. Of these, 232 also had a histopathologic diagnosis of cancer. Some 125 patients were treated for lung cancer on the bases of the clinical, radiographic and cytologic findings. In six patients, follow-up studies failed to confirm a cytologic diagnosis of cancer. Thus, these six patients were considered to have been given false-positive diagnoses.

Table 14–21 shows the patient group on which histopathologic diagnoses of primary or metastatic malignant neoplasms were made. A total of 633 patients had recorded histopathologic diagnoses of malignant neoplasms involving the lungs or adjacent respiratory areas. Of those, 590 patients had histologically confirmed primary malignant neoplasms and 43 patients had metastatic cancers to the lungs or malignant neo-

TABLE 14–21. Total Group of Histologically Confirmed Cancer on Which the Study Was Based

	Number
Primary neoplasms of lungs	590
No cytopathologic specimen	105
Cytopathology diagnostic of cancer	232
Negative cytopathology	159
Inconclusive cytopathology	94
Cancer metastatic to lungs or neoplasms of adjacent sites	43

From Johnston WW: Ten years of respiratory cytopathology at DUMC. I. The cytopathologic diagnosis of lung cancer during the years 1970 to 1974 noting the significance of specimen number and type. Acta Cytol 25:103–107, 1981.

TABLE 14–22. Role of the Number of Cytopathologic Specimens in Diagnosis (516 Patients with at Least One Satisfactory Specimen)

Specimen Number First Diagnostic of Cancer	Number of Patients	Percent of Total Patients (%)*	Cumulative Percent of Total Patients (%)*
1	177	34.3	34.3
2	82	15.9	50.2
3	36	7.0	57.2
4	24	4.6	61.8
5	11	2.1	63.9
6	7	1.4	65.3
7	4	0.8	66.1
8	3	0.6	66.7
9	1	0.2	66.9
10	0	0.0	66.9
11	0	0.0	66.9
12	1	0.2	67.1

*Total number of patients with accepted lung cancer and cytopathology performed = 516.

From Johnston WW: Ten years of respiratory cytopathology at DUMC. I. The cytopathologic diagnosis of lung cancer during the years 1970 to 1974 noting the significance of specimen number and type. Acta Cytol 25:103–107, 1981.

plasms of adjacent sites. Tables 14–22 through 14–25 summarize the relative roles played by specimen number and type in the diagnosis of lung cancer. Of accepted lung cancer, there were 516 cases in which at least one satisfactory cytologic specimen was examined (Table 14–22). The first specimen was diagnostic of cancer in 177 patients, or 34.3% of the total. Examination of five satisfactory specimens resulted in conclusive diagnoses of cancer in 330 patients or 63.9% of the total Tables 14–23 and 14–24 define more specifically the importance of the use of multiple cytologic specimens in establishing a definitive diagnosis of cancer. A total of 424 patients with cytology diagnostic of

TABLE 14–23. Role of Number of Cytopathologic Speciments in Diagnosis (424 Patients with Three or More Satisfactory Specimens)

Specimen Number First Diagnostic of Cancer	Number of Patients	Percent of Total Patients (%)*	Cumulative Percent of Total Patients (%)*
1	177	41.7	41.7
2	82	19.3	61.0
3	36	8.5	69.5
4	24	5.7	75.2
5	11	2.6	77.8
6	7	1.6	79.4
7	4	0.9	80.3
8	3	0.7	81.0
9	1	0.2	81.2
10	0	—	—
11	0	—	—
12	1	0.2	81.4

*Total number of patients with accepted lung cancer and cytopathology diagnostic of cancer on three or more satisfactory specimens = 424.

From Johnston WW: Ten years of respiratory cytopathology at DUMC. I. The cytopathologic diagnosis of lung cancer during the years 1970 to 1974 noting the significance of specimen number and type. Acta Cytol 25:103–107, 1981.

TABLE 14–24. Role of the Number of Cytopathologic Specimens in Diagnosis (381 Patients with Five or More Satisfactory Specimens)

Specimen Number First Diagnostic of Cancer	Number of Patients	Percent of Total Patients (%)*	Cumulative Percent of Total Patients (%)*
1	177	46.5	46.5
2	82	21.5	68.0
3	36	9.4	77.4
4	24	6.3	83.7
5	11	2.9	86.6
6	7	1.8	88.4
7	4	1.0	89.4
8	3	0.8	90.2
9	1	0.3	90.5
10	0	—	—
11	0	—	—
12	1	0.3	90.8

*Total number of patients with accepted lung cancer and cytopathology diagnostic of cancer on five or more satisfactory specimens = 381.

From Johnston WW: Ten years of respiratory cytopathology at DUMC. I. The cytopathologic diagnosis of lung cancer during the years 1970 to 1974 noting the significance of specimen number and type. Acta Cytol 25:103–107, 1981.

cancer had had at least three satisfactory specimens submitted (Table 14–23). The cancers were diagnosed on the first specimen in 41.7% of these cases. The submission of three specimens detected a total of 69.5%. From Table 14–24 one can obtain the diagnostic advantage gained by increasing the satisfactory specimen count to five.

A minimum of five satisfactory cytologic specimens had been obtained from 381 patients with cytology diagnostic of cancer. From five satisfactory specimens a cytologic diagnosis of cancer was made in 86.6% of these patients. The relationship between sputum and bronchial material in the diagnosis of lung cancer is shown in Table 14–25. In 168 patients (41.7% of 357 patients with cytopathology diagnostic of cancer), sputum only revealed malignant cells and bronchial material in only 93 (26.0%). Both sputum and bronchial material were diagnostic of cancer in 96 patients (26.9%). The first specimen of sputum was found to reveal malignant cells in 27.2% of the patients and the

TABLE 14–25. Relationship Betweem Sputum and Bronchial Material in Lung Cancer Diagnosis

Diagnostic Material	Number of Patients	Percent of Patient Group (%)*
Sputum	168	47.1
Bronchial material only	93	26.0
Sputum and bronchial material	96	26.9
First sputum specimen	97	27.2
First bronchial material	80	22.4

*Patient group = 357 patients with cytopathology diagnostic of cancer.

From Johnston WW: Ten years of respiratory cytopathology at DUMC. I. The cytopathologic diagnosis of lung cancer during the years 1970 to 1974 noting the significance of specimen number and type. Acta Cytol 25:103–107, 1981.

first specimen of bronchial material in 22.4%. From these studies the following conclusions were made.

First and most important, diagnostic respiratory cytology had played a significant role in lung cancer diagnosis. Of a total of 715 consecutive patients with accepted primary lung cancer, an unequivocal cytologic diagnosis of cancer was made in 357 patients or approximately 50% of the cases. Second, the examination of multiple specimens of material from the lower respiratory tract was mandatory if the method were to be utilized maximally. From long experience it is now known that some lung cancers, for reasons as yet unknown, will not exfoliate diagnostic cells regardless of the number of specimens collected; however, in those patients who yield diagnostic cytologic specimens, five specimens will make a definitive diagnosis in over 85% of cases. Third, it is worth continued emphasis that no one specimen type was of exclusive importance in lung cancer diagnosis. Both sputum and bronchial material were essential for maximum diagnostic accuracy. It is of interest, however, that in these studies sputum was equal, if not superior, to bronchial material in the percentage of cancers diagnosed. In comparison, 26.0% of the cancers would have been missed had bronchial material not been examined. In our experience, clinicians frequently lose sight of the extreme diagnostic importance of the early-morning deep-cough specimen of sputum. Instead, they tend to regard the specimen obtained from bronchoscopy or fine needle aspiration as the one most likely to provide the cancer diagnosis.

Correlation Between Sputum and Bronchial Cytologic Specimens and the Histologic Specimen

In addition to the high levels of diagnostic accuracy achieved by sputum and bronchial material in the detection of tumor cells, the usefulness of these specimens in the prediction of histologic type of lung cancer has been shown to be impressively high.

Ng and Horak[380, 381] in their bronchial washing study reported in 1975 that the accuracy of diagnosing tumor cell type was 96% for squamous cell carcinoma, 86% for adenocarcinoma, 77% for large-cell carcinoma and below 50% for bronchioloalveolar carcinoma. In their sputum study also published in 1975 their levels of correlation were as follows: squamous cell carcinoma 95.3%, adenocarcinoma 87.8%, bronchioloalveolar carcinoma 65.0%, large-cell carcinoma 81.4%, small-cell carcinoma 96.5% and adenosquamous carcinoma 65.0%.

Johnston and Frable[260] in their 1976 review of respiratory cytology compared the accuracy in cell typing of lung cancer in two major academic hospitals. In the first institution the levels of predictive typing accuracy were squamous cell carcinoma 92%, adenocarcinoma 86%, small-cell undifferentiated carcinoma 88% and large-cell undifferentiated carcinoma 41%. In the second institution the levels were squamous cell carcinoma 75%, adenocarcinoma 83%, small-cell undifferentiated

TABLE 14–26. Prediction of Histologic Type of Primary Lung Cancer from Specimens of Sputum and Bronchial Material

Histologic Diagnosis	Cytologic Diagnosis					
	Squamous Cell Carcinoma	Adenocarcinoma	Large-cell Carcinoma	Small-cell Carcinoma	Adenosquamous Carcinoma	Unclassified Neoplasm
Squamous cell carcinoma	152	6	37	4	0	2
Adenocarcinoma	4	61	24	0	1	2
Large-cell carcinoma	22	9	28	1	6	0
Small-cell carcinoma	0	1	2	64	0	1
Adenosquamous carcinoma	0	0	1	0	3	0
Percent Correlations	152/178 (85%)	61/77 (79%)	28/92 (30%)	64/69 (93%)	3/10 (30%)	NA

Reproduced with permission from Johnston WW. Cytologic correlations. *In* Pulmonary Pathology. Edited by DH Dail, SP Hammar. New York, Springer-Verlag, 1987.

carcinoma 93%, adenosquamous carcinoma 75% and large-cell undifferentiated carcinoma 68%.

Suprun and associates[521] in a 1980 study reported 75% of 232 malignant cytologic specimens as having been correctly typed. In a study published in 1982, Pilotti and associates[417] reported an overall typing accuracy with sputum of 77% in 229 cases. For specific tumors, it was 94% for squamous cell carcinoma, 65% for adenocarcinoma, 20% for large-cell carcinoma and 81% for small-cell carcinoma.[419, 420]

A later study from our laboratory is summarized in Table 14–26. In this study the cytologic and histologic diagnoses were compared from 431 patients. The highest level of cytologic predictive accuracy (93%) was achieved for small-cell undifferentiated carcinoma. The cytologic presentation of this carcinoma is one of the most characteristic and diagnostic of all the various cancers encountered. Because of the high level of specificity of this diagnosis, one is able to proceed with therapy with great confidence without subjecting the patient to the additional trauma of biopsy or thoracotomy. Among the other cancers, the following cytologic-histologic correlations were found: squamous cell carcinoma 85%, adenocarcinoma 79%, large-cell undifferentiated carcinoma 30% and adenosquamous carcinoma 30%.

In reviewing the lower levels of cytologic-histologic correlation obtained with the other varieties of primary lung cancer, major concern occurs in those situations in which the cytologic prediction of specific cellular differentiation was not reflected in the tissues available for diagnosis. Thus, all cases of squamous cell carcinoma and adenocarcinoma designated as such by original cytologic diagnosis, but not sustained by the tissue diagnosis, were reviewed. For the squamous cell carcinoma group diagnosed cytologically, rediagnosis sustained the original interpretation in 83% of the cases and for the adenocarcinoma group in 57% of cases. Undoubtedly, such observations support the significance of the problems inherent in sampling in tissues as well as cytologic specimens. Further, they support the view that in some tumors, the morphologic features of the cells themselves may provide greater information about the true nature of the neoplasm than the histologic material.

Diagnostic Accuracy of Specimens Obtained by Fine Needle Aspiration

The diagnostic accuracy of FNA of lung as reported in the literature has shown sensitivity rates in the range of 75 to 95% of patients with malignant neoplasms correctly diagnosed by this method and specificity rates of 99% or more.

Tables 14–27 and 14–28 show the experience of our laboratory with FNAs from the lung. In nearly 60% of the cases, a malignant neoplasm was detected. Approximately 44% of these were primary lung neoplasms. In approximately 5% of patients, cancer was suspected but could not be conclusively diagnosed by cytologic diagnosis alone (see Table 14–27). In 765 FNAs of the lung, the specimens were interpreted as conclusively diagnostic for a primary malignant neoplasm. These neoplasms are shown in Table 14–28 and have been divided according to their histologic type. Squamous cell carcinoma was the most frequent diagnosis and was made in approximately 38% of patients. The other major diagnoses in descending order of frequency were large-cell undifferentiated carcinoma, 27.2%; adenocarcinoma, 13.5%; small-cell undifferentiated carcinoma, 12.7% and adenosquamous carci-

TABLE 14–27. Distribution by Diagnostic Categories of Fine Needle Aspirates

Diagnostic Category	Number Patients	Percent Patients
Primary lung cancer	765	43.8
Neoplasm metastatic to lung	261	15.0
Inconclusive	82	4.7
Benign	637	36.5
Total	1745	100.0

Reproduced with permission from Johnston WW: Cytologic correlations. *In* Pulmonary Pathology. Edited by DH Dail, SP Hammar. New York, Springer-Verlag, 1987.

TABLE 14–28. Classification of Primary Lung Neoplasms Diagnosed by Fine Needle Aspiration

Diagnostic Category	Number Patients	Percent Patients
Squamous cell carcinoma	290	37.9
Adenocarcinoma	103	13.5
Large-cell undifferentiated carcinoma	208	72.2
Small-cell undifferentiated carcinoma	97	12.7
Adenosquamous carcinoma	26	3.4
Plasmacytoma	2	0.3
Carcinosarcoma	2	0.3
Carcinoid	3	0.3
Lymphomatoid granulomatosis	1	0.1
Unclassified	33	4.2
Total	765	100.0

Reproduced with permission from Johnston WW: Cytologic correlations. *In* Pulmonary Pathology. Edited by DH Dail, SP Hammar. New York, Springer-Verlag, 1987.

TABLE 14–29. Comparison Between Fine Needle Aspiration (FNA) and Histologic Diagnosis in Primary and Secondary Neoplasms of Lungs

Diagnostic Category	Number Patients	Percent Patients
FNA and tissue diagnostic for cancer	246	85.4
FNA negative for cancer and tissue diagnostic for cancer	40	13.9
FNA positive for cancer and tissue negative for cancer	2	0.7
Total	288	100.0

Reproduced with permission from Johnston WW: Cytologic correlations. *In* Pulmonary Pathology. Edited by DH Dail, SP Hammar. New York, Springer-Verlag, 1987.

needle aspiration biopsy was found to be 86% and specificity 99.9%. A 1988 study by Simpson and associates[501] at the Mayo Clinic of 233 consecutive cases reported a sensitivity of 82% and a specificity of 100%.

Fine Needle Aspiration and Non-neoplastic Lesions of the Lung

Table 14–30 is illustrative of the extent to which FNAs that have been diagnosed as negative for cancer contribute useful information. As has been previously noted in Table 14–29, needle aspiration in our laboratory detected cancer in over 85% of histologically confirmed tumors. The primary usefulness, then, of the negative aspirate, is that it gives a reasonable level of confidence that the patient does not have cancer. Unfortunately, it does not conclusively exclude cancer.

In our series, there were 636 patients in whom no malignant neoplasms were seen and in whom no subsequent studies revealed malignant neoplasms (see

noma, 3.4%. In 4.2% of patients, although it was concluded that neoplastic cells were present, no opinion could be reached with respect to their further classification.

Although the cytologic presentation of the major types of lung cancer in FNAs has been discussed here in the appropriate chapter sections, one important point is worthy of special emphasis. The morphology of lung tumors in these specimens is essentially the same as that in sputum and bronchial material but with one additional characteristic: the FNA, because of direct sampling within the tumor by the needle, should contain large numbers of cancer cells and tissue fragments. The cell block becomes a useful vehicle for their study. Not infrequently microbiopsies of tissue will be available for evaluation in these preparations. *Indeed, the presence of only small numbers of putative tumor cells in an FNA should be a significant warning to the pathologist to exert extreme caution in rendering a conclusive cancer diagnosis. This is the setting in which a false-positive diagnosis of cancer is most likely to occur.*

We have studied 288 consecutive patients from whom tissue had been obtained within a reasonably short interval before or following the aspiration. This group of patients was employed to help address the question of effectiveness of detection in our laboratory. The comparison between the FNA diagnosis of cancer and the histologic diagnosis of cancer in these 288 patients is shown in Table 14–29. In 246 patients (85.4%), both the aspirate and the histologic specimen reflected a diagnosis of cancer. In 40 patients (13.9%), the tissue revealed a cancer which had been missed by the needle aspiration. Review of these specimens failed to reveal tumor cells that could have been overlooked previously. In two patients, the histologic examination did not show any cancer. These two cases then, are considered to be false-positive diagnoses for cancer, with a calculated rate of 0.7%. In both of these cases the cardinal error of overinterpretation of only a few atypical cells prompted these errors. Sensitivity of fine

TABLE 14–30. Distribution of Fine Needle Aspiration Patients Without Lung Neoplasm

Diagnostic Category	Number Patients	Percent Patients
Negative for cancer and without inflammation	489	76.9
Negative for cancer and inflammation, nonspecific	90	14.1
Inflammation, specific		
Bacteria (7)		
Tuberculosis (1)		
Nocardiosis (2)		
Blastomycosis (3)		
Cryptococcosis (6)		
Histoplasmosis (3)		
Candidiasis (2)		
Aspergillosis (8)		
Phycomycosis (3)		
Granuloma (18)		
Abscess (3)		
Oxalate crystals (1)	57	9.0
	636	100.0

Reproduced with permission from Johnston, WW: Cytologic correlations. In Pulmonary Pathology. Edited by DH Dail, SP Hammar. New York, Springer-Verlag, 1987.

Table 14–30). This patient group was further divided into the following diagnostic categories: negative for cancer and without cellular evidence of inflammation or infectious agent, negative for cancer with nonspecific inflammation and negative for cancer with evidence of an infectious organism or specific type of inflammatory process. In two patients, coin lesions called negative by aspiration biopsy were shown on resection to be hamartomas.[117, 327, 435] On review of the preparations, isolated fragments of normal-appearing cartilage provided evidence of the hamartomas.

The third category, comprising 57 patients, is of particular interest here because of the highly specific diagnostic information gained from the lung aspiration. In many of those cases in which an infectious organism was identified, it was immediately apparent on the toluidine blue–stained specimen. Upon notice of the presence of such an organism, the radiologist would then make a second needle pass into the lung and submit the aspirate for culture. The morphology of these organisms has been described in a prior section of this chapter.

We previously emphasized the importance of cytologic methods in the evaluation of patients without lung cancer. Of patients in this category, 9.0% benefited from the FNA diagnosis, which either detected an infectious organism or recognized a morphologic manifestation of a specific type of inflammation. Other laboratories have reported favorable experiences with aspiration in the diagnoses of non-neoplastic and infectious diseases of the lungs.[43, 189, 436]

Correlation Between Fine Needle Aspiration and Histology

A number of investigations have studied the correlations between FNA predictive of tumor classification and subsequent histologic diagnosis of the malignant tumor that had been aspirated. Dahlgren[100] in 1967 reported correlations in the range of 67 to 81%. Sinner recorded ranges of 90 to 100%.[502] In all of the aforementioned studies the highest level of predictive accuracy was for squamous cell carcinoma. Taft and associates[527] in 1980 reported 70% correlation; Poe and

Tobin[429] also in 1980 recorded an overall agreement level of 71%. Thornbury and associates[540] reported in 1981 an overall cytologic-histologic correlation level of 86%. Bonfiglio's[49] later study reported that cytologic diagnosis of adenocarcinoma correlated with tissue diagnoses in 87% of cases, squamous cell carcinoma in 77% and large-cell carcinoma in 62%.

The experience of the investigators in correlations between cytologic diagnoses from FNAs and histologic diagnoses is recorded in Table 14–31. In this study 159 patients with primary lung cancer and with both needle aspirates and tumor tissues available were reviewed. In 95% of cases diagnosed as small-cell undifferentiated carcinoma by aspiration, the diagnosis was confirmed by histologic study; 96% of adenocarcinomas so diagnosed by aspiration were confirmed by histologic study. In a similar fashion other levels of correlation were as follows: squamous cell carcinoma, 80% and large-cell undifferentiated carcinomas, 42%.

In those situations in which the cytologic-histologic correlation is not high, it should not be concluded that the cytologic interpretation is obviously an error and the histologic interpretation is correct. Although this was the original thesis on which the discipline of cytology was founded, cytology has matured and come of age and it can now be appreciated that in some situations the cytologic interpretation may be just as correct as the tissue interpretation or, in some cases, more accurately reflective of the nature of the lesion than the tissue examined. This last situation is being supported more and more by investigations into the ultrastructure of lung tumors in which both cytologic and histologic diagnostic interpretations had been rendered.[5, 82, 89, 110, 112, 122, 226, 227, 230, 309, 353] Indeed, some electron microscopic studies are beginning to challenge most of the currently accepted systems of diagnostic nomenclature for lung cancer. A growing general awareness of the cellular heterogeneity present in most of the "nonsmall-cell" lung carcinomas is evident.

Further studies in the literature suggest that the large-cell carcinomas and poorly differentiated carcinomas, whether of adenomatous or squamous differentiation, may show on ultrastructural examination multiple patterns of differentiation. Hess and associates[226, 227] in a series of studies on the histogenesis

TABLE 14–31. Prediction of Histologic Type of Primary Lung Cancer from Specimens Obtained by Fine Needle Aspiration

Histologic Diagnosis	Cytologic Diagnosis						
	Squamous Cell Carcinoma	Adenocarcinoma	Large-cell Carcinoma	Small-cell Carcinoma	Adenosquamous Carcinoma	Carcinoid	Unclassified Neoplasm
Squamous cell carcinoma	47	1	5	1	0	0	2
Adenocarcinoma	8	27	19	0	6	0	4
Large-cell carcinoma	2	0	10	0	1	0	2
Small-cell carcinoma	1	0	0	18	0	0	1
Adenosquamous carcinoma	1	0	0	0	2	0	0
Carcinoid	0	0	0	0	0	1	0
Correlation	47/59 (80%)	27/28 (96%)	10/24 (42%)	18/19 (95%)	2/9 (22%)	100.0%	

Reproduced with permission from Johnston, WW: Cytologic correlations. In Pulmonary Pathology. Edited by DH Dail, SP Hammar. New York, Springer-Verlag, 1987.

of lung cancer have shown that many poorly to well-differentiated squamous cell carcinomas, poorly to well-differentiated adenocarcinomas and giant cell carcinomas, diagnosed as such by conventional light microscopic criteria, were in reality tumors exhibiting dual differentiation towards both squamous cell carcinoma and adenocarcinoma. Horie and Ohta[230] examined by light and electron microscopy 26 human lung tumors classified as large-cell undifferentiated carcinomas. On the basis of their observations, these investigators were able to subclassify all of these tumors into squamous, adenosquamous and giant cell carcinomas. Dingemans and Mooi[112] investigated by electron microscopy a series of 40 lung tumors that had been diagnosed by conventional light microscopy as squamous cell carcinoma. Both at the tissue level and at the cellular level, the tumors showed highly variable ultrastructural details embracing both tonofibrils and desmosomes on one hand and unmistakable adenomatous differentiation on the other.[112]

Comparison of the Diagnostic Accuracy of Sputum and Bronchial Material and Fine Needle Aspirates

Considerable controversy exists regarding the relative roles that sputum and bronchial cytology, on one hand, and FNA, on the other, should play in the diagnostic workup of the patient with suspected lung cancer. One group supports a protocol that insists on a complete series of at least three to five early-morning sputum samples and at least one bronchoscopy before resorting to needle aspiration. An opposing group calls upon accuracy, cost-effectiveness and rapidity of diagnosis of FNA as reasons for advocating this procedure as the primary approach to suspected lung cancer. A third group, to which our institution belongs, takes an intermediate position in advocating a patient-by-patient decision in the relative roles of these procedures. The few studies in the literature in which the more conventional methods of diagnosis by sputum and bronchial material are compared with FNA fail to clarify completely the controversy. Nasiell,[374] in a study of 42 patients with lung cancer, found that sputum and bronchial material alone could have provided the diagnosis in 62% of the patients, whereas needle aspiration could have provided it in 76%.[374] Dahlgren and Lind[101] in a similar study of 101 patients recorded a 93% positive cancer diagnosis with needle aspiration in contrast to a 42% diagnosis with only sputum. Landsman and his associates[300] compared the diagnostic accuracy of bronchial brushings and needle aspirates and found that brushings detected 89% of lung cancers, whereas aspirates detected only 72%.

Johnston[255] reviewed a group of 168 consecutive lung cancer patients in whom a definitive diagnosis of primary lung cancer was established in a conventional cytologic specimen of sputum or bronchial material or in a specimen obtained by FNA. This review's purpose was to compare the relative accuracies between the modalities of sputum and bronchial material with FNA in the diagnosis of lung cancer among these patients. The patients included in this study were selected from a total of 1093 patients who had been diagnosed and treated for lung cancer at our institution over a 5-year period.

In 325 of these patients (29.8%), a definitive cancer diagnosis was established from histopathologic material alone without any cytologic diagnoses. In 420 patients (38.4%), both histologic and cytologic material had been interpreted as being conclusively diagnostic for lung cancer. In 348 patients (31.8%), a cytologic diagnosis of lung cancer was made without a histologic confirmation. Thus, in a total of 768 of 1093 patients (70.3%), a definitive cytologic diagnosis of cancer had been made. Of these 768 patients, a total of 168 (Table 14–32) patients had been evaluated with both conventional respiratory cytologic methods (sputum and bronchial material) and with FNA. In nine patients (5.4%), only conventional respiratory cytologic specimens were conclusively diagnostic for cancer. In 122 patients (72.6%), only the FNA was diagnostic. In 37 patients

TABLE 14–32. Comparison Between Conventional Respiratory Cytology and Fine Needle Aspiration (FNA) in Lung Cancer Diagnosis in 168 Patients

Classification	Only Conventional Cytology Diagnostic*		Only FNA Diagnostic		Conventional Cytology and FNA Diagnostic		Total
Squamous cell carcinoma	6		39		22		67
		9.0%		58.2%		32.8%	
Adenocarcinoma	1		31		7		39
		2.6%		79.5%		17.9%	
Large-cell undifferentiated carcinoma	1		37		3		41
		2.5%		90.2%		7.3%	
Small-cell undifferentiated carcinoma	1		10		4		15
		6.7%		66.7%		26.6%	
Adenosquamous carcinoma	0		5		1		6
				83.3%		16.7%	
All cancers	9		122		37		168
		5.4%		72.6%		22.0%	

*Includes sputum and bronchial material.

From Johnston, WW: Fine needle aspiration biopsy versus sputum and bronchial material in the diagnosis of lung cancer. Acta Cytol 32:641–646, 1988.

(22.0%), both conventional respiratory specimens and FNA yielded a definitive lung cancer diagnosis. FNA was the only cytologic specimen positive in 90.2% of large-cell undifferentiated carcinomas, 79.5% of adenocarcinomas, 66.7% of small-cell undifferentiated carcinomas and 58.2% of squamous cell carcinomas. In 26.5% of patients a diagnosis of cancer could have been established by conventional cytologic specimens without the necessity of proceeding to percutaneous FNA. From this study, it was concluded that the techniques of conventional respiratory cytology and FNA are complementary in the diagnosis of lung cancer. Although the percentage of lung cancers diagnosed by FNA alone was much greater than that by conventional respiratory cytology alone, more than a fourth of these cancers could be detected by the less invasive techniques of sputum and bronchoscopy.

Over the years of development of needle aspiration at our institution, a formal protocol for its utilization has never been formulated. Individualized physician decisions about the diagnostic approaches to lung lesions have resulted in the data as shown in Table 14–29. Information such as this emphasizes the diagnostic effectiveness of conventional respiratory cytologic methods. The question then of whether or not FNA should be the primary diagnostic tool becomes a complex one of balancing such considerations as length of patient's hospital stay, economic factors, reluctance of some patients to permit their lungs to be pierced by needles and morbidity of needle aspiration. In the experience of our laboratory, sputum and bronchial material provide a high diagnostic yield for lung cancer and in most cases should be used before resorting to aspiration. In contrast, however, it is clear that FNA biopsy is the procedure of primary choice for the patient with suspected metastases to the lung.

References

1. Abramson W, Dzenis V, Hicks S: Cytologic study of sputa and exudates using paraffin tubes. Acta Cytol 8:306–310, 1964.
2. Adamson JS, Senior RM, Merrill T: Alveolar cell carcinoma: An electron microscopic study. Am Rev Respir Dis 100:550–557, 1969.
3. Adelstein DJ, Tomashefski JF, Snow NJ, Horrigan TP, Hines JD: Mixed small cell and non-small cell lung cancer. Chest 89:699–704, 1986.
4. Aisner SC, Gupta PK, Frost JK: Sputum cytology in pulmonary sarcoidosis. Acta Cytol 21:394–398, 1977.
5. Albain KS, True LD, Golomb HM, Hoffman PC, Little AG: Large cell carcinoma of the lung: ultrastructural differentiation and clinicopathologic correlations. Cancer 56:1618–1623, 1985.
6. Allen AR, Fullmer CD: Primary diagnosis of pulmonary echinococcosis by the cytologic technique. Acta Cytol 16:212–216, 1972.
7. An SH, Koprowska I: Primary cytologic diagnosis of asbestosis associated with bronchogenic carcinoma. Case report and review of literature. Acta Cytol 6:391–398, 1962.
8. Anderson RJ, Johnston WW, Szpak CA: Fine needle aspiration of adenoid cystic carcinoma metastatic to the lung. Cytologic features and differential diagnosis. Acta Cytol 29:527–532, 1985.
9. Archer PG, Koprowska I, McDonald JR, Naylor B, Papanicolaou GN, Umiker WO: A study of variability in the interpretation of sputum cytology slides. Cancer Res 26:2122–2144, 1966.
10. Arrigoni MG, Woolner LB, Bernatz PE: Atypical carcinoid tumors of the lung. J Thorac Cardiovasc Surg 64:413–421, 1972.
11. Ashley DJB, Davies HD: Cancer of the lung: histology and biologic behavior. Cancer 20:165–174, 1967a.
12. Ashley DJB, Davies HD: Mixed glandular and squamous-cell carcinoma of the bronchus. Thorax 22:431–436, 1967b.
13. Ashton PR, Hollingsworth AS Jr, Johnston WW: The cytopathology of metastatic breast cancer. Acta Cytol 19:1–6, 1975.
14. Auerbach O, Frasca JM, Parks VR, Carter HW: A comparison of World Health Organization (WHO) classification of lung tumors by light and electron microscopy. Cancer 50:2079–2088, 1982.
15. Auerbach O, Garfinkel L, Parks VR: Histologic type of lung cancer in relation to smoking habits, year of diagnosis and site of metastases. Chest 67:382–387, 1975.
16. Auerbach O, Garfinkel L, Parks VR: Scar cancer of the lung: increase over a 21-year period. Cancer 43:636–642, 1979.
17. Auerbach O, Gere JB, Forman JB, Petrick TG, Smolin HJK, Muehsam GE, Kassouny DY, Stout AP: Changes in bronchial epithelium in relation to smoking and cancer of the lungs; a report of progress. N Engl J Med 256:97–104, 1957.
18. Auerbach O, Hammond EC, Garfinkel L: Changes in bronchial epithelium in relation to cigarette smoking 1955–1960 vs 1970–1977. N Engl J Med 300:381–386, 1979.
19. Auerbach O, Hammond EC, Kirman D, Garfinkel L, Stout AP: Histologic changes in bronchial tubes of cigarette smoking dogs. Cancer 20:2055–2066, 1967.
20. Auerbach O, Stout AP, Hammond EC, Garfinkel L: Changes in bronchial epithelium in relation to cigarette smoking and in relation to lung cancer. N Engl J Med 265:253–267, 1961.
21. Auerbach O, Stout AP, Hammond EC, Garfinkel L: Changes in bronchial epithelium in relationship to sex age, residence, smoking and pneumonia. N Engl J Med 267:111–119, 1962.
22. Bailey TM, Akhtar M, Ali MA: Fine needle aspiration in the diagnosis of tuberculosis. Acta Cytol 29:732–736, 1985.
23. Baird JK, Neafie RC, Connor DH: Parasitic Infections. In Pulmonary Pathology. Edited by DH Dail and SP Hammar. New York, Springer-Verlag, 1988.
24. Bamforth J: The examination of the sputum and pleural fluid in the diagnosis of malignant diseases of the lung. Thorax (London) 1:118–127, 1946.
25. Bamforth J, Osborn GR: Diagnosis from cells. J Clin Pathol 11:473–482, 1958.
26. Barach AL, Bickerman HA, Beck GL, Nanda KGS, Pons ER: Induced sputum as a diagnostic technique for cancer of the lungs. Arch Int Med 106:230–236, 1960.
27. Barton RT, Hagetveit AC: Nickel-related cancers of the respiratory tract. Cancer 45:3061–3064, 1980.
28. Bateson EM: The solitary circumscribed bronchogenic carcinoma: a radiological study of 100 cases. Br J Radiol 37:598–607, 1964.
29. Bauer TW, Erozan YS: Psammoma bodies in small cell carcinoma of the lung: a case report. Acta Cytol 26:327–330, 1982.
30. Beale AJ, Campbell W: A rapid cytological method for the diagnosis of measles. J Clin Pathol 12:335–337, 1959.
31. Bedrossian CWM: Iatrogenic and toxic injury. In Pulmonary Pathology. Edited by DH Dail and SP Hammar. New York, Springer-Verlag, 1988.
32. Bedrossian CWM, Corey BJ: Abnormal sputum cytopathology during chemotherapy with bleomycin. Acta Cytol 22:202–207, 1978.
33. Bedrossian CWM, Rybka DL: Bronchial brushing during fiberoptic bronchoscopy for the cytodiagnosis of lung cancer: comparison with sputum and bronchial washings. Acta Cytol 20:446–453, 1976.
34. Bedrossian CWM, Weilbaecher DG, Bentinck DC, Greenberg SD: Ultrastructure of human bronchioloalveolar cell carcinoma. Cancer 36:1399–1413, 1975.
35. Bell WR, Johnston WW, Bigner SP: The cytologic diagnosis of occult small cell undifferentiated carcinoma of the lung. Acta Cytol 26:73–77, 1982.
36. Bennett DE, Sasser WF, Ferguson TB: Adenocarcinoma of the lung in men: A clincopathologic study of 100 cases. Cancer: 23:431–439, 1969.

37. Bennett, DE, Sasser WF: Bronchiolar carcinoma: A valid clinicopathologic entity? A study of 30 cases. Cancer 24:876–887, 1969.

38. Bennett JE: Mycoses. *In* Principles and Practice of Infectious Disease, vol I. Edited by GL Mandel, RG Douglas Jr, JE Bennett. New York, John Wiley & Sons, 1979.

39. Berkheiser JW: Bronchiolar proliferation and metaplasia associated with bronchiectasis, pulmonary infarcts and anthracosis. Cancer 12:499–508, 1959.

40. Berkheiser JW: Bronchiolar proliferation and metaplasia associated with thromboembolism: a pathological and experimental study. Cancer 16:205–211, 1963.

41. Berkson DM, Snider GL: Heated hypertonic aerosol in collecting sputum specimens for cytological diagnosis. JAMA 173:135–138, 1960.

42. Bewtra C, Dewan N, O'Donahue WJ Jr: Exfoliative sputum cytology in pulmonary embolism. Acta Cytol 27:489–496, 1983.

43. Bhatt ON, Miller R, Riche JL, King EG: Aspiration biopsy in pulmonary opportunistic infections. Acta Cytol 21:206–209, 1977.

44. Bibbo M: Bronchial brush cytology: *In* Compendium on Diagnostic Cytology, 6th ed. Edited by GL Wied, CM Keebler, LG Koss, JW Reagan. Chicago, Tutorials of Cytology, 1988.

45. Bibbo M: Look-alikes in sputum cytology: *In* Compendium on Diagnostic Cytology, 6th ed. Edited by GL Weid, CM Keebler, LG Koss, JW Reagan. Chicago, Tutorials of Cytology, 1988.

45a. Bibbo M: Unpublished data.

46. Bibbo M, Fennessy JJ, Lu C-T, Straus FH, Variakojis D, Weid GL: Bronchial brushing technique for the cytologic diagnosis of peripheral lung lesions. Acta Cytol 17:245–251, 1973.

47. Bickerman HA, Sproul EE, Barach AL: An aerosol method of producing bronchial secretions in human subjects: A clinical technique for detection of lung cancer. Dis Chest 33:347–362, 1958.

48. Black H, Ackerman LV: The importance of epidermoid carcinomas *in situ* in the histogenesis of carcinoma of the lung. Ann Surg 136:44–55, 1953.

49. Bonfiglio T: Transthoracic thin needle aspiration biopsy. *In* Masson Series in Diagnostic Cytopathology, vol 4. Edited by WW Johnston. Paris-New York, Masson, 1983.

50. Bonfiglio TA, Dvoretsky PM, Piscioli F, dePapp EW, Patten SF Jr: Fine needle aspiration biopsy in the evaluation of lymphoreticular tumors of the thorax. Acta Cytol 29:548–553, 1985.

51. Bonikos DS, Bensch KG, Jomplis RW: Peripheral pulmonary carcinoid tumors. Cancer 37:1977–1998, 1976.

52. Bonime RG: Improved procedure for the preparation of pulmonary cytology smears. Acta Cytol 16:543–545, 1972.

53. Borsi S: Diagnosis of pulmonary echinococcosis by cytohistological examination of the sputum. Pathologica 66:311–313, 1974.

54. Braman SS, Whitcomb ME: Endobronchial metastasis. Arch Intern Med 135:543–547, 1975.

55. Brenner SA, Lambert RL, Pablo GE: Superheated aerosol-induced sputum in the cytodiagnosis of lung cancer. Acta Cytol 6:405–408, 1962.

56. Brereton HD, Matthews MJ, Costa J, Kent CH, Johnson RE: Mixed anaplastic small cell and squamous cell carcinoma of the lung. Ann Intern Med. 88:805–806, 1978.

57. Broderick PA, Corvese NL, LaChance T, Allard J: Giant cell carcinoma of lung: A cytologic evaluation. Acta Cytol 19:225–230, 1975.

58. Broghamer Jr WL, Collins WM, Mojsejenko IK: The cytohistopathology of a pseudomesotheliomatous carcinoma of the lung. Acta Cytol 22:239–242, 1978.

59. Burke MD, Melamed MR: Exfoliative cytology of metastatic cancer in lung. Acta Cytol 12:61–74, 1968.

60. Byrd RB, Miller WE, Carr DT, Payne WS, Woolner LB: The roentgenographic appearance of squamous cell carcinoma of the bronchus. Mayo Clin Proc 43:327–332, 1968.

61. Cagle PT, Cohle SD, Greenberg SD: Natural history of pulmonary scar cancers: clinical and pathologic implications. Cancer 56:2031–2035, 1985.

62. Carroll R: Changes in the bronchial epithelium in primary lung cancer. Br J Cancer 15:215–219, 1961.

63. Carter D: Small cell carcinoma of the lung: Am J Surg Pathol 7:787–795, 1983.

64. Carter D: Squamous cell carcinoma of the lung: an update. Semin Diagn Pathol 2:226–234, 1985.

65. Carter D, Eggleston JC: Adenoid cystic carcinoma. *In* Tumors of the Lower Respiratory Tract. Washington DC, Armed Forces Institute of Pathology, p 199–202, 1980.

66. Carter D, Eggleston JC: Bronchioloalveolar carcinoma. *In* Tumors of the Lower Respiratory Tract. Washington DC, Armed Forces Institute of Pathology, p 127–147, 1980.

67. Carter D, Eggleston JC: Central carcinoid tumors. *In* Tumors of the Lower Respiratory Tract. Washington DC, Armed Forces Institute of Pathology, p 163–172, 1980.

68. Carter D, Eggleston JC: Combined adenocarcinoma and squamous cell carcinoma. *In* Tumors of the Lower Respiratory Tract. Washington DC, Armed Forces Institute of Pathology, p 161, 1980.

69. Carter D, Eggleston J: Tumors of the Lower Respiratory Tract. Washington, DC, AFIP, 1980.

70. Chalon J, Katz JS, Ramannthon S, Ambirunga M, Orkin LR: Tracheobronchial epithelial multinucleation in malignant diseases. Science 183:525–526, 1974.

71. Chalon J, Tang C-K, Gorstein F, Turndorf H, Katz JS, Klein GS, Patel C: Diagnostic and prognostic significance of tracheobronchial epithelial multinucleation. Acta Cytol 22:316–320, 1978.

72. Chamberlain DW, Braude AC, Rebuck AS: A critical evaluation of bronchoalveolar lavage; criteria for identifying unsatisfactory specimens. Acta Cytol 31:599–605, 1987.

73. Chan JKC, Tsang DNC, Wong DKK: *Penicillium marneffei* in bronchoalveolar lavage fluid. Acta Cytol 33:523–526, 1989.

74. Chandler FW, Watts JC: Fungal infections. *In* Pulmonary Pathology. Edited by DH Dail, SP Hammar. New York, Springer-Verlag, 1988.

75. Chandra P, Delaney MD, Tuazon CU: Role of special stains in the diagnosis of *Pneumocystis carinii* infection from bronchial washing specimens in patients with the acquired immune deficiency syndrome. Acta Cytol 32:105–108, 1988.

76. Chang JP, Aken M, Russell WO: Sputum cell concentration by membrane filtration for cancer diagnosis: a preliminary report. Acta Cytol 5:168–172, 1961.

77. Chaudhuri B, Nanos S, Soco JN, McGrew EA: Disseminated *Strongyloides stercoralis* infestation detected by sputum cytology. Acta Cytol 24:360–362, 1980.

78. Chaudhuri MR: Primary pulmonary cavitating carcinomas. Thorax 28:354–366, 1973.

79. Chen KTK: Cytology of tracheobronchial amyloidosis. Acta Cytol 28:133–135, 1984.

80. Chipps HD, Kraul LH: Cytologic alterations in pulmonary tuberculosis which simulate carcinoma. (Abstr.) Can Res 10:210, 1950.

81. Chopra SK, Genovesi MG, Simmons DH, Gothe B: Fiberoptic bronchoscopy in the diagnosis of lung cancer: comparison of pre- and post-bronchoscopy sputa, washings, brushings and biopsies. Acta Cytol 21:524–527, 1977.

82. Churg A: The fine structure of large cell undifferentiated carcinoma of the lung: evidence for its relation to squamous cell carcinomas and adenocarcinomas. Hum Pathol 9:143–156, 1978.

83. Churg A, Johnston WH, Stulbarg M: Small cell squamous and mixed small cell squamous-small cell anaplastic carcinomas of the lung. Am J Surg Pathol 4:255–263, 1980.

84. Chute CG, Greenberg ER, Baron J, Korson R, Baker J, Yates J: Presenting conditions of 1539 population-based lung cancer patients by cell type and stage in New Hampshire and Vermont. Cancer 56:2107–2111, 1985.

85. Clayton F: Bronchioloalveolar carcinomas: Cell types, patterns of growth, and prognostic correlates. Cancer 57:1555–1564, 1986.

86. Clerf LH, Herbut PA: Diagnosis of bronchogenic carcinoma by examination of bronchial secretions. Ann Otol 55:646, 1946.

87. Clerf LH, Herbut PA: The value of cytological diagnosis of pulmonary malignancy. Am Rev Tuberc 61:60–65, 1950.

88. Clerf LH, Herbut PA: Early diagnosis of cancer of the lung. JAMA 150:793–795, 1952.

89. Coalson JJ, Mohr JA, Pirtle JK, Dee AL, Rhoades ER: Electron microscopy of neoplasms in the lung with special emphasis on the alveolar cell carcinoma. Am Rev Respir Dis 101:181–197, 1970.

90. Collier FC, Blakemore WS, Kyler RH, Enterline HT, Kirby CK, Johnson J: Carcinoma of the lung: factors which influence five-year survival with special reference to blood vessel invasion. Ann Surg 146:417–423, 1957.

91. Conlan AA, Payne WS, Woolner LB, Sanderson DR: Adenoid cystic carcinoma (cylindroma) and mucuopidermoid carcinoma of the bronchus. J Thorac Cardiovasc Surg 76:369–377, 1978.

92. Conant NF, Smith DT, Baker RD, Callaway JM: Manual of Clinical Mycology, 3rd ed. Philadelphia, WB Saunders, 1971.

93. Cooney W, Dzuira B, Harper R, Nash G: The cytology of sputum from thermally injured patients. Acta Cytol 16:433–437, 1972.

94. Covell JL, Feldman PS: Fine needle aspiration diagnosis of aspiration pneumonia (Phytopneumonitis). Acta Cytol 28:77–80, 1984.

95. Cox JD, Yesner RA: Adenocarcinoma of the lung; recent results from the Veterans Administration Lung Group. Am Rev Resp Dis 120:1025–1029, 1979.

96. Craig ID, Desrosiers P, Lefcoe MS: Giant-cell carcinoma of the lung: a cytologic study. Acta Cytol 27:293–298, 1983.

97. Craig ID, Finley RJ: Spindle-cell carcinoid tumor of lung: cytologic, histopathologic and ultrastructural features. Acta Cytol 26:495–498, 1982.

98. Craig ID, Shum DT, Desrosiers P, McLeod C, Lefcoe MS, Paterson NAM, Finley RJ, Woods B, Anderson RJ: Choriocarcinoma metastatic to the lung: a cytologic study with identification of human choriogonadotropin with an immunoperoxidase technique. Acta Cytol 27:647–640, 1983.

99. D'Ablang G III, Bernard B, Zaharov I, Barton L, Kaplan B, Schwinn CP: Neonatal pulmonary cytology and bronchopulmonary dysplasia. Acta Cytol 19:21–27, 1975.

100. Dahlgren SE: Aspiration biopsy of intrathoracic tumors. Acta Pathol Microbiol Scand (B) 70:566–576, 1967.

101. Dahlgren S, Lind B: Comparison between diagnostic results obtained by transthoracic needle biopsy and by sputum cytology. Acta Cytol 16:53–58, 1972.

102. Dahlgren S, Nordenstrom B: Transthoracic Needle Biopsy. Chicago, Year Book Medical Publishers, 1966.

103. Dail DH: Metabolic and other diseases. In Pulmonary Pathology. DH Dail, SP Hammar. New York, Springer-Verlag, 1988.

104. Daniel WC, Nair SV, Bluestein J: Light and electron microscopic observations of Blastomyces dermatitidis in sputum. Acta Cytol 23:222–226, 1979.

105. Daniele RP, Elias JA, Epstein PE, Rossman MD: Bronchoalveolar lavage: Role in the pathogenesis, diagnosis and management of interstitial lung disease. Ann Intern Med 102:93–99, 1985.

106. Davis S, Stanley KE, Yesner R, Kuang DT, Morris JF: Small cell carcinoma of the lung—survival according to histologic subtype: A Veterans Administration Lung Group Study. Cancer 47:1863–1866, 1981.

107. Dao AH: Entamoeba gingivalis in sputum smears. Acta Cytol 29:632–633, 1985.

108. DeFine LA, Saleba KP, Gibson BB, Wesseler TA, Baughman R: Cytologic evaluation of bronchoalveolar lavage specimens in immunosuppressed patients with suspected opportunistic infections. Acta Cytol 31:235–242, 1987.

109. Deirksheide, WC: Medical Decisions: Interpreting Clinical Tests. ASM News 53:677–680, 1987.

110. Delmonte VC, Alberti O, Saldiva PHN: Large cell carcinoma of the lung: ultrastructural and immunohistochemical features. Chest 90:524–526, 1986.

111. DeVita VT Jr, Hellman S, Rosenberg SA: Cancer: Principles and Practice of Oncology, 3rd ed. Philadelphia, JB Lippincott, 1989.

112. Dingemans KP, Mooi WJ: Ultrastructure of squamous cell carcinoma of the lung. Pathol Annu 19:Pt 1:249–273, 1984.

113. Donaldson JC, Kaminsky DB, Elliott RC: Bronchiolar carcinoma: report of 11 cases and review of the literature. Cancer 41:250–258, 1978.

114. Doshi N, Kanbour A, Fujikura T, Klionsky B: Tracheal aspiration cytology in neonates with respiratory distress. Acta Cytol 26:15–21, 1982.

115. Dube VE: Peripheral bronchial carcinoid with a spindle-cell pattern. Arch Pathol 89:374–377, 1970.

116. Dudgeon LS, Wrigley CH: On the demonstration of particles of malignant growth in the sputum by means of the wet-film method. J Laryngol Otol 50:752–763, 1935.

117. Dunbar F, Leiman G: The aspiration cytology of pulmonary hamartomas. Diag Cytopathol 5:174–180, 1989.

118. Dunn D, Hertel B, Norwood W, Nicoloff DM: Bronchioloalveolar carcinoma of the lung: a clinicopathologic study. Ann Thor Surg 26:241–249, 1978.

119. Ehya H: Cytology of mesothelioma of the tunica vaginalis metastatic to the lung. Acta Cytol 29:79–84, 1985.

120. Eisenberg RS, Dunton BL: Hodgkin's disease first suggested by sputum cytology. Chest 65:218–219, 1974.

121. Eisenstein R, Battiforo HA: Malignant giant cell tumor of bone: exfoliation of tumor cells from pulmonary metastases. Acta Cytol 10:130–133, 1966.

122. Elema JD, Keuning HM: The ultrastructure of small cell lung carcinoma in bronchial biopsy specimens. Hum Pathol 16:1133–1140, 1985.

123. Ellis FH Jr, Woolner LB, Schmidt HW: Metastatic pulmonary malignancy: study of factors involved in exfoliation of malignant cells. J Thorac Surg 20:125–135, 1950.

124. Ellis HD, Kernosky JJ: Efficiency of concentrating malignant cells in sputum. Acta Cytol 7:372–373, 1963.

125. Elson CE, Moore SP, Johnston WW: Morphologic and immunocytochemical studies of bronchioloalveolar carcinoma at Duke University Medical Center, 1968–1986. Analyt Quant Cytol Histol 11:261–274, 1989.

126. Elson CE, Roggli VL, Vollmer RT, Greenberg SD, Fraire AE, Spjut HJ, Yesner R: Prognostic indicators for survival in stage I carcinoma of the lung; a histologic study of 47 surgically resected cases. Mod Pathol 1:288–291, 1988.

127. Erozan YS: Cytopathology in the diagnosis of pulmonary disease. In Multiple Imaging Procedures, vol 1, Pulmonary System, Practical Approaches to Pulmonary Diagnosis. Edited by SS Seigelman, FP Stitik, WR Summer. New York, Grune & Stratton, 1979.

128. Erozan YS, Frost JK: Cytopathologic diagnosis of cancer in pulmonary material: a critical histopathologic correlation. Acta Cytol 14:560–565, 1970.

129. Erozan YS, Frost JK: Cytopathologic diagnosis of lung cancer. In Lung Cancer. Clinical Diagnosis And Treatment. Edited by MJ Straus. New York, Grune & Stratton, 1977. p 106.

130. Farber SM: Clinical appraisal of pulmonary cytology. JAMA 175:345–348, 1961.

131. Farber SM, Benioff MA, Frost JK, Rosenthal M, Tobias G: Cytologic studies of sputum and bronchial secretions in primary carcinoma of the lung. Dis Chest 14:633–664, 1948.

132. Farber SM, McGrath Jr AK, Benioff MA, Rosenthal M: Evaluation of cytologic diagnosis of lung cancer. JAMA 144:1–4, 1950.

133. Farber SM, Pharr SL: The practicing physician and pulmonary cytology. Lancet 77:111–113, 1957.

134. Farber SM, Pharr SL, Wood DA, Gorman RD: The mucolytic and digestive action of trypsin in the preparation of sputum for cytologic study. Science 117:687–690, 1953.

135. Farber SM, Rosenthal M, Alston EF, Benioff MA, McGrath Jr AK: Cytologic Diagnosis of Lung Cancer. Springfield, IL, Charles C Thomas, 1950.

136. Farber SM, Wood DA, Pharr SL, Pierson B: Significant cytologic findings in nonmalignant pulmonary disease. Dis Chest 31:1–13, 1957.

137. Farley ML, Mabry L, Munoz LA, Diserens HW: Crystals occurring in pulmonary cytology specimens. Association with Aspergillus infection. Acta Cytol 29:737–744, 1985.

138. Feldman PS, Covell JL: Fine Needle Aspiration Cytology and Its Clinical Applications: Breast and Lung. Chicago, American Society of Clinical Pathologists Press, 1985.

139. Fennessy JJ: Bronchial brushing in the diagnosis of peripheral lung lesions. A preliminary report. Am J Roentgen 98:474–481, 1966.

140. Fennessy JJ: A method for obtaining cytologic specimens from the periphery of the lung. Acta Cytol 10:413–415, 1966.
141. Fennessy JJ: Transbronchial biopsy of peripheral lung lesions. Radiology 88:878–882, 1967.
142. Fennessy JJ: Bronchial brushing and transbronchial forceps biopsy in the diagnosis of pulmonary lesions. Dis Chest 53:377–389, 1968.
143. Fennessy JJ: Bronchial brushing. Ann Otol 79:924–932, 1970.
144. Fennessy JJ, Fry WA, Manalo-Estrella P, Hidvegi DVSF: The bronchial brushing technique for obtaining cytologic specimens from peripheral lung lesions. Acta Cytol 14:25–30, 1970.
145. Fennessy JJ, Kittle CF: The role of bronchial brushing in the decision for thoracotomy. J Thorac Cardiovasc Surg 66:541–548, 1973.
146. Fennessy JJ, Lu CT, Variakojis D, Straus FH, Bibbo M: Transcatheter biopsy in the diagnosis of diseases of the respiratory tract. An evaluation of seven years' experience with 693 patients. Radiology 110:555–561, 1974.
147. Fields MJ, Martin WF, Young BL, Tweeddale DN: Application of the Nedelkoff-Christopherson millipore method to sputum cytology. Acta Cytol 10:220–222, 1966.
148. Fielding JE: Smoking: health effects and control. N Engl J Med 313:491–498, 555–561, 1985.
149. Fitzgibbons PL, Kern WL: Adenosquamous carcinoma of the lung: a clinical and pathologic study of seven cases. Hum Pathol 16:463–466, 1985.
150. Flehinger BJ, Melamed MR, Zaman MB: Resectability of lung cancer and survival in the New York Lung Cancer Detection Program. World J Surg 5:681–687, 1981.
151. Fleming WH, Jove DF: Primary leiomyosarcoma of the lung with positive sputum cytology. Acta Cytol 19:14–20, 1975.
152. Fleury J, Escudier E, Pocholle M-J, Carre C, Bernaudin JF: Cell population obtained by bronchoalveolar lavage in Pneumocystis carinii pneumonitis. Acta Cytol 29:721–726, 1985.
153. Fleury-Feith J, Escudier E, Pocholle MJ, Carre C, Bernaudin JF: The effects of cytocentrifugation on differential cell counts in samples obtained by bronchoalveolar lavage. Acta Cytol 31:606–610, 1987.
154. Fontanna RS, Sanderson DR, Miller WE, Woolner LB, Taylor WF, Uhlenhopp MA: The Mayo lung project. Preliminary report of "early cancer detection" phase. Cancer 30:1373–1382, 1972.
155. Foot NC: The identification of types of pulmonary cancer in cytologic smears. Am J Pathol 28:963–977, 1952.
156. Foot NC: Cytologic diagnosis in suspected pulmonary cancer. Critical analysis of smears from 1,000 persons. Am J Clin Pathol 25:223–240, 1955.
157. Ford DK, Fidler HK, Lock DR: Dysplastic lesions of the bronchial tree. Cancer 14:1226–123, 1961.
158. Fortuny IE, Tempero KF, Amsden TW: Pneumocystis carinii pneumonia diagnosed from sputum and successfully treated with pentamidine isethionate. Cancer 26:911–913, 1970.
159. Frable WJ: The relationship of pulmonary cytology to survival in lung cancer. Acta Cytol 12:52–56, 1968.
160. Frable WJ: Thin Needle Aspiration Biopsy. Philadelphia, WB Saunders, 1983.
161. Frable WJ, Johnston WW: Respiratory Cytology Transparencies, Explanatory Text and Self-Evaluative Test, International Cytology Slide Sets, XIX. Chicago, Tutorials of Cytology, 1974.
162. Frable WJ, Kay S: Herpesvirus infection of the respiratory tract: electron microscopic observation of the virus in cells obtained from a sputum cytology. Acta Cytol 21:391–393, 1977.
163. Francis D, Borgeskov S: Progress in preoperative diagnosis of pulmonary lesions. Acta Cytol 19:231–234, 1975.
164. Francis D, Jacobsen M: Pulmonary blastoma: Preoperative cytologic and histologic findings. Act Cytol 23:437–442, 1979.
165. Frank AL: The epidemiology and etiology of lung cancer. Clin Chest Med 3:219–228, 1982.
166. Freedman SI, Ang EP, Haley RS: Identification of coccidioidomycosis of the lung by fine needle aspiration biopsy. Acta Cytol 30:420–424, 1986.
167. Frierson HF Jr, Covell JL, Mills SE: Fine needle aspiration cytology of atypical carcinoid of the lung. Acta Cytol 31:471–475, 1987.
168. Frost JK: The cell in health and disease. In Monographs in Clinical Cytology, vol 2. Edited by GL Wied. Basel, S Karger, 1986.
169. Frost JK, Gupta PK, Erozan YS, Carter D, Hollander DH, Leven ML, Ball Jr WO: Pulmonary cytologic alterations in toxic environmental inhalation. Hum Path 4:521–53, 1973.
170. Fry WA, Manalo-Estrella P: Bronchial brushing. Surg Gynecol Obstet 130:67–71, 1970.
171. Füezesi L, Höer P-W, Schmidt W: Exfoliative cytology of multiple endobronchial granular cell tumor. Acta Cytol 33:516–518, 1989.
172. Fullmer CD, Morris RP: Primary cytodiagnosis of unsuspected mediastinal Hodgkin's disease. Report of a case. Acta Cytol 16:77–81, 1972.
173. Fullmer CD, Parrish CM: Pulmonary cytology. A diagnostic method for occult carcinoma. Acta Cytol 13:645–651, 1969.
174. Fullmer CD, Short JG, Allen A, Walker K: Proposed classification for bronchial epithelial cell abnormalities in the category of dyskaryosis. Acta Cytol 13:459–471, 1969.
175. Funkhouser JW, Meininger DE: Cytologic aspects of bronchial brushing in a community hospital. Acta Cytol 16:51–52, 1972.
176. Gagneten CB, Geller CE, Saenz MdC: Diagnosis of bronchogenic carcinoma through the cytologic examination of sputum, with special reference to tumor typing. Acta Cytol 20:530–536, 1976.
177. Gail MH, Eagan RT, Feld R, Ginsberg R, Goodell B, Hill L, Holmes EC, Lukeman JM, Mountain CF, Oldham RK, Person FG, Wright PW, Lake WH: Prognostic factors in patients with resected stage I non-small cell lung cancer: a report from the Lung Cancer Study Group. Cancer 54:1802–1813, 1984.
178. Galen RS, Gambino SR: Beyond Normality: The Predictive Value and Efficiency of Medical Diagnoses. New York, John Wiley & Sons, 1975.
179. Garcia LS, Schimizu RY, Bruckner DA: Sinus tract extension of a liver hydatid cyst and recovery of diagnostic hooklets in sputum. Am J Clin Pathol 85:519–521, 1986.
180. Garret M: Cellular atypias in sputum and bronchial secretions associated with tuberculosis and bronchiectasis. Am J Clin Pathol 34:237–246, 1960.
181. Garret M, Herbsman H, Fierst S: Cytologic diagnosis of echinococcosis. Acta Cytol 21:553–554, 1977.
182. Genoe GA: Diagnosis of bronchogenic carcinoma by means of bronchial brushing combined with bronchography. Am J Roentgenol 120:139–144, 1974.
183. Gephardt GN, Belovich DM: Cytology of pulmonary carcinoid tumors. Acta Cytol 26:434–438, 1982.
184. Ghali VS, Garcia RL, Skolom J: Fluorescence of Pneumocystis carinii in Papanicolaou smears. Hum Pathol 15:907–909, 1984.
185. Glant MD, Wall RW, Ransburg R: Endobronchial granular cell tumor: cytology of a new case and review of the literature. Acta Cytol 23:477–482, 1979.
186. Gocek LA, Siekkinen PJ, Lankerani MR: Unsuspected Strongyloides coexisting with adenocarcinoma of the lung. Acta Cytol 29:628–631, 1985.
187. Goldstein J, Leslie H: Immunoblastic lymphadenopathy with pulmonary lesions and positive sputum cytology. Acta Cytol 22:165–167, 1978.
188. Gottleib LS, Husen LA: Lung cancer among Navajo uranium miners. Chest, 81:449–452, 1982.
189. Granberg I, Willems JS: Endometriosis of lung and pleura diagnosed by aspiration biopsy. Acta Cytol 21:295–297, 1977.
190. Greaves TS, Strigle SM: The recognition of Pneumocystis carinii in routine Papanicolaou-stained smears. Acta Cytol 29:714–720, 1985.
191. Greenberg SD: Asbestos. In Pulmonary Pathology. Edited by DH Dail, SP Hammar. New York, Springer-Verlag, 1988.
192. Greenberg SD, Fraire AE, Kinner BM, Johnson EH: Tumor cell type versus staging in the prognosis of carcinoma of the lung. Pathol Annu 22:Pt2:387–405, 1987.
193. Greenberg SD, Smith MN, Spjut HJ: Bronchioloalveolar carcinoma-cell of origin. Am J Clin Pathol 63:153–167, 1975.
194. Greenberg SD, Smith S, Swank PR, Winkler DG, Spjut HJ, Estrada R, Hunter N, Taylor GR: Visual cell profiles for quantitation of premalignant cells in sputum: a preliminary report. Acta Cytol 26:809–813, 1982.

195. Grote TH, Macon WR, Davis B, Greco FA, Johnson DH: Atypical carcinoid: a distinct clinicopathologic entity. Chest 93:370–375, 1988.

196. Grunze H: A critical review and evaluation of cytodiagnosis in chest diseases. Acta Cytol 4:175–198, 1960.

197. Guglietti LC, Reingold IM: The detection of *Coccidioides immitis* in pulmonary cytology. Acta Cytol 12:332–334, 1968.

198. Gupta RK: Value of sputum cytology in the differential diagnosis of alveolar cell carcinoma from bronchogenic adenocarcinoma. Acta Cytol 25:255–258, 1981.

199. Gupta RK: Value of sputum cytology in the diagnosis and typing of bronchogenic carcinomas, excluding adenocarcinomas. Acta Cytol 26:645–648, 1982.

200. Gupta RK: Diagnosis of unsuspected pulmonary cryptococcosis with sputum cytology. Acta Cytol 39:154–156, 1985.

201. Gupta PK: Identification of *Pneumocystis carinii. In* Compendium on Diagnostic Cytology, VI. Tutorials of Cytology, Chicago, 1988.

202. Gupta PK, Verma K: Calcified (psammoma) bodies in alveolar cell carcinoma of the lung. Acta Cytol 16:59–62, 1972.

203. Hajdu SI: A note on the history of carbowax in cytology. Acta Cytol 27:204–206, 1983.

204. Hajdu SI: Editorial. Cytology and pathology of acquired immune deficiency syndrome. Acta Cytol 30:599–602, 1986.

205. Hajdu SI: Cytology of AIDS: Compendium on Cytology, VI. Chicago, Tutorials of Cytology, 1988.

206. Hajdu SI, Huvos AG, Goodner JT, Foote FW Jr, Beattie EJ Jr: Carcinoma of the trachea: Clinicopathologic study of 41 cases. Cancer 25:1448–1456, 1970.

207. Haley LD, Arch R: Use of millipore membrane filter in the diagnostic tuberculosis laboratory. Am J Clin Pathol 27:117–121, 1957.

208. Hamilton C, Bigner SH, Wells S, Johnston WW: Metastatic medullary carcinoma of the thyroid in sputum—a light and electron microscopic study. Acta Cytol 27:49–53, 1983.

209. Hammer SP: Common Neoplasms. *In* Pulmonary Pathology. Edited by DH Dail, SP Hammar. New York, Springer-Verlag, 1988.

210. Hampson F: Exfoliative cytology in diagnosis of lung cancer—examination of one laboratory's results. B Med J 2:1461–1462, 1956.

211. Hansen HH, Dombernowsky P, Hansen M, Hirsch F: Chemotherapy of advanced small-cell anaplastic carcinoma. Ann Intern Med 89:177–181, 1978.

212. Hattori S, Matsuda M, Nishihara H, Horai T: Early diagnosis of small peripheral lung cancer—cytologic diagnosis of very fresh cancer cells obtained by the TV-brushing technique. Acta Cytol 15:460–467, 1971.

213. Hattori S, Matsuda M, Sugiyama T, Matsuda H: Cytologic diagnosis of early lung cancer: brushing method under X-ray television fluoroscopy. Dis Chest 45:129–142, 1964.

214. Hattori S, Matsuda M, Sugiyama T, Terazawa T, Wada A: Some limitations of cytologic diagnosis of small peripheral lung cancers. Acta Cytol 9:431–436, 1965.

215. Hattori S, Matsuda M, Tateiski R, Terazowa T: Electron microscopic studies on human lung cancer cells. Gann 58:283–290, 1967.

216. Hattori S, Matsuda M, Sugiyama T, Wada A, Terazawa T: Cytologic diagnosis of early lung cancer: An improved TV-brushing method and a review of negative results. Dis Chest 48:123–129, 1965.

217. Hayata Y: Lung Cancer Diagnosis. Tokyo, Igaku-Shoin. 1982.

218. Hawkins AG, Hsiu J-G, Smith RM III, Stitik FP, Siddiky MA, Edwards OE: Pulmonary dirofilariasis diagnosed by fine needle aspiration biopsy. A case report. Acta Cytol 29:19–22, 1985.

219. Haynes E: Trypsin as a digestant of sputum and other broth fluids preliminary to examination for acid-fast bacilli. J Lab Clin Med 27:806–809, 1942.

220. Heaston DK, Mills SR, Moore AV, Johnston WW: Percutaneous thoracic needle biopsy. In Pulmonary Disease. Edited by C Putman. New York, Appleton-Century-Crofts, 1981.

221. Hennigar GR: Drug and chemical injury-environmental pathology. *In* Anderson's Pathology, vol 1. Edited by JM Kissan. St. Louis, C. V. Mosby Company, 1990.

222. Herbut PA: Cancer cells in bronchial secretions. Am J Pathol 23:867–868, 1947.

223. Herbut PA: Correlation of cytological with pathological findings in tumors of the lung, 1951. Proc Symp Exfoliative Cytol. New York, American Cancer Society, 1953.

224. Herbut PA, Clerf LH: Bronchogenic carcinoma. Diagnosis by cytologic study of bronchoscopically removed secretions. JAMA 130:1006–1012, 1946.

225. Herbut PA, Clerf LH: Cytology of bronchial secretions: a diagnostic aid in the diagnosis of pulmonary tuberculosis. Am Rev Tuberc 54:488–494, 1946.

226. Hess FG Jr, McDowell EM, Resau JH, Trump BF: The respiratory epithelium. IX. Validity and reproducibility of revised cytologic criteria for human and hamster respiratory tract tumors. Acta Cytol 25:485–498, 1981.

227. Hess FG Jr, McDowell EM, Trump BF: The respiratory epithelium. VIII. Interpretation of cytologic criteria for human and hamster respiratory tract tumors. Acta Cytol 25:111–134, 1981.

228. Hirsch FR, Osterlind K, Hansen HH: The prognostic significance of histopathologic subtyping of small cell carcinoma of the lung according to the classification of the World Health Organization: A study of 375 consecutive cases. Cancer 52:2144–2150, 1983.

229. Hoch-Ligeti C, Eller LL: Significance of multinucleated epithelial cells in bronchial washings. Acta Cytol 7:258–261, 1963.

230. Horie A, Ohta M: Ultrastructural features of large cell carcinoma of lung with reference to the prognosis of patients. Hum Pathol 12:423–432, 1981.

231. Horsley JR, Miller RE, Amy RW, King EG: Bronchial submucosal needle aspiration performed through the fiberoptic bronchoscope. Acta Cytol 28:211–2176, 1984.

232. Houston HE, Payne WS, Harrison EG Jr, Olsen AM: Primary cancers of the trachea. Arch Surg 99:132–140, 1969.

233. Hsiu J-G, Kreuger JK, D'Amato NA, Moris JR: Primary malignant fibrous histiocytoma of the lung; fine needle aspiration cytologic features. Acta Cytol 31:345–350, 1987.

234. Hsiu J-G, Stitik FP, D'Amato NA, Kaplan AS, Burger RL, Hawkins AG: Primary amyloidosis presenting as a unilateral hilar mass. Report of a case diagnosed by fine needle aspiration biopsy. Acta Cytol 30:55–58, 1985.

235. Hsu C: Cytologic diagnosis of lung tumors from bronchial brushings of Chinese patients in Hong Kong. Acta Cytol 27:641–646, 1983.

236. Huang M-S, Colby JR, Martin WJ Jr: Utility of bronchoalveolar lavage in the diagnosis of drug-induced pulmonary toxicity. *In* Principles and Practice of Infectious Disease. GL Mandel, RG Douglas Jr, JE Bennett. John Wiley & Sons, 1979.

237. Humphreys K, Hieger LR: *Strongyloides stercoralis* in routine Papanicolaou-stained sputum smears. Acta Cytol 23:471–476, 1979.

238. Hutter RVP, Collins HS: The occurrence of opportunistic fungus infections in a cancer hospital. Lab Invest 11:1035–1045, 1962.

239. Iglehart JD, Wolfe WG, Vernon WB, Shelburne JD, Sabiston DC Jr: Electron microscopy in selection of patients with small cell carcinoma of the lung for medical versus surgical therapy. J Thorac Cardiovasc Surg 90:351–360, 1985.

240. Ishizuka T, Yoshitake J, Yamada T, Horie S, Koshiishi M, Nagai S, Satou T: Diagnosis of a case of pulmonary carcinosarcoma by detection of rhabdomyosarcoma cells in sputum. Acta Cytol 32:658–662, 1988.

241. Jacques J, Currie W: Bronchioloalveolar cell carcinoma: a Clara cell tumor? Cancer 40:2171–2180, 1977.

242. Jain U, Mani K, Frable WJ: Cytomegalic inclusion disease: cytologic diagnosis from bronchial brushing material. Acta Cytol 17:467–468, 1973.

243. Jarvi OH, Hormia MS, Autio JVK, Kangas SJ, Tilvis PK: Cytologic diagnosis of pulmonary carcinoma in two hospitals. Acta Cytol 11:477–482, 1967.

244. Jay SJ, Wehr K, Nicholson DP, Smith AL: Diagnostic sensitivity and specificity of pulmonary cytology: comparison of techniques used in conjunction with flexible fiber optic bronchoscopy. Acta Cytol 24:304–312, 1980.

245. Johnston WW: The cytopathology of mycotic infections. Lab Med 2:34–40, 1971.

246. Johnston WW: The cytopathology of opportunistic infections of the respiratory tract. Lab Manag 19:43–49, 1981.

247. Johnston WW: Cytopathology of the respiratory tract. *In* Manual of Cytotechnology. Chicago, American Society of Clinical Pathologists, 1982.

248. Johnston WW: Pulmonary cytopathology in the compromised host. *In* Lung Pathology for the Clinician. Edited by SD Greenberg. New York, Thieme-Stratton, Inc., 1982.

249. Johnston WW: Ten years of respiratory cytopathology at Duke University Medical Center. III. The significance of inconclusive cytopathologic diagnoses during the years 1970–1974. Acta Cytol 26:759–766, 1982.

250. Johnston WW: Percutaneous FNAB of the lung. Acta Cytol 28:218–224, 1984.

251. Johnston WW: Cytologic diagnosis of lung cancer. Pathol Res Pract 181:1–36, 1986.

252. Johnston WW: Mycoses in cytopathology. *In* Compendium on Diagnostic Cytology, 6th ed. Edited by GL Wied, CM Keebler, LG Koss, JW Reagan. Chicago, Tutorials of Cytology, 1988.

253. Johnston WW: Cytologic correlations. *In* Pulmonary Pathology. Edited by DH Dail, SP Hammar. New York, Springer-Verlag, 1988.

254. Johnston WW: Cytopathology of the lung. *In* Compendium on Diagnostic Cytology, 6th ed. Edited by GL Weid, CM Keebler, LG Koss, JW Reagan. Chicago, Tutorials of Cytology, 1988.

255. Johnston WW: Fine needle aspiration biopsy versus sputum and bronchial material in the diagnosis of lung cancer: a comparative study of 168 patients. Acta Cytol 32:641–646, 1988.

256. Johnston WW: Histologic and cytologic patterns of lung cancer in 2580 men and women over a 15-year period. Acta Cytol 32:163–168, 1988.

257. Johnston WW, Amatulli J: The role of cytology in the primary diagnosis of North American blastomycosis. Acta Cytol 14:200–204, 1970.

258. Johnston WW, Bossen EH: Ten years of respiratory cytopathology at Duke University Medical Center. I. The cytopathologic diagnosis of lung cancer during the years 1970–1974, noting the significance of specimen number and type. Acta Cytol 25:103–107, 1981.

259. Johnston WW, Bossen EH: Ten years of respiratory cytopathology at Duke University Medical Center. II. A comparison between cytopathology and histopathology in typing of lung cancer during the years 1970–1974. Acta Cytol 25:499–505, 1981.

260. Johnston WW, Frable WJ: Cytopathology of the respiratory tract: a review. Am J Pathol 84:371–424, 1976.

261. Johnston WW, Frable WJ: Diagnostic Respiratory Cytopathology. Paris, Masson, 1979.

262. Johnston WW, Ginn FL, Amatulli JM: Light and electron microscopic observations on malignant cells in cerebrospinal fluid from metastatic alveolar cell carcinoma. Acta Cytol 15:365–371, 1971.

263. Johnston WW, Schlein B, Amatulli J: Cytopathologic diagnosis of fungus infections. I. A method for the preparation of simulated cytopathologic material for the teaching of fungus morphology in cytology specimens. II. The presence of fungus in clinical material. Acta Cytol 13:488–495, 1969.

264. Jones TC: Protozoal disease. *In* Principles and Practice of Infectious Disease. Edited by GL Mandel, RG Douglas Jr, JE Bennett. New YOrk, John Wiley & Sons, 1979.

265. Jordan AG, Predmore L, Sullivan MM, Memoli VA: The cytodiagnosis of well-differentiated neuroendocrine carcinoma; A distinct clinicopathologic entity. Acta Cytol 31:656–670, 1987.

266. Kaminsky DB: Applications of thin-needle aspiration biopsy in a community hospital. In The Masson Series in Diagnostic Cytopathology, vol 2. Edited by WW Johnston. New York, Masson, 1981.

267. Kanbour A, Doshi N, Fujikura T: Neonatal tracheobronchial cytology of bronchopulmonary dysplasia. Acta Cytol 24:60, 1980.

268. Kanhouwa SB, Matthews MJ: Reliability of cytologic typing of lung cancer. Acta Cytol 20:229–232, 1976.

269. Kato H, Konaka C, Ono J, Takahashi M, Hayata Y: Squamous metaplasia. *In* Cytology of the Lung. Tokyo, Igaku-Shoin Ltd, 1983.

270. Kawahara EI, Nakanishi I, Kuroda Y, Morishita T: Fine needle aspiration biopsy of primary malignant fibrous histiocytoma of the lung. Acta Cytol. 32:226–230, 1988.

271. Kenney M, Webber CA: Diagnosis of strongyloidiasis in Papanicolaou-stained sputum smears. Acta Cytol 18:270–273, 1974.

272. Kawecka M: Cytological evaluation of the sputum in patients with bronchiectasis and the possibility of erroneous diagnosis of carcinoma. Acta Union Intern Cancer 15:469–473, 1959.

273. Kern WH: Cytology of hyperplastic and neoplastic lesions of terminal bronchioles and alveoli. Acta Cytol 9:372–379, 1965.

274. Kern WH, Crepeau AG, Jones JC: Primary Hodgkin's disease of the lung. Cancer 14:1151–1165, 1961.

275. Kern WH, Jones JC, Chapman ND: Pathology of bronchogenic carcinoma in long-term survivors. Cancer 21:772, 1968.

276. Kern WH, Schweizer C: Sputum cytology of metastatic carcinoma of the lung. Acta Cytol 20:514–520, 1976.

277. Kierszenbaum AL: Bronchial metaplasia: observations on its histology and cytology. Acta Cytol 9:365–371, 1965.

278. Kim H, Hughs WT: Comparison of methods for identification of *Pneumocystis carinii* in pulmonary aspirates. Am J Clin Pathol 60:462–466, 1973.

279. Kim G, Naylor B, Han IH: Fine needle aspiration cytology of sarcomas metastatic to the lung. Acta Cytol 30:688–694, 1986.

280. Kimula Y: A histochemical and ultrastructural study of adenocarcinoma of the lung. Am J Surg Pathol 2:253–264, 1978.

281. Kinsella DL: Bronchial cell atypias: a report of a preliminary study correlating cytology with histology. Cancer 12:463–472, 1959.

282. Kirsh MM, Orvald T, Naylor B, Kahn DR, Sloan H: Diagnostic accuracy of exfoliative pulmonary cytology. Ann Thorac Surg 9:335–338, 1970.

283. Kjaer T, Dreyer V, Hansen JL: Clinical experiences concerning tumor cells in the sputum. Acta Med Scand (Stock) Suppl 234:177–185, 1949.

284. Knudtson KP: Mucolytic action of hyaluronidase on sputum for the cytological diagnosis of lung cancer. Acta Cytol 7:59–61, 1963.

285. Koprowska I: Intranuclear inclusion bodies in smears of respiratory secretions. Acta Cytol 5:219–228, 1961.

286. Koprowska I, An SH, Corsey D, Dracopoulos I, Vaskelis PS: Cytologic patterns of developing bronchogenic carcinoma. Acta Cytol 9:424–430, 1965.

287. Kory RC: Electron microscopy of sputum. *In* Sputum Fundamentals and Clinical Pathology. Edited by MJ Dulfano. Springfield, IL, Charles C Thomas, 1973.

288. Koss LG: Cellular changes simulating bronchogenic carcinoma. Acta Unio Internat Contra Cancrum 14:501–503, 1958.

289. Koss LG: A quarter of a century of cytology. Acta Cytol 21:639–642, 1977.

290. Koss LG: Diagnostic Cytology and Its Histopathologic Bases, 3rd ed. Philadelphia, JB Lippincott, 1979.

291. Koss LG, Melamed MR, Goodner JT: Pulmonary cytology—a brief survey of diagnostic results from July 1st, 1952 until December 31st, 1960. Acta Cytol 8:104–113, 1964.

292. Koss LG, Richardson HL: Some pitfalls of cytological diagnosis of lung cancer. Cancer 8:937–947, 1955.

293. Koss LG, Woyke S, Olszewski W: Aspiration Biopsy. Cytologic Interpretation and Histologic Bases. Tokyo, Igaku-Shoin, 1985.

294. Kreyberg L: Histological Typing of Lung Tumours, 2nd ed. Geneva, World Health Organization, 1981.

295. Krumerman MS: Leiomyosarcoma of the lung: primary cytodiagnosis in two consecutive cases. Acta Cytol 21:103–108, 1977.

296. Kuhn C: Fine structure of bronchioloalveolar cell carcinoma. Cancer 30:1107–1118, 1972.

297. Kuhn C, Askin FB: Lung and Mediastinum. *In* Anderson's Pathology, vol 1. Edited by JM Kissan. St. Louis, C. V. Mosby Company, 1990.

298. Kyriakos M, Rockoff SD: Brush biopsy of bronchial carcinoid—a source of cytologic error. Acta Cytol 16:261–268, 1972.

299. Lambird PA, Ashton PR: Exfoliative cytopathology of a primary pulmonary malignant histiocytoma. Acta Cytol 14:83–86, 1970.

300. Landsman S, Burgner FA, Lim GHK: Comparison of bronchial brushing and percutaneous needle aspiration biopsy in the diagnosis of malignant lung lesions. Radiology 115:275–278, 1975.

301. Lange E, Koeg K: Cytologic typing of lung cancer. Acta Cytol 16:327–330, 1972.

302. Larsh HW, Goodman NL: Sputum Mycology. *In* Sputum Fundamentals and Clinical Pathology. Edited by MJ Dulfano. Springfield, Ill, Charles C Thomas, 1973.

303. Lavoie RR, McDonald JR, Kling GA: Cavitation in squamous carcinoma of the lung. Acta Cytol 21:210–214, 1977.

304. Lazo BG, Feiner LL, Schriff NS: A study of routine cytologic screening of sputum for cancer in 800 men consecutively admitted to a tuberculosis service. Chest 65:646–649, 1974.

305. Lazzari G, Vineis C, Cugini A: Cytologic diagnosis of primary pulmonary actinomycosis: report of two cases. Acta Cytol 25:299–301, 1981.

306. Lefer L, Johnston WW: Hydrogen peroxide bleach technique in the diagnosis of malignant melanoma. Acta Cytol 16:505–506, 1972.

307. Lefer L, Johnston WW: Electron microscopic observations of sputum in alveolar cell carcinoma. Acta Cytol 20:26–31, 1976.

308. Leiman G, Markowitz S: Asbestos bodies in pulmonary fine needle aspirates: A more sinister finding than in other cytologic specimens? Acta Cytol 30:555–556, 1986.

309. Leong AS: The relevance of ultrastructural examination in the classification of primary lung tumors. Pathology 14:37–46, 1982.

310. Levij IS: A case of primary cavitary Hodgkin's disease of the lungs, diagnosed cytologically. Acta Cytol 16:546–549, 1972.

311. Levine SE, Mossler JA, Johnston WW: The cytopathology of metastatic ameloblastoma. Acta Cytol 25:295–298, 1981.

312. Lieberman MW, Lebovitz RM: Neoplasia. *In* Anderson's Pathology, vol 1. Edited by JM Kissan. St. Louis, C. V. Mosby Company, 1990.

313. Liebow AA: Bronchioloalveolar carcinoma. Adv Intern Med 10:329–358, 1960.

314. Liebow AA, Lindskog GE, Bloomer WE: Cytological studies of sputum and bronchial secretions in the diagnosis of cancer of the lung. Cancer 1:223–233, 1948.

315. Linder J, Radio SJ, Robbins RA, Ghafouri MO, Rennard SI: Bronchoalveolar lavage in the cytologic diagnosis of carcinoma of the lung. Acta Cytol 31:796–801, 1987.

316. Linder J, Rennard SI: Bronchoalveolar lavage. Chicago, American Society of Clinical Pathologists, 1988.

317. Lipford EH, Sears DL, Eggleston JC, Moore GW, Lillemoe KD, Baker RR: Prognostic factors in surgically resected limited-stage, nonsmall cell carcinoma of the lung. Am J Surg Pathol 8:357–365, 1984.

318. Liu W: Concentration and fractionation of cytologic elements in sputum. Acta Cytol 10:368–372, 1966.

319. Llienfeld AM: Some limitations and problems of screening for cancer. Cancer 33:1720–1724, 1974.

320. Lobenthal SW, Hajdu SI, Urmacher C: Cytologic findings in homosexual males with acquired immunodeficiency. Acta Cytol 27:597–604, 1983.

321. Lopes-Cardozo P, DeGraaf S, DeBoer MJ, Doesburg N, Kapsenberg PD: The results of cytology in 1000 patients with pulmonary malignancy. Acta Cytol 11:120–131, 1967.

322. Losner S, Volk BW, Slade WR, Nathanson L, Jacobi H: Diagnosis of lipid pneumonia by examination of sputum. Am J Clin Pathol 20:539–545, 1950.

323. Louria DB, Lieberman PH, Collins HS, Blevins A: Pulmonary mycetoma due to *Allescheria boydii*. Arch Intern Med 121:748–751, 1966.

324. Lozowski W, Hajdu SI: The cytologic diagnosis of primary bronchioloalveolar carcinoma. Acta Cytol 30:569–570, 1986.

325. Lozowski W, Hajdu SI, Melamed MR: Cytomorphology of carcinoid tumors. Acta Cytol 23:360–365, 1979.

326. Lozowski MS, Mishriki YY, Epstein H: Metastatic malignant

327. fibrous histiocytoma in lung examined by fine needle aspiration: case report and literature review. Acta Cytol 24:350–354, 1980.

327. Ludwig ME, Otis RD, Cole SR, Westcott JL: Fine needle aspiration cytology of pulmonary hamartomas. Acta Cytol 26:671–677, 1982.

328. Ludwig RA, Balachandran I: Mycosis fungoides: the importance of pulmonary cytology in the diagnosis of a case with systemic involvement. Acta Cytol 27:198–201, 1983.

329. Madri JA: Inflammation and healing. *In* Anderson's Pathology, vol 1. Edited by JM Kissan. St. Louis, C. V. Mosby Company, 1990.

330. Madri JA, Carter D: Scar cancers of the lung: origin and significance. Hum Pathol 15:625–631, 1984.

331. Malberger E, Lemberg S: Transthoracic fine needle aspiration cytology: a study of 301 aspirations from 221 cases. Acta Cytol 26:172–178, 1982.

332. Mandlebaum FS: The diagnosis of malignant tumors by paraffine sections of centrifuged exudates. J Lab Clin Med 2:580, 1917.

333. Manning JT, Spjut HJ, Tschen JA: Bronchioloalveolar carcinoma: the significance of two histopathologic types. Cancer 54:525–534, 1984.

334. Marchevsky A, Nieburgs HE, Olenko E, Kirschner P, Teirsein A, Kleinerman J: Pulmonary tumorlets in cases of "tuberculoma" of the lung with malignant cells in brush biopsy. Acta Cytol 26:491–494, 1982.

335. Marcial MA, Marcial-Rojas RA: Protozoal and helminthic disease. *In* Anderson's Pathology, vol 1. Edited by JM Kissan. St. Louis, C. V. Mosby Company, 1990.

336. Mark EJ, Quay SC, Dickensin GR: Papillary carcinoid tumor of the lung. Cancer 48:316–324, 1981.

337. Markel SF, Abell MR, Haight C, French AJ: Neoplasms of bronchus commonly designated as adenomas. Cancer 17:590–608, 1964.

338. Marsh BR, Frost JK, Erozan YS, Carter D: Occult bronchogenic carcinoma. Endoscopic localization and television documentation. Cancer 30:1348–1352, 1972.

339. Marsh BR, Frost JK, Erozan YS, Carter D, Proctor DF: Flexible fiberoptic bronchoscopy. Its place in the search for lung cancer. Ann Otol Rhinol Laryngol 82:757–764, 1973.

340. Masin F, Masin M: Frequencies of alveolar cells in concentrated sputum specimens related to cytologic classes. Acta Cytol 10:362–367, 1966.

341. Matsuda M, Nagumo S, Horai T, Yoshino K: Cytologic diagnosis of laryngeal and hypopharyngeal squamous cell carcinoma in sputum. Acta Cytol 32:655–657, 1988.

342. Matsuo T, Kinoshita S, Iwasaki K, Shibata M, Ushio T, Kawata S, Gotanda T: Chrondrosarcoma of the trachea: A case report and literature review. Acta Cytol 32:908–912, 1988.

343. Matthews MJ, Gazdar AF: Pathology of small cell carcinoma of the lung and its subtypes: a clinicopathologic correlation. *In* Lung Cancer. Edited by RD Livingstone. The Hague, Nijhoff M, 1981.

344. Maygarden SJ, Flanders EL: Mycobacteria can be seen as "negative images" in cytology smears from patients with acquired immunodeficiency syndrome. Mod Pathol 2:239–243, 1989.

345. McCallum SM: Ova of the lung fluke *Paragonimus kellicotti* in fluid from a cyst. Acta Cytol 19:279–280, 1975.

346. McCarty SA: Solving the cytopreparation problem of mucoid specimens with a mucoliquefying agent (Mucolexx) and nuclepore filters. Acta Cytol 16:221–223, 1972.

347. McDonald JR: Exfoliative, cytology in genitourinary and pulmonary diseases. Am J Clin Pathol 24:684–687, 1954.

348. McDonald JR: Pulmonary cytology. Am J Surg 89:462–464, 1955.

349. McGrath EJ, Gall EA, Kessler DP: Bronchogenic carcinoma: a product of multiple sites of origin. J Thorac Surg 24:271–283, 1952.

350. McKay DG, Ware PF, Atwood DA, Harken DE: The diagnosis of bronchogenic carcinoma by smears of bronchoscopic aspirations. Cancer 1:208–222, 1948.

351. Melamed MR, Flehinger BJ, Zaman MB: Screening for early lung cancer—Results of the Memorial Sloan-Kettering study in New York. Chest 86:44–53, 1984.

352. Melamed MR, Koss LG, Cliffton EE: Roentgenologically occult lung cancer. Diagnosed by cytology. Cancer 16:1537–1551, 1963.

353. Mennemeyer R, Hammar SP, Wheelis RF, Jones HW, Bartha M: Cytologic, histologic and electron microscopic correlations in poorly differentiated primary lung carcinoma: a study of 43 cases. Acta Cytol 23:297–302, 1979.

354. Meyer EC, Liebow AA: Relationship of interstitial pneumonia and honeycombing and atypical epithelial proliferation to cancer of the lung. Cancer 18:322–351, 1965.

355. Meyer JA, Bechtold E, Jones DB: Positive sputum cytologic test for five years before specific detection of bronchial carcinoma. J Thorac Cardiovasc Surg 57:318–324, 1969.

356. Miller WT, Husted J, Freiman D, Atkinson B, Pietra GG: Bronchioloalveolar carcinoma: Two clinical entities with one pathologic diagnosis. Am J Roentgenol 130:905–912, 1978.

357. Mills SE, Walker AN, Cooper PH, Kron IL: Atypical carcinoid tumor of the lung: a clinicopathologic study of 17 cases. Am J Surg Pathol 6:643–654, 1982.

358. Mitchell ML, King DE, Bonfiglio TA, Patten SF Jr: Pulmonary fine needle aspiration cytopathology: a five-year correlation study. Acta Cytol 28:72–76, 1984.

359. Miyamoto H, Inoue S, Abe S, Murao M, Yasuda S, Sakai E: Relationship between cytomorphologic features and prognosis in small-cell carcinoma of the lung. Acta Cytol 26:429–433, 1982.

360. Moersch HJ, McDonald JR: The significance of cell types in bronchogenic carcinoma. Dis Chest 23:621–633, 1953.

361. Mountain CF: A new international staging system for lung cancer. Chest 89(suppl)4:225(s)–232(s), 1986.

362. Munjal S, Gupta JC, Munjal KR: Microfilariae in laryngeal and pharyngeal brushing smears from a case of carcinoma of the pharnyx. Acta Cytol 29:1009–1010, 1985.

363. Murray JF: Postnatal growth and development of the lung. In The Normal Lung: The Basis for Diagnosis and Treatment of Pulmonary Disease. Philadelphia, WB Saunders, 1976.

364. Mylius EA, Gullvag B: Alveolar macrophage count as an indicator of lung reaction to industrial air pollution. Acta Cytol 30:157–162, 1986.

365. Naib ZM: Giant cell carcinoma of the lung: Cytological study of the exfoliated cells in sputa and bronchial washings. Dis Chest 40:69–73, 1961.

366. Naib ZM: Exfoliative cytology in fungus diseases of the lung. Acta Cytol 6:413–416, 1962.

367. Naib ZM: Pitfalls in the cytologic diagnosis of oat cell carcinoma of the lung. Acta Cytol 8:34–38, 1964.

368. Naib ZM, Stewart JA, Dowdle WR, Casey HL, Marine WM, Nahmias AJ: Cytological features of viral respiratory tract infections. Acta Cytol 12:162–171, 1968.

369. Nash AD, Stout AP: Giant cell carcinoma of the lung; report of 5 cases. Cancer 11:369–376, 1958.

370. Nash G, Foley FD: Herpetic infection of the middle and lower respiratory tract. Am J Clin Pathol 54:857–863, 1970.

371. Nasiell M: The general appearance of the bronchial epithelium in bronchial carcinoma: A histopathological study with some cytological viewpoints. Acta Cytol 7:97–106, 1963.

372. Nasiell M: Metaplasia and atypical metaplasia in the bronchial epithelium: a histopathologic and cytopathologic study. Acta Cytol 10:421–427, 1966.

373. Nasiell M: Abnormal columnar cell findings in bronchial epithelium. A cytologic and histologic study of lung cancer and non-cancer cases. Acta Cytol 11:397–402, 1967.

374. Nasiell M: Diagnosis of lung cancer by aspiration biopsy and a comparison between this method and exfoliative cytology. Acta Cytol 11:114–119, 1967.

375. Nasiell M, Kato H, Auer G: Cytomorphological grading and Feulgen DNA analysis of metaplastic and neoplastic bronchial cells. Cancer 41:1511–1521, 1978.

376. Nasiell M, Roger V, Nasiell K, Enstad I, Vogel B, Bisther A: Cytologic findings indicating pulmonary tuberculosis. I. The diagnostic significance of epithelioid cells and Langerhans giant cells found in sputum or bronchial secretions. Acta Cytol 16:146–151, 1972.

377. Nasiell M, Vogel B: Cytomorphology of benign changes and early carcinoma of the lung. Compendium on Cytology. VI. Chicago, Tutorials of Cytology, 1988.

378. Naylor B, Railey C: A pitfall in the cytodiagnosis of sputum of asthmatics. J Clin Pathol 7:84–89, 1964.

379. Ness MJ, Rennard SI, Vaughn WP, Ghafouri Mo A, Linder JA: Detection of Candida antigen in bronchoalveolar lavage fluid. Acta Cytol 32:347–352, 1988.

380. Ng ABP, Horak GC: Factors significant in the diagnostic accuracy of lung cytology in bronchial washing and sputum samples. I. Bronchial washings. Acta Cytol 27:391–396, 1983.

381. Ng ABP, Horak GC: Factors significant in the diagnostic accuracy of lung cytology in bronchial washing and sputum samples. II. Sputum samples. Acta Cytol 27:397–402, 1983.

382. Nguyen G-K: Exfoliative cytology of angiosarcoma of the pulmonary artery. Acta Cytol 29:624–627, 1985.

383. Nguyen G-K: Cytology of bronchial gland carcinoma. Acta Cytol 32:235–239, 1988.

384. Nguyen G-K: Aspiration biopsy cytology of benign clear cell ("sugar") tumor of the lung. Acta Cytol 33:511–515, 1989.

385. Nguyen G-K, Jennot A: Cytopathologic aspects of pulmonary metastasis of malignant fibrous histiocytoma, myxoid variant: fine needle aspiration biopsy of a case. Acta Cytol 26:349–353, 1982.

386. Nguyen G-K, Shnitka TK: Aspiration biopsy cytology of adenocarcinoid tumor of the bronchial tree. Acta Cytol 31:726–730, 1987.

387. Niewoehner DE, Kleinerman V, Rice DB: Pathologic changes in peripheral airways of young cigarette smokers. N Engl J Med 291:755–758, 1974.

388. Nixon DW, Murphy GF, Sewell CW, Kutner M, Lynn MJ: Relationship between survival and histologic type in small cell anaplastic carcinoma of the lung. Cancer 44:1045–1049, 1979.

389. Nordenstrom BEW: Technical aspects of obtaining cellular material from lesions deep in the lung: a radiologist's view and description of the screw-needle sampling technique. Acta Cytol 28:233–242, 1984.

390. Northway WH Jr, Rosan RC, Porter DY: Pulmonary disease following respiratory therapy of hyaline membrane disease and bronchopulmonary dysplasia. N Engl J Med 276:357–374, 1967.

391. Nōu E: The natural five-year course in bronchial carcinoma: epidemiologic results. Cancer 53:2211–2216, 1984.

392. Ognibere FP, Shelhamer J, Gill V, Marcher AM, Loew D, Parder MM, Gelmann E, Fauci AS, Parrillo JE, Masur H: The diagnosis of Pneumocystis carinii pneumonia in patients with the acquired immunodeficiency syndrome using segmental bronchoalveolar lavage. Am Rev Resp Dis 129:929–932, 1984.

393. Okike N, Bernatz PE, Woolner LB: Carcinoid tumors of the lung. Ann Thorac Surg 22:270–277, 1976.

394. Olson RG, Froeb HF, Palmer LA: Sputum cytology after inhalation of heated propylene glycol. JAMA 178:668–670, 1961.

395. Orenstein M, Webber CA, Heurich AE: Cytologic diagnosis of Pneumocystis carinii infection by bronchoalveolar lavage in acquired immune deficiency syndrome. Acta Cytol 29:727–731, 1985.

396. Osborne PT, Giltman LI, Uthman EO: Trichomonads in the respiratory tract: a case report and literature review. Acta Cytol 28:136–138, 1984.

397. Osburn HS: Lung cancer in a mining district in Rhodesia. S Afr Med J 43:1307–1312, 1969.

398. Paladugu RR, Benfield JR, Pak HY, Ross RK, Teplitz RL: Bronchopulmonary Kulchitzky cell carcinomas: a new classification scheme for typical and atypical carcinoids Cancer 55:1303–1311, 1985.

399. Palva T, Saloheimo M: Observations on the cytologic pattern of bronchial aspirates in pulmonary tuberculosis. Acta Tuberc Sand 31:278–288, 1955.

400. Pak HY, Yokota SB, Friedberg HA: Thymoma diagnosed by transthoracic fine needle aspiration. Acta Cytol 26:210–216, 1982.

401. Pak HY, Yokota SB, Teplitz RL, Shaw SL, Werner JL: Rapid staining techniques employed in fine needle aspirations of the lung. Acta Cytol 25:178–184, 1981.

402. Papanicolaou GN: Atlas of Exfoliative Cytology. Cambridge, Commonwealth Fund, Harvard University Press, 1954.

403. Papanicolaou GN: Degenerative changes in ciliated cells exfoliating from the bronchial epithelium as a cytologic criterion in the diagnosis of diseases of the lung. NY State J Med 56:2647–2650, 1956.

404. Papanicolaou GN, Cromwell HA: Diagnosis of cancer of the lung by the cytologic method. Dis Chest 15:412–418, 1949.

405. Papanicolaou GN, Koprowska I: Carcinoma in situ of the right lower bronchus. Cancer 4:141–146, 1951.

406. Payne WS, Fontana RS, Woolner LB: Bronchial tumors originating from mucous glands: current classification and unusual manifestations. Med Clin North Am 48:945–960, 1968.

407. Pearse AGE, Polak JM: The neural crest origin of endocrine polypeptide cells of the APUD series. In Endocrinology 1971. Edited by S Taylor. London, Heinemann, 1972.

408. Pedersen B, Brons M, Holm K, Pedersen D, Lund C: The value of provoked expectoration in obtaining sputum samples for cytologic investigation. A prospective, consecutive and controlled investigation of 134 patients. Acta Cytol 29:750–752, 1985.

409. Perry MD, Furlong JW, Johnston WW: Fine needle aspiration cytology of metastatic dermatofibrosarcoma protuberans; a case report. Acta Cytol 30:507–512, 1986.

410. Perlman EJ, Erozan YS, Howdon A: The role of the Saccomanno technique in sputum cytopathologic diagnosis of lung cancer. Am J Clin Pathol 91:57–60, 1989.

411. Pett SB Jr, Wernly JA, Aki BF: Lung cancer—Current concepts and controversies West J Med 145:52–64, 1986.

412. Pfitzer P, Knoblich PG: Giant carcinoma cells of bronchiogenic origin. Acta Cytol 12:256–261, 1968.

413. Pharr SL, Farber SM: Cellular concentration of sputum and bronchial aspirations by tryptic digestion. Acta Cytol 6:447–454, 1962.

414. Philps FR: The identification of carcinoma cells in the sputum. Br J Cancer 8:67–96, 1954.

415. Pierce CH, Hirsch JG: Ciliocytophthoria: relationship to viral respiratory infections of human. Proc Soc Exp Biol Med 98:489–492, 1958.

416. Pierce CH, Knox AW: Ciliocytophthoria in sputum from patients with adenovirus infections. Proc Soc Exp Biol Med 104:492–495, 1960.

417. Pilotti S, Rilke F, Gribaudi G, Damascelli B: Fine needle aspiration biopsy cytology of primary and metastatic pulmonary tumors. Acta Cytol 26:661–670, 1982.

418. Pilotti S, Rilke F, Gribaudi G, Damascelli B, Ravasi G: Transthoracic fine needle aspiration biopsy in pulmonary lesions: updated results. Acta Cytol 28:225–232, 1984.

419. Pilotti S, Rilke F, Gribaudi G, Ravasi GL: Sputum cytology for the diagnosis of carcinoma of the lung. Acta Cytol 26:649–654, 1982.

420. Pilotti S, Rilke F, Gribaudi G, Spinelli P: Cytologic diagnosis of pulmonary carcinoma on bronchoscopic brushing material. Acta Cytol 26:655–660, 1982.

421. Pilotti S, Rilke F, Lombardi L: Pulmonary carcinoid with glandular features. Report of two cases with positive fine needle aspiration biopsy cytology. Acta Cytol 27:511–514, 1983.

422. Pintozzi RL, Blecka LJ, Nanos S: The morphologic identification of Pneumocystis carinii. Acta Cytol 23:35–39, 1979.

423. Plamenac P, Nikulin A: Atypia of the bronchial epithelium in wind instrument players and in singers: a cytopathologic study. Acta Cytol 13:274–278, 1969.

424. Plamenac P, Nikulin A, Pikula B: Cytology of the respiratory tract in former smokers. Acta Cytol 16:256–260, 1972.

425. Plamenac P, Nikulin A, Pikula B: Cytologic changes of the respiratory tract in young adults as a consequence of high levels of air pollution exposure. Acta Cytol 17:241–244, 1973.

426. Plamenac P, Nikulin A, Pikula B: Cytologic changes of the respiratory epithelium in iron foundry workers. Acta Cytol 18:34–40, 1974.

427. Plamenac P, Nikulin A, Pikula B, Markovic Z: Cytologic changes in the respiratory tract in children smokers. Acta Cytol 23:389–391, 1979.

428. Plamenac P, Nikulin A, Pikula B, Vujanic G: Cytologic changes of the respiratory tract as a consequence of air pollution and smoking. Acta Cytol 23:449–453, 1979.

429. Poe RH, Tobin RE: Sensitivity and specificity of needle biopsy in lung malignancy. Am Rev Respir Dis 122:725–729, 1980.

430. Pontifex AH, Roberts FJ: Fine needle aspiration biopsy cytology in the diagnosis of inflammatory lesions. Acta Cytol 29:979–982, 1985.

431. Prolla JC, Rosa UW, Xavier RG: The detection of Cryptococcus neoformans in sputum cytology. Report of one case. Acta Cytol 14:87–91, 1970.

432. Radford EP, Renard KG: Lung cancer in Swedish iron miners exposed to low doses of radon daughters. N Engl J Med 310:1485–1494, 1984.

433. Radice PA, Matthews MJ, Ihde DC, Gazdar AF, Carney DN, Bunn PA, Cohen MH, Fussieck BE, Makuch RW, Minna JD: The clinical behavior of "mixed" small cell/large cell, bronchogenic carcinoma compared to "pure" small cell subtypes. Cancer 50:2894–2902, 1982.

434. Radio SJ, Rennard SI, Ghafouri MoA, Linder J: Cytomorphology of Alternaria in bronchoalveolar lavage specimens. Acta Cytol 31:243–248, 1987.

435. Ramzy I: Pulmonary hamartomas: cytologic appearances of fine needle aspiration biopsy. Acta Cytol 20:15–19, 1976.

436. Ramzy I, Geraghty R, Lefcoe MS, Lefcoe NM: Chronic eosinophilic pneumonia: diagnosis by fine needle aspiration. Acta Cytol 22:366–369, 1978.

437. Ranchod M, Levine GD: Spindle-cell carcinoid tumors of the lung. A clinicopathologic study of 35 cases. Am J Surg Pathol 4:315–331, 1980.

438. Rastgeldi S, Tomenius JA, Williams G: The simultaneous separation and concentration of corpuscular elements and bacteria from sputum. Acta Cytol 3:183–187, 1959.

439. Reale FR, Variakojis D, Compton J, Bibbo M: Cytodiagnosis of Hodgkin's disease in sputum specimens. Acta Cytol 27:258–261, 1983.

440. Reid JD, Carr AH: The validity and value of histological and cytological classification of lung cancer. Cancer 14:673–698, 1961.

441. Repsher LH, Schroter G, Hammond WS: Diagnosis of Pneumocystis carinii pneumonitis by means of endobronchial brush biopsy. New Engl J Med 286:340–341, 1972.

442. Reyes CV, Kathuria S, MacGlashan A: Diagnostic value of calcium oxalate crystals in respiratory and pleural fluid cytology: a case report. Acta Cytol 23:65–68, 1979.

443. Riazmontazer N, Bedayat G: Cytology of plasma cell myeloma in bronchial washing. Acta Cytol 33:519–522, 1989.

444. Richardson HL, Hunter WC, Conklin WS, Petersen AB: A cytohistologic study of bronchial secretions. Am J Clin Pathol 19:323–327, 1949.

445. Richardson HL, Koss LG, Simon TR: An evaluation of the concomitant use of cytological and histocytological techniques in the recognition of cancer in exfoliated material from various sources. Cancer 8:948–950, 1955.

446. Risse EKJ, Van't Hof MA, Vooijs GP: Relationship between patient characteristics and the sputum cytologic diagnosis of lung cancer. Acta Cytol 31:159–165, 1987.

447. Risse EKJ, Vooijs GP, Van't Hof MA: Relationship between the cellular composition of sputum and the cytologic diagnosis of lung cancer. Acta Cytol 31:170–176, 1987.

448. Risse EKJ, Vooijs GP, Van't Hof MA: Diagnostic significance of "severe dysplasia" in sputum cytology. Acta Cytol 23:629–634, 1988.

449. Ro JY, Tsakalakis PJ, White VA, Luna MA, Change-Tung EG, Green L, Cribbett L, Ayala AG: Pulmonary dirofilariasis: The great imitator of primary or metastatic lung tumor. A clinicopathologic analysis of seven cases and a review of the literature. Hum Pathol 20(1):69–76, 1989.

450. Roberts TW, Pollak A, Howard R, Howard E: Tracheobronchial cytology utilizing an improved tussilator (cough machine). Acta Cytol 7:174–179, 1963.

451. Roger V, Nasiell M, Linden M, Enstad I: Cytologic differential diagnosis of bronchioloalveolar carcinoma and bronchogenic adenocarcinoma. Acta Cytol 20:303–307, 1976.

452. Roger V, Nasiell M, Nasiell K, Hjerpe A, Enstad I, Bisther

A: Cytologic findings indicating pulmonary tuberculosis. II. The occurrence in sputum of epithelioid cells and multinucleated giant cells in pulmonary tuberculosis, chronic nontuberculous inflammatory lung disease and bronchogenic carcinoma. Acta Cytol 16:538–542, 1972.

453. Roggli VL, Johnston WW, Kaminsky DB: Asbestos bodies in fine needle aspirates of the lung. Acta Cytol 28:493–498, 1984.

454. Roggli VL, Piantadosi CA, Bell DY: Asbestos bodies in bronchoalveolar lavage fluid: A study of 20 asbestos-exposed individuals and comparison to patients with other chronic interstitial lung disease. Acta Cytol 30:470–476, 1986.

455. Roggli VL, Vollmer RT, Greenberg SD, McGavran MH, Spjut HJ, Yesner R: Lung cancer heterogeneity: a blinded and randomized study of 100 consecutive cases. Hum Path 16:569–579, 1985.

456. Roglic M, Jukic S, Damjanov I: Cytology of the solitary papilloma of the bronchus. Acta Cytol 19:11–13, 1975.

457. Rollins SD, Genack LJ, Schumann GB: Primary cytodiagnosis of dually differentiated lung cancer by transthoracic fine needle aspiration. Acta Cytol 32:231–234, 1988.

458. Rome DS: The value of aerosol-produced sputum as a screening technique for lung cancer. Acta Unio Internat Cancr 15:474–476, 1959.

459. Rome DS: Value of aerosol-produced sputum as screening technic for lung cancer. NY State J Med 61:2054–2060, 1961.

460. Rome DS, Olson KB: Sputum specimens versus bronchial aspirates in diagnosis of bronchogenic cancer. JAMA 164:167–171, 1957.

461. Rome DS, Olson KB: A direct comparison of natural and aerosol produced sputum collected from 776 asymptomatic men. Acta Cytol 5:173–176, 1961.

462. Rosa UW, Prolla JC, Gastal ED: Cytology in diagnosis of cancer affecting the lung. Results in 1000 consecutive patients. Chest 63:203–207, 1973.

463. Rosen PP, Martini N, Armstrong D: *Pneumocystis carinii* pneumonia. Diagnosis by lung biopsy. Am J Med 58:794–802, 1975.

464. Rosen SE, Koprowska I: Cytologic diagnosis of a case of pulmonary cryptococcosis. Acta Cytol 26:499–502, 1982.

465. Rosen SE, Vonderheid EC, Koprowska I: Mycosis fungoides with pulmonary involvement: cytopathologic findings. Acta Cytol 28:51–57, 1984.

466. Rosenberg BF, Spjut HJ, Gedney MM: Exfoliative cytology in metastatic cancer of the lung. New Engl J Med 261:226–231, 1959.

467. Rosenblatt MB, Lisa JR, Collier F: Primary and metastatic bronchioloalveolar carcinoma. Dis Chest 52:147–152, 1967.

468. Rosenthal DL: Cytology of inflammatory diseases of the lung. *In* Compendium on Diagnostic Cytology, 6th ed. Edited by GL Weid, CM Keebler, LG Koss, JW Reagan. Chicago, Tutorials of Cytology, 1988.

469. Rosenthal DL: Cytopathology of pulmonary disease. In Monographs in Clinical Cytology. Edited by GL Wied. Basel, Karger SH, 1988.

470. Rosenthal DL, Wallace JM: Fine needle aspiration of pulmonary lesions via fiberoptic bronchoscopy. Acta Cytol 28:203–210, 1984.

471. Rubel LR, Reynolds RE: Cytologic description of squamous cell papilloma of the respiratory tract. Acta Cytol 23:227–230, 1979.

472. Russell WO, Neidhardt HW, Mountain CF, Griffith KM, Chang JP: Cytodiagnosis of lung cancer. A report of a four-year laboratory, clinical, and statistical study with a review of the literature on lung cancer and pulmonary cytology. Acta Cytol 7:1–44, 1963.

473. Saccomanno G: Diagnostic Pulmonary Pathology. Chicago, American Society of Clinical Pathologists, 1978.

474. Saccomanno G, Archer VE, Auerbach O, Saunders RP, Brennan LM: Development of carcinoma of the lung as reflected in exfoliated cells. Cancer 33:256–270, 1974.

475. Saccomanno G, Saunders RP, Archer VE, Auerbach O, Kuschner M, Beckler PA: Cancer of the lung—The cytology of sputum prior to the development of carcinoma. Acta Cytol 9:413–423, 1965.

476. Saccomanno G, Saunders RP, Ellis H, Archer VE, Wood BG, Beckler PA: Concentration of carcinoma or atypical cells in sputum. Acta Cytol 7:305–310, 1963.

477. Saccomanno G, Saunders RP, Klein MG, Archer VE, Brennan L: Cytology of the lung in reference to irritant, individual sensitivity and healing. Acta Cytol 14:377–381, 1970.

478. Saffiotti U, Montesano R, Sellahumar AR, Borg SA: Experimental cancer of the lung—Inhibition by vitamin A of induction of tracheobronchial squamous metaplasia and squamous cell tumors. Cancer 20:857–864, 1967.

479. Saito Y, Imai T, Sato M, Ota S-I, Kanma K, Takahashi S, Usuda K, Sagawa M, Nagamoto N, Suda H Nakada T: Cytologic study of tissue repair in human bronchial epithelium. Acta Cytol 32:622–628, 1988.

480. Sanerkin NG, Evans DMD: The sputum in bronchial asthma: pathognomonic patterns. J Pathol Bact 89:535–541, 1965.

481. Sassy-Dobray G: The evaluation of cytology in the early diagnosis of pulmonary carcinoma. Acta Cytol 14:95–103, 1970.

482. Sassy-Dobray G: Possibilities of early diagnosis of bronchogenic carcinoma. Acta Cytol 19:351–357, 1975.

483. Sawada K, Fukuma S, Seki Y, Tanaka F, Ishida I, Ikeda H, Tanaka N: Cytologic features of primary leiomyosarcoma of the lung: report of a case diagnosed by bronchial brushing procedure. Acta Cytol 21:770–773, 1977.

484. Schmitz B, Pfitzer P: Acellular bodies in sputum. Acta Cytol 28:118–125, 1984.

485. Schreiber H, Saccomanno G, Martin DH, Brennan L: Sequential cytological changes during development of respiratory tract tumors induced in hamsters by benzo(a)pyrene-ferric oxide. Cancer Res 34:689–698, 1974.

486. Schulz H, Meurers H: Diagnosis of pulmonary adenomatosis from the sputum by means of electron microscopy. Acta Cytol 8:242–251, 1964.

487. Schumann GB, DiFiore K, Johnston JL: Sputum cytodiagnosis of disseminated histiocytic lymphoma: a case report. Acta Cytol 27:262–266, 1983.

488. Schwinn CP, Sargent EM, Turner AF, Gordonson J, Pashky O: Cytopathology of percutaneous pulmonary needle aspiration biopsy: *In* Compendium on Cytology, 6th ed. Edited by GL Weid, CM Keebler, LG Koss, JW Reagon Chicago, Tutorials of Cytology, 1988.

489. Shaheen K, Oertel YC: Mycosis fungoides cells in sputum: a case report. Acta Cytol 28:483–486, 1984.

490. Shimosato Y, Suzuki A, Hashimoto T, Nishiwaki Y, Kodama T, Yoneyama T, Kameya T: Prognostic implications of fibrotic focus (scar) in small peripheral lung cancers. Am J Surg Pathol 4:365–373, 1980.

491. Shroff CP: Abrasive bronchial brushing cytology. A preliminary study of 200 specimens for the diagnosis of neoplastic and non-neoplastic bronchopulmonary lesions. Acta Cytol 29:101–107, 1985.

492. Sidhu GS, Forrester EM: Glycogen-rich Clara cell–type bronchioloalveolar carcinoma: light and electron microscopic study. Cancer 40:2209–2215, 1977.

493. Silverberg E, Lubera JA: Cancer statistics, 1989. Cancer 39:3–20, 1989.

494. Silverman JF, Finley JL, Park HK, Norris HT, Strausbauch PH: Psammoma bodies and optically clear nuclei in bronchioloalveolar cell carcinoma: diagnosis by fine needle aspiration with histologic and ultrastructural confirmation. Diag Cytopath 1:205–215, 1985.

495. Silverman JF, Finley JL, Park HK, Strausbauch P, Unverferth M, Carney M: Fine needle aspiration cytology of bronchioloalveolar-cell carcinoma of the lung. Acta Cytol 29:887–894, 1985.

496. Silverman JF, Johnsrude IS: Fine needle aspiration cytology of granulomatous cryptococcosis of the lung. Acta Cytol 29:157–161, 1985.

497. Silverman JF, Marrow HG: Fine needle aspiration cytology of granulomatous diseases of the lung, including nontuberculous *Mycobacterium* infection. Acta Cytol 29:535–541, 1985.

498. Silverman JF, Turner RC, West RL, Dillard TA: Bronchoalveolar lavage in the diagnosis of lipoid pneumonia. Diag Cytopathol 5:3–8, 1989.

499. Silverman JF, Weaver MD, Gardner N, Larkin EW, Park HK: Aspiration biopsy cytology of malignant schwannoma metastatic to the lung. Acta Cytol 29:15–18, 1985.

500. Silverman JF, Weaver MD, Shaw R, Newman WJ: Fine needle aspiration cytology of pulmonary infarct. Acta Cytol 29:162–166, 1985.

501. Simpson RW, Johnson DA, Wold LE, Goellner JR: Transthoracic needle aspiration biopsy; Review of 233 cases. Acta Cytol 32:101–104, 1988.

502. Sinner W: Transthoracic needle biopsy of small peripheral malignant lung lesions. Invest Radiol 8:305–314, 1973.

503. Skitarelic K, von Haam E: Bronchial brushings and washings: A diagnostically rewarding procedure? Acta Cytol 18:321–326, 1974.

504. Smith JH, Frable WJ: Adenocarcinoma of the lung. Cytologic correlation with histologic types. Acta Cytol 18:316–320, 1974.

505. Smith RC, Amy RW: Adenoid cystic carcinoma metastatic to the lung. Report of a case diagnosed by fine needle aspiration biopsy cytology. Acta Cytol 29:535–536, 1985.

506. Sobonya RE: *Pneumocystis* infection. *In* Pulmonary Pathology. Edited by DH Dail, SP Hammar. New York, Springer-Verlag, 1988.

507. Soracci R: Asbestos and lung cancer: an analysis of the epidemiological evidence on the asbestos-smoking interaction. Int J Cancer 20:323–331, 1977.

508. Spahr J, Draffin R, Johnston WW: Cytopathologic findings in pulmonary blastoma. Acta Cytol 23:454–459, 1979.

509. Spjut HJ, Fier DJ, Ackerman LV: Exfoliative cytology and pulmonary cancer. J Thorac Surg 30:90–107, 1955.

510. Sproul EE, Huvos A, Britsch C: A two-year follow up study of 261 patients examined by use of superheated aerosol-induced sputum. Acta Cytol 6:409–412, 1962.

511. Stein B, Zaatari GS, Pine JR: Amiodarone pulmonary toxicity; clinical, cytologic and ultrastructural findings. Acta Cytol 31:357–361, 1987.

512. Stitik FP: Percutaneous lung biopsy. *In* Multiple Imaging Procedures: Pulmonary System, Practical Approaches to Pulmonary Diagnosis, vol 1. Edited by SS Seigelman, FP Stitik, WR Summer. New York, Grune & Stratton, 1979.

513. Stover DE, White DA, Romano PA, Gellene RA: Diagnosis of pulmonary disease in acquired immunodeficiency syndrome (AIDS): Role of bronchoscopy and bronchoalveolar lavage. Am Rev Resp Dis 130:659–662, 1984.

514. Stover DE, Zaman MB, Hajdu SI, Lange M, Gold, J, Armstrong D: Bronchoalveolar lavage in the diagnosis of diffuse pulmonary infiltrates in the immunosuppressed host. Ann Intern Med 101:1–7, 1984.

515. Strang C, Simpson JA: Carcinomatous abscess of the lung. Thorax 8:11–28, 1953.

516. Strigle SM, Gal AA: A review of pulmonary cytopathology in the acquired immunodeficiency syndrome. Acta Cytol 5:44–54, 1989.

517. Strobel SL, Keyhani-Rofagha S, O'Toole RV, Nahman BJ: Nonaspiration-needle smear preparations of pulmonary lesions. A comparison of cytology and histology. Acta Cytol 29:1047–1052, 1985.

518. Subramony C, Cason Z, O'Neal RM: Splendore-Hoeppli phenomenon around *Blastomyces* in cytologic preparation. Acta Cytol 28:684–686, 1984.

519. Suprun H: A comparative filter technique study and the relative efficiency of these sieves as applied in sputum cytology for pulmonary cancer cytodiagnosis. Acta Cytol 18:248–251, 1974.

520. Suprun H, Koss LG: The cytological study of sputum and bronchial washings in Hodgkin's disease with pulmonary involvement. Cancer 17:674–680, 1964.

521. Suprun H, Pedio G, Ruttner JR: The diagnostic reliability of cytologic typing in primary lung cancer with a review of the literature. Acta Cytol 24:494–500, 1980.

522. Swank PR, Greenberg SD, Montalvo J, Hunter NR, Spjut HJ, Estrada R, Winkler DG, Taylor GR: The application of visual cell profiles in the study of premalignant atypias in sputum. Acta Cytol 29:373–378, 1985.

523. Szyfelbein WM, Ross JS: Carcinoids, atypical carcinoids and small cell carcinomas of the lung: differential diagnosis of fine needle aspiration biopsy specimens. Diagn Cytopathol 4:1–8, 1988.

524. Szyfelbein WM, Schiller AL: Cytologic diagnosis of giant cell tumor of bone metastatic to lung: A case report. Acta Cytol 23:460–464, 1979.

525. Tabatowski K, Roggli VL, Fulkerson WJ, Langley RL, Benning T, Johnston WW: Giant cell interstitial pneumonia in a hard-metal worker: Cytologic, histologic and analytical electron microscopic investigation. Acta Cytol 32:240–246, 1988.

526. Tabei SZ, Abdollahi B, Nili F: Diagnosis of metastatic adamantinoma of the tibia by pulmonary brushing cytology. Acta Cytol 32:579–581, 1988.

527. Taft PD, Szyfelbein WM, Greene R: A study of variability in cytologic diagnosis based on pulmonary aspiration specimens. Am J Clin Pathol 73:36–40, 1980.

528. Takahashi M: Color Atlas of Cancer Cytology. Tokyo, Igaku-Shoin, 1971.

529. Takahashi M, Hashimoto K, Osada H: Parenteral administration of chymotrypsin for the early detection of cancer cells in sputum. Acta Cytol 11:61–63, 1967.

530. Takahashi M, Urabe M: A new cell concentration method for cancer cytology of sputum. Cancer 16:199–204, 1963.

531. Takeda M: Virus identification in cytologic and histologic material by electron microscopy. Acta Cytol 13:206–209, 1969.

532. Takenega A, Matsuda M, Horai T, Ikegami H, Hattori S: Giant cell carcinoma of the lung: comparative studies of the same cancer cells by light microscopy and scanning electron microscopy. Acta Cytol 24:190–196, 1980.

533. Tanaka T, Yamamoto M, Tamura T, Moritani Y, Miyai M, Hiraki S, Ohnoshi T, Kimura I: Cytologic and histologic correlation in primary lung cancer. A study of 154 cases with resectable tumors. Acta Cytol 29:49–56, 1985.

534. Tani EM, Franco M: Pulmonary cytology in paracoccidioidomycosis. Acta Cytol 28:571–575, 1984.

535. Tani EM, Schmitt FCL, Oliveira MLS, Gobetti SMP, Decarlis RMST: Pulmonary cytology in tuberculosis. Acta Cytol 31:460–463, 1987.

536. Tao LC, Delarue NC, Sanders D, Weisbrod G: Bronchioloalveolar carcinoma: a correlative clinical and cytologic study. Cancer 42:2759–2767, 1978.

537. Tao LC, Robertson DI: Cytologic diagnosis of bronchial mucoepidermoid carcinoma by fine needle aspiration biopsy. Acta Cytol 22:221–224, 1978.

538. Tao LC, WEisbrod GL, Pearson FG, Sanders DE, Donat EE, Filipetto L: Cytologic diagnosis of bronchioloalveolar carcinoma by fine needle aspiration biopsy. Cancer 57:1565–1570, 1986.

539. Tassoni EM: Pools of lymphocytes: Significance in pulmonary secretions. Acta Cytol 7:168–173, 1963.

540. Thornbury JR, Burke DP, Naylor B: Transthoracic needle aspiration biopsy: Accuracy of cytologic typing of malignant neoplasms. Am J Radiol 136:719–724, 1981.

541. Tweeddale DN, Harbord RP, Nuzum CT, Pielemeier B, Kington E: A new technique to obtain sputum for cytologic study: External percussion and vibration of the chest wall. Acta Cytol 10:214–219, 1966.

542. Tomb JA, Mattosian R: Diagnosis of pulmonary hydatidosis by sputum cytology. Johns Hopkins Med J 139:38–40, 1976.

543. Toomes H, Delphendahl A, Manke HG, Vogt-Moykopf I: The coin lesion of the lung: a review of 955 resected coin lesions. Cancer 51:534–537, 1983.

544. Truong LD, Underwood RD, Greenberg SD, McLarty JW: Diagnosis and typing of lung carcinomas by cytopathologic methods: a review of 108 cases. Acta Cytol 29:379–384, 1985.

545. Tsuboi E, Ikeda S, Tajima M, Shimosata Y, Ishikawa S: Transbronchial biopsy smear for diagnosis of peripheral pulmonary carcinomas. Cancer 20:687–698, 1968.

546. Tsumuraya M, Kodama T, Kameya T, Shimosato Y, Koketsu H, Uei Y: Light and electron microscopic analysis of intranuclear inclusions in papillary adenocarcinoma of the lung. Acta Cytol 25:523–532, 1981.

547. Umiker WO: False-negative reports in the cytologic diagnosis of cancer of the lung. Am J Clin Pathol 28:37–45, 1957.

548. Umiker WO: Diagnosis of bronchogenic carcinoma; an evalu-

ation of pulmonary cytology, bronchoscopy and scalene lymph node biopsy. Dis Chest 37:82–90, 1960.

549. Umiker WO: The current role of exfoliative cytopathology in the routine diagnosis of bronchogenic carcinoma; a five-year study of 152 consecutive, unselected cases. Dis Chest 40:154–159, 1961.

550. Umiker WO: A new vista in pulmonary cytology; aerosol induction of sputum. Dis Chest 39:512–51, 1961.

551. Umiker WO, DeWeese MS, Lawrence GH: Diagnosis of lung cancer by bronchoscopic biopsy, scalene lymph node biopsy, and cytologic smears. A report of 42 histologically proven cases. Surgery 41:705–713, 1957.

552. Umiker WO, Korst DR, Cole RP, Manikas SG: Collection of sputum for cytologic examination. Spontaneous vs. artificially produced sputum. New Engl J Med 262:565–566, 1960.

553. Umiker WO, Sourenne R: A simple method for concentrating carcinoma cells in sputum. Am J Clin Pathol 35:411–412, 1961.

554. Valaitis J, Warren S, Gamble D: Increasing incidence of adenocarcinoma of the lung. Cancer 47:1042–1046, 1981.

555. Valentine EH: Squamous metaplasia of the bronchus. A study of metaplastic changes occurring in epithelium of the major bronchi in cancerous and noncancerous cases. Cancer 10:272–279, 1957.

556. Valicenti JF Jr, Daniell C, Gobien RP: Thin needle aspiration cytology of benign intrathoracic lesions. Acta Cytol 25:659–664, 1981.

557. Valicenti JF Jr, McMaster KR III, Daniell CJ: Sputum cytology of giant cell interstitial pneumonia. Acta Cytol 23:217–221, 1979.

558. Vernon SE: Nodular pulmonary sarcoidosis. Diagnosis with fine needle aspiration biopsy. Acta Cytol 29:473–476, 1985.

559. Vieyra-Herrera G, Becerril-Carmona G, Padua-Gabriel A, Jessurun J, Alonso-de Ruiz P: *Strongyloides stercoralis* hyperinfection in a patient with the acquired immune deficiency syndrome. Acta Cytol 32:277–278, 1988.

560. Vincent RG, Pickren JW, Lane WW, Bross I, Hiroshi T, Houten L, Gutierrez AC, Rzepka T: The changing histopathology of lung cancer: a review of 1682 cases. Cancer 39:1647–1655, 1977.

561. Vincent TN, Satterfield JV, Ackerman LV: Carcinoma of the lung in women. Cancer 18:559–570, 1965.

562. von Haam E: A comparative study of the accuracy of cancer cell detection by cytological methods. Acta Cytol 6:508–518, 1962.

563. Wagner ED, Ramzy I, Greenberg SD, Gonzalez JM: Transbronchial fine-needle aspiration. Am J Clini Pathol 92:36–50, 1989.

564. Wagoner JK, Infante PF, Bayliss DL: Beryllium: an etiologic agent in the induction of lung cancer, non-neoplastic respiratory disease, and heart disease among industrially exposed workers. Environ Res 21:15–34, 1980.

565. Walker AN, Walker GK, Feldman PS: Diagnosis of *Legionella micdadei* pneumonia from cytologic specimens. Acta Cytol 27:252–254, 1983.

565a. Walker KR, Fullmer CD: Observations of eosinophilic extracytoplasmic processes in pulmonary macrophages. Progress report. Acta Cytol 15:363–364, 1971.

566. Walloch J: Pulmonary cytopathology in historical perspective. *In* Lung Cancer. The Evolution of Concepts. Edited by JG Gruhn, ST Rosen. New York, Field & Wood, 1989.

567. Wandall HH: A study on neoplastic cells in sputum as a contribution to the diagnosis of primary lung cancer. Acta Chir Scand 91:1–143, 1944.

568. Wang N-S: Anatomy. *In* Pulmonary Pathology. Edited by DH Dail, SP Hammar. New York, Springer-Verlag, 1988.

569. Wang NS, Seemayer TA, Ahmed MN, Knaack J: Giant cell carcinoma of the lung: a light and electron microscopic study. Hum Pathol 7:3–16, 1976.

570. Wang SE, Nieberg RK: Fine needle aspiration cytology of sclerosing hemangioma of the lung, a mimicker of bronchioloalveolar carcinoma. Acta Cytol 30:51–54, 1985.

571. Wang T, Reyes CV, Kathuria S, Strinden C: Diagnosis of *Strongyloides stercoralis* in sputum cytology. Acta Cytol 24:40–43, 1980.

572. Warner NE, McGrew EA, Nenos S: Cytologic study of the sputum in cytomegalic inclusion disease. Acta Cytol 8:311–315, 1964.

573. Warren KS: Diseases due to helminths. *In* Principles and Practice of Infectious Disease. Edited by GL Mandel, RG Douglas Jr, JE Bennett. New York, John Wiley & Sons, 1979.

574. Watson WL, Cromwell R, Craver L, Papanicolaou GN: Cytology of bronchial secretions. Its role in the diagnosis of cancer. J Thora Surg 18:113–122, 1949.

575. Waxweiler RJ, Smith AH, Falk H, Tyroler HA: Excess lung cancer risk in a synthetic chemicals plant. Environ Health Perspect 41:159–165, 1981.

576. Weiss W, Boucot KR, Cooper DA: Growth rate in the detection and prognosis of bronchogenic carcinoma. JAMA 198:108–114, 1966.

577. Weiss W, Boucot KR, Cooper DA: The histopathology of bronchogenic carcinoma and its relation to growth rate, metastasis and prognosis, Cancer 26:965–970, 1970.

578. Wheeler TM, Johnson ED, Coughlin D, Greenberg SD: The sensitivity of detection of asbestos bodies in sputa and bronchial washings. Acta Cytol 32:647–650, 1988.

579. Wihman G, Bergstrom J: Histological technique for the examination of the cell content of sputum. Acta Med Scand (Stockh) 142:433–440, 1952.

580. Wilkins EW, Grillo HC, Moncure AC, Scannell JG: Changing times in surgical management of bronchopulmonary carcinoid tumor. Ann Thorac Surg 38:339–344, 1984.

581. Willett GD, Schumann GB, Genack L: Primary cytodiagnosis of synchronous small-cell cancer and squamous-cell carcinoma of the respiratory tract. Acta Cytol 28:610–613, 1984.

582. Williams JW: Alveolar metaplasia; its relationship to pulmonary fibrosis in industry and development of lung cancer. Br J Cancer 11:30–42, 1957.

583. Willie SM, Snyder RN: The identification of *Paragonimus westermani* in bronchial washings. Case report. Acta Cytol 21:101–102, 1977.

584. Wilson RA: An unusual second primary tumor: report of a case of atypical carcinoid of the lung. Acta Cytol 22:362–365, 1978.

585. Winn WC Jr, Walker DH: Viral infections. *In* Pulmonary Pathology. Edited by DH Dail, SP Hammar. New York, Springer-Verlag, 1988.

586. Wisecarver J, Nerss MJ, Rennard SI, Thompson AB, Armitage JO, Linder J: Bronchoalveolar lavage in the assessment of pulmonary Hodgkin's disease. Acta Cytol 33:527–532, 1989.

587. Wolfe WG, Johnston WW: Transbronchial brushing through bronchoscope in the diagnosis of pulmonary and esophageal disease. NC Med J 31:297–301, 1970.

588. Woolner LB: Recent advances in pulmonary cytology: Early detection and localization of occult lung cancer in symptomless males. *In* Advances In Clinical Cytology, vol 1. Edited by LG Koss, D Coleman. London, Butterworths, 1981.

589. Woolner LB: Pulmonary cytopathology: *In* Compendium on Diagnostic Cytology, 6th ed. Edited by GL Wied, CM Keebler, LG Koss, JW Reagan. Chicago, Tutorials of Cytology, 1988.

590. Woolner LB, Andersen HA, Bernatz PE: "Occult" carcinoma of the bronchus: A study of 15 cases of *in situ* or early invasive bronchogenic carcinoma. Dis Chest 37:278–288, 1960.

591. Woolner LB, Fontana RWS, Sanderson DR, et al: Mayo Lung Project evaluation of lung cancer screening through December 1979. Mayo Clin Proc 56:544–555, 1981.

592. Woolner LB, McDonald JR: Bronchogenic carcinoma: diagnosis by microscopic examination of sputum and bronchial secretions; preliminary report. Proc Staff Meetings Mayo Clin 22:369–381, 1947.

593. Woolner LB, McDonald JR: Carcinoma cells in sputum and bronchial secretions. Surg Gynecol Obstet 88:273–290, 1949.

594. Woolner LB, McDonald JR: Cytologic diagnosis of bronchogenic carcinoma. Am J Clin Pathol 19:765–769, 1949.

595. Woolner LB, McDonald JR: Diagnosis of carcinoma of the lung; the value of cytologic study of sputum and bronchial secretions. JAMA 139:497–502, 1949.

596. Woolner LB, McDonald JR: Cytologic diagnosis of bronchogenic carcinoma. Dis Chest 17:1–10, 1950.

597. Woolner LB, McDonald JR: Cytology of sputum and bronchial secretions: studies on 588 patients with miscellaneous pulmonary lesions. Ann Intern Med 33:1164–1174, 1950.

598. Wynder EL, Graham EA: Tobacco smoking as a possible etiologic factor in bronchogenic carcinoma: a study of 684 proven cases. JAMA 143:329–336, 1950.

599. Yesner R: Spectrum of lung cancer and ectopic hormones. Pathol Annu 13:(Pt1):217–240, 1978.

600. Yesner R: Small cell tumors of the lung. Am J Surg Pathol 7:775–785, 1983.

601. Yesner R, Carter D: Pathology of carcinoma of the lung; changing patterns. Clin Chest Med 3:257–289, 1982.

602. Yesner R, Gelfman NA, Feinstein AR: A reappraisal of histopathology in lung cancer and correlation of cell types with antecedent cigarette smoking. Am Rev Resp Dis 107:790–797, 1973.

603. Zaharopoulos P, Schnadig VJ, Davie KD, Boudreau RE, Weedn VW: Multiseptate bodies in systemic phaeohyphomycosis diagnosed by fine needle aspiration cytology. 32:885–891, 1988.

604. Zaharopoulos P, Wong JY, Stewart GD: Cytomorphology of the variants of small-cell carcinoma of the lung. Acta Cytol 26:800–808, 1982.

605. Zajicek J: Aspiration biopsy cytology. Part 1. Cytology of supradiaphragmatic organs. *In* Monographs in Clinical Cytology, vol 4. Edited by GL Wied. Basel, Karger, 1974.

606. Zavala DC: Diagnostic fiberoptic bronchoscopy: Techniques and results of biopsy of 600 patients. Chest 68:12–19, 1975.

15

Oral Cavity

Sol Silverman, Jr.

Cancers of the lips, tongue, floor of the mouth, palate, gingiva, buccal mucosa and oropharynx now account for about 4% of all new cancers each year in the United States. Over 90% are squamous carcinomas. Oral cancer occurs in all ethnic groups with some variations. These variations appear to be associated primarily with tobacco and alcohol usage. Oral malignancies occur in about twice as many men as women, and 95% are found in persons older than 40 years.

Oral cancer accounts for approximately 3% of all cancer-related deaths. Although mortality is high among oral cancer patients (less than 50% of the patients are cured), the survival rate increases dramatically when these cancers are detected early, i.e., when the lesions are less than 3 cm in diameter and there is no evidence of involvement in the regional cervical lymph nodes.

EARLY DIAGNOSIS

Currently, the most effective way of combating oral cancer is by early diagnosis followed by adequate treatment.[34] Because most oral cancers are squamous cell carcinomas, the vast majority of oral cancers will be diagnosed from lesions on the mucosal surfaces, which is lined by this type of epithelium (stratified squamous).

The clinician's dilemma is differentiating cancerous lesions from a multitude of other ill-defined, controversial and poorly understood lesions that also occur in the oral cavity.[33] Most oral lesions are benign, but many have an appearance that may be easily confused with a malignant lesion. Some benign lesions are considered premalignant because they have been statistically correlated with subsequent cancerous changes, e.g., leukoplakia. Conversely, malignant lesions seen in an early stage may often be mistaken for a benign change.

Early carcinoma of the oral cavity may remain painless unless the lesion becomes ulcerated. However, some patients do not seek consultation until severe and persistent pain develops. The most frequent complaint is that of a sore or an irritation in the mouth. Infrequently a patient will seek consultation because of a lump in the neck, which may represent metastasis to a lymph node from an oral lesion, of which the patient is unaware.

Oral carcinoma in the early stage may appear as a small, apparently harmless area of induration or localized change such as erosion, erythema or keratosis. Because of the variability in signs and symptoms among oral cancer patients, even excellent clinical judgment and broad experience do not preclude diagnostic errors.

Although apparently benign, any oral lesion that does not respond to the usual therapeutic measures should be considered malignant until histologically shown to be benign. Histologic examination of tissue from a biopsy is the only definitive method of diagnosing oral cancer.

Obviously, immediate biopsy of every oral lesion is impractical and not indicated when other simple, reliable and acceptable techniques are available to support clinical judgment in differentiating benign lesions from early malignant changes. Exfoliative cytologic study is one such technique.

Toluidine blue or vital staining is also a useful technique for supplementing clinical judgment.[5, 14, 15, 19, 21, 31] The mechanism is based upon selective dye binding by dysplastic or malignant cells in the oral epithelium. Its value is based on simplicity, inexpensiveness, noninvasive technique and accuracy. In summary, toluidine blue staining may complement and accelerate a cytologic smear or biopsy or both by further indicating sites likely to reflect the most serious pathologic changes.

Fine needle aspiration (FNA) has a limited but very important role in oral diagnosis. FNA is the technique of choice in the initial microscopic assessment of major salivary gland lesions and palpable cervical (neck) lymph nodes when tumor is suspected.[24] Occasionally FNA is useful in deeply seated extranodal or glandular masses. In these instances, the needle usually has to be directed with imaging techniques.[13]

BIOPSY

Because of the variability of signs and symptoms, even extensive clinical experience will not preclude diagnostic errors. Because oral cancer has such a poor prognosis, early detection and early adequate treatment are essential to the improvement of cure rates. However, because of the large number of benign lesions occurring in the mouth, immediate biopsy of every ill-defined or innocuous-appearing mucosal change is impractical and not indicated. It is obvious, then, that a simple, reliable, and acceptable technique to support clinical judgment in differentiating benign from early malignant neoplasia is highly desirable. Exfoliative cytology serves this purpose, but it must be remembered that cytology is an adjunct to, not a substitute for, biopsy.

CYTOLOGY

Because the oral epithelium renews itself rapidly (probably within 2 weeks) and most superficial epithelial cells of the mouth contain nuclei, surface scrapings may be reliable indicators of dysplastic or neoplastic changes (Fig. 15–1). Direct smears allow for accurate sampling of a lesion and aid in complete screening.[30] Numerous reports substantiate the fact that use of oral cytology has accelerated biopsy of lesions that did not clinically appear to be oral cancers, thus leading to the early diagnosis of malignancies that would otherwise have remained temporarily unsuspected.[1, 9, 11, 23]

Collection of Smear. Label one end of a glass microscope slide with patient's name, date and area from which the material is to be obtained. Use a clean cotton-tipped applicator or wood spatula for collection of the specimen (Fig. 15–2). If the area to be scraped is dry, the applicator or spatula should be moistened. Usually saliva or tissue excretions are sufficient to prevent dehydration. Collect the material from the lesion by using slight rolling and scraping motions. Remember, slides may be inadequate if there is a pseudomembrane, too thick saliva, excess bleeding or

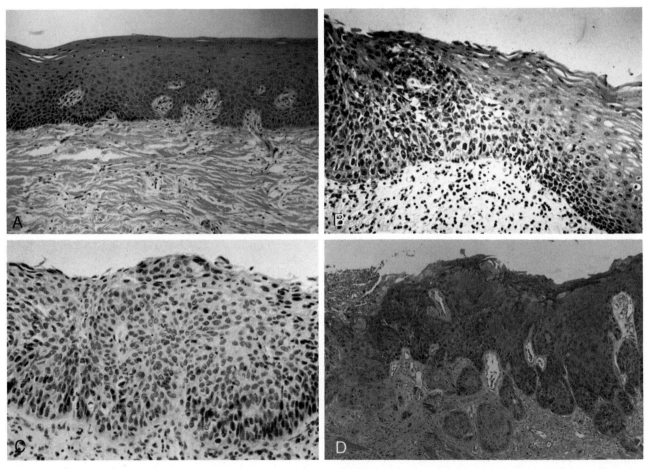

FIGURE 15–1. Transformation of epithelium from normal to malignant. *A*, Normal buccal epithelium (hematoxylin-eosin; ×100). *B*, Transition zone between normal buccal epithelium and severe dysplasia or carcinoma *in situ* (hematoxylin-eosin; ×200). *C*, Intraepithelial carcinoma. Note the apparently intact basal lamina (basement membrane), which is confining all of the abnormal cells to the epithelial layer (hematoxylin-eosin; ×200). *D*, Squamous cell carcinoma. Malignant cells, both individually and in groups, have penetrated the basal lamina and invaded the connective tissue (hematoxylin-eosin; ×100).

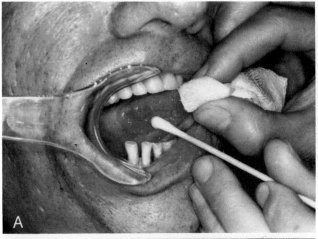

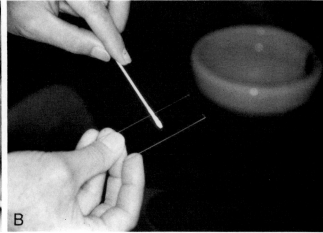

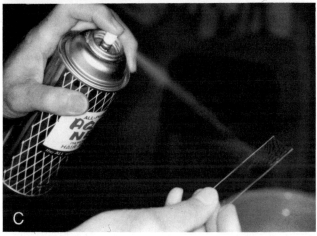

FIGURE 15–2. Exfoliative cytology technique. *A*, Smear is obtained from a tongue ulcer with a cotton-tipped applicator, using a firm, rolling motion. *B*, Cells are transferred, using a streaking, rolling movement, to the central portion of a clean microscope slide. *C*, A short burst of spray adequately fixes the cells to the slide and preserves them for staining.

no moisture. The scrapings should be immediately smeared on the center area of the slide (approximately 2.5 × 2.5 cm).

Fixation of Smear. Alcohol (70%) is adequate for fixation. Commercial spray fixatives or hair sprays are satisfactory and also make it easier to handle the specimen. Do not allow the smear to dry before fixation.

Staining of Smear. The smear is stained by a modified Papanicolaou-Traut technique using Mayer's hemotoxylin, orange G, eosin and light green. The slide can be made ready for screening in less than 1 hour.

Screening of Smears. It should be recalled that the entire oral cavity is lined by stratified squamous epithelium, which varies in thickness and keratinization according to anatomic and functional sites (Table 15–1) (Fig. 15–3).

ORAL HISTOLOGY

The oral cavity is lined with stratified squamous epithelium. The degree of normal surface keratinization (genetically predetermined) varies as follows: hard palate, gingiva and dorsal tongue are keratinized, oropharynx, soft palate, lateral and ventral tongue and floor of mouth are unkeratinized and the buccal and labial mucosae are intermediate between these two extremes. The only specialized epithelia occur in the tongue, which contains papillae (filiform, fungiform and circumvallate) and taste buds.

General features of *normal* intraoral squamous cells are as follows (Fig. 15–4):

1. *Keratinized surface cells* (mature or cornified cells) are more flattened and irregular in appearance and have a small, pyknotic nucleus or are anucleated; the cytoplasm stains pink, yellow or orange (acidophilic).

2. *Unkeratinized surface cells* (intermediate maturity) may be slightly flattened, with somewhat irregular cytoplasmic morphology and some degree of nuclear

TABLE 15–1. Appearance of Surface Cells in Relation to Location

Hard palate, gingiva and dorsal tongue	Mature cells: High degree of cornification and some cells anucleated
Buccal and labial mucosae	Intermediate maturity: Nucleated basophilic and acidophilic staining cells
Floor of mouth, ventral tongue, lateral tongue, soft palate and oropharynx	Least maturity: Predominantly basophilic cells with large nuclei

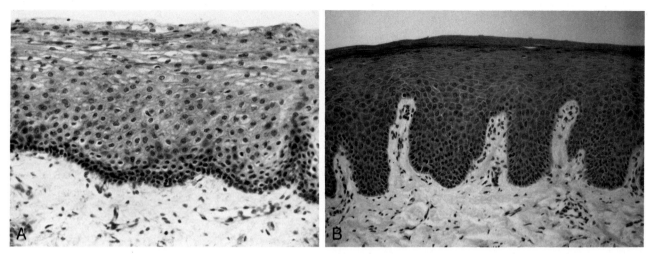

FIGURE 15–3. Variations in **maturation of normal oral epithelium.** A, Nonkeratinized soft palate (hematoxylin-eosin; ×200). B, Keratinized hard palate (hematoxylin-eosin stain; ×100).

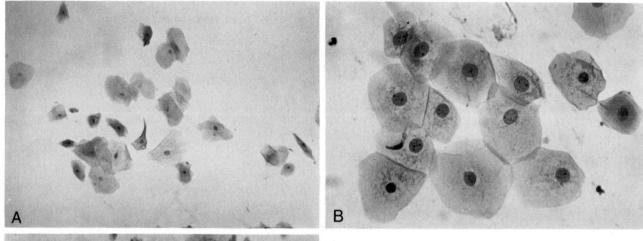

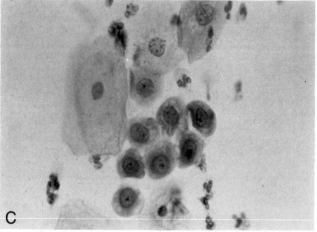

FIGURE 15–4. Surface cells from normal epithelium. A, Mature epithelial cells from the surface of keratinized epithelium. Note that some cells are anucleate. In others, the nuclei are disappearing by proteolytic action (Papanicolaou stain; ×200). B, Squamous cells from nonkeratinized epithelium. Note uniform size, shape and position of nuclei with adequate surrounding cytoplasm (Papanicolaou stain; ×400). C, Cells from a newly healed ulcer. Note the clump of basal cells, characterized by large nuclei and a small amount of surrounding cytoplasm. Compare these with the larger mature squame (Papanicolaou stain; ×400).

contraction; cytoplasm is usually basophilic but may be acidophilic and stain pink or red.

3. *Parabasal and immature prickle cells* are spheric or cuboid and have a centrally placed nucleus with even distribution of chromatin; cytoplasm stains green or blue-green (basophilic).

BENIGN ORAL LESIONS

Benign lesions occurring in the mouth may have a variable clinical appearance that often makes diagnoses difficult.[26] Many of these lesions will initially be examined from cytologic scrapings in the attempt to differentiate them from malignant lesions as well as to help guide clinical management, which may involve medication, the removal of irritants, incisional or excisional biopsies or other modes of care. The cytologic atypias observed in material obtained from benign lesions are sometimes helpful in establishing a diagnosis; experience is necessary in some cases to differentiate these changes from those relating to malignancy.

General Considerations

In patients with pernicious or iron deficiency anemias, the nuclei of oral cells may be enlarged; reduction in nuclear size occurs in response to treatment.[8, 36] This nuclear enlargement is variable, and its diagnostic value and clinical significance are questionable. It is common in screening procedures to find occasionally enlarged nuclei in cells from normal patients. They are also observable in patients who are receiving certain drugs, irradiation treatment or chemotherapy for cancer and in patients who demonstrate a variety of mucosal irritations.[26]

Estrogen Effects

Because of the morphologic similarity between the stratified squamous epithelia of the oral cavity and that of the uterine cervix, a similar estrogenic response has been presupposed. A study in our laboratory[27] showed no alterations in either cytoplasmic staining or nuclear morphology in 24 normal women studied by weekly buccal smears through two menstrual cycles, although there were variations between subjects.

In addition, estrogen administration to a group of postmenopausal women with osteoporosis showed no interval changes in oral scrapings or biopsies, whereas vaginal smears from these women reflected the expected estrogenic effects. Dokumov and Spasov[6] also found no correlations, whereas Anderson and coworkers[2] stated that there was some limited value in smears from specific oral sites regarding oral cytology as an index of estrogenemia.

Chromosomal Sex

Buccal scrapings may reflect the presence of Barr bodies, the heterochromatic X chromosome seen adjacent to the nuclear membrane during interphase. These bodies may be seen in 14 to 56% of squamous cells (average 26%) in normal women.[10, 20] These bodies are essentially absent in normal males. In checking buccal smears against peripheral blood leukocytes, Douglass and Beaver[7] found no Barr bodies when there was only one X chromosome and 2 to 21% demonstrating Barr bodies when two X chromosomes were found.

Viral Lesions

Primary herpetic stomatitis is an acute oral herpesvirus infection characterized by crusting of the lips, intraoral ulcers, pain, lymphadenopathy and fever. It may be confused with bacterial infections, infectious mononucleosis, erythema multiforme, blood dyscrasias or other nonspecific stomatitides. The herpesvirus has a capacity to induce excessive nuclear protein production, chromatin aberrations and abnormal nuclear divisions, thus producing bizarre pseudogiant cells (Fig. 15–5).[29] Recurrent herpetic infections of the lips (cold sores) and mouth can also form these abnormal squamous cells. It should be recalled that the common recurrent aphthous ulcer (canker sore) is not due to the herpesvirus and will usually demonstrate a slightly enlarged nucleus with adequate surrounding acidophilic cytoplasm. Care must be taken to observe carefully all the morphologic changes in viral-infected cells and to correlate them with the clinical findings to avoid false-positives for malignancy.

Pemphigus Vulgaris

The mucosa of the mouth is involved in a large percentage of patients with pemphigus, an autoimmune mucocutaneous disease. The disease frequently begins on the mucosa of the mouth and is usually severe. The type and appearance of the oral lesions is similar to those of the skin. The bullae are rarely seen because they break soon after formation, leaving varying-sized ulcerations.

The vermilion border of the lips adjoining the skin are usually afflicted. The lesions may be covered with a whitish exudate; they bleed easily and are painful.

Acantholytic changes are represented by numerous fairly uniform basal and parabasal cells with an increased nucleocytoplasmic ratio and large singular or multiple irregular nucleoli (Fig. 15–6).[12, 14] The chromatin in some instances may show an abnormal pattern. Perinuclear cytoplasmic halo formation may be seen. The cells may be interpreted mistakenly as suspicious for malignancy when not correlated with clinical descriptions.

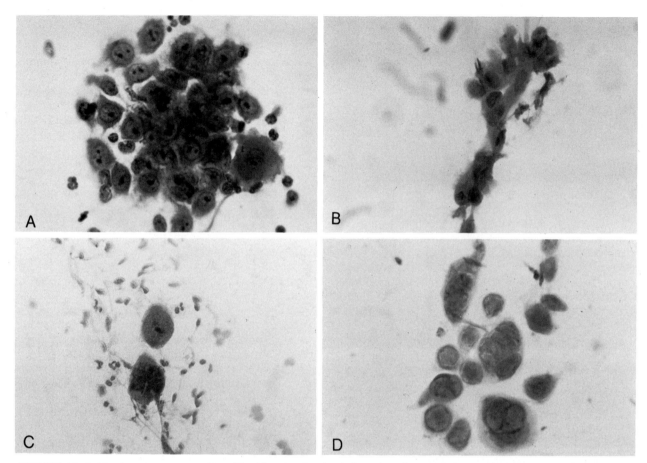

FIGURE 15–5. Varying appearances *(A to D)* of **herpes simplex infected oral squamous cells** (Papanicolaou stain; ×400).

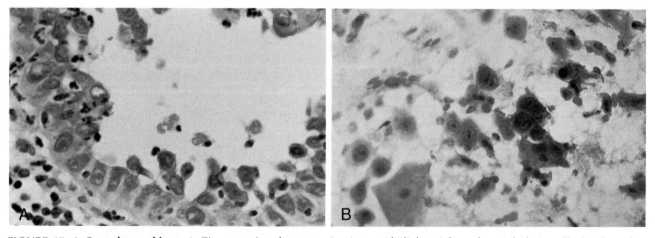

FIGURE 15–6. Buccal pemphigus. *A,* Tissue section demonstrating intraepithelial vesicle and acantholytic cells that have lost their desmosomal attachments from antigen-antibody reactions (hematoxylin-eosin; ×400). *B,* Acantholytic squamous cells (Tzanck) seen in a smear from a broken epithelial vesicle (hematoxylin-eosin; ×400).

Ulcerations and Inflammations

The oral mucosal responses to physical, chemical or biologic agents vary widely in their clinical appearance. Scrapings from these lesions may reveal cells whose cytoplasm is abnormally acidophilic or parabasal-like cells with enlarged nuclei and scanty surrounding cytoplasm or both. Infrequently, prominent and multiple nucleoli, abnormal chromatin patterns and multinucleation will be found. These may account for suspicious-appearing cells and exemplify the importance of correlating clinical and microscopic findings to determine a rational course of patient management. False-positive results are very infrequent. Studies have revealed no significant effects from dentures or cigarette smoking on the morphology of exfoliated cells.[4, 18] However, chronic irritation can increase the degree of keratinization. Presence of white blood cells (polymorphonuclear leukocytes and lymphocytes) can vary greatly in number.

Leukoplakia

Leukoplakia may be defined as any white plaque or patch that cannot be scraped off the oral mucosa. It occurs in less than 5% of the adult population. Leukoplakia has been shown to be a precancerous lesion in some patients.[32, 35] Because dysplasia or an early cancer may appear as a patch of leukoplakia,[3, 34, 38] clinical examination is often supplemented with cytologic scrapings, particularly for cases in which a biopsy is delayed or not considered. Additionally, cytologic supplementation to a biopsy is often helpful because more mucosa can be evaluated.

The most constant histopathologic finding in leukoplakia is hyperkeratosis (formation or increase in thickness of stratum corneum) (Fig. 15–7). Smears from the surface, even prior to ulceration, may yield representative cells if abnormal maturation is occurring. This is based on the fact that hyperparakeratotic surface cells, because of a relatively fast renewal time of probably less than 2 weeks, contain nuclei representative of an abnormal epithelial maturation pattern. Even leukoplakias that appear histologically as hyperorthokeratotic contain, in effect, many tightly packed but intact cells, some of which contain nuclei. Moreover, carcinoma usually does not occur in hyperorthokeratotic stratum corneum, but a transition to hyperparakeratosis will take place first.

Any cytologic atypia from leukoplakic lesions demands a biopsy. Persistence of leukoplakia when removal is not feasible requires constant clinical observation and microscopic follow-up. Studies indicate that most false-negative cytologic findings from oral carcinomas are derived from carcinomas displaying hyperkeratosis (clinical white lesions that microscopically display well-differentiated malignant squamous cells).

In a study of oral lesions resembling leukoplakia, namely, the white sponge nevus, Darier's disease and hereditary benign intraepithelial dyskeratosis, Witkop[39] cites cytologic changes characteristic of these lesions: cell-within-cell inclusions in Darier's disease and hereditary benign intraepithelial dyskeratosis, and eosinophilic condensations in the cytoplasm of cells from the white sponge nevus. However, these changes are

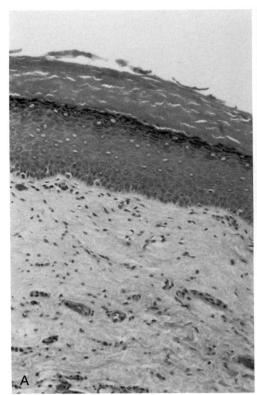

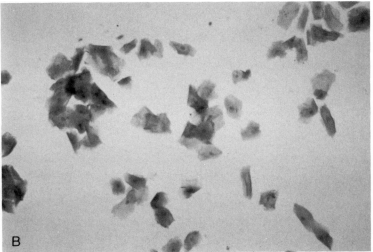

FIGURE 15–7. Oral leukoplakia. *A,* Hyperkeratosis (hematoxylin-eosin, ×100). *B,* Surface scraping that demonstrates mixture of nucleate and anucleate squamous cells (Papanicolaou stain; ×100).

not specific and may also be found in irradiated cells, cells from patients receiving chemotherapy and occasionally in cells from subjects with other benign oral conditions.

Nasal and Antral Oral Fistulae

Openings between the oral cavity and the maxillary antrum or nasal cavity following surgery expose mucosal surfaces that usually exhibit erythematous and granulomatous-like changes that are difficult to interpret clinically. Cytologic smears serve as a useful adjunct in evaluating these changes. The columnar cells obtained often have slightly enlarged, pleomorphic or hyperchromatic nuclei, which may contain prominent nucleoli. They are often interpreted as suspicious, particularly when cilia are not observed or they appear cuboidal rather than elongated or both.

Radiation Changes

Oral radiation for cancer induces numerous cytologic changes that may persist for long periods following completion of the therapy. These changes include nuclear and cytoplasmic enlargement and vacuolization, binucleation and nuclear aberrations (Fig. 15–8).

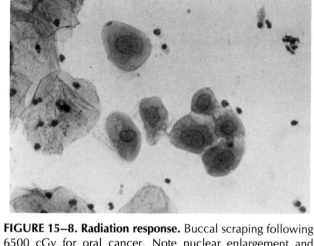

FIGURE 15–8. Radiation response. Buccal scraping following 6500 cGy for oral cancer. Note nuclear enlargement and cytoplasmic vacuolization (Papanicolaou stain; ×400).

Combinations of these morphologic changes may involve as much as 40% of the cells in a representative cytologic scraping. Studies have shown no correlation between cytologic changes and either the radiation dose delivered or the clinical results of treatment.[17, 28] It is also of interest that these same changes, although in a smaller magnitude, may be observed prior to irradiation.

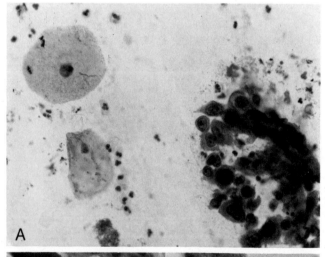

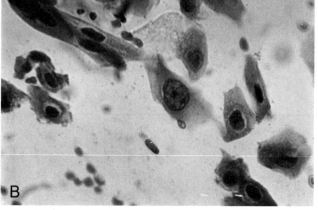

FIGURE 15–9. Malignant cells from surface of **squamous carcinoma.** A, Group of malignant cells and two mature squamous cells (Papanicolaou stain; ×400). B, High-power view of malignant cells. Note the altered nucleocytoplasmic ratio, pleomorphism, enlarged nuclei, irregular nuclear membrane and hyperchromatism (Papanicolaou stain; ×400).

Candidiasis

In normal buccal scrapings, fungal spores and hypha-like structures are not seen. Therefore, their presence indicates a possible candidal infection.

MALIGNANT ORAL LESIONS

The following are criteria upon which cytologic interpretations of *malignant* cells are based (all criteria usually are not found in each specimen) (Fig. 15–9).
1. Enlarged nuclei
2. Variation in nuclear size and shape (pleomorphism)
3. Prominent and irregular nuclear borders
4. Increased nucleocytoplasmic ratio (decreased cytoplasm)
5. Multiple prominent and irregular nuclei
6. Hyperchromatism (increased nucleoproteins)
7. Abnormal chromatin pattern and distribution
8. Discrepancy in maturation (extreme variations).

Table 15–2 describes reporting of oral smears. Cells from benign lesions may have atypical appearances, but they seldom display enough criteria to cause them to be misinterpreted as malignant. Classification of benign diseases from exfoliative cytologic studies has not been forthcoming.

DIAGNOSTIC ACCURACY

False-negative reports have been few.[22, 23, 25, 37] These errors, although undesirable, are not critical because the way cytologic reports are used primarily to supplement and not to replace clinical judgment. The following criteria are observed: (1) If clinical suspicion remains in the face of a negative or atypical report, further smears or biopsy should be performed. (2) A suspicious report indicates a definite need to establish a diagnosis immediately. (3) When smears contain cells consistent with malignancy, biopsy is mandatory. The just-mentioned studies prompt the following conclusions:

1. Cytologic smears indicate the presence of suspicious or malignant-appearing cells in most oral malignancies and are useful in aiding clinical assessment of malignancy and accelerating biopsy.
2. Most false-negatives are derived from tissue that has a marked hyperkeratotic component. This reflects the difficulty of assessing malignant criteria in well-differentiated cells as well as difficulties in sampling.
3. Cytology has a limited value for assessment of potential carcinoma of the vermilion border because of the highly differentiated nature of these lesions and the keratotic characteristic of this epithelium.

References

1. Allegra SR, Broderick PA, Corvese N: Oral Cytology. Seven-year oral cytology screening program in the State of Rhode Island. Analysis of 6,448 cases. Acta Cytol 17:42–48, 1973.
2. Anderson WR, Belding J, Pixley E: Oral cytology. A hormonal evaluation. Acta Cytol 13:81–88, 1969.
3. Banoczy J: Cytologic study of the keratinization pattern in oral leukoplakia. J Dent Res 50:1562–1566, 1971.
4. Brown AM, Young A: The effects of age and smoking on the maturation of the oral mucosa. Acta Cytol 14:566–569, 1970.
5. Dietrich CP, Sampaio LO, DeOrca HM, Nader HB: Role of sulfated mucopolysaccharides in cell recognition and neoplastic transformation. An Acad Bras Cienc 52:179–186, 1980.
6. Dokumov SI, Spasov SA: A comparison of oral and vaginal smears in women with normal menstrual cycles. Acta Cytol 14:31–34, 1970.
7. Douglass LE, Beaver DL: Experience with buccal smears in the general cytopathology laboratory. Acta Cytol 13:595–600, 1969.
8. Farrant PC: Nuclear changes in oral epithelium in pernicious anemia. Lancet 19:830, 1958.
9. Folsom TC, White CP, Bromer L, Canby HF, Garrington GE: Oral exfoliative cytology. Review of the literature and report of a three-year study. Oral Surg Oral Med Oral Pathol 33:61–74, 1972.
10. Hagy GW, Broderick MM: Variation of sex chromatin in human oral mucosa during the menstrual cycle. Acta Cytol 16:314–321, 1972.
11. Hayes RL, Berg GW, Ross WL: Oral cytology: Its value and its limitations. J Am Dent Assoc 79:649–657, 1969.
12. Levin ES, Lunnin M: The oral exfoliative cytology of pemphigus. A report on two cases. Acta Cytol 13:108–110, 1969.
13. Ljung BME, Larsson SG, Hanafee W: Computed tomography–guided aspiration cytologic examination in head and neck lesions. Arch Otolaryngol 110:604–607, 1984.
14. Mashberg A: Reevaluation of toluidine blue application as a diagnostic adjunct in the detection of asymptomatic oral squamous carcinoma: A continuing prospective study of oral cancer, III. Cancer 46:758–763, 1980.
15. Mashberg A: Final evaluation of tolonium chloride rinse for screening of high-risk patients with asymptomatic squamous carcinoma. J Am Dent Assoc 106:319–323, 1983.
16. Medak, H, Burlakow P, McGrew EA, Tiecke R: The cytology of vesicular conditions affecting the oral mucosa: Pemphigus vulgaris. Acta Cytol 14:11–25, 1970.
17. Memon MH, Jafarey NA: Cytologic study of radiation changes in carcinoma of the oral cavity: Prognostic value of various observations. Acta Cytol 14:22, 1970.
18. Meyer J, Rubinstein AS, Medak H: Early effects of smoking on surface cytology of the oral mucosa. Oral Surg Oral Med Oral Pathol 30:700–710, 1970.
19. Nader HB, Dietrick CP: Determination of sulfate after chromatography and toluidine blue complex formation. Anal Biochem 78:112, 1977.
20. Platt LI, Kailin EW: Buccal X-chromatin frequency in numerous diseases. Acta Cytol 13:700–707, 1969.
21. Rosenberg D, Cretin S: Use of meta-analysis to evaluate tolon-

TABLE 15–2. Report of Smear

Positive	Criteria for malignant cellular change are observed.
Negative	No malignant cells are observed in the specimen. These cells may appear atypical but do not demonstrate malignant criteria. In the event of a continued clinical suspicion or persistence of a lesion, a negative report should not be taken as conclusive. This is particularly true in hyperkeratotic lesions.
Suspicious or inconclusive	Cells are seen that do not fulfill the malignant criteria adequately to allow a positive report, yet reveal enough deviation from normal to indicate that follow-up studies should be performed.
Inadequate	Either cellular morphology is not preserved adequately for interpretation, or the presented material is too scanty to be a representative specimen.

ium chloride in oral cancer screening. Oral Surg Oral Med Oral Pathol 67:621–627, 1989.

22. Rovin S: An assessment of the negative oral cytologic diagnosis. J Am Dent Assoc 74:759–762, 1967.

23. Sandler HC: Errors of oral cytodiagnosis. Report of follow-up of 1,801 patients. J Am Dent Assoc 72:851–854, 1966.

24. Scher RL, Oostingh PE, Levine PA, Cantrell RW, Feldman PS: Role of fine needle aspiration in the diagnosis of lesions of the oral cavity, oropharynx, and nasopharynx. Cancer 62:2602–2606, 1988.

25. Shklar G, Cataldo E, Meyer I: Reliability of the cytology smear in the diagnosis of oral cancer. Arch Otolaryng 91:158, 1970.

26. Silverman S Jr: The cytology of benign oral lesions. Acta Cytol 9:287–295, 1965.

27. Silverman S Jr, Shouse C: Estrogen effects on human oral epithelium. Cytologic, histologic and clinical comparisons. J Oral Therapeut Pharmacol 3:87–93, 1966.

28. Silverman S Jr, Sheline GE, Gillooly CJ Jr: Radiation therapy and oral carcinoma. Radiation response and exfoliative cytology. Cancer 20:1297–1300, 1967.

29. Silverman S Jr, Beumer J: Primary herpetic gingivostomatitis of adult onset. Oral Surg Oral Med Oral Pathol 36:496–503, 1973.

30. Silverman S Jr, Bilimoria KF, Bhargava K, Mani NJ, Shah RA: Cytologic, histologic and clinical correlations of precancerous and cancerous oral lesions in 57,518 industrial workers of Gujarat, India. Acta Cytol 21:196–198, 1977.

31. Silverman S Jr, Migliorati C, Barbosa J: Toluidine blue staining in the detection of oral precancerous malignant lesions. Oral Surg Oral Med Oral Pathol 57:379–382, 1983.

32. Silverman S Jr, Gorsky M, Lozada F: Oral leukoplakia and malignant transformation. A follow-up study of 257 patients. Cancer 53:563–568, 1984.

33. Silverman S Jr: Oral Cancer, 3rd ed. Atlanta, American Cancer Society, pp 1–6, 1990.

34. Silverman S Jr: Early diagnosis of oral cancer. Cancer 62:1796–99, 1988.

35. Silverman S Jr, Bhargava K, Mani NJ, Smith LW, Malaowalla AM: Malignant transformation and natural history of oral leukoplakia in 57,518 industrial workers of Gujarat, India. Cancer 38:1790–1795, 1976.

36. Staats OJ, Robinson LH, Butterworth CE Jr: The effect of systemic therapy on nuclear size of oral epithelial cells in folate-related anemias. Acta Cytol 13:84, 1969.

37. Stahl SS, Koss LG, Brown RC Jr, Murray D: Oral cytologic screening in a large metropolitan area. J Am Dent Assoc 75:1385–1388, 1967.

38. Waldron CA, Shafer WG: Leukoplakia revisited. A clinico-pathologic study of 3256 oral leukoplakias. Cancer 36:1386, 1975.

39. Witkop CJ Jr: Epithelial intracellular bodies associated with hereditary dyskeratoses and cancer therapy. *In* Proceedings of the First International Congress of Exfoliative Cytology. Philadelphia, JB Lippincott Co, pp 259–268, 1962.

16

Alimentary Tract (Esophagus, Stomach, Colon, Rectum)

O. A. N. Husain

Cytology of the gastrointestinal tract has never been universally applied in the diagnosis of early or even late cancers, although there has been considerable published evidence of its potential value over the years.

One of the early pioneers of gastrointestinal cytology, Giovanni Marini,[66] illustrated by drawing from gastric washings the benign and malignant cells he encountered. More than thirty years later George N. Papanicolaou[77] was extolling the virtue of lavage techniques and Rudolph Schade[85] in his monograph showed that, even in a low-risk population, he could, by means of a simple automated wash technique, discover a substantial proportion of cancers at an early stage before they were detectable by other means. He established this more demanding area of diagnostic cytology in relation to the improved prognosis of cancers detected at an early stage. It was, however, the advent of the malleable fiberscope,[38] which overcame the restricted use of the rigid gastroscope originally designed by Kussmaul and introduced by Mikulicz in 1868, that led to the rapid increase in cytologic diagnosis.

This was best seen in Japan, whose population has one of the highest rates of gastric cancer in the world. With the malleable fiberscopes came the more purposive directional wash techniques favored by the Japanese, whereas the brush, with its ensheathing Teflon tube, had a greater stimulus from the West. Although it lagged behind, because of its more cumbersome length for maneuvering, the colonic brush is now producing remarkable results.

COLLECTION AND PROCESSING OF SPECIMENS

Meticulous attention to technique is essential in this area of cytology and, because this is in the joint province of both gastroenterologists and pathologists, a close cooperative strategy must be achieved and practiced. It is paramount that a specially trained technician or nurse be involved in the production, collection and preparation of these specimens. It is in this area more than anywhere else that it is a true saying that success in cytologic diagnosis is 80% preparation and 20% interpretation. It is for that reason that we should first consider these important procedures.

Sampling Techniques

Many of these techniques relate to the gastric lesions and are of historic interest only.

1. Blind lavage methods
   a. Simple saline wash
   b. Use of Ringer's or Hartman's solution
   c. Use of chymotrypsin A or papain
   d. Martinez continuous suction (Faucher tube)
2. Blind abrasive methods
   a. Zelltopfsonde
   b. Gastric brush
   c. Abrasive balloon
   d. Antral abrasive balloon
3. Directional brush and wash samples via a fiberscope

The nondirectional abrasive instruments mostly used to collect samples from the stomach and esophagus all were in vogue in the 1940s and acquired mucosal samples by virtue of a protruding and rotating sponge in the case of the Zelltopsonde or by various protruding brushes or inflatable balloons.[85] The large gastric antral balloon, which was shaped to expand to fit the whole of the pyloric antrum, was probably the most disagreeable of all such instruments to swallow and withdraw, even in the deflated state. Only the use of the esoph-

TABLE 16–1. The Efficiency of Various Investigators Using Different Sampling Techniques

Series	Accuracy (%)	Method
Papanicolaou and Cooper (1947)[77]	37	Fasting aspirate
Graham and coworkers (1948)[36]	62	Fasting aspirate
Traut and coworkers (1952)[98]	71	Papain lavage
Crozier and coworkers (1956)[23]	69	Lavage and brush
Seybolt and Papanicolaou (1957)[87]	66	Abrasive balloon
Fakuda (quoted by Tazaki) (1959)[96]	85	Modified balloon
Cabre-Fiol and coworkers (1959)[14]	90	Mandril-sound
Raskin and coworkers (1959)[81]	95	Gastric washings
Schade (1960)[85]	97	Gastric washings
Witte (1959)[102]	65	Zelltopfsonde
MacDonald and coworkers (1963)[62]	93	Chymotrypsin A wash
Taebel and coworkers (1965)[92]	81	Gastric washings
Blendis and coworkers (1967)[9]	81	Gastric washings
Kasugai (1968)[48]	97	Fiberscope brush
Shida (1971)[88]	90	Fiberscope brush
Witzel and coworkers (1976)[103]	84	Fiberscope brush
Thompson and coworkers (1977)[97]	90	Fiberscope brush
Young and Hughes (1980)[106]	92	Fiberscope brush
Mackenzie and coworkers (1977)[63]	94	Fiberscope brush
Boddington (1978)[11]	79	Fiberscope brush
Husain (1986)[41]	83	Fiberscope brush
Moreno-Otero and coworkers (1983)[74]	90	Fiberscope brush
Chambers and Clark (1986)[17]	85	Fiberscope brush
Cook and coworkers (1988)[21]	85	Fiberscope brush

ageal balloon seems to have survived until the present day. The Martinez double-lumen irrigation tube used for continous flow of normal saline solution to act as a washout was also unpleasant and is a thing of the past. The use by cytology of these techniques was more for screening and detection than for diagnosis, and it was not until the development of the flexible fiberscope that more purposive brush, suction and directional lavage samples were collected from hitherto inaccessible sites.[49, 101] This resulted in a better-preserved and more presentable cell sample and improved diagnostic accuracy.[46, 47, 50, 59, 103] The history of improvement is reflected more in improved technique than in time, as is seen from the accuracy rates of the long list of authors listed in Table 16–1.[9, 11, 14, 17, 21, 23, 36, 41, 48, 62, 63, 74, 77, 81, 85, 87, 88, 92, 96–98, 102, 103, 106]

Simple wash techniques are still used in those patients unwilling or unable to undergo esophagoscopy or gastroscopy owing to stenosis of the pharynx or the esophagus, and also for screening because wash techniques are only about half to a third as expensive as fiberscopic brush sampling.[40] Moreover, it may become the simpler mode of sampling for those more refined immunologic or cytochemical techniques in which more specific identification or functional assessment of cell behavior can be achieved.[43]

Patient Preparation and Collection Procedures for Blind and Directional Washes and Brushes for the Upper Gastric Tract

The esophagus lends itself well to simple 20- to 40-ml direct washing with buffered saline solution above any stricture, although almost as much information can

be derived from the collection of stomach contents beyond any lesion or stricture. For this procedure, preparation of the patient for a gastric sample is recommended.

Esophageal Balloon. An up-to-date and atraumatic version of this method and instruments devised by Berry[8] in South Africa is detailed.

The mouth and pharynx of a fasting patient are sprayed with local anesthetic and an "introducing tube," 95 mm in diameter, is swallowed to just beyond the cricopharynx (15 cm from the teeth). The introducing tube is stiffened by an internal stylet, and this is removed to pass a special catheter with a deflated balloon through the cardioesophageal junction (40 cm from teeth). The balloon is inflated with about 5 ml of air and then passed up and down the esophagus three times, causing little patient discomfort. After deflation the balloon and catheter are withdrawn. The collapsed balloon is squeezed like a sponge, and cells are transferred onto two or more glass slides, immediately fixed in 95% alcohol and stained by the Papanicolaou technique. The morphology is excellent and interpretation relatively easy.

Large numbers of cases can be processed using a standard endoscopic nylon brush passed inside a nasogastric tube. There is no doubt that this simpler method of using an indirect (i.e., not endoscopically directed) brush can achieve high levels of accuracy as depicted by Dowlatshahi and coworkers,[25] in which an accuracy rate of 78% for malignant, 95% for potentially premalignant and 100% for nonmalignant cases was achieved. The method is simple, safe, inexpensive and acceptable to the patient (98% compliance).

For blind gastric washings the patient needs to fast overnight, although he or she is encouraged to drink liberal amounts of water because dehydration seriously restricts cell exfoliation and also results in rapid absorption of the wash fluid. A Levin tube, plastic or rubber (12 to 14 French gauge or 3 to 4 mm in diameter), with a few more holes cut out near its end for a broader salvage, is passed through the mouth or, preferably, via the nose to a midgastric position, and the whole of the resting juice is aspirated and kept. About 250 to 300 ml of buffered saline solution is then introduced down the tube, after which the abdomen is ballotted or massaged and the patient made to flex and extend the body so as to induce exfoliation of the surface mucosal cells. This washing is then aspirated; the procedure may then be repeated. If much tenacious mucus is present it may be necessary to repeat the test by giving the patient 7 mg of chymotrypsin A in a glass of water half an hour before the gastric wash, which is then performed using a further 7 mg of chymotrypsin A in a sodium acetate buffer with a pH of 5.6. At this pH the enzyme digests the mucus but not the mucosal cells.

The resting juice and each gastric wash are immediately neutralized with N/10 sodium hydroxide—if necessary with a pH up to 6, but not beyond, because alkali destroys cells more quickly than acid—and the samples centrifuged rapidly, preferably in ice-cold siliconized tubes. The deposit is smeared onto about six clean slides, some of which are immediately wet-fixed for staining by the Papanicolaou technique; a few thinner smears are rapidly air-dried for staining by a Romanowsky method (e.g., May-Grünwald-Giemsa schedule). The screening and checking of such smears calls for much skill and patience in the interpretation of cell changes, which are by no means as clear-cut or as florid as cell changes in smears taken with a brush.

Endoscopic Directional Washes and Brushes. There was a significant improvement in the detection rate in Japan during the 10 years after 1956 as shown by the rise in the proportion of early surface cancers from 3.8% to 34.5% of all cancers found[79] mainly due to the combination of biopsy and directional wash cytology. It is of interest to note that the highest levels of detection by cytology of gastric cancer, with a sensitivity approaching 97%,[48] occurred using a directional jet wash technique, although Halter and associates[37] were only able to achieve a 50% accuracy. In fact, the Japanese were more enthusiastic about directional wash than about brush samples, and it was in the West that the latter found more favor and success. There are only a few major manufacturers of fiberscopes, but we have used the Olympus instruments, either the GFD end-viewing one for the esophagus or the side-viewing one for the stomach. The more versatile oblique-viewing instrument with its ability to move through 180 degrees has, however, become the model of choice because it can be used for both stomach and esophagus. The smaller pediatric version is welcomed by adults as more acceptable and still proves to be an effective instrument, albeit with smaller biopsy samples. The schedule is the same as that used to collect tissue biopsies for histology; in fact, it is becoming the custom to collect both samples in most instances.

Collecting the Gastric Sample (Blind and Directional)

After fasting overnight the patient is sedated with diazepam intravenously and the larynx is anesthetized with 1% lidocaine. The saline- or glycerol-lubricated fiberscope (oily lubricants may obscure cellular detail) is passed with the patient lying in the supine or left lateral position, with or without an airway. After inspection of the stomach any lesion is photographed and both brush and biopsy samples are taken. It is preferable to obtain the brush sample before the biopsy because the latter results in bleeding, which both obscures the lesion and detracts from the quality of a subsequently collected cytologic sample, whereas interpretation of the biopsy is not affected by the reverse order of collection.[97]

Originally the large and robust brush issued by the makers for cleaning the endoscope was used, but this resulted in the restricted practice of using the brush as the last act of a gastroscopy and withdrawing it within the instrument before removing the instrument from the patient. Such a brush is still worthwhile when used to sample the more stenotic esophageal lesions, but nowadays the ranges of smaller brushes are enclosed inside transparent Teflon sheaths, which permit multiple samples to be collected. The brush sample, when obtained, is pulled back just within the Teflon sheath, and the whole sheath is withdrawn.

The collection of a good brush sample usually requires an experienced assistant because the gastroscopist may well be engaged in maneuvering the end of the scope and holding the lesion in focus while the assistant manipulates the brush. The need then is to plunge the brush firmly and briskly into the mucosa five to ten times so that the lamina propria is penetrated. Anything less than this fails to obtain a reliable sample and may lead to a false-negative result. The site and mode of sampling are important, as will be seen from Figure 16–1. In this situation the need to sample from the growing outer edge of a cavitating ulcer is logical, but the areas to sample in the various forms of surface cancer in the stomach are just as important, as is the need to sample straight down into the center of a possible tumorous shallow ulcer when there is a suspicion of a mesodermal tumor (see Fig. 16–1). The most common of these are leiomyosarcoma and lymphoma. Penetration to a depth sufficient to retrieve deeper cell tissue is then paramount.

In Japan and in many centers in the United States and Europe up to ten specimens of both biopsy and brush samples are collected, but in the United Kingdom, laboratories are lucky to get one, perhaps two, cytology samples for examination. Directional wash samples are not often collected outside Japan but the technique is simple. The opening of the Teflon tube is directed at a particular lesion at close quarters and a forceful injection of buffered saline solution is aimed at the site. Immediate suction with the syringe that injected the fluid results in salvage of cells in that area.

Types of Early Gastric Cancer and Their Sampling Sites

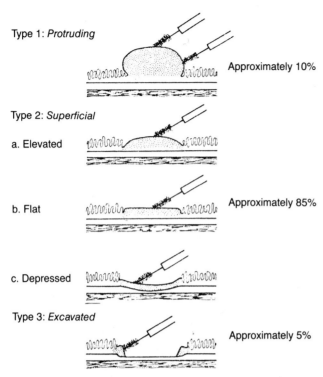

FIGURE 16–1. Mode of sampling by **gastric brush** from early and surface cancers and their approximate incidence in Japan.

Patient Preparation and Collection Procedures from the Lower Bowel and Rectum

The newer regimens of clearing the lower bowel have revolutionized the cytologic diagnosis of colorectal disease, and neoplasia in particular. Such preparation varies considerably, from an elaborate schedule such as that used by Rosenberg and Giles[84] to that of Melville and colleagues.[69] For colonic irrigation cytology the patient is given two senna concentrate (Senokot) tablets 2 days prior to the examination, then 15 ml of castor oil as well as two Senokot tablets on the day before and an enema of oxyphenisatin acetate (Veripaque) in 2 pints of water on the day of the test. A Henderson bowel colonic lavage machine then irrigates the bowel continuously with 20 to 40 ml of fluid over 30 minutes. After resting the bowel for an hour the colonoscope is passed, with the patient in the left lateral position, for 25 cm. The patient is moved into the right lateral position and the bowel irrigated with 300 to 500 ml of Hartman's solution. This is accompanied by abdominal massage with the patient in various positions. The fluid is finally allowed to run back and centrifuged in an ice-cold centrifuge machine. Smears are made in a fashion similar to gastric wash specimens.[84]

A much simpler method of a standard 48-hour bowel preparation using 2 sachets of Picolax (sodium picosulfate, 10 mg; magnesium oxide, 3.5 mg; citric acid,

12.0 mg; excipients and flavors, 9.5 mg.) and one of senna concentrate (X-Prep) seems to suffice for colonoscopy, wash, brush and biopsy specimens.[69]

There is no doubt that, for collection from the esophagus and stomach, brush samples are greatly superior to the wash preparations but, of course, they cannot give such a wide assessment. The maneuvers for collecting brush specimens for cytology are similar to those carried out in the stomach, but more robust brushes are needed for the colon, and these have now been developed.[69]

Preparation of Brush and Wash Samples

Ideally, brush smears should be prepared immediately, but the brush head, if withdrawn just within the Teflon tube, will maintain reasonable cell morphology for 15 to 30 minutes so that the specimen can be rapidly transported to the laboratory where more ideal conditions for processing exist with minimal loss of technician time. The brush is first protruded from the Teflon tube over a small 1-ounce bottle (a "universal container") containing about 10 ml of buffered saline solution. Any drop of fluid containing cells is thus not lost. The brush is then rolled rather than rubbed onto a clean glass slide. About four to six, or even more, smears can be made from each brush sample, most of which are rapidly wet-fixed in alcohol for Papanicolaou staining while one or two of the thinner and later-made smears are rapidly air-dried for staining with a Romanowsky stain. We use May-Gruenwald-Giemsa in our laboratories.

Even after making this number of direct smears the brush retains a considerable amount of material, and cells can be agitated off by a simple vortexer with the brush head immersed in buffered saline solution (Fig. 16–2). Care should be taken during vortexing to avoid

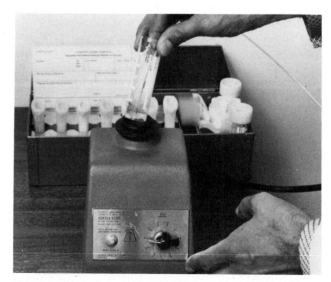

FIGURE 16–2. The use of a **vortexer** to agitate off the residual cells from the brush after making direct smears.

any droplet spray being transmitted to the atmosphere by the simple procedure of inserting a cotton wool plug into the mouth of the vial. In fact, full protective procedures with mask, gown and gloves should be mandatory for staff preparing such specimens because even rolling a brush on a slide creates small droplet particles in the surrounding air. This sample is then aspirated on to a Millipore filter, fixed in alcohol and stained by the Papanicolaou technique. A remarkable number of cells are often displayed and occasionally may be the best, if not the only, evidence of neoplasia.

The brushes are sold as disposable, but with care, they can be reused. After total immersion in 2% glutaraldehyde for half an hour, they can be thoroughly and safely cleaned with the tip of a needle or another firm nylon brush by sweeping the needle or nylon brush towards the tip of the wire under running water, then sterilizing the brush with formalin steam at 70 to 80°C for 4 to 6 hours. In this way, and with microscopic inspection of the bristle ends, these tiny, fragile brushes can be reused ten or more times. The newer, more robust brush for colonic sampling tolerates cleaning, sterilization and reusing.[69] As labor costs go up, and if the price of the mass-produced brush comes down, this exercise may well cease to be cost-effective, but it has been a regular part of our cytology department's responsibilities to ensure removal of any residual material and to preserve the tiny brush heads as long as possible. With the increase of diseases such as acquired immunodeficiency syndrome (AIDS) and the risk of imperfect resterilization, such economies may become unacceptable.

Directional wash samples can be either concentrated in a similar fashion to the blind wash specimen by centrifuging in ice-cold siliconized tubes or aspirated onto a Millipore membrane, or both techniques can be employed. For small fluid samples cytocentrifuge specimens can be made.

Imprint Smear

The use of the biopsy imprint smear technique[105] to achieve cytologic sampling of a deep tissue plane was considered superior to that of directional washes because it gave a degree of structural arrangement of the cells,[95] but the manipulation of this minute biopsy fragment by repeatedly dabbing it onto slides can interfere with its subsequent histologic examination and interpretation and its use for cytology has lost favor with many authorities.

CYTOLOGY OF ESOPHAGEAL, GASTRIC AND COLONIC SPECIMENS

Because each of these sites produces distinctive cell patterns and problems in diagnosis, they will be dealt with separately and sequentially.

ESOPHAGUS

Normal Anatomy, Physiology and Histology

In development, the endoderm or primitive alimentary tract, starting at the buccal cavity and pharynx, buds off the larynx anteriorly to then form the bronchi and lungs of the pulmonary tract, but the gut continues on down through the chest as the esophagus, a hollow, muscular tube some 25 cm long.

Histologically, the esophagus, like the rest of the alimentary tract, is composed of four layers or coats, although it is unique in not possessing a serosal coat. It traverses the mediastinal tissue in front of the spine and behind the trachea while the arch of the aorta curls around in front from right to left ultimately to lie behind the esophagus as they both pass through the diaphragm. There is an outer muscular coat of longitudinal fibers and an inner circular one. The esophagus is composed of voluntary or striated muscle for the upper two thirds; the lower third is composed of smooth or involuntary muscle, which forms the esophageal sphincter that prevents the regurgitation of food. The submucosa is deep and consists of collagenous and elastic fibers, and contained in it is a plethora of blood vessels, nerves and a ramifying lymphatic plexus. It is this plexus that permits a rapid spread of carcinoma into the mediastinum and makes early diagnosis even more necessary. The submucosa contains a number of compound racemose mucus-secreting glands, possessing long ducts drawing towards the mucosal surface. Characteristically, these glands possess basally positioned nuclei and abundant vacuolated mucus-filled cytoplasm.

In addition, there are the esophageal cardiac glands found in the lamina propria of the mucosa itself. These mimic the glands in the cardia of the stomach and occur in both the upper and lower thirds of the esophagus and may extend and express themselves onto the mucosal surface as pits or stretches of glandular epithelium.

The bulk of the esophagus is, however, composed of nonkeratinizing stratified squamous epithelium on a thin basal lamina beneath which lies the fibrous lamina propria. This connective tissue projects into the epithelium in the fashion of narrow papillae with a vascular core. There are no hair follicles or other adnexa present as in the skin, but scattered melanoblasts exist within the squamous epithelium.

Normal Cytology

The normal esophageal brush or wash samples are composed of mature squamous cells of the superficial and intermediate type. The superficial squames possess small, dark, pyknotic nuclei and abundant eosinophilic cytoplasm that may contain some keratohyaline granules, but true keratinization does not normally occur.

An occasional benign epithelial pearl may be present. The intermediate cell has a more azurophilic or greenish-blue cytoplasm, and the nucleus is larger, usually oval, with a vesicular chromatin pattern.

Sometimes cells from a deeper parabasal layer occur. These can be the result of vigorous brushing but are usually due to some degree of friability of the epithelium.

The advent of glandular mucus-secreting cells in an esophageal sample is usually the result of the brush reaching the stomach, but the racemose glands in the upper and lower thirds of the esophagus are another source, and the existence of Barrett's esophagus always has to be considered (see the following).

Diseases of the Esophagus

Inflammatory-Reactive Lesions

These include nonspecific bacterial, fungal and viral infections and granulomata and esophagitis (Fig. 16–3).

Fungal Infections. These are mainly caused by *Candida albicans* and less commonly *Aspergillus.* The organisms can be identified easily in either Papanicolaou or Giemsa stained preparations or one can resort to a periodic acid–Schiff (PAS) or a silver stain to demonstrate them. There is often a purulent exudate present and because both ulceration and plaque formation occur the picture will include squamous cells of all degrees of maturation showing increased nuclear size and density but with a relatively uniform chromatin pattern. There is some polychromasia and hyperkeratosis with brownish-yellow degenerative granules in a disturbed and vacuolated cytoplasm. Intracytoplasmic polymorphs and cell debris are seen; this feature is more common in benign than in malignant lesions.

Viral Infections. These are most commonly due to herpes simplex, in which the characteristic immature

cells showing multinucleation and a ground glass texture of the nucleoplasm, often with large eosinophilic inclusions, is distinctive. Concomitant infections with both *Monilia* and herpes are not uncommon.[72, 83]

Chronic Granulomatous Esophagitis. This is a condition in which tuberculosis and syphilis have been implicated, and special stains together with a culture are needed to reach a diagnosis. The cytologic picture consists of squamous cells showing nuclear and cytoplasmic inflammatory changes accompanied by a subacute or chronic inflammatory exudate of polymorphs, histiocytes, lymphocytes and the occasional giant cell (see Fig. 16–3).

Reflux Esophagitis. This is a distinct entity, although relatively rare, and is often associated with a hiatus hernia accompanied by overeating. Alcoholism, diabetic autonomic neuropathy and scleroderma are also rare associations. The condition results in eventual erosion of the squamous epithelium of the lower esophagus by hydrochloric acid, pepsin or bile salts; in consequence, the cytologic picture is one of an inflammatory exudate with a number of cells from all squamous layers. Active regenerative and metaplastic squamous cells are seen in brush and wash samples.

What causes difficulties is the presence of deep or parabasal squames, originally described by Gephart and Graham,[34] but these usually show good cellular adhesion in contrast to the malignant variety, although even in this situation syncytia occur. Another, but rare, condition is herpetic esophagitis, in which there are large, immature-looking cells showing multinucleation and intranuclear inclusions that can be interpreted as nucleoli; these can cause some concern when seen in benign lesions.[57] A further difficulty is that this condition may be associated with neoplasia.[7]

Premalignant Lesions

Barrett's Esophagus. The presence of glandular cells from the lower end of the esophagus when the brush has not passed through the gastroesophageal sphincter must alert the cytologist to the existence of Barrett's esophagus. Barrett originally stated that a columnar cell–lined lower end of esophagus was a condition denied by some, misunderstood by others and ignored by the majority.[4]

We cannot pursue the etiology in this treatise, but it is suffice to say that the extension of glandular epithelium into the esophagus is probably due to reflux of the gastric contents through a lax or incoordinate sphincter. The consequent erosion of squamous epithelium results in a glandular overgrowth that is itself subject to repeated ulceration and to an increased incidence of carcinoma, both at that site and, curiously, also at the colon. The cytologic picture is one of glandular cells in sheets and clusters showing mild to gross inflammatory and metaplastic changes.

Leukoplakia. This is a debatable lesion, not acknowledged by some, considered to be hyperkeratosis by others and looked upon as a precancerous lesion by yet others. The cytologic picture is one of orangeophilic

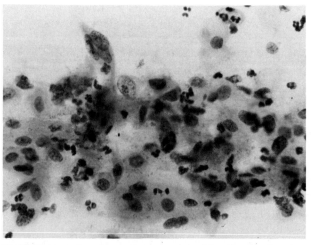

FIGURE 16–3. Esophageal scrape smear. **Esophagitis** showing considerable nuclear enlargement and pleomorphism (Papanicolaou stain; ×160).

and eosinophilic superficial squames, either anucleate or containing pyknotic nuclei. A more common cause of such white patches is glycogenic acanthosis, in which the focal hyperplasia of epithelial squames contains abundant glycogen—it is restricted to the lower third of the esophagus and has no malignant potential.

Benign Neoplasms

Squamous Papillomas. A few genuine squamous papillomas exist but most are inflammatory in origin. In these cases the cytologic picture is that of reactive changes in squamous cells.

Nonepithelial Tumors. The majority of tumors are nonepithelial, namely, lipoma, leiomyoma, hemangioma and lymphangioma. These lie deep to the mucosa, and cytology would be informative only if the brush were to penetrate deep enough to sample the underlying tumor. This procedure is not to be recommended if there is any likelihood of a vascular lesion.

Malignant Neoplasms of the Esophagus

The WHO classification of esophageal tumors is listed next, but only a few are of interest to the cytologist and are considered in detail.

Malignant Epithelial Tumors

- Squamous cell carcinoma
- Adenocarcinoma
- Adenoid cystic carcinoma
- Adenosquamous carcinoma
- Undifferentiated carcinoma.

Malignant Nonepithelial Tumors

- Leiomyosarcoma
- Lymphosarcoma.

Miscellaneous Tumors

- Carcinosarcoma
- Malignant melanoma
- Lymphoreticular tumor
- Sarcoma.

Squamous Cell Carcinoma. Squamous cell carcinoma of the esophagus is the most common malignant tumor. The incidence is quoted as being between 60 and 95% of all esophageal tumors, depending on whether cancers of the postcricoid region and the cardia are included.[75] In 60% of cases the tumor is polypoidal, in 25% it is ulcerative and in 15% it is infiltrating. The last group is detected later, and it can simulate the leather bottle tumors of the stomach (Fig. 16–4).

Cytologically the tumor can be graded as well-differentiated, moderately well differentiated or poorly differentiated squamous cancer. Cells from well-differentiated carcinoma usually display abundant, brightly staining red or orange keratin. This appears either as broad irregular bands across the cells or more often as central islands of keratin around the nucleus. The intercellular bridges are usually prominent, and there is a faint, almost refractile concentric haloing of the cytoplasm around the nucleus. This feature is also seen in less well differentiated tumors when it can be of diagnostic value. There can be difficulties in distinguishing poorly differentiated squamous tumors from glandular tumors because the extreme versions of both forms present almost as a syncytium of lightly staining cells with pale nuclei in a pale, somewhat foamy or even flocculated cytoplasm. The nuclei of both well-differentiated and poorly differentiated squamous tu-

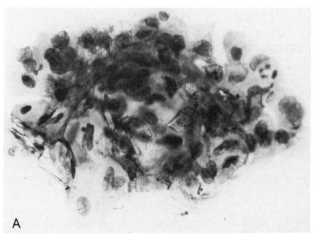
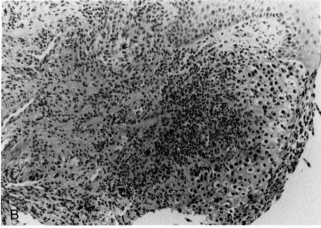

FIGURE 16–4. Squamous cell carcinoma of esophagus. A moderately well-differentiated squamous cell carcinoma showing considerable pleomorphism but still recognizable squamous cells. *A*, Esophageal scrape smear (Papanicolaou stain; ×160). *B*, Esophageal biopsy (hematoxylin and eosin; ×40).

mors are more centrally placed than in adenocarcinomas; they display varying degrees of pleomorphism with irregular chromatin clumping and often with more than one nucleolus, again with marked pleomorphism compared with glandular tumors. These have an eccentrically placed nucleus, single, usually rounded nucleoli and a more frothy cytoplasm. At times it is difficult to decide on the origin, and then the term large-cell undifferentiated tumor is applied (Fig. 16–5).

Adenocarcinoma. The incidence of such tumors in the middle and upper thirds of the esophagus is around 2%, but in the lower third the position is complicated by extension of tumors from the stomach or malignancy developing in Barrett's esophagus, where it arises in an area of metaplastic epithelium. At times tumors appear to be budding off from squamous epithelium, and the fact that reserve cells are multipotential must explain the occurrence of mixed and undifferentiated tumors. The cytologic pattern is often one of marginally positioned, clear, rounded nuclei with a prominent nuclear membrane. Nucleoli can be single or multiple and are usually rounded in comparison with the more angular, variable and multiple nucleoli seen in the squamous cell carcinoma. The cytoplasm is frothy or floccular, sometimes with vacuoles of mucus secretion, reaching at times to a signet-ring formation. Characteristically these cells present in papillary clusters, but single cells can be seen.

The remaining tumors of the esophagus will be considered with those of the stomach because they have similar features and relevance. A number of the rarer nonepithelial lesions such as the lymphoreticular and sarcomatous tumors are probably best referred to elsewhere in this volume because the cellular morphology is similar in whatever organ they occur.

STOMACH

Normal Anatomy, Physiology and Histology

This hourglass-shaped sac, of some 1500-ml volume, where the esophagus enters its right upper margin, produces a bulging fundus above and to the left and then sweeps down towards the midline and right side, with a short lesser curvature to the right and a 4 to 5 times longer greater curvature to the left and below, passing towards the pylorus. In fact, the stomach can be divided into four parts: the **cardia,** some 2 to 3 cm immediately distal to the esophagus; the **fundus,** which is that portion above a gastroesophageal junction; the **body,** nearly two thirds of the remainder; and the **pyloric antrum,** which leads via the pyloric sphincter to the duodenum. The blood supply and lymphatic plexus are prolific and surround the stomach, tracking down both greater and lesser curvatures, and this has a distinct bearing on the spread of tumors from the mucosa to the greater and lesser omenta and to the liver.

The wall of the stomach is again in four layers: the serosa, the muscle coat, the submucosa and the mucosa.

The serosa is the visceral layer of the peritoneum and is contiguous with the greater and lesser omenta. The muscle coat is in three layers, all of smooth muscle arranged from the outside in, as longitudinal, circular and oblique. There is a thin, well-demarcated loose connective tissue submucosa, on top of which lies the mucosa. This is of the most interest to the cytologist and is composed of three general types of gastric glands: the cardiac, the main gastric and the pyloric.

The cardiac glands occur around the cardiac orifice and are simple tubular glands, mostly mucus secreting. It is the main gastric glands that occupy the body and fundus that are of greatest cytologic importance. They cluster in three to seven glands, all opening into a gastric pit. The mucosa of the normal fundus and body can be divided into two zones; the superficial zone (25%) consists of glandular pits or foveolae, and it is in this area in the regenerative phase that mitosis increases in the less well differentiated cells that contain only occasional mucigen granules in the cytoplasm. Completely undifferentiated cells can appear in this region, and these are apparently the source of renewal of all other epithelial cells in the gastric mucosa.

The lower 75% of mucosa consists of straight tubules perpendicular to the surface, extending down from the pits to the muscularis mucosa, where coiling and acinus formation occur. These are so-called mucus neck glands, flask shaped, with a narrow apex and broad

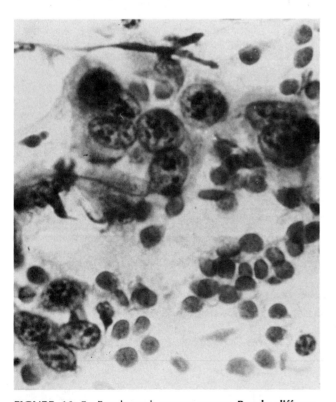

FIGURE 16–5. Esophageal scrape smear. **Poorly differentiated carcinoma** showing sheets of nucleolated cells making the differentiation between glandular and squamous cancer difficult (Papanicolaou stain; ×160).

base; they are strongly PAS positive and found near the pits, and they exist throughout the whole extent of the tubule. The other two main types of cell, the zymogenic or chief cell and the oxyntic cell, are distinctive but not important to recognize for the cytologist, except to identify the source of mucosa from which the sample may have been taken. The parietal or oxyntic cells that secrete hydrochloric acid are concentrated mainly at the center of the gland and are large and spheroid or pyramidal, with abundant, deeply esinophilic granular cytoplasm and a single large nucleus, with perhaps two or more nucleoli. The chief or zymogenic cells, which secrete the proteolytic enzymes, including pepsin, predominate in the body of the glands but also near the neck. Pyramidal in shape, with a single nucleus in abundant basophilic cytoplasm, they are distinctive. Scattered between basement membrane and the zymogenic cells are the argentaffin cells, which are rounded or flattened, with granules that stain with silver salts. These secrete serotonin, which relaxes gastric muscle and may have some role in gastric motility.

The epithelium of the fundus of the body lining the foveolae or pits is composed of tall columnar mucus-secreting cells with nuclei towards the base of the cell. The cytoplasm is finely granular, usually eosinophilic and often vacuolated, but huge vacuoles creating goblet cells are not seen in normal mucosa.

In the pyloric antrum, the mucosa is divided into almost equal halves, the superficial zone being composed predominantly of mucus-secreting epithelial cells, with only an occasional parietal or oxyntic cell to be seen, and no chief cells.

The lamina propria of the mucosa in this area consists of fine connective tissue, which occupies the narrow space between the gland and muscularis mucosa but forms larger areas between the gland elements and contains numerous small lymphocytes, with some eosinophils and plasma cells. There are lymph follicle–like collections in the pyloric region. The muscularis mucosa is deep to these and consists of a thin layer of nonstriated muscle composed of outer longitudinal and inner circular layers, the latter reaching up between the mucosal glands.

This mucosal pattern changes as it traverses the pylorus and enters the duodenum, jejunum, ileum and some 25 feet of intestine, until it enters the cecum and large intestine.

Normal Cytology

As with most normal epithelia, there is little spontaneous exfoliation from undiseased gastric mucosa. Ballottement and massage of the abdomen are needed to release cells when a gastric wash technique is used, and brush samples are needed to obtain a really satisfactory specimen. If inflamed, and this is almost always the case in clinical practice, the epithelium lifts off in small or larger sheets and is seen characteristically as a honeycomb pattern on plane view or as a palisade with closely linked cells that possess eccentric

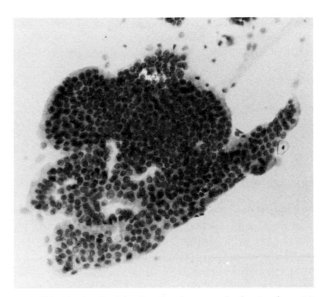

FIGURE 16–6. Gastric brush. A normal sheet of gastric mucosa with cells both in plane view, showing a typical honeycomb pattern, and in side view, showing a palisade pattern (Papanicolaou stain; ×80).

nuclei when the cells are seen in profile (Fig. 16–6). Columnar cell nuclei are situated at the base of the cell adjacent to the basement membrane; the luminal surface shows a terminal plate and cilia that stain red with Papanicolaou stain. The nuclei of healthy cells are round or oval with a uniform, finely granular chromatin pattern and a distinct nuclear membrane; small nucleoli are often present. The cytoplasm is substantial with a finely granular or vacuolated appearance. In addition to presenting as sheets, cells can exfoliate in small clusters that have a characteristic cartwheel appearance with cells joined either by their basal or luminal borders. Single cells are also common, particularly if there is any degree of inflammation or metaplasia present. Rarely whole sheets together with their intact crypts break away even in a gastric wash because of inflammatory loosening of the mucosa (Fig. 16–7).

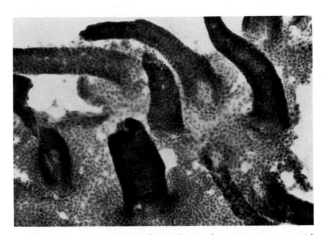

FIGURE 16–7. Gastric wash. A sheet of gastric mucosa with intact crypts giving an "elephant trunk" appearance (Papanicolaou stain; ×40).

Attempts to identify the different constituent cells that are present in gastric mucosa serve little purpose, although the small, cylindric, vacuolated parietal cells and the plump chief cells with their coarse, basophilic cytoplasmic granules can be recognized. The greater need is to identify the cellular changes that are found in the presence of disease. The diseased states of the stomach can be considered under the following headings.

Extraneous Cells and Materials

It can be said by way of introduction that not all that is seen in the smears necessarily originates from the organ in question because both the upper and lower respiratory tract and the buccopharyngeal regions give rise to much swallowed material that will appear in esophageal or gastric samples; this must always be remembered when interpreting such smears. Perhaps the most common "foreign" cell is the "buccal squame," which can arise from the lips backwards and is usually of a mature intermediate cell type, although both parabasal and superficial cells occur. The other common and distinctive cell is the pulmonary macrophage that, with its ingested black carbon or brown blood pigment, should present no difficulty in interpretation. With the wash samples, other contaminants, such as food particles (mostly vegetable and sometimes meat fiber) (Fig. 16–8), dental powder and other ingested material, serve to obscure the cytologic picture, as do the columnar cells, mucus and polymorphs that may well derive from the upper or lower respiratory tract. The nasal mucosal cells appear more as narrow elongated cells than those found in the stomach. At times these extraneous cells may come from a malignant lesion in a lung, buccal cavity or pharynx, as in the case illustrated in Figure 16–9. On the whole, the brush samples do not suffer from these contaminants as much, and preservation of the cells is much

better than in wash specimens. In fact, it is important to know which type of preparation one is examining in both pulmonary and gastrointestinal tract samples because the appearances differ considerably. The washed-off sheets of gastric cells, having been in contact with the saline during the process time, lose quite a lot of cellular detail compared with the fresher cells brushed from the intact mucosa. Here, the chromatin looks more active and the nucleoli more distinct, and there is a greater temptation to call a lesion neoplastic when it is not.

Inflammatory Diseases: Gastritis and Peptic Ulceration

Acute Gastritis. Acute gastritis is usually transitory but can be fulminating and fatal, and consequently is not usually subject to cytologic investigation. It may result from irritation or allergy produced by alcohol, salicylates or ferrous sulphate, and more recently drugs such as naproxen and indomethacin have been implicated.

Histologically the swollen mucosa with the accompanying heavy inflammatory cell infiltration gives rise to conspicuous cytoplasmic and nuclear abnormality, causing difficulty in distinguishing it from cancer.[53] The cytologic features reflect the marked cellular abnormality, with nuclear pleomorphism and prominent large nucleoli. Cells present as disaggregating clusters in a polymorphonuclear exudate. Caution should be practiced in cases of acute gastritis with an explosive onset.

Chronic Gastritis. This can be divided into infective and granulomatous forms. The causes are numerous and include tuberculosis, syphilis, histoplasmosis and rarely giardiasis from an associated duodenitis.[104] In cases in which these are suspected, special stains can be used in an attempt to identify the organism. Multinucleated Langhans giant cells and epithelioid cells are seldom present in wash or brush specimens but if present are quite distinctive. Further differential diagnoses to be considered in such cases are Crohn's disease and sarcoidosis. These can occur but are rare in the stomach.

Chronic Nonspecific Gastritis. This can be subdivided into chronic superficial and chronic atrophic gastritis. The disease can be active or quiescent and can lead to atrophy.[75] Chronic superficial and atrophic gastritis appear to be a natural sequence in the disease state, and the cytologic pictures are indistinguishable. The histologic appearance is one of vascular congestion and a chronic inflammatory infiltrate of the superficial layers of the mucosa, leading later to an extension into the deeper layers, with the lamina propria being more heavily involved and the mucosa becoming atrophic. Consequently the cytologic picture is one of a chronic inflammatory cell exudate in which gastric mucosal cells are seen singly and in sheets and fragments. These show more rounded and cuboid atrophic forms with enlarged and hyperchromatic nuclei sometimes dis-

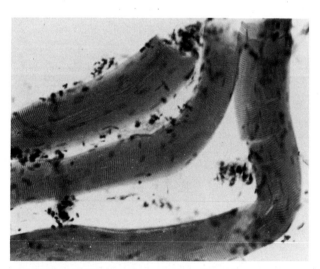

FIGURE 16–8. Gastric wash. Muscle fibers from a previous meal show typical cross striations (Papanicolaou stain; ×160).

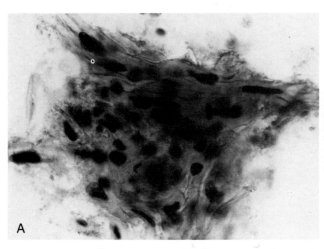

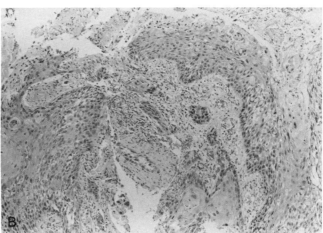

FIGURE 16–9. Malignant squamous cells present in the gastric wash from a patient with a postcricoid squamous cell carcinoma of the esophagus. The patient was 62 years old and survived 10 years following cobalt therapy. *A*, Gastric wash (Papanicolaou stain). *B*, Biopsy of postcricoid region (hematoxylin and eosin; × 25).

playing reactive nucleoli and both inflammatory and degenerative changes in the cytoplasm (Fig. 16–10).

Gastric atrophy is probably the quiescent end stage, with the cytologic picture reflecting the chronicity and with an increase in the lymphocyte component of the exudate. Careful screening is important in these cases because 70% of all gastric cancers appear to arise in atrophic mucosa.[67]

In addition, atrophy of the gastric mucosa also occurs in patients with pernicious anemia. In this genetic disease there is a simple mucosal atrophy that is more or less indistinguishable from the late-stage atrophy described earlier. However, probably reflecting the lack of vitamin B_{12}, the epithelial cell nuclei are enlarged and have an emptiness or blandness, with little linear creases of the delicate nuclear membrane across them. Small, sometimes red staining nucleoli or chromocenters are seen in some of these cells.[12, 94] The significant point about pernicious anemia is that there appears to be a twofold to fivefold increase in the incidence of malignancy in such cases.[55, 100]

Peptic Ulceration. Acute ulceration is associated with the picture of acute gastritis, but chronic ulcers are of more significance and interest cytologically because, as with gastric atrophy, such an ulcer acts as an entity from which neoplasia can develop. On rare occasions gastric ulcers can be multiple, but it is the single ulcers that need attention. These normally vary in size from 1 to 3 cm but can be more than 10 cm in diameter. The edges are clear-cut, in contrast to the everted edges of malignant ulcers, and brush sampling has to be directed to the growing outer edge to obtain the best specimen (Fig. 16–11). Thinned atrophic mucosa surrounds the ulcer, and this also needs careful sampling in case a surface cancer is developing, especially the distal side of the ulcer. The cytologic picture of chronic gastritis and gastric ulceration ranges from marked reactivity of epithelial cells with prominent nucleoli through varying degrees of intestinal metaplasia, atrophy and cell death.

Intestinal Metaplasia. This is a significant feature in the cellular changes in atrophic gastritis and peptic ulceration and progression towards neoplasia and should be considered in some detail.

In intestinal metaplasia, the normal gastric mucosa is replaced by cells of the intestinal type with an increase of goblet cells, Paneth cells and argentaffin cells. The last two varieties are not easy to identify, but the goblet cell with its bulbous content of mucus, producing a compressed, eccentrically positioned nucleus, is easy to discern; engulfment of polymorphs by such cells is characteristic.

Intestinal metaplasia or intestinalization of the gastric mucosa takes two main forms. In the first, in comparison with the round, eccentric, finely granular nucleus of the normal cell, the nucleus is larger, oval, hyperchromatic and more heavily granular, perhaps with a nucleolus. The nucleus adopts a more central position in the columnar cell so that the appearance is very similar to that of a large intestinal columnar cell, and it may still retain a brush border (Fig. 16–12). In

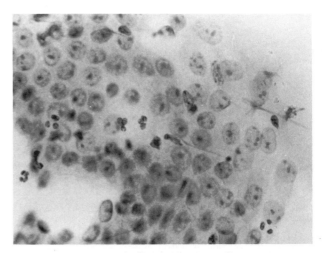

FIGURE 16–10. Gastric brush. Reactive changes in gastric mucosa. Note the mild pleomorphism and nucleolation (Papanicolaou stain; × 160).

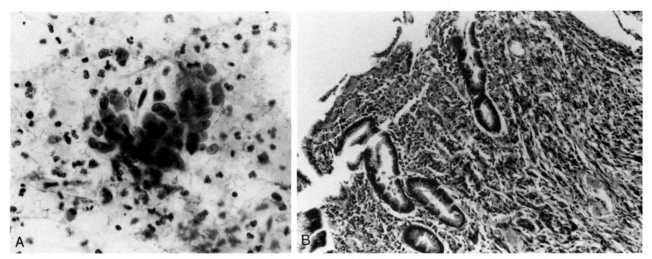

FIGURE 16–11. Poorly differentiated adenocarcinoma arising at the edge of an ulcer (MacroPhotograph). *A,* Gastric brush (Papanicolaou stain; ×160). *B,* Section of edge of ulcer (hematoxylin and eosin; ×40).

the second variety of metaplastic change the cell takes on a more flattened, broader or squared-off look with, again, centralization of the nucleus, which remains relatively round with a distinct nuclear membrane and often a prominent nucleolus. It may be of some interest that intestinal metaplasia appears to occur in the stomach even in newborns, although the significance is difficult to assess. It was discovered in the course of evaluating the cause of neonatal death.[13]

In summary, the cytologic picture of chronic atrophic gastritis and peptic ulceration has to be distinguished from any neoplastic process that may develop, and there are no short cuts—every smear sample has to be examined carefully and judgment given on any significant cell changes. Of particular importance is any increased granularity of the chromoplasm and any irregular condensation of chromatin beneath the nuclear membrane and around the nucleolus; attention should also be paid to the size of nucleoli. This theme is developed in the section on neoplasia.

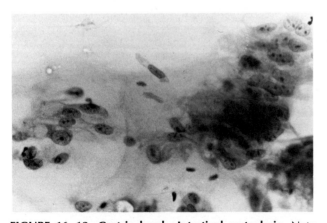

FIGURE 16–12. Gastric brush. Intestinal metaplasia. Note the similarity to the large intestine's columnar cells with goblet cells, a more centrally placed nucleus and nucleoli (Papanicolaou stain; ×160).

Benign Tumors

There are only two major types of benign tumors of the stomach that are worth considering cytologically. These are polyps and leiomyomas.

Benign Epithelial Polyps: Hyperplastic or Regenerative. This type of polyp accounts for nearly 90% of all gastric polyps. They are relatively small, 1 or 2 cm in diameter, usually pedunculated and frequently multiple. The mucosa shed from the surface consists of a single layer of gastric columnar epithelium showing a degree of nuclear crowding. The polyp itself may show cystic dilatation, and sometimes this is reflected in the smear fragments. There is little likelihood of malignancy developing (Fig. 16–13).

Adenomatous Polyp. This is probably a true neoplasm and is not at all common. Adenomatous polyps are usually larger than hyperplastic polyps, single and almost always sessile. Histologically the pattern is papillary, villous or tubulovillous, and the cells exfoliated are tall columnar cells showing varying degrees of atypia that reflect tissue dysplasia. It is necessary to decide whether the cells show only the benign changes of hyperplasia or true malignancy, and when there is any doubt, excision should be advised.

Leiomyoma. The stomach is the most common site for leiomyomas of the gastrointestinal tract. Although these tumors may be asymptomatic they can present with hemorrhage, iron deficiency anemia or abdominal pain and discomfort. Some remain within the stomach wall, but if large, they pedunculate into the cavity, and ulceration of the covering mucosa can produce a characteristic dimple that is used by the radiologist in making an x-ray diagnosis. An exception is illustrated in Figure 16–14; in this situation, the radiologic diagnosis of leiomyoma was corrected to that of malignant epithelial polyp with metastases.

In cases in which there is ulceration of the mucosa overlying the tumor, the cytologic picture shows reactive and metaplastic cells, sometimes with atypia, similar to that seen in peptic ulcer. This may confuse the

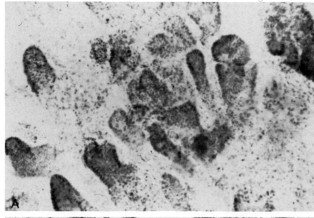

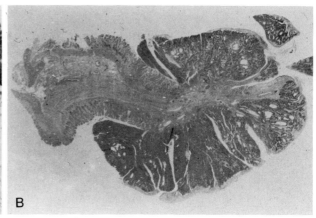

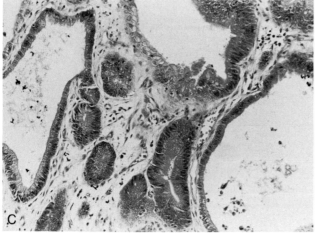

FIGURE 16–13. **Benign papilloma** in a man of 58 years who presented with a small hematemesis. *A,* Gastric wash. A sheet of benign mucosa with intact crypts (Papanicolaou stain; × 40). *B,* The excised polyp that was 2 cm in diameter (hematoxylin and eosin; × 4). *C,* Histology of the polyp showing cystic dilation of the glands (hematoxylin and eosin; × 80).

diagnosis if brushing of the lesion has not penetrated the base of the ulcer or the mucosa to sample the tumor. Cells from the tumor, be they benign or malignant, are polygonal and fusiform in type, but in cytologic material the former may predominate.[15] The cells have large, finely granular nuclei and small nucleoli with soft, ill-defined cytoplasm (Fig. 16–15).

Premalignant Lesions (Surface Cancer)

Carcinoma *in situ* is rarely recognized or diagnosed in gastric epithelium and is held in doubt by some.[2, 10]

Surface cancer, on the other hand, is a well-known entity and has been described by Ewing,[28] Golden and Stout,[35] Bamforth[2] and Friesen and coworkers.[32]

Mason,[63] in a survey of 78 patients, showed that eight (10%) of stomachs with gastric ulcers and other benign lesions displayed surface cancer. These cancers were often multifocal in origin[2, 20, 73] and invisible to the naked eye, except for some degree of slight nodulation or roughening of the mucosa and often an overall thinning of the mucosa, a feature of the loss of normal rugae. When a benign ulcer is present, the surface cancer is usually well away from it and often distal to it.

Surface cancers do metastasize sometimes.[52, 91] Long survival rates have been reported,[67] even when lymph node metastases have occurred. It is possible that surface cancer remains quiescent for many years, and the Japanese have been successful in screening for it at that stage, which appears on average to be about 10 years before true invasive cancer develops. Schade[85] used his automated wash technique to identify these in a series of hospital patients.[85]

The histologic appearance of surface cancer is that of a totally disorganized and cancerous epithelium, but there is no penetration of the muscularis mucosa. It is often found bordering an area of intestinal metaplasia, which many believe is a precancerous state. Consequently there is no difference in the cytologic picture of surface or invasive cancer, except perhaps a greater degree of degenerative and inflammatory changes in the latter (Fig. 16–16).

Malignant Tumors

These are classified according to macroscopic appearance.

- Superficial or surface carcinoma
- Polypoid carcinoma
- Ulcerated infiltrative carcinoma, shallow or deep
- Fungating carcinoma
- Diffusely infiltrating carcinoma.

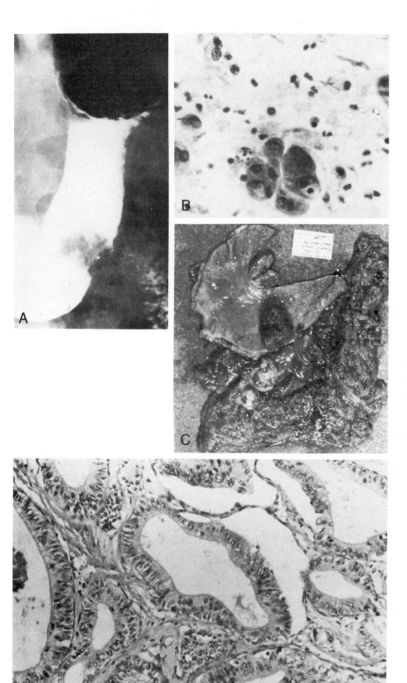

FIGURE 16–14. Malignant papilloma. *A,* Barium meal. Diagnosed by the radiologist as a leiomyoma because of the central dimple. *B,* Gastric wash. Clusters of malignant cells shed from an adenocarcinoma (Papanicolaou stain; ×160). *C,* Gastrectomy specimen opened to show the malignant papilloma and metastases in the omentum. *D,* Section of the malignant papilloma (hematoxylin and eosin; ×80).

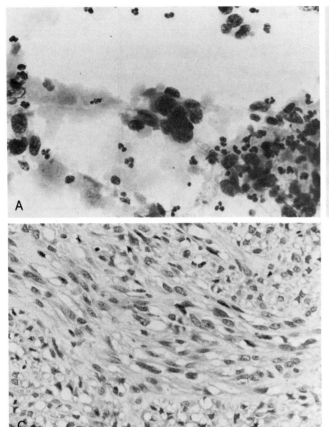

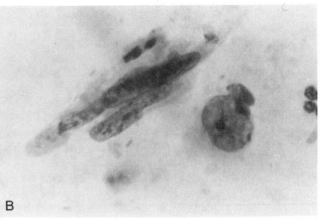

FIGURE 16–15. Leiomyosarcoma. Poorly differentiated malignant cells are present showing polygonal and fiber forms. *A*, Gastric brush. Undifferentiated polygonal cells (Papanicolaou stain; ×160). *B*, Gastric brush. At a higher magnification fiber cells are seen with a single polygonal cell (Papanicolaou stain; ×400). *C*, Section of leiomyosarcoma. An area from the center of the tumor shows a band of fiber cells with surrounding nests of polygonal cells (hematoxylin and eosin; ×80).

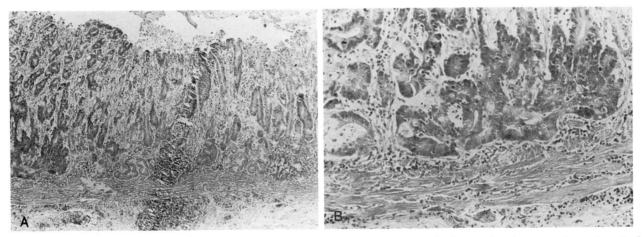

FIGURE 16–16. Surface cancer. *A*, Section of stomach. Note that to one side of the knife's artifact the tissue shows intestinal metaplasia, whereas to the other, there is an adenocarcinoma involving surface epithelium only with an intact muscularis mucosa (hematoxylin and eosin; ×16). *B*, Section of stomach. At a higher magnification the juxtaposition of tumor and intact muscularis mucosa is seen more clearly (hematoxylin and eosin; ×40).

Looking at these groups more practically Lauren[58] attempted to divide gastric tumors into two main varieties—the intestinal type and the diffuse type. In general the proportion of each type in the population differs in various parts of the world, but essentially the intestinal form with its surface glandular pattern of intestinal metaplasia is recognized at an earlier stage cytologically than the diffuse infiltrating type, which is composed of single undifferentiated cells infiltrating the stomach wall. There is, however, a substantial "mixed" group, and many pathologists revert to the World Health Organization classification:

- Adenocarcinoma: papillary, tubular, mucinous and signet-ring cell (a variant of mucinous)
- Adenosquamous carcinoma
- Squamous carcinoma
- Undifferentiated and unclassifiable carcinoma.

To these should be added the malignant mesodermal tumors of the stomach:

- Sarcoma and leiomyosarcoma
- Lymphoma.

The histologic picture of gastric cancer is predominantly that of an adenocarcinoma in which the appearances range from a small to a large cell, with tubular or papillary formation, both in a variable amount of mucus secretion in the more differentiated forms. The signet-ring form is not common, although it is quite distinctive, with a relatively small cell type in which the nuclei are characteristically pressed against the sides of the cell through an excess of mucus. The squamous carcinomas are quite rare, as are the adenosquamous, whereas the undifferentiated carcinomas vary from a relatively large cell down to the small anaplastic carcinoma simplex, infiltrating the stomach wall and causing a solid thickened leather bottle stomach. Each of these are reflected in the cytology, so much so that one could quite effectively match the cytology to the histologic counterpart.

The cytologic appearances in the various types of cancer of the stomach are usually correlated with the histologic pattern; the well-differentiated tumors have substantial cytoplasm and are composed in fairly well formed cell clusters with marginating nuclei displaying irregular chromatin condensation, usually beneath the nuclear membrane and around the nucleoli. These nucleoli are usually large, rounded and single, as opposed to the more pleomorphic and multiple nucleoli seen in squamous cancer. Much floccular cytoplasm is present, usually staining heavily for mucin, both neutral and acid, and often for sulfamucins, as do atypical metaplastic counterparts (Fig. 16–17).

In the case of the undifferentiated cancer, the disaggregation of cells—with the resultant debris—and the large irregular nuclei with heavy chromatin condensation and often little residual cytoplasm can pose a problem of cell type, and in this situation epithelial markers and mucin stains should help. The differentiation between squamous and glandular cancer, especially at the cardia, poses a similar problem, and at

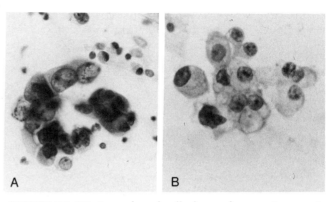

FIGURE 16–17. Examples of cells from **adenocarcinoma of the stomach.** (See also Fig. 16–10A.) *A,* Gastric wash. Well-differentiated adenocarcinoma (Papanicolaou stain; ×160). *B,* Gastric wash. Mucus-secreting adenocarcinoma showing a partial signet-ring formation (Papanicolaou stain; ×160).

times it is almost impossible to make a decision as to which way the multipotent cell is expressing itself as a new clone of neoplasia.

Perhaps the best way to register the diagnostic features of gastric cancer is to review the basic criteria of malignancy that we all use.

The most important distinction to be made is between the often severe cell changes that can occur with gastritis or ulceration and true malignancy. It is therefore relevant to review the criteria of malignancy to identify those that are of most value in gastric cytology and the degree of confidence that can be placed on each individual feature.

Anisocytosis or Pleomorphism. These are not very reliable criteria unless present in an extreme form because glandular cells are notorious for variation in size and shape due to reaction.

Anisonucleosis. Again, one has to allow for considerable variation in glandular cells showing reactive changes.

Hyperchromasia. Glandular nuclei can be pale as well as hyperchromatic in both reaction and neoplasia. The effect of degenerative changes (karyorrhexis) is an additional complication.

Loss of Cytoplasmic Boundaries. In the cytology of many sites this is a valuable criterion, but it is to some extent nullified in gastric material because of autodigestion and autolysis due to acidity.

Nucleocytoplasmic Ratio. The same problem applies in this case because loss of the cytoplasmic boundaries prevents this being one of the most decisive of criteria of malignancy.

One might be dismayed by such a lack of useful criteria were it not for the fact that in many instances they can be used, but in gastrointestinal cytology, other features have to be considered and relied upon.

Nuclear Membrane and Chromatin Pattern. Except in the presence of gross degenerative changes, in benign and reactive states the nuclear outline is essentially smooth and the membrane fine and uniform. In malignancy the nuclear membrane is distinctly finely irregular, both in outline and in the condensation of chromatin seen on the inner aspect of the nuclear membrane. One may have to observe this under high magnification, but this feature as well as the overall texture of the nucleoplasm has a certain coarseness or brightness not present in inflammatory states, in which a degree of blurring due to other nucleoprotein changes occurs. A similar chromatin condensation occurs around the nucleolus, which is often bright red in Papanicolaou stained smears. Nucleoli may be multiple and usually retain a more or less rounded outline, but they are much enlarged.

Nucleonucleolar Ratio. It has been said that in most reactive states nucleoli have a ratio of less than 1:15 of the diameter of the nucleus, but that if this ratio were increased to 1:10, then the finding was distinctly suspicious of neoplasm.[85] Danno,[24] working on my series of cases, effectively demonstrated his "distant index," a factor of nucleonucleolar ratio that clearly separates the benign and reactive from the neoplastic cases. In cases in which there is much loss of cytoplasm due to autodigestion, cytoplasmic evidence is lost but the nucleonucleolar ratio can still be used.

Sarcomas and Lymphomas

The reader is best referred elsewhere in this volume for the classification and cellular detail of these tumors, but pursuing this refined cellular differentiation in a little more detail to distinguish the sarcomas or lymphomas from the epithelial carcinomas, it is worth noting that the lipoleiomyomatous tumors seldom present more specific cellular criteria than lipid-filled globules in the cytoplasm in the former or the more fusiform shape of the latter, although for the most part an irregular pleomorphic undifferentiation characterizes both tumors (see Fig. 16–15). When it comes to the lymphomas it is worth remembering the simple criteria listed by Shida[89] of the features distinguishing the cells of the histocytic lymphomas, the lymphocytic lymphomas and the epithelial gastric carcinomas. The nuclear membrane is thin and almost obscured in the histiocytomas, distinct in the lymphocytic lymphomas and heavy in carcinomas, whereas the chromatin pattern is delicate but closely packed in the histiocytomas, slightly packed in the lymphocytic lymphomas and heavily and irregularly condensed in the carcinomas. There is also more pleomorphism and loss of cytoplasm in the epithelial tumors, but mitosis occurs more frequently in the histocytic lymphomas. The separation into the Hodgkin's and non-Hodgkin's lymphomas by virtue of finding the binuclear Reed-Sternberg giant cells is another useful differential. In cases of real doubt immunochemistry should be resorted to with the use of leukocyte-associated antigens versus the carcinoembryonic antigens and some of the other epithelial markers to separate the lymphoreticular from the epithelial tumor. Gatter and coworkers,[33] using a panel of seven monoclonal antibodies, were successful in distinguishing between anaplastic carcinoma and lymphoma. Finally, recourse to electron microscopy may be made to demonstrate the absence of intercellular junctions in the lymphomas.

COLON AND RECTUM

Normal Anatomy, Physiology and Histology

The large intestine, some 1.5 m (5 feet) long, which runs from the cecum via the ascending, transverse, descending and sigmoid colon and rectum to the anus, has a transverse diameter much greater than the small bowel, but like the latter, it diminishes gradually towards its distal end except for the rectal ampulla.

It is covered by the peritoneum completely at the cecum, anteriorly only for the rest of the colon, on the front and sides for the upper third of the rectum and in front only for the middle third; the lower third is entirely subperitoneal.

The wall of the colon itself is composed from outside in of pouches of fat, the epiploic appendices, two muscle layers, the outer longitudinal fibers—mainly in three narrow bands or teniae coli, which fuse together 6 inches above the peritoneal reflexion at the rectum— and a circular muscle fiber layer consisting of fasciculi as a continuous sheath around the bowel. The rectum has complete layers of circular and longitudinal muscle with anterior and posterior thickenings, and these, as do the teniae coli, act to contract longitudinally in concert with the circular muscle to pass the contents of the lower bowel along. There is a submucosa of loose connective tissue, a thin muscularis mucosa on top of which lies the mucosa.

The blood supply, both arterial and venous, and the lymphatic drainage are complex; lymph nodes exist close to the bowel wall, both paracolic and pararectal, and then along the main blood supply, both in the abdomen and down in the pelvis.

The microanatomy of the mucosa is of most interest to the cytologist. This consists of long epithelial tubules of relatively tall columnar cells interspersed with goblet cells within the crypts; these are embedded directly into the connective tissue (lamina propria) and rest on a muscularis mucosa. The muscularis mucosa is pierced by the capillary and blood supply, lymphatic plexus and lymph follicles which lie astride it in the form of rings of lymphocytes surrounding germinal follicles. These increase from cecum to rectum and become prominent in inflammatory states of the upper as well as the lower gastrointestinal tract.

The function of the lower bowel is to extract water, sodium and chloride from the 500 ml of chyme received from the small intestine and to excrete potassium and bicarbonate with a reduction to 100 ml of fluid contents on defecation.

The cytologic changes in the various diseases of the colon have been well documented over the years,[78] and commendable accuracy began to emerge in skilled hands.[6] The attempt to detect cancer in the markedly inflammatory, reactive and necrotic background of ulcerative colitis has been quite successful,[30] and a much greater involvement of the cytologist in this field is bound to occur. Again, benefits accrue when both biopsy and cytology augment their findings. Accuracies of 97% are being claimed for the combined techniques,[45] whereas either biopsy or cytology alone achieves around 80%.[18]

Normal Cytology

The normal cellular pattern of both wash and brush specimens shows the typical colonic mucosal cell as a tall, fairly large columnar cell with a basally placed, round nucleus that has a distinct nuclear membrane and a finely granular chromoplasm. Nucleoli are not prominent in the resting cell. The cytoplasm is smooth to finely floccular, and there is a prominent end-plate with well-formed cilia. Cells are normally found in regular intact sheets with either a honeycomb or a pallisade pattern depending on whether they are observed from a plane or a side view. Mucus-secreting cells are not very evident in normal mucosa (Fig. 16–18).

Inflammatory Disease

Simple colitis is usually nonspecific, but amebic and schistosomal infection need to be considered and sought for by special stains. Cases of ulcerative colitis are more complex because chronicity with reactive and degenerative changes is superadded.

The cytologic picture of colitis is one of acute on chronic inflammatory exudate, in which the glandular cells are sometimes irregularly enlarged and the nuclei more active and granular with prominent nuclear membrane and nucleoli. There is also an increase in the number and size of mucus-secreting goblet cells, and degenerate changes and cell debris are also evident.

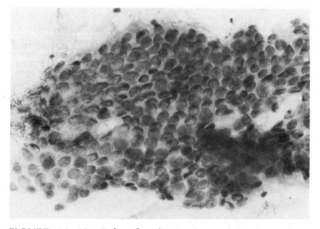

FIGURE 16–18. Colon brush. A sheet of benign colonic mucosa showing a honeycomb pattern with palisading at one edge (Papanicolaou stain; ×160).

Dysplasia

Dysplasia is the term used when cell changes fall short of being diagnostic for malignancy. It can follow the severity and chronicity of inflammatory disease, and cells show some disturbance in the uniformity of staining of the cytoplasm together with a marked irregular increase in nuclear chromatin and prominent nucleoli.

Cancer of the Colorectum

True neoplasia is depicted as a marked exaggeration of the foregoing dysplasia with much enlarged, even giant, hyperchromatic nuclei. It is sometimes evident that only part of a polyp undergoes malignant change. (Fig. 16–19). This is unlike polyps elsewhere in the intestinal tract and in other organs such as the endometrium, where the whole excrescence is neoplastic. The degree of pleomorphism and total lack of any organized cellular pattern that occurs in true cancer are relatively easy to pronounce on, as is seen also in the rectum (Fig. 16–20).

Nonepithelial Tumors

Other tumors of the lower bowel such as lymphoma, not all that rare, and sarcoma, usually leiomyosarcoma, have been detailed elsewhere in this volume and similar diagnostic criteria obtained.

REPORTING ON SMEARS

Reporting of esophageal, gastric and colorectal cytology is both easy and difficult. The negative cases are often the more arduous to screen because a thorough search must be made for any atypical features. On the other hand, a frankly malignant case shows up clearly and quickly, and it does not take long to establish a fairly definitive diagnosis. In this situation, the answer can often be obtained within an hour or two of collecting the specimen.

It is the marginal changes that create problems and require an exhaustive study before a report can be made. This usually means a report delayed to the next day. A rapid reporting system is, however, appreciated because the gastroenterologist or surgeon can then anticipate and arrange for the next move at a much earlier stage and the patient is kept in suspense for a much shorter time.

It is inevitable that categorization of case reports occurs in order to provide a communicative shorthand between pathologist and clinician, and we rely on a Papanicolaou-type grading system for our own and our clinical colleague's usage, which has proved effective and meaningful.

Grade I. This denotes an adequate specimen showing no sign of malignancy.

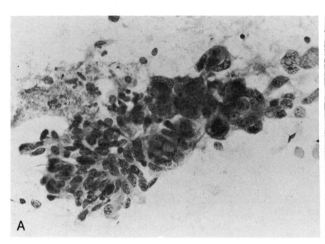
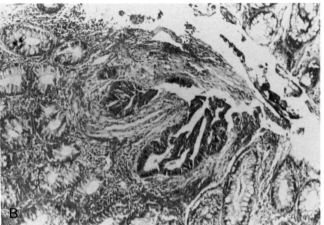

FIGURE 16–19. Partial malignant change in a **colonic polyp.** *A,* Colon brush. This field shows malignant and reactive columnar cells (Papanicolaou stain; ×160). *B,* Section of polyp. One malignant tubule is seen at the center of the field (hematoxylin and eosin; ×40).

Grade II. This is also benign but is accompanied by substantial inflammatory changes in the epithelial cells, mainly reflected in the nuclei.

Grade IIR. We have devised this grade in order to heighten the suspicion of an inflammatory or reactive-like smear pattern in which the changes are bordering on the neoplastic, a so-called borderline lesion. It refers to a markedly atypical picture, requiring a repeat (R) or at least a close follow-up by either brush or biopsy or both. Our laboratory feels a responsibility to ensure a repeat sample is obtained in such cases.

Grade III. In this grade, there are atypical and often dyskaryotic cells that are suspicious of a preneoplastic lesion, or even of invasion, but there is insufficient evidence to provide a confident report. Again it behooves us to keep an eye on the follow-up of such a case.

Grade IV. Malignancy is obvious and diagnostic and, because it is impossible to distinguish a surface from

an invasive cancer, this grade refers to both types of lesions.

Grade O. This denotes an identifiably inadequate or unsatisfactory sample that may exist on its own—a totally unsatisfactory and unreadable sample graded as O—or as O(I), or O(II), or even as O(III), when the specimen, although inadequate and unreliable, is also rated as possessing abnormal cells amounting to the grade number in parentheses. It thus leaves open the possibility of a more severe lesion detectable from a more reliable sample and is accompanied by a recommendation that a repeat sample be obtained.

The Written Report

This should be presented in three parts. Our practice has been *firstly* to present a descriptive cytologic report that is comprehensive but admittedly not always under-

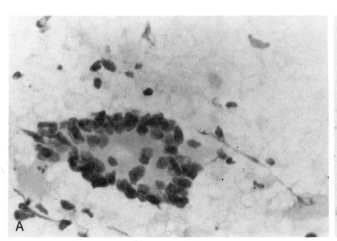
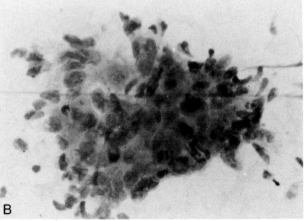

FIGURE 16–20. Rectal touch preparations. These preparations contrast **normal and malignant rectal mucosa.** *A,* A cluster of benign rectal cells (Papanicolaou stain; ×160). *B,* Note the pleomorphism and loss of polarity in this fragment smeared from the glove after a digital examination of an adenocarcinoma of the rectum (Papanicolaou stain; ×160).

TABLE 16–2. Gastric and Esophageal Brush Cytology: Charing Cross and St. Stephen's Hospital Incidence of Lesions and Accuracy of Histology and Cytology

Cytology Categories*					
Normal	*Inflammatory*	*Atypical (to Follow)*	*Suspected Malignancy*	*Malignant*	*Total*
160(17)	285(14)	17(2)	19(2)	75	556

Accuracy of Histology and Cytology						
Total	*Positive Cytology Positive Histology*	*Positive Cytology Negative Histology*	*Negative Cytology Positive Histology*	*Positive Cytology Unsatisfactory Biopsy*	*Positive Histology Unsatisfactory Cytology*	*False-Negative Both*	*False-Positive Both*
110	70	11	9	11	7	1	1

Cytology sensitivity (overall)	92/110 = 83.6%
Cytology sensitivity (minus unsatisfactory)	92/103 = 89.3%
Histology sensitivity (overall)	86/110 = 78.1%
Histology sensitivity (minus unsatisfactory)	86/99 = 86.9%
Combined histology and cytology sensitivity	108/110 = 98.1%

*Unsatisfactory samples in parentheses.

stood by the noncytologist and sadly sometimes not even by another cytologist, *secondly* to give the interpretation of the findings in histologic terms and *thirdly* to give a recommendation for further investigational procedure should the diagnosis not be explicit or the lesion be so suspect as to warrant follow-up. In other words, we do not restrict ourselves to a simple malignant or benign option because the reactive and hyperplastic changes encountered, especially in the glandular lesions, may be so borderline that it would be as much a folly to ignore such changes as to overidentify them. We therefore utilize the category IIR (mentioned earlier) with due circumspection but with a simple explanation of concern.

Diagnostic Accuracy

Table 16–2 shows that the cases from a 4-year survey of gastric cancer in Charing Cross and St. Stephen's Hospitals have produced a scatter of grades, and Table 16–3 expresses the accuracy of both cytologic and histologic biopsies in a few published series. It will be evident that the cytologic samples appear to be marginally more accurate and probably reflect the larger cellular sample obtained with the brush, compared with the small histologic biopsy, sometimes made with compression-distortion and not always sufficiently sectioned to express the full cellular content of the excised fragment.

It is the final column of Table 16–2 summarizing the accuracies of both samples together that provides the more significant message and indicates the value of both techniques being used together, preferably reported by the same pathologist.

It can be seen that there has been one false-positive report in our particular series, although we do have the IIR category that permits us an identity of an atypical borderline picture. This apparent under-reporting, we feel, errs on the right side, and seven of these cases turned out to be malignant on subsequent cytology or histology. Follow-up of the negative cases for over 6 years has not disclosed any missed lesions.

A review of the smears in the cytologically negative–histologically positive cases has not disclosed any atypical or malignant cells, and one can only presume that sampling was at fault. In this situation, multiple biopsies and brushes would help to reduce such an error.

False-positives have been reported by most authorities,[80, 82] and also ourselves in the past, but it is a moot point whether an adequate search for a focus of surface cancer in the excised organ had been made before accepting that the cytology gave a false-positive result.

TABLE 16–3. Accuracy of Endoscopic Cytology and Biopsy in the Diagnosis of Gastric Tumors

Author	Date	Cases	Correct Cytology (%)	Correct Histology (%)	Correct Combined (%)
Kobayashi and coworkers[51]	1970	26	97.0	66.7	100.0
Serck-Hanssen and coworkers[86]	1973	68	94.1	52.9	94.1
Bemvenuti and coworkers[5]	1975	58	77.8	82.2	?
Smithies and coworkers[90]	1975	34	82.4	61.8	97.1
Witzel and coworkers[103]	1976	73	83.6	79.5	95.9
Young and Hughes[106]	1980	61	91.8	68.9	91.8
Boddington (incl. 1969/73 series)[11]	1978	84	78.5	72.6	92.8
Husain (1986)[41]	1986	110	83.6	78.1	98.1
Cook and coworkers[21]	1988	234	85.0	86.0	91.0

SCREENING FOR EARLY AND PRETUMOROUS STATES

Although there are differing degrees of expression of preinvasive phases of *in situ* or surface tumor in the esophagus, stomach and colorectum, all these sites do have such a category, but they vary considerably in their modes of expression, duration and incidence geographically, as witnessed by the very high rates of cancer of the esophagus in China[22] and in Iran[65] and of the stomach in Japan,[76] Iceland and Czechoslovakia with mortalities of three to five times the average. In our more developed communities the higher rate of colonic cancer demands attention. These higher incidences justify attempts at screening for such tumors in the populations. There is, however, a substantial proportion of early stage tumorous disease even in the countries with lower incidence rates, but these have to be skillfully searched for.

For instance, in the United Kingdom it was shown that from 10 to 16% of stomach cancers were in an early stage when so sought.[27] Moreover, there are stages even before a surface cancer develops in which atrophic gastritis, esophagitis and colitis make it imperative to identify such lesions in order to detect cancer early before serious trouble ensues. It is therefore of some importance to apply early diagnostic tests and screening techniques to such organs, at least in the high-risk groups for whom cytology can play a substantial part and also in those needing long-term surveillance following ablative therapy of such conditions.[39]

Screening for Cancer of the Esophagus

Screening for such lesions has been the subject of considerable activity in China and Iran and this has, by and large, been by the use of inflatable balloons and simple brushes and has been quite successful. (See Chapter 3, Cytologic Screening Programs, for additional information.) Berry's[8] tolerable balloon technique, which she used to screen 50 cancer cases and 500 control patients of African origin, is now becoming a standard approach. The simple nasal tube–guided brush[25] is, however, more convenient and appears to

be highly efficient and accurate (see section on sampling methods).

Screening in Early Cancer of the Stomach

This is well established in Japan with its high incidence of disease,[1, 88, 93] although the logic and approach do seem to emphasize the use of double-contrast x-ray more than cytology as an initial technique.[40] The opportunity of detecting a higher proportion of early surface cancers does relate to an increased search of symptomatic patients by improved diagnostic methods.[26, 27, 31, 64, 70] For example, in the series by Evans following the introduction of endoscopy the rate of diagnosis of surface cancers went from 0.5 to 10.0%. Again, in a series from the Massachusetts General Hospital the application of routine gastric cytology on patients attending the gastrointestinal unit resulted in detection of 8 per 1000 cases of early subclinical cancers of the stomach over and above those diagnosed clinically or by other techniques.[40]

The most glaring contrast is seen between the Japanese statistics and the 4-year survival rate of only 9% in a series of seven countries in Europe,[61] in which all patients presented with clinical symptoms, the predominant ones being weight loss, pain, vomiting, anorexia and weakness, and with the diagnosis confirmed by barium meal in 96%, gastroscopy in 28% and cytology in less than 6%. This contrasts with Shida's latest figures,[89] in which the mean 5-year survival rate was 98.8% when the tumor was restricted to the mucosa and submucosa, 74.2% when muscle was invaded, 49.3% when the tumor had reached the serosa and 21.3% when cancer had invaded beyond that. This success is claimed to be largely owing to early detection by screening (Fig. 16–21).

The question of whether some form of screening could be afforded in the so-called low-incidence countries such as the United States or the United Kingdom has been considered in relation to costs[40] and discussed in a Lancet lead article.[56] The article noted that even with screening it was found that a mean time of 7 months existed between first symptoms and operation.[19, 61]

FIGURE 16–21. Survival from **gastric cancer** with differing degrees of invasion. (*m/sm* = cancer cells limited to mucosa and submucosa; *pm* = cancer cells penetrate muscle layer; *ss* = cancer cell invasion reaches to subserosal layer; *s(+)* = cancer cell invasion to beyond serosa; *n* = 365.) (Redrawn from Shida, S. Personal communication, 1989.)

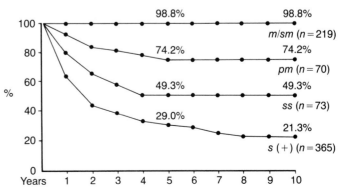

Survival of Gastric Cancer Patients after Gastrectomy

It is obvious that, although cytology is beginning to improve in European centers, the pursuit of double-contrast x-rays, so vital to initial scanning, has not substantially developed in the United Kingdom or in Europe generally as an application in this field.

In Takahashi's[93] screening program, which reflects the logistics of the Japanese experience, for every 1000 people seen in the traveling caravan who are initially screened by a personal interview and double-contrast fluoroscopy, around 200 to 300 demonstrate sufficient abnormality to pass to the next stage clinic, where endoscopy, biopsy and cytology narrow the problem cases down to 50 to 100 persons, consisting of cancers, ulcers, polyps and other pathology needing hospital treatment.

If, however, a greater degree of gastroscopy and double-contrast x-rays were to be undertaken on those with symptoms relating to dyspepsia (which would include those suffering from chronic gastritis, in which more than 75% of stomach cancer cases develop), then some inroads could be made. However, it is estimated by Barnes and coworkers[3] that there are about 4500 dyspeptics in every 300,000 population, that is, those served by one of our District General Hospitals. Many are probably over 45 years of age, and, to be economical, a more searching and simple method of preselection may well have to be implemented.

It is more than likely that primary screening by cytology or even double-contrast radiography is not going to be cost-effective, especially in low-risk countries, and that some other technique, both simple and economical, such as the measurement of the lactate dehydrogenase and its isomers or the glucose-6-phosphate dehydrogenase cytochemical assays, may need to be devised as a prescreening test to provide a group for the more specific radiologic and gastroscopic investigations.[42]

Screening for Colonic Cancer

There is not time or space here to consider in detail the arguments for screening for a disease that is the second most common malignancy in both men and women in the United States with a 5-year survival rate from the time of clinical presentation of 42%. This compares with those whose diagnosis is made prior to the onset of symptoms, when the 5-year survival rate can reach 92%. A full review of the high-risk groups and methods of screening for colorectal cancer has been given by Fath and Winawar.[29] The high-risk groups are those with ulcerative and granulomatous colitis, a past history of colorectal cancer and adenoma[99] and women who have had breast or genital tumors. Also at risk are people with a family history of adenomata, polyposis syndrome, juvenile polyposis, colorectal cancer and adenoma and cancer family syndrome.

The screening tests include digital rectal examination,[54, 60] the simple occult blood test, flexible fiberoptic sigmoidoscopy, barium enema, colonoscopy and polypectomy with examination of biopsy and cytology samples. Use of these different modalities in the armamentarium varies with the risk categories, and colonoscopy for biopsy and cytology may be done at intervals varying from 1 to 5 years.

ADDITIONAL CYTOLOGIC METHODS OF CANCER DETECTION

Various other approaches have demonstrated significant advances in this field. Jass and Filipe[44] have demonstrated that the sulfamycins are increased in metaplasia and neoplasia of gastric mucosa and, in effect, identify a high-risk group. The use of glucose-6-phosphate dehydrogenase assays in oxygen and nitrogen has effectively distinguished neoplastic from nonneoplastic cells in stomach, colon, bladder, cervix and breasts and is worthy of further exploration.[43] In addition, the identification of a substantial labile component of the nuclear DNA by a slowed Feulgen hydrolysis technique[71] has also been successfully demonstrated in gastric samples in my unpublished work. It is expected that immunocytochemistry or the new molecular markers will also achieve some success in this field.

References

1. Aikawa K: Gastric cancer screening in Osaka. Prev Med 4:154–162, 1975.
2. Bamforth J: Early carcinomatous changes in the stomach. Brit J Surg 43:292–296, 1955.
3. Barnes RJ, Gear MWL, Nicol A, Dew AB: Study of dyspepsia in general practice as assessed by endoscopy and radiology. Br Med J 4:214–216, 1974.
4. Barrett NR: The lower esophagus lined by columnar epithelium. Surgery 41:881–894, 1957.
5. Bemvenuti GA, Hattori K, Levin B, Kirsner JB, Reilly RW: Endoscopic sampling tissue diagnosis in gastrointestinal malignancy. Gastrointest Endosc 21:159–161, 1975.
6. Bemvenuti GA, Prolla JC, Kirsner JB, Reilly RW: Direct vision brushing cytology in the diagnosis of colo-rectal malignancy. Acta Cytol 18:477–481, 1974.
7. Berg JW: Esophageal herpes, a complication of cancer therapy. Cancer 8:731–740, 1955.
8. Berry AV, Baskind AF, Hamilton DG: Cytologic screening for esophageal cancer. Acta Cytol 2:135–141, 1981.
9. Blendis LM, Beilby JOW, Wilson JP, Cole MJ, Hadley GD: Carcinoma of the stomach: Evaluation of individual and combined diagnostic accuracy of radiology, cytology and gastrophotography. Br Med J 1:656–659, 1967.
10. Bocian JJ, Geschke AE: Carcinoma in situ of the stomach. Arch Pathol 65:6–12, 1958.
11. Boddington MM: Cytological aspects. In Topics in Gastroenterology, vol 6. Edited by SC Truelove, MR Heyworth. Oxford, Blackwell, pp 165–178, 1978.
12. Brandborg LL, Tanaguchi L, Rubin CE: Exfoliative cytology in non-malignant conditions of the upper intestinal tract. Acta Cytol 5:187–190, 1961.
13. Butler EB: Personal communication, 1971.
14. Cabre-Fiol V, Olo-Garcia R, Vilardell F: Five years of cytological diagnosis of gastric cancer by "exfoliative biopsy." Proceedings of World Congress of Gastroenterology, Washington. Baltimore, Williams & Wilkins, p 1006, 1959.

15. Cabre-Fiol V, Vilardell F, Sala-Cladera E, and Perez Mota A: Pre-operative cytological diagnosis of gastric leiomyosarcoma. Gastroenterology 68:563–566, 1975.
16. Carter KJ, Schaffer HA, Ritchie WP: Early gastric cancer. Ann Surg 199:604–608, 1984.
17. Chambers LA, Clark WE: The endoscopic diagnosis of gastroesophageal malignancy: A cytologic review. Acta Cytol 30:110–114, 1986.
18. Chen YL: The diagnosis of colo-rectal cancer with cytologic brushings under direct vision at fiberoptic colonoscopy. Dis Colon Rectum 30:342–344, 1987.
19. Cohn I: Gastrointestinal cancer. Surgical survey of abdominal tragedy. Am J Surg 135:3–11, 1978.
20. Collins WT, Gall EA: Gastric carcinoma: A multicentric lesion. Cancer 5:62–72, 1952.
21. Cook JJ, de Carlo DJ, Haneman B, Hunt DR, Talley NA, Mellor D: The role of brush cytology in the diagnosis of gastric malignancy. Acta Cytol 32:461–464, 1988.
22. Co-ordinating Group for Research of Esophageal Carcinoma—Chinese Academy of Medical Sciences and Honan Province: The early detection of carcinoma of the esophagus. Sci Sin 16:457–463, 1973.
23. Crozier RE, Middleton M, Ross JR: Clinical application of gastric cytology. N Engl J Med 255:1128–1131, 1956.
24. Danno M: Statistical criteria for the cytology of gastric cancer. A proposal of distance index. Acta Cytol 20:466–468, 1976.
25. Dowlatshahi K, Skinner DB, De Meester TR, Zachary L, Bibbo M, Wied GL: Evaluation of brush cytology as an independent technique for detection of esophageal cancer. J Thorac Cardiovasc Surg 89:849–851, 1988.
26. Elster K, Kolazek F, Shimamoto K, Freitag H: Early gastric cancer. Experience in Germany. Endoscopy 7:5–10, 1975.
27. Evans DMD, Craven JL, Murphy F, Cleary BK: Comparison of "early gastric cancer" in Britain and Japan. Gut 19:1–9, 1978.
28. Ewing J: The beginnings of gastric cancer. Am J Surg 31:20–25, 1936.
29. Fath RB, Winawar SJ: Early diagnosis of colo-rectal cancer. Annu Rev Med 34:501–517, 1983.
30. Festa VI, Hajdu SI, Winawar SJ: Colorectal cytology in chronic ulcerative colitis. Acta Cytol 29:262–268, 1985.
31. Fevre DI, Green PHR, Barratt PJ, Nagy GS: Review of five cases of early gastric cancer. Gut 17:41–47, 1976.
32. Friesen G, Dockerty MB, ReMine WM: Superficial carcinoma of the stomach. Surgery 51:300–312, 1962.
33. Gatter KC, Abdulaziz Z, Beverley P, Corvalan JRF, Ford C, Lane EB, Mota M, Nash JRG, Pulford K, Stein H, Taylor-Papadimitriou J, Woodhouse C, Mason DY: Use of monoclonal antibodies for the histopathological diagnosis of human malignancy. J Clin Pathol 35:1253–1267, 1982.
34. Gephart T, Graham RM: The cellular detection of carcinoma of the esophagus. Surg Gynecol Obstet 108:75–82, 1959.
35. Golden R, Stout AP: Superficial spreading carcinoma of the stomach. AJR 59 157–162, 1948.
36. Graham RM, Ulfelder H, Green TH: The cytologic method as an aid in the diagnosis of gastric carcinoma. Surg Gynecol Obstet 86:257–259, 1948.
37. Halter F, Witzel L, Gretillat PA, Scheurer U, Keller M: Diagnostic value of biopsy guided lavage and brush cytology in esophagogastroscopy. Am J Digest Dis 22:129–131, 1977.
38. Hirschowitz BI, Curtiss LE, Peters CW, Pollard HM: Demonstration of a new gastroscope, "The fibrescope." Gastroenterology 35:50, 1958.
39. Houghton PWJ, Mortensen NJM, Allan A, Williamson RCN, Davis JD: Early gastric cancer, the case for long-term surveillance. Br Med J, 291:305–308, 1985.
40. Husain OAN: Cytological screening for cancer of the stomach. Proc Royal Soc Med 69:489–494, 1976.
41. Husain OAN: Cytology of the esophagus, stomach and duodenum. *In* Biopsy Pathology of the Esophagus, Stomach and Duodenum. Edited by DW Day. Biopsy Pathology Series. London, Chapman and Hall Medical, pp 261–283, 1986.
42. Husain OAN, Zeegen R, Parkins RA, Ibrahim KS, Grainger J, Basu R: Cytodiagnosis of gastric cancer. *In* Recent Advances

in Gastrointestinal Pathology. Edited by R Wright. London, WB Saunders, pp 241–254, 1980.
43. Ibrahim KS, Husain OAN, Bitensky L, Chayan J: A modified tetrazolium reaction for identifying malignant cells from gastric and colonic cancer. J Clin Pathol 36:133–136, 1983.
44. Jass JR, Filipe MI: The mucin profile of normal gastric mucosa, intestinal metaplasia and its variants and gastric carcinoma. Histochem J 13:931–939, 1981.
45. Jeevanandam V, Treat MR, Forde KA: A comparison of direct brush cytology and biopsy in the diagnosis of colo-rectal cancer. Gastrointest Endosc 33:370–371, 1987.
46. Kameya S, Nakamura S, Mizutaric K: Gastrofibrescope for biopsy. Gastroenterol Endosc (Japanese), 6:36–40, 1964.
47. Kasagai T: Gastric biopsy and cytology by the fibre gastroscope. Gastroenterol Endosc (Japanese) 6:187–190, 1964.
48. Kasugai T: Evaluation of gastric lavage cytology under direct vision by the fibergastroscope employing Hanks' solution as a washing solution. Acta Cytol 12:345–351, 1968.
49. Kasugai T: Gastrofibrescopic techniques for cell collections. *In* Compendium on Diagnostic Cytology, vol 4. Edited by GL Wied, LG Koss, JW Reagan. Chicago, Tutorials in Cytology, pp 492–496, 1976.
50. Kidokoro T, Soma S, Seta R, Goto K, Yamakara T, Taniai A, Katayanagi T: Gastric cytology under direct vision with special reference to the suction method. Jpn Soc Clin Cytol 5:31, 1966.
51. Kobayashi S, Prolla JC, Kirsner JB: Brushing cytology of the esophagus and stomach under direct vision by fiberscopes. Acta Cytol 14:219–223, 1970.
52. Konjetzney GE: The superficial cancer of the gastric mucosa. Am J Digest Dis 20:91–96, 1953.
53. Koss LG: Diagnostic cytology and its histopathologic bases, 3rd ed. Philadelphia, JB Lippincott, pp 835–837, 1979.
54. Kune G, Baird L, Lusink C: Rapid cytological diagnosis of rectal cancer. Ann R Coll Surg Engl 66:85–86, 1984.
55. Kuster GGR, Remine WH, Docherty MB: Gastric cancer in pernicious anemia with and without achlorhydria. Ann Surg 175:783, 1972.
56. Lancet leading article (anonymous). Screening for gastric cancer in the West. Lancet I:1023–1024, 1978.
57. Lasser A: Herpes simplex virus esophagitis. Acta Cytol 21:301–302, 1977.
58. Lauren P: The two histological main types of gastric carcinoma: Diffuse and so-called intestinal type carcinoma. An attempt at a histo-clinical classification. Acta Pathol Microbiol Immunol Scand 64:31–49, 1972.
59. Liavag I, Marcussen J, Serck-Hanssen A: Direct vision brush cytology in the diagnosis of gastric disease. Acta Chir Scand 137:682–688, 1971.
60. Linehan JJ, Melcher DH, Strachan CJ: Rapid outpatient detection of rectal cancer by gloved digital scrape cytology. Acta Cytol 27:146–151, 1983.
61. Lundh G, Burn JI, Kolig G, Richard CA, Thompson JWW, van Elk PJ, Oszacki J: A co-operative international study of gastric cancer. Ann R Coll Surg Engl 54:2–12, 1974.
62. MacDonald WC, Brandenborg LL, Taniguchi I, Beh JE, Rubin CE: Exfoliated cytological screening for gastric cancer. Cancer 27:163–169, 1963.
63. MacKenzie JF, Rogers IM, Moule B, Young JA, Hughes HE, Lee FD, Russell RI, Blumgart LH: Comparison of double contrast radiology, standard radiology, endoscopy, also of histology and cytology in the diagnosis of gastric cancer. Gut 18:416–420, 1977.
64. Machado G, Davies JD, Tudway AJC, Salmon PR, Reed AE: Superficial cancer of the stomach. Br Med J 2:77–79, 1976.
65. Mahboubi E, Kmet J, Cook PJ, Day NE, Ghadirian P, Salmasizadeh S: Esophageal cancer studies in the Caspian littoral of Iran; The Caspian Cancer Registry. Br J Cancer 28:197–891, 1973.
66. Marini G: Ancora sulla diagnosi del-carcinoma della stomaco in base all'esame citologico dell'acqua di Lavatura Clin Medica Italia 49:65, 1910.
67. Mason MK: Surface carcinoma of the stomach. Gut 6:185–193, 1965.

68. Mason MK: Surface carcinoma of the stomach. Pathological features and clinical significance. T Gastroent 9:562–571, 1966.

69. Melville DM, Richman P, Shepherd NA, Williams CB, Lennard Jones JE: British cytology of the colon and rectum in ulcerative colitis: An aid to cancer diagnosis. J Clin Pathol 41:1180–1186, 1988.

70. Miller G, Kaufmann M: Das magenfruhkarzinom in Europa. Dtsch Med Wochenschr 100:1964–1949, 1975.

71. Millett JA, Husain OAN: Analysis of chromatin in carcinoma *in situ*. *In* Quantitative Cytochemistry and Its Application. Edited by JR Pattison, L Bitensky, J Chayan. London, Academic Press pp 37–42, 1979.

72. Mirra SS, Bryan JA, Butz WC, Miles ML: Concomitant herpes—monilial esophagitis: Case report with ultra structure study. Hum Pathol 8:760–763, 1982.

73. Moertel CO, Bargen JA, Soule EH: Multiple gastric cancer. Gastroenterology 32:1095–1163, 1957.

74. Moreno-Otero R, Martinez-Raposo A, Cantero J, Pajares JM: Exfoliative cytodiagnosis of gastric adenocarcinoma. Acta Cytol 27:485–488, 1983.

75. Morson BC: Colour Atlas of Gastrointestinal Pathology. The Oxford Colour Atlases of Pathology. Edited by H Miller. Oxford, Oxford University Press pp 20–25 and 41–46, 1988.

76. Murakami H: Fluoroscopy of the stomach in recumbent position with the horizontal radiation. Rinsho Hoshasen 16:336–341, 1971.

77. Papanicolaou GN, Cooper WA: The cytology of the gastric fluid in the diagnosis of carcinoma of the stomach. J Natl Cancer Inst 7:357–360, 1947.

78. Prolla JC, Kirsner JB: Handbook and Atlas of Gastrointestinal Exfoliative Cytology. Chicago, University of Chicago Press, pp 57–60, 1972.

79. Prolla JC, Kobayashi S, Kirsner JB: Gastric cancer: Some recent improvements in diagnosis based upon the Japanese experience. Arch Intern Med 124:238–246, 1969.

80. Prolla JC, Reilly RW, Kirsner JB, Cockerham L: Direct vision endoscopic cytology and biopsy in the diagnosis of esophageal and gastric tumors: Current experience. Acta Cytol 21:399–402, 1977.

81. Raskin HF, Kirsner JB, Palmer WL: Role of exfoliative cytology in the diagnosis of cancer of the digestive tract. JAMA 169:789–791, 1959.

82. Richards WCD, Spriggs AI: Cytology of gastric mucosa. J Clin Pathol 14:132–139, 1961.

83. Rosen P, Hajdn SI: Visceral herpes virus infection in patients with cancer. Am J Clin Pathol 56:459–65, 1971.

84. Rosenberg IL, Giles GR: The value of colonic exfoliative cytology in the diagnosis of carcinoma of the larger intestine. Dis Colon Rectum 20:1–10, 1977.

85. Schade ROK: Gastric Cytology. London, Edward Arnold, pp 7, 10–16 and 37, 1960.

86. Serck-Hanssen A, Marcussen J, Liavag I: Cancer detection and prevention. Edited by C Maltoni. Proceedings of the Second International Symposium on Cancer Detection and Prevention, Bologna. Amersterdam, Excerpta Medica, 1973.

87. Seybolt JF, Papanicolaou GN: The value of cytology in the diagnosis of gastric cancer. Gastroenterology 33:369–377, 1957.

88. Shida S: Biopsy smear cytology with the fibregastroscope for direct observation. *In* Early Gastric Cancer. Gann Monograph on Cancer Research, vol 11. Edited by T Murakami. Tokyo, University of Tokyo Press, pp 223–232, 1971.

89. Shida S: Gastric cytology. Its evaluation for the diagnosis of early gastric cancer. *In* Compendium on Diagnostic Cytology. Edited by GL Wied, LG Koss, JW Reagan. Chicago, Tutorials in Cytology, pp 382–387, 1988.

90. Smithies A, Lovell D, Hishon S: Value of brush cytology in diagnosis of gastric cancer. Gut 16:326–395, 1975.

91. Stout AP: Atlas of Tumor Pathology in Tumors of the Stomach, Section VI. Washington, Armed Forces Institute of Pathology, fascicle 21, section 6, p 72, 1953.

92. Taebel DW, Prolla JC, Kirsner JB: Exfoliative cytology in the diagnosis of stomach cancer. Ann Intern Med 63:1018–1026, 1965.

93. Takahashi K: Outline of gastric mass survey by x-ray. *In* Early Gastric Cancer, Gann Monograph on Cancer Research, vol 11. Edited by T Murakami. Tokyo, University of Tokyo Press, pp 21–26, 1971.

94. Takeda M: Atlas of Diagnostic Gastrointestinal Cytology. New York, Igaku-Shoin, pp 111, 1983.

95. Tamura K, Masuzawa M, Akiyama T, Rukui O: Touch smear cytology for endoscopic diagnosis of gastric carcinoma. Am J Gastroenterol 67:463–467, 1977.

96. Tazaki Y: Clinical aspects of gastric carcinoma in Japan. *In* Proceedings of World Congress of Gastroenterology, Baltimore. Williams and Wilkins, pp 1148, 1959.

97. Thompson H, Hoare AM, Dykes PW, Allan RN, Keighley MRR: A prospective randomised trial to compare brush cytology before and after punch biopsy for endoscopic diagnosis of gastric cancer. Gut 18:398, 1977.

98. Traut HF, Rosenthal M, Harrison JT, Farber SM, Grimes OF: Evaluation of cytologic diagnosis of gastric cancer. Surg Gynecol Obstet 95:709–716, 1952.

99. Tripp MR, Sampline RE, Kogan FJ, Morgan TR: Colorectal neoplasia and Barrett's esophagus. Am J Gastroenterol 81:1063–1064, 1986.

100. Videbach A, Mosbeek J: The etiology of gastric carcinoma elucidated by a study of 302 pedigrees. Acta Med Scand 149:137, 1954.

101. Winawer SJ, Posner G, Lightdale CJ, Sherlock P, Melamed M, Fortner JG: Endoscopic diagnosis of advanced gastric cancer: Factors influencing yield. Gastroenterology 69:1183–1187, 1976.

102. Witte S: Die Zytodiagnostik des magen Karzinomas. Krebsarzt 14:408–411, 1959.

103. Witzel L, Halter F, Gretillat PA, Scheurer U, Keller M: Evaluation of specific value of endoscopic biopsies and brush cytology for malignancies of the esophagus and stomach. Gut 17:375–377, 1976.

104. Wright SG, Tomkins AM, Ridley DS: Giardiasis: Clinical and therapeutic aspects. Gut 18:343–350, 1977.

105. Yoshii Y, Takanashi J, Yamaoka Y, Kasugai T: Significance of imprint smears in cytological diagnosis of malignant tumors of stomach. Acta Cytol 14:249–253, 1970.

106. Young JA, Hughes HE: Report on a three year trial of endoscopic cytology of stomach and duodenum. Gut 21:241–246, 1980.

17

Urinary Tract

William H. Kern

The presence of single renal epithelial cells, cell casts or tissue fragments has been recognized for many decades as an important finding in the evaluation of patients with nephritis or with parenchymal damage as may occur in industrial workers exposed to cadmium or many other chemicals. The findings have been used to monitor renal allograft rejection. These observations remain in the realm of urinalysis and clinical microscopy. Renal tubular epithelial cells are not present in most urine specimens, and tumor cells exfoliate from renal adenocarcinomas only in advanced stages of the disease. Gross or microscopic hematuria is frequently the first symptom of renal adenocarcinoma or of urothelial carcinoma and mandates further studies until a diagnosis is established. Urothelial cells are present in all urines and exfoliate readily from tumors of the urothelial lining. Urine cytology is therefore an important primary or, in combination with cystoscopy and biopsy, adjunct method in the diagnosis of urothelial tumors.

The cytologic examination of urine is performed in screening programs of asymptomatic but high-risk patients for case finding, in the diagnostic evaluation of symptomatic patients and in the follow-up and monitoring of patients with known and treated disease. The clinical history, including any prior surgical procedures, treatment modalities and comparison with previous biopsies or cytologic specimens, is essential for a cytopathologic evaluation. This may permit the diagnosis of recurrent well-differentiated tumors that could not be identified without comparison with previous material and it will prevent overdiagnosis of atypias that may be associated with previous treatment.

SCREENING FOR BLADDER CANCER

Screening programs for bladder cancer by cytologic examination have been undertaken and reported sparingly.[24] Such programs were conducted for individuals considered at high risk, such as industrial workers

exposed to aromatic amines or cadmium, phenacetin or opium abusers and bilharzial populations. Holmquist[18] reported results of screening of 9870 outpatients by routine urinalysis wet preparations. Of these, 148 (1.5%) were considered abnormal. Cytopathologic and histopathologic follow-up studies revealed evidence of cancer in 12 of these patients, for a pickup rate of 1.2 per 1000. Toluidine blue and phase-contrast microscopy have been advocated for rapid screening of a clinic or hospital population. This then must be supplemented by examination of stained slides if there are abnormal findings.

Based on the known high sensitivity of urine cytology for nonpapillary carcinoma *in situ*, which is the usual precursor of invasive bladder cancer, screening programs of carefully chosen high-risk populations should yield significant results. This is indeed the case, and the positive yield in screening programs for high-risk groups ranges from ten to 70 per 1000 persons.[13] The yield is only two per 1000 individuals in a bilharzial population and ten per 1000 in phenacetin users, which still exceeds that in a routinely screened clinic or hospital population. Screening programs clearly lead to detection of bladder cancer at an earlier stage than in patients who present with symptoms in unscreened groups, provided that the screening procedure is applied frequently enough. Nevertheless, existing evidence does not establish that early detection enables treatments to be used that increase the length of survival for screened populations.[19]

Examination of Symptomatic Patients

The most common presenting symptoms in patients with bladder cancer is gross hematuria. Patients with gross or microscopic hematuria must be further evaluated until the source of the bleeding has been securely established. This usually requires an intravenous pyelogram because of the possibility of renal adenocarcinoma and a cytologic examination of the urine that, depending on the findings, may be followed by bladder washings for flow cytometry, cystoscopy and bladder biopsies. Cytologic examination of voided urine is a simple, noninvasive procedure with high sensitivity for nonpapillary and *in situ* urothelial carcinoma and should be performed in all symptomatic patients. If combined with flow cytometry performed on bladder washings the sensitivity of the two modalities for bladder cancer is 98%.[9]

Follow-up After Treatment

Urine cytology is of particular value in the follow-up of patients with known and treated urothelial tumors. Low-grade papillary tumors cannot be readily diagnosed cytologically, whether they are primary or recurrent, but bladder tumors of grade II or III and all *in situ* and nonpapillary carcinomas can be diagnosed with a high degree of accuracy. These are the significant bladder cancers that frequently recur or may be associated with low-grade papillary tumors. Cystoscopy and biopsy are the appropriate procedures for visible tumors, but cytology has the distinct advantage of sampling the entire urothelial mucosa. This permits the detection of clinically occult and *in situ* urothelial tumors. Most patients with superficial nonpapillary bladder carcinoma will develop clinically apparent recurrent carcinoma, yet only 40% have positive urine cytology immediately following transurethral resection and prior to clinically apparent and documented recurrent bladder cancer.[2] This may be due to inflammation and regenerative epithelial atypia in the immediate postoperative period, which may mask minimal cytologic evidence of carcinoma. If recurrence follows positive postoperative cytology, it can be assumed to arise from residual neoplastic epithelium. Recurrence following negative postoperative cytology suggests tranformation within an unstable urothelium and is often multicentric. The sensitivity of flow cytometric examination of irrigation cytology specimens for recurrent bladder cancer is approximately 78% and is higher than that of cytologic examination. It is also higher for well-differentiated papillary tumors than cytologic examination alone. The simplicity, convenience and relative accuracy of voided urine cytology makes it, nevertheless, the first-line diagnostic technique in this setting. Irrigation cytology specimens are more sensitive than voided urinary cytology, and bladder wash flow cytometry is more sensitive than either in diagnosing bladder cancer. Flow cytometry may be more sensitive because of the better sampling of bladder irrigation compared with voided urine and because of the measurement technique itself.[3]

SAMPLING TECHNIQUES

Sample Collection

Voided urine is the specimen of choice for all screening programs and for diagnostic studies in male patients

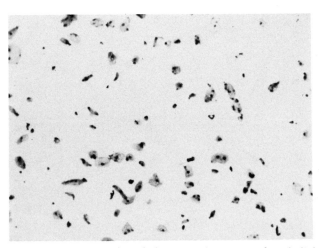

FIGURE 17–1. Normal voided urine with numerous **urothelial and squamous cells** (filter preparation; Papanicolaou stain; ×80).

because of the ease of collection and satisfactory results. Catheterized urine is the preferred specimen from female patients. Hydration of the patients, collection of the second voiding in the morning and collection of three successive morning specimens have been recommended by some authors, but because of the good cellularity that can be uniformly obtained by filter preparations as shown in Figure 17–1 and the significant exfoliation from all nonpapillary tumors of the urothelium, the examination of a single urine specimen is sufficient. What is important is prompt fixation, which can best be accomplished by collection of 50 to 100 ml of urine in an equal amount of 50% alcohol. Ethyl alcohol is preferable but isopropyl or denatured alcohol are acceptable. If the specimen is to be processed by the Saccomanno blending technique, 2% polyethylene glycol (Carbowax) must be added. Urothelial cells remain well preserved for processing for several days, regardless of whether the urine is collected after hydration or not, or during the morning hours or later during the day. Urine osmolality does not significantly influence cell preservation, but a low pH is desirable and the ingestion of 1 g of vitamin C at bedtime before examination has been recommended. This is not practical for screening purposes and we have not followed this procedure in our own laboratory.

Bladder Washings

Bladder washings with normal saline or Ringer's solution performed at cystoscopy, if indicated in combination with biopsies or resections, produce a highly cellular specimen that contains more cell clusters than seen in voided urine. This procedure is recommended whenever a cystoscopy is performed and is the specimen that should be used for flow cytometric studies. The washings should also be collected in equal amounts of alcohol for fixation.

Washings and Brushings of Ureters and Renal Pelvis

If lesions in this region are suspected, washings and brushings can be obtained by retrograde catheterization. These specimens are characterized by the presence of large numbers of multinucleated urothelial cells and by greater variation in their appearance than bladder specimens and must be interpreted conservatively.

Sample Preparation

Smears of Fresh and Fixed Specimens. Direct smears may be prepared after centrifugation of 50 ml of urine for 5 to 10 minutes at 1200 rpm. Albuminized slides or the addition of celloidin solution are recommended for better attachment of cells to the slides. The slides are then stained by the Papanicolaou method. Cytocentrifugation also produces high-quality slides and is used by many laboratories.

Saccomanno Blending Technique

The urine must be collected in Carbowax alcohol fixative for this procedure. In this procedure, the cell button that is obtained after centrifugation is homogenized in an electric shaker for a few seconds and smears of the homogenized sediment are prepared. The air-dried smears must be placed in 95% alcohol for 10 minutes to dissolve the Carbowax and are then stained by the Papanicolaou technique.

Cell Blocks

Urine rarely contains adequate material for the preparation of cell blocks, but if visible sediment or tissue fragments are present, a cell block should be prepared.

Filter Preparations

Filter preparations consistently provide greater cellularity than sediment smears and good cellular detail. The procedure for urine specimen preparation in our laboratory is as follows:

Specimens are collected in 100-ml cups containing 50 ml of 50% isopropyl alcohol. An equal volume of urine should be added. Three 8-μ filters are prepared. They allow red blood cells and bacteria to pass through in order not to obscure cellular detail.

Filter preparation is as follows:

1. Wet a glass grid with saline.
2. Place a filter on the grid.
3. Place a funnel on the grid with a clamp.
4. Mix the specimen well and pour into the funnel. Use approximately one third of the specimen per filter; stop when filtration slows.

5. Break suction before the entire specimen has run through the filter so that the filter is not permitted to dry.
6. Remove the filter and clip it to a glass slide that has been identified with the specimen accession number, and immediately place it in 95% ethyl alcohol. Fix for 20 to 30 minutes.
7. Stain by the Papanicolaou method.
8. After staining, remove the filter from the slide, turn it cell side down on the slide and blot dry. (The filter will be slightly opaque when completely dry.)
9. With the slide on a flat, even surface, rapidly flood the filter with chloroform and cover with a glass Petri dish to allow the filter to evaporate slowly.
10. When the filter is completely dry, dip the slide into xylene and cover with a coverslip. If the filter dries cloudy, reflood it and allow it to dry again. This should remove the cloudiness.

UROTHELIUM AND SPECIALIZED LINING

Histology

Urinary tract cytology is almost exclusively concerned with evaluation of the *urothelium* that lines the urinary bladder and other excretory passages, namely the renal pelves, ureters and portions of the urethra. The epithelium is adaptable to the changing volume and permits the storage and expulsion of the urine. This *transitional cell epithelium* is highly specialized and uniform but does include epithelial buds, subepithelial often centrally cystic nests (the nests of Brunn) and areas of squamous metaplasia or squamous variance. The transitional epithelial cells have unique ultrastructural features including surface folds that are believed to provide additional plasma membrane during bladder expansion and robust junctional complexes that provide a watertight seal (Fig. 17–2). The predominant transitional cell epithelium or urothelium in the calices is two or three cells thick and in the ureters, four or five. The empty bladder is lined by six to eight layers of transitional cells. Three cell types are recognizable by light microscopy. These are the large, often binucleated or multinucleated superficial cells covering the cells that form the lower portions of the epithelium-like umbrellas. The underlying intermediate pyramidal cells are smaller and somewhat elongated. A layer of even smaller cuboidal cells with little cytoplasm is located adjacent to the basement membrane. The three cell types can be distinguished by flow cytometry and by different patterns of lectin binding. These cells can also be well defined by morphologic examination of urine specimens. The superficial cells are characterized by a shape maintained by a rigid surface membrane. They have an acidophilic cytoplasm. Many are binucleated (Fig. 17–3), and some (approximately 3%) are multinucleated (Fig. 17–4). The nuclei are large and are apt to undergo reactive change. The intermediate and basal cells are similar and have well-developed desmosomal connections and a plasma membrane that

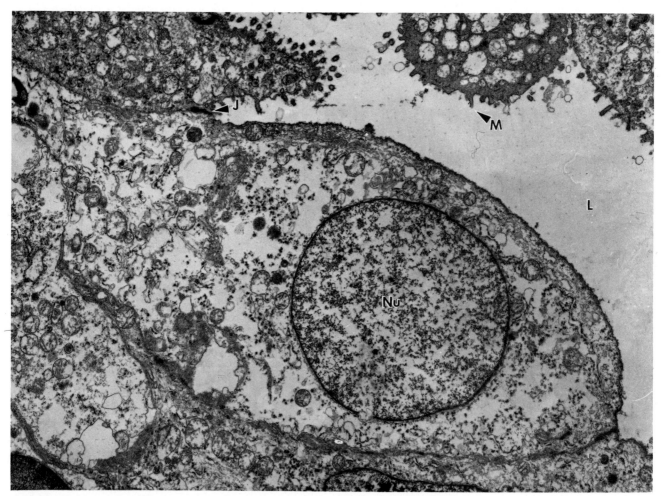

FIGURE 17–2. Electron photomicrograph of an apical portion of **transitional epithelium** showing the lumen (L) of the bladder. The epithelial cell develops villous processes (M) that represent the surface folds thought to provide additional plasma membrane during bladder expansion. In this rather relaxed cell the nucleus (Nu) is rounded and the cytoplasm rather pale. The robust junctional complex (J) is seen to provide a watertight seal just below the lumen (×12,000). (Courtesy of Dr. M.J. Patterson, Department of Pathology, The Hospital of the Good Samaritan, Los Angeles, CA.)

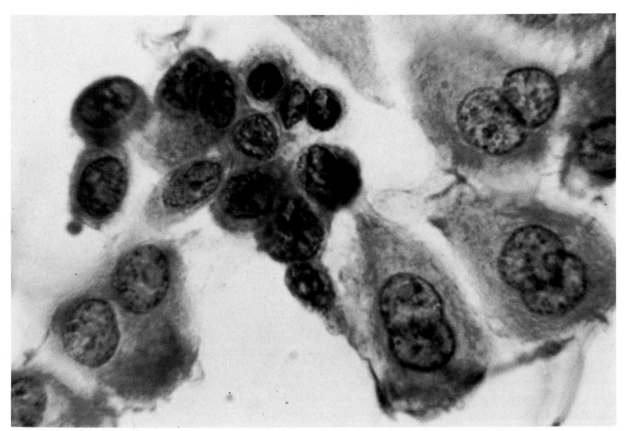

FIGURE 17–3. Normal transitional urothelial cells. The large cells are from the superficial and the small cells from the basal layers (Papanicolaou stain; ×350). (With permission from Gamarra MC and Zeim T: Cytologic spectrum of bladder cancer. Urology 23:(Suppl 3) 23–26, 1984.)

is folded in the empty bladder. It is capable of unfolding when the bladder becomes dilated. The arrangement of these cells is regular with their long axis perpendicular to the basal membrane. Their cytoplasm contains glycogen, often resulting in a clear appearance during processing. The superficial cells also contain glycogen and may contain mucus.

The prostatic segment of the male urethra is lined by transitional epithelium, but the short membranous and long cavernous urethra are lined by stratified or pseudostratified columnar epithelium. The epithelium near the meatus is squamous. Many recesses, namely the lacunae of Morgagni, communicate with deeper branching tubules and the glands of Littre. The epithelium of the female urethra near the bladder is also transitional and in the remaining parts usually squamous, often with interspersed areas of pseudostratified columnar epithelium. Invaginations that are lined by mucus-producing cells similar to those found in the glands of Littre may be present.

Normal Cytology

Transitional epithelial cells are present in all urine specimens. In voided urine they occur singly or in the form of loosely cohesive clusters or sheets. They vary considerably in size (Fig. 17–5), with a cell diameter from 9 to 40 μ and a cell size of 75 to 1400 square μ with a mean of 340 square μ. The cytoplasm is opaque (Fig. 17–6), granular or vacuolated (Fig. 17–7). Renal tubular epithelial cells are rarely found in voided or catheterized urine, except in cases of renal transplant rejection or renal parenchymal disease (Fig. 17–8). The renal tubular epithelial cells have round nuclei and usually a granular cytoplasm. Many transitional

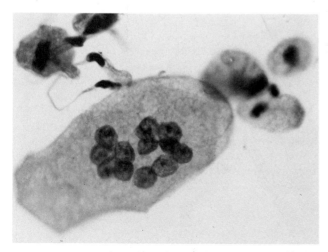

FIGURE 17–4. Multinucleated superficial cell from ureteral catheterization (Papanicolaou stain; ×900).

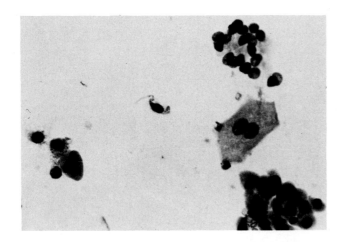

FIGURE 17–5. Large superficial and smaller pyramidal or basal cells (Papanicolaou stain; ×360).

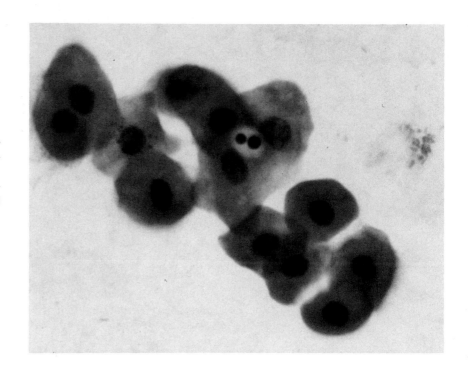

FIGURE 17–6. Clusters of **normal transitional epithelial cells** with dense cytoplasm (Papanicolaou stain; ×900). (With permission from Kern WH: Epithelial cells in urine sediments. Am J Clin Pathol 56:67–72, 1971).

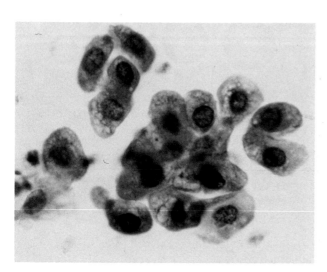

FIGURE 17–7. Transitional epithelial cells with prominently vacuolated cytoplasm (Papanicolaou stain; ×900). (With permission from Kern WH: Epithelial cells in urine sediments. Am J Clin Pathol 56:67–72, 1971.)

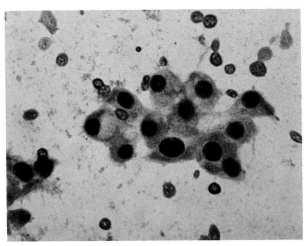

FIGURE 17–8. Renal tubular epithelial cells from imprint smear. The cells are of a size similar to that of transitional epithelial cells and have uniform, round nuclei (Papanicolaou stain; ×1000). (With permission from Kern WH: Epithelial cells in urine sediments. Am J Clin Pathol 56:67–72, 1971.)

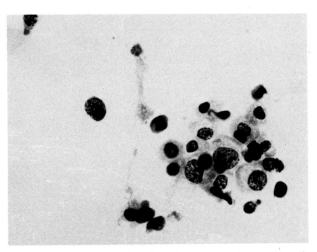

FIGURE 17–10. Ureteral catheterization specimen. **Superficial urothelial cells** showing slight anisonucleosis and "salt-and-pepper" nuclei (Papanicolaou stain; ×320).

cells are elongated or columnar (Fig. 17–9). The nuclei are usually round, but they may be irregular in outline or may appear pyknotic. Large superficial or binucleated cells, often with relatively large nuclei that have a salt-and-pepper appearance, are particularly common in ureteral catheterization specimens (Fig. 17–10). The nuclei average 7.5 μ in diameter and vary from 10 to 90 square μ in size, with a mean of 36 square μ.[21] The nucleoplasm is usually bland or vesicular, and the chromatin pattern of most nuclei is finely granular or has a salt-and-pepper appearance. Small nucleoli are rarely present. The cytoplasmic and nuclear features of 500 normal urothelial cells are shown in Table 17–1 and are compared with those of hyperplastic and neoplastic urothelial cells.

The described three cell types of the urothelium, namely, the large, often multinucleated superficial

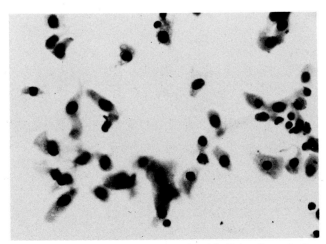

FIGURE 17–9. Normal transitional epithelial cells including many cells of columnar configuration (Papanicolaou stain; ×320).

cells, the intermediate pyramidal cells and the cuboidal cells adjacent to the basement membrane, can be identified in single cell suspensions prepared from tissues and in voided and catheterized urine specimens. Eldidi and Patten[14] reported that the basal cells have a mean cytoplasmic area of 82 square μ, a mean nuclear area of 24 square μ and a relative nuclear area of 29 square μ. They are predominantly oval, with basophilic, dense cytoplasm and single nuclei. The pyramidal cells are larger, with a mean cell area of 229 square μ and a mean nuclear area of 40 square μ. They are also predominantly oval with a basophilic cytoplasm and well-defined cell borders. The nuclei are generally single and oval. The superficial cells are considerably larger, with a mean area of 500 square μ and a mean nuclear area of 64 square μ. The relative nuclear area is 13%. These cells are less basophilic. Binucleation occurs in 19% and 3% are multinucleated. Most nuclei are oval. Nucleoli are more prominent than in the smaller cells. Pyramidal or intermediate cells predominate in voided urine, but 42% of cells in catheterized urine are superficial. They are particularly prominent in ureteral catherization specimens. Cell aggregates and cytoplasmic molding are also more common in catheterized rather than voided specimens. The large multinucleated cells that are prominent in ureteral or renal pelvic washings may contain as many as 20 or 30 centrally crowded nuclei (see Fig. 17–4).

Squamous cells of intermediate and less commonly of superficial type are often present, more commonly in women (Figs. 17–11 and 17–12). They exfoliate from portions of the urethra that are lined by squamous epithelium, from areas of squamous metaplasia in the urinary bladder or from zones of squamous epithelium that may be found in the trigone of women. Some squamous cells may represent vaginal contamination. The squamous cells present do reflect the effect of estrogen. Areas of squamous metaplasia are often regular and well differentiated, and the exfoliated squamous cells cannot be distinguished from those that exfoliate from areas where squamous epithelium is

TABLE 17–1. Cytoplasmic and Nuclear Features

Cytoplasm	Normal	Benign Atypical	Papillary Carcinoma Grade I	Papillary Carcinoma Grade II	Transitional Carcinoma Grade III-IV
Number of cells evaluated	500	1186	3433	2091	1719
Isodiametric cells (%)	21	19	27	19	19
Round	17	17	26	18	18
Polygonal	4	2	1	1	1
Nonisodiametric (%)	79	81	73	81	81
Oval	36	19	13	12	9
Irregular	43	62	60	69	72
Vacuolation (%)					
None	44	36	40	27	32
Diffuse	48	43	44	52	50
Large and discrete	8	21	16	21	18

Nuclei	Normal	Benign Atypical	Papillary Carcinoma Grade I	Papillary Carcinoma Grade II	Transitional Carcinoma Grade III-IV
Number of nuclei evaluated	500	1260	3460	2107	1758
Nuclear shape (%)					
Round	7	19	12	12	9
Oval	50	30	23	25	16
Irregular	43	51	65	63	75
Hyperchromasia (%)					
Bland or vesicular	47	20	13	13	8
Slight	17	27	20	19	18
Moderate	13	29	30	29	31
Marked	23	24	37	39	43
Nucleoli (%)					
Present	1	21	27	27	43
Multiple	—	10	14	16	29
Macro.	—	1	4	7	11
Chromatin pattern (%)					
Opaque	20	20	22	20	15
Finely granular	79	60	30	20	11
Coarsely granular	1	20	48	60	74

(Reproduced with permission from Kern WH: The cytology of transitional cell carcinoma of the urinary bladder. Acta Cytol 19:422, 1975.)

normally found. The Brunn nests are buds or sprouts of transitional epithelium that grow from the surface into the underlying lamina propria and may become centrally cavitated or cystic. The cells lining the cystic spaces may remain flattened or low cuboidal and resemble transitional cells, but they may become columnar and mucinous. These changes are considered to be reactive and metaplastic. When the morphologic appearance is characterized by the presence of mucin-secreting colonic-type epithelium, they are referred to as cystitis glandularis or as intestinal or glandular metaplasia. Many of the columnar cells that are often

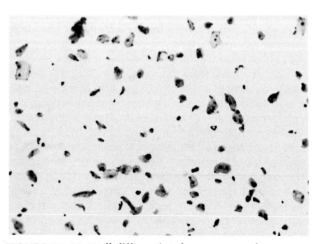

FIGURE 17–11. Well-differentiated squamous and some urothelial cells (Papanicolaou stain; ×80).

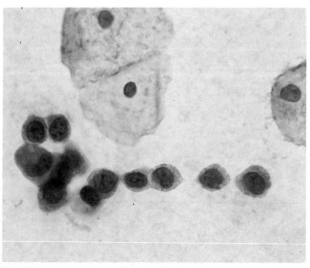

FIGURE 17–12. Normal urothelial and squamous cells (Papanicolaou stain; ×500).

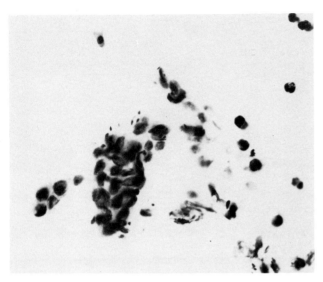

FIGURE 17–13. Prostatic columnar cells and spermatozoa obtained after prostatic massage (Papanicolaou stain; ×320).

seen in urine are cells from the intermediate zone of the transitional epithelium, but they may exfoliate from metaplastic columnar or glandular epithelium, from the urethra and, in males after instrumentation or prostatic massage, from the prostate (Fig. 17–13). Spontaneous exfoliation of prostatic columnar cells or of cells from the seminal vesicles that may contain cytoplasmic pigment is rarely, if ever, observed. The lacunae of Morgagni and glands of Littre are other possible sites of origin. Most columnar cells are non-ciliated but rarely, ciliated cells have been described in voided urine.[39] They may represent cells from the vasa deferentia or the epididymis, structures that are lined by columnar cells with stereocilia, or they may be the result of an unusual differentiation. The morphologic appearance of columnar cells depends on their site of origin. If benign, the nuclei are oval, uniform or bland or have a finely granular chromatin pattern.

Small numbers of polymorphonuclear leukocytes are often present in normal urine. Histiocytes are found in inflammatory conditions but, in small numbers, may be present in normal urine. They have indistinct cell borders, a foamy cytoplasm and eccentric, lobed or bean-shaped nuclei. They are often difficult to differentiate from degenerated epithelial cells. Spermatozoa (see Fig. 17–13), crystals and *Trichomonas* organisms may be seen.

Degenerative changes of exfoliated cells that were suspended in urine, in the bladder or after voiding do occur and may interfere with interpretation. The urine osmolality ranges from 100 to over 1000 mOs per liter, with an average of 500, and is rarely in the normal range for serum (275 to 300 mOs per liter). This suspension in a usually hyper- but sometimes hypotonic fluid should be associated with degenerative changes in the cells, but extensive quantitative studies in our laboratory did not demonstrate a relationship between either cell size or degree of degenerative change with the osmolality. We were also unable to demonstrate

such changes with the urine pH, although medication with ascorbic acid is recommended by some in order to acidify for better cytologic preservation. The most important step to eliminate degenerative changes is immediate fixation of the collected urine with an equal amount of 50% alcohol. If this prompt fixation is then followed by well-controlled cytopreparation, in our laboratory with the filter technique as described, degenerative changes do not interfere with interpretation. Reactive changes may be difficult to differentiate from neoplastic ones, as described later, but the most significant problem in interpretation is the distinction of the large superficial cells from tumor cells. The morphology of these cells must be known. Their prominence in ureteral catheterization specimens is particularly striking. In our own consultative practice, the specimens that are most commonly referred for review are ureteral, with many large superficial cells that were initially incorrectly interpreted as tumor cells. This misinterpretation has led to several nephrectomies of nonneoplastic kidneys.

NONNEOPLASTIC ABNORMALITIES

Developmental Abnormalities

Patency of the urachus at the vesicle end of the structure may lead to a urachal diverticulum or to the presence of remnants of columnar epithelium in this area. This may be a source of exfoliated columnar cells in the urine, and adenocarcinomas are known to develop from this tissue. Exstrophic bladders may also be lined by columnar epithelium that may become the site of adenocarcinomas. Cytology does not play a role in the evaluation of this abnormality.

Endometriosis

Endometriosis is the growth of endometrial glands accompanied by endometrial stroma in abnormal locations. It commonly involves the ovaries and pelvic peritoneum and less commonly the colon, appendix, vagina and umbilicus. Although even less common than at those sites, endometriosis of the urinary tract has been reported and the bladder is the most common site of involvement.[35] The condition usually occurs in women of childbearing age. The symptoms include hematuria which may be cyclic, dysuria and suprapubic pain. If the surface epithelium is involved and the urothelium is penetrated, endometrial stromal and glandular cells may be shed into the urine. The cytologic presentation of these endometrial cells in urine is very similar to that seen in vaginal smears. The presence of small cells with a high nucleocytoplasmic ratio in a urinary specimen raises the possibility of poorly differentiated urothelial carcinoma or lymphoma, but the marked uniformity of the cells and their occurrence in exodus-type clusters should suggest the possibility of endometriosis of the bladder.

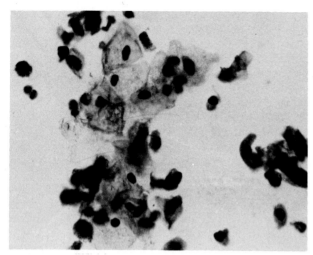

FIGURE 17–14. Metaplastic squamous cells and well-differentiated transitional epithelial cells (Papanicolaou stain; ×320).

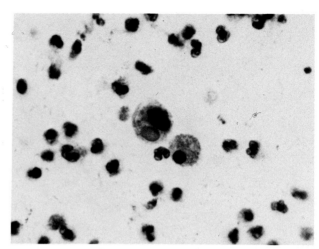

FIGURE 17–15. Acute inflammation (cystitis). An eosinophilic inclusion is present in degenerating urothelial cells (Papanicolaou stain; ×500).

Diverticulosis of the Urinary Bladder

Diverticula of the urinary bladder may be congenital, but they often develop because of partial urinary obstruction in the bladder neck region, most commonly caused by nodular hyperplasia of the prostate. The ostium into the bladder is usually large but may be narrow or pinpoint in size. The bladder mucosa is often chronically inflamed, and in many cases, the urothelium is replaced by metaplastic squamous epithelium. The mere presence of squamous cells in urine obviously does not permit a diagnosis of diverticulum, but if this finding can be combined with the clinical information, it may suggest such a diagnosis (Fig. 17–14). Evidence of hyperkeratosis and of squamous dysplasia must be reported because squamous as well as transitional cell carcinomas may develop in diverticula.

Nonspecific and Bacterial Inflammation

Inflammation of the lower urinary tract is commonly caused by bacteria, usually as a complication of an obstructive process such as prostatic hyperplasia or carcinoma, strictures or calculi (Fig. 17–15). In our institution, positive urine cultures most frequently contain *Escherichia coli* (32%), streptococcus group D (10%), *Proteus mirabilis* (9%), *Pseudomonas aeruginosa* (9%) and *Klebsiella pneumoniae* (6%) organisms. Tuberculosis of the bladder is usually associated with and secondary to tuberculosis of the kidneys.

Regardless of the etiology, cystitis is cytologically characterized by the presence of polymorphonuclear leukocytes, necrotic debris, histiocytes, degenerative changes in urothelial cells, urothelial hyperplasia and often urothelial atypia (Fig. 17–16). The slightly greater irregularity of the cell outlines and the increased percentage of cells that contain generally small nucleoli and occasionally have a coarsely granular

nucleoplasm are illustrated in Table 17–1. Red blood cells are invariably present. The transitional cells are increased in number and are often obscured by the inflammatory cell population. The nuclei tend to be moderately enlarged, to an average nuclear diameter of 8 to 10 µ. They often contain clear zones or chromatin "bars" and may contain nucleoli. The cellular outline is usually hazy (Fig. 17–17). Degenerated cells may be large and may have a clear or vacuolated cytoplasm that contains collections of polymorphonuclear leukocytes. Sizeable clusters of partially necrotic cells may be present. The coarsely granular pattern of malignant urothelial cells or macronucleoli are not seen. A very dense, cellular inflammatory exudate associated with hyperplastic or degenerating urothelial cells or partially necrotic cell clusters without the nuclear characteristic of malignancy or severe dysplasia is of infectious or inflammatory origin. Even extensively ulcerated and necrotic transitional cell carcino-

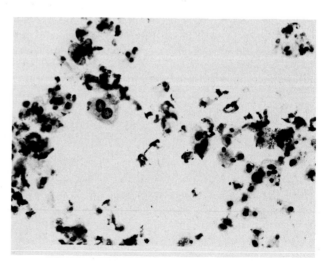

FIGURE 17–16. Acute inflammation. Inflammatory debris and reactive urothelial cells are present (Papanicolaou stain; ×320).

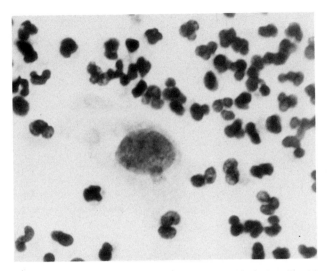

FIGURE 17–17. Acute cystitis. A large urothelial cell with relatively bland nucleus and ill-defined cytoplasm is present (Papanicolaou stain; × 1000). (With permission from Kern WH: Epithelial cells in urine sediments. Am J Clin Pathol 56:67–72, 1971.)

mas of the urinary bladder invariably exfoliate unequivocally malignant cells and a greater amount of necrotic material and relatively fewer leukocytes than is the case in cystitis.

Virus Infections

A number of virus infections cause morphologically characteristic changes in renal cells and in urothelium. Cytomegalic inclusion disease is caused by the *cytomegalovirus* (CMV), a member of the herpesvirus group. It is spread by intrauterine or perinatal transmission to the fetus by an infected mother, sexually or through blood products. Young children and patients who are immunosuppressed because of cancer or acquired immunodeficiency syndrome (AIDS) or who suffer from immunosuppression associated with transplants are at risk. The renal tubular epithelium is frequently involved, and the disease is seen in renal transplant patients. The affected renal tubular cells are enlarged and contain large basophilic or eosinophilic single nuclear inclusions that are surrounded by clear halos. The inclusions are sharply demarcated from the nuclear membrane. Remnants of the chromatin are condensed peripherally. Papovaviruses are divided into two groups: papillomaviruses and polyomaviruses. The polyomavirus is of particular importance in urine cytology because active infection is usually localized to the brain and urinary tract. Urinary excretion of viruses in pregnant women has been reported, showing that the fetus is at risk of infection.[1] Like CMV, the virus also infects or is reactivated if the host's immunity is impaired by immunosuppressive drugs such as those given to renal allograft recipients, in AIDS or in cancer patients. The virus is readily recognized morphologically in cells exfoliated in the urinary tract, and the principal differential diagnosis is with CMV. The inclu-

sion-bearing cells are even larger than those infected with CMV and contain dense, basophilic, homogeneous nuclear inclusion bodies (Fig. 17–18). The nuclear membranes are thickened. In contrast to the CMV-infected cell in which the virus inclusions are surrounded by a clear zone, the basophilic homogeneous inclusion in a polyomavirus-infected cell often completely fills the enlarged nucleus. If a clear halo remains, it is sharply distinguished from the thickened nuclear membrane. Electron-microscopic examination shows the virus particles to be unencapsulated, in contrast to the encapsulation observed in CMV (Fig. 17–19). Immunoperoxidase procedures with simian virus 40 antiserum have been successfully used to confirm infection by polyomavirus (Fig. 17–20). The *human papilloma virus* is responsible for condylomatous lesions in the lower urinary tract, but these lesions are generally confined to the urethra and the mucocutaneous regions of the meatus and are readily accessible for biopsy and excision. Koilocytosis and other morphologic changes characteristic for this condition are described elsewhere.

Malakoplakia

Malakoplakia is a granulomatous disease of the bladder or upper urinary tract. Multiple soft, nodular, often umbilicated yellowish plaques appear in the mucosa and submucosa, frequently in the region of the trigone. They may be mistaken for cancer clinically and are associated with immunodeficiency states. Several cases have been seen in transplant patients.

Histologically, the plaques are found to consist of epithelioid histiocytes with a granular, acidophilic cytoplasm. Some of the cells contain homogeneous or

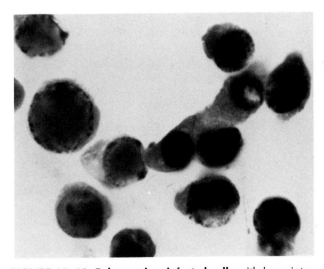

FIGURE 17–18. Polyomavirus-infected cells with large intranuclear inclusions and degenerated cytoplasm (Papanicolaou stain; × 1000). (With permission from Akura K, et al: Use of immunocytochemistry on urinary sediments for the rapid identification of human polyomavirus infection. Acta Cytol 32:247–251, 1988.)

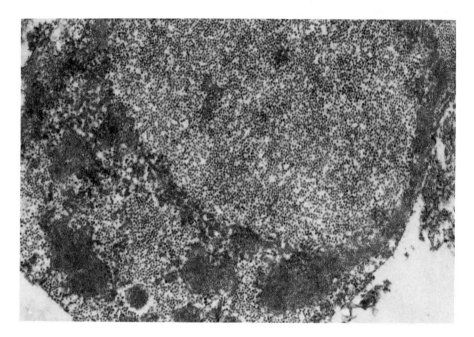

FIGURE 17–19. Electron photomicrograph of **polyomavirus-infected cell.** The nucleus is packed with small round virus particles of 40 nm diameter (×20,000). (With permission from Akura K, et al: Use of immunocytochemistry on urinary sediments for the rapid identification of human polyomavirus infection. Acta Cytol 32:247–251, 1988.)

FIGURE 17–20. Papovavirus nuclear antigen is detected in the nuclei of the two infected cells on the right. The transitional cell at the lower left did not stain (Papanicolaou immunoperoxidase stain; hematoxylin counter stain; ×1000). (With permission from Akura K, et al: Use of immunocytochemistry on urinary sediments for the rapid identification of human polyomavirus infection. Acta Cytol 32:247–251, 1988.)

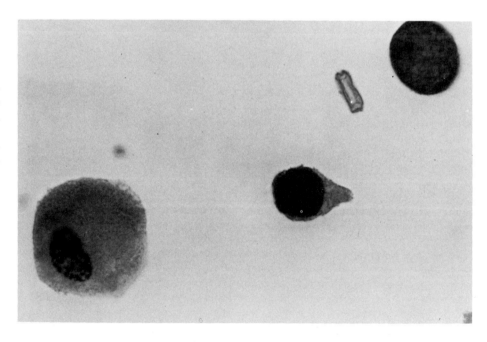

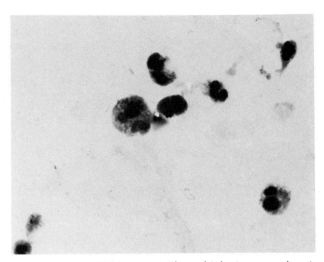

FIGURE 17–21. Histiocytes with multiple intracytoplasmic inclusions consistent with **malakoplakia** (Papanicolaou stain; ×320).

concentrically layered intracytoplasmic inclusions known as Michaelis-Gutmann bodies or calcospherites. The inclusions are basophilic and periodic acid-Schiff positive and stain for iron and calcium. They may represent the end result of bacterial degradation and degenerative changes, and the process is regarded by some as a defect in the host macrophage response to bacterial infection, usually gram-negative bacilli. The urine contains histiocytes of this type, often with multiple granules in a foamy cytoplasm (Fig. 17–21). Some may be found to contain the calcospherites that average 8 μ in diameter. The condition is rare, and finding cells that are diagnostic is exceptional.

Degenerative Changes

Disintegration of the cytoplasm, pyknosis of the nuclei and karyolysis of the nuclei of scattered transitional cells may be seen in urine from healthy individuals as well as in urine containing malignant cells. Because there is often an attached tag of partially preserved cytoplasm, these cells that were initially described by Papanicolaou are referred to as comet cells or decoy cells. They may have some of the characteristics of malignancy, and it is therefore important that they be recognized for what they are.[8] The cells for the most part contain round or oval nuclei that have a coarse chromatin network or are completely hyperchromatic. The previously referred-to tag of cytoplasm may be attached, but it may be absent. Occasional cells are binucleate. They are a major pitfall and can be misinterpreted as malignant. The smooth nuclear outline, evidence of cytoplasmic degeneration, and the usually small number of these abnormal cells in an often hypocellular urine specimen should prevent a false-positive diagnosis. It should be noted that they are rare in immediately fixed urine specimens that are processed by filter preparation.

Intracytoplasmic and Intranuclear Inclusions

Inclusions other than those caused by viruses may be present in epithelial cells in urine. Some studies have concluded that the presence of eosinophilic intracytoplasmic inclusion bodies (EIBs) is not correlated with a specific disease and may be a degenerative phenomenon (see Fig. 17–15). Other studies indicate that many intracytoplasmic and intranuclear inclusion-bearing cells are related to heavy metal toxicity or are related to drugs or chemotherapy, microorganisms, metabolic disorders or immunologic alterations (Fig. 17–22). It has been demonstrated by quantitative studies that the EIBs are significantly associated with degenerative changes. Only rare cells with inclusion bodies have intact nuclei. The inclusions are more common in women over the age of 50 years and in voided rather than catheterized specimens, further indicating the possibility of degenerative change. Increased numbers of EIBs have definitely been demonstrated, however, in industrial workers exposed to lead, in immunosuppressed renal transplant patients and in diverse disease processes, including mucocutaneous lymph node syndrome (Kawasaki disease).

Cytologic Changes Associated with Calculi

Urinary tract calculi may be associated with cytologic changes and atypias that are a major cause of false-positive cytologic diagnoses. The changes are often due to uric acid calculi in the upper urinary tract. If they are thought to be related to a mass lesion in a renal pelvis or ureter, a false-positive diagnosis has at times resulted in an unjustified nephrectomy. Two major studies of this subject[17, 34] showed the cytologic examination of the urine to be normal in 53 and 87% of the cases, respectively. Hematuria and leukocyturia were observed in many of the specimens that showed no other significant abnormalities. The cytologic atypias were characterized by the presence of clusters of

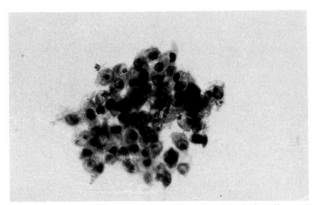

FIGURE 17–22. Cluster of **transitional epithelial cells** with prominent intranuclear inclusions (Papanicolaou stain; ×320).

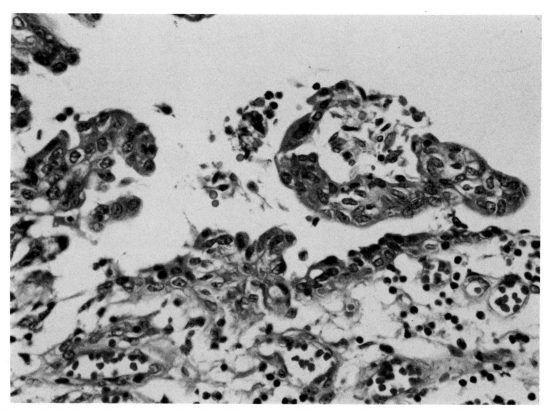

FIGURE 17–23. Urothelium in a calculus-containing kidney with surface ulceration and shedding of papillary transitional cell cluster (original magnification ×100). (With permission from Highman W and Wilson E: Urine cytology in patients with calculi. J Clin Pathol 35:350–356, 1982.)

transitional epithelial cells with smooth borders and 5 to 150 cells per cluster. They were often papillary in shape (Fig. 17–23). Nuclei were centrally located, of normal size and shape and surrounded by an even rim of cytoplasm. The cells that were considered suspicious of carcinoma and, in one of the series, caused a false-positive cytologic diagnosis in 4% of the patients were arranged in irregular clusters of transitional cells with ragged borders. The nuclear morphology was abnormal, with nuclear pleomorphism and variable staining. Some nuclei were large, with prominent nucleoli and a coarse granular chromatin, and others were darker and dense. Occasional mitoses were seen.

The cytologic appearance of these abnormal cells includes many criteria of malignancy. Although it is not possible to distinguish individual cells or a few cell clusters from those exfoliated from malignant tumors, knowledge of the clinical history and the radiologic findings is helpful. The fact that urine specimens from patients with tumors almost invariably contain numerous malignant cells, including many more single malignant cells and, in papillary tumors, cell clusters, should also aid in avoiding a false-positive diagnosis. Furthermore, more than half of urine specimens from patients with calculi show no significant epithelial abnormalities at all, and the only finding may be hematuria. If abnormalities exist they involve relatively few cells, and in a majority of cases, the clusters are smooth bordered and the individual transitional cells may vary in size but are well differentiated as noted previously (Fig. 17–24). The urine of some patients with calculi

contains increased numbers of large but cytologically benign–appearing multinucleated superficial transitional cells. It has been suggested that there may be a relation between calculi and cancer of the upper urogenital tract, but this has not been clearly established.

Iatrogenic Changes

Most of these are related to treatment for cancer of the urinary tract and will be described in that section.

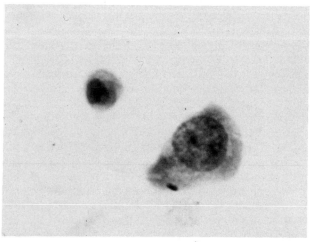

FIGURE 17–24. Size variation in **transitional epithelial cells** (Papanicolaou stain; ×100).

Hyperplasia, Atypia and Dysplasia

These changes are or may be precursors of tumors of the urothelium and will be described in that section.

TUMORS OF THE URINARY TRACT

Approximately 70,000 tumors of the urinary tract are newly diagnosed in the United States annually, including approximately 47,000 carcinomas of the urinary bladder. Between 75 and 85% of these cases are superficial. The urothelial tumors may be papillary or nonpapillary and invasive or *in situ*. Nonpapillary tumors and at least the poorly differentiated papillary tumors arise from areas of atypical urothelial proliferation. Mapping of the urinary bladder in cystectomy specimens clearly demonstrates the association of epithelial atypias and carcinoma *in situ* with invasive nonpapillary carcinoma. Papillary and nonpapillary tumors often coexist in the same patient but the development of well-differentiated papillary tumors from areas of epithelial atypia is not as clearly demonstrable, and these tumors are often surrounded by normal-appearing urothelium. Because of their different biologic behavior and different cytologic presentation, the papillary and nonpapillary tumors will be discussed separately. All tumors of the urothelium exfoliate readily into the urinary stream. The great majority occur in the urinary bladder. Squamous and glandular components may be present. The tumors that arise below the surface epithelium such as in renal parenchyma or in the prostate are unlikely to exfoliate until they have become large and disrupt the urothelial lining. Urine cytology is rarely a means of primary diagnosis in these cases.

Transitional Cell Papilloma

Transitional cell papillomas of the urinary bladder are uncommon benign papillary tumors with thin fibrovascular cores that are covered by cytologically normal or nearly normal urothelium that is less than seven layers in thickness (Fig. 17–25). The tumors are small and may be multiple, and they may arise in areas of the urothelium that, like the tumors themselves, usually show no significant cytologic atypia. Inverted transitional cell papillomas or "Brunnian adenomas" are another variant of benign urothelial tumors that are composed of well-differentiated transitional epithelial cells. These tumors occur mainly in elderly men and are located in the trigone, bladder neck or prostatic urethra. They are composed of invaginated urothelium resembling that of the nests of Brunn and are covered by layers of benign urothelium on the surface. Because of the small size of transitional papillomas and the good cohesion of the near-normal cells, exfoliation is scant. Although there may be increased numbers of clusters of urothelial cells, a cytologic diagnosis is rarely, if ever, possible. The same is true for the inverted papillomas that are covered by normal uro-

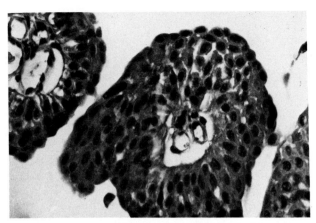

FIGURE 17–25. Transitional cell papilloma. A delicate vascularized stalk is covered by five to seven layers of well-differentiated transitional epithelial cells (Papanicolaou stain; ×160).

thelium. These tumors can be effectively treated by transurethral resection and recur infrequently, and if cytologically malignant cells are found in their presence, they invariably exfoliate from areas of dysplasia or carcinoma *in situ* that may coexist. Because of the good differentiation and minimal deviation from normal of the epithelial cells of papillomas, there are no specific findings that permit a cytologic diagnosis. The specimens from patients with papillomas, nevertheless, are usually not normal.[44] The exfoliated epithelium is abundant in approximately one third of such cases, and few specimens are scantily cellular. However, in one half of 50 cases, the overall cellularity was similar to that of cases without tumors. Red blood cells are present slightly more frequently in patients with papilloma than in other urologic patients. The most common abnormality in papillomas is the presence of elongated epithelial cells (Fig. 17–26). These must be

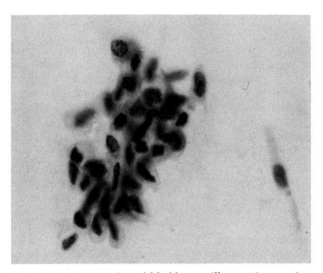

FIGURE 17–26. Imprint of bladder papilloma. Elongated or spindle-shaped cells with somewhat angular and slightly hyperchromatic nuclei (Papanicolaou stain; ×560). (With permission from Wolinska WH, et al: Cytology of bladder papilloma. Acta Cytol 29:817–822, 1985.)

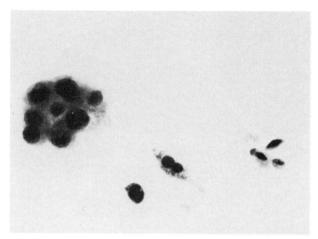

FIGURE 17–27. Cluster of urothelial cells that exfoliated from a **papilloma**. The nuclei appear to be slightly enlarged and hyperchromatic but are very uniform (Papanicolaou stain; ×320).

distinguished from the elongated smooth muscle cells that are sometimes found in catheterized urine specimens or in voided urine after manipulation. Smaller round epithelial cells tend to be loosely clustered (Fig. 17–27), and the elongated cells are usually single. The nuclei of the exfoliated cells are minimally or not at all abnormal, and any significant deviation from normal relates to the cell shape. The minimal cytologic abnormalities that are present are within the range of atypia that may be induced by inflammatory or irritative processes. The cytologic findings may be described as consistent with or suggestive of papilloma, particularly if the clinical history or review of slide material indicates that the patient had such tumors in the past, but a definite cytologic diagnosis cannot be made.

Papillary Transitional Cell Carcinoma

Papillary transitional cell carcinomas include noninvasive papillary tumors that resemble papillomas but are characterized by a thicker (more than seven cell layers) urothelium, slight abnormality in the architecture with occasional broader papillae and greater cytologic atypia than is seen in papillomas. The moderately differentiated (grade II) tumors have even broader and blunter papillae, usually infiltrate the submucosa and have nuclei that are larger and slightly pleomorphic, show increased mitotic activity, are hyperchromatic and may be aneupolid (Fig. 17–28). Most pathologic classifications use only three grades, and if not, grades III and IV should be combined in the assessment of the biologic potential. These higher-grade tumors are invariably invasive and often extend into the muscle layer. Only surface portions may retain a papillary configuration, and the papillary processes are markedly blunted. The nuclei are even larger and more pleomorphic, and the nucleocytoplasmic ratio is high. Mitoses are frequent and bizarre cell forms are present. Squamous and, less commonly, glandular neo-

plastic components may be present in a few of the high-grade papillary tumors, but less commonly so than in nonpapillary carcinomas.

The *cytologic findings* in urine depend on the grade of the tumor and, conversely, the grade can be predicted based on the cytologic findings. Because the grade is also clearly associated with the depth of invasion, the cytologic findings may further provide information concerning the probable stage of the tumor.

Papillary Transitional Cell Carcinomas, Grade I. These differ only slightly from transitional cell papillomas; they are usually somewhat larger and have a slightly greater degree of cytologic atypia. Similarly, the cytologic findings differ only slightly. In most cases, the urine samples are more cellular than normal and an average of 15 cohesive clusters of four or more cells are present per 1000 cells, approximately eightfold the number of clusters found in normal control urine samples (Fig. 17–29). As in papillomas, some of these cells are elongated and have oval but still relatively small and bland, only slightly hyperchromatic nuclei (Fig. 17–30). Nucleoli are present in approximately 25% of the nuclei. The nucleoplasm of slightly more than half of the nuclei is finely granular or opaque. The single cells present also resemble normal or reactive cells and do not show definite criteria of malignancy as seen in higher-grade tumors (Fig. 17–31). Red blood cells may be increased in number. A cytologic diagnosis is only rarely possible, usually in cases in which the urine is particularly cellular and numerous clusters of moderately atypical cells are present. These findings may be considered consistent with low-grade papillary carcinomas, especially if the patient had such lesions in the past and previous biopsies are available for comparison. Particularly in specimens that contain only few clusters, a distinction from reactive papillary

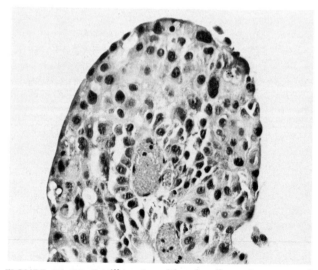

FIGURE 17–28. Papillary transitional cell carcinoma, moderately differentiated (grade II). The papilla is still frond-like, but the tumor cells contain enlarged, moderately irregular and hyperchromatic nuclei (hematoxylin and eosin; ×320).

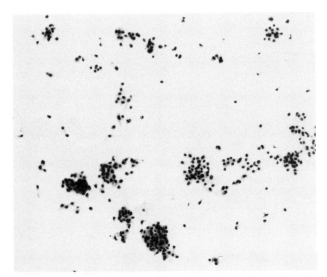

FIGURE 17–29. Voided urine from a patient with **moderately well-differentiated (grade II) papillary transitional cell carcinoma.** Many moderately atypical urothelial cells are present and arranged in clusters (Papanicolaou stain; ×80).

hyperplasia of the type that may be associated with calculi is often not possible (Fig. 17–32). A report may briefly comment on the presence of increased numbers of cells and cell clusters and state that "low-grade papillary tumor must be considered" or "cannot be excluded."

Papillary Transitional Cell Carcinoma, Grade II. This is usually identifiable by cytologic examination. The urine samples are even more cellular, and in over one half of the cases, more than 1000 neoplastic cells will be found in two filter preparations (see Fig. 17–29). The neoplastic cells show more striking nuclear abnormalities and still are frequently arranged in clus-

ters (Fig. 17–33). This considerable cellularity, which is due to the enhanced exfoliation of the neoplastic cells, makes it rarely necessary to examine a second or third specimen. The numerous abnormal cells present must be recognized and interpreted, but the screening that is essential for the interpretation of cervical smears or sputum specimens is generally not required. Table 17–2 shows the number of neoplastic cells present in different categories, ranging from normal to high-grade lesion or grade IV tumor. The nuclei are larger, with a mean nuclear size of 78 square μ, compared with 54 square μ in grade I transitional cell carcinomas, as shown in Figure 17–34. The mean nucleocytoplasmic ratio, which for normal cells is 12 and for papillary carcinomas grade I approximately 37, is further increased to approximately 42.[21] The importance of the nucleocytoplasmic ratio has also been emphasized by Boon and coworkers.[6]

High-Grade (Grade III) Papillary Transitional Cell Carcinomas. These are characterized by highly cellular urine specimens. They are similar to the urine specimens characteristic of high-grade nonpapillary carcinomas, but there are still somewhat larger numbers of cell clusters and minute tissue fragments. The nuclei are more than twice the size of normal nuclei (see Fig. 17–34) and average 90 square μ. They have irregular nuclear outlines and a predominantly coarsely granular chromatin pattern (see Table 17–1). Many contain one or more large or irregularly outlined nucleoli. The degree of hyperchromasia is greater than that of nonneoplastic transitional cells and of cells from welldifferentiated transitional cell carcinomas. This increase in nuclear size, ragged nuclear outlines, coarse chromatin pattern and pleomorphism and the great cellularity permit a diagnosis in almost all cases (Fig. 17–35). Many of these tumors are partially necrotic or ulcerated and red blood cells, leukocytes and necrotic

FIGURE 17–30. Papillary cluster of transitional cells from **low-grade papillary transitional cell carcinoma.** Minimal changes consist of a decreased amount of cytoplasm and slight variability of nuclear size (Papanicolaou stain; ×350). (With permission from Gamarra MC and Zeim T: Cytologic spectrum of bladder cancer. Urology (Suppl 3) 23:23–26, 1984.)

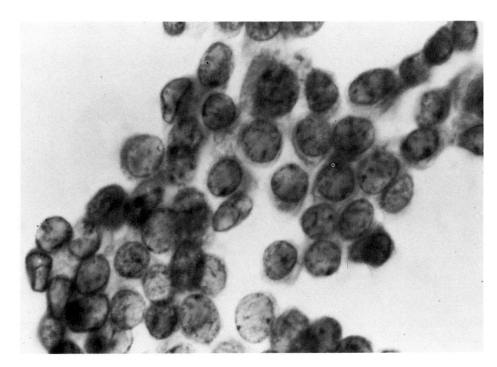

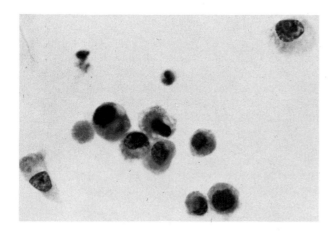

FIGURE 17–31. Transitional epithelial cells that exfoliated from **moderately well-differentiated papillary transitional cell carcinoma.** Slight nuclear pleomorphism and hyperchromasia are seen with a coarse chromatin pattern in some cells (Papanicolaou stain; ×500).

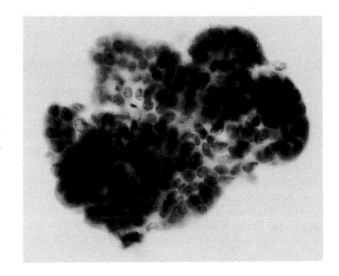

FIGURE 17–32. Papillary cluster of urothelial cells associated with **calculous disease.** A definite cytologic distinction from a low-grade papillary urothelial tumor is not possible (Papanicolaou stain; ×320).

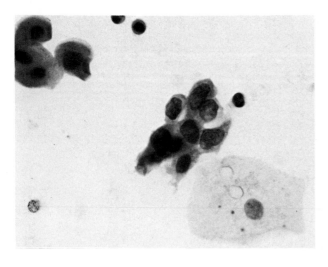

FIGURE 17–33. Cluster of **neoplastic urothelial cells** with moderately enlarged irregular nuclei and increased nucleocytoplasmic (N/C) ratio (Papanicolaou stain; ×500).

TABLE 17–2. Number of Neoplastic Cells in the Different Categories

Neoplastic Cells Present	Normal	Benign Atypical	Papillary Carcinoma Grade I	Papillary Carcinoma Grade II	Transitional Carcinoma Grade III-IV
0	5 (100%)	15 (100%)	—	—	—
<100	—	—	5 (14%)	2 (9%)	2 (11%)
100–500	—	—	12 (32%)	5 (23%)	4 (22%)
500–1000	—	—	5 (14%)	2 (9%)	1 (6%)
>1000	—	—	15 (40%)	13 (59%)	11 (61%)
Ratio normal/atypical/mal cells	94/6/0	79/21/0	48/27/25	44/22/34	40/24/36

(Reproduced with permission from Kern WH: The cytology of transitional cell carcinoma of the urinary bladder. Acta Cytol 19:421, 1975.)

NUCLEAR SIZE
(Nuclear Areas in Square Microns)

Normal, 501 nuclei
Range: 11-89 μ²   Mean: 36 μ²

Benign Atypical, 1328 nuclei
Range: 11-311 μ²   Mean: 52 μ²

FIGURE 17–34. Nuclear size of **normal, atypical and neoplastic cells** as measured by planimetry. (With permission from Kern WH: The cytology of transitional cell carcinoma of the urinary bladder. Acta Cytol 16:424, 1975.)

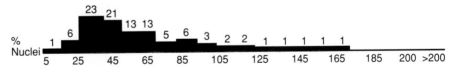

Papillary Transitional Cell Carcinoma, grade I, 3272 nuclei
Range: 11-534 μ²   Mean: 54 μ²

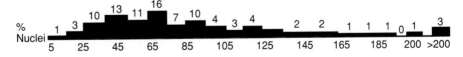

Papillary Transitional Cell Carcinoma, grade II, 1965 nuclei
Range: 11-726 μ²   Mean: 78 μ²

Transitional Cell Carcinoma, grade III and IV, 1389 nuclei
Range: 17-450 μ²   Mean: 90 μ²

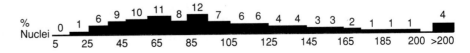

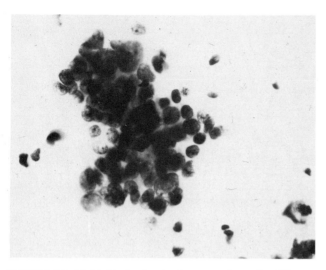

FIGURE 17–35. Voided urine in the case of **poorly differentiated papillary transitional cell carcinoma.** The tumor cells have moderately irregular nuclei with a coarse chromatin pattern, a high nucleocytoplasmic (N/C) ratio and an arrangement in the form of loose clusters (Papanicolaou stain; × 320).

debris are present. Keratinizing malignant squamous cells may also be seen if the tumor includes squamoid zones; sometimes this is the predominant cell type.

Flow cytometry has been applied not only for the diagnosis but for classification of urothelial tumors. Patients with diploid tumors rarely experience progression or recurrence, whereas in aneuploid tumors, the progression rate is 10% for tetraploid lesions and 50% for those with nontetraploid aneuploid lesions.[10] A high histologic grade generally is associated with aneuploidy.

Morphometric studies have also been used to evaluate and differentiate cells that exfoliate from well-differentiated (grade I) and moderately differentiated (grade II) tumors.[6] Normal urothelial cells often cannot be distinguished from cells exfoliated from grade I tumors, but grade I and grade II tumors can be differentiated using this methodology. If such a distinction can be made by means of a noninvasive cytologic examination, it is valuable in the assessment and treatment of these cases. This is because low-grade tumors that often cannot be diagnosed cytologically and sometimes are not even suspected are essentially benign without significant risk of progression.[20] The high-grade neoplasms are aggressive, whether they are papillary, flat or nodular and account for over 90% of tumor-related deaths.

Urothelial Dysplasia and Transitional Cell Carcinoma *In Situ*

Transitional Cell Carcinoma In Situ and Precancerous Lesions

It has long been recognized that transitional cell carcinoma *in situ* of the urothelium may precede

accompany or follow invasive bladder cancer.[28] The association of precancerous lesions with bladder cancer has been well documented by mapping of the urothelium by Koss and associates[26] and by Farrow and colleagues.[15] Carcinoma *in situ* in turn is preceded or accompanied by less severe changes with urothelial abnormalities ranging from normal or near normal to full-fledged carcinoma *in situ*. These changes have been referred to as atypical hyperplasia or as dysplasia. The lesions are not strictly comparable with dysplasia of the uterine cervix or cervical intraepithelial neoplasia, but because dysplasia is recognized as denoting a premalignant condition it is the preferred term for these alterations. The increased exfoliation and at least focal denudation of the urothelium in carcinoma *in situ* causes a "pseudocystitis" (Fig. 17–36).[5] This may become symptomatic, with frequency, dysuria or hematuria. Dysplasia, on the other hand, is not associated with specific symptoms and is therefore recognized primarily in patients with associated symptomatic bladder cancer or in patients who are being followed after treatment. The exceptions are the occasional cases detected in screening programs. Dysplasia of the urothelium, most commonly of the bladder, or "atypical hyperplasia," is customarily further subclassified into mild, moderate or severe. Mild dysplasia closely resembles normal urothelium and severe dysplasia, transitional cell carcinoma *in situ*.

Mild Dysplasia. Mild dysplasia is characterized by normal or near normal thickness of the epithelium, usually less than seven layers, a slight increase in the number and slight crowding of the cells and slight to moderate nuclear enlargement. The nuclear outlines are still fairly uniform. Some of the cells have nuclei with a coarsely granular chromatin. Few mitoses may be seen.

Severe Dysplasia. In this condition, the urothelium is strikingly abnormal. The cells are large, with enlarged, hyperchromatic and more pleomorphic nuclei and an increased nucleocytoplasmic ratio. The nuclear outlines are irregular, and a coarse chromatin pattern is prominent. Mitoses are considerably more common than in mild dysplasia. Moderate dysplasia is characterized by changes between these two extremes.

Transitional Cell Carcinoma *In Situ*. This diagnosis is made if the changes are cytologically those of urothelial carcinoma, with nuclear enlargement, irregularity, hyperchromasia and prominent mitotic activity. It has been proposed that only lesions with cells that contain nuclei larger than 80 square μ should be classified as carcinoma *in situ* and lesions with smaller nuclei that are classified as low-grade carcinomas *in situ* by some should be classified as mild, moderate or severe dysplasias.[5] This is a reasonable histologic classification that also closely relates to cytology because it is the lesions with greater nuclear size and pleomorphism that show particular lack of cellular cohesion and are associated with extensive exfoliation. This exfoliation of the abnormal bladder epithelium can be of such a degree that the stroma reaches the surface. The changes cause a pseudocystitis that is often symptomatic.

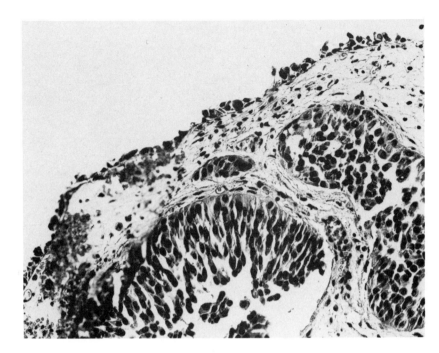

FIGURE 17–36. Transitional cell carcinoma *in situ* involving nests of von Brunn. The surface epithelium is partially denuded (hematoxylin and eosin; ×160).

The cytology of carcinoma *in situ* is characterized by the presence of numerous abnormal cells that are moderately larger than normal transitional cells and have hyperchromatic, enlarged and irregularly outlined nuclei (Figs. 17–37 and 17–38). The chromatin is usually coarsely granular (Fig. 17–39). Large nucleoli are prominent. The pattern is relatively monotonous and bizarre, and very pleomorphic cancer cells are rare. Many of the cells exfoliate singly, but a few occur in small fragments or clusters. In many cases there is no ulceration or inflammation and the background is usually clean. Some leukocytes or red blood cells are present if the epithelium is denuded. Because of the extensive exfoliation from these lesions, the cytologic accuracy is high and a diagnosis can be made in most cases.

Urine samples from patients with *dysplasias* also contain abnormal cells, corresponding to the dysplastic changes described. The exfoliation is less extensive and fewer abnormal cells are present. The nuclei are smaller, less pleomorphic and hyperchromatic, and the background is clean (Fig. 17–40). The principal cytologic differential diagnosis includes the atypical changes caused by inflammation, calculi or instrumentation. In these cases and particularly in calculous disease, individual cells may be impossible to differentiate from those exfoliated in severe dysplasia or carcinoma *in situ*, but the cellularity is never as great as in the latter conditions. As noted, this is due to the lack of cohesion of cells in areas of carcinoma *in situ* and, to a lesser degree, dysplasias. This appears to be associated with the decrease in numbers of desmosomes that has been found with increasing tumor grade.

Carcinoma *in situ* and urothelial dysplasia are con-

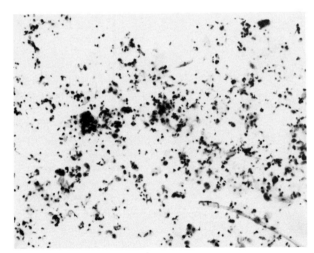

FIGURE 17–37. Hypercellular urine specimen in a case of **transitional cell carcinoma** *in situ*. Many abnormal cells with enlarged nuclei are present. The background is relatively clean (Papanicolaou stain; ×80).

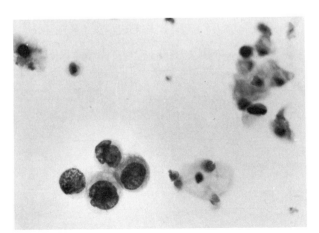

FIGURE 17–38. **Abnormal urothelial cells** with enlarged and irregular nuclei, a coarse chromatin pattern and a high nucleocytoplasmic (N/C) ratio. The background is clean (Papanicolaou stain; ×300).

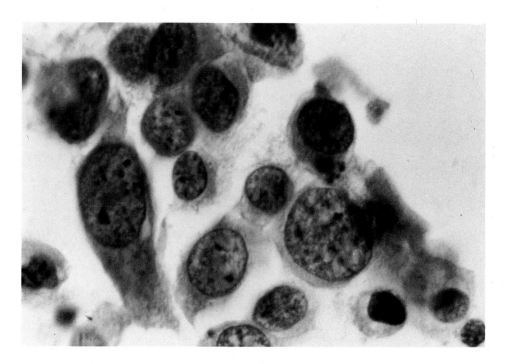

FIGURE 17–39. Loose group of anaplastic epithelial cells from **transitional cell carcinoma *in situ* of bladder.** The chromatin pattern is coarse (Papanicolaou stain; ×350). (With permission from Gamarra MC and Zeim T: Cytologic spectrum of bladder cancer. Urology (Suppl 3) 23:23–26, 1984.)

ditions most often found in middle-aged or elderly men. They occur predominantly in the urinary bladder but may involve all other portions of the urothelium and not infrequently extend into prostatic ducts. The changes precede invasion but can involve nests of Brunn (see Fig. 17–36).

Invasive Nonpapillary Transitional Cell Carcinoma

The noninvasive phase of nonpapillary transitional cell carcinoma is flat, transitional cell carcinoma *in situ* as described previously. Because the epithelium in *in situ* carcinoma is frequently not significantly thickened, the diagnosis is made by evaluating the cytologic features and therefore, there is no well-differentiated or grade I nonpapillary carcinoma. Most *in situ* transitional cell carcinomas, by definition, are high grade, as are most infiltrating nonpapillary carcinomas. Grossly, these carcinomas are often ulcerated, nodular or bulky and infiltrate the bladder wall. Histologically, the tumors are composed of irregular nests, sheets and cords of cells with enlarged, irregular, hyperchromatic nuclei and relatively scant cytoplasm. Undifferentiated small-cell forms are also seen. Glandular and squamoid

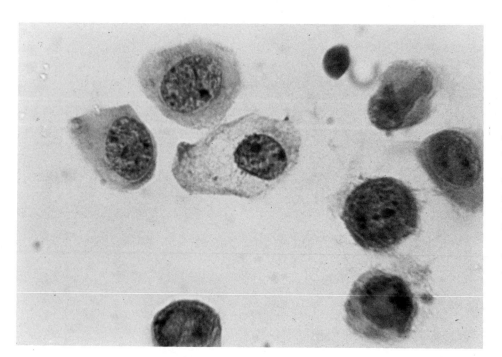

FIGURE 17–40. Atypical transitional cells with moderately enlarged, fairly uniform nuclei containing small nucleoli. The pattern is consistent with **mild to moderate urothelial dysplasia** (Papanicolaou stain; ×350). (With permission form Gamarra MC and Zeim T: Cytologic spectrum of bladder cancer. Urology (Suppl 3) 23:23–26, 1984.)

TABLE 17–3. Grade and Pathologic Stage of Bladder Cancer Cases*

Classification and Grade		Cases	P-0	PIS	PA	P-1	P-2	P-3A	P-3B	P-4
Cystectomies										
TCIS		10		9						1
PTCC	I	2			2					
	II	10	21 (18%)		1	3	5			1
	III	9				5	2	1	1	
TCC	I	0								1
	II	13	70 (61%)			8	2	1	1	11
	III	41				8	4	7	11	8
	IV	16						3	5	
Sq ca		5				1		2	1	1
Adenocarcinoma		3						1	2	
Sarcoma		1						1		
No tumor		4	4							
Total		114	4	9	3	25	13	16	21	23

*TCIS = transitional cell carcinoma *in situ;* PTCC = papillary transitional cell carcinoma; TCC = transitional cell carcinoma; Sq ca = squamous carcinoma. (Reproduced with permission from Kern WH: The grade and pathologic stage of bladder cancer. Cancer 53:1187, 1984.)

components may be included but, as will be described, may also occur in a pure form. Lymphatic infiltration is common.

Because of the correlation of the cell type and degree of differentiation to the depth of infiltration, the probability of such infiltration may be anticipated not only by examination of biopsies but also by the cytologic findings in these tumors. The correlation of the grade and pathologic stage based on the examination of radical cystectomy specimens is shown in Table 17–3.[23]

The nonpapillary transitional cell carcinomas in this series are of a higher grade, but whether the tumors are papillary or nonpapillary, the depth of invasion is directly related to the grade. Muscle invasion, either superficial (P-2) or deep (P-3A), was observed only in grade II or less-differentiated tumors, and deep invasion with extension into perivesical tissues (P-3B and P-4) is largely restricted to poorly differentiated, grade III carcinomas.

In this same group of cases, the cytologic findings in turn closely correlated to the grade of the tumor. Only five of 16 grade I papillary carcinomas could be classified as positive, but 75% of grade II and 81% of grade III and IV transitional cell carcinomas were definitely identified as cancer and furthermore, in all instances, as carcinomas of a medium or high grade. This permits a prediction of the probable extent of invasion (Table 17–4).

TABLE 17–4. Correlation of Cytologic and Histologic Classification in 125 Bladder Cancer Cases*

Cytologic Diagnosis	Cases	CIS	PTCC I	PTCC II	PTCC III	TCC II	TCC III	TCC IV	Other
Negative	14 (11%)	0	7	4	0	0	1	1	1
Suspicious	22 (18%)	4	4	3	3	1	0	3	4
Positive	89 (71%)	12	5	20	7	3	21	7	14
All cases	125	16	16	27	10	4	22	11	19

*PTCC = papillary transitional cell carcinoma; TCC = transitional cell carcinoma; CIS = carcinoma *in situ.* (Reproduced with permission from Kern WH: The grade and pathologic stage of bladder cancer. Cancer 53:1188, 1984.)

The cytologic findings in voided urine and bladder washings from patients with invasive transitional cell carcinoma are similar for high-grade papillary tumors and for nonpapillary tumors except for less frequent clustering in the latter. It is exceptional to find only few malignant cells (see Table 17–2). The urine cellularity is greatly increased, and in most cases, over one fourth of the cells present are neoplastic. The tumor cells contain large (75 to 90 square μ), irregular and pleomorphic nuclei that are hyperchromatic, have a coarsely granular chromatin pattern and contain multiple or macronucleoli (Figs. 17–41 to 17–44). Even if poorly differentiated, the transitional cells still retain some of their morphologic characteristics (Fig. 17–45).

Application of morphometric measurements and a judgment of the degree of nuclear enlargement and pleomorphism permit an evaluation of the probable grade of the tumor. Reports may be worded, "Malig-

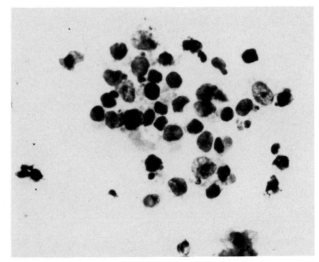

FIGURE 17–41. Poorly differentiated (grade III) transitional cell carcinoma. Considerable nuclear pleomorphism and hyperchromasia are seen. The nucleocytoplasmic (N/C) ratio is high (Papanicolaou stain; ×360).

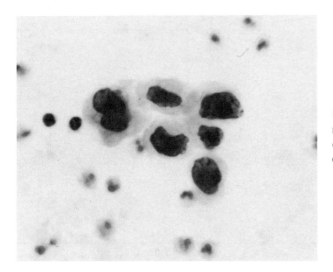

FIGURE 17–42. Poorly differentiated transitional cell carcinoma. The nuclei are large, pleomorphic and markedly hyperchromatic. The background includes necrotic and inflammatory debris (Papanicolaou stain; ×300).

nant urothelial cells present—consistent with high-grade, ulcerated transitional cell carcinoma."

The sensitivity of urine cytology for these tumors is high, and the described morphologic differences from normal and reactive cells can be readily resolved in most cases.[29] If glandular or squamous components are included in the tumor, cells indicating these changes may be present. Cells from urothelial carcinoma usually have a homogeneous cytoplasm, but vacuolation may be present and does not necessarily indicate glandular differentiation. Cell clusters with well-defined outlines and unequivocally columnar-type cells should be present to make such a diagnosis.

Urine cytology is especially helpful in the follow-up of patients with known and previously conservatively treated bladder tumors. Papillary tumors rarely progress to more aggressive forms but are often associated with dysplasia or carcinoma *in situ* and concurrent or

subsequent aggressive nonpapillary tumors. Positive cytologic findings in patients whose biopsies show low-grade papillary tumors are characteristic of such a process. At first presentation, 90% of patients with invasive carcinoma have such tumors,[30] but this is often associated with the simultaneous presence or a previous occurrence of low-grade tumors.

Flow cytometry has proved to be of particular value in following these patients and is slightly more sensitive but also slightly less specific than urine cytology. Badalament and coworkers[2] demonstrated this in a series of cases (Table 17–5). The highest sensitivity for the detection of bladder cancer was obtained by combining cytologic and flow cytometric examinations.

Aneuploid stemlines are associated with recurrence in 85% of patients who were treated with surgery alone, and tetraploidy with a 79% recurrence rate. Diploid and tetraploid cell populations are less reliable

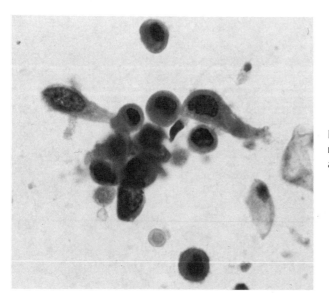

FIGURE 17–43. Poorly differentiated transitional cell carcinoma. Large pleomorphic tumor cells with irregular nuclei and a coarsely granular chromatin pattern (Papanicolaou stain; ×500).

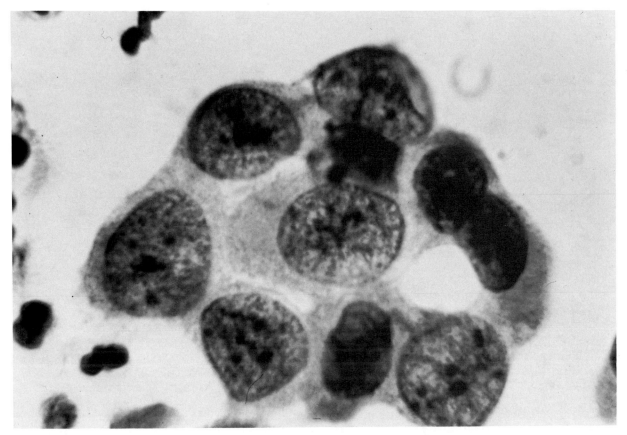

FIGURE 17–44. Group of malignant cells from **high grade (III) transitional cell carcinoma of bladder.** The nuclei display an irregular chromatin pattern and contain nucleoli. The amount of cytoplasm is small (Papanicolaou stain; ×350). (With permission from Gamarra MC and Zeima T: Cytologic spectrum of bladder cancer. Urology (Suppl 3) 23:23–26, 1984.)

TABLE 17–5. The Sensitivity of Bladder Wash Flow Cytometry Versus Bladder Wash Cytology Versus Voided Urinary Cytology*

Tumor Category	Test Type and Cases Detected (%)				
	One VUC	*Two VUC*	*Three VUC*	*One BWC*	*One BWFCM*
Papilloma (n = 11)	2/11 (18)	1/10 (10)	0/3 (0)	4/11 (36)	9/11 (82)
Ta (n = 14)	8/14 (57)	6/12 (50)	3/5 (60)	10/14 (71)	13/14 (93)
TIS (n = 18)	7/18 (39)	5/14 (36)	7/13 (54)	10/18 (56)	14/18 (78)
T1 (n = 19)	9/19 (47)	10/18 (56)	8/10 (80)	15/19 (79)	17/19 (89)
T2 (n = 8)	3/8 (38)	3/7 (43)	3/4 (75)	4/8 (50)	5/8 (62)
Combined (n = 70)	29/70 (41)	25/61 (41)	21/35 (60)	43/70 (61)	58/70 (83)
Papilloma excluded (n = 59)	27/59 (46)	24/51 (47)	21/32 (66)	39/59 (66)	49/59 (83)
Papilloma and T2 excluded (n = 51)	24/51 (47)	21/44 (48)	18/28 (64)	35/51 (69)	44/51 (86)

*VUC = voided urinary cytology; BWC = bladder wash cytology; BWFCM = bladder wash flow cytometry; TIS = tumor *in situ.* (Reproduced with permission from Badalament RA, et al: The sensitivity of bladder wash flow cytometry, bladder wash cytology, and voided cytology in the detection of bladder carcinoma. Cancer 60:1425, 1987.)

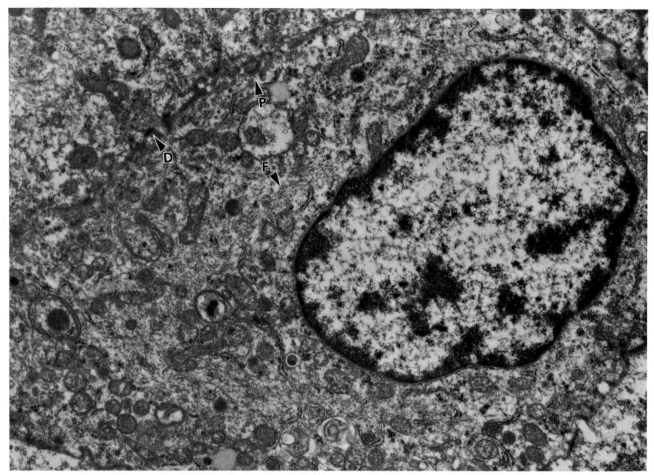

FIGURE 17–45. Electron photomicrograph of **poorly differentiated transitional cell carcinoma, metastatic to the lung.** Some of the normal features have been lost, but the plasmalemmal interdigitations (P), intermediate filaments (F) and stout desmosomes (D) seen in normal transitional cell epithelium have been retained (×14,000). (Courtesy of Dr. M.J. Patterson, Department of Pathology, The Hospital of the Good Samaritan, Los Angeles, CA.)

predictors of recurrent cancer in patients who were previously treated with local chemotherapy or radiation.[38]

Squamous Cell Carcinoma

Squamous cell carcinoma may represent a component of poorly differentiated transitional cell carcinoma, but in 2 to 3% of patients it is the principal primary tumor. The percentage is much higher in regions of the world in which *Schistosoma haematobium* commonly infects the bladder and where over one half of bladder cancers are squamous in type. Many of the squamous cell carcinomas occurring in other regions are associated with squamous metaplasia and occasionally with the squamous metaplasia found in bladder diverticula. Most tumors are keratinizing. Cytologically, the urine specimens contain keratinizing malignant epithelial cells (Fig. 17–46). If the tumor is high grade and if keratinization is not readily apparent in malignant cells, they are often associated with atypical metaplastic squamous cells.

Adenocarcinoma

Glandular components of transitional cell carcinomas are less common than squamous areas. Pure adenocarcinomas are relatively rare and represent approximately 2% of all primary urothelial tumors. Some tumors are mucin secreting and resemble colonic adenocarcinoma, probably arising from metaplastic differentiation to this type of epithelium as is often observed in bladder exstrophy. Some of these patients have a history of urinary tract lithiasis or infection, which may have caused glandular metaplasia.[40] The cytology is characterized by the presence of clusters of columnar or cuboidal cells with large, hyperchromatic, irregular nuclei. The cytoplasm is usually vacuolated, with large single vacuoles that push the nucleus towards the periphery. The nuclei tend to be vesicular and contain large nucleoli and dense chromatin strands. Signet-ring cell (colloid) adenocarcinomas and clear cell (mesonephric) adenocarcinomas have also been described. Tumors arising from remnants of the allantoic duct or urachus in the dome of the bladder are other rare variants.

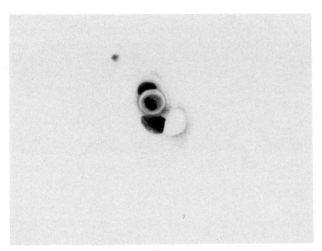

FIGURE 17–46. Keratinizing neoplastic squamous cells in the urine of a patient with **squamous cell carcinoma of the urinary bladder** (Papanicolaou stain; ×320).

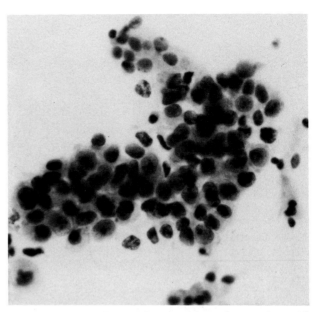

FIGURE 17–48. Cells in catheterized urine from patient with **advanced, poorly differentiated adenocarcinoma of prostate.** The tumor cells are arranged in loose sheets. Nucleoli are prominent (Papanicolaou stain; ×320).

Adenocarcinomas of the Kidney. In late stages, these adenocarcinomas invade the renal pelvis and then exfoliate into the urine. This is invariably preceded by hematuria. The renal adenocarcinomas are often well differentiated and usually of a clear cell type. If tumor cells are present in urine, they are large with irregular cell borders. The cytoplasm is abundant, well defined and prominently vacuolated. The cells are usually clustered (Fig. 17–47). A cytologic diagnosis is occasionally made, but only in late or advanced stages. Cytology is not a useful diagnostic tool for this condition. Wilms' tumor or nephroblastoma, one of the most common tumors of young children, rarely exfoliates into urine, and cytology is not useful or indicated.

Adenocarcinomas of the Prostate. These are common and are often well differentiated. Exfoliated malignant cells may be seen and are occasionally diagnos-

tic after prostatic massage or instrumentation, or in far-advanced disease when the bladder is extensively infiltrated (Fig. 17–48). Cytologic examination of urine is rarely, if ever, a means of primary diagnosis and should not be relied upon. Fine needle aspiration is well established as a diagnostic procedure and is discussed in another chapter.

The cytologic appearance of neoplastic urothelial cells frequently suggests the possibility of adenocarcinoma. This is due to prominent clustering, particularly of papillary tumors, and to the fact that the cytoplasm is often vacuolated and that the nuclei may contain large nucleoli. Such findings in a sputum specimen would definitely suggest that the neoplasm is an adenocarcinoma. In the great majority of positive urine specimens, this is not the case and the tumor will be subsequently found to be a transitional cell carcinoma. Good evidence of adenocarcinoma must therefore exist, preferably in the form of smooth-surfaced tissue fragments and clear characteristic of adenocarcinoma. Mucicarmine and immunoperoxidase stains may at times help in the differential diagnosis.

Miscellaneous Tumors

Nephrogenic Adenomas of the Urinary Bladder. These are rare tumors or metaplastic lesions of the urinary bladder that may develop in response to trauma, chronic irritation and infection, radiation or intravesical bacillus Calmette-Guerin installation for transitional cell carcinoma. The lesions consist of papillary or metaplastic glandular structures, often with an abrupt transition from the adjacent normal transitional mucosa.[41] Depending on the histologic pattern of the lesion, the corresponding urinary cytology is charac-

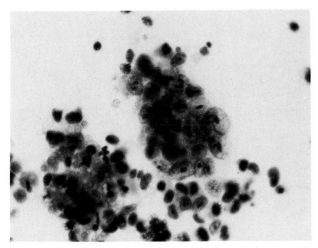

FIGURE 17–47. Cluster of neoplastic cells with large nuclei containing prominent nucleoli. The cytoplasm is scant and slightly vacuolated. The cells exfoliated from an **advanced clear cell type adenocarcinoma of the kidney** (Papanicolaou stain; ×320).

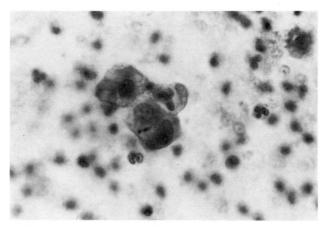

FIGURE 17–49. Cluster of abnormal vacuolated cells representative of urine cytology of **nephrogenic adenoma.** Inflammatory cells are present in the background (hematoxylin and eosin; ×520). (With permission from Stilmant M, et al: Cytology of nephrogenic adenoma of the urinary bladder. Acta Cytol 30:35–40, 1986.)

terized by the presence of papillary fragments, sometimes with palisading, or by the presence of cells with a vacuolated cytoplasm (Fig. 17–49). The features may resemble those of low-grade papillary carcinoma or adenocarcinoma. Tumor cells are usually present in small numbers, and the findings must be correlated with the clinical history.

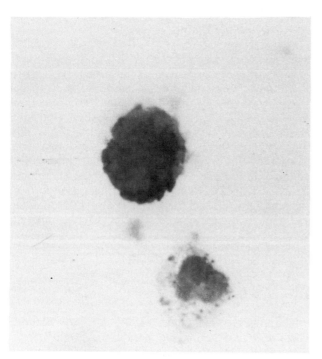

FIGURE 17–50. Malignant cell in urine sediment that exfoliated from a **malignant lymphoma.** It stained strongly for kappa light chain immunoglobulin. A neutrophil also shows weak enzyme staining. (Immunoalkaline phosphatase method; ×1320). (With permission from Yan LT, et al: Immunocytochemical diagnosis of lymphoma from urine sediment. Acta Cytol 29:827–832, 1985.)

Sarcomas. Sarcomas of the lower urinary tract include rhabdomyosarcoma in children, adult-type rhabdomyosarcomas, carcinosarcomas and lymphomas. These tumors are rare, and the diagnosis may be suggested by cytologic findings. Immunocytochemical studies may permit classification of malignant lymphomas from the urine sediment (Fig. 17–50).

Special Aspects of Anatomic Sites Other than Urinary Bladder

Urethra

Primary malignancies of the male and female urethra that are unassociated with bladder tumors are rare. Squamous cell carcinomas are relatively most common, and most of the rest are adenocarcinomas (Fig. 17–51) or transitional cell carcinomas.[31] Primary malignant melanomas (Fig. 17–52) and clear cell adenocarcinoma have also been described and have cytologic features similar to these tumors occurring at other sites.

The most commonly required examination of a urethral specimen is that after cystectomy for bladder carcinoma.[45] Approximately 10% of patients who are treated for invasive transitional cell carcinoma of the bladder develop neoplastic lesions in the urethra, and periodic, regular follow-up examinations are therefore indicated. The specimens are best collected by saline lavage of the urethra and collection of the efflux in an equal amount of 50% alcohol. Many of the cases detected are transitional cell carcinomas *in situ*. The cytologic morphology is similar to that of bladder tumors. Invasive carcinoma may also be found.

Condylomata acuminata and rarely flat condylomata occur in the urethra, usually near the meatus. The cytologic findings correspond to those of condylomata at other sites.

Urethral caruncles are urethral lesions of elderly

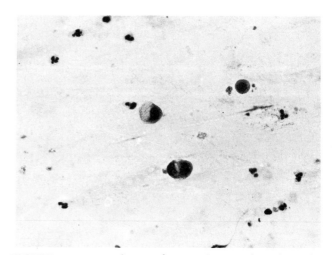

FIGURE 17–51. Mucinous adenocarcinoma of urethra. The tumor cells contain moderately large eccentric hyperchromatic nuclei and large cytoplasmic mucin vacuoles (Papanicolaou stain; ×320).

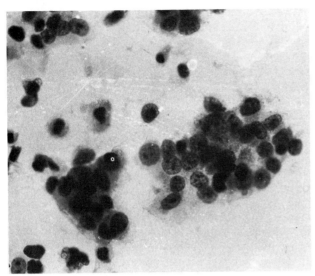

FIGURE 17–52. Neoplastic cells with nuclei that have a coarse chromatin pattern and contain prominent nucleoli from a patient with **malignant melanoma of the urethra** (Papanicolaou stain; ×320).

women. They are also located near the meatus and are polypoid. Cleft-like spaces are lined by hyperplastic urothelial cells and the stroma is characterized by chronic inflammatory changes. The epithelium may be hyperplastic, but it is rarely the source of an erroneous false-positive diagnosis.

Upper Collecting System of the Urinary Tract

Urothelial tumors of the upper urinary tract histologically resemble those of the urinary bladder. Tumors of the pelvis are twice as common as those of the ureter. They are often associated with bladder tumors, and many are multifocal or extensive and invasive.[16] The tumors of the renal pelvis may infiltrate deeply into the kidney and form large masses that grossly resemble renal adenocarcinoma.

Urinary cytology is usually diagnostic, particularly in high-grade tumors. In well-differentiated papillary transitional cell carcinomas, the urine samples may be hypercellular but there are no significant cytologic deviations and a definite diagnosis is usually not possible. In high-grade tumors the nuclei are enlarged and pleomorphic. Nucleoli are present and mitoses may be seen. The tumor cells occur singly and in small or large irregular clusters. Caution and conservatism in interpretation are necessary because catheterized specimens from the upper urinary tract contain large numbers of superficial cells and often show a degree of atypia that is not seen in voided or catheterized bladder urine and could be mistakenly interpreted as carcinoma of the upper urinary tract. Good cell preservation and adherence to clear-cut nuclear criteria of malignancy are necessary to make a positive diagnosis.

Kidneys

As noted previously, urinary cytology is unsatisfactory as a means of detecting renal adenocarcinoma. Some authors report a positive diagnosis in over 40% of patients with renal adenocarcinoma,[32] but the results obtained by most other laboratories indicate a lesser sensitivity. If malignant cells are present in advanced cases, they are usually large, with distinct nucleoli and have a clear or vacuolated cytoplasm (see Fig. 17–47). Granular eosinophilic cells with pyknotic nuclei and distinct or ill-defined cytoplasmic borders are also seen and are probably the result of degenerative changes.

Prostate

As described elsewhere, fine needle aspiration of the prostate is a recognized procedure for the diagnosis and classification of prostatic adenocarcinoma. Cells characteristic of adenocarcinoma may be present in voided urine spontaneously or after prostatic massage, particularly if the carcinoma is high grade or advanced (see Fig. 17–48). The sensitivity of urine examination is only approximately 20%,[37] and this procedure is therefore not appropriate for the early detection of prostatic carcinoma.

IATROGENIC CHANGES

Instrumentation and in particular catheterization of the ureters and renal pelves is followed by reactive changes and produces large numbers of superficial cells that may be misinterpreted as dysplastic or neoplastic, as described previously. The major iatrogenic changes, however, are those that follow treatment of cancer and transplant procedures with immunosuppression. Just as modern therapy of leukemias and malignant lymphomas is effective but causes a host of significant early and late pathologic changes, so does the therapy of tumors of the urinary tract. Treatment of other sites, such as irradiation of the rectum or systemic chemotherapy, similarly may cause significant pathologic and cytologic changes of the urinary tract.

Irradiation Changes

Irradiation of the urinary bladder or other portions of the collecting system initially causes mucosal congestion and localized edema. This progresses to edema of the lamina propria with vasculitis, inflammatory changes and ulceration. The epithelium adjacent to the ulcers is often hyperplastic and may undergo squamous metaplasia.

Cytologically, the urothelial cells exfoliating from this mucosa have moderately irregular, enlarged, mildly to moderately hyperchromatic and sometimes multiple nucleoli (Fig. 17–53). The cytoplasm shows polychromasia, is often frothy and contains fine to

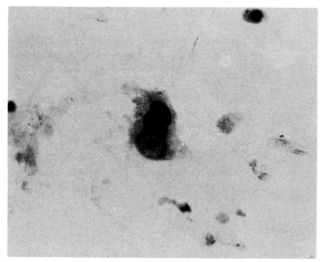

FIGURE 17–53. Irradiation changes with nuclear enlargement, hyperchromasia and moderate pleomorphism (Papanicolaou stain; ×320).

large vacuoles. The most reliable criterion of radiation effect is the marked cellular enlargement. The cells measure up to 2500 square μ, averaging approximately 900 square μ. Irradiated malignant cells from transitional cell carcinomas show similar changes but have a relatively scanty cytoplasm with enlarged, irregular and hyperchromatic nuclei. Irregular jagged macronucleoli are sometimes present. The described irradiation changes appear at a predictable dose level after approximately 2800 rads.[27]

Chemotherapy Effects

The bladder epithelium is affected by chemotherapeutic agents that may be given systemically for the treatment of malignancies of various organ systems and by alkylating agents that are administered intravesically by catheter. *Cyclophosphamide* is an alkylating agent given systemically for various cancers. Active metabolites are excreted in the urine, where they often cause enlargement of the urothelial cells, with nuclear enlargement, irregularity and hyperchromasia and a salt-and-pepper nuclear chromatin distribution. Nucleoli may be seen, and multinucleated cells are often present (Fig. 17–54). This is usually associated with a hemorrhagic cystitis and increased exfoliation of the epithelial cells. The patient's history and the degenerative changes that are associated with the cytologic effect should permit correct interpretation. It must be noted, however, that epithelial cancers and in particular transitional cell carcinoma may develop in patients after treatment with cyclophosphamide, and the presence of cytologically malignant cells that appear viable should therefore not be dismissed as being merely secondary to chemotherapy.

In contrast to cyclophosphamide, triethylenethiophosphoramide (thio-TEPA) and mitomycin C are polyfunctional alkylating agents that are used for treatment of superficial transitional cell carcinoma of the

bladder by intravesical installation. The changes introduced by thio-TEPA mimic those of neoplastic cells but differ in several respects.[11] The nuclei become enlarged to a slight or moderate degree. There is moderate hyperchromasia, but often the chromatin is smudgy and lacks a sharply detailed pattern. The nuclei become slightly or moderately enlarged without a significant increase in chromatin. They are round or ovoid with smooth, thin chromatinic rims that may be wrinkled. Large multinucleated cells are often present. Small and sometimes multiple nucleoli occur. The cytoplasm of these cells shows degenerative changes including vacuolation and frayed borders. The cytologic diagnosis of transitional cell carcinoma often remains the same after thio-TEPA treatment. If a transitional cell carcinoma is present, it can be diagnosed before as well as after therapy and, as after treatment with cylophosphamide, the presence of preserved, malignant cells indicates neoplasia rather than reactive changes.

Mitomycin C is also used intravesically for the treatment of superficial transitional cell carcinoma and is effective in one third to one half of the patients. Like thio-TEPA, mitomycin C acts to abrade vesical mucosa of visible superficial tumors and may be followed by nuclear and cytoplasmic changes similar to those observed with thio-TEPA.[7] They mimic neoplastic changes, and degeneration is readily apparent. Cytologic examination of urine is useful in the follow-up of patients so treated and permits diagnosis of persistent *in situ* or high-grade transitional cell carcinomas. The benefits of intravesical chemotherapy as well as tumor recurrence can be well demonstrated by flow cytometry.

Cytology of Ileal Conduits

Ileal conduits or other enteric pouches are created at the time of cystectomy. The ureters empty into the pouch and examination of the urine is a sensitive means

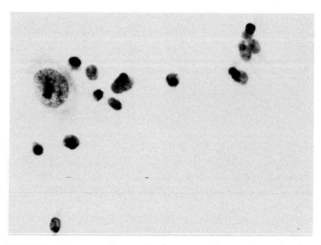

FIGURE 17–54. Nuclear enlargement and prominent nucleolus in cell exfoliated from a patient who was treated with 5-FU, mitomycin and vincristine (Papanicolaou stain; ×320).

of diagnosing additional or multicentric carcinoma of the upper urinary tract.[16]

The small intestinal mucosa of the pouch becomes flattened after 2 years, but the epithelial cells remain columnar.[43] The mucosal stroma invariably becomes chronically inflamed and contains numerous macrophages and lymphocytes. The cell turnover rate of the intestinal epithelium exceeds that of the bladder, resulting in abundant exfoliation of intestinal-type epithelial cells and histiocytes. Both single cells and clusters are numerous. Most of the cells are rounded, with dark-staining, moderately irregular nuclei and an amphophilic cytoplasm. Nuclear pyknosis, karyorrhexis and cytoplasmic inclusions are common. The cytoplasm is often vacuolated. Red blood cells are occasionally and leukocytes are invariably present. Special organisms such as *Candida* or *Aspergillus* may be found.

Malignant cells from recurrent or multicentric carcinoma can be readily diagnosed in this background of normal or degenerating cells if the diagnosis is based on the presence of well-preserved, viable cells. The nuclear hyperchromasia in the ileal epithelial cells is due to degeneration and must be differentiated from malignant changes.

Direct involvement of an ileal conduit with a recurrent transitional cell carcinoma is relatively rare, but several cases of direct neoplastic involvement of the ileal pouch have been reported.[33]

Renal Allograft Monitoring

Examination of urine to evaluate renal abnormalities preceded the use of urine cytology for cancer diagnosis and is still an important component of clinical microscopy. Renal tubular epithelial cells and renal tubular casts can be recognized in routinely processed cytologic material. These elements exfoliate in renal inflammatory or degenerative as well as in neoplastic disease. Renal epithelial fragments must be differentiated from urothelial cells as well as from renal casts. They are defined as structures containing at least three cells of collecting duct origin (Fig. 17–55). They may encase casts, have a honeycomb arrangement or be attached to a cast. The cytoplasm may be pigmented and may contain crystals or lipid vacuoles.

Urine cytology has become an important means of monitoring for acute allograft rejection. Renal transplantation is the accepted therapy for end-stage renal failure and cytologic examination of urine has been performed since this procedure was developed.[12, 42] The most common complications are acute allograft rejection and CMV infection. Both can be diagnosed and monitored by cytologic examination.

During the first postoperative hours, a macrohematuria is observed, which is reduced to microhematuria during the following days and usually ceases after 10 days. Some casts, oxalate crystals and slightly increased

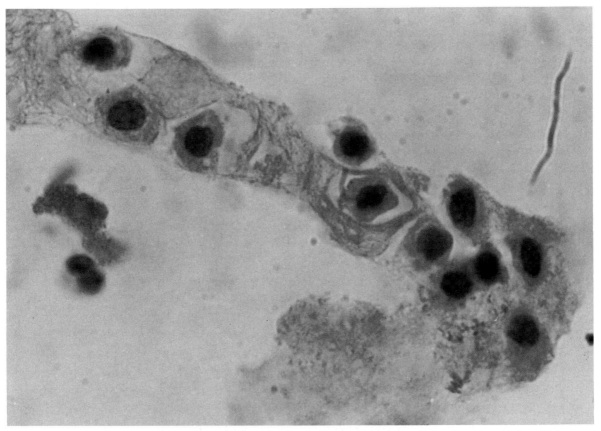

FIGURE 17–55. Renal tubule cell cast in case of **allograft injury.** The cast is composed of collecting cells in a fibrinous protein matrix (Papanicolaou stain; ×304). (With permission from Eggensberger D, et al: The utility of cytodiagnostic urinalysis for monitoring renal allograft injury. Am J Nephrol 8:27–34, 1988.)

number of polymorphonuclear leukocytes are found during the first 3 days. Macrophages are more frequent than urothelial cells, and lymphocytes and degenerated renal tubular cells are common (Fig. 17–56). If there are no further complications the cytologic findings return to normal.

The diagnosis of an *acute rejection crisis* can be made based on the presence of increased numbers of renal tubular cells that occur singly or in clusters. Two types of cells are present. These are normal tubular cells of round or oval shape with eccentric nuclei and tubular cells with nuclear alterations including prominent nucleoli, degenerative changes and pyknosis. Casts are increased in number and the background is dirty. Erythrocytes are often present. Lymphocytes may be seen but in some series are reported in only one fourth of the cases.[42] The presence of epithelial fragments has been emphasized as an important criterion.[36] On occasion, the exfoliation site of the fragments cannot be determined by the cytologic presentation, but recognition of morphologic features of renal epithelial fragments does permit a diagnosis of ischemic necrosis. Such fragments and pathologic casts are a characteristic background. In the clinical setting of renal transplantation, their presence is diagnostic of an acute allograft rejection. Other pathologic conditions that may cause exfoliation of fragments including cells from collecting ducts include severe tubular injury, renal infarction and papillary necrosis. Additional conditions that are known to cause exfoliation of tissue fragments such as instrumentation, lithiasis and papillary transitional cell carcinoma should be excluded on both clinical grounds and the cytologic appearance.

After long-term immunosuppressive medication there may be transient episodes of urothelial cell atypia. Numerous cases of urothelial cancer have been reported following systemic cyclophosphamide therapy. This usually occurs after years of treatment with doses of 100 mg or higher. Rare cases of transitional cell carcinoma have also been reported in patients with renal transplants after immunosuppression.

Specific infections occur in allograft recipients and fungi may be seen in their urine. CMV infection is particularly common. The cytologic findings are as described previously. They are characterized by the presence of epithelial cells with large eosinophilic nuclear inclusions or cells with dense inclusions surrounded by a halo and a thickened nuclear membrane, so-called owl's eye cells.[42]

SPECIAL TECHNIQUES

Flow Cytometry

The reader is referred to Chapter 37, Flow Cytometry, for details concerning the principles and methods.

Voided urine is generally not adequate and the cell samples must be obtained by the vigorous flushing of the bladder through a soft rubbery catheter five to ten times with 50 ml of saline solution or during cystoscopy by lavage.

A number of methodologies are being used. The procedure recommended by Melamed and coworkers[28] and Badalament and colleagues[4] is as follows:

Bladder irrigation specimens are centrifuged at 1500 rpm for 10 minutes, the supernatant discarded and the cell pellet resuspended in Hank's balanced salt solution without Ca^{2+} and Mg^{2+}. The cell suspension is sieved

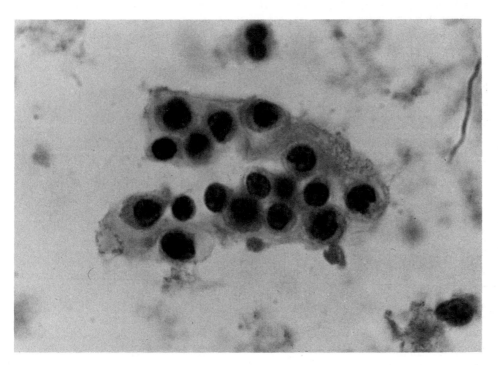

FIGURE 17–56. Lymphocyte cast. The distinct nuclear chromatin pattern of lymphocytes is evident (Papanicolaou stain; ×304). (With permission from Eggensberger D, et al: The utility of cytodiagnostic urinalysis for monitoring renal allograft injury. Am J Nephrol 8:27–34, 1988.)

through a 53-μ nylon mesh filter to remove tissue fragments and cell groups and adjusted to a concentration of approximately 10^6 cells/ml. A two-step acridine orange (AO) technique is used to stain the cells. Briefly, a 0.2-ml aliquot of the cell suspension is incubated with 0.4 ml of acid detergent (0.1% vol/vol Triton X-100, 0.08 N HCl and 0.15 M NaCl) for 30 seconds at room temperature. To this is added 1.2 ml of an AO-staining solution consisting of 6.0 mg of chromatographically purified AO in 100 ml of buffer (10^{-3} M ethylenediaminetetraacetic acid [EDTA], 0.15 M NaCl and 0.1 M citrate-phosphate pH 6.0). The stained sample is run immediately on a flow cytometer equipped with an argon ion laser operating at a wavelength of 488 nm. AO binds to double-helical DNA by intercalation and fluoresces green in blue (488 nm) light, and binds to single-stranded RNA by electrostatic forces to fluoresce red. Any double-stranded RNA is denatured to its single-stranded form by the EDTA in the staining solution. Fluorescence emission at the green and red wavelength bands is quantified for each cell and measurements stored in a minicomputer interfaced to the flow cytometer. Peripheral blood lymphocytes from healthy donors are used as a control to establish the 2c (normal) diploid content of DNA (DNA index of 1).

A total of 5000 cells per sample are measured. The green (DNA) and red (RNA) fluorescence intensities and green pulse width (nuclear diameter) for each cell are recorded in list mode. Cell doublets and larger groups are identified by their increased green pulse width measurements and eliminated. The DNA-RNA data are then displayed as scattergrams for the remaining single-cell population. Subpopulations of bladder epithelial cells are identified by interactive computer analysis and distinguished from dead cells, squamous cells and granulocytes. A positive diagnosis of cancer is made in cases with an aneuploid stemline or 16% or more of the measured cells with hyperdiploid DNA (i.e., greater than 2c DNA content) or both. A specimen is considered negative for cancer if no aneuploid stemline is detected and fewer than 11% of the cells measured by flow are hyperdiploid. If 11 to 15.9% of the cells measured are hyperdiploid and no aneuploid stemline is detected, the samples are considered suspicious.

Immunocytochemistry

Immunoperoxidase stains can be performed on urine specimens including Papanicolaou stained smears after removal of the coverslips. This procedure can provide positive cytologic diagnoses, identify viruses (e.g., polyomavirus) and permit classification of malignant lymphomas as B or T cell types. For additional information, see Chapter 38, Immunocytochemistry.

Morphometry

Morphometry using a microscope equipped with a television camera attachment and a computer can generate accurate data of the nuclear perimeter, nuclear area and the nucleocytoplasmic ratio. These measurements permit classification of the various groups of urothelial cells, and the nuclear measurements correlate closely to the grade of tumor. See Chapter 35, Morphometry, for technical details. Boon and coworkers[6] were unable to distinguish normal urothelial cells from cells that exfoliated from grade I tumors because of similar cellular and nuclear dimensions. They did demonstrate that, when compared with grade II tumors, the nucleocytoplasmic ratio of grade I tumor cells is smaller. They found grade II tumor cells to be larger and associated with anisocytosis.

Blood Group Antigen Predictors

The deletion of A, B and H blood group antigens is associated with biochemical and structural changes of the cell surface in neoplastic transformation and in particular with alterations of glycolipid and glycoprotein components. The A, B and H blood group substances are decreased in high-grade and aggressive tumors. This deletion is accompanied by the appearance of precursors or cryptic antigens. The antigen reactivity is determined by a modified specific erythrocyte adherence test and correlates with prognosis but, at this time, is not widely used or of clinical significance.

Other Tumor Markers

Carcinoembryonic antigen has been used in the evaluation of exfoliated urothelial tumor cells without significant clinical correlation. Urothelial organ antigen is present in carcinoma cells to a lesser degree than in normal urothelium. Lactate dehydrogenase, alkaline phosphatase and beta glucuronidase have been used in evaluation of urine for the presence of malignancy, and galactosyl transferase isoenzyme is reportedly present to a greater degree in neoplastic than in normal urothelial cells. These tumor markers are of considerable interest in the understanding of bladder cancer but at this time are not important in the diagnostic evaluation of patients.

DIAGNOSTIC ACCURACY

The purpose and goals of cytologic examination of urine were discussed in the beginning of this chapter. Predictably, the yield is low in screening programs but is high in the diagnostic evaluation of patients who are

TABLE 17–6. Cytologic Classification of 898 Tumors of the Urinary Tract

Tumor Type	Cases	Urine Cytology		
		Negative	Suspicious	Positive
Transitional cell carcinoma, *in situ* (75–88)	63	1 (2%)	21 (33%)	41 (65%)
Transitional cell carcinoma, grade I	159	56 (35%)	54 (34%)	49 (31%)
Transitional cell carcinoma, grade II	268	54 (20%)	97 (36%)	117 (44%)
Transitional cell carcinoma, grade III or IV	242	14 (6%)	54 (22%)	174 (72%)
Squamous cell carcinoma, bladder	16	1 (6%)	3 (19%)	12 (75%)
Adenocarcinoma, bladder	16	2 (12%)	4 (25%)	10 (63%)
Squamous cell carcinoma, urethra	3	0	1 (33%)	2 (67%)
Adenocarcinoma, urethra	1	0	0	1 (100%)
Adenocarcinoma, kidney	36	29 (81%)	7 (19%)	0
Adenocarcinoma, prostate	64	35 (55%)	14 (22%)	15 (23%)
Metastatic carcinoma	29	6 (21%)	8 (27%)	15 (52%)
Malignant melanoma	1	0	0	1 (100%)
Total	898	198 (22%)	263 (29%)	437 (49%)

symptomatic or who are being followed after being previously diagnosed with and treated for bladder cancer. The reported results vary considerably because of differences in the patient population, in the method of examination and in the diagnostic criteria and nomenclature employed. All reports of series of bladder tumors indicate that papillomas and well-differentiated papillary carcinomas cannot be reliably diagnosed. If these tumors are included, the results will differ significantly from those of series that are confined to invasive bladder tumors. Nevertheless, the sensitivity for transitional cell carcinoma is high. The overall sensitivity of urine cytology for primary carcinoma of the bladder, namely, the ability to identify correctly patients with malignant disease as measured by the rate of cytologic diagnoses in cases of cancer, has been reported to range from 47 to 97%. The sensitivity in our own cases (Table 17–6) is 83%.

In our own laboratory, 8093 urine specimens were obtained from 5092 patients over a 28-year period of time, averaging 1.6 specimens per patient. We rarely feel the need for examination of multiple specimens because filter preparations provide a cellular specimen of good quality, and if there are difficulties in interpretation, this is rarely, if ever, resolved by examination of repeat specimens. Approximately one third of the well-differentiated, grade I papillary carcinomas were considered negative and one third were considered abnormal or suspicious on the basis of increased cellularity and prominent clustering. The sensitivity of this examination is not adequate for a diagnostic test of papillomas or grade I papillary carcinomas, but these tumors are for all practical purposes benign. The sensitivity increases to 80% for grade II and to 94% for grade III transitional cell carcinomas. Transitional cell carcinomas *in situ* similarly can be diagnosed as suspicious or positive in all instances.

It is of interest to note that this sensitivity and an acceptable specificity of urine cytology, with an only 3% false-positive rate in our material, is very similar to that obtainable in sputum cytology.[22] Voided urine is the material that is most suitable for examination but, as noted, bladder washings are slightly more sensitive and may provide even better results. These, however, must be obtained in connection with cystos-

copy, usually during follow-up examination of patients with known bladder cancer. Flow cytometry has been used extensively for follow-up examination of patients with known bladder cancer as well. Positive urine cytology often corresponds to aneuploidy by flow cytometric examination.[25]

The grade of urothelial tumors is associated with the stage, and a similar correlation exists between cytologic findings and the stage of the disease.[23] Recurrences relate more to the stage than the grade and are often characterized by a higher grade than was noted when the tumor was first diagnosed. Positive urine cytology has been reported to be associated with a poor prognosis and is a separate risk factor. This is undoubtedly due to the fact that high-grade tumors tend to be more often positive than low-grade papillary and therefore nonaggressive tumors. Increased nuclear size and pleomorphism and the greater exfoliation in poorly differentiated carcinomas have been documented by morphometric measurements and account for the high rate of positive diagnoses in these cases. The nuclear size, irregular and coarse chromatin pattern and pleomorphism can be correlated with the grade of tumors. An exact grade need not be indicated in a cytopathologic report, but a comment that the findings are consistent with poorly differentiated, probably invasive transitional cell carcinoma should be made if justified by the findings and may be of value in clinical management.

In summary, urine cytology is an established diagnostic procedure in the primary diagnosis and follow-up of patients with urothelial carcinoma and has an acceptable sensitivity and specificity. It is not reliable in the diagnosis of adenocarcinomas of the kidneys or prostate. Screening programs for high-risk populations may be useful, but the experience with such programs is still limited.

References

1. Akura KA, Hatakenake M, Kawai K, Takenaka M, Kato K: Use of immunocytochemistry on urinary sediments for the rapid identification of human polyomavirus infection: A case report. Acta Cytol 32:247–251, 1988.
2. Badalament RA, Gay H, Cibas ES, Herr HW, Whitmore WF Jr, Fair WR, Melamed MR: Monitoring endoscopic treatment

of superficial bladder carcinoma by postoperative urinary cytology. J Urol 138:760–762, 1987.

3. Badalament RA, Hermansen DK, Kimmel M, Gay H, Herr HW, Fair WR, Whitmore WF Jr, Melamed MR: The sensitivity of bladder wash flow cytometry, bladder wash cytology, and voided cytology in the detection of bladder carcinoma. Cancer 60:1423–1427, 1987.

4. Badalament RA, Kimmel M, Gay H, Cibas ES, Whitmore WF Jr, Herr HW, Fair WR, Melamed MR: The sensitivity of flow cyometry compared with conventional cytology in the detection of superficial bladder carcinoma. Cancer 59:2078–2085, 1987.

5. Boon ME, Blomjous CEM, Zwartendijk J, Heinhuis RJ, Ooms ECM: Carcinoma in situ of the urinary bladder: Clinical presentation, cytologic pattern and stromal changes. Acta Cytol 30:360–366, 1986.

6. Boon ME, Kurver PHJ, Baak JPA, Ooms ECM: Morphometric differences between urothelial cells in voided urine of patients with grade I and grade II bladder tumours. J Clin Pathol 34:612–615, 1981.

7. Cant JD, Murphy WM, Soloway MS: Prognostic significance of urine cytology in initial follow-up after intravesical mitomycin C for superficial bladder cancer. Cancer 57:2119–2122, 1986.

8. Crabbe JGS: "Comet" or "decoy" cells found in urinary sediment smears. Acta Cytol 15:303–305, 1971.

9. Dean PJ, Murphy WM: Importance of urinary cytology and future role of flow cytometry. Urology [Suppl] 26:11–15, 1985.

10. deVere White RW, Deitch AD, West B, Fitzpatrick JM: The predictive value of flow cytometric information in the clinical management of stage O (Ta) bladder cancer. J Urol 139:279–282, 1988.

11. Droller MJ, Erozan YS: Thiotepa effects on urinary cytology in the interpretation of transitional cell cancer. J Urol 134:671–674, 1985.

12. Eggensperger D, Schweitzer S, Ferriol E, O'Dowd G, Light JA: The utility of cytodiagnostic urinalysis for monitoring renal allograft injury. Am J Nephrol 8:27–34, 1988.

13. El-Bolkainy MN: Cytology of bladder carcinoma. J Urol 124:20–22, 1980.

14. Eldidi MM, Patten SF Jr: New cytologic classification of normal urothelial cells: An analytical and morphometric study. Acta Cytol 26:725, 1982.

15. Farrow GM, Utz DC, Rife CC: Morphological and clinical observations of patients with early bladder cancer treated with total cystectomy. Cancer 36:2495, 1976.

16. Highman WJ: Transitional carcinoma of the upper urinary tract: A histological and cytopathological study. J Clin Pathol 39:297–306, 1986.

17. Highman W, Wilson E: Urine cytology in patients with calculi. J Clin Pathol 35:350–356, 1982.

18. Holmquist ND: Detection of urinary tract cancer in urinalysis specimens in an outpatient population. Am J Clin Pathol 89:499–504, 1988.

19. Jacobs R: A review of the effectiveness of urinary cytology as a screening technique for occupational bladder cancer. J Soc Occup Med 37:24–26, 1987.

20. Jordan AM, Weingarten J, Murphy WM: Transitional cell neoplasms of the urinary bladder: Can biologic potential be predicted from histologic grading? Cancer 60:2766–2774, 1987.

21. Kern WH: The cytology of transitional cell carcinoma of the urinary bladder. Acta Cytol 19:420–428, 1975.

22. Kern WH: The diagnostic accuracy of sputum and urine cytology. Acta Cytol 32:651–654, 1988.

23. Kern WH: The grade and pathologic stage of bladder cancer. Cancer 53:1185–1189, 1984.

24. Kern W: Screening tests for bladder cancer. In Screening for cancer. Edited by AB Miller. Orlando, Academic Press, pp 121–140, 1985.

25. Koss LG, Deitch D, Ramanathan R, Sherman AB: Diagnostic value of cytology of voided urine. Acta Cytol 29:810–816, 1985.

26. Koss LG, Tiamson EM, Robbins MD: Mapping of cancerous and precancerous bladder changes. JAMA 227:281–285, 1974.

27. Loveless KJ: The effects of radiation upon the cytology of benign and malignant bladder epithelium. Acta Cytol 17:355–360, 1973.

28. Melamed MR, Koss LG, Ricci A, Whitmore WF: Cytohistological observations on developing carcinoma of the urinary bladder in man. Cancer 13:67–74, 1960.

29. Murphy WM, Soloway MS, Jukkola AF, Crabtree WN, Ford KS: Urinary cytology and bladder cancer: The cellular features of transitional cell neoplasms. Cancer 53:1555–1565, 1984.

30. Newman LH, Tannenbaum M, Droller MJ: Muscle-invasive bladder cancer: Does it arise de novo or from preexisting superficial disease? Urology 32:58–62, 1988.

31. Peven DR, Hidvegi DF: Clear-cell adenocarcinoma of the female urethra. Acta Cytol 29:142–146, 1985.

32. Piscioli F, Detassis C, Polla E, Pusiol T, Reich A, Luciani L: Cytologic presentation of renal adenocarcinoma in urinary sediment. Acta Cytol 27:383–390, 1983.

33. Rosvanis TK, Rohner TJ, Abt AB: Transitional cell carcinoma in an ileal conduit. Cancer 63:1233–1236, 1989.

34. Rubben H, Hering F, Dahm HH, Lutzeyer W: Value of exfoliative urinary cytology for differentiation between uric acid stone and tumor of upper urinary tract. Urology 22:571–573, 1982.

35. Schneider V, Smith MJV, Frable WJ: Urinary cytology in endometriosis of the bladder. Acta Cytol 24:30–33, 1980.

36. Schumann GB, Weiss MA, Johnston JL: Cytodifferentiation of urinary epithelial fragments. Papillary transitional cell carcinoma in a renal allograft recipient. Acta Cytol 25:302–306, 1981.

37. Sharifi R, Shaw M, Ray V, Rhee H, Nagubadi S, Guinan P: Evaluation of cytologic techniques for diagnosis of prostate cancer. Urol 21:417–420, 1983.

38. Tetu B, Katz RL, Kalter SP, von Eschenbach AC, Barlogie B: Acridine-orange flow cytometry of urinary bladder washings for the detection of transitional cell carcinoma of the bladder. Cancer 60:1815–1822, 1987.

39. Thomson HDP: Ciliated cells in voided urine. Acta Cytol 26:263–264, 1982.

40. Trillo AA, Kuchler LL, Wood AC, Prater T: Adenocarcinoma of the urinary bladder: Histologic, cytologic and ultrastructural features in a case. Acta Cytol 25:285–290, 1981.

41. Troster M, Wyatt JK, Alen-Halagah J: Nephrogenic adenoma of the urinary bladder: Histologic and cytologic observations in a case. Acta Cytol 30:41–44, 1986.

42. Winkelmann M, Grabensee B, Pfitzer P: Differential diagnosis of acute allograft rejection and CMV infection in renal transplantation by urinary cytology. Pathol Res Pract 180:161–168, 1985.

43. Wolinska WH, Melamed MR: Urinary conduit cytology. Cancer 32:1000–1006, 1973.

44. Wolinska WH, Melamed MR, Klein FA: Cytology of bladder papilloma. Acta Cytol 29:817–822, 1985.

45. Wolinska WH, Melamed MR, Schellhammer PF, Whitmore WF Jr: Urethral cytology following cystectomy for bladder carcinoma. Am J Surg Pathol 1:225–234, 1977.

18

Central Nervous System

Sandra H. Bigner

Although cerebrospinal fluid (CSF) is often discussed as one of the body cavity fluids, several major differences exist between this fluid and effusions. First, CSF is a fluid that is normally present, whereas an effusion is always a pathologic finding. Second, the pial and arachnoidal cells that line the subarachnoid space (SAS) rarely shed into the CSF, whereas the mesothelial cells that line the pleural, peritoneal and pericardial cavities frequently proliferate and are often major cellular components of effusions. Third, because the presence of an effusion is abnormal, cytologic evaluation of this fluid is most often performed to determine whether or not the accumulation has a neoplastic etiology. Sampling of CSF, in contrast, is performed in a variety of clinical situations. For example, examination of this fluid is among the most direct and effective means of diagnosing conditions that primarily involve the SAS space, such as leptomeningitis, subarachnoid hemorrhage and meningeal carcinomatosis. In addition, the contact of the SAS with the entire brain and spinal cord as well as its continuity with the ventricular system means that CSF often indirectly reflects disorders located primarily within the parenchyma of the central nervous system (CNS). Therefore, cytologic evaluation of a sample of CSF requires knowledge of the clinical findings of the patient from whom it was obtained. An understanding of the cytologic presentation of the spectrum of CNS disorders, which can be manifested in CSF, is also required.

Fine needle aspiration of the brain, like fine needle aspiration of other body sites, is generally performed as one step in the evaluation of mass lesions. As in other locations, the differential diagnosis includes inflammatory masses, such as abscesses, tuberculomas and other types of granulomas, and neoplasms, such as lymphomas, metastatic tumors and primary brain tumors.

The application of cytologic techniques to diagnoses of conditions that are manifested in CSF are discussed here with emphasis on disorders that occur primarily in the SAS. The presentation of intracranial lesions in

needle aspirates and cyst fluids are also described, including the cytologic characteristics of the most common types of primary brain tumors.

PREPARATORY METHODS

Cerebrospinal Fluid

Because of the low cellularity of CSF, cytopreparatory methods have been developed that allow concentration of the cells with preservation of their morphologic characteristics. The two methods that are most widely used today are membrane filtration and cytocentrifugation.

The types of membranes used in preparations of CSF are Millipore filters, nucleopore filters and Gelman filters. Filters have the advantage, when used correctly, of retention of virtually every cell in the sample. One disadvantage is that staining with methods other than the Papanicolaou stain is generally not satisfactory. In addition, good results require considerable skill and experience as well as attention to detail, as too much pressure produces unacceptable distortion of the cells; air drying and unevenness in the mounting medium are also common errors.

Cytocentrifugation has advantages in that the preparatory method is simpler and less time consuming than filters. Air-dried slides also can easily be made for staining with a variety of stains as well as immunohistochemical methods. The main disadvantage is that some degree of cell loss is practically inevitable.

Choice of method of preparation should be determined by the number and types of cases of CSF processed in an individual laboratory as well as the overall specimen volume and distribution. For example, in a small laboratory, which is not accustomed to preparing filters, cytocentrifugation is usually the method of choice. Filters are more appropriately used in the laboratory in which a high volume of CSF samples are processed or one in which filters are routinely used for other specimen types. In our laboratory both membrane filters and cytocentrifuged slides are prepared on each case.[8] The Millipore filters give the best cell yield, whereas the cellular detail on Papanicolaou-stained cytocentrifuged slides is often superior. Air-dried slides prepared by this method are employed for Diff-Quik staining and immunohistochemistry.

Fine Needle Aspiration Biopsy

Method of preparation of samples obtained by needle aspiration depends on the size and consistency of the tissue. Large pieces of firm tissue are best processed for histologic evaluation as cell blocks. Small fragments of firm tissue are often utilized for squash preparations, and loosely aggregated cells may be smeared.[37, 38] In any case, additional cellular material may be obtained by washing the needle with a balanced salt solution, which may be used for filters or cytocentrifuged preparations. It is critical that the observer be familiar with the presentation of common brain lesions in the type of preparation that is being examined. For example, because the perceived cellularity is one of the most important parameters in distinguishing normal brain cells from gliosis and low-grade astrocytomas, experience in judging thickness of the smeared or squashed material is necessary in making this determination.

These preparations may be stained with a variety of methods. Hematoxylin and eosin are standard for cell blocks, whereas the Papanicolaou stain is generally applied to other types of slides. In addition, it is frequently helpful to prepare air-dried slides, which may be utilized for immunohistochemistry, particularly in high-grade tumors in which malignant gliomas must be distinguished from metastasis and lymphoma.

NORMAL CEREBROSPINAL FLUID AND HISTOLOGY

The CSF is formed in the ventricles of the brain, and it travels posteriorly to exit into the SAS, which covers the brain and spinal cord. The SAS is lined externally by the thin arachnoid membrane composed of meningothelial cells and internally by the pial surface of the brain. The only cellular elements normally seen in the SAS are blood vessels and strands of loose connective tissue. Although CSF is theoretically acellular, small numbers of lymphocytes and occasional monocytes are seen in most samples of CSF (Fig. 18–1). Based on evaluation of samples from patients in whom no neurologic disorders are found, as well as from patients with seizures and those undergoing myelography, cell counts of less than 5 or 10 cells per mm³ are considered to be normal in adults. Slightly higher cell counts may be seen in neonates, although

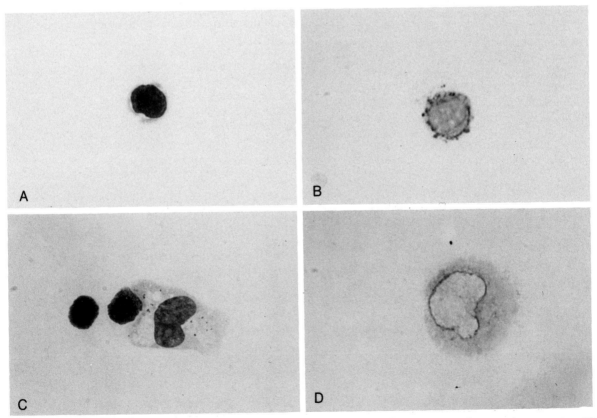

FIGURE 18–1. Normal components of cerebrospinal fluid (CSF) include lymphocytes, *(A)* and *(B)*, and monocytes, *(C)* and *(D)*. A and C, Diff-Quik stain; ×1000. B and D, Immunoperoxidase using panleukocyte antibody 2D1; ×1000.

there are seldom opportunities to examine fluid from neurologically uninvolved individuals in this age group.

The composition of the cellular component and the morphology of the individual cells are critical factors in determining whether the cells in a sample of CSF are normal or pathologic. Mature lymphocytes of small or intermediate size and a few monocytes, presumably derived from blood, are the cell types seen in normal CSF (see Fig. 18–1). The presence of polymorphonuclear leukocytes; enlarged, atypical lymphocytes or monocytes that have become phagocytic, as well as an increase in absolute cell number, are all indications that a pathologic condition exists. In some reports these atypical, reactive elements have been termed "pia arachnoid cells," suggesting that they are derived from proliferations of the lining cells of the SAS in a manner analogous to the reactive mesothelium of effusions. The demonstration that these cells express either lymphoid or monocytic antigens, however, and their morphologic resemblance to inflammatory cells rather than meningothelial cells support the interpretation that they are of hematogenous origin (see Fig. 18–1).

Most normal brain and spinal cord elements, such as neurons and glia, are rarely if ever detected in CSF derived by lumbar puncture.[51] Papillary fragments of cuboidal cells probably originating in the choroid plexus are, however, occasionally seen. Because fragments of choroid plexus cannot be reliably distinguished cytologically from ependymal cells, these elements are termed "ependymal-choroidal cells" by some observers. Regardless of the histogenesis of these cells in an individual case, it is important to recognize this normal cellular component to avoid mistaking these fragments for neoplasia. Other normal elements that are sometimes encountered in CSF obtained by lumbar puncture are chondrocytes from the intervertebral disk (Fig. 18–2). The presence of these cells is probably a physical phenomenon related to direct contact of the sampling needle with the disk and carries no known pathologic significance.[31] Rarely isolated, benign spindle-shaped cells are encountered. Although some observers have considered them to represent astrocytes, others believe that they are fibroblasts from the loose connective tissue of the SAS.

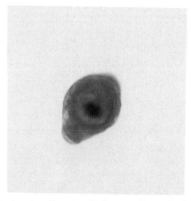

FIGURE 18–2. Cartilage cell in cerebrospinal fluid (CSF) derived by lumbar puncture (Papanicolaou stain; × 1000).

VENTRICULAR FLUID

The insertion of ventricular shunts and the introduction of radiopaque material into ventricles are procedures frequently performed in patients with hydrocephalus. If a neoplastic condition is suspected ventricular fluid may be obtained throught the shunt or needle for cytologic evaluation. In a patient with known meningeal tumor spread, an intraventricular cannula attached to the Omaya reservoir may be placed to allow installation of chemotherapeutic agents. Fluid is sometimes withdrawn through the tube for examination. Ventricular fluids obtained by this means differ from lumbar puncture–derived CSF in that they frequently contain choroid plexus cells in large numbers (Fig. 18–3A).[57] Fragments of normal gray and white matter containing neurons and glia and portions of capillaries are also often seen (Fig. 18–3B and C). Recognition that these cell types are characteristic of ventricular fluids is critical so that they are not misinterpreted as being neoplastic in origin.

INFECTIOUS CONDITIONS

Increased numbers of inflammatory cells in a sample of CSF, particularly if a component of polymorphonuclear leukocytes or enlarged and atypical lymphocytes is observed, suggests that an infectious process may be present. Although higher cell counts are more likely to occur if the disorder is occurring predominantly in the SAS, meningeal infections cannot be reliably distinguished from meningeal infiltrates secondary to primary parenchyma disease of the brain or spinal cord. The composition of the cellular infiltrate may suggest that the process in an individual patient is likely to be infectious rather than a reaction to a noninfectious disorder and may suggest a bacterial, viral or fungal etiology. Nevertheless, diagnosis of an infection requires demonstration of the responsible organism by direct visualization, culture or antibody titer.

The most typical cellular presentation of acute bacterial meningitis is an infiltrate composed predominantly of polymorphonuclear leukocytes. This pattern is not specific for this disorder, however, as an acute inflammatory infiltrate can also be seen in the CSF or acute cerebral infarctions and, occasionally, in the early stages of viral and fungal infections.

Viral meningoencephalitis most frequently produces a predominantly lymphocytic response in CSF. The cells often show atypical features, such as clumped chromatin and prominent nucleoli, and distinguishing between a viral infection and lymphoma may be difficult.[11] The viruses that usually produce this disorder are the enteroviruses, which do not display characteristic cellular inclusions in cells of CSF. Other viruses that involve the parenchyma of the brain and spinal cord and produce a meningeal infiltrate are cytomegalovirus (CMV), herpes simplex, herpes zoster and JC virus and SV40-PML virus of progressive multifocal leukoencephalopathy (PML). Although cells contain-

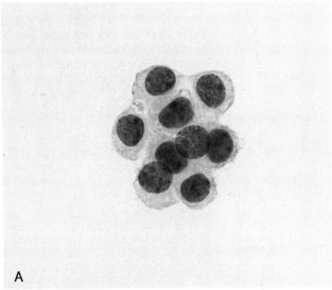

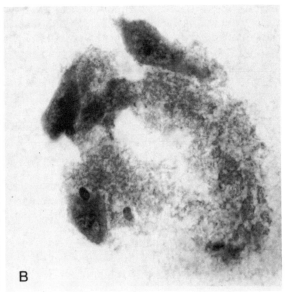

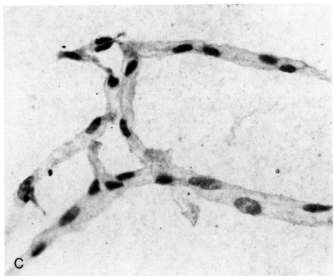

FIGURE 18–3. Components frequently seen in ventricular fluids. *A*, Choroid plexus cells (Papanicolaou stain; ×1000). *B*, Gray matter containing neurons (Papanicolaou stain; ×680). *C*, Capillary (Papanicolaou stain; ×680).

ing the characteristic nuclear inclusions of these viruses can be demonstrated in open biopsy and needle biopsy specimens of the parenchymal lesions, inclusion-bearing cells are only rarely identified in CSF. To date, the literature contains only two reported cases of herpes encephalitis and one case of CMV infection in a patient with acquired immune deficiency syndrome (AIDS) in whom cells with typical inclusions were seen in CSF.[8, 21, 29]

A nonspecific lymphocytosis may be seen due to CNS infections of other etiologies. Wilber and colleagues[56] have described an atypical lymphocytic proliferation with plasmacytosis in the CSF of patients with cerebral cysticercosis. Similar findings have also been reported in the CSF of patients with Lyme disease.[44]

Three types of CNS disorders are seen in patients with AIDS. First is AIDS encephalopathy resulting directly or indirectly from infection of cells within the brain or spinal cord by the AIDS virus. Histologically, the lesions consist of glial nodules, chronic inflamma-

tion, gliosis and sometimes multinucleated giant cells. The CSF from these patients usually contains only a nonspecific chronic inflammatory infiltrate, although rarely, multinucleated giant cells may be encountered. The second group of abnormalities consists of opportunistic infections that are most frequently produced by *Cryptococcus neoformans*, *Toxoplasma gondii*, mycobacteria, *Candida* and viruses such as CMV and PML. Although these organisms or their characteristic cellular inclusions can frequently be demonstrated by open-brain biopsy specimens or needle aspirates of the cerebral lesions,[25] their manifestations in CSF are usually nonspecific with the exception of rare cases of CMV inclusion–bearing cells in CSF.[29] Among these infections, cryptococcal meningitis is the only process in which examination of CSF yields a specific diagnosis in a high percent of cases. The third disorder involving the CNS of patients with AIDS is neoplasia that is most frequently lymphoma. Examination of the CSF often reveals the characteristic malignant cells of lymphoma both in AIDS patients with primary CNS lymphoma involving the subarachnoid space and in patients with systemic lymphoma and CNS metastases. Because the majority of these lymphomas are of the B-cell type, immunohistochemical markers are often helpful in establishing the diagnosis.

Cryptococcus neoformans is the most frequent cause of fungal meningitis. This organism usually enters the body through the respiratory system and disseminates to the CNS hematogenously.[17] Cryptococcal meningitis may be a complication of immunosuppression as is seen in recipients of organ transplants, in patients with lymphoma and leukemia and in patients with AIDS. This disease occasionally occurs, however, in otherwise healthy individuals. In the immunosuppressed patient, in particular, there may be very little cellular reaction and the CSF may contain multitudes of organisms. In some cases, however, a brisk inflammatory reaction may occur. The cells can be mainly lymphocytes, although occasionally polymorphonuclear leukocytes or macrophages predominate. The organisms are frequently demonstrable morphologically as round yeast forms of variable diameters, which produce thin-necked buds (Fig. 18–4).[3, 46] Commonly, the organisms have a refractile appearance, possibly due to the mounting medium which is trapped between the capsule of the organism and the coverslip (see Fig. 18–4). Organisms with this presentation can be mistaken for particles of glove powder, which are also refractile.

Cryptococci often possess a thick, mucopolysaccharide capsule that stains readily with mucicarmine, Alcian blue and colloidal iron stains. Organisms without a prominent capsule are sometimes encountered, however, and these structures may be difficult to distinguish from partially lysed erythrocytes or even bubbles of air or water, which may be trapped under the coverslip. The presence of true buds are useful in distinguishing the organisms from these other structures.

Cryptococci must also be distinguished from other types of budding yeasts, such as *Blastomyces dermititidis* and *Histoplasma capsulatum*, which occur only rarely in CSF. In addition to the thin-necked buds and mucopolysaccharide capsule that is characteristic of *Cryptococcus*, this organism usually displays a wide range of diameters within an individual specimen.

Blastomyces is uniformly large with diameters of 8 to 12 μ and *Histoplasma* is uniformly small, generally 1 to 5 μ in size. In addition to diagnosing cryptococcal meningitis cytologically, the organism may be identified by its growth characteristics in culture and by demonstration of cryptococcal antigen by radioimmunoassay.

DEMYELINATING DISEASES

The cellular components in CSF from patients with demyelinating diseases are variable, depending on the specific diagnosis and the phase and extent of the disease. In multiple sclerosis (MS), for example, the cell counts and constitution may be normal during quiescent phases of the disease. Immunophenotyping of the lymphocyte populations generally reveals T cell predominance with mature T cells expressing either the helper or suppressor phenotype.[39] Some observers have described a decreased suppressor/helper cell ratio in both CSF and peripheral blood of MS patients during exacerbation due to an absolute decline in the number of suppressor cells.[47] Other studies, however, have failed to demonstrate differences in suppressor/helper cell ratios between CSF from patients with MS and patients with other CNS disorders, such as Guillain-Barré syndrome (GBS) and CNS infections.[42] Rarely, in acute, rapidly progressive cases other cell types including polymorphonuclear leukocytes and macrophages may be seen.

In most cases of GBS, the CSF is acellular, but when inflammatory cells are present a lymphocytic response predominates. The clinical picture is similar to that seen in viral meningoencephalitis with a polyclonal lymphocytic population with T cell predominance. For the other diseases in which demyelination is a component, the nature and extent of cellular elements in CSF reflect the nature of the infiltrate within the parenchyma of the brain and spinal cord.

VASCULAR DISORDERS

The two general categories of vascular disorders that occur in the CNS are hemorrhage and infarction and both processes may be reflected in the CSF. In cases of pure hemorrhage due to a ruptured aneurysm, bleeding vascular malformation or intracerebral hemorrhage with rupture into the SAS, the appearance of blood in the CSF is followed within hours by the appearance of macrophages that rapidly begin engulfing the erythrocytes. Within several days degeneration of the red blood cells to hemosiderin produces the characteristic hemosiderin-laden macrophages associated with this process (Fig. 18–5). This sequence of events is a general response to the presence of blood in CSF and is irrespective of the etiology of the bleeding. For example, blood introduced into CSF during lumbar puncture or a "traumatic tap" elicits an identical reaction.

Cerebral infarction frequently produces a secondary inflammatory response in CSF. Whether or not cells

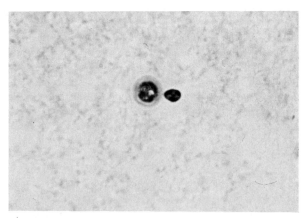

FIGURE 18–4. Budding yeast of cryptococcus in cerebrospinal fluid (CSF) (Papanicolaou stain; ×1700).

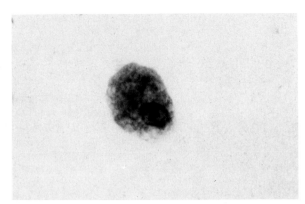

FIGURE 18–5. Hemosiderin-laden macrophage in cerebrospinal fluid (CSF) from a patient with **subarachnoid hemorrhage** (Papanicolaou stain; ×1000).

appear in CSF is a function of the size of the infarct and its proximity to the surface of the brain or spinal cord. The type of cellular reaction is related to the stage and character of the infarct and in general reflects the histologic appearance of the intraparenchymal lesion. In the early stages polymorphonuclear leukocytes, sometimes with a hemorrhagic component, are seen. This picture rapidly shifts to a predominantly macrophage response in which fragments of degenerated myelin fill the cytoplasm of the cells. At this stage the fluid may be extremely hypercellular and can be confused with a neoplasm if the observer does not consider the possibility of a destructive lesion.

TRAUMA

Cellular infiltrates in CSF from victims of CNS trauma are indistinguishable from the cells seen in subarachnoid hemorrhage and destructive lesions of other etiologies. Thus, red blood cells and macrophages containing hemosiderin or myelin debris are the most common manifestions of trauma in CSF. Patients with sinus and basilar skull fractures with tears in the meninges are at risk for developing leakage of sinus contents into the SAS. The CSF in this setting contains a marked acute inflammatory reaction. Bacteria and other elements, such as fragments of *Candida* and ciliated respiratory epithelial cells from the sinus lining, may also be seen.[9]

REACTIONS TO INTRAVENTRICULAR SHUNTS

Occasionally, highly cellular samples of CSF containing reactive ependymal cells, epithelioid cells and multinucleated giant cells are obtained through intraventricular shunts (Fig. 18–6).[10] They may be associated with a history of a malfunctioning shunt and in some cases have been correlated with a histologically documented granulomatous process occluding the shunt tip. Recognition that this type of reaction may

be associated with a malfunctioning shunt is important in aiding the surgeon in deciding whether or not a shunt revision is necessary. In addition, awareness of this presentation will avoid confusing this reaction with a granulomatous process of infectious etiology or neoplasm. In addition to this type of foreign-body reaction, the presence of an intraventricular shunt is one of the etiologies of eosinophilia in CSF.[52]

NEOPLASIA

A variety of neoplastic processes, including leukemia, lymphoma, carcinoma, melanoma and primary CNS tumor can be detected by examination of CSF when they involve the ventricles or SAS. Because the majority of patients with meningeal tumor have a known tumor diagnosis at the time of subarachnoid dissemination, the question is usually whether or not cells similar to those in the original biopsy sample are present in the CSF. In the few cases in which patients without a previous diagnosis of neoplasia present with neoplastic cells in CSF, knowledge of the age of the patients, locations of other tumor masses in the body and morphology of the cells, including their expression of specific antigens using immunohistochemistry, will usually allow an accurate diagnosis.

Leukemia

Because the most common pattern of leukemic involvement of the CNS is infiltration of the SAS with little or no parenchymal disease, examination of CSF is the most practical means of establishing this diagnosis. This process is particularly common in childhood leukemia with acute lymphocytic leukemia (ALL) and undifferentiated stem cell leukemia being among the most prevalent types. With the advent in the 1960s of chemotherapeutic protocols capable of producing systemic remission, CNS relapse occurred in more than

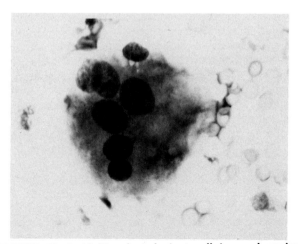

FIGURE 18–6. Multinucleated giant cell in cerebrospinal fluid (CSF) obtained from an intraventricular shunt (Diff-Quik stain; ×680).

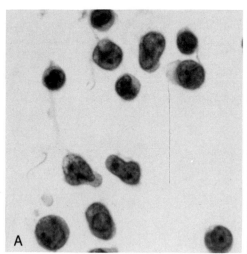
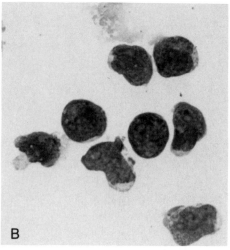

FIGURE 18–7. Blast forms in cerebrospinal fluid (CSF) from a child with **acute lymphocytic leukemia (ALL).** *A,* Papanicolaou stain; ×1000. *B,* Diff-Quik stain; ×1000.

50% of patients with ALL. This observation led to the routine administration of CNS prophylaxis with radiation or chemotherapy, a practice that has dramatically reduced the incidence of CNS disease.[12, 16, 28] Nevertheless, this complication still occurs in 5 to 15% of cases, making periodic examination of the CSF in patients with ALL a component of standard protocols.[27, 45]

The cells of ALL are typical blast forms with high nucleocytoplasmic ratios and round or convoluted nuclei (Fig. 18–7). All varieties of ALL, including null, B, T and pre-B cell types, can involve the CSF with a possible tendency for T-cell disorders to behave in this fashion most frequently. When large numbers of blast forms are present, they can be readily identified on routine preparations making immunohistochemical procedures for lymphoid antigens unnecessary (see Fig. 18–7). Occasionally, a problem in differential diagnosis arises between recurrent leukemia and pleocytosis due to infection in a patient with ALL. In this case, immunohistochemical demonstration of polyclonality or of a monoclonal population, expressing the same phenotype as was seen in the marrow, may resolve the problem.

Diagnostic difficulties may also arise when only a few abnormal cells are encountered in a mixed cellular population in CSF from a patient with ALL. Although some observers have used antibodies against common acute lymphoblastic leukemia antigen (CALLA) or expression of terminal deoxynucleotidyltransferase in this setting to identify small populations of blast forms, recurrent ALL should probably not be diagnosed using this criterion alone because rare CALLA-positive cells can be seen in individuals without leukemia.[27, 53] Another problem area is where abnormal cells are seen in a specimen of low cellularity. Even if a few blast forms can be identified with certainty, these patients so affected present a difficult clinical problem in that conflicting evidence exists as to whether or not they should be treated for CNS relapse. Although earlier studies suggested that the presence of only rare blast forms in CSF samples of normal cell counts should result in aggressive intrathecal therapy, further studies in which such patients have been treated conservatively

have shown spontaneous clearing of the abnormal cells in some of them. The approach suggested by McIntosh and Ritchey[33] for patients with ALL is to treat them for CNS relapse if the CSF contains more than 10 cell/μl with blast forms or with less then 10 cells/μl if blast forms predominate. For patients in whom only rare blast forms are seen in CSF samples with less than 5 white blood cells/μl, however, their policy is only to repeat the examination of CSF every few months to 1 year provided that the patient is in systemic remission and lacks CNS symptoms.

Involvement of the CNS is also seen in patients with acute myelogenous leukemia (AML), acute promyelocytic leukemia (APML) (Fig. 18–8), acute monocytic leukemia (AMoL) and acute myelomonocytic leukemia (AMMoL). Patients with AMMoL and inversions of chromosome 16, in particular, are at risk for having meningeal involvement at the time of presentation.[34] The absolute incidence of CSF leukemia is lower than in ALL due to the shorter survival times of these patients, but with increased survival times of these patients, as new therapeutic protocols are developed, the incidence of this complication can be expected to increase.[43] Central nervous system leukemia may occur either at initial presentation or at relapse. The cells resemble the blast forms seen in the marrow and peripheral blood and can be readily identified on routine preparations. In contrast to the acute leukemias, CNS involvement is unusual in the chronic phase of myelogenous leukemia (CML). When patients enter the accelerated phase or blast crisis, however, immature myeloid forms may be observed in the CSF of some patients.[8]

Symptomatic CNS involvement is so rare in patients with chronic lymphocytic leukemia (CLL) and prolymphocytic leukemia, that an infectious process should be considered first when they develop signs of meningeal disease.[18] Because of their immunocompromised status, viral and cryptococcal meningitides are common in this group of patients, and the lymphocytosis that is sometimes produced may be difficult to distinguish from leukemic involvement.[11] Application of immunohistochemical lymphoid markers often resolves the

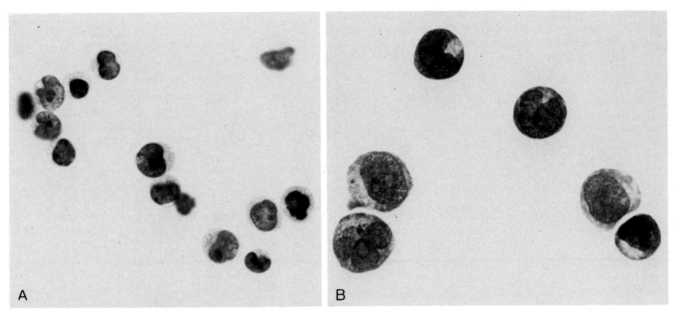

FIGURE 18–8. Immature myeloid cells in cerebrospinal fluid (CSF) from a patient with **acute promyelocytic leukemia (APML).** *A*, Papanicolaou stain; ×1000. *B*, Diff-Quik stain; ×1000.

problem. If these procedures are not available, a careful search for cryptococcal infection and a conservative position of awaiting spontaneous resolution of a viral infection are approaches that may establish the diagnosis.

Lymphoma

As with leukemia, the most common pattern of CNS involvement from systemic lymphoma is subarachnoid dissemination with little or no parenchymal disease. Occasionally, however, multifocal infiltrates occur within the brain and spinal cord of patients with bulky disease elsewhere. Although primary CNS lymphoma generally presents as a solitary mass lesion, CSF dissemination is common during the course of this disease.

The varieties of lymphoma that tend to seed the SAS are among the most aggressive histologic types and include large-cell lymphoma and immunoblastic sarcoma in the adult as well as lymphoblastic lymphoma, Burkitt's lymphoma and undifferentiated lymphoma in the child. Detection of these cells is based on the presence of a monomorphous population with cellular characteristics of the lymphoma type demonstrated elsewhere in the patient. Because the majority of lymphomas involving the CSF are the B-cell type, whereas reactive lymphocytoses contain mainly T cells, the demonstration of a monoclonal population expressing one type of light chain and one type of heavy chain is a helpful diagnostic adjunct in difficult cases.[36] If the phenotype has previously been demonstrated in nodal tissue, documentation of the same pattern in cells in CSF allows a specific and definitive diagnosis. For T-cell lymphoma, interpretation of lymphoid marker panels may be more difficult owing to the mixture of neoplastic and reactive T cells that is frequently encountered.[30]

The better differentiated forms of lymphoma, including nodular lymphoma, and small-cell lymphoma of the cleaved and noncleaved varieties, in contrast, uncommonly produce symptomatic CNS involvement. As in the case with CLL, infectious processes should be considered in patients with these disorders who develop neurologic problems. The immunohistochemical application of lymphoid antibodies is often definitive in distinguishing lymphoma from reactive conditions in samples of CSF from these patients. Hodgkin's disease, also, rarely involves the CNS directly and is almost never seen in the SAS or CSF.

Metastatic Carcinoma and Meningeal Carcinomatosis

The ability to diagnose metastatic carcinoma to the CNS by examination of CSF is directly proportional to the extent to which the process involves the ventricular system and SAS. In cases in which the metastatic lesions are confined to the brain and spinal cord parenchyma or to the bones and extradural space of the skull or spine, cells have no access to the CSF. In many cases of brain metastases, however, large lesions or small multiple foci impinge upon the surface of the brain, cord and ventricles and shed diagnostic cells into CSF.[19] The cells may be few in number and are frequently mixed with a dense infiltrate of lymphocytes and macrophages making multiple samplings and careful study of the fluid necessary to establish the diagnosis. The application of anticytokeratin or anticarcinoma antibodies can be extremely useful in these situations to highlight rare malignant cells within an inflammatory background.[4]

In approximately 5% of cases of brain metastases a pattern consisting almost entirely of subarachnoid involvement is encountered.[20] This condition, termed meningeal carcinomatosis or carcinomatous meningitis, may be difficult to diagnose clinically, particularly in the patient without previous documentation of cancer. The demonstration of cranial nerve palsies or compression of spinal nerve roots may lead to suspicion of this process and examination of CSF is the most practical and definitive means of establishing this diagnosis.

Carcinoma of the lung and the breast, with their tendency to disseminate hematogenously, are the tumor types encountered most frequently in CSF, both as the result of multifocal metastases and of meningeal carcinomatosis.[5, 7, 8, 15, 32, 40] Although adenocarcinoma of the stomach is considerably less common than it was in the early part of this century, cases of meningeal carcinomatosis from this source are still seen, and this tumor type remains responsible for many cases of meningeal carcinomatosis that appear with an occult primary.[5] Other tumor types that are reasonably frequent in the population, including renal cell carcinoma, adenocarcinoma of the colon and transitional cell carcinoma of the bladder, are uncommonly seen in CSF as they tend to produce solitary brain metastases rather than multifocal lesions or meningeal carcinomatosis. In addition to these tumor types that involve the SAS hematogenously, some neoplasms arising in the head and sinuses, such as squamous cell carcinoma in the adult and embryonal rhabdomyosarcoma in the child, enter the CSF by direct invasion of bone or travel along cranial nerves. Rarely, a similar process occurs in the pelvis when squamous cell carcinoma of the uterine cervix or adenocarcinoma of the colon grows directly into the subarachnoid space of the spinal cord.[8, 55]

The morphology of these cells is generally the same as their presentation in other types of cytologic specimens (Fig. 18–9) except, however, for a greater tendency for carcinoma cells to shed singly or in loose clusters rather than in cohesive tissue fragments. This characteristic is particularly obvious with breast carcinoma, which usually occurs in CSF as single cells and only rarely forms balls and morula.

Cutaneous melanoma is among the tumor types with the greatest liklihood of CNS metastasis. The majority of fatal cases of disseminated melanoma had nervous system involvement found at the time of autopsy.[1] Cells can be identified in CSF from patients with multifocal lesions of the brain and cord if the SAS space is invaded, and tumor spread is readily diagnosed in cases of diffuse subarachnoid melanomatosis. In a patient who presents with melanoma in the CSF in the absence of an identified primary tumor in the skin or mucous membranes, it may be impossible to determine whether or not the process actually began in the meninges as a primary meningeal melanoma.[49]

Cells of malignant melanoma are characteristically large with coarse nuclear chromatin and prominent macronucleoli (Fig. 18–10). When cytoplasmic melanin pigment is present, a specific diagnosis of melanoma can be made, even in the absence of previous documentation of melanoma elsewhere in the body.[5] In the absence of pigment it may be difficult to distinguish

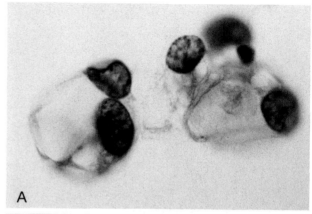

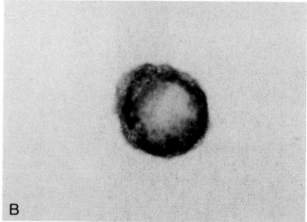

FIGURE 18–9. Adenocarcinoma metastatic to cerebrospinal fluid (CSF) from the breast. A, Papanicolaou stain; ×1000. B, Positive immunoperoxidase reaction using anticytokeratin antibody; ×1000.

these cells from other large-cell malignancies, such as large-cell undifferentiated carcinoma of the lung and large-cell lymphoma. Here, positive reactivity with antimelanoma antibodies, such as HM-15 and ME 1-14 with absence of cytoplasmic cytokeratin, and lack of expression of anticarcinoma antibodies and panleukocyte reagents are useful in helping to establish the diagnosis (see Fig. 18–10).[50]

Although the majority of patients with meningeal carcinomatosis have a known primary tumor at the time they develop this CNS complication, occasional patients present first with meningeal symptoms and an occult tumor. When cytologically malignant cells are demonstrated in CSF from such a patient, lymphoma, metastatic carcinoma, melanoma and primary brain tumors should all be considered. Although the morphologic features of the cells may be sufficiently characteristic to allow a specific diagnosis, we have found a panel of antibodies to be helpful in making these distinctions (Table 18–1).[54] Primary brain tumors express panneuroectodermal antigens such as the one detected by monoclonal antibody UJ13A. Malignant gliomas express glial fibrillary acidic protein (GFAP) in addition. Metastatic carcinomas, in contrast, are negative with these reagents but generally express cytokeratins (Fig. 18–9B), and many express carci-

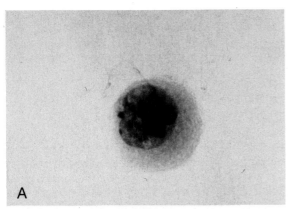

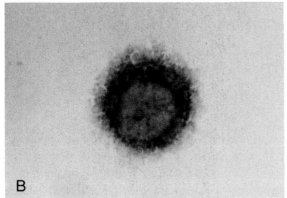

FIGURE 18–10. Cells of **malignant melanoma in cerebrospinal fluid (CSF).** *A,* Papanicolaou stain; ×1000. *B,* Positive immunoperoxidase reaction using antimelanoma antibody Mel-14; ×1000.

noma-associated antigens such as CEA or TAG-72 detected by antibody B72.3 as well. Melanomas are negative for the reagents described but express S-100 protein and react with melanoma-associated antibodies. The use of anti-S-100 protein antibodies alone, however, is insufficient to distinguish melanoma from the other tumor types, because these reagents react with many primary brain tumors and a subset of carcinomas in addition to melanoma.[50] Lymphomas are negative for the reagents described but are detected by panleukocyte reagents as well as antibodies against T-cell and B-cell antigens. Because no single reagent will reliably distinguish metastases from other tumor types, antibody panels when used in conjunction with clinical history and cytologic features allow an accurate diagnosis in the majority of cases.

In many cases one can establish that the meningeal tumor is likely to be metastatic based either on the presence of an extracranial mass or the pattern of an antigen expression in the tumor cells. Here the problem may be to determine the site of the primary tumor. With the exception of antimelanoma reagents and a small number of organ-specific markers, such as prostatic-specific antigen in prostatic carcinoma, no reliable antibodies exist that can be employed to distinguish among metastases from various sites. In this setting, it is useful to consider that the majority of cases of meningeal carcinomatosis with occult primary tumors originate in the lung. Breast carcinoma, in contrast, only rarely appears first with subarachnoid dissemination before the discovery of a breast mass.[5, 13, 24] Carcinoma of the stomach should also be considered in this situation, although the incidence of this tumor type spreading in the meninges is considerably lower than that of carcinoma of the lung.

Primary Central Nervous System Tumors

Gliomas. As with metastatic tumors, the only primary CNS tumors that are detectable by examination of CSF are those that involve the ventricles or SAS by direct extension and those that disseminate through the spinal fluid pathways. Although any histologic type of malignant adult glioma may produce this finding, advanced glioblastoma multiforme is the tumor type that most frequently spreads in this fashion. The morphology of the cells seen in CSF in these cases is as varied as the histologic spectrum.[8] Cells may be anaplastic ranging from small to large in size, or may retain their resemblance to astrocytes. However, even the most poorly differentiated tumors usually retain the expression of GFAP in at least some cells allowing for a specific diagnosis using antibodies against GFAP.[54] Another tumor type also exhibiting this type of behavior is the malignant ependymoma, which also sheds into CSF as morphologically undifferentiated cells. Low-grade gliomas including astrocytomas, ependymomas and oligodendrogliomas may also metastasize throughout the ventricular system and SAS.[2, 26, 35] These tumors are not always demonstrable by cytologic examination of CSF, however, because they often produce cohesive implants, which exfoliate poorly. In addition, because these cells are cytologically benign, they can be difficult to distinguish from macrophages and monocytes unless specific antibodies are employed.

The most common malignant primary brain tumor of childhood, the medulloblastoma, commonly spreads through the neuroaxis by way of the spinal fluid path-

TABLE 18–1. Antibodies Useful in Distinguishing Among Lymphoma/Leukemia, Metastatic Carcinoma, Melanoma and Primary Brain Tumors

	Anticytokeratin	B72.3	S-100	Mel-14	UJ13A	GFAP	2D1
Carcinoma	+	+	−/+	−	−	−	−
Melanoma	−	−	+	+	−	−	−
Lymphoma/Leukemia	−	−	−	−	−	−	+
Glioblastoma	−	−	+	+	+	+	−
Medulloblastoma	−	−	+	+	+	−	−

GFAP = glial fibrillary acidic protein.

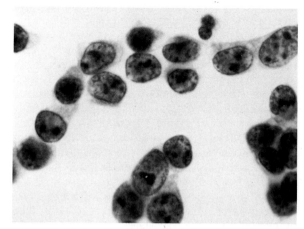

FIGURE 18–11. Small undifferentiated malignant tumor cells of medulloblastoma in cerebrospinal fluid (CSF) (Papanicolaou stain; × 1000).

way.[22, 41] This tumor appears as cell clusters and isolated cells with high nucleocytoplasmic ratios, hyperchromatic nuclei and scant cytoplasm (Fig. 18–11). These cells express panneuroectodermal antigens such as those detected by monoclonal antibodies UJ13A, are usually negative for GFAP and sometimes express neurofilament proteins.[23] Gliomas represent another relatively large group of childhood brain tumors. Although most of these neoplasms are low grade and slow growing, the most malignant variety of astrocytic glioma, glioblastoma multiforme, is capable of disseminating in the SAS. This pattern of behavior is particularly characteristic of malignant brain stem gliomas. These cells are frequently small in size and anaplastic in their cellular characteristics, making them difficult to distinguish from other small-cell neoplasms, such as medulloblastoma and ependymoblastoma. Precise localization of the primary tumor in the brain stem as opposed to the fourth ventricle or cerebellum is helpful in making this distinction. In addition, the expression of large amounts of GFAP while characteristic of gliomas is unusual in medulloblastomas.

Another group of childhood tumors that are relatively uncommon, but share the tendency to disseminate through spinal fluid pathways, are tumors of the pineal gland and hypothalamic region.[14] The germinoma is the tumor type that is most notorious for CSF spread, but the other types of malignant germ cell tumors and the primary pineal tumor, the pineoblastoma, behave in a similar manner.[48]

Although the majority of primary brain tumors that spread in the CSF are histologically malignant and biologically aggressive, choroid plexus tumors of all grades, ranging from the choroid plexus papilloma to the choroid plexus carcinoma, exhibit this behavior. This pattern of spread is undoubtedly because of the location of these tumors in the ventricles with ready access to the CSF as well as the friable, papillary nature of the tissue. The morphology of these papillary fronds is usually sufficiently characteristic to allow diagnosis of these tumors.[8] The malignant variety is

cytologically similar to metastatic papillary adenocarcinoma, but the extremely young age of these infants with the typical large, intraventricular masses that are produced allow this distinction to be readily made.

DIAGNOSTIC ACCURACY IN CEREBROSPINAL FLUID CYTOLOGY

Because the meninges are seldom biopsied the only data concerning rate of falsely negative cases of CSF are derived from autopsy findings. Glass and associates[19] observed that the likelihood of obtaining positive CSF findings in patients with meningeal dissemination is directly proportional to the extent of meningeal disease. Thus, malignant cells are detected in about a third of patients with only focal meningeal infiltration, whereas approximately two thirds of cases of diffuse meningeal carcinomatosis can be detected cytologically.[19] Olson and associates[40] also point out that multiple examinations of CSF increase the overall rate of detection to 80% of cases, presumably because of better sampling.

A series of 225 samples of CSF reported by Bigner and Johnston[5] had a false-positive rate of five in 225. Cases of falsely positive diagnoses include (1) a case of herpes meningoencephalitis that was misinterpreted as adenocarcinoma, (2) a case that probably represented cross contamination of a filter with adenocarcinoma from another patient, (3) a case in which a filter containing reactive mesothelium from an effusion was mislabeled as CSF and misinterpreted as adenocarcinoma, (4) a case of a foreign-body reaction in a sample obtained postoperatively that was erroneously thought to contain tumor cells and (5) a case of bacterial meningitis in a child with leukemia that was incorrectly diagnosed as malignant. In the series of 117 cases studied post-mortem by Glass and associates,[19] there were three cases of falsely positive diagnoses (2.6.%). All three cases involved patients with lymphoma in whom infectious meningitis was erroneously interpreted as being neoplastic.

Borowitz and associates[11] assessed the accuracy of the diagnosis of leukemia and lymphoma in CSF by reviewing the morphology and clinical outcome of 45 patients. They reported an overall false-positive rate of 10/72 or 14% of the samples. Diagnostic accuracy was highest for acute leukemia, but all patients with CLL had falsely positive diagnoses due to misinterpretation of reactive lymphocytes in cases of fungal or viral meningitis. Because these data were acquired prior to the availability of lymphocyte marker studies, one would anticipate that this source of falsely positive diagnoses could largely be eliminated by the application of immunohistology to identify lymphocytic subsets.

These studies demonstrate that the rate of falsely positive diagnoses in CSF is low for metastases and primary brain tumors but is a significant problem in CNS leukemia and lymphoma. In general the incidence of false-positive diagnoses in CSF can be reduced by awareness of three areas of diagnostic pitfalls. Because normal CSF is practically acellular, laboratory contamination of these samples with benign or malignant cells from other patients presents a major problem in CSF cytology, particularly when membrane filters are used. Contamination of staining dishes or the instruments used in preparation with malignant cells can lead to an erroneous diagnoses of malignancy. In addition, contamination of CSF with benign cells, such as bronchial epithelium, squamous cells or reactive mesothelium, can cause diagnostic difficulties and can be misinterpreted as representing a pathologic or neoplastic process.

A second pitfall is the misinterpretation of normal brain elements. Thus, chondrocytes, ependymal-choroidal cells, and neurons and glia, particularly in ventricular fluids, can cause a problem if the observer is unaware of the cytologic appearance of these elements.

A third major pitfall is the misinterpretation of reactive lymphocytes as representing leukemia or lymphoma. This situation is frequently encountered both in patients who are known to have leukemia or lymphoma and in patients who have meningeal symptoms and no prior history of neoplasia. This problem can largely be eliminated by the application of immunohistochemical markers as discussed previously.

NEEDLE ASPIRATES OF INTRACRANIAL LESIONS

The most common application of fine needle aspiration to the CNS is in the evaluation of a supratentorial mass in an adult. Table 18–2 lists the lesions that should be considered in this clinical setting. A general approach is to divide preparations into those of low cellularity and high cellularity and within the latter category to distinguish specimens containing cells with benign cytologic features from those with malignant ones.

Because aspiration of brain lesions is performed to evaluate mass lesions, samples of normal brain should theoretically not be encountered. In reality, however, the lesion may be missed on the first attempt yielding only normal brain tissue containing sparse numbers of neurons or glia (Fig. 18–12). In these cases normal brain must be distinguished from other processes yielding samples of low cellularity, such as reactive gliosis and low-grade astrocytomas (Figs. 18–13 and 18–14).

TABLE 18–2. Supratentorial Masses in the Adult

Low Cellularity	
Normal brain	
Reactive gliosis	
Low-grade astrocytoma	

High Cellularity (Cytologically Benign)	High Cellularity (Cytologically Malignant)
Abscess	Lymphoma
Granuloma	Metastatic carcinoma
Infarct	Melanoma
Hemorrhage	Sarcoma
Oligodendroglioma	Glioblastoma multiforme
Ependymoma	

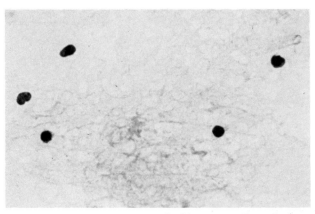

FIGURE 18–12. Smear of **normal white matter** (Papanicolaou stain; ×680).

In both gliosis and low-grade tumors the sample is more cellular than is normal brain. In smear preparations, however, thickness of the sample influences the cellularity so that this factor must be considered in judging the cellular density. In smears of normal brain stained with hematoxylin and eosin or Papanicolaou stain, only the nuclei of glia are visible (see Fig. 18–12). Silver impregnation stains or immunohistochemistry using antibodies against GFAP are necessary to demonstrate the cell bodies and processes. In gliosis, however, the cytoplasm of the astrocytes is often dense and becomes visible in routine preparations. Low-grade astrocytomas may have either inconspicuous or visible cytoplasm, but in addition to increased cellularity the nuclei become more hyperchromatic and irregular in shape than do normal cells or those in gliosis (see Fig. 18–14).

Aspiration of many mass lesions produces a hypercellular smear. These processes include abscesses, granulomas, infarctions, hemorrhages, lymphomas, metastases and many types of primary brain tumors (see Table 18–2). The distinctions between these lesions depend to a large extent on individual cellular morphology, but additional factors such as age of the patient, precise location of the lesion within the brain and clinical history, especially the presence of a known primary tumor, may be critical in making the correct diagnosis. Identification of inflammatory and reactive conditions is possible when neutrophils, granulomatous inflammation or macrophages containing red blood cells, hemosiderin or myelin debris are seen (Fig. 18–15). The presentation of lymphoma and metastatic tumors is essentially the same as in other types of cytologic specimens. Therefore the remainder of this discussion focuses on primary brain tumors.

In contrast to low-grade astrocytomas, the other types of low-grade primary brain tumors, oligodendrogliomas and ependymomas are hypercellular.[37, 38] Oligodendrogliomas have round, regular nuclei with delicate chromatin and moderate amounts of cytoplasm (Fig. 18–16). The uniformity of the cells and the occasional presence of calcifications are useful features in identifying these tumors. Cells of ependymomas are also uniform but the nuclei are slightly oval and the

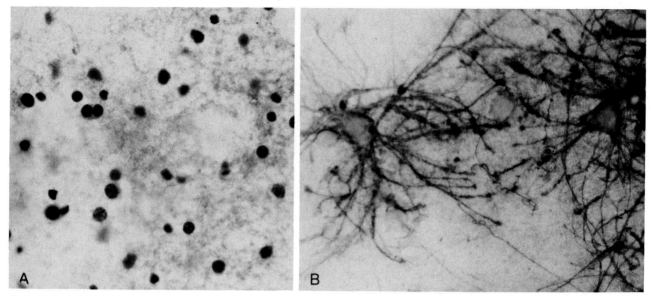

FIGURE 18–13. Needle aspirate of **reactive gliosis.** A, Papanicolaou stain; ×680. B, Immunoperoxidase using antibody against glial fibrillary acidic protein (GFAP); ×680.

cytoplasm often has a columnar shape (Fig. 18–17). Perivascular pseudorosettes and true rosettes are occasionally seen. Many ependymomas and oligodendrogliomas express GFAP (Fig. 18–16B), and these tumors are usually positive for panneuroectodermal reagents such as antibody UJ13A. The lymphoid and hematopoietic cell types seen in reactive conditions, in contrast, are usually negative with these markers, but react with panleukocyte reagents as well as antibodies against the specific types of inflammatory cells. Thus, antibodies can be helpful in distinguishing these low-grade neoplasms from non-neoplastic conditions, but reagents are not yet available that reliably distinguish between oligodendrogliomas and ependymomas.

As shown in Table 18–2, when highly cellular, cytologically malignant lesions are encountered, primary malignant brain tumors, including glioblastoma multiforme, primary CNS lymphoma and primary sarcomas, should be considered in addition to metastases from

systemic carcinoma, lymphoma, melanoma and sarcoma. Cells from glioblastomas may range from large to small and may exhibit pleomorphism. Nuclei are typically hyperchromatic and irregular but generally lack the pronounced clumping and clearing and macronucleoli that are characteristic of metastatic carcinoma (Fig. 18–18). The cytoplasm may be dense or wispy but generally lacks distinct cell borders, and excentrically placed nuclei with cytoplasmic tails and processes are common. In addition, most of these tumors contain at least some cells that express GFAP, making this marker useful in establishing the diagnosis of high-grade astrocytoma (Fig. 18–18B). A limitation in most cytologic preparations, however, is in distinguishing between anaplastic astrocytoma (an astrocytic neoplasm of intermediate grade) and glioblastoma multiforme. Generally, focal necrosis is the most reliable feature in separating glioblastoma from the lower grade tumors in histologic sections of biopsy samples and cell

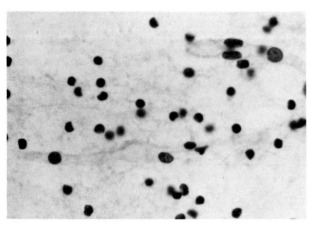

FIGURE 18–14. Needle aspirate of **low-grade astrocytoma** (Papanicolaou stain; ×880).

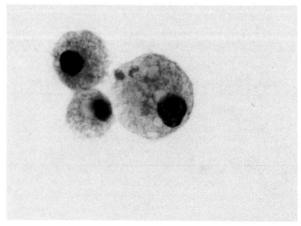

FIGURE 18–15. Needle aspirate of **cerebral infarct** shows numerous macrophages (Papanicolaou stain; ×1000).

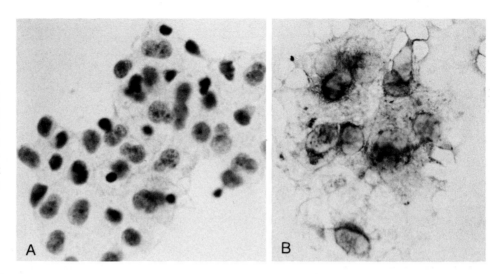

FIGURE 18–16. Needle aspirate of **oligodendroglioma** is hypercellular containing cells with round nuclei and wispy cytoplasm. *A,* Papanicolaou stain; ×680. *B,* Immunoperoxidase using antibody against glial fibrillary acidic protein (GFAP); ×680.

blocks, but it is usually difficult, if not impossible, to distinguish necrosis from fibrin and other types of debris in needle aspirates. Although the cytologic features of the neoplastic cells in hypercellular aspirates may be sufficiently characteristic to distinguish among glioblastoma, sarcoma metastasis and lymphoma, the application of an antibody panel, such as the one described in Table 18–1, can be utilized to make these distinctions.

As shown in Table 18–3, many of the same neoplasms occur in children as in adults. The distribution of astrocytic neoplasms is different, however, as the majority of childhood gliomas occur in the posterior fossa, whereas they predominate supratentorially in the adult. Furthermore, brain stem gliomas are one of the more common astrocytic tumors in childhood, whereas they are rare after age 25. In addition to the tumors discussed thus far, malignant small-cell neoplasms constitute a large proportion of brain tumors in children. These neoplasms have been termed primitive neuroectodermal tumors by some observers who note the morphologic similarities of these tumors in various intracranial locations. Others retain the older terminology that distinguishes medulloblastomas that occur in the cerebellum from cerebral neuroblastomas

and pineoblastomas. In all locations these tumors resemble adrenal neuroblastomas and retinoblastomas, being composed of small cells with round, hyperchromatic nuclei, inconspicuous nucleoli and scant cytoplasm occurring in diffuse sheets.[38] Rosettes can be

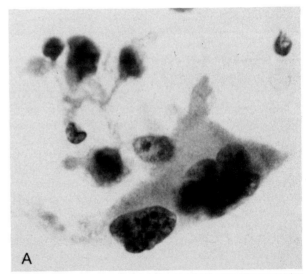

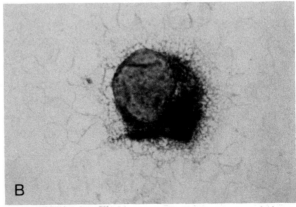

FIGURE 18–18. Needle aspirate of **glioblastoma multiforme.** *A,* Papanicolaou stain; ×1000. *B,* Immunoperoxidase using antibody against glial fibrillary acidic protein (GFAP); ×1000.

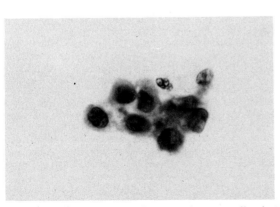

FIGURE 18–17. Smear of **ependymoma** shows small cuboidal cells with bland oval nuclei (Papanicolaou stain; ×680).

TABLE 18–3. Primary Brain Tumors in the Child

Supratentorial Tumors	Cerebellar Tumors
Astrocytoma	Astrocytoma
Ependymoma	Medulloblastoma (PNET)
Oligodendroglioma	
Glioblastoma multiforme	**Brain Stem Tumors**
Cerebral neuroblastoma	Astrocytoma
(PNET)	Glioblastoma multiforme
Tumors of the Pineal Region	**Intraventricular Tumors**
Germinoma	Ependymoma
Teratoma	Choroid plexus papilloma
Endodermal sinus tumor	Choroid plexus carcinoma
Embryonal carcinoma	
Pineocytoma	
Pineoblastoma	

PNET = Primitive neuroectodermal tumor.

seen in any of these tumors but are less commonly seen in medulloblastomas than in the other tumor types. As discussed previously, this group of neoplasms typically expresses panneuroectodermal markers, and many tumors contain neurofilament protein negating their value in distinguishing these tumors from one another. The absence of GFAP, however, is useful in differentiating these tumors from malignant gliomas, and the lack of lymphoid antigens and markers of epithelial and mesenchymal cells help distinguish these tumors from lymphoma, carcinoma and sarcoma.

DIAGNOSTIC ACCURACY OF NEEDLE ASPIRATION

Comparison of diagnoses of intercranial masses sampled by needle aspiration with histologically processed biopsy specimens has shown a diagnostic accuracy of 87.5 to 90%.[37, 38] In one series of 56 tumors the precise histologic diagnosis was made cytologically in 43 cases (77%).[38] A major problem was produced by nonrepresentative sampling. Thus, a common pitfall in needle aspiration of cerebral masses is the misinterpretation of reactive astrocytes as representing low-grade glioma. Reactive gliosis is commonly present around abcessess, infarcts and metastases. If the needle fails to sample the lesion itself and instead touches the periphery, reactive gliosis may be obtained.

Another pitfall is the misclassification of primary CNS tumors. In the absence of necrosis, one cannot confidently distinguish glioblastomas from anaplastic astrocytomas, and oligodendrogliomas can be confused with anaplastic astrocytomas. Although the distinction between metastases and high-grade gliomas may occasionally be difficult on routine cytologic preparations, antibody panels are helpful in this situation.

References

1. Amer MH, Al-Sarraf M, Baker LH, Vaitkevicius VK: Malignant melanoma and central nervous system metastases: Incidence, diagnosis, treatment and survival. Cancer 42:660–668, 1978.
2. Balhuizen JC, Bots GTAM, Schaberg A, Bosman FT: Value of cerebrospinal fluid cytology for the diagnosis of malignancies in the central nervous system. J Neurosurg 48:747–753, 1978.
3. Bigner SH: Cytologic diagnosis of cryptococcal meningitis. American Society of Clinical Pathologists check sample. Cytopathology 11:1–5, 1983.
4. Bigner SH: The application of immunocytochemical techniques to specimens derived from the central nervous system (CNS). American Society of Clinical Pathologists check sample. Cytopathology 14:1–5, 1986.
5. Bigner SH, Johnston WW: The diagnostic challenge of tumors manifested initially by the shedding of cells into cerebrospinal fluid. Acta Cytol 28:29–36, 1984.
6. Bigner SH, Johnston WW: The cytopathology of cerebrospinal fluid. I. Non-neoplastic conditions. Lymphoma and leukemia. Acta Cytol 25:335–353, 1981.
7. Bigner SH, Johnston WW: The cytopathology of cerebrospinal fluid. A review. Part II. Metastatic cancer, meningeal carcinomatosis and primary central nervous system neoplasms. Acta Cytol 25:461–480, 1981.
8. Bigner SH, Johnston WW: Cytopathology of The Central Nervous System. New York, Masson Publishing Company, Inc., pp 39–44; 59–62; 65–70; 75–124; 1983.
9. Bigner SH, Elmore PD, Dee AL, Hoffman M, Johnston WW: Unusual presentations of inflammatory conditions in cerebrospinal fluid. Acta Cytol 29:291–296, 1985.
10. Bigner SH, Elmore PD, Dee AL, Johnston WW: The cytopathology of reactions to ventricular shunts. Acta Cytol 29:391–396, 1985.
11. Borowitz MJ, Bigner SH, Johnston WW: Diagnostic problems in the cytologic evaluation of cerebrospinal fluid for lymphoma and leukemia. Acta Cytol 25:665–674, 1981.
12. Dahl GV, Simone JV, Hustu HO, Mason C: Preventive central nervous system irradiation in children with acute nonlymphocytic leukemia. Cancer 42:2187–2192, 1978.
13. Dee AL: Carcinoma of the breast presenting initially in cerebrospinal fluid. Acta Cytol 29:909–910, 1985.
14. DeGirolami U, Schmidek H: Clinicopathological study of 53 tumors of the pineal region. J Neurosurg 39:455–462, 1973.
15. Ehya H, Hajdu SL, Melamed MR: Cytopathology of nonlymphoreticular neoplasms metastatic to the central nervous system. Acta Cytol 25:599–610, 1981.
16. Evans AE, Gilbert ES, Zandstra R: The increasing incidence of central nervous system leukemia in children. (Children's Cancer Study Group A.) Cancer 26:404–409, 1970.
17. Fetter BF, Klintworth GK, Hendry WS: Mycoses of the Central Nervous System. Baltimore, Williams & Williams, p 131, 1967.
18. Getaz EP, Miller GJ: Spinal cord involvement in chronic lymphocytic leukemia. Cancer 43:1858–1861, 1979.
19. Glass JP, Melamed MR, Chernik NL, Posner JB: Malignant cells in cerebrospinal fluid (CSF): The meaning of a positive CSF cytology. Neurology 29:1369–1375, 1979.
20. Gonzalez-Vitale JC, Garcia-Bunuel R: Meningeal carcinomatosis. Cancer 37:2906–2911, 1976.
21. Gupta PK, Gupta PC, Roy S, Banerji AK: Herpes simplex encephalitis cerebrospinal fluid cytology studies—Two case reports. Acta Cytol 16:563–565, 1972.
22. Harisiadis L, Chang CH: Medulloblastoma in children: A correlation between staging and results of treatment. Int J Radiat Oncol Biol 2:833–841, 1977.
23. He X, Skapek SX, Wikstrand CJ, Friedman HS, Trojanowski JQ, Kemshed JT, Coakham HB, Bigner SH, Bigner DD: Phenotypic analysis of four human medulloblastoma cell lines and transplantable xenografts. J Neuropathol Exp Neurol 48:48–68, 1989.
24. Heimann A, Merino MJ: Carcinomatous meningitis as the initial manifestation of breast cancer. Acta Cytol 30:25–28, 1986.
25. Hinnanti K, Perchick A, Koslow M, Burstein DE: Cytologic findings in brain biopsy crush preparations from 16 patients with AIDS or AIDS risk factors. Acta Cytol 32:774, 1988.
26. Ho KL, Hoschner JA, Wolfe DE: Primary leptomeningeal gliomatosis. Arch Neurol 38:662–666, 1981.
27. Homans AC, Forman EN, Baker BE: Use of monoclonal antibodies to identify cerebrospinal fluid lymphocytes in children with acute lymphoblastic leukemia. Blood 66:1321–1325, 1985.
28. Hustu HO, Aur RJA, Verzosa MS, Simone JV, Pinkel D:

Prevention of central nervous system leukemia by irradiation. Cancer 32:585–597, 1973.

29. Katz RL, Alappattu C, Glass PJ, Bruner JM: Cerebrospinal fluid manifestations of the neurologic complications of human immunodeficiency virus infection. Acta Cytol 33:233–244, 1989.

30. Knowles DM: Immunophenotypic and antigen receptor gene rearrangement analysis in T-cell neoplasia. Am J Pathol 134:761–785, 1989.

31. Leiman G, Klein C, Berry AV: Cells of nucleus pulposus in cerebrospinal fluid: A case report. Acta Cytol 24:347–349, 1980.

32. Little JR, Dale ADJ, Okazaki H: Meningeal carcinomatosis: Clinical manifestations. Arch Neurol 30:138–143, 1974.

33. McIntosh S, Ritchey AK: Diagnostic problems in cerebrospinal fluid of children with lymphoid malignancies. Am J Pediatr Hematol Onc 8(1):28–31, 1987.

34. Meyer RJ, Ferreira PPC, Cuttner JG, Treenberg ML, Goldberg J, Holland JF: Central nervous system involvement at presentation in acute granulocytic leukemia, a prospective cytocentrifuge study. Am J Med 68:691–694, 1980.

35. Miller RR, Lin F, Mallonee MM: Cytologic diagnosis of gliomatosis cerebri. Acta Cytol 25:37–39, 1981.

36. Moser RP, Robinson JA, Prostko ER: Lymphocyte subpopulations in human cerebrospinal fluid. Neurology 26:726–728, 1976.

37. Mouriquand C, Benabid AL, Breyton M: Stereotaxic cytology of brain tumors. Review of an eight-year experience. Acta Cytol 31:756–764, 1987.

38. Nguyen GK, Johnston ES, Mielke BW: Cytology of neuroectodermal tumors of the brain in crush preparations. Acta Cytol 33:67–73, 1989.

39. Noronha A, Richman DP, Arnason GW: Multiple sclerosis: Activated cells in cerebrospinal fluid in acute exacerbations. Ann Neurol 18(6):722–725, 1985.

40. Olson ME, Chernik NL, Posner JB: Infiltration of the leptomeninges by systemic cancer: A clinical and pathological study. Arch Neurol 30:122–137, 1974.

41. Packer RJ, Siegel KR, Sutton LN, Litmann P, Bruce DA, Schut L: Leptomeningeal dissemination of primary central nervous system tumors of childhood. Ann Neurol 18:217–221, 1985.

42. Polman CH, de Groot CJA, Koestsier JC, Sminia T, Veerman AJP: Cerebrospinal fluid cells in multiple sclerosis and other neurological diseases: an immunocytochemical study. J Neurol 234:19–22, 1987.

43. Pui C-H, Dahl GV, Kalwinsky DK, Look A, Mirro T, Dodge J, Richard K, Simone JV: Central nervous system leukemia in children with acute nonlymphoblastic leukemia. Blood 66:1062–1067, 1985.

44. Razavi-Encha F, Fleury-Feith J, Gherandi R, Bernaudin JF: Cytologic features of cerebrospinal fluid in Lyme disease. Acta Cytol 31:439–440, 1987.

45. Ricevuti G, Savoldi F, Piccolo G, Marchioni E, Rizzo SC: Meningeal leukemia diagnosed by cytocentrifuge study of cerebrospinal fluid: A study of 631 cerebrospinal fluid samples from 87 patients. Arch Neurol 43:466–470, 1986.

46. Saigo P, Rosen PP, Kaplan MH, Solan G, Melamed MR: Identification of *Cryptococcus neoformans* in cytologic preparations of cerebrospinal fluid. Am J Clin Pathol 67:141–145, 1977.

47. Santoli D, DeFreitas EC, Sandberg-Wollheim M, Koprowski H: Phenotypic and functional characterization of T cell clones derived from the cerebrospinal fluid of multiple sclerosis patients. Am Assoc Immunol 132:2386–2391, 1984.

48. Schmidek HH: Pineal Tumours. New York, Masson Publishing Company Inc., p 43, 1977.

49. Schmidt P, Neuen-Jacob E, Blanke M, Arendt G, Wechsler W, Pfitzer P: Primary malignant melanoblastosis of the meninges. Clinical, cytologic and neuropathologic findings in a case. Acta Cytol 32:713–717, 1988.

50. Shoup SA, Johnston WW, Seigler HF, Tello JW, Schlom J, Bigner DD, Bigner SH: A panel of antibodies useful in the cytologic diagnosis of metastatic melanoma. Acta Cytol 34:385–392, 1990.

51. Trojanowski JQ, Atkinson B, Lee VM: An immunocytochemical study of normal and abnormal human cerebrospinal fluid with monoclonal antibodies to glial fibrillary acidic protein. Acta Cytol 30:235–239, 1986.

52. Tzvetanova EM, Tzekov CT: Eosinophilia in the cerebrospinal fluid of children with shunts implanted for the treatment of internal hydrocephalus. Acta Cytol 30:277–280, 1986.

53. Veerman AJP, Hismans LDR, Van Zantwijk ICH: Diagnosis of meningeal leukemia using immunoperoxidase methods to demonstrate common acute lymphoblastic leukemia cells in cerebrospinal fluid. Leukemia Res 9:1195–1200, 1985.

54. Vick WW, Wikstrand CJ, Bullard DE, Kemshead J, Coakham HB, Schlom J, Johnston WW, Bigner DD, Bigner SH: The use of a panel of monoclonal antibodies in the evaluation of cytologic specimens from the central nervous system. Acta Cytol 31:815–824, 1987.

55. Weed JC Jr, Creasman WT: Meningeal carcinomatosis secondary to advanced squamous cell carcinoma of the cervix: A case report. Gynecol Oncol 3:201–204, 1975.

56. Wilber RR, King EB, Howes EL Jr: Cerebrospinal fluid cytology in five patients with cerebral cysticercosis. Acta Cytol 24:421–426, 1980.

57. Wilkins RH, Odom GL: Ependymal-choroidal cells in cerebrospinal fluid: Increased incidence in hydrocephalic infants. J Neurosurg 41:555–560, 1974.

19

Eye

Dorothy L. Rosenthal
Diane B. Mandell
Ben J. Glasgow

Cytopathologists have had minimal experience with specimens from the eye and surrounding tissues until recently. A search of the cytology literature reveals very few articles dealing with only a few types of lesions, predominantly infectious conjunctivitis, melanoma and retinoblastoma.[22, 37, 50, 51, 53, 60, 68] Interest now is probably due to improved noninvasive imaging techniques and greater confidence by ophthalmologists in obtaining samples by needle aspiration and vitreous washing.[61]

With improved sampling capabilities and the increasing numbers of immunocompromised patients, the diagnostic cytology laboratory will predictably be challenged with unfamiliar, sight- and life-threatening diseases. The major experience presented in this chapter is gathered from the archives of the University of California, Los Angeles (UCLA) Cytology Service and the Jules Stein Eye Institute (JSEI).[26] Clearly, the population is unusual, in that it represents a referral practice, with lesions and disease situations that general ophthalmic practices rarely encounter or treat.

When the UCLA Cytology Service was asked to process the vitrectomy washings obtained in the JSEI operating theater, we were perplexed by the cells and found no help in the literature. Processing of the sample was difficult, owing to the variation in viscosity of the washing product. After conquering the preparation of the specimens, we obtained autopsy eyes for simulated washing to obtain samples that would contain undiseased cells and tissue fragments. The eyes were then embedded and histologically prepared so that we could correlate the histology with the cytology. The result was a library of standards to which we could refer and from which we were able to learn.[45] This experience is shared later in the chapter.

Because many lesions that are found in this area are common to other parts of the body, they will be mentioned briefly in this chapter, with reference to the appropriate chapter where the lesion is more fully described. Only those lesions that have unique features referrable to the eye and its adnexa are explored here in depth.

SAMPLING AND CYTOPREPARATORY TECHNIQUES

Most lesions of the eyelid, eye and orbit are approached by fine needle aspiration (FNA). Diseases of the conjunctiva and cornea are usually scraped (S). If the process involves the vitreous, vitrectomy with ocutome washing (OW) is generally performed. These abbreviations are used to indicate the most common method of sampling as each lesion or disease process is described.

Scraping. Lesions appropriate for scraping require local anesthesia, followed by forceful scraping with a small platinum spatula. The cellular yield is then smeared onto one or more slides, depending on the amount of material. To avoid air drying, the slide can be positioned horizontally and flooded with 95% alcohol before smearing. The alcohol is allowed to evaporate from the cell spread for a few minutes before immersing the slide completely into a container of the fixative.[52]

Fine Needle Aspiration. FNA of the eye must be undertaken by a skilled and trained ophthalmologic surgeon. Depending on the location of the target lesion, localization by imaging techniques may be required.

Intraocular (Vitrectomy) Washing. The pars plana (closed) vitrectomy was initially described by Machemer and colleagues[41–44, 55] in the early 1970s. The original vitrectomy instrument had cutting, suction and infusion capabilities. It was able to remove intraocular tissues, e.g., vitreous, blood, fibrovascular membranes,

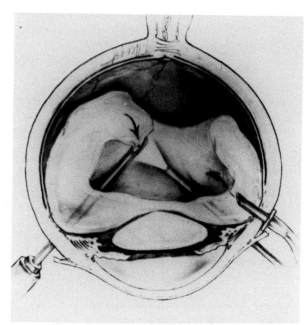

FIGURE 19–1. Divided system vitrectomy instrumentation.

lens material and inflammatory debris. Continual refinements have led to the development of new instruments with scissors capability, a self-contained fiberoptic light source and intraocular photocoagulation with diathermy capabilities (Fig. 19–1).

The underlying surgical goal of vitrectomy is removal of either vitreal opacities, such as hemorrhage, or intravitreal fibrous strands. If not removed, fibrous strands may contract, causing tractional retinal detachments,[46] with resultant decreased vision or blindness. Vitrectomy is most often performed on patients with proliferative diabetic retinopathy.[7, 48, 57] The vitrectomy instrument is able to remove nonresorbed vitreous hemorrhage, fibrovascular tissue and preretinal and epiretinal membranes commonly seen as severe complications of diabetes mellitus.[47] Vitrectomy is also used to remove intraocular hemorrhage caused by trauma, sickle-cell disease and branch retinal vein occlusion,[70] and to remove intraocular foreign bodies. Endophthalmitis may respond to treatment by vitrectomy.

In addition to these therapeutic indications, vitrectomy has been performed for diagnostic purposes. Engel and coworkers[25] and Green[29] have reviewed numerous cases in which diagnostic vitrectomies were performed. Engel's group divided diagnostic vitrectomies into three categories: (1) those performed to make specific diagnoses; (2) those performed to confirm a presumed but clinically unproven diagnosis and (3) those performed to diagnose a previously unsuspected condition. The cases reviewed by Engel's group and by Green included neoplastic lesions, e.g., malignant melanoma, metastatic tumors and histiocytic lymphomas. Piro and colleagues[58] described its use in confirming metastatic breast carcinoma to the eye.

Several methods of processing intraocular fluids have been described in the literature.[16, 24, 30, 65] Green reviewed the membrane filter technique. Chess and associates[16] compared the cytocentrifugation technique to the celloidin-bag technique. The method to be described was developed by one of us (DBM) to process the vitrectomy specimens received by the UCLA Cytology Service.[45]

Method. Intraocular specimens processed in the UCLA Cytology Service are collected in the operating rooms of the JSEI. The intraocular surgical instrument is the ocutome-fragmatome. It features a 20-gauge suction-cutter probe. The specimens are collected in sterile cups and delivered by messenger to the cytology laboratory. If there is any delay, the specimens are refrigerated.

Appearance and volume of the specimen are described. The entire specimen is centrifuged in a large standing centrifuge for 5 minutes at 3500 rpm. The supernatant is carefully pipetted off, and the gross appearance of the sediment is evaluated. If the sediment is bloody or appears to be composed of lens fragments, care must be taken in approximating the amount of material needed to prepare a monolayer Cytospin slide preparation.

Cytocentrifuge Preparation. The Cytospin chambers are prepared according to the manufacturer's instructions.[30] If sediment is scant, four Cytospin slides are prepared. If an adequate amount of material is left in the centrifuge tube, about 0.5 ml or more, a cell block is made (see subsequent discussion).

The specimen is cytocentrifuged at 650 rpm for 5 minutes. After cytocentrifugation, all slides are fixed in 95% ethyl alcohol. One wet-fixed slide is stained with a modified Papanicolaou stain, and three fixed slides are saved for special stains if and when necessary.

Cell Block Preparation. The supernatant is removed with a disposable pipette. Approximately 5 ml of 95% ethyl alcohol is slowly added to the centrifuge tube. Care is needed not to disturb the sediment. The 95% ethyl alcohol is employed to harden the sediment so that the sediment can be removed from the centrifuge tube as a pellet on the next day. The sediment is carefully loosened with an angle pick and gently teased onto a piece of lens paper, which is then folded and placed into a cassette. The labeled cassette is put into a container of 10% formalin. After histologic processing, hematoxylin-stained cell block sections are returned to the cytology laboratory, where they are screened and described by the cytotechnologist. These sections may also be utilized for special stains.

Culture is the best method for bacterial identification, but air-dried smears may be employed as a preliminary demonstration of bacteria. Papanicolaou-stained slides and the cell block are used for identification of neoplastic or inflammatory processes. Cell block sections demonstrate large tissue fragments (Fig. 19–2) better than do Cytospin preparations. After screening by the cytotechnologist, the cell block section and the Cytospin slides are delivered to the ocular pathologist for final evaluation.

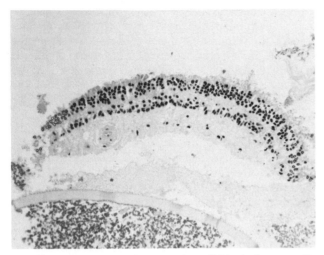

FIGURE 19–2. Retinal fragment in cell block (hematoxylin and eosin; ×400).

Special Techniques

To detect *Chlamydia* organisms

1. Perform standard conjunctival scraping.
2. Direct fluorescent antibody (DFA) technique uses a monoclonal antibody and can be performed on a routinely made smear.[4] The preparation time is 15 minutes, after which the smear is ready for screening.
3. *Chlamydia* culture is the best method.[66] The cultured cells are grown on a coverslip for 48 hours and then stained by DFA as in 2.
4. Giemsa stain is no longer used for *Chlamydia* identification, as the DFA method is far more sensitive and specific.[4]

To detect viral cytopathic effect (CPE)

1. Each viral group has CPE changes specific for that family of viruses and, sometimes, specific for the individual virus, e.g., herpes and cytomegalovirus (CMV).
2. The specimen can be obtained by corneal scrape, conjunctival scrape, retinal biopsy or subretinal fluid.
3. After culturing the specimen, viral specific CPE is noted and can be confirmed by DFA. If CPE is subtle or not found DFA can indicate early subvisual changes.[63]

ANATOMY AND HISTOLOGY

The first three compartments are referred to as the adnexa, relative to the eye or globe: eyelid, conjunctiva, orbit and eye (globe).

The eyelids are bifaced, functioning as protective skin externally and as lubricating membranes on their inner surfaces. As such, they will be involved with lesions identical to those of the skin and mucous membranes elsewhere. Unique to the area are the lacrimal and the Meibomian glands. The lacrimal gland is histologically a tubuloalveolar serous gland and its function is to produce tears. The Meibomian glands are specialized sebaceous glands.

The conjunctiva is a thin membrane, in need of the lubrication supplied by the lid glands, and is divided into palpebral (eyelid) and bulbar ("white" of the eye") portions. By itself it is capable of producing some lubricant from its stratified columnar and mucus-secreting goblet cells.

The bony orbit has four walls forming a pear-shape open on opposite sides. The walls are named roof, floor, and lateral and medial walls, and are related anatomically to the frontal, maxillary, ethmoid and sphenoid sinuses. Therefore, diseases affecting the sinuses can involve the orbit and vice versa. Contained within the orbital cavity are the lacrimal glands, extra-ocular muscles, arteries and veins to the area, various nerves, fibrofatty tissue, optic nerve and the eye. For a more graphic understanding, the reader is referred to any standard textbook of anatomy.

The wall of the globe (Fig. 19–3) is divided into an outer coat (sclera and cornea), a middle coat or uvea (choroid, ciliary body and iris) and the inner coat (retina). Of the outer coat, only the cornea participates in vision and, therefore, must be transparent and avascular. The ciliary body is intimately associated with the lens and is responsible for its support and contour. At the back of the globe, the retina is thickest (ten layers) and is the functional peripheral neurologic portion of sight.

The optic nerve is an extension of the brain and ends in the optic nerve's head at the back of the globe. The meninges covering the brain are contiguous with the optic nerve as it enters the bony orbit.

The contents of the globe are the lens, supported and controlled by the uvea, and two liquid-filled compartments that are separated by the lens. The anterior chamber contains a thin fluid, the aqueous humor; the major portion of the globe contains a viscous gel, the vitreous body. Both fluids must be free of cells and color in order to optimally transmit light to the retina. Cornea, lens, aqueous humor and vitreous body compose the refracting media of the eye.

LESIONS ACCESSIBLE FOR CYTOLOGIC SAMPLING DIVIDED ACCORDING TO ANATOMIC COMPARTMENT

Although many diseases of the eye, orbit, surrounding tissue and lids are also found elsewhere, the normal cytologic components and terminology of structures of the eye are unfamiliar to most pathologists. Obviously, before disease can be recognized, the normal cell constituents must be learned in order to avoid incorrect diagnoses (Table 19–1).

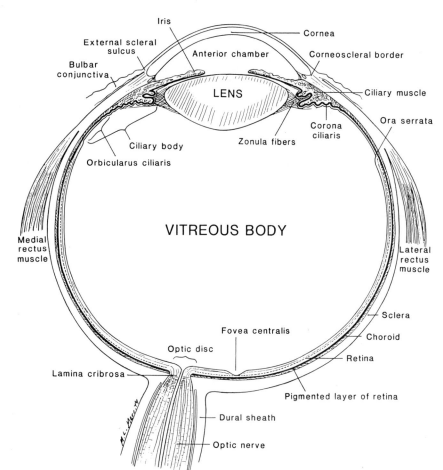

FIGURE 19–3. Anatomic landmarks of the globe.

TABLE 19–1. Compartments of the Globe Suitable For Cytologic Examination

Normal Histology and Cytology		
Compartment	*Histology*	*Cytology*
Cornea (S)	Stratified squamous	Intermediate squamous
	Ulceration	Repair epithelium
Conjunctiva (S)	Stratified columnar	(1) Basal columnar cells: single or sheets, excentric nuclei, small nucleoli, variable pigment
		(2) Goblet cells: secretory vacuoles, crescentic nucleus
Uvea (FNA)	Choroid	Retinal pigment and epithelial cells
	Ciliary body	
	Iris	
Retina (FNA)	Rods and cones	Clusters of small, dark nuclei at the edge of neurofibril mesh
	Neurons	Large, pale nuclei with attenuated fibrils
Ocular chambers (OW)	Amorphous fluid	Lymphs, histiocytes, rare

Lesions Common to All Three Compartments

Developmental (Benign) Tumors

Lesions common to all three adnexal compartments include *developmental (benign) tumors (FNA)*: dermoid cysts, epithelial inclusion cysts and ectopic lacrimal glands.

Contents of dermoid and epithelial (epidermoid) inclusion cysts are identical to those found in these same lesions elsewhere in the body. The reader is referred to the discussion of dermal cysts in Chapter 21, Skin. Ectopic lacrimal glands may be aspirated and are composed of clusters of acinar cells, obviously secretory, and with small nuclei. These glandular groups should not be confused with adenocarcinomas, in which the nuclei have malignant criteria.

Inflammatory Lesions

Inflammatory lesions (FNA) include granulomatous inflammation. The mention of granuloma immediately conjures the features of tuberculosis. Other infectious diseases characteristically provoke similar inflammatory responses, but usually without caseous necrosis. In the eye, similar cellular constituents may be present but do not necessarily indicate a causative infectious organism. Nonspecific granulomas may reflect systemic sarcoidosis (compact noncaseating granulomas), Wegener's granulomatosis (granulomas and angiitis) and juvenile xanthogranuloma (with Touton giant cells). Each lesion in the eye reflects the characteristics of the disease elsewhere in the body.

Selsky and coworkers[62] were able to diagnose ocular involvement in a patient with Whipple's disease, a chronic multisystem malady, involving predominantly the wall of the small intestine, but viritually every tissue in the body is susceptible to deposits of fat and foamy macrophages. Characteristic vitreous opacities and retinitis, with consequent compromised visual acuity, are a result of infiltration of the tissue with foamy macrophages. These benign histiocytes contain intracytoplasmic periodic acid–Schiff-positive material. Electron micrographs disclose bacillary bodies. Further studies have failed to incriminate and causally relate specific organisms with the disease, but many patients respond favorably to antibiotics.

Benign Neoplasms

Benign neoplasms (FNA) include lymphoid hyperplasia. Benign lymphoproliferative disease is a diagnostically difficult entity and can be histologically and cytologically mistaken for a malignant lymphoid neoplasm. Architectural and cellular detail are critical to distinguish between those malignant processes and those reactive to a benign stimulus. Mixed mononuclear cell populations and germinal center cells, especially tingible body macrophages, favor a benign diagnosis. Immunocytochemistry may be useful to settle conflicts.[12, 33, 40] However, one should be aware that even immunoglobulin gene rearrangement and immunochemical evidence of monoclonality do not always correlate with the clinical course in lymphoid lesions of the orbit.

Malignant Neoplasms

Malignant neoplasms (FNA) include lymphoma, melanoma, squamous carcinoma and metastatic lesions. Whereas melanoma and lymphoma can be found anywhere in the body, their morphology and clinical behavior when they occur primarily in the eye possess some unique characteristics. Careful clinical history is mandatory to determine whether the lesion in the eye is primary or metastatic. Such critical information will dictate the treatment and influence the outcome. At each discussion pertinent to the anatomic location, tumor behavior specific to the area will be noted. Otherwise, the cytologic features are discussed elsewhere in this book.

Lesions Specific to Each Compartment

Eyelids

As noted, lesions affecting the lids are similar to skin lesions in general, with similar histologic and cytologic characteristics. Only a few diseases are unique to this area or require extra care to obtain the samples without unnecessarily damaging the delicate tissues of the eye and surrounding structures.

Viral Diseases (S). Molluscum contagiosum, verruca vulgaris, herpes zoster and herpes types 1 and 2 can infect the lids and conjunctiva. These diseases are frequently sexually transmitted and will be present in the genital tracts of the patient, sexual partner or both. Diagnosis and treatment, therefore, should be directed towards all likely sources, so that reinoculation does not occur, as these infections can be sight threatening. Morphologic characteristics can be diagnostic if the eye specimen is well preserved and not air dried, which is easier to say than to do because of minimal moisture in the area. (For detailed cytologic features, the reader is referred to the appropriate sections in this text and to the illustrated chapter by Naib in another work.[52]) Advances in viral diagnosis, e.g., *in situ* hybridization, various "blot" methods and improved culture techniques, are welcome aids to confirming these lesions.

Xanthelasmas (FNA). These lesions are so clinically characteristic that the need for cytologic diagnosis is remote. However, if a xanthelasma were to be aspirated, only lipid-filled macrophages would be recovered.

Melanocytic tumors (FNA or S). Little experience is reflected in the literature regarding cytology of benign nevi in any location. However, if a melanoma is suspected, then an aspirate[19] or a scraping[11] of the lesion would contain cells in which the nuclear features and size would clearly define the lesion as malignant. Pigmented lesions are usually completely excised for cosmesis, diagnosis and potential cure, without employing an intermediate cytologic diagnosis.

Chalazion (FNA). These painful swellings are caused by retained secretions of the Meibomian glands and are characterized by a mixture of lipogranulomatous and suppurative inflammation. The process is usually grossly diffuse, occasionally nodular and can clinically mimic a sebaceous carcinoma. An aspirate contains granulomas with lipid-laden macrophages and neutrophils.

The additional lesions listed subsequently may be found in the lid and are accessible to the aspirating needle or by scraping. Their cellular characteristics in this location are no different than elsewhere in the body. (The reader is referred to the summary articles on FNA cytology of eyelid lesions by Arora[2] and of skin lesions by Canti in Chapter 21 and to the comprehensive chapter on the last topic in Koss's text on aspiration cytology.[39])

> Juvenile xanthogranuloma
> Amyloid deposits
> Skin adnexal tumors
> Neurilemoma
> Pilomatrixoma
> Adenocarcinoma
> Basal cell carcinoma
> Sebaceous carcinoma

Conjunctiva

This mucous membrane is composed predominantly of tall columnar cells, occasionally interrupted by goblet cells. The latter will be increased if the need for more mucus is present. Both cell types contain single round or oval nuclei with finely granular chromatin and small inconspicuous nucleoli. The cytoplasmic vacuole in the goblet cell displaces the nucleus towards the basement membrane. When these cells are scraped, the nonsecretory columnar cells appear as a honeycomb with centrally placed nuclei, or as a palisading clusters. Goblet cells will be intermixed, the nuclei excentrically placed by the adjacent vacuole. No cilia or terminal bars are present on either cell type.

The following list includes infrequently encountered lesions by the cytopathologist. However, their easy access predicts that cytologic diagnosis may be attempted (FNA).

> Choristomas
> Ephelis
> Neurofibroma
> Nevi, blue and nevocellular
> Infectious inflammations[38]
> Ligneous conjunctivitis
> Mooren's ulcer
> Sarcoid[6]
> Keratoacanthoma[9]

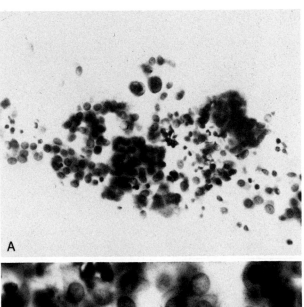

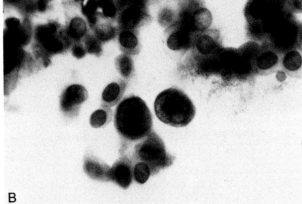

FIGURE 19–4. Herpetic conjunctivitis (conjunctival scrape; Papanicolaou stain; A, ×400; B, ×1000).

Bacterial and Viral Conjunctivitis (S). These are best diagnosed by culture, but the exudate can contain cells in distinctive patterns to provide a screening procedure. When classic viral inclusions are identified in conjunctival cells (Fig. 19–4), a presumptive diagnosis can be provided.[67]

Vernal Conjunctivitis (S). This is thought to be a recurrent hypersensitivity reaction of the conjunctiva, occurring in atopic-allergy patients. It is produced by mucosal presentation of an antigen, such as common ragweed. Increased levels of IgE have been found in the serum and tears of such patients.[34]

Although not usually a target for cytologic evaluation, this condition may mimic other causes of "red eye" and may be subjected to microscopic evaluation. The resulting smears will contain inflammatory cells, including eosinophils, mast cells or basophils and lymphocytes (Fig. 19–5A and 19–5B).[10] If the condition is chronic, goblet cells may be abundant (Fig. 19–5C and 19–5D). Careful search for signs of *Chlamydia* is important, as the treatment of the two diseases is significantly different, and the outcome of untreated chlamydial conjunctivitis is more serious than an allergic reaction.

Chlamydial Conjunctivitis (Tracoma and TRIC— Trachoma Inclusion Conjunctivitis) (S). Unfortunately, the characteristic inclusions of *Chlamydia* are

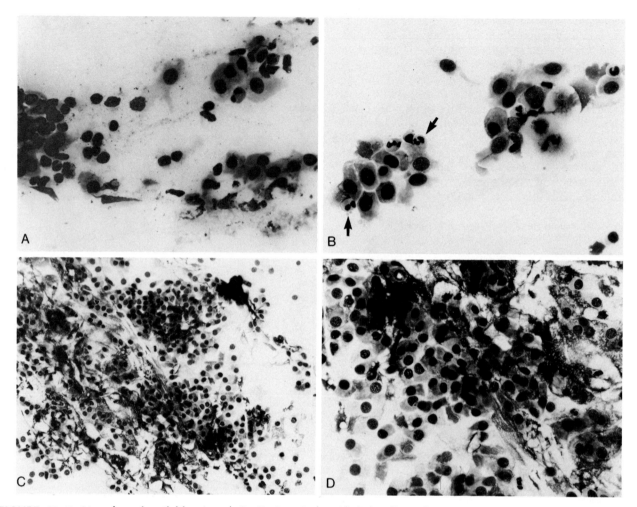

FIGURE 19–5. Vernal conjunctivitis. *A* and *B*, Conjunctival epithelial cells with assorted inflammatory cells. Note the eosinophils (arrows). *C* and *D*, Abundant goblet cells (conjunctival scrape; *A*, hematoxylin and eosin; *B* to *D*, May-Gruenwald Giemsa stain; *A, B* and *D*, ×400; *C*, ×200).

not frequently found in conjunctival smears.[8] Wilhelmus and associates[69] detected only 8% inclusions in culture-positive cases of chlamydial conjunctivitis, with an inconsistent and, therefore, diagnostically unreliable inflammatory pattern. They stress the importance of immunochemical confirmation of suspected disease and recommend that Giemsa-stained smears be utilized as a screening procedure. Since the availability of monoconal antibodies to *Chlamydia*, we no longer use Giemsa-stained smears for *Chlamydia* screening. An article by Dean and associates[20] demonstrates the diagnostic sensitivity of DNA-probe technology for this difficult morphologic diagnosis. Naib[50] correlated perinatal ocular and maternal genital infections, concluding that 61% of 54 mothers of a set of infected newborns had diagnosable *Chlamydia* in recent cervical smears, further emphasizing the need for reliable identification of this organism.

Orbit

Most lesions of the orbit are approached by FNA. It requires an ophthalmologist very familiar with the anatomy of the orbit and adnexa and capable of treating the complications. The experience of Kennerdell's group with 156 orbital FNAs is summarized in Table 19–2.[36] Kennerdell admits that insufficient aspirates usually are a consequence of a fibrous lesion, an orbital apical location or a lymphocytic tumor with insufficient cells for a definitive diagnosis.[35] Successful FNA of this relatively unfamiliar area depends on a team of skilled individuals: ophthalmologist, radiologist, ophthalmologic pathologist and cytopathologist.

Hematoma. This lesion would rarely be subjected to cytologic investigation. Fibrinated blood, macrophages and perhaps fibroblasts would be recovered in an aspiration.

Mucocele. Similar to the salivary gland lesion, this simple cyst contains mucus, scattered inflammatory cells and occasional nondescript cuboidal epithelial cells (Fig. 19–6).

Meningioma. Although meningioma can involve the orbit by extension from the intracranial space, the lesion may also arise from the meninges covering the optic nerve and appear as a retrobulbar mass within the orbit. In either situation, the cytomorphology is identical, composed of small ovoid nuclei with scant cytoplasm. Nuclear chromatin is fine, nucleoli are inconspicuous and nuclear pseudoinclusions may be

TABLE 19–2. Fine Needle Aspirates of Orbital Lesions

Type of Lesion	Number
Carcinoma	44 (28%)
Undifferentiated	20
Adenocarcinoma	15
Adenoid cystic	4
Prostatic	1
Renal cell	2
Transitional cell	2
Neural Tumors	9 (6%)
Meningioma	5
Juvenile histiocytoma	3
Malignant astrocytoma	1
Inflammations	30 (19%)
Nonspecific	21
Abscess	9
Other Neoplasms	10 (6%)
Rhabdomyosarcoma	2
Plasmacytoma	5
Leukemia	1
Malignant melanoma	2
Lymphoid Lesions	27 (17%)
Miscellaneous	5 (3%)
Hematoma	1
Eosinophilic granuloma	1
Dermoid cyst	2
Hemangioma	1

Reproduced with permission from Kennerdell JS, et al: Orbital fine-needle aspiration biopsy. Am J Ophthalmol 99:547–551, 1985.

found. The classic three-dimensional concentric whorls of these cells (noncalcified psammoma bodies) provide the conclusive diagnosis (Fig. 19–7).[18, 36] Dispersed tumor cells interconnect the psammoma bodies by their fine cytoplasmic processes.

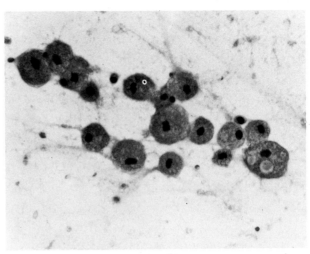

FIGURE 19–6. Mucocele of orbit. Numerous macrophages are suspended in fibrinous mucus (Papanicolaou stain; ×400).

Metastatic Lesions. While metastates to the orbit usually reflect disseminated disease, the occurrence of a metastatic deposit in this region may rarely be the first presentation of the patient's illness.[39] When metastases do occur in the region of the eye, they are commonly from the breast in women, from the lung in men, and from neuroblastomas in children. Needless to say, distinguishing retinoblastoma from neuroblastoma is cytologically impossible[59] and is determined only by history and gross presentation of the tumor.

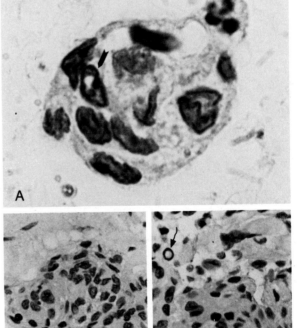

FIGURE 19–7. Orbital meningioma. The whorls of small meningothelial cells are characteristic. Note the intranuclear inclusions (arrows) (*A*, fine needle aspiration (FNA); hematoxylin and eosin stain; ×300; *B* and *C*, tissue sections; hematoxylin and eosin stain; ×250). (Courtesy of E. G. Cristallini.)

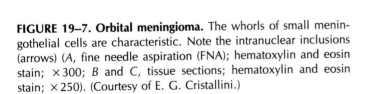

Invasion from adjacent structures is also commonly seen (Fig. 19–8).

The remainder of the list includes those lesions encountered in our surgical pathology experience. Any of the lesions could be aspirated without difficulty. Their diagnoses are dependent not only on the pathologist's familiarity with the cytology of the lesions but on the realization that the lesions might be expected in this location (Fig. 19–9).

Neurofibroma
Nodular fasciitis
Wegener's granulomatosis
Juvenile xanthogranuloma
Eosinophilic granuloma
Fibrous histiocytoma
Granular cell myoblastoma
Nonchromaffin paraganglioma
Schwannoma
Fibrosarcoma
Malignant fibrous histiocytoma
Granulocytic sarcoma
Myxoid sarcoma
Plasmacytoma
Rhabdomyosarcoma
Spindle-cell sarcoma

Globe

When diagnosing lesions of the various compartments of the eye, access needs to be considered. Superficial lesions, such as infections of the cornea, are cytologically diagnosed by scraping. Lesions within the eyeball are usually approached by noninvasive imaging techniques for localization and then aspirated with a very thin needle (25-gauge or smaller).[32] If larger-bore needles are used, the chances of excessive bleeding and needle track seeding by malignant tumors are too high to make the procedure worth the risk. Such was the situation in the 1950s when the technique of eye FNA was all but abandoned.[14] Intraocular washings during vitrectomy will be addressed subsequently.

Benign Conditions. Normal corneal cells are almost identical to intermediate squamous cells of the female genital tract. If corneal ulceration has occurred, parabasal cells will be present, as well as cells displaying features of repair. If the scrape has been too vigorous, parabasal cells may also be identified, but repair changes will be absent. Keratinized squamous cells are pathologic and require a diagnosis akin to the intraepithelial lesions of the uterine cervix, depending upon the severity of nuclear abnormalities.[9] Keratinized cells

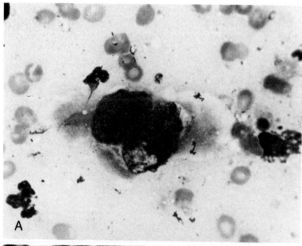

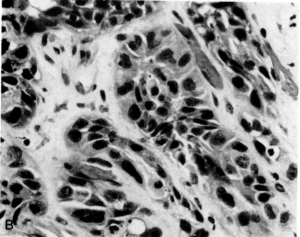

FIGURE 19–8. **Squamous carcinoma** of the skin extending into the orbit (*A, B,* fine needle aspiration (FNA); May-Gruenwald-Giemsa stain; ×1000; *B,* resection; hematoxylin and eosin stain; ×400).

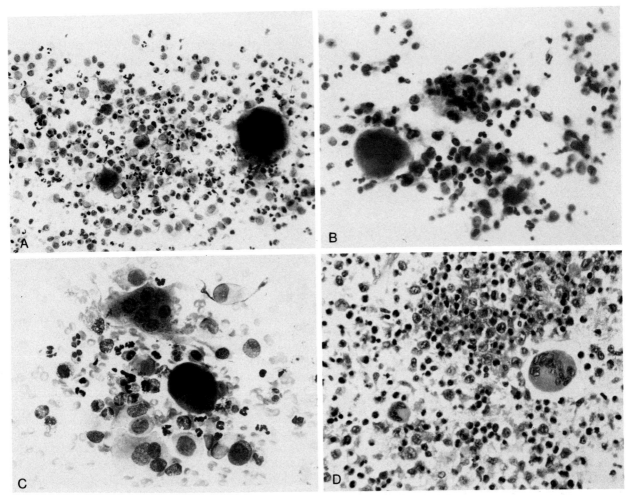

FIGURE 19–9. **Histiocytosis X** involving the orbit and adjacent soft tissues (fine needle aspiration (FNA), *A* to *C*; *A*, May-Gruenwald-Giemsa stain; × 200; *B*, hematoxylin and eosin stain; × 400; *C*, May-Gruenwald-Giemsa stain; × 400; biopsy, *D*; hematoxylin and eosin; × 400).

without dysplasia should also be noted, and their cause, e.g., keratoconjunctivitis sicca and vitamin A deficiency, determined.[54]

Infections. As the acquired immune deficiency syndrome (AIDS) epidemic spreads away from major cities, the infections that these patients develop will demand diagnosis.[23] For example, until a few years ago, CMV retinitis was rare, and when discovered, was untreatable, resulting in blindness and death. Currently, the infection is a common one in immunocompromised patients but is effectively treated if diagnosed early. A case of orbital aspergillosis diagnosed by FNA was described by Austin and coworkers.[3] An anterior chamber aspirate confirmed the clinical diagnosis of ocular coccidioidomycosis in the eye of a patient treated at UCLA (Fig. 19–10).[45]

Diagnosis of either bacterial endophthalmitis or phacoanaphylactic response to retained lens material should be considered in severely inflamed eyes following extracapsular cataract extraction. Endophthalmitis is characterized by acute and chronic inflammatory cells, including histiocytes, multinucleated histiocytes and lymphocytes (Fig. 19–11). Clinically, it is extremely important to differentiate phacoanaphylaxis

from postoperative bacterial endophthalmitis because endophthalmitis requires immediate antibiotic therapy.

Noninfectious Inflammatory and Post-traumatic Conditions. Cellular material obtained during vitrectomy or anterior chamber aspiration assumes definite

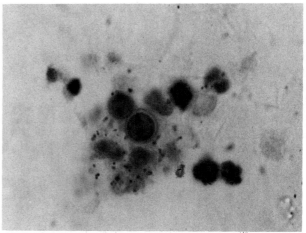

FIGURE 19–10. **Coccidioidomycosis.** Direct smear made from anterior chamber aspirate (Papanicolaou stain; × 400).

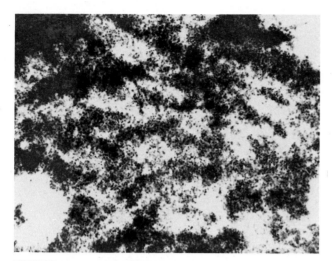

FIGURE 19–11. Endophthalmitis in vitrectomy washing (Cytospin preparation; Papanicolaou stain; ×100).

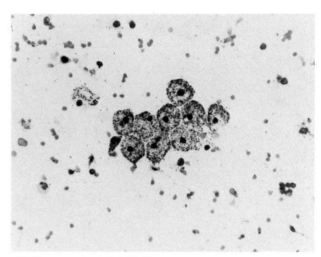

FIGURE 19–13. Retinal pigment epithelium in vitrectomy washing (Cytospin preparation; Papanicolaou stain; ×400).

patterns reflecting the disease processes.[33, 47–49, 56] Proliferative diabetic retinopathy is the most common condition requiring vitreous surgery.[47, 48] Extraretinal fibrovascular tissue proliferates along the posterior vitreous surface. When portions of the posterior vitreous separate from the retina, the fibrovascular tissue may continue to proliferate, covering parts of the retina or causing such secondary complications as vitreous hemorrhage and tractional retinal detachment. Cytologic examination of vitrectomy fluid from patients with proliferative diabetic retinopathy often contains fibrovascular membranes (Fig. 19–12).

Retinal pigment epithelial (RPE) cells are frequently seen in cytologic preparations (Fig. 19–13). They appear as cuboidal cells containing numerous melanin granules in the cytoplasm.[31, 52] These RPE cells are believed to enter the vitreous cavity through retinal tears or holes, by migration or sometimes dispersion following retinal cryotherapy. The RPE cells have been found in intravitreal fibrous strands.

Fragments of retinal cells may be present in vitrectomy specimens (Figs. 19–14 and 19–15). Cytologically, these cells are found singly and in groups or tissue-like fragments. They are slender, elongated cells, often arranged in parallel rows. At the opposite end from the nucleus, the cytoplasm is ill-defined and attenuated. Often there is an area of perinuclear clearing, which is characteristic of retinal cells. They may be confused with lymphocytes if poorly preserved.

Melanin pigment can be found both in cells and free floating (Fig. 19–16) and should not be confused with bacteria or blood pigment. The histiocytes seen in vitreous washing specimens can have their cytoplasm packed with melanin granules, but their usually excentric, bean-shaped nuclei will separate them from RPE cells, in which the nuclei are round and centrally placed.

Blood-induced glaucoma can be confirmed by cytologic evaluation of vitreous fluid. In this condition, red blood cells that have been present in the vitreous for

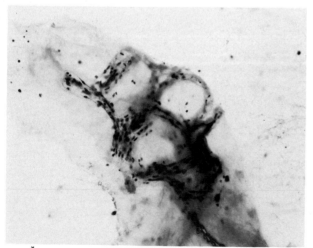

FIGURE 19–12. Fibrovascular membrane in vitrectomy washing (Cytospin preparation; Papanicolaou stain; ×200).

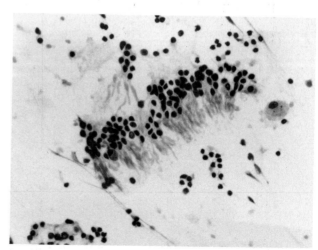

FIGURE 19–14. Retina in vitrectomy washing (Cytospin preparation; Papanicolaou stain; ×400).

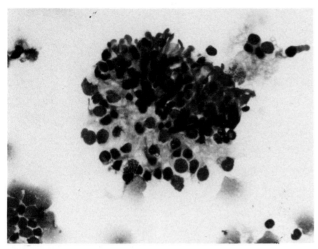

FIGURE 19–15. Retina in vitrectomy washing (Cytospin preparation; May-Gruenwald-Giemsa stain; ×400).

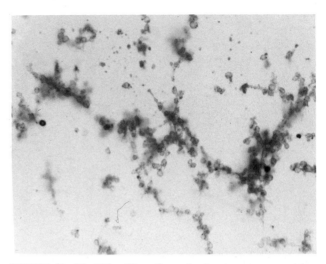

FIGURE 19–17. "Ghost" erythrocytes in vitrectomy washing (Cytospin preparation; Papanicolaou stain; ×400).

an extended period of time lose their hemoglobin and become "ghost erythrocytes." If these ghost erythrocytes pass forwards into the anterior chamber, they can mechanically obstruct the trabecular meshwork, blocking aqueous outflow and thereby causing a secondary glaucoma. This condition is most commonly seen following trauma in which damage to anterior hyaloid (the most anterior portion of the vitreous) has occurred. Eyes with blood-induced glaucoma show a spectrum of pathologic findings that suggest that obstruction of aqueous outflow is caused by a combination of ghost erythrocytes (Fig. 19–17), hemolytic cells (Fig. 19–18) and hemosiderin. Engel and associates[25] considered hemolytic cells to be histiocytes or macrophages with engulfed red blood cells.

It is now recognized that mechanical blockade of the anterior chamber angle structures is caused by proteinaceous debris and characteristic large macrophages that have ingested lens material. Phacolytic cells are swollen histiocytes with lightly eosinophilic granular cytoplasm

and lens material. These cells can be seen in anterior chamber aspirate specimens.

Phacolytic glaucoma and phacoanaphylaxis may produce lens fragments and inflammatory cells in both anterior and vitreous fluids (Fig. 19–19).[27] The characteristic appearance of lens epithelium may have nuclei (Fig. 19–20). Lens capsule may also be present in the vitreous washing specimen; this capsule appears as a well-demarcated fragment of transparent material (Fig. 19–21).

Neoplasms

Melanomas and retinoblastomas are the most common primary neoplasms of the area, but metastatic tumors are more common. Malignancies most frequently metastasizing to the eye are breast in women and lung in men.[39, 64] Neuroblastomas in children often travel to the eye, making distinction from a retinoblas-

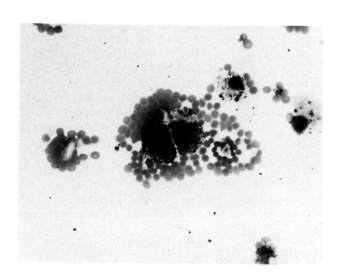

FIGURE 19–16. Macrophage with pigment in vitrectomy washing (Cytospin preparation; Papanicolaou stain; ×400).

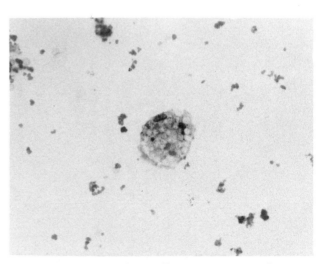

FIGURE 19–18. Hemolytic cells in vitrectomy washing (Cytospin preparation; Papanicolaou stain; ×400).

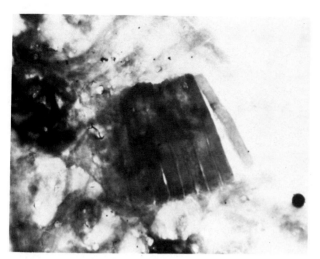

FIGURE 19–19. Lens fragment in vitrectomy washing (Cytospin preparation; May-Gruenwald-Giemsa stain; ×400).

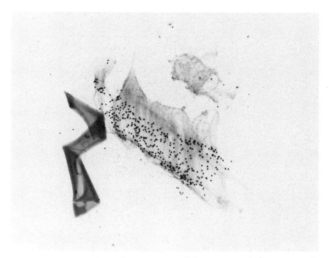

FIGURE 19–21. Lens fragment and fragment of glass capsule in vitrectomy washing (Cytospin preparation; Papanicolaou stain; ×100).

toma impossible on cytologic grounds;[59] accurate history and anatomic location are necessary for diagnosis.

Ocular melanomas are usually located in the choroid, causing visual deficits, or more rarely in the iris or ciliary body, where they are obvious to the careful observer. Their diagnosis is dependent on the skills of the aspirator and diagnostician and the quality of the specimen. Char and colleagues[15] aspirated 28 uveal melanomas and correctly diagnosed 25 (89%). Two of their cases that were incorrectly diagnosed were very difficult to classify histologically, and the third case was inadequate. They conclude that "The safety of orbital or intraocular fine needle biopsy has not been definitively established, and as others have noted this technique should not be used unless the information gained is important for clinical management."

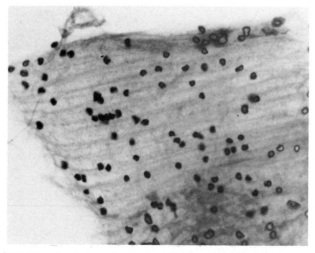

FIGURE 19–20. Lens fragment with lens epithelium in vitrectomy washing (Cytospin preparation; Papanicolaou stain; ×400).

Histologically, intraocular melanomas may be divided into epithelial and spindle cells (Fig. 19–22). As the biologic behavior is not necessarily reflected in the cytomorphologic features, the treatment tends to be more conservative than that for melanomas elsewhere, in order to preserve sight, whenever possible.

Smears of aspirates of epithelial type contain freely dispersed large, variably shaped cells, usually polygonal, but occasionally spindle. Cytoplasm is generally opaque but can contain small vacuoles and, usually, melanin granules. Free melanin pigment can be seen in the background and ingested in benign macrophages. Nuclei are large and pleomorphic, especially in the truly epithelioid cells, are frequently excentric and sometimes multiple. Nucleoli are prominent and large, and intranuclear cytoplasmic invaginations can be found, as in melanomas elsewhere. This cytohistologic pattern is not diagnostically difficult, especially if the cells are pigmented.

The spindle-cell type is composed of slender cohesive cells, connected by bipolar cytoplasmic processes. Melanin pigment and intranuclear inclusions are not as common as in the other variant. These cells may be intermixed with epithelioid cells. Immunochemical verification is not always helpful in defining the tumor as being of melanocytic origin and cannot reliably distinguish between primary and metastatic lesions.[17]

Retinoblastoma, the most common intraocular tumor of children,[1, 14, 59] may be genetically transmitted as an autosomal dominant. Therefore, family history is significant. Its bilaterality in approximately a third of cases makes it all the more tragic. Early diagnosis and treatment are critical to save the patient. The lesion may appear as a subretinal mass or in the vitreous (Fig. 19–23).

The small tumor cells with invisible cytoplasm have cytologic features characteristic of all the neural ectodermal (neural crest) tumors and, therefore, cannot be distinguished morphologically. Clinical presentation and history are essential to confirm the diagnosis. As

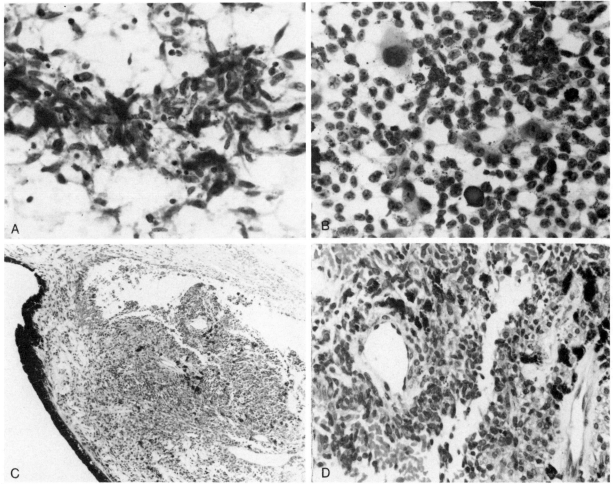

FIGURE 19–22. Uveal melanoma. *A,* Spindle type. *B,* Epithelioid type. (Smears provided by Dr. Britt-Marie Ljung.) (Fine needle aspiration (FNA) *A* and *B,* Papanicolaou stain; ×400. Exenteration specimen of spindle type. *C* and *D,* Hematoxylin and eosin; *C,* ×100; *D,* ×400.)

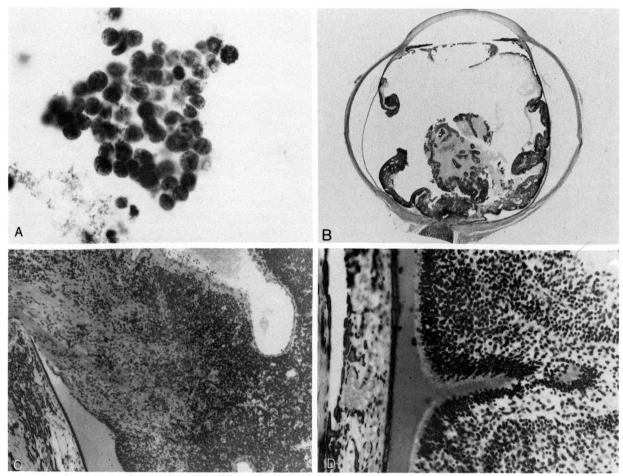

FIGURE 19–23. Retinoblastoma. (*A*, Fine needle aspiration (FNA); Papanicolaou stain; ×1000. *B*, Whole mount of eye; hematoxylin and eosin; ×12.5. *C*, and *D*, Sections of tumor; hematoxylin-eosin; *C*, ×100; *D*, ×200.)

these tumors frequently extend into the central nervous system (CNS), a spinal tap for cytologic examination of cerebrospinal fluid (CSF) is critical to preoperative staging and postoperative treatment.[59] In both FNA and CSF examinations, scant cytoplasm; dark polygonal nuclei of almost identical size; smudged nuclear chromatin; inconspicuous nucleoli and nuclear molding, requiring cell clusters in the sample, are mandatory criteria. In FNA preparations, the presence of rosettes and particularly fleurettes may be diagnostic. Flexner-Wintersteiner rosettes are formed by peripheral arrangement of nuclei with finely fibrillar cytoplasmic processes radiating to the center of the circle. Fleurettes demonstrate photoreceptor-cell differentiation and are found only in well-differentiated retinoblastomas.

Lymphomas rarely involve the eye, but when they do, approximately 75% of the patients will develop CNS involvement, resulting in death.[28] The diagnosis of intraocular lymphoma is difficult and often delayed, because the disease is misdiagnosed as idiopathic uveitis. Ljung and coworkers[40] retrospectively reviewed 14 patients with intraocular lymphoma to establish the relative value of cytologic features and immunologic markers. These investigators concluded that morphology, e.g., irregular nuclear outlines, prominent nucleoli and coarsened chromatin, is still the most sensitive parameter for accurate diagnosis. Only one of the nine lymphomas expressed monoclonality. This seeming contradiction can be explained by the frequently observed mixture of benign inflammatory cells with malignant lymphoid cells. Usefulness of immunologic analysis of these specimens is therefore severely limited. These workers point out that frequently more than one specimen is necessary to confirm the diagnosis and that although most studies conclude that ocular lymphoma is invariably fatal, subsequent to CNS spread, if diagnosed and treated early, the patient can be cured.[13]

Other tumors of the eye are considered as medical curiosities and can be found in the literature as infrequent singular case reports.[21] Our experience dictates that when a cytologic sample from the eye does not fit the criteria of commonly expected lesions, the cytopathologist must rely on careful patient history, the clinical impression and a search of comprehensive ophthalmologic pathology texts. Consultation with an experienced ophthalmic pathologist will usually result in a "ballpark" diagnosis, sufficient to direct the clinical management of the patient.

DIAGNOSTIC ACCURACY

At least, cytologic diagnosis of lesions of the eye and adnexa can confirm the clinical impression. At best, the opinion rendered can be equivalent to a tissue diagnosis. Our collective experience unfortunately is small, and a review of the literature identifies very few papers with a patient population large enough to reach statistically valid conclusions. To date, the three papers that analyze diagnostic reliablity deal with fine needle samples of intraocular and orbital/periorbital lesions.

Kennerdell and colleagues[36] emphasize that the primary reason for aspirating a lesion is its nonresectability. Their experience is summarized in Table 19–2 and is discussed above under diagnosis of orbital lesions. They emphasize the morbidity associated with the procedure, which includes, commonly, retrobulbar hemorrhage and, rarely, blindness and death. However, despite these risks, these workers strongly support the importance of this diagnostic modality, quoting an 80% positive identification rate, 18% insufficient rate and 2% false diagnoses (one false-negative, two false-positive results).

This same paper includes an anecdotal report by Liu who surveyed 138 orbital FNAs. Seven patients had diffuse retrobulbar hemorrhages that resorbed. However, ten patients had severe sequelae, including blindness, and three patients died from brain-related complications. All serious complications resulted from faulty technique, further emphasizing the importance of experience on the part of the surgeon. If performed carefully, the procedure is clearly beneficial if it avoids extensive surgery to arrive at a diagnosis.

The article by Char and associates discusses their experience with uveal melanomas.[15] Fine needle aspirates of 29 uveal melanomas resulted in correct diagnoses in 26 patients (89%). Morbidity was minimal. In an attempt to improve prognostic accuracy, a subset of this group of tumors was also subjected to bromodeoxyuridine (BrdUrd) analysis. More experience with this technique and DNA estimates of intraocular melanomas needs to be accumulated before such information can be confidently factored into patient management and prognosis.

The relatively new technique of fine needle sampling without aspiration is advocated by Zajdela and colleagues.[71] Their published experience of 62 cases of orbital and periorbital neoplasms disclosed the following: 49/56 (87%) cytologically diagnosed tumors were confirmed histologically; three of the tumors (5%) required diagnosis by surgical procedure; the false-positive diagnoses (4%) were of a meningioma and a reactive lymphoid hyperplasia; the solitary false-negative case (2%) resulted from a non-Hodgkin's lymphoma.

In the remaining six patients, biochemical studies or examination of nodal metastases in biopsy material contributed to the final cytologic diagnosis. None of these patients experienced orbital hemorrhage, presumably because suction was not used to obtain the cell sample.

We gratefully acknowledge the archival research efforts of Catherine Minick and the photographic expertise of Carol Appleton.

References

1. Akhtar M, Ali MA, Sabbah R, Sackey K, Bakry M: Aspiration cytology of retinoblastoma: light and electron microscopic correlations. Diagn Cytopathol 4:306–311, 1988.
2. Arora R, Rewari R, Betheria SM: Fine needle aspiration of lid tumors. Acta Cytol 34:227–232, 1990.
3. Austin P, Dekker A, Kennerdell J: Orbital aspergillosis: Report of a case diagnosed by fine needle aspiration biopsy. Acta Cytol 27:166–169, 1983.

4. Bell TA, Kuo C, Stamm WE, Tam MR, Stephens RS, Holmes KK, Grayston JT: Direct fluorescent monoclonal antibody stain for rapid detection of infant *Chlamydia trachomatis* infections. Pediatrics 74:224–228, 1984.

5. Benson WE: Vitrectomy. *In* Clinical Ophthalmology, vol 5. Edited by TD Duane, EA Jaeger. Philadelphia, Harper & Row, 1984, pp 1–23.

6. Bienfait MF, Hoogsteden HC, Baarsma GS, Adriaansen HJ, Verheijen-Breemhaar L: Diagnostic value of bronchoalveolar lavage in ocular sarcoidosis. Acta Ophthalmol 65:745–748, 1987.

7. Blakenship GW: Stability of pars plana vitrectomy results for diabetic retinopathy complications. Arch Ophthalmol 99:1009–1012, 1981.

8. Blodi BA, Byrne KA, Tabbara KF: Goblet cell population among patients with inactive trachoma. Int Ophthalmol 12:41–45, 1988.

9. Brown HH, Glasgow BJ, Holland GN, Foos RY: Keratinizing corneal intraepithelial neoplasia. Cornea 8:220–224, 1989.

10. Butrus SI, Abelson MB: Laboratory evaluation of ocular allergy. Int Ophthalmol Clin 28:324–328, 1988.

11. Canti G: Rapid cytological diagnosis of skin lesions. *In* Advances in Clinical Cytology, volume 2. Edited by LG Koss, DV Coleman. New York, Masson Publishing Co., Inc., 1984.

12. Char DH, Ljung BM, Deschenes J, Miller TR: Intraocular lymphoma: immunological and cytological analysis. Br J Ophthalmol 72:905–911, 1988.

13. Char DH, Margolis L, Newman AB: Ocular reticulum cell sarcoma. Am J Ophthalmol 91:480–483, 1981.

14. Char DH, Miller TR: Fine needle biopsy in retinoblastoma. Am J Ophthalmol 97:686–690, 1984.

15. Char DH, Miller TR, Ljung B-M, Howes EL, Stoloff A: Fine needle aspiration biopsy in uveal melanoma. Acta Cytol 33:599–605, 1989.

16. Chess J, Sebag J, Tolentino F, Schepens CL, Calderone JP, Coughlin-Wilkinson E, Albert DM: Pathological processing of vitrectomy specimens. Ophthalmology 90:1560–1564, 1983.

17. Cochran AJ, Foulds WS, Damato BE, Trope GE, Morrison L, Lee WR: Assessment of immunological techniques in the diagnosis and prognosis of ocular malignant melanoma. Br J Ophthalmol 69:171–176, 1985.

18. Cristallini EG, Bolis GB, Ottaviano P: Fine needle aspiration biopsy of orbital meningioma. Report of a Case. Acta Cytol 34:236–238, 1990.

19. Czerniak B, Woyke S, Domagala W, Kryzysztolik Z: Fine needle aspiration cytology of intraocular malignant melanoma. Acta Cytol 27:157–165, 1983.

20. Dean D, Palmer L, Pant CR, Courtright P, Falkow S, O'Hanley P: Use of a *Chlamydia trachomatis* DNA probe for detection of ocular Chlamydiae. J Clin Microbiol 27:1062–1067, 1989.

21. De Juan, Green WR, Gupta PK, Baranano EC: Vitreous seeding by retinal astrocytic hamartoma in a patient with tuberous sclerosis. Retina 4:100–102, 1984.

22. Dykstra PC, Dykstra BA: The cytologic diagnosis of carcinoma and related lesions of the ocular conjunctiva and cornea. Trans Am Acad Ophthalmol Otolaryngol 73:979–995, 1969.

23. Elovaara I, Iivanainen M, Valle SL, Suni J, Tervo T, Lahdevirta J: CSF protein and cellular profiles in various stages of HIV infection related to neurological manifestations. J Neurol Sci 78:331–342, 1987.

24. Engel HM, de la Cruz ZC, Jimenez-Abalahin LD, Green WR, Michels RG: Cytopreparatory techniques for eye fluid specimens obtained by vitrectomy. Acta Cytol 26:551–560, 1982.

25. Engel HM, Green WR, Michels RG, Rice TA, Erozan YS: Diagnostic vitrectomy. Retina 1:121–149, 1981.

26. Foos RY: The eye and adnexa. *In* Surgical Pathology, 2nd ed. Edited by WF Coulson. Philadelphia, JB Lippincott, 1988.

27. Goldberg MF: Cytological diagnosis of phacolytic glaucoma utilizing Millipore filtration of the aqueous. Br J Ophthalmol 51:847–853, 1967.

28. Graham E: Intraocular involvement of T and B cell lymphomas. Eye 1:691–698, 1987.

29. Green WR: Diagnostic cytopathology of ocular fluid specimens. Ophthalmology 91:726–749, 1984.

30. Havener VR: Processing aqueous taps and vitrectomies using the Shandon Southern Cytospin SCA-0031. Sewickley, Shandon Southern Instruments, 1978.

31. Hogan MJ, Zimmerman LE: Ophthalmic Pathology: An Atlas and Textbook. Philadelphia, WB Saunders, pp 469–473, 1962.

32. Jakobiec FA, Coleman DJ, Chattock A: Ultrasonographically guided needle biopsy and cytologic diagnosis of solid intraocular tumors. Ophthalmology 86:1662–1678, 1979.

33. Kaplan HJ, Meredith TA, Aaberg TM, Keller RH: Reclassification of intraocular reticulum cell sarcoma (histiocytic lymphoma): Immunologic characterization of vitreous cells. Arch Ophthalmol 98:707–710, 1980.

34. Khatami M, Donnelly JJ, John T, Rockey JH: Vernal conjunctivitis. Model studies in guinea pigs immunized topically with fluoresceinyl ovalbumin. Arch Ophthalmol 102:1683–1688, 1984.

35. Kennerdell JS, Dekker A, Johnson BL, Dubois PJ: Fine-needle aspiration biospy: its use in orbital tumours. Arch Ophthalmol 97:1315–1317, 1979.

36. Kennerdell JS, Slamovits TL, Dekker A, Johnson BL: Orbital fine-needle aspiration biopsy. Am J Ophthalmol 99:547–551, 1985.

37. Kimura SJ, Thygeson P: The cytology of external ocular disease. Am J Ophthalmol 39:137–154, 1955.

38. Koss LG: Diagnostic Cytology and Its Histopathologic Bases, Third ed. Philadelphia, JB Lippincott, pp 984–986, 1979.

39. Koss LG, Woyke S, Olszewski W: Aspiration Biopsy: Cytologic Interpretation and Histologic Bases. Tokyo, Igaku-Shoin, 1984.

40. Ljung BM, Char D, Miller TR, Deschenes J: Intraocular lymphoma. Cytologic diagnosis and the role of immunologic markers. Acta Cytol 32:840–847, 1988.

41. Machemer R: A new concept for vitreous surgery. Part 2. Am J Ophthalmol 74:1022–1033, 1972.

42. Machemer R: A new concept for vitreous surgery. Part 7. Arch Ophthalmol 92:407–412, 1974.

43. Machemer R, Norton EWD: A new concept for vitreous surgery. Part 3. Am J Ophthalmol 74:1034–1056, 1972.

44. Machemer R, Parel JM, Buettner H: A new concept for vitreous surgery. Part 1. Am J Ophthalmol 73:1–7, 1972.

45. Mandell DB, Levy JJ, Rosenthal DL: Preparation and cytologic evaluation of intraocular fluids. Acta Cytol 31:150–158, 1987.

46. May DR, Wang WJ, Yeh M, Parel JM, Mannis MJ, Chu FN: Results of 110 vitrectomies with a portable vitrectomy system. Am J Ophthalmol 96:775–782, 1983.

47. Michels RG: Vitrectomy for complications of diabetic retinopathy. Arch Ophthalmol 96:237–246, 1978.

48. Michels RG: Proliferative diabetic retinopathy. Retina 1:1–17, 1981.

49. Michels RG: Vitreous Surgery. San Francisco, American Academy of Ophthalmology Manuals Programs, pp 1–126, 1982.

50. Naib ZM: Cytology of TRIC agent infection of the eye of newborn infants and their mothers' genital tracts. Acta Cytol 14:390–395, 1970.

51. Naib ZM: Cytology of ocular lesions. Acta Cytol 16:178–185, 1972.

52. Naib ZM: Cytology of ophthalmological diseases. *In* Advances in Clinical Cytology. Edited by LG Koss, DV Coleman. London, Butterworths, 1981.

53. Naib ZM, Clepper AS, Elliott SR: Exfoliative cytology as an aid in the diagnosis of ophthalmic lesions. Acta Cytol 11:295–303, 1967.

54. Nelson JD: Impression cytology. Cornea 7:71–81, 1988.

55. Parel JM, Machemer R, Aumayr W: A new concept for vitreous surgery. Part 4. Am J Ophthalmol 77:6–12, 1974.

56. Peretz W, Ettinghausen S, Gray G: Oncocytic adenocarcinoma of the lacrimal sac. Arch Ophthalmol 96:303–304, 1978.

57. Peyman GA, Huamonte FU, Goldberg MF, Sanders DR, Nagpal KC, Raichand M: Four hundred consecutive pars plana vitrectomies with the vitrophage. Arch Ophthalmol 96:45–50, 1978.

58. Piro P, Pappas H, Erozan YS, Michels RG, Sherman SH, Green WR: Diagnostic vitrectomy in metastatic breast carcinoma in the vitreous. Retina 2:182–188, 1982.

59. Rosenthal DL: Cytology of the Central Nervous System, vol 8. *In* Monographs in Clinical Cytology. Edited by GL Wied, Basel, S Karger, 1984.

60. Sagiroglu N, Ozgonul T, Muderrris S: Diagnostic intraocular cytology. Acta Cytol 19:32–37, 1975.
61. Sanderson T, Pustai W, Shelley L, Gelender H, Ng ABP: Cytologic evaluation of ocular lesions. Acta Cytol 24:391–400, 1980.
62. Selsky EJ, Knox DL, Maumenee AE, Green WR: Ocular involvement in Whipple's disease. Retina 4:103–106, 1984.
63. Stenkvist EO, Brege KG: Application of immunofluorescent technique in the cytologic diagnosis of human herpes simplex keratitis. Acta Cytol 19:411–419, 1975.
64. Sternberg P Jr, Tiedman J, Hickingbotham D, McCuen BW II, Proia AD: Controlled aspiration of subretinal fluid in the diagnosis of carcinoma metastatic to the choroid. Arch Ophthalmol 102:1622–1625, 1984.
65. Stulting RD, Leif RC, Clarkson JG, Bobbitt D: Centrifugal cytology of ocular fluids. Arch Ophthalmol 100:822–825, 1982.
66. Tam MR, Stamm WE, Handsfield HH, Stephens R, Kou C, Holmes KK, Ditzenberger K, Krieger M, Nowinski RC: Culture-independent diagnosis of *Chlamydia trachomatis* using monoclonal antibodies. New Eng J Med 310:1146–1150, 1984.
67. Thelmo W, Csordas J, Davis P, Marshall KG: The cytology of acute bacterial and follicular conjunctivitis. Acta Cytol 16:172–177, 1972.
68. Thygeson P: The cytology of conjunctival exudates. Am J Ophthalmol 29:1499–1513, 1946.
69. Wilhelmus KR, Robinson NM, Tredici LL, Jones DB: Conjunctival cytology of adult chlamydial conjunctivitis. Arch Ophthalmol 104:691–693, 1986.
70. Yeshaya A, Treister G: Pars plana vitrectomy for vitreous hemorrhage and retinal vein occlusion. Ann Ophthalmol 15:615–617, 1983.
71. Zajdela A, de Maublanc MA, Schlienger P, Haye C: Cytologic diagnosis of orbital and periorbital palpable tumors using fine-needle sampling without aspiration. Diagn Cytopathol 2:17–20, 1986.

20

Soft Tissue and Bone

Steven I. Hajdu

Soft tissue and bone tumors arise from derivatives of the embryonic mesoderm and are composed of heterologous cellular elements, neoplastic cells and entrapped cells of local host tissues, at different stages of differentiation.[14, 17] Some of these are primitive "arrested" forms and others are highly differentiated, forming specific tissue patterns, containing complex cytoplasmic organelles and capable of depositing biochemically and immunologically active products. The cell morphology, tissue pattern and overall composition of tumors are subject to modulation and can be influenced by local tissue conditions and an endless number of other factors. Hence, it is apparent that soft tissue and bone tumors (primary, recurrent and metastatic) may assume, permanently or temporarily, misleading and overlapping cell morphology and histologic pattern.[3, 13, 15, 18, 29, 40, 42, 45]

Ascertaining the cell of origin (histogenesis) for many soft tissue and bone tumors is still problematic, but it is almost certain that most soft tissue and bone tumors originate from primitive pluripotential mesenchymal cells. It is estimated that over 6000 new cases of soft tissue sarcomas and approximately 2000 of bone sarcomas are diagnosed annually in the United States. Over 200, more or less well-defined, microscopic forms of soft tissue and bone tumors are known, of which more than 70 are malignant neoplasms, nearly 70 are benign neoplasms and over 80 are reactive, non-neoplastic lesions that may resemble benign or malignant neoplasms.[18] It must be kept in mind that non-neoplastic (reactive) lesions and benign neoplasms outnumber malignant neoplasms (sarcomas) by a margin of about 100 to 1. Immunocytochemical reactions and electron microscopy, despite continuous efforts, have not fulfilled most expectations because soft tissue and bone tumors present a broad range of ultrastructural appearances and immunocytochemical reactions. But perhaps the most disappointing is that immunocytochemical and ultrastructural techniques are not helpful in distinguishing malignant neoplasms from benign ones.[3, 7, 15, 35]

Practically all malignant neoplasms occurring in patients under 15 years of age are nonepithelial in origin. The three most common malignant soft tissue and bone neoplasms that account for 90% of the sarcomas in patients under 15 years of age are embryonal rhabdomyosarcoma, Ewing's sarcoma and intraskeletal osteosarcoma. The three most common non-neoplastic lesions are fibromatosis, aneurysmal bone cyst and fibrous dysplasia; the three most common benign neoplasms are lipoblastoma, nonossifying fibroma and osteoid osteoma. Among patients 60 years old and older, the most common non-neoplastic lesions include elastofibroma, lipogranuloma and Paget's disease. Primary intraskeletal benign neoplasms in this age group are extremely rare, but benign soft tissue neoplasms such as benign fibrous histiocytomas, various lipomas and leiomyoma are not uncommon. In elderly patients, the most commonly seen malignant neoplasms are liposarcoma, leiomyosarcoma, plasma cell myeloma, Paget's sarcoma, extraskeletal chondrosarcoma and extraskeletal osteosarcoma.[14, 17, 25]

Although many soft tissue and bone sarcomas are ubiquitous in their anatomic distribution, most show a predilection for certain sites. Approximately half of the soft tissue and bone sarcomas have a unique site preference for the extremities.[13, 14]

Caution in the interpretation of aspiration smears and exfoliated cells from soft tissue and bone tumors, particularly in a primary diagnostic setting, cannot be sufficiently emphasized (Tables 20–1 and 20–2). Those cytopathologists who seldom see such tumors should be extremely cautious in interpreting cytologic smears from such lesions; in most cases, they would do well to limit themselves to listing the pathologic entities that should be considered in the differential diagnosis (Table 20–3) and to defer definitive diagnosis until the results of further studies or formal tissue biopsy become available.[16, 18, 21, 22, 28] Cytopathologists should take care to use sound judgment and should rely on their experience in surgical pathology with soft tissue and bone tumors when they are called on to make a

502

TABLE 20–1. Cytologic Diagnosis of 100 Consecutive Primary Soft Tissue and Bone Sarcomas in Aspiration Smears

Histologic Types of Sarcomas	Total Number of Cases	Positive for Sarcoma	Nonspecific Malignant Cells	Nonspecific Atypical Cells
Malignant fibroblastic fibrous histiocytoma	3	2	—	1
Malignant pleomorphic fibrous histiocytoma	12	3	9	—
Fibrosarcoma	4	2	2	—
Tendosynovial sarcoma	6	3	3	—
Epithelioid and clear cell sarcoma	3	—	2	1
Well-differentiated liposarcoma	6	—	—	6
Myxoid liposarcoma	10	8	1	1
Lipoblastic liposarcoma	2	—	2	—
Pleomorphic liposarcoma	4	2	2	—
Leiomyosarcoma	3	2	1	—
Rhabdomyosarcoma	9	4	4	1
Angiosarcoma	2	—	2	—
Chondrosarcoma	7	3	2	2
Osteosarcoma	10	4	6	—
Malignant peripheral nerve tumor	7	3	3	1
Ewing's sarcoma	8	—	8	—
Alveolar soft part sarcoma	2	—	2	—
Chordoma	2	1	1	—
Total	100	37	50	13

TABLE 20–2. Cytologic Diagnosis of 100 Consecutive Metastatic Soft Tissue and Bone Sarcomas*

Histologic Types of Primary Sarcomas	Total Number of Cases	Positive for Sarcomas	Nonspecific Malignant Cells	Nonspecific Atypical Cells
Malignant fibroblastic fibrous histiocytoma	1	1	—	—
Malignant histiocytic fibrous histiocytoma	1	—	1	—
Malignant pleomorphic fibrous histiocytoma	13	12	1	—
Fibrosarcoma	1	1	—	—
Tendosynovial sarcoma	11	8	2	1
Epithelioid and clear cell sarcoma	4	1	3	—
Myxoid liposarcoma	1	1	—	—
Fibroblastic liposarcoma	2	2	—	—
Lipoblastic liposarcoma	1	—	1	—
Pleomorphic liposarcoma	6	6	—	—
Leiomyosarcoma	8	7	1	—
Rhabdomyosarcoma	11	8	3	—
Angiosarcoma	2	1	1	—
Hemangiopericytoma	1	—	1	—
Kaposi's sarcoma	2	1	—	1
Chondrosarcoma	6	4	2	—
Osteosarcoma	15	12	3	—
Malignant peripheral nerve tumor	5	4	—	1
Ewing's sarcoma	9	8	1	—
Total	100	77	20	3

*In most cases, the diagnosis of the primary sarcoma was known at the time of cytologic diagnosis. The most common source of specimens were effusions, sputa, bronchial brushings and aspirates.

TABLE 20–3. Classification of the Most Common Soft Tissue and Bone Tumors According to Cell Morphology and Growth Pattern*

Cells	Patterns of Growth					
	Arranged	Spreading	Lacy	Epithelioid	Alveolar	Disarranged
Slender spindle	Fasciitis Fibroblastic fibrous histiocytoma Fibroblastic liposarcoma Neurofibroma Neurofibrosarcoma Schwannoma	Fibromatosis Kaposi's sarcoma Monophasic tendosynovial sarcoma Neurofibroma Neurofibrosarcoma	Fibroblastic liposarcoma Myxoid rhabdomyosarcoma		Biphasic tendosynovial sarcoma Hemangiopericytoma	Fibromatosis Osteosarcoma Pleomorphic fibrous histiocytoma
Plump spindle	Fasciitis Fibrosarcoma Leiomyoma Leiomyosarcoma Neurofibroma Neurofibrosarcoma Schwannoma	Desmoid Fasciitis Fibromatosis Fibrosarcoma Kaposi's sarcoma Leiomyoma Leiomyosarcoma Myositis ossificans Neurofibroma Osteosarcoma Schwannoma				Fibromatosis Fibrosarcoma Leiomyosarcoma Osteosarcoma
Granular epithelioid	Histiocytic fibrous histiocytoma Neuroepithelioma	Myositis ossificans	Chondroblastoma Eosinophilic granuloma Histiocytic fibrous histiocytoma Leiomyoblastoma Lipoblastic liposarcoma Osteoblastoma Tendosynovitis	Clear cell sarcoma Embryonal rhabdomyosarcoma Eosinophilic granuloma Ewing's sarcoma Hemangiosarcoma Histiocytic fibrous histiocytoma Leiomyoblastoma Lipoblastic liposarcoma Lymphangiosarcoma	Alveolar rhabdomyosarcoma Alveolar soft part sarcoma Biphasic tendosynovial sarcoma Epithelioid sarcoma Ewing's sarcoma Hemangioma Hemangiosarcoma Hibernoma Leiomyoblastoma Lymphangiosarcoma Osteoblastoma Osteosarcoma	Granular cell tumor Hemangiosarcoma Lymphangiosarcoma Osteoblastoma Osteosarcoma Rhabdomyosarcoma
Clear epithelioid	Pleomorphic fibrous histiocytoma Schwannoma	Schwannoma	Chondroma Chondrosarcoma Chordoma Clear cell sarcoma Fat necrosis Leiomyoblastoma Lipoma Myxoid liposarcoma Osteochondroma Osteosarcoma Schwannoma Well-differentiated liposarcoma	Chondroma Chondrosarcoma Chordoma Clear cell sarcoma Epithelioid sarcoma Leiomyoblastoma	Chordoma Clear cell sarcoma Leiomyoblastoma Well-differentiated liposarcoma	Chondroblastoma Leiomyoblastoma
Isomorphic giant	Histiocytic fibrous histiocytoma	Myositis ossificans Osteosarcoma	Histiocytic fibrous histiocytoma Tendosynovitis	Histiocytic fibrous histiocytoma Osteoblastoma		Foreign body granuloma Osteoblastoma Osteosarcoma Pleomorphic fibrous histiocytoma
Pleomorphic giant	Leiomyosarcoma Neurofibrosarcoma Pleomorphic fibrous histiocytoma Pleomorphic lipoma Schwannoma	Fibrosarcoma Leiomyoma Leiomyosarcoma Neurofibrosarcoma Osteosarcoma Pleomorphic liposarcoma Pleomorphic rhabdomyosarcoma Schwannoma	Fat necrosis Hibernoma Leiomyoblastoma Osteosarcoma Pleomorphic lipoma Pleomorphic liposarcoma	Leiomyoblastoma Rhabdomyoma	Alveolar soft part sarcoma Hemangiosarcoma Lymphangiosarcoma	Callus Fat necrosis Fibrosarcoma Foreign body granuloma Hemangiosarcoma Leiomyoblastoma Leiomyosarcoma Lymphangiosarcoma Myositis ossificans Osteosarcoma Pleomorphic fibrous histiocytoma Pleomorphic rhabdomyosarcoma Proliferative myositis Rhabdomyoma

*Modified from Hajdu SI: Differential Diagnosis of Soft Tissue and Bone Tumors. Philadelphia, Lea & Febiger, 1986.

definitive diagnosis. The diagnostic assessment should end with a written report by using appropriate pathologic and cytologic descriptions. Because it is the microscopic diagnosis that determines therapy, pathologists, cytopathologists and cytologists assume a great responsibility when they recommend radical therapy, but they assume a still greater responsibility when they advise against it.[18]

SAMPLING TECHNIQUES

Technically, the aspiration smears are prepared from materials obtained from soft tissues by 20- to 22-gauge needle and from bone by 18- to 20-gauge needle. Most of the deep soft tissue and bone tumors and all metastatic sarcomas are aspirated under radiologic control. Aspiration smears are placed in 95% ethyl alcohol and stained with hematoxylin and eosin or Papanicolaou stain.

Smears from specimens other than aspirates, e.g., sputa and effusion, are prepared by using standard, nonfilter, preparatory techniques and are stained according to the Papanicolaou method.

UNDIFFERENTIATED CONNECTIVE TISSUE TUMORS

Aneurysmal bone cyst affects females somewhat more commonly than males and occurs almost exclusively during the first and second decades of life. This cyst is a solitary intraskeletal lesion that involves most commonly the vertebrae and the metaphasis, i.e., the distal end, of long bones. Microscopically, aneurysmal bone cyst is composed of clear, slender and plump cytoplasmic epithelioid, foamy histiocytes and hemosiderin-containing granular forms in a myxovascular or myxofibrillar stroma (Fig. 20–1). Similar microscopic elements can be seen in simple bone cyst, reparative granuloma of jaw bones and other granulomas, histiocytic fibrous histiocytoma and telangiectatic osteosarcoma.[14, 18]

Foreign body granuloma is induced by intrinsic or extrinsic trauma or a foreign object, e.g., suture material. The microscopic appearance is influenced by the duration and location of the lesion. In the acute-phase mononucleated inflammatory cells, lymphocytes and histiocytes in congested reticular matrix dominate. In advanced chronic lesions large multinucleated and mononucleated forms are ubiquitous; the matrix is fibrous, sclerotic and, not uncommonly, locally calcified or ossified. Microscopically, in the differential diagnosis, an almost endless number of non-neoplastic lesions, fasciitis, fat necrosis, proliferative myositis, myositis ossificans, pleomorphic lipoma, pleomorphic liposarcoma and osteosarcoma should be considered.[18]

Benign fibroblastic fibrous histiocytoma is usually a solitary, cutaneous extremity lesion, but in about 30% of the cases it is multiple and, rarely, it can be found in deep soft tissues, parenchymal organs and bone. Microscopically, it is composed of short fibroblasts

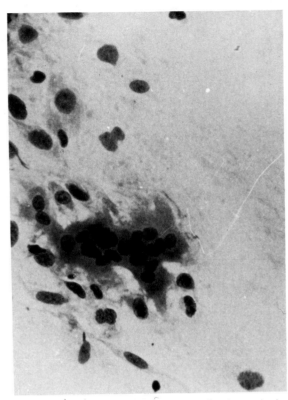

FIGURE 20–1. Aneurysmal bone cyst. Slender and plump spindle cells with poorly preserved cell processes and epulis-type multinucleated giant cells (bone aspirate; hematoxylin and eosin; ×450).

with finely reticular cell processes that are arranged in a "cartwheel" or storiform pattern. The fibroblasts and oval or round nucleated histiocytes later become inconspicuous components and are arranged about thin-walled capillary vessels. In the differential diagnosis all tumors that microscopically contain short arranged fibroblasts, e.g., fasciitis, malignant fibroblastic fibrous histiocytoma, neurofibroma and leiomyoma should be considered.[18]

Malignant fibroblastic fibrous histiocytoma is, most often, located in the shoulder and the trunk, but the soft tissues of the extremities and long bones can also be occasionally the primary site. Microscopically, it is composed of fairly uniform slender fibroblasts with reticular cytoplasmic processes arranged in whorls or bundles around thin-walled capillary vessels. The individual neoplastic cells are slender or plump fibroblasts, which tend to spread out in round or oval histiocytic forms as tissue space and matrix substance permit (Fig. 20–2).[18, 38] Mononucleated or multinucleated giant cells as well as foam cells are not a feature of these tumors and mitotic figures are rare. In the differential diagnosis, fibroblastic tumors and other tumors composed of slender or plump spindle cells, e.g., benign fibroblastic fibrous histiocytoma, fibrosarcoma, benign and malignant smooth muscle tumors and benign and malignant peripheral nerve tumors should be considered.[18]

Benign histiocytic fibrous histiocytoma is a rare neo-

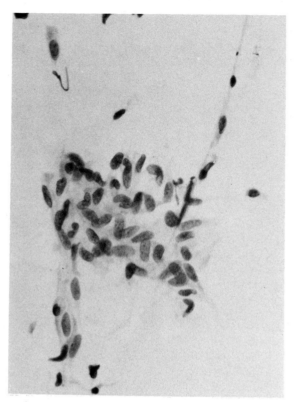

FIGURE 20–2. Malignant fibroblastic fibrous histiocytoma (dermatofibrosarcoma protuberans). Slender spindle cells in arranged storiform pattern (soft tissue aspirate; hematoxylin and eosin; ×450).

Microscopically, the bulky part is made up of slender or plump spindle cells with finely reticular or collagenous cell processes, a few epulis-type multinucleated giant cells (so-called osteoclasts) and occasional pleomorphic tumor giant cells (Fig. 20–4).[18, 41] Because of the dominance of sarcomatous "stromal" elements, sarcomas, e.g., fibrosarcoma, malignant pleomorphic fibrous histiocytoma, malignant peripheral nerve tumors and osteosarcoma, must be considered in the differential diagnosis.

Benign pleomorphic fibrous histiocytoma is a rare neoplasm and composed of a spectrum of histiocytes, fibroblasts and multinucleated Touton and epulis-type giant cells. Nests of lipophages and a variable number of pigmented foam cells and chronic inflammatory cells are usually admixed with the other elements. Identical or similar cells can be seen in scores of benign and malignant primary soft tissue and bone lesions, e.g., fat necrosis, granulomas and malignant pleomorphic fibrous histiocytoma and osteosarcoma, just to mention a few. Also, one must include in the differential diagnosis clear cell neoplasms, e.g., renal cell carcinoma and clear cell, so-called balloon-cell, melanoma.[14, 18]

Malignant pleomorphic fibrous histiocytoma occurs mostly in adults after the age of 40 and often reaches considerable size.[13, 14] The microscopic appearance of malignant pleomorphic fibrous histiocytoma varies according to a combination of five basic elements: mono-

plasm; less than 0.1% of all soft tissue tumors and less than 8% of all bone tumors belong to this category.[18] Patients having this neoplasm in the soft tissues are usually between 30 and 50 years of age, and those who present with bone primary are usually 40 to 60 years of age. Septa of thin and broad connective tissue between brownish cystic cavities contain two distinct cell types: multinucleated epulis-type giant cells (so-called osteoclasts) and oval, round or somewhat elongated mononuclear stromal cells. The giant cells dominate the microscopic appearance, and the nuclei of the giant cells are often a dozen or more in number. The cytoplasm of the giant cells as well as the stromal cells is granular, dense and rich in glycogen. The cell processes are fine and can be demonstrated with silver stain. Lipid and hemosiderin-containing mononucleated foam cells can also be seen (Fig. 20–3).[17, 18] With consideration of the aforementioned, the diagnosis of benign histiocytic fibrous histiocytoma can be rendered in an aspiration smear, but it must be kept constantly in mind that similar elements, though in different ratio, are often seen in solitary bone cyst, aneurysmal bone cyst, malignant histiocytic fibrous histiocytoma, giant cell reparative granuloma and nodular tendosynovitis.[18]

Malignant histiocytic fibrous histiocytoma is rare; approximately 0.5% of all soft tissue and bone sarcomas are malignant histiocytic fibrous histiocytoma.

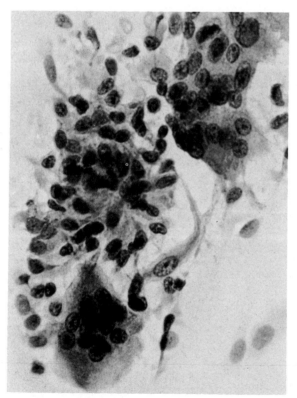

FIGURE 20–3. Benign histiocytic fibrous histiocytoma (benign giant cell tumor). Large multinucleated epulis-type giant cells and oval and spindle "matrix" cells (bone aspirate; hematoxylin and eosin; ×450).

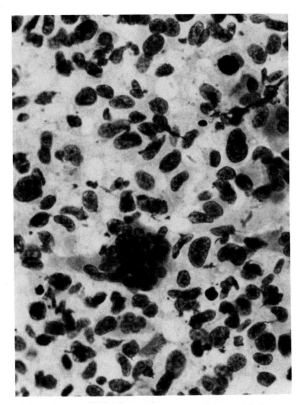

FIGURE 20–4. Malignant histiocytic fibrous histiocytoma (malignant giant cell tumors). Many round, epithelioid and plump, fibroblastic spindle cells in a disarranged pattern and a solitary epulis-type giant cell (bone aspirate; hematoxylin and eosin; ×450).

nuclear histiocytic round cells, multinucleated Touton-type giant cells, slender or plump fibroblasts, bizarre polymorphic tumor giant cells and stromal components such as vessels.[18] The mononuclear cells, particularly the ones resembling histiocytes, usually have well-defined cytoplasm and nuclei with prominent nucleoli. Clusters of seemingly unrelated cells, chronic inflammatory cells and lymphocytes are often present (Fig. 20–5). Several tumors composed of giant pleomorphic cells should be considered in the differential diagnosis, e.g., benign pleomorphic fibrous histiocytoma, pleomorphic lipoma, pleomorphic fibrosarcoma, pleomorphic liposarcoma, proliferative myositis, myositis ossificans, osteosarcoma, malignant melanoma and desmoplastic large-cell carcinoma such as renal cell carcinoma (Fig. 20–6).[14, 18]

FIBROUS TISSUE TUMORS

Fasciitis is a common reactive lesion. Over 50% of these lesions are located in the upper extremity, particularly in the forearm and near the axillary fold. Microscopically, fasciitis is composed of slender and plump spindle cells, fibroblasts, mostly in an arranged pattern. The cell processes are slender, elaborate and interdigitating with a resemblance to monolayer tissue culture.[8, 15] The matrix is richly vascular and myxoid.

Cellularity may vary from one microscopic field to another, but chronic inflammatory cells, lymphocytes, histiocytes and extravasated red blood cells are constant findings (Fig. 20–7). In the differential diagnosis, numerous benign and malignant entities should be considered, e.g., fibroblastic fibrous histiocytoma, fibromatosis, fibrosarcoma, myxoid and fibroblastic adipose tissue tumors, smooth muscle tumors and peripheral nerve tumors.[18]

Fibromatosis is a relatively uncommon lesion and may be multiple and familiar and may be complicated by contractures and other deformities. Most fibromatoses are painless, subcutaneous or submucosal, poorly circumscribed, infiltrative, firm nodules. The dominant cells in fibromatosis are well-differentiated, fairly uniform fibroblasts and myofibroblasts with vesicular, plump nuclei and fibrillar or broad cytoplasmic processes.[12] Calcification and formation of metaplastic cartilage and bone are rare findings, but certain forms, e.g., mesenteric fibromatosis, may exhibit great cellularity and poor differentiation. The most common tumors that should be considered in the differential diagnosis are fasciitis, desmoid tumor, fibrosarcoma, scar tissue and peripheral nerve tumors.[14, 18]

Desmoid fibrosarcoma is a low-grade malignant neoplasm with scar-like consistency and may occur at any age, but it is diagnosed most often in patients in the third and fourth decades. The back, chest wall, head

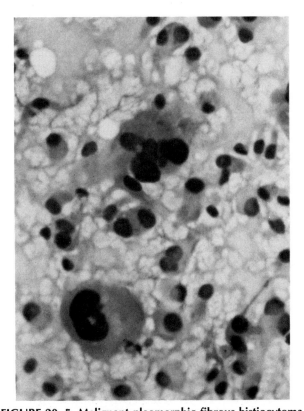

FIGURE 20–5. Malignant pleomorphic fibrous histiocytoma. Isolated spindle cells with round and oval nuclei. Note the multinucleated tumor giant cells (soft tissue aspirate; hematoxylin and eosin; ×450).

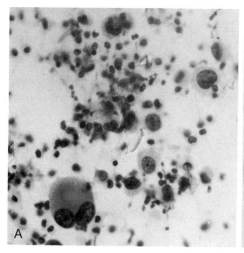

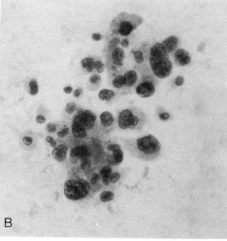

FIGURE 20–6. Metastatic malignant pleomorphic fibrous histiocytoma. *A,* Multiple isolated mononuclear and multinuclear round cells in inflammatory background (pleural effusion; Papanicolaou; ×450). *B,* Clusters of granular cytoplasmic neoplastic cells in clean background (pleural effusion; Papanicolaou; ×450).

and neck areas and the extremities, particularly the lower extremities, are the most common primary sites.[12] Microscopically, desmoid tumor is composed of well-differentiated and uniform fibroblasts and fibrocytes. The neoplastic cells are plump, with elongated monochromatic and vesicular nuclei that are dispersed between well-formed, Trichrome-positive collagen fibers. The degree of cellularity is variable. No evidence exists of mitotic activity or necrosis. Tumor giant cells, inflammatory cells and other reactive cells are practically never seen in untreated desmoid tumor. In the differential diagnosis other fibroblastic lesions, e.g., scar, fibromatosis, fibrosarcoma and benign and malignant peripheral nerve tumors, should be considered.[18]

Fibrosarcoma is mainly a soft tissue neoplasm but may also occur in bone. It is estimated that 6% of all primary malignant bone tumors are fibrosarcomas. Fibrosarcoma is a disease of adults, usually between 35 and 55 years of age.[14, 18] The cellular composition of low-grade fibrosarcoma is similar to that of desmoid

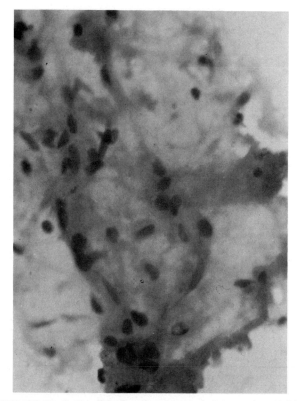

FIGURE 20–7. Fasciitis. Poorly preserved elongated nuclei in a mesh of tangled slender cytoplasmic processes in myxoid background (soft tissue aspirate; hematoxylin and eosin; ×450).

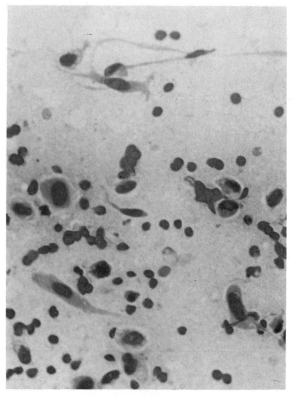

FIGURE 20–8. Fibrosarcoma. Oval nuclei in plump or slender cytoplasmic processes in nonmyxoid, hemorrhagic background (soft tissue aspirate; hematoxylin and eosin; ×450).

tumor. Microscopic evidence of bundle or fascicle formation is seen. The neoplastic cells are fairly uniform, nongiant cell–forming fibroblasts with elongated and broad cytoplasmic processes and separated by an intercellular collagenous matrix. Areas of necrosis, cysts and mitotic figures are absent or sparse. High-grade fibrosarcoma, microscopically, is composed of fibroblasts at different stages of maturation. The neoplastic fibroblasts vary in size and shape from oval and spindle forms to polygonal, and distorted and multinucleated forms are common. The intercellular matrix is variable, and in many cases it is minimal (Fig. 20–8). Irregular areas of necrosis and cystic spaces are common, and mitotic figures can be found with ease. Because of the almost ubiquitous presence of fibroblasts and fibrocytes in various soft tissue and bone tumors, the number of lesions one should consider in the differential diagnosis, microscopically, is seemingly endless. Fibroblastic and pleomorphic fibrous histiocytomas, fibromatosis, desmoid fibrosarcoma, fibroblastic and pleomorphic liposarcomas, smooth muscle tumors, peripheral nerve tumors and desmoplastic epithelial neoplasms are perhaps the most common tumors to be considered in the differential diagnosis (Fig. 20–9).[18]

TENDOSYNOVIAL TUMORS

Tendosynovitis is a reactive process that may affect the synovial membrane, tendon sheath and bursae and

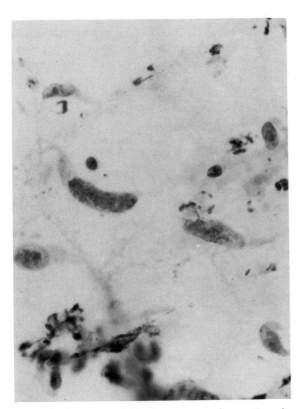

FIGURE 20–9. Postradiation fibrosarcoma metastatic to lung. Elongated and oval nuclei with whip-like poorly outlined cytoplasmic processes (transthoracic aspirate; Papanicolaou; ×450).

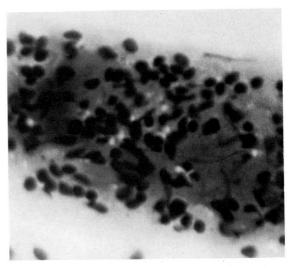

FIGURE 20–10. Tendosynovitis. A mixture of poorly preserved round histiocytic forms and slender spindle cells in myxoid background (soft tissue aspirate; hematoxylin and eosin; ×450).

is most commonly seen in older adult patients and elderly patients. Specific forms are granulomatous tendosynovitis, gouty arthritis and rheumatoid arthritis.[32] Granulomatous tendosynovitis may be caused by acid-fast bacilli or various fungi. In gouty arthritis the urate crystals are demonstrable with polarizing filters and because of the water-soluble nature of urate crystals, smears and tissue sections should be placed in absolute alcohol. In rheumatoid arthritis, a nonspecific excessive proliferation of tendosynovial lining cells in the form of hypertrophic villi is seen in association with the formation of follicle-free lymphoid nodules. Similar changes plus the deposit of epulis-type giant cells and hemosiderin-containing foam cells are found to excess in the so-called pigmented villonodular synovitis (Fig. 20–10).[18]

Biphasic tendosynovial sarcoma is usually of considerable size and is predominantly found in the proximity of major joints. It is diagnosed predominantly during the fourth and fifth decades of life.[12, 13] Microscopically, biphasic tendosynovial sarcoma is composed of slender and monomorphic tumor cells arranged in two distinct patterns: alveolar or pseudoglandular and spreading. The neoplastic cells are uniform round or oval cells with minute cytoplasm and uniform nuclei and are arranged in clusters, cords and cellular sheets. Rarely, papillary or villous arrangements near cystic spaces and at the edge of the tumor can be seen (Fig. 20–11). The lining cells of pseudoglandular or tubular units show a positive reaction for cytokeratins and vimentin and a negative reaction for carcinoembryonic antigen (CEA); they contain no intracytoplasmic mucicarminophilic material. In the differential diagnosis malignant histiocytic fibrous histiocytoma, malignant epithelioid mesothelioma, glandular schwannoma, Wilms' tumor and skin adnexal tumors should be considered (Fig. 20–12).[18, 33]

Monophasic tendosynovial sarcoma is the most common form of the tendosynovial sarcomas and amounts to 5% of all soft tissue sarcomas. It is predominantly

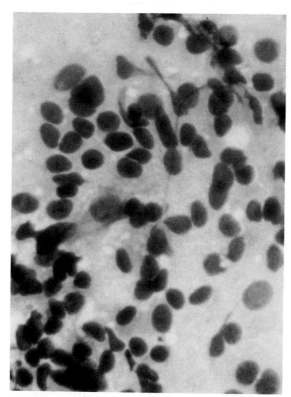

FIGURE 20–11. Biphasic tendosynovial sarcoma. Oval and round cells with poorly outlined cytoplasm in pseudoglandular arrangement and in single form (soft tissue aspirate; hematoxylin and eosin; ×450).

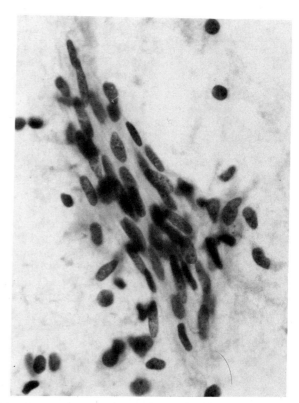

FIGURE 20–13. Monophasic tendosynovial sarcoma. Monotonous slender cells with uniform elongated nuclei (soft tissue aspirate; hematoxylin and eosin; ×450).

a disease of young adults in the third and fourth decades; the extremities, including the foot, lower leg, thigh and forearm, are the most common sites.[13, 14] Microscopically, it is predominantly composed of uniform slender spindle cells with short reticulin stain–positive cytoplasmic processes and oval or small cigar-shaped nuclei. The elongated neoplastic cells are arranged in sheets, fascicles and parallel cords. Mitotic figures, tumor giant cells and necrosis are extremely rare (Fig. 20–13). Immunohistochemical reactions for cytokeratins and vimentin may color the cytoplasm of some of the neoplastic epithelioid cells. The monoto-

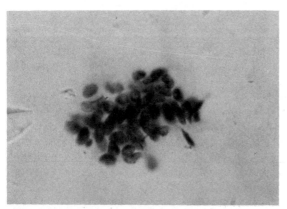

FIGURE 20–12. Biphasic tendosynovial sarcoma metastatic to lung. A cluster of naked-appearing uniform round and oval nuclei (pleural effusion; Papanicolaou; ×350).

nous uniformity of the neoplastic cells, short slender cytoplasmic processes and absence of giant cells warrant inclusion of monophasic tendosynovial sarcoma in the differential diagnosis with malignant fibroblastic fibrous histiocytoma, fibroblastic fibrosarcoma, peripheral nerve tumors, spindle cell mesothelioma, desmoplastic melanoma and desmoplastic carcinoma (Fig. 20–14).[14, 18]

Epithelioid sarcoma usually appears in the form of multiple cutaneous and paratendinous nodules and has a tendency to spread to regional lymph nodes (Fig. 20–15).[14, 33] Approximately 1% of soft tissue sarcomas are epithelioid sarcoma. It is a disease most often diagnosed in patients who are in the late teens and during the third decade. Microscopically, the hallmark of epithelioid sarcoma is the centrally necrotic, fused, epithelioid nodules. The nodules exhibit various stages of maturation, differentiation and cellularity. The granular and clear cytoplasmic, round and oval, epithelioid cells merge imperceptibly with finely reticular slender and plump spindle cells.[1, 14] The epithelioid cells give a nonhomogenous positive reaction for cytokeratins and vimentin and a negative reaction for S-100 protein and mucin. This pattern of immunohistochemical reactivity and the presence of clear and dark cells, junctional complexes, scanty rough endoplasmic reticulum (RER) and few Golgi and mitochondria, ultrastructurally, support a tendosynovial origin.[35] In the differential diagnosis granulomatous lesions, such as granuloma annulare, rheumatoid nodule and foreign body

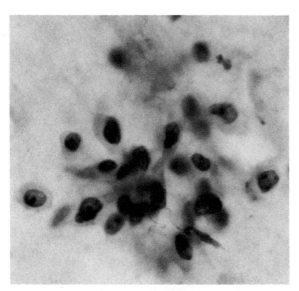

FIGURE 20–14. Monophasic tendosynovial sarcoma metastatic to lung. Small dark cells in a loose cluster show some variation in size and shape of nuclei and cytoplasm (pleural effusion; Papanicolaou; ×450).

granuloma, must be considered along with neoplasms, such as malignant melanoma, skin adnexal tumors and non-neoplastic tumors like fasciitis.[18]

Clear cell sarcoma is also known as aponeurotic clear cell sarcoma and clear cell sarcoma of tendons.[12, 14] In the pure form it is extremely rare, less than 0.5% of the soft tissue sarcomas, but it is not uncommon in combination with epithelioid sarcoma and biphasic or monophasic tendosynovial sarcoma. Microscopically, to a certain extent, it has an overlapping morphology with epithelioid sarcoma except for the zones of central necrosis.[18] The neoplastic cells are predominantly round or oval, clear epithelioid cells with round well-defined vesicular nuclei and prominent nucleoli arranged in nests or fascicles. With immunohistochemical stains, the neoplastic cells react positively for cytokeratins and vimentin and negatively for S-100 protein, CEA and mucin. Some of the reported cases of clear cell sarcoma are misdiagnosed malignant melanoma, without apparent cutaneous or mucosal primary. Cytologically, the diagnosis of clear cell sarcoma can be entertained provided other neoplasms that may appear with clear cell features, e.g., leiomyosarcoma, renal cell carcinoma, skin adnexal tumors and malignant melanoma, are kept in mind.[18]

ADIPOSE TISSUE TUMORS

Fat necrosis is far more common than it appears from clinical experience. Fat necrosis may develop at the site of physical trauma or contact with bile or pancreatic secretion. The combination of atrophic and degenerating adipocytes with pyknotic nuclei, nests of proliferating granular cytoplasmic lipoblasts, lipid-filled mononucleated and multinucleated macrophages and assorted acute and chronic inflammatory cells is the hallmark of fat necrosis (Fig. 20–16). Because no

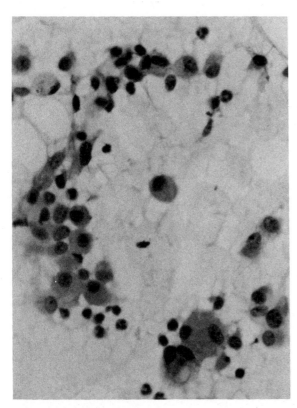

FIGURE 20–15. Epithelioid sarcoma. Granular, cytoplasmic, round cells with sharply outlined cytoplasm and nuclei (soft tissue aspirate; hematoxylin and eosin; ×450).

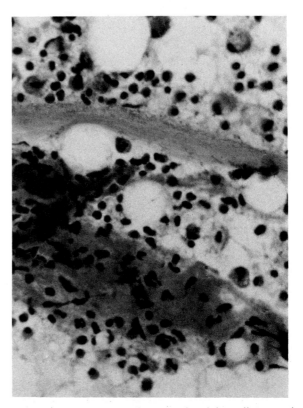

FIGURE 20–16. Fat necrosis. Vacuolated fat cells, granular cytoplasmic histiocytes, lymphocytes and amorphous debris (soft tissue aspirate; hematoxylin and eosin; ×450).

specific single cell characterizes fat necrosis, the clue to the suggestive cytologic diagnosis is its inclusion in the differential diagnosis with other entities, e.g., lipogranuloma, pleomorphic lipoma, hibernoma and fibrous histiocytoma.[18]

Lipoma is the most common neoplasm of adipose tissue. Lipoma may occur in any location and any organ, but the subcutaneous tissues of the shoulder, back, chest, neck and thigh are the most common sites.[12] The size may vary from a few millimeters to several centimeters, and the number can be solitary or multiple. The consistency and microscopic appearance of lipomas vary according to histologic type and cellularity. The most consistent and dominant cells are mature fat cells, adipocytes, fibrous connective tissue elements and nonbranching capillary vessels. Most of the fat cells are spheric and distended, uniform, monovacuolated adipocytes with pyknotic excentrically placed nuclei, but it is not uncommon to find a few small polyhedral multivacuolated preadipocytes and finely granular round lipoblasts (Fig. 20–17).[18, 44] In infiltrating lipoma, the cell membranes of many adipocytes are disrupted, giving a myxoid of myxoma appearance. In sclerosing or fibroblastic lipoma the intercellular matrix is mostly acellular, sclerosing collagenous tissue. Myelolipoma shows a unique combination of adipose tissue and hematopoietic cells and is found most commonly in the adrenal. Lipoma can be diagnosed in an aspiration smear with certainty owing to the characteristic uniform adipocytes in tightly adherent lobular arrangement. However, lipomas, partic-

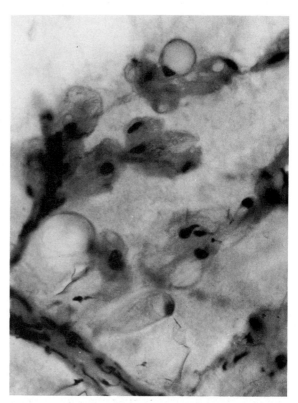

FIGURE 20–18. Hibernoma. Well-differentiated granular cytoplasmic fat cells in an angiomyxomatous background (soft tissue aspirate; hematoxylin and eosin; ×450).

ularly the long-standing and bulky ones, may transform focally or in several areas into liposarcoma; therefore, a definitive diagnosis should be rendered after the histologic examination of the excised tumor.[18]

Hibernoma, also called lipoma of brown fat, is found most commonly in the subcutaneous tissues of the back, shoulder, axilla and occasionally in the retroperitoneum and mediastinum. Microscopically, it is mainly composed of mononucleated globoid or polygonal lipochrome pigment-rich adipocytes with centrally placed dark nuclei and coarsely granular cytoplasm. The tumor cells are often arranged in tightly composed nests and lobules (Fig. 20–18).[18, 24] The microscopic resemblance of hibernoma to histocytic fibrous histiocytoma, proliferative myositis, granular cell myoblastoma, alveolar soft part sarcoma and oncocytoma may cause, in limited tissue or aspiration biopsy, a diagnostic problem.

Well-differentiated liposarcoma is also called lipoma-like liposarcoma. Although a pure form of well-differentiated liposarcoma is a nonmetastasizing, low-grade, malignant neoplasm, the bulky size makes it worrisome.[12, 13] It is a disease of adults over 40. Microscopically, it is composed of well-differentiated globoid, monovacuolated distended adipocytes not too different from those commonly seen in lipomas. However, the neoplastic adipocytes show variation in size of cytoplasm and nuclei. The microscopic diagnosis depends on pattern recognition with consideration of cellular elements. Therefore, it is most unlikely that this neo-

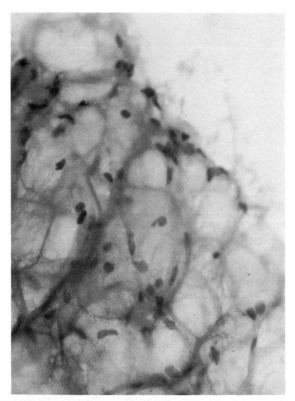

FIGURE 20–17. Lipoma. Well-differentiated adipocytes in a cohesive cluster (soft tissue aspirate; hematoxylin and eosin; ×450).

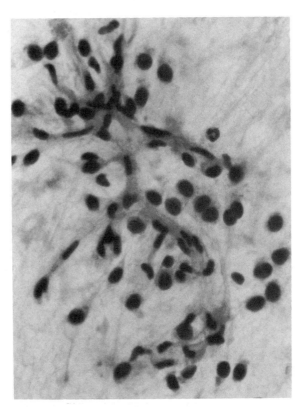

FIGURE 20–19. Myxoid liposarcoma. Round and slender neoplastic fat cells are held together by a trabecular network of fine capillary vessels (soft tissue aspirate; hematoxylin and eosin; ×450).

plasm can be accurately diagnosed using an aspiration biopsy sample. Because of the borderline or lipoma-like nature of this neoplasm, atypical or cellular lipoma, pleomorphic lipoma and liposarcomas of other types must be considered in the differential diagnosis.[18]

Myxoid liposarcoma is usually a bulky pseudoencapsulated neoplasm and found most commonly in adults in the deep thigh, buttock and retroperitoneum. Microscopically, the fine, interconnected capillary vessels forming a network that appears like chicken wire is the hallmark of this neoplasm.[10, 12, 17] The dominant cell types are multivacuolated preadipocytes with excentrically placed round or oval nuclei and a few granular or monovacuolated round lipoblasts. These elements are tightly adherent to the outer wall of branching capillary vessels and extending fine reticular cell processes giving a lacy appearance to the sarcoma. The distinct and elaborate trabecular vascular pattern is retained even in minute tissue fragments and aspirates (Fig. 20–19).[18] In the differential diagnosis, fibrous histiocytoma, myxoid lipoma, myxoid smooth muscle tumors, myxoid peripheral nerve tumors and myxoid chondrosarcoma must be considered.

Lipoblastic liposarcoma is an uncommon neoplasm and is mainly found in the deep tissues of the thigh of young adults during the third and fourth decades. Microscopically, it is predominantly composed of oval or round cells, lipoblasts and preadipocytes, in a myxomucinous or fibrillar background. The individual cells

are most commonly uniform round cells with granular, occasionally vacuolated, ill-defined cytoplasm. The nuclei may vary slightly in size and shape, most being round or oval with prominent nucleoli.[18] The nuclei may be scalloped and pushed peripherally by lipid droplets (Fig. 20–20). No specific product of organelles can be identified with the electron microscope or immunocytochemistry. Tumors that are predominantly composed of uniform round cells, malignant histiocytic fibrous histiocytoma, clear cell sarcoma, leiomyoblastoma, chondroblastic tumors and lymphoreticular neoplasm should be considered in the differential diagnosis.

Fibroblastic liposarcomas as to sex and site distribution correspond to those of myxoid liposarcomas. Microscopically, the dominant cells are slender, fibroblast-like, fat- and glycogen-containing prolipoblasts. The neoplastic cells follow the paths of the ubiquitous and branching, thin-walled capillary vessels.[12] Occasional areas containing signet ring–type or stellate preadipocytes and granular cytoplasmic lipoblasts can be seen. In avascular areas the prolipoblasts with their slender cytoplasmic processes may show storiform arrangement and may resemble fibroblastic fibrous histiocytoma, peripheral nerve tumor and desmoplastic melanoma.[18]

Pleomorphic liposarcoma is a bulky, deep-seated relatively rare soft tissue neoplasm. Proximal parts of the extremities, buttock and retroperitoneum are the most common primary sites.[13, 14] It is a disease of adults, predominantly in the sixth and seventh decades. Microscopically, the neoplastic cells vary in size and shape from small round lipoblasts and elongated slen-

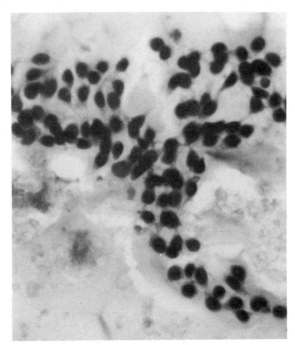

FIGURE 20–20. Lipoblastic liposarcoma. Uniform lipoblast with round nuclei and minute granular cytoplasm in cell cords and clusters (soft tissue aspirate; hematoxylin and eosin; ×450).

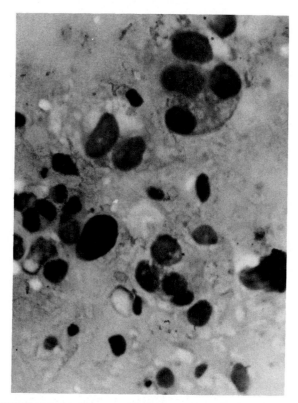

FIGURE 20–21. Pleomorphic liposarcoma. Pleomorphic neoplastic fat cells ranging in size from small to giant forms, with granular and vacuolated cytoplasm (soft tissue aspirate; hematoxylin and eosin; ×450).

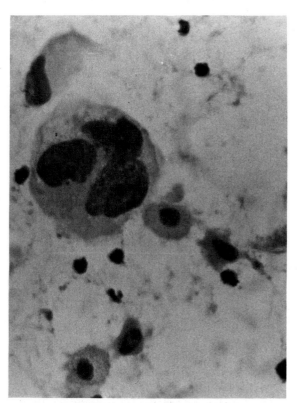

FIGURE 20–22. Pleomorphic liposarcoma metastatic to lung. Mononucleated and multinucleated neoplastic cells without specific features (pleural effusion; Papanicolaou; ×450).

der fibroblastic forms to monovacuolated distended adipocytes and multinucleated, granular cytoplasmic, neoplastic giant cells.[10, 18] The neoplastic cells grow in loosely formed clusters and ill-formed, disarranged sheets (Fig. 20–21). Pleomorphic liposarcoma is a highly vascular neoplasm, and pools of extravasated red blood cells are common findings. In advanced or neglected cases, there is a clear tendency in differentiation towards pleomorphic fibrosarcoma. In the differential diagnosis other pleomorphic neoplasms, e.g., pleomorphic fibrous histiocytoma, fibrosarcoma, rhabdomyosarcoma and osteosarcoma, must be considered (Fig. 20–22).

MUSCLE TUMORS

Proliferative myositis is a rare, rapidly enlarging, painful inflammatory pseudotumor of skeletal muscle and may assume several centimeters in size. Microscopically, in the proliferative phase, the two chief microscopic components are proliferating granular cytoplasmic epithelioid cells and loosely arranged polygonal, ganglion cell-like giant histiocytes (Fig. 20–23).[18] Because of its cellular composition and intramuscular location, myositis ossificans must also be included in the differential diagnosis with several giant cell–containing tumors, e.g., pleomorphic lipomas and pleomorphic sarcomas.

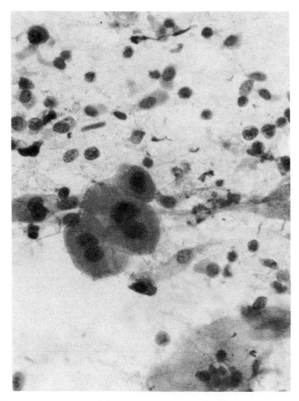

FIGURE 20–23. Proliferative myositis. Ganglion cell-like binucleated histiocytic forms in the background of nonspecific elements (soft tissue aspirate; hematoxylin and eosin; ×450).

Myositis ossificans is a self-limited, non-neoplastic lesion of skeletal muscle and found most commonly in young adults in the thigh and buttock. Microscopically, it is characterized by deposits of orderly, radially oriented and partially calcified trabeculae of ectopic and metaplastic bone. The intertrabecular matrix varies in cellularity from florid fibrohistiocytic to sclerosing, according to duration of the lesion. In addition to bone-forming lesions, e.g., callus and osteoblastoma, osteosarcoma should be included in the differential diagnosis.[18]

Leiomyoma is one of the most common benign soft tissue tumors. It can grow in any place where muscle is found, e.g., the skin, lung, intestines, uterus and retroperitoneum. Because of the location or some other features several specific forms are distinguished. Cutaneous leiomyoma is thought to originate from blood vessel walls or from arrectores pilorum.[12] Angiomyoma arises in the walls of vessels usually in the area of the ankle joint in females of childbearing age. Peritoneal leiomyomatosis is characterized by the development of multiple peritoneal nodules. The fact that almost all cases have been associated with pregnancy implicates hormonal stimulus as an etiologic factor.[14] Despite variation in site and size, microscopically, leiomyomas appear similar but may exhibit some variation in differentiation and cellularity, according to the duration of the tumor. Tumors of short duration tend to be cellular and composed of fairly uniform plump spindle cells. Leiomyomas of long duration, in comparison, may show areas of sclerosis and calcification. Some of the tumors that should be considered in the differential diagnosis are fibromatosis, leiomyosarcoma, desmoid fibrosarcoma and desmoplastic melanoma.

Rhabdomyoma is an exceedingly rare tumor and is predominantly a disease of adult males between the ages of 25 and 40. The most common site is the head and neck region. Microscopically, two forms, the so-called adult type and fetal type, are distinguished.[12] The fetal form consists of haphazardly oriented bundles of undifferentiated mesenchymal cells and fairly typical, cross-striated, strap cells in a loosely arranged and sparsely cellular matrix. The adult type of rhabdomyoma is predominantly composed of fairly uniform, closely packed polygonal rhabdomyoblasts with granular and vacuolated cytoplasm. The tumor cells show positive reaction for muscle common antigen, desmin, myoglobin and vimentin. With the help of these immunohistochemical reactions and electron microscopy, rhabdomyoma can be differentiated from granular cell tumor, hibernoma, alveolar soft part sarcoma and oncocytic tumors.[5]

Leiomyosarcoma is a ubiquitous pseudoencapsulated malignant neoplasm of smooth muscle. Most of the leiomyosarcomas are primary neoplasms of the uterus and gastrointestinal tract, particularly the stomach. The origin of leiomyosarcomas in soft tissues, cutaneous and deep tissues, is rare.[12] The microscopic appearance varies to a large extent according to histologic grade of the sarcoma. Low-grade leiomyosarcoma is mainly composed of fairly uniform, well-differentiated, elon-

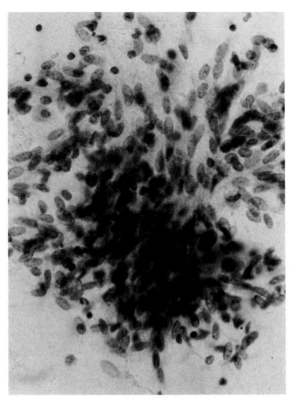

FIGURE 20–24. Metastatic leiomyosarcoma. Plump spindle cells with poorly outlined cytoplasmic processes and oval nuclei (liver aspirate; hematoxylin and eosin; ×350).

gated, plump, spindle cells with blunt-end nuclei. The tumor cells show little or no pleomorphism. High-grade leiomyosarcoma may contain low-grade histologic areas, but the sarcoma is predominantly composed of well-differentiated, uniform leiomyocytes and poorly differentiated, round, epithelioid polygonal or pleomorphic leiomyoblasts. Mononucleated and multinucleated giant cells are often seen. In cytologic smears aspirated and exfoliated neoplastic smooth muscle cells retain a striking resemblance to leiomyosarcoma in histologic sections (Figs. 20–24 and 20–25).[6, 18, 31] Low-grade or high-grade leiomyosarcoma may appear, partly or completely, as a round cell neoplasm. If the round or epithelioid leiomyoblasts are the main or exclusive cellular elements of the sarcoma, the term leiomyoblastoma is an appropriate one. The dominant cells are round, often vacuolated, leiomyoblasts with clear round nuclei (Fig. 20–26).[18] Because of an almost endless number of spindle cell tumors, e.g., fibromatosis, leiomyoma, fibrosarcoma, fibrous mesothelioma, peripheral nerve tumors and desmoplastic melanoma, attempts should be made to carry out ultrastructural examination and immunohistochemical studies if malignant smooth muscle tumor is suspected.[7, 35]

Embryonal rhabdomyosarcoma in adults is extremely rare. Nearly 80% of all soft tissue sarcomas during childhood are embryonal rhabdomyosarcoma. The extremities, head and neck areas and genitourinary organs are the most common sites.[12, 14] Microscopically, the botryoid sarcoma seen in infants and young chil-

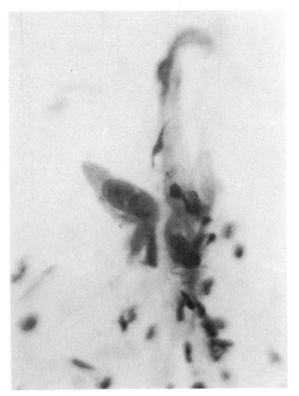

FIGURE 20–25. Gastric leiomyosarcoma. Poorly preserved tangled whip-like cell processes and a well-outlined oval nucleus (gastric brushing; Papanicolaou; ×450).

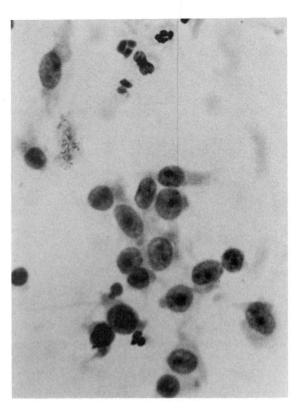

FIGURE 20–26. Gastric leiomyoblastoma. Round and oval nuclei in delicate, interlinked, cytoplasmic material (gastric brushing; Papanicolaou; ×450).

dren, mainly in the vagina and uterus and urinary bladder, and in young adults, in the nose and nasopharynx, is mostly composed of short slender cells with fragile cytoplasmic processes and dark pyknotic nuclei and occasionally round or oval cells with round nuclei and minute cytoplasm in abundant, sparsely vascular, myxoid matrix (Fig. 20–27). The epithelioid rhabdomyosarcoma consists of small round or oval cells with somewhat excentrically placed round or oval nuclei in small granular cytoplasm. The cells show no cohesion, but clusters, nests or sheet formations in an epithelioid arrangement are common features (Figs. 20–28 and 20–29). Alveolar rhabdomyosarcoma is composed, microscopically, of uniform, mostly mononucleated granular epithelioid cells with round nuclei and prominent nucleoli. The neoplastic cells are arranged in tubules and rosette-forming nests (Fig. 20–30).[18, 19] Alveolar rhabdomyosarcoma is usually found in older children and young adults in deep soft tissues of the extremities. A rare form of rhabdomyosarcoma named rhabdomyoblastoma appears with a unique microscopic picture that is dominated by granular, round, ganglion cell-like cells with hourglass-appearing prominent cytoplasm and excentrically placed nuclei. The demonstration of intracellular cross-striated filaments has as much a possibility with light microscopy as electron microscopy.[12, 35] Immunohistochemical reactions for vimentin are consistently positive, and well-differentiated rhabdomyoblast may exhibit positive reaction for muscle common antigen, myosin, desmin and rarely

myoglobin.[7, 18] Most embryonal rhabdomyosarcoma can be readily diagnosed in cytologic preparations. In the differential diagnosis, several round cell neoplasms must be considered including, for example, neuroblas-

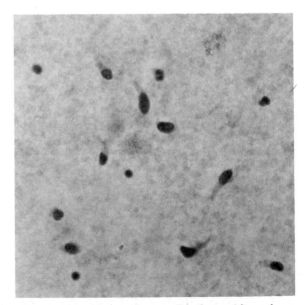

FIGURE 20–27. Metastatic myxoid (botryoid) embryonal rhabdomyosarcoma. Isolated fragile cells with solitary minute nuclei and cell processes (peritoneal effusion; Papanicolaou; ×450).

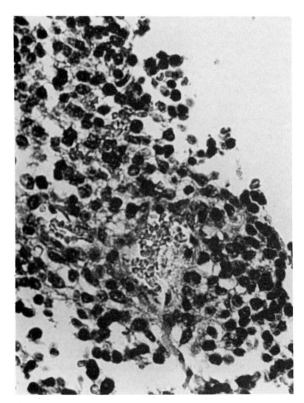

FIGURE 20–28. Embryonal rhabdomyosarcoma, epithelioid type. Mononucleated and binucleated, uniform round cells in loosely attached clusters. Note the granular and clear round cytoplasms (soft tissue aspirate; hematoxylin and eosin; ×450).

toma, primitive neuroectodermal tumor, hemangiopericytoma, granulocytic sarcoma, malignant lymphoma and Ewing's sarcoma.

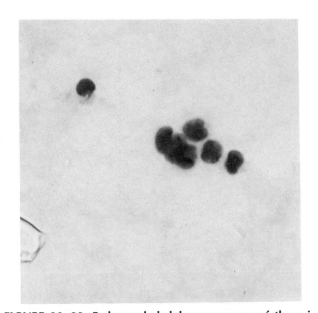

FIGURE 20–29. Embryonal rhabdomyosarcoma of the urinary bladder. Naked appearing mononucleated and binucleated forms in a cluster (urine sediment; Papanicolaou; ×450).

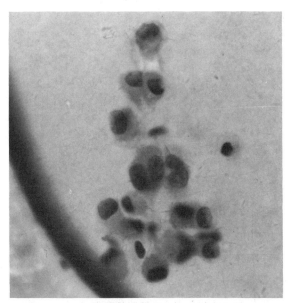

FIGURE 20–30. Metastatic alveolar rhabdomyosarcoma. Mononucleated and binucleated cells with finely granular cytoplasm in a pseudoalveolar unit (pleural effusion; Papanicolaou; ×450).

Pleomorphic rhabdomyosarcoma is a rare soft tissue sarcoma of adults. It affects most commonly adults over 50 years of age, and proximal parts of the extremities are the most common sites. The shape of cells ranges from round and oval embryonal rhabdomyoblasts to polygonal multinucleated giant cells to slender strap cells with well-defined, whip-like cytoplasmic processes. Because of the only occasional assembly of intracytoplasmic filaments, in a few rare cells, into the characteristic cross-striation, specific light-microscopic and ultrastructural diagnoses can be difficult and time consuming (Fig. 20–31).[12, 18] Immunohistochemical demonstration of muscle common antigen, myosin and desmin are helpful but only positive reaction for myoglobin can be regarded as specific for rhabdomyosarcoma (Fig. 20–32).

TUMORS OF VESSELS

Hemangiomas can be found at any age and at any site but roughly 25% are discovered in children under 10 years of age and about 5% are multifocal. The trunk, extremities and head and neck regions are the most common sites. Microscopically, capillary hemangioma is composed of capillary vessels lined by a single layer of flattened, nonproliferating, endothelial cells surrounded by a discontinuous layer of pericytes and reticulum fibers.[12, 14] Cavernous and venous hemangiomas are composed of dilated, distended and interconnected blood vessels. Vascular spaces are lined by thin fibrillar or sclerosed walls. Hypertrophic hemangioma occurs almost exclusively in children and infants. It is characterized by proliferation of capillary blood vessels in lobular or acinar arrangement, endothelial

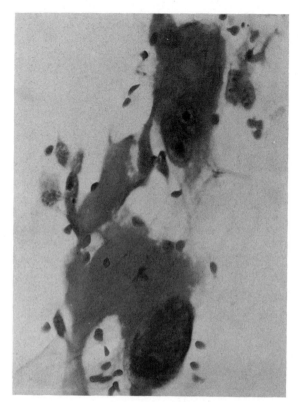

FIGURE 20–31. Pleomorphic rhabdomyosarcoma. Pleomorphic tumor giant cells with broad cell processes. Note the giant nucleoli (soft tissue aspirate; hematoxylin and eosin; ×450).

common forms, but parenchymal organs such as the spleen, liver and breast can on rare occasions be the primary sites.[12] In bone, hemangiosarcoma can be unifocal or occasionally multifocal but is an exceedingly rare neoplasm.[14] Although, microscopically, several forms ranging from angiomatous and cribriform to solid spindle cell and epithelioid type are distinguished, a deliberate attempt should be made to differentiate the histologically low-grade sarcomas from the high-grade ones.

Because of the variable histologic patterns and cell morphology one can find in hemangiosarcomas, ultrastructural and immunohistochemical studies are a must for definitive diagnosis. Ultrastructural demonstration of Weibel-Palade bodies in a malignant neoplasm is a sine qua non of endothelial origin.[12] Immunohistochemical demonstration of a positive reaction for factor VIII–related antigen and positive cytoplasmic staining with *Ulex europaeus* agglutinin (UEA) can occasionally be helpful.[18] In a cytology smear some of the most bizarre neoplastic endothelial cells can be recognized as malignant cells, but further classification as to type or histologic grade of the tumor would be too much to expect (Fig. 20–33). Tumors that cause the most problems in differential diagnosis are hypertrophic hemangioma, pleomorphic fibrous histiocytoma, biphasic tendosynovial sarcoma and Kaposi's sarcoma (Fig. 20–34).

Lymphangiosarcoma is often associated with lymphedema that can be congenital or acquired, e.g., caused

hyperplasia and atypia. Cytologic examination plays a limited role in the diagnosis of hemangiomas because any attempt to biopsy or aspirate lesions that are suspected to be of vascular nature should be discouraged.

Hemangiopericytoma is a rare malignant neoplasm of soft tissues and may occur at any age but is most common during the fourth and fifth decades. It may arise in almost any part of the body, but the most common sites are the lower extremities. Microscopically, hemangiopericytoma is composed of flat, endothelial cell–lined, fine capillary vessels. These ubiquitous round or distended vascular units are surrounded by uniform, round epithelioid pericytes in fibrillar and loosely arranged stroma.[18, 34] Ultrastructurally, neoplastic hemangiopericytes possess basement membranes, occasional pinocytic vesicles and fine cytoplasmic filaments. Because of a lack of specific or suggestive microscopic features of neoplastic pericytes, the diagnosis of hemangiopericytoma cannot be rendered with any certainty in an aspiration smear or in a limited tissue biopsy. The diagnosis is made by exclusion of other tumors, e.g., paraganglioma, monophasic tendosynovial sarcoma and lipoblastic liposarcoma.

Hemangiosarcoma is usually a solitary, firm neoplasm with a brownish-red cut section. Hemangiosarcoma shows no particular site preference but roughly a third are diagnosed in the head and neck areas. Cutaneous, superficial primaries are one of the most

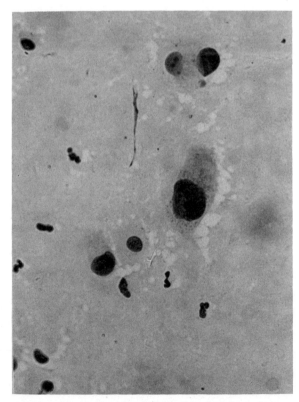

FIGURE 20–32. Metastatic pleomorphic rhabdomyosarcoma. Nonspecific pleomorphic tumor cells (pleural effusion; Papanicolaou; ×450).

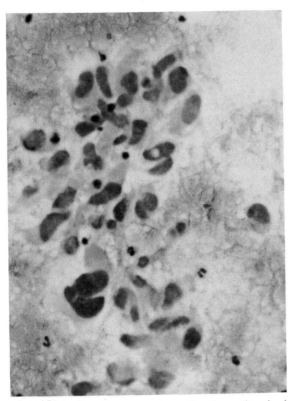

FIGURE 20–33. Hemangiosarcoma. Poorly outlined pleomorphic cells in loose clusters show considerable variation in shape and size of nuclei (bone aspirate; hematoxylin and eosin; ×450).

by surgery for groin hernia, filarial infection and axillary node dissection and irradiation for mammary carcinoma.[12] Microscopically, the neoplastic cells in lymphangiosarcoma are the endothelial-lining cells of lymphatic vessels. No specific distinction is seen between the cellular composition of lymphangiosarcoma and hemangiosarcoma. It is doubtful whether lymphangiosarcoma can ever be specifically diagnosed from cytologic samples. However, undoubtedly, the possibility can be entertained in the right clinical setting. In the differential diagnosis one should consider those tumors that are listed in the differential diagnosis of hemangiosarcoma.[18]

Kaposi's sarcoma appears most commonly on the skin as solitary or multiple reddish-brown or bluish-red slightly elevated nodules of a few millimeters in size and may spread all over the body, including into the regional lymph nodes, visceral and parenchymal organs and bone marrow. In patients without acquired immune deficiency syndrome (AIDS), the process usually begins in the lower extremities.[12, 14] Kaposi's sarcoma develops in about a third of the patients with AIDS and can appear anywhere in the body except in the brain. The exact cell of origin of Kaposi's sarcoma is still debated, but immunohistochemical, factor VIII and UEA reactivity and ultrastructural studies suggest an endothelial origin. The tumor cells are short or elongated with fibrillar cytoplasmic processes, pyknotic oval or spindle-shaped nuclei (Fig. 20–35).[18, 23] Tumor

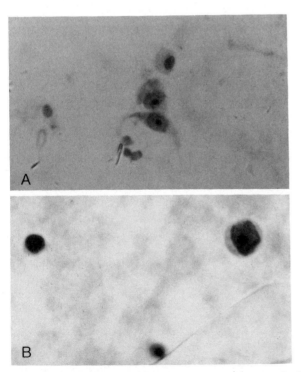

FIGURE 20–34. Metastatic angiosarcoma. *A,* Giant nucleoli, round nuclei and ill-defined granular cytoplasm (sputum; Papanicolaou; ×450). *B,* Note the giant nucleolus in an odd-shaped nucleus (pleural effusion; Papanicolaou; ×450).

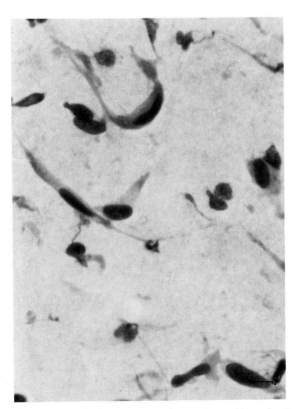

FIGURE 20–35. Recurrent Kaposi's sarcoma. Note the isolated cells with long cell processes and mostly solitary cigar-shaped nuclei (soft tissue aspirate; hematoxylin and eosin; ×450).

cells assembled in clusters, cords or tubules in a loosely arranged hemorrhagic background give the appearance of abortive capillary vessels. In the confluent stage of the disease cavernous and distended hemorrhagic spaces dominate. In the advanced solid forms, the tumor cells are long with attenuated cell processes and cigar-shaped nuclei, tightly packed in spreading pattern and only focally hemorrhagic, resembling poorly differentiated leiomyosarcoma. The diagnosis in cytologic smear and in limited, needle biopsy must be made with caution with full understanding that in patients who tested positive for human immunodeficiency virus (HIV), microscopic diagnosis of Kaposi's sarcoma is an unequivocal confirmation of AIDS.[18] In the differential diagnosis other vascular and hemorrhagic lesions, e.g., fasciitis, granulomatous lesions, hemangioma, bacillary angiomatosis, hemangiosarcoma and smooth muscle tumors, should be considered.

CARTILAGE-PRODUCING TUMORS

Chondroblastoma, in most cases, is found in the region of the knee in the epiphyseal cartilage of long bones. Microscopically, it is composed of zonal deposits of poorly differentiated chondroblasts and chondrocytes, which may be partially calcified, and epulis-type multinucleated giant cells.[14] The chondroid elements possess a single round or oval nucleus that may be slightly indented and may contain a nuclear groove. The cytoplasm is well-defined and may contain granular calcified material giving a peppery appearance. Because of focal cystic areas, histiocytic fibrous histiocytoma should be considered in the differential diagnosis. Chondroma, chondrosarcoma and osteosarcoma must also be considered in the differential diagnosis.

Chondroma in soft tissues or so-called enchondroma in bone is usually a solitary well-defined lesion. In soft tissues the tendinous synovial tissues of the knee area and the hands are affected most commonly. Over a third of the intraskeletal chondromas occur in the small tubular bones of the hand.[14] The chondrocytes of chondroma are poorly outlined cells with indistinct cell borders, abundant clear or vacuolated cytoplasm and small round pyknotic nuclei.[17] Binucleated forms and mitotic figures are extremely rare with sclerosed matrix. Chondrocytes can be part of almost innumerable tumors, e.g., chondroid metaplasia, pleomorphic adenoma, pulmonary hamartoma, osteochondroma, callus, chondrosarcoma and osteosarcoma.

Osteochondroma is the most common benign neoplasm. It is a radiologically distinct tumor of children and is diagnosed in most cases during the second decade. The distal end of the femur and proximal end of the tibia and humerus are the most common sites. Microscopically, it is composed of well-differentiated chondrocytes similar to those of chondroma, but a distinct, trabecular, endochondral ossification makes it different. The chondrocytes are either in cohesive nests or in rows in a usually hyalinized matrix.[18] In the differential diagnosis, all tumors that contain cartilage, e.g., callus, chondroid metaplasia, myositis ossificans,

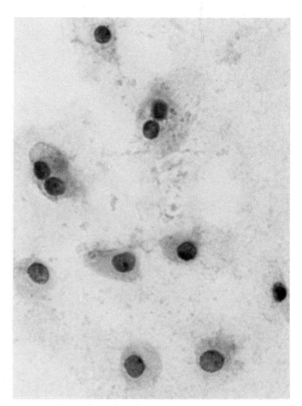

FIGURE 20–36. Chondrosarcoma. Mononucleated and binucleated chondrocytes of well-differentiated chondrosarcoma with abundant finely granular cytoplasm (soft tissue aspirate; hematoxylin and eosin; × 450).

tendosynovial chondromatosis, chondrosarcoma and osteosarcoma, must be considered.

Chondrosarcoma can be primary in soft tissue or bones. Nearly three quarters of the intraskeletal chondrosarcomas are found in the trunk and proximal end of the femur and humerus. Those in soft tissues are, in most cases, in deep parts of the extremities. Extraskeletal and intraskeletal chondrosarcomas are found most commonly during the fifth to seventh decades of life.[14] Microscopically, four major and distinct forms are recognized: well-differentiated, myxoid, chondroblastic and pleomorphic.[18, 37] Well-differentiated chondrosarcoma is composed largely of poorly defined chondrocytes with vesicular or clear cytoplasm and prominent or plump oval or round nuclei and, invariably, a few small round epithelioid cells and chondroblasts in an abundant myxoid matrix (Fig. 20–36). Myxoid chondrosarcoma is composed of delicate chondroid elements with fragile and indistinct cell borders in short cords or small coalescent lobules. The nuclei are round, oval or slightly elongated or crescent-shaped, and the matrix is richly myxoid. Chondroblastic chondrosarcoma is composed almost exclusively of round or oval granular cytoplasmic chondroblasts. Sheets and nests of chondroblasts are held together by the finely reticular and myxoid matrix. Some neoplastic cells are distended with abundant clear cytoplasm. In pleomorphic or so-called dedifferentiated chondrosarcoma, the dominant elements may show no resem-

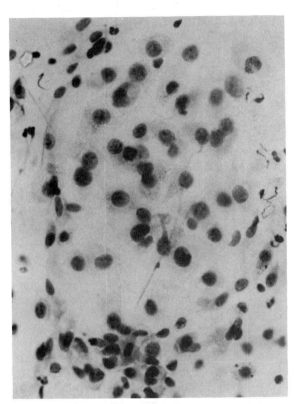

FIGURE 20–37. Chondrosarcoma metastatic to lung. Poorly differentiated chondroblastic forms in a loose cluster and in a myxoid background (bronchial brushing; Papanicolaou; ×450).

blance to chondrocytes and chondroblasts.[2, 18] Pleomorphic fibrous histiocytic forms and spindle cells resembling neoplastic fibroblasts are usually admixed with vaguely outlined pleomorphic neoplastic chondrocytes and chondroblasts. In all forms of chondrosarcoma microscopic evidence of binucleation, focal calcification and cystic degeneration can be detected. No specific immunohistochemical markers, beyond the S-100 protein reaction, exist.[7, 35] The most common neoplasms that should be considered in the differential diagnosis are chondroblastoma, chondroma, liposarcoma, osteosarcoma and chordoma (Fig. 20–37).

OSTEOID-PRODUCING TUMORS

Callus is a benign, reparative lesion of bone at the site of a fracture. Microscopically, callus may mimic, at different stages of growth, several forms of benign and malignant neoplasms. Up to about 2 weeks the dominant elements are atypical mononucleated and multinucleated histiocytes and disarranged slender reticular fibroblasts in myxoid and necrotic stroma. As the ossification advances, about 6 weeks after the fracture, calcium deposition in the osteoid begins and lamellar bone appears; osteoblasts transform to polygonal osteocytes and the chondroblasts to chondrocytes. Bizarre forms and mitotic figures are constant findings and the callus process may extend through the periosteum into surrounding soft tissues, including muscle.

It is difficult to visualize a callus that would permit precise microscopic diagnosis in material obtained by a needle. Osteoid metaplasia, myositis ossificans, osteoblastoma, chondroblastoma and osteosarcoma should be included in the differential diagnosis.

Osteoblastoma is a rare benign neoplasm of bone. It is found most commonly during the second and third decades and has a predilection for the vertebral column.[14] It is composed, almost exclusively, of osteoblasts lined by interlacing and disrupted, partly calcified, bone trabeculae and islands of osteoid. The osteoblasts are uniform, round cells with granular cytoplasm. The intertrabecular matrix is an essential component and is composed of small epulis-type giant cells, slender spindle cells in a vascular and myxoid background. In the differential diagnosis aneurysmal bone cyst, histiocytic fibrous histiocytoma and osteosarcoma should be considered.[18]

Osteosarcoma, excluding plasma cell myeloma, is the most common primary malignant bone tumor. An estimated 30% of malignant bone tumors are osteosarcoma.[14, 18] In soft tissue it is extremely rare—less than 1% of soft tissue sarcomas are classified as osteosarcoma. Intraskeletal osteosarcoma occurs most commonly during the second decade and in soft tissue during the sixth decade. The metaphyseal ends of long bones in this order—distal femur, proximal tibia, proximal humerus and proximal femur—are the most common sites. Microscopically, a wide variety of growth patterns, cells and matrix materials characterize osteosarcoma.

The single most important diagnostic criterion is the identification of malignant cells producing osteoid bone.[17] Because of a variety of dominant cellular elements, several microscopic forms are distinguished.[2, 20, 30] Osteoblastic osteosarcoma is composed of round epithelioid osteoblasts with prominent granular cytoplasm and round nuclei, containing granular chromatin and nucleoli. Chondroblastic osteosarcoma is dominated by islands of poorly differentiated neoplastic cartilage that merges with areas composed of sheets of neoplastic fibroblasts. Osteosarcoma growing as malignant fibrous histiocytoma contains a wide spectrum of malignant fibrous histiocytic forms, from mononucleated epithelioid and spindle cells to mononucleated and multinucleated tumor giant cells (Fig. 20–38). Osteoid production is often focal and limited to small irregular areas. Fibroblastic osteosarcoma produces a combination of broad sheets and fascicles of poorly differentiated collagenous fibrosarcoma mainly composed of plump spindle cells and malignant osteoblasts. Telangiectatic osteosarcoma is a hemorrhagic neoplasm, and the loose mesh of the vascular matrix is partitioned by malignant osteoblasts lined with irregular and interlinked trabeculae of osteoid. Sclerosing osteosarcoma is composed of anastomosing trabeculae of partly calcified osteoid and minimal or no appreciable intertrabecular matrix. Malignant osteoblasts are identifiable only by a diligent search around the rim and in the lacunae of lamellar bony trabeculae. Osteosarcoma, purely on microscopic grounds, must be distinguished from all those tumors that contain or

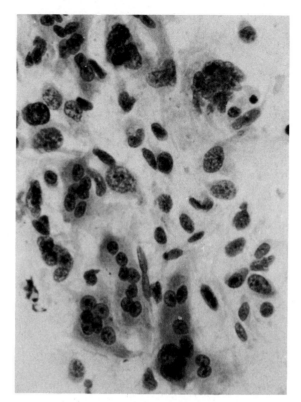

FIGURE 20–38. Osteosarcoma. Mononucleated and multinucleated pleomorphic cells are admixed with epulis-type giant cells (Bone aspirate; hematoxylin and eosin; ×450).

may contain osteoid bone, e.g., callus, myositis ossificans, aneurysmal bone cyst, fibrous histiocytoma, fibrosarcoma, osteoblastoma, chondrosarcoma and metaplastic ossification (Fig. 20–39).[14, 18]

TUMORS OF PERIPHERAL NERVE

Benign peripheral nerve tumors, so-called schwannomas, are almost always solitary lesions, and this is a disease of young adults and may appear anywhere in the body. Neurofibromas can be solitary or multiple. Any part of the body can be affected, and neurofibromas may appear at any age. Neurofibromatosis is a slowly progressive hereditary disease and appears in the form of multiple tumor nodules throughout the body; it may be found in association with cutaneous café-au-lait spots.[14] Microscopically, the composition of benign peripheral nerve tumors varies according to their size, location and duration. The most common single cell that is ubiquitous in every form of benign peripheral nerve tumors is a slender spindle cell with long hair-like cytoplasmic processes and a solitary oval or elongated pyknotic nucleus. The cytoplasmic processes of several cells may form bundles and can be tangled. The nuclei often form a parallel row or palisade.

Occasionally, one may find orderly palisading, Antoni A, areas merging with, Antoni B, areas composed of finely granular small epithelioid cells in a myxoid

background.[18, 39] Undoubtedly, because of the monomorphic nature of benign peripheral nerve tumors, limited biopsy sample and even aspirate may be sufficient for a tentative diagnosis (Fig. 20–40). However, because of the potential overlapping in microscopy with other tumors, the following tumors must be included in the differential diagnosis: fasciitis, fibromatosis, fibroblastic fibrous histiocytoma, leiomyoma, fibroblastic liposarcoma, monophasic tendosynovial sarcoma, melanoma, parosteal osteosarcoma and malignant peripheral nerve tumors.

Malignant peripheral nerve tumor is usually a solitary neoplasm. The primary site can be anywhere in the body, but the deep soft tissues of the proximal parts of the extremities, pelvis and retroperitoneum are the most commonly affected sites. This tumor is seen most commonly during the third and fourth decades. Most of the malignant peripheral nerve tumors can be traced upon dissection to a major nerve, usually branches of the sciatic or brachial nerves.[14] Microscopically, they are composed of a wide spectrum of cellular elements but malignant fibrous histiocytic cells are the most dominant.[18, 26] So-called low-grade malignant schwannomas are predominantly composed of slender fibroblasts in a storiform and spreading pattern. Necrosis is minimal and the overall appearance has a resemblance to malignant fibroblastic fibrous histiocytoma.

High-grade malignant schwannomas are predominantly composed of malignant pleomorphic fibrous histiocytic elements, ranging from spindle cells to multinucleated tumor giant cells. The mitotic count is

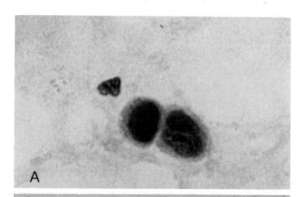

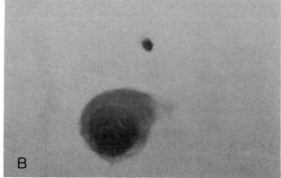

FIGURE 20–39. Metastatic osteosarcoma. A, Large, nonspecific, neoplastic cells with granular cytoplasm (pleural effusion; Papanicolaou; ×450). B, A solitary granular cytoplasmic tumor giant cell (bronchial brushing; Papanicolaou; ×450).

usually high (more than five mitoses per ten high-power microscopic fields), and substantial tumor necrosis is seen. Microscopically, neurofibrosarcomas can also be divided into low-grade and high-grade forms.[14, 18] The low-grade neurofibrosarcoma is composed of slender and plump collagenous fibroblasts and fibrocytes that are assembled in a spreading pattern in abundant fibrillar or sclerosed matrix (Fig. 20–41). High-grade neurofibrosarcoma is very similar to high-grade fibrosarcoma except for the neurofibromatous areas. Some of the various forms of malignant peripheral nerve tumors retain focally some of the ultrastructural features that characterize benign peripheral nerve tumors, and they may also show a positive reaction with S-100 protein and may be complicated by contractures and other deformities.[12, 14] Rarely, malignant peripheral nerve tumors may contain areas of embryonal rhabdomyosarcoma. Such highly malignant neoplasms are singled out by the distinct name, Triton tumor. An equally rare and a highly malignant neoplasm, the so-called epithelioid peripheral nerve tumor, is predominantly composed of poorly differentiated small and uniform cells with ill-defined cytoplasmic borders and round or oval nuclei. Because of the complex, heterogenous composition of malignant peripheral nerve tumors, in the differential diagnosis many tumors should be considered, e.g., desmoid tumor, fibrosarcoma, leiomyosarcoma, monophasic tendosynovial sarcoma and benign or atypical peripheral nerve tumors.

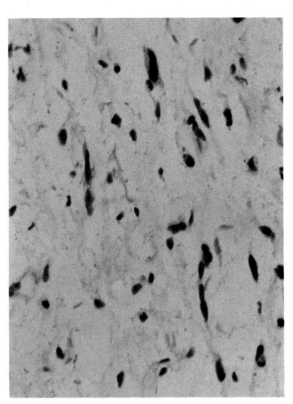

FIGURE 20–41. Malignant peripheral nerve tumor, low-grade neurofibrosarcoma. Widely separated cells with long and branching hair-like cytoplasmic processes exhibit long pyknotic nuclei (soft tissue aspirate; hematoxylin and eosin; ×450).

MISCELLANEOUS TUMORS

Osteomyelitis seldom appears without the signs and symptoms of an acute feverish illness. It affects the ends of long bones in children and the diaphysis, midportion, in adults. Microscopically, in the acute phase the diagnosis can be made without difficulty, even in limited material, such as aspirates, because of a pure culture of polymorphonuclear granulocytes and a few lymphocytes admixed with marrow elements. Chronic or longstanding osteomyelitis can be difficult to diagnose microscopically, particularly in smears, because of the variation and combination of cells that may include plasma cells, lymphocytes, fibroblasts, histiocytes, various amounts of necrotic debris and bone fragments, so-called sequestra. Malignant lymphoma, Ewing's sarcoma and, in the presence of eosinophils, eosinophilic granuloma should be considered in the differential diagnosis.[18]

Eosinophilic granuloma is a reactive, proliferative process that may involve any bone, but the skull, mandible, ribs, vertebrae, femur and humerus are the most common sites. Microscopically, it is a hemorrhagic lesion containing a large number of eosinophils, mononucleated histiocytes, occasional foam cells and pigmented multinucleated forms. Variable numbers of proteinaceous crystalline structures, the so-called Charcot-Leyden crystals, are a by-product of the de-

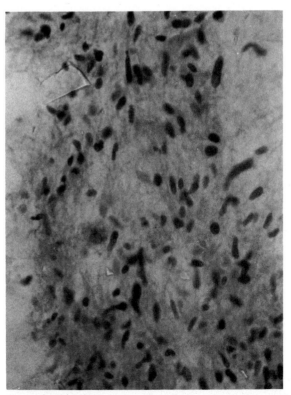

FIGURE 20–40. Benign peripheral nerve tumor, so-called cellular schwannoma. Tangled wire-like cell processes holding the naked-appearing nuclei together (soft tissue aspirate; hematoxylin and eosin; ×450).

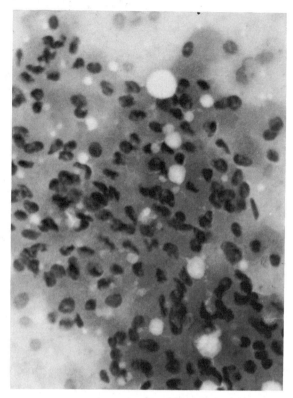

FIGURE 20–42. Benign granular cell tumor. Uniform mostly round cells with large granular cytoplasm in a cohesive cluster (soft tissue aspirate; hematoxylin and eosin; ×450).

struction of eosinophils. With the electron microscope, cytoplasmic inclusions, the Langerhans or Birbeck granules, are demonstrable in some of the cells and regarded as pathognomonic. Tumors such as ossifying fibroma, fibrous histiocytoma and malignant lymphoma should be considered in the differential diagnosis.

Benign granular cell tumors may occur anywhere in the body, but nearly 50% are found in the submucosal and subcutaneous tissues of the head and neck and have a special affinity to the tongue. It is predominantly a disease during the fourth and fifth decades. Microscopically, the predominant elements are ill-defined globoid cells with large granular cytoplasm. The cytoplasmic granules stain positive with periodic acid–Schiff (PAS) before and after distase digestion. The nuclei are uniform in size and shape and excentrically located in the cytoplasm (Fig. 20–42).[9, 11, 43] Any lesion that shows considerable cellular pleomorphism, multinucleation, and contains neoplastic spindle cells and giant cells should be regarded as a malignant granular cell tumor. In the differential diagnosis, storage disease, rhabdomyoma, rhabdomyoblastoma, hibernoma and alveolar soft part sarcoma should be considered.

Ewing's sarcoma may affect any bone but long bones of the lower extremity, vertebrae and ribs are the most common sites. Ewing's sarcoma has a male predilection and is most commonly diagnosed during the second decade.[14] Microscopically, Ewing's sarcoma is composed of solidly packed small round cells with well-defined minute granular cytoplasm. Little or no variation is found in shape and size of the tumor cells, but

a few mononucleated larger forms can occasionally be found. The tumor cells are in large clusters or in sheets partitioned by slim reticular fibers (Fig. 20–43). The presence of intracytoplasmic glycogen, in many cells, is demonstrable with the PAS reaction and with electron microscopy.[4, 18, 21] The cytologic diagnosis is possible with some reservation and exclusion of other small-cell neoplasms, e.g., malignant lymphoma, leukemia, primitive neuroectodermal tumor, eosinophilic granuloma, plasmacytoma, neuroblastoma, embryonal rhabdomyosarcoma and metastatic small-cell carcinomas (Fig. 20–44).

Alveolar soft part sarcoma is a slowly progressive malignant neoplasm. Most alveolar soft part sarcomas are found in the extremities, but chest wall and abdominal wall primaries are not uncommon.[12, 14] Microscopically, the most prominent feature is the repetitious alveolar arrangement of large polygonal cells with distinct cell borders. The cytoplasm is abundant, granular and may contain small vacuoles. The excentrically placed vesicular nuclei usually assume a centripetal position in the alveoli and contain distinct nucleoli. Binucleated or multinucleated forms are rare, and mitoses are uncommon. The cytoplasmic granules of neoplastic cells stain positive with PAS and are undigestible with distase.[18, 27] Some of the cells may also contain protein-carbohydrate crystals that are light microscopically and ultrastructurally demonstrable. Alveolar rhabdomyosarcoma, epithelioid mesothelioma,

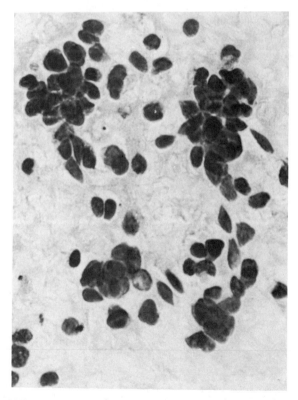

FIGURE 20–43. Ewing's sarcoma. Granular cytoplasmic round cells with round, oval and spindle-shaped nuclei, singly and in clusters (bone aspirate; hematoxylin and eosin; ×450).

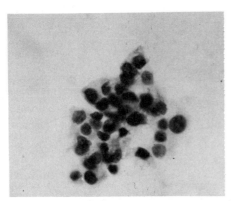

FIGURE 20–44. Metastatic Ewing's sarcoma. A cluster of neoplastic cells with dark round and oval nuclei resembling small cell carcinoma (sputum; Papanicolaou; ×350).

oncocytoma and skin adnexal apocrine tumors should be considered in the differential diagnosis.

Chordoma is an uncommon malignant neoplasm of the proximal and distal axial skeleton. Sacrococcygeal chordoma is predominantly found during the fifth and sixth decades. The spheno-occipital form is less common and can be found in patients of any age, including children and young adults.[14] Microscopically, the main cellular forms are the so-called physaliphorous cells. These are ill-defined vacuolated cells of variable sizes with distended mucus droplets containing cytoplasm. The size of the nuclei may vary but giant forms are rare (Fig. 20–45). Chondroblasts and chondrocytes in nest and zonal arrangements are most common in the spheno-occipital forms. The tumor cells show consis-

tently positive reaction with cytokeratins, vimentin and S-100 protein.[18, 36] Neoplasms that should be considered in the differential diagnosis are chondrosarcoma, myxopapillary ependymoma, pleomorphic adenoma and adenocarcinoma.

References

1. Ahmed MN, Feldman M, Seemayer TA: Cytology of epithelioid sarcoma. Acta Cytol 18:459–461, 1974.
2. Akerman M, Berg NO, Persson BM: Fine needle aspiration biopsy in the evaluation of tumor-like lesions of bone. Acta Orthop Scand 47:129–136, 1976.
3. Akerman M, Rydholm A, Persson B: Aspiration cytology of soft tissue tumors. Acta Orthop Scand 56:407–412, 1985.
4. Akhtar M, Ali MA, Sabbah R: Aspiration cytology of Ewing's sarcoma. Light and electron microscopic correlations. Cancer 56:2051–2060, 1985.
5. Bondeson L, Andreasson L: Aspiration cytology of adult rhabdomyoma. Acta Cytol 30:679–682, 1986.
6. Boram LH, Erlandson RA, Hajdu SI: Mesodermal mixed tumors of the uterus. Cancer 30:1295–1306, 1982.
7. Chess Q, Hajdu SI: The role of immunoperoxidase staining in diagnostic cytology. Acta Cytol 30:1–7, 1986.
8. Dahl I, Akerman M: Nodular fasciitis. A correlative cytologic and histologic study of 13 cases. Acta Cytol 25:215–222, 1981.
9. Franzen S, Stenkvist B: Diagnosis of granular cell myoblastoma by fine needle aspiration biopsy. Acta Pathol Microbiol Scand 72:391–395, 1968.
10. Geisinger KR, Naylor B, Beals TF, Novak PM: Cytopathology including transmission and scanning electron microscopy of pleomorphic liposarcoma in pleural fluids. Acta Cytol 24:435–441, 1980.
11. Glant MD, Wall RW, Ransburg R: Endobronchial granular cell tumor. Cytology of a new case and review of the literature. Acta Cytol 23:477–482, 1979.
12. Hajdu SI: Pathology of Soft Tissue Tumors. Philadelphia, Lea & Febiger, 1979.
13. Hajdu SI: The paradox of sarcomas. Acta Cytol 24:373–383, 1980.
14. Hajdu SI: Differential Diagnosis of Soft Tissue and Bone Tumors. Philadelphia, Lea & Febiger, 1986.
15. Hajdu SI, Bean MA, Fogh J, Hajdu EO, Ricci A: Papanicolaou smear of cultured human tumor cells. Acta Cytol 18:327–332, 1974.
16. Hajdu SI, Ehya H, Frable WJ, Geisinger KR, Gompel CM, Kern WH, Lowhagen T, Oertel Y, Ramzy I, Rilke F, Saigo PE, Suprun HZ, Yazdi HM: The value and limitations of aspiration cytology in the diagnosis of primary tumors. Acta Cytol 33:741–790, 1989.
17. Hajdu SI, Hajdu EO: Cytopathology of Sarcomas and Other Nonepithelial Malignant Tumors. Philadelphia, WB Saunders, 1976.
18. Hajdu SI, Hajdu EO: Cytopathology of Soft Tissue and Bone Tumors. Basel, S Karger, 1989.
19. Hajdu SI, Koss LG: Cytologic diagnosis of metastatic myosarcomas. Acta Cytol 13:545–551, 1969.
20. Hajdu SI, Melamed MR: Needle biopsy of primary malignant bone tumors. Surg Gynecol Obstet 133:829–832, 1971.
21. Hajdu SI, Melamed MR: The diagnostic value of aspiration smears. Am J Clin Pathol 59:350–356, 1973.
22. Hajdu SI, Melamed MR: Limitations of aspiration cytology in the diagnosis of primary neoplasms. Acta Cytol 28:337–345, 1984.
23. Hales M, Bottles K, Miller T, Donegan E, Ljung BM: Diagnosis of Kaposi's sarcoma by fine-needle aspiration. Cancer 88:20–25, 1987.
24. Hashimoto CH, Cobb CJ: Cytodiagnosis of hibernoma. A case report. Diagn Cytopathol 3:326–329, 1987.
25. Helson L, Krochmal P, Hajdu SI: Diagnostic value of cytologic specimens obtained from children with cancer. Ann Clin Lab Sci 5:294–297, 1975.

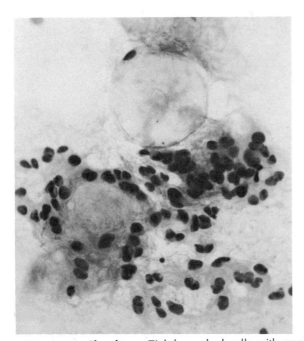

FIGURE 20–45. Chordoma. Tightly packed cells with small granular or distended clear cytoplasm in fibromyxoid background (bone aspirate; hematoxylin and eosin; ×350).

26. Hood IC, Qizilbash AH, Young JEM, Archibald SD: Fine needle cytology of a benign and a malignant schwannoma. Acta Cytol 28:157–164, 1984.

27. Kapila K, Chopra P, Verma K: Fine needle aspiration cytology of alveolar soft part sarcoma. A case report. Acta Cytol 29:559–561, 1985.

28. Katz RI, Silva EG, Santos LA de, Lukeman JM: Diagnosis of eosinophilic granuloma of bone biopsy by cytology, histology and electron microscopy of transcutaneous bone aspiration biopsy. J Bone Joint Surg 62:1284–1290, 1980.

29. Kim K, Naylor B, Han IH: Fine needle aspiration cytology of sarcomas metastastic to the lung. Acta Cytol 30:688–694, 1986.

30. Layfield LJ, Glasgow BJ, Du Puis MH, Bhuta S: Aspiration cytology of primary bone lesions. Acta Cytol 31:177–184, 1987.

31. Massoni EA, Hajdu SI: Cytology of primary and metastatic uterine sarcomas. Acta Cytol 28:93–100, 1984.

32. Naib ZM: Cytology of synovial fluid. Acta Cytol 17:299–309, 1973.

33. Nguyen GK, Jeannot A: Cytology of synovial sarcoma metastases in pleural fluid. Acta Cytol 26:517–520, 1982.

34. Nickels J, Koivuniema A: Cytology of malignant hemangiopericytoma. Acta Cytol 23:119–125, 1979.

35. Nordgren H, Akerman M: Electron microscopy of fine needle aspiration biopsy from soft tissue tumors. Acta Cytol 26:179–188, 1982.

36. O'Dowd G, Schumann GB: Aspiration cytology and cytochemistry of coccygeal chordoma. A case report and review of the literature. Acta Cytol 27:178–183, 1983.

37. Olszewski W, Woyke S, Musiatowicz B: Fine needle aspiration biopsy cytology of chondrosarcoma. Acta Cytol 27:345–349, 1983.

38. Perry MD, Furlong JW, Johnston WW: Fine needle aspiration cytology of metastatic dermatofibrosarcoma protuberans. A case report. Acta Cytol 30:507–513, 1986.

39. Ramzy I: Benign schwannoma demonstration of Verocay bodies using fine needle aspiration. Acta Cytol 21:316–319, 1978.

40. Sears D, Hajdu SI: The cytologic diagnosis of malignant neoplasms in pleural and peritoneal effusions. Acta Cytol 31:85–97, 1987.

41. Sneige N, Ayala AG, Carrasco CH, Murray J, Raymond AK: Giant cell tumor of bone. A cytologic study of 24 cases. Diagn Cytopathol 1:111–117, 1985.

42. Stormby N, Akerman M: Cytodiagnosis of bone lesions by means of fine-needle aspiration biopsy. Acta Cytol 17:166–172, 1983.

43. Sussman EB, Hajdu SI, Gray GF: Granular cell myoblastoma of the breast. Am J Surg 126:669–670, 1973.

44. Walaas L, Kindblom LG: Lipomatous tumors: a correlative cytologic and histologic study of 27 tumors examined by fine needle aspiration cytology. Human Pathol 16:6–18, 1985.

45. Yazdi HM, Hajdu SI, Melamed MR: Cytopathology of pericardial effusions. Acta Cytol 24:401–412, 1980.

21

Skin

Gordon Canti

It has been about 60 years since Dudgeon and coworkers[9, 10] described a wet film technique for the rapid diagnosis of various tumors. Some basal cell carcinomas were included in this series. The preparations were fixed while still wet in Schaudinn's fluid and stained with hematoxylin and eosin. Another "wet" fixation technique using methanol and 1% toluidine blue was described by Russell and associates[29] for the rapid intraoperative diagnosis of brain tumors. The so-called wet film technique was a milestone in cytologic diagnosis because it preserved morphologic detail for staining with conventional histologic stains. The method attracted little attention, however, until Papanicolaou introduced his alcohol-based polychromatic stains, which further enhanced the transparency and appearance of the preparations. Although these stains were originally designed for investigation of the cervix, the Papanicolaou technique has since spread into all fields of cytologic diagnosis.

The more specific application of cytology to the diagnosis of skin diseases was pioneered by Tzanck and Aron-Brunetiere[35, 36] in 1947 and 1949, who published articles on the differential diagnosis of bullous lesions employing air-dried film and Romanowsky staining. A steady flow of reports have been published since then,[12, 13, 15, 17, 18, 20, 28, 31, 34, 37, 39, 40, 45] using a variety of fixation and staining techniques. In spite of the enthusiasm of these individual investigators, dermatologic cytology is not widely practiced—surely because its practical advantages have not been fully communicated.

The majority of skin diseases are associated with nonspecific inflammatory and reactive changes and are therefore not amenable to cytologic diagnosis. Cytology is of no avail when the diagnosis is dependent on histologic pattern. A few diseases are characterized by specific changes at the cellular level and are therefore particularly suitable for sampling by scraping or, in the case of deeper lesions, by fine needle aspiration (FNA).

TECHNIQUE

The majority of lesions with specific cytomorphologic features are on the skin surface and therefore accessible to scraping. In order to ensure that adequate material is obtained and suitably prepared, it is essential that the pathologist personally takes the sample. Scalpel blades can be utilized, but they are not ideally shaped and might cause unnecessary damage or bleeding. Curettes have been recommended, but they are unsatisfactory for transferring small fragments of tissue onto a glass slide. The light model double-ended dissector has advantages over other instruments (Fig. 21–1). The small rounded end can be sharpened to provide a good scraping, but not cutting, edge, and the smooth convex surface facilitates the transfer of tissue onto the slide. Soft or small fragments can be spread with the instrument; larger and more solid fragments should be squashed between slides. The instrument can be quickly sterilized by light flaming. Alternatively, when surface scraping is not possible, samples can be obtained by FNA.

The sample must be fixed immediately in an alcohol fixative for Papanicolaou staining. In addition, if preferred, and especially when a lymphoma is suspected, a smear should be dried for Romanowsky staining or the Diff-quik technique may be applied for rapid diagnosis. It is also advantageous to examine a vitally stained wet preparation immediately, so that in the event of an inadequate sample, another can be taken while the patient is still available. The wet preparation is made by covering the smear with a drop of 1% methylene blue and applying a coverslip. Examination

DOWN. ENGLAND
JD 015-01-T

FIGURE 21–1. Swedish light-model, double-ended dissector.

under the microscope must be immediate, as cloudy swelling will occur within a few minutes.

Diagnosis can often be made based on the wet preparation and reported immediately, thus enabling the clinician to take appropriate action at the first consultation and saving the patient a second visit.[4, 5] The fixed preparation can be examined later for confirmation and filed for permanent record.

HISTOLOGY

The skin is composed of two layers—the epidermis and the dermis. The epidermis is composed of stratified squamous epithelium. For descriptive purposes it can be divided into five layers: the stratum germinativum, stratum spinosum, stratum granulosum, stratum lucidum and stratum corneum (Fig. 21–2). The stratum germinativum or germinal layer is composed of a single layer of small columnar cells attached to and orientated vertically to the basement membrane. They have basophilic cytoplasm and deeply staining elongated nuclei. Cells produced by mitotic division in the germinal epithelium move up into the next layer, forming the stratum spinosum or prickle cell layer. Here the cells are polyhedral and firmly attached to each other by short cytoplasmic spines, the intercellular bridges. The cytoplasm remains basophilic. As the cells progress towards the skin surface they become flattened, the nuclei become vesicular and the nucleocytoplasmic ratio decreases. Nearer the surface in the stratum granulosum the cells are even more flattened and contain keratohyalin granules, which are thought to be the precursors of keratin. These cells degenerate as they move upwards into the stratum lucidum—an ill-defined layer in which the cells lose their identity and the nuclei fade. The cytoplasm contains eosinophilic keratohyalin. In the outermost layer, the stratum corneum, the dead cells are replaced by keratinized scales, which stain pink with eosin or orange with Papanicolaou stain. Wedged between the cells of the germinal layer are small cells with clear cytoplasm—these are the melanocytes, which produce pigment granules. The latter migrate through the epidermis in keratinocytes or in melanophages. The amount of pigment in the skin varies according to site, race or sun exposure. The epidermis is avascular.

The dermis is a dense connective tissue composed of collagenous, reticular and elastic fibers arranged in an irregular network. It is thrown up into ridges that protrude into the epidermis and produce the fine lines on the skin surface. Below, it merges imperceptibly with the superficial fascia. The dermis contains fibroblasts, fibrocytes, histiocytes, fat cells and pigmented connective tissue cells, the chromatophores. Blood vessels, lymphatics and nerve cells course through the dermis, and it contains the hair follicles, sebaceous glands and sweat glands.

Hair Follicle

The outer sheath of the hair follicle is a downwards extension of the surface epidermis into the dermal and subdermal tissue. At the base of the follicle is the hair bulb constituting the undifferentiated hair matrix cells, which give rise to a variety of cells forming the hair and its sheath.

Sebaceous Gland

Sebaceous glands are saccular glands located in the dermis. Each lobule possesses a peripheral layer of small cuboidal cells that give rise by division to larger cells containing lipid granules. The lipid-laden cells fill the lobule and progress towards the secretory duct where they disintegrate, releasing the sebaceous material into the hair follicle.

Sweat Gland

The sweat glands are coiled tubular glands lying in the dermal and subdermal tissues. They are lined by a single layer of cuboidal cells, of which there are two types—serous and mucus secreting. The secretory duct, which is also lined by cuboidal epithelium, takes a spiral course through the epidermis to open directly onto the skin surface.

Cytologic preparations of normal skin, obtained by scraping, contain anucleate superficial squamous cells. A few nucleated cells and intermediate cells can be obtained if pressure is applied. Parabasal cells from the strata spinosum are obtained only in inflammatory and hyperplastic lesions.

Intercellular bridges cannot be seen in fixed smears, but they can be seen in wet preparations by closing the substage diaphragm. Cells from the germinal layer are so firmly adherent that they are seldom dislodged.

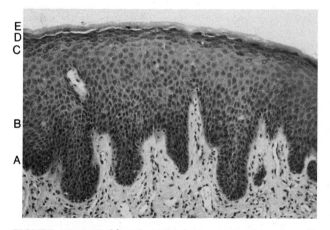

FIGURE 21–2. Epidermis. Histologic section showing (A) stratum germinativum, (B) stratum spinosum, (C) stratum granulosum, (D) stratum lucidum and (E) stratum corneum (hematoxylin and eosin; ×120).

CYTOLOGIC APPEARANCES OF SOME COMMON SKIN LESIONS

Basal Cell Carcinoma

In medical centers where a diagnostic cytologic service is available to the dermatologist, the commonest and most useful cytologic investigation is for the differential diagnosis of basal cell carcinoma (BCC, synonyms—basal cell epithelioma; rodent-ulcer) from keratoses and other skin lesions, which may imitate it.[4, 5, 38]

The majority of BCCs are of the nodular type and are either ulcerated or covered by such an attenuated epidermis that no difficulty is encountered in obtaining adequate material by scraping. Any clot, crust or necrotic material is first removed, exposing the soft translucent tumor (Fig. 21–3). A fragment of this material when crushed between slides breaks up so characteristically into small visible fragments that microscopic examination in many cases is almost superfluous (Fig. 21–4). Microscopy shows the fragments to consist of syncytial sheets of small closely packed cohesive cells that tend to spread in a monolayer (Fig. 21–5). The cells are evenly spaced and usually there is little polarity within the cell mass, but characteristic palisading occurs at the periphery of some of the clumps producing a smooth scalloped perimeter (Fig. 21–6). The appearance is very similar to that in the histologic section. The nuclei are round or oval and sometimes elongated. They are typically monomorphic and hyperchromatic with a fine granular chromatin pattern and one or two small chromocenters. Pleomorphism, nucleoli and occasional mitotic figures are seen in the more active tumors, especially when there is superimposed infection.

Frequent mitotic figures, coarse chromatin clumping and conspicuous nucleoli may arouse the suspicion of

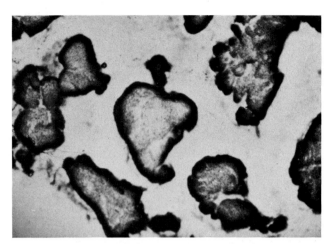

FIGURE 21–4. Basal cell carcinoma. Numerous small fragments with scalloped borders visible to the naked eye. The peripheral cells in each clump are more heavily stained (wet film methylene blue; ×12).

squamous cell carcinoma. Basal cell carcinoma, however, is distinguished by the absence of intercellular bridges (Fig. 21–7).[22] This feature can be verified only in a fresh wet preparation by closing the substage diaphragm and varying the focus. The presence of intercellular bridges in all the clusters precludes BCC (Fig. 21–8).

The methylene or toluidine blue preparation is also useful for demonstrating the metachromatic pink staining of the mucopolysaccharide, which is commonly present in the stroma. The numerous discrete single cells seen in some preparations are of little diagnostic value as they so closely resemble nevus cells, but typical cohesive sheets of cells will almost always be present. Fusiform and stellate cells sometimes predominate, especially in the more cystic tumors (Fig. 21–9). Another distinguishing feature of BCC is hyperchromasia,

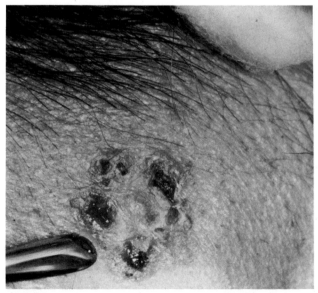

FIGURE 21–3. Scraping a **basal cell carcinoma.** Note the translucent material on the tip of the instrument.

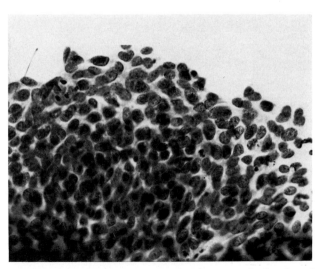

FIGURE 21–5. Basal cell carcinoma smear. Evenly distributed almost monomorphic nuclei with little cytoplasm between them; no visible cell border (Papanicolaou stain; ×560).

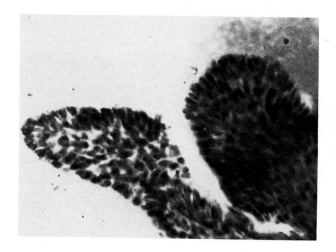

FIGURE 21–6. Basal cell carcinoma. Lobule of tumor showing hyperchromasia and palisading of peripheral cells (Papanicolaou stain; ×420).

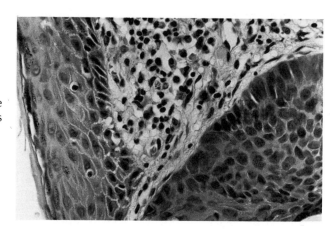

FIGURE 21–7. Histologic section of basal cell carcinoma. Note the absence of intercellular bridges compared with the basal cells of the overlying epidermis (hematoxylin and eosin; ×420).

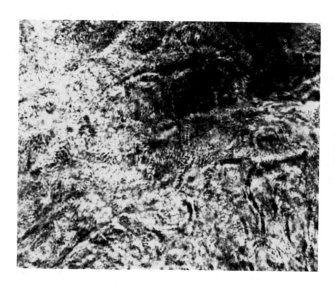

FIGURE 21–8. Prickle cells from a keratotic lesion. The intercellular bridges are best seen in an unstained area of the cell cluster with the substage diaphragm closed. Only a few of the bridges show in any one focal plain (wet film methylene blue; ×700).

FIGURE 21–9. Basal cell carcinoma. Spindle cells from cystic lesion (Papanicolaou stain; ×420).

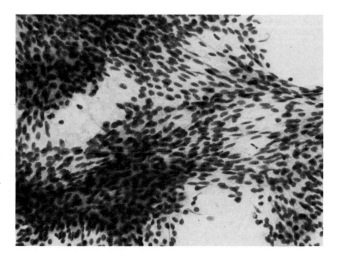

which is enhanced by the close packing of the cells and the basophilic cytoplasm. This feature is shown best in the Papanicolaou stained preparations and contrasts with the wider spacing, paler nuclei and eosinophilic cytoplasm of keratotic lesions.

Although not of great clinical significance, the histologic variants of BCC can occasionally be distinguished in cytologic preparations. The pigmented tumors contain intracellular and extracellular melanin granules, which are best displayed in the wet methylene blue preparations. In the keratotic (basisquamous, metatypical) variant, some squamous differentiation is seen with prickle cells, keratinization, whorling and, sometimes, horny cysts, but intercellular bridges will be absent in at least some of the cell clusters. Sebaceous cells may be incorporated in some cystic lesions, but typical undifferentiated basal cell clusters will also be present. The morphea-like or fibrosing BCC is distinguished by its hardness. Some difficulty may be encountered in obtaining an adequate sample by scraping. In these cases and those in which the overlying epidermis is intact, a small incision with the point of a scalpel blade exposes the tumor material; alternatively, fine needle aspiration may be preferred.[24]

Numerous cutaneous lesions may arouse a clinical suspicion of BCC. Those most commonly encountered are senile and solar keratoses, a solitary molluscum contagiosum vesicle, sebaceous gland hyperplasia or adenoma and keratoacanthoma and squamous cell carcinoma. The cytology of these lesions is described under separate headings. The lesion that causes the most difficulty is the basisquamous type of BCC, which can be confused with squamous cell carcinoma. The same problem sometimes confronts the histologist.

Squamous Cell Carcinoma

Squamous cell carcinoma (SCC) usually occurs as shallow indurated ulcers with a raised edge, or they may take the form of a raised fungating growth that bleeds easily. Abundant cellular material is usually obtained without difficulty owing to the loss of cell cohesion. Microscopic examination in the majority of cases demonstrates unequivocal malignant cells in the wet film or Papanicolaou stained smear (Fig. 21–10).

A few lesions may present a problem in the differential diagnosis, however. The basisquamous type of BCC has been referred to. The small-cell type of SCC in particular can resemble BCC (Fig. 21–11), but the presence of intercellular bridges is an important aid to the correct diagnosis. In addition, clusters of malignant squamous cells possess a ragged border with no evidence of palisading. Loss of polarity occurs, and the cells tend to overlie each other more than in BCC. The nuclei of malignant squamous cells are more vesicular with coarse chromatin clumping and conspicuous nucleoli. The nucleocytoplasmic ratio is lower than in the BCC, and the cytoplasm stains pink or orange with the Papanicolaou stain. Some difficulty may also be encountered with the very well-differentiated tumors that occur most frequently on the lips or

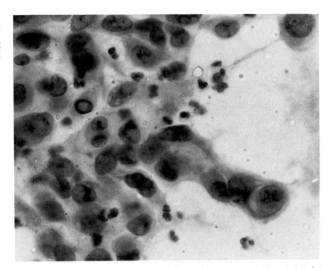

FIGURE 21–10. Squamous cell carcinoma. Rather poorly differentiated (Papanicolaou stain; × 560).

in the mouth. Often no cytomorphologic evidence of malignancy is seen apart from a slight dyskaryosis and pleomorphism in the superficial cells (Fig. 21–12). The healing edge of an inflammatory ulcer will contain very active squamous cells and even mitotic figures. It is therefore important to sample different areas. The base of an inflammatory ulcer is soft and will yield inflammatory cells and granulation tissue, whereas the base of a malignant ulcer is hard and will yield atypical squamous cells.

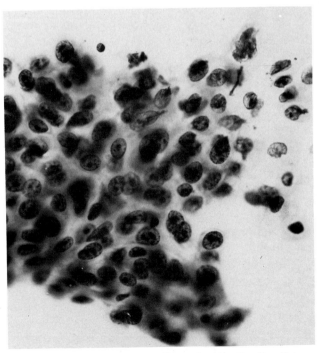

FIGURE 21–11. Squamous cell carcinoma. Small-cell type for comparison with basal cell carcinoma (see Fig. 21–5). Note nucleoli and irregular chromatin clumping. There is loss of polarity and a more three-dimensional configuration (Papanicolaou stain; × 560).

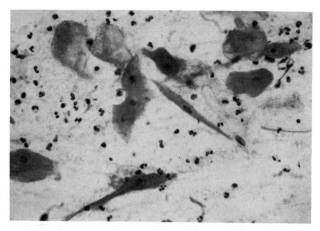

FIGURE 21–12. Squamous cell carcinoma. Scraping from the hard base of a very well differentiated malignant ulcer. Dyskariosis is slight; pleomorphism is more significant (Papanicolaou stain; ×350).

Senile and Solar Keratoses

Malignant transformation not infrequently occurs in areas of keratosis. This is seen most commonly in patients who have been exposed to sunlight over a long period. The lesions are often multiple, rendering numerous biopsies impractical. Cytologic investigation is most useful for investigating these patients for the earliest evidence of malignant transformation.

Superficial scraping is not very productive and yields highly keratinized superficial squamous cells and tight clusters of acanthotic cells, together with varying quantities of inflammatory cells. In the majority of cases no evidence of neoplasia exists, but deep scraping of the more active lesions may produce suspicious-looking cells. The failure to recognize malignancy at this stage does not have serious consequences for the patient, as carcinomas arising in keratotic lesions rarely metastasize.[23] Many of these lesions heal after a diagnostic scraping, but the persistent lesion may eventually require biopsy to exclude carcinoma.

Carcinoma *In Situ*

The microscopic appearance in smears is similar to that seen in cervical cancer *in situ* (Bowen's disease and erythroplasia of Queyrat). Depending on the degree of surface differentiation, the cells range from the atypical superficial to the small undifferentiated basal type (Fig. 21–13), which is so characteristic of the cervical lesion. These small basal cells individually resemble those of BCC, but because of the loss of cohesion, they do not remain in syncytial sheets, and they are accompanied by more obviously atypical squamous cells. Whereas in cervical smears the experienced cytologist can usually distinguish between *in situ* and invasive carcinoma, in the skin the difference is not so pronounced. Evidence of invasion is therefore more likely to depend on the clinical appearance or subsequent biopsy.

Seborrheic Keratosis (Basal Cell Papilloma)

These lesions are usually distinct clinically, but when flattened or ulcerated they may be mistaken for BCC or SCC. Scraping yields a few degenerate and keratinized superficial squamous cells and sometimes horny cysts. Deeper tissue is not easily detached. Microscopy of the wet film shows acanthosis with intercellular bridges in all the cell clusters.

Keratoacanthoma

The macroscopic appearance of keratoacanthoma is usually distinctive (Fig. 21–14), but some lesions are not typical and may resemble BCC or SCC. Scrapings from the central crater consist of abundant anucleate and keratinized squamous cells showing no atypical forms (Fig. 21–15). Scrapings from the lip of the crater or from the papillae in the depths of the crater yield clusters of hyperplastic squamous epithelium but no evidence of malignancy. It is possible therefore to exclude BCC by cytology and to report the cytologic findings only as consistent with keratoacanthoma. Well-differentiated carcinoma cannot always be excluded; therefore, a biopsy will be required if there is any doubt clinically.

Sebaceous Gland Hyperplasia

Nodular enlargement of sebaceous glands due to blockage of ducts (comedones) and hyperplasia can closely mimic BCC clinically. Microscopy of scrapings shows oily sebaceous material in the wet film, together with clusters of large foamy sebaceous cells containing fat globules. Fixation in alcohol dissolves the sebum, giving a clearer view of the cells (Fig. 21–16). Occa-

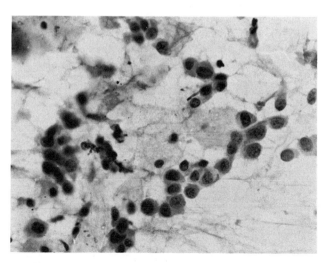

FIGURE 21–13. Bowen's disease. Small mainly monomorphic undifferentiated cells lying singly or in loose clusters (Papanicolaou stain; ×560).

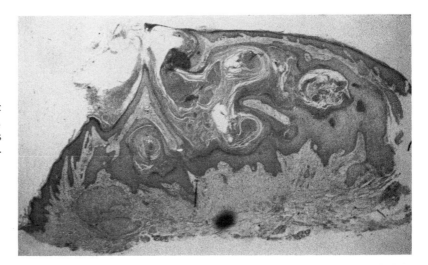

FIGURE 21–14. Keratoacanthoma. Histologic section through the raised edge of the lesion. Note the exfoliated superficial cells and debris trapped in the cavities and between the papillae (hematoxylin and eosin; ×12).

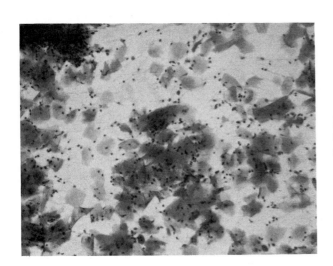

FIGURE 21–15. Keratoacanthoma. Scrapings from the central cavity consisting of superficial squamous cells and one cluster of deeper acanthotic cells (Papanicolaou stain; ×120).

FIGURE 21–16. Sebaceous cells. Large cells with abundant foamy cytoplasm (Papanicolaou stain; ×560).

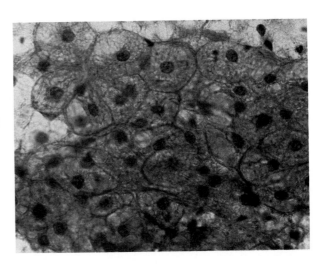

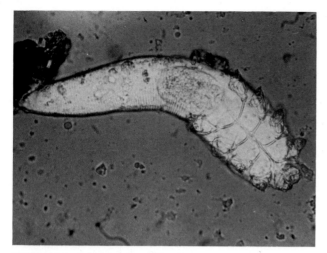

FIGURE 21–17. Demodex folliculorum. Note the eight sucker feet and the cross striations on the abdomen (wet film methylene blue; ×560).

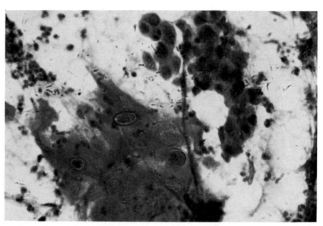

FIGURE 21–19. Paget's disease of the nipple. Showing three vacuolated Paget's cells within the fragment of epidermis. A cluster of poorly differentiated adenocarcinoma cells is adjacent to the fragment (Papanicolaou stain; ×420).

sionally sebaceous cells are found in association with BCC.

Demodex folliculorum is a normal inhabitant of sebaceous glands on the face. The mite is seen best in a methylene blue–stained wet film (Fig. 21–17). It is sometimes present in large numbers and may be the cause of some persistent comedones.

Paget's Disease of the Nipple

Paget's disease of the nipple is a cutaneous manifestation of an underlying duct carcinoma (Fig. 21–18). The clinical picture is characteristic, but even so a tissue diagnosis is essential before surgery. A confirmatory cytologic diagnosis is particularly valuable in this context, as it is such a simple test to perform and interpret. The eczematous lesion is usually soft and friable so that a good sample of the deeper layer of the epidermis is readily obtainable. The characteristic swollen Paget's cells within the epidermis are not well displayed in cytologic preparations owing to the cohe-

siveness and density of the epidermal fragments (Fig. 21–19), but the ectopic malignant cells from the deeper layers are conspicuous. The morphology varies according to the degree of differentiation; the histologic type of the malignant cells may not always be distinct. Immunocytochemical staining can be useful in differentiating from SCC and is particularly important when the disease occurs on the vulva.[8, 14, 25]

Malignant Melanoma

Malignant melanoma usually appears as a soft hemorrhagic or ulcerated lesion, which may or may not be pigmented. Recent onset of irritation, enlargement, hemorrhage or ulceration in a preexisting mole may arouse the suspicion of a malignant change.

Surgical biopsy is generally regarded as carrying the risk of dissemination, yet a tissue diagnosis is essential before proceeding with a treatment protocol that is bound to be more drastic than for other skin lesions. Cytologic diagnosis can therefore make an important contribution to the management of a suspect lesion. With an open lesion it is possible to obtain satisfactory specimens with an imprint or gentle scraping without any risk of dissemination. If this is not possible, fine needle aspiration is equally satisfactory. Numerous publications confirm that this method is widely practiced with apparent safety.[16, 19, 33, 41, 43, 44]

The loss of cell cohesion, which is a characteristic of melanoma, ensures an abundance of cells. The cytomorphology varies considerably from case to case and within the same tumor. In the less differentiated lesions marked pleomorphism occurs, including multinucleate giant cells (Fig. 21–20). At the other end of the spectrum, the tumor may be composed of comparatively benign-looking nevoid or fusiform cells. In general, the cells are of moderate size with a normal or slightly raised nucleocytoplasmic ratio. The nuclei are usually of the open vesicular type with coarse chromatin granules and a well-defined nuclear membrane,

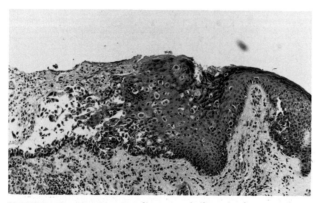

FIGURE 21–18. Paget's disease of the nipple. Histologic section showing the large vacuolated Paget's cells within the epidermis (hematoxylin and eosin; ×45).

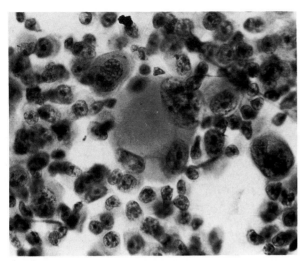

FIGURE 21–20. Malignant melanoma. A poorly differentiated tumor with multinucleated malignant giant cells. Note the macronucleoli (Papanicolaou stain; ×560).

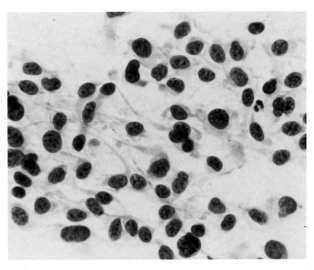

FIGURE 21–22. Malignant melanoma. A well-differentiated tumor with dense hyperchromatic nuclei, coarse chromatin pattern, indefinite cell borders and loss of cohesiveness (Papanicolaou stain; ×560).

which may be irregular. A characteristic feature in a high proportion of tumors is a large eosinophilic nucleolus, which is exceptionally conspicuous in Papanicolaou-stained smears (Fig. 21–21). Cell outline is often ill-defined in smear preparations; the cytoplasm is palely basophilic.

Cell size and outline often vary within narrower limits than might be expected with nuclei of such malignant aspect, thus imparting a certain uniform appearance which the experienced cytologist learns to recognize (Fig. 21–22). The amount of pigment, which is best seen in methylene blue preparations, varies considerably from heavily laden cells, wherein the nucleus may be obscured, to complete absence. The melanin granules may be found within the tumor cells or in the accompanying melanophores. The presence of pigment, though seen in only a minority of cytologic preparations, is virtually diagnostic, but both BCC and dermatofibroma protruberens[11] can also be pigmented. Rarely, the clinical appearance of a nonpigmented

melanoma may resemble Bowen's disease clinically, and the cell morphology may not be dissimilar.

Cutaneous Metastases

Breast cancer provides the majority of cases referred for cytologic investigation—either ulcerated primary tumors or localized recurrences in skin or scar following treatment. Scraping or fine needle aspiration (FNA) will depend on the type of lesion. Specific morphologic features are described elsewhere

Diffuse infiltration of the dermis can be investigated by FNA. Cell yield will be small but only a few ectopic malignant cells are required for a diagnosis.

In suspected cases of lymphoma and mycosis fungoides, priority should be given to air-dried smears for Romanowsky staining.

Pemphigus Vulgaris

The basic pathologic lesion of pemphigus is the dissolution of the intercellular bridges (acantholysis),[6] causing a cleft in the epidermis that fills with fluid containing the partially lysed cells.[27] The superficial cell layer remains intact resulting in a raised bulla, the base of which is composed of very actively regenerating squamous epithelium (Fig. 21–23).

A sample of fluid is easily obtained by needle aspiration of a fresh bulla. Cell yield is increased by allowing the needle to rest on the base during aspiration. Films can be made from the centrifuge deposit of the fluid or, in the case of older collapsed bullae, from scrapings of the base.

The presence of abundant single acantholytic cells is the key to the differentiation of pemphigus from other bullous lesions (Fig. 21–24).[1, 2, 35] In the fluid the cells

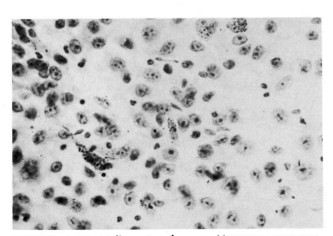

FIGURE 21–21. Malignant melanoma. Numerous macronucleoli and melanin granules are shown in some of the cells (Papanicolaou stain; ×420).

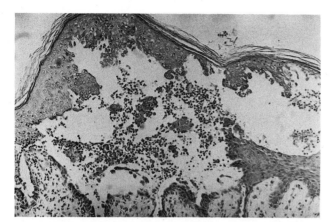

FIGURE 21–23. Pemphigus vulgaris. Histologic section of bulla showing acantholysis with separation of the superficial epidermis and accumulation of acantholytic cells in the fluid beneath. Note how the basal cells are exfoliating directly into the bulla (hematoxylin and eosin; ×45).

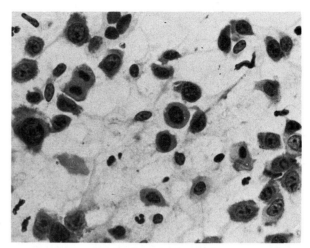

FIGURE 21–25. Pemphigus vulgaris. Scraping from base of bulla. Smear comprises very active basal and parabasal cells showing lysis of intercellular bridges and loss of cohesion. Abnormal chromatin clumping and mitotic figures contribute to the appearance of malignancy (Papanicolaou stain; ×560).

are mostly single, but scrapings yield a higher proportion of loosely attached cell clusters (Fig. 21–25). The most striking morphologic feature is the well-preserved nucleus surrounded by degenerating cytoplasm giving a false impression of a raised nucleocytoplasmic ratio. In inflammatory lesions nuclear degeneration usually precedes that of the cytoplasm and cell membrane. In Romanowsky-stained preparations, the cell tends to round up with condensation of the peripheral cytoplasm, resulting in a perinuclear halo as described by Tzanck and others (Fig. 21–26).[1, 2, 7, 21, 26, 30, 35, 36]

In a wet fixed preparation, the remains of the cytoplasm, which are basophilic, have a fuzzy outline. The nuclei are vesicular and hyperchromatic with coarse granular chromatin and enlarged chromocenters and nucleoli. Mitotic figures may be present (see Fig. 21–25). The appearance is very similar to that seen in SCC in which a minor degree of acantholysis may also be present. Confusion is unlikely to occur except in

vaginal smears when the nature of the lesion may not have been observed or the diagnosis of pemphigus suspected. Tzanck had placed undue emphasis on the presence of multinucleate giant cells ("monstrosités cellulares"). They are actually not of diagnostic significance, but it is important to recognize them in order to avoid confusion with the multinucleate cells of herpes (Fig. 21–27). Cell size has been reported as smaller than normal,[2] but it is not of particular significance as it varies with the degree of lysis and shrinkage and the level of the cleft in the epidermis.

Acantholysis occurs in pemphigus vulgaris and its variants pemphigus vegetans and pemphigus foliaceus.[2] It is also seen in benign familial pemphigus (Hailey-Hailey disease) and keratosis follicularis (Darier's dis-

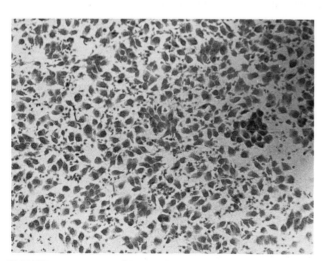

FIGURE 21–24. Pemphigus vulgaris. Aspiration from bulla; numerous discrete acantholytic cells and one small cluster (Papanicolaou stain; ×130).

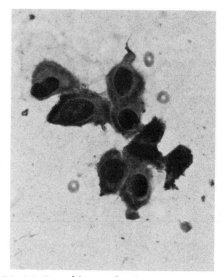

FIGURE 21–26. Pemphigus vulgaris. A Romanowsky preparation showing condensation of the peripheral cytoplasm (May-Grünwald-Giemsa; ×560).

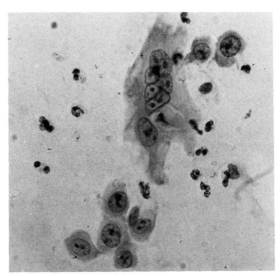

FIGURE 21–27. Pemphigus vulgaris. Multinucleated giant cell with prominent nucleoli. The acantholysis in the adjacent cells and the active chromatin pattern help to avoid confusion with herpes (Papanicolaou stain; ×560).

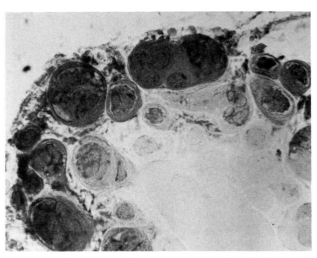

FIGURE 21–29. Herpes simplex. Aspiration from bulla, showing complete disorganization of chromatin. This phenomenon is seen in only the acute stage (wet film methylene blue; ×560).

ease). All other bullous dermatoses are subepidermal and do not contain acantholytic cells. Late bullous pemphigoid eruptions may become intraepidermal, but there is no acantholysis.

Herpes Simplex, Herpes Zoster, Varicella

As with pemphigus, specimens can be obtained either by aspiration of a vesicle, if still intact, or by scraping the base of an ulcer. Tzanck[35] employed the Romanowsky stain, but modern cytologists are more familiar with the characteristic multinucleation and intranuclear inclusions as seen in the Papanicolaou-stained cervical smears (Fig. 21–28). Rapid diagnosis

can be made with wet preparations stained with methylene blue (Fig. 21–29).

The cytologic appearance must not be confused with that of pemphigus. In both diseases multinucleation and some acantholysis are seen, but in pemphigus the chromatin pattern is well-preserved in all the nuclei and the cell borders are indistinct (see Fig. 21–27). In herpes the nuclei appear as empty rings; the cell borders may be ill defined but only a small proportion of cells are affected. In herpes, one occasionally sees small solid intranuclear inclusions resembling macronucleoli, but the majority of cells show the typical cytomorphology. A recently erupted herpetic vesicle can contain cells with such disorganized chromatin structure as to suggest malignancy (see Fig. 21–29), but typical intranuclear inclusions are also present.

Herpes zoster and varicella present a similar cytologic picture,[3] but the lesions are often dry and characteristic morphology has to be sought.

Molluscum Contagiosum

The clinical picture of multiple small white vesicles is unequivocal, but when only one vesicle is present, cytologic diagnosis may be required. The milky white fluid is easily expressed. Microscopy shows enormous numbers of "molluscum bodies" (Fig. 21–30). These are degenerate superficial squamous cells, so loaded with virus particles that the pyknotic nucleus is compressed against the cell wall and not easily seen (Fig. 21–31).

Lupus Vulgaris and Sarcoid

Cutaneous manifestations of sarcoid are probably seen more frequently today in developed countries than those of tuberculosis. Scrapings yield inflamma-

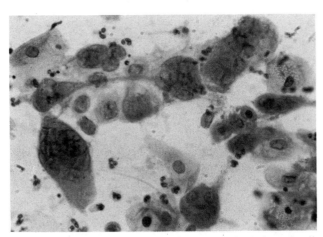

FIGURE 21–28. Herpes simplex. Typical multinucleated cells with chromophobic nuclear inclusions (Papanicolaou stain; ×560).

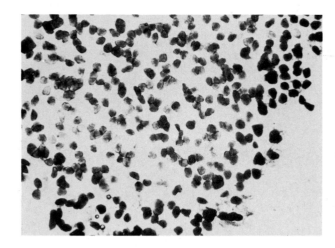

FIGURE 21–30. Molluscum contagiosum. Molluscum bodies expressed from vesicle (wet film methylene blue; ×90).

FIGURE 21–31. Molluscum contagiosum showing compression of nucleus against the cell membrane (Papanicolaou stain; ×560).

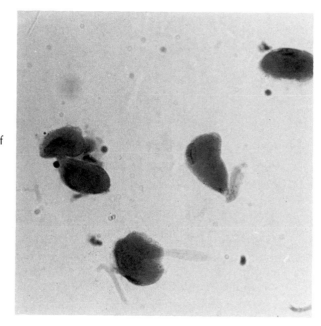

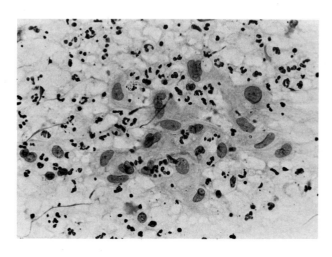

FIGURE 21–32. Sarcoid. Epithelioid histiocytes. Langhans's type giant cells (not shown) were also present in the same smear (Papanicolaou stain; ×560).

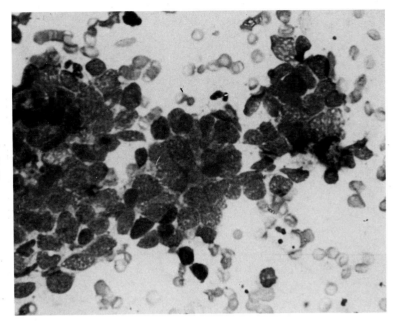

FIGURE 21–33. Pilomatrixoma. Fine needle aspiration showing undifferentiated basal cells. There is a deceptive similarity to small-cell carcinoma (May-Grünwald-Giemsa; × 800).

tory cells consistent with granuloma. Identification is not difficult when Langhans's giant cells are present, but in their absence the diagnosis depends on the recognition of epithelioid histiocytes (Fig. 21–32).

Pilomatrixoma (Calcifying Epithelioma of Malherbe)

This hard subcutaneous tumor is a diagnostic pitfall for the unwary.[42]

As the name implies it is a benign tumor of the hair follicle. The neoplastic cells reflect the cellular components of the matrix, which is a modified squamous epithelium derived from the epidermis. To complicate the picture, there is frequently a granulomatous reaction around the islands of neoplastic tissue, which may also include areas of calcification.

Samples of the tumor must be obtained by FNA. The cellular elements can be divided into three types. In the first type, the basal or basaloid cells from the germinal layer are small and hyperchromatic with little or no cytoplasm. They closely resemble the cells of BCC. When degenerate and pyknotic and especially when seen in tightly packed clusters, they can be mistaken for small-cell or undifferentiated carcinoma (Fig. 21–33). In the second type, the more mature cells are identifiable as squamous; they are generally small, have a vesicular nucleus, scanty or absent cytoplasm and a prominent nucleolus. The loss of cohesion and the admixture of cells from different layers and the numerous naked nuclei contribute to a pleomorphic picture, suggestive of undifferentiated or squamous cell carcinoma. In the third type of cell, a modified form of keratinization has taken place that stains only faintly yellow with Papanicolaou stain. Furthermore, the nucleus has faded completely, leaving an empty space, hence the term "shadow" cells (Fig. 21–34). To add to the confusion, the aspirate may contain numerous granuloma cells, amorphous debris and calcified material.

These tumors, although more frequently seen in young people, often occur deep in the neck, raising a clinical suspicion of disease in a lymph node and thus lowering the objectivity of the clinician and the cytologist. Erroneous diagnosis can be avoided by awareness of the possibility of a pilomatrixoma and by observing the wide range of differentiation present in one smear.[32] Shadow cells are highly characteristic, but unfortunately they are not always conspicuous owing to their poor affinity for stain and the presence of amorphous debris.

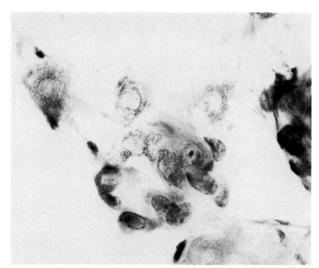

FIGURE 21–34. Pilomatrixoma. FNA showing the small nucleated squamous cells and anucleate shadow cells (Papanicolaou stain; × 800). (Courtesy of Dr. I. Ramzy.)

References

1. Brennan JG: Contributions to the study of pemphigus. AMA Arch Dermatol 68:481–498, 1953.
2. Blank H, Burgoon CF: Abnormal cytology in epithelial cells in pemphigus vulgaris: A diagnostic aid. J Invest Dermatol 18:213–221, 1952.
3. Blank H, Burgoon CF, Baldridge G, Urbach F: Cytologic smears in diagnosis of herpes simplex, herpes zoster and varicella. JAMA 146:1410–1412, 1951.
4. Brown CL, Klaber MR, Robertson MG: Rapid cytological diagnosis of basal cell carcinoma of skin. J Clin Pathol 32:361–367, 1979.
5. Canti G: Rapid cytological diagnosis of skin lesions. In Advances in Clinical Cytology, Vol 2. Edited by LG Koss and DV Coleman. New York, Masson Publishing, 1984.
6. Civatte A: Structure histologique de la bulle des pemphigus vrais. Ann Dermatol Syph 8:16–24, 1943.
7. Cordero AAJ: Valor del citodiagnostico en las dermatosis ampollares. Rev Argent Dermatosif 31:578–585, 1947.
8. Creasman WT, Gallager HS, Rutledge F: Paget's disease of the vulva. Gynaecol Oncol 3:133–148, 1975.
9. Dudgeon LS, Barrett NR: Examination of fresh tissues by the wet film method. Br J Surg 22:4–22, 1934.
10. Dudgeon LS, Patrick CV: A new method for the rapid microscopical diagnosis of tumours. Br J Surg 15:250–261, 1927.
11. Dupree WB, Langloss JM, Weiss SW: Pigmented dermatofibroma protruberens. Am J Surg Pathol 9:630–639, 1985.
12. Goldman L, McCabe RM, Sawyer F: The importance of cytology technique for the dermatologist in office practice. AMA Arch Dermatol 81:359–368, 1960.
13. Graham JH, Bingul O, Urbach F, Burgoon CF, Jr, Helwig EB: Papanicolaou smears and frozen sections on selected cutaneous neoplasms. JAMA 178:380–385, 1961.
14. Guldhammer B, Norgaard T: The differential diagnosis of intradermal malignant lesions using immunohistochemistry. Am J Dermatol 8:295–301, 1986.
15. Haber H: Cytodiagnosis in dermatology. Br J Dermatol 66:79–94, 1954.
16. Hajdu SI, Sarino A: Cytological diagnosis of malignant melanoma. Acta Cytol 17:320–327, 1973.
17. Hauser W: Die Zytodiagnostik in der Dermatologie. Handbuch der Hautund Geschlechtskrankheiten. Berlin, Springer Verlag, J Jadassohn, 1964.
18. Hitch JM, Wilson TB, Scoggin A: Evaluation of rapid method of cytologic diagnosis in suspected skin cancer. South Med J 44:407–414, 1951.
19. Kline TS, Kannan V: Aspiration biopsy cytology and melanoma. Am J Clin Pathol 77:597–601, 1982.
20. Koss LG, Woyke S, Oeszewski W: The skin and soft tissue. In Aspiration Biopsy: Cytological Interpretation and Histologic Bases. Tokyo, Igaku-Skoin, 1984.
21. Kuhn BH, Iverson L: Pemphigus vulgaris, a clinicoanatomic study. Arch Dermatol Syph 57:891–899, 1948.
22. Lever WF, Schaumberg-Lever G: Histopathology of the Skin, 5th ed. Philadelphia, JB Lippincott, p 539, 1975.
23. Lund HZ: How often does squamous cell carcinoma of the skin metastasize? Arch Dermol 92:635–637, 1965.
24. Malberger E, Tillinger R, Lichtig C: Diagnosis of basal cell carcinoma with aspiration cytology. Acta Cytol 28:301–304, 1984.
25. Masukawa T, Friedrich EG: Cytopathology of Paget's disease of the vulva. Diagnostic abrasive cytology. Acta Cytol 22:476–478, 1978.
26. Nelemans TC: Pemphigus Vulgaris en Dermatitis Herpetiformis Duhring; een Aetiologisch, Histologisch en Cytologisch Onderzoek. The Netherlands, Te Assen Bij, 1951.
27. Percival G, Hannay PW: Observations on the structure and formation of bullae. Parts I and II. Br J Dermatol Syph 61:41–54, 77–89, 1949.
28. Ruocco V: Cytodiagnoss in Dermatology. Napoli, Italy, Co-operative Libraria Universitaire, Soc. Coup. a.r.l., 1980.
29. Russell DS, Krayenbuhl H, Cairns H: The wet film technique in the histological diagnosis of intracranial tumours. A rapid method. J Pathol Bact 45:501–505, 1937.
30. Santoianni G: Cytology of blisters according to modern methods: Bullous dermatoses with particular interest in the pemphigus group. Ann Ital Dermatol Sif 5:335–340, 1951.
31. Selbach G, Heisel E: The cytological approach to skin disease. Acta Cytol 6:439–442, 1962.
32. Solanki P, Ramzy I, Durr N, Henkes D: Pilomatrixoma. Cytological features with differential diagnostic considerations. Arch Pathol Lab Med 111:294–297, 1987.
33. Svejda J, Mechl Z, Sopkova B: Cytology in the diagnosis of malignant melanoma. Tumori 64:229–232, 1978.
34. Traenkle HL, Burke EM: Currettement technique for biopsy. Use in detection of cutaneous cancer. JAMA 143:429–430, 1950.
35. Tzanck A: Le cyto-diagnostic immediat en dermatologie. Ann Dermatol Syph 7:68–70, 1947.
36. Tzanck A, Aron-Brunetiere R: Le "cytodiagnostic immediat" des dermatoses bulleuses. Gaz Med Port 2:667–675, 1949.
37. Urbach F, Burke EM, Traenkle HL: Cytodiagnosis of cutaneous malignancy. AMA Arch Dermatol 76:343–350, 1957.
38. Vilanova X, Aguade JP, Rueda LA: The cytological aspects of basal cell carcinoma. J Invest Dermatol 39:123–131, 1962.
39. Wilson GT: Cutaneous smears: Diagnostic aid in certain malignant lesions of skin. J Invest Dermatol 22:173–187, 1954.
40. Woodburne AR, Philpott OS, Philpott JA: Cytology studies in skin cancer. Arch Dermatol 82:992–997, 1960.
41. Woyke S, Domegala W, Czerniak B, Strokoska M: FNAC of malignant melanoma of skin. Acta Cytol 24:529–538, 1980.
42. Woyke S, Olszewski W, Eichelkraut A: Pilomatrixoma. A pitfall in the aspiration cytology of skin tumours. Acta Cytol 2:189–194, 1982.
43. Yamada T, Itou U, Watanabe Y, Okashi S: Cytological diagnosis of malignant melanoma. Acta Cytol 16:70–76, 1972.
44. Zajicek J: Cytology of supradiaphragmatic organs. Basel, S Karger, 1974.
45. Zoon JJ, Mali JWH: Remarks on cell diagnostics in normal and some pathological conditions of the skin. Dermatologica 101:145–153, 1950.

22

Pleural, Peritoneal and Pericardial Fluids

Bernard Naylor

Cytologic examination of a serous fluid is of paramount importance because the finding of cancer cells in such a specimen denotes that the patient has cancer that is not only advanced but also almost always incurable. With the exception of cerebrospinal fluid, in no other type of cytologic specimen does the finding of exfoliated cancer cells have such ominous prognostic significance. Apart from the finding of cancer cells, cytologic examination of pleural, peritoneal and pericardial fluids may also reveal information about inflammatory conditions of the serous membranes, parasitic infestations, infection with bacteria, fungi or viruses and the presence of a fistulous connection with a serous cavity.

SAMPLING TECHNIQUE

Although a serous effusion may be removed at the time of surgical exploration, it is usually removed by the relatively simple procedure of inserting a wide bore needle (under local anesthesia) through the body wall into the fluid-containing cavity. Peritoneal fluid is removed by abdominal paracentesis, colloquially referred to as paracentesis, pleural fluid by thoracentesis and pericardial fluid by pericardiocentesis.

Specimens may be obtained by instilling physiologic saline solution into the various recesses of the peritoneal cavity, then withdrawing the fluid and submitting it for cytologic examination as a peritoneal "washing." This procedure has acquired a considerable literature[211] and is now part of orthodox gynecologic practice. It is virtually confined to patients undergoing abdominal exploration for gynecologic neoplasms in order to detect peritoneal dissemination of cancer cells. Peritoneal dialysate from patients undergoing long-term peritoneal dialysis for renal failure is occasionally submitted for cytologic examination.

Collecting Serous Fluids

The fluid is collected into a clean, dry container, which need not be sterile, and sent to the laboratory as soon as possible. If it is not possible to send the fluid immediately it should be stored in a refrigerator at 4°C and not allowed to freeze. We do not require anticoagulant or fixative to be added to the fluid. Anticoagulation by adding heparin to the receptacle before the fluid is collected does not interfere with cytologic detail.

Formalin, alcohol or any other kind of cellular preservative must not be added to specimens of serous fluid sent to our laboratory. Not only does formalin prevent cells from adhering well to a slide, but it also interferes with the quality of staining by the Papanicolaou method. Adding alcohol causes some precipitation of protein in virtually all specimens, thereby interfering with adherence of the cells to the slide. Apart from these criticisms of the use of formalin or alcohol, neither is necessary because keeping the specimen at refrigerator temperature, even for several days, will preserve cells well (Fig. 22–1).

Gross Appearance of Serous Fluids

The appearance to the naked eye of a serous fluid sometimes reveals clues as to the cause of an effusion and the nature of its cellular contents. Therefore, for every serous fluid received by the laboratory, note should be made of its volume, color and clarity and any unusual physical features, such as malodor, opalescence or high viscosity.

Many serous fluids are noticeably bloodstained. In a survey carried out in our laboratory 46% of pleural (n = 179) and 27% of peritoneal (n = 104) fluids were visibly bloodstained, a term used for fluids whose color

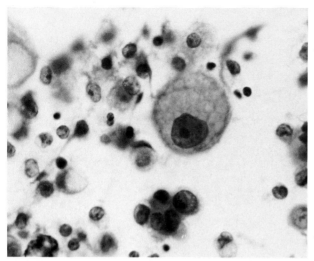

FIGURE 22–1. Well-preserved **adenocarcinoma cells** prepared from a specimen that had been stored at 4°C for 14 days after collection. Smear of pleural fluid (Papanicolaou stain; ×208).

ranged from orange to deep red. It is a commonly held belief that heavily bloodstained effusions are likely to be caused by cancer and that such fluids are more likely to contain cancer cells. However, of the 60 deep red fluids in the combined series (n = 283), only 13 contained cancer cells. Furthermore, of the 58 fluids that contained cancer cells, 30 were bloodstained and 28 were not, which denotes that fluids containing cancer cells are just as likely as not to be bloodstained, an observation described previously.[19, 26]

Occasionally a fluid contains so many cancer cells that if allowed to stand and sediment spontaneously they will form a thick whitish yellow layer at the bottom of the container. Similar spontaneously occurring sediment may develop in fluids containing numerous neutrophilic leukocytes. Such purulent fluids may be malodorous owing to a high bacterial content. Pleural fluid from a patient with rheumatoid pleuritis may contain a heavy, whitish, flocculent sediment, and the supernatant may have the appearance of fruit juice, such as lime or pineapple juice.

Individual particles of cancer in a serous fluid may occasionally be so large as to be visible to the naked eye. Such particles, strikingly illustrated by de Vries,[41] may be spheroids, ellipsoids or similar shapes. Figure 22–2 is a striking example of particles of metastatic squamous cell carcinoma in pleural fluid in which the particles were about the size and shape of sesame seeds. Such particles provide excellent material for cell blocks.

Fluids containing numerous pigmented melanoma cells may be chocolate brown; when centrifuged they form a dark brown sediment and a clear yellow supernatant. Of a much lighter brown hue are fluids containing many hemosiderophages, a manifestation of old hemorrhage within the serous cavity. Fluids from jaundiced patients may have a rather dark brown-orange or greenish appearance that remains with the supernatant after the specimen has been centrifuged.

Serous effusions caused by diffuse malignant mesothelioma of epithelial type often contain a high concentration of hyaluronic acid,[31, 152] increasing the viscosity of the fluid so much that it may have a honey-like consistence. We have also observed such high viscosity due to hyaluronic acid in a pleural fluid containing cells of metastatic Wilms' tumor. Fluid from the peritoneal cavity of a patient with pseudomyxoma peritonei is extremely difficult to aspirate because of its heavy mucoid consistence. Processing this material is difficult because the cells it contains do not sediment during centrifugation.

Fluids containing numerous cholesterol crystals are yellow and turbid and have a swirling, shimmering, "gold paint" appearance, especially when agitated. The presence of cholesterol crystals can be confirmed by using a stained wet film (see the following), but the crystals will not be seen in the permanent preparation stained by the Papanicolaou method, having been dissolved in the staining circuit. Chylous fluids have a milky white appearance with a creamy topmost layer due to their high concentration of emulsified lipid.

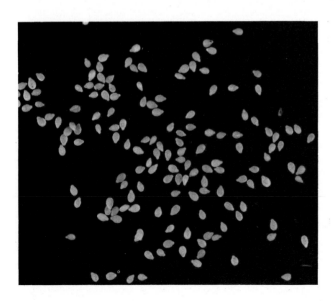

FIGURE 22–2. Particles of **squamous cell carcinoma** visible to the naked eye. Pleural fluid (unstained; natural size).

CYTOPREPARATORY TECHNIQUE

For every serous fluid we routinely use three techniques: a toluidine blue stained wet film, wet-fixed smears stained with the Papanicolaou stain and cell blocks stained with hematoxylin and eosin. The immunoperoxidase technique and other special stains are occasionally used, usually on cell block material, although it is possible to apply the immunoperoxidase technique to Papanicolaou stained smears without having to destain them. Electron microscopy is not routinely used. Its major practical application has been in attempting to discriminate between cells of mesotheliomas and adenocarcinomas; however, its usefulness in this and other respects has been eclipsed by immunocytochemistry.

Preliminary Steps

1. Remove any clots and extract all fluid from them by pressing them against the side of the container with a spatula or tongue blade until left with a firm, rubbery mass. If the shrunken clot is large, put it into a Petri dish and cut it into small fragments. Put the clot into 10% buffered formalin (as used for surgical specimens), allow it to fix for at least 30 minutes and process the fragments as tissue.

2. Shake up the remaining fluid to disperse cells. Pour off an aliquot (up to 50 ml) into a centrifuge tube and centrifuge the sample for 5 minutes at 2000 rpm.

3. If the sediment is firm, pour off the supernatant by completely inverting the tube. If the sediment is bloody or loose, pipette off the supernatant.

4. Prepare a toluidine blue–stained wet film as described subsequently.

Wet Film Technique

1. With a wire loop (as used in microbiology), remove a drop of the topmost layer of the sediment and transfer it onto the center of a glass slide.

2. Put an approximately equal sized drop of toluidine blue stain (see the following) on the slide next to the drop of sediment.

3. Mix the two drops together with the corner of a coverslip and then place the coverslip over the mixture. This wet film can be examined immediately.

4. Prepare the permanent smears as described subsequently.

Permanent Smears

1. With the wire loop, remove one or two drops of the topmost layer of the sediment. Transfer these drops onto the center of a glass slide.

2. Using the loop, quickly spread the material on the slide in a longitudinal and crisscross manner.

3. Before any drying of the smeared material takes place, quickly immerse the slide in 95% ethanol. If this movement is carried out slowly, a distinctive "ribbing" artifact will appear in the smeared material.[158] Several smears may be put in the same container of fixative. To prevent cells of one slide from adhering to the back of another keep them separated by attaching a paper clip to one end of alternate slides.

As an alternative fixative, one may use 95% methanol, 95% propanol or any of the commercially available spray fixatives. Spray fixatives tend to create a "pooling" artifact in bloody smears, which may detract from the evenness of the smear and be visually annoying.

An alternative method of spreading the sediment, especially when it is thick, is to place one or two drops of the sediment near one end of a slide (slide A). Then place another slide (slide B) over this, and after the sediment has spread spontaneously, pull the two apart quickly. Slide A will have almost all of the cellular material and should be fixed immediately, whereas slide B has only a little material and should be discarded or used as an additional A slide.

Cell Block Technique

After preparing the wet film and smears for the Papanicolaou stain, prepare a cell block of the residual sediment.

1. Add two or three drops of plasma to the remaining sediment. Mix the two together. (Outdated plasma from a blood bank is used for this purpose.)

2. Add three or four drops of thrombin solution (see the following) to the mixture. Mix again.

3. Allow the mixture to clot; this usually takes only a few seconds.

4. Add tinted (see the following) 10% buffered formalin to the clot. Pour the clot and the formalin into a Petri dish that contains any spontaneously formed clot.

5. Cut the newly formed clot into small pieces and allow them to fix for 30 minutes.

6. Process the fragments (spontaneous and induced clot) as tissue.

The technical sequence for preparing permanent smears and cell blocks is illustrated in Figure 22–3.

Tinted Formalin

The formalin used to fix the cell block material should be colored pink-orange by adding a small amount of powdered eosin. The embedded specimen will then stand out tinted in the paraffin wax, and the histotechnologists will find it much easier to cut the sections. Adding eosin to the formalin does not alter the appearance of the stained sections.

Thrombin Solution

This is prepared by adding 10 ml of distilled water to a vial containing 5000 units of powdered thrombin.

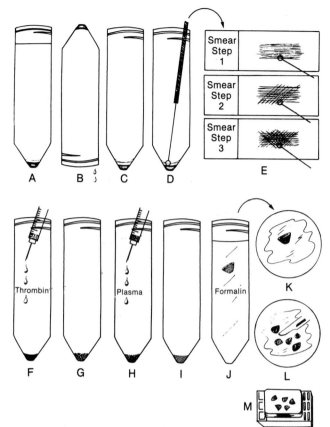

FIGURE 22–3. Technical sequence for **preparation of a permanent smear and a cell block** up to paraffin embedding.

Toluidine Blue Stain

This is a modification of the stain described by McCormack and coworkers[148] for examination of bronchial secretions:

- Toluidine blue   (0.5 g)
- 95% ethanol   (20.0 ml)
- Distilled water   (80.0 ml)

Store the stain in the refrigerator to prevent fungal growth.

Usefulness of Stained Wet Films

The preparation of a wet film is extremely simple and quick, and the film is ready to be examined immediately. After viewing, the wet film is discarded. The advantages of this preparation are several.

1. Frequently a wet film reveals a distinctly diagnostic cellular picture, enabling a report to be issued within 10 to 15 minutes after receiving the specimen in the laboratory.

2. Wet films enable one to identify the "super-positive" serous fluids, those teeming with cancer cells. Not only are such specimens easily identified, but it is also possible to eliminate them from the routine stain-

ing circuit in order to avoid cross-contamination of other specimens.

We do not permanently stain such super-positive fluids until immediately before the whole staining circuit is changed each week. Even though they may have been in the laboratory for several days, a report will have already been issued on them based on the wet film evaluation. By using the stained wet film technique, we have avoided the (questionable) need for separate staining circuits for gynecologic and nongynecologic specimens.

3. A stained wet film may enable one immediately to identify unusual or interesting cytologic specimens, thereby providing the opportunity to prepare more smears before the sediment is clotted for preparation of the cell block.

A large, solid fragment of neoplasm may absorb the toluidine blue stain very slowly or only at its periphery (Fig. 22–4). Such fragments are easily overlooked.

Apart from these advantages stained wet films may reveal certain constituents in sediments obtained by centrifugation that will not be seen in the permanent smears, such as cholesterol crystals, which are brilliantly highlighted by polarized light (Fig. 22–5). Another crystalline curiosity revealed by the wet film technique are Charcot-Leyden crystals (Fig. 22–6), which may be found in fluids containing numerous eosinophilic leukocytes.[164] Bloody effusions may contain sheaves of hematoidin crystals (Fig. 22–7), formed by the breakdown of hemoglobin. The cellular fragments known as detached ciliary tufts (DCTs), found in certain types of peritoneal fluid, are vigorously motile in the fresh state, a property that is detectable only by using a wet film. Wet films will reveal psammoma bodies, not because they take up the stain, but because they do not react with toluidine blue and therefore stand out unstained against the surrounding stained cells (Fig. 22–8).

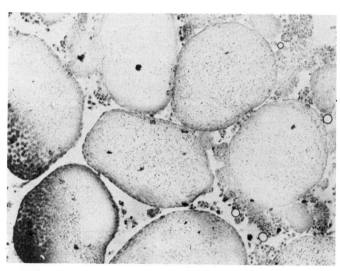

FIGURE 22–4. Large, partly stained spheroids ("proliferation spheres") of **metastatic ductal carcinoma of the breast** that the stain had not completely penetrated (wet film of pleural fluid; toluidine blue; × 83).

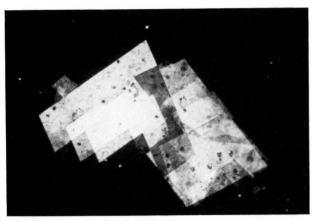

FIGURE 22–5. Flat, angulated **cholesterol crystals**, a manifestation of long-standing effusion, in this case due to **rheumatoid pleuritis** (wet film of pleural fluid; toluidine blue; polarized light; ×528).

Usefulness of Cell Block Preparations

Although the use of cell blocks is not standard practice in all laboratories, we find it indispensable. Specimens that are not anticoagulated frequently contain a clot that may be voluminous. Such a clot may have developed rapidly after the fluid was aspirated to enmesh virtually all of the neoplastic cells in the specimen. Consequently smears prepared from the remaining fluid after the clot was removed may be devoid of neoplastic and other cells. In such a situation, sections of the spontaneously formed clot frequently reveal numerous obvious neoplastic cells. In a series of 863 serous fluids that contained cancer cells and that we had examined by both smear and cell block techniques, both techniques gave positive results in 696 cases. With 113 specimens, only the smears were positive, and with 54 specimens, only the cell block

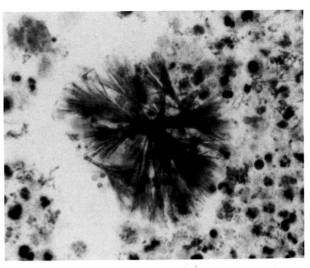

FIGURE 22–7. Sheaves of **hematoidin crystals** in a background of viable and necrotic leukocytes (wet film of pleural fluid; toluidine blue; ×660).

was positive. Cell blocks therefore enhanced our positive results by 6.7%.

The discrepancy of negative smears and positive cell blocks is explained by the fluid spontaneously and rapidly clotting before it was processed, thereby entrapping the neoplastic cells. Such a spontaneously formed clot in cell blocks is composed of dense, deep magenta and often laminated fibrin (Fig. 22–9), whereas the induced clot of the sediment obtained by centrifugation is composed of delicate, hardly visible fibrin (Fig. 22–10). The appearance of a spontaneously formed fibrin clot is due to its having had time to contract and become dense. With an induced clot this does not take place because it is fixed in formalin within seconds or minutes after it has formed.

Cell block preparations may also reveal certain histologic aspects of a neoplasm such as papillary, acinar or duct-like formations. Cell blocks also demonstrate psammoma bodies and other calcific concretions extremely well (Fig. 22–11), which may be difficult or impossible to detect in the permanent smears.

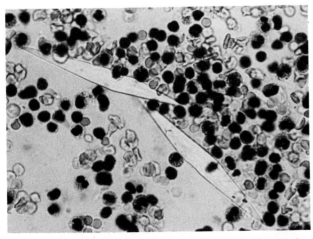

FIGURE 22–6. Charcot-Leyden crystals in a background of eosinophils, lymphocytes and red blood cells (wet film of pleural fluid; toluidine blue; ×528). (Reproduced with permission from Naylor B, Novak PM: Charcot-Leyden crystals in pleural fluids. Acta Cytol 29:781–784, 1985.)

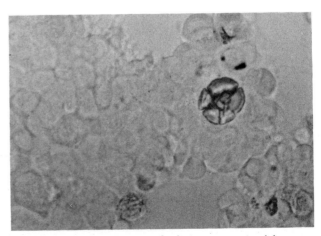

FIGURE 22–8. A psammoma body in an unstained fragment of **metastatic papillary adenocarcinoma of thyroid gland** (wet film of pleural fluid; toluidine blue; ×528).

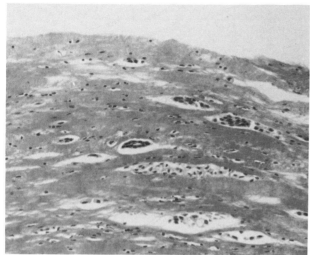

FIGURE 22–9. Spontaneously formed clot composed of dense laminated bands of fibrin containing a few fragments of **metastatic adenocarcinoma** (cell block of pleural fluid; hematoxylin and eosin; ×33).

Cell blocks reveal other interesting histologic or cytologic entities, some mere curiosities, others of importance. Figure 22–12 illustrates a fragment of liver in the cell block of peritoneal fluid due to the paracentesis needle transversing the liver on its way to the peritoneal cavity. Retrospective analysis of the smears revealed only an occasional hepatocyte (Fig. 22–13). In our material cell blocks have also revealed granulation tissue (Fig. 22–14), cholesterol clefts (Fig. 22–15), epidermis (Fig. 22–16), lung (Fig. 22–17), squamous epithelial cells (Fig. 22–18), skeletal muscle (Fig. 22–19), cartilage (Fig. 22–20), vegetable matter (Fig. 22–21), colonies of microorganisms (Fig. 22–22), accessory skin structures in subcutaneous adipose tissue (Fig. 22–23), fragments of hyperplastic peritoneal mesothelium with collagenous stroma (Fig. 22–24) and fibroblastic tissue. Many of these entities were either not present or were unrecognizable in the smear preparations.

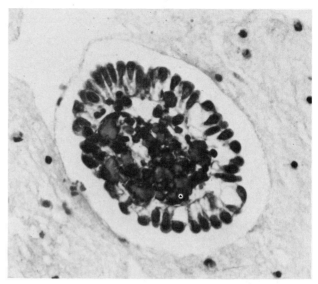

FIGURE 22–11. A cluster of small **psammoma bodies** in a fragment of **papillary ovarian serous cystadenocarcinoma** of low malignant potential (cell block of peritoneal fluid; hematoxylin and eosin; ×330).

THE SEROUS CAVITIES

The embryonic coelomic cavity gives rise to the serous cavities: pleural, peritoneal and pericardial. The term *serous* refers to the small amount of serum-like

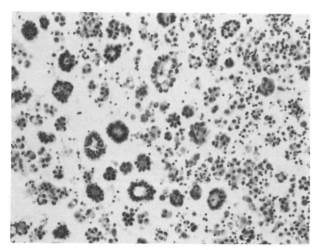

FIGURE 22–10. Same specimen as in Figure 22–9. This was prepared by clotting the sediment obtained by centrifugation. The **newly formed fibrin network** holding these particles of **adenocarcinoma** together is virtually invisible. This fluid had clotted spontaneously but before it did so most of the fragments of adenocarcinoma settled to the bottom of the container. Therefore, the spontaneously formed clot (see Fig. 22–9) contained only a small number of fragments of carcinoma, whereas the specimen obtained by centrifugation contained numerous fragments (cell block of pleural fluid; hematoxylin and eosin; ×10).

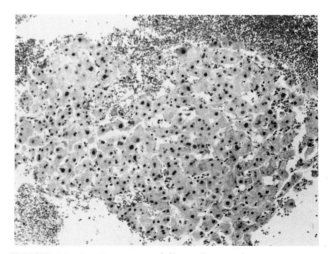

FIGURE 22–12. Fragment of liver due to the paracentesis needle traversing the liver en route to the peritoneal cavity (cell block of peritoneal fluid; hematoxylin and eosin; ×132).

FIGURE 22–13. Same specimen as in Figure 22–12. **Hepatocyte** (smear of the fluid; Papanicolaou stain; ×825).

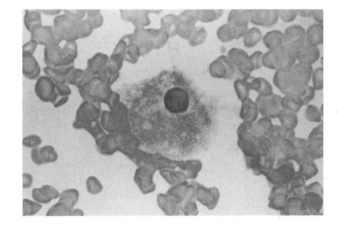

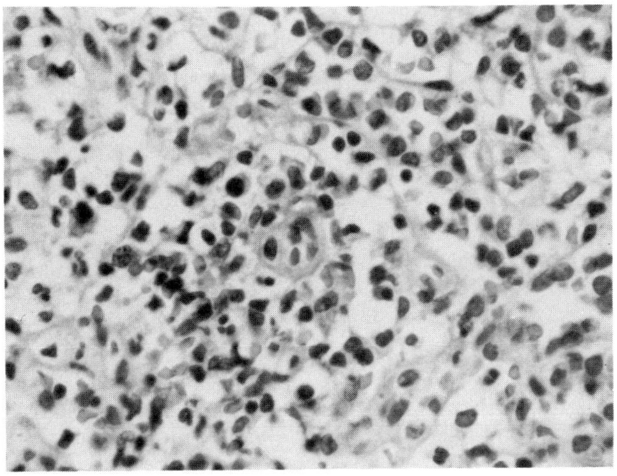

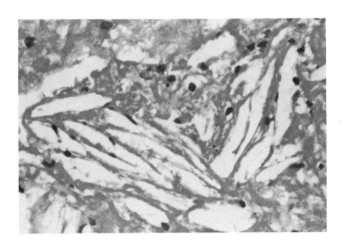

FIGURE 22–14. **Granulation tissue** presumably from the surface of inflamed pleura (cell block of pleural fluid; hematoxylin and eosin; ×528).

FIGURE 22–15. **Cholesterol clefts in fibrin**, a manifestation of long-standing effusion, in this case due to rheumatoid pleuritis (cell block of pleural fluid; hematoxylin and eosin; ×330). (Reproduced with permission from Naylor B: The pathognomonic cytologic picture of rheumatoid pleuritis. Acta Cytol 34:465–473, 1990.)

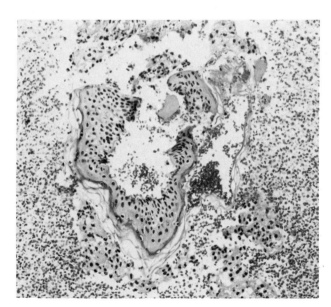

FIGURE 22–16. A fragment of **epidermis** detached by the thoracentesis needle (cell block of pleural fluid; hematoxylin and eosin; ×132).

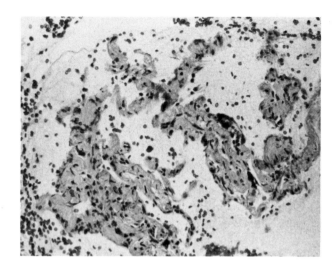

FIGURE 22–17. Fragments of **pulmonary parenchyma**. The thoracentesis needle penetrated a part of the lung that was adherent to the parietal pleura by neoplastic adhesions (cell block of pleural fluid; hematoxylin and eosin; ×208).

FIGURE 22–18. Stratified squamous epithelial cells that entered the pleural cavity through an esophagopleural fistula (cell block of pleural fluid; hematoxylin and eosin; ×330).

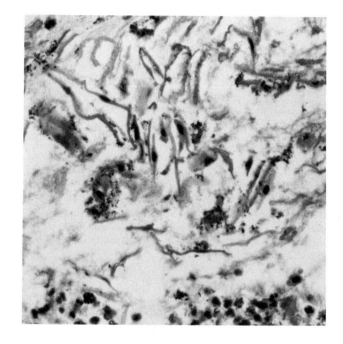

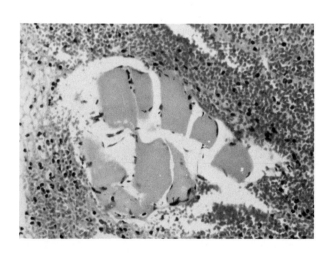

FIGURE 22–19. Fragment of **intercostal skeletal muscle** detached by the thoracentesis needle (cell block of pleural fluid; hematoxylin and eosin; ×208).

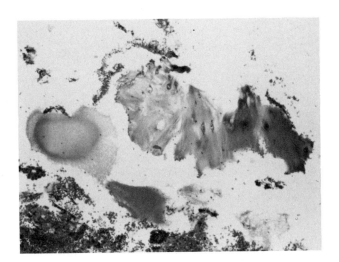

FIGURE 22–20. Fragment of **costal cartilage** detached by the pericardiocentesis needle (cell block of pericardial fluid; hematoxylin and eosin; ×83).

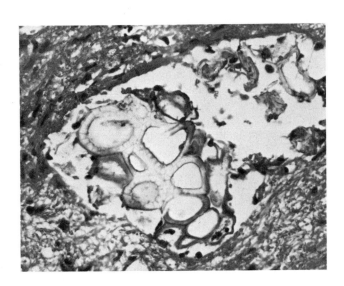

FIGURE 22–21. Fragment of **vegetable matter** presumably a contaminant after the specimen had been collected. The patient had no evidence of fistula (cell block of pleural fluid; hematoxylin and eosin; ×330).

FIGURE 22–22. Colonies of **cocci** in a background of inflammatory cells: evidence of bacterial pleuritis (cell block of pleural fluid; hematoxylin and eosin; ×825).

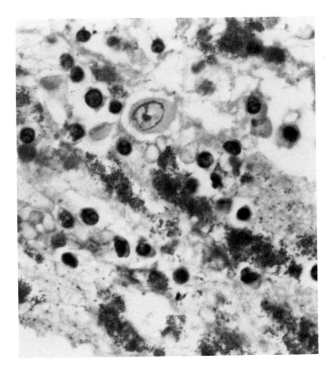

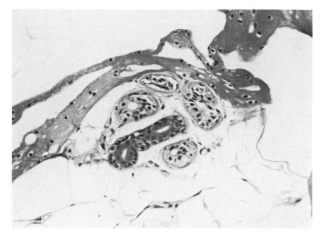

FIGURE 22–23. Fragment of **subcutaneous adipose tissue** detached by the thoracentesis needle. It contains a sweat gland (cell block of pleural fluid; hematoxylin and eosin; ×208).

fluid each cavity contains. The term is also applied to the cavity partly surrounding each testis formed by the tunica vaginalis testis, an embryonic extension of the peritoneal cavity. Because our experience with fluid from the tunica vaginalis testis is virtually nonexistent, this type of specimen will not be dealt with, except for brief reference. For an account of the cytology of this cavity, the reader should consult the monograph of Spriggs and Boddington.[215] The serous cavities are commonly (and somewhat imprecisely) referred to as *body cavities*. Under normal conditions the cavities are collapsed sacs invaginated by the heart, lungs or intestines. Each cavity is completely closed (except the peritoneal cavity at the point at which it receives the fimbriated ends of the fallopian tubes), and each contains a small amount of fluid. The outer layer of each serous cavity is the parietal layer; the layer directly in contact with the enveloped organ is the visceral layer.

Apart from a thin film of fluid, these layers are in contact with each other; thus, under normal conditions, each cavity is only a potential cavity. When a cavity contains an excess of fluid, it becomes an actual cavity. Each cavity is lined by a monolayer of mesothelial cells beneath which is a layer of connective tissue, supplied with blood vessels, lymphatics and nerves (Fig. 22–25). The close proximity of blood and lymphatic vessels to mesothelium may partly account for the ready spread of neoplastic cells into a serous cavity.

TYPES OF EFFUSIONS

Accumulation of fluid in a serous cavity above the normal small amount is referred to as an effusion. Effusions are designated according to their location: pleural, peritoneal or pericardial. The condition of peritoneal effusion is frequently referred to as ascites and the fluid as ascitic fluid. Air may sometimes be introduced into a serous cavity either by trauma (including surgical trauma), for radiologic diagnostic purposes, for therapy or secondary to a pathologic process, producing the condition of pneumothorax, pneumoperitoneum or pneumopericardium. When these conditions are accompanied by effusion, the terms are expanded to indicate its presence: pneumohydrothorax, pneumohydroperitoneum and pneumohydropericardium.

Transudates and Exudates

The number and type of non-neoplastic cells commonly found in serous effusions depend to a large extent on the pathogenetic mechanisms of fluid formation, which determine whether a fluid is classified as a transudate or an exudate. Transudates are fluids characterized by a low protein content, usually less

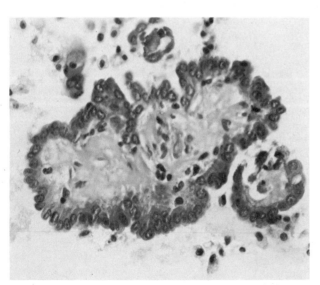

FIGURE 22–24. Fragments of **hyperplastic pericardial mesothelium** with a collagenous stroma (cell block of pericardial fluid; hematoxylin and eosin; ×330).

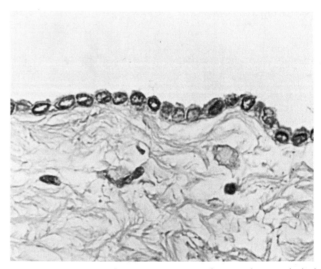

FIGURE 22–25. Peritoneum. A monolayer of mesothelial cells beneath which is a layer of fibrous connective tissue (hematoxylin and eosin; ×235).

than 3.0 g/dl, and low specific gravity, usually below 1.015. Transudates accumulate by the filtration of serum across physically intact capillary walls under conditions in which the outflow of fluid through a serous membrane exceeds the normal reabsorptive process. This may take place as a result of increased venous pressure, as in congestive heart failure or cirrhosis of the liver, or in hypoproteinemia in renal failure. Transudates generally have a lower cellular content than exudates, and their fibrin content is also lower. The cellular content usually consists of mesothelial cells and macrophages, with an occasional lymphocyte or neutrophilic leukocyte.

Exudates result from damage to the capillary walls that ramify in the serosal connective tissue. This damage allows escape of protein and various cellular constituents of the blood into the serous cavity, resulting in a fluid that has a higher protein content (3.0 g/dl or more) and specific gravity (>1.015) than that of the typical transudate. Furthermore, the cellular content is higher and is likely to contain many inflammatory cells in exudates caused by inflammation or, in exudates caused by neoplasm on the serosal surface, many neoplastic cells.

Pleural inflammatory exudates are likely to be caused by pneumonia, pulmonary infarct, pulmonary abscess, pleuritis or secondary bacterial infection of a transudate. Peritoneal inflammatory exudates are likely to be caused by peritonitis, either spontaneous bacterial or secondary to infarct or inflammation of the bowel, spontaneous or traumatic rupture of a viscus or pelvic inflammatory disease in women. Pericardial effusions that are exudates are likely to be caused by viral or bacterial inflammation of the pericardium or uremic pericarditis. In the less prosperous nations of the world, tuberculous inflammation of a serous membrane is always foremost in the minds of clinicians, whereas in affluent societies it is far less frequent.

Serous effusions caused by neoplasm may be transudates, resulting from failure of resorption of serous fluid due to mechanical interference by neoplasm, or they may be exudates caused by neoplasm damaging the capillaries of the serous membranes.

NORMAL CELLS

Every pleural, peritoneal and pericardial fluid contains cells, often numerous, occasionally scanty. The non-neoplastic cells commonly found in serous fluids are those derived from blood (erythrocytes and leukocytes) and from the serosal lining, the mesothelial cells. The proportion of the different types of these cells varies considerably, depending on certain circumstances such as the cause and the duration of the effusion and the presence or absence of inflammation.

Examples of normal cells that are rarely found in spontaneously occurring serous fluids are megakaryocytes, hepatocytes and cells derived from the alimentary or respiratory tract via a fistula. Cells detached from the fimbriated end of the fallopian tubes are occasionally found in peritoneal fluid obtained by culdocentesis, laparoscopy, laparotomy or dialysis catheter.

Range of Normal Cells

It is difficult to ascertain what is a normal range for cells in serous fluids because normally the serous cavities contain only a small amount of fluid. It is only when there is an excess of fluid, an abnormal situation, that it is possible to aspirate it. It is known, however, that the cellular content of peritoneal fluid varies considerably in different animal species.[172] Attempts to obtain normal peritoneal and pleural fluid from humans at the time of surgical exploration are nullified by the fluid becoming contaminated by blood and fragments of mesothelium detached from the underlying connective tissue by surgical trauma. Yamada[253] aspirated pleural fluid from healthy soldiers and found that the cellular content ranged from 1700 to 6200 cells per ml, with most of the cells being classified as large mononuclear cells and the remainder as mesothelial cells and lymphocytes. Specimens of normal peritoneal fluid may be obtained at the time of laparoscopy and also by culdocentesis. In our experience, culdocentesis has seldom provided more than 1 or 2 ml of peritoneal fluid, containing mainly cells that appeared to be macrophages (histiocytes) with an occasional mesothelial cell and lymphocyte. However, culdocentesis specimens from apparently normal subjects may contain papillary clusters of mesothelial cells in which there are psammoma bodies.[117, 197]

Pericardial fluid may be easily obtained by aspirating the pericardial sac at the time of thoracotomy. Spriggs and Boddington[213] examined the sediment of 14 samples of pericardial fluid obtained in this way. The cells were classified as mesothelial or macrophages, and mitotic figures were found in some of the cells. They also noted that serous fluids collected at autopsy generally contained large numbers of mesothelial cells that had exfoliated postmortem, an observation confirmed by our own experience. Ramsey and colleagues[184] obtained pericardial fluid from patients undergoing thoracotomy, some for cardiac surgery. These fluids contained small macrophages and mesothelial cells, some in papillary clusters.

In spite of the uncertainty as to what is a normal range of the various cell types in serous fluids, it is common practice to send these fluids to the hematology laboratory for total and differential cell counts. Such counts should be performed only on fluids that have been anticoagulated; otherwise, any clot that forms is likely to entrap cells and give spurious results.

Only a few characteristic (though not specifically diagnostic) cytologic pictures are demonstrated by total and differential cell counts, such as the cytologic pictures of acute purulent inflammation, eosinophilic effusion and lymphocytic effusion. In non-neoplastic conditions the cytologic picture is usually that of a mixed population that, when analyzed quantitatively, does not give any specific diagnostic findings. It is clear from published studies that total and differential cell counts on pleural and peritoneal fluids are of little or no diagnostic value;[44, 138, 173] in fact, the presence of neoplastic cells was regarded by Light and coworkers[138] as the only useful finding.

Mesothelial Cells

Mesothelial cells readily undergo hypertrophy and hyperplasia in response to a wide variety of stimuli, such as inflammation of the serous membrane, inflammation or necrosis of underlying parenchyma, the presence of foreign substances in the serous cavity such as blood or air and even the presence of a long-standing sterile effusion such as may occur in the peritoneal cavity in hepatic cirrhosis. It is not possible to tell from microscopic examination of mesothelial cells what the stimulus was that gave rise to their hypertrophy or hyperplasia; this has to be determined from clinical and other information.

In the presence of an effusion, whatever its cause, mesothelial cells exfoliate, often in large numbers, either as single cells or as clusters of cells or both. It is entirely possible that mesothelial cells exfoliated into a serous fluid continue to proliferate because they are in a natural medium. In fact, of all the benign cells seen in cytopathologic practice, mesothelial cells are the most likely to show mitotic figures, evidence of their ability to proliferate in a serous fluid.

Cytology

The prototypic mesothelial cell exfoliated into a serous fluid (Fig. 22–26) is round, about 25 μ in diameter and has a single central or excentric nucleus. With the Papanicolaou stain, the cytoplasm is dense and gray-green and tends to become less dense at the periphery of the cell, imparting an indistinct foamy or

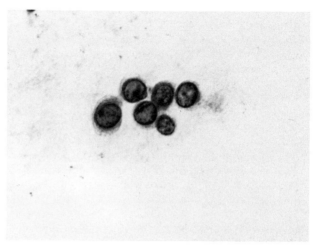

FIGURE 22–27. A group of small **mesothelial cells** with a high nucleocytoplasmic ratio (smear of pleural fluid; Papanicolaou stain; ×750).

even scalloped appearance to the cell membrane. The nucleus is round or oval and possesses a well-defined, smoothly contoured membrane. The chromatin is uniformly granular, and nucleoli are readily identified. (The electron-microscopic appearance of mesothelial cells is dealt with elsewhere in this text.)

Mesothelial cells vary considerably in size, from small cells about 9 μ in diameter with relatively little cytoplasm (Fig. 22–27) to giant cells, more than 60 μ in diameter. Frequently, large hypertrophied and much smaller mesothelial cells are seen joined to each other. Giant mesothelial cells are almost always multinucleated, often with ten or more nuclei (Fig. 22–28). Morphologic evaluation of 1000 mesothelial cells in ten serous fluids received in our laboratory revealed that two cells had three nuclei, 36 had two, and 962 (96.2%)

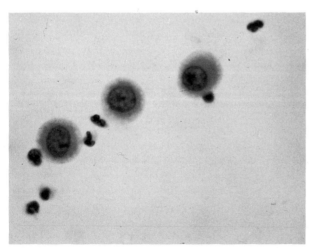

FIGURE 22–26. Three prototypical **mesothelial cells**. Note the dense cytoplasm, which tends to fade at the periphery; the smoothly contoured, central or slightly eccentric nuclei; the smooth nuclear membrane and the readily visible nucleoli (smear of pleural fluid; Papanicolaou stain; ×528).

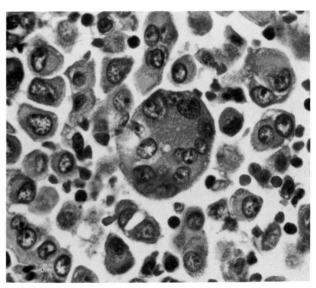

FIGURE 22–28. A giant multinucleated **mesothelial cell** possessing about 17 nuclei. It is accompanied by numerous hypertrophied mesothelial cells (cell block of pleural fluid; hematoxylin and eosin; ×528).

had only one nucleus. Mitotic figures were found in only 3 out of 1000 cells.

Cytoplasmic vacuolation, when present, may take several forms: (1) one or more tiny, unobtrusive vacuoles scattered throughout the cytoplasm but more likely to be near the nucleus, (2) a large, solitary vacuole that seems to displace the nucleus to the periphery of the cell and (3) an elongated perinuclear vacuole that curves around a segment of the nuclear membrane like a tiny sausage. It is not uncommon to find a mesothelial cell with a large, solitary vacuole and an excentric nucleus joined to a typical nonvacuolated mesothelial cell, clearly denoting the mesothelial lineage and benign nature of the vacuolated cell (Fig. 22–29).

Mesothelial cells articulate with each other in a characteristic manner. One form of articulation consists of cells joined at flattened apposing surfaces. Groups composed of two to four mesothelial cells are frequently seen with this type of articulation. Between the apposing cellular surfaces, clefts or "windows" may develop suggesting that the conjoined cells are about to become detached from each other (Fig. 22–30). Less commonly seen, although with the same type of articulation, are larger sheets of mesothelial cells with a mosaic appearance composed of up to about ten cells. Another articulation characteristic of mesothelial cells is illustrated in Figure 22–31, in which the cytoplasm of one cell appears to be "grasping" an adjacent cell. This type of articulation is carried a stage further when the cytoplasm of the grasping cell seems to be about to pinch off the cytoplasm of the cell being grasped. The final scene in this visual sequence is the appearance of one mesothelial cell within another. It should be mentioned that all of these types of articulation can be seen, although much less frequently, in adenocarcinoma cells in serous fluids.

Tissue fragments composed of mesothelial cells characteristically have knobby contours due to individual

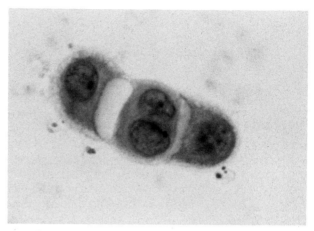

FIGURE 22–30. A short chain of **mesothelial cells** joined at flattened apposed surfaces. "Windows" are forming between the cells (smear of pleural fluid; Papanicolaou stains; × 1320).

cells protruding from the periphery (Figs. 22–32 and 22–33). In smears, it is the presence of these more-visible protruding cells that allows the mass of cells to be identified as mesothelial. Occasionally, however, large, round, smoothly contoured clusters of mesothelial cells are found (Fig. 22–34), a situation in which it is more difficult to determine the mesothelial nature of the cells. It should be possible, however, to detect a fine rim of cytoplasm at the edge of the cluster showing the peripheral cytoplasmic fading characteristic of mesothelial cells. Furthermore, it should be possible to discern that the nuclei are smoothly contoured, a feature against a diagnosis of adenocarcinoma. Cell block preparations can be extremely useful in this situation because they may more readily reveal the benign nature of these fragments. Should any doubt remain as to whether the cells are mesothelial or adenocarcinomatous, immunocytochemistry applied to cell block material will usually enable one to distinguish between mesothelial and adenocarcinoma cells (see section on mesothelioma, later in this chapter).

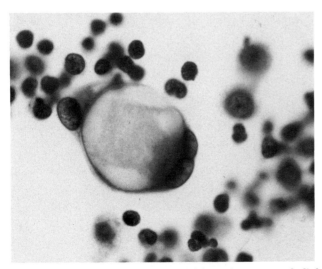

FIGURE 22–29. A large vacuolated binucleate **mesothelial cell** attached to a small, nonvacuolated mesothelial cell (smear of pleural fluid; Papanicolaou stain; × 825).

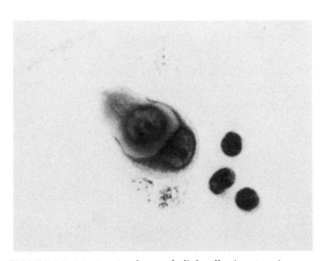

FIGURE 22–31. A pair of **mesothelial cells** showing the type of articulation where one cell seems to be clasping another (smear of pleural fluid; Papanicolaou stain; × 1320).

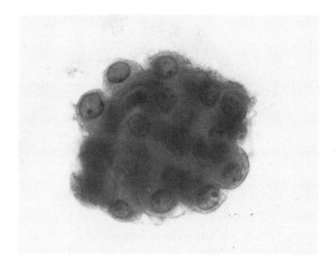

FIGURE 22–32. A tissue fragment composed of **mesothelial cells**. The fragment has a "knobby" contour. The protruding cells at the periphery show mesothelial characteristics (smear of pericardial fluid; Papanicolaou stain; ×825). (Courtesy of Dr. Sudha R. Kini, Detroit, Michigan.)

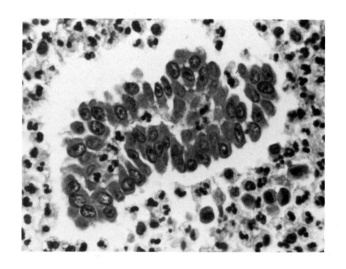

FIGURE 22–33. A tissue fragment composed of **mesothelial cells**. Note the characteristic scalloped contour (cell block of pleural fluid; hematoxylin and eosin; ×528).

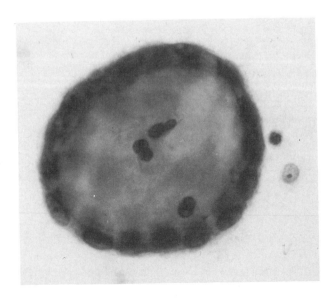

FIGURE 22–34. A smoothly contoured tissue fragment covered by **mesothelial cells**. This fragment has an "empty" appearance due to its acellular core of collagen. By focusing up and down on the center it is possible to detect an upper and lower plane of cells (smear of pericardial fluid; Papanicolaou stain; ×825).

Giant multinucleated mesothelial cells are not uncommon, having been reported in 26% of 396 serous fluids.[140] They may be misinterpreted as giant multinucleated macrophages. However, such macrophages are a rarity in serous fluids, being found almost exclusively in specimens from patients with rheumatoid pleuritis or pericarditis.[161] Furthermore, the cytoplasm of giant multinucleated mesothelial cells does not exhibit the fine, diffuse vacuolation typical of macrophages. It may contain several well-defined vacuoles, with the residual nonvacuolated cytoplasm being typical of mesothelial cells in general. In contrast to the nuclei of macrophages, the nuclei of giant multinucleated mesothelial cells are smoothly contoured with well-defined membranes, and they contain prominent nucleoli. Giant multinucleated mesothelial cells are always accompanied by numerous smaller cells whose mesothelial lineage is obvious (see Fig. 22–28).

In light-microscopic preparations it may sometimes be difficult to distinguish between vacuolated mesothelial cells and macrophages because mesothelial cells may acquire large solitary vacuoles or numerous small cytoplasmic vacuoles similar to those seen in macrophages. A useful point of discrimination is that when such a vacuolated cell is joined to a cell that is obviously mesothelial (see Fig. 22–29), then the former cell is also undoubtedly mesothelial. In reality, having to make such a distinction is not of great practical importance.

"Atypical" and "Reactive" Mesothelial Cells

We commonly come across reports from other laboratories of "atypical" or "reactive" mesothelial cells, overused and inappropriate designations given to mesothelial cells that are merely hypertrophic (Fig. 22–35) and usually hyperplastic. Furthermore, meso-

thelial cells that are not well spread and well stained, especially if the serous fluid is bloody, may appear dark, thereby creating diagnostic uncertainty; hence, the use of the terms atypical and reactive. Perhaps it is the quality of the preparation that should be regarded as atypical rather than the state of the mesothelial cells. Furthermore, the use of this term is misleading to clinicians because they may misinterpret it as signifying a precursor of mesothelial neoplasia. If hypertrophic and hyperplastic mesothelial cells are recognized as such and are a nonspecific finding, then there is no point in reporting their presence, which merely denotes that something has stimulated the cells to undergo enlargement and proliferation.

Mesothelial Cells in Wet Films

The morphologic features of mesothelial cells seen in Papanicolaou stained smears are also visible in toluidine blue stained wet films, with several important differences. First, mesothelial cells in wet films are noticeably larger than those in permanent, wet fixed preparations. (This size difference applies to all types of cells examined in wet films.) Another difference is that mesothelial cells in wet films frequently contain tiny, glistening, golden, cytoplasmic lipidic inclusions that are not seen in the permanent preparations because they are dissolved by solvents in the fixative or staining circuit. Finally, the types of articulation characteristic of mesothelial cells are usually more difficult to discern in wet films, although careful observation will reveal that they are present.

Cell Block Preparations

Mesothelial cells in cell block preparations generally do not present any particular diagnostic difficulty. Because these preparations are stained with hematoxylin and eosin, the cytoplasmic staining reaction is one of various shades of pink. Except for this, all of the previously mentioned morphologic features of mesothelial cells seen in Papanicolaou stained smears are discernible in cell block preparations, although not as readily as in smears. Large fragments of mesothelium may be seen in cell block preparations that, because of their size, could be mistaken for fragments of carcinoma. However, apart from any nuclear features that signify benignity or malignancy, fragments of carcinoma tend to occur in solid, two-dimensional masses, whereas fragments of mesothelium present as monolayer strips of cells,[142] seen in their most exuberant form in peritoneal washings (see the following).

Peritoneal Washings and Culdocentesis Specimens

Mesothelial cells collected by culdocentesis or peritoneal washing present some morphologic features different from those of mesothelial cells exfoliated into

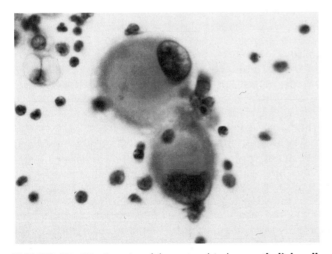

FIGURE 22–35. A pair of hypertrophied **mesothelial cells** from a patient with hepatic cirrhosis. Mesothelial cells such as these are frequently reported as "atypical" or "reactive" (smear of peritoneal fluid; Papanicolaou stain; × 528).

spontaneously occurring effusions. Apart from specimens obtained by culdocentesis, these intraoperative specimens are virtually all obtained during laparotomy for gynecologic surgery. Such specimens may consist of only a few milliliters of fluid found in the cul-de-sac (pouch of Douglas) when the abdomen is opened. On the other hand, the volume of the peritoneal washings sent to our laboratory ranges from about 25 to 50 ml.

Mesothelium obtained by this procedure is frequently seen as large, flat sheets of cells fitting together in an orderly mosaic (Fig. 22–36). The size of these sheets should, in itself, indicate that they are benign fragments of mesothelium, detached either by surgical trauma or by the washing procedure (which includes suction of the fluid used for the washing). Flatness of the sheets, the orderly mosaicism of their cells and the absence of nuclear features of malignancy are further indications of their benignity.

Specimens obtained at laparotomy may contain large fragments of mesothelium presenting as coiled monolayer strips of cells, especially well seen in cell blocks. A commonly seen variant of detached mesothelium in these intraoperative specimens, especially in cell block preparations, is a monolayer of mesothelium folded over on itself to give the appearance of a papillary frond, such as might become detached from a papillary ovarian carcinoma (Fig. 22–37). However, because they are composed of monolayers of cells apposed to each other, these pseudopapillations do not possess a connective tissue core. No matter what configurations these detached fragments of mesothelium acquire, careful attention to morphologic detail will fail to reveal convincing evidence of malignancy.

Diagnostic Pitfalls

Papillary fragments of mesothelium that become detached from the serosa, especially during peritoneal

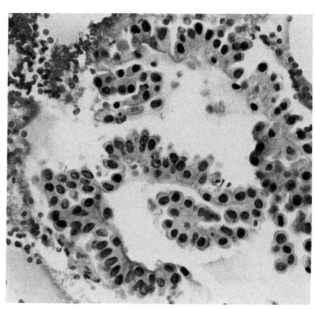

FIGURE 22–37. Coiled monolayer strips of **mesothelium** resembling fragments of papillary neoplasm. Note the absence of any connective tissue core (cell block of peritoneal washing; hematoxylin and eosin; × 330).

washing, may consist of a connective tissue core covered by a layer of mesothelial cells (see Fig. 22–24); such connective tissue cores may become calcified. Kern[117] described a specimen obtained by culdocentesis that contained psammoma bodies and that was reported as being consistent with papillary hyperplasia of ovarian capsular tissue (germinal epithelium) or papillary adenocarcinoma. Subsequent hysterectomy and bilateral salpingo-oophorectomy revealed only periovarian fibrous adhesions associated with small papillary mesothelial proliferations containing psammoma bodies. This and other reported examples,[197] combined with our own experience of finding psammoma bodies in peritoneal washings from patients with no evidence of cancer, illustrate that malignancy must not be diagnosed on the presence of psammoma bodies alone. The diagnosis must be based on the accepted nuclear changes of malignancy in any accompanying cells.

Becker and coworkers[12] reported an example of overdiagnosis due to the presence in pericardial fluid of exfoliated micropapillary excrescences covered by mesothelial cells. The original diagnosis of adenocarcinoma was proved to be erroneous by necropsy, when the source of the mesothelial cell–covered papillary fragments was shown to be a benign fibrous "papilloma" on the parietal pericardium about one eighth of an inch in diameter. Such benign papillary proliferations may develop on any serous surface and are usually attributed, especially in the female pelvis, to the effects of previous inflammation, including that induced by surgical operation. They do not cause effusion.

With the Papanicolaou stain, such fragments of collagenous connective tissue covered by mesothelium appear as smoothly contoured, homogeneous, pale green bodies covered by a layer of flattened cells (Fig.

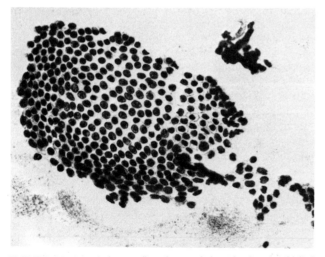

FIGURE 22–36. A large, flat sheet of detached **mesothelial cells**. Apart from the appearance of individual cells, the large size of this sheet and its orderly mosaicism are against the diagnosis of carcinoma (smear of peritoneal washing; Papanicolaou stain; × 165).

22–38). Such fragments are most frequently seen in washings obtained at the time of gynecologic surgery or in culdocentesis specimens. The three-dimensional, spheroid nature of these fragments is detected by focusing up and down on the fragment and finding that the covering cells are visible at different planes. An inexperienced observer might regard these characteristic fragments as adenocarcinoma cells distended by mucin. Apart from their nuclei not possessing indisputable features of malignancy, any doubt as to the composition of these fragments can be settled by cell block preparations, which show the characteristic eosinophilic collagenous cores.

To anyone embarking on cytopathology it soon becomes obvious that the mesothelial cell in all of its variations offers the greatest potential for being misinterpreted as metastatic adenocarcinoma. Probably every seasoned cytopathologist has at sometime or other misinterpreted mesothelial cells as adenocarcinoma. The important question is how can one eliminate or at least diminish the chance and frequency of such error. The first step is to rely only on well-prepared specimens in which the cells are wet fixed (if the Papanicolaou stain is being used), not overstained and easily visible. With such preparations the mesothelial nature of individual cells should be obvious. Smears that are too thick or very bloody increase the potential for overdiagnosis. In such smears the staining reaction of mesothelial cells is darker, with the consequence that their nuclei appear hyperchromatic and suggestive of malignancy. However, the benign nature of mesothelial cells in the thicker areas of the smear may be deduced by finding at the periphery of the smear, where the staining reaction is not as dark, that none of the cells look malignant; instead, they appear mesothelial and benign. This is an important practical point in dealing with thick, overstained preparations. If one can be satisfied that cells at the periphery of the smear are not malignant, one should assume that less visible but similar cells elsewhere in the smear are also benign.

When, because of inexperience or diffidence, the cytologic picture remains unsolved or ambiguous or when mesothelial cells appear to be hypertrophic or hyperplastic (atypical or reactive), we prefer to adopt a pragmatic approach and report such specimens as negative for neoplastic cells. As mentioned previously, a report of atypical or reactive mesothelial cells may introduce an element of uncertainty about whether neoplastic cells are really present or absent in a specimen. Therefore, we do not report the presence of such cells. If doubt remains whether cells are mesothelial or carcinomatous, this should be stated in straightforward terms, leaving it to the clinician to decide if further investigation is necessary.

Red Blood Cells

The sediment obtained by centrifugation of most serous fluids, even those that appear not to be bloodstained, contains a layer of red blood cells visible to the naked eye. When the centrifuged deposit contains a deep layer of red cells, dipping the loop only a millimeter or so too deeply into the deposit may result in smears having a high proportion of red cells and very few cells from the buffy layer.

Cytology

Red blood cells are readily recognized in Papanicolaou stained smears as neatly round, orange-red discoids about 7 μ in diameter, although many may become distorted into elongated forms in the process of spreading the cellular sample. Fixation may cause red cells to undergo lysis, leaving residual empty cell membranes with a slightly cyanophilic staining reaction. Hemoglobin released from these cells may remain as part of the proteinaceous background of a smear, thereby imparting a reddish cast to the smeared material, both to the naked eye and under the microscope. In the toluidine blue stained wet films red blood cells are unstained, remaining a light straw yellow.

Apart from these artifacts, normal red cells generally show little morphologic variation. Spherocytic forms have been described in air-dried preparations of pleural fluid from patients with hemothorax.[213, 215] Heinz bodies, globules of degraded hemoglobin formed in stagnant collections of blood, may be seen in Papanicolaou stained smears, but they are more readily identified in the stained wet films (Fig. 22–39).

Immature red cells may be present in serous fluids when they are present in circulating blood, as, for example, in leukoerythroblastic anemia, chronic myelogenous leukemia and myeloproliferative disorders.[215] However, we have found it virtually impossible to discern these immature forms in smears prepared by the Papanicolaou method; air-dried Romanowsky stained smears are far superior for this purpose. Neutrophilic leukocytes may undergo degenerative changes

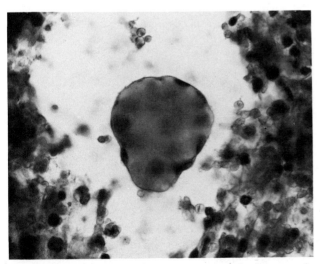

FIGURE 22–38. A tissue fragment composed of a smooth, acellular collagenous core covered by flattened **mesothelial cells** (smear of peritoneal washing; Papanicolaou stain; ×412).

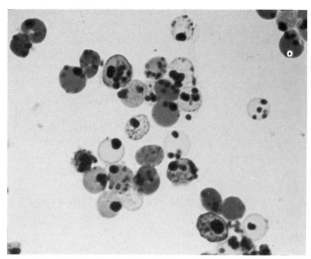

FIGURE 22–39. Red blood cells, many containing Heinz bodies, globules of degraded hemoglobin (wet film of pleural fluid; toluidine blue; ×825).

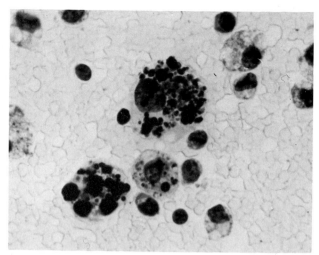

FIGURE 22–40. Red blood cells, lymphocytes and macrophages. Several macrophages contain dark granules of hemosiderin. In wet films hemosiderin stains dark blue (wet film of pleural fluid; toluidine blue; ×528).

in which their nuclei become pyknotic, a change that simulates normoblasts.

Intraerythrocytic crystallization of hemoglobin, a result of polymerization of the hemoglobin molecules, may occur in peripheral blood in certain hemoglobinopathies, being more pronounced in hemoglobin C disease. Zaharopoulos and Wong[260] described two examples of such crystallization in red cells in pleural fluids in patients who had neither clinical nor other evidence of hemoglobinopathy. Under laboratory conditions they produced intraerythrocytic crystallization of hemoglobin in specimens of hemorrhagic pleural fluid by subjecting them to agents that induced decreased oxygen concentration and osmotic dehydration of the cells. They suggested that a similar process takes place in fluid accumulated in confined body spaces such as the pleural cavity.

Intact red blood cells may be phagocytosed by macrophages. When the red cells disintegrate their hemoglobin is converted into hematoidin or hemosiderin which, if present in a large enough amount, will impart a distinctly yellow (xanthochromic) appearance to the supernatant. In stained wet films, hematoidin pigment may occasionally be seen as sheaves of fine, elongated, yellow-brown extracellular crystals (see Fig. 22–7), whereas hemosiderin is seen as dark blue granules in the cytoplasm of macrophages (Fig. 22–40). In Papanicolaou stained smears hematoidin retains the same appearance, but the staining reaction of hemosiderin is golden brown to olive green. Hemosiderin gives a positive staining reaction for iron (Perls' test), whereas hematoidin does not.

Neutrophil Leukocytes

Almost every specimen of serous fluid contains neutrophil leukocytes. Their number varies from just the occasional cell to highly cellular purulent fluids in which all or almost all of the cells are neutrophils. Purulent fluids are of a light yellow turbidity and a creamy

consistency. If infected, they may be malodorous. Neutrophils are readily recognized in toluidine blue stained wet films, Papanicolaou stained permanent smears and cell block preparations.

Inflammation, infarction or rupture of an organ are the principal causes of serous effusion containing numerous neutrophils. Hypertrophied mesothelial cells may also be present in the early stages of acute inflammation, but as the neutrophils dominate the picture, the mesothelial cells die and disintegrate. Even in purulent effusions a small percent of the cells may be macrophages or lymphocytes or both.

Cytology

In wet films, the cytoplasm remains unstained or weakly stained (Fig. 22–41). It is finely granular, and

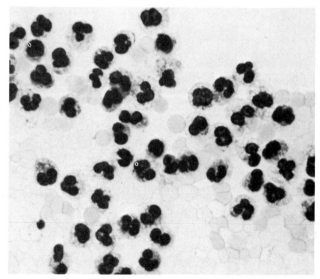

FIGURE 22–41. Neutrophilic leukocytes. Their cytoplasmic granularity is hardly visible (wet film of peritoneal fluid; toluidine blue; ×528).

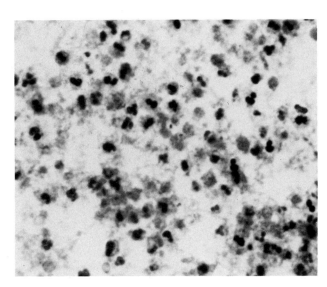

FIGURE 22–42. Empyema fluid containing numerous **neutrophilic leukocytes**. Many have become necrotic and appear as light gray particles that are disintegrating to form the granular background (smear of pleural fluid; Papanicolaou stain; ×528).

the granules may exhibit brownian movement. Their nuclei are usually trilobed, although two-, four- and five-lobed nuclei are not uncommon. In Papanicolaou stained smears, neutrophils are smaller, and their cytoplasm exhibits a faintly cyanophilic staining reaction. In these preparations, as in cell blocks, the cytoplasmic granules are virtually impossible to discern, although a suggestion of cytoplasmic granularity may be detected.

Neutrophils in noninfected fluids are generally well preserved. In infected purulent fluids neutrophils degenerate; in some fluids virtually every neutrophil is necrotic. Necrotic neutrophils become transformed into ill-defined, light gray to gray-blue particles without any visible nuclear material or cytoplasmic granularity (Fig. 22–42). Nuclei of necrotic cells may also condense into round, solitary, deeply cyanophilic masses, or each lobe may become pyknotic (Fig. 22–43) to give the picture of "mercury drop" karyorrhexis.

In stained wet films, neutrophils may contain well-defined, light yellow, glistening, refractile cytoplasmic granules of lipid (Fig. 22–44). These granules may be so numerous that they crowd the cytoplasm. We have observed lipid-containing neutrophils in serous fluids from patients with a wide variety of neoplastic and non-neoplastic conditions, an observation confirmed by reports describing them in pleural fluids caused by tuberculosis, rheumatoid disease and a variety of neoplasms.[57, 58, 167] Whenever neutrophils contain lipid droplets, they are also likely to be found in macrophages and mesothelial cells in the fluid. These lipidic granules are not visible in Papanicolaou stained smears or cell block preparations.

Eosinophilic Leukocytes

Eosinophilic Pleural Effusion

Several comprehensive reviews going back to the early days of cytodiagnosis attest to the fascination that eosinophilic effusions, especially pleural effusions,

have held for clinicians.[15, 222] However, the arbitrary criterion for designating a pleural fluid as "eosinophilic" has varied from a fluid with as few as 5% to one with at least 50% of the cells being eosinophils. For the sake of argument, we have adopted a criterion of a concentration of 10% or more as used by Koss.[126]

Eosinophilic pleural effusion has been reported in association with a wide variety of conditions: allergy, autoimmune disorders, pneumonia (including viral pneumonia), pulmonary infarct, fungal infection, parasitic infection, malignant neoplasms, pulmonary tuberculosis, artificial and spontaneous pneumothorax and hemothorax, including that induced by thoracic trauma.[15, 213, 231] Eighty-one of the 127 (64%) cases of eosinophilic pleural effusion analyzed by Spriggs and Boddington[213] and 8 of 30 (27%) analyzed by Veress and coworkers[231] were associated with some form of thoracic trauma. Apart from accidental trauma, these series include the trauma associated with therapeutic

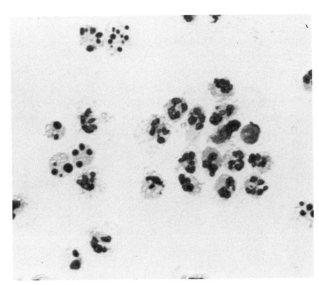

FIGURE 22–43. Neutrophilic leukocytes. The nuclei of several have degenerated to form neatly round dense cyanophilic particles (wet film of pleural fluid; toluidine blue; ×528).

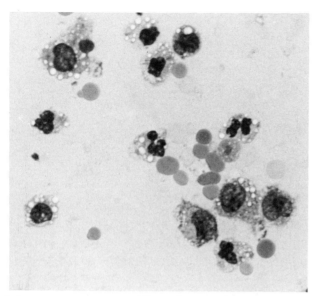

FIGURE 22–44. Neutrophils and macrophages containing lipid vacuoles, a nonspecific finding (wet film of pleural fluid; toluidine blue; ×528).

pneumothorax, thoracotomy and that associated with repeated aspiration of pleural fluid.

Most of these examples of trauma would have been associated with some degree of hemothorax, suggesting that red blood cells exert a chemotactic influence on eosinophil migration into the pleural cavity. However, Spriggs and Boddington,[213] noting that hemothorax, frequently mentioned as a cause of pleural eosinophilia, is often associated with pneumothorax, raised the question of whether the eosinophilia is induced by air in the pleural cavity. Even if blood does stimulate pleural eosinophilia, it is important to remember that a high proportion of eosinophilic pleural effusions are not bloodstained.[125]

In keeping with air being the stimulator of pleural eosinophilia, the literature from the era of therapeutic pneumothorax well documents the appearance of eosinophils in the resulting effusions.[50, 188, 196] This observation prompted Spriggs[209] to re-examine pleural fluids from seven cases of spontaneous pneumothorax, of which five were eosinophilic. He concluded that pleural eosinophilia is the normal reaction of the pleura to the introduction of air into the pleural cavity and suggested that the reaction is more likely due to suspended particles of animal or vegetable origin than to the air itself.

When pneumothorax can be excluded, the commonest causes of eosinophilic pleural effusion seem to be pulmonary infarct, pneumonia and neoplasm.[215] Hodgkin's disease is rarely associated with eosinophilic pleural effusion. Only a minority of cases can be attributed to recognizable hypersensitivity states, including parasitic infestation. Another cause of pleural eosinophilic effusion is the benign type of effusion associated with the inhalation of asbestos;[1] in a series of 60 cases, 26% showed eosinophilia of various degrees.[92]

When all of the possible causes of eosinophilic pleural effusions have been eliminated, there is a substantial residue of cases in which the cause can not be identified. For example, in 11 of 30 cases of Veress and coworkers[231] and 11 of 23 consecutive cases of eosinophilic pleural effusion in our laboratory (an aggregate of 42%), there were no data that adequately accounted for the effusions.

Despite the uncertainty surrounding the pathogenesis of idiopathic eosinophilic pleural effusions, they seem to have a good prognosis even in patients with a previous history of cancer. This was well illustrated by Veress and coworkers[231] who found that in 22 of their 30 patients, including six with a past history of cancer, the effusions eventually disappeared. Six of the 30 patients died from myocardial infarction, and two were lost to follow-up. Their series also showed a predominance of males with eosinophilic pleural effusions, in keeping with previous observations.[25, 77, 105, 125, 213]

Because it has been impossible to identify a single linking pathologic mechanism behind the formation of eosinophilic pleural effusion, it has been suggested that these effusions exists in two forms: an effusion of relatively acute onset related to an allergic reaction or to thoracic trauma,[14, 130] and the more chronic form with a longer clinical course.[231]

Eosinophilic Peritoneal Effusion

Eosinophilic peritoneal effusions are rare. We have no record of such an effusion in our laboratory. Examples have been reported of eosinophilic peritoneal effusion associated with malignant neoplasm,[228] various allergic states,[87, 88] parasitic infection,[190] eosinophilic gastroenteritis[67, 89, 100, 132, 157, 202] and chronic peritoneal dialysis.[38, 95, 121, 135] It is possible that one or more of the agents used in peritoneal dialysis, such as antiseptic, talc, particles of tubing and peritoneal catheters provoke a hypersensitivity reaction characterized by an efflux of eosinophils. In addition to eosinophilia, chronic peritoneal dialysis may stimulate mesothelial hypertrophy and hyperplasia.[60, 95]

Eosinophilic Pericardial Effusion

Eosinophilic pericardial effusion is even rarer than eosinophilic peritoneal effusion. We have never seen an example in our laboratory. A few examples have been reported in association with pulmonary eosinophilia,[42, 84, 109] including one associated with the use of the drug cromolyn sodium.[203] Examples of Hodgkin's disease[151] and of lymphocytic lymphoma[90] first manifesting themselves by eosinophilic effusion have been reported.

Cytology

Most serous fluids contain at least the occasional eosinophilic leukocyte, recognizable in toluidine blue stained wet films, Papanicolaou stained permanent smears and cell block preparations. Compared with neutrophils, eosinophils are slightly larger, their nuclei are generally bilobed and their cytoplasmic granules are larger and more readily visible. These morphologic features are recognizable in wet films (Fig. 22–45). Because the granules are not stained by toluidine blue they appear colorless or a pale yellow. Most eosinophils have bilobed nuclei, although many nuclei have three or occasionally four lobes. The lobes are slightly larger and more neatly round than those of neutrophils. A pyknotic form in which the nucleus is represented by a solitary chromatinic mass with no lobes is occasionally seen, especially in fluids that have stood for some time after aspiration.[213]

In Papanicolaou stained smears, eosinophils are smaller than in wet films and the cytoplasmic granules are much less obvious, frequently being manifested by only a fine eosinophilic granularity. In Papanicolaou stained smears the cytoplasmic staining reaction may be a light green with little or no granularity; such cells are recognized as eosinophils by their size and the bilobation of their nuclei. Cell block preparations demonstrate eosinophils well (Fig. 22–46). Eosinophils undergo necrosis, although we have not observed widespread necrosis of eosinophils in smears similar to that seen in neutrophils in empyema fluids. On a rare occasion we have seen a large aggregate of necrotic eosinophils in the cell block of an eosinophilic effusion.

Basophil Leukocytes and Mast Cells

Basophil leukocytes and mast cells are small, round cells whose cytoplasm contains round granules about 0.5 μ in diameter that stain purple with basic dyes. In

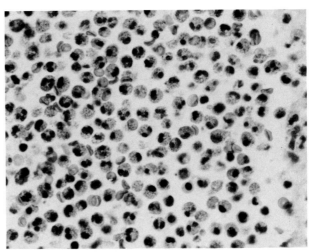

FIGURE 22–46. Eosinophilic effusion. Virtually all of the cells in this field are eosinophils (cell block of pleural fluid; hematoxylin and eosin; ×528).

staining, these granules often change the shade of the dye, the phenomenon of metachromasia. Mast cells presumably originate in connective tissues of the body, whereas basophils originate with other leukocytes in the bone marrow from which they enter the blood stream.

In our routinely prepared wet films, it is not uncommon to see the occasional basophil or mast cell. We have never found them in large numbers, although Spriggs and Boddington[213] recorded several examples in which the basophil content was 10% or more. In one of their cases (chronic myeloid leukemia) the percent of basophils was 27.

Cytology

Mast cells and basophils are readily recognized with a Romanowsky stain, but they are not recognizable in Papanicolaou stained smears or in cell blocks stained with hematoxylin and eosin. They can be recognized in toluidine blue stained wet films (Fig. 22–47) in which the granules are a delicate purple-pink, quite different from the deep blue of the stain itself.

Mast cells, slightly larger than basophils, are about the size of small mesothelial cells. Their nuclei are round or oval and centrally placed, whereas the nuclei of basophils are usually bilobed. The cytoplasm of mast cells is entirely occupied with granules; the cytoplasm of basophils contains far fewer.

Macrophages

Cytology

Macrophages are found in various proportions in almost every serous fluid. Their size varies considerably, from about 15 to 100 μ in diameter, with most within the range of 20 to 40 μ. In smears the typical macrophage is easily identified by its size, excentric

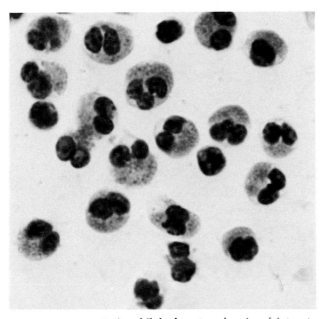

FIGURE 22–45. Eosinophil leukocytes showing faint cytoplasmic granularity, typical with the Papanicolaou stain. Note that most of the nuclei are bilobed (smear of pleural fluid; Papanicolaou stain; ×1320).

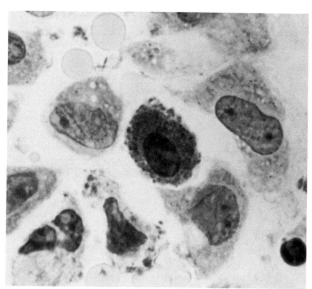

FIGURE 22–47. A **mast cell** surrounded by macrophages. The cytoplasmic granules of the mast cell are metachromatic and show a delicate purple-pink staining reaction (wet film of peritoneal fluid; toluidine blue; ×1320).

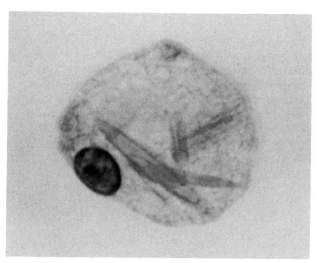

FIGURE 22–49. A **macrophage** containing needle-like crystals in its cytoplasm, probably immunoglobulins synthesized by plasma cells. The patient had an indolent plasma-cell dyscrasia, resulting in excessive production of a monoclonal immunoglobulin (smear of peritoneal fluid; Papanicolaou stain; ×320). (Reproduced with permission from Martin AW, Karstens PHB, Yam LT: Crystalline deposits in ascites in a case of cryoglobulinemia. Acta Cytol 31:631–636, 1987.)

round or bean-shaped nucleus and lightly stained lacy cytoplasm (Fig. 22–48). Because macrophages are phagocytic, their cytoplasm may contain leukocytes, nuclear particles, red blood cells, carbon particles, lipid droplets, melanin or hemosiderin (see Fig. 22–40). Crystalline cytoplasmic inclusions (Fig. 22–49) in macrophages in ascitic fluid from a patient with an indolent plasma cell dyscrasia, resulting in excessive production of immunoglobulin, have been reported.[146]

Macrophages tend to be discrete but may appear to coalesce, presumably due to their long microvilli becoming entangled. This gives a loose, sheet-like ap-

pearance to a group of macrophages (Fig. 22–50). Such sheets do not have the tight cohesiveness and sharp definition of sheets of mesothelial cells; they tend to straggle at the periphery, and the overall cohesiveness of the group has a loose quality, with spaces between individual cells. Furthermore, the lacy, porous appearance of the cytoplasm contrasts sharply with the dense cytoplasm of mesothelial cells.

Macrophages may contain large solitary or loculate cytoplasmic vacuoles that appear to displace the nucleus to the periphery of the cell (Fig. 22–51), a picture suggestive of signet-ring adenocarcinoma. This type of

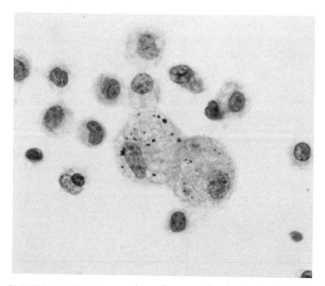

FIGURE 22–48. Large and small **macrophages**. Several appear to be cohesive. Note the round to bean-shaped nuclei, the "lacy" cytoplasm and the phagocytosed dark cytoplasmic particles in two of the cells (smear of pleural fluid; Papanicolaou stain; ×528).

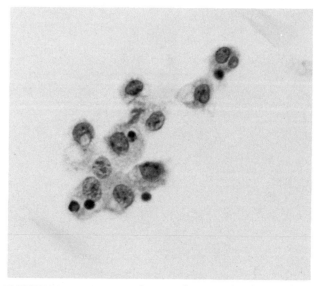

FIGURE 22–50. A group of **macrophages** with a loose, sheet-like appearance (smear of pleural fluid; Papanicolaou stain; ×528).

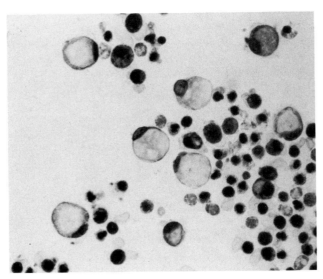

FIGURE 22–51. Lymphoid cells and highly vacuolated **macrophages** with a signet-ring appearance (smear of pleural fluid; toluidine blue; ×330).

vacuolation may be seen not only in macrophages and adenocarcinoma cells but also in mesothelial cells. In cell block preparations of a spontaneously formed clot, groups of macrophages that have become tightly packed against each other as the clot contracted may be seen (Fig. 22–52). These compact groups of macrophages may be readily mistaken for fragments of adenocarcinoma.

Degenerating mesothelial cells with finely vacuolated cytoplasm resemble macrophages. It is not uncommon to find a group of cells consisting of obvious mesothelial cells, cells that appear to be macrophages and cells that seem to be intermediate forms. This observation, combined with electron-microscopic and experimental observations, has been adduced to support the transformation of mesothelial cells into macrophages.[215] Whether this does or does not happen is not a matter of great diagnostic importance.

Macrophages usually have a single nucleus, although binucleation is not uncommon. The finding of giant multinucleated macrophages formed by fusion of a number of macrophages or by mitotic division of a nucleus is a rarity, virtually confined to effusions caused by rheumatoid pleuritis or rheumatoid pericarditis (see subsequently). Giant multinucleated mesothelial cells are seen with much more frequency, and whenever a cell is regarded as a giant multinucleated macrophage, the question should be raised as to whether it is really a mesothelial cell. The presence of giant multinucleated macrophages in peritoneal fluid should raise the question of the paracentesis needle having entered an ovarian cyst. Ovarian cysts frequently contain numerous macrophages, many of the giant multinucleated type.

Lymphoid Cells

Lymphoid cells in effusions are similar to those in lymphoid tissue in general, with most being of the small, mature type. T and B lymphocytes cannot be distinguished in routine preparations, but can be identified by immunocytochemical staining using monoclonal antibodies. Most lymphoid cells in benign effusions are of T cell origin.

Cytology

Almost every serous fluid contains at least a few lymphoid cells, readily recognized in Papanicolaou stained smears as small cells with little or no cytoplasm dominated by round deeply staining nuclei (Fig. 22–53). Their size varies according to the amount of drying occurring during preparation of the smear and prior to

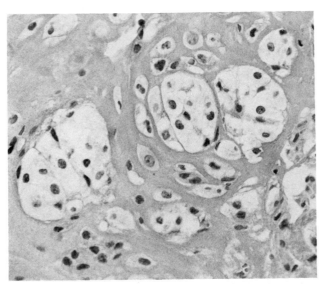

FIGURE 22–52. Groups of cohesive **macrophages** that had become packed against each other as the spontaneously formed clot contracted. This specimen had been mistakenly diagnosed as metastatic adenocarcinoma (cell block of pleural fluid; hematoxylin and eosin; ×330).

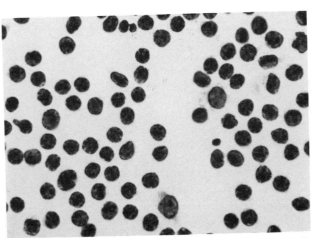

FIGURE 22–53. Numerous **lymphoid cells.** Most are small, mature lymphocytes. Others, with larger, paler nuclei, are immunoblasts, some with prominent nucleoli (smear of pleural fluid; Papanicolaou stain; ×825).

fixation. In the thicker parts of a smear, where air-drying is minimal, the lymphoid cells are smaller, whereas at the periphery of a smear, where some air-drying is almost inevitable, lymphoid cells have a larger diameter and appear flatter and less darkly stained. This variation in size and staining reaction is not seen in cell block preparations.

The nuclei of mature lymphocytes are neatly round, although some may be slightly indented or notched. Nucleoli are difficult to find in the Papanicolaou smears, although they are frequently visible in wet films. When lymphocytes are present in large numbers it is customary to find a few less mature, slightly larger lymphoid cells. In these less mature forms the chromatin is paler and nucleoli are visible (see Fig. 22–53). Cytoplasm, although scanty, is most readily seen in stained wet films and in Papanicolaou stained smears in which they had undergone momentary drying before they were fixed. The cytoplasm appears usually as a small, eccentric tag, although in the air-dried cells it may be seen to circumscribe the nucleus completely. Lymphoid cells with endoplasmic reticulum distended by immunoglobulin in the form of hyaline droplets (Mott cells[155]) are occasionally found (Fig. 22–54). Intracytoplasmic droplets of immunoglobulin have also been described in cells of lymphoplasmacytoid lymphoma in effusions.[257]

Mature plasma cells similar to those in bone marrow may be found, usually in effusions containing many lymphoid cells (Fig. 22–55). Larger, less mature appearing plasmacytoid cells are also frequently seen in such effusions; they may contain two or more nuclei.

Apart from their size and shape, one of the most important features distinguishing lymphoid cells from those of small-cell carcinoma is their property of remaining separated from each other. In contrast, the cells of small-cell carcinomas form cohesive clusters. A small number of lymphoid cells will be found that touch each other, but the contact, involving only a small segment of the periphery of each cell, is reminiscent of a kiss, whereas the contact between cells of small-cell carcinoma is more of an embrace. This

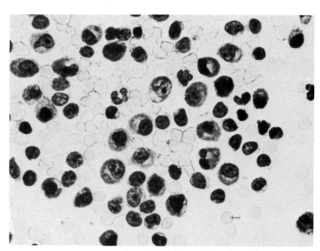

FIGURE 22–55. Mixed inflammatory picture consisting of **lymphocytes, plasma cells** and the occasional **neutrophil** (wet film of pleural fluid; toluidine blue; ×528).

property of lymphoid cells being separated is even obvious in cell block preparations.

In contrast to purulent effusions, those dominated by non-neoplastic lymphoid cells contain only a very small percent of necrotic cells. A prolonged search under high power is usually needed to find what seems to be a necrotic lymphocyte. Such a necrotic lymphocyte may show the type of karyorrhexis consisting of tiny round particles reminiscent of a dispersed drop of mercury (mercury drop karyorrhexis). This type of karyorrhexis, difficult to find in benign lymphocytic effusions, is frequently seen in effusions containing lymphoma cells.[149]

Megakaryocytes

Morphologically normal megakaryocytes are a rare finding in serous fluids. Almost all of the reported examples were associated with a myeloproliferative disorder, lymphoma or metastatic carcinoma, situations in which bone marrow was replaced either by neoplastic cells or fibrous connective tissue, resulting in extramedullary hemopoiesis immediately adjacent to a serous cavity.[129, 177, 213, 215, 220, 232, 233, 256]

We know of only one reported case in which the presence of megakaryocytes in a serous fluid was clearly not associated with extramedullary hemopoiesis.[11] The patient developed hemorrhagic pleural effusion due to an overdose of anticoagulant, and the pleural fluid contained megakaryocytes. Because necropsy did not reveal myeloid metaplasia or a myeloproliferative disorder, their presence in the effusion was attributed to the hemorrhagic condition of the lung, which enabled megakaryocyte-containing blood from pulmonary capillaries (where megakaryocytes are normally found) to enter the pleural cavity. The megakaryocytes in this case, as in most cases associated with extramedullary hemopoiesis, were of the classic giant cell type, with abundant cytoplasm and multilobed nuclei (Fig. 22–56), similar to those in bone marrow.

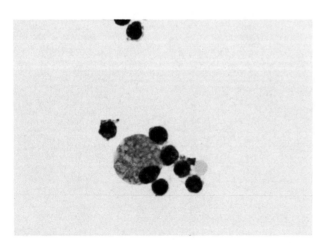

FIGURE 22–54. A Mott cell. A lymphoid cell with endoplasmic reticulum distended by droplets of immunoglobulin (wet film of pleural fluid; toluidine blue; ×528).

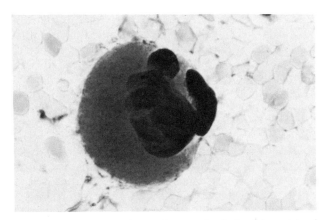

FIGURE 22–56. Normal **megakaryocyte** derived from blood that had oozed from the pulmonary parenchyma into the pleural cavity (wet film of pleural fluid; toluidine blue; ×660).

Detached Ciliary Tufts (DCTs)

In 1953, Ebner[51] described motile ciliated cellular fragments in fluid obtained from benign ovarian cysts; other authors have also described the presence of such cellular fragments, DCTs, in nonascitic fluid aspirated from the peritoneal cavity by laparotomy or laparoscopy[34, 166, 182, 200] or in peritoneal dialysate.[192] The phenomenon has been likened to *ciliocytophthoria* (CCP), a term Papanicolaou coined to describe degenerated ciliated respiratory epithelial cells in sputum.[175] CCP is morphologically somewhat different from DCTs. DCTs consist of anucleated fragments of ciliated columnar epithelial cells derived from the fallopian tube. In contrast, cells described under the term CCP may still contain nuclei, and frequently they contain eosinophilic cytoplasmic inclusions, a manifestation of degeneration. Neither nuclei nor cytoplasmic inclusions are seen in DCTs.

Cytology

In all of the reported cases of DCTs in fluid from the peritoneal cavity the patients were female, and all of them had their fallopian tubes in place, evidence of the tubal origin of DCTs. Very occasionally a peritoneal washing may contain a large fragment of ciliated glandular epithelium, presumably derived from a fallopian tube.

DCTs are visible in toluidine blue stained wet films as tiny, ciliated, non-nucleated cellular fragments. If the specimen is fresh, they may be seen to execute a jerky rotating and linear movement. Because of this they have been mistaken for a parasite.[134, 192]

DCTs are extremely difficult to find in wet fixed, Papanicolaou stained smears even when they are known to be present, having been seen in a wet film. Figure 22–57 illustrates DCTs in a stained wet film of fluid from the cul-de-sac of a woman undergoing laparotomy for a tubal ectopic pregnancy. Figure 22–58 is a scanning electron micrograph of fluid from the cul-de-sac of a woman undergoing laparotomy for a ruptured hydrosalpinx.

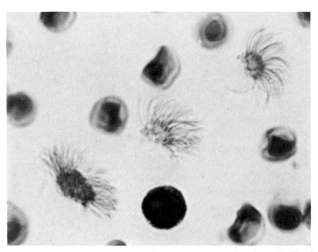

FIGURE 22–57. Three **detached ciliary tufts** (DCTs) in fluid obtained at the time of laparotomy performed because of a ruptured tubal pregnancy. These DCTs were highly mobile in the wet film (wet film of fluid from the cul-de-sac; toluidine blue; ×1320).

NON-NEOPLASTIC EFFUSIONS

Nonspecific Inflammation

Inflammation of a serous cavity is usually a complication of an underlying lesion, although not necessarily an inflammatory lesion. For example, pulmonary neo-

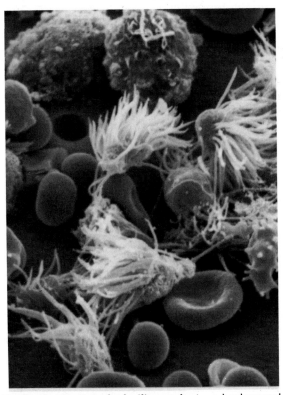

FIGURE 22–58. **Detached ciliary tufts** in a background of red blood cells and a lymphocyte. This fluid was obtained from the cul-de-sac at the time of laparotomy for ruptured hydrosalpinx (scanning electron micrograph; ×3400). (Courtesy of Dr. Theodore F. Beals, Ann Arbor, Michigan.)

plasms often induce inflammation of the surrounding pulmonary parenchyma (pneumonia), which frequently extends to the pleura. This results in pleuritis, clinically manifested as pleurisy, which may be accompanied by effusion showing a cytologic picture of inflammation with or without neoplastic cells. Another frequently occurring situation is when a sterile, noninflammatory effusion develops as, for example, in congestive heart failure. In this situation, the cytologic picture is devoid of any inflammatory component but, sooner or later, because of secondary infection of the pulmonary parenchyma, a frank inflammatory picture develops.

Almost all inflammatory pictures in serous fluids are nonspecific in that they do not reveal the etiologic background of the effusion. The cause of any effusion showing a nonspecific inflammatory picture must be determined by considering the clinical background of the patient, together with radiologic, biochemical, immunologic and microbiologic findings. Generally, all that one can determine on cytologic examination of a serous fluid showing an inflammatory picture is that the patient has, to a greater or lesser degree, inflammation of the serous cavity.

In addition to inflammatory cells, an inflammatory reaction also frequently results in a fibrinous exudate on the serosal surface. In smears this is seen as long, cyanophilic strands (Fig. 22–59); in cell blocks spontaneously formed fibrin forms dense fibrillary eosinophilic masses (see Fig. 22–9). Inflammation of a serous membrane frequently induces hypertrophy and hyperplasia of mesothelial cells so that the inflammatory cells are mixed with many enlarged, exfoliated mesothelial cells. On the other hand, some inflammatory pictures may be devoid of mesothelial cells either because the inflammatory reaction has caused the mesothelial cells to degenerate and disintegrate or because the inflammatory exudate so extensively covers and adheres to the mesothelium that mesothelial cells are prevented from exfoliating.

Nonspecific inflammatory pictures may show two extremes: acute purulent inflammation in which vir-

tually all of the cells are neutrophils or chronic inflammation in which the picture is virtually all lymphoid cells. Other markers of the various stages of inflammation, such as fibroblastic tissue, organizing fibrin or granulation tissue (see Fig. 22–14) are not seen in smears but may occasionally be found in cell block preparations.

In our experience, virtually all purulent effusions, with their creamy yellow-white consistency (and sometimes foul-smelling odor) have been derived from the pleural cavity. Purulent pericardial and peritoneal effusions have been rare; the former were caused by carcinomas metastatic to the pericardium, the latter by infarct of the small intestine. Most of the frankly purulent pleural effusions (pleural empyema) were secondary to primary bacterial pneumonias. The second most common cause was pneumonia secondary to neoplasm in the lungs; the third was pulmonary tuberculosis in which, presumably, secondary bacterial infection of an initially nonpurulent effusion had taken place. Other causes included esophageal carcinoma, thoracic surgery, pulmonary infarct and fistula.

The frankly purulent effusions are extremely cellular, with virtually all of their viable-appearing cells recognizable as neutrophils. Frequently a high proportion of the leukocytes undergo degeneration, resulting in individual cells appearing as smudgy anucleated blobs; it may need a careful search to find the occasional viable-appearing neutrophil. In some degenerate neutrophils the nuclei become extremely pyknotic, ending up as neatly rounded chromatinic masses, or the nuclei may fragment into tiny spheroid particles. Occasionally in such fluids it is possible to see microorganisms, either dispersed or in cloud-like cyanophilic colonies (see Fig. 22–22).

At the other extreme of the cytologic spectrum of nonspecific inflammation is the effusion in which the cytologic picture is dominated by lymphoid cells. This cytologic manifestation of chronic inflammation of the serous membrane may, as in the case of purulent effusions, be secondary to a variety of underlying conditions. Virtually all of our lymphocytic effusions have been pleural, and the underlying cause of most of these effusions was neoplasm in the lung, either primary or metastatic. The next most frequent cause was pulmonary tuberculosis in which, presumably, the tuberculous process in the pulmonary parenchyma had extended to the pleura. Next, were pleural lymphocytic effusions whose causes remained unknown and, finally, a small group of lymphocytic effusions with miscellaneous underlying causes.

It is well recognized that the presence of a uniform population of small lymphocytes in an effusion may be due to chronic lymphocytic leukemia or malignant lymphoma of the small-cell type as well as a chronic inflammatory process. Because these two neoplasms are more likely to be a manifestation of neoplastic change in B lymphocytes rather than T lymphocytes, enumeration of the two types of lymphocytes in a lymphocytic effusion might contribute to distinguishing between non-neoplastic and neoplastic lymphocytic effusions. This approach has been used with some

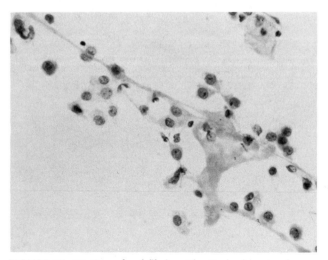

FIGURE 22–59. Strands of fibrin with attached **macrophages** (smear of pleural fluid; Papanicolaou stain; ×330).

success in making this discrimination.[45, 68] Most of the cells in non-neoplastic lymphocytic effusions were T cells, in contrast to the predominance of B cells in effusions of patients with lymphoma or leukemia. A different, nonimmunologic approach was used by Pettersson,[178] who demonstrated that the presence of acid alpha-naphthyl acetate esterase can also be used as a criterion to distinguish between T and B lymphocytes and that non-neoplastic lymphocytes in pleural effusions were usually of the T type.

The cytologic extremes of inflammation in serous effusions, purulent and lymphocytic, are the exception. Effusions showing any type of inflammatory component are more likely to show a mixed, less monotonous picture of inflammation, one composed of neutrophils, macrophages and lymphoid cells, including plasma cells. In addition, various numbers of mesothelial cells are likely to be present. In these mixed inflammatory effusions it is not possible to deduce the nature of the underlying histopathologic process causing the effusion. Furthermore, one cytologic picture of inflammation may become transformed into another as a result of treatment or the natural course of events, such as when an acute purulent inflammatory picture becomes transformed into one of lymphocytic effusion. We seldom have had the opportunity to witness such a transformation.

Specific Inflammatory Pictures

Two specific inflammatory pictures, that of rheumatoid disease and the other of systemic lupus erythematosus (SLE), may be seen in serous fluids. The cytologic picture of SLE has been reported in fluids from all three serous cavities, whereas the picture of rheumatoid serositis has been reported only in pleural and pericardial fluids.

Rheumatoid Disease

Rheumatoid disease acquires cytologic significance when the necrotizing granulomatous inflammation found in the synovium and subsynovial tissue of rheumatoid arthritic joints develops on the pleura or pericardium, resulting in effusion. A cytologic picture may be seen in the effusions that is not only unique but also pathognomonic of rheumatoid serositis,[161] a picture consisting of three elements: elongated spindle-shaped macrophages, multinucleated giant macrophages and necrotic granular background material. This triad is composed of cellular elements exfoliated from areas of inflammation of the serous membrane that are morphologic replicas of the necrotizing granulomatous inflammatory reaction composed of a palisade of macrophages that characterizes rheumatoid arthritis and rheumatoid subcutaneous nodules.

Histopathology. Figure 22–60 illustrates a needle biopsy specimen of parietal pleura of a woman with long-standing rheumatoid arthritis and a pleural effusion of 6 months' duration. It depicts the typical

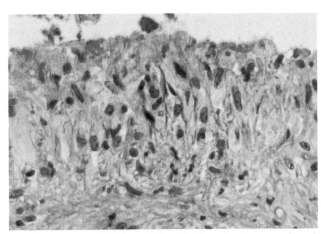

FIGURE 22–60. The pleural mesothelium has been replaced by a **palisade of macrophages**, the classic histologic picture of **rheumatoid pleuritis** (needle biopsy specimen; hematoxylin and eosin; × 400). (Reproduced with permission from Nosanchuk JS, Naylor B: A unique cytologic picture in pleural fluid from patients with rheumatoid arthritis. Am J Clin Pathol 50:330–335, 1968. Copyright by Williams & Wilkins, 1968.)

granulomatous inflammatory reaction of rheumatoid pleuritis, consisting of a palisade of elongated macrophages on the pleural surface. Such specimens may also contain multinucleated giant macrophages, a common manifestation of granulomatous inflammatory reactions in general. The unique cytologic picture of rheumatoid serositis in an effusion consists of viable and necrotic cells exfoliated from such areas.

Cytology. The number of elongated and giant multinucleated macrophages in rheumatoid effusions varies; they may be abundant, but generally they are not, and occasionally they are absent. The most striking examples of elongated macrophages are up to about 150 μ in length and are fairly uniform in thickness except for their tapering ends (Fig. 22–61).

Their cytoplasm is moderately dense, acidophilic or cyanophilic (depending on the thickness of the smear and the quality of the stain) and often has a finely granular ground glass appearance. The nuclei of these cells are frequently multiple and are usually round or oval, although they may be quite elongated as they conform to the shape of the cell. The giant multinucleated round or oval macrophages have a diameter of up to about 70 μ and may contain 20 or more nuclei (Fig. 22–62). Apart from the size and shape of these cells and their large number of nuclei, their morphologic features are the same as those of the elongated macrophages. In addition, various cellular forms can be found that are morphologically transitional between these elongated slender macrophages and the giant, round, multinucleated macrophages. A detailed scanning- and electron-microscopic and immunocytochemical study of cells in a pleural fluid showing the picture of rheumatoid pleuritis strongly supported the belief that all of the various types of cells described previously are macrophages.[65]

Necrotic Background Material. The granular necrotic background material, formed by necrosis and

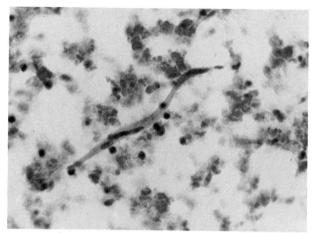

FIGURE 22–61. Rheumatoid pleuritis. An elongated, **multinucleated macrophage** in a background of **amorphous granular material** (smear of pleural fluid from the same patient as in Figure 22–60; Papanicolaou stain; ×350). (Reproduced with permission from Nosanchuk JS, Naylor B: A unique cytologic picture in pleural fluid from patients with rheumatoid arthritis. Am J Clin Pathol 50:330–335, 1968. Copyright by Williams & Wilkins, 1968.)

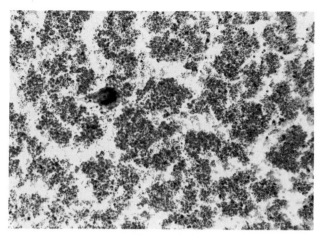

FIGURE 22–63. Rheumatoid pleuritis. A field dominated by **amorphous granular material** in which there is a solitary giant multinucleated macrophage (smear of pleural fluid from the same patient as in Figure 22–61; Papanicolaou stain; ×150). (Reproduced with permission from Nosanchuk JS, Naylor B: A unique cytologic picture in pleural fluid from patients with rheumatoid arthritis. Am J Clin Pathol 50:330–335, 1968. Copyright by Williams & Wilkins, 1968.)

disintegration of the macrophages, may be so abundant that it dominates the microscopic picture (Fig. 22–63). Its staining reaction in Papanicolaou stained smears is various shades of red, pink, orange or green, depending on the thickness of the smear and the quality of the stain. In smears the granules range from about 5 to 50 μ in diameter. They are amorphous and possess "soft," fluffy outlines. In cell blocks stained with hematoxylin and eosin the granular material is seen as large, well-defined, distinctly eosinophilic, dense, island-like aggregates (Fig. 22–64), which may have been formed by compaction of the granules during

centrifugation of the specimen. It is obvious that this granular material consists of necrotic cells because some particles retain the elongated form of viable macrophages. Figure 22–65 illustrates a necrotic giant multinucleated macrophage before it disintegrated to blend with the surrounding granules.

Rheumatoid effusions may also contain various other cells such as neutrophils, lymphocytes and small mononuclear macrophages. Because of the long-standing nature of rheumatoid effusions, many of these back-

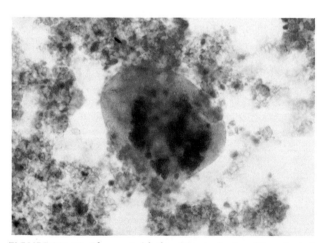

FIGURE 22–62. Rheumatoid pleuritis: A giant multinucleated macrophage in a background of **amorphous granular material** (smear of pleural fluid from the same patient as in Figure 22–61; Papanicolaou stain; ×600). (Reproduced with permission from Nosanchuk JS, Naylor B: A unique cytologic picture in pleural fluid from patients with rheumatoid arthritis. Am J Clin Pathol 50:330–335, 1968. Copyright by Williams & Wilkins, 1968.)

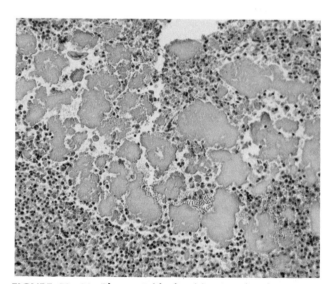

FIGURE 22–64. Rheumatoid pleuritis. Angulated, compact islands of **eosinophilic granular material** in a background of inflammatory cells (cell block of pleural fluid; hematoxylin and eosin; ×150). (Reproduced with permission from Nosanchuk JS, Naylor B: A unique cytologic picture in pleural fluid from patients with rheumatoid arthritis. Am J Clin Pathol 50:330–335, 1968. Copyright by Williams & Wilkins, 1968.)

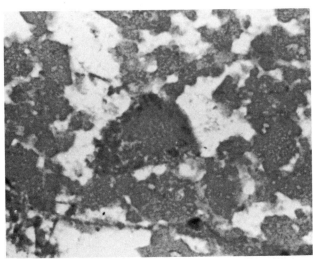

FIGURE 22–65. Rheumatoid pleuritis. Compact islands of **eosinophilic granular material** in which there is a **necrotic giant multinucleated macrophage** (cell block of pleural fluid; hematoxylin and eosin; × 400). (Reproduced with permission from Naylor B: The pathognomonic cytologic picture of rheumatoid pleuritis. Acta Cytol 34:465–473, 1990.)

ground cells also become necrotic to contribute to the granular material. Many of these necrotic cells undergo karyorrhexis before the cell disintegrates to produce a picture that, at first glance, resembles a purulent effusion (Fig. 22–66). Mesothelial cells were noticeably absent from almost all our rheumatoid effusions that showed the cytologic picture of rheumatoid serositis, being found (in small numbers) in only one of our 24 specimens.

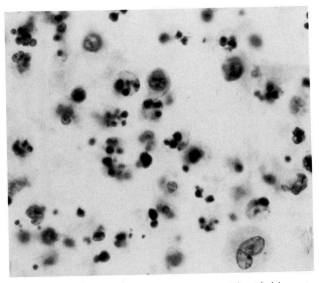

FIGURE 22–66. Numerous **leukocytes**, not identifiable as to type, contain neatly round, cyanophilic particles with a staining reaction of pyknotic nuclei. The patient had rheumatoid pleuritis. Such cells have been referred to inappropriately as either "ragocytes" or "RA cells" (smear of pleural fluid; Papanicolaou stain; × 825). (Reproduced with permission from Naylor B: The pathognomonic cytologic picture of rheumatoid pleuritis. Acta Cytol 34:465–473, 1990.)

The complete cytologic triad of rheumatoid serositis may not be present in every cytologically diagnosable specimen. However, it may be possible to make the correct diagnosis when only one or two of the three components is present. All three components were present in only 12 of 24 cytologically diagnosable pleural fluids, two components were present in seven of the fluids and one component, the granular necrotic material, was found in 23 of the 24 fluids. The three cytologic components are equally discernible in smears and cell block preparations.

The cytologic picture just described is not only unique, but it is also pathognomonic of rheumatoid pleuritis or pericarditis. This observation has been amply confirmed by our own experience and by other reports in the literature.[161] We are unaware of any recorded example of rheumatoid peritonitis with effusion showing the cytologic picture of rheumatoid disease, although the possibility exists that such a case will present itself because rheumatoid nodules have been described on the peritoneum.[54, 185]

Almost all of the patients whose pleural or pericardial fluid showed the cytologic picture of rheumatoid disease had clear clinical evidence of rheumatoid arthritis. Because the pleural manifestations of rheumatoid disease may precede the arthralgia,[99, 239] the possibility exists of diagnosing rheumatoid pleuritis or pericarditis by cytologic examination of serous fluid *before* a patient develops rheumatoid arthritis. In the series of Boddington and coworkers[22] pericardial effusion showing the cytologic picture of rheumatoid disease developed in one patient 2 months before the onset of arthritis.

Any account of the pathognomonic cytologic picture of rheumatoid pleural and pericardial effusion requires mention of the so-called ragocyte and rheumatoid arthritis (RA) cell. The term ragocyte was coined by Delbarre and colleagues[40] to refer to small, spheric cytoplasmic inclusions in neutrophils and occasionally in monocytes in *unstained wet films* of cells from synovial fluid from patients with various type of arthritis. These authors observed that ragocytes were most likely to be found in synovial fluids from patients with rheumatoid arthritis, an observation confirmed by Astorga and Bollet[8] and also by Hollander and associates,[97] who adopted the term RA cells for these inclusion-bearing leukocytes.

Such cells were subsequently described in pleural and pericardial fluids from patients with rheumatoid effusions.[18, 30, 56, 145] The inclusions are easily seen in toluidine blue stained wet films and give the staining reaction for neutral fat.[22] Neutrophilic leukocytes containing fat droplets are certainly common in rheumatoid pleural effusion; however, they may be seen in effusions caused by a variety of other conditions,[57, 58, 167] including effusions caused by malignant neoplasm. It is a mistake to rely on the presence of RA cells in pleural and pericardial fluids to confirm or even suggest the diagnosis of rheumatoid disease.

The pleural fluid of five of our 24 cases of cytologically diagnosable rheumatoid pleuritis contained cholesterol crystals (see Fig. 22–5), a manifestation of the breakdown of cell membranes, due to widespread necrosis of macrophages and other cells in an effusion of long duration. Cell block preparations from such fluids may exhibit acicular clefts (see Fig. 22–15), denoting the presence of cholesterol crystals that were dissolved when the specimen was processed.

Unless the full-blown cytologic picture of rheumatoid pleuritis is present, it is easy to overlook the significance of the partial cytologic picture, which is what initially happened in our own laboratory. It is important to diagnose rheumatoid pleuritis or pericarditis cytologically; otherwise, patients will be subjected to useless investigation, including thoracotomy, to find out the cause of their effusion, or they may be subjected to useless therapy, such as therapy against tuberculosis, such as happened with some of our patients.

Systemic Lupus Erythematosus

In 1948, Hargraves and coworkers[85] reported the serendipitous discovery of the lupus erythematosus (LE) cell in bone marrow. The LE cell is a neutrophil or, occasionally, a macrophage that has engulfed the denatured nucleus of an injured cell, the injury having been caused by circulating antinuclear antibodies present in excessive amounts in the serum of patients with SLE. These antibodies are presumed to cause the homogenization of nuclei of dead or injured cells that are subsequently phagocytosed to form LE cells.

Such altered nuclear material in histologic specimens from patients with SLE was recognized long before the discovery of the LE cell. In this form the nuclear material is referred to as a *hematoxylin body,* a dense, homogeneous cyanophilic particle about the size of a neutrophil, probably consisting mainly of altered nuclear material with a small cytoplasmic component. When a hematoxylin body is phagocytosed, the phagocytic cell with its engulfed contents is known as an LE cell.

Since the discovery of the LE cell in bone marrow and subsequently in peripheral blood, it has also been described in serous fluids. Most of the well-documented and illustrated examples of LE cells in serous fluids from patients with SLE were in pleural fluids, with the next most frequent source being pericardial fluid and the least common being peritoneal fluid.[163]

The formation of LE cells is generally regarded as an *in vitro* phenomenon; however, several authors reported finding LE cells in pleural fluids very shortly after the fluids had been aspirated,[186, 215] which supports the idea that LE cells can develop *in vivo.* Furthermore, a serous fluid that has been allowed to stand at room temperature may contain far more LE cells than the same fluid examined shortly after it was aspirated,[186, 215] evidence that LE cells continue to form spontaneously *in vitro.*

A comprehensive cumulative review[49] of various manifestations of SLE in 962 patients with the disease revealed that at some stage pleural effusion developed in 29% and peritoneal effusion in 11%; pericarditis, with or without effusion, developed in 33%. The same review showed that up to 3% of patients with SLE developed pleural effusion or pericarditis as an initial manifestation of the disease. Ascites as the presenting feature of SLE is less common, although a few cases have been reported.[111]

Apart from the reported examples of LE cells in serous fluids of patients with SLE, there are reports of LE cells in pleural and peritoneal fluid from patients who developed an SLE-like syndrome as a result of taking certain drugs.[113] In these drug-induced examples of the LE phenomenon, the LE cells were morphologically indistinguishable from those found in patients with nondrug-induced SLE. We have not seen such an example in our laboratory.

In several of our examples of LE cells in serous fluids, the cells were not observed until the time of retrospective review of the specimens, which illustrates how readily LE cells can be overlooked. A history of a patient having SLE may facilitate the finding of LE cells, but it is important to bear in mind that any unexplained serous effusion in a young person, especially if the patient is female, may be caused by SLE, and a deliberate search for LE cells should be carried out. It is also important to realize that a serous effusion may be the first clinical manifestation of SLE and that a fluid containing LE cells may be sent to the laboratory unaccompanied by a clinical history of SLE.

The cytologic literature records two examples of atypical cells in pleural fluids from patients with SLE. The earlier of these reports depicted cells that were mistaken for neoplastic cells.[4] It is obvious from the illustrations that the atypical cells were hypertrophied mesothelial cells, a nonspecific finding. Equally nonspecific were the atypical cells depicted, in a later publication in which, again, the illustrated cells had the morphologic features of hypertrophied mesothelial cells.[116] Similar cells were also illustrated in pleural fluids from two patients with SLE by Butler and Stanbridge.[29]

It would be most imprudent to allow the presence of hypertrophied mesothelial cells in serous fluids to suggest a diagnosis of SLE. They are a nonspecific finding, one that is extremely prevalent in serous fluids from patients with a wide variety of inflammatory and other diseases. Only one cell has any diagnostic significance in the diagnosis of SLE: the LE cell, with or without hematoxylin bodies in the background.

Cytology. We have found LE cells in serous fluids not only in routinely prepared Papanicolaou stained smears (Fig. 22–67) but also in cell block preparations and in toluidine blue–stained wet films (Fig. 22–68). LE cells may be so numerous that they are seen in virtually every microscopic field, or they may be so few that several minutes of deliberate searching are required to find just one. A specimen containing LE cells may also contain unengulfed hematoxylin bodies. In Papanicolaou stained smears phagocytosed or non-phagocytosed hematoxylin bodies show a variety of staining reactions: various shades of gray, green, purple and blue. In LE cells the nucleus is pushed over to the side and may seem to be a continuous crescentic band,

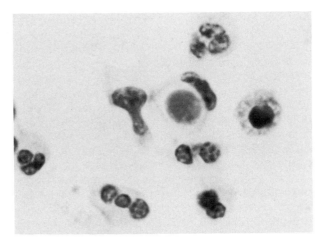

FIGURE 22–67. A lupus erythematosus (LE) cell accompanied by several **leukocytes** (smear of pleural fluid; Papanicolaou stain; ×1320).

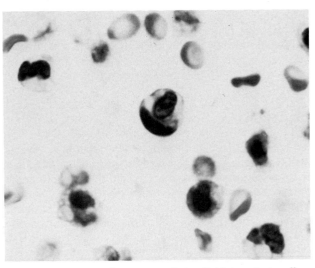

FIGURE 22–69. In the center of the field is a **tart cell**, a leukocyte that has engulfed a nucleus that still exhibits internal structure. If this were a lupus erythematosus (LE) cell, the engulfed nucleus would be homogeneous (cell block of pleural fluid; hematoxylin and eosin; ×1320).

or it may retain lobar divisions. Some smears containing LE cells, especially when they are numerous, show a background heavy in nuclear fragments and necrotic cells (see Fig. 22–68), presumably neutrophils. All of the serous fluids in which we have found LE cells also contained readily found, although not necessarily predominating, neutrophils, cells that are the virtual prerequisite for the formation of LE cells.

Tart Cells. When searching for LE cells one may come across small macrophages that have phagocytosed a nonhomogenized nucleus, presumably a bare nucleus of a cell that died and underwent cytolysis (Fig. 22–69). These cells were named *tart cells,* not because they were likened to a small piece of pastry, but because the last name of the patient in whose bone marrow they were first found in tremendous numbers was Tart.[85] Some tart cells can be found in virtually every serous fluid. The difference between tart cells

and LE cells is that in the former the phagocytosed nuclear material is not homogeneous, still showing some chromatinic structure, whereas in LE cells the phagocytosed hematoxylin bodies are homogeneous.

Congestive Heart Failure

One of the most frequent manifestations of congestive heart failure is pleural effusion, which may be accompanied by peritoneal or pericardial effusion, and even though the clinical diagnosis may be obvious, serous fluid from patients with congestive heart failure is frequently submitted for cytologic examination. Typically, such effusions are transudates, although later, with inflammatory complications, they may become exudates. In a series of 18 pleural and two ascitic fluids from 20 patients with effusions attributable to congestive heart failure, we found that the cellularity ranged from low to high, being moderate to low in most specimens. Those with the highest cellularity tended to contain the highest number of neutrophils, evidence of the effusion having changed from a transudate to an exudate.

Most of these fluids seemed to have remained sterile, however, with a low number or a virtual absence of neutrophils. Twelve of the 20 fluids contained very few or no mesothelial cells. The specimen with the highest number of mesothelial cells also contained the highest number of neutrophilic leukocytes. The number of macrophages and leukocytes varied; in some specimens they were entirely or virtually absent. Four of the effusions contained large numbers of lymphocytes and would be considered lymphocytic effusions. Two of the effusions contained hemosiderophages, a manifestation of the breakdown of red blood cells that had passed into the serous cavity. The cytologic picture of serous effusions caused by congestive heart failure is, there-

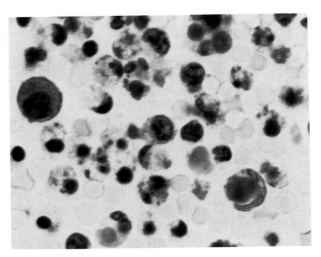

FIGURE 22–68. A lupus erythematosus (LE) cell (bottom right corner) accompanied by other **leukocytes**. Some are disintegrating, and others appear to contain particles of homogeneous material (hematoxylin bodies) (wet film of pleural fluid; toluidine blue; ×1320).

fore, nonspecific. The contribution of the cytology laboratory is mainly to rule out the presence of neoplastic cells and to determine if the cytologic picture is specific for any particular non-neoplastic disease or entity.

Pneumonia

Pneumonia (inflammation of the pulmonary parenchyma), whatever its cause, does not always result in pleural effusions. However, when the inflammatory process extends to the pleura, it may induce a similar type of inflammatory reaction thereon, resulting in effusion. The types of inflammatory reaction range from the acute purulent, dominated by neutrophils, to the chronic, dominated by lymphocytes, with all variety of inflammatory exudate in between. In addition, strands of fibrin may form part of the background, either as cyanophilic strands in smears or as dense eosinophilic masses in cell blocks. Acute bacterial pneumonia is most likely to give acute purulent pleuritis, although in the resolving phase the purulent component diminishes to become complemented by macrophages and lymphocytes. Eventually, if the process becomes chronic, lymphocytes will predominate. On the other hand, viral pneumonias typically evoke a lymphoid response from the beginning, and any resulting effusion contains an abundance of lymphoid cells, possibly including plasma cells. Should the effusion become secondarily infected, neutrophils will also enter the cytologic picture.

Because a cytologic picture dominated by a heavy exudate of neutrophils or lymphocytes or a mixture of both is not specific for any particular type of lesion, it is not possible to determine on cytologic examination whether the patients has pneumonia; all that can be stated is that the cytologic picture is consistent with pneumonia.

Infarct

Pulmonary infarct is characterized by a subpleural zone of hemorrhagic necrosis of the pulmonary parenchyma, usually in a cone shape with the base of the cone formed by the pleura. The necrotic parenchymal tissue induces an inflammatory reaction on the overlying pleura, which retains a thin zone of viability owing to its own separate blood supply. It is the area of pleural inflammation that is responsible for any ensuing exudative effusion. We have also seen examples of peritoneal effusion from patients with infarct of the small intestine or of the liver.

In pleural effusions from patients with pulmonary infarcts, the cellularity ranged from slight to profuse, with most specimens being classified as moderate to profusely cellular. In many of the pleural fluids there was no dominant cytologic picture, with mesothelial cells, macrophages (including hemosiderophages), lymphocytes and neutrophils being present. Some fluids were eosinophilic, with eosinophil counts ranging

from 15 to 66%. Other fluids were highly cellular, with most cells being neutrophils, and some fluids showed a heavy lymphocytosis. In our cases of small intestinal infarct resulting in effusion, two of the four specimens contained numerous neutrophils, one contained numerous lymphocytes and the fourth contained only a few neutrophils. Again, we have situations in which cytologic examination of serous fluid does not provide a diagnosis of a specific pathologic entity, although it may be useful to rule out the presence of cancer cells.

Pneumothorax

Pneumothorax is frequently accompanied by effusion, possibly induced by the presence of air and its impurities in the pleural cavity as well as any pulmonary parenchymal contents that also entered the cavity. The cytologic picture of pneumothorax is nonspecific, but one feature we have noted in our specimens and that has been noted by others[215] is a high proportion of eosinophils, possibly due to allergenic impurities in the air.[209] The presence of air in the pleural cavity may also stimulate mesothelial cells to enlarge, manifested by the presence of numerous hypertrophic mesothelial cells in an accompanying effusion.

Tuberculosis

It has long been known that the typical pleural effusion caused by tuberculosis has a high proportion of lymphocytes and very few or no mesothelial cells,[101, 212, 246, 247] although in tuberculous pleuritis of short duration the effusion may contain some neutrophils and mesothelial cells. The scarcity or absence of mesothelial cells in tuberculous pleural effusions is attributable to deposition of fibrin on the pleural surface, either sealing off the mesothelial cells or destroying them or both. The presence of numerous mesothelial cells in a pleural fluid should be regarded as strong evidence that the effusion is not caused by tuberculosis. Nontuberculous confluent inflammatory exudates and neoplastic deposits may either cover or occupy so much of the mesothelium that effusions caused by these processes may also be devoid of mesothelial cells. Most tuberculous pleural effusions contain 80 to 100% lymphocytes. They may contain small numbers of neutrophils, macrophages, plasma cells and red blood cells. Multinucleated giant macrophages and epithelioid cells have been recorded in tuberculous effusions but must be considered a rarity.[75, 103]

A reported study analyzed T cell subsets and activation markers on T cells in pleural fluids in an attempt to distinguish between tuberculous pleurisy and other lymphocyte-rich effusions.[79] However, significant differences were not observed, leading to the conclusion that phenotypic analysis of lymphocytes is of limited diagnostic usefulness in such situations.

At some stage of the tuberculous process an effusion may become secondarily infected, possibly by rupture of a tuberculous cavity of the lungs into the pleural space. In such cases pleural empyema may ensue in which the cytologic picture changes to one of virtually all neutrophils. When empyema is of long duration, pleural fibrosis may develop, causing it to become encysted. In this situation the empyema fluid may lose its cellularity, resulting in a fluid of low cellularity containing cholesterol crystals due to the breakdown of cell membranes.

In peritoneal tuberculosis the predominant cellular picture is likely to be lymphocytic, although macrophages and neutrophils and, sometimes, mesothelial cells may also be present. In contrast to tuberculous pleuritis, the presence of mesothelial cells does not exclude peritoneal tuberculosis. In tuberculous pericarditis, the cytologic picture is similar to that of tuberculous pleuritis.

Hepatic Cirrhosis

The long-standing transudates occupying the peritoneal cavity of patients with hepatic cirrhosis are typically sterile, with few or no acute inflammatory cells. In our analysis of 20 such fluids, the cellularity was generally low, although six were profusely cellular with the dominating cell being mesothelial. In six of the fluids mesothelial cells were very few or absent. The other cells consisted almost entirely of lymphocytes and macrophages in small numbers. Peritoneal fluid of a patient with hepatic cirrhosis containing more than a few neutrophils should raise the question of whether the patient is developing spontaneous bacterial peritonitis, a complication of decompensating hepatic cirrhosis.

For some reason, ascitic fluids from patients with hepatic cirrhosis seem to pose a problem in cytodiagnosis owing to the presence of hypertrophied mesothelial cells, either solitary or in clusters. Analysis of these cells is no different from the analysis of such cells found in different circumstances. In fact, because ascitic fluids of patients with cirrhosis are less likely to be bloody or to contain a dominant inflammatory exudate, analysis of these mesothelial cells should, if anything, be straightforward. If careful attention is paid to the morphologic details of mesothelial cells mentioned previously, errors of overdiagnosis can be avoided.

Parasitic Infections

Although parasitic infections are endemic throughout the world they have seldom been recorded in specimens of serous fluid sent for cytologic examination. In our laboratory we have seen the following parasites in pleural or peritoneal fluids: *Echinococcus granulosus*, *Paragonimus westermani*, *Strongyloides stercoralis* and *Trichomonas* species. This small group, collected over a 33-year period, illustrates the infrequency of such specimens in a North American practice. Of the five patients whose specimens contained these parasites, three were immigrants to the United

States, one was a migrant from the southern to the northern half of the United States and one had always lived in Michigan. In this era of widespread and rapid travel, parasitic infections are likely to appear in the most unexpected manner as exemplified by some of our cases.

Echinococcosis (Hydatid Disease). Echinococcosis is an infection by larval tapeworms of the genus *Echinococcus*, with infections by *E. granulosus* being the most common. Today, echinococcosis is probably most prevalent in East Africa but is common in the Mediterranean countries and in the Middle East. Echinococcosis in humans results from our accidental role as intermediate host in the life cycle of the dwarf tapeworm *E. granulosus*.

In 1973, Jacobson[102] reported from our laboratory a case of echinococcosis diagnosed by cytologic examination of pleural fluid. The patient, a resident of Michigan, suddenly developed a large pleural effusion that contained scolices of *E. granulosus* (Fig. 22–70). He was subsequently discovered to have a large hydatid cyst in the liver that, while he was playing soccer, had ruptured through the diaphragm to give instant pleural effusion. In this case, the patient's disease might be regarded as occupational because, as a former shepherd in Yugoslavia, he had been in contact with both

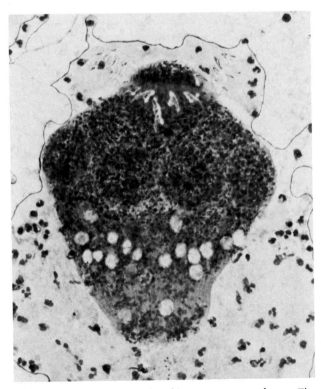

FIGURE 22–70. Scolex of *Echinococcus granulosus*. The patient had a hydatid cyst in the liver that ruptured through the diaphragm to cause pleural effusion. When this photograph was taken, this sealed wet film had been stored at 4°C for 10 years (wet film of pleural fluid; toluidine blue; ×330). (Reproduced with permission from Jacobson ES: A case of secondary echinococcosis diagnosed by cytologic examination of pleural fluid and needle biopsy of pleura. Acta Cytol 17:76–79, 1973.)

definitive (dog) and intermediate hosts (sheep). The diagnosis was greatly facilitated by the use of a toluidine blue–stained wet film. Smears stained by the Papanicolaou method also demonstrated the scolices, but they were far less striking.

Paragonimiasis. Paragonimiasis is infection by trematodes of the genus *Paragonimus*, with most infections of humans with flukes of this genus attributed to *P. westermani*. It is an important human disease in South Asia and parts of Latin American and Africa. The use of raw or incompletely cooked crabs or crayfish and their juices for food or medicine is the most important method of transmission.

We have examined specimens of pleural fluid containing the ova of *P. westermani* from two patients, both Koreans who had immigrated to the United States and were residents of Michigan. Eggs of *P. westermani* (Fig. 22–71) are easily seen in the Papanicolaou stained permanent smears and in toluidine blue stained wet films. In Papanicolaou stained preparations they are ovoid, yellow-brown, thick walled and birefringent and have a flattened operculum at one end and a lateral fold. They can be readily mistaken for a contaminant, such as a pollen grain or other type of vegetable cell.

Strongyloidiasis. Strongyloidiasis, infection by the nematode *Strongyloides stercoralis*, is prevalent through the tropical and temperate climates, but is most common in warm, wet regions. In the United States the parasite is more prevalent in the south. Healthy individuals tolerate infection by *S. stercoralis* well, but in immunosuppressed patients filariform larvae resident in the intestine may penetrate the intestinal wall and spread to other organs in the body and in doing so provoke the formation of pleural or peritoneal effusion.

We have seen one example of *S. stercoralis* in a serous fluid.[137] The patient, a man from Kentucky who was being treated with prednisone for membranoproliferative glomerulonephritis, developed abdominal symptoms and was found to have ascites. The ascitic fluid contained larvae of *S. stercoralis*. The patient died, with necropsy revealing disseminated strongyloidiasis. Other examples of the cytologic detection of *S. stercoralis* in serous fluids have been reported.[9, 139, 181] In the case of Lintermans,[139] a child died of peritonitis, with *S. stercoralis* being found in the peritoneal fluid. The diagnosis of infection with *S. stercoralis* is very important because lifesaving therapy can be instituted, in some cases resulting in a cure.

Trichomoniasis. Trichomonads rarely infect serous fluids, and the only fluids in which they have been reported have been pleural.[150, 153, 238] In two of the three reported cases as well as in our own case, invasion of the pleural cavity by the organism was attributable to an abnormal connection between the respiratory or alimentary tract and a pleural cavity through a leaking suture line in patients who had undergone gastrectomy and partial esophagectomy for gastric adenocarcinoma. In one reported case the patient developed *Trichomonas* empyema as a consequence of aspiration pneumonia, but there was no evidence of any connection between the respiratory tract and the pleural space.[238] In none of the reported cases of *Trichomonas* infections of serous fluid, as in our own case, was it possible to culture the organism. The significance of trichomonads in a pleural fluid is unknown. However, it appears that the organism can be eliminated by treatment with metronidazole.

The organism is easily demonstrated by direct microscopic examination of fresh, unfixed material. In our own case, an unstained wet film of pleural empyema fluid contained a scattering of highly mobile trichomonads executing a jerky rolling movement. We were not able to find the organism in our Papanicolaou stained smears.

Giardiasis. Giardiasis is infection of the small intestine by the protozoan *Giardia lamblia*, a harmless commensal in most subjects. The parasite is worldwide, with higher rates of infection found in warmer climates and in crowded, unsanitary environments. Giardiasis may be epidemic and has achieved some notoriety on the medical scene by infecting travelers to areas of high endemicity.

G. lamblia occurs as trophozoites and cysts. The former are flat, pear-shaped, binucleated, flagellate organisms, which are most numerous in the duodenum and upper jejunum. Our experience of *G. lamblia* in duodenal aspirates has shown that the organism is quite recognizable in Papanicolaou stained material, being about as visible as *Trichomonas vaginalis* in vaginal specimens. However, because of its rarity in peritoneal fluids it could easily be overlooked. Recently, examples of *G. lamblia* have been described in a peritoneal "aspirate" and in two peritoneal lavage specimens (Fig. 22–72).[21, 48] In these three patients the peritoneal specimens were obtained as part of an investigation to diagnose ruptured intestines secondary to abdominal trauma. The three specimens contained trophozoites of *G. lamblia* and one contained cysts. The significance of finding the parasite in peritoneal fluid is that it is evidence of perforation of the intestine.

Balantidiasis. Balantidiasis, infection by the protozoan *Balantidium coli*, is worldwide, but infections are more common in tropical and subtropical regions. In

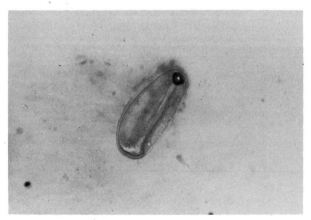

FIGURE 22–71. Ovum of *Paragonimus westermani*. The patient, a resident of the United States, was originally from Korea (smear of pleural fluid; Papanicolaou stain; ×330).

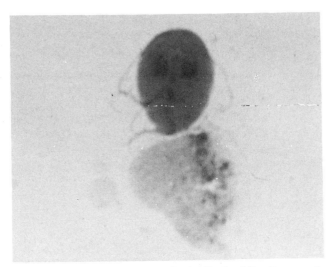

FIGURE 22–72. Trophozoite of **Giardia lamblia**. Cytocentrifuge preparation of peritoneal lavage (Wright stain; ×2000). (Reproduced with permission from Drew PA, Krauss JS: Identification of *Giardia lamblia* in peritoneal fluid of trauma patients. Acta Cytol 33:283–284, 1989.)

temperate zones higher rates of infection develop where there is crowding and poor personal hygiene.

Trophozoites of *B. coli* live in the large intestine where they may invade the mucosa, causing ulcers. Perforation of the bowel wall with accompanying peritonitis is a rare but sometimes fatal complication. Lahiri and associates[133] described a case of fatal balantidium peritonitis that was diagnosed by cytologic examination of peritoneal fluid (Fig. 22–73).

Schistosomiasis (Bilharziasis). Schistosomiasis is infection caused by flukes (trematodes) of any species of the genus *Schistosoma*. The geographic distribution of schistosomiasis in humans depends on the distribution of snail hosts and opportunity for infection for both snail and human. The basic lesions of schistosomiasis are circumscribed granulomas or eosinophilic and neu-

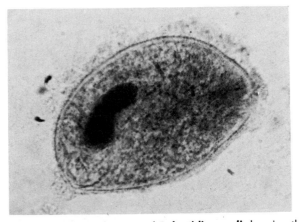

FIGURE 22–73. Trophozoite of **Balantidium coli** showing the large macronucleus and the thin cell membrane covered with cilia (smear of peritoneal fluid; Papanicolaou stain; ×820). (Reproduced with permission from Lahiri VJ, Elhence BR, Agarwal BM: Balantidium peritonitis diagnosed on cytologic material. Acta Cytol 21:123–124, 1977.)

trophilic infiltrates around eggs. The eggs frequently become calcified and surrounded by hyalinized scar tissue. Recently Okuyama and coauthors[169] described an ovum of *S. japonicum* in ascitic fluid of an elderly woman who died with hepatic cirrhosis in which the hepatic scar tissue contained numerous schistosomal ova.

Amebiasis. Amebiasis is invasion of tissue by the protozoan *Entamoeba histolytica*. Infection takes place when trophozoites of *E. histolytica* invade the colonic mucosa, where the infection may remain localized and be minimal for years or may extend to the liver and other organs. Amebiasis is found worldwide but varies greatly in severity from patient to patient and from one geographic area to another.

Complications of colonic amebiasis include peritonitis from perforation and amebic abscess of the liver. Complications of liver abscess include perforation and peritonitis and extension through the diaphragm to the pleural cavity and pericardium. Therefore, it is entirely possible that a cytologic specimen from any of the serous cavities could contain *E. histolytica*.

We have not seen amebae in any of our specimens of serous fluid, but they have been described in pericardial fluid in patients with suppurative amebic pericarditis. The presence of liver cells in the pericardial fluid of one patient was in keeping with the amebic pericarditis being secondary to an amebic liver abscess that had spread through the diaphragm into the pericardial cavity.[144] In most of the patients the pericardial fluid had the typical granular gray-pink ("anchovy sauce") appearance.

Filariasis. The type of filariasis usually manifested in serous fluids is bancroftian filariasis, an infection by the filarial worm *Wuchereria bancrofti* that causes disease by blocking lymphatic vessels. Generally the disease is diagnosed by finding the microfiliarial larvae in peripheral blood. However, instances have been reported, both in endemic and nonendemic areas, of microfilariae, presumably of *W. bancrofti*, in pleural, pericardial and hydrocele fluids, all emanating from the Indian subcontinent or from Asiatic Indians living in nonendemic areas.[32, 93, 194, 229, 237] A different species of microfilaria, *Mansonella ozzardi*, has also been described in ascitic fluid.[59]

Fungal Infections

Disseminated fungal disease is usually confined to patients whose immunologic defenses are diminished by some recognized underlying disease (such as cancer) or by cytotoxic and immunosuppressive chemotherapy. Other risk factors include the excessive use of broad-spectrum antibiotics, high-dose corticosteroids, indwelling venous and peritoneal catheters and prosthetic devices (such as artificial heart valves). In addition to these risky situations there is the latter-day affliction, acquired immune deficiency syndrome (AIDS). In view of the widespread prevalence of these conditions it surprising that cytopathology laboratories do not receive more serous fluids showing evidence of opportunistic fungal infection.

We have seen examples of serous fluids showing opportunistic infections with *Candida* species, *Cryptococcus* species, *Coccidioides immitis* and *Aspergillus niger*. In the case of candidiasis, the specimen was from a child receiving chemotherapy for neuroblastoma. This overwhelming infection was diagnosed in peritoneal fluid (Fig. 22–74) a few days before the child died and was singularly devoid of any accompanying inflammatory cells. Gronemeyer and coworkers[74] described opportunistic *Candida tropicalis* in purulent pericardial fluid examined postmortem from a patient with Hodgkin's disease being treated with chemotherapy. The patient died with disseminated candidiasis.

In the case of cryptococcosis the specimen was ascitic fluid from a patient being treated with corticosteroids for SLE. The microorganisms were abundant but could be easily overlooked because of their small size and tendency to blend with the background. Many were engulfed by macrophages (Fig. 22–75).

The patient with *C. immitis* infection had lived in the extreme southwest of Colorado, an area endemic for *C. immitis*. He was being treated with chemotherapy for leukemia when he developed bronchopneumonia with pleural effusion, in which there were large fungal spherules containing endospores. Many of the spherules exhibited the Splendore-Hoeppli effect,[96, 207] consisting of a hyaline, eosinophilic, radiate precipitate around the organism (Fig. 22–76). It is believed to be a result of an immune response resulting in deposition of immunocomplexes around the fungus.[234]

Covell and colleagues[36] described two examples of nonopportunistic North American blastomycosis in which cytologic examination of pleural fluid played a primary role in determining the nature of the effusion. In both cases, pleural fluid contained the typical thick-walled, budding yeast form of *Blastomyces dermatitidis* (Fig. 22–77). Spriggs and Boddington[213] illustrated an

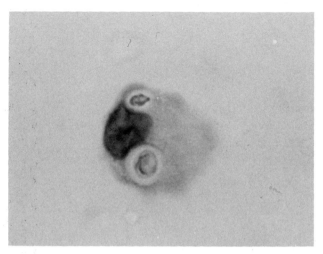

FIGURE 22–75. A macrophage containing *Cryptococcus* species. The patient had systemic lupus erythematosus (SLE) and was being treating with corticosteroids (smear of peritoneal fluid; Papanicolaou stain; ×1320). (Courtesy of Dr. Prabodh K. Gupta, Philadelphia, Pennsylvania.)

example of the yeast form of *Blastomyces brasiliensis* in a giant multinucleated macrophage in pleural fluid of a Brazilian patient.

Reyes and coauthors[187] reported a case of pulmonary and pleural infection with *A. niger* in a known case of pulmonary tuberculosis. In addition to the fungus (Fig. 22–78), the bronchial biopsy specimen and pleural fluid contained sheaves of birefringent calcium oxalate crystals (Fig. 22–79), a metabolic product of *Aspergillus* species, especially *A. niger*. These authors suggested that the presence of such crystals in a background of inflammatory cells should be a clue to infection with *A. niger*.

Pulmonary infection with *Pneumocystis carinii*, now regarded as probably fungal,[52] has long been recognized as a cause of pneumonia in immunosuppressed

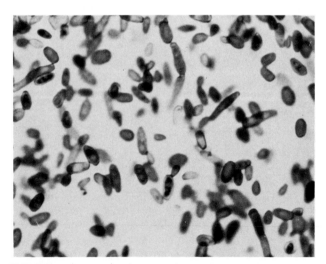

FIGURE 22–74. Yeast forms and pseudohyphae of *Candida* species. The patient was being treated by chemotherapy for neuroblastoma. Note the lack of an inflammatory response (smear of peritoneal fluid; methenamine silver; ×825).

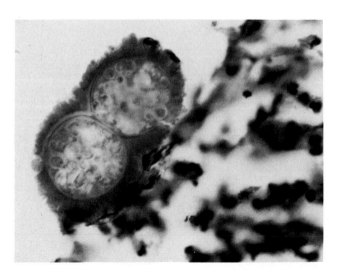

FIGURE 22–76. Large spherules of *Coccidioides immitis* containing endospores. The radiate precipitate around the organism is the Splendore-Hoeppli effect (cell block of pleural fluid; hematoxylin and eosin; ×825).

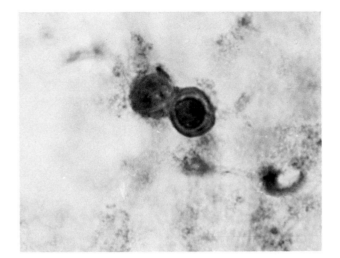

FIGURE 22–77. Budding yeast forms of ***Blastomyces dermatitidis*** (smear of pleural fluid; Papanicolaou stain; ×1320). (Courtesy of Ms. Jamie L. Covell, Richmond, Virginia.)

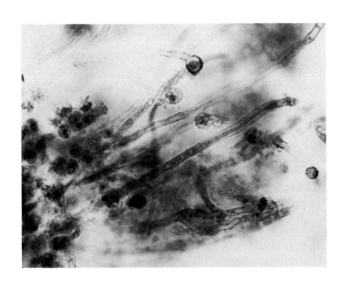

FIGURE 22–78. Hyphae of ***Aspergillus niger*** in fluid from a patient with pulmonary tuberculosis. Presumably the fungus was a secondary invader of the tuberculous lung (smear of pleural fluid; Papanicolaou stain; ×528). (Courtesy of Dr. Cesar V. Reyes, Hines, Illinois.)

FIGURE 22–79. Sheaves of **calcium oxalate crystals** in a background of inflammatory cells (smear of pleural fluid from the same specimen as in Figure 22–78; Papanicolaou stain; ×40).

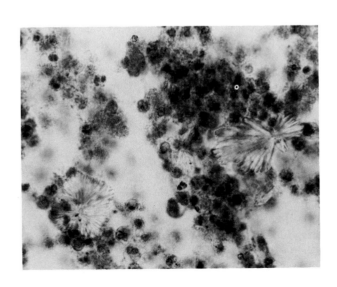

patients. Examples of extrapulmonary infection with the organism have rarely been described, although with the increased number of patients undergoing organ transplantation and the epidemic of AIDS, more examples of extrapulmonary infection are likely to be recognized. Bedrossian and coworkers[13] illustrated the typical organisms in a methenamine silver stained specimen of pleural fluid from an AIDS patient.

Viral Infection

Viral infection, especially of the lung, frequently causes an effusion containing numerous lymphoid cells, the type of cellular exudate generally associated with such infections. However, to diagnose with certainty viral infection of a serous cavity it is essential to find cells bearing inclusions specific for a particular type of virus, so-called virocytes. Such changes in serous fluids are a rarity.

Goodman and associates,[72] in a retrospective analysis of serous fluids from patients who had definite evidence of infection with *Herpesvirus simplex* or *Cytomegalovirus*, found virocytes diagnostic of herpetic infection (presumably by *Herpesvirus simplex*) in a pleural fluid and changes consistent with *Cytomegalovirus* infection in a pleural and a pericardial fluid. Their illustrations of herpetic virocytes, with typical multinucleated giant cells exhibiting nuclear molding, sharp nuclear membranes and smooth chromatin, or smaller uninucleated cells with prominent intranuclear inclusions and heavy nuclear membranes, are diagnostic of herpetic infection. In the case of patients with necropsy-proven *Cytomegalovirus* infection, the cytologic evidence of infection consisted of sheets of mesothelial cells with homogeneous, degenerated, gelatinous chromatin and occasional multinucleated cells, presumably mesothelial, with a similar appearance. Intracytoplasmic inclusions were not seen.

We have seen two pleural fluids containing herpetic virocytes. One patient had pleural empyema with a thoracotomy drainage tube *in situ*. Because this patient had cutaneous herpes simplex near the thoracotomy incision, it is possible that the virocytes came from this lesion. The other patient had nerpetic stomatitis and probably also had a ruptured esophagus. The herpetic virocytes in the resulting pleural fluid may have been derived from swallowed saliva (Fig. 22–80).

We have seen one specimen of serous fluid with cells showing changes attributable to *Cytomegalovirus* infection. The patient was receiving immunosuppressive drugs for a renal transplant when she developed ascites. The peritoneal fluid contained cells that were apparently mesothelial but that contained enlarged nuclei with smooth chromatin and what appeared to be cytoplasmic inclusion material. It was difficult to detect the classic morphologic picture of *Cytomegalovirus* infection in these cells; however, application of the immunoperoxidase technique using a monoclonal antibody against *Cytomegalovirus* demonstrated that these cells were indeed infected with the virus.

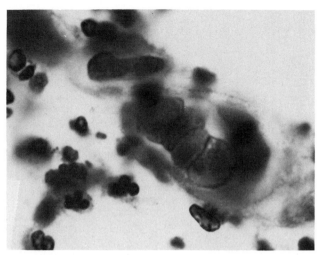

FIGURE 22–80. Herpetic virocytes from a patient with herpetic stomatitis and possibly a ruptured esophagus (smear of pleural fluid; Papanicolaou stain; ×1320).

Fistula

Fistula may result in bizarre cytologic pictures characterized by the paradoxical presence in a serous fluid of non-neoplastic cells and nonhuman cellular elements that normally have no access to a serous cavity. The most striking cytologic picture in a serous effusion due to fistula is one containing vegetable cells, cells that may simulate various pathologic conditions and entities.[242] Spriggs and Boddington[213, 215] and Lopes Cardozo[140] depicted squamous epithelial cells and vegetable cells in serous fluids from patients with bronchopleural fistula, esophagopleural fistula and gastric perforation.

We have examined four serous fluids, all pleural, that developed as a result of fistula. The most striking was from a patient with gastropleural fistula due to gastric lymphoma that had eroded through the diaphragm to give a pleural effusion replete with vegetable cells, squamous epithelial cells, fungi and amorphous debris, all derived from the respiratory and alimentary tracts (Fig. 22–81). The other three specimens were due to esophagopleural fistulas. One contained vegetable cells, another herpetic virocytes and the third motile trichomonads. The finding of such cells in a serous fluid may be an important clue that a patient has developed a fistula or ruptured a viscus or that a surgical anastomosis is leaking.

Red Blood Cell Changes

Dekker and coworkers[39] described sickle cells in pleural fluid from a patient with sickle cell anemia (hemoglobin S disease) caused by the presence of a genetic variant of the normal adult hemoglobin molecule. Their patient developed pleural effusions, presumably secondary to pleuritis associated with pulmonary infarction attributable to the sickling of red blood

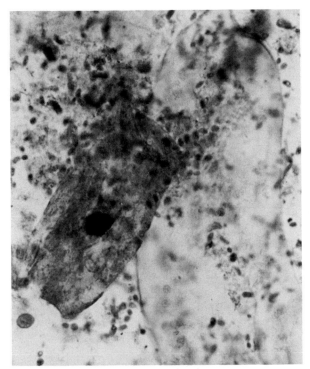

FIGURE 22–81. **Vegetable cells**, unidentified fungus and amorphous granular background material all derived from the respiratory and alimentary tracts of a patient with gastropleural fistula due to lymphoma (smear of pleural fluid; Papanicolaou stain; ×528). (Courtesy of Dr. James N. Landers, Detroit, Michigan.)

cells in blood incompletely saturated with oxygen. Their review of the current literature indicated that pleural effusion occurs in about 28% of patients with sickle cell disease. These authors postulated that the sickle shape of the red cells could be caused by artifactual distortion in the process of smearing and fixing the specimen. However, they excluded this possibility by examining a series of serous fluids from patients without sickle cell anemia. In these fluids they did not find the same sickle cell shapes seen in fluids from patients with sickle cell disease.

Since becoming aware of the possibility of finding sickle cells in serous fluids prepared by the Papanicolaou method, we have discovered examples in our own specimens (Fig. 22–82). It is entirely possible that we (and others) have overlooked other examples of this characteristic morphologic change in red blood cells because it is not common practice in diagnostic cytopathology to pay too close attention to the shapes of red blood cells.

We have seen rouleau formation of red cells in toluidine blue–stained wet films (Fig. 22–83) in patients with Waldenström's macroglobulinemia, which is characterized by the presence of a monoclonal IgM paraprotein in the blood that initiates rouleau formation. The phenomenon was easily detected in the stained (and unstained) wet films, whereas in the Papanicolaou stained smears it was manifested as a massive clumping of the red cells in which it was impossible to discern

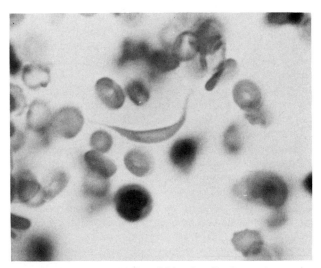

FIGURE 22–82. A **sickled red blood cell**. The patient, who was of the Negroid race, had no symptoms or clinical signs related to the sickling of red blood cells (smear of pleural fluid; Papanicolaou stain; ×1320).

the rouleau change, and the change was hardly discernible in the cell block preparations.

Endometriosis

Endometriosis, the presence outside the endometrial cavity of tissue that replicates endometrium, is not uncommon in the ovaries and, to a lesser extent, on the pelvic peritoneum. It is found with less frequency in the abdomen as the distance from the pelvis increases, and it becomes a rarity above the diaphragm. Three examples of endometriosis manifested in spontaneously occurring serous effusions, two pleural and one peritoneal, have been recorded.[63, 259] The pleural effusions occurred in women who were found by thoracotomy to have pleural endometrial implants, and the patient with peritoneal effusion was found by laparotomy to have peritoneal endometrial implants.

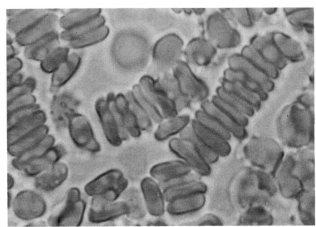

FIGURE 22–83. **Rouleau formation of red blood cells**. The patient had Waldenström's macroglobulinemia (wet film of pleural fluid; toluidine blue; ×1320).

One of the pleural fluids was hemorrhagic, and the peritoneal fluid was described as being brown. The cytologic manifestation of endometriosis was based on the presence of small columnar-shaped cells accompanied by small round cells, some of which were cohesive. Hemosiderin-containing macrophages were also present. In the case of peritoneal endometriosis, histochemistry demonstrated the presence of hemosiderin and hematoidin in the exfoliated cells.[63]

Otherwise, endometrial cells, either from foci of endometriosis or from tubal reflux, are most likely to be seen in specimens obtained by culdocentesis or in peritoneal washings.[29, 215] Butler and Stanbridge[29] described cells consistent with endometrial stroma and epithelium in aspirates obtained from the cul-de-sac (pouch of Douglas); the presence of these cells was believed to be due to reflux menstrual fluid. The cells believed to be of endometrial stromal origin were very similar to the macrophage-like cells seen in postmenstrual cervical smears.

The diagnosis of endometriosis from cells in spontaneously occurring serous effusions, culdocentesis specimens or peritoneal washings is fraught with difficulty. Individual endometrial stromal cells may be similar in shape and size to lymphoid cells, or they may closely resemble macrophages or small mesothelial cells. Furthermore, endometrial cells of epithelial type in a serous effusion or peritoneal washing may, unless their epithelial architecture is extremely well preserved, resemble small fragments of mesothelium. In fact, in the three reported cases of endometriotic cells in spontaneously occuring effusions referred to previously, there is no record of a cytologic diagnosis of endometriosis being reported prior to biopsy; it appears that the cytologic presentation of endometriosis was recognized retrospectively. Probably the most reliable method of diagnosing endometriosis in a serous fluid is to demonstrate endometriotic fragments in a cell block preparation, which would allow identification of both epithelial and stromal components.

Curschmann's Spirals

Curschmann's spirals are common in cytologic specimens from the respiratory tract and have also been recorded in cervical smears.[168] In these situations their presence could be explained by their being formed from mucus normally present in the environment. However, a paradoxical source of Curschmann's spirals was reported by Wahl,[236] who found them in peritoneal washings, pleural fluids and peritoneal dialysate.

We have observed five examples of Curschmann's spirals in smears and cell blocks of spontaneously occurring pleural and peritoneal fluids of five patients.[162] On the whole, these spirals were much shorter than those usually seen in respiratory or cervical secretions (Fig. 22–84), although some were similar in size to those seen in sputum (Fig. 22–85). Some spirals were rather poorly formed and were regarded as incipient spirals. Three of the five patients had serous effusions containing mucus-secreting carcinoma cells;

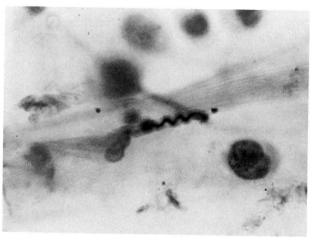

FIGURE 22–84. A tiny **Curschmann's spiral** that at one end appears to blend with a streak of mucus. The fluid also contained metastatic gastric adenocarcinoma cells (smear of pleural fluid; Papanicolaou stain; ×825). (Reproduced with permission from Naylor B: Curschmann's spirals in pleural and peritoneal fluids. Acta Cytol 34:474–478, 1990.)

in fact, one patient had pseudomyxoma peritonei, characterized by mucoid ascitic fluid. Of the other two patients, one had pleural empyema and the other possibly had spontaneous bacterial peritonitis associated with hepatic cirrhosis.

Based on the observation that Curschmann's spirals in the female genital tract have been recorded only in patients who had a uterus *in situ*, thereby providing a source of mucus, we believe that the presence of mucus in serous fluids can account for spiral formation. But where there were no epithelial cells producing mucus to give rise to spiral formation, as in Wahl's[236] cases

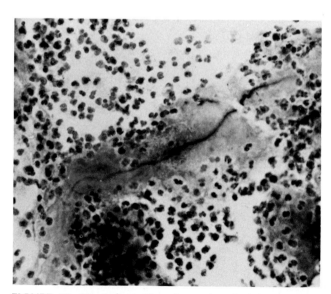

FIGURE 22–85. A long **Curschmann's spiral** in empyema fluid. The patient had no evidence of fistula or carcinoma (smear of pleural fluid; Papanicolaou stain; ×208). (Reproduced with permission from Naylor B: Curschmann's spirals in pleural and peritoneal fluids. Acta Cytol 34:474–478, 1990.)

and some of ours, we suggest that mucosubstances normally present in submesothelial tissue account for spiral formation, especially if there is an overlay of inflammation. Such inflammation may increase mesothelial permeability, thereby facilitating transport of mucosubstances into a serosal cavity. Whatever the mode of formation of Curschmann's spirals is, they are a rarity of no known clinical significance.

Charcot-Leyden Crystals

Charcot-Leyden crystals have been described in serous fluids, both in the 1980s and in publications from almost a century earlier,[164] although from the scarcity of reported examples it appears to be a rarely observed phenomenon. However, crystal formation can be readily induced in pleural fluids by artificial means, such as adding one of a variety of detergents.[10]

In all of the spontaneously occurring examples of Charcot-Leyden crystals in serous fluids in which a description of the accompanying cells was provided, it is obvious that the fluids were classifiable as eosinophilic.[128, 164, 179] This is understandable because the extensive literature on eosinophilic leukocytes clearly indicates that Charcot-Leyden crystals develop from degenerating eosinophilic leukocytes.[15] That the crystals are so rarely seen in serous fluids is the result of the fluids being processed while they are fresh and relatively warm, before crystals have time to form from the cytoplasmic granules released from degenerating eosinophils.

In all our cases the crystals were observed only in the toluidine blue stained wet films, never in the permanent smears or cell blocks. Either the wet films or the specimens of fluid from which they had been prepared had stood in the refrigerator at 4°C for at least 24 hours. The crystals were typical Charcot-Leyden crystals: slender birefringent needles of uniform shape but of variable length and width, consisting of two hexagonal pyramids joined base to base (see Fig. 22–6). Eosinophil leukocytes were readily found in these wet films. Some crystals lay free in the fluid medium, some were alongside eosinophilic leukocytes, and some seemed to be emerging from eosinophilic leukocytes.

The most likely situation for Charcot-Leyden crystals to be found in a serous fluid is when a stained wet film is prepared from an eosinophilic effusion that has been stored in a refrigerator, particularly over a weekend when the laboratory is closed. We have observed Charcot-Leyden crystal formation in serous effusions only in such circumstances. Except for this crystal formation being an expression of at least a local eosinophilia, which may result from a wide variety of stimuli, it is not of any known significance. It is merely a curiosity.

Ferruginous Bodies

The literature records two examples of what appear to be typical asbestos bodies in pleural fluid;[29, 140] one

of the patients was described as having a history of asbestos exposure. It is possible that asbestos bodies could enter the pleural cavity through a bronchopleural fistula, although in neither of these cases was the presence of such a fistula mentioned. Without such a history, it is presumed that the thoracentesis needle penetrated the pulmonary parenchyma.

The rare finding of such bodies in a pleural fluid should be regarded as significant of a heavy asbestos burden in the lung. It is well recognized that virtually all inhabitants of modern urban societies have ferruginous bodies in their lungs,[204] but the concentration of ferruginous bodies in members of the general population is so low that they are rarely found in routinely prepared sections of lung.[43] Therefore, without a clear history of bronchopleural fistula, the finding of even one ferruginous body in a pleural fluid should indicate that not only has the thoracentesis needle penetrated the pulmonary parenchyma but also that the asbestos burden in the lung is heavy.

Radiation Reaction

Unlike radiation reaction seen in squamous and glandular epithelial cells from a variety of organs, we have never been able to identify an indisputable response to ionizing radiation in benign cells in serous fluids, although anecdotal accounts of radiation reaction of mesothelial cells in peritoneal and pleural fluids exist.[126, 140, 233] Von Haam's[233] account of radiation reaction of mesothelial cells and carcinoma cells in pleural fluids is quite unconvincing. The mesothelial cells illustrated as showing morphologic changes secondary to radiation are poorly illustrated and, assuming that they are hypertrophic owing to the effect of irradiation, their enlargement is well within the bounds of hypertrophy induced by a wide variety of other agents. The same stricture applies to the carcinoma cells illustrated as showing a reaction to irradiation. It is our impression that mesothelial cells in serous fluids show little or no detectable reaction to ionizing radiation, and that if they do show a reaction, it is not recognizable as such.

NEOPLASTIC EFFUSIONS

General

Many effusions associated with cancer are a result of some form of indirect mechanism, such as when a transudate develops as the result of venous obstruction caused by neoplasm or when an exudate develops as a result of inflammatory changes in an organ secondary to the presence of neoplasm. These are extremely common situations, and in such effusions neoplastic cells are not to be found. Even when a serous fluid contains neoplastic cells, the number of such cells may vary considerably, from a specimen that consists almost 100% of neoplastic cells to one that contains only a few. In the former situation, neoplasm presumably erupted through the mesothelium, perhaps in many areas, whereas when neoplastic cells are few the neoplasm may be confined mainly to subserosal connective tissue, penetrating the overlying mesothelium in only small areas.

Effusions containing neoplastic cells usually contain benign cells, which frequently outnumber the neoplastic cells. Mesothelial cells may be stimulated to undergo hypertrophy and hyperplasia, and their number may greatly exceed that of the neoplastic cells. In addition, such an effusion may contain macrophages and lymphocytes. Occasionally, such an effusion, apart from the presence of neoplastic cells, is entirely lymphocytic. Purulent effusions containing neoplastic cells are not common and denote coexisting inflammation of either the serous membrane or the underlying parenchyma or both. Hemorrhagic effusions are a result of vascular congestion of the subserosal connective tissue caused by the presence of neoplasm and are approximately twice as common in neoplastic effusions as in non-neoplastic effusions.[26]

Identification of Neoplastic Cells

In most situations, such as in cervicovaginal cytology, the cytologic diagnosis of cancer is carried out against a background of benign cells of the type that gave rise to the cancer cells. Furthermore, often there is an accompanying range of cells intermediate between the benign and malignant. In such a situation identification of cells that are cancerous depends on knowing the range of deviation of cells normal to the specimen. In serous fluids the situation is different in that, with the exception of mesotheliomas and a few ovarian carcinomas, neoplastic cells have a totally different appearance from any benign cells that accompany them.

It is well recognized that the diagnosis of neoplastic cells in an effusion does not depend on any single morphologic criterion or constellation of criteria. One may gain the impression from textbooks that the diagnosis of neoplasm in an effusion depends on finding cells that are large with a high nucleocytoplasmic ratio and that possess large, hyperchromatic, irregularly shaped nuclei with prominent nucleoli, and on the presence of abnormal mitotic figures. However, these criteria cannot always be applied to the diagnosis of neoplastic cells in effusions. For example, the cells of oat-cell carcinoma and some adenocarcinomas are small, the cells of mesotheliomas and some adenocarcinomas may possess profuse cytoplasm with a resulting low nucleocytoplasmic ratio and the nuclei of mesotheliomas and some adenocarcinomas may not be irregular in shape or hyperchromatic. Obviously, in making a diagnosis of neoplastic cells in a serous effusion the observer subconsciously employs a large number of criteria, some subtle, in arriving at a correct diagnosis, and the application of these criteria depends on familiarity with the type of specimen, the type of preparation and the context in which the diagnosis is being made. Essentially, one is attempting to recognize cells that are alien to the type of specimen, a finding that with few exceptions allows them to be recognized as cancerous.

Almost all examples of neoplastic cells in serous effusions are recognizable on routine preparations. Supplementary methods of identifying cancer cells are occasionally employed. However, they are virtually never used to make the decision as to whether the cells are neoplastic or non-neoplastic; instead, they are applied to demonstrate certain characteristics of particular types of neoplasm. Immunocytochemistry has its most fruitful application in distinguishing between adenocarcinoma and malignant mesothelioma and in confirming a suspected diagnosis of melanoma in cells that are amelanotic. The use of histochemistry is more or less limited to the demonstration in certain cells of mucin, glycogen, melanin or hemosiderin; however, it rarely has any real practical value. Electron microscopy does not enable one to discriminate between neoplastic and non-neoplastic cells, although it may have some use in this respect in selected cases.[46] Its use is to demonstrate distinctive features of certain types of neoplastic cells, such as osmiophilic bodies in metastatic bronchioloalveolar cell carcinoma, melanosomes in the cells of amelanotic melanoma, dense core granules in neuroendocrine neoplasms, intracytoplasmic lumina in certain metastatic adenocarcinomas and short microvilli with central filaments in gastric and colonic adenocarcinomas. Cytogenetic analysis can demonstrate abnormal karyotypes in neoplastic cells, but it is too laborious and expensive for routine application.

Differential Diagnosis of Types of Neoplasms and Determination of Primary Sites of Neoplasms

Most neoplasms in serous fluids are readily classifiable as to the type of neoplasm that gave rise to them. This especially true of adenocarcinomas, oat-cell carcinomas, keratinizing squamous cell carcinomas, melanomas and lymphomas. Adenocarcinomas are by far the commonest type of neoplastic cells to be found in serous fluids and, with experience, it may be possible to suggest with accuracy the primary site of the neoplasm, especially if given information about the sex of the patient and the site from which the fluid was obtained. Several studies[61, 156, 206] attested to this, but it is not clear how much success in this type of divination rests solely on morphologic features of the adenocarcinoma cells and how much depends on a knowledge of probabilities when supplied with the sex of the patient and the site of origin of the fluid. Despite some success in deducing the origin of adenocarcinomas from their cells exfoliated into effusions, there are always cases in which the deduction turns out to be wrong. From a practical point of view, determining the site of origin of adenocarcinoma cells is an interesting but largely redundant exercise because the clinical background of a patient usually provides the best clues about the origin of the cells.

Adenocarcinoma

Most adenocarcinoma cells in serous fluids originate in neoplasms of breast, lung or ovary. The cells may show the classic features of adenocarcinoma: a tendency to form smoothly contoured cohesive groups composed of large cells with eccentric, malignant-appearing nuclei, prominent nucleoli and vacuolated cytoplasm. However, adenocarcinoma cells in effusions exhibit great morphologic variation, not only in individual cells but also in their degree of organization, with some represented by groups of cells so large that they are visible to the naked eye, whereas others consist almost exclusively of isolated cells that have no contact with their neighboring carcinoma cells.

Cell Clusters

Adenocarcinoma cells may be single, or they may form clusters composed of only a few cells or large papillary fragments or spheroids composed of hundreds of cells. Neatly circumscribed, nonvacuolated spheroids (Fig. 22–86, see also Fig. 22–4), dubbed "proliferation spheres" by Foot,[61] are frequently seen with metastatic breast cancer and to a lesser extent with ovarian and pulmonary carcinomas and carcinomas from other sites.

As mentioned previously, mesothelial cells may form such spheres (see Fig. 22–34), but careful attention to nuclear and cytoplasmic detail, particularly at the periphery of the sphere, will reveal their mesothelial nature. Neoplastic proliferation spheres are frequently hollow but may be solid. The hollowness is readily demonstrated in cell blocks (Fig. 22–87). In smears the hollowness is discernable by a rather empty appearance at the center of the sphere (see Fig. 22–86).

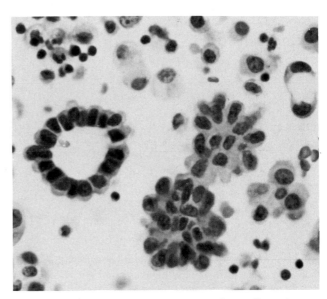

FIGURE 22–87. Fragments of **metastatic duct cell carcinoma** of the breast, one hollow and others solid (cell block of pleural fluid; hematoxylin and eosin; ×528).

By focusing on this empty center it is possible to find cells in two focal planes: an upper and a lower plane. Spriggs[210] demonstrated that most of these hollow clusters are not forming acini because their cells are nearly always oriented with their distal surface, often bearing microvilli, at the periphery and their basal surface next to the cavity, sometimes on a basal lamina. Clusters of adenocarcinoma cells that are not hollow are usually composed entirely of neoplastic cells, but collagen may occasionally be demonstrated at the center of a cluster, either by light microscopy or electron microscopy.[143, 210, 243]

Vacuolation of Adenocarcinoma Cells

Cell clusters exhibiting cytoplasmic vacuolation are common and may be seen in adenocarcinomas from all primary sites. The degree of vacuolation varies; in its extreme form it is particularly common in carcinomas of the ovary and the lung. Many of the vacuoles do not give the staining reaction of mucin because they contain glycogen or are a manifestation of degeneration. In toluidine blue stained wet films some vacuoles may contain a magenta-pink metachromatic substance, presumably mucin. However, most of the vacuoles in adenocarcinoma cells in the same specimen will not contain this metachromatic substance.

With some adenocarcinomas the cytologic picture is more likely to be one of virtually all isolated cells rather than one of clusters of cells. This is especially true with adenocarcinoma of the stomach (Fig. 22–88) and carcinoma of the breast, especially of the lobular type (Fig. 22–89). The isolated cells of gastric adenocarcinoma are frequently of the signet-ring type, with their nuclei displaced by large solitary cytoplasmic vacuoles (see Fig. 22–88). Some adenocarcinomas (see Fig. 22–89), as well as the occasional mesothelial cell,

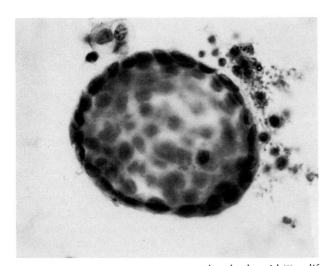

FIGURE 22–86. A compact, nonvacuolated spheroid ("proliferation sphere") of **metastatic ductal adenocarcinoma of the breast.** The empty appearance of the center of this spheroid denotes that it is hollow. Focusing in the center reveals two planes of cells, a lower and an upper (smear of pleural fluid; Papanicolaou stain; ×600).

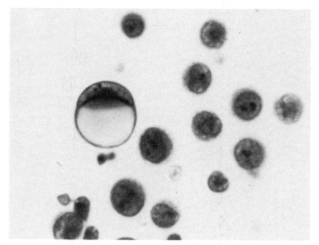

FIGURE 22–88. Metastatic gastric adenocarcinoma. All of the carcinoma cells in this field are discrete. One cell is highly vacuolated, imparting a signet-ring appearance (smear of pleural fluid; Papanicolaou stain; ×825).

contain in their cytoplasm one or more sharply defined clear areas in the center of which is a dense spot, like the bull's eye of a target. These spots are periodic acid–Schiff (PAS) positive and electron dense, and the spaces that contain them are lined by abundant microvilli (Fig. 22–90). Such cells correspond to the cells with intracytoplasmic lumina seen in histologic section of certain adenocarcinomas, especially lobular carcinoma of the breast.[217]

Ciliated Adenocarcinoma Cells

We have never seen in a serous fluid an adenocarcinoma cell bearing cilia. In Romanowsky stained preparations it may be possible to find adenocarcinoma cells, especially of ovarian carcinoma, bearing tufts of

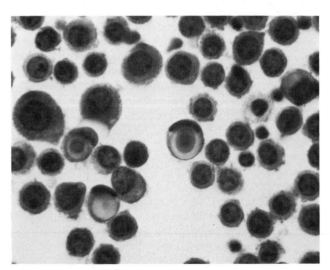

FIGURE 22–89. Metastatic lobular carcinoma of the breast. Almost all of the cells are discrete. Some contain cytoplasmic vacuoles in which there are dark central droplets of mucus (smear of peritoneal fluid; Papanicolaou stain; ×528).

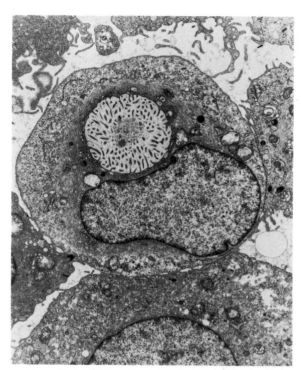

FIGURE 22–90. Cell of **metastatic lobular adenocarcinoma in peritoneal fluid** with a cytoplasmic vacuole lined by microvilli and containing a central droplet of mucus (transmission electron micrograph of same specimen as Figure 22–89; ×4300).

microvilli that superficially resemble cilia. Such cells were first described by Ebner[51] in peritoneal fluid containing cells of ovarian cystadenocarcinoma. The same publication also depicted cells that were truly ciliated; however, they were obtained from a benign ovarian cyst and were an example of DCTs, described previously.

Tufts of microvilli on ovarian adenocarcinoma cells in serous fluids have been well illustrated by Spriggs and Boddington.[213, 215] They are much more readily demonstrated in air-dried preparations stained by the Romanowsky method than in Papanicolaou stained preparations. However, Papanicolaou stained smears may reveal ill-defined tufts of microvilli, especially when situated on the end of a tiny cytoplasmic protrusion, as illustrated by Spriggs and Boddington.[215]

True cilia have rarely been demonstrated on adenocarcinoma cells in serous effusions.[51, 78, 122] Ebner's[51] case 1 may have been one of these in that the ovarian adenocarcinoma cells bearing long slender processes were motile. Gupta and coworkers[78] also illustrated cells of a widespread ovarian adenocarcinoma in pleural and peritoneal fluid that bore eosinophilic processes with terminal plates, evidence that they were truly cilia.

Ghadially[66] published an electron micrograph showing a compound cilium on a cell from a peritoneal effusion caused by ovarian carcinoma. An occasional benign mesothelial cell may also bear tufts of microvilli, a phenomenon well illustrated in Romanowsky stained smears by Spriggs and Boddington.[215] They also illustrated an example of mesothelioma cells that bore not only tufts of microvilli but also surface hairs that had the internal structure of true cilia.

Squamous Cell Carcinoma

The finding of squamous carcinoma cells in a serous fluid is an uncommon event. Furthermore, it has been difficult to glean from the literature which organs give rise to the squamous carcinomas whose cells are found in serous fluids and what their morphologic features are likely to be. To find an answer to this we reviewed the records of 7389 patients whose serous effusions had been examined cytologically.[205] Squamous carcinoma cells were found in serous fluids from only 46 patients (pleural 34, peritoneal 8, pericardial 4), with most of the cells originating in primary neoplasms of the lung, the female genital tract or the larynx.

Cytology

All of the recognized types[73] of squamous carcinoma cells were found in these fluids, with the most frequent being the nonkeratinizing third-type cell (Fig. 22–91), present in 50% of the fluids. In descending order of frequency were undifferentiated carcinoma cells, polygonal anucleated squamous carcinoma cells, malignant pearls and vacuolated third-type cells, keratinizing third-type and polygonal cells (Fig. 22–92) and tadpole cells. Fiber cells were found very infrequently.

At least a few squamous carcinoma cells that were vacuolated were found in 28% of the specimens, cells that could be misinterpreted as adenocarcinoma. However, it is well recognized in histologic sections that squamous cell carcinomas frequently contain cells that are vacuolated. In fact, in our review of the routinely

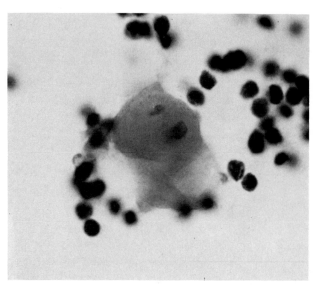

FIGURE 22–92. Metastatic squamous cell carcinoma from the larynx. Polygonal squamous carcinoma cell in which the nucleus is undergoing lysis (smear of peritoneal fluid; Papanicolaou stain; ×800). (Reproduced with permission from Smith-Purslow MJ, Kini SR, Naylor B: Cells of squamous cell carcinoma in pleural, peritoneal and pericardial fluids. Origin and morphology. Acta Cytol 33:245–253, 1989.)

prepared histopathologic sections of the 46 squamous carcinomas in this series, some degree of cytoplasmic vacuolation of the carcinoma was found in 37 (80%). In contrast to the cells of adenocarcinomas, the cells of squamous carcinomas in serous fluids, both vacuolated and nonvacuolated, tended to be discrete.

Tissue fragments of squamous cell carcinoma were found in 40% of the specimens, and they tended to have a more flat, two-dimensional appearance than those of adenocarcinoma. Within the fragments it was possible to discern well-defined cell boundaries (Fig. 22–93), and the central position of the nuclei in the cells composing the fragments was sometimes discernable. The typing of squamous cell carcinoma in a serous fluid may be facilitated by the cell block preparation, which often contains large fragments of carcinoma that are clearly of squamous cell type (Figs. 22–94 and 22–95).

Some squamous carcinoma cells in serous fluids may be similar in size, shape and staining reaction to normal superficial or intermediate squamous cells, but their nuclei are larger and darker and their chromatin is coarser (Fig. 22–96). As such polygonal carcinoma cells mature, their nuclei undergo lysis to produce a carcinoma cell that is anucleated or that contains only a trace of residual nucleus (see Fig. 22–92). The latter could be mistaken for a contaminant derived from the epidermis of a patient, clinician or technologist. However, such contaminant cells are few in serous fluids. Their borders are not sharply defined and their staining reaction is pale yellow, in contrast to the sharper definition and cytoplasmic orangeophilia or eosinophilia of polygonal anucleated squamous carcinoma cells.

Other possible sources of polygonal anucleated squa-

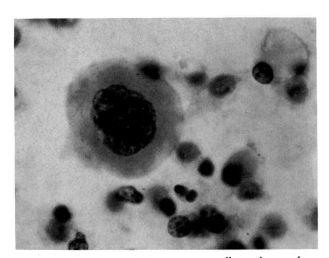

FIGURE 22–91. Metastatic squamous cell carcinoma from the larynx. Third type cell (smear of pleural fluid; Papanicolaou stain; ×800). (Reproduced with permission from Smith-Purslow MJ, Kini SR, Naylor B: Cells of squamous cell carcinoma in pleural, peritoneal and pericardial fluids. Origin and morphology. Acta Cytol 33:245–253, 1989.)

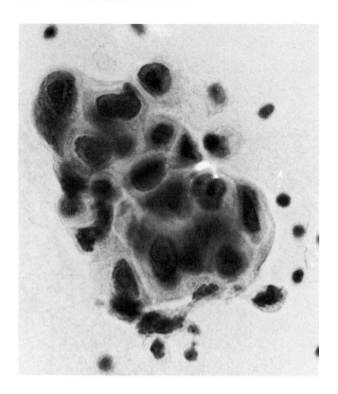

FIGURE 22–93. Metastatic squamous cell carcinoma from the lung. Fragment of carcinoma composed of third type cells. Note that it is possible to discern the borders of individual cells within the fragment (smear of peritoneal fluid; Papanicolaou stain; ×800). (Reproduced with permission from Smith-Purslow MJ, Kini SR, Naylor B: Cells of squamous cell carcinoma in pleural, peritoneal and pericardial fluids. Origin and morphology. Acta Cytol 33:245–253, 1989.)

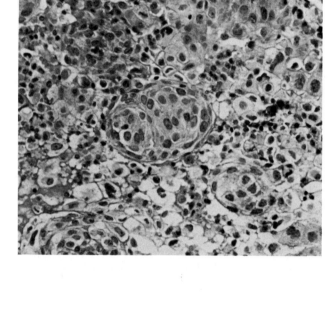

FIGURE 22–94. Metastatic squamous cell carcinoma from the uterine cervix. Moderately differentiated nonkeratinizing squamous cell carcinoma (cell block of peritoneal fluid; hematoxylin and eosin; ×200). (Reproduced with permission from Smith-Purslow MJ, Kini SR, Naylor B: Cells of squamous cell carcinoma in pleural, peritoneal and pericardial fluids. Origin and morphology. Acta Cytol 33:245–253, 1989.)

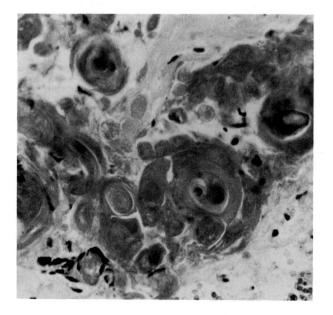

FIGURE 22–95. Metastatic squamous cell carcinoma from skin of the penis manifested by masses of virtually anucleate keratin (cell block of pleural fluid; hematoxylin and eosin; ×800). (Reproduced with permission from Smith-Purslow MJ, Kini SR, Naylor B: Cells of squamous cell carcinoma in pleural, peritoneal and pericardial fluids. Origin and morphology. Acta Cytol 33:245–253, 1989.)

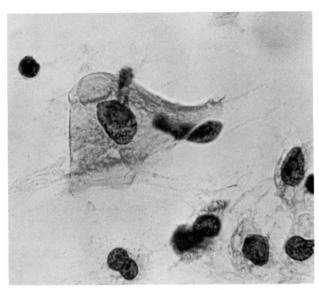

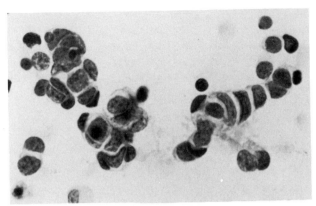

FIGURE 22–97. Oat-cell carcinoma appearing as amorphous clusters and a chain of cells with an angulated side extension. The nuclei are angulated and show more variation in size and shape than those of lymphocytes. The tight cohesiveness of these cells would never be seen in lymphoid cells. The chain is reminiscent of a silhouette of a vertebral column or a stack of coins of different denominations (smear of pleural fluid; Papanicolaou stain; ×825).

FIGURE 22–96. Metastatic squamous cell carcinoma from skin of the penis. Polygonal-type squamous carcinoma cell, similar in size and shape to an intermediate squamous cell; however, the nucleus is larger and irregular in shape, and the chromatin is coarse (smear of pleural fluid; Papanicolaou stain; ×800). (Reproduced with permission from Smith-Purslow MJ, Kini SR, Naylor B: Cells of squamous cell carcinoma in pleural, peritoneal and pericardial fluids. Origin and morphology. Acta Cytol 33:245–253, 1989.)

mous cells in serous fluids are (1) a metastatic or ruptured teratoma,[33, 76] (2) a fistula between the serous cavity and the alimentary or respiratory tract, (3) a fragment of skin introduced into the serous cavity during the aspiration procedure, (4) an ovarian acanthoadenocarcinoma or adenosquamous carcinoma[226] and (5) a focus of squamous metaplasia of the mesothelium. We have experienced all of these except the last mentioned.

The incidence of squamous carcinoma cells in serous fluids is not high, and if these cells do not show clear evidence of keratinization it is easy to overlook their squamous origin. However, one should expect that virtually every example of metastatic squamous cell carcinoma in a serous fluid will, as in our series, be derived from a patient known to have or have had squamous cell carcinoma.

Anaplastic Carcinoma

The anaplastic carcinomas are best exemplified by the small-cell anaplastic carcinoma (oat-cell carcinoma) of the lung, a major histologic type of lung cancer. The cytologic presentation in serous fluids of this highly aggressive carcinoma is well documented.[29, 126, 140, 193, 213, 215]

Cytology

The cells of oat-cell carcinoma in smears stained by the Papanicolaou method appear discretely or in small clusters (Figs. 22–97 and 22–98). The cells are small, about twice the size of lymphocytes. They also show a degree of nuclear angulation not seen in lymphocytes. Like lymphocytes they possess very little cytoplasm or may seem to possess none at all, often appearing to be composed entirely of hyperchromatic nuclei.

Another important distinction is that oat cells in serous fluids are cohesive, a feature not seen in lymphoid cells. Cohesive oat cells form tiny groups, frequently in the form of chains with side arms coming off at various angles (see Fig. 22–97), or they may form larger clusters. Smaller groups frequently exhibit a characteristic type of articulation in which one oat

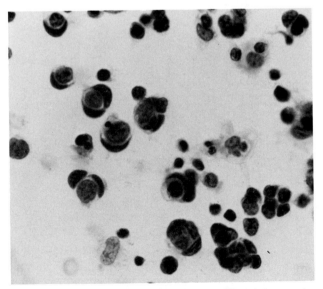

FIGURE 22–98. Small groups of **oat cells** exhibiting the characteristic type of articulation where one cell seems to be capping the other with its nucleus thus acquiring a quarter-moon shape (smear of pleural fluid; Papanicolaou stain; ×825).

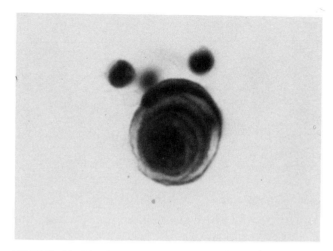

FIGURE 22–99. A compact group of **oat cells** that has acquired an "onion skin" appearance (smear of pleural fluid; Papanicolaou stain; ×1320).

cell seems to be capping another, with its nucleus acquiring a quarter-moon shape (see Fig. 22–98) or, in its extreme form, in which a tiny, compact group of cells acquires an "onion skin" appearance (Fig. 22–99).

The chains of oat cells are reminiscent of a stack of coins of different denominations or of the silhouette of a vertebral column (see Fig. 22–97). These configurations and the cells composing them are virtually diagnostic of metastatic bronchogenic oat-cell carcinoma. If seen, they should be regarded as diagnostic of this condition unless it can be proved that the neoplasm has arisen in a different organ because small-cell carcinomas, histogenetically akin to bronchogenic oat-cell carcinomas, occasionally arise in other organs.

Because oat cells in serous fluids are so small, it is easy to overlook their presence. Spriggs and Boddington[214] recommended use of Romanowsky stained air-dried smears for diagnosing oat-cell carcinoma because in this type of preparation the cells are larger and more frequently show a small amount of cytoplasm. Oat cells do stand out more in the air-dried preparations; however, once familiarity with these cells in Papanicolaou stained preparations is acquired, they should not be overlooked. They may be readily identified in cell block preparations as well as in toluidine blue stained wet films. In cell block preparations the cells frequently show more cytoplasm, and their nuclei may retain their elongated form (Fig. 22–100), as seen in sections of tissue.

A serous fluid containing oat cells may be mistaken for one containing lymphoma cells and vice versa. Lymphoma cells do not cluster, in either small or larger aggregates, as do oat cells. Furthermore, their angulated outline and absence of prominent nucleoli should prevent oat cells from being misinterpreted as lymphoma. Many oat cells become necrotic, producing faintly staining cellular particles as the cells undergo lysis or dense hyperchromatic pyknotic nuclei that simulate lymphocytes. Other small-cell, nonlymphomatous malignant neoplasms in serous fluids, such as

neuroblastoma or Wilms' tumor may resemble oat-cell carcinoma. Apart from any subtle difference between the cells of these neoplasms and oat-cell carcinoma, their clinical presentation is quite different from that of oat-cell carcinoma.

Small-cell anaplastic carcinoma of the lung may be composed of cells that are slightly larger than those of oat-cell carcinoma, being an anaplastic carcinoma of intermediate cell subtype. Apart from the increased size of the cells, this carcinoma is in every other respect similar to the small-cell carcinoma of oat-cell type. Various other types of carcinomas, such as adenocarcinoma or squamous cell carcinoma, may be so poorly differentiated that they are regarded as anaplastic or undifferentiated carcinomas. In these neoplasms the cells tend to be even larger than those of the intermediate cell type of small-cell anaplastic carcinoma of the lung; furthermore, their different histogenetic background may be detected by immunocytochemistry. Generally, the more the cells of anaplastic carcinomas of the lung and other organs increase in size, the more they acquire visible cytoplasm and prominent nucleoli, but in other respects they may retain morphologic features of cells of small-cell anaplastic carcinoma of the lung.

Urothelial Carcinoma

Urothelial (transitional cell) carcinomas seldom produce effusions containing carcinoma cells. For example, in the statistical series of Spriggs and Boddington[213] only ten of 2186 serous effusions were considered to be due to carcinoma of the bladder, and in only six of these ten were neoplastic cells found. These six cases accounted for only 1.1% of all positive reports of cancer cells in serous fluids.

The cells of urothelial carcinoma in serous fluids do

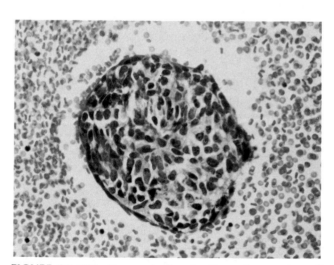

FIGURE 22–100. Fragment of **oat-cell carcinoma.** In cell block preparations the neoplasm tends to show more cytoplasm than is seen in smears, and the nuclei are more elongated, as in tissue sections (cell block of pleural fluid; hematoxylin and eosin; ×330).

not have any distinctive features. They may occur in clusters or singly and be vacuolated, probably due to degeneration, or nonvacuolated, in which case they may resemble mesothelial cells, except that their nuclei show features of malignancy.[213, 215, 223] Rarely can neoplasms of this type be accurately identified in serous fluids without knowledge of the patient's previously having urothelial carcinoma.

Melanoma

Patients with advanced melanoma, usually of cutaneous origin, frequently develop a serous effusion. Such an effusion may be the first manifestation of metastatic melanoma several years after treatment of the primary neoplasm. The cytologic picture of melanoma in serous fluids has been well described.[29, 81, 83, 126, 140, 213, 215, 254] The typical cytologic picture that emerges from these publications is of a fluid containing numerous obviously malignant cells that tend to be discrete, although small clusters may be present. The cells are round with abundant cytoplasm that contains brown pigment (Fig. 22–101). The nuclei are eccentric and oval and frequently contain large nucleoli. Multinucleated forms are frequently seen, and some nuclei may contain a vacuole that is an intranuclear invagination of cytoplasm.

Rarely, a fluid containing melanoma cells is chocolate brown; when the fluid is centrifuged the cellular deposit is dark brown and the supernatant is clear light

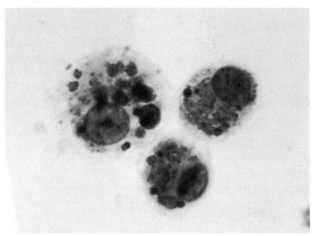

FIGURE 22–102. Melanophages. The fluid also contained pigmented melanoma cells. Melanophages frequently contain more pigment than the melanoma cells they accompany. Melanophages may be present even when the melanoma cells appear to be amelanotic (smear of pleural fluid; Papanicolaou stain; ×1320).

yellow. The cytoplasm of the melanoma cells in such a fluid is heavily pigmented, so much so that it may be difficult to discern the nuclei. However, such heavily pigmented melanoma cells in a serous fluid are the exception; most are either lightly pigmented or do not contain any pigment visible in routine preparations. In some melanoma cells the pigment is manifested as a light gray-brown dusting of the cytoplasm without the formation of obvious granules. Other cells in a fluid containing melanoma cells, such as macrophages and mesothelial cells, may also contain cytoplasmic melanin (Fig. 22–102).

In some serous fluids all of the melanoma cells are amelanotic and may resemble mesothelial cells (Fig. 22–103). However, attention to the morphologic char-

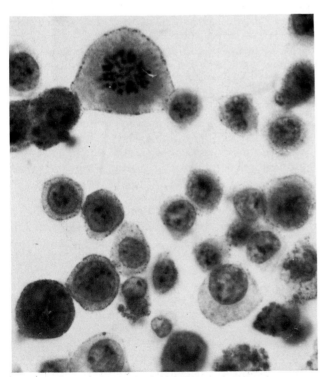

FIGURE 22–101. Metastatic melanoma cells from a cutaneous melanoma. The cells show a tendency to be discrete or to form small clusters. Cytoplasm is pigmented. Many nuclei are excentric and nucleoli are prominent (smear of pleural fluid; Papanicolaou stain; ×825).

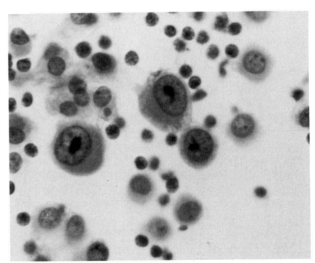

FIGURE 22–103. Metastatic amelanotic melanoma cells from a cutaneous melanoma. Apart from their large, irregularly shaped nucleoli, these cells could be misinterpreted as mesothelial cells (smear of pleural fluid; Papanicolaou stain; ×528).

acteristics of melanoma in general, albeit without cytoplasmic pigment, should enable one to at least suspect that the neoplastic cells are melanoma. Further characterization of melanoma cells can almost always be successfully carried out by the use of immunoperoxidase staining, using the monoclonal antibodies S-100 and HMB-45.[171, 180] S-100 protein is an acidic protein of unknown function normally found in a wide variety of neurogenous and non-neurogenous cells as well as in a variety of neoplasms. S-100 protein is not a melanoma-specific marker. On the other hand, monoclonal antibody HMB-45, as used on decolorized smears previously stained by the Papanicolaou method, was shown to have a high specificity for melanoma cells.[171] In addition to the reactions to anti–S-100 and anti–HMB-45, melanoma cells give a positive reaction to antivimentin and anti–NKI/C3 and anti–NKI/BTEV.[3]

It may be possible by transmission electron microscopy to demonstrate the melanomatous nature of neoplastic cells by revealing melanosomes. However, this technique cannot be applied retrospectively to smears or paraffin-embedded cell block material. Furthermore, it is time consuming and expensive.[69, 251]

Mesothelioma

Mesothelioma has attracted a great deal of international attention since Wagner and coauthors[235] in South Africa described an association between this neoplasm and the inhalation of asbestos. Apart from the epidemiologic and etiologic aspects of mesothelioma that this publication introduced, it opened up anew the question of whether the neoplasm mesothelioma really exists, a controversial subject at that time.[248] The controversy existed because diffuse malignant mesothelioma of the epithelial type frequently shows morphologic features similar to those of adenocarcinoma metastatic to a serous membrane. It was felt, therefore, that unless an occult adenocarcinoma could be excluded by complete necropsy, the diagnosis of mesothelioma was never justified, and even when adenocarcinoma was excluded, the diagnosis had to be viewed with a degree of skepticism. Any doubts about the existence of mesothelioma have now been dispelled by a large body of literature that has accumulated over 3 decades dealing with epidemiologic, etiologic, clinical, routine morphologic, histochemical, electron microscopic and immunocytochemical aspects of the neoplasm, largely summarized by the reviews of Antman[5] and Hillerdal,[91] the monograph of McCaughey and associates[147] and the articles of Ordoñez[170] and Johnston and colleagues.[108]

Primary neoplasms of the serous membranes classified as mesotheliomas may be divided into two types: diffuse and localized. The diffuse mesotheliomas are malignant; the localized neoplasms are either benign or malignant, mostly the former. In fact, some variants of localized mesotheliomas should, perhaps, be designated as either fibromas or fibrosarcomas. From the point of view of the cytology of serous effusions, it is only the diffuse malignant mesotheliomas that contribute cells of diagnostic significance and, even then, it is virtually only the epithelial variant that gives rise to a distinctive cytologic picture.

In this context the term *mesothelioma* does not include the rare primary papillary serous neoplasm of the peritoneum that occurs in women.[16] This neoplasm, which may be disseminated throughout the peritoneal cavity, is morphologically similar to ovarian papillary serous neoplasms and is quite distinct from mesothelioma. No account of the cytologic manifestation of this condition in ascitic fluid appears to have been published.

Diffuse malignant mesothelioma may arise on pleura, peritoneum, pericardium or tunica vaginalis of the testis. It most commonly arises from pleura or peritoneum, especially the former; it rarely arises from the pericardium or tunica vaginalis testis. The neoplasm usually affects men in their 6th and 7th decades of life and may develop multifocally in more than one serous cavity. Even though it may appear to develop in only one serous cavity, by the time a patient dies it frequently involves more than one.

In the earliest stages of their disease, most patients with diffuse malignant mesothelioma develop symptoms and signs of effusion. A pleural effusion may be clinically silent, being discovered only on a routine x-ray film of the chest; on the other hand, the patient may experience breathlessness or an aching pain in the chest. A patient with peritoneal mesothelioma may complain of abdominal swelling. Consequently, one of the first specimens received by the laboratory from a patient with diffuse malignant mesothelioma is likely to be pleural or peritoneal fluid.

Histologically, the diffuse form of malignant mesothelioma has either an epithelial or a sarcomatous appearance. The epithelial variant is either a well-differentiated papillary form (hence, its similarity to metastatic adenocarcinoma) or a medullary form or a combination of these, whereas the sarcomatous variant is composed of spindle cells, sometimes accompanied by a great amount of collagen. The epithelial type of mesothelioma is the more common; however, the two types frequently coexist.

As to the histogenesis of these two types of mesothelioma, it is easy to imagine the monolayer of mesothelial cells undergoing neoplastic transformation to produce mesothelioma of the epithelial type. In histologic sections of mesotheliomas it is not uncommon to find segments of mesothelium that appear to have undergone such a transformation to form neoplastic papillary fronds. On the other hand, accumulating evidence now suggests that the submesothelial mesenchyma retains the potential to differentiate into either epithelial or sarcomatous types of neoplasm or both.[37]

As mentioned earlier, the earliest manifestation of diffuse malignant mesothelioma is usually pleural or peritoneal effusion. At this stage both layers of the serosa are studded with innumerable tiny neoplastic nodules. As the disease progresses the nodules increase in size and coalesce to produce a thick rind of neoplasm on each serosal surface. Eventually the two layers fuse so that the amount of space available for effusion is considerably diminished or even completely obliterated. As the neoplasm continues to grow it causes bulging of either the hemithorax or abdomen, with displacement or constriction of underlying organs.

Cytology

Many accounts have been given of the cytologic manifestations of diffuse malignant mesothelioma in serous fluids. [17, 27, 29, 53, 81, 104, 110, 120, 123, 126, 140, 159, 160, 176, 215, 222, 225, 244, 245] They dealt almost exclusively with the cytology of diffuse malignant mesothelioma of the epithelial type, the type more readily recognizable from cells exfoliated into serous cavities.

The cytologic diagnosis of diffuse malignant mesothelioma of the epithelial type is a two-step process. First, the cells in the fluid must be recognized as being of mesothelial lineage, and second, they must be recognized as neoplastic. The first step is usually not difficult because mesothelioma cells of the epithelial type retain the morphologic features of benign mesothelial cells with such fidelity that they are recognized as being of a mesothelial nature. [159] In smears the morphologic features of non-neoplastic mesothelial cells, recapitulated in their neoplastic form, are those of shape, cytoplasmic staining reaction, nuclear position, size and shape, nucleolar prominence and types of intercellular articulation, as well as the formation of small or large mosaic sheets of cells and irregularly shaped clusters with knobby contours.

Malignant mesothelioma cells should show these morphologic characteristics to be recognized as mesothelial, but they should also be different enough from the normal or hypertrophic mesothelial cells to appear neoplastic. Generally it is not difficult to perceive their

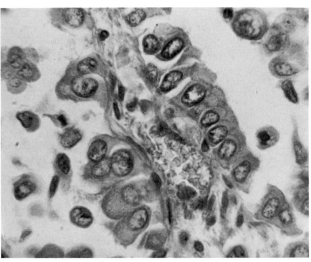

FIGURE 22–105. Papillary diffuse malignant **mesothelioma**. Same specimen as in Figure 22–104. This illustrates the typical neoplastic cells of a well-differentiated, papillary, diffuse malignant mesothelioma of the epithelial type (hematoxylin and eosin; ×600).

mesothelial origin, but it may be difficult to decide that they are malignant because the standard nuclear feature of malignancy may be poorly represented. [160] Nevertheless, our experience with cytologic preparations of pleural and peritoneal fluids from patients with diffuse malignant mesothelioma has enabled us to reach the point at which we can usually definitely diagnose or at least suspect the presence of mesothelioma.

Figure 22–104 illustrates a histologic section of a well-differentiated papillary diffuse malignant mesothelioma of pleura, and Figure 22–105 illustrates the cells composing this neoplasm. Figures 22–106 through 22–110 illustrate cells exfoliated from this mesotheli-

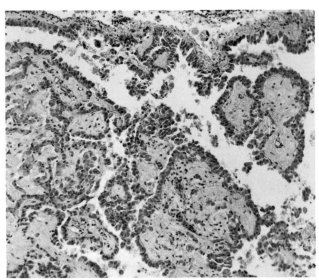

FIGURE 22–104. Papillary diffuse malignant **mesothelioma** arising from the parietal pleura, shown at the top (hematoxylin and eosin; ×150). (Reproduced with permission from Naylor B: The exfoliative cytology of diffuse malignant mesothelioma. J Pathol Bacteriol 86:293–298, 1963.)

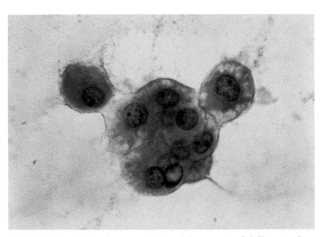

FIGURE 22–106. A large exfoliated fragment of diffuse malignant **mesothelioma** of the epithelial type. This specimen and those illustrated in Figures 22–107 to 22–110 are from the pleural effusion associated with the mesothelioma illustrated in Figure 22–104 (smear of pleural fluid; Papanicolaou stain; ×600). (Reproduced with permission from Naylor B: The exfoliative cytology of diffuse malignant mesothelioma. J Pathol Bacteriol 86:293–298, 1963.)

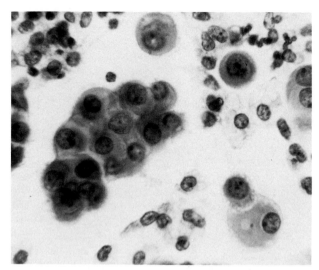

FIGURE 22–107. A large cluster of **mesothelioma cells** accompanied by two smaller clusters and a discrete mesothelioma cell (smear of pleural fluid; Papanicolaou stain; ×600).

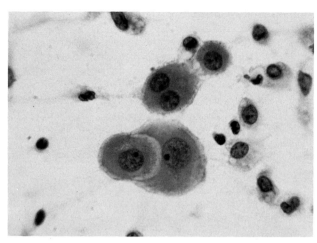

FIGURE 22–109. Two pairs of **mesothelioma cells**. One pair exhibits very prominent nucleoli (smear of pleural fluid; Papanicolaou stain; ×600). (Reproduced with permission from Naylor B: The exfoliative cytology of diffuse malignant mesothelioma. J Pathol Bacteriol 86:293–298, 1963.)

oma into the accompanying pleural effusion. In contrast to the picture of mesothelial hypertrophy and hyperplasia, the cells of mesotheliomas tend to be more profuse, often extremely so, and to form large clusters (see Fig. 22–106) usually accompanied by many smaller clusters and discrete cells (see Fig. 22–107), all exhibiting the morphologic characteristics of mesothelial cells. Furthermore, the individual cells are enlarged, although their nucleocytoplasmic ratio is about the same or even smaller than that usually seen in benign mesothelial cells (see Fig. 22–108). The nuclei also tend to be smoothly round or oval (see Figs. 22–106 to 22–108), in contrast to the more angulated nuclear outline typical of adenocarcinoma. On the whole, the nucleoli are prominent (see Fig. 22–109), and the nuclear chromatin is slightly increased

in density and more coarsely granular than in benign mesothelial cells, subtle features that seldom can be relied on to reveal the malignant nature of the cells.

Such neoplastic mesothelial cells may be so similar to benign mesothelial cells that it takes an experienced eye to perceive the differences between them. From experience, we have found that once we have determined that the cells in question are of mesothelial lineage, the most significant features pointing to the diagnosis of mesothelioma are the following: the large number of cells, the numerous clusters of cells, the increased size of the cells and the prominence of their nucleoli. These and other morphologic differences between benign mesothelial and mesothelioma cells have been analyzed quantitatively by Kwee and coauthors.[131] Vacuolated mesothelioma cells may be seen,[159, 216] but in all other respects they resemble the nonvacuolated

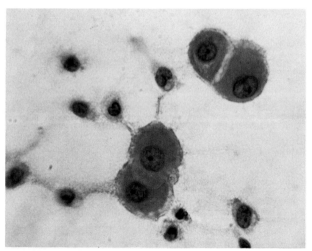

FIGURE 22–108. Two pairs of **mesothelioma cells**. In contrast to typical benign mesothelial cells, these cells are larger and have a lower nucleocytoplasmic ratio (smear of pleural fluid; Papanicolaou stain; ×600). (Reproduced with permission from Naylor B: The exfoliative cytology of diffuse malignant mesothelioma. J Pathol Bacteriol 86:293–298, 1963.)

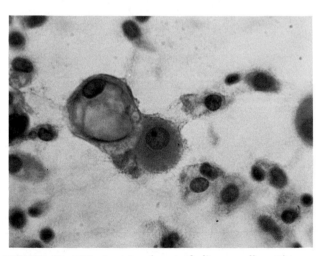

FIGURE 22–110. A pair of **mesothelioma cells** with one exhibiting marked vacuolation (smear of pleural fluid; Papanicolaou stain; ×600). (Reproduced with permission from Naylor B: The exfoliative cytology of diffuse malignant mesothelioma. J Pathol Bacteriol 86:293–298, 1963.)

mesothelioma cells that accompany them (see Fig. 22–110).

The ability to diagnose mesothelioma without resort to major surgery is a desirable goal because this neoplasm has a tendency to grow into thoracotomy and laparotomy wounds. It may even spread along the track of a thoracentesis needle. As with cytologic (or histopathologic) diagnoses in general, it is always advisable to render diagnostic opinions in conjunction with clinical information and any information derived from ancillary tests, especially that of pleural needle biopsy, which is commonly carried out at the time of thoracentesis.

Morphologic Variants

Apart from the "standard" cytologic features of diffuse malignant mesothelioma described previously, various other morphologic features have been emphasized. For example, Whitaker[243] pointed out the relatively high frequency of a central core of collagen within aggregates of mesothelioma cells in cell blocks (Fig. 22–111), much higher than in aggregates of metastatic adenocarcinoma cells. However, this phenomenon is not confined to malignant mesothelial cells; it has also been demonstrated in clusters of spontaneously exfoliated benign mesothelial cells[12, 218] and is frequently seen in smears and cell blocks of peritoneal washings (see Fig. 22–38).

Highly vacuolated or ballooned forms of mesothelioma cells have been occasionally described.[120, 136, 159, 189, 216] Some vacuolated mesothelioma cells may be seen in almost every cytologic preparation of mesothelioma; however, we have not seen an example in which a high proportion or almost all of the cells are highly vacuolated, macrophage-like, as described by Spriggs and

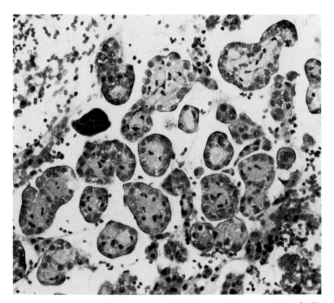

FIGURE 22–111. Fragments of diffuse malignant **mesothelioma** of the epithelial type with collagenous cores (cell block of pleural fluid; hematoxylin and eosin; × 41). (Courtesy of Dr. John D. Schaldenbrand, Ann Arbor, Michigan.)

Grunze.[216] This type of vacuolation is quite different from the diffuse, fine, lipid-containing cytoplasmic vacuoles found in some mesotheliomas, best demonstrated with air-dried films stained with one of the Romanowsky stains.[2, 23, 24] This pattern of vacuolation in mesotheliomas has been found to differ from that seen in benign mesothelial proliferations.[2, 23]

Special Techniques

Because it is important to distinguish between mesothelioma and metastatic adenocarcinoma in serous fluids, not only from the epidemiologic and therapeutic aspects but also from the aspect of asbestos-related litigation, immunocytochemistry and electron microscopy have been widely used to make this distinction. Whitaker[243] also pointed out the usefulness of using cell blocks in the diagnosis of mesothelioma. Not only do they demonstrate the presence of collagen cores in some clusters, but they also provide a readily available medium for immunocytochemical investigation.

Electron Microscopy. Transmission electron microscopy of surgical specimens demonstrated that mesotheliomas, in contrast to adenocarcinomas, have a significantly greater microvillus length-to-diameter ratio and more abundant intermediate filaments.[240] Mesotheliomas also have more complex microvilli than adenocarcinomas. These and other investigators' results on the ultrastructure of mesothelioma have been summarized by Coleman and coworkers.[35]

The ultrastructural approach to distinguishing between mesothelioma and adenocarcinoma, applied in a prospective study of cells in serous fluids, demonstrated that transmission electron microscopy can discriminate between adenocarcinoma and mesothelioma, but that it cannot be used to distinguish neoplastic from non-neoplastic mesothelial cells.[124] Similarly, scanning electron microscopy of serous effusions may distinguish between mesothelial cells and cells of metastatic adenocarcinoma.[47, 70] However, it does not discriminate between single benign and malignant mesothelial cells either.[28] Although electron microscopy seems in theory to have some value in the diagnosis of diffuse malignant mesothelioma, in practice it seldom needs to be used because most diagnoses of mesothelioma can be made on the basis of cytologic findings using light microscopy, especially in combination with immunocytochemistry.

Histochemistry. In an attempt to improve the distinction between mesothelioma and adenocarcinoma, histochemistry can be applied to cytologic specimens, with the aim of demonstrating in mesotheliomas the mucopolysaccharide hyaluronic acid and the lack of neutral mucosubstance, which could be produced by adenocarcinoma cells. Paraffin-embedded cell block material is especially useful for this purpose. This approach was first adopted in histopathologic material by Kannerstein and associates,[112] who found that the better differentiated mesotheliomas were more likely to produce hyaluronic acid. The alcian blue or colloidal iron reactions may demonstrate positively staining material in cytoplasmic vacuoles, tubular lumina or spaces within clusters of mesothelioma cells, material that is largely or entirely removed by prior treatment with hyaluronidase. Diffuse cytoplasmic staining or a rare positive vacuole is nondiagnostic. Mucus-bearing carcinomas generally contain material that stains with alcian blue or colloidal iron but that is not removed by hyaluronidase.

The PAS reaction may be positive in benign or neoplastic mesothelial cells owing to the presence of cytoplasmic glycogen. After treatment with diastase the reaction is negative in mesothelioma, whereas it remains positive in the presence of epithelial mucin of adenocarcinoma. Triol and coworkers[225] applied histochemical stains to cell block material from 55 mesotheliomas and found that a combination of stains was diagnostically useful in 42% of cases in which the original impression of mesothelioma was uncertain or equivocal, and it provided an added confirmatory finding in 64% of the diagnosable mesotheliomas. Overall, the staining results were "actively supportive" in 47% of the cases. Although the mucicarmine stain was included in their study, it was no longer routinely used because it had proved to be unpredictable, being neither as sensitive nor as reliable as the PAS reaction for demonstrating epithelial mucin. In our laboratory we have used these histochemical reactions to discriminate between mesothelioma and adenocarcinoma only sporadically because we find that in general these reactions are not too easy to interpret and that we diagnose mesothelioma just as well without them. Furthermore, we believe that conventional cytochemistry has been superceded by immunocytochemistry.

Immunocytochemistry. The 1980s has seen a burst of articles dealing with the use of immunocytochemistry to discriminate between mesothelioma and adenocarcinoma; these have been summarized and analyzed by Ordoñez[170] and Johnston and colleagues.[108] Essentially, what has emerged from the plethora of publications is that the greatest sensitivity in distinguishing mesothelioma from adenocarcinoma can be achieved by immunostaining using anticarcinoembryonic antigen, anti–TAG-72 (B72.3) and anti–Leu-M1. Furthermore, both neoplasms are likely to give a reaction to low-molecular-weight keratin monoclonal antibody. When there is a question of discriminating between adenocarcinoma and mesothelioma it has become the routine practice in our laboratory to apply immunohistochemistry to tissues or cytologic specimens (usually cell block preparations) using four monoclonal antibodies. In doing so, we have obtained satisfactory corroboration of our original impressions based on routinely prepared smears or cell block preparations. The point of testing for low-molecular-weight cytokeratin, which is likely to give a positive reaction with both neoplasms, is to obtain at least one positive result, thereby indicating antigenic integrity. Deserving of further investigation on cytologic specimens from serous fluids is the application of a polyclonal antibody to mesothelial cells. This has been applied with some success in verifying histologic diagnoses of malignant mesothelioma.[47, 201]

A diagnosis of mesothelioma should take into ac-

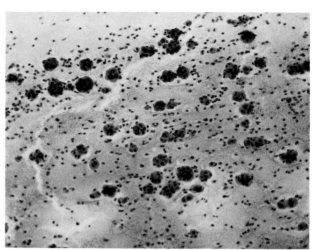

FIGURE 22–112. Numerous clusters of **mesothelioma cells** in a dense, granular, eosinophilic background due to the high concentration of hyaluronic acid in the specimen. To the naked eye the specimen was noticeably viscous (smear of pleural fluid; Papanicolaou stain; ×150). (Reproduced with permission from Naylor B: The exfoliative cytology of diffuse malignant mesothelioma. J Pathol Bacteriol 86:293–298, 1963.)

count all of the clinical findings and radiologic and other investigations as well as the routinely prepared cytologic and histologic preparations. Most mesotheliomas are diagnosable without resort to immunohistochemistry. In this era of asbestos-related litigation, however, it may sometimes be advantageous to support a diagnosis of mesothelioma by this technique.

Viscosity of the Fluid. It has long been known that effusions caused by diffuse malignant mesothelioma of the epithelial type may contain a high concentration of hyaluronic acid,[31, 86, 94, 152] a finding that may be used to corroborate a diagnosis of mesothelioma. A serous fluid with a high concentration of hyaluronic acid may show increased viscosity visible to the naked eye. Such increased viscosity due to hyaluronic acid may also be manifested in smears of the cellular sediment as a diffuse, granular, acidophilic or cyanophilic background (Fig. 22–112).

Flow cytometry has been applied to the diagnosis of mesothelioma and is dealt with in a later chapter.

In all of the previous discussion concerning the diagnosis of mesothelioma, only diffuse malignant mesothelioma of the epithelial type is considered. Sarcomatous mesotheliomas or the sarcomatous portions of mixed mesotheliomas may exfoliate their cells in any accompanying effusion, although it is our impression that the purely sarcomatous mesothelioma is much less likely to cause effusion. Their exfoliated cells appear as elongated malignant cells typical of many types of spindle cell sarcoma. A few examples of this type of cell have been reported.[29, 81, 120, 123, 126, 225] We have not seen such cells in our material.

Carcinoma of the Lung

In about 40% of pleural fluids containing cancer cells, the cells are derived from a primary carcinoma of the lung. In most cases they are adenocarcinoma cells, with the rest being squamous cell carcinoma or small-cell anaplastic carcinoma, subjects dealt with previously. It is well recognized that some lung cancers defy precise histologic typing into one of these categories; however, this residue of histologically nonclassifiable lung cancers when exfoliated into serous fluids generally exhibit the morphologic characteristics of adenocarcinoma and are thus classified. Consequently, the range of morphologic variation of adenocarcinoma in fluids is quite striking, with the most well-differentiated adenocarcinomas, such as bronchioloalveolar cell carcinoma at one extreme and pleomorphic giant cell carcinomas at the other.

The typical adenocarcinoma of the lung is characterized by large, obviously malignant cells occurring singly and in clusters (which may be papillary). Many cells show various degrees of vacuolation (Fig. 22–113). Some of the most differentiated examples of adenocarcinoma of the lung in serous fluids are derived from bronchioloalveolar cell carcinomas, and in these cases the clusters of adenocarcinoma cells are composed of cells with a low nucleocytoplasmic ratio and highly vacuolated, mucin-containing cytoplasm (Fig. 22–114). At the other extreme are the pleomorphic giant cell carcinomas which, when exfoliated into a serous fluid, exhibit morphologic features of adenocarcinoma, such as the tendency of their cells to cluster and of their nuclei to be excentric, although cytoplasmic vacuolation may be absent (Fig. 22–115). Psammoma bodies may occasionally be seen in clusters of adenocarcinoma cells derived from a primary carcinoma of the lung.

Woyke and colleagues[250] demonstrated by transmission electron microscopy numerous lamellar osmiophilic bodies in the cytoplasm of adenocarcinoma cells in pleural fluid, a finding that enabled the histologic type of the tumor, bronchioloalveolar cell carcinoma,

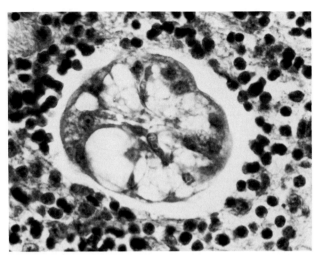

FIGURE 22–114. Bronchioloalveolar cell carcinoma. Note the vacuolated cytoplasm and low nucleocytoplasmic ratio (cell block of pleural fluid; hematoxylin and eosin; ×528).

to be established because some of these carcinomas are believed to be derived from type II pneumocytes. Osmiophilic bodies without lamination were also described in a similar case by Gondos and coworkers.[71]

Carcinoma of the Breast

Metastatic breast carcinoma is an important contributor to the cytology of serous fluids because of the high incidence of the disease and the frequency with which it metastasizes to a serous membrane, especially pleura, to cause effusion. Metastatic breast cancer cells are most often found in pleural fluids, although occasionally they are found in ascitic and pericardial fluids. In many cases of recurrent carcinoma of the breast, the first manifestation of persistent neoplasm will be a

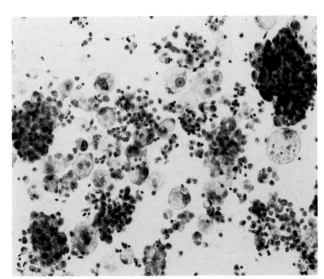

FIGURE 22–113. Metastatic bronchogenic adenocarcinoma. Numerous large, obviously malignant cells occurring singly and in clusters, with many of the cells showing various degrees of vacuolation (smear of pleural fluid; Papanicolaou stain; ×208).

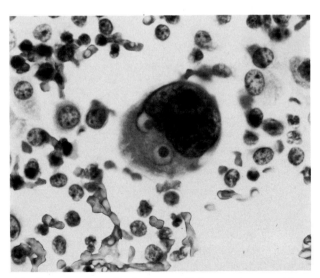

FIGURE 22–115. Cell of gigantocellular carcinoma of lung. Note the excentricity of the nucleus, indicative of its adenocarcinomatous nature. The cytoplasm contains two ingested nuclei (smear of pleural fluid; Papanicolaou stain; ×412).

pleural effusion. Such effusion may not develop until a decade or more after treatment of the primary neoplasm. The presence of metastatic breast carcinoma cells in a serous fluid does not always mean that death is imminent. We have records of patients with pleural effusion who survived from 2 to 4 years after the diagnosis of adenocarcinoma in the fluid.

Cytology

The cytologic picture of metastatic breast carcinoma has been well documented.[7, 29, 126, 140, 213, 233] Breast carcinoma cells in a serous fluid are usually abundant and of medium to small size. One classic presentation of breast carcinoma is as compact, dense, smoothly round, so-called proliferation spheres,[61] which may represent a multiplication of free cells in the fluid. Because of the high optical density of these spheres in smears (see Fig. 22–4 and 22–86), it is generally impossible to discern the individual cytologic features characteristic of malignancy; however, cell block preparations of such fluids clearly reveal the carcinomatous nature of the spheres (see Fig. 22–87). Even though in some of these fluids most of the carcinoma cells are forming these dense spheres, careful inspection will reveal isolated adenocarcinoma cells in the background.

Cell block preparations reveal that some proliferation spheres are solid, whereas others are hollow (see Fig. 22–87). This hollowness may be only partial, thereby imparting a cribriform pattern to the fragment of adenocarcinoma (Fig. 22–116) similar to that frequently seen in histopathologic sections of ductal carcinoma. In smears their hollowness can be discerned by the rather empty appearance of the center of the

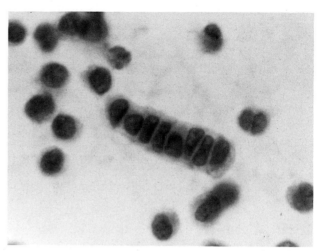

FIGURE 22–117. Metastatic lobular carcinoma of breast. All of the cells in this field are carcinoma cells. They are very small and form a caterpillar-like chain (smear of pericardial fluid; Papanicolaou stain; ×825).

sphere (see Fig. 22–86), and careful focusing will reveal that the cells in the center of the sphere are on two different planes. Proliferation spheres are characteristic of duct cell carcinoma of the breast.[7] They may occasionally be seen in effusions containing adenocarcinoma cells from other sources. We have seen them with ovarian adenocarcinoma, oat-cell carcinoma and squamous cell carcinoma as well as with several other types of neoplasm that are rarely found in serous fluids, such as carcinoid tumor.

Lobular carcinomas are typically manifested as numerous small, isolated carcinoma cells that could be mistaken for macrophages or small mesothelial cells, especially the latter (see Fig. 22–89). However, apart from the great number of fairly uniform isolated cells, individual cells show irregularity of nuclear shape, heavy nuclear membranes and prominent nucleoli. In addition, the cytoplasm of cells of lobular carcinomas (like that of some duct cell carcinomas) frequently displays one or more cytoplasmic vacuoles (see Fig. 22–89) lined by microvilli (see Fig. 22–90) and containing a mass of mucus.[217]

Cells of lobular carcinoma also have a tendency to form small, caterpillar-like or "Indian file" chains (Fig. 22–117) similar to those commonly seen with oat-cell carcinoma. They are quite different from oat-cell carcinoma; the cells are larger and possess readily visible cytoplasm, the nuclei are not as hyperchromatic and the nucleoli are visible.

The picture of a hypercellular specimen containing numerous small, round, neoplastic cells of fairly uniform shape and size could be mistaken for lymphoma. However, in virtually every example of metastatic lobular carcinoma it is possible to find small groups of cohesive cells denoting their epithelial nature. We have seen only one example in which such groups were not present. In such a case it would be possible to distinguish between metastatic adenocarcinoma and lymphoma by the use of immunocytochemistry.

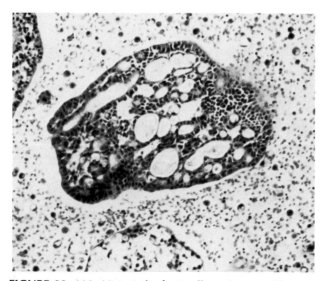

FIGURE 22–116. Metastatic duct cell carcinoma of breast. The partly hollow fragment of carcinoma has a cribriform appearance similar to that frequently seen in histologic sections of ductal carcinoma of the breast (cell block of pleural fluid; hematoxylin and eosin; ×132).

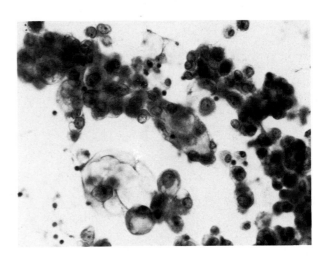

FIGURE 22–118. Metastatic ovarian papillary adenocarcinoma. This highly cellular specimen containing large papillary fragments of neoplasm, highly vacuolated cells and numerous single cells is typical of many ovarian carcinomas in serous fluids (smear of peritoneal fluid; Papanicolaou stain; ×330).

Carcinoma of the Ovary

Ovarian glandular neoplasms show a wide range of differentiation, from benign cystadenomas through ovarian tumors of low malignant potential to frankly invasive adenocarcinomas of various degrees of differentiation. Ovarian carcinoma is a frequent cause of ascites and, to a lesser extent, pleural effusion. In fact, the first clinical manifestation of ovarian carcinoma often is abdominal swelling due to peritoneal effusion, with the ascitic fluid containing carcinoma cells.

Cytology

Generally, ovarian carcinoma is readily recognizable in serous fluid, not necessarily as ovarian but certainly as metastatic adenocarcinoma. The number of neoplastic cells is usually high, with the cells presenting as large, acinar or papillary clusters mixed with numerous single cells, many of them vacuolated (Fig. 22–118). The papillary clusters may contain psammoma bodies; however, they are easily overlooked in Papanicolaou stained smears, being much more readily seen in cell block preparations (see Fig. 22–11) and even in unstained wet films. Cell block preparations often show the clusters of highly vacuolated cells in smears as fragments of tissue with a rather crumpled, cribriform appearance (Fig. 22–119).

Individual carcinoma cells show the morphologic features characteristic of adenocarcinoma. Usually they are quite large, even gigantic, and frequently they are hypervacuolated. Such vacuolation does not necessarily signify that the cytoplasm contains mucin; it may be due to glycogen or a degenerative change. Ascitic fluid taken from a woman that contains numerous large, hypervacuolated adenocarcinoma cells in papillary groups and singly is usually a manifestation of ovarian carcinoma.

The prognosis of ovarian tumors of low malignant

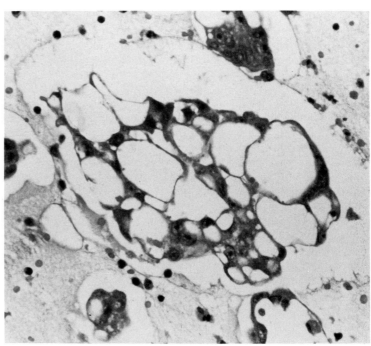

FIGURE 22–119. A fragment of highly vacuolated **metastatic ovarian adenocarcinoma** with a rather crumpled cribriform pattern (cell block of peritoneal fluid; hematoxylin and eosin; ×330).

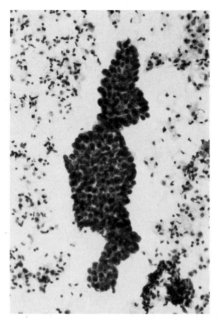

FIGURE 22–120. Papillary fragment of **metastatic ovarian serous cystadenocarcinoma** of low malignant potential. The fragment has a fairly smooth border, and the neoplastic cells are relatively small and uniform, with a high nucleocytoplasmic ratio and no intracytoplasmic vacuoles (smear of peritoneal fluid; Papanicolaou stain; ×185). (Reproduced with permission from Johnson TL, Kumar NB, Hopkins M, Hughes JD: Cytologic features of ovarian tumors of low malignant potential in peritoneal fluid. Acta Cytol 32:513–518, 1986.)

potential, neoplasms with some of the histologic features of carcinoma, is significantly better than that of invasive ovarian carcinoma and generally requires a less aggressive therapeutic approach. Distinguishing between the two types of carcinoma in a peritoneal fluid may therefore have some practical application. Johnson and coworkers[107] compared the cytologic presentation in peritoneal fluids of ovarian tumors of low malignant potential with that of invasive ovarian carcinoma. Cytologic preparations from the former contained large, cohesive papillary fragments with smooth borders (Fig. 22–120). The neoplastic cells were relatively small and uniform, with a high nucleocytoplasmic ratio, few intracytoplasmic vacuoles and inconspicuous nucleoli. Mitotic figures were rare. In contrast, peritoneal fluids from patients with invasive ovarian carcinoma contained smaller papillary fragments that were not cohesive and had irregular borders. The neoplastic cells were relatively large and pleomorphic, with low nucleocytoplasmic ratios, abundant intracytoplasmic vacuoles and prominent nucleoli. Most preparations contained many single cells and mitotic figures.

Some serous adenocarcinomas present with relatively small cells that are single or arranged in small groups. Their cytoplasm may show little vacuolation, and the nuclei do not exhibit pronounced deviation from those of mesothelial cells (Fig. 22–121). Such cells are likely to be derived from a fairly well differ-

entiated serous adenocarcinoma, and their morphologic similarity to mesothelial cells is a reflection of their origin from germinal epithelium of the ovary, which shares an embryonic origin with mesothelium.

Pseudomyxoma Peritonei

A well-differentiated, mucin-producing ovarian adenocarcinoma may rupture, spilling its mucoid contents into the abdominal cavity, where the carcinoma cells continue to proliferate and produce mucin. The patient develops a slowly accumulating but ultimately massive peritoneal effusion that is extremely difficult to aspirate because of its thick mucoid consistency. Furthermore, the aspirated fluid is difficult to smear and, except for the occasional macrophage, may appear to be devoid of cells. However, if enough fluid is examined, especially by the smear and cell block techniques, it is possible to find groups of well-differentiated, vacuolated adenocarcinoma cells in honeycomb-like sheets or strips[208, 223] as illustrated in Figure 22–122.

This condition, known as pseudomyxoma peritonei, is rare. It is extremely difficult to treat because the viscosity of the intraperitoneal fluid does not permit intraperitoneal antineoplastic drugs to diffuse through the peritoneal cavity. Ultimately the condition is fatal, usually owing to intestinal obstruction. The condition may also be brought about by dissemination of a well-differentiated, mucin-producing adenocarcinoma of the large intestine, particularly the appendix.[183] In such a situation, the condition also occurs in males.

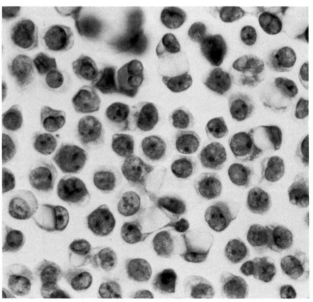

FIGURE 22–121. Metastatic ovarian serous cystadenocarcinoma. The cells are fairly small and uniform in shape and size and occur singly or in small groups. Vacuolation is not prominent. Such cells might readily be mistaken for mesothelial cells (smear of peritoneal fluid; Papanicolaou stain; ×528).

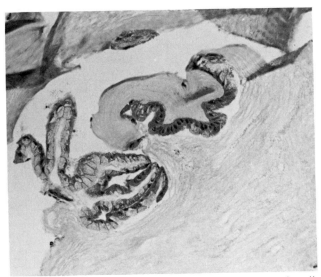

FIGURE 22–122. Pseudomyxoma peritonei. Strips of well-differentiated adenocarcinoma in a background of mucus. The patient was a man. The primary neoplasm was in the vermiform appendix. Because of its mucoid nature this fluid was extremely difficult to aspirate and to smear (cell block of peritoneal fluid; hematoxylin and eosin; ×165).

Carcinoma of the Gastrointestinal Tract

Despite the frequency of colonic adenocarcinoma as a cause of death, the finding of cells from this neoplasm in a serous fluid is not a common event. Usually they are found in ascitic fluid. As the incidence of gastric carcinoma declines, cells from this lesion in serous fluids are now being seen with less frequency. Most are seen in peritoneal fluids. The cytologic presentation of colonic and gastric carcinomas has, in our experience, been similar. Most of these lesions presented mainly with single cells in the fluids, although in the colonic carcinomas, they were usually few, whereas with the gastric carcinomas, the fluids usually contained a large number of single carcinoma cells, many of the signet-ring type (see Fig. 22–88).

In cell block preparations, fragments of colonic carcinoma frequently are composed of elongated columnar cells with dark nuclei (Fig. 22–123), typical of such neoplasms in biopsy specimens. Because these carcinomas as well as the gastric carcinomas are usually mucin producing, the background of the preparation may also contain streaks of mucus, reaching its extreme form in pseudomyxoma peritonei, discussed earlier.

Miscellaneous Carcinomas

We have seen examples of adenocarcinomas of endometrial, prostatic, pancreatic, biliary, cervical, thyroid, renal and hepatic origin in serous fluids. Their appearance varied greatly from small cells of fairly uniform size and shape, not unlike macrophages, to large, multinucleated cells that were obviously malignant. Some came almost exclusively as single cells, others almost entirely as cell clusters; most were a combination of both. One of our cases of endometrial carcinomas contained psammoma bodies. Our only example of hepatocellular carcinoma had dense granular eosinophilic cytoplasm similar to that of hepatocytes. The few examples of prostatic adenocarcinoma consisted of small neoplastic cells. Otherwise, the cells of this heterogenous group of adenocarcinomas had on the whole no distinguishing features that would enable one to determine their site of origin. Such a determination relied heavily on the clinical background and, to some extent, a review of any previously obtained histopathologic material from the patient.

Lymphoma and Leukemia

Serous effusions are a common complication of lymphomas and leukemias, especially the former, and the frequency with which lymphoma and leukemia cells can be found in these fluids is rivaled only by carcinoma cells metastatic from neoplasms of the breast, the lung or the ovary. In almost every case in which lymphoma or leukemia cells are found in a serous fluid, the patient is known to have the disease. Rarely, however, the finding of lymphoma cells in an effusion is the first morphologic manifestation of the disease.

Earlier analyses of lymphoma and leukemia cells in serous effusions dealt with cytologic preparations prepared exclusively by the Papanicolaou method.[20, 81, 149] Their depiction of cells as neoplastic was sound; however, the method does not allow the same degree of correlation with the various types of lymphoma and leukemia that can be achieved by the use of air-dried Romanowsky stained preparations. The latter approach to the diagnosis of lymphomas and leukemias

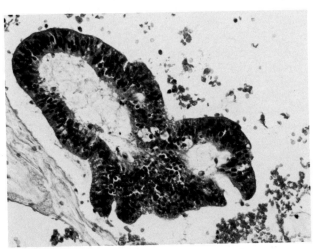

FIGURE 22–123. Fragment of **metastatic colonic adenocarcinoma** composed of elongated columnar cells with dark nuclei, typical of such neoplasms in biopsy specimens. The background contains a streak of mucus (cell block of peritoneal fluid; hematoxylin and eosin; ×208).

in serous fluids, addressed in later publications,[215, 219] demonstrated that a high degree of correlation can be achieved between the typing of lymphoma cells in serous fluids and the histologic typing of the neoplasm (using the Kiel classification). It is our impression, however, that for the detection of lymphoma or leukemia cells in serous fluids, without any need for refinement of classification, the two techniques give similar results, and that persons experienced with either method have similar difficulties when confronted with cytologic pictures that are equivocal.

In reality, not being able to precisely type lymphoma or leukemia cells in serous fluids is rarely a disadvantage because virtually all of the patients have already been diagnosed as having one or the other condition, and the type of neoplasm is already known. Apart from routine morphologic examination, immunologic and cytometric methods have been applied with some success to the diagnosis and typing of non-Hodgkin's lymphomas in serous fluids.[115, 146, 252]

Most effusions due to lymphoma are clear, slightly bloodstained or occasionally chylous. In fact, lymphoma is the commonest cause of a chylous effusion.[215] The cytologic picture is frequently dominated by lymphoma cells; often virtually every cell in the effusion is lymphoma (Fig. 22–124). Not all effusions caused by lymphoma or leukemia contain neoplastic cells; such effusions may be the result of inflammation secondary to the neoplasm or to neoplastic occlusion of vascular channels.

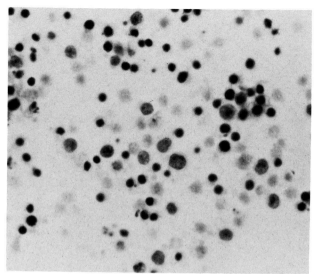

FIGURE 22–125. Stem cell leukemia. A high proportion of the cells is necrotic, manifested by light gray cells with no internal structure or cells with pyknotic nuclei, resembling lymphocytes. A few of the cells are still viable (smear of pleural fluid; Papanicolaou stain; ×528).

One of the most important aspects of the cytology of non-Hodgkin's lymphomas and leukemia is that the neoplastic cells do not exhibit genuine attachment to each other. If such attachment can be found, the neoplasm is neither lymphoma nor leukemia. Another striking feature of these neoplasms in serous fluids is that they frequently exhibit massive necrosis, a feature rarely observed with carcinomas. Widespread necrosis is virtually confined to the higher grade lymphomas and some leukemias and may be seen in several forms: obvious necrosis of the entire cell (Fig. 22–125), lysis of cells with subsequent disintegration to form granular background material (Fig. 22–126), pyknosis of nuclei

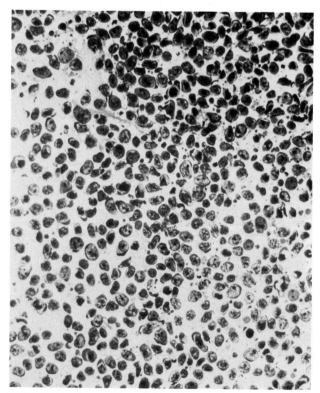

FIGURE 22–124. Large-cell lymphoma, intermediate grade. Virtually every cell in this crowded field is lymphomatous. None of the cells show genuine attachment to each other (wet film of pleural fluid; toluidine blue; ×160).

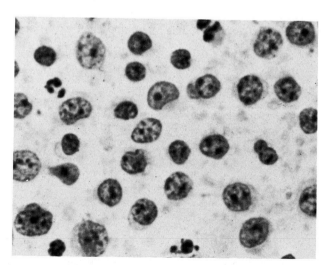

FIGURE 22–126. Large cell lymphoma, intermediate grade. A few of the cells are necrotic, as evidenced by nuclear fragmentation. The background contains light gray particles, formed from cells that have disintegrated (smear of pleural fluid; Papanicolaou stain; ×512).

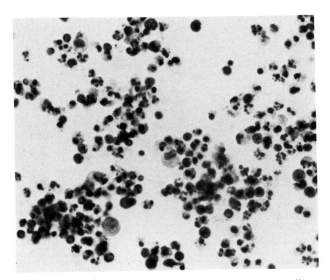

FIGURE 22–127. Burkitt's lymphoma. Most of the cells in this field are necrotic. Their nuclei have fragmented into tiny cyanophilic particles (mercury-drop karyorrhexis). At first glance these necrotic cells resemble neutrophils (smear of pleural fluid; Papanicolaou stain; ×330).

to form cells that resemble lymphocytes (see Fig. 22–125) and fragmentation of nuclei in the cytoplasm to form tiny, round cyanophilic cytoplasmic particles reminiscent of a dispersed drop of mercury (mercury drop karyorrhexis). At first glance, a smear exhibiting mercury drop karyorrhexis may appear to contain numerous neutrophilic leukocytes (Fig. 22–127). It has been suggested that this type of necrosis is secondary to chemotherapy[149]; however, we have seen it on several occasions before treatment was begun.

In our laboratory we have used the Papanicolaou method exclusively for our smears. Consequently, we do not claim to be able to achieve the accuracy of typing of lymphomas or leukemias that may be possible with smears prepared by the Romanowsky method. In contrast to the situation with carcinomas, cell block preparations of serous fluids containing lymphoma or leukemia cells have seldom contributed any additional diagnostic information. On the other hand, stained wet films have frequently demonstrated with remarkable

clarity the lymphomatous or leukemic nature of an effusion (Fig. 22–128; see also Fig. 22–124). Generally, the cytologic features of non-Hodgkin's lymphomas in serous fluids and the accuracy that may be achieved in their diagnosis depends on the morphologic type of lymphoma: low grade, intermediate grade or high grade (Working Formulation for Clinical Usage).

Cytology

Low-grade lymphomas are exemplified by small-cell lymphocytic lymphoma, which is composed of cells that in routine preparations are morphologically indistinguishable from benign lymphocytes. Such cells may also be seen with chronic lymphocytic leukemia. Demonstrating the neoplastic nature of these cells may require flow cytometry to show their monoclonality.

Spriggs and Boddington[213, 215] illustrated a distinctive clumping of chromatin in cells of chronic lymphocytic leukemia in pleural fluids. Cells with these clumps of chromatin, likened to clots, have been referred to as cellules grumelees (clotted cells).[221] The phenomenon seems to be virtually confined to cells of low-grade lymphocytic lymphoma (Fig. 22–129) or chronic lymphocytic leukemia, and its appearance can be influenced by the method of fixing the smear. It has been shown to be more likely to occur in smears that have been fixed by methanol,[198] the usual fixative for Romanowsky stained smears, although it has been illustrated in a Papanicolaou stained smear that presumably was fixed with ethanol.[215] We have also observed the phenomenon in toluidine blue stained wet films.

Enumeration of T and B lymphocytes in such effusions may aid in distinguishing those that are inflammatory from those that are neoplastic. In inflammatory lymphoid effusions most of the cells are of the T type, whereas in lymphomas and leukemias a high proportion of the cells are of the B type.[146] A high proportion of B cells is strong evidence of lymphoma, especially

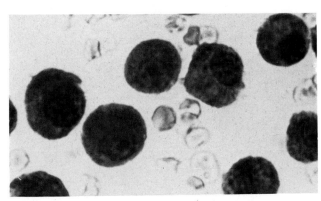

FIGURE 22–128. Myelomatosis. Except for the red blood cells, every cell in this field is a myeloma cell (wet film of pleural fluid; toluidine blue; ×640).

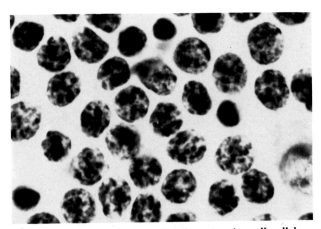

FIGURE 22–129. Cells of well-differentiated **small-cell lymphocytic lymphoma** (low grade) exhibiting coarse clumps of chromatin, so-called cellules grumelées (smear of pleural fluid; Papanicolaou stain; ×660). (Courtesy of Mr. Tarring A. Seidel, Danville, Pennsylvania.)

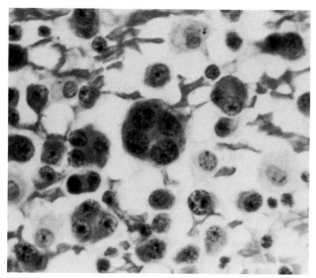

FIGURE 22–130. Myeloma cells (smear of pleural fluid; Papanicolaou stain; ×528).

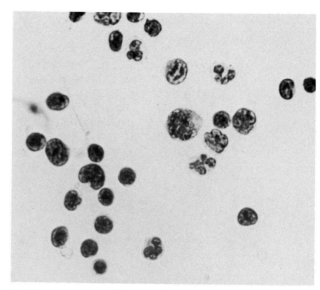

FIGURE 22–132. Malignant lymphoma, mixed small- and large-cell type, intermediate grade (smear of pleural fluid; Papanicolaou stain; ×528).

if only a single light chain is present. Usually in chronic lymphocytic leukemia the proportion of B cells approximates 100%, provided that the effusion is due to leukemic infiltration of the serosa and not to intercurrent inflammation.

Because of the low turnover of cells in myelomatosis, this condition is classified as a low-grade lymphoma. Myeloma cells are rarely seen in serous fluids, but when they are present, they are numerous. They possess morphologic features of plasma cells but are larger and more often multinucleated and possess prominent nucleoli (Fig. 22–130; see also Fig. 22–128). These features and their large number distinguish them from plasma cells in mixed inflammatory reactions.

Lymphoma cells of the higher grades are generally not difficult to recognize. The cells are larger, as are their nuclei, which may show various degrees of poly-

morphism, and their nucleoli are more prominent (Figs. 22–131 and 22–132). Furthermore, necrosis of individual cells is more likely to occur and may dominate the cytologic picture. The cytologic extreme of the high-grade lymphomas is exemplified by large-cell immunoblastic lymphoma of polymorphous type (Fig. 22–133).

Cells of all types of leukemia may be found in serous fluids. Their recognition is best accomplished by using air-dried Romanowsky stained smears, and the cells are recognized according to the usual morphologic criteria featured in atlases of hematology. As in lymphomatous effusions, necrosis may be widespread (see Fig. 22–125). The unusual leukemia, hairy cell leukemia, has a rather characteristic appearance in the Papanicolaou stained smears.[127] Superficially the cells resembled lymphocytes, except they are slightly larger,

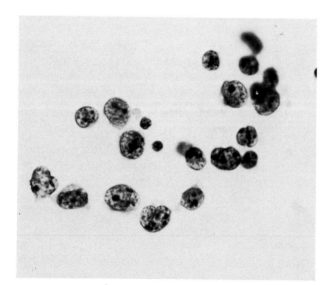

FIGURE 22–131. Large-cell lymphoma, intermediate grade. Same specimen as Figure 22–124 (smear of pleural fluid; Papanicolaou stain; ×330).

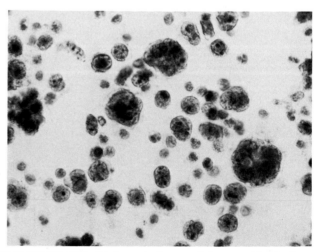

FIGURE 22–133. High-grade large-cell **immunoblastic lymphoma** of the polymorphous type (smear of pleural fluid; Papanicolaou stain; ×330).

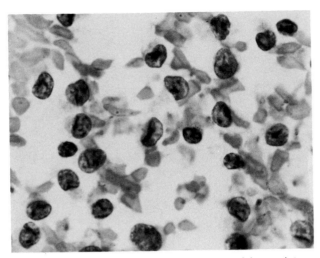

FIGURE 22–134. Hairy cell leukemia. Many of the nuclei are slightly indented, and in some of the cells nucleoli are prominent (smear of pleural fluid; Papanicolaou stain; × 825).

their nuclei are paler and many are slightly indented and their nucleoli are more prominent (Fig. 22–134). In Papanicolaou stained preparations the projecting cytoplasmic "hairs" are not visible.

Hodgkin's Disease

Serous effusion are fairly common in patients with Hodgkin's disease, especially in the pleural cavity. Whenever we have examined fluid from a patient with Hodgkin's disease, the diagnosis had already been established.

Generally, the cytologic picture is nonspecific, consisting mainly of lymphocytes and plasma cells with macrophages and mesothelial cells. Pleural eosinophilia may be present, but in our experience this a rare event. The only diagnostic feature of Hodgkin's disease in effusion is the multinucleated Reed-Sternberg cell (Fig. 22–135), which may be accompanied by mononuclear variants known as Hodgkin's cells. It has been our experience as well as that of others[149, 215] that effusions due to Hodgkin's disease are not likely to contain Reed-Sternberg cells. If present, they are usually in small numbers, and it may require careful scrutiny of several smears before finding one convincing example. In Romanowsky stained preparations Reed-Sternberg cells are large with two or more nuclei exhibiting a "butterfly" or "mirror image" configuration. In Papanicolaou stained preparations they are much smaller and more difficult to find, although it should be possible to find them with about the same frequency as with the air-dried Romanowsky stained preparations.[249]

Myelofibrosis with Myeloid Metaplasia

Myelofibrosis with myeloid metaplasia is a neoplastic disorder of the common hematologic precursor cell accompanied by prominent fibrosis of the marrow. The condition is characterized by myeloid metaplasia, especially at the sites of fetal extramedullary hematopoiesis (Fig. 22–136), but this may also develop immediately beneath the mesothelium in many other locations to cause effusion. These foci of myeloid metaplasia may be of only microscopic size, but they may be so large that they are visible to the naked eye just beneath the mesothelium or they may form mesothelium-covered masses bulging into the serous cavity (Fig. 22–137). Leukemic conversion may take place with the production of leukemic cells in the serous fluid. However, the most distinctive feature of the effusions associated with this condition is the presence of large, atypical, neoplastic megakaryocytes (Fig. 22–138).[129] These megakaryocytes are larger than normal and are frequently accompanied by megakaryocytes that have extruded their nuclei to leave only an anucleated cytoplasmic mass (Fig. 22–139).

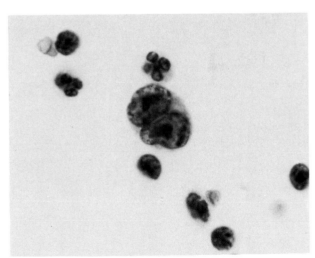

FIGURE 22–135. Hodgkin's disease. A binucleate Reed-Sternberg cell with prominent nucleoli (smear of pleural fluid; Papanicolaou stain; × 528).

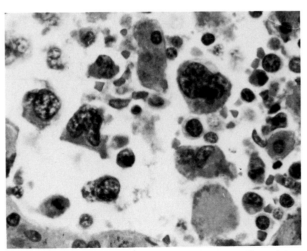

FIGURE 22–136. Liver invaded by **leukemic cells** and large **neoplastic megakaryocytes** (section from the specimen illustrated in Figure 22–137; hematoxylin and eosin; × 528).

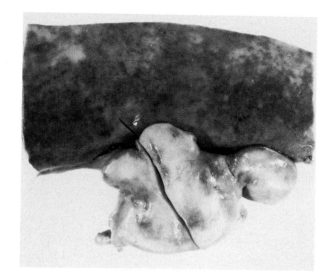

FIGURE 22–137. Lower border of liver from the necropsy of a patient who died from myelofibrosis with **myeloid metaplasia**. The liver shows numerous submesothelial pale foci of myeloid metaplasia. A large mesothelium-covered nodule of myeloid metaplastic tissue bulges from the surface of the liver (natural size).

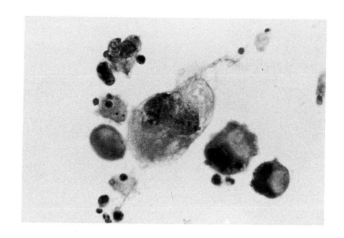

FIGURE 22–138. Neoplastic megakaryocytes. Smear of peritoneal fluid from the same case as illustrated in Figures 22–136, 22–137 and 22–139 (Papanicolaou stain; ×330). (Reproduced with permission from Kumar NB, Naylor B: Megakaryocytes in pleural and peritoneal fluids; prevalence, significance, morphology, and cytohistological correlation. J Clin Pathol 33:1153–1159, 1980.)

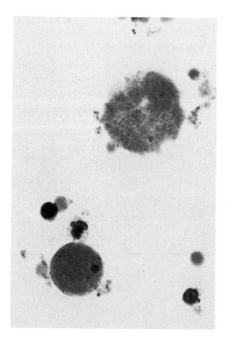

FIGURE 22–139. Two anucleate **megakaryocytes.** Both contain residual nuclear material (smear of peritoneal fluid from the same case as Figures 22–136 through 22–138; Papanicolaou stain; ×660). (Reproduced with permission from Kumar NB, Naylor B: Megakaryocytes in pleural and peritoneal fluids: prevalence, significance, morphology, and cytohistological correlation. J Clin Pathol 33:1153–1159, 1980.)

Neoplasms Rarely Seen in Serous Fluids

Certain neoplasms are rarely seen in serous effusions, with the result that outside the major specialist centers most laboratories accumulate no more than a few examples. Consequently, most descriptions of these neoplasms are single case reports. The largest published description of such cases is in the book of Hajdu and Hajdu,[81] whose material was derived from a major cancer hospital. Neoplasms in this category include nonlymphomatous sarcomas, thymoma, neuroendocrine tumors, nephroblastomas, neuroblastomas and germ cell neoplasms.

In virtually all of the reported examples of these neoplasms in serous fluids, the diagnosis of cancer, including its type, was already known because the patient had an obvious primary neoplasm or a previously removed neoplasm. In such cases the role of the laboratory is, essentially, to report on the presence or absence of malignant cells in a serous fluid and, if possible, to state that they are morphologically similar to, or consistent with, cells composing the known primary neoplasm. It is seldom necessary to deal further with the typing of these neoplasms.

Cells of these neoplasms in serous fluids generally fall into four groups: (1) malignant cells that are generally large, pleomorphic and multinucleated, frequently with a fiber shape, (2) cells that are small and apparently undifferentiated with scanty cytoplasm, (3) cells of germ cell neoplasms and (4) cells of malignant histiocytoses.

Pleomorphic and Spindle Cell Neoplasms

Cells in the first group correspond to many of the well-recognized spindle cell and pleomorphic sarcomas. In this category we have seen examples of malignant fibrous histiocytoma, liposarcoma (Fig. 22–140), neurofibrosarcoma (Fig. 22–141), angiosarcoma (Fig. 22–142) and rhabdomyosarcoma (Fig. 22–143). Apart from those recorded in the book of Hajdu and Hajdu,[81] other examples in the literature include those of osteosarcoma,[126] angiosarcoma,[62, 215, 258] clear cell sarcoma,[165] chondrosarcoma,[233] malignant ganglioneuroma,[140] endometrial stromal sarcoma,[98] malignant fibrous histiocytoma,[195, 255] liposarcoma, [64, 223, 233] fibrosarcoma,[140, 215] cystosarcoma phyllodes,[140] myosarcoma[82, 126, 215, 223, 233] and thymoma.[230, 261]

Small-Cell "Undifferentiated" Neoplasms

The small, undifferentiated-appearing cells with scanty cytoplasm of the second group frequently exhibit molding. Such cells are reminiscent of oat-cell carcinoma. This picture has been illustrated in cases of carcinoid tumor,[141] Merkel cell tumor,[241] myosar-

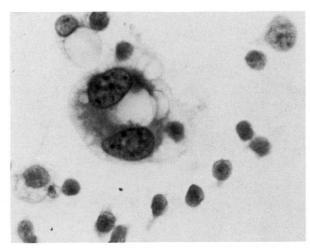

FIGURE 22–140. Pleomorphic liposarcoma. The cytoplasm is dominated by a large vacuole and the nuclei have the typical peripheral location (smear of pleural fluid; Papanicolaou stain; ×660). (Reproduced with permission from Geisinger KR, Naylor B, Beals TF, Novak PM: Cytopathology, including transmission and electron microscopy, of pleomorphic liposarcoma in pleural fluids. Acta Cytol 24:435–441, 1980.)

coma,[81, 82, 126] Ewing's tumor,[81] synovial sarcoma[140] and neuroblastoma.[55, 106, 140, 215, 223] Larger cells of similar appearance were also illustrated for neurofibrosarcoma, leiomyosarcoma and synovial sarcoma by Spriggs and Boddington.[215] Cells of nephroblastoma (Wilms' tumor) in serous fluids have also been illustrated.[80, 81, 140, 213, 215]

In this category we have seen examples of Ewing's sarcoma, Wilms' tumor, carcinoid tumor (Fig. 22–144) and neuroblastoma (Fig. 22–145). Because the cells of these neoplasms in serous fluids are so uncommon and the morphologic differences between the cells of these neoplasms are so subtle, no attempt will be made to

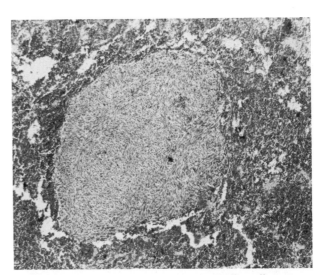

FIGURE 22–141. A large fragment of **spindle cell sarcoma**, probably neurofibrosarcoma (cell block of pleural fluid; hematoxylin and eosin; ×83).

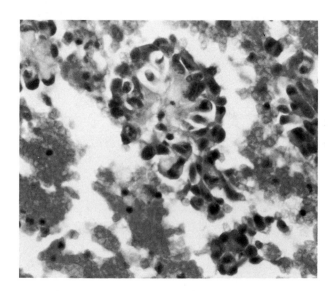

FIGURE 22–142. Fragments of **hemangiosarcoma**. The fragments have a central collagenous core covered by neoplastic cells. This appearance is typical for this neoplasm in serous fluids (cell block of pleural fluid; hematoxylin and eosin; ×330).

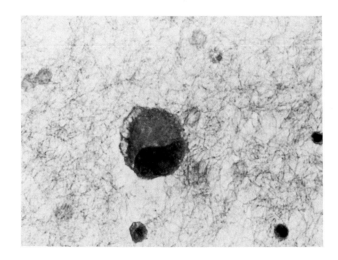

FIGURE 22–143. Metastatic nasopharyngeal rhabdomyosarcoma. The cytoplasmic staining reaction is pink. Cross striations not seen (cell block of pleural fluid; hematoxylin and eosin; ×528).

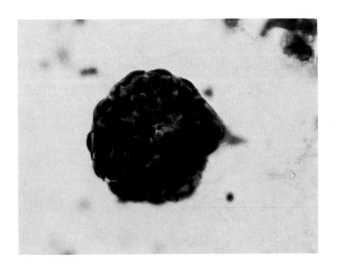

FIGURE 22–144. Fragment of **metastatic thymic carcinoid tumor** composed of small cells with scanty cytoplasm (smear of pleural fluid; Papanicolaou stain; ×52). (Courtesy of Dr. Dorothy L. Rosenthal, Los Angeles, California.)

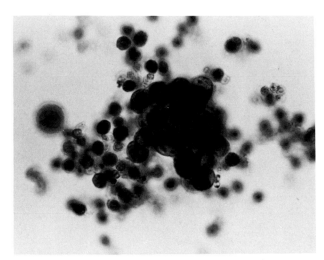

FIGURE 22–145. Fragment of **metastatic neuroblastoma** composed of small, apparently undifferentiated cells with scanty cytoplasm (smear of pleural fluid; Papanicolaou stain; × 528).

distinguish between them. One possibility, however, is that neuroblastoma may form identifiable rosettes, a phenomenon we have not seen but that has been described by Hajdu and Hajdu.[81] We have seen one striking example of non-neoplastic cells diagnosed as neuroblastoma, a misdiagnosis caused by inflammatory cells aggregating around particles of foreign material in a peritoneal fluid to form rosettes (Fig. 22–146).

Germ Cell Neoplasms

Cells of germ cell neoplasms are occasionally seen in serous fluids. Probably the most frequently seen are

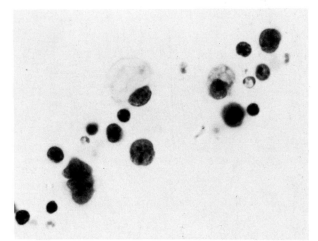

FIGURE 22–147. Metastatic ovarian dysgerminoma. This field shows a small cluster of dysgerminoma cells and three isolated dysgerminoma cells (one out of focus). The other cells in this field are macrophages and lymphoid cells (smear of pleural fluid; Papanicolaou stain; × 750).

those of seminoma or dysgerminoma, which are morphologically exactly alike. These cells may occur singly or in small groupings (Fig. 22–147). The cells are somewhat larger than the average mesothelial cell and show little variation in size and shape. They have a high nucleocytoplasmic ratio and prominent nucleoli.[114, 215, 223]

Endodermal sinus tumor (yolk sac tumor) has been described in serous fluids as small, tightly packed, uniform, cells in clusters[81] or as clusters of larger cells resembling adenocarcinoma (Fig. 22–148) and as giving a positive immunocytochemical reactions for alpha-fetoprotein.[154, 191] Takahashi[223] recorded positive immunofluorescent staining of cells in ascitic fluid from

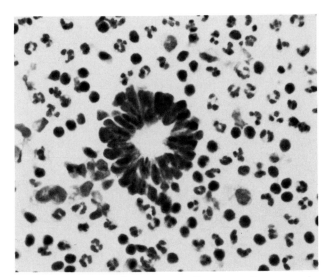

FIGURE 22–146. Inflammatory cells aggregating around a particle of foreign material (not visible in this plane of focus) to form a rosette. The fluid contained many such formations, which had been misinterpreted as metastatic neuroblastoma. The patient, a 54-year-old man, was ultimately proved to have tuberculous peritonitis (smear of peritoneal fluid; Papanicolaou stain; × 528).

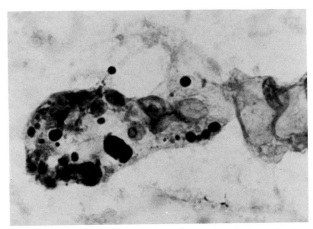

FIGURE 22–148. Fragment of **ovarian endodermal sinus tumor** appearing as vacuolated adenocarcinoma. Hyaline globules, characteristic of alpha-fetoprotein synthesizing cells, are present in the cytoplasm as darkly staining periodic acid–Schiff (PAS)–positive globules (smear of peritoneal fluid; PAS stain; × 400). (Reproduced with permission from Morimoto N, Ozawa M, Amano S: Diagnostic value of hyaline globules in endodermal sinus tumor. Report of two cases. Acta Cytol 25:417–420, 1981.)

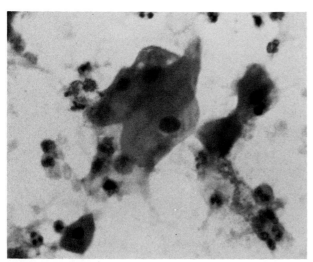

FIGURE 22–149. Benign-appearing squamous epithelial cells derived from **metastatic testicular teratoma**. Elsewhere in the smear were cells that appeared to be adenocarcinoma (smear of peritoneal fluid; Papanicolaou stain; × 528). (Courtesy of Dr. Maria C. Gamarra, Buffalo, New York.)

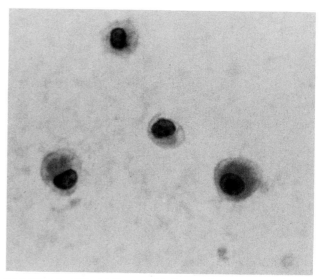

FIGURE 22–150. **Malignant histiocytosis**, type unspecified. Almost all of the cells in this fluid consisted of these benign-appearing, nonphagocytic macrophage-like cells (smear of pleural fluid; Papanicolaou stain; × 825).

an ovarian embryonal carcinoma using an antibody against alpha-fetoprotein.

When malignant teratoma causes a serous effusion, the type of cell found in the fluid depends on the type of tissue that has undergone malignant transformation. We have seen examples of malignant teratoma represented by cells similar to those of small-cell anaplastic carcinoma or sarcoma, whereas others appeared to be adenocarcinoma. One of our examples (testicular teratoma) contained not only cells that appeared to be adenocarcinoma but also cells that had the appearance of benign squamous epithelial cells (Fig. 22–149). Similar-appearing squamous cells derived from benign and malignant teratomas have been previously illustrated.[33, 76, 81, 223] Takahashi[223] illustrated rosettes of neural tissue cells and benign-appearing squamous cells from pleural fluid in a case of metastatic ovarian teratoma.

We have not seen examples of choriocarcinoma cells in effusions, although they have been illustrated by several authors.[140, 174, 227] Luse and Reagan[143] illustrated a villus-like structure accompanied by irregular aggregates of cells resembling syncytial cells in ascitic fluid from a patient with testicular teratocarcinoma. Granulosa cell tumor in ascitic fluid has been illustrated as rather small cells with little or no cytoplasm.[215, 223] Examples of germ cell tumors of the pineal gland that have metastasized to the peritoneal cavity via a ventriculoperitoneal shunt have been described.[118, 119]

Malignant Histiocytosis

True histiocytic neoplasms exhibit a cytology spectrum ranging from cells that have the appearance of normal macrophages to malignant forms that have a

similar general appearance but in which the cytoplasm is much reduced. These conditions have rarely been reported in serous fluids,[6, 126] and we have seen only two examples in our laboratory. In each case the neoplastic cells had the appearance of benign macrophages (Figs. 22–150 and 22–151); however, in both patients the condition was fatal, and at necropsy numerous organs were infiltrated by these benign-appearing cells (Fig. 22–152).

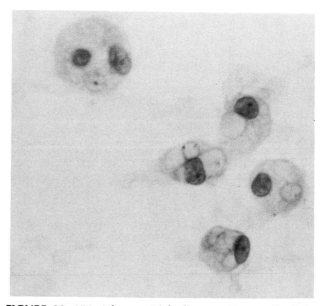

FIGURE 22–151. **Niemann-Pick disease**. Almost all of the cells in this fluid consisted of these benign-appearing, slightly phagocytic macrophage-like cells (smear of peritoneal fluid; Papanicolaou stain; × 825).

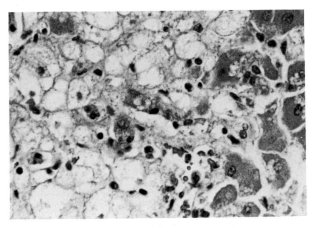

FIGURE 22–152. Niemann-Pick disease. Same case as Figure 22–151. The liver is extensively infiltrated by cells similar to those in the peritoneal fluid. Residual hepatic parenchyma on the right (necropsy liver; hematoxylin and eosin; ×330).

REPORTING OF RESULTS AND STATISTICS

Reporting

To be of diagnostic value to clinicians, reports on the presence or absence of neoplastic cells in serous fluids should be expressed as unequivocally as possible. When neoplastic cells are present in a fluid, they are usually present in large numbers and are readily recognizable as such. Seldom should it be necessary to resort to special technical methods to determine if neoplastic cells are present. The incremental yield of "positive" results from the use of such methods is extremely small, scarcely affecting the statistical analysis of results.

We have never employed a numeric classification, such as the Papanicolaou system, in our reporting of cytologic specimens, preferring to use telegraphic English prose rather than Roman numerals. Typical examples of our reporting are as follows:

- Examination for neoplastic cells: Positive, for adenocarcinoma
- Examination for neoplastic cells: Negative. Numerous neutrophilic leukocytes
- Examination for neoplastic cells: Negative. This fluid shows the pathognomonic cytologic picture of rheumatoid pleuritis.

It should be understood by clinicians that reporting a specimen as being "negative" for neoplastic cells does not exclude neoplasm as the cause of the effusion. As mentioned previously, effusions may be caused by neoplastic obstruction of lymphatic or blood vessels or inflammation secondary to the presence of neoplasm or both. The only time we comment with any frequency with respect to non-neoplastic cells is when numerous neutrophilic leukocytes are present. We do not comment on the presence of mesothelial cells, macrophages or lymphoid cells, believing that to do so would be providing the clinician with useless information.

We do not report the presence of cells that are "consistent with neoplasm," which is merely a way of stating that cells are present that may be neoplastic but that, on the other hand, may not be neoplastic. As much as possible we avoid reporting cells as "suspicious" of being neoplastic, believing that such a report is not much more useful to the clinician than no report at all. When we have been driven to issuing a "suspicious" report, it is because of the presence of only one or two cells that are strongly suggestive of neoplasm. Such a report implies that we are almost certain that the fluid contains neoplastic cells, and in such cases examination of additional material has generally enabled us to make a definite diagnosis of neoplasm.

Reliability of Positive and Negative Reports

In their monograph, Spriggs and Boddington[215] analyzed the statistical results of six published series, which were the only large series published in the previous 25 years from which relevant figures could be extracted. Some of these series dealt exclusively with pleural or peritoneal effusions, whereas the others dealt with both types of effusion. The number of specimens in the six series ranged from 159 to 2198. The total number of cases covered by these series was 6001, with an average of 1000.

In their analysis of these series, Spriggs and Boddington calculated sensitivity, specificity, predictive value of positive reports and predictive value of negative reports. The reader is referred to Chapter 3, Cytologic Screening Programs, for definitions of these terms.

To give examples, *sensitivity* of 0.70 means that in cases of cancer, 70% were given unequivocal positive reports and 30% were reported as either negative or suspicious. *Specificity* of 0.95 means that in cases without cancer 95% were reported as negative and 5% were given false-positive or suspicious reports. A *predictive value of positive* of 0.97 means that 3% of positive reports were false, and a *predictive value of negative* of 0.80 means that 20% of negative reports were from cases with cancer.

Analysis of the 6001 specimens gave the following:	
Total cases	6001
Total with malignant disease	2558
Cytology positive	1489
Cytology negative	860
Total without malignant disease	3443
Cytology positive	10
Cytology negative	3340
Sensitivity	0.58
Specificity	0.97
Predictive value of positive	0.993
Predictive value of negative	0.80

Cases reported as suspicious ranged from 2.9 to 5.8% in peritoneal fluids and 1.8 to 7.7% in pleural fluids, with an average for all specimens of 5.6%. In the early days of our laboratory 36 (3.9%) of the first

935 cases were reported as suspicious. The percent of suspicious reports has diminished over the years and is now below 1%. The number of cases reported as suspicious are not included in this table.

References

1. Adelman M, Albelda S, Gottlieb J, Haponik EF: Diagnostic utility of pleural fluid eosinophilia. Am J Med 77:915–920, 1984.
2. Alons CL, Veldhuizen RW, Boon ME: Learning from quantitation. Anal Quant Cytol Histol 3:178–181, 1981.
3. Angeli S, Koelma IA, Fleuren GJ, Van Steenis GJ: Malignant melanoma in fine needle aspirates and effusions. An immunocytochemical study using monoclonal antibodies. Acta Cytol 32:707–712, 1988.
4. Anikin BS, Myshentsiva LP: A case of systemic lupus erythematosus with atypical cells in the pleural exudate (in Russian). Ter Arkh 39:108–110, 1967.
5. Antman KH: Malignant mesothelioma. N Engl J Med 303:200–202, 1980.
6. Aozasa K, Kurokawa K, Kabori Y, Sawashi Y, Sawada M: Malignant histiocytosis showing ascites and recurrent meningeal infiltration. Acta Cytol 24:228–231, 1980.
7. Ashton PR, Hollingsworth AS, Johnston WW: The cytopathology of metastatic breast cancer. Acta Cytol 19:1–6, 1975.
8. Astorga G, Bollet AJ: Diagnostic specificity and possible pathogenetic significance of inclusion-body cells in synovial fluid. Arthritis Rheum 7:288–289, 1964.
9. Avagnina MA, Elsner B, Iotti RM, Re R: *Strongyloides stercoralis* in Papanicolaou-stained smears of ascitic fluid. Acta Cytol 24:36–39, 1980.
10. Ayres WW: Production of Charcot-Leyden crystals from eosinophils with aerosol MA. Blood 4:595–602, 1949.
11. Bartziota EV, Naylor B: Megakaryocytes in a hemorrhagic pleural effusion caused by anticoagulant overdose. Acta Cytol 30:163–165, 1986.
12. Becker SN, Pepin DW, Rosenthal DL: Mesothelial papilloma. A case of mistaken identity in a pericardial effusion. Acta Cytol 30:266–268, 1976.
13. Bedrossian CWM, Mason MR, Gupta PK: Rapid cytologic diagnosis of *Pneumocystis*: A comparison of effective techniques. Semin Diagn Pathol 6:245–261, 1989.
14. Beekman JF, Bosniak S, Canter HG: Eosinophilia and elevated IgE concentration in a serous pleural effusion following trauma. Am Rev Respir Dis 110:484–489, 1974.
15. Beeson PB, Bass DA: The Eosinophil. Philadelphia, WB Saunders, 1977.
16. Bell DA, Scully RE: Benign and borderline serous lesions of the peritoneum in women. *In* Pathology Annual, 1989. II. Edited by PP Rosen, RE Fechner. East Norwalk, Appleton and Lange, pp 1–21, 1989.
17. Berge J, Grontöft O: Cytologic diagnosis of malignant pleural mesothelioma. Acta Cytol 9:207–212, 1965.
18. Berger HW, Seckler SG: Pleural and pericardial effusions in rheumatoid disease. Ann Intern Med 64:1291–1296, 1966.
19. Berliner K: Hemorrhagic pleural effusion: An analysis of 120 cases. Ann Intern Med 14:2266–2284, 1941.
20. Billingham ME, Rawlinson DG, Berry PF, Kempson RL: The cytodiagnosis of malignant lymphomas and Hodgkin's disease in cerebrospinal, pleural and ascitic fluids. Acta Cytol 19:547–556, 1975.
21. Bloch T, Davis TE, Schwenk GR: *Giardia lamblia* in peritoneal fluid. Acta Cytol 31:783–784, 1987.
22. Boddington MM, Spriggs AI, Morton JA, Mowat AG: Cytodiagnosis of rheumatoid pleural effusion. J Clin Pathol 24:95–106, 1971.
23. Boon ME, Kwee HS, Alons CL, Morawetz F, Veldhuizen RW: Discrimination between primary pleural and primary peritoneal mesotheliomas by morphometry and analysis of the vacuolization pattern of the exfoliated mesothelial cells. Acta Cytol 26:103–108, 1982.
24. Boon ME, Veldhuizen RW, Ruinaard C, Snieders MW, Kwee

WS: Qualitative distinctive differences between the vacuoles of mesothelioma cells and of cells from metastatic carcinoma exfoliated in pleural fluid. Acta Cytol 28:443–449, 1984.
25. Bower G: Eosinophilic pleural effusion. A condition with multiple causes. Am Rev Respir Dis 95:746–751, 1967.
26. Broghamer WL, Richardson ME, Faurest SE: Malignancy-associated serosanguinous pleural effusions. Acta Cytol 28:46–50, 1984.
27. Butler EB, Berry AV: Diffuse mesothelioma: Diagnostic criteria using exfoliative cytology. *In* Biological Effects of Asbestos. Edited by P Bogovske, JC Gilson, V Timbrell, JC Wagner. Lyon, IARC Sci Publ No. 8, pp 68–73, 1973.
28. Butler EB, Johnson NF: The use of electron microscopy in the diagnosis of diffuse mesotheliomas using human pleural effusions. *In* Biological Effects of Mineral Fibres. Edited by JC Wagner. Lyon, IARC Sci Publ No. 30, pp 409–418, 1980.
29. Butler EB, Stanbridge CM: Cytology of Body Cavity Fluids. A Colour Atlas. London, Chapman and Hall, 1986.
30. Carmichael DS, Golding DN: Rheumatoid pleural effusion with "RA cells" in the pleural fluid. Br Med J 1:814, 1967.
31. Castor WC, Naylor B: Acid mucopolysaccharide composition of serous effusions. Study of 100 patients with neoplastic and non-neoplastic conditions. Cancer 20:462–466, 1967.
32. Charan S, Sinha K: Constrictive pericarditis following pericardial effusions. Indian Heart J 25:213–215, 1973.
33. Cobb CJ, Wynn J, Cobb SR, Duane GB: Cytologic findings in an effusion caused by rupture of a benign cystic teratoma of the mediastinum into a serous cavity. Acta Cytol 29:1015–1020, 1985.
34. Coleman DV: Ciliated organisms in dialysis fluid. Lancet 1:1030, 1986.
35. Coleman M, Henderson DW, Mukherjee TM: The ultrastructure of malignant pleural mesothelioma. *In* Pathology Annual, 1989. I. Edited by PP Rosen, RE Fechner. East Norwalk, Appleton and Lange, pp 303–353, 1989.
36. Covell JL, Lowry EH, Feldman PS: Cytologic diagnosis of blastomycosis in pleural fluid. Acta Cytol 26:833–836, 1982.
37. Craighead JE: Current pathogenetic concepts of diffuse malignant mesothelioma. Hum Pathol 18:544–557, 1987.
38. Daugirdas JT, Leehey DJ, Popli S, Gandhi VC, Zayas I, Hoffman W, Ing TS: Induction of peritoneal-fluid eosinophilia by intraperitoneal air in patients on continuous ambulatory peritoneal dialysis. N Engl J Med 313:1481, 1985.
39. Dekker A, Graham T, Bupp PA: The occurrence of sickle cells in pleural fluid: Report of a patient with sickle cell disease. Acta Cytol 19:251–254, 1975.
40. Delbarre F, Kahan A, Amor B, Krassinine G: Le ragocyte synovial. Son interêt pour le diagnostic des maladies rheumatismales. Presse Méd 72:2129–2132, 1964.
41. de Vries MW: Über freie Metastasen in der Bauchhohle bei Ovarialkrebs. Beitr Pathol Anat 93:198–208, 1934.
42. Dickie HA, Grimm E: Löffler's syndrome with associated eosinophilic polyserositis. Am J Med 7:690–693, 1949.
43. Dickie TE, Naylor B: Prevalence of "asbestos" bodies in human lungs at necropsy. Chest 56:122–125, 1969.
44. Dines DE, Pierre RV, Franzen SJ: The value of cells in the pleural fluid in the differential diagnosis. Mayo Clin Proc 50:571–572, 1975.
45. Domagala W, Emerson EE, Koss LG: T and B lymphocyte enumeration in the diagnosis of lymphocyte-rich pleural fluids. Acta Cytol 25:108–110, 1981.
46. Domagala W, Woyke S: Transmission and scanning electron microscopic studies of cells in effusions. Acta Cytol 19:214–223, 1975.
47. Donna A, Betta P-G, Jones JSP: Verification of the histologic diagnosis of malignant mesothelioma in relation to the binding of an antimesothelial cell antibody. Cancer 63:1331–1336, 1989.
48. Drew PA, Krauss JS: Identification of *Giardia lamblia* in peritoneal fluid of trauma patients. Acta Cytol 33:283–284, 1989.
49. Dubois EL: Lupus Erythematosus, 2nd ed. Los Angeles, University of Southern California Press, 1974.
50. Dumarest F, Parodi F, Lelong J: Sur la pathogénie des épanchements pleuraux du pneumothorax artificiel. Ann Méd Interne 8:367–391, 1920.

51. Ebner H-J: Untersuchungen zur Cytologie and Cytochemie cilioepithelialer Tumorzellen im Punktat seroser Ovarialcystome und Cystadenocarcinome. Z Krebsforsch 59:581–593, 1953.

52. Edman JC, Kovacs JA, Masur H, Santi DV, Elwood HJ, Sogin ML: Ribosomal RNA sequence shows *Pneumocystis carinii* to be a member of the fungi. Nature 334:519–522, 1988.

53. Ehya H: The cytologic diagnosis of mesothelioma. Semin Diagn Pathol 3:196–203, 1986.

54. Ellman P, Cudkowicz L, Elwood JS: Widespread serous membrane involvement by rheumatoid nodules. J Clin Pathol 7:239–244, 1954.

55. Farr GH, Hajdu SI: Exfoliative cytology of metastatic neuroblastoma. Acta Cytol 16:203–206, 1971.

56. Faurschou P: Rheumatoid pleuritis and thoracoscopy. Scand J Resp Dis 55:277–283, 1974.

57. Faurschou P, Faarup P: Granulocytes containing cytoplasmic inclusions in human tuberculous pleuritis. Scand J Resp Dis 54:341–346, 1973.

58. Faurschou P, Faarup P: Pleural granulocytes with cytoplasmic inclusions from patients with malignant lung tumors and mesothelioma. Eur J Respir Dis 61:151–155, 1980.

59. Figueroa JM: Presence of microfilariae of *Mansonella ozzardi* in ascitic fluid. Acta Cytol 17:73–75, 1973.

60. Fok FK, Bewtra C, Hammeke MD: Cytology of peritoneal fluid from patients on continuous ambulatory peritoneal dialysis. Acta Cytol 33:595–598, 1989.

61. Foot NC: Identification of types and primary sites of metastatic tumors from exfoliated cells in serous fluids. Am J Pathol 30:661–677, 1954.

62. Gaba AR, Fine G, Raju UB: Malignant angioendothelioma. Cytologic, histologic and ultrastructural findings. Acta Cytol 27:76–80, 1983.

63. Gaulier A, Jouret-Mourin A, Marsan C: Peritoneal endometriosis. Report of a case with cytologic, cytochemical and histopathologic study. Acta Cytol 27:446–449, 1983.

64. Geisinger KR, Naylor B, Beals TF, Novak PM: Cytopathology, including transmission and electron microscopy, of pleomorphic liposarcoma in pleural fluids. Acta Cytol 24:435–441, 1980.

65. Geisinger KR, Vance RP, Prater T, Semble E, Disko EJ: Rheumatoid pleural effusion. A transmission and scanning electron microscopic evaluation. Acta Cytol 29:239–247, 1985.

66. Ghadially F: Ultrastructural Pathology of the Cell and Matrix, 2nd ed. London, Butterworths, 1982.

67. Ghai OP, Khetarpal SK: Eosinophilic peritonitis. Indian J Child Health 11:568–571, 1962.

68. Ghosh AK, Spriggs AI, Mason DY: Immunocytochemical staining of T and B lymphocytes in serous effusions. J Clin Pathol 38:608–612, 1985.

69. Gibson LE, Goellner JR: Amelanotic melanoma: Cases studied by Fontana stain, S-100 immunostain, and ultrastructural examination. Mayo Clin Proc 63:777–782, 1988.

70. Gondos B, Lai CE, King EB: Distinction between atypical mesothelial cells and malignant cells by scanning electron microscopy. Acta Cytol 23:321–326, 1979.

71. Gondos B, McIntosh KM, Renston RH, King EB: Application of electron microscopy in the definitive diagnosis of effusions. Acta Cytol 22:297–304, 1978.

72. Goodman ZD, Gupta PK, Frost JK, Erozan YS: Cytodiagnosis of viral infections in body cavity fluids. Acta Cytol 23:204–208, 1979.

73. Graham RM: The Cytologic Diagnosis of Cancer, 3rd ed. Philadelphia, WB Saunders, 1972.

74. Gronemeyer PS, Weissfeld AS, Sonnenwirth AC: Purulent pericarditis complicating systemic infection with *Candida tropicalis*. Am J Clin Pathol 77:471–475, 1982.

75. Grunze H: Klinische Zytologie der Thoraxkrankheiten. Stuttgart, Ferdinand Enke, 1955.

76. Grunze H: The comparative diagnostic accuracy, efficiency and specificity of cytologic techniques used in the diagnosis of malignant neoplasms in serous effusions of pleural and pericardial cavities. Acta Cytol 8:150–159, 1964.

77. Guhl R: Über pleurale Eosinophilie. Die sogenannte "Eosinophile Pleuritis." Schweiz Med Wochenschr 87:838–842, 1957.

78. Gupta PK, Albritton N, Erozan YS, Frost JK: Occurrence of cilia in exfoliated ovarian adenocarcinoma cells. Diagn Cytopathol 1:228–231, 1985.

79. Guzman J, Bross KJ, Wurtemberger G, Freudenberg N, Costabel U: Tuberculous pleural effusions: Lymphocyte phenotypes in comparison with other lymphocyte-rich effusions. Diag Cytopathol 5:139, 1989.

80. Hajdu SI: Exfoliative cytology of primary and metastatic Wilms' tumors. Acta Cytol 15:339–342, 1971.

81. Hajdu SI, Hajdu EO: Cytopathology of Sarcomas and Other Nonepithelial Malignant Tumors. Philadelphia, WB Saunders, 1976.

82. Hajdu SI, Koss LG: Cytologic diagnosis of metastatic myosarcomas. Acta Cytol 13:545–551, 1969.

83. Hajdu SI, Savino A: Cytologic diagnosis of malignant melanoma. Acta Cytol 17:320–327, 1973.

84. Hall JW, Kozak M, Spink WW: Pulmonary infiltrates, pericarditis and eosinophilia. A unique case of pulmonary infiltration and eosinophilia syndrome. Am J Med 36:135–143, 1964.

85. Hargraves MM, Richmond H, Morton R: Presentation of two bone marrow elements: The "tart" cell and the "LE" cell. Proc Staff Meet Mayo Clin 23:25–28, 1948.

86. Harington JS, Wagner JC, Smith M: The detection of hyaluronic acid in pleural fluids of cases with diffuse pleural mesotheliomas. Br J Exp Pathol 44:81–83, 1963.

87. Harkavy J: Vascular allergy. Pathogenesis of bronchial asthma with recurrent pulmonary infiltrations and eosinophilic peritonitis. Arch Intern Med 67:709–734, 1941.

88. Harkavy J: Vascular allergy. III. J Allergy 14:507–537, 1943.

89. Harley JB, Glushien AS, Fisher ER: Eosinophilic peritonitis. Ann Intern Med 51:301–308, 1959.

90. Henderson AH, Mejia G: Malignant lymphoma presenting with a high eosinophilia, eosinophilic pleurisy, and pericarditis. Thorax 24:124–125, 1969.

91. Hillerdal G: Malignant mesothelioma 1982: Review of 4710 published cases. Br J Dis Chest 77:321–343, 1983.

92. Hillerdal G, Özesmi M: Benign asbestos pleural effusion: 73 exudates in 60 patients. Eur J Respir Dis 71:113–121, 1987.

93. Hira PR, Lindberg LG, Ryd W, Behbehani K: Cytologic diagnosis of bancroftian filariasis in a nonendemic area. Acta Cytol 32:267–269, 1988.

94. Hjerpe A: Liquid-chromatographic determination of hyaluronic acid in pleural and ascitic fluids. Clin Chem 32:952–956, 1986.

95. Hoeltermann W, Schlotmann-Hoeller E, Winkelmann M, Pfitzer P: Lavage fluid from continuous ambulatory peritoneal dialysis. A model for mesothelial cell changes. Acta Cytol 33:591–594, 1989.

96. Hoeppli R: Histological observations in experimental schistosomiasis japonica. Chin Med J 46:1179–1186, 1932.

97. Hollander JL, McCarty DJ, Astorga G, Castro-Murillo E: Studies on the pathogenesis of rheumatoid joint inflammation. I. The "RA" cell and a working hypothesis. Ann Intern Med 62:271–280, 1965.

98. Hong IS: The exfoliative cytology of endometrial stromal sarcoma in peritoneal fluid. Acta Cytol 25:277–281, 1981.

99. Horler AR, Thompson M: The pleural and pulmonary complications of rheumatoid arthritis. Ann Intern Med 51:1179–1203, 1959.

100. Hunt CE, Papermaster TC, Nelson EN, Krivit W: Eosinophilic peritonitis. Report of two cases. Lancet 87:473–476, 1967.

101. Hurwitz S, Leiman G, Shapiro C: Mesothelial cells in pleural fluid: TB or not TB? S Afr Med J 57:937–939, 1980.

102. Jacobson ES: A case of secondary echinococcosis diagnosed by cytologic examination of pleural fluid and needle biopsy of pleura. Acta Cytol 17:76–79, 1973.

103. Jager J: Epithelioidzellen in tuberkulösen Pleuragüssen. Z Erk Atmungsorgane 157:85–89, 1981.

104. Japko L, Horta AA, Schreiber K, Mitsudo S, Karwa GL, Singh G, Koss LG: Malignant mesothelioma of the tunica vaginalis testis: Report of first case with preoperative diagnosis. Cancer 49:119–127, 1982.

105. Jarvinen KAJ, Kahampaa A: Prognosis in cases with eosinophilic pleural effusion. 17 cases followed for five to twelve years. Acta Med Scand 164:245–251, 1959.

106. Jobst SB, Ljung B-M, Gilkey FN, Rosenthal DL: Cytologic diagnosis of olfactory neuroblastoma. Report of a case with multiple diagnostic parameters. Acta Cytol 27:299–305, 1983.

107. Johnson TL, Kumar NB, Hopkins M, Hughes JD: Cytologic features of ovarian tumors of low malignant potential in peritoneal fluids. Acta Cytol 32:513–518, 1986.

108. Johnston WW, Szpak CA, Thor A, Simpson J, Schlom J: Antibodies to tumor-associated antigens: Applications in clinical cytology. In Compendium on Diagnostic Cytology, 6th ed. Edited by GL Wied, CM Keebler, LG Koss, JW Reagan. Chicago, Tutorials of Cytology, pp 567–578, 1988.

109. Jolobe OMP, Melnick SC: Asthma, pulmonary eosinophilia, and eosinophilic pericarditis. Thorax 38:690–691, 1983.

110. Jones JSP, Lund C, Planteydt HT, Butler EB: Colour Atlas of Mesothelioma. Hingham, MTP Press, 1985.

111. Jones PE, Rawcliffe P, White N, Segal AW: Painless ascites in systemic lupus erythematosus. Br Med J 1:1513, 1977.

112. Kannerstein M, Churg J, Magner D: Histochemistry in the diagnosis of malignant mesothelioma. Ann Clin Lab Sci 3:207–211, 1973.

113. Kaplan AI, Zakher, F, Sabin S: Drug-induced lupus erythematosus with in vivo lupus erythematosus cells in pleural fluid. Chest 73:875–876, 1978.

114. Kashimura M, Tsukamoto N, Matsuyama T, Kashimura Y, Sugimori H, Taki I: Cytologic findings of ascites from patients with ovarian dysgerminoma. Acta Cytol 27:59–62, 1983.

115. Katz RL, Raval P, Manning JT, McLaughlin P, Barlogie B: A morphologic, immunologic, and cytometric approach to the classification of non-Hodgkin's lymphoma in effusions. Diagn Cytopathol 3:91–101, 1987.

116. Kelley S, McGarry P, Hutson Y: Atypical cells in pleural fluid characteristic of systemic lupus erythematosus. Acta Cytol 15:357–362, 1971.

117. Kern WH: Benign papillary structures with psammoma bodies in culdocentesis fluid. Acta Cytol 13:178–180, 1969.

118. Kim K, Koo BC, Delaflor RR, Shaikh BS: Pineal germinoma with widespread extracranial metastases. Diagn Cytopathol 1:118–122, 1985.

119. Kimura N, Namiki T, Wada T, Sasano N: Peritoneal implantation of endodermal sinus tumor of the pineal region via a ventriculoperitoneal shunt. Cytodiagnosis with immunocytochemical demonstration of alpha-fetoprotein. Acta Cytol 28:143–147, 1984.

120. Klempman S: The exfoliative cytology of diffuse pleural mesothelioma. Cancer 15:691–704, 1962.

121. Knight KR, Polak A, Crump J, Maskell R: Laboratory diagnosis and oral treatment of CAPD peritonitis. Lancet 2:1301–1304, 1982.

122. Kobayashi TK, Teraoka S, Tsujioka T, Yoshida Y: Ciliated ovarian adenocarcinoma cells in ascitic fluid cytology: Report of a case with immunocytochemical features. Diagn Cytopathol 4:234–238, 1988.

123. Kobayashi Y, Takeda S, Yamamoto T, Goi S: Cytologic detection of malignant mesothelioma of the pericardium. Acta Cytol 22:344–349, 1978.

124. Kobzik L, Antman KH, Warhol MJ: The distinction of mesothelioma from adenocarcinoma in malignant effusions by electron microscopy. Acta Cytol 29:219–225, 1985.

125. Kokkola K, Valta R: Aetiology and findings in eosinophilic pleural effusion. Scand J Resp Dis [Suppl] 89:159–165, 1974.

126. Koss LG: Diagnostic Cytology and Its Histopathologic Bases, 3rd ed. Philadelphia, JB Lippincott, 1979.

127. Krause JR, Dekker A: Hairy cell leukemia (leukemic reticuloendotheliosis) in serous effusions. Acta Cytol 22:80–82, 1978.

128. Krishnan S, Statsinger AL, Kleinman M, Bertoni MA, Sharma P: Eosinophilic pleural effusion with Charcot-Leyden crystals. Acta Cytol 27:529–532, 1983.

129. Kumar NB, Naylor B: Megakaryocytes in pleural and peritoneal fluids: Prevalence, significance, morphology, and cytohistological correlation. J Clin Pathol 33:1153–1159, 1980.

130. Kumar UN, Varkey B, Matthai G: Posttraumatic pleural fluid and blood eosinophilia. JAMA 234:625–626, 1975.

131. Kwee W-S, Veldhuizen RW, Alons CA, Morawetz F, Boon ME: Quantitative and qualitative differences between benign and malignant mesothelial cells in pleural fluid. Acta Cytol 26:401–406, 1982.

132. Laederich L, Mamou H: Péritonite ascitique fugace à éosinophiles. Presse Méd 55:789, 1947.

133. Lahiri VL, Elhence BR, Agarwal BM: Balantidium peritonitis diagnosed on cytologic material. Acta Cytol 21:123–124, 1977.

134. Lecestre MJ, Engelmann, P, Rochard F, Ferand-Lougnon J: Observation de corps ciliaires dans les liquides du cul-de-sac de Douglas: A propos de deux cas. Arch Anat Cytol Pathol 27:160–162, 1979.

135. Lee S, Schoen I: Eosinophilia of peritoneal fluid and peripheral blood associated with chronic peritoneal dialysis. Am J Clin Pathol 47:638–640, 1967.

136. Legrand M, Pariente R: Ultrastructural study of pleural fluid in mesothelioma. Thorax 29:164–171, 1974.

137. Liepman M: Disseminated Strongyloides stercoralis: A complication of immunosuppression. JAMA 231:387–389, 1975.

138. Light RW, Erozan YS, Ball WC: Cells in pleural fluid. Their value in differential diagnosis. Arch Intern Med 132:854–860, 1973.

139. Lintermans JP: Fatal peritonitis, an unusual clinical complication of Strongyloides stercoralis infestation. Clin Pediatr 14:974–978, 1975.

140. Lopes Cardozo P: Atlas of Clinical Cytology. Leiden's-Hertogenbosch, Targa bv, 1976.

141. Lozowski W, Hajdu SI, Melamed MR: Cytomorphology of carcinoid tumors. Acta Cytol 23:360–365, 1979.

142. Luse SA, Reagan JW: A histocytological study of effusions. I. Effusions not associated with malignant tumors. Cancer 7:1155–1166, 1954.

143. Luse SA, Reagan JW: A histocytological study of effusions. II. Effusions associated with malignant tumors. Cancer 7:1167–1181, 1954.

144. Macleod IN, Wilmot AJ, Powell SJ: Amoebic pericarditis. Q J Med 35:293–311, 1966.

145. Mandl MAJ, Watson JI, Henderson JAM, Wang N-S: Pleural fluid in rheumatoid pleuritis: Patient summary with histopathologic studies. Arch Intern Med 124:373–376, 1969.

146. Martin SE, Zhang H-Z, Magyarosy E, Jaffe ES, Hsu S-M, Chu EW: Immunologic methods in cytology: Definitive diagnosis of non-Hodgkin's lymphomas using immunologic markers for T- and B-cells. Am J Clin Pathol 82:666–673, 1984.

147. McCaughey WTE, Kannerstein M, Churg J: Tumors and Pseudotumors of the Serous Membranes. Atlas of Tumor Pathology, second series, fascicle 20. Washington, DC, Armed Forces Institute of Pathology, 1985.

148. McCormack LJ, Hazard JB, Effler DB, Groves LK, Belovich D: Experience with cytologic examination of bronchial swabbings in diagnosis of cancer of lung: Study of 602 cases. J Thorac Surg 29:277–282, 1955.

149. Melamed MR: The cytological presentation of malignant lymphomas and related diseases in effusions. Cancer 16:413–431, 1963.

150. Memik F: Trichomonads in pleural effusion. JAMA 204:1145–1146, 1968.

151. Mérab A, Taleb N, Saliby E, Eliane E, Naffah MJ, Kyriakos S: Les péricardites hodgkiniennes. A propos d'un cas de malade de Hodgkin revelée par un péricardite avec épanchement et presence de cellules de Sternberg dans le liquide de ponction. Semin Hôp Paris 35:2590–2594, 1959.

152. Meyer K, Chaffee E: Hyaluronic acid in pleural fluid associated with malignant tumor involving pleura and peritoneum. J Biol Chem 133:83–91, 1940.

153. Miller MJ, Leith DE, Brooks JR, Fencl V: Trichomonas empyema. Thorax 37:384–385, 1982.

154. Morimoto N, Ozawa M, Amano S: Diagnostic value of hyaline globules in endodermal sinus tumor. Acta Cytol 25:417–420, 1971.

155. Mott FW: The cerebro-spinal fluid in relation to disease of the nervous system. Br Med J 2:1954–1960, 1904.

156. Murphy WM, Ng ABP: Determination of primary site by examination of cancer cells in body fluids. Am J Clin Pathol 58:479–488, 1972.

157. Navarrenne P, Sultan C: Une ascite fugace à éosinophiles. Presse Méd 70:2515–2517, 1962.

158. Naylor B: The elimination of a "ribbing" effect in cytologic smears. Am J Clin Pathol 30:143–144, 1958.

159. Naylor B: The exfoliative cytology of diffuse malignant mesothelioma. J Pathol Bacteriol 86:293–298, 1963.

160. Naylor B: The role of the cytology laboratory in the diagnosis of diffuse malignant mesothelioma. *In* International Konferenz uber die biolgischen Wirkungen des Asbestes. Edited by Holstein, Anspach. Dresden, pp 288–295, 1973.

161. Naylor B: The pathognomonic cytologic picture of rheumatoid pleuritis. Acta Cytol 34:465–473, 1990.

162. Naylor B: Curschmann's spirals in pleural and peritoneal fluids. Acta Cytol 34:474–478, 1990.

163. Naylor B: Cytologic aspects of pleural, peritoneal and pericardial effusions in patients with systemic lupus erythematosus (in preparation).

164. Naylor B, Novak PM: Charcot-Leyden crystals in pleural fluids. Acta Cytol 29:781–784, 1985.

165. Nguyen G-K, Schnitka TK, Jewell LD, Wroblewski JA: Exfoliative cytology of clear-cell sarcoma metastases in pleural fluid. Diagn Cytopathol 2:144–149, 1986.

166. Nicoli RM, Quilici M: Un pseudoparasite animé en milieu peritoneal. Ann Parasitol Hum Comp 57:101–104, 1982.

167. Nielsen MH, Faurschou P, Faarup P: Fine structure of granulocytes with cytoplasmic inclusions in pleural effusions from patients with rheumatoid pleuritis, tuberculous pleuritis and pleural carcinomatosis. Acta Pathol Microbiol Scand [A] 83:433–442, 1975.

168. Novak PM, Kumar NB, Naylor B: Curschmann's spirals in cervicovaginal smears. Prevalence, morphology, significance and origin. Acta Cytol 28:5–8, 1984.

169. Okuyama T, Imai S, Tsubura Y: Egg of *Schistosoma japonicum* in ascitic fluid. Acta Cytol 29:651–652, 1985.

170. Ordoñez NG: The immunohistochemical diagnosis of mesothelioma: Differentiation of mesothelioma and lung adenocarcinoma. Am J Surg Pathol 13:276–291, 1989.

171. Ordoñez NG, Sneige N, Hickey RC, Brooks TE: Use of monoclonal antibody HMB-45 in the cytologic diagnosis of melanoma. Acta Cytol 32:684–688, 1988.

172. Padawer J, Gordon AS: Cellular elements in the peritoneal fluid of some mammals. Anat Rec 124:209–222, 1956.

173. Paddock FK: The diagnostic significance of serous fluids in disease. N Engl J Med 223:1010–1015, 1940.

174. Pagès A, Marsan C: Cytopathologie des épanchements des sereuses. *In* Atlas de Cytologie, vol 3. Edited by A Sicard, C Marsan. Paris, Varia, 1968.

175. Papanicolaou GN: Degenerative changes in ciliated cells exfoliating from the bronchial epithelium as a cytologic criterion in the diagnosis of disease of the lung. NY State J Med 56:2647–2650, 1956.

176. Papanicolaou GN: Atlas of Exfoliative Cytology. Supplements 1 and 2. Cambridge, Harvard University Press, 1956, 1960.

177. Patel NM, Kurtides ES: Ascites in agnogenic myeloid metaplasia: Association with peritoneal implant of myeloid tissue and therapy. Cancer 50:1189–1190, 1982.

178. Pettersson T: Acid alpha-napthyl acetate esterase staining of lymphocytes in pleural effusions. Acta Cytol 26:109–114, 1982.

179. Pfitzer P: Eosinophilic pleural effusion with Charcot-Leyden crystals. Acta Cytol 29:906–908, 1985.

180. Pinto MM: An immunoperoxidase study of S-100 protein in neoplastic cells in serous effusions. Use as a marker for melanoma. Acta Cytol 30:240–244, 1986.

181. Pollock TW, Perencevich EN: Hyperinfection with *Strongyloides stercoralis* in a patient with Hodgkin's disease. J Am Osteopath Assoc 76:171–175, 1976.

182. Poropatich C, Ehya H: Detached ciliary tufts in pouch of Douglas fluid. Acta Cytol 30:442–444, 1986.

183. Rammou-Kinia R, Sirmakechian-Karra T: Pseudomyxoma peritonei and malignant mucocele of the appendix. A case report. Acta Cytol 30:169–172, 1986.

184. Ramsey SJ, Tweeddale DN, Bryant LR, Braunstein H: Cytologic features of pericardial mesothelium. Acta Cytol 14:283–290, 1970.

185. Raven RW, Parkes Weber F, Woodhouse Price L: The necrobiotic nodules of rheumatoid arthritis. Case in which the scalp, abdominal wall (involving striped muscle), larynx, pericardium (involving myocardium), pleurae (involving lungs), and peritoneum were affected. Ann Rheum Dis 7:63–75, 1948.

186. Reda MG, Baigelman W: Pleural effusion in systemic lupus erythematosus. Acta Cytol 24:553–557, 1980.

187. Reyes CV, Kathuria S, MacGlashan A: Diagnostic value of calcium oxalate crystals in respiratory and pleural fluid cytology. A case report. Acta Cytol 23:65–68, 1979.

188. Rist E, Veber T: Les pleurésies tuberculeuses du pneumothorax artificiel. Etude pathogénique et expérimentale. Ann Méd Interne 24:153–177, 1928.

189. Roberts GH, Campbell GM: Exfoliative cytology of diffuse mesothelioma. J Clin Pathol 25:577–582, 1972.

190. Rolleston HD: A case of eosinophile ascites: With remarks. Br Med J 1:238–239, 1914.

191. Roncalli M, Gribaudi G, Simoncelli D, Servida E: Cytology of yolk-sac tumor of the ovary in ascitic fluid. Report of a case. Acta Cytol 32:113–116, 1988.

192. Roxby CM, Wood M, Martin AM, McHugh M: Ciliated organisms seen in fluid following dialysis. Lancet 1:916, 1986.

193. Salhadin A, Nasiell M, Nasiell K, Silfversward C, Hjerpe A, Wadas AM, Enstad I: The unique cytologic picture of oat cell carcinoma in effusions. Acta Cytol 20:298–302, 1976.

194. Samantaray SK, Pulimood BN: Filarial pericardial effusion. J Assoc Physicians India 23:349–351, 1975.

195. Satake T, Matsuyama M: Cytologic features of ascites in malignant fibrous histiocytoma of the colon. Acta Pathol Jpn 38:921–928, 1988.

196. Schwartz S, Broadbent M: Eosinophiles and other components of pleural fluids. Am Clin Climatol Assoc Trans 55:96–105, 1939.

197. Schwinn CP, Berstein GS, Willie S: Culdocentesis. *In* Compendium on Diagnostic Cytology, 6th ed. Edited by GL Wied, CM Keebler, LG Koss, JW Reagan. Chicago, Tutorials of Cytology, pp 216–227, 1988.

198. Seidel TA, Garbes AD: Cellules grumelees: Old terminology revisited. Regarding the cytologic diagnosis of chronic lymphocytic leukemia and well-differentiated lymphocytic lymphoma in pleural effusions. Acta Cytol 29:775–780, 1985.

199. Shih L-Y, Lin F-C, Kuo T-T: Cutaneous and pericardial extramedullary hematopoiesis with cardiac tamponade in chronic myeloid leukemia. Am J Clin Pathol 89:693–697, 1988.

200. Sidawy MK, Chandra P, Oertel YC: Detached ciliary tufts in female peritoneal washings. A common finding. Acta Cytol 31:841–844, 1987.

201. Singh G, Whiteside TL, Dekker A: Immunodiagnosis of mesothelioma: Use of antimesothelial cell serum in an indirect immunofluorescence assay. Cancer 43:2288–2296, 1979.

202. Sison ABM, Dionisio SA, Silva JA, Chavez PC: Allergic peritonitis. Report of a case. JAMA 134:1007–1010, 1947.

203. Slater EE: Cardiac tamponade and peripheral eosinophilia in a patient receiving cromolyn sodium. Chest 73:878–879, 1978.

204. Smith MJ, Naylor B: A method for extracting ferruginous bodies from sputum and pulmonary tissue. Am J Clin Pathol 58:250–254, 1972.

205. Smith-Purslow MJ, Kini SR, Naylor B: Cells of squamous cell carcinoma in pleural, peritoneal and pericardial fluids. Origin and morphology. Acta Cytol 33:245–253, 1989.

206. Spieler P, Gloor F: Identification of types and primary sites of malignant tumors by examination of exfoliated tumor cells in serous fluids. Comparison with the diagnostic accuracy on small histologic biopsies. Acta Cytol 29:753–767, 1985.

207. Splendore A: Sobre a cultura d'uma nova especie de cogumello pathogenico (Sporotrichose de Splendore). Riv Sci São Paulo 3:62, 1908.

208. Spriggs AI: The Cytology of Effusions in the Pleural, Pericardial and Peritoneal Cavities. New York, Grune and Stratton, 1957.

209. Spriggs AI: Pleural eosinophilia due to pneumothorax. Acta Cytol 23:425, 1979.

210. Spriggs AI: The architecture of tumor cell clusters in serous effusions. *In* Advances in Clinical Cytology, vol 2. Edited by LG Koss, DV Coleman. New York, Masson, pp 267–290, 1984.

211. Spriggs AI: Cytology of peritoneal aspirates and washings. Br J Obstet Gynaecol 94:1–3, 1987.

212. Spriggs AI, Boddington MM: Absence of mesothelial cells from tuberculous pleural effusions. Thorax 15:169–171, 1960.

213. Spriggs AI, Boddington MM: The Cytology of Effusions, Pleural, Pericardial and Peritoneal, and of Cerebrospinal Fluid, 2nd ed. London, William Heinemann, 1968.

214. Spriggs AI, Boddington MM: Oat-cell bronchial carcinoma. Identification of cells in pleural fluid. Acta Cytol 20:525–529, 1976.

215. Spriggs AI, Boddington MM: Atlas of Serous Fluid Cytopathology. A Guide to the Cells of Pleural, Pericardial, Peritoneal and Hydrocele Fluids. *In* Current Histopathology Series, vol 14. Edited by GA Gresham. Dordrecht, Kluwer Academic Publishers, 1989.

216. Spriggs AI, Grunze H: An unusual cytologic presentation of mesothelioma in serous effusions. Acta Cytol 27:288–292, 1983.

217. Spriggs AI, Jerrome DW: Intracellular mucous inclusions. A feature of malignant cells in effusions in the serous cavities, particularly due to carcinoma of the breast. J Clin Pathol 28:929–936, 1975.

218. Spriggs AI, Jerrome DW: Benign mesothelial proliferation with collagen formation in pericardial fluid. Acta Cytol 23:428–430, 1978.

219. Spriggs AI, Vanhegan RI: Cytological diagnosis of lymphoma in serous effusions. J Clin Pathol 34:1311–1325, 1981.

220. Stephenson RW, Britt DA, Schumann GB: Primary cytodiagnosis of peritoneal extramedullary hematopoiesis. Diagn Cytopathol 2:241–243, 1986.

221. Strunge T: La Ponction des Ganglions Lymphatiques. Copenhagen, Ejnar Munksgaard, 1944.

222. Sulavik S, Katz S: Pleural Effusions. Some Infrequently Emphasized Causes. Springfield, Charles C Thomas, 1963.

223. Takahashi M: Color Atlas of Cancer Cytology, 2nd ed. New York, Igaku-Shoin, 1981.

224. Tao LC: The cytopathology of mesothelioma. Acta Cytol 23:209–213, 1979.

225. Triol JH, Conston AS, Chandler SV: Malignant mesothelioma. Cytopathology of 75 cases seen in a New Jersey community hospital. Acta Cytol 28:37–45, 1984.

226. Tsukamoto N, Matsukuma K, Daimauru Y, Ota M: Cytologic presentation of ovarian adenosquamous carcinoma in ascitic fluid. A case report. Acta Cytol 28:703–705, 1984.

227. Uei Y, Koketsu H, Konda C, Kimura K: Cytodiagnosis of HCG-secreting choriocarcinoma of the stomach. Report of a case. Acta Cytol 17:431–434, 1973.

228. Vargas-Suarez J: Uber Ursprung und Bedeutung der in Pleuraergussen vorkommenden Zellen. Beitr Klin Tuberk 2:201–224, 1904.

229. Vassilakos P, Cox JN: Filariasis diagnosed by cytologic examination of hydrocele fluid. Acta Cytol 18:62–64, 1974.

230. Venegas RJ, Sun NC: Cardiac tamponade as a presentation of malignant thymoma. Acta Cytol 32:257–262, 1988.

231. Veress JF, Koss LG, Schreiber K: Eosinophilic pleural effusions. Acta Cytol 23:40–44, 1979.

232. Vilaseca J, Arnau JM, Tallada N, Salas A: Megakaryocytes in serous effusions. J Clin Pathol 34:939, 1981.

233. von Haam E: Cytology of Transudates and Exudates, vol 5. Monographs in Clinical Cytology. Edited by GL Wied. Basel, S Karger, 1977.

234. von Lichtenberg F, Smith JH, Cheever AW: The Hoeppli phenomenon in schistosomiasis: Comparative pathology and immunopathology. Am J Trop Med Hyg 15:886–895, 1966.

235. Wagner JC, Sleggs CA, Marchand P: Diffuse pleural mesothelioma and asbestos exposure in the Northwestern Cape Province. Br J Ind Med 17:260–271, 1960.

236. Wahl RW: Curschmann's spirals in pleural and peritoneal fluids. Report of 12 cases. Acta Cytol 30:147–151, 1986.

237. Walter A, Krishnaswami H, Cariappa A: Microfilariae of *Wuchereria bancrofti* in cytologic smears. Acta Cytol 27:432–436, 1983.

238. Waltzer PD, Rutherford I, East R: Empyema with *Trichomonas* species. Am Rev Respir Dis 118:415–418, 1978.

239. Ward R: Pleural effusion and rheumatoid disease. Lancet 2:1336–1338, 1961.

240. Warhol MJ, Hickey WF, Corson JM: Malignant mesothelioma. Ultrastructural distinction from adenocarcinoma. Am J Surg Pathol 6:307–314, 1982.

241. Watson CW, Friedman KJ: Cytology of neuroendocrine (Merkel-cell) carcinoma in pleural fluid. A case report. Acta Cytol 29:397–402, 1985.

242. Weaver KM, Novak PM, Naylor B: Vegetable cell contaminants in cytologic specimens. Their resemblance to cells associated with various normal and pathologic states. Acta Cytol 25:210–214, 1981.

243. Whitaker D: Cell aggregates in malignant mesothelioma. Acta Cytol 21:236–239, 1977.

244. Whitaker D, Shilkin KB: The cytology of malignant mesothelioma in Western Australia. Acta Cytol 22:67–70, 1978.

245. Whitaker D, Shilkin KB: Diagnosis of pleural malignant mesothelioma in life—A practical approach. J Pathol 143:147–175, 1984.

246. Widal, Ravaut: Applications cliniques de l'étude histologique des épanchements sérofibrineux de la plèvre (pleuresies tuberculeuses). Comp Rend Soc Biol 52:648–651, 1900.

247. Widal, Ravaut: Applications cliniques de l'étude histologique des épanchements sérofibrineux de la plèvre (pleuresies mecaniques). Comp Rend Soc Biol 52:651–653, 1900.

248. Willis RA: Pathology of Tumours, 2nd ed. London, Butterworths, 1953.

249. Wilson MS, Theil KS, Goodwin RA, Brandt JT: Comparison of Papanicolaou's and Wright-Giemsa stains in the examination of body fluids for Hodgkin's disease. Arch Pathol Lab Med 112:612–615, 1988.

250. Woyke S, Domagala W, Olszewski W: Alveolar cell carcinoma of the lung: An ultrastructural study of the cancer cells detected in the pleural fluid. Acta Cytol 16:63–69, 1972.

251. Wuerker RB, Guglietti LC, Nations ED: Comparison of light and transmission electron microscopy for the evaluation of body cavity effusions. Acta Cytol 27:614–624, 1983.

252. Yam LT, Lin DG, Janckila AJ, Li C-Y: Immunocytochemical diagnosis of lymphoma in serous effusions. Acta Cytol 29:833–841, 1985.

253. Yamada S: Über die seröse Flüssigkeit in der Pleurahohle der gesunden Menschen. Z Gesamte Exp Med 90:342–348, 1933.

254. Yamada T, Itou U, Watanabe Y, Ohashi S: Cytologic diagnosis of malignant melanoma. Acta Cytol 16:70–76, 1972.

255. Yang H-Y, Weaver LL, Foti PR: Primary malignant fibrous histiocytoma of the pleura. A case report. Acta Cytol 27:683–687, 1983.

256. Yazdi HM: Cytopathology of extramedullary hemopoiesis in effusions and peritoneal washings: A report of three cases with immunohistochemical study. Diagn Cytopathol 2:326–329, 1986.

257. Young JA, Crocker J: Pleural fluid cytology in lymphoplasmacytoid lymphoma with numerous intracytoplasmic immunoglobulin inclusions. A case report with immunocytochemistry. Acta Cytol 28:419–424, 1984.

258. Young JA, Crocker J: Colour Atlas of Pulmonary Cytopathology. Oxford, Harvey Miller, 1985.

259. Zaatari GS, Gupta PK, Bhagavan BS, Jarboe BR: Cytopathology of pleural endometriosis. Acta Cytol 26:229–232, 1982.

260. Zaharopoulos P, Wong JC: Hemoglobin crystals in fluid specimens from confined body spaces. Acta Cytol 31:777–782, 1987.

261. Zirkin HJ: Pleural fluid cytology of invasive thymoma. Acta Cytol 29:1011–1014, 1985.

Fine Needle Aspiration of Various Organs and Body Sites

23

Imaging Techniques

Stephen R. Ell

Fine needle aspiration for cytologic diagnosis has become an indispensable component of the workup of many abnormalities. Once fraught with dangers because of the risks of large bore needles and inadequate imaging capabilities, such procedures are now essentially free of mortality and involve minimal morbidity.[1, 8, 9, 12, 13, 17, 18, 20] In many cases, such procedures obviate surgery by either demonstrating a benign etiology or proving a metastatic disease.

In discussing imaging techniques in fine needle aspiration, it is important to remember the skill of the cytopathologist. With no difference in technique of biopsy, I have experienced a diagnostic rate of only 20% in one hospital and nearly 90% in another. Although many fine needles do provide cores, surgical pathology is not always of help, and it is crucial to recognize the level of the ability of the pathologists with whom one works.

Radiology has yet to provide an ideal imaging device for biopsy. Yet it is valuable to consider what would constitute such a device, for its components bear on the choice of modality in the majority of cases.

Perhaps most important is first the ability to perform the procedure on a critically ill patient, who cannot cooperate. Many biopsies cannot be performed at all because of patient condition, yet these are often cases in which a relatively noninvasive diagnostic procedure would be immensely beneficial.

Second, biopsy without the use of contrast agents is highly desirable. Not only do such agents provoke significant reactions in a small number of patients, but the osmolar load from the contrast agents may turn borderline renal function into frank failure. The new crop of nonionic contrast agents can prevent most, if not all, of these problems, but their current cost is extremely high for routine use.

Third, the ideal imaging modality for biopsy would not expose the patient to ionizing radiation. Fluoroscopy often results in 2 to 5 rads per minute, and procedures of the complexity considered here often consume large amounts of time. Likewise computed tomography (CT) typically requires multiple slices of the same or very close level, resulting in a significant accumulated dose.

Fourth, such a device would not of itself determine the direction from which the biopsy was attempted. The shortest path to a lesion that does not traverse a structure at risk from a fine needle is always optimal, because it decreases the number of passes necessary to place a needle in a lesion, a factor that becomes exponential when several passes are made.

Fifth, our ideal imaging system would permit real-time visualization of the procedure. Both CT and magnetic resonance imaging (MRI) are made somewhat clumsy by this problem. Ultrasound and fluoroscopy provide this capability.

Sixth, an ideal imaging device would allow biopsy of small parts and very small lesions without additional difficulty.

Seventh, an ideal device should be capable of producing images that demonstrate unequivocally that the specimen came from the lesion in question. This is not merely for legal purposes—legitimate questions arise when a biopsy shows tissue normal for a given organ as to from where the specimen came. Thus, documentation of needle position is crucial to the avoidance of surgical biopsy. The evidence of the origin of an aspirate must be conclusive.

Lastly, the ideal imaging technique would be inexpensive. As pressure mounts to contain health care costs, this factor will come to the fore.

At this time, no single modality comes close to fulfilling all of these requirements. In the following discussion of available choices, we direct our argument along the lines of which of the strengths each modality offers and therefore for what purposes it is best suited.

BASIC TECHNIQUE

Although the method of guidance may vary, certain aspects of fine needle aspiration are essentially constant. Many excellent small bore biopsy needles are available (Fig. 23–1), and personal preference as much as anything else plays a major role in choosing one or two for routine use. The gauge of the needle is central, however, to the safety of the procedure. Both on the bases of personal experience and published results of numerous investigators, a reasonable generalization is that a 22-gauge needle can traverse bowel and if necessary even major vessels (in extreme circumstances when no other approach is possible) without significant risk, whereas a 20-gauge needle in the same circumstance may produce peritonitis or major hemorrhage. The use of 22-gauge biopsy needles is strongly recommended as a safety precaution in aspiration biopsies. In specific instances, even smaller needles are advisable.

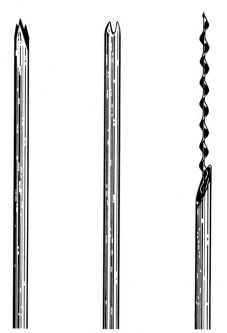

FIGURE 23–1. Three examples, from among many, of excellent **22-gauge cutting and aspiration biopsy needles.** They are, from left to right, **Franseen, EZM,** and **Rotex** needles.

Before the biopsy, notification is given to the cytopathology laboratory and the presence of a technologist from that laboratory is extremely helpful during the procedure to optimize handling of the biopsy specimens. Should the presence of such a technologist be impossible, it is advisable to inquire of the pathologist how the specimen is optimally handled at the time of biopsy, and the appropriate materials should be made available.

Informed consent is obtained from the patients or their representatives if they cannot give it personally. We generally mention vasovagal responses, infection, hematoma or hemorrhage, if the approach is risky in that regard, plus other possibilities particular to the organ in question. We state that, although we will use local anesthetic for the skin and subcutaneous tissues, the patient will experience some pain from the biopsy. If the approach involves passing near a rib we inform the patient that the pain may be much greater because of the sensitivity of the bone and is not a cause for alarm. We have found it inadvisable to indicate that pain will be trivial, because the experience is highly subjective and the experience of more pain than anticipated may induce a vasovagal or other undesirable response. In practice, we rarely use intravenous contrast material, but occasionally, as for a hepatic lesion, we inform the patient of the risks attendant upon its administration. Realistically, to know that contrast agent is needed, the patient will have undergone contrast agent administration before, making the risk more apparent. Once consent is obtained, we offer the patient sedation, usually diazepam, 2 to 3 mg, intravenously, repeated as needed, if he or she appears very anxious. A peripheral intravenous line is established in case sedation is needed later or in case a complication or change in status requires venous access.

The approach to the lesion should be chosen before the patient enters the room, insofar as possible. The skin is prepared with an iodine solution and allowed to dry. Isopropyl alcohol is used to remove the iodine, which is often irritating to the skin if left. Infiltration with local anesthetic of the skin and subcutaneous tissues is then performed. A tiny incision is made through the skin with a scalpel to ease the entry and manipulation of the biopsy needle. All biopsy needles employ a stylet, which is left in place until the needle is in the lesion. It is important to gauge the depth of the lesion from the skin, and a Steri-strip can be placed around the needle to prevent the needle's being advanced too far. Whenever possible, a needle insertion perpendicular to the skin is preferable to another angled approach, because the last is much more difficult to judge. The patient is asked to hold his or her breath during needle insertion. Once the needle is placed, its position is established by whatever imaging modality is being employed. Once the needle is in the lesion its position is documented with a film image.

With the needle tip in the lesion, the stylet is removed and extension tubing attached to a 10- or 20-cc syringe is connected to the needle. The tubing is filled with normal saline and the syringe filled with 2 to 3 ml as well. The needle is then rotated back and forth, while short (4 to 5 mm) advances and withdrawals of the needle are made. Suction is applied to the syringe during this procedure. Some biopsy sets come with syringes with stops, which permit a constant suction. The syringe is observed for the appearance of tissue and blood. If none is seen, we inject 1 ml of normal saline and repeat the process. A second or third pass can be made, depending on what tissue is observed to have been recovered and the risk.

The specimen is then prepared under the guidance of a cytopathologist or cytotechnologist. In a case in which infection is a major concern, we may divide the sample, but usually all is given to cytopathology. Some medical centers have microscopes and other apparatus for immediate viewing to determine if the biopsy should be repeated.

FLUOROSCOPY

Before CT and ultrasound, fluoroscopy was the only method of imaging available for needle biopsy. Now its use is mainly confined to chest lesions, where air gives adequate contrast to identify a soft tissue structure.[12, 16]

Fluoroscopy has much to recommend it. Pulmonary nodules should be viewed fluoroscopically before biopsy in order to determine whether or not they contain calcification. Sometimes an appropriate obliquity with ideal collimation will demonstrate calcification in a nodule, which is accepted as proof of benignity. If no calcification is identified, biopsy can proceed.

Ideally, bi-plane fluoroscopy should be employed. In practice, a C-arm unit, which can image at right angles without moving the patient, is more than adequate. Single plane fluoroscopy is also acceptable, especially if it is possible to "feel" the needle enter the lesion. If the patient can easily turn on his or her side, conventional fluoroscopy can be employed, although, with the main use of fluoroscopy being for pulmonary nodules, it is wise to restrict motion when a needle traverses the pleura.

Fluoroscopy is, in most medical centers, relatively inexpensive. The main disadvantages lie in the limited number of sites in the body for which fluoroscopic guidance can be provided and in the radiation dose. A C-arm can often be brought to the bedside, but unless a lesion is outlined by air or has an identifiable calcification within it, fluoroscopy is limited in its range of applications. Further, each minute of fluoroscopic time requires something on the order of 2 to 5 rads. When biopsy is performed under fluoroscopy, a time should be set to determine what dose the patient received. During a difficult biopsy, strenuous effort is required to limit radiation dosage.

ULTRASOUND

Ultrasonic guidance of biopsies offers many advantages. Ultrasound units themselves, or at least the current generation of sector or real-time scanners, are portable, permitting bedside biopsy capability. No biohazard results from the type of imaging necessary for biopsy. Ultrasound is currently the best modality for biopsy of extremely ill patients, who can neither come to the radiology department nor remain still. Most units have videotape recorders attached, so that the entire procedure can be kept for review. Specialized transducers are available for the biopsy of small lesions, particularly in the prostate. Indeed, only specialized MRI studies and ultrasound have the capacity to identify very small lesions in such locations.[2, 6, 10, 11, 15] No better way exists to image pleural fluid, determine whether it is loculated and guide aspiration than with ultrasound.

Yet certain limitations apply in ultrasound-guided biopsy, which can be obtrusive. Ultrasound cannot image through bone or air. Ribs may interfere with visualization of the liver, for example. Many needles produce so many artifacts that lesions cease to be identifiable when the needle approaches or enters them. The features of the needles that produce these effects have been elucidated and the problem should decrease in the future.[3] In this situation, documentation and identification of actual needle position become problematic. Further, ultrasound may dictate the route of biopsy, which is undesirable. For example, biopsy of retroperitoneal nodes, particularly para-aortic nodes, can usually be done by a ventral approach because such nodes cannot typically be imaged from the back because of interference from the spine and attenuation by the back musculature and fat. Air in the bowel may make reproduction of imaging of abdominal structures impossible.

Ultrasound has been used to biopsy anterior mediastinal masses.[19] I have had no experience with this technique, although the results reported are encouraging. The only reservation I would express at this point in the development of this method is that the unit employed have Doppler capability, lest an ascending aortic aneurysm be biopsied inadvertently. Anecdotes from the days when syphilitic aneurysms were common suggest that such a biopsy could prove quite dramatic.

COMPUTED TOMOGRAPHY

Computed tomography, or CT, is the most versatile of currently available imaging modalities.[7, 9, 12–14, 20] Not only does it give the most anatomically detailed images (although they are, in fact, not anatomic images at all but mathematic reconstructions based on complex calculations of the x-ray attenuation coefficient of voxels—volume elements—included in the area examined), but CT permits the widest choice of approaches. All current CT scanners can calculate angles and distances for all approaches and permit assessment of which approach requires traversing the least tissue or which allows the avoidance of structures best not traversed at all (e.g., the aorta). Because of features of most reconstruction algorithms, the sudden change

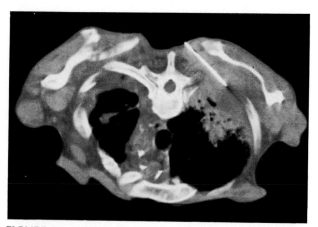

FIGURE 23–2. Image from a computed tomography biopsy. Note the very black area at the end of the needle. This is a so-called overshoot artifact, which reliably demonstrates that the needle tip is indeed in the image.

in relative density between the needle tip and the adjacent tissue produces a telltale artifact that locates the needle tip precisely (Fig. 23–2). Documentation of the biopsy site with CT is superior to that of any other modality. Computed tomography is also the least limited in terms of what can be imaged. From bone to air, no other modality can display so much detail in so many structures.

Computed tomography is not perfect as an imaging modality for biopsy, however. Patient cooperation is extremely important, and even with sedation, it is sometimes not realistic to attempt biopsy of patients unable or unwilling to follow instructions. Most important for lesions in the chest, slightly less so for those in the abdomen, and least for those in the pelvis, the patient's capacity to reproduce a given level of inspiration can determine the success of a biopsy attempt. Not that such concerns are unimportant in other types of biopsy guidance, but CT is somewhat unique in requiring an appreciable interval from needle placement to image of the result. A CT image is narrowly collimated and typically is about 1 cm thick, or at biopsy 4 to 5 mm. Dose to the tissue in the slice is in the range of 1 to 4 rads per image. The amount of scatter outside the slice thickness must also be taken into account, although generalizable dosimetry studies in this regard are lacking. If only three or four scans of the same level are needed to document needle placement, the radiation dose may be from 3 to about 16 rads. When the correct level is selected and the placement is extremely difficult, up to ten images at the same level may be required with a potential 40 rads exposure. Beyond that level (knowledge of the dosimetry of the scanner used for biopsy is crucial), continuation of the procedure should be questioned. In many cases (e.g., proof of metastatic disease), there is still a benefit in continuing, but cumulative radiation dose to the patient must be considered in CT-guided biopsy.

Another significant problem comes from the approach. It is most desirable with CT guidance to biopsy

in such a way that the needle enters the patient at right angles to the plane of the skin. If the needle is angled even a few degrees, it may require several additional images with the associated waiting time and radiation to find the needle tip. In addition, a needle tip only partly in the scanned field, because of an oblique approach, can be difficult to demonstrate adequately, although at least in theory the gantry of the scanner could be tilted to compensate for this. In practice, however, the degree of obliquity is usually difficult to determine, and I have had no real success with this method.

The anticipated advent of portable CT will make the importance of this modality even greater as a biopsy tool, as such units will bring CT guidance to the bedside.

COMPUTERIZED STEREOTACTIC BIOPSY IN BREAST LESIONS

Mammography has been shown to be one of the few tools available to decrease mortality from breast cancer. An example of the new technology available for the biopsy of breast lesions has been reported.[4] The device, which has shown considerable value (i.e., its false-negative rate is trivial), when compared with excision biopsy uses two views of the breast taken at different obliquities and computes the angles of a needle holder directed toward the compressed breast.[12] This device employs trigonometric functions to determine the angles and its "computer" is handheld or can be. Similar devices, aimed at avoiding the previous trial-and-error needle placement with radiographs obtained after every needle placement, are reaching the market. The first such device described is limited to lesions not close to the chest wall and employs a table over 1-cm thick through an opening in which the patient allows one breast to fall. Although far from perfect, the device brings the advantages of aspiration cytology to breast lesions, which previously were subjected to needle placement only for localization of lesions and which were then surgically excised.

MAGNETIC RESONANCE IMAGING

Magnetic resonance imaging (MRI) is undergoing explosive growth. Without describing the immense complexities associated with this modality, a few salient points are worth noting. When its qualities are compared with our list for an "ideal" imaging modality, MRI offers much. It permits reconstruction of an image in essentially any view desired (e.g., axial, sagittal, coronal), which would permit the widest latitude in choosing a needle approach. Differentiation of normal from abnormal tissue is potentially greater than with any other modality. No known biohazard exists from MRI, which promises the benefits of CT without the hazards.

As currently used, however, MRI is generally impractical for biopsy. The reason is twofold. The very long pulse sequences employed to obtain images results in unacceptably long procedures. The degree of patient cooperation necessary is higher than with any other modality. In addition to reproducing respiration, the patient is confined in an extremely small space, and an appreciable number cannot tolerate the psychologic stress and demonstrate claustrophobia. Together, the combination leaves MRI as a rarely used modality for biopsy, although the lengthy imaging process is not inherent to the modality and improves with technologic change.[5] At another level, the long scan times result in artifact-degraded views of moving structures, making much chest and abdominal imaging of limited value.

Another problem, which is much less serious, is inherent to the modality as currently utilized. Magnetic resonance imaging does not image cortical bone, largely because most returned signal is from water. Flowing blood or other moving fluid also returns no signal. The use of surface coils for imaging, although the resultant images are often spectacularly detailed, makes biopsy impractical for regions thus scanned.

Currently, MRI is the most expensive imaging modality available for biopsy guidance.

Thus, MRI shows great promise as an aid in biopsy, but much of that promise remains to be fulfilled, especially when its cost is considered.

CONCLUSION

Aspiration biopsy is an indispensable part of modern diagnosis, obviating surgical intervention in many cases and giving accurate preoperative information in many others. The technique of biopsy is relatively simple, whereas the skill of the individual pathologist is absolutely crucial to the utility of the method.

Biopsy kits and needles are many, but very little harm can be done below the neck with a 22-gauge needle, whereas a 20-gauge or larger needle in identical circumstances can result in fatal complications. This factor is particularly important when considering paths near or through either bowel or blood vessels. With this in mind, the older distinction between cutting needles and aspiration biopsies is insignificant, and many excellent 22-gauge cutting needles are available, which, unless carelessly used, can be employed routinely.

No current imaging modality is perfect for all biopsies. The main points outlined in this chapter regarding what biopsy is best handled by which imaging modality are summarized in Table 23–1.

One of the surest ways to prove oneself wrong is to predict the future. Ten years ago very few radiologists had ever heard of MRI or nuclear magnetic resonance—NMR—as it was then known. (The "nuclear" was removed to make it clear that no radiation was involved.) What is written here is believed appropriate for the time it was written and holds no wisdom for the future.

Nonetheless, the future of guided aspiration needle biopsy appears bright. In many situations, this rela-

TABLE 23–1. Biopsy Sites and Recommended Methods of Guidance

Type of Biopsy	Best Imaging Modality
Pulmonary nodule	Fluoroscopy, CT
Hilar or mediastinal mass or adenopathy	CT with IV contrast material
Pleural fluid	Ultrasound
Pleural mass	CT, Ultrasound
Liver lesion	CT, Ultrasound
Pancreas	CT
Retroperitoneal nodes	CT
Pelvic structures	CT, Ultrasound
Prostatic lesions	Endorectal ultrasound
Thyroid lesions	Ultrasound
Masses in superficial soft tissues or in extremities	Ultrasound, CT
Kidney (when assessing organ status as a whole, e.g., transplant)	Ultrasound
Kidney mass	CT
Adrenal mass	CT

This list is neither exhaustive nor are the recommendations intended to be absolute. Ultrasound can be used in many situations that do not appear on this list. Modalities are listed as best, *in general*, for a particular site based on the criteria discussed in this chapter. (CT = computed tomography; IV = intravenous.)

tively safe procedure can determine whether a patient requires major surgery or not. Aspiration biopsy is an indispensable part of modern diagnosis and seems likely to remain so.

References

1. Ballard GL, Boyd WR: A specially designed cutting aspiration needle for lung biopsy. Am J Radiol 130:889–903, 1978.
2. Bockish A, Jager N, Biersack HJ: Magnetic resonance (MR) imaging of prostatic tumours, a comparison with x-ray, CT, and transrectal ultrasound (TRS). Eur J Radiol 8:54–62, 1988.
3. Bondestam S, Kreula J: Needle tip echogenicity: a study with real time ultrasound. Invest Radiol 24:555–560, 1988.
4. Dowlatshahi K, Schmidt RA, Jokich PM, Bibbo M, Springer E, Gent HJ: Diagnosis of nonpalpable breast tumors using stereotaxic needle cytology. Radiology: RSNA Scientific Program [Suppl] 165:172, 1987.
5. Duckwiler G, Lufkin RB, Hanafee WN: MRI-directed needle biopsies. Radiol Clin North Am 17:255–264, 1989.
6. Gefter WB, Spritzer CE, Eisenberg B, LiVolsi VA, Axell L, Velchik M, Alavi A, Schenck J, Kressel HY: Thyroid imaging with high-field-strength surface-coil MR. Radiology 164:483–489, 1987.
7. Goldstein H, Zornoza J, Wallace S: Percutaneous fine needle aspiration biopsy of pancreatic and other abdominal masses. Radiology 123:319–326, 1977.
8. Harter LP, Moss AA, Goldberg HI: Computed tomographic-guided fine needle aspirations for neoplastic and inflammatory diseases. Am J Radiol 140:363–370, 1983.
9. House AJS, Thomson KR: Evaluation of a new transthoracic needle for biopsy of benign and malignant lung lesions. Am J Radiol 129:215–220, 1977.
10. Lee F, Littrup PJ, Kumasaka GH, Borlaza GS, McLeary RD: Use of transrectal ultrasound in the diagnosis, guided biopsy, staging and screening of prostate cancer. Radiographics 7:627–640, 1987.
11. Lee F, Littrup PJ, McLeary RD, Kumasaka GH, Borlaza GS,

McHugh TA, Soiderer MR, Roi LD: Needle aspiration and core biopsy of prostate cancer: comparative evaluation with biplanar transrectal US guidance. Radiology 163:515–521, 1987.

12. MacMahon H, Ell SR, Ferguson MK: Diagnostic methods in lung cancer. *In* Lung Cancer: A Comprehensive Treatise. Edited by JD Bitran, HM Golomb, KAG Little, RR Weichselbaum. New York, Grune & Stratton, 1988.

13. Moss AA: Interventional computed tomography. *In* Computed Tomography of the Body. Edited by AA Moss, G Gamsu, HK Genant. Philadelphia, WB Saunders, 1983.

14. Mueller PR, Wittenberg J, Ferrucci JT: Fine needle aspiration of abdominal masses. Semin Roentgenol 16:52–68, 1981.

15. Noma S, Kanaoka M, Minami S, Sagoh T, Yamashita K, Nishimura K, Togashi K, Itoh K, Kujisawa I, Nakano Y, Oomura M, Tasaka Y, Itoh H, Konishi J: Thyroid masses: MR imaging and pathologic correlation. Radiology 168:759–766, 1988.

16. Pereiras RV, Meiers W, Kunhards B, Troner M, Hutson D, Barkin JS, Viamonte M: Fluoroscopically guided thin needle aspiration biopsy of the abdomen and retroperitoneum. Am J Radiol 131:197–204, 1978.

17. Sinner WN: Complications of percutaneous transthoracic needle aspiration biopsy. Acta Radiol Diagn 17:813–827, 1976.

18. Sinner WN: Transthoracic needle biopsy of small peripheral malignant lung lesions. Invest Radiol 8:305–314, 1973.

19. Wernecke K, Vassallo P, Peters PE, von Bassewitz DB: Mediastinal tumors: Biopsy under US guidance. Radiology 172:473–476, 1989.

20. Westcott JL: Percutaneous needle aspiration of hilar and mediastinal masses. Radiology 141:323–329, 1981.

24

Salivary Glands and Rare Head and Neck Lesions

Torsten Löwhagen
Edneia Miyki Tani
Lambert Skoog

Salivary Glands

A nodule or diffuse enlargement of the salivary glands may be caused by a cystic lesion, an inflammation, a degenerative process or a benign or malignant neoplasm. For adequate management, the exact nature of the process has to be revealed. Only microscopic evaluation can determine the nature of the lesion. Incisional or cutting needle biopsies have not been accepted as the procedure of choice to obtain tissue for diagnostic purposes because of various complications. Fine needle aspiration (FNA), however, has a negligible risk of complications, and in medical centers where the technique is routinely used, approximately a third of all patients with salivary gland lesions are spared surgery.[38] Of equal importance is that an FNA diagnosis will allow an individualized treatment plan, when surgery is required. The clinical impact of FNA has been demonstrated in several studies.[12, 34, 36, 41, 43, 53]

TECHNIQUE

The technique of aspiration does not differ from that used for other superficial sites.[56] The FNA procedure employing a 23- or 25-gauge needle is rarely painful to the degree that it prevents successful sampling. Rarely, a small hematoma may occur or some blood may be seen in the saliva after aspiration.

In our clinic, slides of aspirates are air dried and alcohol fixed, routinely. The slides are stained with May-Grünwald-Giemsa and Papanicolaou stains, respectively. We find both stains helpful as each method places emphasis on different features.

ANATOMY AND HISTOLOGY

The parotid, the submandibular and the sublingual glands compose the major salivary glands. The parotid gland is of ectodermal origin and its secretion is serous and drains through Stensen's duct into the oral cavity. The submandibular gland is of endodermal derivation and secretes a mixed but predominantly serous substance. It drains via Wharton's duct at the sublingual caruncle close to the frenulum of the tongue. The sublingual gland lies in the floor of the mouth adjacent to the midline and produces a mixed, primarily mucus secretion.

Minor salivary glands are nonencapsulated aggregates of mucus or mixed mucous-serous glands located superficially over the lips, throughout the oral cavity, nasopharynx, sinuses, trachea and bronchi.

The glands are organized into lobules. Each lobule consists of a cluster of acini around a terminal duct system. The acini are made up of pyramid-shaped epithelial cells, which have excentric round nuclei (Fig. 24–1). The cytoplasm is abundant, finely granular and acidophilic in serous glands and clear in mucus-secreting glands. Flat myoepithelial cells with elongated nuclei form an outer layer around each acinus. From the lobules, the secretion is conveyed via interlobular ducts to the main secretory ducts. The smallest excretory ducts are lined by cuboidal cells, whereas those lining larger ducts are tall and columnar. Near the orifice in the oral cavity, the ducts are lined by stratified squamous epithelium. A layer of myoepithelial cells is present between the lining epithelial cells and the basement membrane.

With increasing age the cells of acini and ducts occasionally transform into oncocytes.[21] An oncocytic cell is a large epithelial cell with distinct cell borders, eosinophilic finely granular cytoplasm and a round nucleus, often with a central prominent nucleolus.

The parotid gland normally contains small lymphoid aggregates and one or more nodes. Salivary ducts and acini have also been found in lymph nodes outside the capsule of the parotid gland.[20]

CYTOLOGY

Aspiration of normal or near normal salivary glands usually gives only a small amount of epithelial cells. Normal structures are often seen as "contamination" in aspirates from pathologic lesions. The normal structures are viewed as basically acinar cells in well-preserved cohesive ball-like formations (Fig. 24–2), and ductal cells in monolayered sheets.

The acinar cells have a central or excentric, small rounded nucleus with a small nucleolus. The cytoplasm is abundant, granular and rather foamy (Fig. 24–3). Bare cell nuclei are usually observed in the background. Terminal secretory ducts appear as short tubular structures, and larger ducts appear as flat clusters or sheets of cuboidal or columnar cells with evenly spaced monomorphous nuclei. Myoepithelial cells are only occasionally noted as small dark nuclei superimposed in the clusters. Lymphoid cells may be aspirated from intrasalivary lymphoid tissue.

The lesions that cause enlargement of salivary glands are listed in Table 24–1.

TABLE 24–1. Lesions Causing Salivary Gland Enlargement

Non-neoplastic lesions	Neoplastic lesions
Cysts	**Benign**
Simple cyst	Pleomorphic adenoma (mixed tumor)
Mucocele or retention cyst	Adenolymphoma (Warthin's tumor)
Epidermoid cyst	Basal cell adenoma
Branchial cleft cyst	Oncocytoma
Inflammatory lesions	Hemangioma
Acute sialoadenitis	Other benign mesenchymal tumors (e.g., lipomas)
Chronic sialoadenitis (sialolithiasis)	
Granulomatous sialoadenitis	**Malignant**
Intraglandular lymph node hyperplasia	Adenoid cystic carcinoma
	Mucoepidermoid carcinoma
Autoimmune disorders	Acinic cell carcinoma
Benign lymphoepithelial lesions (Mikulicz-Sjögren's syndrome)	Adenocarcinoma (not otherwise specified)
	Squamous cell carcinoma
	Undifferentiated carcinoma
	Carcinoma ex pleomorphic adenoma
	Malignant lymphoma
	Others

NON-NEOPLASTIC LESIONS

Cysts

Most benign and malignant salivary gland lesions may have a cystic component. Cystic aspirates therefore cause a special problem because the cyst fluid alone does not allow for a morphologic evaluation. The most common cyst is a ductal retention cyst due to obstruction (sialolithiasis), and it contains watery fluid or in cases of inflamed cysts, a cloudy fluid.

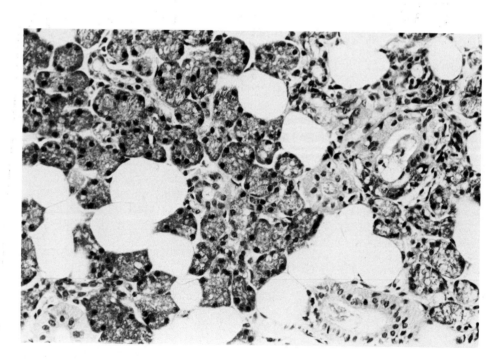

FIGURE 24–1. Normal salivary gland. Tissue section (hematoxylin and eosin; ×80).

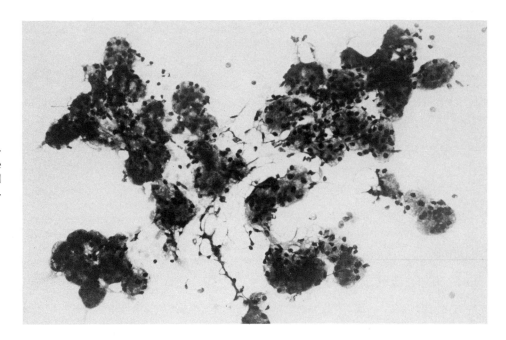

FIGURE 24–2. Aspirate of **normal salivary gland.** Cohesive ball-like formations constituted by acinar cells (May-Grünwald-Giemsa; ×50).

Retention cysts of the major salivary glands that are deep seated are at palpation felt to be rather firm. They are therefore likely to be diagnosed clinically as solid neoplasms. Fine needle aspiration will, however, readily disclose the nature of the lesion. In such cases, a clinical follow-up after a few weeks should suffice. If the cyst recurs, it should be reaspirated to attempt a cure and to obtain a further sample for cytologic evaluation.

If a residual mass persists, however, the aspiration should be repeated because some benign and malignant salivary gland tumors may have a cystic component. An initial sampling from a cystic portion of the tumor may therefore be misleading, and a repeat biopsy should be performed from the walls of the cyst to help establish a diagnosis.

Branchial cleft cysts can occasionally appear in the anterior portion of a parotid gland and on clinical examination be mistaken for a salivary gland lesion.

Small superficial cysts are often encountered in minor salivary glands of the lips and the oral mucosa. They are in general accurately diagnosed clinically. At aspiration such cysts yield a clear, mucous fluid and leave no residual mass.

Cytology

An aspirate from a benign retention cyst is usually clear with a watery to viscous consistency. It can, however, be cloudy and yellowish when secondary inflammation has taken place. The smear usually contains only a few histiocytes and degenerative epithelial

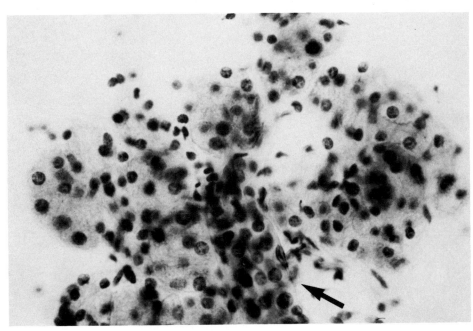

FIGURE 24–3. A duct (arrow) surrounded by groups of cells with abundant granular and well-demarcated cytoplasm. The nuclei are round and centrally located (Papanicolaou; ×160).

cells. Epithelial cells of cuboidal, columnar or squamous type can occur together with inflammatory cells and histiocytes. The cytologic features of non-neoplastic cystic lesions are summarized subsequently.

If the palpatory findings normalize after aspiration and the smear contains only a few phagocytes or occasional epithelial cells, the lesion is probably a retention cyst.

Non-neoplastic Cysts: Common Cytologic Features

- Water-like or viscous mucoid aspirate
- Histiocytes and other inflammatory cells
- Epithelial cells—cuboidal and squamoid

Inflammatory Lesions

Acute Sialoadenitis

In young individuals, viral infections have a predilection for involving the parotid glands, which become diffusely enlarged. The diagnosis is usually obvious on clinical grounds and rarely requires morphologic confirmation.

Acute bacterial sialoadenitis is characterized by diffuse painful enlargement of the salivary gland. It occurs with equal frequency in the parotid and submandibular salivary glands, mostly in elderly patients. Poor oral hygiene with dehydration, sialolithiasis and impaired immune response are generally thought to be immediate or contributory causes of this condition. Acute sialoadenitis with or without abscess formation can clinically simulate a malignant tumor.

Aspirates from acute inflammatory salivary gland lesions contain fibrin, cellular debris, neutrophils, lymphocytes and histiocytes (Fig. 24–4). In cases with sialolithiasis, calculi may also be encountered.

Chronic Sialoadenitis

Nonspecific chronic sialoadenitis is often secondary to stricture and obstruction of the ducts. In elderly patients, a decreased secretion of saliva and retrograde infections may result in a gradual diffuse enlargement of the salivary glands. It is frequently seen after radiotherapy of the oral cavity. Symptoms include recurrent mild pain and diffuse swelling related to eating. In more chronic cases of sialoadenitis, the gland becomes fibrotic and hard with secondary atrophy of acini and proliferation of ductal epithelium. In obstructive sialoadenitis caused by calculi, the epithelium may undergo squamous and mucoid metaplasia and the ducts become dilated by mucous material.

Cytology

Aspirates from nonobstructive sialoadenitis contain sparse cellular elements. The acinic cells are atrophic and may barely be seen in the smears. The duct cells that predominate are often small and tightly packed in clusters. Scattered fibroblasts, lymphocytes and granulocytes may also be seen.

In some cases of clinically suspected chronic sialoadenitis, the aspiration may yield only normal salivary gland structures.

Aspirates from the obstructive type of chronic sialoadenitis may contain mucus, ductal cells with evidence of squamous metaplasia and cylindric cells some of which may even have cilia. In addition, macrophages

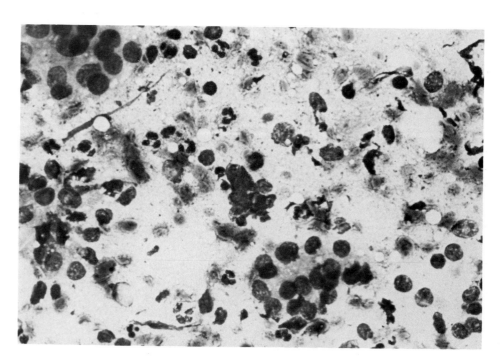

FIGURE 24–4. Acute sialoadenitis. Clusters of epithelial cells admixed with cellular debris and neutrophils (May-Grünwald-Giemsa; ×160).

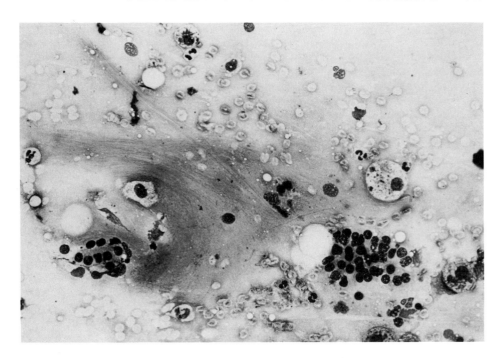

FIGURE 24–5. Obstructive chronic sialoadenitis showing mucus, macrophages and clusters of epithelial cells (May-Grünwald-Giemsa; ×80).

with vacuolated cytoplasm imitating mucus-producing cells, lymphocytes, granulocytes and crystals of various shapes may be observed (Fig. 24–5).

Chronic Non-obstructive Sialoadenitis: Common Cytologic Features

- Ductal epithelium in clusters and sheets
- Scanty acinar groups with atrophy of epithelium
- Occasional fibroblasts, lymphocytes, neutrophils and macrophages

Lymphadenitis

Small lymph nodes are often found within the parotid gland. When such lymph nodes enlarge they can clinically be difficult to differentiate from neoplasms. Fine needle aspiration will identify the lymphoid nature of the lesion and often differentiates among reactive lymph node hyperplasia, nonspecific lymphadenitis, granulomatous lymphadenitis and lymphoma. The cytology pertaining to intraparotid lymph nodes does not differ from that of lymph nodes from other sites and is described elsewhere.

Benign Lymphoepithelial Lesion and Related Conditions

The benign lymphoepithelial lesions, of which Mikulicz-Sjögren's syndrome is the most common, are characterized by insidious swelling of one or several salivary and lacrimal glands. These swellings can become quite large and are usually bilateral and symmetric (Fig. 24–6). This condition results in decreased secretion from the lacrimal and salivary glands causing keratoconjunctivitis and xerostomia. Some investigators believe that the disease has an autoimmune etiology, and rheumatoid arthritis and hypergammaglobulinemia are other common components of this syndrome.

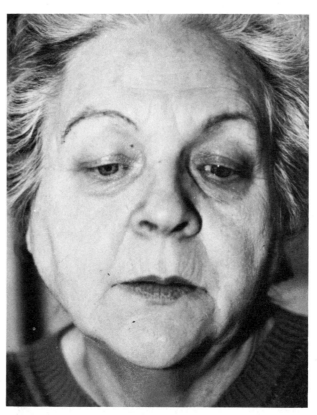

FIGURE 24–6. Benign lymphoepithelial lesion. Bilateral swelling of parotid glands.

Cytology

The aspirates contain lymphoid cells with the same morphologic variability as that seen in reactive hyperplasia of lymph nodes. Small mature lymphocytes are admixed with follicular center cells, plasma cells and histiocytes (Fig. 24–7). This appearance corresponds to the histology of such affected glands, which have abundant lymphoid tissue with large germinal centers. The tissue contains scattered solid epithelial rests, which represent myoepithelial proliferations, but cytologically few, if any, epithelial or epithelioid cells are encountered.

A careful cytologic evaluation of the lymphoid infiltrate will be needed to exclude a low-grade lymphoma. In fact, an immunocytochemical evaluation of the lymphoid cells may be the only possible way to differentiate a reactive from a neoplastic infiltrate.

Salivary Gland Lesions Containing Lymphocytes

- Intraparotid lymph nodes
- Lymphoepithelial lesion
- Chronic sialoadenitis
- Malignant lymphoma
- Warthin's tumor
- Mucoepidermoid carcinoma
- Undifferentiated carcinoma
- Others

The cell pattern of a reactive intraparotid lymph node and a lymphoepithelial lesion is essentially the same. It ranges from small lymphocytes to centroblasts and immunoblasts. Scanty ductal and epithelioid histiocytic elements may be seen in aspirates from lymphoepithelial lesions. Therefore, the diagnosis of lymphoepithelial lesion is dependent on the correlation of clinical features and cytopathologic findings.

In chronic sialoadenitis, the lymphoid cells are less numerous and are generally accompanied by a mixture of plasma cells, granulocytes, macrophages and fragments of benign salivary ducts.

Several investigators have reported the possibility of transition from benign lymphoepithelial lesions to malignant lymphomas.[2] Low-grade malignant lymphomas can have either a monotonous or a mixed-cell pattern, whereas smears from high-grade lymphomas are dominated by blasts. The cytologic diagnosis of malignant lymphoma should be confirmed using immunocytochemical methods to determine whether the lymphoid cells are polyclonal (benign) or monoclonal (malignant).[50, 51]

Aspirates from a Warthin's tumor or a mucoepidermoid carcinoma often contain numerous lymphoid elements. These tumors are often cystic, and the lymphoid cells usually appear in a background precipitate admixed with mucoid material. An abundance of lymphocytes should not cause diagnostic problems, as the aspirates in general contain sheets and clusters of oncocytic or vacuolated mucus-producing cells. A massive lymphoid infiltration also has been observed in association with an undifferentiated carcinoma.[1]

NEOPLASMS

The incidence of salivary gland neoplasms is approximately 2 per 100,000 persons annually.[9] Tumors are more frequent in the parotid glands than in the other salivary glands, whether major or minor.[52] A 4:1 ratio is found between benign and malignant tumors.[14] In addition, enlargement of the salivary glands is more often due to a non-neoplastic disorder than to the presence of neoplasms.

Benign Tumors

Pleomorphic Adenoma (Mixed Tumor)

Pleomorphic adenomas constitute about 75% of major salivary gland tumors.[18] Mixed tumors can occur in minor salivary glands as well. The tumors usually occur as a well-circumscribed, solitary, painless and slow-growing nodule. Most of the tumors arise in the superficial portion of the the parotid gland.

Histologically, pleomorphic adenomas have a capsule that often is incomplete, a fact that explains recurrences after apparent "complete" excision. The tumors are composed of epithelial and myoepithelial elements and a sparse to abundant stroma. The epithelial component may have a trabecular, glandular,

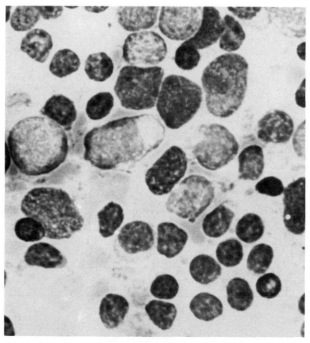

FIGURE 24–7. Cytology of **lymphoepithelial lesion.** Small lymphocytes mixed with follicle center cells (May-Grünwald-Giemsa; ×200).

solid or adenoid cystic (cylindromatous) pattern. Foci of squamous metaplasia, oncocytic changes, mucus production and cells with sebaceous differentiation may be encountered within the same tumor. The stromal component can be myxoid, chondroid or myxochondroid.

The ratio of epithelial to mesenchymal components varies widely. Some pleomorphic adenomas may be quite cellular, composed almost entirely of epithelial or spindly myoepithelial cells, whereas others have predominantly mesenchymal components with very few epithelial cells. The variability in histologic pattern is typically reflected in fine needle aspirates.

Cytology. Aspirates from pleomorphic adenomas have a thick, gelatinous consistency. In May-Grünwald-Giemsa–stained smears, the mesenchymal fragments appear as an intensively red to dark purple, fibrillar, mucoid substance (Fig. 24–8). Rounded, monomorphous epithelial cells with a well-defined, sometimes excentric cytoplasm occur together with spindled myoepithelial cells (Fig. 24–9). They are seen dispersed or in groups within or separated from the stromal substance. The epithelial and myoepithelial cells can be difficult to identify because the May-Grünwald-Giemsa stain penetrates the mucoid tissue poorly giving only a pale blue color to the nuclei.

In Papanicolaou-stained smears, the mesenchymal substance is gray to pale pink and usually has a distinct fibrillar structure (Fig. 24–9).

Pleomorphic Adenoma: Common Cytologic Features

- Fibrillary, myxoid stromal substance
- Uniform, medium-sized epithelial cells, dispersed and in loosely cohesive groups
- Clusters and single cells gradually merging with the mucoid mesenchymal elements

Cystic change may occur in pleomorphic adenomas and cause diagnostic difficulties. Such aspirates may contain cellular debris and squamous as well as mucus-producing cells. Enlargement of some epithelial cells in an otherwise typical aspirate of pleomorphic adenoma does not generally indicate a malignant tumor.[11] However, any features suggestive of pleomorphic adenoma should overrule occasional findings that may be suggestive of malignancy. This is the "dogma of pleomorphic adenoma," which is practiced in our clinic.

The distinction between pleomorphic adenoma and adenoid cystic carcinoma can be difficult. Aspirates from pleomorphic adenomas may also contain structures characteristic of adenoid cystic carcinoma, such as mucus globules surrounded by monomorphous epithelial cells. Sampling performed from different parts of the tumor should reduce this risk of diagnostic error.

If the aspirate is evaluated with only a Papanicolaou stain, the myxoid material of pleomorphic adenoma may be mistaken for epithelial mucus.

Malignant transformation (carcinoma ex pleomorphia) within a pleomorphic adenoma can occur. It is then most often an invasive, undifferentiated carcinoma with markedly abnormal, anaplastic malignant cells.

Monomorphic Adenomas

If the epithelial cells predominate in a pleomorphic adenoma, the tumor may be diagnosed as a monomorphic adenoma. The distinction, however, does not seem to be important because the management of these neoplasms is the same.

Benign tumors in which uniform cells form glandular or solid patterns without a myxoid stroma are sometimes referred to as monomorphic adenomas. The

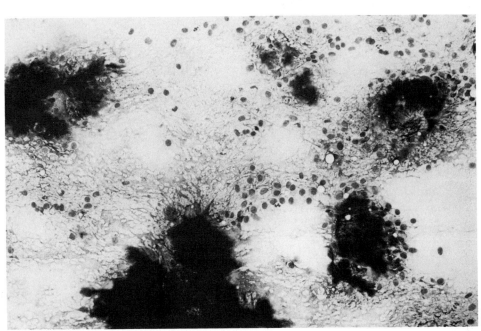

FIGURE 24–8. Pleomorphic adenoma. Aspirate showing the dense chondromyxoid stroma and monomorphous epithelial cells (May-Grünwald-Giemsa; ×40).

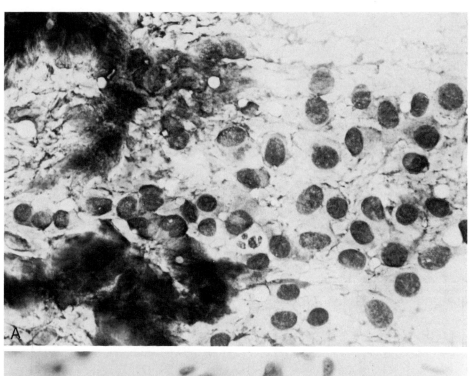

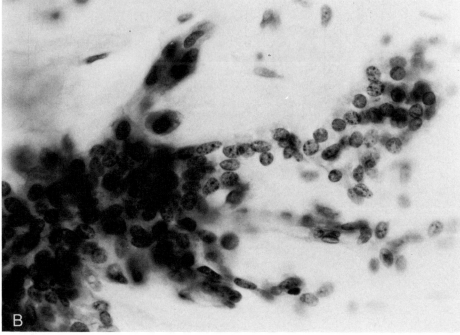

FIGURE 24–9. Pleomorphic adenoma. Epithelial cells with round or oval nuclei with evenly distributed chromatin and tiny nucleoli *(A)*. The fibrillar myxoid stroma is easily identified in May-Grünwald-Giemsa (pink) (×160), whereas it is barely visible *(B)* in Papanicolaou stain (×160).

group of monomorphic adenomas includes adenolymphoma (Warthin's tumor), oxyphilic adenoma (oncocytoma), basal cell adenoma and other rare types such as clear cell, trabecular, tubular and sebaceous adenoma.

Adenolymphoma (Warthin's Tumor, Papillary Cyst-adenolymphoma)

Adenolymphomas usually occur within the lower portion of the parotid gland and are thought to develop from salivary gland inclusions in lymph nodes adjacent to the lower pole of the parotid gland (Fig. 24–10). They constitute approximately 5% of all parotid tumors and are rarely found outside the parotid area. Adenolymphomas are bilateral in 5 to 10% of cases. Previously, these tumors were found usually in men; however, later reports of tumor incidence cite a male to female ratio of about 1.4:1.

Physical examination usually reveals a soft, doughy, painless swelling with poorly defined borders. The tumors vary in size. Without treatment, they tend to reach a certain size of about 3 to 5 cm and then stop growing. Adenolymphomas are in most cases cystic.

Histologically, the cystic spaces are lined by a double-layered, oncocytic epithelium often forming papillary projections. The epithelium is usually double-layered and in case of inflammation, the epithelium may undergo squamous metaplasia. Occasionally, mucus-producing goblet cells are observed. The contents of the cystic portion of the tumor vary in consistency from thin watery fluid to thick viscous fluid. It may have an admixture of cholesterol crystals, inflammatory cells, histiocytes and desquamated epithelial cells with pyknotic nuclei. The supporting stroma contains lymphoid elements, which often form large germinal centers.

Cytology. Cystic material with a thin watery to mucoid appearance predominates in aspirates from adenolymphoma. The smears contain a granular and amorphous substance, sheets of cells with oncocytic changes, cellular debris and macrophages. A lymphoid component is almost always present but the amount varies.

The characteristic and diagnostic feature in adenolymphoma is the presence of flat irregular sheets of polyhedral, finely granular oncocytic cells with well-defined cellular borders (Fig. 24–11). With Papanicolaou stain, these sheets have a honeycomb arrangement (Fig. 24–11). Occasionally, papillary fragments with the lymphoid stroma and overlying oncocytic cells can be observed. The nuclei of the oncocytic cells are round, with a granular chromatin pattern and a central, small nucleolus. Mast cells are a frequent finding in May-Grünwald-Griemsa–stained material but are not easily seen in Papanicolaou-stained smears. They are found in association with the sheets of oncocytic cells. Mast cells may also occur, but less frequently, in mucoepidermoid carcinoma and pleomorphic adenomas.[5]

Adenolymphoma (Warthin's Tumor): Common Cytologic Features

- Monolayered sheets of oncocytic cells with distinct cell borders
- Mixed population of lymphocytes often in tissue tangles
- Precipitate of thin-to-mucoid material containing a granular, amorphous substance and cellular debris

An aspirate containing only fluid or mucoid material is obviously not diagnostic but raises the possibility of adenolymphoma if the aspiration is made in the parotid gland region.

Cystic, well-differentiated mucoepidermoid carcinomas may also yield aspirates of abundant mucoid material containing small clusters of epithelial cells with minimal nuclear atypia and numerous lymphocytes. The epithelial cells in this case usually are superimposed and have a finely vacuolated cytoplasm, a sign of mucus production. These cells do not usually appear in monolayered sheets, and the cellular borders are indistinct.

Metaplastic epidermoid cells in adenolymphomas can be quite atypical but rarely show true keratinization. They can, however, be confused with squamoid carcinoma cells. We advocate that a conclusive diagnosis of metastatic squamous cell carcinoma in the parotid area should be made only if a primary carcinoma can be found in the oral or upper respiratory tract.

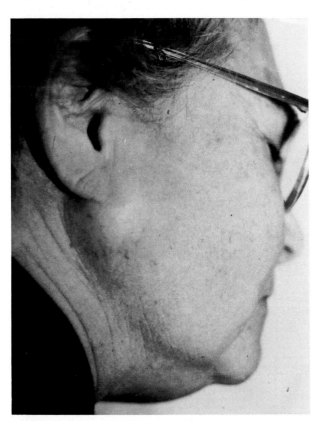

FIGURE 24–10. Cystadenolymphoma (Warthin's tumor) swelling of the lower portion of the parotid gland.

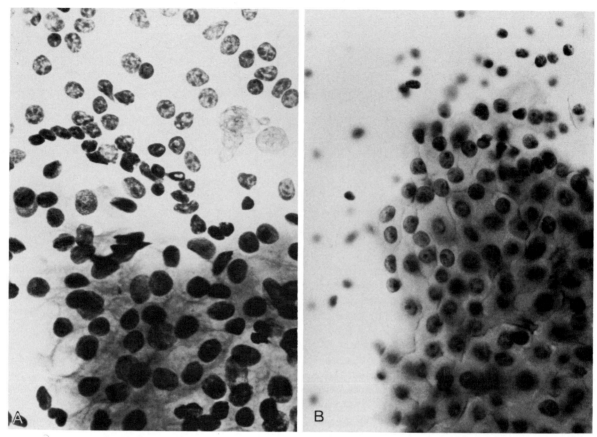

FIGURE 24–11. Cystadenolymphoma. Aspirate showing lymphoid cells and flat sheet of polyhedral oncocytic cells with well-defined cellular borders in a honeycomb arrangement (A) May-Grünwald-Giemsa (×132) and (B) Papanicolaou (×132).

Aspirates from a predominantly solid adenolymphoma with only a few lymphocytes may be indistinguishable from oncocytoma. Distinction between these two neoplasms is not critical as their management should be identical. Some workers believe that these two tumors are actually the same entity.[17]

Oncocytoma (Oxyphilic Adenoma)

Oncocytomas are rare benign tumors, which typically appear as a hard nodule. They are most often found in the parotid gland but can be found in all major salivary glands. The tumor is composed of cells with abundant granular eosinophilic cytoplasm and round central or excentric nuclei with distinct nucleoli. The cells are uniform and arranged in solid acinar groups or parallel columns with sparse delicate supporting stroma (Fig. 24–12). Unlike most Warthin's tumors, oncocytomas lack lymphoid infiltrates.

Cytology. In aspirates from oncocytomas, the principal feature is solid plugs and sheets of polygonal, monomorphous oncocytic cells in a clean or slightly bloody background (Fig. 24–13). These cells are identical to the oncocytes of Warthin's tumor. Lymphoid cells and a proteinaceous precipitate are not observed in oncocytomas.

Oncocytoma: Common Cytologic Findings

- Numerous uniform large cells with abundant finely granular cytoplasm (oncocytes)
- Round nuclei usually centrally located within the cell and containing distinct nucleoli
- Absence of fluid, debris and lymphoid cells

Oncocytomas may be confused with non-neoplastic oncocytic nodular hyperplasia, acinic cell carcinoma and Warthin's tumor. A precise cytologic distinction between various benign lesions containing oncocytic cells does not seem important as all are cured by simple surgical excision. It is more important to differentiate between a benign oncocytic lesion and a malignant tumor, which requires a different type of surgery. In aspirates from acinic cell carcinoma, the cells tend to be more granular and finely vacuolated than typical cells from oncocytoma. In May-Grünwald-Giemsa, the cytoplasm of cells from acinic cell carcinoma usually stains slate-gray and exhibits a fine red granulation not seen in benign oncocytic cells.

Pleomorphic adenoma and mucoepidermoid carcinoma may have focal oncocytic changes. This problem is overcome by adequate sampling of material from different parts of these tumors.

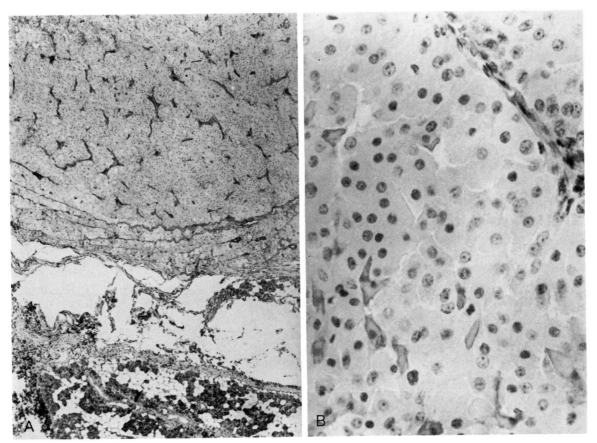

FIGURE 24–12. Oncocytoma. *A*, Tissue section showing a well-circumscribed solid tumor (hematoxylin and eosin; ×10). *B*, Uniform cells with abundant cytoplasma and round cental nuclei (hematoxylin and eosin; ×100).

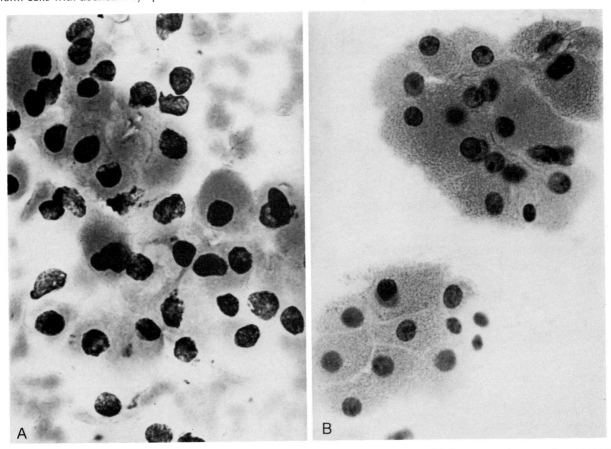

FIGURE 24–13. Oncocytoma. Aspirate showing sheets of polygonal oncocytic cells with large granular cytoplasm *(A)* May-Grünwald-Giemsa (×132) and *(B)* Papanicolaou (×132).

Basal Cell Adenoma

Neoplasms of this type account for about 2% of all primary tumors of the major salivary glands.[17, 24] The term basal cell adenoma is used to identify a neoplasm with a single, well-defined, basaloid histologic pattern, which can have a diverse architecture such as trabecular, tubular, papillary and solid patterns.[3, 17] Cystic changes may be superimposed on these patterns. The mesenchymal chondromyxoid elements of the type encountered in pleomorphic adenomas are generally lacking.

Cytology. The fine needle aspiration features of basal cell adenoma have been described by several investigators.[22, 56] Smears are cellular and show cohesive, solid groups and irregularly branching cords. The individual cells are uniform with scant cytoplasm, oval nuclei and finely granular chromatin. Nucleoli may be seen in occasional cells. Single cells usually appear as naked nuclei, and small amounts of amorphous material may be seen at the edges of cell clusters. This matrix is homogeneous, stains bright red with May-Grünwald-Giemsa stain and is almost translucent in Papanicolaou-stained slides.

Basal Cell Adenoma: Common Cytologic Findings

- Small clusters of branching cords composed of small uniform cells with round to oval nuclei
- Individual cells appear as naked nuclei or have a scant amount of cytoplasm
- Sparse homogeneous background material

Fine needle aspirates from basal cell adenomas and from the solid form of adenoid cystic carcinomas have similar cytologic features. The size and configuration of cell groups, as well as the individual cell morphology and the presence of single cells, are virtually identical. The solid adenoid cystic carcinoma is lacking the metachromatic globules or cylinders that characterize cribiform adenoid cystic carcinoma.

As evidenced by several investigators, the distinction between these two prognostically quite different tumor entities is very difficult.[22, 27, 46, 56] Clinically, pain or nerve damage indicates malignancy.

The cytologic differentiation from pleomorphic adenoma is sometimes difficult but seems to be less important because the management is similar.

Clear Cell Adenoma

Clear cell adenomas are composed of prominent clear cells that form tubular structures. The differential diagnosis in tissue sections includes acinic cell tumor and mucoepidermoid tumor.[6] Although we have not encountered this uncommon tumor, we assume that the same differential diagnostic problem would occur in fine needle aspirates.

Sebaceous Cell Adenoma

Sebaceous cell adenoma is a neoplasm made up of flat polygonal cells similar to the sebaceous cells usually seen in smears from epidermoid cysts.[56]

Sebaceous cells are occasionally seen in tissue specimens from major salivary glands and within neoplasms such as pleomorphic adenoma and Warthin's tumor.[17]

Malignant Tumors

Adenoid Cystic Carcinoma

Adenoid cystic carcinoma accounts for 3 to 5% of all salivary gland tumors and occurs in both the minor and major salivary glands.[14] It is a slow-growing malignant tumor (formerly known as cylindroma). Neural invasion occurs early, producing paralysis of motor nerves in about a third and pain in about half of the patients.[11, 44] The remainder of the patients affected by this tumor usually present with asymptomatic swelling.

Adenoid cystic carcinoma has a high tendency for recurrence after surgical removal probably due to its infiltrative growth pattern. Distant metastases usually occur in the lungs and in bone, whereas lymphatic metastases are less frequent.

The histologic picture of adenoid cystic carcinoma is variable. In a classic case, the tumor is composed of small uniform cells arranged concentrically in a cribiform pattern around the gland-like spaces filled with homogeneous material produced by the tumor cells.[49] A continuous spectrum is found from this classic pattern to an equal mixture of cribiform and solid structures to a predominantly solid, basaloid pattern.

Cytology. Despite its name, this tumor is more commonly solid and aspiration of cystic fluid is exceptional. The smear contains round or branching multilayered clusters of cohesive small uniform epithelial cells. They occasionally may be arranged around globules of homogeneous acellular material (Fig. 24-14). These mucoid globules were considered to be the key to establishing a diagnosis of adenoid cystic carcinoma in aspirates.[13] In some cases they may be prominent, whereas in others they may be very few or single globules. The individual cells are small and have round or ovoid nuclei and a narrow rim of cytoplasm (Fig. 24-15). The nuclei show little variation in size and shape. The nucleoli are usually readily visible and sometimes prominent. The homogeneous acellular material is referred to as the main cytologic feature.

Adenoid Cystic Carcinoma: Principal Cytologic Features

- Small uniform cohesive cancer cells with minimal cytoplasm and distinct nucleoli
- Spheric aggregates, rosette-like groups of cancer cells or both

FIGURE 24–14. Adenoid cystic carcinoma. *A*, Clusters of small uniform epithelial cells surrounding globules of homogeneous, acellular material (May-Grünwald-Giemsa; ×50). *B*, Uniform epithelial cells arranged around translucent poorly visible globules (Papanicolaou; ×50).

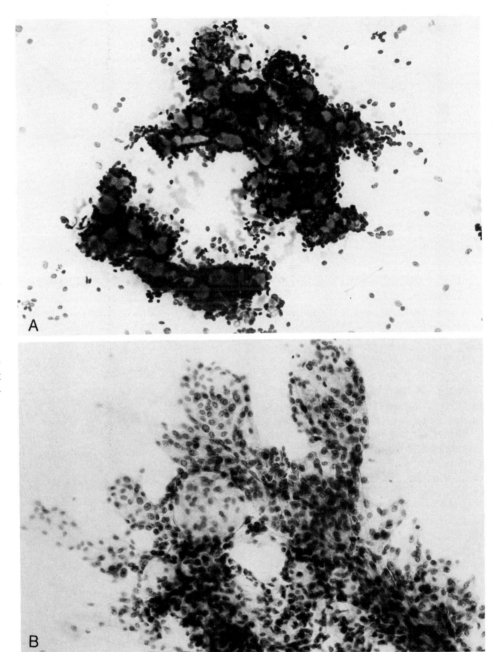

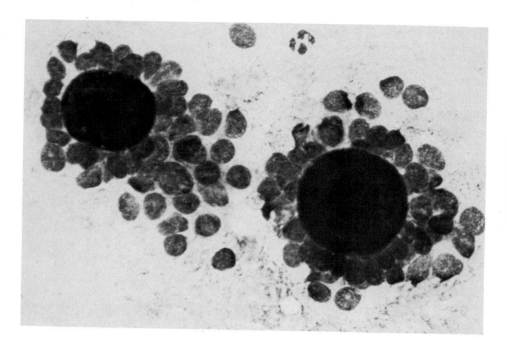

FIGURE 24–15. Adenoid cystic carcinoma. Spheric globules surrounded by epithelial cells with round to oval nuclei and scanty cytoplasm (May-Grünwald-Giemsa; ×200).

- Magenta-stained mucoid globules, cylinders of homogeneous acellular material (May-Grünwald-Giemsa) or both

A true differential diagnostic problem lies in the fact that a pleomorphic adenoma, as a part of its pattern, may occasionally possess classic adenoid cystic cytologic features. If these structures appear together with any other features of pleomorphic adenoma, these last findings should be emphasized more; a diagnosis of pleomorphic adenoma should be rendered with a note to the clinician to rule in or out pleomorphic adenoma.

The majority of smears from adenoid cystic carcinomas contain mucoid globules even if these are present in only one microscopic field. In the absence of such mucoid globules, however, the distinction between the solid type of adenoid cystic carcinoma, which is a poorly differentiated tumor, and basal cell adenoma becomes difficult. The cellular patterns of both tumors have similar basaloid cells arranged in cohesive, nonorganoid structures. In such a case, a close evaluation of nuclear details may be of help in suggesting the correct diagnosis. The nuclei of basal cell adenoma have evenly distributed chromatin and no nucleoli, whereas adenoid cystic carcinomas, especially of the solid, poorly differentiated type, more often have a marked chromatin pattern and prominent nucleoli.

The cytologic identification of adenoid cystic carcinoma rests on adequate sampling and careful inspection of all material to rule out the possibility of benign pleomorphic adenoma or basal cell adenoma. If radical surgery is planned based upon the cytologic diagnosis, our rule is that the diagnosis should be made taking into account the cytologic findings and the patient's symptoms. If signs and symptoms of nerve damage are present and a smear displays the typical cytologic findings of adenoid cystic carcinoma, a conclusive diagnosis can be made. In our institution, we refuse to take the full diagnostic responsibility for a radical surgical procedure in which sacrifice of the fascial nerve may be necessary in cases where there may be classic cytologic findings of adenoid cystic carcinoma but the patient is symptom free.

Other small-cell malignant tumors, either primary or metastatic, such as small-cell undifferentiated carcinoma, neuroendocrine carcinoma and lymphoma rarely pose any differential diagnostic problems providing both Papanicolaou and May-Grünwald-Giemsa stains are used.

Mucoepidermoid Carcinoma

Mucoepidermoid carcinomas derive from ductal cells and occur only in the major salivary gland where they constitute approximately 5% of all neoplasms.[15, 47] The tumors occur in all age groups and may be slowly developing, painless, nonsymptomatic low-grade carcinomas or rapidly growing, symptomatic, high-grade tumors.

Histologically, low-grade tumors typically have cystic spaces filled with mucoid material. The cysts are lined by tall, mucus-secreting cells with finely vacuolated cytoplasm and intermediate cells that vary in their degree of epidermoid differentiation (Fig. 24–16). These intermediate cells characteristically stain positively with mucin stains.

The high-grade tumors are predominantly solid. They are composed of markedly atypical epidermoid cells with few mucus-producing cells.

Cytology. Zajicek and coworkers were largely responsible for the cytologic criteria to diagnose mucoepidermoid carcinoma.[57]

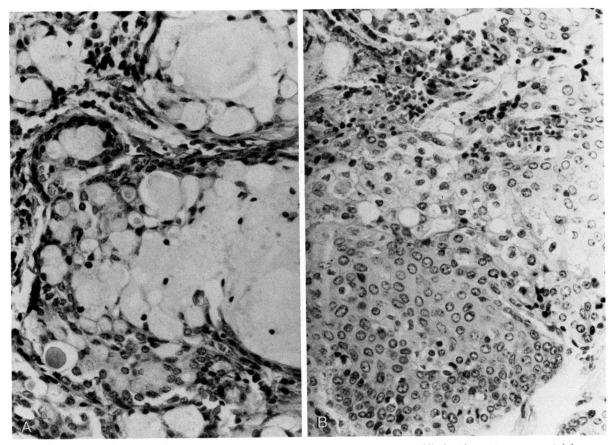

FIGURE 24–16. Mucoepidermoid carcinoma. Tissue section showing (A) cystic spaces filled with mucinous material (hematoxylin and eosin; ×66) and (B) epidermoid differentiation (hematoxylin and eosin; ×66).

Aspirates from low-grade tumors contain both clusters of epithelial cells and a mucoid substance. The diagnosis is mainly based on the identification of mucus-producing cells and intermediate epidermoid tumor cells, which are usually arranged in irregular, multilayered clusters.

The mucus-producing cells can be round, columnar or polyhedral with large, well-defined, finely vacuolated cytoplasm. The nuclei are small, uniform and usually lack atypia. An isolated mucus-producing cell may be difficult to distinguish from a macrophage.

The intermediate epidermoid cells usually appear in tightly packed clusters. These cells have small, round, uniform nuclei with small nucleoli and a well-defined, homogeneous cytoplasm. Paranuclear vacuoles may indicate a gradual transition to mucus-secreting cells (Fig. 24–17). Fully keratinized epidermoid cells are rarely encountered in the well-differentiated mucoepidermoid carcinoma.

At times aspirate smears may contain only mucoid material, dispersed phagocytes, cellular debris and inflammatory cells. In such a case, a repeat aspiration should be performed if the lesion persists or recurs after aspiration.

Occasionally, dense accumulation of lymphocytes is seen and may produce a background pattern similar to that of a Warthin's tumor.

High-grade mucoepidermoid carcinomas are solid, and aspiration yields a semisolid material containing large, polymorphic cells with dark nuclei and prominent nucleoli. Sometimes signet ring–type cells are present. Differentiation between a high-grade mucoepidermoid carcinoma and other types of poorly differentiated carcinomas is sometimes not feasible cytologically.

Mucoepidermoid Carcinoma: Principal Cytologic Features

Low-grade

- Background of mucus and debris
- Coexisting mucus-producing cells with finely vacuolated cytoplasm and intermediate epidermoid tumor cells
- Clusters of cells with a gradual transition from intermediate to mucus-producing cells can be observed

High-grade

- Semisolid aspirate with numerous markedly atypical cells
- Epidermoid or mucus-producing cells

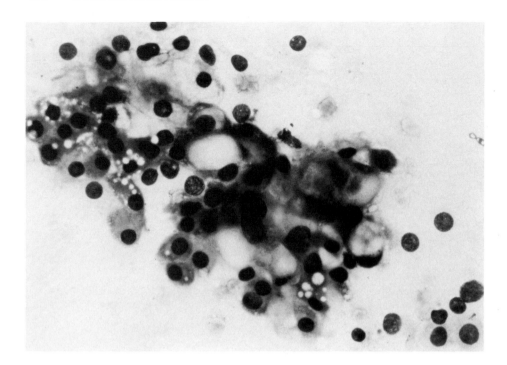

FIGURE 24–17. Mucoepidermoid carcinoma. Fine needle aspiration smear with cluster of epithelial cells, some of an epidermoid nature and others with vacuoles in the cytoplasm, indicating mucus production (May-Grünwald-Giemsa; ×132).

Aspirates from benign lesions, such as retention cysts, obstructive sialoadenitis and Warthin's tumor, may contain mucus, debris, glandular and neoplastic squamous cells in a combination that may mimic mucoepidermoid carcinoma. Numerous inflammatory cells can obscure the evaluation of the epithelial elements essential for proper diagnosis. If the cytologic findings are less than characteristic, it is advisable that the cytopathologist render a descriptive report with a discussion of alternative diagnoses.

Acinic Cell Carcinoma

Acinar cells both in major and minor salivary glands can give rise to the acinic cell carcinoma, a rare neoplasm constituting about 1% of salivary gland tumors. In general, these are asymptomatic, solid neoplasms with a slow growth rate.

The microscopic appearance includes solid, microcystic, papillary-cystic or follicular growth patterns (Fig. 24–18). Well-differentiated tumors are characterized by "hypernephroid" cells with varying amounts of eosinophilic cytoplasmic granular cells that may resemble normal serous acinar cells (see Fig. 24–18). The nuclei are uniform, normochromatic with very small nucleoli. In poorly differentiated variants, the nuclei are polymorphic, large and hyperchromatic with prominent central nucleoli.

Lymphoid aggregates with germinal centers may be prominent at the periphery and in the stroma of some tumors. Invasion and metastatic spread can occur independent of a tumor's morphologic appearance.[10]

Cytology. Aspirate smears from acinic cell carcinoma contain regular and cohesive cells without an admixture of fat or ductal epithelium. These cells are similar to but larger than acinar cells of the normal salivary gland and sometimes adhere to fibrovascular cores giving them a papillary appearance. Poorly formed acinic structures are also often discernible. In May-Grünwald-Giemsa stain, the cytoplasm appears either finely vacuolated or dense gray. The nuclei are uniform, round or oval with a small, central nucleolus (Fig. 24–19). Numerous naked nuclei are usually found. Lymphocytes may be encountered in rare variants of carcinomas with lymphoid infiltrates of the stroma.[35] Smears from the papillary-cystic variant of acinic cell carcinoma can sometimes contain laminated calcifications resembling psammoma bodies.[4]

In the case of poorly differentiated acinic cell carcinomas, the aspirates contain large cells with dark, pleomorphic nuclei and prominent nucleoli. Because of a marked anaplasia, it may be difficult to ascertain the origin of these tumor cells.

Acinic Cell Carcinoma (Well-differentiated): Common Cytologic Features

- Abundant tumor cells resembling normal acinar cells in bloody but "clean" background
- Cohesive clusters of cells sometimes with a fibrovascular core
- Tendency to form acinar-like groups
- Plentiful cytoplasm containing medium-sized, slightly atypical nuclei with tiny nucleoli
- Occasional bare tumor cell nuclei

Non-neoplastic salivary gland tissue should not be confused with well-differentiated acinic cell carcinoma. Normal acinar cells appear in typical round, basket-like arrangements with attached ductal structures and fat cells as opposed to acinic cell carcinoma cells.

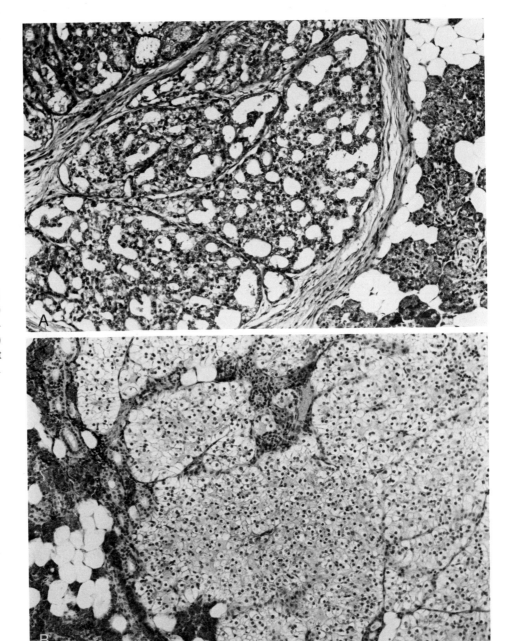

FIGURE 24–18. Acinic cell carcinoma tissue section *(A)* follicular growth pattern (hematoxylin and eosin; ×33) and *(B)* hypernephroid variant (hematoxylin and eosin; ×33).

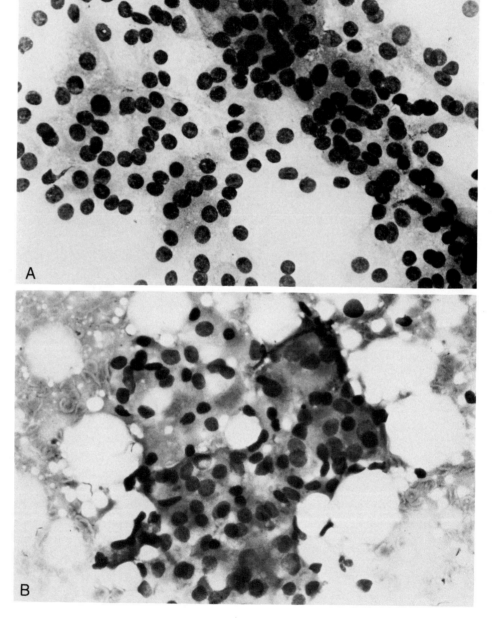

FIGURE 24–19. Acinic cell carcinoma. *A,* Clusters showing acinar formations composed of cells with indistinct cytoplasm and uniform round nuclei. Tissue section revealed follicular growth pattern (May-Grünwald-Giemsa; ×132). *B,* Solid clusters of tumor cells with indistinct cytoplasm from a hypernephroid type of acinic cell carcinoma (May-Grünwald-Giemsa; ×132).

Occasionally, the acinic cells may resemble oncocytes and this may cause problems in differentiating acinic cell carcinomas from Warthin's tumors or oncocytomas.[56] Observations of acinic structures and cells with foamy cytoplasm in the background material should lead the examiner to a correct diagnosis in most cases.

Large cells with abundant finely vacuolated or clear cytoplasm are also seen in aspirates from mucoepidermal carcinomas. Notation of the absence of intracellular mucus in acinic cell tumors should prevent mistakes in classification.

Carcinoma Ex Pleomorphic Adenoma (Adenocarcinoma Arising in a Mixed Tumor)

Adenocarcinoma in a preexisting pleomorphic adenoma typically appears with a rapid increase in size in a previously slow-growing tumor. Histologically, one finds a pleomorphic adenoma with a distinct focus of adenocarcinoma, adenoid cystic carcinoma, epidermal carcinoma or undifferentiated carcinoma. A patient with a malignant focus of this kind, which is entirely confined within a pleomorphic adenoma, usually does not have symptoms of a malignant lesion.[29] Only when invasion occurs in surrounding salivary gland tissue does the tumor behave clinically as a malignant tumor.

The cytologic features obviously depend on the subtype of carcinoma within the pleomorphic adenoma. The malignant cell population is readily identified in most cases. If a benign component typical for pleomorphic adenoma coexists with a cytologically malignant component, we suggest that a definite diagnosis be deferred until histologic examination of the lesion.

Malignant Mixed Tumor

This tumor has the overall configuration of a pleomorphic adenoma, but the epithelial cells display the morphologic features of cancer. Only two reports of fine needle aspiration of malignant mixed tumor have been published.[26, 28]

Primary Epidermoid Cell Carcinoma

The criteria for diagnosis of epidermoid cell carcinomas, which occur in salivary glands, are the same as for other sites. In typical cases, the individual tumor cells have abundant homogeneous, sharply demarcated cytoplasm. Keratin formation, epithelial pearls and fragments of keratinized cytoplasm and intercellular bridges are typical findings.

The distinction among the poorly differentiated adenocarcinomas, the solid type of mucoepidermoid carcinomas and the metastatic squamous cell carcinomas sometimes may not be feasible. History, physical findings and further investigations may be helpful in determining whether the tumor is primary or metastatic.

Undifferentiated Carcinoma

This tumor grows rapidly giving a painful mass, and the patient often presents with facial nerve paralysis. Histologically a large-cell undifferentiated carcinoma and a small-cell carcinoma similar to oat cell carcinoma of the bronchi have been described.[18, 25, 54] Within these, tumor necrosis and hemorrhage appear along with frequent mitoses.

Aspirates contain loose clusters of carcinoma cells and usually many individual cells without morphologic characteristics that permit their further classification into any of the accepted subtypes of salivary gland carcinoma.

The small-cell variant of undifferentiated carcinoma shows small, round or oval nuclei and small nucleoli. The cytoplasm is very sparse, and most cells appear as naked nuclei. In our experience, this tumor is difficult to distinguish from metastatic nasopharyngeal carcinoma.

Mesenchymal Tumors

Benign and malignant soft tissue tumors occur also in salivary glands. Cytologic diagnoses of such neoplasms have been reported.[31] The cytologically diagnosed tumors included lipoma, neurofibroma, neurofibrosarcoma and lymphoma. The cytologic features of these and other mesenchymal tumors are similar to those in other sites.

Metastatic Tumors

The clinical presentation of a metastatic tumor may not differ from that of a primary neoplasm. Malignant lesions that most commonly metastasize to the parotid region are squamous cell carcinoma and malignant melanoma.[34] Less frequent metastases are from kidney and breast carcinomas.

DIAGNOSTIC ACCURACY

The cytologic diagnosis of salivary gland tumors requires a great deal of experience partly because of the great diversity of tumor types and because of the complexity of cytologic patterns of individual tumors.[56] The literature in this field has expanded considerably providing excellent guides to improved diagnostic accuracy. This is illustrated by the results presented in Table 24–2. In the early work of Eneroth and associates,[12] a low sensitivity was recorded. This is to a large extent explained by the underdiagnosis of adenoid cystic and acinic cell carcinomas. At that time, the cytologic criteria for these tumors were poorly defined.

TABLE 24–2. Diagnostic Accuracy of Fine Needle Aspiration of Salivary Gland Tumors

Study*	Number of Cases	Sensitivity† (%)	Specificity† (%)
Eneroth, Franzén, Zajicek[12]	632	66.3	98.8
Persson, Zettergren[36]	216	87.5	99.4
Webb[53]	38	100	96.2
Qizilbash, Young[39]	155	90.7	98.0

*Based on studies with histologically confirmed diagnoses.
†According to Galen RS, Gambino SR: Beyond Normality. The Predictive Value of Medical Diagnosis. New York, John Wiley & Sons, 1975.

Later studies could benefit from the pioneer work of Zajicek and his colleagues, and the figures for sensitivity increased considerably to vary between 87.5 and 100% (see Table 24–2).

The accuracy of benign diagnoses was in all studies high, varying between 96.2 and 99.4%.

In our opinion, it should be possible to correctly diagnose a majority of benign and high-grade malignant tumors with only a modest experience with FNA. In contrast, some diagnoses should be made with caution even by the most experienced cytopathologists. Adenoid cystic carcinoma is such a tumor. The cytologic features of this tumor can be shared with structures found in some pleomorphic adenomas, which makes a conclusive diagnosis of adenoid cystic carcinoma difficult.

Cystic mucus-containing lesions of the salivary gland are a special problem. Fluid or mucus obtained from Warthin's tumor, obstructive sialoadenitis and well-differentiated mucoepidermoid carcinoma may appear very similar on smears. The cytologic evaluation of cells may be difficult if the smears contain only few cells.

Rare Head and Neck Lesions

At the Division of Clinical Cytology, Karolinska Hospital, Sweden, approximately 8000 patients are seen every year. They are referred mainly by those in the fields of general practice; internal medicine; surgery; ear, nose and throat and oncology. The lesions discussed in this chapter have all been encountered among these patients during the last 10 years. Some of these tumors or tumor-like lesions have been diagnosed only once during this period, whereas others may have been seen annually. We have chosen to describe primary lesions only. Thus, metastases and lymph-node disorders are not included. We have not attempted to provide a comprehensive presentation based on literature studies but rather we based the selection of rare neck lesions on our own clinical experience.

The lesions as discussed are given in Table 24–3.

BENIGN LESIONS

Cervical Rib

This anatomic variant is a congenital overdevelopment of the lateral process of the seventh cervical

TABLE 24–3. Rare Lesions of the Head and Neck

Benign	Malignant
Cervical rib	Papillary thyroid carcinoma in thyroglossal cyst
Chondroma	
Nodular fasciitis	Neuroendocrine carcinoma (Merkel cell) of the skin
Proliferative myositis	
Parathyroid adenoma/cyst	
Carotid body tumor	
Pilomatrixoma (calcifying epithelioma of Malherbe)	

vertebra. Prominent lateral processes can also be found in the other cervical vertebrae. These large processes often exist without causing symptoms but may produce neurologic or vascular disturbances. On physical examination they may appear as fixed hard lumps, which even by the experienced examiner may be mistaken for a metastatic tumor. Fine needle aspiration biopsy attempts will disclose their bony nature, but the cortical bone is thin and may be penetrated even with a thin needle. Aspiration will then yield bone marrow cells. In rare instances, the smears contain only scattered megakaryocytes, which can superficially resemble polymorphic tumor cells.

Cervical Rib: Cytologic Features

- Fine needle aspiration biopsy attempts will identify the osseous nature of the process
- Smears may contain marrow cells

Chondromas

This benign cartilaginous tumor arises in the periosteum and appears as a swelling of the bones in the extremities. Local resection usually results in successful treatment, but recurrences are experienced.[45] The hyoid bone has been described as an excessively rare site of chondroma. One patient with a hyoid chondroma was examined at the Division of Clinical Cytology, Karolinska Hospital. The patient had a multilobated firm submandibular mass, indistinguishable from a primary salivary gland tumor. Histologically, this tumor is more cellular than ordinary cartilaginous tissue. Slight nuclear atypia as well as binucleate cells may be observed.

Fine needle aspiration smears are dominated by

fibrillar chondroid fragments. Nucleated cells are only rarely observed. They have indistinct cellular borders, weakly stained nuclei and pale blue cytoplasm (May-Grünwald-Giemsa). The cytologic distinction between chondroma and pleomorphic adenoma with extensive chondroid metaplasia may be impossible.

Chondroma: Cytologic Features

- Chondroid fragments
- Few free-lying monomorphous cells
- Cells with indistinct pale blue cytoplasm

Parathyroid Lesions

Cysts and tumors arising in the parathyroid glands may appear as palpable lesions in the neck. Most commonly they are found in close proximity to the thyroid gland but may appear as high as in the submandibular region.

The cysts are thin walled and contain a watery clear fluid, which in most instances is free of cells. As much as 10 ml of fluid can be aspirated from a large parathyroid cyst. Aspiration of watery clear fluid from a neck cyst should produce the clinical suspicion of a parathyroid cyst. Parathormone analysis of the fluid may elucidate the nature of the cyst. Parathyroid cysts are rarely associated with hyperparathyroidism.

Adenomas are solid tumors that in rare cases may be as large as 7 to 8 cm in diameter. The patient usually presents with clinical signs of hyperparathy-roidism. Serum levels of calcium and parathormone are elevated. Sections show chief cells or oxyphilic cells in trabeculae or cords in a vascular stroma.

Fine needle aspiration smears contain many naked nuclei either dissociated or in loosely attached groups (Fig. 24–20). Anisokaryosis is usually prominent. When present, the cytoplasm is large, oxyphilic or pale blue, sometimes vacuolated.[30, 33] The absence of colloid is a helpful feature. The cytologic pattern of parathyroid adenoma in most instances allows a conclusive diagnosis. A follicular tumor of the thyroid or a carotid body tumor may, however, show a cytologic pattern similar to that of a parathyroid adenoma.[30, 33]

Parathyroid Adenoma: Cytologic Features

- Mostly dissociated cells; some loosely attached cell groups may occur
- Naked nuclei are common; anisokaryosis
- Oxyphilic or pale blue, sometimes vacuolated cytoplasm

Nodular Fasciitis

This lesion commonly appears as a rapidly growing hard tumor of the neck, trunk or extremities in young patients, although no sites or age groups seem to be spared. The tumor that usually is less than 5 cm often has fascial attachment but can be found in the subcutaneous tissue. Spontaneous regression occurs within 2 to 3 months.

Sections show monomorphous fibroblasts arranged in bundles with collagen in a loose "feathery" pattern. Mitotic figures are common. Large plump myofibroblasts are found as well as lymphocytes and plasma cells.

Fine needle aspiration smears characteristically show ovoid fibroblasts and plump myofibroblasts dispersed in a granular eosinophilic (May-Grünwald-Giemsa) background (Fig. 24–21). Collagen fragments or myxoid substances can often be observed. The fibroblasts have an ovoid nucleus, an elongated basophilic cytoplasm with tapering ends. The larger myofibroblast has a polygonal or triangular basophilic cytoplasm and an ovoid excentrically positioned nucleus (Fig. 24–21). Neutrophils, eosinophils, lymphocytes and plasma cells are present in varying proportions.

In most instances the cytologic pattern is characteristic and allows a conclusive diagnosis.[7] The differential diagnosis should include fibrosarcoma, malignant fibrous histiocytoma and schwannoma. In case of large or deep lesions diagnosed as nodular fasciitis, clinical control and repeat biopsy are advisable. In extreme cases we have followed patients using biopsies at 2-week intervals for 2 months before the lesion started to regress.

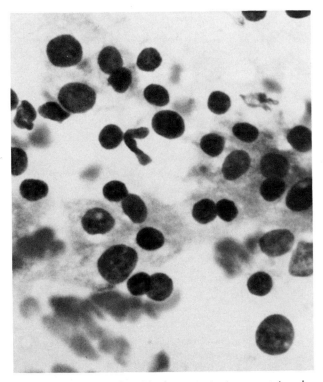

FIGURE 24–20. Parathyroid adenoma. Aspirate contains clusters of loosely attached cells. Note anisokaryosis and indistinct granular cytoplasm (May-Grünwald-Giemsa; × 200).

Nodular Fasciitis: Cytologic Features

- Fibroblasts with ovoid nuclei
- Plump myofibroblasts with polyhedral or triangular basophilic cytoplasm; excentric nucleus

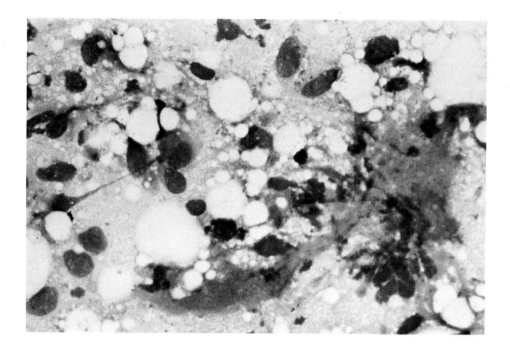

FIGURE 24–21. Nodular fasciitis. Smear with fibroblasts and large plump cells in a granular background. Collagen fragment and some lymphocytes are also present (May-Grünwald-Giemsa; ×160).

- Collagen or myxoid substance
- Inflammatory cells

Proliferative Myositis

This process is an intramuscular counterpart of proliferative fasciitis. It grows rapidly without causing significant pain. No sex predilection occurs. The pa-

tients are often middle aged. The muscles of the trunk are most frequently affected. In rare cases, the sternocleidomastoid is involved (Fig. 24–22).

Surgical biopsy samples disclose a fibroblastic proliferation in the stromal tissue. Giant cells with an excentric nucleus, distinct nucleoli and a large polyhedral cytoplasm are frequent. The muscular tissue shows atrophy without regeneration.

The cytologic smears contain fibroblast-like spindle

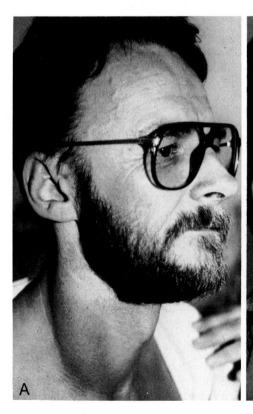
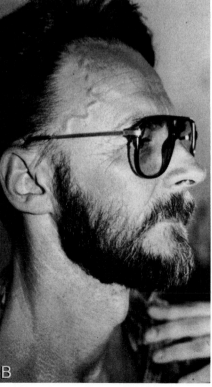

A

B

FIGURE 24–22. Proliferative myositis. Firm tumor of one week's duration in the sternocleidomastoid. *A,* Aspiration resulted in a conclusive diagnosis of proliferative myositis. *B,* Same patient 10 days after initial biopsy. No palpable tumor left.

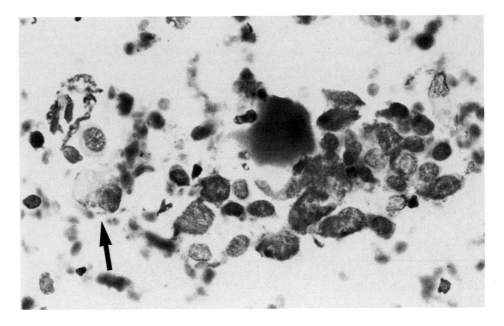

FIGURE 24–23. Proliferative myositis. Fine needle aspiration smear from the patient shown in Figure 24–22. Atrophic muscle fragment (center), immature fibroblasts, ganglion-like cell (arrow) and inflammatory cells (May-Grün-wald-Giemsa; ×160).

cells and numerous giant cells, which have a sharply outlined, polygonal cytoplasm (Fig. 24–23). Binucleate giant cells and inflammatory cells are also present.[40] In addition, muscle fibers with signs of atrophy are a constant finding. The differential diagnostic considerations should be the same as those for nodular fasciitis.

Proliferative Myositis: Cytologic Features

- Fibroblast-like cells with ovoid nuclei
- Giant cells, sometimes binucleated, with large polyhedral cytoplasm ("ganglion cell")
- Muscle fibers with signs of atrophy

Carotid Body Tumor

The carotid body is the origin of this tumor, which usually appears as a firm ovoid mass in front of the sternocleidomastoid. Bilateral tumors are extremely rare (Fig. 24–24). The clinical presentation may vary, and the tumor can sometimes be positioned posterior to the sternocleidomastoid muscle or at the base of the skull. On physical examination, it is a tumor that is mobile horizontally but not vertically. Pulsations can sometimes be distinct. It is recommended that caution be exercised when aspirating a suspicious-looking carotid body tumor. Local hemorrhage may compress the artery resulting in a cerebral catastrophy.[16] Using a 25-gauge needle, we have so far not observed any complications.

Histologically, carotid body tumor is composed of nests of cells in a vascular stroma of reticulin fibers. Anisokaryocytosis can be marked, but mitoses are rare. Foci of hemorrhage are frequent findings.

Fine needle aspiration smears are bloody and contain cells in a loosely follicular arrangement (Fig. 24–25).

Moderate anisokaryocytosis is common, and the nuclei may vary in shape from round to spindle.[16] The cytoplasm is pale, poorly defined and contains eosinophilic granules (May-Grünwald-Giemsa). The cytologic pattern is typical and allows a confident diagnosis.

Carotid Body Tumor: Cytologic Features

- Dispersed tumor cells sometimes in follicular arrangement
- Diffuse pale cytoplasm with eosinophilic granules
- Round to spindle-shaped nuclei

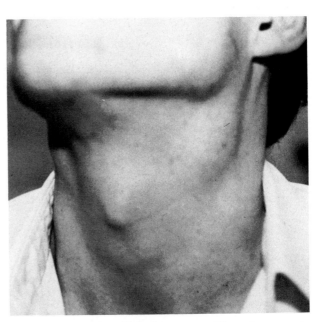

FIGURE 24–24. Carotid body tumors. Bilateral tumors in typical setting.

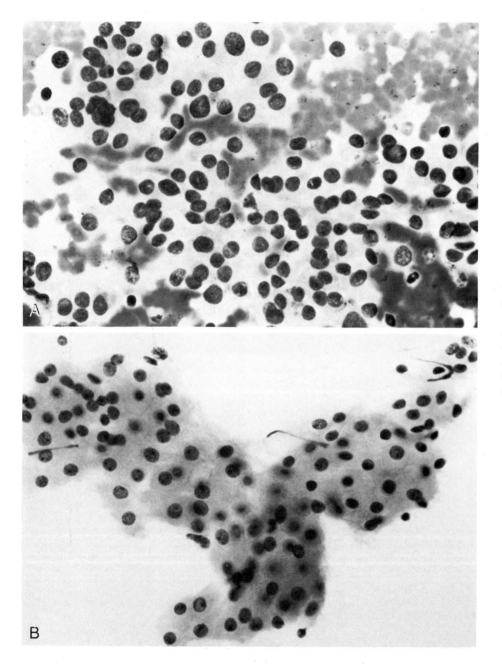

FIGURE 24–25. Carotid body tumor. Fine needle aspiration smear contains single cells and loose follicular formations. Moderate anisokaryosis. The cytoplasm is poorly defined in May-Grünwald-Giemsa (×132) (A), finely granular in Papanicolaou (×132) (B).

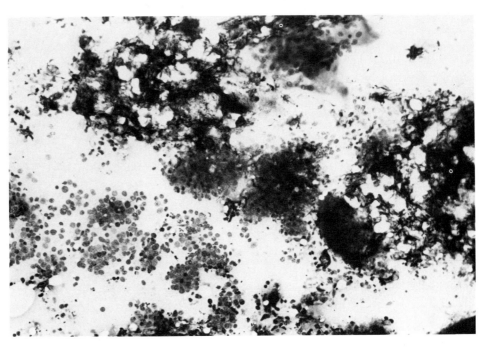

FIGURE 24–26. Pilomatrix-oma (calcifying epithelioma of Malherbe). Aspirate contains tumor cells, multinucleated foreign-body giant cells, amorphous calcium deposit and sheets of shadow cells. The tumor cells, single or in clusters, have round monotonous nuclei and poorly defined cytoplasm (May-Grünwald-Giemsa; ×40).

Pilomatrixoma (Calcifying Epithelioma of Malherbe)

This slow-growing benign skin adnexal tumor occurs both in children and adults. The head, neck and upper extremities are the most common sites. Clinically, the lesion appears as an irregular firm subcutaneous mass, less than 3 cm in diameter.

The histologic pattern of pilomatrixoma is characterized by irregular islands of epithelial cells in a cellular stroma. The epithelial cells, which have round-to-oval nuclei and scanty cytoplasm, are found in the periphery of the tumor. In the central areas anucleated "shadow" cells dominate. Granular or amorphous calcium deposit is present.

Aspirates contain free lying and clusters of monomorphous cells with round nuclei and poorly defined cytoplasm. A delicate pink (May-Grünwald-Giemsa) stroma is present in the clusters (Fig. 24–26). Mitoses are rare. Inflammatory cells and foreign body giant

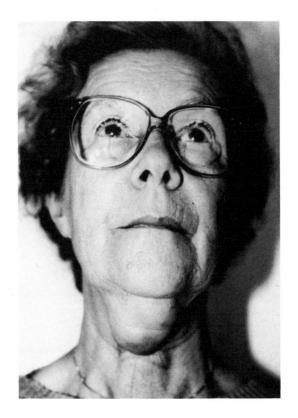

FIGURE 24–27. Carcinoma in thyroglossal cyst.

cells are important features. The cytologic pattern may simulate a small-cell, undifferentiated carcinoma.[55] The identification of calcium deposits, sheets of "shadow" cells and clusters of tumor cells surrounded by a delicate stroma allow a conclusive diagnosis.

Pilomatrixoma: Cytologic Features

- Epithelial cells in solid clusters with delicate stroma
- Sheets of anucleated cells
- Calcium debris
- Foreign body giant cells

MALIGNANT TUMORS

Carcinomas in Thyroglossal Cysts

Thyroglossal cysts usually occur in the anterior midline between the hyoid and the mandible. The cyst walls, which are lined by columnar epithelium, may contain thyroid tissue. Colloid goiter and thyroiditis can afflict this aberrant thyroid tissue when the thyroid gland is involved. Primary malignant thyroid neoplasms are rarely observed in the thyroglossal cyst (Fig. 24–27).[23, 37] Papillary and follicular carcinomas yield aspirates with a characteristic cytologic pattern (Fig. 24–28).

A normal physical examination and scintigram of the thyroid gland will rule out metastasis from a carcinoma in the gland to the submental lymph node. This finding is of importance to allow adequate primary surgery.

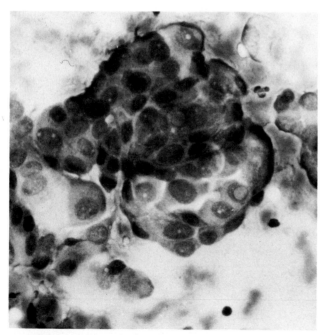

FIGURE 24–28. Carcinoma in thyroglossal cyst. Fine needle aspiration biopsy specimen from lesion shown in Figure 24–27. Aspirate with cytologic features consistent with papillary carcinoma of the thyroid (May-Grünwald-Giemsa; ×132).

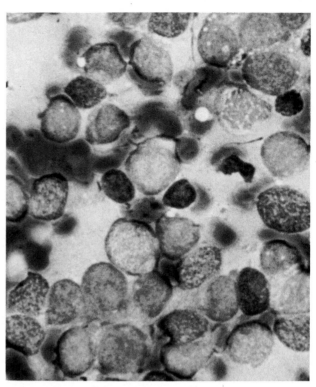

FIGURE 24–29. Neuroendocrine carcinoma (Merkel cell tumor) of the skin. Aspirate shows small round tumor cells with scanty cytoplasm. Note tendency to microacinar arrangements (May-Grünwald-Giemsa; ×200).

Papillary Thyroid Carcinoma of the Thyroglossal Duct: Cytologic Features

- Papillary clusters
- Cells with dense cytoplasm and intranuclear invagination
- Psammoma bodies; viscous colloid

Neuroendocrine Carcinoma of the Skin (Merkel Cell Tumor)

The Merkel cell of the skin is the origin of this aggressive tumor. It occurs in elderly individuals; the face, neck and extremities are the most common sites. The rapidly growing skin tumor is sometimes ulcerated and has a violaceous hue. Surgery is recommended because the tumor responds poorly to radiation and chemotherapy.

Histologic sections are characterized by monotonous round tumor cells with a trabecular growth pattern. The tumor cell has a scanty cytoplasm and can be mistaken for a lymphoma cell. Mitoses are common.

Cytologic evaluation of FNA smears shows a dispersed tumor cell population dominated by naked nuclei. A few small-cell clusters can usually be detected as well as a tendency towards molding (Fig. 24–29).[32, 42, 48] When present, the cytoplasm is sparse and weakly basophilic. The chromatin is finely granular, and the nucleoli are indistinct.

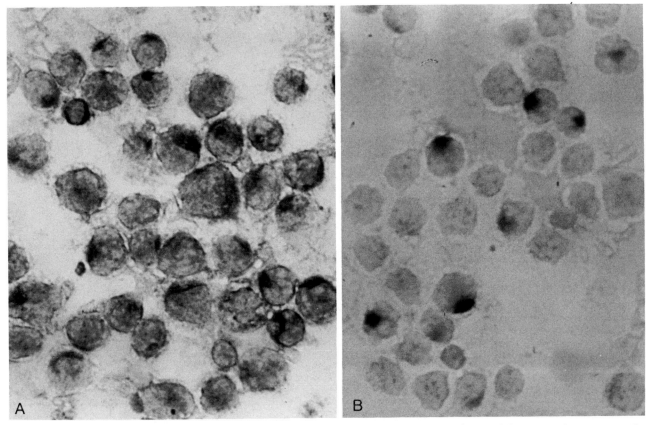

FIGURE 24–30. Neuroendocrine carcinoma (Merkel cell tumor) of the skin. Immunocytochemical detection of neuron-specific enolase *(A)* and cytokeratin *(B)* (Alkaline phosphatase; ×200).

The cytologic identification of a Merkel cell tumor requires considerable experience. From a clinical point of view it is important to exclude the possibility of a high-grade lymphoma and a metastasis from a small-cell lung carcinoma. Absence of lymphoglandular bodies and the finding of small-cell clusters rule out malignant lymphoma. Immunocytochemistry will identify cytokeratin and neuron-specific enolase concentrated in a paranuclear dot in Merkel tumor cells (Fig. 24–30).[8, 42] On cytologic grounds it seems impossible to differentiate a Merkel cell tumor from a metastasis of an undifferentiated small-cell lung carcinoma. However, the clinical presentation should differ between these two disorders.

Neuroendocrine Carcinoma of the Skin: Cytologic Features

- Dispersed tumor cells often without cytoplasm
- Few small clusters
- Monotonous fragile nuclei
- Frequent mitoses

References

1. Arthaud JB: Anaplastic parotid carcinoma ("malignant lympho-epithelial lesion") in seven Alaskan natives. Am J Clin Pathol 57:275–286, 1972.
2. Azzopardi JG, Evans TJ: Malignant lymphoma of parotid associated with Mikulicz's disease (benign lymphoepithelial lesion). J Clin Pathol 24:744–752, 1971.
3. Batsakis JG: Basal cell adenoma of the parotid gland. Cancer 29:226–230, 1972.
4. Bottles K, Löwhagen T: Psammoma bodies in the aspiration cytology smears of an acinic cell tumour. Acta Cytol 29:191–192, 1985.
5. Bottles K, Löwhagen T, Miller TR: Mast cells in the aspiration cytology differential diagnosis of adenolymphoma. Acta Cytol 29:513–515, 1985.
6. Corridan M: Glycogen-rich clear cell adenoma of the parotid gland. J Pathol Bacteriol 72:623–627, 1956.
7. Dahl I, Åkerman M: Nodular fasciitis. A correlative cytologic and histologic study of 13 cases. Acta Cytol 25:215–222, 1981.
8. Domagala W, Lubinski J, Lasota J, Giryn I, Weber I, Osborn M: Neuroendocrine (Merkel cell) carcinomas of skin; cytology, intermediate filament typing and ultrastructure of tumor cells in fine needle aspirates. Acta Cytol 31:267–275, 1967.
9. Eneroth C-M: Histological and clinical aspects of parotid tumours. Acta Otolaryngol 191 [Suppl]:5–99, 1964.
10. Eneroth C-M, Hamberger CA, Jakobsson P: Malignancy of acinic cell carcinoma. Ann Otol Rhinol Laryngol 75:780–793, 1966.
11. Eneroth C-M, Zajicek J: Aspiration biopsy of salivary gland tumors. III. Morphologic studies on smears and histologic sections from 368 mixed tumors. Acta Cytol 10:440–454, 1966.
12. Eneroth C-M, Franzén S, Zajicek J: Cytologic diagnosis on aspirates from 1000 salivary gland tumours. Acta Otolaryngol 224 [Suppl]:168–172, 1967.
13. Eneroth C-M, Zajicek J: Aspiration biopsy of salivary gland tumors. IV. Morphologic studies on smears and histologic sections from 45 cases of adenoid cystic carcinoma. Acta Cytol 13:59–63, 1969.
14. Eneroth C-M: Salivary gland tumors in the parotid gland, submandibular gland, and the palate region. Cancer 27:1415–1418, 1971.

15. Eneroth C-M, Hjertman L, Moberger G, Söderberg G: Muco-epidermoid carcinomas of the salivary gland. Acta Otolaryngol 73:68–74, 1972.

16. Engzell U, Franzén S, Zajicek J: Aspiration biopsy of tumors of the neck. II. Cytologic findings in 13 cases of carotid body tumour. Acta Cytol 15:25–30, 1971.

17. Evans RW, Cruickshank AH: Epithelial Tumors of the Salivary Glands. Philadelphia, WB Saunders, 1970.

18. Evans RW, Cruickshank AH: Epithelial Tumors of the Salivary Glands. Major Problems in Pathology, vol 1. Philadelphia, WB Saunders, 1970.

19. Galen RS, Gambino SR: Beyond Normality: The Predictive Value of Medical Diagnosis. New York, John Wiley & Sons, 1975.

20. Godwin JT: Benign lymphoepithelial lesion of the parotid gland. Cancer 5:1089–1103, 1952.

21. Hamperl H: Ueber das Vorkommen von Onkozyten in verschiedenen Organen und ihren Geschwülsten. Virch Arch Path Anat 298:327–375, 1936.

22. Hood IC, Qizilbash AH, Salama SSS, Alexopoulou I: Basal cell adenoma of parotid. Difficulty of differentiation from adenoid cystic carcinoma on aspiration biopsy. Acta Cytol 27:515–520, 1983.

23. Joseph TJ, Komorowski RA: Thyroglossal duct carcinoma. Hum Pathol 6:717–729, 1975.

24. Kleinsasser O, Klein HJ: Basalzelladenome der Speichel drüsen. Arch Klin Exp Nasen Kehlkopfheilkd 189:302–316, 1967.

25. Koss LG, Spiro RH, Hajdu SI: Small cell (oat cell) carcinoma of minor salivary gland origin. Cancer 30:737–741, 1972.

26. Koss LG, Woyke S, Olszewski W: Aspiration Biopsy. Cytologic Interpretation and Histologic Bases. Tokyo, Igaku-Shoin, pp 214–220, 1984.

27. Layfield LJ: Fine needle aspiration cytology of a trabecular adenoma of the parotid gland. Acta Cytol 29:999–1002, 1985.

28. Linsk JA, Franzén S, Perrone-Donnorso R: Aspiration biopsy cytology of the salivary glands. In: Clinical Aspiration Cytology. Edited by JA Linsk, S Franzén. Philadelphia, JB Lippincott, 1983.

29. LiVolsi VA, Perzin KH: Malignant tumors arising in salivary gland. Carcinoma arising in benign mixed tumors. A clinico-pathologic study. Cancer 39:2209–2230, 1977.

30. Löwhagen T, Sprenger E: Cytologic presentation of thyroid tumors in aspiration biopsy smears. Acta Cytol 18:192–197, 1974.

31. Mavec P, Eneroth C-M, Franzén S, Moberger G, Zajicek J: Aspiration biopsy of salivary gland tumors. I. Correlation of cytologic reports from 652 aspiration biopsies with clinical and histologic findings. Acta Otolaryngol, 58:472–484, 1964.

32. Mellblom L, Akerman M, Carlén B: Aspiration biopsy of neuroendocrine (Merkel cell) carcinoma of the skin: report of a case. Acta Cytol 28:297–300, 1984.

33. Mincione G, Borrelli D, Cicchi P, Ipponi P, Fiorini A: Fine needle aspiration cytology of parathyroid adenoma. Acta Cytol 30:65–69, 1986.

34. O'Dwyer P, Farrar WB, James AG, Finkelmeier W, McCabe DP: Needle aspiration biopsy of major salivary gland tumors. Cancer 57:554–557, 1986.

35. Palma O, Torri AM, deCristofaro JA, Fiaccavento S: Fine needle aspiration cytology in two cases of well-differentiated acinic cell carcinoma of the parotid glands. Discussion of diagnostic criteria. Acta Cytol 29:516–521, 1985.

36. Persson PS, Zettergren L: Cytologic diagnosis of salivary gland tumors by aspiration biopsy. Acta Cytol 17:351–354, 1973.

37. Pitts W, Tani E, Skoog L: Papillary carcinoma in fine needle aspiration smears of a thyroglossal duct lesion. Acta Cytol 32:599–601, 1988.

38. Qizilbash AH, Sianos J, Young JEM, Archibald SD: Fine needle aspiration biopsy cytology of major salivary glands. Acta Cytol 29:503–512, 1985.

39. Qizilbash AH, Young EJ: Guides to Clinical Aspiration Biopsy. Head and Neck. Tokyo, Igaku-Shoin, 1988.

40. Reif RM: The cytologic picture of proliferative myositis. Acta Cytol 26: 376–377, 1982.

41. Sismanis A, Merriam JM, Kline TS, Davis RK, Shapshay SM, Strong MS: Diagnosis of salivary gland tumors by fine needle aspiration biopsy. Head Neck Surg 3:482–489, 1981.

42. Skoog L, Schmitt F, Tani E: Neuroendocrine (Merkel cell) carcinoma of the skin: Immunocytochemical and cytomorphologic analysis on fine needle aspirates. Diagno Cytopathol 6:53–57, 1990.

43. Söderström N: Fine Needle Aspiration Biopsy. Stockholm, Almqvist & Wiksell, 1966.

44. Spiro RH, Huvos AG, Strong EW: Adenoid cystic carcinoma of salivary origin. A clinicopathologic study of 242 cases. Am J Surg 128:512–520, 1974.

45. Spjut H, Dorfman H, Fechner R, Ackerman L: Tumors of bone and cartilage. In Atlas of Tumor Pathology. Washington, DC, Armed Forces Institute of Pathology, 1971.

46. Stanley MW, Horwitz CA, Henry MJ, Burton LG, Löwhagen T: Basal-cell adenoma of the salivary gland: A benign adenoma that cytologically mimics adenocystic carcinoma. Diagn Cytopathol 4:342–346, 1988.

47. Stewart FW, Foote FW, Becker WF: Mucoepidermoid tumors of the salivary glands. Ann Surg 122:820–844, 1945.

48. Szpak CA, Bossen EH, Linder J, Johnston WW: Cytomorphology of primary small-cell (Merkel cell) carcinoma of the skin in fine needle aspirates. Acta Cytol 28:280–286, 1984.

49. Tandler B: Ultrastructure of adenoid cystic carcinoma. Lab Invest 24:504–512, 1971.

50. Tani EM, Christensson B, Porwit A, Skoog L: Immunocyto-chemical analysis and cytomorphological diagnosis on fine needle aspirates of lymphoproliferative diseases. Acta Cytol 32:209–215, 1988.

51. Tani EM, Skoog L: Fine needle aspiration cytology and immu-nocytochemistry in the diagnosis of lymphoid lesions of the thyroid. Acta Cytol 33:48–52, 1989.

52. Thackray AC, Lucas RB: Tumors of the major salivary glands. In Atlas of Tumor Pathology, fascicle 10, second series. Washington DC, Armed Forces Institute of Pathology, 1974.

53. Webb AJ: Cytologic diagnosis of salivary gland lesions in adult and pediatric surgical patients. Acta Cytol 17:51–58, 1973.

54. Wirman JA, Battifora HA: Small cell undifferentiated carcinoma of salivary gland origin. Cancer 37:1840–1848, 1976.

55. Woyke S, Olszewski W, Eichelkraut A: Pilomatrixoma: A pitfall in the aspiration cytology of skin tumors. Acta Cytol 26:189–194, 1982.

56. Zajicek J: Aspiration biopsy cytology. I. Cytology of supradia-phragmatic organs. Monogr Clin Cytol 4:37–39, 1974.

57. Zajicek J, Eneroth C-M, Jakobsson P: Aspiration biopsy of salivary gland tumors. VI. Morphologic studies on smears and histologic sections from mucoepidermoid carcinoma. Acta Cytol 20:35–41, 1976.

25

Thyroid

Hugo Galera Davidson
Ricardo Gonzalez Campora

The fine needle aspiration (FNA) method for studying the thyroid was first developed in Sweden in the Radiunhelmet Hospital of Stockholm in the 1950s. The Swedish investigators established its utility in the diagnostic protocol of the patient with thyroid problems and its correlations with the clinical manifestations of various pathologic entities.[49, 111–113, 115, 116, 131–136, 143, 169–171, 173–175] In the United States, FNA came into use at a later date.[72, 95, 123, 124, 126, 127] At present, FNA of the thyroid is a first-line diagnostic procedure that is fully accepted in the diagnostic work-up of patients in most hospitals in conjunction with more traditional methods. The main purpose of thyroid FNA is to distinguish between patients with malignant, or possibly malignant, thyroid nodules from those with benign nodules that can be followed clinically. Studies of the precision, efficiency, indications, diagnostic criteria, relation to other diagnostic techniques and clinical-pathologic correlations have generated many published reports (see references 2, 3, 6, 9–11, 16, 17, 36, 38, 39, 46, 53, 56, 64, 70, 71, 76, 79, 84, 100–102, 110, 114, 122, 123, 125, 128, 138, 140, 145, 151, 152, 159, 177, 178, 182, 184, 189, 192).

In principle, any thyroid enlargement can be studied by FNA; nonetheless, the maximum benefits are obtained in the evaluation of the thyroid nodule. The prevalence of thyroid nodules depends on the population studied and increases linearly with age by a mean of 0.08% per year. In the general adult population it ranges from 4 to 7%, and in children, from 0.2 to 1.5%.[148] Thyroid cancer occurs in only a small proportion of patients with thyroid nodules, ranging from 10 to 20%[34, 183] for the general population and from 18 to 30% for the population exposed to ionizing radiation.[42, 151] When a comparison is made of the incidence of malignant tumors in surgical pieces excised according to classic criteria (clinical history, palpation, echography and scintigraphy) with that of tumors excised according to cytologic indications, there is a net numeric predominance of the second group and an appreciable reduction in the economic cost of the disease.[24] As such, with FNA the number of thyroidectomies has been halved, whereas the incidence of malignant lesions has doubled.[71, 124] Nonetheless, the consequences of this conservative methodology have yet to be evaluated definitively, because certain benign diseases (nodular goiter, lymphocytic thyroiditis) coexist with, or eventually develop into, follicular carcinoma, papillary carcinoma or lymphoma.[73, 78]

Other specific indications of FNA are the evaluation of diffuse goiter, the follow-up of individuals exposed to irradiation of the head and neck, screening for familial medullary carcinoma and therapeutic drainage of cystic lesions.

TECHNIQUE

The technique of FNA of the thyroid follows the general guidelines of FNA as in other organs. Preferably, 22- to 23-gauge needles are used with disposable 10- or 20-cc syringes mounted on a mechanical device to facilitate aspiration.[114] To obtain an optimal output certain points must be taken into account. The patient should be placed in the supine position with the neck extended; a pillow under the patient's neck is helpful. The aspiration should be performed by a physician experienced in palpating thyroid nodules, and he or she should be on the side contralateral to the lesion. During the puncture, the patient should remain immobile and contain respiration. The gland is immobilized against the trachea with one hand while the aspiration is done rapidly, maintaining a negative pressure until blood appears at the cone of the needle. The number of aspirations made in each patient depends on the characteristics of the lesion. Generally speaking, two aspirations suffice in single nodular lesions less than 3 cm in diameter. When the lesion is larger, three or four aspirations can be performed. The central zones should be avoided because they often possess regressive changes. In multinodular goiter, several nodules should be sampled. In diffuse goiter, material is obtained from both thyroid lobes. When the lesion is cystic, an attempt is made to extract the contents of the cyst and the thyroid is then palpated to search for intracapsular nodular lesions. No specific contraindication to thyroid FNA is reported. Nonetheless, special care should be taken in children and in incapacitated adults, in whom the immobility of the neck cannot be ensured. The material aspirated is extended and fixed using standard techniques.[116] Three to six slides per case should be made to obtain air-dried, alcohol- or spray-fixed material to stain with the May-Grünwald-Giemsa (MGG) and Papanicolau (P) methods.

NORMAL THYROID

Histology

The thyroid gland is constituted by two symmetric oval lobes situated on each side of the neck and connected medially by an isthmus. Each lobe contains multiple lobules composed of 20 to 40 follicles enmeshed in a fine, capillary-rich connective network. In histologic sections, the follicles usually appear as ringlike structures lined by cuboidal cells with round nuclei. Sections made tangential to the follicular epithelium usually exhibit a honeycomb aspect, with well-defined cell margins and central nuclei. The height of the follicular epithelium varies between 3 and 20 μm, depending on the secretory activity and age of the subject. The colloid contains thyroglobulin in concentrated solution. C, or parafollicular, cells differ from the follicular cells in their topography, form and function. They are larger, triangle-shaped with clear cytoplasm, and they secrete calcitonin. In the postnatal thyroid, these cells are located on the inner side of the follicular basement membrane, isolated or in small groups, and they are separated from the colloid by follicular cells.[45]

Cytology

The cytologic appearance of the normal thyroid gland produces small variations related to age and functional state. It is often similar to that observed in some diffuse and nodular goiters and it is very difficult to differentiate it, on a strictly cytologic basis, from the parathyroid glands.[172] Aspirations of the normal thyroid gland generally yield little blood-stained material. The smears contain few follicular cells and scant colloid, with follicular cells dispersed or in small clusters. Rarely are well-constituted follicles recovered. The cytoplasm is pale and poorly delimited. The nucleus is centrally located, oval or round, and contains fine granular chromatin and one or two small nucleoli. With the May-Grünwald-Giemsa technique, the cytoplasm is grayish and the nucleus has an inconspicuous nucleolus; sometimes the cytoplasm contains numerous

vacuoles with coarse dark blue granules (paravacuolar granules).[170] Bare nuclei are often present that are similar in size and characteristics to those of normal lymphocytes. The colloid has the aspect of proteidic material, appearing as a fine film of variable color, from gray-green to rose with Papanicolaou staining and red-violet with May-Grünwald-Giemsa staining.

METABOLIC DISORDERS

Amyloidosis

Thyroid involvement in primary amyloidosis is exceptional, but in secondary amyloidosis it occurs in up to 80% of cases.[8] The amyloid deposit commences at the perivascular level and discretely affects the interstice; on rare occasions it is massive, originating a euthyroid goiter.[89] The aspiration material contains few cells and small fragments of cyanophilic amyloid, including a few oval nuclei. Congo red produces a characteristic reddish color with yellowish green birefringence. The presence of amyloid in a thyroid aspiration is not pathognomonic of medullary carcinoma.

Hemochromatosis

Thyroid involvement is secondary to the massive iron overload. The thyroid has a brown color and conserves its usual form and function. The deposit of iron pigment is particularly intense in the cytoplasm of the follicular cells, as well as in the macrophages and fibroblasts of the struma. In the aspiration, hemosiderin has a yellowish-brown color and is located in the form of coarse birefringent granules in the cytoplasm of follicular cells and macrophages.

Black Thyroid Syndrome

The black thyroid syndrome is associated with administration of minocycline and tetracycline.[11] The majority of cases reported are of post-mortem findings in which there was no alteration in thyroid function. The gland adopts this coloring because of intracytoplasmic deposits in follicular cells of a brown pigment having the characteristics of neuromelanin and lipofuscin, which are also apparent on cytologic smears.[188]

THYROIDITIS

With the exception of Hashimoto's thyroiditis, inflammatory thyroid processes are uncommon entities that are classified according to their clinical course.

Acute Thyroiditis

This is a suppurative lesion that begins abruptly with swelling and intense pain of the anterior cervical region, fever and tachycardia. Generally, patients do not present functional alterations and they rarely undergo FNA.[14] The gland is enlarged by multiple abscesses. Aspirated material contains abundant neutrophils and macrophages, scant follicular cells, with degenerative changes, cellular debris and fibrin (Fig. 25–1A). Biologic agents are occasionally identified (e.g. staphylococcus).

The differential diagnosis must be made with other lesions that course with copious inflammatory infiltrate, such as infected thyroglossal cysts, cervical inflammations and some anaplastic carcinomas.

Subacute Thyroiditis

This includes two well-defined anatomoclinical entities.

Subacute Granulomatous Thyroiditis of Quervain. This is a nonspecific self-limited inflammation, probably of viral origin. It occurs most frequently in middle-aged women and commonly resolves spontaneously in the course of 2 or 3 months. It appears slowly or abruptly after a respiratory infection and is manifested by fever, asthenia, myalgia and painful swelling.

Thyroid involvement can be focal or diffuse. It commences with necrosis of the follicular epithelium, edema and infiltration of neutrophils, lymphocytes, macrophages and multinucleate giant cells. Sometimes epithelioid granulomas are seen. The findings progress to interstitial fibrosis and follicular regeneration.

Cytologic findings depend on the disease stage. At the onset are observed degenerated follicular cells, multinucleate giant cells, epithelioid cells, mature lymphocytes and neutrophils on a dirty background containing cellular debris and abundant colloid. The cytoplasm of the giant cells may contain remains of colloid (Fig. 25–1B).[143] In advanced stages, the aspirations are small and contain scant inflammatory cells and fibroblasts with active nuclei.[46, 143, 184]

Subacute Lymphocytic Thyroiditis (Silent Thyroiditis). This form of hyperthyroidism courses with painful swelling of the neck that resolves spontaneously. Sometimes it appears in women during postpartum. The histologic picture includes follicular destruction and a moderate lymphocytic infiltrate, without germinal centers or Hürthle cells. In contrast to Hashimoto's thyroiditis, the hyperthyroid crises are related to follicular destruction and not stimulation.[130] Although no reports have been published of the utility of FNA in this entity, it could be helpful in the differential diagnosis of hyperthyroidism.

Chronic Thyroiditis

The term chronic thyroiditis groups histologically heterogeneous lesions in which the extension of the glandular involvement varies.

Chronic Granulomatous Thyroiditis. These are relatively uncommon lesions that are characterized by the existence of numerous disseminated granulomas or large solitary lesions with central necroses. The etiology is tuberculous, syphilitic or mycotic, and they are not usually studied by FNA.

Riedel's Thyroiditis. This is a chronic, fibrosing multifocal inflammation, probably of autoimmune origin. The disease is rare and courses without serious involvement of thyroid function. The patient develops a painless mass on a previous goiter, which produces dysphagia or dyspnea. The thyroid gland presents a diffuse, fibrous and petrous appearance that extends to the extrathyroid structures. The lesion commences with degenerative follicular changes, endophlebitis and an intense inflammatory infiltrate consisting of lymphocytes, plasmacytes, neutrophils and eosinophils. Intense fibrosis that destroys the thyroid parenchyma later develops.[158]

Diagnosis by FNA is difficult because aspiration

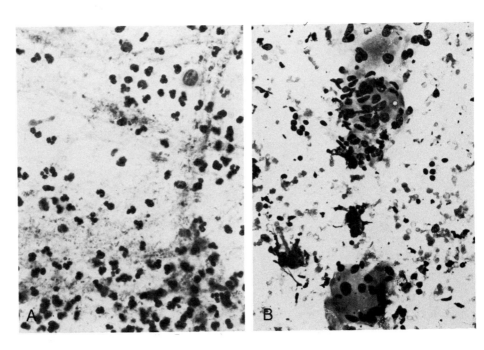

FIGURE 25–1. *A,* **Acute suppurative thyroiditis.** Abundant neutrophilic granulocytes, macrophages and cell debris. (Papanicolaou; ×250). *B,* **Subacute thyroiditis of Quervain.** Multinucleated giant cells grouped in granuloma-like arrangements. Lymphocytes, neutrophilic granulocytes and cell debris are also present (May-Grünwald-Giemsa; ×250.)

specimens are usually poor in cells, and the cellularity is nonspecific. In the smear can be seen mature lymphocytes, degenerated follicular cells, neutrophils and fibroblasts.[46]

Focal Lymphocytic Thyroiditis. This banal lesion occurs on a normal or pathologic thyroid (nodular goiter, primary hyperplasia and papillary carcinoma). Sometimes it coexists with extrathyroid disease (Addison's disease, Simmond's cachexia and cirrhosis). Histologically, it is characterized by lymphoplasmacytic clusters associated with degenerated thyroid follicles. It is usually unapparent on FNA, but it is sometimes recognized by the presence of groups of mature lymphocytes in relation to follicular cells.[143]

Hashimoto's Thyroiditis. At present, this is the most common form of noniatrogenic hypothyroidism. Three anatomoclinical entities, probably corresponding to different stages of the same lesion, have been identified.

Acute lymphocytic thyroiditis is viewed as the incipient stage of Hashimoto's thyroiditis because it is observed in young patients, coursing with euthyroidism and discrete glandular enlargement.[197] Moreover, in some patients serum antibody titers are low or normal.[69] The gland has marked lymphocytic infiltration, slight oncocytic changes and mild follicular destruction. The aspiration contains little colloid, numerous lymphoid cells and a variable amount of follicular cells. Oncocytic or Hürthle's cells are sporadic.[143] The lymphoid cells correspond mainly to mature lymphocytes, but stimulated lymphocytes and plasmacytes can be seen. The lymphocytes often have artifacts produced by extension. To establish the differential diagnosis with malignant lymphoma it is occasionally necessary to demonstrate the polyclonal nature of the infiltrate by using immunocytochemical techniques.[179]

Hypertrophic lymphocytic thyroiditis is the florid form of the entity and is generally observed in women. It is manifested by a picture of hypofunctional goiter (unilateral or diffuse), often accompanied by high serum levels of antithyroid antibodies.[57, 93] In the histologic study, the lymphoplasmacytic infiltrate forms germinal centers and tends to disorganize the lobar architecture. Regenerative follicles and interstitial fibrosis are also seen, and the follicular cells frequently present oncocytic transformation. Sometimes hyperplastic nodules of these oncocytic cells are seen.

On FNA, there is usually a variable amount of bloody fluid. Smears contain scant colloid and abundant cellularity, predominantly lymphoid or epithelial. Most of the lymphoid cells are mature lymphocytes and plasmacytes; nonetheless, centrofollicular lymphoid cells and macrophages are observed. Often the lymphocytes appear to have artifacts by extension, presenting a nuclear prolongation or tail (Fig. 25–2A and B). Although the presence of a lymphoid infiltrate is an important finding for the diagnosis of lymphocytic thyroiditis, this type of infiltrate is also seen in other entities, such as inflammation (tuberculosis), Graves's disease, papillary carcinoma and lymphoma. The follicular cells vary considerably in number and morphology and can exhibit changes characteristic of "mitochondrion-rich cells" or even Hürthle cells,[66] as well as signs of cytoplasmic hyperstimulation (marginal vacuoles) (Fig. 25–2C). The typical Hürthle cell is large, with well-defined margins, fine granular eosinophilic cytoplasm and a large, hyperchromatic and pleomorphic nucleus. Although aspirated material containing a predominance of epithelial cells can have a cytologic appearance very similar to that of oncocytic tumors, the inflammatory nature of the lesion is apparent from the presence of cellular detritus on the grounds of the extension and the absence of macronucleoli in the Hürthle cells.[46, 94] Aside from lymphoid and epithelial cells, the aspiration also yields macrophages, multinucleate cells and epithelioid cells. The multinucleate cells are usually scant in number, with few nuclei, and the cytoplasm sometimes contains

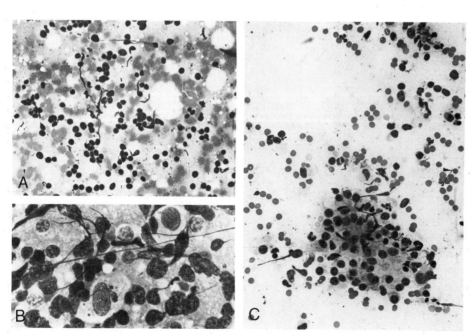

FIGURE 25–2. Hashimoto's thyroiditis. *A*, Abundant lymphocytes and cell debris in a background rich in red blood cells and colloid (May-Grünwald-Giemsa; ×100). *B*, Detail showing centrofollicular cells, macrophages and cell debris (May-Grünwald-Giemsa; ×1000). *C*, Monolayer of Hürthle cells in a background rich in lymphocytes and cell debris (May-Grünwald-Giemsa ×400).

colloid material. Exceptionally, psammoma bodies have been described.[48]

Atrophic lymphocytic thyroiditis is characterized by hypothyroidism associated with fibrous goiter. Histologically, marked follicular atrophy, oncocytic cells, squamous metaplasia and lymphocytic infiltration are noted.[88] Although rarely studied by FNA, aspiration yields little material and is constituted of fibroblasts, lymphocytes, follicular cells and oncocytic cells.[46]

In a patient with the classic clinical form of presentation and a mixed cytologic picture containing lymphoid and epithelial cells, the diagnosis of Hashimoto's thyroiditis is relatively simple. Diagnostic difficulties appear when an unusual clinical picture is accompanied by a cytologic specimen with predominance of a cellular type (lymphoid or epithelial). In these situations, the lesion may bring to mind other inflammatory diseases (Quervain's thyroiditis and Riedel's thyroiditis) and neoplasms (Hürthle cell tumors, papillary carcinoma and lymphoma). This problem is compounded if, as is frequent, Hashimoto's thyroiditis coexists with a malignant epithelial tumor (follicular or papillary carcinoma).[141] Moreover, many lymphomas develop on a prior lymphocytic thyroiditis.[197] In Hashimoto's thyroiditis, the oncocytic cells are arrayed alone or in layers, presenting bland chromatin with regressive atypias and small nucleoli, often mixed with lymphocytes. In contrast, Hürthle cell tumors tend to form three-dimensional clusters of syncytial appearance and the cellular nuclei exhibit granular chromatin and a macronucleolus. Nuclear pleomorphism and the number of lymphoid cells should not be considered important differential signs.[83, 93, 147]

HYPERPLASIA

The term goiter is used to designate clinically any thyroid enlargement, but in pathology it is restricted to hyperplastic processes, whether nodular or diffuse, and these can course with hyper-, normo- or hypofunction.

Toxic Diffuse Hyperplasia (Graves's Disease)

This autoimmune disorder typically courses with diffuse goiter, hyperthyroidism and exophthalmos. It usually appears in women of 20 to 50 years and is the most common cause of thyroid hyperfunction. Glandular enlargement is due to the action of a circulating antibody, long-acting thyroid stimulator (LATS), that stimulates specific thyroid-stimulating hormone (TSH) receptors in follicular cells.[187]

The gland has moderate, symmetric enlargement, intense congestion and accentuated lobar pattern. The follicles are lined by columnar or cuboidal cells, the largest ones showing papillary projections, pale colloid and numerous resorption vacuoles. Lymphoid infiltrates, Hürthle cells and granulomas are seen occasionally. Farbota and colleagues[51] report coexistent carcinoma and Graves's disease in 5% of cases, the most common histologic variant being papillary carcinoma.

The utility of FNA in Graves's disease is limited because the diagnosis is generally made on the basis of clinical features and laboratory data. Aspiration usually yields little material, of a blood-stained appearance. The smear shows numerous follicular cells mixed with blood and scant colloid. The follicular cells are dispersed or arrayed in loose monolayers or follicles (Fig. 25–3A). Papillae are not usually observed. The cytoplasm is pale and finely granular; it often contains marginal cytoplasmic vacuoles (Fig. 25–3C). The vacuoles are optically clear in preparations stained with the Papanicolaou stain; however, when stained with the May-Grünwald-Giemsa technique they contain rose-colored granular material.[132] These cells are also

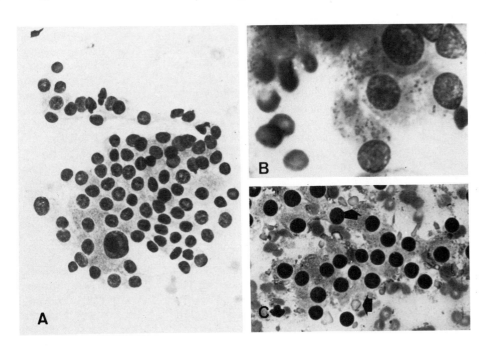

FIGURE 25–3. Graves's disease. *A,* Monolayer follicular cells' cluster. The cells show abundant fine granular cytoplasm and anisonucleosis (May-Grünwald-Giemsa; ×400). *B,* Detail showing paravacuolar granules (May-Grünwald-Giemsa; ×1000). *C,* Cluster of follicular cells showing marginal vacuoles (May-Grünwald-Giemsa; ×400).

called "flare cells" or "flame cells." On electron microscopy, the vacuolar content has been identified as phagolysosomes generated by hyperactivity.[143, 174] The nuclei have discrete variations in form and size that are enhanced after the use of antithyroid drugs.[46, 131] Marginal cytoplasmic vacuoles, although suggestive of a diagnosis of thyrotoxicosis, are nonspecific because they are also encountered in nontoxic goiter, Hashimoto's thyroiditis and follicular carcinoma.[132, 144] Other, less constant, cytologic findings are the presence of a lymphocyte component, Hürthle cells and paravacuolar cytoplasmic granules (Fig. 25–3B). The existence of multinucleate cells and epithelioid granulomas has been reported.[85, 133]

To evaluate the smear, the clinical and exploratory findings must be considered because the cytologic picture is not specific of Graves's disease but is common to all the states with a course of thyroid hyperfunction (hot nodular goiter, toxic adenoma and primary hyperthyroidism).

The differential diagnosis of hyperthyroidism must be made with other entities that have highly cellular aspiration material, such as follicular proliferation, nodular goiter and papillary carcinoma, as well as Hashimoto's thyroiditis when Hürthle cells and lymphoid infiltrates are found.

Diffuse Colloidal Hyperplasia

This represents the initial form of response of the thyroid gland to a peripheral thyroxine deficit, and it is seen mainly in young women. The gland is translucid, yellowish and uniformly enlarged. The follicles are swollen with pale colloid and lined by flat epithelium. Focally, small active follicles that protrude into adjacent follicles are observed, corresponding to the areas of active hormonal synthesis.

In diffuse colloidal goiter, aspiration yields abundant colloid and scant follicular cells of normal aspect. The cells are dispersed or form small loose monolayers; occasionally, well-formed follicular structures are seen. From a practical point of view, the combination of a discretely enlarged gland with a smear rich in colloid and follicular cells of normal appearance is suggestive of colloidal goiter. Although aspirations with abundant colloidal material are indicative of a benign lesion, some papillary and follicular carcinomas also contain abundant colloid.[56, 121] C cells are rarely observed in a smear from a normal or hyperplastic thyroid gland, and when they exist the morphology is similar to that of cells of a medullary carcinoma.[134]

Nodular Hyperplasia

Nodular colloidal hyperplasia represents a form of sustained thyroid stimulation due to peripheral hormonal deficit. The nodules can be single, but more often they are multiple. Most nodules do not capture radioactive contrast and are called cold nodules, whereas those that capture contrast (hot nodules) are

functional. In the hot nodules, the clinical picture is euthyroid in 80% of the cases; only 20% of the cases exhibit hyperthyroidism (*toxic nodular hyperplasia*). The low incidence of malignancy reported in hot nodules usually precludes FNA; nonetheless, it is occasionally associated with papillary carcinoma.[168] The multinodular gland generally has involutional changes and a thickened capsule. Histologic study discloses nodules with dilated follicles lined with flat epithelium (colloid nodules) alternating with others constituted by small follicles lined with tall cylindric cells and with scant colloid (adenomatous nodules). Frequently, regressive phenomena secondary to hemorrhage and ischemic necrosis are seen, such as cholesterol crystals, foamy macrophages and siderophages, fibrosis, calcification and even ossification. Oncocytic transformation can also be observed. The cystic spaces contain necrotic debris, cholesterol crystals and numerous macrophages. The hot nodules usually have medium size follicles lined with a tall columnar epithelium.

Thyroid cancer is more common in patients with nodular goiters than in the general population, with an incidence ranging from 5 to 25%.[160] The histologic carcinoma variant most often associated with nodular goiter is follicular carcinoma.

In *dyshormonogenic nodular hyperplasia* due to an enzymatic defect in the biosynthesis of thyroid hormone, the goiter develops in the first months of life or later, according to the severity of the deficit. Regressive changes are common and the follicles are small and contain little colloid. The follicular cells usually have mitoses and anisokaryosis. Although this picture can be confused with that of follicular carcinoma, the association of the two entities is infrequent.[185]

Cystic nodules represent from 15 to 25% of all thyroid nodules, and it is estimated that FNA cures 20 to 65% of them by evacuating their contents and considerably reduces their size in 30%.[33, 37] The incidence of malignancy is close to 1% of all cystic lesions, and 10% of those treated surgically. The probability of malignant transformation increases progressively with the size of the lesion; therefore, any cystic nodule more than 3 cm in diameter may require surgery.[9]

In nodular goiter, FNA provides material of highly variable characteristics, sometimes bloody or viscous, other times corresponding to a brown translucent fluid typical of a cystic lesion. In *colloidal nodular goiter* the aspiration contains abundant colloid and scant follicular cells, inflammatory cells and hematic material. The colloid can be mixed with blood or form a protein film with folds[1] or a mosaic-like crackling (Fig. 25–4A and B). Less often, they appear as dense spheric clusters (Fig. 25–4D). Follicular cells can be dispersed or grouped into small monolayers or microfollicles. In the monolayers, the cells have a cylindric or cuboid form and a central nucleus. The cytoplasm is pale and the nuclei, more or less homogeneous, exhibit fine chromatin distributed uniformly. The isolated cells have marked cytoplasmic fragility, speckled cytoplasm often being seen, as well as intracytoplasmic vacuoles and bare, hyperchromatic nuclei (Fig. 25–5A). Some specimens contain Hürthle cells, isolated or in monolayers,

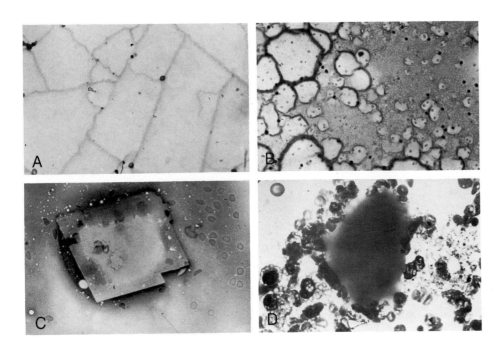

FIGURE 25–4. Nodular goiter. *A,* Cracked colloid forming a mosaic pattern (May-Grünwald-Giemsa; ×100). *B,* Abundant colloid forming irregular foldings of different sizes and sparse cellular component (May-Grünwald-Giemsa; ×100). *C,* Cholesterol crystal (May-Grünwald-Giemsa; ×100). *D,* Dense inspissated colloid surrounded by an aggregate of macrophages (May-Grünwald-Giemsa; ×400).

mixed with the usual follicular cells and with cells of characteristics intermediate between follicular and Hürthle cells.

In *adenomatous nodules,* aspiration specimens exhibit little colloid and numerous follicular cells that are arranged mainly in monolayers and follicles. Three-dimensional clusters are also observed and, more rarely, papillary structures (Fig. 25–5B). As in colloidal nodules, Hürthle cells can be found. Although the nuclear pleomorphism of the follicular cells is usually mild, it can be intense and accompanied by prominent nucleoli.[52] Because of the lack of cytologic criteria for differentiating true neoplastic follicular cell proliferation, surgical excision of the hypercellular nodules is advisable.

In almost all nodular goiters, the aspiration yields diverse inflammatory cells. Macrophages are almost constantly present and have vacuolated cytoplasm and hemosiderin or lipofuchsin granules or both. The nucleus is vesicular and central or excentric (Fig. 25–6A). On occasion, the macrophages have lengthened forms and nuclei with marked pleomorphism. The nuclear changes can become so intense as to suggest a diagnosis of anaplastic carcinoma. The follicular cells can demonstrate vacuolar cytoplasmic degeneration, making them indistinguishable from macrophages (Fig. 25–6B). Few lymphocytes and neutrophils are seen. Although the nuclei of the lymphocytes and follicular cells are different, when the latter are bare and hyperchromatic they cannot be differentiated from lymphocyte nuclei. Sometimes, goiters with degenerative changes exhibit giant multinucleate cells, calcified par-

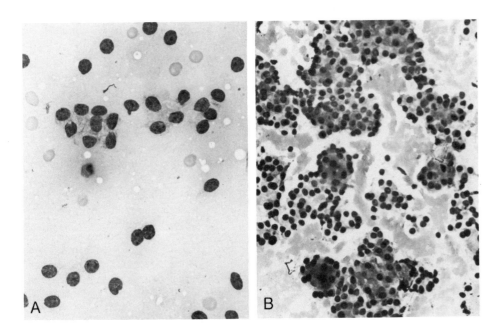

FIGURE 25–5. Nodular goiter. *A,* Colloid nodule. Uniform follicular cells both singly and forming monolayered cluster. Cell boundaries are not discernible. Notice bare lymphocyte-like nuclei in background of thin colloid (May-Grünwald-Giemsa; ×400). *B,* **Adenomatoid nodule**. Abundant follicular cells forming follicles. The nuclei are small, uniform and contain evenly distributed chromatin (May-Grünwald-Giemsa; ×250).

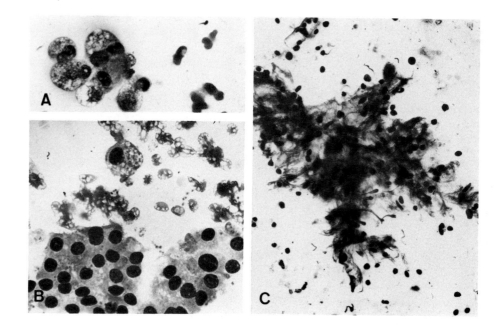

FIGURE 25–6. Regressive changes in **nodular goiter**. *A*, Cluster of thyroid macrophages with vacuolated cytoplasm (May-Grünwald-Giemsa; ×400). *B*, Degenerated follicular cells with cytoplasmic vacuoles and thyroid phagocytes (May-Grünwald-Giemsa; ×400). *C*, Fragment of hyalinized stroma with bare nuclei (May-Grünwald-Giemsa; ×100).

ticles, cholesterol crystals (see Fig. 25–4C), fragments of connective tissue and active fibroblasts (Fig. 25–6C).

The cytologic picture of *toxic nodular hyperplasia* is similar to that observed in Graves's disease[46, 132] and basically consists of numerous follicular cells with signs of hyperstimulation and scant colloid. In patients treated with antithyroid drugs, the cytology can be confused with that of a neoplasm because of the cellularity and marked nuclear variations.[46] In contrast, the cytologic picture of a hot nodule in euthyroid patients is that of a benign nodular colloidal lesion.[108]

Aspirations from *cystic nodules* yield a variable amount of liquid that can be blood-stained, dark brown or transparent yellow. The smears contain few follicular cells, which have degenerative changes, and abundant macrophages. Although the majority of cystic lesions of the thyroid are benign, they eventually develop follicular or papillary carcinomas.[9, 65, 74] Other cystic lesions of the neck that should be considered in the differential diagnosis of thyroid cysts are thyroglossal and branchial cysts and cystic lymph node metastases of papillary carcinoma.

In aspiration specimens of *dyshormonogenic nodular hyperplasia* (congenital hypothyroidism) and in histologic studies, the cytology is usually confused with that of follicular neoplasm owing to the scant colloid, wealth of follicular cells arranged in groups and follicles and marked anisokaryosis.[46]

FOLLICULAR NEOPLASIA

The cytologic diagnosis of follicular tumors (adenoma and carcinoma) is difficult because the criteria do not rest fundamentally on cellular characteristics but on other aspects, such as capsular or vascular invasion and metastases at a distance.[55, 121, 195] Although it has been said that certain morphometric and cyto-

metric data permit the separation of adenomas and well-differentiated follicular carcinomas,[20–22, 60, 103, 117, 176, 198] in practice this is not feasible; therefore, the use of generic labels such as "follicular proliferation" or "follicular neoplasm"[46, 49, 53, 61, 100, 112–116, 123, 152, 184] and surgical excision of the tumor are recommended.

Follicular adenoma is a benign encapsulated tumor that shows evidence of follicular differentiation.[77] Generally, it is a solitary cold nodule that corresponds to a lesion that can reach 10 cm in diameter. Follicular adenoma often has central involuted areas similar to those seen in goiters. Microscopically, the follicular cells have a uniform aspect and can be arrayed in follicles, trabeculae and solid nests. In accordance with the architectural pattern and the cellular characteristics, the following histologic varieties are recognized: normofollicular (simple), macrofollicular (colloid), microfollicular (fetal), trabecular and solid (embryonic), hyalinizing trabecular, toxic (functional), atypical, clear-cell, Hürthle cell, mucus-producing signet ring cell and adipose cell with struma metaplasia.[77, 149]

Of special interest in the differential diagnosis are hyalinizing trabecular adenoma, atypical adenoma and toxic adenoma.

Hyalinizing trabecular adenoma is constituted by polygonal, oval and fusiform cells arranged in solid nests or trabeculae separated by connective tracts with marked hyalinization of the perivascular stroma. Although the general structure of the tumor brings to mind medullary carcinoma, the tumoral cells are similar to those of papillary carcinoma because they contain cytoplasmic nuclear inclusions and nuclei with longitudinal folds.[28]

Atypical adenoma is an encapsulated, highly cellular tumor with numerous bizarre nuclei and scant mitotic figures,[104] which has been considered as a follicular carcinoma *in situ* because it lacks the vascular and capsular invasion typical of follicular carcinoma.[91]

Toxic adenoma is an infrequent lesion that manifests

as a hot nodule and generally courses with mild hyperthyroidism.

Histologically, these are composite lesions consisting of follicles lined with tall cylindric cells and signs of colloid resorption, sometimes tending to form papillary structures.[142] Although the existence of total encapsulation, compression of adjacent parenchyma and uniformity in the internal structure have been reported as being differential signs of adenoma, the distinction with adenomatoid nodules is not always possible because these findings are inconstant.

Follicular carcinoma is a malignant tumor that shows follicular differentiation and lacks the diagnostic signs of papillary carcinoma.[77] It represents 15% of thyroid carcinomas.[195] In areas of endemic goiter or with iodine deficit, it is the most common variant of thyroid carcinoma.[40, 190] Follicular carcinoma occurs above all in women over 30 years. It appears as a slowly growing mass that tends to metastasize by blood to distant organs, usually bone and lung.[195] Two well-defined anatomoclinical forms are known: encapsulated, or microinvasive, with little tendency to metastasize, and a very invasive form with marked vascular invasion and a tendency to metastatic dissemination. The mean 10-year survival rates of the two types of tumor are about 85% and 50%, respectively.[55, 195] Follicular carcinoma can have a follicular (micro-, macro- or normofollicular) or trabecular pattern. The cells generally show scant or moderate nuclear atypia, and the criteria for malignancy rely on demonstration of capsular or vascular invasion, or metastases at a distance.[55, 121, 195] Two other cytologic varieties are the Hürthle cell and clear cell carcinomas.[77]

Poorly differentiated thyroid carcinoma (insular carcinoma) seems to represent an intermediate tumor between differentiated follicular cell carcinoma (follicular carcinoma and papillary carcinoma) and anaplastic carcinoma.[26] It is a highly invasive neoplasm that has abundant necrotic foci. The tumoral cells have a variable degree of pleomorphism and tend to be arrayed into solid, well-defined nests. The prognosis is much more somber than that of extremely invasive follicular carcinoma, and insular carcinoma demonstrates regional lymphatic invasion more frequently.

Generally, in the usual *follicular adenomas and well-differentiated follicular carcinomas* (microfollicular and solid trabecular), the cytologic picture is similar. The aspiration specimen is rich in follicular cells and has little or no colloid. The follicular cells are arranged in small three-dimensional clusters with a certain syncytial aspect, forming loose monolayers and microfollicular structures. Although the presence of isolated cells is a constant finding, their number is relatively small. In general, the follicular cells are monomorphic. The cytoplasm is pale, with poorly defined limits, and the nucleus is round and excentric. The chromatin is finely granular and the nucleolus is uniform and unobtrusive (Fig. 25–7). On occasion, the nuclei have marked anisokaryosis, hyperchromasia and prominent nucleolus. Exceptionally, nuclei with cytoplasmic inclusions have been reported.[62]

Among the cytologic findings suggestive of well-differentiated follicular carcinoma are increased cellularity, scant tendency to form microfollicles, numerous isolated cells, increased nuclear diameter and prominent nucleolus or macronucleolus.[11, 91, 97, 100, 101, 114, 128] Miller and associates[128] and Kini[91] report that by using several of these criteria, 70 to 82% of the follicular carcinomas can be diagnosed.

Difficulties appear when an attempt is made to correlate the cytologic findings of follicular proliferation with the biologic behavior. Colloidal follicular carcinomas (normo- and macrofollicular) exhibit aspiration material with follicular cells arranged in loose monolayers and forming follicles, together with abundant colloid, the aspect being similar to that of colloidal goiter. This differential diagnosis is complicated still more in neoplasms that, like goiters, have regressive

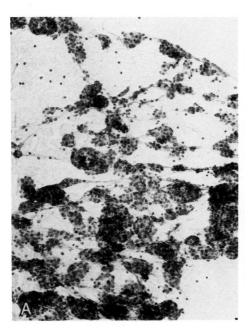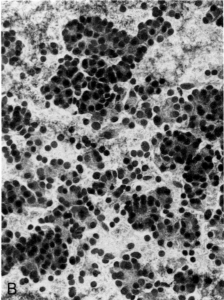

FIGURE 25–7. *A,* **Follicular adenoma**. Tissue fragments with follicular pattern. Nuclei are round and uniform in size and shape. Colloid is absent in the background (Papanicolaou; ×100). *B,* **Well-differentiated follicular carcinoma**. Tissue fragments with follicular pattern and numerous isolated cells. Nuclei are round and enlarged in size (Papanicolaou stain; ×250).

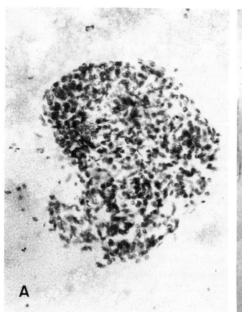

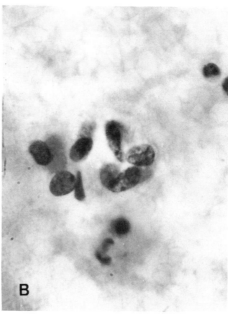

FIGURE 25–8. Hyalinizing trabecular adenoma. *A,* Tissue fragment with smooth external contour and three-dimensional configuration (Papanicolaou; ×100). *B,* Detail showing oval nuclei with nuclear grooves (Papanicolaou; ×1000).

changes. On the other hand, there are adenomas with smears that show marked cellularity and nuclear pleomorphism, which can lead to a cytologic diagnosis of malignancy. This is the case of the so-called atypical adenoma and hyalinizing trabecular adenoma. In specimens of *atypical adenoma* the cells have little cohesiveness and are arranged forming three-dimensional clusters. The nuclei have anisokaryosis and discrete irregularities but conserve a finely granular chromatinic pattern and lack a macronucleolus. Fusiform and pleomorphic cells are often identified.[103] Material from *hyalinizing trabecular adenoma* contains a moderate number of cells arranged in irregular clusters. The cells are oval or elongated. The cytoplasm has poorly defined margins and sometimes has a filamentous aspect. Occasionally, cells are arranged in a parallel curved

pattern that seems to irradiate from a hyaline and acellular center. Nuclei are oval or elliptic, contain bland chromatin and often have nuclear folds and cytoplasmic inclusions (Fig. 25–8).[63]

The cytologic picture of *toxic adenoma* is similar to that described previously in Graves's disease and toxic nodular goiter.

Poorly differentiated follicular carcinoma does not present problems of differential diagnosis with adenoma and nodular goiter, because the signs of malignancy are marked. Usually hypercellularity is seen with a notable loss of cellular cohesion, necrosis with cellular debris and absence of colloid. The nuclei exhibit anisokaryosis, irregular contour, thick-grain chromatin and prominent nucleolus[91, 114] (Fig. 25–9).

The differential diagnosis of follicular neoplasm in-

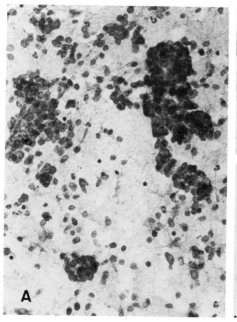

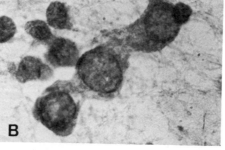

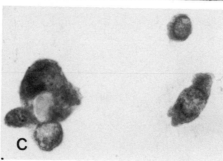

FIGURE 25–9. Poorly differentiated follicular carcinoma. *A,* Low power view showing numerous isolated cells and syncytial type of tissue fragment (Papanicolaou; ×250). *B,* The follicular cells contain enlarged round to oval nuclei with coarse granular chromatin and a single micronucleus (Papanicolaou; ×1000). *C,* Detail showing a cluster of follicular cells delineating a follicle (Papanicolaou; ×1000).

cludes adenomatous hyperplasia, papillary carcinoma of follicular pattern and parathyroid adenoma and carcinoma. It has been suggested that the best differential criterion between goiter and follicular neoplasm is the architecture, because the presence of three-dimensional clusters of follicular cells with overlapping nuclei is usually an almost constant finding in follicular proliferation.[91, 97]

HÜRTHLE CELL NEOPLASIA (ONCOCYTIC NEOPLASMS)

The biologic behavior and the rationale for considering these lesions (adenoma and carcinoma) as a distinctive clinicopathologic entity are debated.[19, 66, 68, 77, 121, 150, 180] However, cytologically, they represent a well-defined diagnostic category.[46, 91, 94, 100, 101, 114]

Hürthle cell tumors constitute 5% of thyroid tumors. Independent of their benign or malignant nature, they are solid, homogeneous, brown and with frequent regressive areas. The cells are arrayed in follicles, cords or solid masses. Oncocytic change seems to be a secondary phenomenon that occurs in both adenomas and in follicular and papillary carcinoma.[66, 77, 121] The frequency of malignant transformation and the biologic aggressiveness of the oncocytic tumors is superior to that observed in other differentiated follicular cell tumors.[66, 150]

Aspirations are usually very cellular, with little or no colloid. In general, the cells show little cohesiveness and can be dispersed, or form loose monolayers, or even three-dimensional clusters of follicular structure. The general aspect of the smear is monomorphic, because almost all the tumoral cells have similar cytoplasmic and nuclear features. The number of ordinary follicular cells is usually fairly scarce. The Hürthle cells are polygonal, large and more or less uniform, with granular eosinophilic cytoplasm and well-defined margins. The nucleus is large, generally excentric and sometime pleomorphic. The nucleolus is prominent and cherry red in color (Fig. 25–10). Although no cytologic[46, 83, 115] or cytometric[19, 59] criteria permit a clear separation between adenoma and carcinoma of the Hürthle cells, some signs help to establish a diagnosis of malignancy, such as hypercellularity, presence of syncytia, predominance of isolated cells, increase in nucleocytoplasmic ratio, nuclear pleomorphism, nuclear membrane irregularities, nuclear cytoplasmic inclusions and multiple nucleolus or cherry-red macronucleolus.[91, 94] By applying several of these criteria, a diagnostic precision of 60% can be achieved.[91]

Eventually, the tumors can demonstrate central ischemic necrosis after FNA, leaving a thin peripheral ring of tumoral tissue. This phenomenon is much more common in Hürthle cell tumors than in any other thyroid neoplasm.[92]

The differential diagnosis is made fundamentally with benign lesions that contain Hürthle cells (nodular goiter, Hashimoto's thyroiditis, Graves's disease and with papillary and medullary carcinomas. The most important cytologic data that suggest that a lesion is a Hürthle cell tumor are the monomorphic aspect of the smear, the exiguous cellular cohesiveness, the presence of macronucleoli and the absence of lymphocytic infiltrates and filamentous cellular debris. It has been reported that the Hürthle cells in Hashimoto's thyroiditis possess more pleomorphism than that observed in malignant neoplasm.[46, 91] Likewise, it has also been reported that the Hürthle cells contain nuclear-cytoplasmic inclusions,[181] but this finding should not be considered as a sign of papillary carcinoma with oncocytic transformation.

As occurs with thyroid follicular proliferation and parathyroid tumors, the oncocytic varieties of these tumors cannot be differentiated on the basis of cytology; immunocytochemical techniques are needed.

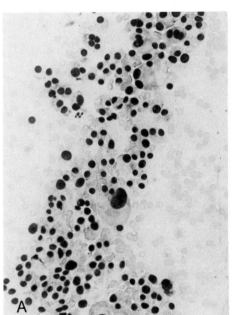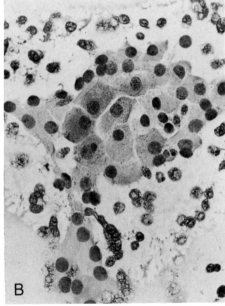

FIGURE 25–10. Hürthle cell neoplasm. *A,* Monomorphic cell population of Hürthle cells forming loosely cohesive sheets. There is marked anisonucleosis (May-Grünwald-Giemsa; ×250). *B,* Hürthle cells are large oval to polygonal cells, with abundant granular cytoplasm and well-defined contours. Nuclei are slightly excentric and contain fine granular chromatin. Colloid is absent (Papanicolaou; ×400).

PAPILLARY CARCINOMA

This is a malignant epithelial tumor that forms papillary and follicular structures and exhibits characteristic nuclear changes.[77] Papillary carcinoma is the most common histologic variant of thyroid carcinoma,[195] and it is the thyroid tumor most often associated with irradiation of the head and neck. It is commonly diagnosed in adolescent and younger females.[119, 194, 195] The proportion of multicentric tumors varies between 20 and 80%, depending on the extension of the thyroid examination.[15] The tumor has a notable propensity to lymphatic dissemination. In more than 50% of the patients, regional cervical lymph nodes are affected at the time of surgery. Although metastatic spread, particularly to the lung and bones, occurs in approximately 10% of the cases, the global 10-year survival is 80%.[120, 186, 195]

The tumor usually appears as a cold nodule, with or without palpable lymph nodes. In 20% of cases, the first sign is a metastatic cervical lymph node in the absence of a palpable mass in the neck.[27] This is designated *occult carcinoma (microcarcinoma)* and is a lesion less than 1 cm in diameter that is usually found post-mortem or in surgical pieces from Graves's disease, nodular goiter and Hashimoto's thyroiditis. Microcarcinoma's course is almost always asymptomatic, but it occasionally appears in the form of local or distant metastases; the prognosis is always excellent.[80] The usual aspect of papillary carcinoma is a firm, grayish, nonencapsulated nodule of 1 to 5 cm in diameter. Approximately 10% of cases correspond to *encapsulated papillary carcinoma* that has developed over a previous adenoma.[27, 157]

Most papillary carcinomas are composed, at least in part, by papillary structures centered around a connective vascular axis covered with a single row of tumoral cells. In a third of the cases, the central axis contains inflammatory cells (lymphocytes and macrophages), and in almost half, psammoma bodies.[54, 99] The nuclei of the tumoral cells are oval shaped with an irregular contour; they tend to overlap, but no true stratification exists. The nuclear membrane is reinforced, and the nucleoplasm is hypochromatic (optically clear, bare, pale or ground-glass nuclei). Nuclei with cytoplasmic inclusions and longitudinal folds are often seen. The nucleolus is generally small and excentric. The pale or bare nuclei are artifacts that are only seen in paraffin-included sections. Although none of these cytologic features is pathognomonic of papillary carcinoma, their association is fairly representative of this tumoral variety.[120] The cytoplasm of the papillary carcinoma cells is abundant, and produce mild eosinophilia, amphophilia or oncocytic changes may occur. Sometimes areas of squamous metaplasia are identified.[27]

A special histologic form of papillary carcinoma with a prognosis similar to that of the typical form is the *follicular variant*. This lesion is easily confused with follicular adenoma and carcinoma, and its diagnosis depends on recognition of the cytologic features of papillary carcinoma, because papillary structures are generally absent.[31] Another form, with a less favorable prognosis, is *diffuse sclerosing papillary carcinoma*. This lesion affects one or both thyroid lobes and consists of multiple foci of papillary carcinoma immersed in a fibrous stroma with lymphoid infiltration. Frequently, the cells have squamous metaplasia, and numerous psammoma bodies are visible.[186] Other peculiar and less common variants are *oncocytic papillary carcinoma, clear cell papillary carcinoma, tall cell papillary carcinoma and solid papillary carcinoma.*[27, 75, 87, 186]

Aspirations of papillary carcinoma have a peculiar cytologic picture with abundant cells and scant colloid. Cells are arranged into papillary structures or monolayers with digitiform projections or are dispersed. The papillary structures can have varied morphology and dimensions. Occasionally, large tissue fragments with prominent vascular networks and frequent digitiform projections are seen (Fig. 25–11A). In contrast, in other instances, the cellular fragments are spheric, with smooth contour and palisading of nuclei (Fig. 25–11B), or they constitute syncytial structures with abundant overlapping nuclei. Isolated cells are generally few in number; when they predominate, the diagnosis of papillary carcinoma should be made with care because the cytologic features may be similar to those of medullary carcinoma.[81, 127] Individually, papillary carcinoma cells are larger than those of follicular proliferations; they have a polygonal contour with well-defined margins and a central nucleus.

The cytoplasm, generally abundant, can be of variable density. Sometimes it is dense and homogeneous, recalling the cells of squamous metaplasia, or it is granular, as in cells with oncocytic transformation (Fig. 25–11C). At other times, particularly in cystic forms, it contains numerous vacuoles. The nuclei are oval, moderately polymorphic and discretely hypochromatic with the Papanicolaou technique and hyperchromatic with May-Grünwald-Giemsa. The chromatin is finely granular, and the nucleolus is generally small and unobtrusive. The optically clear or ground-glass nuclei so characteristic of the histologic sections are not noted in the smears.[43, 129] Nonetheless, nuclear cytoplasmic inclusions and longitudinal folds are often identified (Fig. 25–12A). Nuclear cytoplasmic inclusions are present in more than 5% of the cells in 90% of cases.[32, 43, 153, 173] They are characterized by a precise contour and a density and texture similar to those of cytoplasm.

The longitudinal nuclear folds, which are particularly prominent with the Papanicolaou technique, can appear as multiple longitudinal furrows or superficial notches, giving the nucleus a lobed appearance.[162] The nuclear folds are usually identified in isolated cells and in monolayers, being more difficult to recognize in tissue fragments because of nuclear overlap. The coexistence of longitudinal folds and nuclear inclusions in the same nucleus is very improbable.[43, 67] Although the nuclear features are important for the diagnosis of papillary carcinoma, when seen in the proper context, they are not constant or specific. Nuclear inclusions are cited in thyroid disease, in both primary tumors (anaplastic carcinoma, medullary carcinoma, follicular neoplasm, hyalinizing trabecular adenoma, Hürthle

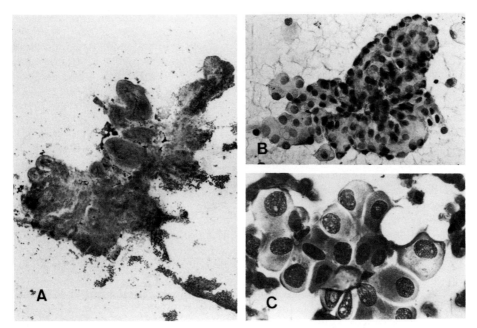

FIGURE 25–11. Papillary carcinoma. *A,* Tissue fragment with complex branching pattern. Some appear monolayered, and another has a syncytial pattern (May-Grünwald-Giemsa; ×50). *B,* Single papillary tissue fragment with smooth contour and palisading of nuclei (May-Grünwald-Giemsa; ×100). *C,* Group of loosely cohesive cells with features of Hürthle cells (May-Grünwald-Giemsa; ×1000).

cell carcinoma) and secondary tumors (metastases of renal carcinoma), and in nontumoral lesions (Hashimoto's thyroiditis).[46, 53, 62, 95, 107, 181, 199] Although nuclear folds are more constant than nuclear inclusions,[95, 162] they have also been reported in other entities, such as follicular adenoma, follicular carcinoma, nodular goiter, Hashimoto's thyroiditis and medullary carcinoma.[30, 43, 67, 153] Nonetheless, the following tetrad of nuclear features is of diagnostic value in papillary carcinoma: large hypochromatic nucleus, small nucleo-

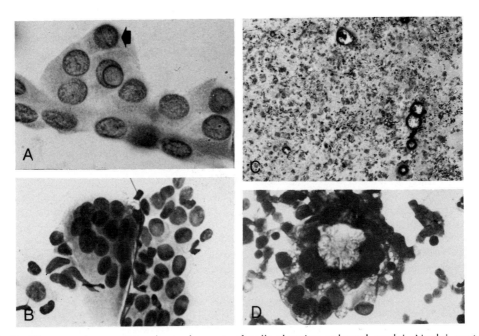

FIGURE 25–12. Papillary carcinoma. Monolayered group of cells showing enlarged nuclei. Nuclei contain fine granular chromatin and occasionally show intranuclear cytoplasmic inclusion and linear grooves (Papanicolaou; ×1000). *B,* Detail showing a multinucleated foreign body–type giant cells close to a monolayer of tumor cells (May-Grünwald-Giemsa; ×400). *C,* Low power view showing several psammomas bodies in a background with numerous lymphocytes (May-Grünwald-Giemsa; ×100). *D,* Detail showing a psammoma body "decorated" by tumor cells (May-Grünwald-Giemsa; ×450).

lus, nuclear folds and intranuclear cytoplasmic inclusions.[91]

The colloid in papillary carcinoma is scant but fairly characteristic; it is viscous and appears as threads of irregular thickness.[115] Although foamy macrophages and cellular detritus are found in most papillary carcinomas, they are particularly abundant in encapsulated and cystic forms.

Multinucleate cells are not constant findings, but they are sometimes abundant. Their presence should be evaluated in the general context of the aspiration to avoid confusion with other entities having giant cells (Fig. 25–12B).[81] Lymphoid cells are often part of the picture of papillary carcinoma and should be evaluated in conjunction with the presence of epithelial cells to avoid confusion with Hashimoto's thyroiditis. Psammoma bodies are observed in a small number of cases.[43, 85, 153, 162] These calcified structures of concentric laminas measure about 100 μ, stain dark blue with May-Grünwald-Giemsa and red with Papanicolaou stains and are found within the papillary formations or surrounded by a single row of tumoral cells (see Fig. 25–12C and D). Psammoma bodies are not specific of papillary carcinoma of the thyroid, because they have also been described in other lesions, such as toxic diffuse goiter and Hashimoto's thyroiditis.[48]

In *papillary carcinoma with a follicular pattern,* the aspiration specimen frequently exhibits syncytial fragments with occasional follicular structures, similar to those seen in follicular proliferation. Its diagnosis rests on the identification of the nuclear features of papillary carcinoma, for which smears stained with Papanicolaou or hematoxylin-eosin are particularly useful. The nuclear hypochromatism, fine-grain chromatin, cytoplasmic folds and inclusions and moderate nuclear polymorphism are much more evident with these stains than with May-Grünwald-Giemsa.[82, 127]

In *diffuse sclerosing papillary carcinoma,* a dense lymphocytic inflammatory component is particularly prominent, together with monolayers of squamous metaplasic cells and numerous psammoma bodies (see Fig. 25–12C).

In *cystic papillary carcinoma,* aspiration yields abundant brown fluid with numerous hemosiderin-laden macrophages and neoplastic cells. This tumor should always be suspected in cystic lesions of more than 3 cm diameter that contain fluid rich in follicular cells or in cysts that remain palpable after evacuation. Taking into account that the lymph node metastases of papillary carcinoma should eventually also undergo cystic transformation, the differential diagnosis should include other nonthyroid lesions that course with a cystic morphology (metastases of epidermoid carcinoma and branchial cyst).

The differential diagnosis of papillary carcinoma must be made with non-neoplastic lesions (intrathyroid lesions, nodular hyperplasia, Hashimoto's thyroiditis) and neoplastic lesions (oncocytic tumors, follicular carcinoma, medullary carcinoma). Likewise, it must be kept in mind that papillary carcinoma can coexist with other pathologies and certain clinical, radiologic and cytologic discrepancies can appear.[13]

MEDULLARY CARCINOMA

This is a malignant tumor consisting of cells that have parafollicular differentiation.[77] Its incidence ranges from 12 to 17% of all thyroid carcinomas.[154] In contrast to the other varieties of differentiated carcinoma (papillary and follicular), thyroid medullary carcinoma does not show any predilection for sex or age. It can appear sporadically or as a familial disease with a dominant autosomal inheritance. In the familial form it can appear as an isolated lesion or in conjunction with other endocrinal neoplasms constituting the type II multiple endocrinal neoplasm syndrome (MEN). In MEN IIA, the thyroid lesion (carcinoma or C cell hyperplasia) is associated with pheochromocytoma and hyperparathyroidism. The IIB form is accompanied by pheochromocytoma, mucosal neuromas, intestinal ganglioneuromatosis and Marfan's habitus.[167]

This tumor is usually small, clearly delimited, almost never encapsulated and exhibits a predilection for the superior poles of the thyroid lobes. In familial cases the lesions are multicentric, and they originate from microscopic hyperplasia foci.[4, 77] In the classic histologic picture of medullary carcinoma, cells are arrayed in an organoid pattern into nests and cords. The connective struma often contains amyloid. Cells are generally polygonal or fusiform and contain uniform, round or oval nuclei and granular, amphophilic or eosinophilic cytoplasm. In the cytoplasm, calcitonin and many other substances have been found (e.g., katacalcin, somatostatin, chromogranin, adrenocorticotropic hormone, serotonin, bombesin, glucagon, neurotensin, catecholamines, insulin, carcinoembryonic antigen.[4] Numerous histologic varieties have been described in accordance with the predominant cell type, gross features and histochemical properties.[4]

Sporadic tumors appear after 40 years of age and evidence a slowly progressive growth curve with early metastases in cervical lymph nodes, liver and bone. In familial forms, which represent 15 to 30% of all medullary carcinomas, the clinical presentation is much earlier. The prognosis is related to the form of clinical presentation and the disease stage.[154]

The cytologic picture of medullary carcinoma varies widely from one case to another. The classic polygonal and fusiform cell varieties are the most common and those most easily recognized. The aspiration generally contains abundant blood and numerous dispersed cells. Loose monolayers or three-dimensional cell clusters are seen less often (Fig. 25–13). The isolated cells have well-defined margins and vary notably in form and size. Marked cellular polymorphism is usually evident, with round, oval, triangular, polygonal and fusiform cells (Fig. 25–13A). The cytoplasm is moderately dense and eosinophilic and occasionally contains granules that stain metachromatically red with the May-Grünwald-Giemsa technique (Figs. 25–14A and C).[115] Although these cytoplasmic granules have diagnostic value, they are not pathognomonic, having been described in follicular tumors, anaplastic carcinoma and metastatic carcinoma of the breast.[46, 111, 115] Moreover, they are not seen in all cases or in all cells.[175] The

FIGURE 25–13. Medullary carcinoma. *A*, Cellular smear showing isolated cells and a loosely cohesive group of cells. The cells varied notably in shape: round, oval, cuboidal, spindle and plasmacytoid (Papanicolaou; ×250). *B*, Isolated cells and syncytial type of tissue fragment composed of uniform round to oval cells. (May-Grünwald-Giemsa; ×200).

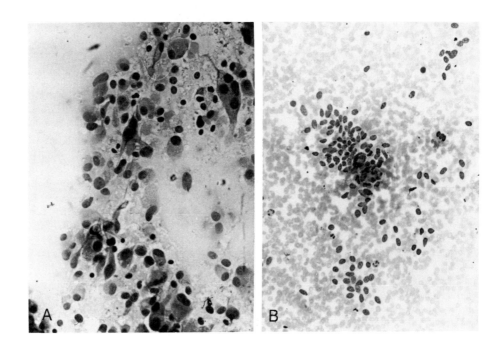

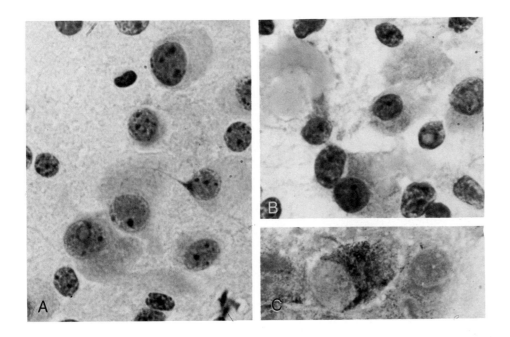

FIGURE 25–14. Medullary carcinoma. *A*, Plasmacytoid isolated cells. The nuclei are round to oval and contain coarse granular chromatin with several nucleoli (May-Grünwald-Giemsa; ×1000). *B*, Detail showing a globular, pale, aggregate of extracellular amyloid (Papanicolaou; ×1000). *C*, Detail showing intracytoplasmic fine granules (May-Grünwald-Giemsa; ×1000).

nuclei are usually oval, moderately pleomorphic, with coarse granular chromatin and one or two small nucleoli (Figs. 25–14A and B).

Binucleate or multinucleate cells are sometimes seen. The excentric situation of the nucleus gives the cell a certain plasmacytic appearance (see Fig. 25–14A). Occasionally, nuclear cytoplasmic inclusions similar to those of papillary carcinoma are observed.[96, 155] In some cases, a dense amorphic material is found that stains similarly to colloid. It demonstrates a characteristic birefringence of the amyloid when stained with Congo red and examined under polarized light (see Fig. 25–14B). Exceptionally, reports have been made of melanin pigment in the cytoplasm of tumoral cells[90] and intracytoplasmic vacuoles suggestive of mucus production.[114]

The differential diagnosis should be established fundamentally with Hürthle cell tumor, papillary carcinoma and anaplastic carcinoma, particularly in cases that exhibit a monomorphic cellular population. The most characteristic findings to support the diagnosis of medullary carcinoma are abundant isolated cells with marked variations in size and form, plasmacytic-like cells and presence of metachromatic cytoplasmic granules. In case of doubt, ultrastructural and histochemical studies should be made of the aspiration material,[146, 155] because both methods provide definitive information.

ANAPLASTIC CARCINOMA

This highly malignant tumor consists partly or totally of undifferentiated cells.[77] Anaplastic carcinoma represents 10% of all thyroid carcinomas[25, 195] and is the most aggressive neoplasm of this gland: more than 85% of patients die within a year of diagnosis.[5] This carcinoma occurs above all in older women (average age 65 years), and it is exceptional in patients under 50 years.[25] In 80% of cases a previous history of "goiter" due to nodular hyperplasia, follicular adenoma, papillary carcinoma or follicular carcinoma is evident; less frequently, anaplastic carcinoma develops on a Hürthle or a medullary carcinoma.[25, 137] The disease is usually manifested by rapid thyroid enlargement, regional lymphadenopathy, dyspnea, dysphonia, dysphagia and pain. Visceral metastases are common and primarily affect the lung and liver.[5, 25]

The tumor is generally large and fleshy, with extensive areas of necrosis. Three basic types of anaplastic cells (fusiform, giant and squamous) can coexist in different proportions, without the predominance of one type over another having any prognostic significance.[25] The fusiform cells are arrayed in compact fascicles in such a way that the lesion can be confused with fibrosarcoma, hemangiopericytoma and malignant fibrohistiocytoma. Giant cells (uninucleate or multinucleate) often coexist with a neutrophilic inflammatory infiltrate. This histologic picture brings to mind those of malignant inflammatory fibrohistiocytoma and angiosarcoma. The squamous cell type suggests nonkeratinizing epidermoid carcinoma. Regardless of the cell type, all the anaplastic carcinomas have marked nuclear pleomorphism, numerous atypical mitoses, frequent and extensive areas of necrosis and elevated capacities for local infiltration and vascular invasion. Immunohistochemistry and electron microscopy can help in the differential diagnosis with primitive sarcomas and in establishing the histogenic origin of the tumor.[25, 85] In almost 10% of cases, a differentiated neoplastic component is discovered (follicular, papillary or medullary tumor).

The cytologic picture depends on the histologic type. In most cases, the lesion consists of giant or mixed cells (giant and fusiform cells). Aspiration yields numerous tumoral cells on a background rich in necrotic debris and hematic material. The tumoral cells vary widely in form and size and are usually dispersed;

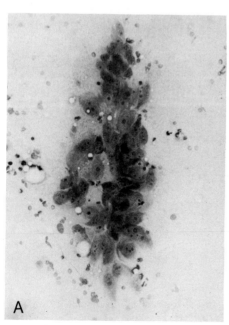

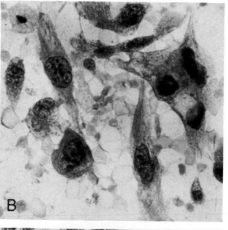

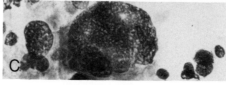

FIGURE 25–15. Anaplastic carcinoma. *A,* Tissue fragment formed by large ovoid pleomorphic cells with enlarged nuclei and prominent nucleoli (May-Grünwald-Giemsa; ×450). *B,* Isolated fusiform cells with extremely pleomorphic nuclei (Papanicolaou; ×1000). *C,* Detail showing a giant polygonal pleomorphic cell (May-Grünwald-Giemsa; ×1000).

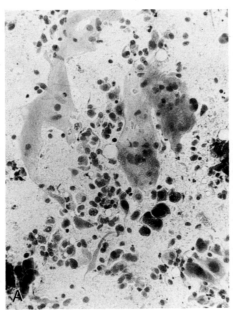 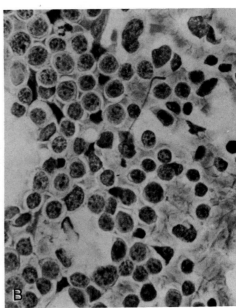

FIGURE 25–16. *A,* **Anaplastic carcinoma with osteoclast-like cells**. Isolated pleomorphic, round polygonal and spindle cells intermingled with large cells with numerous, relatively small and uniform nuclei (Papanicolaou; ×250). *B,* **Primary lymphoma of the thyroid**. Monomorphic cell population of isolated cells (Papanicolaou; ×450).

nonetheless, some monolayers and three-dimensional clusters can also be found (Fig. 25–15A). The cytoplasm can be densely granular or contain tiny vacuoles. The nucleus, round or oval, often has an irregular contour and can even be multiple (Fig. 25–15B and C). The nuclear membrane is thick, and the coarse-grain chromatin is irregularly distributed. The nucleoli are always prominent, and mitoses are frequent and atypical.[46, 114, 156] Nuclear cytoplasmic inclusions can be seen occasionally. Tumoral cells may be accompanied by an inflammatory component rich in neutrophils, with images of neutrophilic cannibalism. Sometimes multinucleate giant cells of the osteoclastic type are visible (Fig. 25–16A).[193]

The differential diagnosis must be made with other primary lesions (suppurative thyroiditis, Quervain's thyroiditis, fibrosarcoma, Hürthle cell carcinoma, medullary carcinoma, malignant hemangioendothelioma and epidermoid carcinoma) and with metastases of giant-cell carcinoma of the lung, melanoma and renal carcinoma. Nonetheless, the clinical findings are always significant (a rapidly growing nodule that usually develops over a previous thyroid lesion, in an older person) as are the characteristics of the aspiration specimen (epithelial cells with marked pleomorphism and nuclear atypias, a tendency to dissociation and a dirty inflammatory and hematic background). The diagnostic precision is practically 100%.[84, 156] On rare occasions, aspiration specimens from nodular goiters reveal pleomorphic, fusiform and hyperchromatic cells, which can lead to a false diagnosis of fusiform cell carcinoma. Alternatively, the cytologic picture of malignant hemangioendothelioma is quite similar to that of anaplastic carcinoma, the only differential feature being the presence of erythrophagocytosis in the vascular tumor.[46]

LYMPHOMA

Primitive thyroid lymphomas are tumors that have been underestimated in frequency because they overlap partially with the category of small-cell anaplastic carcinoma. Nonetheless, in two series their incidence is estimated at 2 to 8% of malignant tumors of the thyroid.[23, 35] Because 15% of patients with systemic malignant lymphomas present with thyroid involvement,[161] systemic disease must be excluded before diagnosing primitive thyroid lymphoma. Almost all cases correspond to non-Hodgkin's lymphoma[41] and affect mainly patients of advanced age, predominantly females. The tumor occurs as a firm cervical mass of rapid evolution (weeks), that in a third of the cases is accompanied by compressive symptoms (hoarseness, dyspnea, dysphagia, obstruction of the vena cava). In some patients (15%), lymphoma appears after a lengthy history of goiter. Often the presentation is accompanied by regional lymph node enlargement.[7, 23, 196] The association with lymphocytic thyroiditis of the adjacent thyroid parenchyma is frequent, and it is thought that this form of thyroiditis increases the risk of thyroid lymphoma.[78]

The tumor is grayish, fleshy and firm, does not exhibit necrosis and tends to affect both lobes. Its growth is diffuse, with frequent necrosis of isolated cells, a tendency to capsular and extrathyroid infiltration, invasion and destruction of follicles and invasion of vascular walls. With rare exceptions[47] the lymphoid proliferation corresponds to a monoclonal growth of B lymphocytes, preferably of the large, undivided cell type.[7, 23, 35, 166, 196] At present, primitive lymphoma of the thyroid is considered as a lymphoid neoplasm of mucus surfaces,[17] which explains why the gastrointestinal tract is often simultaneously involved as well as the tendency of the tumor to remain localized for a long time. The mean 5-year survival is 50%.

The aspiration specimen lacks epithelial cell clusters, consisting of a monomorphic population of lymphoid cells that are dispersed or, sometimes, arranged into lymphoid tissue fragments. The nuclei of the tumoral cells are uniform and occupy most of the cytoplasm. The nuclear details vary according to the type of lymphoma (Fig. 25–16B). The background is dirty, with tumoral diathesis[46, 73, 118]; karyorrhexis, mitoses and lymphoglandular bodies are common. The immunocytochemical study generally reveals a monoclonal immune phenotype.[179]

The differential diagnosis must be made with Hashimoto's thyroiditis and with diffuse small-cell carcinoma of the thyroid. The findings that enable Hashimoto's thyroiditis to be diagnosed are mixed cellularity (reactive), polyclonal lymphoid population, lymphoid clusters corresponding to germinal centers and Hürthle cell clusters. At present, the so-called small-cell anaplastic carcinomas are considered generally as primitive lymphomas, metastatic and medullary carcinomas being less common. True, diffuse, anaplastic carcinomas of follicular small cells are exceptional. To typify these entities, immunocytochemical techniques or electron microscopy is required.[150]

THYROID METASTASES

These are less important clinically, although they are more common than primary malignant lesions. The majority correspond to the direct spread of primary neoplasms of the pharynx, larynx and upper third of the esophagus. The thyroid is affected by hematogenous dissemination, usually in the advanced stages of carcinoma of the breast, lung or kidney, or of melanoma, leukemia and lymphoma. It is generally a postmortem finding; nonetheless, on occasions it can be clinically manifest.[161, 191] Fine needle aspiration is of interest in all these circumstances. Although the appearance of the thyroid nodule in the case of disseminated tumoral disease usually is suggestive of metastatic disease, this is not always so. Approximately 71% of the thyroid nodules of patients with extrathyroid cancer correspond to benign lesions, 17% to metastatic tumors, 6% to primary tumors, 1% to Hashimoto's thyroiditis and the rest to lesions with inconclusive cytologic findings.[50]

The aspiration fluid is usually fairly cellular, with tumoral diathesis; the malignant cells are mixed with normal follicular cells.[98] Only on rare occasions can the histologic type be determined from the smear study; in the majority of cases it is necessary to exclude primitive anaplastic carcinoma because dispersed cells or groups of cells without signs of specific differentiation are found. The presence of melanin and bile or the disposition of the cells in molds or in palisades is suggestive of an origin in the melanic cells, liver, lung or intestine. Some metastatic tumors (clear cell carcinoma of the kidney, anaplastic carcinoma of the lung) can bring to mind primary carcinomas, particularly clear cell follicular carcinomas and anaplastic carcinomas.[29, 50, 98, 105, 106, 109]

DIAGNOSTIC ACCURACY

The cytologic study of the smears should be carried out keeping in mind the clinical features and other ancillary data of the patient. Certain lesions (e.g., colloidal goiter) yield specimens with few cells and abundant colloid. Although, in principle, this material would be considered as cytologically useless, it is concordant with the clinical impression. Approximately 2 to 15% of the smears are unsatisfactory for evaluation.[17] This percentage increases greatly when the aspiration is performed in an unskilled manner.[182]

In satisfactory smears, the tumor is diagnosed as benign in more than 60% of cases, malignant in 5% and suspicious in the rest. Approximately 20% of the suspicious cases followed by surgery correspond to malignant tumors.[17] In the cytologic diagnosis an attempt should be made to establish the type of lesion. Sufficient criteria to do so exist in the majority of entities, the exceptions being follicular proliferation and Hürthle cell tumors. New technologies have been developed to resolve this problem, but both planimetry and DNA quantitation present overlapping values on comparing benign with malignant lesions.[18, 20–22, 59, 60, 86, 117, 176, 198] Immunocytochemical techniques have been very useful in identifying primary and metastatic lesions but not in differentiating benign from malignant lesions.[44, 58, 139, 146, 179]

The predictive value of FNA of the thyroid changes notably if lesions that look suspicious for malignancy are categorized as malignant: the true incidence of malignant disease increases, but the percentage of patients who undergo surgery ranges from 15 to 40%.[61, 70, 152] On the other hand, by initially categorizing suspicious cases as positive, sensitivity is enhanced but specificity falls. On the other hand, if tumors that look suspicious for malignancy are not included in the malignant group, the sensitivity falls sharply and specificity rises.

References

1. Abele JS, Miller TR: Fine needle aspiration of the thyroid nodule: clinical application. *In* Endocrine Surgery of the Thyroid and Parathyroid Glands. Edited by OH Clark. St. Louis, CV Mosby Co, 1985.
2. Aggarwal SK, Jayaran G, Kakar A, Goel GD, Prakash R, Pant S: Fine needle aspiration cytologic diagnosis of the solitary cold thyroid nodule. Comparison with ultrasonography radionuclide perfusion study and xeroradiography. Acta Cytol 33:41–47, 1989.
3. Akerman M, Tennvall J, Biŏklund A, Måatensson H, Mŏller T: Sensitivity and specificity of fine needle aspiration cytology in the diagnosis of tumors of the thyroid gland. Acta Cytol 29:850–855, 1985.
4. Albores-Saavedra J, Livolsi VA, Williams ED: Session IV: Medullary carcinoma. Semin Diagn Pathol 2:137–146, 1985.
5. Aldinger KA, Samaan NA, Ibanez M, Hill CR, Jr: Anaplastic carcinoma of the thyroid. Cancer 41:2267–2275, 1978.

6. Al-Sayer HM, Krukowski ZH, Williams VMM, Matherson NA: Fine needle aspiration cytology in isolated thyroid swellings: A prospective two-year evaluation. Br Med J 290:1490–1492, 1985.

7. Anscombe AM, Wright DH: Primary malignant lymphoma of the thyroid—a tumor of mucosa-associated lymphoid tissue: review of seventy-six cases. Histopathology 9:81–97, 1985.

8. Arean VM, Klein RE: Amyloid goiter. Am J Clin Pathol 36:341–355, 1961.

9. Aschcraft MW, VanHerle AJ: Management of thyroid nodules. II. Scanning techniques, thyroid suppressive therapy, and fine needle aspiration. Head Neck 3:297–322, 1981.

10. Astorga R, Garcia-Canton JA, Rodriguez JR, Leal A, Acosta D, Gavilan I, Garcia-Luna PP, Leon J: Fiabilidad de la punción aspiración con aguja fina en el bocio nodular no tóxico. Correlación con los hallazgos quirúrgicos y punciones repetidas. Med Clin (Barc) 85:733–736, 1985.

11. Atkinson B, Ernst CS, Livolsi VA: Cytologic diagnoses of follicular tumors of the thyroid. Diagn Cytopathol 2:1–3, 1986.

12. Attwood HD, Dennett X: A black thyroid and minocycline treatment. Br Med J 2:1109–1110, 1976.

13. Beecham JE: Coexistent disease as a complicating factor in the fine needle aspiration diagnosis of papillary carcinoma of the thyroid. Acta Cytol 30:435–438, 1986.

14. Berger SA, Zonszein J, Villamera P, Mittaman N: Infectious diseases of the thyroid gland. Rev Infect Dis 5:108–122, 1983.

15. Black BM, Virk TA, Woolner LB: Multicentricity of papillary adenocarcinoma of the thyroid: Influence on treatment. J Clin Endocrinol Metab 20:130–135, 1960.

16. Blum M: Managing the solitary thyroid nodule: Role of needle biopsy. Ann Intern Med 87:375–377, 1977.

17. Boey J, Hsu C, Collins RJ: False-negative errors in fine-needle aspiration biopsy of dominant thyroid nodules. A prospective follow-up study. World J Surg 10:623–630, 1986.

18. Bondeson L, Bondeson AG, Lindholm K, Ljungberg O, Tibblin S: Morphometric studies on nuclei in smears of fine needle aspirates from oxyphilic tumors of the thyroid. Acta Cytol 27:437–440, 1983.

19. Bondeson L, Bondeson AG, Ljungberg O, Tibblin S: Oxyphil tumors of the thyroid. Follow-up of 42 surgical cases. Am Surg 196:677–680, 1981.

20. Boon ME, Baak JPA: Thyroid: morphometry for the preoperative diagnosis of follicular adenoma and carcinoma. In A Manual of Morphometry in Diagnostic Pathology. Berlin, Springer-Verlag, 1983.

21. Boon ME, Löwhagen T, Cardozo PL, Blonk DI, Kurver PJH, Baak JPA: Computation of preoperative diagnosis probability for follicular adenoma and carcinoma of the thyroid on aspiration smears. Anal Quant Cytol 4:1–5, 1982.

22. Boon ME, Löwhagen T, Willems JS: Planimetric studies on fine needle aspirates from follicular adenomas and follicular carcinomas of the thyroid. Acta Cytol 24:145–148, 1980.

23. Burke JS, Butler JJ, Fuller LM: Malignant lymphoma of the thyroid. A clinicopathological study of 35 patients including ultrastructural observations. Cancer 39:1587–1602, 1977.

24. Caplan RH, Wester S, Kisken WA: Fine needle aspiration biopsy of solitary thyroid nodules. Effect on cost of management, frequency of thyroid surgery, and operative yield of thyroid malignancy. Minn Med 69:189–192, 1986.

25. Carcangiu ML, Steeder T, Zampi G, Rosai J: Anaplastic thyroid carcinoma. A study of 70 cases. Am J Clin Pathol 83:135–158, 1985.

26. Carcangiu ML, Zampi G, Rosai J: Poorly differentiated ("insular") thyroid carcinoma. A reinterpretation of Langhans' "wuchernde struma." Am J Surg Pathol 8:655–668, 1984.

27. Carcagiu ML, Zampi G, Rosai J: Papillary thyroid carcinoma: a study of its many morphologic expressions and clinical correlates. Part 1. Pathol Annu 20: 1–44, 1985.

28. Carney JA, Ryan J, Goellner JR: Hyalinizing trabecular adenoma of the thyroid gland. Am J Surg Pathol 11:583–591, 1987.

29. Chacho MS, Greenebaum E, Moussouris MF, Schreiber K, Koss LG: Value of aspiration cytology of the thyroid in metastatic disease. Acta Cytol 31:705–712, 1987.

30. Chan JKC, Saw D: The grooved nucleus a useful diagnostic criterion of papillary carcinoma of the thyroid. Am J Surg Pathol 10:672–679, 1986.

31. Chen KTK, Rosai J: Follicular variant of thyroid papillary carcinoma. A clinicopathological study of six cases. Am J Surg Pathol 1:123–130, 1977.

32. Christ M, Haja J: Intranuclear cytoplasmic inclusions (invaginations) in thyroid aspirations, frequency and specificity. Acta Cytol 23:327–331, 1979.

33. Clark OH, Okerlund MD, Cavalieri RR, Greenspan FS: Diagnosis and treatment of thyroid, parathyroid, and thyroglossal duct cyst. J Clin Endocrinol Metabol 48:983–988, 1979.

34. Cole WH, Majarakis JD, Slaughter DP: Incidence of carcinoma of the thyroid in nodular goiter. J Clin Endocrinol Metabol 9:1007–1011, 1949.

35. Compagno J, Oertel JE: Malignant lymphoma and other lymphoproliferative disorders of the thyroid gland: a clinicopathologic study of 245 cases. Am J Clin Pathol 74:1–11, 1980.

36. Cornillot M, Granier AM, Houcke M: La cytopunction des lésions thyroidiennes; confrontations anatomopathologiques; lesions benignes (600 observations). Arch Anat Cytol Pathol 26:219–228, 1978.

37. Crile G Jr: Treatment of thyroid cyst by aspiration. Surgery 59:210–212, 1966.

38. Crile G Jr, Hawk WA: Aspiration biopsy of the thyroid nodules. Surg Gynecol Obstet 136:241–247, 1973.

39. Crockford PH, Bain GO: Fine needle aspiration biopsy of the thyroid. Cancer Med Assoc J 110:1029–1032, 1974.

40. Cuello C, Correa P, Eisenberg H: Geographic pathology of thyroid carcinoma. Cancer 23:230–239, 1969.

41. De Baets M, Vanholder R, Eeckhaut W, Hamers J, Van Hove W, De Roose J, Vermeulen A, Roels H, Van Breda Vriesman PJC: Primary Hodgkin's disease of the thyroid. Report of a case demonstrated by immunoperoxidase-positive Reed-Sternberg cells. Acta Haematol 65:54–59, 1981.

42. DeGroot LJ, Reilly M, Pinnamenemi K, Refetoff S: Retrospective and prospective study of radiation induced thyroid disease. Am J Med 74:852–862, 1983.

43. Deligeorgi-Politi H: Nuclear crease as a cytodiagnostic feature of papillary thyroid carcinoma in fine-needle aspiration biopsies. Diagn Cytopathol 3:307–310, 1987.

44. Domagala W, Lasota J, Wolska H, Lubinski J, Weber K, Osborn M: Diagnosis of metastatic renal cell and thyroid carcinoma by intermediate filament typing and cytology of tumor cells in fine needle aspirates. Acta Cytol 32:415–421, 1988.

45. Doniach I: The thyroid gland. In Systemic Pathology, 2nd ed, vol 4. Edited by W St C Symmers. New York, Churchill Livingstone, 1978.

46. Droesse M: Cytological Aspiration Biopsy of the Thyroid Gland. F.K. Stuttgart, Schattauer Verlag, 1980.

47. Dunbar JA, Lyall MH, MacGillivray JB, Potts RC: T-cell lymphoma of the thyroid. Br Med J 2:679, 1977.

48. Dugan JM, Atkinson BF, Avitabile A, Schimmel M, Livolsi A VA : Psammoma bodies in fine needle aspirate of the thyroid in lymphocytic thyroiditis. Acta Cytol 31:330–334, 1987.

49. Einhorn J, Franzen S: Thin-needle biopsy in the diagnosis of the thyroid disease. Acta Radiol 58:321–336, 1962.

50. Fanning TV, Katz RL: Evaluation of thyroid nodules in cancer patients. Acta Cytol 30:572, 1986.

51. Farbota LM, Calandra DB, Lawrence AM, Paloyan E: Thyroid carcinoma in Graves's disease. Surgery 98:1148–1153, 1985.

52. Feichter GE, Gderttler K: Age-related nuclear size variability of thyrocytes in thyroid aspirates. Anal Quant Cytol 5:75–78, 1983.

53. Frable WJ: The thyroid. In Thin Needle Aspiration Biopsy. Major Problems in Pathology, vol 14. Edited by JL Bennington. Philadelphia, WB Saunders, 1983.

54. Franssila KD: Is the differentiation between papillary and follicular thyroid carcinoma valid? Cancer 32:853–864, 1973.

55. Franssila KO, Ackerman LV, Brown CL, Hedinger CE: Session II: Follicular carcinoma. Semin Diagn Pathol 2:101–122, 1985.

56. Friedman M, Shimaoka K, Getaz P: Needle aspiration of 310 thyroid lesions. Acta Cytol 23:194–203, 1979.

57. Friedman H, Shimaoka K, Rao V, Tsakada Y, Gavilan M,

Tamura K: Diagnosis of chronic lymphocytic thyroiditis (nodular presentation) by needle aspiration. Acta Cytol 25:513–522, 1981.

58. Gal R, Aronof A, Gertzmann H, Kessler E: The potential value of the demonstration of thyroglobulin by immunoperoxidase techniques in fine needle aspiration cytology. Acta Cytol 31:713–716, 1987.

59. Galera-Davidson H, Bibbo M, Bartels PH, Dytch HE, Puls JH: Correlation between automated DNA ploidy measurements of Hürthle-cell tumors and their histopathologic and clinical features. Anal Quant Cytol Histol 8:157–166, 1986.

60. Gershengorn MC, McClung MR, Chu EW, Weintraub BD, Robbins J: Fine needle aspiration cytology in the preoperative diagnosis of thyroid nodules. Ann Intern Med 87:265–269, 1977.

61. Gharib H, Goellner JR, Zinsmeister AR, Grant CS, Van Heerden JA: Fine needle aspiration biopsy of the thyroid. The problem of suspicious cytologic findings. Ann Intern Med 101:25–28, 1984.

62. Glant MD, Berger EK, Davey DD: Intranuclear cytoplasmic inclusions in aspirates of follicular neoplasms of the thyroid. A report of two cases. Acta Cytol 28:576–580, 1984.

63. Goellner JR, Carney JA: Cytologic features of fine-needle aspirates of hyalinizing trabecular adenoma of the thyroid. Am J Clin Pathol 91:115–119, 1989.

64. Goellner JR, Gharib H, Grant CS, Johnson DA: Fine needle aspiration cytology of the thyroid: 1980 to 1986. Acta Cytol 31:587–590, 1987.

65. Goellner JR, Johnson DA: Cytology of cystic papillary carcinoma of the thyroid. Acta Cytol 26:797–799, 1982.

66. Gonzalez-Campora R, Herrero-Zapatero A, Lerma E, Sanchez F, Galera H: Hürthle cell and mitochondrion-rich cell tumors. A clinicopathologic study. Cancer 57:1154–1163, 1986.

67. Gould E, Watzak L, Chamizo W, Albores-Saavedra J: Nuclear grooves in cytologic preparations. A study of the utility of this feature in the diagnosis of papillary carcinoma. Acta Cytol 33:16–20, 1989.

68. Gundry SR, Burney RE, Thompson NW, Lloyd R: Total thyroidectomy for Hürthle cell neoplasm of the thyroid. Arch Surg 118:529–532, 1983.

69. Gutteridge DH, Orell SR: Non-toxic goiter: diagnostic role of aspiration cytology, antibodies and serum thyrotrophin. Clin Endocrinol 9:505–514, 1978.

70. Hamaker RC, Singer MI, DeRossi RV, Shockley WW: Role of needle biopsy in thyroid nodules. Arch Otolaryngol 109:225–228, 1983.

71. Hamburger JI, Gharib H, Melton LJ III, Goellner JR, Zinsmeister AR: Fine needle aspiration biopsy of the thyroid nodules: impact on thyroid practice and cost of care. Am J Med 73:381–384, 1982.

72. Hamburger JI, Miller JM, Kini SR: Clinical-pathological evaluation of thyroid nodules. *In* Handbook and Atlas. Minnesota, Southfield, 1979.

73. Hamburger JI, Miller JM, Kini SR: Lymphoma of the thyroid. Ann Intern Med 99:685–693, 1983.

74. Hammer M, Wortsman J, Folse R: Cancer in cystic lesions of the thyroid. Arch Surg 117:1020–1023, 1982.

75. Hawk WA, Hazard JB: The many appearances of papillary carcinoma of the thyroid. Cleve Clin Q 43:207–216, 1976.

76. Hawkins F, Bellido D, Bernal C, Rigopoulou D, Ruiz-Valdepeñan MP, Lazaro E, Perez-Barrios A, Agustin P: Fine needle aspiration biopsy in the diagnosis of thyroid cancer and thyroid disease. Cancer 59:1206–1209, 1987.

77. Hedinger C, Williams ED, Sobin LH: Histological typing of thyroid tumours. World Health Organization. International Histological Classification of Tumours, 2nd ed. Berlin, Springer-Verlag, 1988.

78. Holm LE, Blombren H, Löwhagen T: Cancer risks in patients with chronic lymphocytic thyroiditis. N Engl J Med 312:601–604, 1985.

79. Hsu CH, Boey J: Diagnostic pitfalls in the fine needle aspiration of thyroid nodules. Acta Cytol 31:699–704, 1987.

80. Hubert JP Jr, Kiernan PD, Bearhs OH, McConahey WM, Woolner LB: Occult papillary carcinoma of the thyroid. Arch Surg 115:394–398, 1980.

81. Hudvegi DF, Heltgren S, Gallagher L: Origin of giant cells from papillary carcinoma of the thyroid: immunologic, enzymatic and ultrastructural aspects of cytopreparations. Acta Cytol 25:742–745, 1981.

82. Hugh JC, Duggan MA, Chang-Poon V: The fine-needle aspiration appearance of the follicular variant of thyroid papillary carcinoma. A report of three cases. Diagn Cytopathol 4:196–201, 1988.

83. Jayaram G: Problems in the interpretation of Hürthle populations in fine needle aspirates from the thyroid. Acta Cytol 27:84–85, 1983.

84. Jayaram G: Fine needle aspiration cytologic study of the solitary thyroid nodule; profile of 308 cases with histologic correlation. Acta Cytol 29:967–973, 1985.

85. Jayaram G, Singh B, Marwaha RK: Graves's disease. Appearance in cytologic smears from fine needle aspirates of the thyroid gland. Acta Cytol 33:36–40, 1989.

86. Joensuu H, Klemi P, Eerola E: DNA aneuploidy in follicular adenomas of the thyroid gland. Am J Pathol 124:373–376, 1986.

87. Johnson TL, Lloyd RV, Thompson MW, Beierwaltes WH, Sisson JC: Prognostic implications of the tall cell variant of papillary thyroid carcinoma. Am J Surg Pathol 12:22–27, 1988.

88. Katz SM, Vickery AL: The fibrous variant of Hashimoto's thyroiditis. Hum Pathol 5:161–170, 1974.

89. Kennedy JS, Thompson JA, Buchanan WM: Amyloid in the thyroid. Quant J Med 43:127–143, 1974.

90. Kimura N, Ishioka K, Miura Y, Sasano N, Takaya K, Mouri T, Kimura T, Nakazato Y, Yamada R: Melanin-producing medullary thyroid carcinoma with glandular differentiation. Acta Cytol 33:61–66, 1989.

91. Kini SR: The thyroid. *In* Guides to Clinical Aspiration Biopsy. Edited by TS Kline. Tokyo, Igaku-Shoin, 1987.

92. Kini SR, Miller M: Infarction of thyroid neoplasms following aspiration biopsy (Abst). Acta Cytol 30:591, 1986.

93. Kini SR, Miller JM, Hamburger JI: Problems in the cytologic diagnosis of the cold thyroid nodule in patients with lymphocytic thyroiditis. Acta Cytol 25:506–512, 1981.

94. Kini SR, Miller JM, Hamburger JI: Cytopathology of Hürthle cell lesions of the thyroid gland by fine needle aspiration. Acta Cytol 25:647–652, 1981.

95. Kini SR, Miller JM, Hamburger JI, Smith MJ: Cytopathology of papillary carcinoma of the thyroid by fine needle aspiration. Acta Cytol 24:511–521, 1980.

96. Kini SR, Miller JM, Hamburger JI, Smith MJ: Cytopathologic features of medullary carcinoma of the thyroid. Arch Pathol Lab Med 108:156–159, 1984.

97. Kini SR, Miller JM, Hamburger JI, Smith MJ: Cytopathology of follicular lesions of the thyroid gland. Diagn Cytopathol 1:123–132, 1985.

98. Kini SR, Smith MJ, Miller JM, Hamburger JI: Fine needle aspiration cytology of tumors metastatic to the thyroid gland (Abst). Acta Cytol 26:743, 1982.

99. Klinck GH, Winship T: Psammoma bodies and thyroid cancer. Cancer 12:656–662, 1959.

100. Kline T: The thyroid. *In* Handbook of Fine Needle Aspiration Biopsy Cytology, 2nd ed. Edited by TS Kline. New York, Churchill Livingstone, 1988.

101. Koss LG, Woykes S, Olszewski W: The thyroid. *In* Aspiration Biopsy. Cytologic Interpretation and Histologic Bases. Tokyo, Igaku-Shoin, 1984.

102. Kung IJM, Yuen RWS: Fine needle aspiration of the thyroid. Distinction between colloid nodules and follicular neoplasms using cell blocks and 21-gauge needles. Acta Cytol 33:53–60, 1989.

103. Lang W, Atay Z, Georgii A: Die cytologische unterscheidung follikulären tumoren in der Schilddrüse. Virchows Arch (Pathol Anat) 378:199–211, 1978.

104. Lang W, Georgii A, Stauch G, Kienzle E: The differentiation of atypical adenoma and encapsulated follicular carcinoma in the thyroid glans. Virchow Arch (Pathol Anat) 385:125–141, 1980.

105. Lasser A, Rothman JG, Calahia VJ: Renal cell carcinoma metastatic to the thyroid. Aspiration cytology and histologic findings. Acta Cytol 29:856–858, 1985.

106. Lennard TWJ, Wadehra V, Farndon JR: Fine needle aspiration biopsy in diagnosis of metastates to thyroid gland. J Royal Soc Med 77:196–197, 1984.

107. Lew W, Orell S, Henderson DW: Intranuclear vacuoles in nonpapillary carcinoma of the thyroid. Acta Cytol 28:581–586, 1984.

108. Liel Y, Zirkin HJ, Sobel R: Fine needle aspiration of the hot thyroid nodule. Acta Cytol 32:866–867, 1988.

109. Linsk JA, Franzen S: Aspiration cytology of metastatic hypernephroma. Acta Cytol 28:250–254, 1984.

110. Lipton RF, Abel MS: Aspiration biopsy of the thyroid in the evaluation of thyroid dysfunction. Am J Med Sci 208:736–742, 1944.

111. Ljungberg O: Cytologic diagnosis of medullary carcinoma of the thyroid gland with special regard to the demonstration of amyloid in smears of fine needle aspirates. Acta Cytol 16:253–255, 1972.

112. Löwhagen T: Thyroid. *In* Aspiration Biopsy Cytology. Part 1. Cytology of Supradiaphragmatic organs. Edited by J Zajizek. Basel, S. Karger, 1974.

113. Löwhagen T, Granberg P-O, Lundell G, Skinnari P, Sundbland R, Willems JS: Aspiration biopsy cytology (ABC) in nodules of the thyroid gland suspected to be malignant. Surg Clin North Am 59:3–18, 1979.

114. Löwhagen T, Linsk JA: Aspiration biopsy cytology of the thyroid gland. *In* Clinical Aspiration Cytology, 2nd ed. Edited by J Linsk, S Franzen. Philadelphia, JB Lippincott, 1988.

115. Löwhagen T, Sprenger E: Cytologic presentation of thyroid tumors in aspiration biopsy smears: A review of 60 cases. Acta Cytol 18:192–197, 1974.

116. Löwhagen T, Willems JS, Lundell G, Sundblad R, Granberg PO: Aspiration biopsy cytology in the diagnosis of thyroid cancer. World J Surg 5:61–73, 1981.

117. Luck JB, Mumaew UR, Frable WJ: Fine needle aspiration biopsy of the thyroid. Differential diagnosis by videoplan image analysis. Acta Cytol 26:793–796, 1982.

118. Matsuda M, Sone H, Koyama H, Ishiguro S: Fine needle aspiration cytology of malignant lymphoma of the thyroid. Diagn Cytopathol 3:244–249, 1987.

119. Mazzaferri EL: Thyroid carcinoma following therapeutic and accidental radiation exposure. *In* Special Topics in Endocrinology and Metabolism. Edited by MP Cohen, PP Foa. New York, Alan R Liss, 1981.

120. Mazzaferri EL, Oertel JE: The pathology and prognosis of thyroid cancer. *In* Surgery of the Thyroid and Parathyroid Glands. Edited by EL Kaplan. New York, Churchill Livingstone, 1983.

121. Meissner WA, Warren S: Tumor of the thyroid gland, fascicle 4, 2nd series. *In* Atlas of Tumor Pathology. Washington DC, Armed Forces Institute of Pathology, 1969.

122. Miller JM: Evaluation of thyroid nodules: Accent on needle biopsy. Med Clin North Am 69:1063–1077, 1985.

123. Miller JM, Hamburger JI, Kini SR: Diagnosis of thyroid nodules. Use of fine-needle aspiration and needle biopsy. JAMA 241:481–484, 1979.

124. Miller JM, Hamburger JI, Kini SR: The impact of needle biopsy on the preoperative diagnosis of thyroid nodules. Henry Ford Hosp Med J 28:145–148, 1980.

125. Miller JM, Hamburger JI, Kini SR: Needle biopsy of the thyroid: An update. Surg Rounds 72–81, January, 1984.

126. Miller JM, Kini SR, Hamburger JI: Needle biopsy diagnosis of papillary thyroid carcinoma. Cancer 48:989–993, 1981.

127. Miller JM, Kini SR, Hamburger JI: Needle biopsy of the thyroid. New York, Praeger Publishers, 1983.

128. Miller JM, Kini SR, Hamburger JI: The diagnosis of malignant follicular neoplasms of the thyroid by needle biopsy. Cancer 55:2812–2817, 1985.

129. Miller TR, Bottles K, Holly E, Friend NF, Abele JS: A stepwise logistic regression analysis of papillary carcinoma of the thyroid. Acta Cytol 30:285–293, 1986.

130. Mizukami Y, Michigishi TI, Hashimoto T, Tonami N, Hisaba K, Matsubara F, Takazakura E: Silent thyroiditis: A histologic and immunohistochemical study. Hum Pathol 19:423–431, 1988.

131. Nilsson G: Nuclear sizes in fine needle aspirates from toxic goiters. Acta Endocrinol 70:273–288, 1972.

132. Nilsson G: Marginal vacuoles in fine needle aspiration biopsy smears of toxic goiters. Acta Pathol Microbiol Scand Sect A 80:289–293, 1972.

133. Nilsson G: Lymphoid infiltration in toxic goiters; studies with fine needle aspiration biopsy. Acta Endocrinol 71:480–490, 1972.

134. Nilsson G: C cells in non-malignant human goiters studied in fine needle aspiration biopsy specimens. Acta Med Scand 191:249–256, 1972.

135. Nilsson LR, Persson PS: Cytological aspiration biopsy in adolescent goiter. Acta Paediatr 53:333–338, 1964.

136. Nilsson G, Söderström N, Telenius-Berg M: Diagnosing thyroid carcinoma. Lancet 2:666–667, 1970.

137. Nishiyama RH, Dunn EL, Thompson NW: Anaplastic spindle cell and giant cell tumors of the thyroid gland. Cancer 30:113–127, 1972.

138. Norton LW, Wangensteen SL, Davis JR, Paplanus SH, Werner SC: Utility of thyroid biopsy aspiration. Surgery 90:700–705, 1982.

139. Ordoñez NG, Katz R, Luna M, Samaan NA: Medullary thyroid carcinoma metastatic to breast diagnosis by fine-needle aspiration biopsy. Diagn Cytopathol 4:254–257, 1988.

140. Orell SR, Sterrett GF, Walters MNI, Whitaker D: The thyroid. *In* Manual and Atlas of Fine Needle Aspiration Cytology. New York, Churchill Livingstone, 1986.

141. Ott RA, Calandra DB, McCall A, Shah KH, Lawrence AM, Paloyan E: The incidence of thyroid carcinoma in patients with Hashimoto's thyroiditis and solitary cold nodules. Surgery 98:1202–1206, 1985.

142. Panke TW, Croxson MS, Parker JW, Carriere DP, Rosoff L, Warner NE: Triiodothyronine-secreting (toxic) adenoma of the thyroid gland. Light and electron microscopic characteristics. Cancer 41:528–537, 1978.

143. Persson PS: Cytodiagnosis of thyroiditis. Acta Med Scand 483:8–100, 1968.

144. Pitts WC, Berry GJ: Marginal vacuoles in metastatic thyroid carcinoma. Diagn Cytopathol 5:200–202, 1989.

145. Ramacciotti CE, Pretorius HT, Chu EW, Barsky SH, Brennan MF, Robbins J: Diagnostic accuracy and use of aspiration biopsy in the management of thyroid nodules. Arch Intern Med 144:1169–1173, 1984.

146. Rastad J, Wilander E, Lindgren PG, Ljunghall S, Stenkvist BG, Akerström G: Cytologic diagnosis of medullary carcinoma of the thyroid by Sevier-Munger silver staining and calcitonin immunocytochemistry. Acta Cytol 31:45–47, 1987.

147. Ravinsky E, Safneck JR: Differentiation of Hashimoto's thyroiditis from thyroid neoplasms in fine needle aspirates. Acta Cytol 32:854–861, 1988.

148. Risgway EC: Clinical evaluation of solitary thyroid nodules. *In* Werner's The Thyroid. A Fundamental and Clinical Text, 5th ed. Edited by SH Ingbar, LE Braverman. Philadelphia, JB Lippincott, 1986.

149. Rosai J: The thyroid gland. *In* Ackerman's Surgical Pathology, 7th ed, vol 1. St. Louis, CV Mosby Co, 1989.

150. Rosai J, Carcagiu ML: Pathology of thyroid tumors. Some recent and old questions. Hum Pathol 15:1008–1012, 1984.

151. Rosen IB, Palmer JA, Bain J, Strawbridge H, Walfish PG: Efficacy of needle biopsy in postradiation thyroid disease. Surgery 94:1002–1007, 1983.

152. Rosen IB, Wallace O, Strawbridge HG, Walfish PG: Reevaluation of needle aspiration cytology in detection of thyroid cancer. Surgery 90:747–756, 1981.

153. Rupp M, Ehya H: Nuclear grooves in the aspiration cytology of papillary carcinoma of the thyroid. Acta Cytol 33:21–26, 1989.

154. Saad MF, Ordoñez NG, Rashid RK, Guido JJ, Hill CS Jr, Hickey RIC, Samaan NA: Medullary carcinoma of the thyroid. A study of the clinical features and prognostic factors in 161 patients. Medicine 63:319–342, 1984.

155. Schäffer R, Müller HA, Pfeiffer V, Orhanns W: Cytologic findings in medullary carcinoma of the thyroid. Pathol Res Pract 178:461–466, 1984.

156. Schneider V, Frable WJ: Spindle and giant cell carcinoma of the thyroid. Acta Cytol 24:184–189, 1980.

157. Schröder S, Bocker W, Dralle H, Kortmann K, Stern C: The encapsulated papillary carcinoma of the thyroid. A morphologic

subtype of the papillary thyroid carcinoma. Cancer 54:90–93, 1984.

158. Schwaegerle SM, Bauer TW, Esselstyn CB: Riedel's thyroiditis. Am J Clin Pathol 90:715–722, 1988.

159. Schwartz AE, Weieburgs HE, Davies TF, Gilbert PL, Friedman EW: The place of fine-needle biopsy in the diagnosis of nodules of the thyroid. Surg Gynecol Obstet 155:54–58, 1982.

160. Selenkow HA, Karp PJ: An approach to diagnosis and therapy of thyroid tumors. Semin Nucl Med 1:461–468, 1971.

161. Shimaoka K, Sokal JE, Pickern J: Metastatic neoplasms in the thyroid gland. Cancer 15:557–565, 1962.

162. Shurbaji MS, Gupta PK, Frost JK: Nuclear grooves: A useful criterion in the cytopathologic diagnosis of papillary thyroid carcinoma. Diagn Cytopathol 4:91–94, 1988.

163. Silverman JF, West RL, Finley JL, Larkin EW, Park HK, Swanson MS, Fore WW: Fine-needle aspiration versus large needle or cutting biopsy in evaluation of thyroid nodules. Diagn Cytopathol 2:25–30, 1986.

164. Silverman JF, West RL, Larkin EW, Park K, Finley JL, Swanson MS, Fore WW: The role of fine-needle aspiration biopsy in the rapid diagnosis and management of thyroid neoplasm. Cancer 57:1164–1170, 1986.

165. Silverman SH, Nussbaum M, Rausen AR: Thyroid nodules in children. A ten-year experience at one institution. Mt Sinai J Med 46:460–463, 1979.

166. Sirota DK, Segal RL: Primary lymphomas of the thyroid gland. JAMA 242:1743–1746, 1979.

167. Sizemore GW, Heath H III, Carney JA: Multiple endocrine neoplasia type 2. Clin Endocrinol Metab 9:299–315, 1980.

168. Sobel RJ, Liel Y, Goldstein J: Papillary carcinoma and the solitary autonomously functioning nodule of the thyroid. Israel J Med Sci 21:878–882, 1985.

169. Söderström N: Puncture of goiters for aspiration biopsy. A preliminary report. Acta Med Scand 144:237–244, 1952.

170. Söderström N: Identification of normal tissue and tumors by cytologic aspiration biopsy. Acta Soc Med 65:53–87, 1958.

171. Söderström N: Fine-needle aspiration biopsy. Stockholm, Almquist och Wiksell, Förlag, 1966.

172. Söderström N: Identification of normal tissue by aspiration cytology. In Clinical Aspiration Cytology. Edited by JA Linsk, S Franzen. Philadelphia, JB Lippincott, 1983.

173. Söderström N, Björklund A: Intranuclear cytoplasmic inclusions in some types of thyroid cancer. Acta Cytol 17:191–197, 1973.

174. Söderström N, Nilsson C: Cytologic diagnosis of thyrotoxicosis. Acta Med Scand 205:263–265, 1979.

175. Söderström N, Telenius-Berg M, Akerman M: Diagnosis of medullary carcinoma of the thyroid by fine-needle aspiration biopsy. Acta Med Scand 197:71–76, 1975.

176. Sprenger E, Löwhagen T, Vogt-Schaden M: Differential diagnosis between follicular adenoma and follicular carcinoma of the thyroid by nuclear DNA determination. Acta Cytol 21:528–530, 1977.

177. Stavric SD, Karanfilski BT, Kalamaras AK, Serafimov NZ, Georgievska BS, Korubin VH: Early diagnosis and detection of clinically non-suspected thyroid neoplasia by the cytologic method. Cancer 45: 340–344, 1980.

178. Suen KC, Quenville NF: Fine needle aspiration biopsy of the thyroid gland: A study of 304 cases. J Clin Pathol 36:1036–1045, 1983.

179. Tani E, Skoog L: Fine needle aspiration cytology and immunocytochemistry in the diagnosis of lymphoid lesions of the thyroid gland. Acta Cytol 33:48–52, 1989.

180. Thompson NW, Dunn EL, Batsakis JG, Nishiyama RH: Hürthle cell lesions of the thyroid gland. Surg Gynecol Obstet 139:555–560, 1974.

181. Thranov I, Francis D, Olsen J: Intranuclear cytoplasmic invaginations in a Hürthle cell carcinoma of the thyroid. Acta Cytol 27:341–344, 1983.

182. Varhaug JE, Segadal E, Heimann P: The utility of fine needle aspiration biopsy cytology in the management of thyroid tumors. World J Surg 5:573–577, 1981.

183. Veith FT, Brooks JR, Grigsby WP, Selenkow HA: The nodular thyroid gland and cancer: a practical approach to the problem. N Engl J Med 270:431–436, 1964.

184. Vickery AL: Needle biopsy pathology. Clin Endocrinol Metab 10:275–293, 1981.

185. Vickery AL: The diagnosis of malignancy in dyshormonogenetic goiter. Clin Endocrinol Metab 10:317–335, 1981.

186. Vickery AL Jr, Cancangiu ML, Johannessen JV, Sobrinho-Simoes M: Papillary Carcinoma: Session I. Semin Diagn Pathol 2:90–100, 1985.

187. Volpe R: The pathogenesis of Graves's disease: an overview. Clin Endocrinol Metab 7:3–29, 1978.

188. Wajda KJ, Wilson MS, Lucas J, Marsh WL: Fine needle aspiration cytology findings in the black thyroid syndrome. Acta Cytol 32:862–865, 1988.

189. Walfish PG, Hazani E, Strawbridge HTG, Miskin M, Rosen IB: A prospective study of combined ultrasonography and needle aspiration biopsy in the assessment of the hypofunctioning thyroid nodule. Surgery 83:474–482, 1977.

190. Williams ED, Doniach I, Bjarnason O, Michie W: Thyroid cancer in an iodine rich area. A histopathological study. Cancer 39:215–222, 1977.

191. Willis RA: The spread of tumors in the human body. London, Butterworth, 1951.

192. Willems JS, Löwhagen T: The role of fine needle aspiration cytology in the management of thyroid disease. Clin Endocrinol Metab 10:267–292, 1981.

193. Willems JS, Löwhagen T, Palombini L: The cytology of a giant cell osteoclastoma like malignant thyroid neoplasm: a case report. Acta Cytol 23:214–216, 1979.

194. Winship T, Rosvoll RV: Thyroid carcinoma in childhood. Final report on a 20-year study. Clin Proc Child Hosp Natl Med Cancer 26:327–348, 1970.

195. Woolner LB, Beahrs OH, Black B, McConahey W, Keating FR: Classification and prognosis of thyroid carcinoma, a study of 885 cases observed in a 30-year period. Am J Surg 102:354–387, 1961.

196. Woolner LB, McConahey WM, Beahrs OH, Black BM: Primary malignant lymphoma of the thyroid. Am J Surg 111:502–523, 1966.

197. Woolner LB, McConahey WH, Beahrs OH: Struma lymphomatosa and related thyroidal disorders. J Clin Endocrinol Metab 19:53–83, 1959.

198. Wright RG, Castles H, Mortimer RH: Morphometric analysis of thyroid cell aspirates. J Clin Pathol 40:443–445, 1987.

199. Zirkin MJ: Follicular adenoma of the thyroid with intranuclear vacuoles and clear nuclei: a case report. Acta Cytol 28:587–592, 1984.

26

Lymph Nodes

Dilip K. Das

As components of peripheral or secondary lymphoid organs, lymph nodes are an important part of the immune system. Because lymph nodes become enlarged in a wide spectrum of diseases, including infection and malignancy, enlarged lymph nodes are a quite common finding in clinical practice. Management of such cases depends on lymph node pathology, which can be studied by collecting material from the lymph node through fine needle aspiration (FNA) or excision biopsy. The simple procedure of needle aspiration of the lymph node possibly dates back to 1904 when Greig and Gray[49] were investigating cases of trypanosomiasis. Nearly two decades later, in 1921, Guthrie[53] systematically performed lymph node aspiration for diagnostic purposes. In 1930, Martin and Ellis[83] published their experience with the technique. Since then FNA of the lymph node has become increasingly accepted and has been described often in the literature.[9, 12, 39, 54, 64, 65, 78, 84, 87, 88, 101, 111]

SAMPLING TECHNIQUES

Clinical history, physical examination, correct performance of FNA and proper handling of the aspirate are the four essential components in the management of patients with lymphadenopathy.[44]

The technique of FNA from lymph nodes may vary depending upon the sites.

Superficial Lymph Nodes

Fine needle aspiration from palpable lymph nodes under direct vision yields an adequate sample in most cases. A few studies claim that ultrasonography helps in the aspiration of nonpalpable superficial lymph nodes in 4 to 18% of cases when confirming the diagnosis of benign, lymphomatous or metastatic lesions.[5, 15]

Deep-Seated Lymph Nodes

Imaging aids such as computed-tomographic (CT) scan, fluoroscopy and ultrasonography have been utilized for the FNA of deep-seated lymph nodes in the abdominal cavity and thorax. Computed tomography–guided aspiration has been performed in abdominal/retroperitoneal lymph nodes by Jeffrey[57] and Bandy and coworkers.[7] Numerous studies have been conducted on the preoperative evaluation of pelvic lymph node metastasis in gynecologic malignancies[86] and urologic malignancies, including bladder and prostatic carcinoma,[13, 47, 48, 94, 95] using bipedal lymphangiography and fluoroscopic-guided fine needle aspiration cytology. Accurate prediction of nodal involvement in these studies resulted in the avoidance of staging lymph node dissection and even radical surgical procedures, such as prostatectomy and cystectomy.

Transbronchial Aspiration

Flexible transbronchial aspiration of mediastinal nodes and transcarinal needle aspiration have been performed as a supplement to bronchoscopic evaluation of neoplastic lung diseases with satisfactory results.[16, 114]

Proper handling of aspirate is very important for subsequent cytodiagnosis. The quantity and the appearance of aspirated material helps to determine if it is representative or if the FNA needs to be repeated. In guided aspiration of deep-seated lymph nodes, rapid staining should be used to determine whether representative material has been obtained. In doing so additional punctures and possible associated complications can be avoided.[23] The quality of aspirated material may also give a clue to the likely diagnosis and to the special staining techniques, if any, to be employed. For example, a necrotic aspirate may suggest necrosis in tuberculous lymph node or in metastatic squamous cell carcinoma; a mucoid aspirate suggests a metastatic mucin-secreting adenocarcinoma and a dark-colored aspirate suggests a metastatic malignant melanoma.

At least two smears, one air dried for May-Grünwald-Giemsa (MGG) and another wet fixed for Papanicolaou stain, should be prepared. Additional smears may be prepared for special staining whenever necessary. Material can also be collected for other special techniques, which are discussed further on in the chapter.

NORMAL LYMPH NODE ANATOMY AND HISTOLOGY

Lymph nodes are organized collections of lymphoreticular tissue in the form of pink-gray kidney-shaped encapsulated organs. They are located at anatomically constant points along the course of lymphatic vessels;

the common sites of distribution for clinical consideration are the cervical, axillary, mediastinal, retroperitoneal, iliac and inguinal regions.

Anatomically a lymph node is divided into an outer cortex and an inner medulla (Fig. 26–1A). The cortex is predominantly a B-dependent area and contains primary and secondary lymphoid follicles. The primary follicles are compact collections of inactive or resting lymphocytes. The secondary follicles, which develop from an antigenic stimulus, show a pale central area of lymphocytes at various stages of differentiation: small and large and cleaved and noncleaved cells. In between these cells can be seen scattered phagocytic histiocytes (starry-sky macrophages) (Fig. 26–1B and C). The central pale area is surrounded by a mantle or corona of small dark-staining lymphocytes.

The large noncleaved cell leaves the germinal center for the interfollicular area, where it is designated as a B immunoblast. The B immunoblast forms plasma cells. The area in between the cortex and medulla is called the paracortical or T-dependent area. The de-

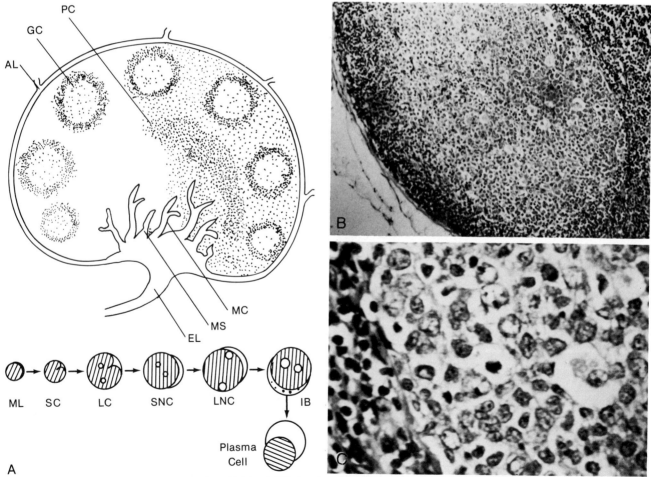

FIGURE 26–1. Structure of a **lymph node.** Diagrammatic representation. B-dependent area showing germinal centers (GC), T-dependent paracortical area (PC) and medulla. (AL = afferent lymphatics; MC = medullary cord; MS = medullary sinus; EL = efferent lymphatic; ML = mature lymphocyte; SC = small cleaved cell; LC = large cleaved cell; SNC = small noncleaved cell; LNC = large noncleaved cell; IB = immunoblast.) *B*, Histology of reactive lymph node showing a secondary reactive follicle (germinal center) (hematoxylin and eosin; ×110). C, Histology of **reactive lymph node.** Higher magnification of a germinal center showing cleaved and noncleaved cells (hematoxylin and eosin; ×440).

velopment of resting T cells into T immunoblasts and activated T cells appears to occur in a manner similar to that of B cells.[81] The medulla contains medullary cords with string-like arrays of both B and T cells, plasma cells and macrophages that converge on the hilus.

CYTOLOGY

A normal lymph node is barely palpable and thus rarely a target for fine needle aspiration cytology (FNAC). Therefore, the cytomorphologic characteristics of cells from a normal lymph node, as described here, are essentially based on the morphology of individual cells as observed in the aspirate from a reactive lymph node (Fig. 26–2). The lymphocytes, plasma cells, histiocytes, mast cells, eosinophils and neutrophils are the various cell types observed. The lymphocytes constitute 87.0 to 99.0%, the plasma cells 0 to 5% and the remainder of the cells 1 to 3% of the total population in the aspirate from a normal lymph node.[42, 79, 113]

Mature Lymphocytes or Resting Lymphocytes

The small, round lymphocytes measure 7 to 9 μm in May-Grünwald-Giemsa–stained smears[60] and 4 to 6 μm in Papanicolaou technique.[63] A thin rim of pale blue cytoplasm is often visible at one edge of the cell. The nuclei are characterized by blocks or clumps of dense chromatin.

Follicular Center Cells

These cells may be cleaved (small and large) or noncleaved (small and large). Lennert[71] has described them as centrocytes and centroblasts. Small cleaved cells (centrocytes) are somewhat larger than small round lymphocytes and possess indented nuclei with fine regular chromatin. Large cleaved cells are about two times the size of small lymphocytes. The nuclei are indented and contain two or more small nucleoli. Noncleaved cells are two to three times larger than small lymphocytes. The chromatin is even and finely granular. Multiple nucleoli are usually found near the nuclear membrane in large noncleaved cells.

Immunoblasts

These are large cells, three times larger than small lymphocytes. The nuclei are round with irregular, finely granular chromatin and one or more excentrically placed nucleoli. The surrounding cytoplasm is abundant and deeply basophilic and often contains cytoplasmic vacuolizations.

Plasma Cells

In plasma cells the nucleus is excentrically placed and possesses densely packed coarse chromatin that may be arranged in a typical cartwheel-like pattern. The cytoplasm is deeply basophilic and contains a paranuclear clear area.

Macrophages

Also described as tingible body cells, germinal center histiocytes and phagocytes, these cells show wide variation in size. In the resting phase, the cells measure 14 to 34 μm in diameter. Those containing phagocytosed fragments of degenerated cells (tingible bodies) may measure up to 50 μm.[79] The nucleus is about 13 μm in diameter and contains evenly distributed reticulated chromatin. One to three small nucleoli may be present. At times such macrophages possess two or more nuclei.

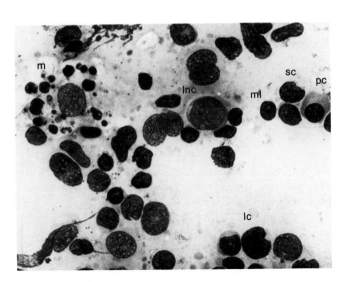

FIGURE 26–2. Lymph node aspirate showing various cell types. (ml = mature small round lymphocytes; sc = small cleaved cell; lc = large cleaved cells; lnc = large noncleaved cells; pc = plasma cell and m = tingible body macrophages.) (May-Grünwald-Giemsa; ×640.)

TABLE 26–1. Causes of Lymphadenopathy

I. Lymphadenitis and hyperplasia
  A. Nonspecific
  B. Specific
    1. Infectious diseases: tuberculosis, leprosy, cat-scratch disease, streptococcal and staphylococcal infections, histoplasmosis, coccidioidomycosis, actinomycosis, cryptococcosis, infectious mononucleosis, AIDS, toxoplasmosis, trypanosomiasis, leishmaniasis and filariasis.
    2. Immunologic disorders and diseases: autoimmune disorders, SLE and rheumatoid arthritis, and prelymphomatous conditions, e.g., AILD.
    3. Miscellaneous diseases (diseases of unknown etiology): sarcoidosis, dermatopathic lymphadenitis.
II. Lymphomas and leukemias
  A. Non-Hodgkin's lymphoma
  B. Plasma cell tumor
  C. Nonlymphoid leukemia
  D. Hodgkin's disease
III. Metastatic neoplasms
  A. Carcinomas
    1. Squamous cell carcinoma
    2. Adenocarcinoma
    3. Anaplastic carcinoma
    4. Carcinoma from specific sites such as kidney, thyroid, breast, salivary gland, liver and testis
  B. Malignant melanoma
  C. Soft tissue and bone tumors
  D. Germ cell tumors

AIDS = acquired immune deficiency syndrome; SLE = systemic lupus erythematosus; AILD = angioimmunoblastic lymphadenopathy.

Other Histocytic Cells

In smears, histiocytes with clear to light eosinophilic cytoplasm and round, vesicular, kidney-shaped, or, at times, epithelioid nuclei may be found singly scattered or in sheets. These cells are called interdigitating cells or epithelioid histiocytes depending on cell morphology.

LESIONS OF LYMPH NODES

As shown in Table 26–1, cytodiagnosis of lymph node aspirate can be grouped under three major categories: lymphadenitis and hyperplasia, lymphomas and leukemias and metastatic neoplasms. Assessment of overall cellularity and pattern of cell arrangement and identification of predominant cell type and background elements constitute the most important components of the microscopic assessment of a lymph node aspirate.[44] The lymph node aspirate should be examined under lower magnification, which will give an impression about cellularity, polymorphic versus monomorphic appearance of cells and presence of specific cell types, such as epithelioid cells, Reed-Sternberg cells and alien cells of a metastatic lesion. It may also help in selecting a specific area for detailed examination under higher magnification.

Lymphadenitis and Hyperplasia

Three cytologic patterns can be described under lymphadenitis and hyperplasia: reactive hyperplasia, suppurative lymphadenitis and granulomatous lymphadenitis.

Reactive Hyperplasia

High cell density, polymorphic cytologic pattern and tingible bodies are the three important characteristics of follicular hyperplasia according to Stani.[110] The smear usually contains lymphocytes at different stages of maturation, a varying number of tingible body macrophages and an increased number of plasma cells (Fig. 26–3). A few neutrophils and eosinophils can be seen. The lymphoid cells consist of small mature lymphocytes, small and large cleaved cells, small and large noncleaved cells and immunoblasts (Fig. 26–4). The ratio is estimated to be 80:20 for small to large cells.[88] Lymphohistiocytic aggregates are also found very frequently in reactive hyperplasia.[92]

Suppurative Lymphadenitis

In the initial phase a mixture of lymphocytes and neutrophils may be seen in the smear. This phase is followed by a florid state in which frank purulent material is aspirated; the smear contains both well-preserved and degenerated neutrophils and cell debris (Fig. 26–5). With organization of the inflammatory exudate, especially in antibiotic-treated cases, the smear contains polymorphs, lymphocytes, plasma cells

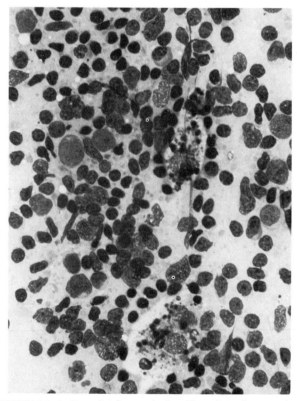

FIGURE 26–3. Reactive hyperplasia of lymph node. Lymphocytes at various stages of differentiation and tingible body macrophages (May-Grünwald-Giemsa; × 400).

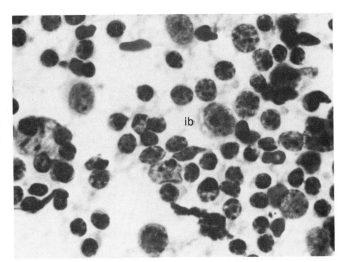

FIGURE 26–4. Reactive hyperplasia. Lymphocytes in various stages of differentiation and immunoblasts (IB) (Papanicolaou; ×1000).

and histiocytes along with cell debris (Fig. 26–6A). This mixed inflammatory exudate may be found in close relationship to a capillary network (Fig. 26–6B).

Granulomatous Lymphadenitis

The characteristic feature is the clustering of epithelioid cells in a lymphoid smear (Fig. 26–7A). The epithelioid cell has an elongated nucleus with fine

granular chromatin and a small nucleolus (Fig. 26–7B). Often, the demarcation between cytoplasm of adjacent cells cannot be discerned. Multinucleated foreign body or Langhans's giant cells with typical

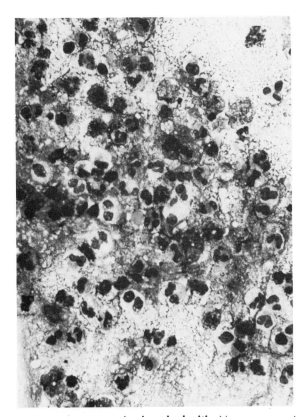

FIGURE 26–5. Suppurative lymphadenitis. Numerous neutrophils and cell debris from a case of tuberculous lymphadenitis. No epithelioid granuloma seen (May-Grünwald-Giemsa; ×400).

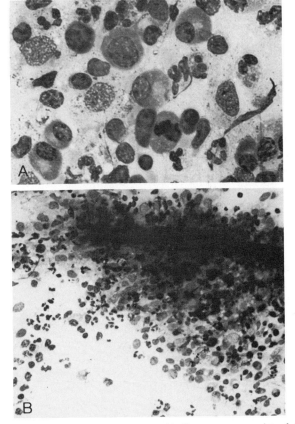

FIGURE 26–6. *A,* Organization of inflammatory exudate following **suppurative lymphadenitis.** A mixture of lymphocytes, neutrophils, plasma cells and histiocytes is seen (May-Grünwald-Giemsa; ×600). *B,* Mixed inflammatory exudate in relation to a capillary in the smear from a lymph node showing **organizing suppurative lymphadenitis** (May-Grünwald-Giemsa; ×400).

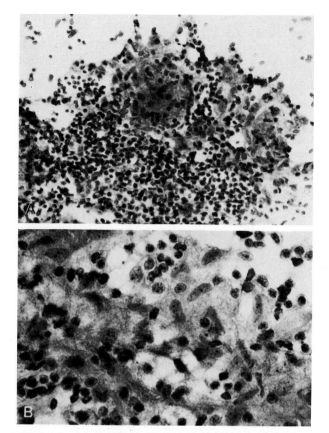

FIGURE 26–7. *A*, Noncaseating epithelioid granuloma in **tuberculous lymphadenitis** (Papanicolaou; ×200). *B*, Higher magnification of **epithelioid cells** having elongated nuclei and small nucleoli. Cytoplasmic outline is indistinct (Papanicolaou; ×400).

peripheral arrangement of nuclei and necrotic material may or may not be present.

These patterns may be nonspecific, e.g., in most of the smears showing reactive hyperplasia. They may also indicate one or more specific diseases that may or may not be infectious. More than one pattern can be observed in some diseases, e.g., tuberculosis.

INFECTIOUS DISEASES

Mycobacterial Infections

Tuberculosis and leprosy are the mycobacterial infections that may affect lymph nodes. The role of FNA in the diagnosis of tuberculous lymphadenitis has been discussed in numerous studies.[6, 100, 105] The cytologic picture in tuberculous lymphadenitis can be divided into three patterns.[35]

1. *Epithelioid granuloma without necrosis.* Groups of epithelioid cells are found along with a variable number of lymphoid cells (Fig. 26–8A). Foreign body or Langhans's giant cells may or may not be present (Fig. 26–8B).
2. *Epithelioid granuloma with necrosis.* In addition to epithelioid cells, the smears contain clumps of pink amorphous cellular debris or necrotic material (Fig.

26–9A). Lymphocytes and Langhans's giant cells may be found. With the initiation of liquefaction in necrotic foci, neutrophils begin appearing in increasing numbers (Fig. 26–9B).
3. *Necrotic material without epithelioid granuloma.* Clumps of amorphous acellular material can be seen. At times liquefied necrotic material with marked polymorphonuclear infiltration gives rise to the observation of suppurative lymphadenitis (see Fig. 26–5).

Acid-fast bacilli (AFB) positivity in aspiration smears of tuberculous lymphadenitis is between 40.6 and 56.4%.[35, 100, 105] In a study by Das and colleagues[35] the AFB positivity in the three aforementioned cellular patterns was 9.1%, 64.7% and 77.4%, respectively. It appears that these groups are similar to the various stages of tissue response described in progressive tuberculous lesions of the lung: formation of epithelioid granuloma, necrosis in granuloma and liquefaction of necrotic foci with dissemination of the disease.[3, 68]

The characteristic cell in lymph node aspirate of lepromatous leprosy is a syncitial histiocyte (Virchow's

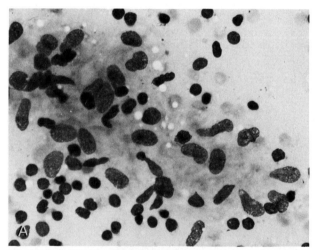

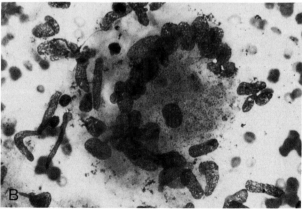

FIGURE 26–8. *A*, **Tuberculous lymphadenitis.** Aspirate from right cervical lymph node in a 25-year-old female shows lymphocytes and a group of epithelioid cells (May-Grünwald-Giemsa; ×400). *B*, **Tuberculous lymphadenitis.** Typical Langhans's giant cells with peripherally arranged nuclei and epithelioid cells. Aspiration from abdominal lymph node (May-Grünwald-Giemsa; ×400).

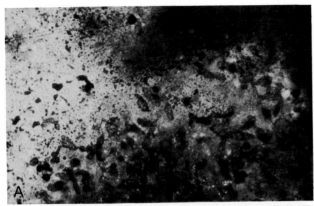

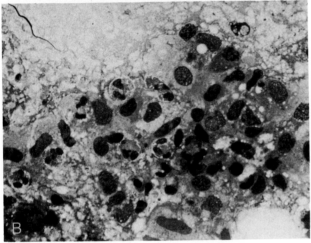

FIGURE 26–9. A, **Tuberculous lymphadenitis.** Degenerated epithelioid cells and necrotic material (May-Grünwald-Giemsa; ×160). B, **Tuberculous lymphadenitis.** Epithelioid cells and polymorphs along with liquefied necrotic material in the background (May-Grünwald-Giemsa; ×400).

cell or globus cell) with vacuolated cytoplasm and a poorly defined outline (Fig. 26–10A).[19, 51, 59] This histiocyte contains numerous lepra bacilli in the form of globi when stained by modified Ziehl-Neelsen stain described by Fite and associates.[41] Four cytologic types (I to IV) have been described by Gupta and associates[51] in a study of lymph node aspirates in leprosy cases. In correlating lymph node histology, types I and II corresponded to lepromatous lesions; type III corresponded to borderline lesions, towards the lepromatous end of the spectrum, and type IV corresponded well to borderline lesions, towards the tuberculoid end of the spectrum. An increasing number of lymphocytes are noticed from types I to IV smears, with a change in appearance from classic foamy histiocytes in types I and II smears to atypical histiocytes in type III smears and epithelioid histiocytes in type IV smears (Fig. 26–10B).

Bacterial Infections

Streptococcal and staphylococcal infections may result in typical suppurative lymphadenitis. The cocci can be better demonstrated with Gram's stain.

Regional lymphadenopathy is a cardinal sign of cat-scratch disease. Close contact with a cat is cited by 90% of patients, and 75% of patients cite being scratched by a cat.[17] The histologic appearance of the lymph node is characterized by suppurative granulomas.[104] The cytologic picture is of granulomas with peripheral palisading of epithelioid histiocytes and central neutrophilic infiltration. The associated cell population is polymorphic.[108] The process has been described as subacute suppurative lymphadenitis by Linsk and Franzen.[75]

Fungal Infections

Common fungal infections affecting the lymph nodes are histoplasmosis and coccidioidomycosis. *Histoplasma capsulatum* occurs as oval yeast forms in macrophages (Fig. 26–11A). In coccidioidomycosis an acute inflammatory exudate is aspirated, indicating abscess formation. The endospore form of the organism can be found. In cryptococcosis the lymph node aspirate shows the organisms in histiocytes (Fig. 26–11B) and in multinucleated giant cells.

Cervicofacial actinomycosis may appear as a mass

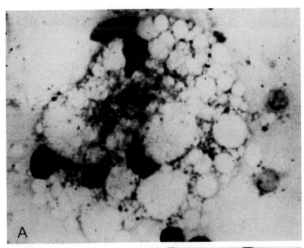

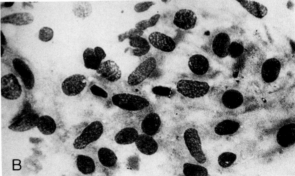

FIGURE 26–10. A, **Syncytial histiocyte** showing distention of the cytoplasm by coarse vacuoles. Many of the vacuoles are lying free in the periphery (May-Grünwald-Giemsa; ×400). (Courtesy of Prof. S. K. Gupta.) B, Lymph node aspirate in **leprosy.** A group of epithelioid histiocytes (May-Grünwald-Giemsa; ×540). (Courtesy of Dr. A. Rajwanshi.)

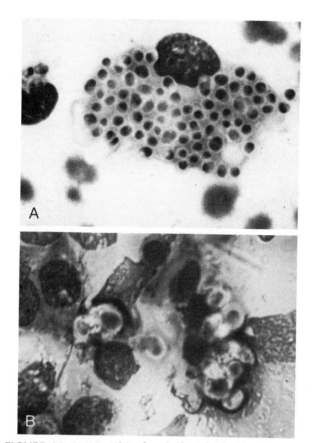

FIGURE 26–11. *A,* **Histoplasmic lymphadenitis.** Numerous oval yeast forms of *Histoplasma capsulatum* seen in macrophages (May-Grünwald-Giemsa; ×1340). (Courtesy of Dr. A. Rajwanshi.) *B,* **Lymph node aspirate** showing rounded bodies of cryptococcus (May-Grünwald-Giemsa; ×1340). (Courtesy of Dr. A. Rajwanshi.)

simulating lymphadenopathy.[25] The aspirate shows an inflammatory exudate consisting predominantly of neutrophils along with a few histiocytes and occasional lymphocytes. *Actinomyces* are seen as balls or aggregates of fine granules and radiating filaments with occasional branching (Fig. 26–12).

Parasitic Infections

Parasitic infections affecting lymph nodes are toxoplasmosis, trypanosomiasis, leishmaniasis and filariasis.[20]

Toxoplasmic lymphadenitis is a relatively common cause of lymph node enlargement, accounting for an estimated 15% of cases of unexplained lymphadenopathy.[67] Yet there are very rare reports of utilization of FNA as a diagnostic method in these cases.[21] A polymorphic lymphoid cell population, tingible body macrophages and epithelioid cells in small and loose aggregates form the characteristic cytologic picture. The crescent-shaped organism is an endozoite measuring 4 to 6 μm in length and 2 μm in breadth having a central nucleus. The causative organism has rarely been described in smears.[4]

Lymph node enlargement, particularly of the posterior triangle of the neck, is a feature of the Gambian form of disease caused by *Trypanosoma gambiense.* Lymph node aspirate in the early phase of the disease may demonstrate the trypomastigotes, which are elongated rather flattened, spindle-shaped flagellated organisms with blunted posterior and pointed anterior ends. The nucleus is central, and the small kinetoplast is situated at the posterior end.

In leishmaniasis, the lymph node aspirate shows a polymorphous population of lymphocytes and epithelioid histiocytes.[69] The histiocytes contain the amastigote forms of *Leishmania donovani* (Fig. 26–13). These are found as oval bodies measuring 2 to 4 μm along the long axis with a kinetoplast lying tangentially or at right angles to the nucleus.

Lymphadenitis is also a frequent accompaniment of classic filariasis.[89] Sheathed microfilaria of *Wucheria bancrofti* with a pointed tail end free of nuclei can be observed in the lymph node aspirate (Fig. 26–14). The parasite is sometimes seen in the lymph node aspirate as the first indication of occult filariasis, and efforts to detect the parasite in the blood may not be successful.

Viral Infections

Infectious mononucleosis syndrome (cytomegalovirus, Epstein-Barr (EB) virus), acquired immune defi-

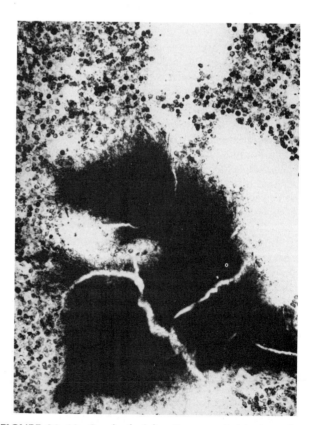

FIGURE 26–12. Cervicofacial actinomycosis. Aspirate from submandibular swelling showing balls of actinomyces and an acute inflammatory exudate. Fine radiating filaments can be seen at the periphery (May-Grünwald-Giemsa; ×160).

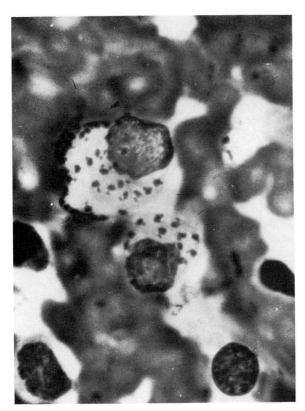

FIGURE 26–13. Lymph node aspirate showing *Leishmania donovani* (LD) bodies in histiocytes (May-Grünwald-Giemsa; ×1340). (Courtesy of Dr. A. Rajwanshi.)

ciency syndrome (AIDS), varicella-herpes zoster and vaccinia are some common viral causes of lymphadenopathy.

In infectious mononucleosis, the lymph node aspirate reveals a high proportion of cells with relatively abundant cytoplasm that stains pale to deep blue with May-Grünwald-Giemsa. These cells range in size from that of small lymphocytes to that of immunoblasts.[63] Many of these cells have plasmacytoid features and prominent nucleoli. Plasma cells and multinucleated giant cells resembling Reed-Sternberg cells of Hodgkin's disease have been noticed.[58, 99] The peripheral blood also shows atypical lymphocytes. The cytodiagnosis should be confirmed by positive findings in the heterophil agglutination test and positive findings in the serologic test for the Epstein-Barr virus antibody. Fine needle aspiration has also been described as a useful and cost effective initial method to evaluate lymphadenopathy in those who are treated at AIDS outpatient departments.[14]

IMMUNOLOGIC DISEASES

Lymphadenopathy has been found in immunologic disorders such as systemic lupus erythematosus (SLE), rheumatoid arthritis and angioimmunoblastic lymphadenopathy (AILD).

Angioimmunoblastic lymphadenopathy has been described as a prelymphomatous condition.[82, 91] Patients usually present with generalized lymphadenopathy, hepatosplenomegaly, cutaneous rash and constitutional symptoms. The FNA smear shows marked proliferation of pleomorphic lymphoid cells including immunoblasts and plasma cells (Fig. 26–15A). Binucleation in the immunoblasts is frequent. An arborizing capillary network supporting the immunoblasts can be seen at times (Fig. 26–15B). The cytologic picture correlates well with the histology, which is characterized by diffuse effacement of lymph node architecture, abundance of small vessels and marked proliferation of pleomorphic lymphoid cells comprised of lymphocytes, plasma cells and immunoblasts.[46]

MISCELLANEOUS DISORDERS

Lymph node aspiration can be of use in certain miscellaneous disorders such as sarcoidosis and dermatopathic lymphadenitis.

The utility of FNA in the diagnosis of sarcoidosis in the lymph nodes has been described adequately.[43, 62] The smear shows lymphocytes and groups of epithelioid cells without any necrotic material. Occasionally, cytoplasmic inclusions in the form of asteroid bodies and Schaumann's bodies can be found.[76] Cytodiagnosis of sarcoidosis needs support from both the clinical

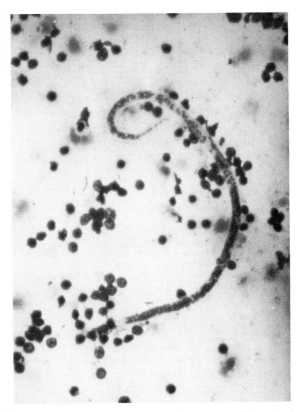

FIGURE 26–14. Filarial lymphadenitis. Fine needle aspiration smear shows lymphocytes and a sheathed microfilaria of *Wuchereria bancrofti* with the pointed, tail end free of nuclei (May-Grünwald-Giemsa; ×540). (Courtsey of Dr. A. Rajwanshi.)

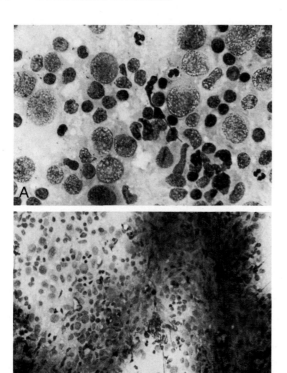

FIGURE 26–15. *A,* Lymph node aspirate from **angioimmuno-blastic lymphadenopathy.** A pleomorphic cytology showing numerous immunoblasts with frequent binucleation (May-Grünwald-Giemsa; ×640). *B,* Angioimmunoblastic lymphadenopathy. Same aspirate as shown in *A.* Arborizing capillary network supports the immunoblasts and other lymphoid cells (May-Grünwald-Giemsa; ×160).

findings and biochemical investigations. In a case of noncaseating granuloma, which is negative for acid-fast bacilli, sarcoid may be a strong possibility in developed countries. However, in developing countries where tuberculosis is very common and acid-fast bacilli are rarely demonstrated in epithelioid granulomas without necrosis, tuberculosis may be considered as the first possibility unless proved otherwise.[100]

LYMPHOMAS AND LEUKEMIAS

The technique of FNA has been used extensively for diagnosis of non-Hodgkin's lymphoma and Hodgkin's disease. The lymphatic and nonlymphoid leukemias infiltrating the lymph nodes can also be studied by this technique.

NON-HODGKIN'S LYMPHOMAS

Cytodiagnosis of non-Hodgkin's lymphoma (NHL) depends on finding a relatively monomorphic popula-

tion of lymphoid cells, whereas its differentiation or grading is predicted by cell size, nuclear size and shape, presence of nucleoli, mitotic activity and so forth.

Subtyping of lymphoma has always been influenced by the histopathologic classification prevalent during the period. This has been reflected in a number of reports,[10, 40, 50] which came to light after publication of Rappaport's morphologic classification.[102] Better understanding of the immune system led to the emergence of classifications such as the Kiel classification[72] and the functional classification of Lukes and Collins[80] in the 1970s. These classifications also found a place in the cytodiagnosis of lymphoma.[26, 109] In the early 1980s, a working formulation on NHL evolved as a compromise and a means of translation among six important classifications,[8, 38, 72, 80, 85, 90, 102] which has since been adopted in the cytodiagnosis of NHL.[66, 97] In the following discussion, the cytologic features of NHL are described as in the working formulation. It is based on knowledge from existing literature and from our experience with 240 cases (Table 26–2). Realizing the limitations of cytology in the diagnosis of histologic characteristics such as nodularity, the grouping of the various cytologic types under low, intermediate and high grades has been slightly modified.

Small Lymphocytic Malignant Lymphomas Consistent with Chronic Lymphocytic Leukemia

The smear is composed of a monotonous population of cells similar to but slightly larger than red blood

TABLE 26–2. Working Formulation of Non-Hodgkin's Lymphoma: Cytologic Diagnosis of 240 Cases

Cytologic Types	No. of Cases
Low Grade	
ML—small lymphocytic (CLL)	8
ML—small lymphocytic (plasmacytoid type)	5
ML—small cleaved cell type	9
Intermediate Grade	
ML—mixed small and large cell	
Cleaved cell type (FCC)	14
with epithelioid histiocytes	9
ML—large-cell (cleaved cell) type	21
High Grade	
ML	
Large cell	
Noncleaved cell	16
Immunoblastic	27
ML	
Lymphoblastic	
Convoluted cell	30
Nonconvoluted cell	29
ML	
Small noncleaved	
Burkitt-type	33
Non-Burkitt-type	28
Miscellaneous Types	11
	240

ML = malignant lymphoma; FCC = follicular center cell; CLL = chronic lymphocytic leukemia.

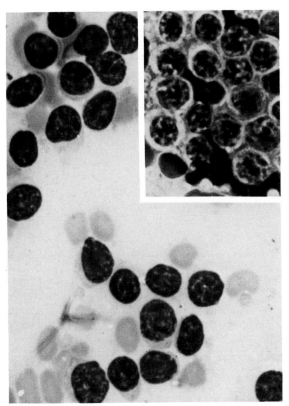

larger than red blood cells and possess scanty cytoplasm and nuclei with cleaving or creases, which often look like a small notch in the nuclear outline (Fig. 26–18). The cytologic picture is monotonous, although a small number of large cleaved and noncleaved cells may be found.

Mixed Small and Large Cells: Follicular Center Cell Type (Centrocytic-Centroblastic Lymphoma)

The smear shows an intimate mixture of small and large cleaved cells (Fig. 26–19A). The large cleaved cells usually have one to two nucleoli. The variation in cell size may impart a superficial resemblance to reactive hyperplasia. However, nuclei of both small cells and large cells look uniformly immature.

Mixed Small and Large Cells with Epithelioid Histiocytes

A variable mixture of atypical small and large lymphoid cells are found to be interspersed with epithelioid

FIGURE 26–16. Malignant lymphoma of small lymphocytes (consistent with chronic lymphocytic leukemia). A monotonous population of lymphoid cells slightly larger than red blood cells (May-Grünwald-Giemsa; ×1000). *Inset*, Multiple coarse chromatin (cellules grumelees) (Papanicolaou; ×1000).

cells (Fig. 26–16). The cells have scanty light blue cytoplasm and round nuclei with multiple coarse chromatin or chromocenters dispersed throughout (inset, Fig. 26–16). The characteristic clumping of chromatin has been described as cellules grumelees.[106] Mitotic activity is extremely rare in this type of lymphoma.

Small Lymphocytic—Plasmacytoid (Lymphoplasmacytic Lymphoma, Immunocytoma)

This is a tumor similar to small lymphocytic lymphoma but having abnormal plasmacytoid differentiation of variable prominence. The plasmacytoid cells are slightly larger than the small round lymphoid cells. Their cytoplasmic characteristics resemble those of plasma cells, but the nucleus is more similar to a lymphocyte (Fig. 26–17).

Small Cleaved Cell (Centrocytic Lymphoma)

Small cleaved cells form the predominant component of the lymph node aspirate. These cells are slightly

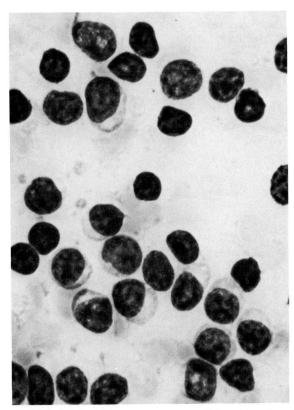

FIGURE 26–17. Malignant lymphoma small lymphocytic cells (plasmacytoid). Small lymphoid cells with plasmacytoid appearance. Lymph node aspirate from a 45-year-old male with a clinical diagnosis of Hodgkin's disease (May-Grünwald-Giemsa; ×1000).

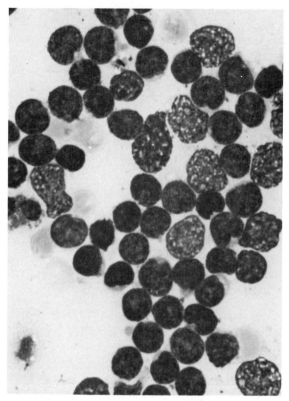

FIGURE 26–18. Malignant lymphoma small cleaved cells. Numerous small lymphoid cells slightly larger than red blood cells. Typical nuclear cleaving or notch is appreciated in many cells (May-Grünwald-Giemsa; ×1000).

histiocytes that are present in small groups, in isolated forms or in both (Fig. 26–19B). These epithelioid histiocytes possess abundant clear cytoplasm and a pale staining, oval or elliptic nucleus. They do not show any evidence of phagocytosis. A small percentage of immunoblasts, plasma cells and eosinophils are present in the majority of cases. Cytologic features of these cases have been described under lymphoepithelioid lymphoma and Lennert's lymphoma.[33]

Large Cleaved Cell Type (Centroblastic Lymphoma)

Large cleaved cells are the predominant cell type. They are twice the diameter of red blood cells. Cytoplasm is minimal and ill-defined, and the nucleus is large with irregular outline or indentation, often imparting a bean- or kidney-shaped appearance (Fig. 26–20). The nucleoli are small but conspicuous. A few mitotic figures may be seen.

Large Cell: Noncleaved Type (Centroblastic Lymphoma)

The smear is composed of large cells with a narrow rim of amphophilic or basophilic cytoplasm and a round-to-oval nucleus with prominent nucleoli situated at or near the nuclear membrane (Figs. 26–21A and 26–21B). The cells are two to three times larger than red blood cells. Mitotic figures are frequent.

Large Cell: Immunoblastic (Immunoblastic Sarcoma or Lymphoma)

Two common variants of this neoplasm are known: plasmacytoid type and clear cell type. The plasmacytoid variant possesses abundant deep basophilic cytoplasm with varying degrees of cytoplasmic vacuolizations. Nuclei are usually excentric and possess coarse chromatin (Fig. 26–22A). A huge, prominent central nucleolus is a characteristic feature. The clear cell variant, as the name indicates, shows large cells with abundant clear or light blue cytoplasm and cytoplasmic vacuolizations. The nuclei are irregular or lobulated and possess evenly distributed chromatin and one to two small but distinct nucleoli (Fig. 26–22B). The plasmacytoid and clear cell type possibly represent B

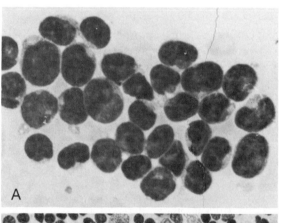
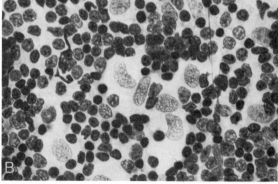

FIGURE 26–19. *A,* **Malignant lymphoma. Mixed small and large cells (follicular center cell type).** A mixture of small and large cleaved cells with an almost uniform degree of nuclear maturation (May-Grünwald-Giemsa; ×1000). *B,* Lymph node aspirate shows a group of **epithelioid histiocytes** with clear cytoplasm, among small and large lymphoid cells (May-Grünwald-Giemsa; ×400). Both cytologic and histopathologic diagnoses were non-Hodgkin's lymphoma with epithelioid histiocytes (Lennert's lymphoma).

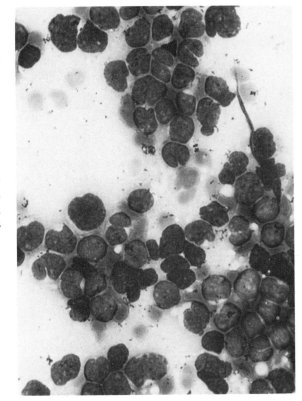

FIGURE 26–20. Malignant lymphoma large cleaved cell type. The lymphoid cells are about twice the size of red blood cells and possess cleaved nuclei with small nucleoli. Lymph node aspirate is from a 42-year-old male who presented with cervical and epigastric masses (May-Grünwald-Giemsa; ×640).

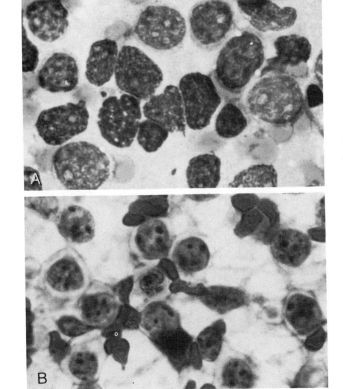

FIGURE 26–21. *A,* **Malignant lymphoma large cell (noncleaved) type.** Aspirate from cervical lymph node in a 28-year-old male. Large cells with round nuclei and prominent nucleoli situated at or close to the nuclear membrane (May-Grünwald-Giemsa; ×1000). *B,* **Malignant lymphoma, large noncleaved type.** Presence of nucleoli at nuclear membrane is striking. Similar finding is described for *A* (Papanicolaou; ×1000).

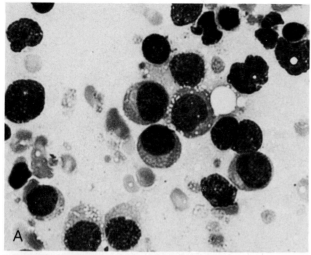

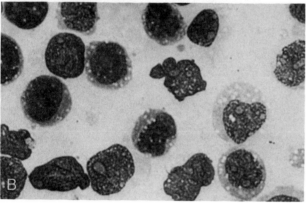

FIGURE 26–22. *A,* **Malignant lymphoma. Large (immunoblastic) cell.** Large lymphoid cells with plasmacytoid differentiation. The nuclei are excentric, and cytoplasm shows vacuolization (May-Grünwald-Giemsa; ×640). *B,* **Malignant lymphoma. Large (immunoblastic) cell.** The large lymphoid cells have abundant clear cytoplasm with vacuolization. The nuclei are irregular and have reticular chromatin (May-Grünwald-Giemsa; ×640).

and T immunoblastic sarcomas as indicated in some earlier studies.[30, 81]

Lymphoblastic: Convoluted Cell Type (Malignant Lymphoma of Convoluted Lymphocytes)

Mediastinal adenopathy and pleural effusions are common findings in these cases. The smear consists of neoplastic lymphoid cells with marked variation in size and shape of nuclei. The cytoplasm is usually scanty. The nuclei are round or angulated with convolutions and gyrations (Fig. 26–23A and B). In a study of 31 cases, Das and associates[31] found nuclear convolutions in an average of 47% of the cells. A variable number of non-neoplastic histiocytes may be present, imparting a pseudo-starry sky–appearance to the smear. Mitotic figures are frequent.

Lymphoblastic: Nonconvoluted Type (Lymphoblastic Lymphoma)

The smear contains lymphoblasts that are usually uniform in size being smaller than cells of immuno-

blastic and large noncleaved cell lymphomas but larger than cells of small lymphocytic cell lymphomas. Nuclei are round, and nucleoli are inconspicuous. A few nuclei may show indentations or fine nuclear grooves. Cytoplasm is scanty and mitotic activity brisk (Fig. 26–24).

Small Noncleaved (Burkitt's Type)

Lymphadenopathy is said to be uncommon in African[115] and American-type[73] Burkitt's lymphomas, whereas it is common in cases in Europe studied by Lennert.[71] The smear is composed of an almost monotonous population of lymphoid cells, which are about twice the size of red blood cells and possess noncleaved nuclei. Cytoplasm is scanty to moderate. Cytoplasmic or nuclear, or both, types of vacuolization are seen (Fig. 26–25A and B). In a study of 40 cases, Das and associates[32] found an average of 60% cells with noncleaved nuclei and 71% cells with cytoplasmic or nuclear, or both, types of vacuolizations. Scattered non-neoplastic histiocytes with engulfed nuclear debris, which imparts a starry sky–appearance to paraffin sections, are present in variable numbers.

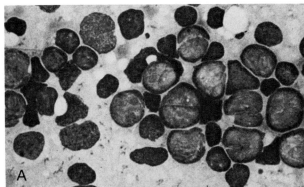

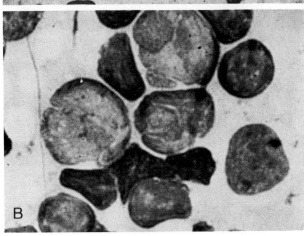

FIGURE 26–23. *A,* **Malignant lymphoma. Lymphoblastic convoluted cell type.** The lymphoid cells show marked variation in size. The nuclei show nuclear convolutions or gyrations (May-Grünwald-Giemsa; ×640). *B,* Higher magnification of *A* to show the nuclear convolutions (May-Grünwald-Giemsa; ×1000).

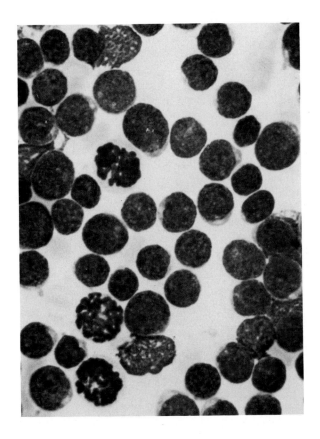

FIGURE 26–24. Malignant lymphoma. Lymphoblastic (nonconvoluted) cell. Lymphoblasts in the range of 10 to 12 μm with mitotic figures frequently seen. (May-Grünwald-Giemsa; ×1000).

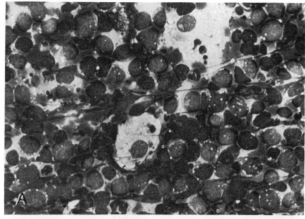

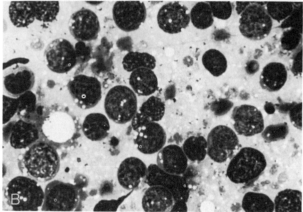

FIGURE 26–25. *A,* **Malignant lymphoma. Small noncleaved (Burkitt's type) cells.** A non-neoplastic histiocyte with nuclear debris (starry sky–macrophage) seen among lymphoma cells (May-Grünwald-Giemsa; ×400). *B,* **Malignant lymphoma. Small noncleaved (Burkitt's type) cells.** Monotonous population of lymphoma cells with noncleaved nuclei and cytoplasmic or nuclear vacuolizations, or both (May-Grünwald-Giemsa; ×640).

Small Noncleaved (Non-Burkitt's Type)

Cytology of this type is more pleomorphic when compared with Burkitt's type lymphoma. The population of cleaved and noncleaved cells is greater, and the cytoplasmic vacuolization is absent in this neoplasm.

Fine Needle Aspiration

From the existing literature it appears that hardly any difference of opinion occurs among cytopathologists regarding the useful role of cytology in the diagnosis of lymphoma. However, it is said that distinguishing well-differentiated lymphocytic lymphoma from florid reactive hyperplasia may be difficult.[63] Reservations have also been expressed about the subtyping of NHL by cytology.[36] Some believe that only limited cytologic types can be diagnosed, but nodular and diffuse patterns cannot be differentiated by cytology.[11, 66] No doubt exists that nodular versus diffuse patterns, which are of strict histologic criteria, cannot

be discerned by FNA. The other difficulties are very minimal if the aspirate is excellent technically and the cytopathologist has adequate experience.

The utility of FNA for diagnosis of NHL has been discussed by a number of investigators.[18, 31, 32, 97] The initial diagnosis of lymphoma by FNA facilitates an efficient staging approach by identifying appropriate tissues for biopsy. In a patient whose medical condition precludes surgical intervention, FNA may be the only means of diagnosing intra-abdominal, intrathoracic or intrapelvic malignancies. In a recurrence, FNA is particularly helpful in obviating biopsy.

In a patient with a history of lymphoma, who develops additional enlarged lymph nodes, FNA can identify the presence of an infectious disease or a second malignancy. It is of help not only in subtyping lymphoma[93] but also in identifying progression of a low-grade lymphoma to a high-grade lymphoma. Special techniques, such as immunocytochemistry[74] and Southern blot hybridization,[56] can be performed on lymph node aspirates to diagnose the functional character and clonal nature of the lymphoma.

PLASMA CELL TUMORS

Plasma cell tumor can primarily involve a lymph node (extramedullary plasma cell tumor) or lymph node involvement can be a sequela of multiple myeloma. Of the nine cases of plasma cell tumor studied by Das and associates,[34] four had lymph node involve-

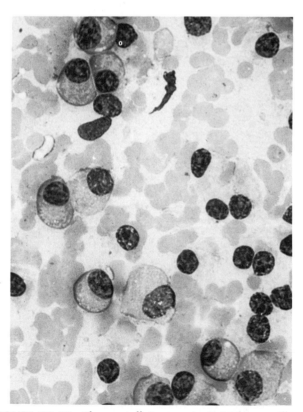

FIGURE 26–26. Plasma cell tumor. Aspirate from axillary lymph node shows abnormal plasma cells with excentric nuclei and a few bare nuclei (May-Grünwald-Giemsa; ×640).

ment. Fine needle aspiration of lymph nodes done in three cases revealed typical myeloma cells in two cases (Fig. 26–26), whereas most of the myeloma cells were of the undifferentiated type in the third case.

NONLYMPHOID LEUKEMIAS

The lymphadenopathy of nonlymphoid leukemia can be due to infiltration of cells of chronic myeloid leukemia (CML) and acute myeloid leukemia (AML) or to blast crisis in CML. Granulocytic leukosarcoma or chloroma can also take its origin in a lymph node.

Lymph node aspirates in CML show immature myeloid cells in various stages of differentiation, especially the myelocytes and metamyelocytes, mixed with lymphocytes of the lymph node (Fig. 26–27). In blast crisis of CML, a variable number of myeloblasts is seen along with the more differentiated myeloid cells of CML (Fig. 26–28). In granulocytic leukosarcoma of the lymph nodes or in AML infiltrating the lymph node, a mixture of myeloblasts and lymphoid cells can be found in the lymph node aspirate (Fig. 26–29).

HODGKIN'S DISEASE

The cytodiagnosis of Hodgkin's disease is based on the demonstration of Hodgkin's cells or Reed-Stern-

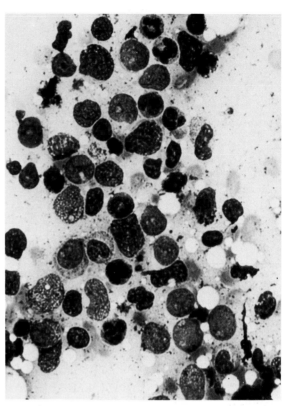

FIGURE 26–28. Blast crisis in **chronic myeloid leukemia.** Lymph node aspirate shows many myeloblasts along with myeloid cells in various stages of maturation (May-Grünwald-Giemsa; ×640).

berg cells, or both, among the appropriate reactive cellular components. Subtyping of Hodgkin's disease is done by a subjective evaluation of the relative proportion of neoplastic cells (Hodgkin's cells and Reed-Sternberg cells) and reactive cellular components.[29, 45, 77]

The Reed-Sternberg cell is a large cell with two or more nuclei or prominent nucleoli. The size usually ranges from 50 to 100 μm. At times, the nuclei are incompletely separated into lobes or joined with each other by thin chromatin threads. The Hodgkin's cell is a large mononucleated cell (30 to 50 μm) with a prominent nucleolus. The cytoplasm of the cell is abundant and usually pale blue in color. The lacunar cells, a variant of Reed-Sternberg cells, are relatively small (30 to 40 μm) with clear cytoplasm and a hypersegmented nucleus.

Lymphocytic Predominance Type

The smear shows an overwhelming population of lymphocytes. Reed-Sternberg cells or Hodgkin's cells are occasional (Fig. 26–30). Often, the Reed-Sternberg cells show nuclear convolutions or lobulations instead of binucleation or multinucleation. Eosinophils and plasma cells are rare, but sometimes many non-neoplastic histiocytes or epithelioid histiocytes are observed in groups or in a dissociated form.

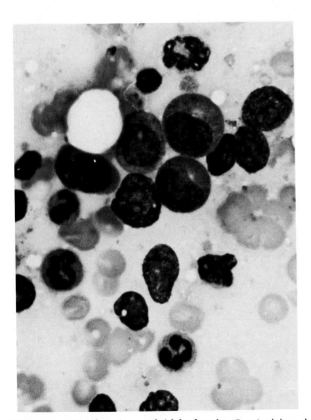

FIGURE 26–27. Chronic myeloid leukemia. Cervical lymph node aspirate from a known case of chronic myelocytic leukemia. Many myelocytes and neutrophils seen (May-Grünwald-Giemsa; ×1000).

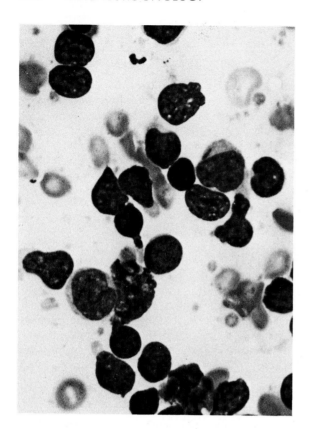

FIGURE 26–29. Acute myeloid leukemia. Lymph node aspirate from a 19-year-old male with acute myelocytic leukemia and generalized lymphadenopathy. Smear shows a few myeloblasts in addition to lymphocytes. An Auer rod is seen in one of the myeloblasts (May-Grünwald-Giemsa; ×1000).

FIGURE 26–30. Hodgkin's disease (lymphocytic predominance). Smear shows numerous lymphocytes and one Reed-Sternberg cell with a convoluted nucleus (May-Grünwald-Giemsa; ×640).

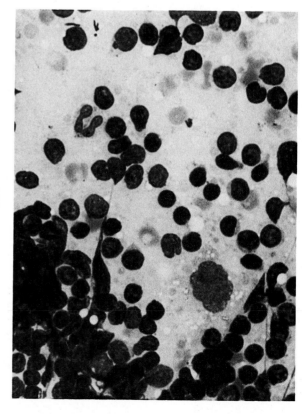

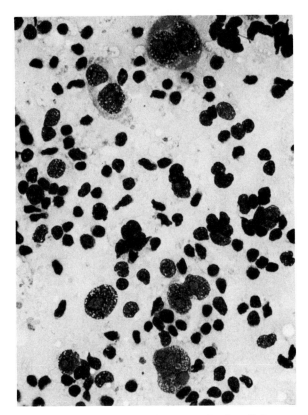

FIGURE 26–31. Hodgkin's disease (mixed cellular type). Smear shows a few classic binucleated Reed-Sternberg cells with prominent nucleoli and Hodgkin's cells (May-Grünwald-Giemsa; × 400).

Mixed Cellular Type

An appreciable number of classic Reed-Sternberg cells and Hodgkin's cells are encountered in the smear (Fig. 26–31). Other reactive components, such as eosinophils, plasma cells and benign histiocytes, are also present.

Lymphocytic Depletion Type

Marked increase in Reed-Sternberg cells and Hodgkin's cells and corresponding decrease in the lymphocytic population are seen. The Reed-Sternberg cells are often pleomorphic (Fig. 26–32).

Nodular Sclerosis Type

A cytologic variant of Reed-Sternberg cells, corresponding to lacunar cells, can be found (Fig. 26–33A and B), but it is not specific for the nodular sclerosis subtype. Fibrocollagenous tissue, giving rise to a nodular pattern in paraffin sections, is rarely aspirated. In our experience most of the nodular sclerosis types are either diagnosed as lymphocytic depletion or mixed cellular type.

Some investigators have expressed reservations about the role of FNA in the subtyping of Hodgkin's disease.[45, 66, 99] Through a differential count of FNA smears, Das and Gupta[28] have shown that the percentage of Reed-Sternberg cells, Hodgkin's cells and lymphocytes in three major subtypes (lymphocytic predominance, mixed cellular, lymphocytic depletion) differ significantly, and the neoplastic cells remain within distinct ranges in these subtypes. These observations support the concept that Hodgkin's disease can be subtyped based on a subjective impression of neoplastic cells and reactive cell population.

METASTATIC NEOPLASMS

The accessibility of enlarged lymph nodes for palpation and puncture, the rich cellularity of the smears due to the high yield of aspirated material and the ease with which alien tumor cells can be differentiated from lymphocytes make the technique of FNA very useful in the investigation of metastatic lymphadenopathy.

The circumstances under which a patient with secondary findings in the lymph nodes may be referred for FNA are the following:

1. For confirmation of a secondary lesion in cases of a known or an occult primary.
2. For diagnosis of a secondary lesion during follow-up of treated primary malignancy.

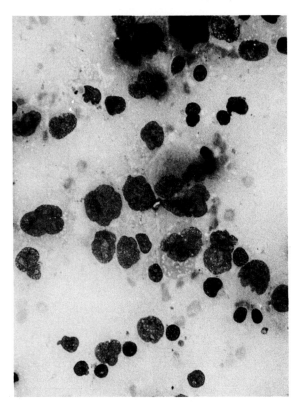

FIGURE 26–32. Hodgkin's disease (lymphocytic depletion type). Smear shows numerous pleomorphic Reed-Sternberg cells, Hodgkin's cells and marked decrease in lymphocytes (May-Grünwald-Giemsa; × 400).

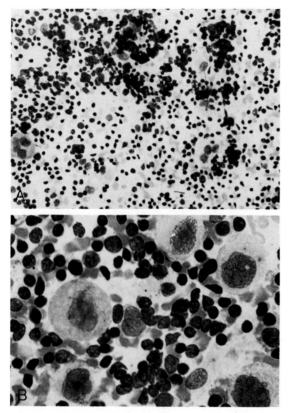

FIGURE 26–33. *A*, **Hodgkin's disease (nodular sclerosis).** Smear contains lymphocytes and two Reed-Sternberg cells with small overlapping nuclei (lacunar cells) (May-Grünwald-Giemsa; ×160). *B*, **Hodgkin's disease (nodular sclerosis).** Lymphocytes and many Reed-Sternberg cells with lobulated nuclei are likely to be cytologic counterparts of lacunar cells (May-Grünwald-Giemsa; ×400).

3. Cases with clinical diagnoses other than metastatic lymphadenopathy, e.g., lymphoma; specific infections, such as tuberculous lymphadenitis or lymphadenopathy and not otherwise specified.
4. For staging of malignancies, such as carcinoma of the bladder and prostate by fluoroscopically guided puncture of the pelvic chain of lymph nodes.

Ideally FNA should be done from both the primary and suspected secondary lesions. This practice not only helps in confirming that primary and secondary lesions have identical cytomorphology but detects any altered differentiation of the secondary or even metastasis from a second primary. Infectious lesions instead of malignancy can also be detected. When the primary is not accessible without difficulty, as in a deep-seated lesion, the diagnosis of metastasis in a superficial lymph node plays a decisive role in management. In case of an occult primary, the cytologic characteristics of a metastatic lesion, a thorough knowledge of lymphatic drainage and common lymph node groups involved by metastasis from various organs help in locating the primary. Hendrick[54] has shown how the frequency of an occult primary was reduced from 36.2% at or before FNA to 9.0% following cytodiagnosis and reexamination of cases. Engzell and associates[39] also had a similar

experience. In their study, the rate of occult primary was reduced from 34.7% (prior to FNA) to only 7.2%, in those who died without known primaries. Similarly, when a patient is referred for aspiration of a primary tumor, the cytopathologist should look for lymph node chains likely to have a secondary. Occasionally, metastatic lymph nodes may be missed by the referring physician or surgeon, and the timely detection of them by the cytopathologist may help in the proper staging of the malignancy. At times, FNA of deep-seated lesions can be avoided.

A number of studies on the role of FNA in metastatic lymphadenopathies have been published.[9, 39, 54, 61, 84] The FNA smears in metastatic lymphadenopathies usually contain malignant alien cells with very little or no lymphoid cell component (Fig. 26–34A). Only in a few cases can an appreciable number of lymphocytes be found (Fig. 26–34B).

METASTATIC CARCINOMAS

Squamous cell carcinomas, adenocarcinomas and undifferentiated carcinomas are the common metastatic carcinomas encountered in lymph node aspirates. Engzell and associates[39] found 40.0%, 38.6% and

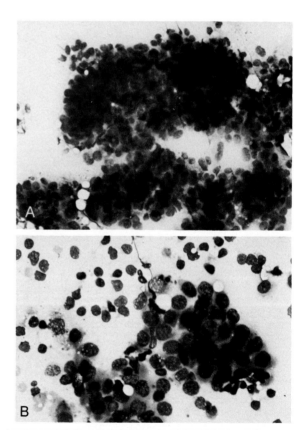

FIGURE 26–34. *A*, Aspirate from supraclavicular lymph node shows **numerous malignant cells in compact papillary clusters** and no lymphocytes (May-Grünwald-Giemsa; ×160). *B*, Fine needle aspiration smear from axillary lymph node in **breast carcinoma.** Groups of malignant cells and lymphocytes (May-Grünwald-Giemsa; ×400).

21.4% as squamous, adenocarcinoma and undifferentiated carcinoma, respectively, among 962 patients with cervical lymph node metastases and histopathologically verified primary tumors. The cytologic features of some of the common metastatic lesions in lymph nodes are discussed in the following sections.

Squamous Cell Carcinoma

Cytologic features of a metastatic squamous cell carcinoma vary, depending on the degree of differentiation of neoplasm and the associated degenerative changes.

The smear of metastatic keratinizing epidermoid carcinoma contains groups of malignant cells and a variable number of keratinized tumor cells (Fig. 26–35A). Tadpole-like cells, fiber cells and structures

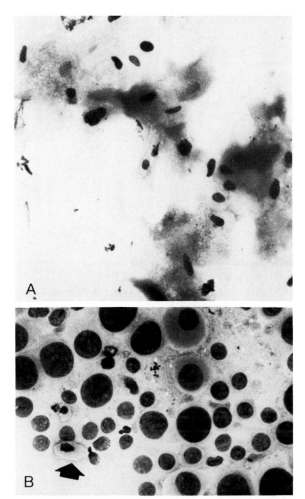

FIGURE 26–36. *A,* **Metastatic well-differentiated (keratinizing) epidermoid carcinoma from a carcinomatous penis.** Aspirate from the inguinal lymph node shows only keratinized cells with hyperchromatic atypical nuclei (May-Grünwald-Giemsa; ×400). *B,* **Metastatic poorly differentiated epidermoid carcinoma.** Occasional cells show evidence of keratinization (arrow) among numerous dissociated malignant cells (May-Grünwald-Giemsa; ×400).

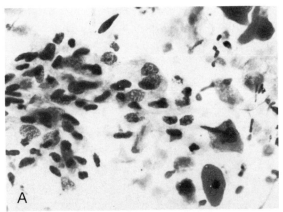

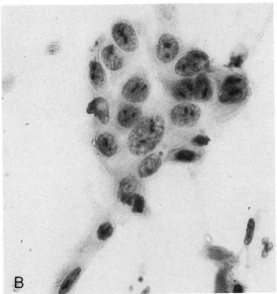

FIGURE 26–35. *A,* **Metastatic squamous cell carcinoma from a carcinomatous bronchus.** Aspirate from supraclavicular lymph node shows a group of malignant cells with round to elongated nuclei and a few keratinized tumor cells (May-Grünwald-Giemsa; ×400). *B,* **Metastatic squamous cell carcinoma.** Tumor cells showing distinct chromocenters or small nucleoli (Papanicolaou; ×640).

suggesting epithelial "pearls" can be seen. In a Papanicolaou-stained smear, the nuclear outline of the tumor cell is well-defined and the nuclear chromatin shows distinct clumping. Nucleoli or chromocenters can be seen occasionally (Fig. 26–35B). The cytoplasm of keratinized cells in Papanicolaou-stained smears reveals organgeophilia. In sharp contrast the cytoplasm of such cells stains royal blue with May-Grünwald-Giemsa staining.

In well-differentiated squamous cell carcinoma, the neoplastic cells may have close resemblance to normal squamous cells (Fig. 26–36A), whereas in poorly differentiated neoplasms, an intensive search may reveal occasional keratinized cells (Fig. 26–36B). The anucleated squames in a well-differentiated case may create confusion with branchiogenic cysts or epidermal inclusion cysts. The presence of hyperchromatic and atypical nuclei and the absence of cholesterol crystals help in the diagnosis of squamous cell carcinoma.

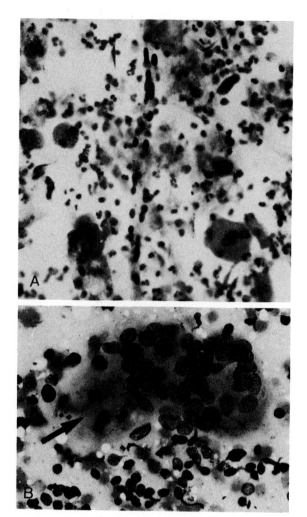

FIGURE 26–37. *A,* **Metastatic (keratinizing) squamous cell carcinoma.** In addition to keratinized malignant cells, dense inflammatory cell infiltration and cell debris indicate tumor necrosis (Papanicolaou; ×400). *B,* **Metastatic squamous cell carcinoma with giant cell reaction.** Aspirate from right cervical lymph node shows lymphocytes, multinucleated giant cells and a few keratinized squamous cells (arrow) (May-Grünwald-Giemsa; ×400).

Metastatic lymph nodes in keratinizing squamous cell carcinoma frequently undergo degenerating changes and liquefaction. In such smears, acute inflammatory cells appear in large number (Fig. 26–37A). Sometimes, inflammatory cell reaction and cell degenerations are so intense that malignant cells are difficult to detect and a false-negative report of suppurative lymphadenitis may be offered. Similarly, reaction to keratin may induce formation of multinucleated giant cells and thus create confusion with granulomatous lymphadenitis (Fig. 26–37B). Careful search for keratinized neoplastic cells or repeat FNA on clinical suspicion of malignancy can be of help in arriving at a correct diagnosis.

Adenocarcinoma

Tumor cells in metastatic adenocarcinoma reveal certain patterns, e.g., monolayer sheets and papillary

formation (Fig. 26–38A) and microacinar formation (Fig. 26–38B). The nuclei in these tumor cells are excentric or basal (Fig. 26–39A). The nucleoli are usually prominent and are appreciated very clearly in Papanicolaou-stained smears (Fig. 26–39B).

Metastasis from specific sites can also be recognized in smears because of certain cytologic features. The presence of magenta bodies in metastatic tumor cells may suggest a primary tumor in the breast. Metastasis from papillary carcinoma of the thyroid may contain typical intranuclear cytoplasmic inclusions (Fig. 26–40). Similarly, occult follicular carcinoma in the thyroid can be recognized by finding a typical microacinar formation and medullary carcinoma from the plasmacytoid, triangular or spindle-shaped cells with intracytoplasmic granules (Fig. 26–41). Extensive vacuolizations due to neutral lipids (Fig. 26–42A and B) in malignant cells from a lymph node may help in the diagnosis of meibomian gland carcinoma of the eyelid, even if it is small and difficult to puncture with the needle. Adenoid cystic can be diagnosed from the small monomorphic tumor cells surrounding mucus globules or cylinders.

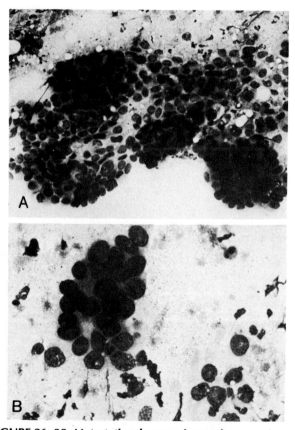

FIGURE 26–38. Metastatic adenocarcinoma from carcinoma of gallbladder. *A,* Aspirate from left supraclavicular lymph node shows tumor cells in monolayer sheets and compact papillary clusters (May-Grünwald-Giemsa; ×160). *B,* Left supraclavicular lymph node aspirate in 20-year-old male with clinical possibilities of lymphoma, tuberculosis and carcinoma of the stomach. Tumor cells showing microacinar formation led to the diagnosis of **metastatic adenocarcinoma from stomach.** (May-Grünwald-Giemsa; ×400).

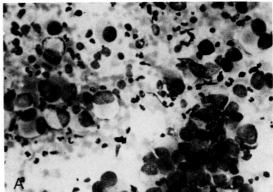

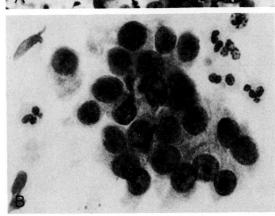

FIGURE 26–39. *A,* **Metastatic adenocarcinoma** in a case of bronchogenic carcinoma. Aspirate from axillary lymph node shows tumor cells in groups and discrete forms with excentric nuclei (May-Grünwald Giemsa; ×200). *B,* **Metastatic adenocarcinoma** showing prominent nucleoli in tumor cells (same case as shown in Fig. 26–38*B*) (Papanicolaou; ×640).

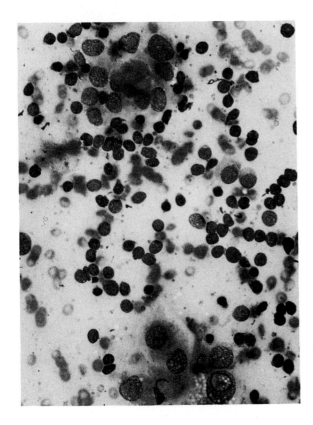

FIGURE 26–40. Lymph node metastasis in **papillary carcinoma thyroid.** Lymphocytes and groups of tumor cells. Intranuclear cytoplasmic inclusions seen in one cell (May-Grünwald-Giemsa; ×400).

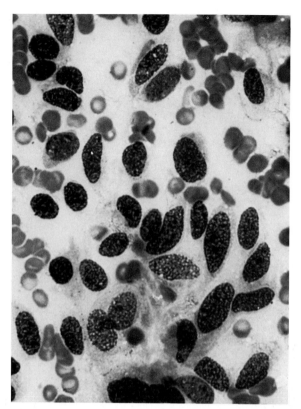

FIGURE 26–41. Lymph node metastasis in **medullary carcinoma thyroid.** Mostly spindle-shaped tumor cells are seen. A few granules are present in a triangular-shaped tumor cell (May-Grünwald-Giemsa; ×640).

Anaplastic Carcinoma

Smears in undifferentiated carcinoma can be the large-cell type or small-cell type. Many large-cell anaplastic carcinomas may indeed be poorly differentiated epidermoid carcinomas or adenocarcinomas. The cells in small-cell anaplastic carcinoma, which can be confused with malignant lymphoma in paraffin sections, appear much larger in May-Grünwald-Giemsa–stained smears compared with lymphoid cells. Although occasional dissociated cells may resemble lymphoid cells, the cohesiveness between the tumor cells and the characteristic nuclear moldings (Figs. 26–43 and 26–44) helps in arriving at a diagnosis.

Transitional Cell Carcinoma

The sources of metastasis of transitional cell carcinoma are usually the renal pelvis, ureter and bladder. The useful role of FNA in the staging and subsequent management of carcinoma of the bladder has been described in a few reports.[13, 95] The tumor cells are cuboidal to low columnar and are present in loosely textured sheets or in isolated form. The nucleoli are usually prominent. A few cells may have a plasmacytoid appearance. Arrangement of the cells around central capillaries gives rise to a papillary formation (Fig. 26–45).

MALIGNANT MELANOMAS

Metastatic malignant melanomas show marked variation in their cytomorphology. Five cytologic patterns, e.g., cells with an abundance of melanin pigment, pleomorphic cytology, round cell type, epithelial-like cells and spindle-shaped cells have been described by Gupta and associates.[52] The cases with melanin pigment are diagnosed without difficulty (Fig. 26–46). Difficulty does arise when the melanin pigment is very scanty or absent. This problem is partly due to occult primaries and lack of clinical suspicion in the majority of cases. Of the 16 cases of lymph node metastasis reported by Gupta and colleagues,[52] the clinical diagnosis was malignant melanoma in only seven cases.

METASTATIC SOFT TISSUE AND BONE TUMORS

Although the diagnosis of a metastatic soft tissue sarcoma or bone tumor in lymph node is not a difficult one to determine, its subtyping may be difficult to determine.

Tumors, such as neuroblastoma and retinoblastoma, show frequent lymph node metastasis. Of the eight

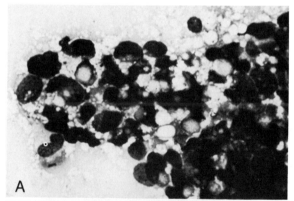
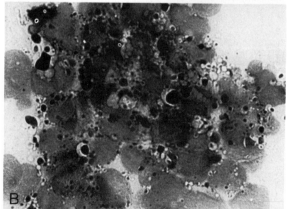

FIGURE 26–42. Metastasis in submandibular lymph node from **meibomian gland carcinoma of eyelid.** *A,* Aspirate shows groups of tumor cells with richly vacuolated cytoplasm (May-Grünwald-Giemsa; ×400). *B,* Demonstration of neutral lipids by oil red O staining (×640).

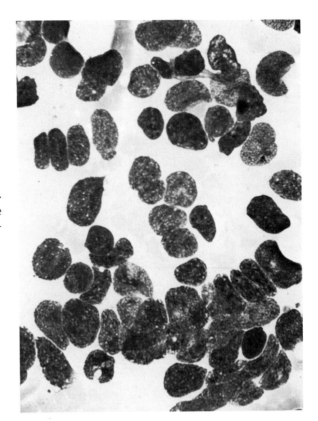

FIGURE 26–43. Metastatic cells from **small-cell anaplastic carcinoma of the bronchus.** Right supraclavicular lymph node aspirate shows small tumor cells with nuclear molding (May-Grünwald-Giemsa; ×640).

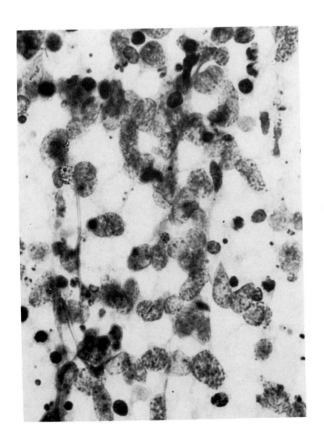

FIGURE 26–44. **Metastatic small-cell anaplastic carcinoma** showing nuclear molding, fine chromatin but no nucleoli (Papanicolaou; ×640).

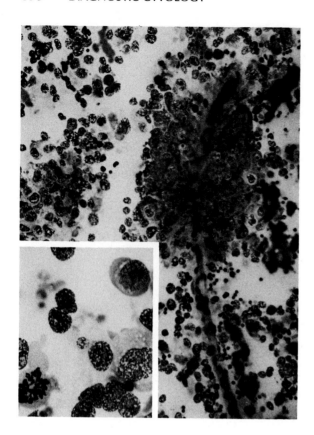

FIGURE 26–45. Metastatic transitional cell carcinoma from carcinoma bladder. Aspirate from right cervical lymph node shows papillary formation by tumor cells. *Inset,* Higher magnification of tumor cells showing plasmacytoid appearance and a mitotic figure (May-Grünwald-Giemsa; ×400).

FIGURE 26–46. Metastatic malignant melanoma. Aspirate from inguinal lymph node shows tumor cells packed with dark melanin pigments (May-Grünwald-Giemsa; ×400).

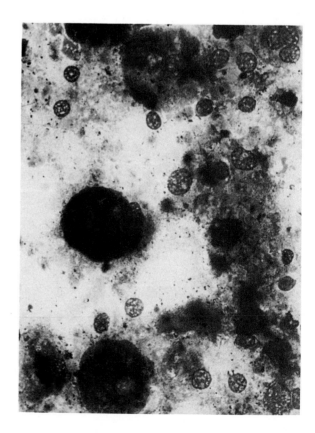

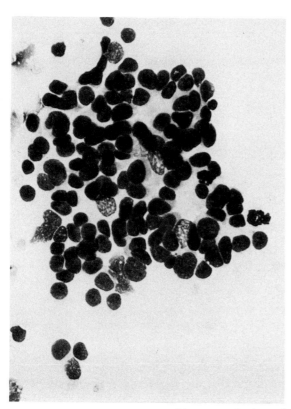

FIGURE 26–47. Metastatic neuroblastoma. Aspirate from cervical lymph node shows rosette formation by tumor cells (May-Grünwald-Giemsa; ×400).

cases of metastatic retinoblastomas reported by Akhtar and associates,[1] five were in the cervical lymph nodes. Although the individual cells can resemble lymphoma cells, their cohesiveness and rosette formation (Fig. 26–47) help one in arriving at the diagnosis of neuroblastoma or retinoblastoma.

GERM CELL TUMORS

Fine needle aspiration can be utilized to confirm metastasis from known primary germ cell tumors of the ovary and testis. Many times the aspirate from a huge retroperitoneal lymph node mass indicates an occult primary in the testis or an overt primary concealed by the patient.

The malignant cells have a typical cytomorphology in the form of a large nucleus with reticulated chromatin and a prominent nucleolus and vacuolated cytoplasm due to glycogen. The stripped off cytoplasm with glycogen imparts a tigroid appearance to the background (Fig. 26–48). The typical teratomas and embryonal carcinomas can also be diagnosed, but when these tumors are undifferentiated difficulty can arise in the diagnosis.[55]

SPECIAL TECHNIQUES

The various special techniques that can be applied to the aspirate from the lymph nodes as an aid in the diagnosis are cytochemistry, bacteriologic culture, immunocytochemistry, ultrastructural studies and molecular hybridization.

Cytochemistry

A wide variety of cytochemical stains can be of help in the diagnosis of benign conditions and malignancy in the lymph node aspirate (Table 26–3). The role of Ziehl-Neelsen stain for demonstration of AFB in tuberculosis and leprosy is well known. Acid-fast bacilli positivity in necrotic material with neutrophilic infiltration has been found to be as high as 80.0%.[100] Smears showing features of suppurative lymphadenitis should be subjected to both Gram and Ziehl-Neelsen staining. Although the former can detect gram-positive streptococcus or staphylococcus and radiating filaments of *Actinomyces*, the latter can detect AFB. The presence of *Actinomyces* can be further confirmed by Gomori's silver methenamine. Even if negative results are obtained by all these staining techniques, a sample sent for bacteriologic culture can be of help in detection of the etiologic agent.

Cytochemical stains, such as acid phosphatase (AcPase), alpha-naphthyl acetate esterase (ANAE) and periodic acid–Schiff (PAS), have been applied to lymph node aspirates of non-Hodgkin's lymphoma cases by Das and Gupta.[27] Focal AcPase and ANAE

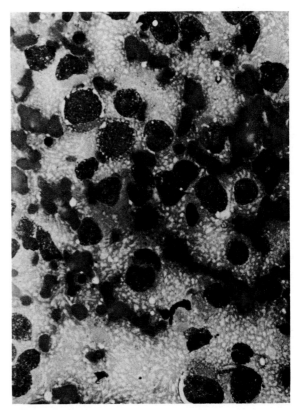

FIGURE 26–48. Metastatic seminoma. Aspirate from abdominal lymph node shows tumor cells with vacuolated cytoplasm and reticular chromatin in nuclei. Background demonstrates a tigroid appearance (May-Grünwald-Giemsa; ×400).

TABLE 26–3. Cell and Microorganism Specificity of Cytochemical Reactions

Cytochemical Reactions	Cell and Microorganism Specificity	Clinical Application
Gram's stain	*Streptococcus* and *Staphylococcus* *Actinomyces*	Suppurative lymphadenitis
Ziehl-Neelsen stain	*Mycobacterium tuberculosis*	TB lymphadenitis
Modified Ziehl-Neelsen stain[41]	*M. leprae*	Lymphadenitis due to lepra bacilli
Alpha-naphthyl acetate esterases	Helper T cells	T-CLL
		T-IBS
		Lymphoepithelioid lymphoma
Acid phosphatase	T lymphoblasts	T-cell lymphomas and leukemias
	T lymphocytes	
Tartrate resistant acid phosphatase	Hairy cell	Hairy cell leukemia
Alkaline phosphatase	Neutrophils	CML
Myeloperoxidase	Granulocytes	AML
Sudan black B	Granulocytes	AML
Chloroacetate esterases	Granulocytes	AML
Periodic acid–Schiff (PAS)	Erythroblasts	Di Guglielmo syndrome
PAS with diastase	Cytoplasmic glycogen in tumor cells	Ewing's sarcoma
		Seminoma
		Embryonal carcinoma
		Renal cell carcinoma
Mucicarmine or Alcian blue	Mucin	Mucin-secreting adenocarcinoma
		Adenoid cystic carcinoma
Schmorl reaction	Melanin	Melanoma (especially amelanotic type)
Oil red O	Neutral lipid	Burkitt-type lymphoma
		Renal cell carcinoma
		Liposarcoma
Feulgen reaction	Nuclear DNA	Various solid tumors (DNA ploidy pattern)

TB = tuberculosis; T-CLL = T chronic lymphocytic leukemia; T-IBS = T immunoblastic sarcoma; CML = chronic myelogenous leukemia; AML = acute myelogenous leukemia.

positivity were found to be reliable markers for T-cell lymphomas. Similarly, for cytochemical confirmation of nonlymphoid leukemias, myeloperoxidase, Sudan black B and chloroacetase esterase have been used.

Periodic acid–Schiff with diastase sensitivity can be of use for demonstration of glycogen in metastasis from Ewing's sarcoma, seminoma and renal cell carcinoma. Mucicarmine and Alcian blue demonstrate mucus in mucin-secreting adenocarcinoma and adenoid cystic carcinoma. Schmorl's reaction is of help in demonstration of melanin in metastatic malignant melanoma, especially the amelanotic ones.[52]

Nuclear DNA ploidy can be measured following Feulgen stain in lymphomas and metastatic/primary epithelial tumors by microphotometric methods, and lymph node aspirates can also be subjected to flow cytometric study.

Culture

As mentioned, an inflammatory exudate that is found to be negative for any microorganism by special cytochemical stains could still help in the detection of the etiologic agent if sent for culture. Bailey and associates[6] employed routine culture for AFB in tuberculous lymphadenopathy to obtain a positive rate of 82.4%. Layfield and colleagues[70] subjected lymph node aspirate to culture in 44 cases with clinical features of inflammation or grossly purulent aspirate and isolated fungi, bacteria or mycobacteria in 30.0% of cases.

Immunocytochemistry

These techniques have been utilized extensively for confirming the cytodiagnosis of lymphoma and characterization of the functional types in 91 to 93% of the cases.[74, 112] For differentiating lymphoma from epithelial neoplasm and for subtyping of epithelial malignancies by intermediate filament typing, immunocytochemical staining has also been applied.[37, 98]

Electron Microscopy

Aspirated material from lymph nodes can be processed for ultrastructural studies. This technique can further aid the cytodiagnosis, especially in undifferentiated tumors. Akhtar and associates[1, 2] have employed this technique in the diagnosis of childhood tumors, including lymphoma, neuroblastoma and retinoblastoma. In a study by Cinti and associates,[22] the tissue structure was found to be better preserved if the aspirate was processed for electron microscopy, but because of the high cost of the ultrastructural study these investigators advise that it should be performed only in limited cases.

Molecular Hybridization

A great potential exists for the lymph node aspirate in the study of gene rearrangement by molecular

TABLE 26–4. Comparison of Clinical Diagnosis and Cytodiagnosis (Lymph Node Aspiration Smears)

Clinical Diagnosis	Total No. of Cases	Cytodiagnosis						
		Lymphoma	Nonlymphoid Leukemia	Secondaries	TB	Reactive	Inflammatory and Necrotic	Not Represented
Lymphoma/Leukemia	394	255 (64.7)	13 (3.3)	30 (7.6)	19 (4.8)	36 (9.1)	13 (3.3)	28 (7.1)
Lymphoma/Secondary	46	23 (50.0)	—	11 (23.9)	4 (8.7)	6 (13.0)	—	2 (4.2)
Lymphoma/TB	27	19 (70.4)	—	—	2 (7.4)	5 (18.5)	1 (3.7)	—
Lymphoma/Secondary TB	8	6 (75.0)	—	2	—	—	—	—
Secondary	1085	25 (2.3)		776 (71.5)	12 (1.1)	154 (14.2)	21 (1.9)	97 (8.9)
TB	106	5 (4.7)	—	3 (2.8)	64 (60.4)	22 (20.8)	6 (5.7)	6 (5.7)
Lymphadenopathy (No.)	426	17 (4.0)	1 (0.2)	168 (39.4)	51 (12.0)	101 (23.7)	36 (8.5)	52 (12.0)
TOTAL	2092	350 (16.7)	14 (0.7)	990 (47.3)	152 (7.3)	324 (15.5)	77 (3.7)	185 (8.8)

hybridization. The material has been found suitable and sufficient for accurately determining clonal proliferation of B cells by analyzing immunoglobulin gene rearrangements.[56]

DIAGNOSTIC ACCURACY

For determination of the diagnostic accuracy of FNA, it is the usual practice to correlate cytodiagnoses with subsequent histologic reports of excised biopsy specimens. However, it should be realized that FNA not only offers tissue diagnosis but serves as a preliminary screening procedure for a number of clinical considerations, e.g., lymphoma, leukemia, metastasis, tuberculosis and lymphadenopathy not otherwise specified. Following the cytodiagnostic decision regarding biopsy from appropriate sites if necessary, other relevant investigations can be decided.

The role of FNA is of immense value in patients who are not suitable candidates for excisional biopsies.

As the confidence of the clinician increases, as indicated on the cytologic reports, the excision biopsy is avoided. Therefore, while correlating the cytologic diagnosis with the histopathologic report, one should not forget the contributions of FNA in relation to clinical diagnoses. In this connection, the correlation between the clinical diagnoses and cytology reports of 2092 consecutive cases of lymphadenopathy subjected to FNA at the Postgraduate Institute of Medical Education and Research, Chandigarh, India,[24] is shown in Table 26–4. Of the cases clinically diagnosed as lymphoma/leukemia, tuberculosis and secondary lesions, 64.7%, 60.4% and 71.5%, respectively, were found to be correct by FNA. An altogether different pathology was detected in the remaining cases. Moreover, in 426 (20.4%) cases no specific clinical diagnoses were offered. Of these, in 374 (87.8%) cases, FNA offered a specific tissue diagnosis.

Statistics from accumulated literature (Table 26–5) reveal that the overall diagnostic accuracy in cases of all types of lymphadenopathy varies from 82 to

TABLE 26–5. Diagnostic Accuracy of Fine Needle Aspiration in Lymphadenopathies

Diagnosis	Authors	No. of Cases	Diagnostic Accuracy (%)
Lymphadenopathy (all types)	Kline et al (1984)	340	83.0
	Ramzy et al (1985)	350	94.0
	Shaha et al (1986)	140	96.0
Lymphoma (Hodgkin's disease and non-Hodgkin's lymphoma)	Carter et al (1988)	133	88.0
	Gupta et al (1977)	50	84.0
	Morrison et al (1952)	101	80.0
			83.0
	Qizilbash et al (1985)	49	86.0
	Russel et al (1983)	59	90.0
Metastatic carcinoma	Engzell et al (1971)	257	90.0
	Kline and Neal (1976)	376	96.0
	Piscioli et al (1985)*	71	93.0
	Zadelza et al (1976)	722	96.0

*Fluoroscopy guided FNA of pelvic lymph node chains in urologic malignancies (bladder and prostatic carcinoma) and other pelvic cancers following bipedal lymphangiography.

96%.[64, 101, 107] For lymphoma (Hodgkin's disease and non-Hodgkin's lymphoma), the diagnostic accuracy varies between 80 and 90%.[18, 50, 88, 99, 103] In cases of metastatic carcinoma, the diagnostic accuracy is 90 to 96%.[39, 65, 96, 116]

In conclusion, it may be realized that FNA and histology are not competitive but complementary to each other in the diagnosis of a case of lymphadenopathy. Whenever required, one technique may supplement the other for increasing the accuracy in tissue diagnosis that is vital for deciding the patient's management.

References

1. Akhtar M, Ali A, Sabbah RS, Bakry M, Sackey K, Nash EJ: Aspiration cytology of neuroblastoma. Light and electron microscopic correlations. Cancer 57:797–803, 1986.
2. Akhtar M, Ali A, Sabbah R, Bakry M, Nash JE: Fine needle aspiration biopsy diagnosis of round cell malignant tumors of childhood. A combined light and electron microscopic approach. Cancer 55:1805–1817, 1985.
3. Anderson JR: Muir's Textbook of Pathology, 11th ed. Edited by JR Anderson, London, Edward Arnold Ltd, 1980.
4. Argyle JC, Schumann GB, Kjeldsberg CR, Athens JW: Identification of a *Toxoplasma* cyst by fine needle aspiration. Am J Clin Pathol 80:256–258, 1983.
5. Baatenburg-de-Jong RJ, Rongen RJ, De-Jong PC, Lameris JS, Knegt P: Screening for lymph nodes in the neck with ultrasound. Clin Otolaryngol 13:5–9, 1988.
6. Bailey TM, Akhtar M, Ali MA: Fine needle aspiration biopsy in the diagnosis of tuberculosis. Acta Cytol 29:732–736, 1985.
7. Bandy LC, Clarke-Pearson DL, Silverman PM, Creasman WT: Computed tomography in evaluation of extrapelvic lymphadenopathy in carcinoma of cervix. Obstet Gynecol 65:73–76, 1985.
8. Bennet MH, Farrer-Brown G, Henry K, Jelliffe AM: Classification of non-Hodgkin's lymphoma. Lancet 2:405–406, 1974.
9. Betsill WL Jr, Hajdu SI: Percutaneous aspiration biopsy of lymph nodes. Am J Clin Pathol 73:471–479, 1980.
10. Billingham ME, Rawlinson DG, Berry PF, Kempson RL: The cytodiagnosis of malignant lymphoma and Hodgkin's disease in cerebrospinal, pleural and ascitic fluids. Acta Cytol 19:547–556, 1975.
11. Bizjack-Schwarzbartl M: Cytologic characteristics of non-Hodgkin's lymphoma. Acta Cytol 32:216–220, 1988.
12. Bloch M: Comparative study of lymph node cytology by puncture and histopathology. Acta Ctyol 11:139–144, 1967.
13. Boccon-Gibod L, Katz M, Cochand B, Le Portz B, Steg A: Lymphography and percutaneous fine needle node aspiration biopsy in the staging of bladder carcinoma. J Urol 132:24–26, 1984.
14. Bottles K, McPhaul LW, Volberding P: Fine needle aspiration biopsy of patients with acquired immunodeficiency syndrome (AIDS): Experience in an outpatient clinic. Ann Intern Med 108:42–45, 1988.
15. Bruneton JN, Normand F, Balu-Maestro C, Kerboul P, Santini N, Thyss A, Schneider M: Lymphomatous superficial lymph nodes: US detection. Radiology 165:233–235, 1987.
16. Brynitz S, Struve-Christensen E: Transcarinal mediastinal needle biopsy as supplement to bronchoscopic evaluation of neoplastic lung diseases. Endoscopy 17:18–20, 1985.
17. Campbell J: Cat-scratch disease. Pathology 12:277–292, 1977.
18. Carter TR, Feldman PS, Innes DJ Jr, Frierson HF Jr, Frigy AF: The role of fine needle aspiration cytology in the diagnosis of lymphoma. Acta Cytol 32:848–853, 1988.
19. Cavett JR III, McAfee R, Ramzy I: Hansen's disease (leprosy). Diagnosis by aspiration biopsy of lymph nodes. Acta Cytol 30:189–193, 1986.
20. Chatterjee KD: Parasitology (Protozoology and Helminthology) in Relation to Clinical Medicine, 12th ed. Edited by KD Chatterjee. Calcutta, Chatterjee Medical Publishers, 1980.
21. Christ ML, Feltes-Kennedy M: Fine needle aspiration of toxoplasmic lymphadenitis. Acta Cytol 26:425–428, 1982.
22. Cinti S, Ferratti M, Amati S, Balercia G, Vecchi A, Osculati F: Electron microscopy applied to fine needle aspiration. A report of six cases from various sites. Tumori 69:423–435, 1983.
23. Civardi G, Fornari F, Cavanna L, DiStasi M, Sbolli G, Buscarini L: Value of rapid staining and assessment of ultrasound-guided fine needle aspiration biopsies. Acta Cytol 32:552–554, 1988.
24. Das DK: Cytomorphological, Cytochemical and Immunological Characterization of Lymphomas. Doctoral Thesis, Postgraduate Institute of Medical Education and Research, Chandigarh, India, 1983.
25. Das DK, Bhatt NC, Khan VA, Luthra UK: Cervicofacial actinomycosis: Diagnosis by fine needle aspiration cytology. Acta Cytol 33:278–280, 1989.
26. Das DK, Gupta SK: Morphological and functional classification of non-Hodgkin's lymphomas: Frequency of distribution of subtypes. Indian J Med Res 81:591–601, 1985.
27. Das DK, Gupta SK: Cytochemical studies in non-Hodgkin's lymphoma. Indian J Med Res 83:19–26, 1986.
28. Das DK, Gupta SK: Cytodiagnosis of Hodgkin's disease: A study of its subtypes by differential cell count in fine needle aspiration smear. Acta Cytol 34:337–341, 1990.
29. Das DK, Gupta SK, Datta BN, Sharma SC: Diagnosis of Hodgkin's disease and its subtypes. Scope and limitation of fine needle aspiration cytology. Acta Cytol 34:329–336, 1990.
30. Das DK, Gupta SK, Datta U, Banerjee CK: Cytodiagnosis of immunoblastic sarcomas (IBS). Bull Postgrad Instit 20:11–20, 1986.
31. Das DK, Gupta SK, Datta U, Sharma SC, Datta BN: Malignant lymphoma of convoluted lymphocytes: Diagnosis by fine needle aspiration cytology and cytochemistry. Diagn Cytopathol 2:307–311, 1986.
32. Das DK, Gupta SK, Pathak IC, Sharma SC, Datta BN: Burkitt-type lymphoma. Diagnosis by fine needle aspiration cytology. Acta Cytol 31:1–7, 1987.
33. Das DK, Gupta SK, Sharma SC, Banerjee CK, Datta U, Datta BN: Cytodiagnosis of Lennert's lymphoma. Indian J Pathol Microbiol 27:161–168, 1984.
34. Das DK, Gupta SK, Sehgal S: Extramedullary plasma cell tumor. Diagnosis by fine needle aspiration cytology. Diagn Cytopathol 2:248–251, 1986.
35. Das DK, Pant JN, Chachra KL, Murthy NS, Satyanarayanan L, Thankamma TC, Kakkar PK: Tuberculous lymphadenitis: Correlation of cellular components and necrosis in lymph node aspirate with AFB positivity and bacillary count. Indian J Pathol Microbiology (in press).
36. DeVita VT Jr, Jaffe ES, Hellman S: Hodgkin's disease and non-Hodgkin lymphoma. *In* Cancer: Principle and Practice of Oncology. Edited by VT DeVita Jr, S Hellman, SA Rosenberg. Philadelphia, JB Lippincott, 1985.
37. Domagala W, Weber K, Osborn M: Differential diagnosis of lymph node aspirates by intermediate filament typing of tumor cells. Acta Cytol 30:225–234, 1986.
38. Dorfman RF: Classification of non-Hodgkin's lymphomas. Lancet 1:1295–1296, 1974.
39. Engzell U, Jacobsson PA, Sigurdson A, Zajicek J: Aspiration biopsy of metastatic carcinoma in lymph nodes of neck: A review of 1101 consecutive cases. Acta Otolaryngol 72:138–147, 1971.
40. Feinberg MR, Bhaskar AG, Bourne P: Differential diagnosis of malignant lymphoma by imprint cytology. Acta Cytol 24:16–25, 1980.
41. Fite GL, Cambre PJ, Turner MH: Procedure for demonstrating lepra bacilli in paraffin sections. Arch Pathol 43:624–625, 1947.
42. Forkner CE: Material from lymph nodes of man. II. Studies on living and fixed cells withdrawn from lymph node of man. Arch Intern Med 40:647–661, 1927.
43. Frable MA, Frable WJ: Fine needle aspiration biopsy: Efficacy in the diagnosis of head and neck sarcoidosis. Laryngoscope 94:1281–1283, 1984.
44. Frable WJ, Kardos TF: Fine needle aspiration biopsy. Application in the diagnosis of lymphoproliferative diseases. Am J Surg Pathol 12[Suppl I]:62–72, 1988.
45. Friedman M, Kim U, Shimaoka K, Panahon A, Han T,

Stutzman L: Appraisal of aspiration cytology in management of Hodgkin's disease. Cancer 45:1653–1663, 1980.

46. Frizzera G, Moran EM, Rappaport H: Angioimmunoblastic lymphadenopathy: Diagnosis and clinical course. Am J Med 59:803–818, 1975.

47. Fujioka T, Koike H, Aoki H, Ohhori T, Chiba R, Okamoto S: Significance of staging pelvic lymphadenectomy for prostatic cancer. Urol Int 42:380–384, 1987.

48. Gothlin JH: Prostatic carcinoma: Staging with percutaneous lymph node biopsy. Bull Cancer 72:462–466, 1985.

49. Greig EDW, Gray ACH: Note on lymphatic glands in sleeping sickness. Lancet 1:1570, 1904.

50. Gupta SK, Datta TK, Aikat BK: Lymph node aspiration biopsy in diagnosis of lymphoma. Indian J Pathol Microbiol 20:231–237, 1977.

51. Gupta SK, Kumar B, Kaur S: Aspiration cytology of lymph nodes in leprosy. Int J Lepr 49:9–15, 1981.

52. Gupta SK, Rajwanshi AK, Das DK: Fine needle aspiration cytology smear pattern of malignant melanoma. Acta Cytol 29:983–988, 1985.

53. Guthrie CG: Gland puncture as a diagnostic measure. Bull Johns Hopkin's Hosp 32:266–269, 1921.

54. Hendrick JW: Occult cancer with cervical lymph node metastasis. In Cancer of the Head and Neck. Edited by J Conley. Washington DC, Butterworth, 1967.

55. Highman WJ, Oliver RT: Diagnosis of metastatic testicular germ cell tumors using fine needle aspiration cytology. J Clin Pathol 40:1324–1333, 1987.

56. Hu E, Horning S, Flynn S, Brown S, Warnke R, Sklar J: Diagnosis of B-cell lymphoma by analysis of immunoglobulin gene rearrangements in biopsy specimen obtained by fine needle aspiration. J Clin Oncol 4:278–283, 1986.

57. Jeffrey RB Jr: Coaxial technique for CT-guided biopsy of deep-seated retroperitoneal lymph nodes. Gastrointest Radiol 13:271–272, 1988.

58. Kardos TF, Kornstein MJ, Frable WJ: Cytology and immunocytology of infectious mononucleosis in fine needle aspiration of lymph nodes. Acta Cytol 32:722–726, 1988.

59. Kaur S, Kumar B, Gupta SK: Fine needle aspiration of lymph nodes in leprosy. A study of bacteriological and morphological indices. Int J Lepr 45:369–372, 1977.

60. Khoory MS: Disease of lymph node and spleen. In Clinical Aspiration Cytology. Edited by KM Koship. Philadelphia, JB Lippincott Co, 1983.

61. Kinsey DL, James AG, Bonta JA: A study of metastatic carcinomas of neck. Ann Surg 147:366–374, 1958.

62. Klemi PJ, Elo JJ, Joensuu H: Fine needle aspiration biopsy of granulomatous disorders. Sarcoidosis 4:38–41, 1987.

63. Kline TS: Lymph nodes and superficial masses. In Handbook of Fine Needle Aspiration Cytology, Second ed. Edited by TS Kline. New York, Churchill Livingstone, 1988.

64. Kline TS, Kannan V, Kline IK: Lymphadenopathy and aspiration biopsy cytology: Review of 376 superficial nodes. Cancer 54:1076–1081, 1984.

65. Kline TS, Neal HS: Needle aspiration biopsy: Diagnosis of subcutaneous nodules and lymph nodes. JAMA 235:2848–2850, 1976.

66. Koss LG, Woyke S, Olszewski W: In Aspiration Biopsy Cytology: Interpretation and Histologic Bases. Edited by LG Koss, S Woyke, W Olszewski. Tokyo, Igaku-Shoin, 1984.

67. Krick JA, Remington JS: Current concepts in parasitology: Toxoplasmosis in adults—An overview. N Engl J Med 298:550–553, 1978.

68. Kuhn III C, Askin FB: In Anderson's Pathology. Edited by JM Kissane. St. Louis, CV Mosby Co, 1985.

69. Kumar PV, Hambarsoomina B, Vaezzadeh K: Fine needle aspiration cytology of localized Leishmania lymphadenitis. Acta Cytol 31:14–16, 1987.

70. Layfield LJ, Glasgow BJ, DuPuis MH: Fine needle aspiration of lymphadenopathy of suspected infectious etiology. Arch Pathol Lab Med 109:810–812, 1985.

71. Lennert K: Malignant lymphomas other than Hodgkin's disease. Berlin-Heidelburg, Springer Verlag, 1978.

72. Lennert K, Mohri N, Stein H, Kaiserling E: The histopathology of malignant lymphoma. Br J Hematol 31[Suppl]:193–203, 1975.

73. Levine PH, Kamaraju LS, Canelly RR, Berard CW, Dorfman RF, Magrath I, Easton JM: The American Burkitt's lymphoma registry: Eight years experience. Cancer 49:1016–1022, 1982.

74. Levitt S, Cheng L, DuPuis MH, Layfield LJ: Fine needle aspiration diagnosis of malignant lymphoma with confirmation by immunoperoxidase staining. Acta Cytol 29:895–902, 1985.

75. Linsk JA, Franzen S: The enlarged lymph nodes. In Fine Needle Aspiration for Clinicians. Edited by JA Linsk, S Franzen. Philadelphia, JB Lippincott Co, 1986.

76. Lopes-Cardozo P: Clinical cytology. Edited by P Lopes-Cardozo, L Stafleu, Leyden, 1954.

77. Lopes-Cardozo P: In Atlas of Clinical Cytology. Edited by P Lopes-Cardozo. The Netherlands, Verlag Chemi, 1975.

78. Lucas PF: Diagnostic value of lymph node aspiration biopsy. Postgrad Med J 30:544–548, 1954.

79. Lucas PF: Lymph node smears in the diagnosis of lymphadenopathy. A review. Blood 10:1030–1054, 1955.

80. Lukes RJ, Collins RD: Immunologic characterization of human malignant lymphomas. Cancer 34:1488–1503, 1974.

81. Lukes RJ, Parker JW, Taylor CR, Tindle BH, Cramer AD, Lincoln TL: Immunologic approaches to non-Hodgkin's lymphomas and related leukemias. Analysis of multiparameter study in 425 cases. Semin Hematol 5:322–351, 1978.

82. Lukes RJ, Tindle BH: Immunoblastic lymphadenopathy: A prelymphomatous state of immunoblastic lymphoma. In Lymphoid Neoplasia. I. Recent Results Cancer Res 64:241–246, 1978.

83. Martin HE, Ellis EB: Biopsy by needle puncture and aspiration. Ann Surg 92:169–181, 1930.

84. Martin HE, Morfit HM: Cervical lymph node metastasis as first symptom of cancer. Surg Gynecol Obstet 78:133–159, 1944.

85. Mathe G, Rappaport H, O'Conor GT, Torloni H: Histological and cytological typing of neoplastic disease of hemopoietic and lymphoid tissue. International Histological Classification of Tumors No. 14, Geneva, 1976.

86. McDonald TW, Shepherd JH, Morley GW, Naylor B, Ruffolo EH, Cavanagh D: Role of needle biopsy in the investigation of gynecologic malignancy. J Reprod Med 32:287–292, 1987.

87. Meatherigham RE, Ackerman LV: Aspiration biopsy of lymph nodes. Surg Gynecol Obstet 84:1071–1076, 1947.

88. Morrison M, Samwick AA, Rubinstein J, Stitch M, Loewe L: Lymph node aspiration. Clinical and hematologic observations in 101 patients. Am J Clin Pathol 22:255–262, 1952.

89. Narasimham MVVL, Rao Ch K, Rao CK: Some clinical aspects of bancroftian filariasis in east Godavari district of Andhra Pradesh. Indian J Med Res 78:631–635, 1983.

90. Nathwani BN, Kim H, Rappaport H: Malignant lymphoma, lymphoblastic. Cancer 38:964–983, 1976.

91. Nathawani BN, Rappaport H, Moran EM, Pangalis GA, Kim H: Evolution of immunoblastic lymphoma in angioimmunoblastic lymphadenopathy. Lymphoid neoplasia I. Recent Results Cancer Res 64:235–240, 1978.

92. O'Dowd GJ, Frable WJ, Behm FG: Fine needle aspiration cytology of benign lymph node hyperplasia. Diagnostic significance of lymphohistiocytic aggregates. Acta Cytol 29:554–558, 1985.

93. Orell SR, Skinner JM: The typing of non-Hodgkin's lymphoma using fine needle aspiration cytology. Pathology 14:389–394, 1982.

94. Piscioli F, Leonardi E, Reich A, Luciani L: Percutaneous lymph node aspiration biopsy and tumor grade in staging of prostatic carcinoma. Prostate 5:459–468, 1984.

95. Piscioli F, Pusiol T, Leonardi E, Luciani L: Role of percutaneous pelvic node aspiration cytology in the management of bladder carcinoma. Acta Cytol 29:37–43, 1985.

96. Piscioli F, Scappini P, Luciani L: Aspiration cytology in the staining of urologic cancer. Cancer 56:1173–1180, 1985.

97. Pontifex AH, Klimo P: Application of aspiration biopsy cytology to lymphomas. Cancer 53:553–556, 1984.

98. Putts JJ, Vooijs GP, Huymans A, Van-Aspert A, Ramaekers FC: Cytoskeletal proteins as tissue specific markers in cytopathology. Exp Cell Biol 54:73–79 1986.

99. Qizilbash AH, Elavathil LJ, Chen V, Young JEM, Archibald SD: Aspiration biopsy cytology of lymph nodes in malignant lymphoma. Diagn Cytopathol 1:18–22, 1985.

100. Rajwanshi A, Bhambhani S, Das DK: Fine needle aspiration cytology diagnosis of tuberculosis. Diagn Cytopathol 3:13–16, 1987.

101. Ramzy I, Rone R, Schultenover SJ, Buhaug J: Lymph node aspiration biopsy: Diagnostic reliability and limitations—an analysis of 350 cases. Diagn Cytopathol 1:39–45, 1985.

102. Rappaport H: Tumors of haemopoietic system. *In* Atlas of Tumor Pathology, Section 3, Fascicle 8. Washington, DC, Armed Forces Institute of Pathology, 1966.

103. Russel J, Orell S, Skinner J, Sehsadri R: Fine needle aspiration cytology in the management of lymphoma. Aust NZ J Med 13:365–368, 1983.

104. Rywlin AM: Hemopoietic system. *In* Anderson's Pathology, 8th ed. Edited by JM Kissane, WAD Anderson. St Louis, CV Mosby Co, 1985.

105. Sadanah-Metre M, Jayaram G: Acid-fast bacilli in aspiration smears from tuberculous lymph nodes. An analysis of 255 cases. Acta Cytol 31:17–19, 1981.

106. Seidel TA, Garbes AD: Cellules grumelees. Old terminology resisted. Regarding the cytologic diagnosis of chronic lymphocytic leukemia and well-differentiated lymphocytic lymphoma in pleural effusions. Acta Cytol 29:775–780, 1985.

107. Saha A, Weber C, Marti J: Fine needle aspiration in the diagnosis of cervical lymphadenopathy. Am J Surg 152:420–423, 1986.

108. Silverman JF: Fine needle aspiration cytology of cat-scratch disease. Acta Cytol 29:542–547, 1985.

109. Spriggs AI, Vanhegan RI: Cytological diagnosis of lymphoma in serous effusions. J Clin Pathol 34:1311–1325, 1981.

110. Stani J: Cytologic diagnosis of reactive lymphadenopathy in fine needle aspiration biopsy specimens. Acta Cytol 31:8–13, 1987.

111. Stewart FW: Diagnosis of tumors by aspiration. Am J Pathol 9:801–812, 1933.

112. Tani EM, Christensson B, Porwit A, Skoog L: Immunocytochemical analysis and cytomorphologic diagnosis on fine needle aspirates of lymphoproliferative disease. Acta Cytol 32:209–215, 1988.

113. Tempka T, Kubiczek M: Normal and pathologic lymphadenogram in light of own research. Acta Med Scand 131:434–450, 1948.

114. Wang KP: Flexible transbronchial needle aspiration biopsy for histologic specimen. Chest 88:860–863, 1985.

115. Wright DH: Gross distribution and haematology. *In* Burkitt's Lymphoma. Edited by DP Burkitt, DH Wright. Edinburgh, E & S Livingstone, 1970.

116. Zadelza A, Ennuyer A, Bataini P, Poncent P: Valeu du diagnostic cytologique des adenopathies par ponction. Confrontations cyto-histologique de 1756 cas. Bull Cancer 63:327–340, 1976.

27

Breast

Jan F. Silverman

Fine needle aspiration (FNA) biopsy of the breast was first used in the 1930s by Martin, Ellis and Stewart,[146, 147, 200] followed in the late 1940s and early 1950s by Adair and Godwin.[2, 77] However, it was not until others in Europe reported a large series of FNA of the breast was aspiration cytology shown to be a valuable and accurate diagnostic procedure.[70, 222, 224, 226, 227] With the rebirth of FNA biopsy in general, aspiration of breast lesions began to gain acceptance in the United States.[54, 64, 67, 121, 133] The advantages of the procedure include accurate diagnosis, low cost, excellent patient acceptance and minimal or no morbidity.[126, 128] However, there was some hesitation in accepting the procedure because of apprehension about needle-tract seeding and because of the need for an experienced cytopathologist to interpret the aspirated material.[1, 54, 118] Another major concern regarding breast FNA biopsy has been that mastectomy might be performed based on a false-positive cytologic diagnosis,[54] with attendant clinical and medicolegal implications.[217] This fear has been heightened by those who advocate that mastectomy be performed based solely on the cytologic report without frozen-section confirmation.[15, 50, 65, 74, 78, 194, 217] However, some investigators advise frozen-section confirmation.[161, 202] Eisenberg and colleagues[50] suggested that the real safeguard lies in the use of very strict criteria for making an accurate diagnosis of malignancy on a breast aspirate.

It has been argued that FNA biopsy followed by excisional biopsy with frozen section for confirmation may actually increase the cost of the workup of a breast mass.[65, 82, 161, 194] Bauermeister,[14] in a discussion of the roles and limitations of both frozen section and FNA biopsy, implied that the procedures are mutually exclusive in the workup of breast masses. This pervasive attitude has perhaps contributed to the slow implementation of FNA biopsy of breast lesions in medical centers having a pathologist who is initially inexperienced with interpreting the material.[1] We have shown that the FNA biopsy is cost-effective by accurately triaging the patient to an outpatient or inpatient setting, rather than by eliminating the frozen section.[190] Our cost analysis demonstrated considerable savings per case, even when combined with the cost of frozen section.

In our practice, the FNA biopsy triage role is defined in the following manner (Fig. 27–1). If a benign FNA biopsy is obtained, the lesion can be excised using a local anesthesia in an outpatient setting. When the FNA biopsy findings are positive, the patient can be hospitalized for both the excisional biopsy and definitive treatment. In many cases in which an unequivocal diagnosis of malignancy is rendered, a frozen section may not be needed, which would further decrease the cost. However, we believe that by utilizing FNA biopsy with frozen-section confirmation in a specific situation, a more accurate diagnosis can be rendered with the virtual elimination of false-positive diagnoses and, thereby, unnecessary mastectomies.[190]

Frozen-section confirmation is especially needed when the FNA results conflict with the clinical impression in atypical or suspicious cases or when atypical cells are present in scanty number or ill prepared material or both. Another situation in which FNA biopsy can be combined with frozen-section confirmation occurs when pathologists are learning and mastering the techniques of FNA biopsy and smear interpretation or when a large volume of cases is not available to allow development of a sufficient level of expertise. With increasing experience and volume of cases, less reliance on frozen-section confirmation will be needed.[190]

TECHNIQUE

For most FNA biopsies, we use a 22-gauge, 1.5-inch needle, attached to a disposable 20-ml syringe fitted in a commercially available holder. Approximately half the smears are immediately wet fixed with sprayed 95% ethyl alcohol and the remaining smears are air dried and stained by a modified rapid Wright stain (Diff-Quik stain).[63, 224, 225] The staining process can be performed within 30 seconds and therefore lends itself to a "quick-read" interpretation of the material. In general, at least two separate passes per lesion are

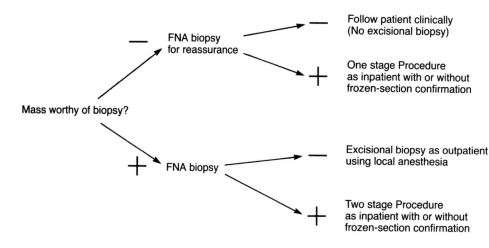

Follow patient clinically
(No excisional biopsy)

One stage Procedure
as inpatient with or without
frozen-section confirmation

Excisional biopsy as outpatient
using local anesthesia

Two stage Procedure
as inpatient with or without
frozen-section confirmation

FIGURE 27–1. Algorithm for workup of a **breast mass** using fine needle aspiration. (Modified from Lannin DR, Silverman JF, Pories WJ, Walker C: Cost-effectiveness of fine needle biopsy of the breast. Ann Surg 203:474–450, 1986.)

initially made and then examined for assessment of adequacy of the specimen and rapid interpretation. If insufficient material is present, additional aspirations are performed. Occasionally, more FNA biopsies are performed when an unusual lesion is encountered, so that material can be submitted for immunocytochemical or electron microscopic studies or both. Currently, additional passes are also obtained for immunocytochemical studies for estrogen receptor protein by Estrogen Receptor Assay Immunocytochemical Analysis (ERA-ICA) and flow cytometry in selective cases. We believe that aspiration for ERA-ICA and flow cytometry may become a more routine procedure.

The most common complication is hematoma formation, which can be decreased if firm pressure is applied after performance of each biopsy. Pneumothorax is a very rare complication.[1, 25] For deep-seated lesions a lateral rather than a vertical approach should be taken. The FNA procedure is usually tolerated well with little pain. However, percutaneous aspirations through the areola for central lesions should be avoided, if possible, because these can be quite painful. Either local anesthesia should be utilized or a lateral approach via the nonareolar skin should be attempted.

Fine needle aspiration biopsy can be utilized for the evaluation of all palpable breast lesions and has the potential for evaluation of nonpalpable mammographically evident lesions. The advantages of the procedure include (1) rapid accurate diagnosis, (2) cost-effective triage role in the treatment of breast masses,[127] (3) differentiation of cysts from solid tumors and a therapeutic procedure when a cyst is encountered, (4) involvement of the patient in the decision-making process when malignancy is encountered, (5) psychological help in the relief of anxiety for a patient with a benign breast lesion, (6) evaluation of local chest wall recurrences[28] and (7) ancillary studies. These last studies include estrogen-receptor analysis, flow cytometry, electron microscopy, image analysis and oncogene assessment that can be performed on the aspirated material.

ANATOMY AND HISTOLOGY

The female mammary gland is a modified sweat gland consisting of a functional epithelial component and surrounding stroma. The breast is composed of 15 to 25 lobes or segments that converge on the nipple in a radial pattern. Each segment consists of a lactiferous duct, lactiferous sinus, segmental collecting duct, subsegmental duct, ductule (terminal duct) and secretory acini (terminal ductules). The collecting ducts are lined by columnar cells, which can be multilayered in the larger ducts. The terminal portions of the lactiferous sinus and the lactiferous duct are lined by stratified squamous epithelium. The secretory acini consist of a single layer of cuboidal or cylindric epithelial cells, with surrounding elongated-to-flat myoepithelial cells resting on a basement membrane. The acini are set within a loose specialized stroma, which defines the lobular unit (Fig. 27–2). The surrounding lobular connective tissue contains increased numbers of capillaries and a few lymphocytes, histiocytes, plasma cells and mast cells. The lobular connective tissue is sharply separated from the more dense periductal fibrous tissue and abundant fat, which makes up the majority of the breast tissue.[10, 90, 164]

After puberty, the breasts are a resting organ undergoing minor repeated stimulations associated with the menstrual cycle.[164] During pregnancy, the breasts undergo lobular and ductal proliferation into the fully differentiated state of lactation. By the end of the second trimester of pregnancy, secretory activity is quite evident. Following lactation, there is involution to the "resting state," which usually takes approximately 3 months but may be longer.[164] With aging, changes occur in the breasts including atrophy of the parenchymal cells, increase in the intralobular fibrous tissue and hyalinization of the stroma. The postmenopausal breasts show an increased amount of fat, a diminished connective tissue component, a persistence of mammary ducts and a disappearance of lobules. The cytologic cellular changes of mammary gland epithelium during the menstrual cycle have been studied with image analysis.[143]

BENIGN LESIONS

Breast Cysts

Single or multiple breast cysts are the most prevalent lesions of the female mammary gland.[116] Although

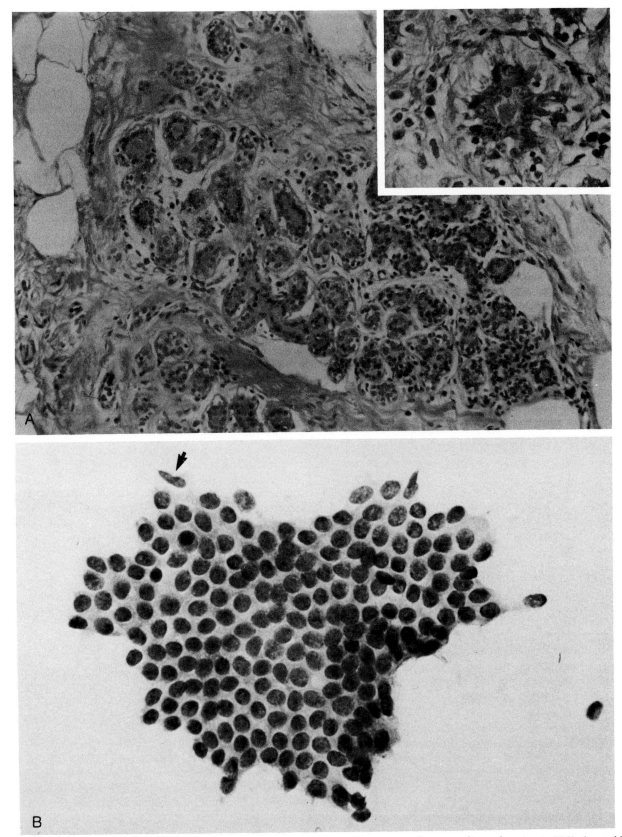

FIGURE 27–2. *A,* **Breast acini** set within a loose stroma defining the lobular unit (hematoxylin and eosin; ×100). *Inset,* High power of terminal ductules consisting of a single layer of cuboidal epithelial cells with surrounding pale, elongated to flat, myoepithelial cells resting on a basement membrane (hematoxylin and eosin; ×400). *B,* Single honeycomb cluster of **benign ductal cells** having a uniform appearance along with a few attached myoepithelial cells at the periphery (arrow) and in the background (Papanicolaou stain; ×200).

aspiration of breast cysts is an ideal procedure for both diagnosis and treatment, some have questioned the utility of cytologically examining all cyst fluid.[27, 63, 206] A lesion is considered to be a breast cyst when greater than 1 ml of fluid is aspirated.[121] The aspirated cyst fluid may be clear, opaque or turbid and may vary from yellow to green or brown to blood stained.[121] Fluid that is clear or light yellow almost always is acellular or quite limited in cellularity, consisting of a few epithelial cells including apocrine cells. Apocrine cells occur almost exclusively in benign cystic lesions.[206] Foam cells are usually present; they are believed to be most likely modified epithelial cells.[121] Intracytoplasmic eosinophilic inclusions have been noted in breast cyst fluid; these are believed to be giant lysosomes.[155]

Following complete aspiration of the cyst, it is especially important to repalpate the area in order to determine if a residual breast lesion is present.[63] If a residual mass is found, a second aspiration should be performed. Ciatto and associates[27] reported the results of aspiration cytologic examinations of 6782 consecutive breast cyst fluids. These investigators noted that the presence of most intracystic lesions and especially intracystic carcinomas was suspected based on physical examination, mammography or aspirated blood-stained fluid. These observations strongly suggest that cytologic examination of cyst fluid should be limited to those that are blood stained.[27, 206] We have encountered examples of intracystic breast carcinomas that were clinically considered to be benign. The aspiration of bloody cyst fluid prompted the submission of specimens for cytologic examination.

Inflammatory Lesions

Most inflammatory lesions of the breast are secondary to bacterial infections, although rarely the breast can be involved with tuberculosis (TB), fungal and viral infections.[10, 90]

Acute Mastitis and Abscess Formation

Fine needle aspiration biopsy of acute mastitis or breast abscess, or both, will reveal increased numbers of neutrophils and foamy macrophages, including evidence of cytophagocytosis (Fig. 27–3). Abundant cell debris will be in the background. Evidence of epithelial atypia may be present in any inflammatory cell process, especially when acute inflammation is present. Atypical epithelial cells may show features of regeneration and repair, including nuclear enlargement and prominent nucleoli (Fig. 27–4). However, in inflammatory atypia, the nucleocytoplasmic ratio is usually within normal limits. One should suspect inflammatory atypia when numerous acute inflammatory cells are seen in the background and neutrophils are found infiltrating the epithelial groupings (see Fig. 27–4).

Cytologic features not supportive of the diagnosis of carcinoma include limited epithelial cellularity and degenerating atypical cells in an inflammatory set-

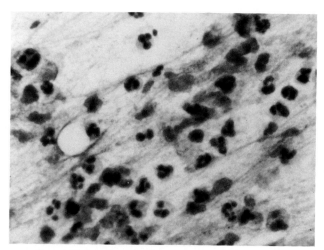

FIGURE 27–3. Acute mastitis consisting of sheets of neutrophils (Papanicolaou stain; × 400).

ting.[63, 115–117, 191] In comedomastitis, a greater number of ductal cells may be present, including those showing a variable degree of inflammatory atypia.[63] In any process demonstrating inflammatory atypia, the degree of atypia appears greater in the Romanovsky-stained air-dried smears (i.e., Diff-Quik stain) than in the Papanicolaou-stained alcohol-fixed smears. Appreciation of the inflammatory background, in which the atypia is present, and a more conservative cytologic interpretation, based on the findings in the Papanicolaou-stained smears, serve as checks in order to avoid a false-positive diagnosis of malignancy.

Plasma Cell Mastitis

Plasma cell mastitis is a common chronic inflammatory condition of the breast characterized by the presence of numerous lymphocytes and plasma cells surrounding ducts filled with inspissated secretion in the acute phase. During the healing phase of this lesion, fibrosis and scar formation occur.[121] The cytologic findings reflect the phase or stage of the process.

Lipomas

Adipose tissue is commonly appreciated in breast aspirates. However, the diagnosis of breast lipoma is made reluctantly in most cases, because the presence of fat in the smears is usually secondary to inadequate sampling of the palpable mass; the fat represents inadvertent sampling of the surrounding adipose tissue (Fig. 27–5). However, if a soft circumscribed freely movable mass is aspirated and the only finding with repeated biopsies is the presence of fat, lipoma can be a suggested diagnosis. The confidence level of making the diagnosis of lipoma is enhanced when the individual interpreting the cytologic material has also performed the aspiration.

FIGURE 27–4. *A,* Cluster of **benign ductal cells** showing atypical features including prominent nucleoli. Note the neutrophils infiltrating the group of epithelial cells (Papanicolaou stain; ×400). *B,* Atypical sheet of **epithelial cells** showing features of regeneration and repair including nuclear enlargement and prominent nucleoli (Papanicolaou stain; ×600).

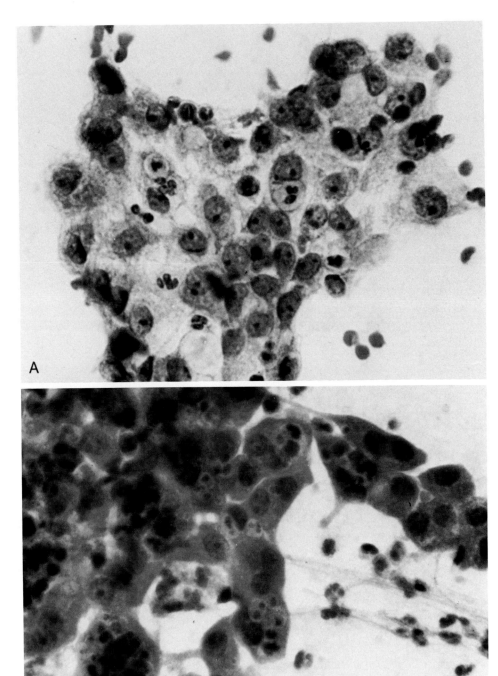

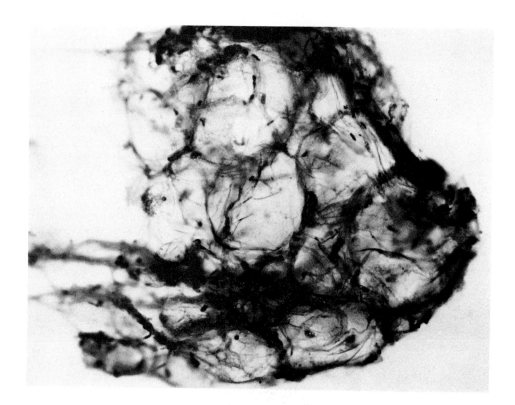

FIGURE 27–5. Cluster of adipose tissue that represents inadvertent sampling of fat surrounding a **discrete breast lesion**. The findings are indistinguishable from those in an aspirate of lipoma (Papanicolaou stain; ×400).

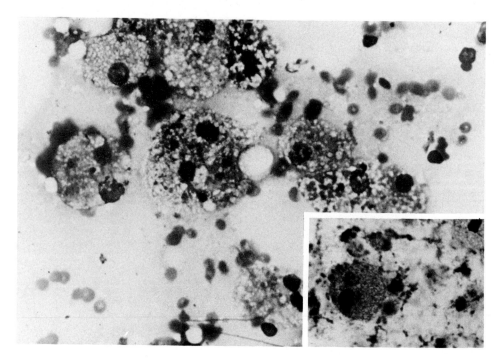

FIGURE 27–6. Aspirate of fat necrosis consisting of lipid-laden macrophages (lipophages) having abundant vacuolated cytoplasm (Diff-Quik stain; ×400). *Inset,* Degenerating histiocytes in fat necrosis having opaque pyknotic nuclei that should not be confused with atypical degenerating ductal cells (Papanicolaou stain; ×200).

Fat Necrosis

Fat necrosis occurs following trauma, foreign body reaction or response to breast malignancy, especially if tumor necrosis is present. Fat necrosis can radiologically, grossly and histologically, especially at frozen section, mimic malignancy. The FNA of fat necrosis consists of fat; amorphous debris (degenerating fat); inflammatory cells, including neutrophils, plasma cells and lymphocytes; and numerous lipid-laden macrophages (lipophages). The lipophages have abundant vacuolated cytoplasm (Fig. 27–6). Multinucleated macrophages and spindle-shaped stromal cells (fibroblasts) can also be present. The rare hibernoma of the breast should be considered in the differential diagnosis when finely and coarsely vacuolated cells are encountered.[96]

Subareolar Abscess

Subareolar abscess of the breast is a specific clinicopathologic entity well known to surgeons but until relatively recently not well described in cytology literature.[72, 191] The lesion is a low-grade infection occurring in the subareolar region. It often begins as a localized area of inflammation beneath the nipple and progresses to form an abscess; this is followed by subsequent cycles of sinus tract formation, drainage, partial healing and recurrence (Fig. 27–7).[191] With the presence of nipple retraction and a mass, the lesion can be clinically confused with a neoplasm such as adenoma of the nipple or breast carcinoma.

We reported the cytomorphologic findings of eight cases of subareolar abscess of the breast diagnosed by FNA biopsy.[191] A spectrum of cytomorphologic findings was appreciated including diagnostic anucleated squames associated with numerous neutrophils, keratinous debris, cholesterol crystals, parakeratosis and strips of squamous epithelium (Fig. 27–8). A foreign body reaction, with sheets of histiocytes and multinucleated foreign body–type giant cells, was noted in some of the cases (Fig. 27–9).

Cytomorphology of Subareolar Abscess

- Anucleated squamous cells
- Acute and chronic inflammation
- Foreign body reaction or granulation tissue or both may be present.
- Epithelial atypia can be a potential pitfall for false-positive diagnosis.

Subareolar abscess of the breast demonstrates some of the potential diagnostic pitfalls for a false-positive diagnosis of malignancy that can occur in any inflammatory process including those involving the breast. These include the presence of groups of atypical ductal cells (Fig. 27–10), squamous atypia and fragments of exuberant granulation tissue (Fig. 27–11). Four of our initial eight cases demonstrated some of these findings, which could potentially lead to a false-positive diagnosis of malignancy, if the other cytologic features of

subareolar abscess were not appreciated.[24, 117, 118, 163, 191] A ruptured epidermal inclusion cyst arising in the skin of the breast shares similar cytologic and histologic features with subareolar abscess, but the peripheral location of the epidermal inclusion cyst should clearly separate that lesion from the central subareolar abscess.

Proposed theories concerning the pathogenesis of subareolar abscess include (1) part of comedomastitis, (2) squamous metaplasia of columnar epithelium of large lactiferous ducts and (3) congenital anomaly of the ductal system.[191, 228] The most likely explanation is squamous metaplasia of the epithelium of the lactiferous duct with filling of the lumen of the duct with keratinous debris, which then ruptures (see Fig. 27–7). A surrounding inflammatory cell reaction occurs including a foreign body reaction to keratinous type debris (see Fig. 27–7). The FNA biopsy can influence the management of the patient because chronic subareolar abscess needs complete surgical excision of the abscess, sinus tract and dilated duct for cure; the early lesion may be treated adequately by aspiration of gross pus and antibiotic therapy.[189, 191]

Fibrocystic Disease

Fibrocystic disease is the most common mass-producing lesion in females over the age of 30 years. The lesions are generally multifocal and may be bilateral. The histologic components of fibrocystic disease include dilation of ducts (cysts), apocrine metaplasia, stromal fibrosis, chronic inflammation and duct hyperplasia.[90] Haagensen believes that the initial insult of fibrocystic disease is periductal mastitis, which results in periductal scarring.[90] The fibrosis produces functional or permanent stasis with retrograde duct dilation and subsequent formation of small-to-large cysts. Aspirations from fibrocystic disease can have limited cellularity due to the fibrotic nature of many of the lesions.[116] In the Linsk and Franzen series,[133] 82% of 210 cases showed few or no cells. Kline's series[116] demonstrated 47% of 214 cases having limited cellularity.[116]

In fibrocystic disease the epithelial cells are generally arranged in tight, cohesive honeycomb-like groups. In general, the cells have round-to-oval nuclei, finely dispersed granular chromatin and imperceptible-to-small nucleoli (Fig. 27–12). Apocrine cells are also arranged in flat sheets or, occasionally, singly and are characterized by abundant granular cytoplasm and hyperchromatic nuclei with prominent nucleoli (Fig. 27–13). Foam cells and stromal fragments can also be present. An important component of fibrocystic disease and an excellent indicator of benignity is the presence of stripped (naked) bipolar nuclei (Fig. 27–14).[65, 67] Naked nuclei are very common in fibroadenomas but are also present in fibrocystic disease. They have a uniform hyperchromatic to smudged chromatin pattern without nucleoli. Occasionally, some wispy cytoplasmic tags can be present. According to some investigators, bipolar nuclei are believed to be derived from myoepithelial cells.[178, 180]

Text continued on page 714

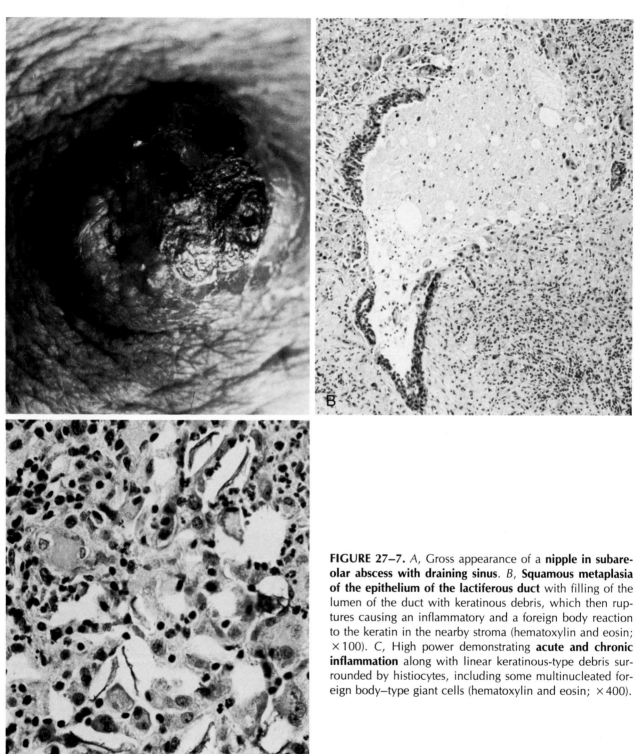

FIGURE 27–7. *A*, Gross appearance of a **nipple in subareolar abscess with draining sinus**. *B*, **Squamous metaplasia of the epithelium of the lactiferous duct** with filling of the lumen of the duct with keratinous debris, which then ruptures causing an inflammatory and a foreign body reaction to the keratin in the nearby stroma (hematoxylin and eosin; ×100). *C*, High power demonstrating **acute and chronic inflammation** along with linear keratinous-type debris surrounded by histiocytes, including some multinucleated foreign body–type giant cells (hematoxylin and eosin; ×400).

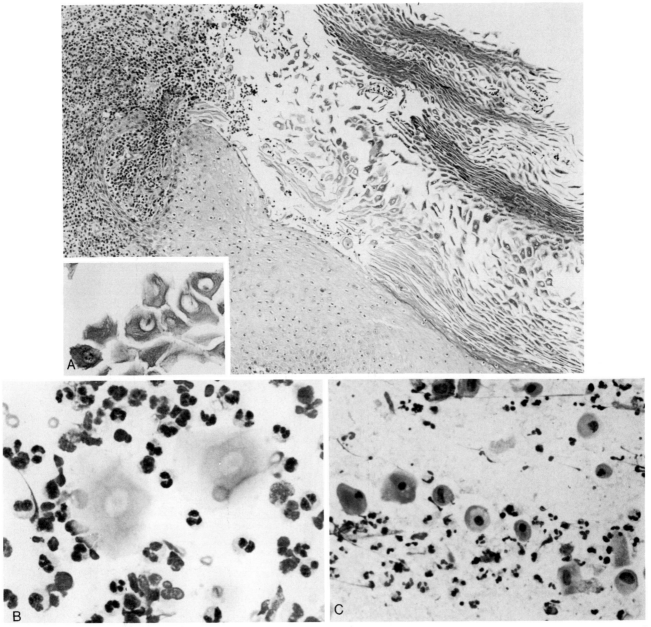

FIGURE 27–8. *A,* **Squamous metaplasia of lactiferous duct** with overlying anucleated squames and keratinous debris and surrounding chronic inflammation (hematoxylin and eosin; ×200). *Inset,* High power of anucleated squames in lumen of lactiferous duct from a case of subareolar abscess (hematoxylin and eosin; ×400). *B,* Fine needle aspiration of subareolar abscess revealing diagnostic **anucleated squames and associated acute inflammation** (Diff-Quik stain; ×400). Note similarity of anucleated squames in aspirate with anucleated squames seen in the inset. *C,* **Parakeratosis and acute inflammation** in aspirate of subareolar abscess (Papanicolaou stain; ×200).

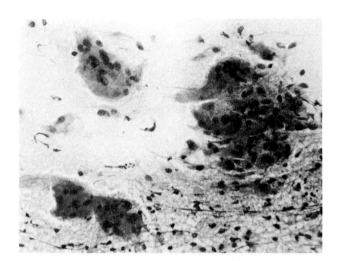

FIGURE 27–9. Prominent foreign body reaction to keratinous debris in aspirate of **subareolar abscess** (Papanicolaou stain; ×200).

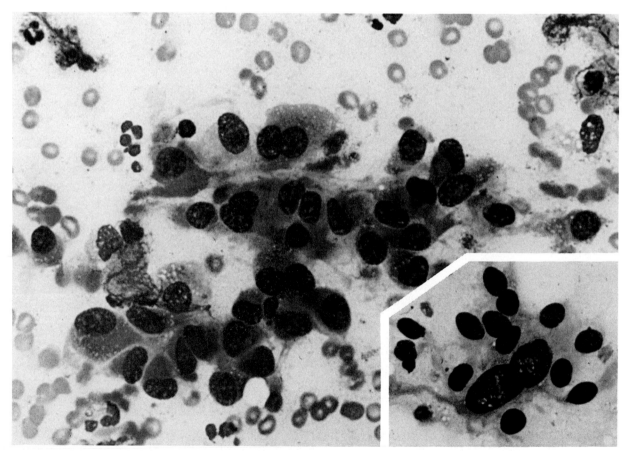

FIGURE 27–10. Atypical group of ductal cells in case of **subareolar abscess**. The group is loosely cohesive and consists of cells showing anisonucleosis, binucleation and slight nuclear enlargement (Diff-Quik stain; ×200). These features of epithelial atypia can be seen in any inflammatory process involving the breast. *Inset,* Loose cluster of atypical cells in subareolar abscess showing marked anisonucleosis (Diff-Quik stain; ×200).

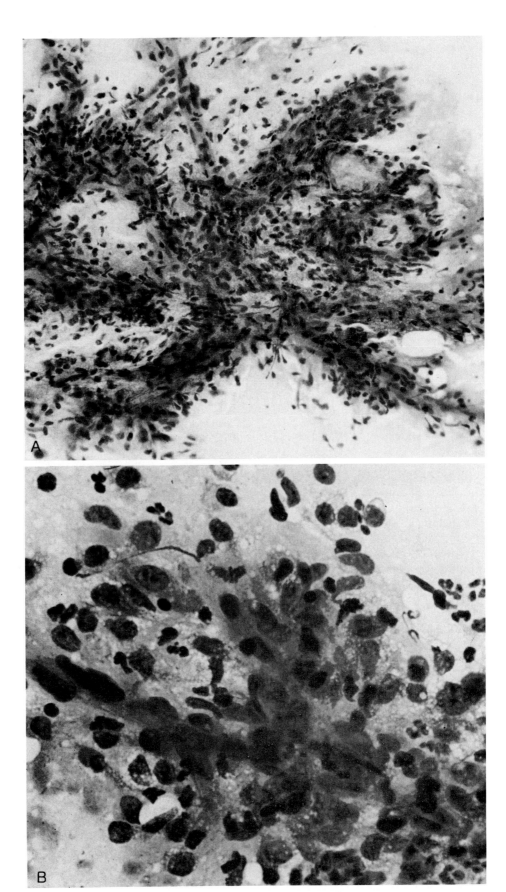

FIGURE 27–11. *A*, Fragment of **exuberant granulation tissue** demonstrating traversing capillaries with adherent histiocytes and inflammatory cells (Papanicolaou stain; ×200). *B*, High power of **granulation tissue** showing the presence of atypical endothelial cells and histiocytes that could potentially lead to a false-positive diagnosis of malignancy. Note the associated acute inflammatory process (Diff-Quik stain; ×400).

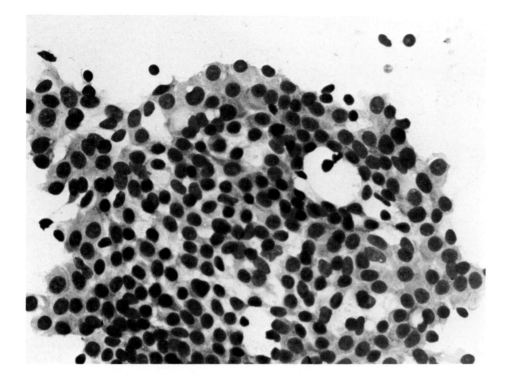

FIGURE 27–12. Aspirate of **fibrocystic change** consisting of a honeycomb group of uniform ductal cells with adherent bipolar naked nuclei and stripped nuclei in the background (Diff-Quik stain; ×200).

Cytomorphology of Fibrocystic Change

- Low-to-moderate cellularity
- Cohesive sheets of benign ductal cells arranged in a honeycomb pattern.
- Bipolar (naked) nuclei; myoepithelial cells dispersed in background and within or attached to sheets of epithelial cells.
- Apocrine cells—variable numbers
- Foam cells—variable numbers
- Fat and stroma—variable
- High cellularity or mild epithelial atypia, or both, may be present in proliferative benign breast lesions, but bipolar nuclei will also be seen.

Proliferative epithelial changes accompanying fibrocystic disease include duct papillomatosis, duct hyperplasia and atypical ductal hyperplasia (Fig. 27–15). In aspirates from proliferative lesions, increased numbers of cohesive groups of ductal cells and naked nuclei are present. However, a potential for a false-positive diagnosis of malignancy exists when there is increased cellularity, including the presence of benign apocrine cells with marked anisonucleosis and macronucleoli, which could be misinterpreted for malignant cells.[122] Ductal cells may also be arranged in groups with slight nuclear overlapping and mild loss of polarity.[117] The benign nature of these lesions should be considered by the presence of diverse cell types, including apocrine, ductal and histiocytic cells, and especially by bipolar naked nuclei in the background.[117]

Although FNA is highly predictive of separating benign from malignant breast lesions, it is less reliable in adequately subclassifying prognostically significant premalignant lesions including moderate, florid and atypical hyperplasias.[47, 113, 164] In some cases, atypical ductal changes may be suspected when there is increased cellularity associated with some atypical cells in a case otherwise showing conventional features of fibrocystic disease (Fig. 27–16). Peterse and coworkers'[170] semiquantitative analysis of cytomorphologic criteria was an attempt to differentiate benign proliferative atypical breast lesions from well-differentiated carcinomas. These investigators found that the features of malignancy were cell dissociation, arrangement in small epithelial clusters, nuclei greater than 16 μ, irregular nuclear membranes, anisonucleosis and necrosis. Benign features were large monolayers, nuclei less than 16 μ without significant variation in nuclear size or contours and the presence of bipolar nuclei in the monolayers.

Using these criteria, atypical benign cases were better separated from malignant cases, although cases still remained with uncertain diagnoses. These investigators recommended surgical biopsies to resolve cases with uncertain cytomorphologic criteria. We routinely recommend either close clinical follow-up or surgical biopsy in these types of cases. King and colleagues[113] utilized image cytometry for the classification of premalignant breast disease present in FNAs. Atypical hyperplasia characteristically showed increased cellularity with cohesive groupings of cells demonstrating mild nuclear and cellular atypia with an occasional isolated atypical intact cell. These workers noted that although FNA is highly predictive of separating benign from malignant breast lesions, it is less so in subclassifying prognostically significant premalignant lesions. They were able to identify six of seven proliferative lesions (atypical hyperplasia and moderate hyperplasia) using image analysis, but none of these cases were recognized using conventional microscopic parameters.

Text continued on page 719

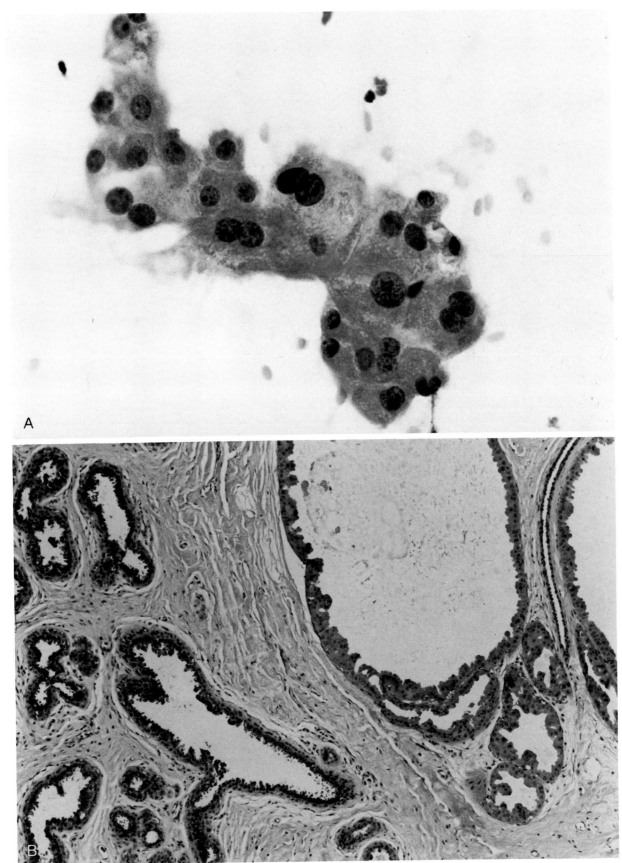

FIGURE 27–13. *A,* **Apocrine cells** arranged in flat sheets. Note the anisonucleosis with prominent nucleoli. However, the cells have abundant granular cytoplasm with a relatively low nucleocytoplasmic ratio (Papanicolaou stain; ×400). *B,* **Fibrocystic change** consisting of a cyst lined by apocrine cells along with stromal fibrosis and mild hyperplasia of the ductal cells (hematoxylin and eosin; ×100).

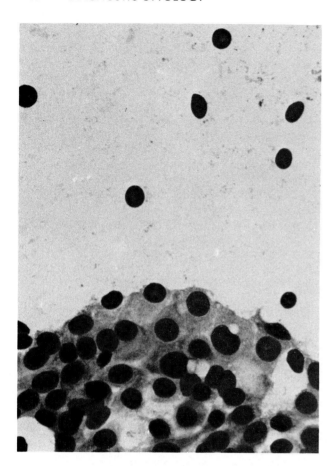

FIGURE 27–14. High power of **stripped (naked) bipolar nuclei** with nearby cluster of benign ductal cells. Note a few spindle-shaped bipolar nuclei at the edge of the ductal cells (Diff-Quik stain; ×400).

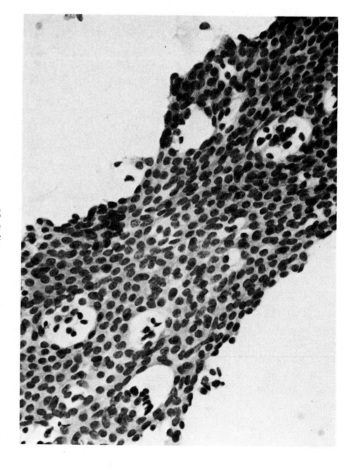

FIGURE 27–15. Sheet of **benign epithelial cells** showing proliferative features including pseudocribriforming. Note the uniform cohesive nature of the epithelial cells with no loss of polarity (Papanicolaou stain; ×200).

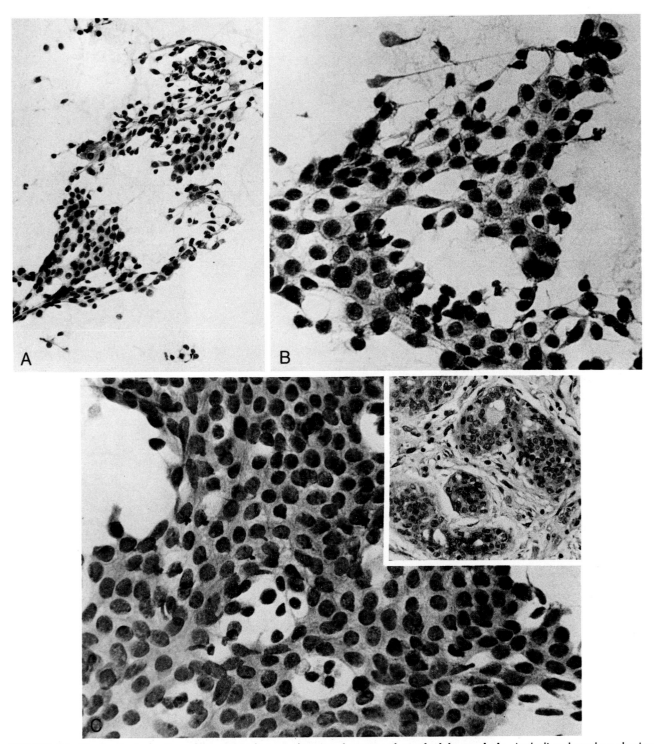

FIGURE 27–16. *A,* Aspirate from fibrocystic disease showing features of **atypical hyperplasia**, including loosely cohesive grouping of the ductal cells. A helpful feature for benignity is the presence of stripped bipolar nuclei in the background (Papanicolaou stain; ×100). *B,* High power of **mildly atypical ductal cells** arranged in a loosely cohesive fashion (Papanicolaou stain; ×400). *C,* Pseudocribriforming in aspirate from fibrocystic change showing **atypical hyperplasia**. Although there is some slight nuclear irregularity and overlapping, bipolar naked nuclei are present, and the cells still maintain their polarity (Papanicolaou stain; ×400). *Inset,* Corresponding surgical biopsy specimen demonstrating florid hyperplasia of the ductules (hematoxylin and eosin; ×200).

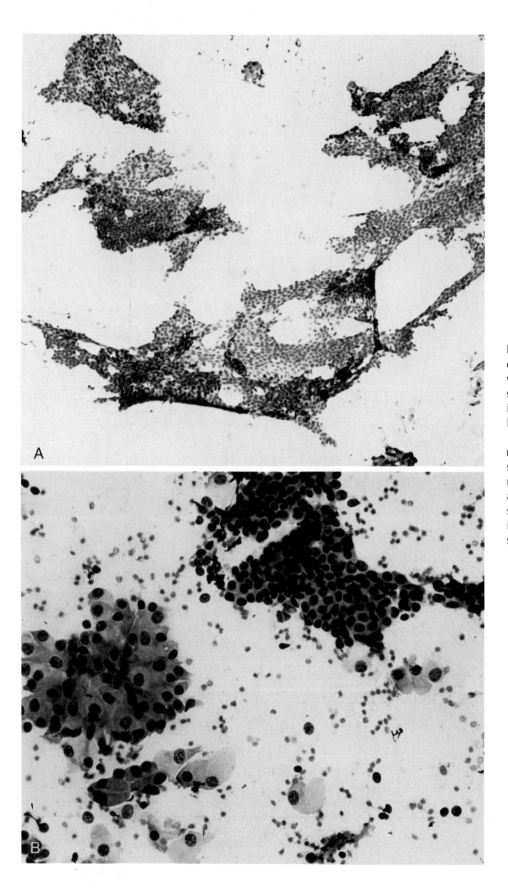

FIGURE 27–17. *A,* Low power of aspirate from a case of **juvenile papillomatosis** demonstrating the increased cellularity that can be seen in this lesion (Papanicolaou stain; ×100). *B,* Aspirate from **juvenile papillomatosis** demonstrating cohesive groups of benign ductal cells, numerous apocrine cells and scattered stripped bipolar naked nuclei in the background (Diff-Quik stain; ×200).

Identification of moderate, florid and atypical hyperplasia in FNA biopsies is especially important because there is a significantly increased risk of developing breast carcinoma in these patients.[164] The consensus statement of the Cancer Comittee of The College of American Pathologists[100] discourages the use of the term "fibrocystic disease" and proposed the term "fibrocystic change or condition." Slightly increased risk (1.5 to 2 times) for cancer was associated with solid or papillary metaplasia of moderate or florid degree (greater than four cells deep) present in histologic material. Moderately increased risk (five times) was associated with atypical ductal or lobular hyperplasia.[100] Additional studies establishing the cytologic criteria for the diagnosis of atypical hyperplasia in FNA biopsies are obviously needed, because identification of these lesions has a bearing on the clinical management of benign breast disease.

Juvenile Papillomatosis

Juvenile papillomatosis is a proliferative breast lesion that occurs almost exclusively in younger females in the age range of 10 to 40 years (mean, 21 years). The patient presents with a discrete breast mass not unlike fibroadenoma, but aspiration often produces cyst fluid.[177] Cytologic findings include increased cellularity with occasional apocrine groupings and numerous naked nuclei in the background (Fig. 27–17). It is impor-

tant to suspect this diagnosis in a young woman, because juvenile papillomatosis may be a marker for breast cancer in the patient's family and may indicate a need for continued long-term follow-up of the patient with juvenile papillomatosis who may herself be at increased risk.[177]

Fibroadenoma

Fibroadenomas are the most frequent benign breast tumors that may occur in all age groups but are especially common in younger females (20 to 35 years old).[90] Palpation will reveal a dominant, movable discrete mass generally measuring less than 4 cm in diameter. Most often a single lesion is identified, although up to 20% of patients present with multiple lesions. Fibroadenomas often increase in size with pregnancy. Aspiration generally produces a hypercellular specimen consisting of large sheets of epithelial cells arranged in tightly cohesive honeycomb groupings (Fig. 27–18). Bottles and associates[22] and others believe that the branching "antler-horn" cluster pattern of the epithelial cells is fairly characteristic but not absolutely specific for the diagnosis of fibroadenoma (Fig. 27–19). The epithelial cells have round nuclei with occasional small nucleoli. Numerous naked bipolar nuclei are seen, including some associated with sheets of epithelial cells, and many lie free in the background.[22, 121]

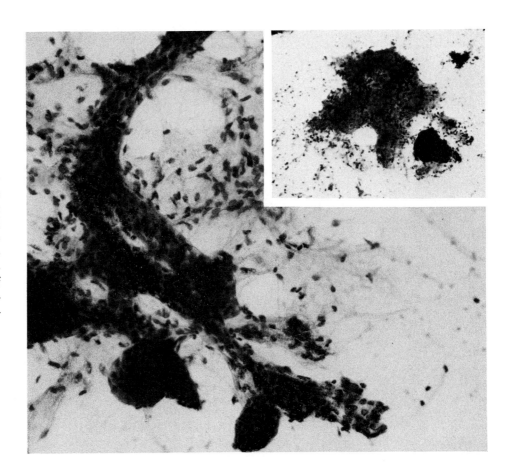

FIGURE 27–18. Aspirate from **fibroadenoma** showing tightly cohesive groups of ductal cells having a branching pattern along with loose stroma and some bipolar naked nuclei (Papanicolaou stain; ×400). *Inset*, Low power of fibroadenoma showing fragments of stroma and associated cohesive groups of ductal cells (Papanicolaou stain; ×100).

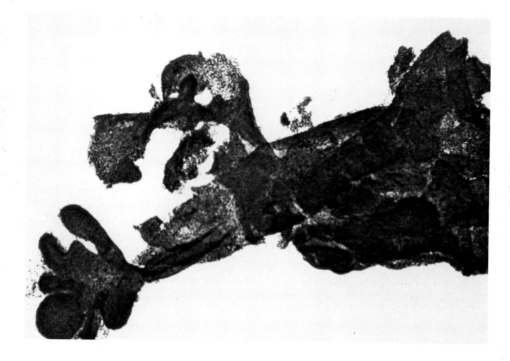

FIGURE 27–19. Large "antler-horn" cluster of epithelial cells seen in **fibroadenoma** (Papanicolaou stain; ×100).

Cytomorphology of Fibroadenomas

- Moderate-to-high cellularity
- Sheets of cohesive epithelial cells
- Branching antler-horn or finger-like projections of epithelial cells
- Numerous bipolar (naked) nuclei
- Stromal fragments; occasional myxoid change seen.
- Few or no foam and apocrine cells
- Freely movable circumscribed discrete mass in contrast to ill-defined indurated lesion of fibrocystic change (clinically helpful feature)
- Ductal atypia can be potential source for false-positive diagnosis.

Although some workers believe that the naked nuclei are derived from myoepithelial cells,[67] others favor a stromal cell origin based on light microscopic, ultrastructural and cytochemical evidence (Fig. 27–20).[211] The cytologic features of fibroadenoma cannot always be distinguished from those of fibrocystic disease.[116] Bottles and coworkers,[22] using stepwise logistic regression analysis, demonstrated that the presence of stromal fragments, antler-horn clusters and marked cellularity were the three most useful variables to distinguish fibroadenoma from fibrocystic disease. A separate analysis demonstrated that honeycomb sheets, antler-horn clusters and stroma were the most useful variables in distinguishing fibroadenoma from ductal

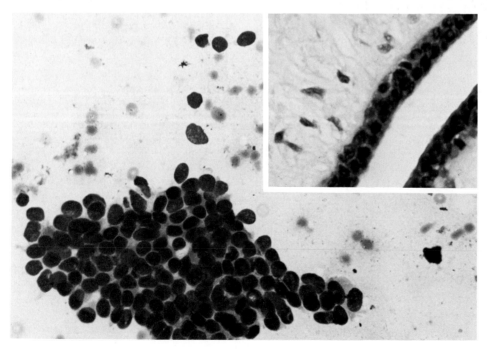

FIGURE 27–20. Cluster of **ductal cells** with nearby naked nuclei (Diff-Quik stain; ×400). *Inset,* Ductal cells with surrounding myoepithelial cells and spindle-shaped stromal cells in the nearby stroma (hematoxylin and eosin; ×400).

carcinoma.[22] We have noted that many cases of fibro-adenoma do not demonstrate the antler-horn clusters. We often rely on the clinical presentation of fibroadenoma as a freely movable circumscribed discrete mass in contrast to the ill-defined indurated lesion of fibrocystic disease.

A potential exists for a false-positive diagnosis of malignancy in aspirates from some cases of fibroadenoma owing to the hypercellularity seen in many of the specimens.[117] Errors usually occur in those cases also showing loose cohesion of the cell groupings with some anisonucleosis and prominent nucleoli (Fig. 27–21). The presence of the finger-like projections or fronds (antler horn–like clusters) and bipolar naked nuclei in the background should suggest the correct diagnosis of fibroadenoma.[117] Naked nuclei and myoepithelial cells, especially when bordering intact epithelial clusters, are especially helpful in defining the benign nature of these lesions.[219] Other changes that can be seen in fibroadenoma include myxoid degeneration of the stroma, foam cells, apocrine cells, single cells with cytoplasm and mitotic figures (Fig. 27–22).[22]

Adenosis Tumor

Adenosis tumor is an unusual palpable breast mass that can be clinically and histologically confused with breast carcinoma, especially at the time of frozen section.[90, 185] The lesion occurs in a wide age range from 20 to 67 years (mean, 37 years). The average size of an adenosis tumor is approximately 2.5 cm, and the histologic appearance is quite similar to that of sclerosing adenosis. Treatment consists of local excision with close clinical follow-up.[90, 185] Aspiration cytology will reveal changes of proliferative fibrocystic disease and stromal fibrosis (Fig. 27–23). Numerous uniform groups of ductal cells, stromal fragments and many stripped bipolar naked nuclei were present in the single case we encountered. A specific diagnosis of adenosis tumor was not made, although a correct interpretation of a benign proliferative breast lesion was possible. Immunoperoxidase studies for muscle actin (HHF) demonstrated positive staining of many bipolar spindle-shaped cells supportive of a myoepithelial origin for these cells. Immunohistochemical studies on the resected specimen showed actin positivity of myoepithelial cells and intact linear staining of type IV collagen around the ductules. Ultrastructural examination revealed ductal cells with surrounding myoepithelial cells resting on a delicate basal lamina with surrounding bundles of collagen. Fine needle aspiration cytologic examination may more clearly identify the benign nature of this unusual breast mass, which at times can be confused with malignancy at frozen section owing to the markedly distorted proliferation of ducts and stroma. The cytologic findings of adenosis tumor are essentially the same as those of an aspirate from sclerosing adenosis.[121, 185] Also considered in the differential diagnosis is the unusual myoepithelioma of the

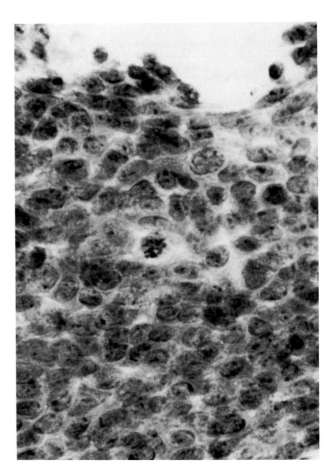

FIGURE 27–21. High power of aspirate from **fibroadenoma** demonstrating nuclear atypicality including overlapping nuclei, mild hyperchromasia, prominent nucleoli and rare mitotic figures that could potentially cause a false-positive diagnosis of malignancy (Papanicolaou stain; ×400).

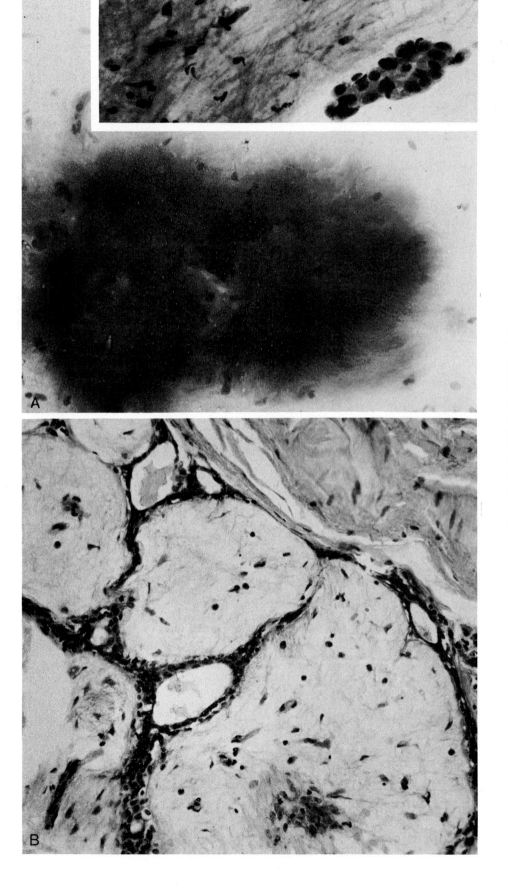

FIGURE 27–22. *A*, Prominent myxoid change seen in occasional cases of **fibroadenoma** (Diff-Quik stain; ×200). *Inset*, Small cluster of benign ductal cells with nearby fibrillary change to the stroma seen in an aspirate of fibroadenoma (Papanicolaou stain; ×200). *B*, Histologic confirmation of fibroadenoma showing prominent myxoid change to the stroma (hematoxylin and eosin; ×200).

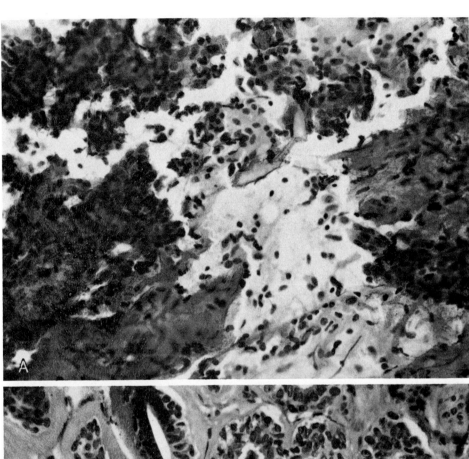

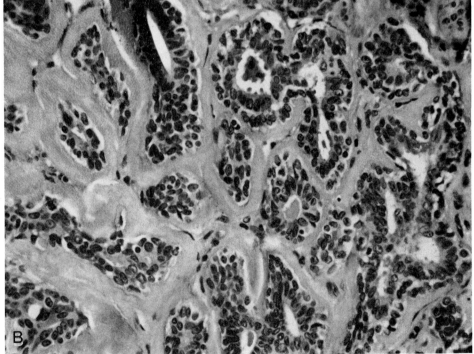

FIGURE 27–23. *A,* Aspirate from **adenosis tumor** showing proliferative lesion with numerous ductal cells and cellular stromal fragment. The cytomorphologic findings are identical to those in aspirates of sclerosing adenosis (Papanicolaou stain; × 200). *B,* Histologic appearance of adenosis tumor showing proliferation of ductules with surrounding dense hyalinized fibroconnective tissue (hematoxylin and eosin; × 200).

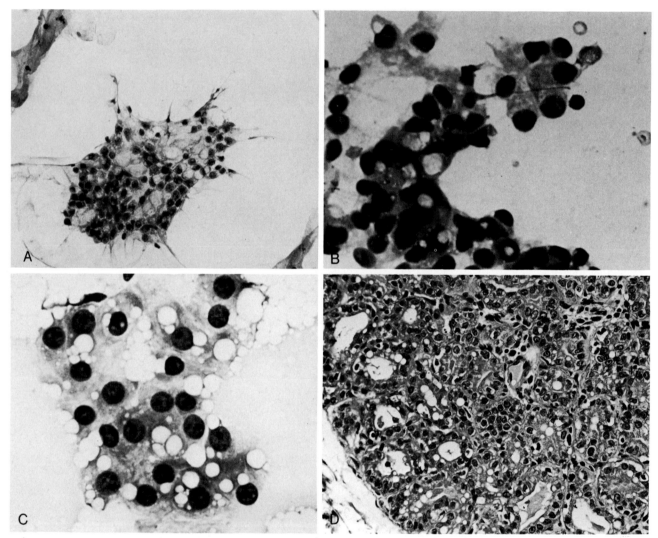

FIGURE 27–24. *A,* Aspirate from **lactating adenoma** consisting of a uniform group of epithelial cells having vacuolated frayed cytoplasm and background secretion (Papanicolaou stain; ×100). *B,* Loose cluster of acinar cells showing intranuclear and cytoplasmic vacuolization with fraying of cytoplasm (Diff-Quik stain; ×200). *C,* Group of acinar cells showing prominent cytoplasmic vacuolization. Note the prominent nucleoli that can be present in cells from aspirates of lactating adenomas (Diff-Quik stain; ×200). *D,* Lactating adenoma showing some intraluminal secretion and cytoplasmic vacuolization of the acinar cells (hematoxylin and eosin; ×100).

breast,[158] which is a neoplasm of myoepithelial cells demonstrating cohesive irregular clusters of spindle-shaped cells.

Adenoma

Few FNA cytologic reports have been made of true adenomas of the breast because of the uncommon nature of this lesion.[67, 225] Zajicek[225] reported a case having a cytologic appearance identical to that of fibroadenoma with no stromal elements. Adenoma of the nipple can be cellular, consisting of clusters of uniform ductal cells and dissociative bipolar naked nuclei.[201]

Benign Lesions During Pregnancy

Most breast lesions in pregnant and postpartum patients are benign and are secondary to the hormonal stimulation of the breast tissue by the pregnancy. Pregnancy produces breast masses *de novo* or enlarges preexisting small breast masses, most of which are fibroadenomas. Although most breast masses in pregnancy are benign, breast carcinoma in the pregnant female needs to be excluded because it is an extremely aggressive lesion with a high mortality rate. Most benign breast lesions associated with pregnancy regress completely by 6 months post partum. Fine needle aspiration cytologic findings of lactating adenomas or fibroadenomas showing lactational change generally produce a cell-rich smear containing a uniform population of epithelial cells, which are usually dispersed with occasional cell clusters.[23, 121] Fibroadenoma of pregnancy may be suspected when the biphasic pattern of epithelial clusters and naked nuclei are appreciated. Lactating adenomas have a "dirty" background caused by disruption of the delicate secretory cytoplasm and spillage of the secretory product into the background caused by the action of smearing the slides (Fig. 27-24).[67]

Cytomorphology of Lactating Adenomas

- Cellular smears
- Dispersed and poorly cohesive cell clusters
- Epithelial cells with fragile, frayed granular-to-foamy-to-vacuolated cytoplasm
- Mildly enlarged, well-dispersed hyperchromatic nuclei with prominent nucleoli; greater numbers of stripped epithelial (acinar) nuclei present in contrast to bipolar naked nuclei of myoepithelial cells.
- Dirty background of cytoplasmic fragments and secretory material

The secretory component can be demonstrated in air-dried smears with periodic acid–Schiff and lipid staining. A potential exists for a false-positive diagnosis of malignancy owing to the pattern of dissociated epithelial cells stripped of cytoplasm coupled with larger epithelial cells demonstrating nuclear atypicality

and prominent irregular nucleoli (Fig. 27–25).[58] The presence of cytoplasmic secretion characterized by cytoplasmic foaminess or vacuolization with fraying of cytoplasmic borders must be appreciated in order to avoid a false-positive diagnosis of malignancy in the occasional aspirate from a lactating adenoma having atypical nuclear features. Although unusual in young women, carcinoma should be considered in the differential diagnosis because it is second only to cervical cancer as the most common newly diagnosed malignant neoplasm in pregnant patients.[91] However, most ductal carcinomas show a greater degree of nuclear atypicality, necrosis, hyperchromasia, loss of polarity and discohesion. Lobular hyperplasia can also occur in the pregnant female and potentially be confused with lobular carcinoma *in situ,* if the presence of a myoepithelial layer surrounding the acinar cells is not appreciated (Fig. 27–26). The major advantage of FNA biopsy in the pregnant woman is avoidance of surgical trauma and anesthesia, which can be an unnecessary risk to both fetus and mother in the work-up of breast masses. Surgery may be followed by poor wound healing in the lactating breast. Fine needle aspiration biopsy may also decrease delays in the diagnosis of breast cancer in pregnancy.[58, 86]

Granular Cell Tumor

Granular cell tumor is an uncommon breast lesion, which is more frequent and more likely to be multifocal in black patients.[36, 102] Granular cell tumors of the breast can closely mimic scirrhous carcinoma, both clinically and at gross examination. Fine needle aspiration cytologic examination usually reveals a cellular specimen consisting of scattered groups of cells with abundant granular cytoplasm and indistinct cell borders with the Romanovsky stains (Fig. 27–27).[136] The nuclei are oval to round, uniform in size and have an evenly dispersed chromatin pattern. Occasional nucleoli may be present. Granular cells stain red with Papanicolaou stain. The cells are also periodic acid–Schiff positive, which accentuates the granules. Immunoperoxidase stains on cytologic material demonstrate S-100 and carcinoembryonic antigen positivity, although the S-100 staining intensity may be decreased in alcohol-fixed smears.[54] Electron microscopic examination shows granules resembling autophagosomes and angulate bodies.[36]

Granulomas

Sarcoidosis of the breast is quite rare. The differential diagnosis includes infectious granulomas secondary to tuberculosis, fungi, leprosy and brucellosis. Granulomas can also be present as a reaction to tumor,[162] a component of fat necrosis or a foreign body reaction (Fig. 27–28). Grossly, the lesion can mimic carcinoma.[73] Doria and colleagues[39] reported the FNA cytologic findings of sarcoidosis involving the breast.

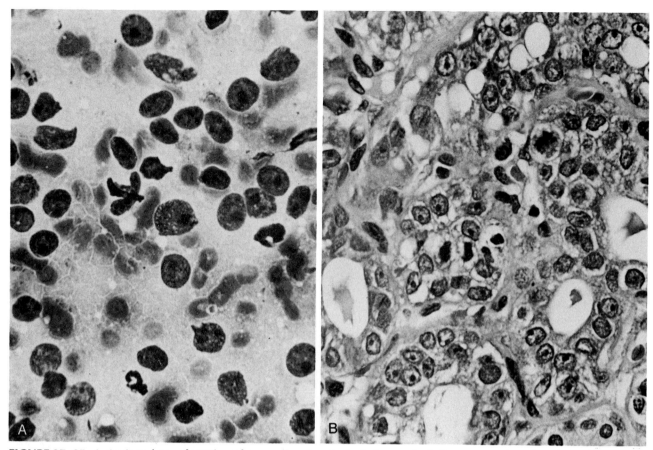

FIGURE 27–25. *A*, Aspirate from a **lactating adenoma** showing atypical changes including many stripped nuclei with prominent nucleoli and some anisonucleosis. The findings could potentially lead to a false-positive diagnosis of malignancy if other features of lactating adenoma are not appreciated (Diff-Quik stain; ×400). *B*, Corresponding histologic section of lactating adenoma showing nuclear irregularity of the acinar cells with prominence of nucleoli (hematoxylin and eosin; ×400).

The smears were cellular and consisted of clusters of epithelioid histiocytes, multinucleated giant cells, lymphocytes and plasma cells. The epithelioid histiocytes were elongated with folded nuclei and ill-defined cytoplasm. No evidence of necrosis was seen, and ductal cells were present. Jayaram[103] reported the cytomorphologic findings of nine cases of tuberculous mastitis diagnosed by FNA biopsy. Three of the patients clinically were thought to have carcinomas. Epithelioid cell granulomas were found in all cases along with Langhans's giant cells and occasional foreign body giant cells. Helpful cytologic features were the presence of a necrotic background and numerous degenerating neutrophils. The diagnosis was confirmed by identifying acid-fast bacilli in the smears. Aspirated material should also be submitted for culture in all cases suspected to have a granulomatous component.

Localized Amyloid Tumor

Localized amyloid tumor of the breast is an exceedingly rare lesion. We have encountered two examples of this entity including one case of metachronous bilateral lesions.[186] This unusual lesion occurs predominantly in elderly females and can be mammographically and clinically confused with carcinoma.[131, 186] Fine needle aspiration biopsy can be a useful procedure to make a preliminary diagnosis when amyloid is appreciated in the smears. Cytologic findings of amyloid include irregular clumps of metachromatic homogeneous material in the modified Wright's stain (Diff-Quik) and irregular cylindric fragments of refractile to glassy eosinophilic material in the Papanicolaou-stained smears (Fig. 27–29). Some interspersed spindle-shaped cells are present at the periphery and within the substance of the amyloid material.[186] Congo red staining with prior potassium permanganate incubation confirmed the amyloid light chain (AL) type of amyloid in both of our cases. Immunofluorescent studies demonstrated IgA, with kappa and lambda light chain deposition within the amyloid foci in one case. Intracytoplasmic IgG with both light chains within plasma cells and amyloid deposits were shown in the second case. Ultrastructural confirmation of one of the cases showed characteristic findings of straight, nonbranching fibrils measuring 4 to 9 nm, diagnostic of amyloid (see Fig. 27–29). Amyloid tumors of the breast can occur in three separate settings: secondary amyloidosis, systemic or multiple myeloma associated amyloidosis and localized primary tumor having a benign course.[186]

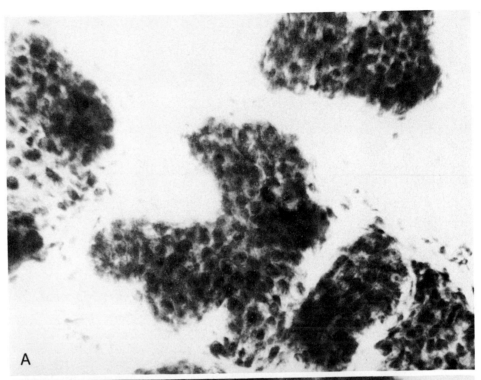

FIGURE 27–26. *A*, **Lobular hyperplasia** showing numerous groups of acinar cells having a uniform appearance (Papanicolaou stain; ×200). *B*, High power showing lobular hyperplasia. A benign feature is the presence of spindle-shaped myoepithelial cells at the peripheral portion of the clusters (Papanicolaou stain; ×400).

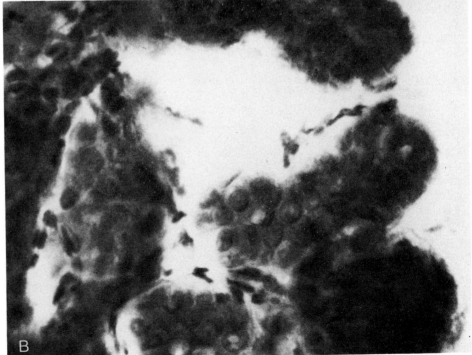

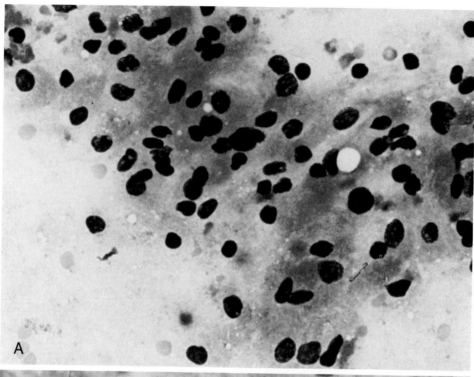

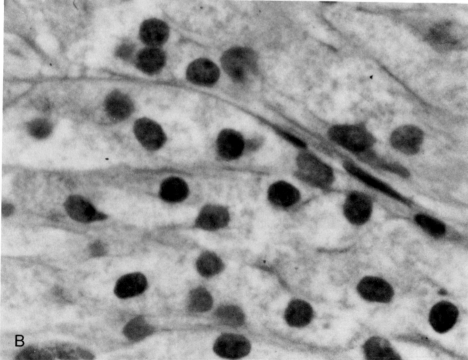

FIGURE 27–27. *A,* Aspirate from **granular cell tumor** of the breast showing scattered oval- to spindle-shaped cells having a relatively low nucleocytoplasmic ratio with surrounding granular cytoplasm (Diff-Quik stain; ×200). *B,* Corresponding histologic section demonstrating characteristic granular cells (hematoxylin and eosin; ×400).

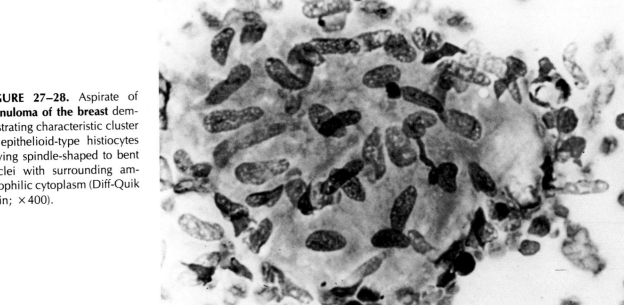

FIGURE 27–28. Aspirate of **granuloma of the breast** demonstrating characteristic cluster of epithelioid-type histiocytes having spindle-shaped to bent nuclei with surrounding amphophilic cytoplasm (Diff-Quik stain; × 400).

Papilloma

Solitary papillomas occur most frequently in women from 50 to 60 years of age.[116] Often the patient presents with a serous or bloody nipple secretion that can be cytologically examined. If a palpable lesion is aspirated, examination would reveal epithelial cells arranged in tight sheets or three-dimensional clusters with a depth of focus (Fig. 27–30). Occasionally, spindle-shaped stromal cells are also present. Because distinguishing a benign papilloma from a well-differentiated papillary carcinoma can be difficult, surgical excision is advised. Another lesion that occurs centrally beneath the nipple and subareolar region is adenoma of the nipple.[201] Aspiration reveals cellular smears with numerous clusters of uniform epithelial cells and scattered naked nuclei.

Gynecomastia

Gynecomastia is a hormonally dependent lesion that occurs most frequently in adolescents and elderly patients. It is more often unilateral although bilateral cases occur (2:1 unilateral to bilateral). Gynecomastia can be classified as juvenile, idiopathic, secondary or drug related (digitalis, reserpine, phenytoin). Aspiration reveals a proliferative lesion in which many groups and clusters of epithelial cells and naked nuclei are seen. Occasional cases show epithelial atypia including some nuclear molding and nucleoli (Fig. 27–31). The diagnosis of malignancy should be avoided unless an aspirate from a male patient shows frankly malignant cytologic features.[87, 105, 193]

MALIGNANT LESIONS

Infiltrating Ductal Carcinoma

Infiltrating ductal carcinoma is the most common histologic type accounting for up to three fourths of the invasive mammary carcinomas in some series.[164] Approximately 55 to 65% experience a five-year survival. In general, aspirations of infiltrating duct carcinomas show features common to all breast carcinomas with a few exceptions. Diagnostic malignant features include abundant cellularity with groups of loosely cohesive malignant cells and individually scattered tumor cells (Fig. 27–32). The background can be bloody with occasional necrotic debris or, rarely, clean. The cellular pattern shows considerable variability, with tumor cells present in three-dimensional clusters, syncytial groupings or occasionally acinar (gland-like) arrangements. The malignant clusters show evidence of loss of polarity and nuclear molding (Fig. 27–33). Considerable variability is observed in tumor cell size, with most of the aspirates consisting of cells larger than normal ductal cells, but occasionally small cancer cells can be present. Individual tumor cells demonstrate malignant cytologic features including increased nucleocytoplasmic ratio, hyperchromatic coarsely granular chromatin and small-to-prominent nucleoli (Fig. 27–34).

Infrequently, the nuclei can be excentric, which lends a plasmacytoid appearance to the cells, most notably in the Diff-Quik preparations. This pattern is most often seen in aspirates of ductal carcinomas from older women (Fig. 27–35). In general, the cytoplasm of ductal carcinoma tends to be basophilic and varies from lacy, finely to coarsely granular or finely vacuo-

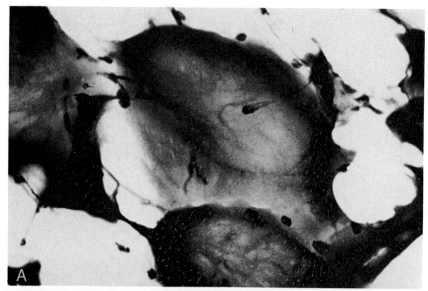

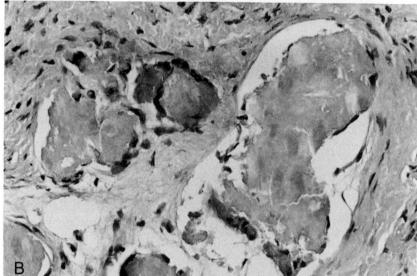

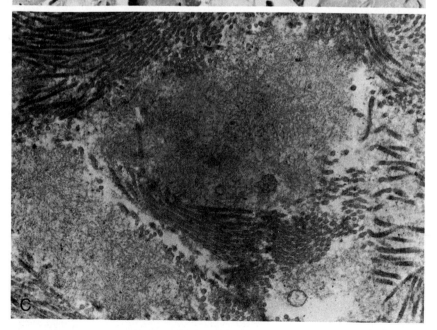

FIGURE 27–29. *A,* Fine needle aspiration of **amyloid tumor of the breast** demonstrating irregular clumps of metachromatically staining homogeneous material along with some associated interspersed spindle-shaped cells (Diff-Quik stain; ×400). *B,* Histologic section of amyloid tumor of the breast revealing similar changes of homogeneous clumps of refractile amyloid material with nearby foreign body reaction (hematoxylin and eosin; ×400). *C,* Ultrastructural confirmation of amyloid showing characteristic findings of straight non-branching fibrils measuring 4 to 9 nm. Note the admixed larger collagen fibrils for comparison (×30,000).

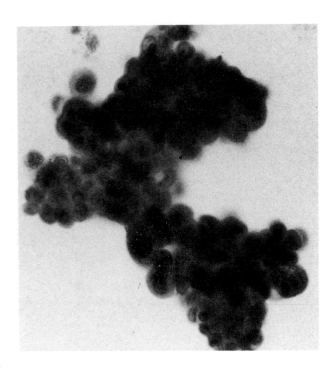

FIGURE 27–30. Three-dimensional cluster of uniform ductal cells consistent with a **papilloma** (Papanicolaou stain; ×400).

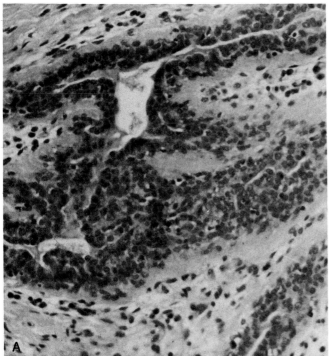

FIGURE 27–31. *A*, Low power view of **gynecomastia** showing ductal hyperplasia with surrounding loose periductal stroma (hematoxylin and eosin; ×100). *B*, High power of epithelial cells showing features similar to those appreciated in the cytology smears including prominent nucleoli (hematoxylin and eosin; ×600). *C*, High power view of aspirate from gynecomastia showing sheet-like arrangement of ductal cells with atypical features including some nuclear irregularity and prominent nucleoli (Papanicolaou stain; ×600).

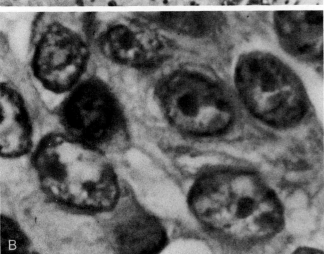

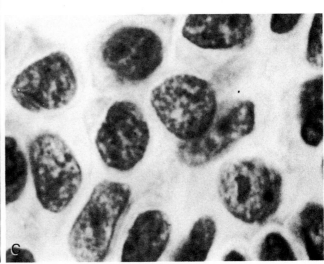

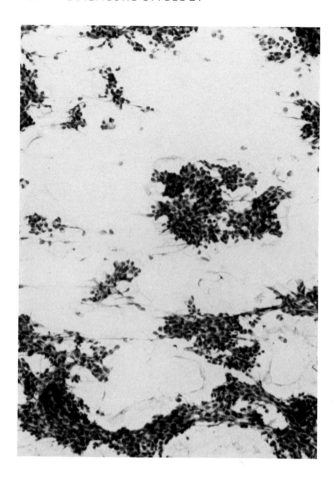

FIGURE 27–32. Low power of aspirate from **ductal carcinoma** demonstrating abundant cellularity with groups of loosely cohesive malignant cells (Papanicolaou stain; ×100).

lated. Sometimes, cases demonstrate coarse cytoplasmic vacuolization or intracellular lumina or both (Fig. 27–36). Some very poorly differentiated breast carcinomas show bizarre pleomorphic cells, including multinucleated tumor cells (see Fig. 27–34). Aspirates from infiltrating ductal carcinoma of small size show features merging with lobular carcinoma, although the cellularity is usually greater and the nuclei tend to be more hyperchromatic. In general, bipolar naked nuclei and benign epithelial groupings are not present, unless the surrounding benign parenchyma is also aspirated. Rarely, benign groups can be appreciated admixed with malignant clusters in an aspirate from a carcinoma arising in a benign papilloma or other benign lesion.

Infiltrating Ductal Carcinoma

- Cellular smears
- Loosely cohesive and individually scattered malignant cells
- Malignant epithelial cells arranged in three-dimensional clusters, syncytial groupings and occasional acinar patterns.
- No bipolar naked nuclei
- Tumor diathesis

Morphologic classification of breast cancer can be applied to FNA specimens. Using the classification schema based on Fisher and the World Health Organization's criteria,[164] we have attempted to differentiate the various histologic types of invasive breast carcinoma based on cytomorphologic criteria. This classifi-

cation may have some bearing on prognosis because favorable breast carcinomas include pure mucinous (colloid), true medullary, tubular carcinoma, adenoid cystic carcinoma, papillary carcinoma and secretory carcinoma, seen predominantly in children and adolescents. Unfavorable breast malignancies include metaplastic carcinoma, inflammatory carcinoma and sarcomas.[164]

Medullary Carcinoma

Medullary carcinoma comprises 5 to 10% of all breast carcinomas and presents grossly as a well-demarcated soft lesion. A pure medullary carcinoma has a better 5-year and 10-year survival than the usual infiltrating duct carcinoma. Histologically, the lesion is characterized by solid masses of very poorly differentiated malignant cells arranged in a syncytial fashion with admixed lymphocytes and plasma cells (Fig. 27–37). Cytologically, numerous malignant cells are present arranged in clusters and syncytial groupings along with individually scattered malignant cells (Fig. 27–38). Tumor cells have enlarged nuclei with considerable variation in size and shape and an increased nucleocytoplasmic ratio; tumor cells usually have multiple macronucleoli with irregular shapes. The surrounding basophilic to finely granular or vacuolated cytoplasm is scant to abundant. Occasionally, large stripped tumor nuclei may be seen (Fig. 27–39).

Frequently, numerous admixed lymphocytes and

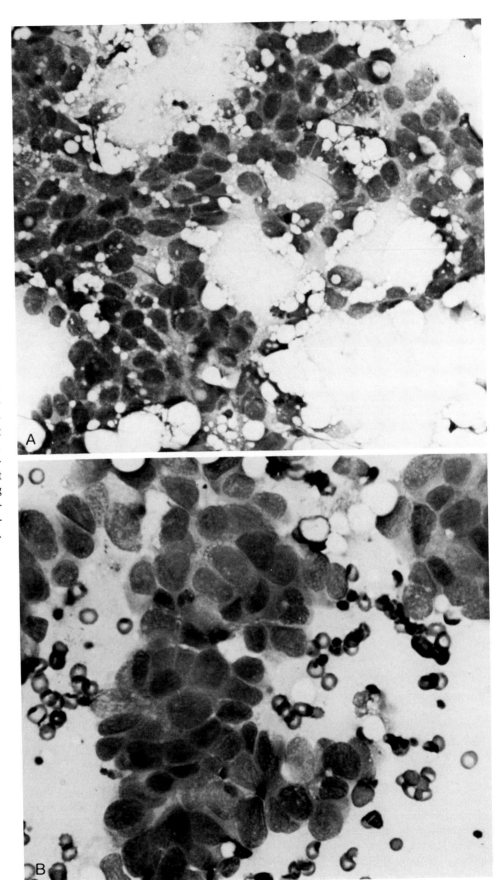

FIGURE 27–33. *A,* Aspirate from **infiltrating ductal carcinoma** showing clusters of malignant cells infiltrating the fat (Diff-Quik stain; ×200). *B,* High power of ductal carcinoma demonstrating malignant cytologic features including anisonucleosis with hyperchromasia and prominent nucleoli (Diff-Quik stain; ×400).

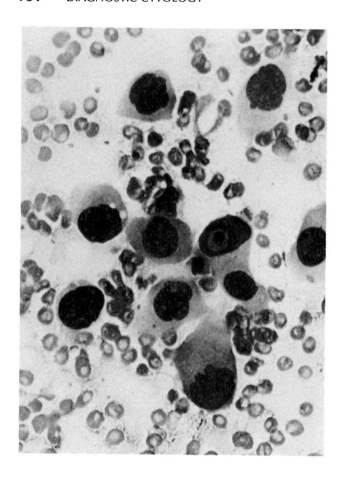

FIGURE 27–34. Fine needle aspiration of **poorly differentiated ductal carcinoma** revealing numerous individually scattered malignant cells (Diff-Quik stain; ×400).

some plasma cells are characteristically present. In any aspirate of a breast mass demonstrating lymphoid cells, a diligent search for malignant epithelial cells should be made in order to avoid a false-negative diagnosis. The diagnosis of medullary carcinoma can often be suspected when a circumscribed soft mass is aspirated and high-grade malignant cells and admixed lymphocytes or plasma cells are present.

Medullary Carcinoma

- Cellular smears
- Loose syncytial aggregates and single cells
- Bizarre tumor cells with prominent nucleoli; occasional stripped tumor nuclei
- Benign lymphoid cells

Mucinous (Colloid) Carcinoma

Mucinous carcinoma comprises about 5% of all breast carcinomas and has a better 5-year to 10-year survival than the usual infiltrating duct carcinoma, although late recurrences are not unusual.[164] Mucinous carcinoma is more common in older women. Mucin-producing carcinomas can be divided into three histologic categories: signet-ring, pure and mixed.[184]

Signet-ring carcinoma has a poor prognosis, and some believe this subtype should be considered a separate entity. Fine needle aspiration of mucinous carcinoma often produces gelatinous material with variable cellularity (Fig. 27–40).[167, 216]

In the pure common variant of mucinous carcinoma, three-dimensional clusters of tumor cells are present surrounded by abundant extracellular mucinous material, which stains metachromatically with the Diff-Quik stain (Fig. 27–41). Some cases demonstrate only a slight degree of atypia of the tumor cells.[44] The nuclei may have a vesicular chromatin pattern with little anisonucleosis or nuclear irregularity. The relatively bland appearance of the tumor cells coupled with decreased cellularity secondary to the abundant extracellular mucinous material can potentially lead to a false-negative diagnosis of malignancy. The diagnosis should be suspected when extracellular mucinous material is seen and individually scattered malignant cells are present.

Mixed mucinous carcinomas show some features of the pure type along with cytologic findings of infiltrating ductal carcinoma.[216] The mucinous background can often be appreciated with special stains (e.g., periodic acid–Schiff, Alcian blue, mucicarmine). A fibroadenoma should be considered in a differential diagnosis because a myxoid change to the stroma can be present. However, fibroadenoma generally occurs in a younger age group and has the cytologic features of cell clusters, with finger-like branching and naked nuclei in the background.

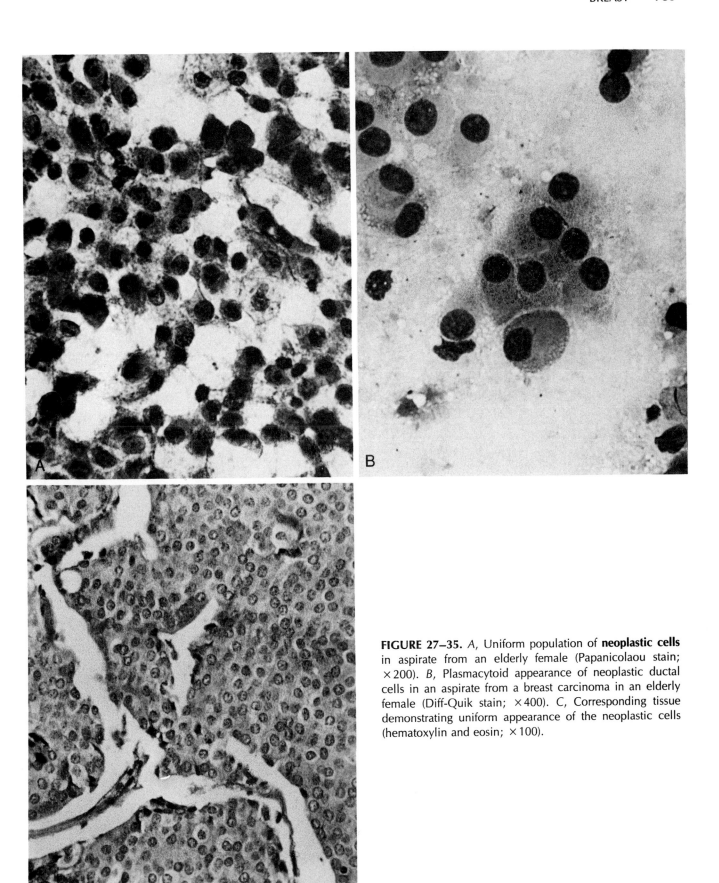

FIGURE 27–35. *A*, Uniform population of **neoplastic cells** in aspirate from an elderly female (Papanicolaou stain; ×200). *B*, Plasmacytoid appearance of neoplastic ductal cells in an aspirate from a breast carcinoma in an elderly female (Diff-Quik stain; ×400). *C*, Corresponding tissue demonstrating uniform appearance of the neoplastic cells (hematoxylin and eosin; ×100).

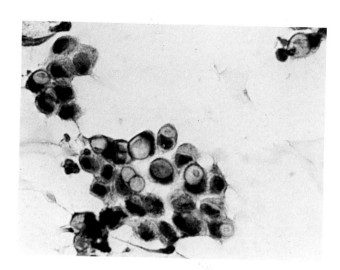

FIGURE 27–36. Cells of **infiltrating ductal carcinoma** demonstrating coarse cytoplasmic vacuolization with targetoid mucin-type globules (Papanicolaou stain; × 200).

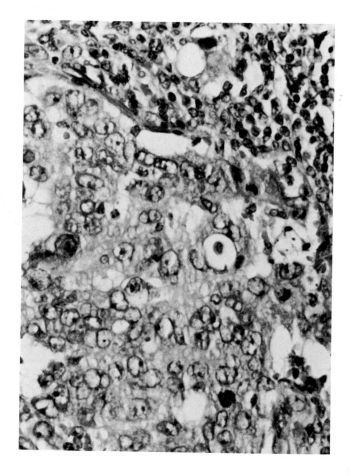

FIGURE 27–37. Histologic appearance of **medullary carcinoma** characterized by syncytial grouping of poorly differentiated malignant cells admixed with lymphocytes and plasma cells (hematoxylin and eosin; × 200).

FIGURE 27–38. *A,* Loose syncytial cluster of malignant cells with admixed chronic inflammatory cells in aspirate of **medullary carcinoma of the breast** (Diff-Quik stain; ×400). *B,* Dual population of malignant ductal cells arranged in a syncytial fashion with admixed chronic inflammatory cells in fine needle aspiration of medullary carcinoma (Papanicolaou stain; ×400).

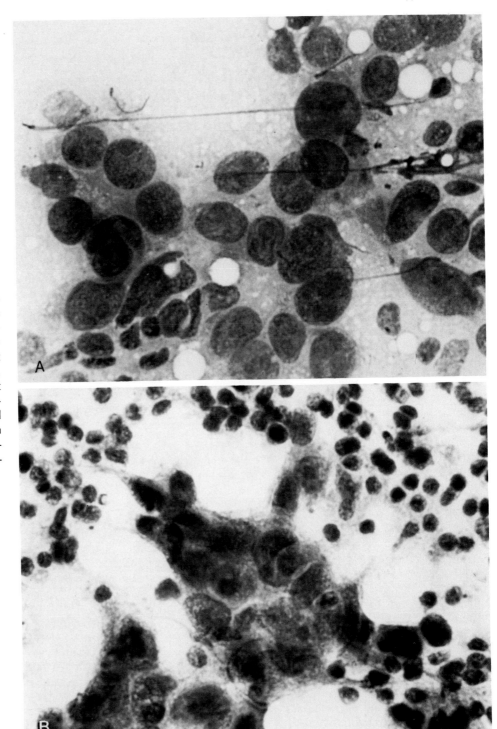

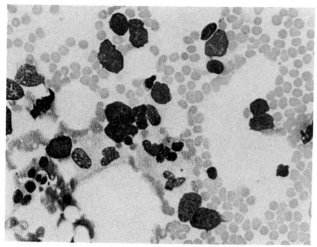

FIGURE 27–39. Scattered stripped malignant nuclei in aspirate of **medullary carcinoma** (Diff-Quik stain; ×200).

Mucinous (Colloid) Carcinoma

- Abundant pools, strands of mucin or both
- Aggregates and cell balls of tumor cells, often uniform in appearance, along with isolated tumor cells
- Occasional signet-ring malignant cells

Tubular (Well-differentiated) Carcinoma

Tubular carcinoma in its pure form tends to be relatively small, in the range of 1 cm. The lesion can be multicentric and bilateral. Lymph node metastasis occurs in one third of the patients, but the overall prognosis even with metastatic disease is excellent. This is another breast carcinoma that can be underdiagnosed in FNA biopsy owing to the relatively uniform appearance of the tumor cells, which may show only mild atypia.[68] The diagnosis may be suspected when groups of atypical cells are arranged in angulated glandular or tubular structures, including some having a comma-shaped projection (Fig. 27–42). Bipolar naked nuclei will also not be present. Because an unequivocal diagnosis of tubular carcinoma often cannot be rendered, this diagnosis will often need frozen-section confirmation before definitive treatment.

Tubular Carcinoma

- Low-to-moderate cellularity
- Angulated, pointed open tubules and glands with comma-shaped projections
- Little or no cellular atypia but no bipolar nuclei (myoepithelial cells) present.

Adenoid Cystic Carcinoma

This rare variant has an excellent prognosis and often does not have lymph node metastasis. The cytologic features are similar to the FNA findings of salivary gland lesions. Morphologically, the tumor consists of nests of small uniform basaloid cells set within a loose stroma. The basaloid cells can be arranged in cribriform cylinders or tubules with intraluminal mucoid material that is mucicarmine positive.[116, 121] Isolated cells stripped of cytoplasm can also be present.

Papillary Carcinoma

Papillary carcinoma in its pure form occurs in approximately 0.3% of breast malignancies, although a papillary component can be seen in up to 3 to 4% of all mammary carcinomas.[156] The tumor often occurs in postmenopausal non-white patients. Characteristically, aspiration cytologic features include the presence of cell groups in the form of three-dimensional papillary groups, along with scattered high columnar cells and a bloody diathesis with hemosiderin-laden macrophages (Fig. 27–43).[119, 156] Kline and Kannon[119] reported minimal nuclear abnormality in some of their cases. Naked nuclei may also be present. These features may make it difficult to separate a papillary carcinoma from either a fibroadenoma or papilloma.[116, 119] However, the naked nuclei from papillary carcinoma are often larger, more elongated and rounder than the benign bipolar nuclei of fibroadenoma.

Papillary Carcinoma

- Cellular smears
- Three-dimensional papillary clusters of uniform atypical cells
- Tall columnar cells
- Naked enlarged atypical nuclei
- Blood and hemosiderin-laden macrophages

Infiltrating Lobular Carcinoma

Infiltrating lobular carcinomas account for 3 to 15% of all breast carcinomas.[164] Lobular carcinoma has a greater degree of bilaterality than the common infiltrating ductal carcinoma. Cytologically, the specimen can be hypocellular and consists of a monomorphic population of mildly atypical cells arranged individually, in small aggregates, "Indian file" or in thin cords. The cells are relatively small with an increased nucleocytoplasmic ratio (Fig. 27–44).[3] The nuclei tend to be finely granular and vary from hypochromatic to mildly hyperchromatic. A mild degree of nuclear irregularity may be present, and a small micronucleolus can be identified. A helpful feature is the presence of cuboidal cells with excentric nuclei and cytoplasmic vacuoles, which can distort the nucleus (Fig. 27–45). However, because of the limited cellularity of some of the cases and the mild atypia of the cells, a false-negative diagnosis of malignancy is quite possible (Fig. 27–46). The most common causes of false-negative diagnoses in breast FNA biopsies are probably the aspirations from lobular carcinomas. However, Kline and associates,[116, 120] using strict cytologic criteria, correctly identified lobular carcinoma in up to 75% of their cases.

Text continued on page 746

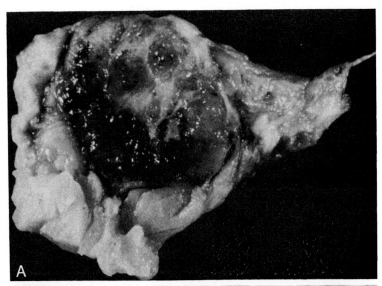

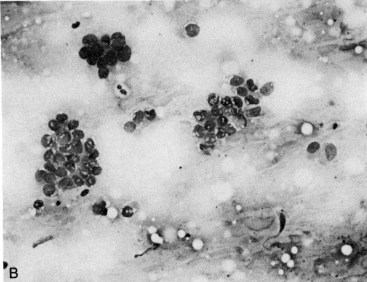

FIGURE 27–40. *A,* Gross appearance of **mucinous carcinoma of the breast** demonstrating the gelatinous quality of the tissue, along with some focal hemorrhage within the neoplasm. *B,* Aspirate from colloid carcinoma of the breast consisting of small groups of uniform cells with surrounding metachromatically staining mucinous material (Diff-Quik stain; ×100). *C,* Corresponding histologic section showing uniform group of vacuolated atypical cells with surrounding stringy mucinous material (hematoxylin and eosin; ×200).

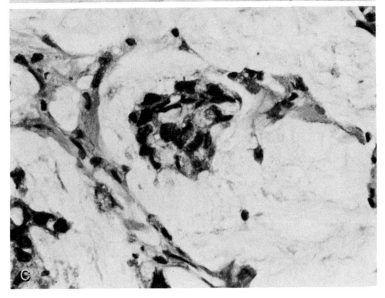

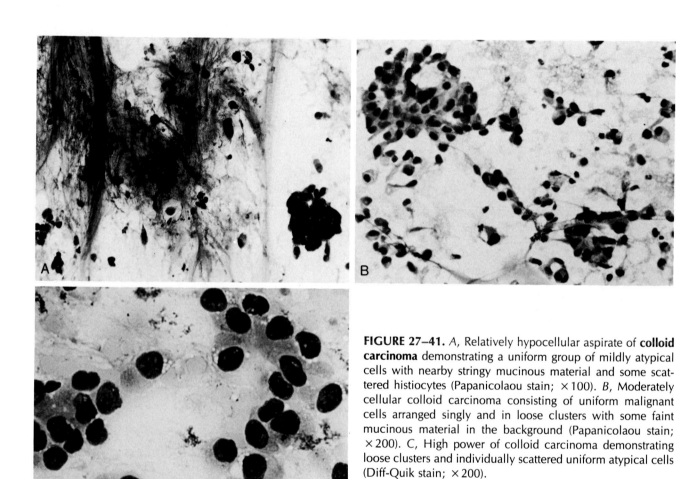

FIGURE 27–41. *A,* Relatively hypocellular aspirate of **colloid carcinoma** demonstrating a uniform group of mildly atypical cells with nearby stringy mucinous material and some scattered histiocytes (Papanicolaou stain; ×100). *B,* Moderately cellular colloid carcinoma consisting of uniform malignant cells arranged singly and in loose clusters with some faint mucinous material in the background (Papanicolaou stain; ×200). *C,* High power of colloid carcinoma demonstrating loose clusters and individually scattered uniform atypical cells (Diff-Quik stain; ×200).

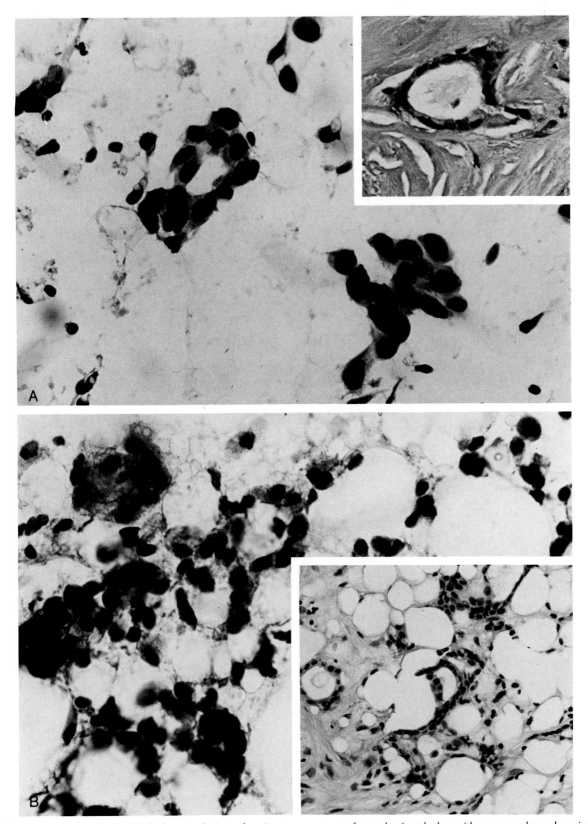

FIGURE 27–42. *A,* Aspirate of **tubular carcinoma** showing two groups of neoplastic tubules with comma-shaped projections. Note the minimal degree of cellular atypia (Papanicolaou stain; ×400). *Inset,* Corresponding histology showing infiltrating neoplastic tubules with prominent desmoplastic fibrosis. Note the open lumina and comma-shaped projections from the neoplastic tubules (hematoxylin and eosin; ×200). *B,* Neoplastic tubules in fat (Papanicolaou stain; ×200). *Inset,* Neoplastic tubules infiltrating the fat (hematoxylin and eosin; ×100).

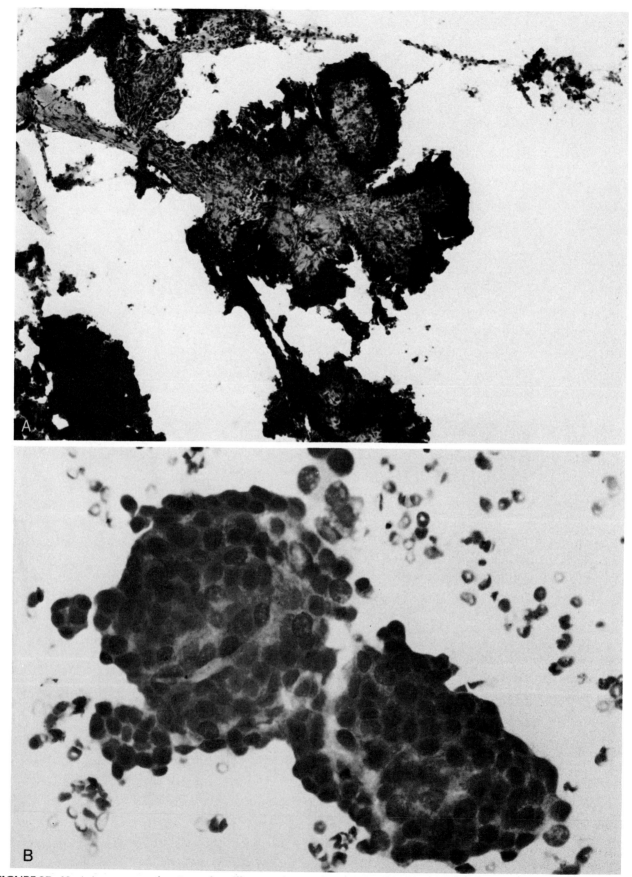

FIGURE 27–43. *A,* Low power of aspirate of **papillary carcinoma** showing papillary fronds with fibrovascular cores (Papanicolaou stain; ×100). *B,* Neoplastic papillary clusters showing depth of focus (Diff-Quik; ×200).

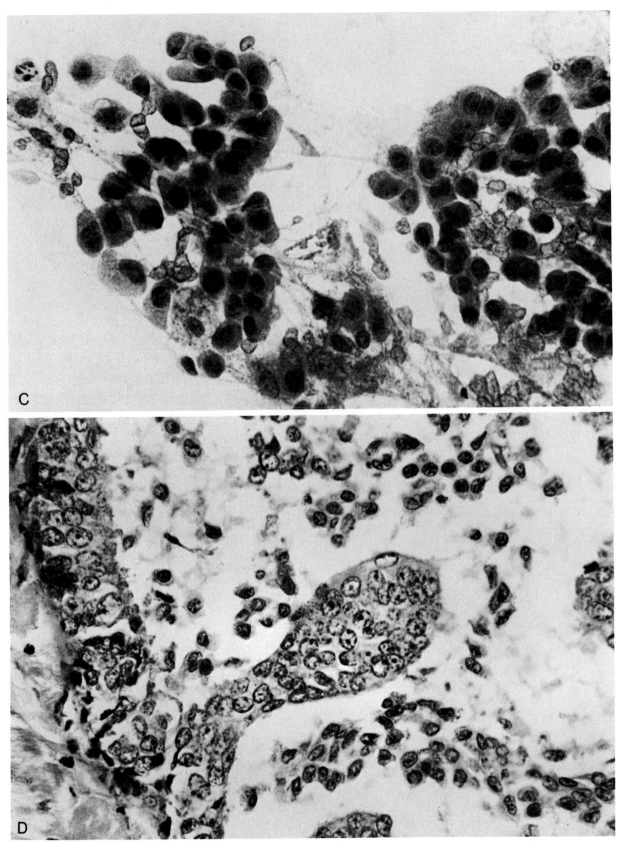

FIGURE 27–43 *Continued C*, Dissociative pattern consisting of uniform atypical cuboidal- to columnar-shaped neoplastic cells in an aspirate of papillary carcinoma (Papanicolaou stain; ×200). *D*, Histologic section demonstrating papillary carcinoma. Note the attached intraluminal papillary cluster along with individually scattered cuboidal- to columnar-shaped neoplastic cells corresponding to cells noted in *C* (hematoxylin and eosin; ×100).

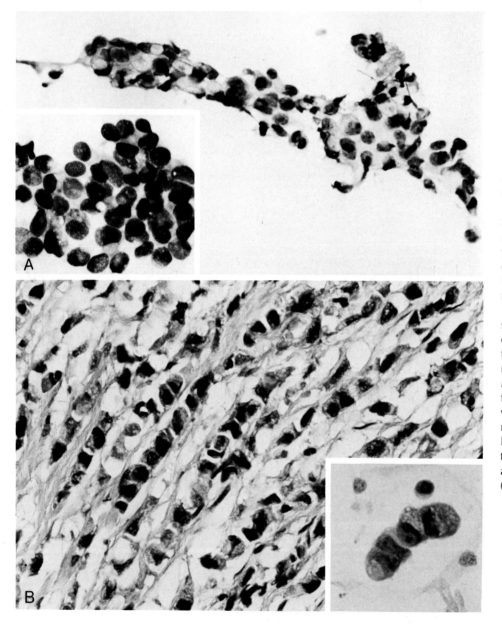

FIGURE 27–44. *A*, Diff-Quik–stained smear from an aspirate of **lobular carcinoma** demonstrating minimal atypia of the neoplastic cells (×200). *Inset*, Small neoplastic cells having a high nucleocytoplasmic ratio with excentrically placed nuclei and cytoplasmic vacuoles in an aspirate of lobular carcinoma (Papanicolaou stain; ×200). *B*, Histologic section showing characteristic "Indian-file" arrangement of infiltrating lobular carcinoma (hematoxylin and eosin; ×400). *Inset*, Occasional cases of infiltrating lobular carcinoma will demonstrate Indian-file arrangement of neoplastic cells. Note nuclear atypicality with the presence of small nucleoli and cytoplasmic vacuolization (Papanicolaou stain; ×400).

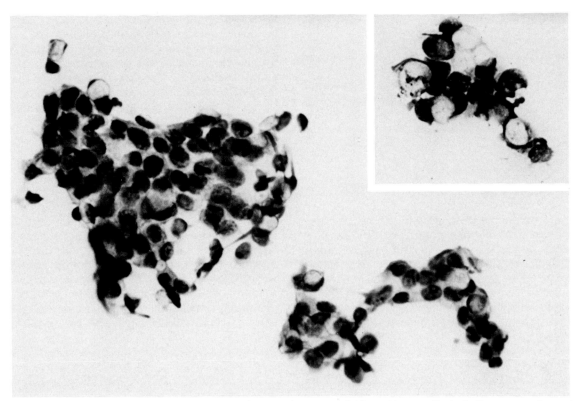

FIGURE 27–45. Lobular carcinoma consisting of cohesive clusters of fairly uniform cells including some signet-ring cells (Papanicolaou stain; ×200). *Inset,* Small cluster of neoplastic cells showing excentrically placed nuclei distorted by coarse cytoplasmic vacuoles in an aspirate of lobular carcinoma (Diff-Quik stain; ×200).

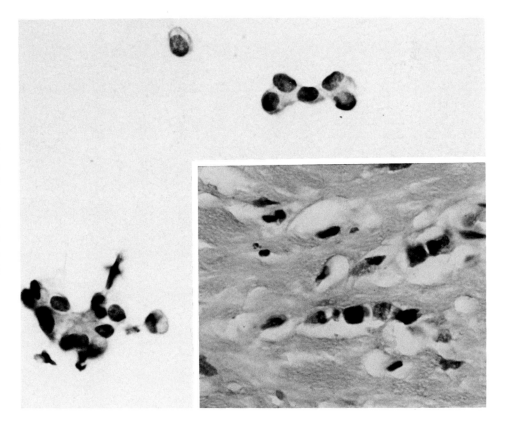

FIGURE 27–46. Aspirate of **lobular carcinoma** demonstrating minimal atypia of the cells and sparse cellularity (Papanicolaou stain; ×200). *Inset,* Resected lobular carcinoma demonstrating sparse cellularity and prominent desmoplastic fibrosis (hematoxylin and eosin; ×200).

Infiltrating Lobular Carcinoma

- Low-to-moderate cellularity
- Single cells and small clusters, cords and strands of atypical cells
- Fairly uniform mildly atypical cells with increased nucleocytoplasmic ratio, hypo- to hyperchromatic, oval-to-irregular nuclei and small nucleoli
- Signet-ring cells and intracytoplasmic mucin helpful features
- No bipolar nuclei

Apocrine Carcinoma

Apocrine carcinoma is an unusual variant of breast carcinoma possibly of sweat duct[116] or ductal origin.[67] The biologic behavior is similar to that of the common invasive ductal carcinoma. Cytologic features include the presence of numerous cells both individually scattered and arranged in syncytial fragments having apocrine features. The features include abundant basophilic-to-eosinophilic granular cytoplasm and large nuclei with prominent nucleoli (Fig. 27–47).[45, 89, 152] The cytologic features of a variant of apocrine carcinoma with lipid-rich giant cells has been described.[45] Secretory carcinoma may also be considered in the differential diagnosis.[157] The aspirated cytologic features of secretory breast carcinoma include irregular large sheets of malignant polygonal cells with granular and vacuolated cytoplasm.[157]

Squamous Cell Carcinoma

Squamous cells in breast aspirates can be derived from epidermoid cysts, cystosarcoma phyllodes, fibroadenomas and infarcted papillomas. Pure squamous cell carcinomas of the breast are quite rare, although squamous cell carcinomas mixed with ductal carcinomas are more common.[49, 83] Cytologically, sheets of well-differentiated or poorly differentiated malignant squamous cells are present, including some cases demonstrating intracytoplasmic keratinization of the cells and intercellular bridges (Fig. 27–48). Tumor cells are

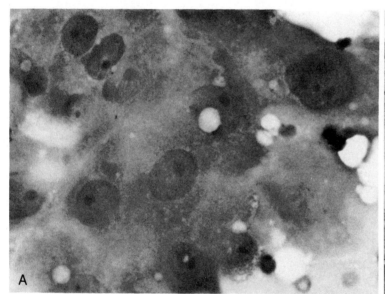

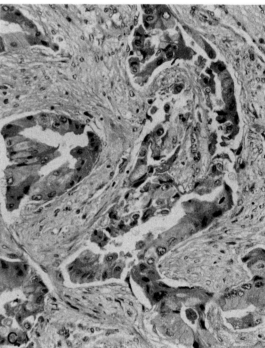

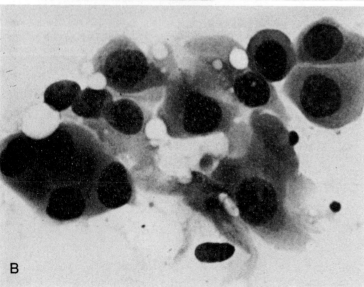

FIGURE 27–47. *A,* Loose cluster of malignant cells in **apocrine carcinoma** demonstrating nuclear enlargement with prominent nucleoli and abundant granular cytoplasm (Diff-Quik stain; ×400). *B,* Apocrine carcinoma with neoplastic cells having malignant cytologic features including hyperchromasia, prominent nucleoli and abundant granular cytoplasm (Papanicolaou stain; ×400). *C,* Infiltrating apocrine carcinoma consisting of malignant cells with apocrine features (hematoxylin and eosin; ×200).

FIGURE 27–48. *A,* **Squamous cell carcinoma** consisting of some cells demonstrating intracytoplasmic keratinization and sharp cytoplasmic borders (Papanicolaou stain; ×400). *B,* Corresponding histologic section showing malignant squamous cells in aspirate of primary squamous cell carcinoma of the breast (hematoxylin and eosin; ×400).

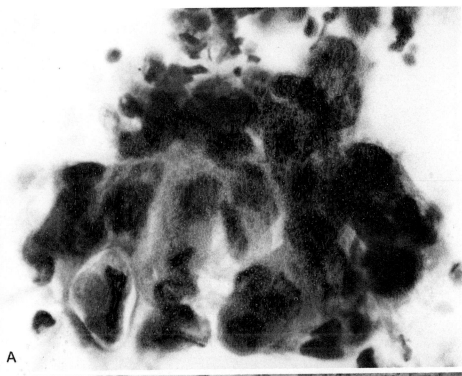

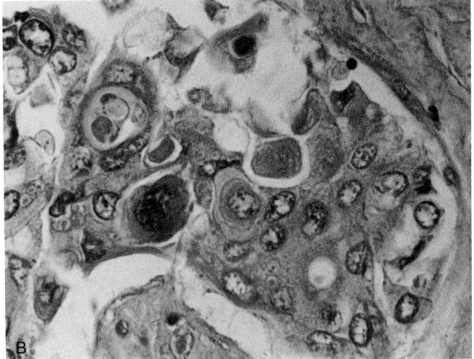

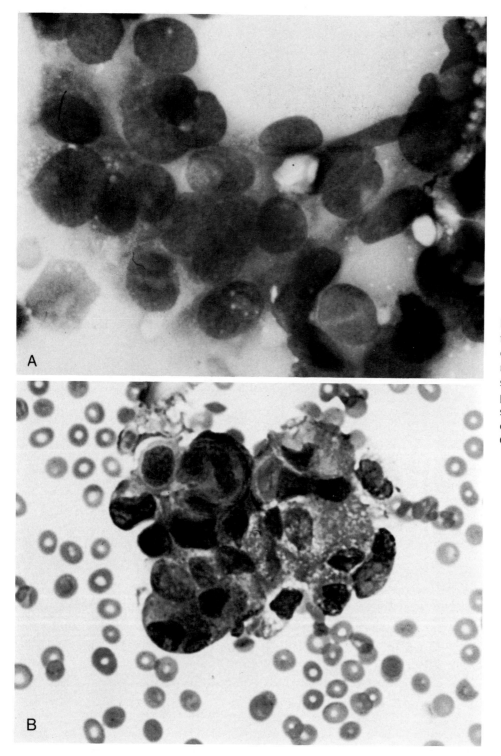

FIGURE 27–49. *A,* Aspirate from an **intracystic carcinoma** consisting of loose clusters of neoplastic cells (Diff-Quik stain; ×400). *B,* Cytospin preparation from the cyst fluid showing a three-dimensional cluster of neoplastic cells (Diff-Quik stain; ×200).

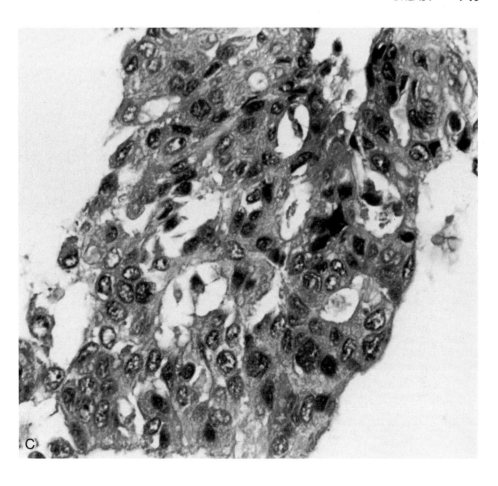

FIGURE 27–49 *Continued C,* Cell block from the same case of intracystic carcinoma demonstrating neoplastic cells (hematoxylin and eosin; ×200).

arranged in sheets, syncytial groupings and individually scattered malignant squamous cells. Some of the tumor cells may show a spindle-shaped tendency. Although some workers classify squamous cell carcinoma as a metaplastic carcinoma, it has a better prognosis than a metaplastic carcinoma having a pseudosarcomatous stroma. An occasional case of squamous cell carcinoma appears as a cystic mass. The behavior and prognosis of squamous cell carcinoma are similar to those of an infiltrating duct carcinoma or worse.[99, 130]

Intracystic Carcinoma

True intracystic carcinoma is an unusual breast malignancy accounting for approximately 0.7% of all breast carcinomas.[196] The typical patient is an obese elderly black female. The aspirated specimen usually consists of hemorrhagic fluid with persistence of a mass following the procedure. Cytologic findings may include scanty cellularity with mildly atypical cells arranged in loosely cohesive groups and papillary clusters (Fig. 27–49).[196] Colandrea and associates[31] reported a case of cystic hypersecretory duct carcinoma of the breast diagnosed by FNA biopsy. Cytologic findings include the presence of mildly atypical epithelial cells arranged singly and in small groups and sheets set in a background of abundant, intensely staining, pink-to-purple thyroid-like colloid material, which had a bub-

bling, fracturing appearance with cracking artifact in the smears.

Inflammatory Carcinoma

This clinicopathologic entity is an aggressive form of breast carcinoma accounting for approximately 2 to 4% of cases. Clinically, the breast appears hyperemic, engorged and edematous with peau d'orange skin changes and histopathologic findings of malignant cells, within the lymphatics of the overlying skin and breast parenchyma. Aspiration of the dermis, subcutaneous tissue or underlying breast tissue reveals cytologic findings of the usual infiltrating ductal carcinoma.

Paget's Disease

Paget's disease appears with an eczema-like change of the nipple and areola, occasionally associated with an underlying breast mass. Cytologic diagnosis can be made by scraping the nipple or by FNA biopsy. Tumor cells consist of clusters of malignant cells along with individually scattered malignant cells. Differentiation from malignant melanoma can be enhanced with an immunocytochemical panel, which will demonstrate positive staining of malignant cells in Paget's disease for (1) estrogen receptor protein, (2) carcinoembryonic

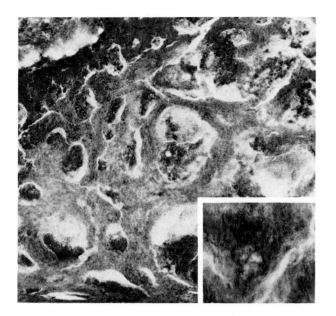

FIGURE 27–50. Low power of aspirate of **intraductal carcinoma** demonstrating cohesive branching of neoplastic cells (Diff-Quik stain; ×100). *Inset,* High power of calcified material in aspirate of intraductal carcinoma staining in a bas-relief fashion (Diff-Quik stain; ×400).

protein, (3) epithelial membrane antigen (EMA) and (4) cytokeratin versus cytoplasmic staining for (a) S-100 protein and (b) HMB in malignant melanoma.

Intraductal Carcinoma

Definite separation of intraductal carcinoma from infiltrating ductal carcinoma is not possible in our experience, although a tendency exists for aspirates of intraductal carcinomas to have a more cohesive arrangement of the malignant cells (Fig. 27–50). However, the cytologic features overlap with the usual invasive ductal carcinomas.[47] Comedocarcinomas consist of numerous malignant cells associated with abundant necrotic debris (Fig. 27–51). Similar findings can be present in invasive carcinomas (Fig. 27–52). Cor-

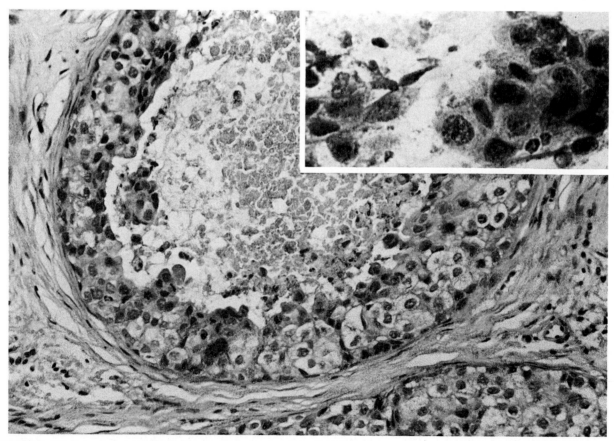

FIGURE 27–51. Resected comedocarcinoma demonstrating intraductal carcinoma with extensive central necrosis (hematoxylin and eosin; ×200). *Inset,* Aspirate from a corresponding lesion showing a loose cluster of neoplastic cells with tumor diathesis in the background (Papanicolaou stain; ×400).

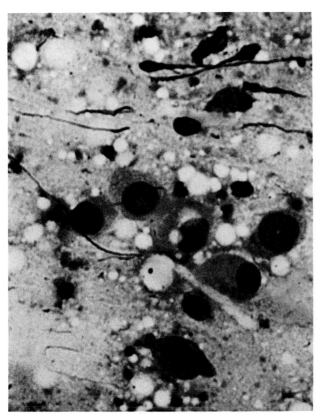

FIGURE 27–52. Fine needle aspiration of **infiltrating ductal carcinoma** showing similar features, namely, neoplastic cells with prominent tumor diathesis in the background indistinguishable from those of an aspirate of comedocarcinoma (Diff-Quik stain; ×200).

relation of the mammography findings may help in differentiating intraductal from invasive ductal carcinomas in some cases. However, additional studies are needed to establish better criteria for an accurate diagnosis of intraductal carcinomas because treatment protocols for invasive carcinoma differ significantly from those for *in situ* breast malignancies.

Radiation-Induced Changes

We expect that the pathologist will be called upon to examine breast aspirates from patients who have received radiation therapy for prior breast cancer. Histologic changes of irradiated breast include epithelial atypia in the terminal duct lobular unit and larger ducts along with stromal and vascular changes.[179] Bondeson[21] reported FNA cytologic findings of severe atypia of the dissociated epithelial cells derived from normal breast epithelium. Knowledge of prior irradiation therapy is crucial in order to avoid a potential false-positive diagnosis of malignancy in these patients presenting with new breast masses.[21, 85, 169] In the reported cases, FNA cytology specimens were generally hypocellular although scattered markedly atypical cells were present. A conservative approach is recommended in this setting.

Cystosarcoma Phyllodes

Cystosarcoma phyllodes is a biphasic tumor composed of both epithelial elements and fibrosarcomatous stroma. Cystosarcoma phyllodes accounts for less than 0.3% of all breast carcinomas.[4] The average age of patients with cystosarcoma phyllodes is 45, about 20 years older than the average age of patients with fibroadenoma.[10] Considerable controversy exists concerning the diagnostic and prognostic histologic parameters that should be used in separating benign from malignant cystosarcomas phyllodes. Tumor size, mitotic activity and stromal atypia and the status of the tumor margin to the surrounding parenchyma are the most useful guidelines in assessing the behavior of cystosarcoma phyllodes.[160, 172] However, the behavior of any specific tumor is unpredictable. Cystosarcoma phyllodes, having a benign histologic appearance, rarely metastasizes but can recur, whereas approximately 12% of malignant cystosarcoma phyllodes metastasize. The assessment of the patient begins with the clinical examination because those with cystosarcoma phyllodes often present with large tumors greater than 4 cm in diameter. Cytologic separation of cystosarcoma phyllodes from fibroadenoma is predominantly based on assessment of the cellularity of the stromal fragments (Fig. 27–53).[188, 192] Linsk and colleagues[133, 134] commented that highly cellular stromal fragments indicate cystosarcoma phyllodes in contrast to the relatively acellular stroma of fibroadenoma in FNA specimens. Another helpful criterion indicating cystosarcoma phyllodes is the presence of spindle-shaped cells enmeshed in pink stroma by metachromatic stains.[133, 134] The cytologic separation of benign from malignant cystosarcoma phyllodes is based on the presence of atypical stromal cells (Fig. 27–54). If orderly bundles of cells with small nuclei without atypia are seen, the lesion is most likely benign. If there is

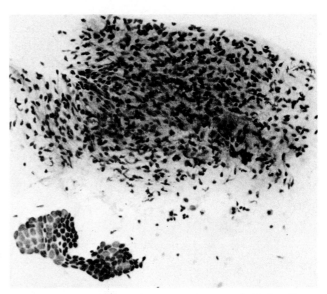

FIGURE 27–53. Aspirate from **cystosarcoma phyllodes** showing hypercellular stromal fragment and nearby cluster of benign ductal cells (Papanicolaou stain; ×100).

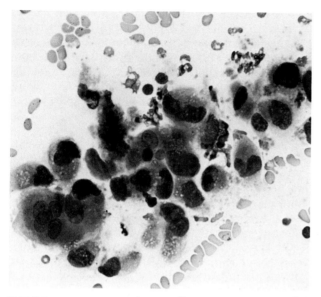

FIGURE 27–54. Aspirate from **malignant cystosarcoma phyllodes** showing dissociative pattern of malignant cells. Other areas in the aspirate demonstrated more conventional hypercellular stromal fragments and benign ductal groups (Diff-Quik stain; × 200).

increased cellularity with atypia, malignant cystosarcoma phyllodes should be considered.[121, 198]

Cystosarcoma Phyllodes

- Cellular smears
- Biphasic population of epithelial and stromal cells
- Hypercellular stromal fragments consisting of spindle-shaped cells enmeshed in metachromatically staining stroma
- Stromal cell atypia is a feature of malignant cystosarcoma phyllodes.
- Epithelial hyperplasia can be present.
- Numerous bipolar naked nuclei
- Occasional cases indistinguishable from fibroadenoma

In our initial experience with cystosarcoma phyllodes, varying degrees of epithelial proliferation were encountered, including three cases showing significant atypical epithelial hyperplasia that could potentially lead to a misdiagnosis of carcinoma (Fig. 27–55).[188] This experience is similar to Norris and Taylor's surgical pathology study of 94 cases of cystosarcoma phyllodes in which 15 cases had significant epithelial

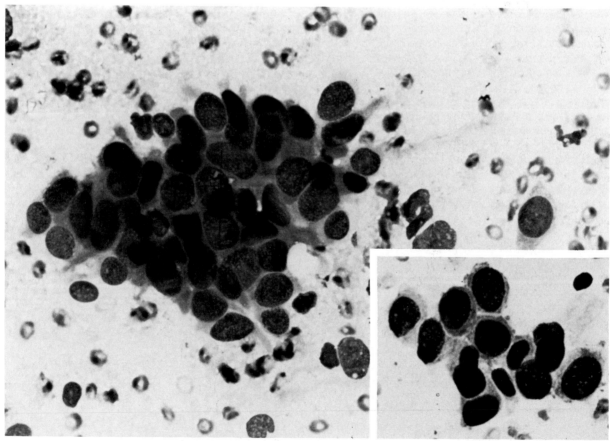

FIGURE 27–55. Aspirate of **benign cystosarcoma phyllodes** showing atypical epithelial hyperplasia that could potentially lead to a misdiagnosis of carcinoma (Diff-Quik stain; × 200). *Inset,* Loose cluster of atypical epithelial cells in an aspirate of cystosarcoma phyllodes (Diff-Quik stain; × 200).

hyperplasia with varying degrees of atypia.[160] Because a prominent epithelial component can be seen in both benign and malignant cystosarcoma phyllodes and in occasional cases the degree of epithelial proliferation could potentially lead to a false-positive diagnosis of breast carcinoma, we believe that frozen-section confirmation should be obtained in cases clinically or cytologically suspected of being cystosarcoma phyllodes. Helpful cytologic features suggestive of cystosarcoma phyllodes and unusual for breast carcinoma include increased numbers of naked nuclei and hypercellular stromal fragments. Potential for a false-negative diagnosis of cystosarcoma phyllodes exists because occasional cases may show a cytologic pattern indistinguishable from fibroadenoma.[121, 188]

Metaplastic Carcinomas (Carcinomas with Pseudosarcomatous Metaplasia) and Pure Sarcomas

Metaplastic carcinoma (carcinoma with pseudosarcomatous metaplasia) is a heterogeneous group of breast malignancies characterized by a mixture of carcinoma with areas of spindle, squamous, chondroid or osseous metaplasia.[20, 40, 76, 88, 101, 107] Metaplastic carcinomas are quite unusual, accounting for only 0.2% of breast malignancies.[107] The average age of patients is 54.3 years, similar to the average age of patients with ordinary infiltrating duct carcinomas. The overall survival is approximately 44% at 5 years, but if there is a predominance of pseudosarcomatous metaplasia, the survival decreases to 28% at 5 years.[107] Primary pure sarcomas of the breast are even less common with malignant fibrous histiocytoma (MFH) of the breast most often encountered.[125, 197]

A case report of an FNA biopsy of a postirradiation MFH of the breast demonstrated spindle-shaped and pleomorphic cells with large bizarre nuclei and foamy-to-vacuolated cytoplasm, including some cells showing evidence of phagocytosis.[139] The cytologic features of pure breast sarcoma and metaplastic carcinoma are similar to those of sarcomas encountered in soft tissue.[110, 111, 215] In our experience, FNA biopsies of MFH of breast were hypercellular and consisted of cells with extreme pleomorphism, including numerous atypical mono-, bi- and multinucleated histiocyte-like and fibroblastic cells. Occasionally, some bland-appearing vacuolated and xanthomatous cells were encountered.[215] Frequent atypical mitotic figures were readily identified. The atypical mononucleated to multinucleated histiocyte-like cells occurred singly and in small unorganized groups lacking any tight cohesion or glandular arrangement (Fig. 27–56). The histiocytes had indistinct cell borders with intracytoplasmic vacuoles, phagocytic debris or scattered acidophilic granules (Fig. 27–57). Touton-like and osteoclast-like giant cells were occasionally seen.

Occasional cases consisted of atypical spindle-shaped fibroblast-like cells, which were arranged singly or in loose clusters without well-formed fascicles.[215] Loosely cohesive groups of atypical cells in MFH can cytologically be arranged in suggestive storiform patterns (Fig. 27–58). Our one example of metastatic fibrosarcoma to the breast consisted of loose aggregates of fibroblastic-like cells showing a tendency to form parallel rows. The aspiration of the metaplastic carcinoma showing chondrosarcomatous differentiation demonstrated scattered bizarre cells set in a myxoid stroma (Fig. 27–59).

In general, we found that Giemsa-stained smears demonstrated cytoplasmic vacuoles, granules and ingested materials along with the extracellular metachromatic stromal elements more clearly than Papanicolaou-stained smears.[188, 215] Other types of breast sarcomas reported in the literature include angiosarcoma and osteogenic sarcoma[54, 148, 151] and primary rhabdomyosarcoma.[210]

The differential diagnosis of metaplastic breast carcinomas should include pseudosarcomatous fasciitis, fibromatosis and large-cell carcinomas.[51, 71, 188, 208, 215] Fine needle aspiration specimens of pseudosarcomatous fasciitis and fibromatosis can be hypocellular to hypercellular and consist of microtissue fragments and individually arranged spindle-shaped cells having a relatively bland appearance.[18, 51, 71] Pleomorphic large-cell carcinomas tend to occur in more cohesive sheets and clusters and do not demonstrate the degree of pleomorphism and phagocytosis that is seen in sarcomas such as MFH.[67, 121, 188, 215] Another unusual variant of breast carcinoma encountered in FNA biopsies is breast carcinoma with osteoclast-like giant cells.[171, 203] Ancillary studies including immunocytochemistry and electron microscopy can be helpful in making a more specific diagnosis of metaplastic carcinoma and pure sarcomas of the breast.[57, 112, 132, 188, 215]

Metastatic Neoplasms

Metastatic neoplasms to the breast are unusual with approximately 250 cases reported in the literature.[187] The incidence at autopsy varies from 1.4 to 6.6% of cases with breast malignancy, excluding those with contralateral primary breast carcinoma. In contrast, metastatic malignancies to the breast have a clinically observed rate of 0.4 to 2% of all breast malignancies.[187] In rare cases, metastatic cancers to the breast can be the initial presenting feature of malignancy and therefore simulate a primary breast carcinoma (Fig. 27–60). The most common metastatic cancers to involve the breast in women are, in decreasing frequency, melanoma, lymphoma, lung cancer, ovarian carcinoma and soft tissue sarcomas followed by gastrointestinal and genitourinary tumors (Fig. 27–61).[93] In men, metastatic carcinoma from the prostate is the most common primary (Fig. 27–62).

Extramedullary hematopoiesis has also been observed in FNA specimens from the breast and may not be associated with an underlying hematologic disorder.[144] In our initial experience with FNA diagnosis of metastatic neoplasms to the breast we encountered 18 examples.[187] These cases include four lung carcinomas,

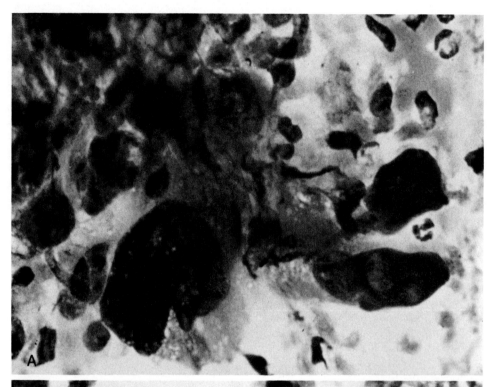

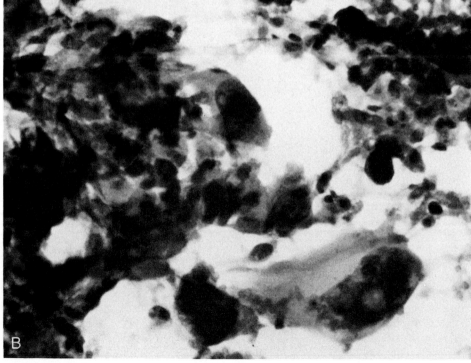

FIGURE 27–56. *A,* Individually scattered bizarre tumor cells in an aspirate of **metaplastic carcinoma** showing features of malignant fibrous histiocytoma (Diff-Quik stain; ×400). *B,* Corresponding alcohol-fixed material showing scattered bizarre tumor giant cells in a metaplastic carcinoma (Papanicolaou stain; ×400).

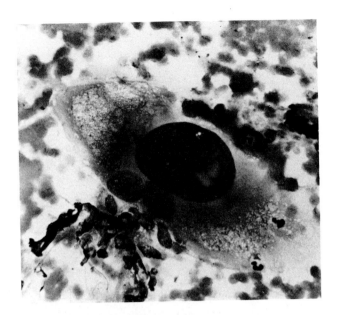

FIGURE 27–57. Malignant tumor giant cell in an aspirate of **metaplastic carcinoma** showing features of malignant fibrous histiocytoma. Note the intracytoplasmic vacuoles with cytophagocytosis and acidophilic granules (Diff-Quik stain; ×600).

two malignant melanomas, three ovarian malignancies and three hematopoietic malignancies. These cases were discovered in a combined series of 2529 breast FNA biopsies of which 666 were malignancies; the metastatic neoplasms to the breast thus constituted 2.7% of all of the malignant breast tumors.[187]

Some 16 biopsy samples confirmed metastatic malignancies in patients with known extramammary primaries. The prebiopsy clinical diagnoses in six of the patients, however, were benign breast lesions. In eight patients, the clinical differential diagnosis was a benign or malignant primary breast lesion versus a metastatic malignancy. Moreover, in two additional patients, the FNA biopsy specimens demonstrated metastatic neoplasms from unsuspected extramammary primaries. Recognition of unusual cytologic patterns raised the suspicion or confirmed the diagnosis of malignancy in all cases. Fine needle aspiration diagnosis of metastatic malignancy of the breast is essential in order to avoid

an unnecessary mastectomy and to assure appropriate chemotherapy and irradiation treatment (Fig. 27–63). Ancillary studies can be performed on the FNA material including immunocytochemistry and electron microscopy in order to make a more definitive diagnosis.[187]

SPECIAL TECHNIQUES

Mammography and Fine Needle Aspiration Biopsy of Nonpalpable Lesions

The combination of clinical examination, mammography and aspiration biopsy has been shown to yield the best diagnostic results in the workup of breast masses.[19, 38, 92, 98, 209] Mammography is believed to be

Text continued on page 761

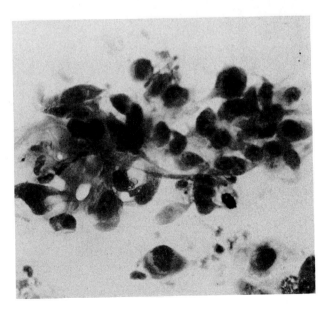

FIGURE 27–58. Loosely cohesive group of spindle-shaped cells in an aspirate of **malignant fibrous histiocytoma of the breast** showing suggestive storiform pattern (Papanicolaou stain; ×400).

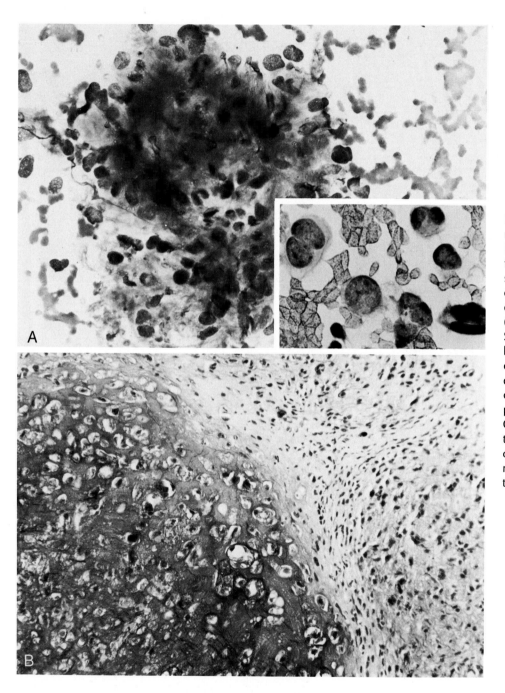

FIGURE 27–59. *A,* Aspirate of **metaplastic carcinoma** showing chondrosarcomatous differentiation characterized by scattered oval malignant cells enmeshed in a metachromatically staining myxoid stroma (Diff-Quik stain; × 200). *Inset,* Scattered mononuclear and binucleated oval malignant cells in metaplastic carcinoma demonstrating chondrosarcomatous differentiation (Papanicolaou stain; × 400). *B,* Corresponding histologic sections showing chrondrosarcomatous differentiation in a metaplastic carcinoma (hematoxylin and eosin; × 250).

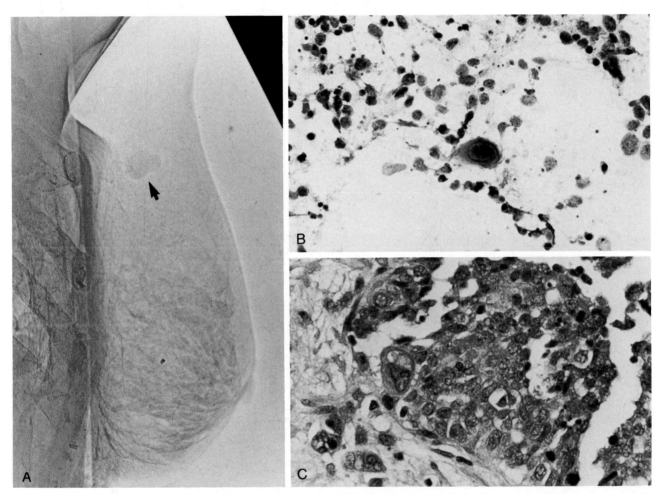

FIGURE 27–60. *A,* Mammogram of patient with **metastatic small-cell carcinoma of the lung to the breast**. Characteristic circumscribed nature of the lesion is demonstrated (arrow). *B,* Aspirate of the breast showing dual population of malignant cells including small cells having features of undifferentiated small-cell carcinoma along with a rare larger cell having squamoid features (Papanicolaou stain; ×200). *C,* Corresponding bronchial biopsy showing small-cell carcinoma, intermediate type, with rare cell demonstrating squamous differentiation (hematoxylin and eosin; ×400).

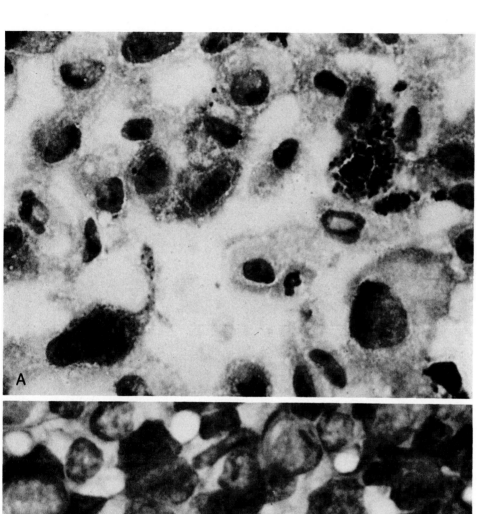

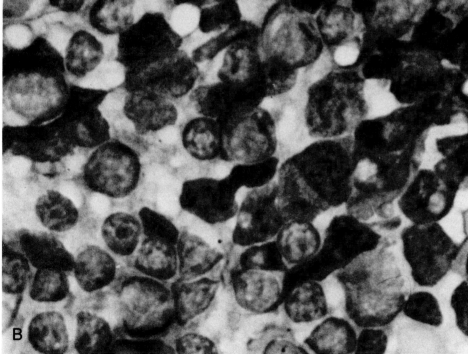

FIGURE 27–61. *A*, Aspirate from **metastatic malignant melanoma to the breast** showing dissociative cell pattern consisting of polygonal to spindle-shaped cells including some that demonstrate intracytoplasmic melanin pigment (Papanicolaou stain; ×400). *B*, Aspirate of **malignant lymphoma** showing dissociative pattern of large atypical lymphoid cells (Diff-Quik stain; ×400).

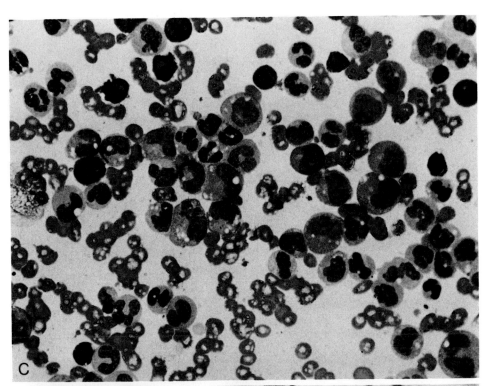

FIGURE 27–61 *Continued C*, Aspirate from **granulocytic sarcoma** of the breast showing spectrum of immature myeloid cells (Diff-Quik stain; ×200). *D*, Metastatic **keratinizing squamous cell carcinoma** in the breast (Papanicolaou stain; ×400).

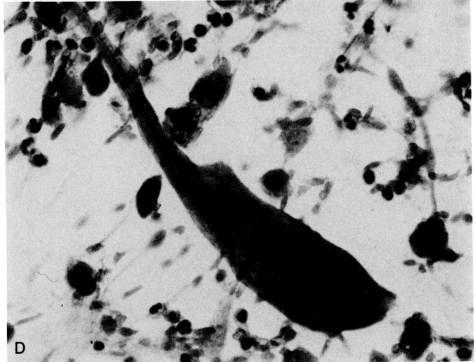

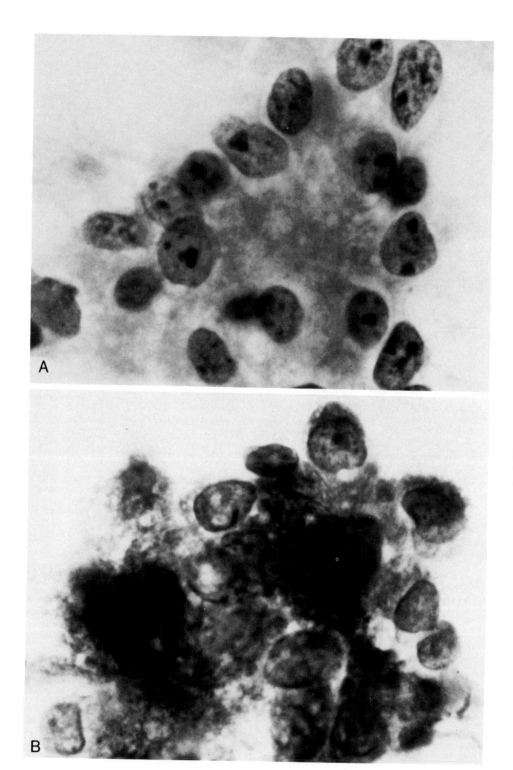

FIGURE 27–62. *A*, Aspirate of **metastatic prostate carcinoma to the breast** showing neoplastic epithelial cluster that would be indistinguishable from a primary breast carcinoma (Papanicolaou stain; × 600). *B*, Positive staining for acid phosphatase confirming the prostatic origin of the metastatic carcinoma (immunoperoxidase stain; × 600).

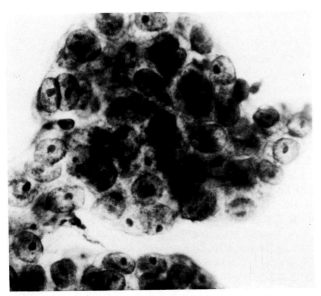

FIGURE 27–63. Metastatic papillary carcinoma of the ovary to the breast. Although most metastatic carcinomas have cytologic patterns unusual for primary breast carcinoma, occasional cases are indistinguishable from a breast primary carcinoma (Papanicolaou stain; ×600).

the best method for detection of nonpalpable breast lesions having a sensitivity of up to 80%.[17] However, its specificity remains relatively low, in the range of 15 to 25%.[17] An interest has developed in performing FNA biopsy of nonpalpable lesions at the time of mammographic examination using specialized localization guidance systems, including two-dimensional coordinate grids,[135] compression cones,[54] ultrasound[62, 94] and stereotaxic guidance.[17, 41, 75, 159, 204, 205] Fine needle aspiration biopsy of nonpalpable mammographically evident lesions may increase the specificity of the mammographic examination. Bibbo and colleagues[17] reported that stereotaxic FNA biopsy of mammographic lesions has a sensitivity in the range of 92 to 93% and a specificity of 93 to 95%.[17] With a positive preoperative diagnosis, additional procedures can be eliminated and the patient can undergo definitive therapy. However, negative biopsy findings should be evaluated in concert with the mammographic appearance of the lesion, because the nonpalpable mass may not have been adequately sampled. If the mammographic lesion has a stellate or ill-defined appearance with microcalcifications, open biopsy utilizing a needle localization procedure should be performed even with negative cytologic findings.[17]

For palpable lesions, it has been recommended that mammographic examination be performed prior to FNA biopsy because the subsequent hematoma or edema can mimic a mass or produce irregularities in an otherwise benign-appearing lesion that can potentially cause a false-positive mammographic diagnosis of malignancy.[114] In one study, this potential for false-positive interpretation was seen exclusively in mammographic examinations done within 1 week of aspiration biopsy. Therefore, these investigators rec-

ommended that if FNA biopsy is performed first, mammographic studies should be postponed at least 2 weeks.[100, 114] However, this study did not document the needle size, which may have a bearing on whether significant hematoma or edema resulted from the FNA biopsy.[114, 182] Additional systematic studies are needed in order to better define the timing of the mammographic examination in relationship to FNA biopsy using 22-gauge needles in the evaluation of palpable breast masses.

Estrogen Receptor Determinations

The determination of the presence of estrogen receptors (ER) of excised breast carcinomas by biochemical means is now a standard practice in the evaluation of the hormonal dependency of breast carcinoma.[104] Some 55 to 60% of ER-positive tumors respond to hormonal therapy, whereas less than 10% of ER-negative tumors respond.[109] A number of studies have been done demonstrating that ER determination using monoclonal antibodies can be applied in FNA biopsy specimens of breast carcinoma.*

Different methodologies have included isoelectric focusing in polyacrylamide gel[183] and single concentration dextran-coated charcoal (DCC) assay on fine-needle specimens. However, more recent studies have employed commercially available immunocytochemical methods (Abbott Laboratories, ER-ICA) on cytologic material using immunocytochemical staining of cells by a peroxidase-antiperoxidase technique (Fig. 27–64).†

Review of the literature shows excellent correlation of ER-ICA on FNA specimens with immunocytochemical studies performed on histologic biopsy samples. The ER-ICA on FNA aspirates also correlates well with biochemical analysis of the excised tumor mass.‡

The sensitivity and specificity of ERA-ICA of FNA specimens when compared with the biochemical method ranged from 71 to 95%. The qualitative ER-ICA determination on the cytology specimen generally uses a semiquantitative assessment, counting the percent of positive cells and intensity of staining in most series.[218] Microcomputer-based image analysis has been utilized to more objectively evaluate the intensity of staining with generation of a histogram.[11, 69]

The traditional biochemical assay is time-consuming and expensive and a less than perfect predictor of response to hormonal therapy. However, it has been traditionally used as the "gold standard" to compare the qualitative immunocytochemical analysis using monoclonal antibodies in both cytologic and histologic material. The ER-ICA method has some advantages over the quantitative biochemical assay.[37, 168, 214, 218] False-negative biochemical assay due to altered ER

---

*See references 26, 32, 34, 35, 37, 48, 61, 84, 109, 124, 137, 140, 142, 145, 149, 150, 153, 154, 168, 173, 174, 183, 207, 214, 218.
†See references 37, 61, 69, 84, 109, 118, 140, 151, 154, 168, 173, 174, 214, 218.
‡See references 6, 9, 37, 69, 84, 109, 118, 137, 140, 154, 168, 173–175, 214, 218.

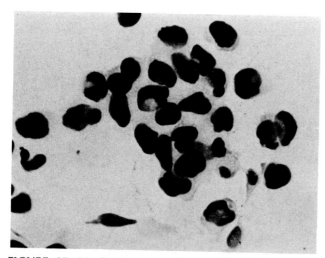

FIGURE 27–64. Estrogen receptor protein demonstrating intense nuclear staining of the malignant cells (immunoperoxidase stain; ×400).

molecules may be determined, which may be recognized by immunoperoxidase study but not by DCC assay. Tamoxifen also blocks the active sites of receptors, thereby preventing biochemical analysis by DCC but detected by the immunoperoxidase procedure.[37, 168, 214, 218] False-positive quantitative studies are possible when an ER-negative tumor is contaminated by ER-positive fibrocystic disease in the specimen. This occurrence is not likely with ER-ICA because one can visualize which cells are being studied.[218] In addition, heterogeneity of the tumor can also be appreciated by the immunocytochemical technique.[168, 218] Other potential sources for a false-negative quantitative biochemical analysis of ER are the lack of prompt tissue processing before freezing or delay in processing frozen specimens; the lack of quality control in assay methodology; the high circulating endogenous estradiol levels, especially in premenopausal women; the low protein content in the specimen; no tumor or low tumor or viable malignant cells in the specimen; the low tumor-to-stroma ratio; the tumor heterogeneity and the preceding irradiation therapy to the biopsy area.[214]

Immunocytochemical studies for ER performed on histologic or FNA biopsy specimens eliminate many of the aforementioned potential causes for a false-negative quantitative study. Therefore, correlation of biochemical ER tests with immunocytochemical studies could increase the reliability of a receptor determination. Parl and Posey[168] believe that the ER-ICA assay is more accurate than the biochemical assay in identifying the presence of ER protein in malignant cells. We believe that both studies are complementary and not mutually exclusive.

Immunocytochemical studies for ER on FNA material also have a role in the workup of metastatic breast cancer and the immediate evaluation of the ER status of the patient when only a small amount of tissue is present for ER study or when the patient refuses surgical biopsy and therefore quantitative studies cannot be performed.[56]

DNA Analysis

The reader is referred to Chapters 36 and 37 on Cell Image Analysis and Flow Cytometry for technical details and additional information. Although not well established, performance of DNA analysis on breast carcinoma specimens using flow cytometric and static image analyses may have clinical prognostic value.[5, 7, 81, 99, 213] Approximately 60 to 92% of malignant breast neoplasms are aneuploidy, whereas benign breast lesions are diploid. Although not universally accepted, there has been some correlation with DNA content and histologic and nuclear grade, ER status and stage of the disease.[12, 33, 106] DNA flow cytometry[8, 175] and static cytometric studies[16, 52, 53, 195] have been applied to FNA biopsy specimens of the breast.[8, 115, 165, 175] Although additional studies are needed to better define the relationship of DNA analysis to prognosis in breast carcinoma, some have suggested that performance of DNA analysis using flow cytometry on FNA biopsy specimens can render prognostic information that may have some bearing on therapeutic decisions.[42, 43, 53, 97] Trials are under way evaluating the relevance of DNA results in node-negative breast cancer patients in an attempt to identify high-risk groups that may benefit from preoperative adjuvant therapy.[29, 59, 60, 138, 141] Clark and colleagues[29] have demonstrated that node-negative patients with aneuploid tumors or diploid tumors with a high S-phase have an increased risk of recurrence. The National Surgery Adjuvant Breast Project is evaluating a protocol (B-18) using preoperative chemotherapy following a malignant diagnosis established by FNA cytology, preferably, or core-needle biopsy. This protocol also includes obtaining cells by FNA biopsy for flow cytometry DNA analysis in order to better define specific groups of patients having a greater risk of recurrence.

DIAGNOSTIC ACCURACY

Fine needle aspiration biopsy of the breast has been shown to be a diagnostically accurate procedure with

TABLE 27–1. Accuracy of Fine Needle Aspiration of the Breast

Authors	Year	Sensitivity (%)	Specificity (%)	Accuracy (%)
Rimsten	1975	84	99	95
Kline	1979	89	98	97
Gardecki	1980	87	95	90
Strawbridge	1981	70	96	87
Bell	1983	73	98	92
Abele	1983	95	97	96
Wanebo	1984	90	95	92
Norton	1984	84	83	84
Ulanow	1984	85	87	86
Frable	1984	89	97	94
Lannin	1985	87	100	96

Reproduced with permission from Lannin DR, Silverman JF, Pories WJ, Walker C: Cost-effectiveness of fine needle biopsy of the breast. Ann Surg 203:474–480, 1986.

a rate ranging from 77 to 99% (Table 27–1).[13, 46, 55, 66, 67, 80, 95, 118, 120, 166, 176, 180, 190, 212, 217, 220, 222, 226] In a cytology literature review, analyzing the results of over 3000 breast aspirations with histologic follow-ups, a sensitivity of 72 to 99% (average, 87%), a specificity of 98 to 100%, a positive predictive value of approximately 100%, a negative predictive value of 87 to 99% and an efficiency of 89 to 99% were found for the procedure. The number of specimens judged insufficient for diagnosis varied from 4 to 13%.[95] Some studies have demonstrated greater accuracy of FNA biopsy when compared with TruCut needle biopsy of the breast.[181] This is especially the case when the cytopathologist examines the patient and performs the FNA biopsy.[67]

Utilization of the so-called triple diagnostic procedures of clinical examination, mammography and FNA cytology increases the accuracy for the diagnosis of breast cancer.[38, 92, 98, 209] A diagnostic accuracy of 99% for breast carcinoma was achieved when all three screening tests were in agreement.

False-negative rates vary, with a range from 1 to 31%[30, 54, 79, 80, 116, 121, 129, 133, 217] and an average rate of 10% in a literature review.[212] False-negative diagnoses are usually due to poor technique, missing the lesion, fibrotic or necrotic nature of the tumor or incorrect interpretation of malignant lesions (Fig. 27–65). Malignant lesions that have the highest potential for false-negative diagnosis include lobular carcinoma, tubular carcinoma, colloid carcinoma, papillary carcinoma and the monomorphic type of ductal carcinoma seen in some elderly patients (Table 27–2).[116, 123, 221] Tumor size also has a bearing on the ability to adequately sample a breast carcinoma. A greater false-negative rate occurs with tumors less than 1 cm[116, 123] and with some very large lesions due to tumor necrosis.[223]

False-positive rates range from 0 to 4.1%.[15, 54, 65, 70, 74, 80, 108, 116, 133, 190, 202, 212, 220] Feldman and Covell[54] reviewed 14 series in which 42 false-positive diagnoses were rendered out of a total of 25,180 FNA biopsies of the breast, for a false-positive rate of 0.17%. In another review, Frable[65] commented that a small number of false-positive diagnoses have occurred in almost all reported series. However, his review included a greater number of false-positive diagnoses, since he included "suspicious diagnosis" in the malignant category. Frable has commented that European series of FNA biopsy of the breast tend to report a greater sensitivity of the procedure with a concomitant higher false-positive rate when compared with American series.[67] Frable implies that this difference may be due to Europeans practicing in a less litigious environment or perhaps relying more on tissue or frozen-section confirmation for all positive cases. The conservative trend in American series is likewise reflected by the greater number of reported suspicious cases with few or no false-positive diagnoses.[67]

In Kline's review of 3809 benign breast lesions, 69 cases were interpreted as suspicious for malignancy.[117] These included 33 examples of fibrocystic disease, nine fibroadenoma, five granulation tissue, three gynecomastia, four papilloma, four periareolar hyper-

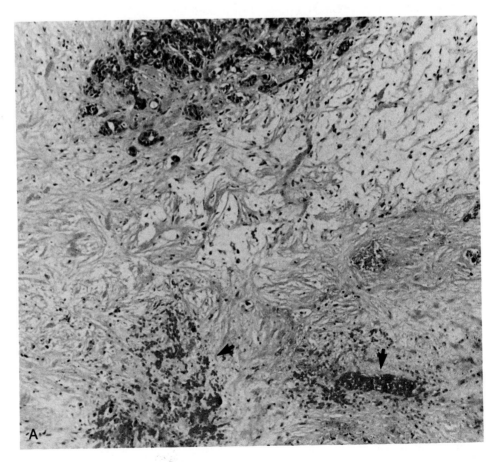

FIGURE 27–65. *A,* Histologic section showing extensive **tumor necrosis** with small group of neoplastic cells at the periphery. Note the hemorrhage in the lower portion of the field (arrows) corresponding to the aspirated site (hematoxylin and eosin; ×100).

Illustration continued on following page

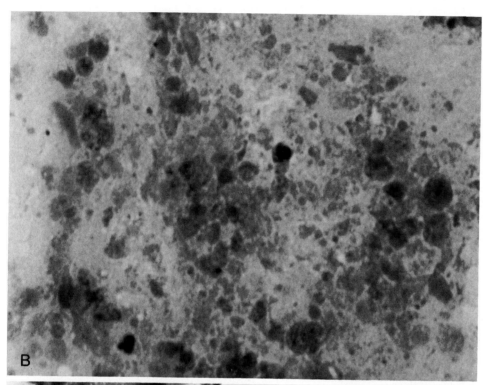

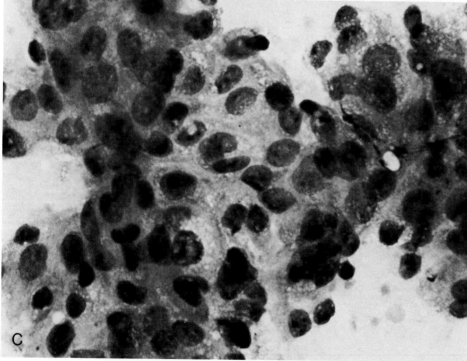

FIGURE 27–65 *Continued B,* **Aspirated carcinoma** consisting exclusively of necrotic cells and background debris with no viable diagnostic tumor cells (Papanicolaou stain; ×400). *C,* Reaspiration of the peripheral portion of the mass demonstrating **diagnostic malignant cells** (Diff-Quik stain; ×200).

TABLE 27–2. Breast Carcinomas Having the Highest Potential for False-Negative Diagnosis When Neoplasm Is Aspirated

Carcinoma	Reason
Lobular carcinoma	Hypocellular due to desmoplastic fibrosis with presence of small cells showing little atypia; note signet-ring cells have excentrically placed atypical nuclei.
Tubular carcinoma	Low to moderate cellularity with minimal atypia of cells; note atypical tubules.
Ductal carcinoma in the elderly	Hypercellular specimen with uniform, atypical cells having plasmacytoid features in Diff-Quik stained material.
Colloid carcinoma	Hypocellular specimen due to abundant extracellular mucinous material and small clusters of mildly atypical cells.
Papillary carcinoma	Mild atypia of epithelial cells; difficult to differentiate from intraductal papilloma.

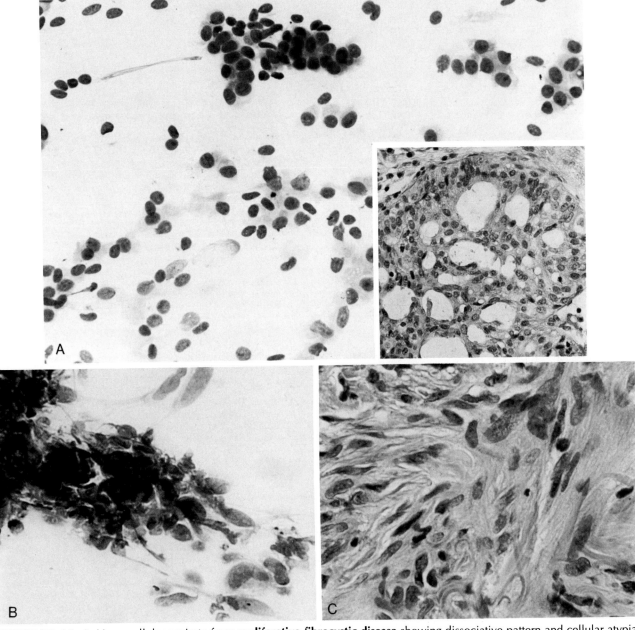

FIGURE 27–66. *A,* Hypercellular aspirate from **proliferative fibrocystic disease** showing dissociative pattern and cellular atypia that could potentially be misdiagnosed as carcinoma. Considerable air-drying artifact also contributes to the atypical features (Diff-Quik stain; ×200). *Inset,* Corresponding histologic sections showing florid intraductal hyperplasia (hematoxylin and eosin; ×200). *B,* Scattered groups of atypical spindle-shaped cells showing considerable air-drying artifact in the aspirate from a nodule arising in a mastectomy scar. Clinically, recurrent breast carcinoma was suspected (Diff-Quik stain; ×200). *C,* Surgical confirmation demonstrating **leiomyoma** rather than recurrent breast carcinoma in the mastectomy scar. The case demonstrates that a definitive diagnosis should not be rendered on ill-prepared material with limited cellularity (hematoxylin and eosin; ×400).

plasia and three pregnancy-related hyperplasia. Sources of the malignant diagnosis include hypercellularity with mild focal atypia including atypia of benign apocrine cells (Fig. 27–66). Occasional cases also showed mild discohesion, anisonucleosis and prominent nucleoli of the ductal cells. We have also found that epithelial hyperplasia in cystosarcoma phyllodes could be potentially misinterpreted as breast carcinoma.[188] Misinterpreting epithelial atypia in inflammatory lesions is also a potential pitfall for a false-positive diagnosis of malignancy.[189] Although the overall false-positive rate in the literature is relatively low, any false-positive diagnosis is unacceptable because in many institutions a mastectomy will be performed based solely on the cytologic interpretation. In any questionable case or in any pathology practice in which the pathologist may be inexperienced in interpreting FNA biopsy or in which the volume of FNA breast biopsies is low, frozen-section confirmation is recommended before definitive treatment.[190]

References

1. Abele JS, Miller TR, Goodson WH III, Hunt TK, Hohn DC: Fine needle aspiration of palpable breast masses: A program for staged implementation. Arch Surg 118:859–863, 1983.
2. Adair FE: Surgical problems involved in breast cancer. Ann Royal Coll Surg Engl 4:360–380, 1949.
3. Antoniades K, Spector HB: Similarities and variations among lobular carcinoma cells. Diagn Cytopathol 3:55–59, 1987.
4. Ariel I: Skeletal metastasis in cystosarcoma phylloides. Arch Surg 82:275–280, 1961.
5. Auer G, Eriksson E, Azavedo E, Caspersson T, Wallgren A: Prognostic significance of nuclear DNA content in mammary adenocarcinomas in humans. Cancer Res 44:394–396, 1984.
6. Auer G, Tribukait B: Comparative single cell and flow DNA analysis in aspiration biopsies from breast carcinomas. Acta Pathol Microbiol Scand 88:355–358, 1980.
7. Auer GU, Caspersson TO, Wallgren AS: DNA content and survival in mammary carcinoma. Anal Quant Cytol 2:161–165, 1980.
8. Auer GU, Askensten U, Erhardt K, Fallenius A, Zetterberg A: Comparison between slide and flow cytophotometric DNA measurements in breast tumors. Analyt Quant Cytol 9:138–146, 1987.
9. Azavedo E, Baral E, Skoog L: Immunohistochemical analysis of estrogen receptors in cells obtained by fine needle aspiration from human mammary carcinomas. Anticancer Res 6:263–266, 1986.
10. Azzopardi JG: Problems in breast pathology, vol. 11. In Major Problems in Pathology. Edited by James L. Bennington. Philadelphia, WB Saunders, 42–55, 346–378, 1979.
11. Bacus S, Flowers JL, Press MF, Bacus JW, McCarty KS: The evaluation of estrogen receptor in primary breast carcinoma by computer-assisted image analysis. Am J Clin Pathol 90:233–239, 1988.
12. Bakke AC, Sahin A, Braziel RM: Applications of flow cytometry in surgical pathology. Lab Med 18:590–596, 1987.
13. Barrows GH, Anderson TJ, Lamb JL, Dixon JM: Fine-needle aspiration of breast cancer: Relationship of clinical factors to cytology results in 689 primary malignancies. Cancer 58:1493–1498, 1986.
14. Bauermeister DE: The role and limitations of frozen section and needle aspiration biopsy in breast cancer diagnosis. Cancer 46:947–949, 1980.
15. Bell DA, Hajdu SI, Urban JA, Gaston JP: Role of aspiration cytology in the diagnosis and management of mammary lesions in office practice. Cancer 51:1182–1189, 1983.
16. Berryman IL, Harvey JM, Sterrett GF, Papadimitrious JM: The nuclear DNA content of human breast carcinoma. Asso-

ciations with clinical stage, axillary lymph node status, estrogen receptor status and outcome. Anal Quant Cytol Histol 9:429–434, 1987.
17. Bibbo M, Scheiber M, Cajulis R, Keebler CM, Wied GL, Dowlatshahi K: Stereotaxic fine needle aspiration cytology of clinically occult malignant and premalignant breast lesions. Acta Cytol 32:193–201, 1988.
18. Bigelow R, Smith R, Goodman PA, Wilson GS: Needle localization of nonpalpable breast masses. Arch Surg 120:565–569, 1985.
19. Bjurstam N, Hedberg K, Hultborn KA, Johansson NT, Johnsen C: Diagnosis of breast carcinoma: An evaluation of clinical examination, mammography, thermography and aspiration biopsy in breast disease. Progr Surg 13:1–65, 1974.
20. Boccato P, Briani G, d'Atri C, Pasini L, Blandamura S, Bizzaro N: Spindle cell and cartilaginous metaplasia in a breast carcinoma with osteoclast-like stromal cells. A difficult fine needle aspiration diagnosis. Acta Cytol 32:75–78, 1988.
21. Bondeson L: Aspiration cytology of radiation-induced changes of normal breast epithelium. Acta Cytol 31:309–310, 1987.
22. Bottles K, Chan JS, Holly EA, Chiu S-H, Miller TR: Cytologic criteria for fibroadenoma: A stepwise logistic regression analysis. Am J Clin Pathol 89:707–713, 1988.
23. Bottles K, Taylor RN: Diagnosis of breast masses in pregnant and lactating women by aspiration cytology. Obstet Gynecol 66:76S–78S, 1985.
24. Carney M, Unverferth M, Silverman JF: Fine needle aspiration cytology of subareolar abscess. Cytotechnol Bull 22:60–64, 1985.
25. Catania S, Boccato P, Bono A, DiPietro S, Pilotti S, Ciatto S, Ravetto C: Pneumothorax: A rare complication of fine needle aspiration of the breast. Acta Cytol 33:140, 1989.
26. Cavailles V, Garcia M, Salazar G, Domergue J, Simony J, Pujol H, Rochefort H: Immunodetection of estrogen receptor and 52,000-Dalton protein in fine needle aspirates of breast cancer tumors. J Natl Cancer Instit 79:245–252, 1987.
27. Ciatto S, Cariaggi P, Bulgaresi P: The value of routine cytologic examination of breast cyst fluids. Acta Cytol 31:301–304, 1987.
28. Ciatto S, Cecchini S, Grazzini G, Iossa A: Fine needle aspiration cytology of clinically suspected local recurrences in breast cancer. Acta Cytol 33:140–141, 1989.
29. Clark GM, Dressler LG, Owens MA, Pounds MT, Oldaker T, McGuire WL: Prediction of relapse or survival in patients with node-negative breast cancer by DNA flow cytometry. N Engl J Med 320:627–633, 1989.
30. Cohen MB, Rodgers RPC, Hales MS, Gonzales JM, Ljung BME, Beckstead JH, Bottles K, Miller TR: Influence of training and experience in fine needle aspiration biopsy of breast: Receiver operating characteristics curve analysis. Arch Pathol Lab Med 111:518–520, 1987.
31. Colandrea JM, Shmookler BM, O'Dowd GJ, Cohen MH: Cystic hypersecretory duct carcinoma of the breast. Report of a case with fine-needle aspiration. Arch Pathol Lab Med 112:560–563, 1988.
32. Coombes RC, Powles TJ, Berger U, Wilson P, McClelland RA, Gazet JC, Trott PA, Ford HT: Prediction of endocrine response in breast cancer by immunocytochemical detection of oestrogen receptor in fine needle aspirates. Lancet 2:701–703, 1987.
33. Coulson PB, Thornthwaite JT, Wooley TW, Sugarbaker EV, Sickinger D: Prognostic indicators including DNA histogram type, receptor content, and staging related to breast cancer patient survival. Cancer Res 44:4187–4196, 1984.
34. Crawford DJ, Lope-Pihie A, Cowan S, George WD, Leake RE: Preoperative determination of oestrogen receptor status in breast cancer by immunocytochemical staining of fine needle aspirates. Br J Surg 72:991–993, 1985.
35. Curtin C, Pertschuk LP, Mitchell V: Histochemical determination of estrogen and progesterone binding in fine needle aspirates of breast cancer. Acta Cytol 26:841–846, 1982.
36. DeMay RM, Kay S: Granular cell tumor of the breast. Pathol Annu 19:121–148, 1984.
37. Devleeschouwer N, Faverly D, Kiss R, Legros N, de Launoit Y, Ryckaert C, Andry M, Lenglet G, Paridaens R, Gompel CM: Comparison of biochemical and immunoenzymatic macromethods and a new immunocytochemical micromethod for

assaying estrogen receptors in human breast carcinomas. Acta Cytol 32:816–824, 1988.

38. Dixon JM, Anderson TJ, Lamb J, Nixon SJ, Forrest APM: Fine needle aspiration cytology in relationships to clinical examination and mammography in the diagnosis of a solid breast mass. Br J Surg 71:598–596, 1984.

39. Doria MI, Tani EM, Skoog L: Sarcoidosis presenting initially as a breast mass: Detection by fine-needle aspiration biopsy. Acta Cytol 31:378–379, 1987.

40. Douglas-Jones AG, Barr WT: Breast carcinoma with tumor giant cells: Report of a case with fine needle aspiration cytology. Acta Cytol 33:109–114, 1989.

41. Dowlatshahi K, Jokich PM, Schmidt R, Bibbo M, Dawson PJ: Cytologic diagnosis of occult breast lesions using stereotaxic needle aspiration: A preliminary report. Arch Surg 122:1343–1346, 1987.

42. Dressler L, Clark G, Owens M, Pounds G, Oldaker T, McGuire W: DNA flow cytometry predicts for relapse in node negative breast cancer patients. Am Soc Clin Oncol 6:57, 1987.

43. Dressler LG, Seamer LC, Owens MA, Clark GM, McGuire WL: DNA flow cytometry and prognostic factors in 1331 frozen breast cancer specimens. Cancer 61:420–427, 1988.

44. Duane GB, Kanter MH, Branigan T, Chang C: A morphologic and morphometric study of cells from colloid carcinoma of the breast obtained by fine needle aspiration: Distinction from other breast lesions. Acta Cytol 31:742–750, 1987.

45. Duggan MA, Young GK, Hwang WS: Fine needle aspiration of an apocrine breast carcinoma with multivacuolated lipid-rich giant cells. Diagn Cytopathol 4:62–66, 1988.

46. Dundas SAC, Sanderson PR, Matta H, Shorthouse AJ: Fine needle aspiration of palpable breast lesions: Results obtained with cytocentrifuge preparation of aspirates. Acta Cytol 32:203–206, 1988.

47. Dziura B, Bonfiglio T: Needle cytology of the breast. A quantitative and qualitative study of the cells of benign and malignant ductal neoplasia. Acta Cytol 23:332–340, 1979.

48. Earl M: Cell collection from fine needle aspirates for estrogen receptor immunocytochemical assay. Acta Cytol 31:377, 1987.

49. Eggers JW, Chesney TM: Squamous cell carcinoma of the breast: A clinicopathologic analysis of eight cases and review of the literature. Hum Pathol 15:526–531, 1984.

50. Eisenberg AJ, Hajdu SI, Wilhelmus J, Melamed MR, Kinne D: Preoperative aspiration cytology of breast tumors. Acta Cytol 30:135–145, 1986.

51. El-Naggar A, Abdul-Karim FW, Marshalleck JJ, Sorensen K: Fine needle aspiration of fibromatosis of the breast. Diagn Cytopathol 3:320–322, 1987.

52. Fallenius AG, Auer GU, Carstensen JM: Prognostic significance of DNA measurements in 409 consecutive breast cancer patients. Cancer 62:331–341, 1988.

53. Fallenius AG, Franzen SA, Auer GU: Predictive value of nuclear DNA content in breast cancer in relation to clinical and morphologic factors. Cancer 62:521–530, 1988.

54. Feldman PS, Covell JL: Breast and lung. *In* Fine Needle Aspiration Cytology and Its Clinical Application. Chicago, American Society of Clinical Pathologists Press, 1985.

55. Fessia L, Botta G, Arisio R, Verga M, Aimone V: Fine needle aspiration of breast lesions: Role and accuracy in a review of 7495 cases. Diagn Cytopathol 3:121–125, 1987.

56. Finley JL, Silverman JF, Chaplinski TJ, Shurlow C: The utility of monoclonal estrogen receptor protein assay on fine needle aspiration biopsies of primary and metastatic breast carcinomas. Acta Cytol 30:588, 1986.

57. Finley JL, Silverman JF, Dabbs DJ, West, Dickens A, Feldman PS, Frable WJ: Chordoma. Diagnosis by fine needle aspiration biopsy with histologic, immunocytochemical, and ultrastructural confirmation. Diagn Cytopathol 2:330–337, 1986.

58. Finley JL, Silverman JF, Lannin DR: Fine needle aspiration cytology of breast masses in pregnant and lactating women. Diagn Cytopathol 5:255–259, 1989.

59. Fisher B, Costantino J, Redmond C: A randomized clinical trial evaluating tamoxifen in the treatment of patients with node-negative breast cancer who have estrogen receptor–positive tumors. N Engl J Med 320:479–484, 1989.

60. Fisher B, Redmond C, Dimitrov NV: A randomized clinical trial evaluating sequential methotrexate and fluorouracil in the treatment of patients with node-negative breast cancer who have estrogen-receptor negative tumors. N Engl J Med 320:473–478, 1989.

61. Flowers J, Burton GV, Cox EB, McCarty KS Sr, Dent GA, Geisinger KR, McCarty KS Jr: Use of monoclonal antiestrogen receptor antibody to evaluate estrogen receptor content in fine needle aspiration breast biopsies. Ann Surg 203:250–254, 1986.

62. Fornage BD, Faroux MJ, Simatos A: Breast masses: US-guided fine needle aspiration biopsy. Radiology 162:409–414, 1987.

63. Frable W: Thin needle aspiration biopsy. *In* Major Problems in Pathology, vol. 14. Philadelphia, W. B. Saunders, 1983.

64. Frable WJ: Fine needle aspiration biopsy: A review. Hum Pathol 14:9–28, 1983.

65. Frable WJ: Needle aspiration of the breast. Cancer 53:671–676, 1984.

66. Frable WJ: Thin needle aspiration biopsy. A personal experience of 469 cases. Am J Clin Pathol 65:168–182, 1976.

67. Frable WJ: Needle aspiration biopsy: Past, present, and future. Hum Pathol 20:504–517, 1989.

68. Frable W, Bonfiglio T, Kaminsky DB, Murphy WM: Diagnostic cytology seminar, case 8: carcinoma, tubular type, of the breast. Acta Cytol 24:90–136, 1980.

69. Franklin WA, Bibbo M, Doria MI, Dytch HE, Toth J, DeSombre E, Wied GL: Quantitation of estrogen receptor content and Ki-67 staining in breast carcinoma by the microTICAS image analysis system. Analyt Quant Cytol Histol 9:279–286, 1987.

70. Franzen S, Zajicek J: Aspiration biopsy in diagnosis of palpable lesions of the breast. Critical review of 3479 consecutive biopsies. Acta Radiol Ther Phys Biol 7:241–262, 1968.

71. Fritsches HG, Muller EA: Pseudosarcomatous fasciitis of the breast: Cytologic and histologic features. Acta Cytol 27:73–75, 1983.

72. Galblum LI, Oertel YC: Subareolar abscess of the breast diagnosed by fine needle aspiration. Am J Clin Pathol 80:496–499, 1983.

73. Gansler TS, Wheeler JE: Mammary sarcoidosis. Two cases and literature review. Arch Pathol Lab Med 108:673–675, 1984.

74. Gardecki TM, Hogbin BM, Melcher DH, Smith RS: Aspiration cytology in the preoperative management of breast cancer. Lancer 2:790–792, 1980.

75. Gent HJ, Sprenger E, Dowlatshahi K: Stereotaxic needle localization and cytological diagnosis of occult breast lesions. Ann Surg 204:580–584, 1986.

76. Gersell DJ, Katzenstein AL: Spindle cell carcinoma of the breast. A clinicopathologic and ultrastructural study. Hum Pathol 12:550–561, 1981.

77. Godwin JT: Aspiration biopsy: Technique and application. Ann NY Acad Sci 63:1348–1373, 1956.

78. Gonzalez E, Grafton WD, Morris DM, Barr LH: Diagnosing breast cancer using frozen sections from TruCut needle biopsies. Ann Surg 202:696–701, 1985.

79. Goodson WH, Mailman RM, Miller TR: Three-year follow-up of benign fine needle aspiration biopsies of the breast. Am J Surg 154:58–61, 1987.

80. Grant CS, Goellner JR, Welch JS, Martin JK: Fine needle aspiration of the breast. Mayo Clin Proc 61:377–381, 1986.

81. Greenebaum E, Koss LG, Sherman AB, Elequin F: Comparison of needle aspiration and solid biopsy technics in the flow cytometric study of DNA distributions of surgically resected tumors. Am J Clin Pathol 82:559–564, 1984.

82. Griffith CN, Kern WH, Mikkelsen WP: Needle aspiration cytologic examination in the management of suspicious lesions of the breast. Surg Gynecol Obstet 162:142–144, 1986.

83. Gubin N: A case of pure primary squamous-cell carcinoma of the breast diagnosed by fine needle aspiration biopsy. Acta Cytol 29:650–651, 1985.

84. Gunduz N, Zheng S, Fisher B: Fluoresceinated estrone binding by cells from human breast cancers obtained by needle aspiration. Cancer 52:1251–1256, 1983.

85. Gupta RK: Radiation-induced cellular changes in the breast: A potential diagnostic pitfall in fine needle aspiration cytology. Acta Cytol 33:141–142, 1989.

86. Gupta RK, Naran S, Buchanan A, Fauck R, Simpson J: Fine

needle aspiration cytology of breast: Its impact on surgical practice with an emphasis on the diagnosis of breast abnormalities in young women. Diagn Cytopathol 4:206–209, 1988.

87. Gupta RK, Naran S, Simpson J: The role of fine needle aspiration cytology (FNAC) in the diagnosis of breast masses in males. Eur J Surg Oncol 14:317–320, 1988.

88. Gupta RK, Wakefield SJ, Holloway LJ, Simpson JS: Immunocytochemical and ultrastructural study of the rare osteoclast-type carcinoma of the breast in a fine needle aspirate. Acta Cytol 32:79–82, 1988.

89. Gupta RK, Wakefield SJ, Naran S, Dowle CC: Immunocytochemical and ultrastructural diagnosis of a rare mixed apocrine-medullary carcinoma of the breast in a fine needle aspirate. Acta Cytol 33:104–108, 1989.

90. Haagensen CD: Diseases of the Breast. Philadelphia, WB Saunders, 1986.

91. Haas JF: Pregnancy in association with a newly diagnosed cancer: A population based epidemiologic assessment. Int J Cancer 34:229, 1984.

92. Hahn P, Hallberg O, Schurer LB: Combination of clinical examination, mammography and aspiration cytology in the diagnosis of carcinoma of the breast (179 cases). Strahlenther Onkol 156:475–479, 1980.

93. Hajdu SI, Urban JA: Cancers metastatic to the breast. Cancer 29:1691–1696, 1972.

94. Hall FM: US-guided aspiration biopsy of the breast. Radiology 164:285–286, 1987.

95. Hammond S, Keyhani-Rofagha S, O'Toole RV: Statistical analysis of fine needle aspiration cytology of the breast. A review of 678 cases plus 4265 cases from the literature. Acta Cytol 31:276–280, 1987.

96. Hashimoto CH, Cobb CJ: Cytodiagnosis of hibernoma: A case report. Diagn Cytopathol 3:326–329, 1987.

97. Hedley DW, Rugg CA, Gelber RD: Association of DNA index and S-phase fraction with prognosis of nodes positive early breast cancer. Cancer Res 47:4729–4736, 1987.

98. Hermansen C, Poulsen HS, Jensen J, Langfeldt B, Steenskov V, Frederiksen P, Jensen OM: Diagnostic reliability of combined physical examination, mammography, and fine-needle puncture ("Triple-Test") in breast tumors. Cancer 60:1866–1871, 1987.

99. Hsiu J-G, Hawkins AG, D'Amato NA, Mullen JT: A case of pure primary squamous cell carcinoma of the breast diagnosed by fine needle aspiration biopsy. Acta Cytol 29:650–651, 1985.

100. Hutter RVP: Is "fibrocystic disease" of the breast precancerous? Arch Pathol Lab Med 110:171–173, 1986.

101. Huvos AG, Lucas JC, Foote FW: Metaplastic breast carcinoma. Rare form of mammary cancer. NY State J Med 12:550–561, 1973.

102. Ingram DL, Mossler JA, Snowhite J, Leight GS, McCarty KS Jr: Granular cell tumors of the breast. Steroid receptor analysis and localization of carcinoembryonic antigen, myoglobin, and S-100 protein. Arch Pathol Lab Med 108:897–901, 1984.

103. Jayaram G: Cytomorphology of tuberculous mastitis. A report of nine cases with fine needle aspiration cytology. Acta Cytol 29:974–978, 1985.

104. Jensen EV, Greene GL, DeSombre ER: The estrogen-receptor immunoassay in the prognosis and treatment of breast cancer. Lab Manag 24:25–42, 1986.

105. Johnson TL, Kini SR: Significance of bloody breast nipple discharge in men. American Society of Clinical Pathologists Check Sample, vol. 15, no. C-87-11 (C-173), 1987.

106. Kallioniemi O-P, Blanco G, Alavaikko M, Hietanen T, Mattila J, Lauslahti K, Lehtinen M, Koivula T: Improving the prognostic value of DNA flow cytometry in breast cancer by combining DNA index and S-phase fraction. A proposed classification of DNA histograms in breast cancer. Cancer 62:2183–2190, 1988.

107. Kaufman MW, Marti JR, Gallager HS, Hoehn JL: Carcinoma of the breast with pseudosarcomatous metaplasia. Cancer 53:1908–1917, 1984.

108. Kern WH: The diagnosis of breast cancer by fine needle aspiration smears. JAMA 241:1125–1127, 1979.

109. Keshgegian AA, Inverso K, Kline TS: Determination of estrogen receptor by monoclonal antireceptor antibody in aspiration biopsy cytology from breast carcinoma. Am J Clin Pathol 89:24–29, 1988.

110. Kim K, Goldblatt PJ: Malignant fibrous histiocytoma. Cytologic, light microscopic and ultrastructural studies. Acta Cytol 26:507–511, 1982.

111. Kim K, Naylor B, Han IH: Fine needle aspiration cytology of sarcomas metastatic to the lung. Acta Cytol 30:688–694, 1986.

112. Kindblom LG, Walaas L, Widehn S: Ultrastructural studies in the preoperative cytologic diagnosis of soft tissue tumors. Semin Diagn Pathol 3:317–344, 1986.

113. King EB, Chew KL, Duarte L, Hom JD, Mayall BH, Miller TR, Petrakis NL: Image cytometric classification of premalignant breast diseases in fine needle aspirates. Cancer 62:114–124, 1988.

114. Klein DL, Sickles EA: Effects of needle aspiration on the mammographic appearance of the breast: A guide to the proper timing of the mammography examination. Radiology 145:44, 1982.

115. Klemi PJ, Joensuu H: Comparison of DNA ploidy in routine fine needle aspiration biopsy samples and paraffin-embedded tissue samples. Anal Quant Cytol Histol 10:195–199, 1988.

116. Kline TS: Handbook of Fine Needle Aspiration Biopsy Cytology. St. Louis, CV Mosby, 1988.

117. Kline TS: Masquerades of malignancy: A review of 4241 aspirations from the breast. Acta Cytol 25:263–266, 1981.

118. Kline TS, Joshi LP, Neal HS: Fine needle aspiration of the breast: Diagnoses and pitfalls: A review of 3545 cases. Cancer 44:1458–1464, 1979.

119. Kline TS, Kannan V: Papillary carcinoma of the breast: A cytomorphologic analysis. Arch Pathol Lab Med 110:189–191, 1986.

120. Kline TS, Kannan V, Kline IK: Appraisal and cytomorphologic analysis of common carcinomas of the breast. Diagn Cytopathol:188–193, 1985.

121. Koss LG, Woyke J, Olszewski W: Aspiration Biopsy: Cytologic Interpretation and Histologic Bases. Tokyo, Igaku-Shoin, 1984.

122. Kreuzer G: Aspiration biopsy cytology in proliferating benign mammary dysplasia. Acta Cytol 22:128–132, 1978.

123. Kreuzer G, Zajicek J: Cytologic diagnosis of mammary tumors from aspiration biopsy smears. III. Studies on 200 carcinomas with false negative or doubtful cytologic reports. Acta Cytol 16:249–252, 1972.

124. Lampertico P, Stagni F: Cytology and hormonal receptors in breast cancer. Diagn Cytopathol 3:17–23, 1987.

125. Langham MR, Mills AS, Demay RM, O'Dowd JG, Grathwohl MA, Horsley JS: Malignant fibrous histiocytoma of the breast. Cancer 54:558–563, 1984.

126. Langmuir VK, Cramer SF, Hood ME: Fine needle aspiration cytology in the management of palpable benign and malignant breast disease: Correlation with clinical and mammographic findings. Acta Cytol 33:93–98, 1989.

127. Lannin DR, Silverman JF, Walker C, Pories WJ: Cost effectiveness of fine needle aspiration of the breast. Ann Surg 203:474–480, 1986.

128. Lee GF: Fine needle aspiration of the breast: The outpatient management of breast lesions. Am J Obstet Gynecol 156:1532–1537, 1987.

129. Lee KR, Foster RS, Papillo JL: Fine needle aspiration of the breast: importance of the aspirator. Acta Cytol 31:281–284, 1987.

130. Leiman G: Squamous carcinoma of the breast: Diagnosis by aspiration cytology. Acta Cytol 26:201–209, 1982.

131. Lew W, Seymour A: Primary amyloid tumor of the breast, case report and literature review. Acta Cytol 29:7–11, 1985.

132. Lindhohm K, Nordgren H, Akerman M: Electron microscopy of the needle aspiration biopsy from a malignant fibrous histiocytoma. Acta Cytol 23:399–401, 1979.

133. Linsk JA, Franzen S: Clinical Aspiration Cytology. Philadelphia, JB Lippincott, 1983.

134. Linsk J, Kreuzer G, Zajicek J: Cytologic diagnosis of mammary tumors from aspiration biopsy smears. II. Studies on 210 fibroadenomas and 210 cases of benign dysplasia. Acta Cytol 16:130–138, 1972.

135. Lofgren M, Andersson I, Bondeson L, Lindholm K: X-ray guided fine needle aspiration for the cytologic diagnosis of nonpalpable breast lesions. Cancer 61:1032–1037, 1988.

136. Lowhagen T, Rubio C: The cytology of the granular cell myoblastoma of the breast. Acta Cytol 21:314–345, 1977.

137. Lozowski MS, Mishriki Y, Chao S, Grimson R, Pai P, Harris

MA, Lundy J: Estrogen receptor determination in fine needle aspirates of the breast: Correlation with histologic grade and comparison with biochemical analysis. Acta Cytol 31:557–562, 1987.

138. The Ludwig Breast Cancer Study Group: Prolonged disease-free survival after one course of perioperative adjuvant chemotherapy for node-negative breast cancer. N Engl J Med 320:491–496, 1989.

139. Luzzatto R, Grossmann S, Scholl JG, Recktenvald M: Postradiation pleomorphic malignant fibrous histiocytoma of the breast. Acta Cytol 30:48–50, 1986.

140. McCarty KS Jr, Miller LS, Cox EB, Konrath J, McCarty KS Sr: Estrogen receptor analyses. Arch Pathol Lab Med 109:716–721, 1985.

141. McGuire WL: Adjuvant therapy of node-negative breast cancer (editorial). N Engl J Med 320:525–527, 1989.

142. Magdelenat H, Laine-Bidron C, Merle S, Zajdela A: Estrogen and progestin receptor assay in fine needle aspirates of breast cancer: Methodological aspects. Eur J Cancer Clin Oncol 23:425–431, 1987.

143. Malberger E, Gutterman E, Bartfeld E, Zajicek G: Cellular changes in the mammary gland epithelium during the menstrual cycle: A computer image analysis study. Acta Cytol 31:305–308, 1987.

144. Malberger E, Hazzani A, Lemberg S: Extramedullary hematopoiesis in breast aspirates. Acta Cytol 32:835–837, 1988.

145. Marchetti E, Bagni A, Querzoli P, Durante E, Marzola A, Fabris G, Nenci I: Immunocytochemical detection of estrogen receptors by staining with monoclonal antibodies on cytologic specimens of human breast cancer. Acta Cytol 32:829–834, 1988.

146. Martin HE, Ellis EB: Aspiration biopsy. Surg Gynecol Obstet 59:578–589, 1934.

147. Martin HE, Ellis EB: Biopsy by needle puncture and aspiration. Ann Surg 92:169–181, 1930.

148. Masin M, Masin F: Cytology of angiosarcoma of the breast. Acta Cytol 22:162–164, 1978.

149. Masood S: Use of monoclonal antibody for assessment of estrogen receptor content in fine-needle aspiration biopsy specimen from patients with breast cancer. Arch Pathol Lab Med 113:26–30, 1989.

150. Masood S, Johnson H: The value of imprint cytology in cytochemical detection of steroid hormone receptors in breast cancer. Am J Clin Pathol 87:30–36, 1987.

151. Mertens HH, Langnickel D, Staedtler F: Primary osteogenic sarcoma of the breast. Acta Cytol 26:512–515, 1982.

152. Mossler JA, Barton TK, Brinkhous AD, McCarty KS, Moylan JA, McCarty KS Jr: Apocrine differentiation in human mammary carcinoma. Cancer 46:2463–2471, 1980.

153. Mossler JA, McCarty KS, Johnston WW: The correlation of cytologic grade and steroid receptor content in effusions of metastatic breast carcinoma. Acta Cytol 25:653–658, 1981.

154. Mossler JA, McCarty KS, Woodard BH, Mitchener LM, Johnston WW: Correlation of mean nuclear area with estrogen receptor content in aspiration cytology of breast carcinoma. Acta Cytol 26:417–421, 1982.

155. Nagy GK, Jacobs JB, Mason-Savas A, Pomerantz SN, DeCiero GJ: Intracytoplasmic eosinophilic inclusion bodies in breast cyst fluid are giant lysosomes. Acta Cytol 33:99–103, 1989.

156. Naran S, Simpson J, Gupta RK: Cytologic diagnosis of papillary carcinoma of the breast in needle aspirates. Diagn Cytopathol 4:33–37, 1988.

157. Nguyen G-K, Neifer R: Aspiration biopsy cytology of secretory carcinoma of the breast. Diagn Cytopathol 3:234–237, 1987.

158. Nguyen G-K, Shnitka TK, Jewell LD: Aspiration biopsy cytology of mammary myoepithelioma. Diagn Cytopathol 3:335–338, 1987.

159. Nordenstrom B, Zajicek J: Stereotaxic needle biopsy and preoperative indication of nonpalpable mammary lesions. Acta Cytol 21:350–351, 1977.

160. Norris HG, Taylor HB: Relationship of histologic features to behavior of cystosarcoma phyllodes. Cancer 20:2090–2099, 1967.

161. Norton LW, Davis JR, Wiens JL, Trego DC, Dunnington GL: Accuracy of aspiration cytology in detecting breast cancer. Surgery 96:806–814, 1984.

162. Oberman HA: Invasive carcinoma of the breast with granulomatous response. Am J Clin Pathol 88:718–721, 1987.

163. Oertel YC, Galblum LI: Fine needle aspiration of the breast: Diagnostic criteria. Pathol Annu Part I, 375–407, 1983.

164. Page DL, Anderson TJ: Diagnostic Histopathology of the Breast. New York, Churchill Livingstone, 1987.

165. Palmer JO, McDivitt RW, Stone KR, Rudloff MA, Gonzalez JG: Flow cytometric analysis of breast needle aspirates. Cancer 62:2387–2391, 1988.

166. Palombini L, Fulciniti F, Vetrani A, De Rosa G, Di Benedetto G, Zeppa P, Troncone G: Fine needle aspiration biopsies of breast masses: A critical analysis of 1956 cases in 8 years (1976-1984). Cancer 61:2273–2277, 1988.

167. Palombini L, Fulciniti F, Vetrani A, Galligioni A, Montaguti A, Pennelli N: Mucoid carcinoma of the breast on fine needle aspiration biopsy sample: Cytology and ultrastructure. Appl Pathol 2:70–75, 1984.

168. Parl FF, Posey YF: Discrepancies of the biochemical and immunohistochemical estrogen receptor assays in breast cancer. Hum Pathol 19:960–966, 1988.

169. Pedio G, Landolt U, Zobeli L: Irradiated benign cells of the breast: A potential diagnostic pitfall in fine needle aspiration cytology. Acta Cytol 32:127–128, 1988.

170. Peterse JL, Koolman-Schellekens MA, van de Peppel-van de Ham T, van Heerde P: Atypia in fine needle aspiration cytology of the breast: A histologic follow-up study of 301 cases. Semin Diagn Pathol 6:126–134, 1989.

171. Pettinato G, Petrella G, Manco A, di Prisco B, Salvatore G, Angrisani P: Carcinoma of the breast with osteoclast-like giant cells: Fine needle aspiration cytology, histology and electron microscopy of 5 cases. Appl Pathol 2:168–178, 1984.

172. Pietruzka M, Barnes L: Cystosarcoma phyllodes. Cancer 41:1974–1983, 1979.

173. Reiner A, Reiner G, Spona J, Teleky B, Kolb R, Holzner JH: Estrogen receptor immunocytochemistry for preoperative determination of estrogen receptor status on fine needle aspirates of breast cancer. Am J Clin Pathol 88:399–404, 1987.

174. Reiner A, Spona J, Reiner G, Schemper M, Kolb R, Kwasny W, Fugger R, Jakesz R, Holzner JH: Estrogen receptor analysis on biopsies and fine needle aspirates from human breast carcinoma: Correlation of biochemical and immunohistochemical methods using monoclonal antireceptor antibodies. Am J Pathol 125:443–449, 1986.

175. Remvikos Y, Magdelenat H, Zajdela A: DNA flow cytometry applied to fine needle sampling of human breast cancer. Cancer 61:1629–1634, 1988.

176. Rosen P, Hajdu S, Robbins G, Foote FW: Diagnosis of carcinoma of the breast by aspiration biopsy. Surg Gynecol Obstet 134:837–838, 1972.

177. Rosen PP, Cantrell B, Mullen DL, DePalo A: Juvenile papillomatosis (Swiss-cheese disease). Am J Surg Pathol 4:3–12, 1980.

178. Russ JE, Winchester DP, Scanlon EF, Christ MA: Cytologic findings of aspiration of tumors of the breast. Surg Gynecol Obstet 146:407–411, 1978.

179. Schnitt SJ, Connolly JL, Harris JR, Cohen RB: Radiation-induced changes in the breast. Hum Pathol 16:545–550, 1984.

180. Schondorf H: Aspiration Cytology of the Breast. Translated by V Schneider. Philadelphia, WB Saunders, p 17, 1978.

181. Shabot M, Goldberg IM, Schick P, Nieberg R, Pilch YH: Aspiration cytology is superior to TruCut needle biopsy in establishing the diagnosis of clinically suspicious breast masses. Ann Surg 196:122–126, 1982.

182. Sickles E, Klein DL, Goodson WH, Hunt TK: Mammography after needle aspiration of palpable breast masses. Am J Surg 145:395–397, 1983.

183. Silfversward C, Humla S: Estrogen receptor analysis on needle aspirates from human mammary carcinoma. Acta Cytol 24:54–57, 1980.

184. Silverberg SG, Kay S, Chitale AR, Levitt SH: Colloid carcinoma of the breast. Am J Clin Pathol 55:355–363, 1971.

185. Silverman JF, Dabbs DJ, Gilbert CF: Adenosis tumor of the breast: Cytologic, histologic, immunocytochemical and ultrastructural observations. Acta Cytol 33:181–187, 1989.

186. Silverman JF, Dabbs DJ, Norris HT, Pories WJ, Legier J, Kay S: Localized primary (AL) amyloid tumor of the breast: Cy-

tologic, histologic, immunocytochemical and ultrastructural observations. Am J Surg Pathol 10:539–545, 1986.

187. Silverman JF, Feldman PS, Covell JL, Frable WJ: Fine needle aspiration cytology of neoplasms metastatic to the breast. Acta Cytol 31:291–300, 1987.

188. Silverman JF, Geisinger KR, Frable WJ: Fine needle aspiration cytology of mesenchymal tumors of the breast. Diagn Cytopathol 4:50–58, 1988.

189. Silverman JF, Lannin DR, Meelheim D, Pories WJ: Subareolar abscess of the breast: The role of fine needle biopsy in the diagnosis and management. Contemp Surg 28:45–48, 1986.

190. Silverman JF, Lannin DR, O'Brien K, Norris HT: The triage role of fine needle aspiration biopsy of palpable breast masses: Diagnostic accuracy and cost effectiveness. Acta Cytol 31:731–736, 1987.

191. Silverman JF, Lannin DR, Unverferth M, Norris HT: Fine needle aspiration cytology of subareolar abscess of the breast: Spectrum of cytomorphologic findings and potential diagnostic pitfalls. Acta Cytol 30:413–419, 1986.

192. Simi U, Moretti D, Iacconi P, Arganini M, Roncella M, Miccoli P, Giacomini G: Fine needle aspiration cytopathology of phyllodes tumor: Differential diagnosis with fibroadenoma. Acta Cytol 32:63–66, 1988.

193. Skoog L: Aspiration cytology of a male breast carcinoma with argyrophilic cells. Acta Cytol 31:379–381, 1987.

194. Smallwood J, Herbert A, Guyer P, Taylor I: Accuracy of aspiration cytology in the diagnosis of breast disease. Br J Surg 72:841–843, 1985.

195. Spyratos F, Briffod M, Gentile A, Brunet M, Brault C, Desplaces A: Flow cytometric study of DNA distribution in cytopunctures of benign and malignant breast lesions. Analyt Quant Cytol 9:485–494, 1987.

196. Squires E, Betsill W: Intracystic carcinoma of the breast: A correlation of cytomorphology, gross pathology, microscopic pathology and clinical data. Acta Cytol 25:267–271, 1981.

197. Stanley MW, Tani EM, Horwitz CA, Tulman S, Skoog L: Primary spindle cell sarcomas of the breast: Diagnosis by fine needle aspiration. Diagn Cytopathol 4:244–249, 1988.

198. Stawicki M, Hsiu J: Malignant cystosarcoma phyllodes. Acta Cytol 23:61–64, 1979.

199. Stenkvist B, Bengtsson E, Eriksson O, Jarkrans T, Nordin B: Image cytometry in malignancy grading of breast cancer: Results in a prospective study with seven years of follow-up. Analyt Quant Cytol 8:293–300, 1986.

200. Stewart FW: The diagnosis of tumors by aspiration. Am J Pathol 9:801–812, 1933.

201. Stormby N, Bondeson L: Adenoma of the nipple. Acta Cytol 28:729–732, 1984.

202. Strawbridge HTG, Bassett AA, Foldes I: Role of cytology in management of lesions of the breast. Surg Gynecol Obstet 152:1–7, 1981.

203. Sugano I, Nagao K, Kondo Y, Nabeshima S, Murakami S: Cytologic and ultrastructural studies of a rare breast carcinoma with osteoclast-like giant cells. Cancer 52:74–78, 1983.

204. Svane G: Stereotaxic fine needle biopsy of nonpalpable breast lesions performed by the mammotest. Recent Results Cancer Res 105:95–96, 1987.

205. Svane G, Silfversward C: Stereotaxic needle biopsy of nonpalpable breast lesions: Cytologic and histopathologic findings. Acta Radiol Diagn 24:283–288, 1983.

206. Takeda T, Suzuki M, Sato Y, Hase T, Yamada S: Aspiration cytology of breast cysts. Acta Cytol 26:37–43, 1982.

207. Tani EM, Skoog L: Immunocytochemical detection of estrogen receptors in mammary Paget cells. Acta Cytol 32:825–828, 1988.

208. Tani EM, Stanley MW, Skoog L: Fine needle aspiration cytology presentation of bilateral mammary fibromatosis: Report of a case. Acta Cytol 32:555–558, 1988.

209. Thomas JM, Fitzharris BM, Redding WH, Williams JE, Trott PA, Powles TJ, Ford HT, Gazet JC: Clinical examination, xeromammography, and fine needle aspiration cytology in diagnosis of breast tumours. Br Med J 2:1139–1141, 1978.

210. Torres V, Ferrer R: Cytology of fine needle aspiration biopsy of primary breast rhabdomyosarcoma in an adolescent girl. Acta Cytol 29:430–434, 1985.

211. Tsuchiya S, Maruyama Y, Koike Y, Yamada K, Kobayashi Y, Kagaya A: Cytologic characteristics and origin of naked nuclei in breast aspirate smears. Acta Cytol 31:285–290, 1987.

212. Ulanow R, Galblum L, Canter JW: Fine needle aspiration in the diagnosis and management of solid breast lesions. Am J Surg 148:653–657, 1984.

213. Uyterlinde AM, Schipper NW, Baak JPA, Peterse H, Matze E: Limited prognostic value of cellular DNA content to classical and morphometrical parameters in invasive ductal breast cancer. Am J Clin Pathol 89:301–307, 1988.

214. Vogel CL, East DR, Voigt W, Thomsen S: Response to tamoxifen in estrogen receptor-poor metastatic breast cancer. Cancer 60:1184–1189, 1987.

215. Walaas L, Angervall L, Hagmar B, Save-Soderbergh J: A correlative cytologic and histologic study of malignant fibrous histiocytoma: An analysis of 40 cases examined by fine needle aspiration cytology. Diagn Cytopathol 2:46–54, 1986.

216. Wall RW, Glant MD: The cytomorphology of mucinous carcinoma of the breast by fine-needle aspiration. American Society of Clinical Pathologists Check Sample vol. 15, no. C-87-12 (C-174), 1987.

217. Wanebo HJ, Feldman PS, Wilnelm MC, Covell JL, Binns RL: Fine needle aspiration cytology in lieu of open biopsy in management of primary breast cancer. Ann Surg 199:569–579, 1984.

218. Weintraub J, Weintraub D, Redard M, Vassilakos P: Evaluation of estrogen receptors by immunocytochemistry on fine needle aspiration biopsy specimens from breast tumors. Cancer 60:1163–1172, 1987.

219. Whitlatch SP, Panke TW: Myoepithelial cells in needle aspirations of two cases of unusual breast lesions: An aid in differential diagnosis. Diagn Cytopathol 2:77–81, 1987.

220. Young GP, Somers RG, Young K, Kaplan M, Cowan DF: Experience with a modified fine needle aspiration biopsy technique in 533 breast cases. Diagn Cytopathol 2:91–98, 1986.

221. Zajdela A, De LaRiva LS, Ghossein NA: The relation of prognosis to the nuclear diameter of breast cancer cells obtained by cytologic aspirations. Acta Cytol 23:75–80, 1979.

222. Zajdela A, Ghossein NA, Pilleron JP, Ennuyer A: The value of aspiration cytology in the diagnosis of breast cancer: Experience at the Foundation Curie. Cancer 35:499–506, 1975.

223. Zajdela A, Zillhardt P, Voillemot N: Cytological diagnosis by fine needle sampling without aspiration. Cancer 59:1201–1205, 1987.

224. Zajicek J: Aspiration Biopsy Cytology. Part II. Cytology of Infradiaphragmatic Organs. Monographs in Clinical Cytology, vol. 7, New York, S Karger, 1974.

225. Zajicek J: Aspiration Biopsy Cytology. Part I. Monographs in Clinical Cytology, vol. 4. New York, S Karger, 1974.

226. Zajicek J, Caspersson T, Jakobsson P, Linsk J, Us-Krasovec M: Cytologic diagnosis of mammary tumors from aspiration biopsy smears. Comparison of cytologic and histologic findings in 2111 lesions and diagnostic use of cytophotometry. Acta Cytol 14:370–376, 1970.

227. Zajicek J, Franzen S, Jakobsson P, Robio C, Unsgaard B: Aspiration biopsy of mammary tumors in diagnosis and research: A critical review of 2200 cases. Acta Cytol 11:169–175, 1967.

228. Zuska JJ, Crile G Jr, Ayres WW: Fistulas of lactiferous ducts. Am J Surg 81:312–317, 1951.

28

Kidney, Adrenal and Retroperitoneum

Ruth L. Katz

KIDNEY

In 1946, Lindblom,[68] a Swedish radiologist, described percutaneous puncture of renal cysts and tumors. Subsequently, during the 1950s, beginning in the Scandinavian countries, the increasing use of fine needle aspiration (FNA) of mass lesions in the kidneys, adrenals and retroperitoneum paralleled the technologic advances in imaging techniques, particularly ultrasound and computed tomography (CT). Because these techniques in themselves have a high degree of diagnostic accuracy and additionally can be used for staging, the inclusion of FNA in the diagnostic triage must be justified by a high degree of accuracy, few complications and low additional cost.[8] The ability of FNA to render an accurate pathologic diagnosis of a primary tumor has assumed increasing significance in the treatment of renal neoplasms owing to the advent of therapies such as intra-arterial embolization, biologic response modification and preoperative radiation and chemotherapy. The main indications for performing FNA of the kidney are for the pathologic identification of a mass lesion, nonsurgical confirmation of advanced neoplasia, confirmation of metastases, staging of tumors and, in some cases, therapeutic aspiration of cystic lesions. More recently, FNA has been used for monitoring the outcome of renal transplantation, obtaining tumorous tissue for ancillary techniques to aid in diagnosis, such as immunocytochemistry and ultrastructural studies, and grading tumors using morphometric and flow cytometric methods.[73]

Imaging Techniques

Procurement of renal tissue for cytology has been performed using intravenous pyelography, selective renal angiography and fluoroscopy and following excretory urography.[53] More recently ultrasonically guided FNA[50] has become the preferred method because it permits the point of entry, angle of incident path and depth of the needle to be defined in absolute terms.[49] The lesion is located with ultrasound and its position relative to surface landmarks memorized. CT can also be used and has the advantage of being able to localize accurately small lesions by verifying the position of the needle tip in a lesion, but it lacks the speed and greater scanning flexibility of ultrasound. FNA is performed following local anesthesia, with the patient in a prone or decubitus position, using a guiding needle with a stylet, 20-gauge spinal needle or 22-gauge Chiba needle. For more details concerning the techniques, see Chapter 23, Imaging Techniques. Immediate cytologic assessment of specimen adequacy is desirable and may require the performance of multiple passes until an adequate specimen has been procured. The contents of the needle and syringe are rinsed into a tissue culture solution (RPMI 1640) if tissue should be required for immunocytochemistry, cell block analysis or flow cytometry. It is our practice to make cell blocks on all FNA specimens, tissue permitting. For ultrastructural studies, the needle is rinsed directly into glutaraldehyde.

Complications of FNA are extremely rare and range from 0 to 4%,[64, 85] in comparison with a reported incidence of serious surgical complications of 1.6 to 8% in patients undergoing open renal biopsy.[60] Occasionally, abscess formation following therapeutic cyst aspiration[71] or bleeding following aspiration[88] has been reported. Needle tract seeding is extremely rare to nonexistent.[54] Other complications from renal aspiration may include arteriovenous fistula, bile peritonitis, colon perforation with abscess and urinoma.[60]

Anatomy and Histology

In the adult, the paired kidneys, located on either side of the great vessels and overlying the lower thoracic and upper lumbar vertebrae (T12 to L3),

771

measure up to 13 cm in length and have an average weight of 150 to 160 g. They are surrounded by perirenal adipose tissue and lie within Gerota's fascia. The left kidney is bounded anteriorly by the pancreas, left adrenal, stomach, splenic flexure of the colon, jejunum and posteroinferior border of the spleen. The right kidney's anterior relationships are with the right adrenal, posterior surface of the liver and hepatic flexure of the colon. Knowledge of the anatomic relationships of the kidneys with other organs is essential for the interpretation of percutaneous renal aspirations because the trajectory of the needle tip may result in the procurement of parenchymal cells from these organs.

The kidney is composed of the cortex and the medulla. The medulla comprises eight to 18 renal pyramids, or lobes, which contain radial striations caused by the straight part of the collecting ducts or uriniferous tubules and their accompanying blood vessels. The uriniferous tubules converge onto the apex, or papilla, of a minor calix that is continuous with one of two or more major calices of the renal pelvis, which continues distally as the ureter. The glandular portion of the kidney resides within the cortex and is composed of a secretory portion, or nephron (derived from metanephrogenic blastema), that unites with the excretory duct system (derived from the wolffian duct). The nephron begins at the renal corpuscle with Bowman's capsule and is continuous with the proximal convoluted tubule, the descending and ascending loops of Henle and the distal convoluted tubule. The renal corpuscle comprises the glomerulus, a tuft of blood capillaries supplied by an afferent and an efferent arteriole that invaginates and invests itself of the inner (visceral) layer of Bowman's capsule. The visceral epithelial cells adhere closely to the endothelial cells and on ultrastructural analysis demonstrate fine processes or pedicels that project onto the basement membrane separating the endothelial cells from the epithelial cells. The outer parietal layer of Bowman's capsule is continuous with the proximal convoluted tubule, whose epithelium consists of a single layer of cells with abundant eosinophilic cytoplasm, a large nucleus and a microvillous brush border. The descending (thin) loop of Henle is lined by pale, flat squamous epithelium, whereas the epithelium lining the ascending limb is cuboid and stains more darkly. The epithelium of the distal convolution is lower, stains less intensely with hematoxylin and eosin and contains more cells on cross section than the proximal convoluted tubule. Microvilli can be seen by electron microscopy on the luminal surface. The cells of the collecting ducts are cuboid and well defined, with a dark nucleus and clear cytoplasm. The cells of the larger collecting ducts are tall and columnar.

Cytology of the Normal Kidney

Normal renal parenchymal components, which usually derive from the renal cortex (Fig. 28–1), may be aspirated during FNA of the kidney. Occasionally,

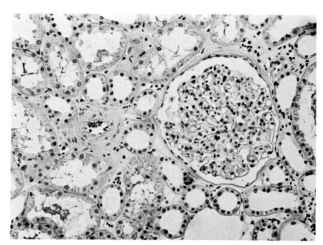

FIGURE 28–1. Normal renal cortex showing a glomerulus, proximal convoluted tubules with ill-defined granular cytoplasm and distal convoluted tubules with well-defined cuboidal cells with conspicious nuclei (hematoxylin and eosin; ×110).

glomeruli may be aspirated. These are large, sharply demarcated, multilayered clusters of epithelial and endothelial cells, which may be continuous with a short segment of proximal convoluted tubule (Fig. 28–2). The proximal convoluted tubules compose most of the substance of the renal cortex and have abundant granular but ill-defined eosinophilic cytoplasm and large, oval nuclei.[6, 82] At high power (×400), careful examination may reveal small, inconspicuous nucleoli (Fig. 28–3). Unlike their histologic counterpart, brush borders cannot be seen in cytologic smears. The cells of Henle's loop and the distal convoluted tubules are much smaller than cells from the proximal tubules. Distal convoluted tubules may be removed intact, appearing as multilayered tubules or cast-like structures (Fig. 28–4). Distal convoluted tubular epithelium is flatter, with more numerous and conspicuous nuclei

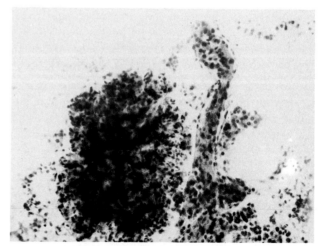

FIGURE 28–2. Cytology of kidney in fine needle aspirate showing a **normal renal glomerulus** continuous with a proximal convoluted tubule and loop of Henle (Papanicolaou stain; ×110).

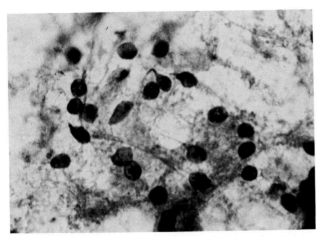

FIGURE 28–3. High power view of aspirate of **normal proximal convoluted tubular cells** showing uniform round nuclei, inconspicuous nucleoli and abundant ill-defined granular cytoplasm. This appearance may be confused with well-differentiated renal cell carcinoma (nuclear grade I) (Papanicolaou stain; ×265).

than the cells of the proximal tubules. Dark cytoplasmic granules may be demonstrated on Romanowsky stains in cells, most probably derived from the ascending loop of Henle or distal convoluted tubules. The cells of the collecting tubules of the medulla are cuboid and sharply defined.

Renal Cysts

Cysts of the kidney are among the most common mass lesions to be aspirated, their incidence, in three large consecutive FNA series, ranging in frequency from 15 to 43%.[23, 96, 117]

Renal cysts may be congenital or acquired, the former resulting from disordered embryogenesis involving cystic enlargement at various sites of the renal tubular system.[90] The diagnosis of congenital cysts rests largely on evidence of genetic transmission, age of the patient, associated congenital abnormalities and the gross and microscopic features of the renal cysts.[94]

Congenital Cysts

Polycystic disease of the kidney may be of the infantile or adult type, both being inherited forms of cystic disease, usually involving both kidneys. Numerous thin-walled unilocular cysts of various sizes lined by flattened epithelial cells involve the renal parenchyma and contain clear fluid. The adult form is usually clinically silent until the 4th decade of life, when the patient may present with gradual onset of renal failure. Occasionally, the disorder may be manifested clinically as lithiasis, flank pain caused by bleeding into a cyst or ureteral obstruction caused by a blood clot.

FNA results in variable amounts of clear or pale amber fluid, containing a few foamy macrophages.

Acquired or Simple Cysts

Most simple cysts are clinically insignificant; they are discovered incidentally during the course of radiologic studies such as intravenous urograms for unrelated urologic symptoms.[106] Because these lesions are amenable to conservative therapy and may not be accurately diagnosed radiologically, FNA has been advocated for all renal masses thought to be renal cysts. They are commonly located subcapsularly, may be multiple and may be several centimeters or more in size. Histologically, they are lined by a flat epithelium overlying a thin fibrous wall[94] and contain fluid that is usually clear and amber colored, consistent with a transudate. Cytologic examination of the fluid usually reveals a few benign cuboid cells and an occasional neutrophil (Fig. 28–5).[106] Fragments of degenerated epithelial cells should not be mistaken for carcinoma. Rarely, simple cysts are discolored or grossly bloody,

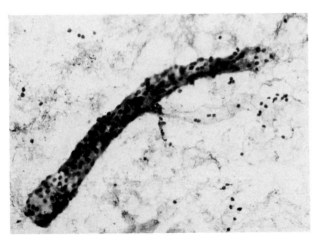

FIGURE 28–4. **Cells of the distal convoluted tubule,** aspirate of normal kidney, shows a multilayered tubular structure with numerous nuclei (Papanicolaou stain; ×110).

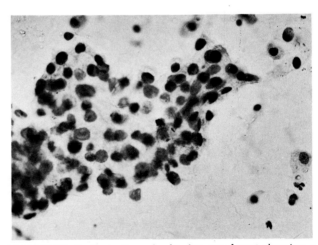

FIGURE 28–5. Aspiration of a **benign renal cyst** showing a fragment of degenerated epithelial cells in a background of cyst fluid containing neutrophils and histiocytes (Papanicolaou stain; ×265).

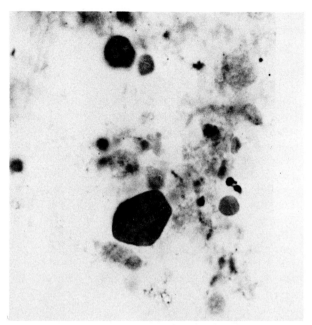

FIGURE 28–6. Aspirate of a **hemorrhagic renal cyst** containing Liesegang-like structures that contain radial striations (Papanicolaou stain; ×650). (Courtesy of Dr. Nour Sneige, MD Anderson Cancer Center, Houston, Texas.)

in which case hemosiderin-laden macrophages may be seen in addition.

Very rarely, rings resembling parasitic ova and characterized as Liesegang structures have been encountered in FNAs of renal hemorrhagic cysts (Fig. 28–6).[111] Numerous spheric double-walled structures with radial striations ranging in size from 8 to 200 μ may be encountered. It is most important from a therapeutic standpoint to differentiate these structures from kidney parasites such as *Dioctophyma renale*, which they may simulate. Unlike *D. renale*, Liesegang structures are cytokeratin negative and are seen to have a fibrillary composition on ultrastructural analysis.

Association of Renal Malignancy with Renal Cysts

The coexistence of a cyst and carcinoma in the same kidney has been reported in approximately 2.3 to 7% of surgically explored renal cysts.[59] Four possible associations of a renal tumor and a cyst within the same kidney have been proposed:[36] (1) The two lesions are widely separated and unrelated in origin. (2) The cyst originates within the tumor. (3) The tumor originates within the cyst. (4) The cyst occurs distal to the tumor. The most commonly observed interrelationship is that of a cyst arising within a tumor secondary to tumor necrosis.

The majority of renal cysts can be treated conservatively by percutaneous renal puncture with avoidance of surgical intervention, provided that the criteria for the diagnosis of a benign cyst are fulfilled, namely that (1) clear, straw-colored fluid is aspirated, (2) there are

no biochemical anomalies, (3) no cytologically atypical cells are aspirated and (4) a regular, smooth cyst cavity (as demonstrated on a double-contrast cystogram) is perfectly superimposable on the space-occupying lesion.[115]

An extraordinarily high incidence of papillary renal neoplasms associated with acquired cysts in renal dialysis patients has been reported.[29] Malignancy is to be strongly suspected in cysts that contain bloody fluid, with an incidence of 30% of carcinomas being reported in a series of hemorrhagic renal cysts.[134] Renal cell carcinomas (RCCs) have also been associated with the presence of clear cyst fluid.[59] Because of the potentially disastrous results of inaccurately differentiating between these two lesions by radiology, FNA, followed by cytologic examination of cyst contents, is recommended.

Inflammatory Disorders of the Kidney

Xanthogranulomatous Pyelonephritis

Xanthogranulomatous pyelonephritis (XPN) is an uncommon chronic inflammatory kidney disease associated with recurrent urinary tract infections, flank pain and a nonfunctioning renal mass or kidney on intravenous pyelography that may mimic a carcinoma.[70] Frequently there may be an associated renal calculus.

Clinically, patients present with symptoms related to renal pain, hematuria, a flank mass or recurrent urinary tract infections with the most common organisms cultured being *Escherichia coli, Pseudomonas* and *Proteus*.[105]

Xanthogranulomatous pyelonephritis may be difficult to distinguish from a hypovascular renal tumor by intravenous pyelogram or arteriography. Plain abdominal films may reveal renal enlargement and staghorn calculi, a retrograde pyelogram may show hydronephrosis or staghorn calculi and a partially or totally nonfunctioning kidney may be demonstrated by renal scans. Sease and coworkers[105] described four patients with XPN who had characteristic ultrasound findings supportive of abscess formation, with FNA findings supportive of XPN. A preoperative diagnosis of XPN can spare the patient a radical nephrectomy; a partial nephrectomy may be the procedure of choice if there is only focal involvement of the kidney. There have been two reports of erroneous preoperative FNA diagnosis of "clear cell carcinoma" and "hypernephroma" in two patients with XPN.[65] Histologically, there may be focal or diffuse replacement of renal parenchyma by sheets of histiocytes with foamy or granular or eosinophilic cytoplasm and small, regular nuclei that may mimic renal adenocarcinoma.[12] Necrosis, multinucleated cells, cholesterol clefts and lymphocytes are commonly seen.

Cytology. Very few cytologic descriptions of XPN exist. Zajicek[135] described the FNA appearance of XPN as an inflammatory process, composed of a proliferation of histiocytes with a lymphocytic infiltrate and areas of necrosis. Nguyen[82] described the presence of single histiocytes and clusters of histiocytes and multinucleated macrophages.

Clusters of histiocytes may be confused with RCC.

Abscesses of the Kidney

Both intrarenal and perinephric abscesses can be accurately localized and aspirated under ultrasound guidance. At the time of aspiration, if turbid fluid or pus is aspirated, a Gram stain on the smears and cultures for microbacteriology are obtained. In the majority of cases, gram-negative organisms are isolated. In many instances, surgery can be avoided and percutaneous drainage may be all the treatment that is required.[64]

Cytology. The smears are characterized by an abundant acute inflammatory exudate. The results of cytology, Gram stain and bacteriology can rapidly confirm the presence of an abscess so that appropriate antibiotic therapy can be instituted.

Tumors of the Kidney

The incidence of primary malignancies of the kidney is relatively low, composing only 1.5% of all human cancers, with the ratio of renal parenchymal to renal pelvic tumors being 4:1. In the adult age group, in order of decreasing frequency, the most common renal neoplasms are renal adenocarcinomas (80 to 90%), followed by urothelial malignancies of the renal pelvis, renal sarcomas, adult Wilms' tumor and sarcomatoid RCCs (carcinosarcomas).[94] In children, renal malignancy is most commonly due to Wilms' tumor, with malignant rhabdoid tumor and clear cell sarcoma of the kidney together accounting for about 6% of pediatric renal tumors.

Classification of Renal Tumors

Renal parenchymal tumors may be broadly classified as being derived from the proximal convoluted tubule, metanephric blastema or mesenchymal structures. Renal pelvic tumors are either epithelial or mesenchymal in derivation.

Awareness of the radiologic appearance of a tumor is vital in the interpretation of renal FNAs because most tumors will display characteristic radiographic features.

RCC is most frequently detected initially by intravenous urography, on which it is characterized as a mass with decreased or heterogeneous staining quality, the latter often being caused by cystic degeneration or necrosis within the tumor.[64] Approximately 75% of RCCs are hypervascular and display characteristic arteriographic features that permit the diagnosis of RCC with a high degree of confidence.[64] The 25% of RCCs that are hypovascular may be attributed to those tumors that are extensively cystic or necrotic, arise within a cyst or demonstrate a predominantly papillary architecture (papillary RCC).[64] The differential diagnosis of a hypovascular renal mass also includes benign renal cysts, abscesses, oncocytoma, transitional cell carcinoma (TCC) of the renal pelvis, renal lymphoma, XPN, sarcomatoid RCC and metastatic renal neoplasms. Renal oncocytomas are well-encapsulated, hypovascular masses, with a distinctive arrangement of internal vessels in a pattern like the spokes of a wheel.[64] Angiomyolipomas may be differentiated by CT and ultrasound on the basis of their fat content; however, they are generally hypervascular and sharply demarcated from the uninvolved kidney.

Benign Renal Tumors

Benign mesenchymal tumors such as leiomyomas, fibromas, lipomas, hemangiomas and lymphangiomas are found at autopsy in the kidneys of 8 to 11% of patients.[12] These are usually asymptomatic and rarely diagnosed during the patient's lifetime.

Angiomyolipoma. Angiomyolipomas are fairly uncommon benign tumors that are composed of a mixture of mature tissue components comprising mature adipose tissue, tortuous, thick-walled blood vessels and fascicles of smooth muscle (Fig. 28–7). They are generally regarded as hamartomas or benign mesenchymomas.[94] Although there is a strong association of angiomyolipomas occurring in patients with tuberous sclerosis, less than 40% of patients with angiomyolipomas demonstrate features of the tuberous sclerosis complex (cutaneous lesions, retinal phakomas, angiomas and cerebellar neoplasm).[12] Patients with tuberous sclerosis may have multiple small and bilateral angiomyolipomas. Patients who present with solitary tumors are frequently younger women who show no stigmata of tuberous sclerosis. The presenting symptom is usually flank or abdominal pain or a palpable mass.[12] The tumors are generally large, with a mean diameter of 9.4 cm.[99] Despite their characteristic radiologic appearance on CT and ultrasound, they may be confused preoperatively with RCC on intravenous urogram.

Cytology. The leiomyomatous component is composed of single cells and clusters of mesenchymal-like cells that may vary in size and shape[82, 83] but are usually small, with ample but indistinct delicate cytoplasm (see Fig. 28–7B).[121] The overlapping nuclei may appear to form syncytial groups because cell borders may not be visible. Nuclear chromatin may vary from finely to coarsely granular. Some cells may show prominent nucleoli. The vascular component is characterized by thick-walled blood vessels lined by endothelial cells.[38] This component may not be seen on cytology but may be demonstrated in cell block preparations (see Fig. 28–7A). The fatty component is composed of mature adipose tissue, which may be abundant. Areas of fat necrosis with histiocytes and multinucleated giant cells may be found.

The pitfalls in diagnosis are as follows:

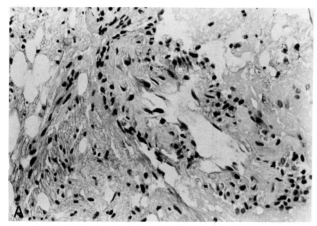

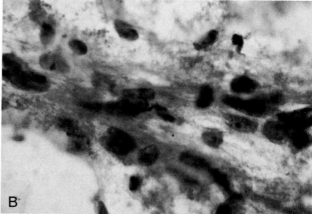

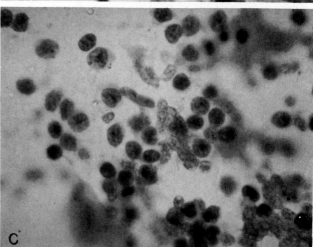

FIGURE 28–7. *A,* Cell block from a fine needle aspiration of a **renal angiomyolipoma** showing mature adipose tissue, thick-walled blood vessels and smooth muscle (hematoxylin and eosin; ×265). *B,* Syncytial sheets of smooth muscle cells representing the **leiomyosarcomatous component of angiomyolipoma.** Note the ill-defined cytoplasm and the somewhat atypical nuclear features (Papanicolaou stain; ×425). *C,* Example of an **angiomyolipoma,** which showed areas of hypercellularity composed of predominantly round cells (Papanicolaou stain; ×425). (Figures 28–7B and 28–7C courtesy of Dr. L. Tao, University of Indiana.)

1. The pleomorphic mesenchymal or smooth muscle cells of angiomyolipoma may be so atypical that they are confused with the sarcoma or sarcomatoid component of sarcomatoid RCC.[82, 94]

2. An atypical pattern may be seen in which highly cellular areas have a predominantly round cell pattern that may be confused with a granular cell RCC (see Fig. 28–7C).[87]

Renal Adenoma. Well-differentiated cortical glandular tumors, less than 3 cm in diameter, have been termed adenomas[10] and have a very low propensity to metastasize. Most of the tumors are found incidentally at autopsy. These lesions are best imaged with CT. Because of their derivation from the proximal tubule and their morphologic similarity to RCC, most authors now accept the view that these are, in fact, small RCCs with a low risk for metastases.[11]

Cytology. Reports on the cytologic appearance of these tumors are rare[5]; however, because the tumor is indistinguishable from well-differentiated RCC by histology, it follows that the cytologic appearance is identical to that of well-differentiated RCC.

Oncocytoma. These tumors are composed of oncocytes, which are large epithelial cells with abundant eosinophilic cytoplasm. Oncocytomas were originally described by Hamperl[43, 44] in the salivary gland in 1931 and were previously recognized in the thyroid and

parathyroid. They were only recently recognized in the kidney when Klein and Valensi[61] reported on 14 patients with oncocytic tumors and emphasized their benign behavior. These tumors are regarded as variants of renal adenomas, derived from proximal convoluted tubular cells, and in spite of attaining a large size, they generally show no tendency to invade or metastasize. The reported average incidence is 5% of all renal neoplasms; they occur predominantly in men, with a peak incidence in the 6th to 8th decades.[94]

The gross features of this neoplasm are quite characteristic; they include a well-demarcated, well-encapsulated tumor that is a mahogany or reddish brown color on the cut surface. The tumors range in size from several millimeters to 25 cm in diameter, with a median diameter of 8 cm. There is often a central fibrous scar (Fig. 28–8). Tumors are usually solitary; however, they may be bilateral or multicentric.

The tumor may be composed of nests or cords of oncocytic cells separated by edematous stroma. Typical cells are polygonal, with round to oval, hyperchromatic nuclei and minimal pleomorphism.[94] Binucleated cells may frequently be seen (Fig. 28–9). Lieber and colleagues[67] described six cases that metastasized and led to the ultimate demise of the patients. These tumors were characterized by nuclei that showed greater nuclear pleomorphism than in the usual oncocytoma.

Cytology. There is a monotonous population of

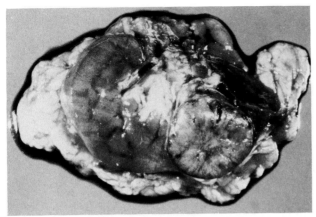

FIGURE 28–8. Gross appearance of an **oncocytoma** characterized by a well-encapsulated reddish-brown tumor with a central fibrous scar.

polygonal single cells or small clusters of cells with defined cell borders and abundant eosinophilic cytoplasm. Nuclei are round to oval, single or multiple and hyperchromatic or so clumped that they appear pyknotic (Fig. 28–10).

Oncocytoma may be confused with well-differentiated granular cell RCC.

Renal Cell Carcinoma

RCC occurs more commonly in men than in women with the peak age at presentation being in the 6th decade. It is predominantly a disease of adults, with few cases being reported in children or adolescents under the age of 20.[94]

Like renal adenoma and oncocytoma, RCC derives from the proximal convoluted tubule, as evidenced ultrastructurally by the demonstration of a number of common characteristics, including a microvillus brush border and numerous elongated and unusually configured mitochondria.[11]

The most common clinical presentation of RCC is

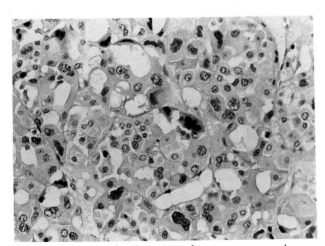

FIGURE 28–9. Histologic section of an **oncocytoma** demonstrating single nuclei and multiple hyperchromatic and pyknotic nuclei (hematoxylin and eosin; ×265).

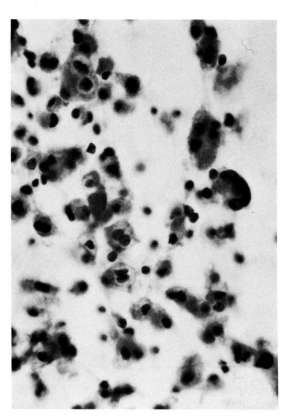

FIGURE 28–10. Aspirate from an **oncocytoma** showing similar cytologic features as the histology. Note that some nuclei may be densely hyperchromatic (Papanicolaou stain; ×265).

hematuria, followed by flank pain and a palpable mass. Up to 25% of RCCs may be asymptomatic,[94] with discovery of the tumor being incidental to a routine physical examination and unrelated radiologic study. Fever, anemia or a high erythrocyte sedimentation rate or symptoms related to metastases, most frequently involving the lungs, bones or central nervous system, may result in the detection of a hitherto undiagnosed primary RCC.

The average size of RCC at nephrectomy is 7.6 cm,[11] with the majority of resected tumors measuring 3.1 to 8 cm.[33] Tumors less than 3 cm in diameter rarely metastasize, and if well differentiated, encapsulated and devoid of hemorrhage and necrosis, have been termed adenomas.[10, 61] There is much controversy, however, regarding this terminology because these tumors are histogenetically and morphologically identical to RCC (see section on renal adenoma). At the MD Anderson Cancer Center the term "adenoma" is not used for any clinically detected lesion, regardless of the size. The majority of RCCs are of an intermediate size (>3 cm and <8 cm) category in which prognosis on the basis of size cannot be predicted.[33]

Staging of RCC based on the extent of disease spread is widely adopted and prognostically significant. In 1969, Robson proposed a staging protocol that is widely accepted.[94] Although Stage I tumors (tumor confined to the kidney) account for 40% of total cases, 25% of patients have distant metastases (Stage IV) at initial presentation, and approximately one third of patients present with regional spread of tumor (Stages II and III).[94]

Histology. At least four different cell types have been described by histology: a clear cell, a granular cell, an intermediate cell (possessing features intermediate between the clear and the granular cells) and an oncocytic cell. RCCs are composed either exclusively of one of these types of cells or of a mixture of these types of cells. The ultrastructural appearance of the cell types demonstrates the clear cells of RCC to have abundant lipid droplets and particulate glycogen and few organelles.[119] Loss of lipid and glycogen occurs during processing, imparting a "plant-like, water clear" appearance.[11] The granular cells contain numerous mitochondria, developed Golgi apparatus, endoplasmic reticulum and only small amounts of lipid and glycogen; hence, their granular eosinophilic cytoplasmic appearance. Oncocytes contain such tightly packed mitochondria and cell organelles that their granularity becomes obscured, so that by light microscopy their cytoplasm appears homogeneously dark and dense.

A number of architectural patterns have been described, most notably tubular, acinar, alveolar, papillary, tubulocystic, solid and mixed. With the exception of the papillary-cystic variety, which is reported to be associated with a less aggressive course,[74] there appears to be no prognostic information associated with pattern.[94]

Grading of RCC. Various histologic grading systems have been proposed based on a combination of nuclear, cytoplasmic and architectural features.[110, 127] A nuclear grading system based on four nuclear grades defined in order of increasing nuclear size, irregularity and nucleolar prominence, proposed by Fuhrman and coworkers,[33] showed that nuclear grade was more effective than tumor size, cell type and cell arrangement in predicting development of metastases following nephrectomy. The importance of nuclear grade in predicting survival has been corroborated by DNA flow cytometry studies comparing ploidy with both survival and nuclear grade. Ploidy has been shown to be a significant predictor of outcome.[41] A significant association between nuclear grade and nuclear DNA content has been reported, the degree of ploidy being felt to be a reflection of the nuclear grade in most instances. Nuclear grading based on the highest nuclear grade (most malignant), even if focal, has been shown to be an independent prognostic variable and may be substituted for flow cytometric analysis of ploidy.[41]

Cytology. For optimal interpretation both smears and cell blocks should be prepared and examined. FNAs of RCC are often very bloody, obscuring cellular detail, and frequently scantly cellular smears may have corresponding cell blocks that demonstrate surprisingly large, well-preserved tissue fragments diagnostic of RCC. In a series of 124 renal aspirates the only diagnostic material available in 9% of cases was on the cell blocks prepared from the FNAs.[96]

Three distinct cell types, the clear cell, the granular cell and the oncocyte, occurring either exclusively or admixed, can be recognized on FNA. The clear cells

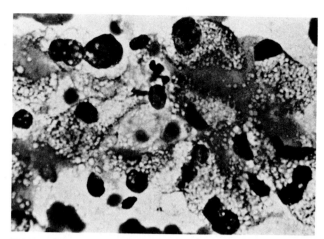

FIGURE 28–11. Renal cell carcinoma air-dried smear demonstrating multivacuolated cytoplasm (Diff-Quik; ×425).

of RCC have abundant, fragile, finely vacuolated cytoplasm, best appreciated on the Diff-Quik stain.[31] A variety of vacuoles have been described,[69] including the large "paper punch" and small punctate varieties as well as vacuoles of irregular size and shape that impart a lacy or web-like appearance (Fig. 28–11). The cell borders may be well defined but are usually indistinct (Fig. 28–12). Some nuclei that are totally or partially stripped of cytoplasm may lie in a loose alveolar pattern in a bubbly or vacuolated background. Granular cells have eosinophilic or cyanophilic cytoplasm, which is moderately dense and granular (Fig. 28–13). Oncocytic cells have extremely dense, eosinophilic, compact cytoplasm with well-defined cell borders. Rarely, RCCs may show a diffuse spindled appearance. It is controversial whether these should be considered a high-grade variant of RCC (Fuhrman's nuclear grade IV) or be classified as a sarcomatoid renal cell carcinoma.

The cells may be single or arranged loosely in flat

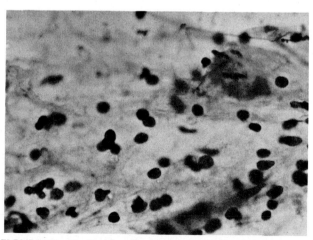

FIGURE 28–12. Renal cell carcinoma, nuclear grade I. Note the clear cytoplasm with indistinct margins, overlapping nuclei imparting an aveolar pattern and perfectly round nuclei without nucleoli. Compare with the similar cytology features of normal proximal tubular cells (Papanicolaou stain; ×265).

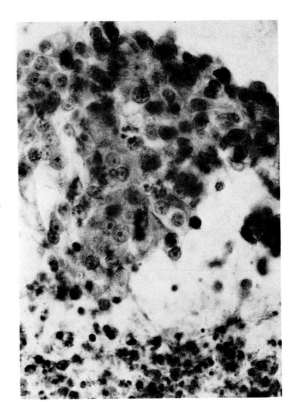

FIGURE 28–13. Renal cell carcinoma, nuclear grade III showing both vacuolated and granular cytoplasm in a background of inflammatory cells and debris (Papanicolaou stain; ×265).

sheets, clusters or an alveolar pattern. Occasionally the smear pattern is mixed, showing cells arranged in clusters or sheets with a focal papillary arrangement characterized by cells arrayed in papillary fronds on well-developed fibrovascular cores. Tumors with a predominantly papillary architecture compose a distinct subgroup (see the following). The nucleocytoplasmic ratio is characteristically low, even in the less-differentiated (higher nuclear grade) RCCs (see the following).

Cytologic grading of RCCs on FNAs has been infrequently utilized[27, 86] and may be limited by the scantiness of the specimen and by how adequately the tumor is represented on just a few needle passes. A recent study at the MD Anderson Cancer Center demonstrated that by using Fuhrman's[33] nuclear grade system, an extremely high concordance between FNAs and subsequent nephrectomy was possible.[20]

Grading of the tumor is done on alcohol-fixed Papanicolaou-stained smears and should be based on the least differentiated or most high-grade cells. It has been shown that multiple grades may coexist in 15% of tumors.[73] Four cytologic grades are proposed, based on Fuhrman's nuclear grading system,[33] which is easily applicable to cytologic specimens (Table 28–1) (Fig. 28–14; see also Figs. 28–12 and 28–13).

Tumors composed of clearly defined areas of high-grade spindle cells interspersed with cells of RCC are

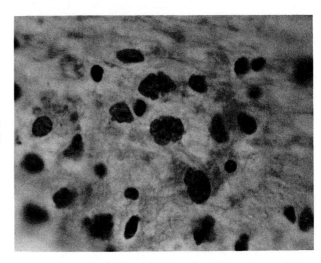

FIGURE 28–14. Aspirate of **renal cell carcinoma, nuclear grade IV,** showing large multilobulated irregular nuclei with prominent nucleoli (Papanicolaou stain; ×425).

TABLE 28–1. A Cytologic Grading System for RCC*

Grade†	Nucleoli at Low Magnification (×100)	Nucleoli at High Magnification (×400)	Nuclear Shape and Size	Cytoplasm
I	–	–	Small, round	Clear
II	–	+	Larger, irregular	Clear, granular
III	+	+	Larger, irregular	Clear, granular
IV‡	+	+	Pleomorphic, larger, bizarre forms; multilobation and hyperchromasia, spindle cells	Clear, granular

*Based on Furhman's nuclear grading system.
†Uses alcohol-fixed smears stained with Papanicolaou stain.
‡Worst-differentiated (most high-grade) cells.
− = absent; + = present.

designated sarcomatoid renal cell carcinomas and considered a separate entity (see the following).

Papillary Renal Cell Carcinoma

Histologically, papillary RCC is defined as a tumor that displays a papillary architecture in at least 50% of the neoplastic areas examined. These tumors are characteristically avascular on intravenous pyelogram and low stage at presentation.[74] They are reported to be less aggressive than the usual RCCs; however, this has not always been a consistent finding.[30, 33]

In two cytology studies,[24, 30] approximately 15% of RCCs fulfilled the criteria for designation as papillary RCCs.

Cytology. At low power, there is frequently a complex papillary architecture, with thick, multilayered fragments of tissue. The fragments are composed of neoplastic cells, which may be cuboid or columnar in shape, arrayed in papillae on central fibrovascular cores (Figs. 28–15 and 28–16). In contrast to the usual RCC, the smears are invariably hypercellular. Necrosis is frequently present. The nucleocytoplasmic ratio is

moderate to high, the nuclear chromatin is often finely granular and the nuclear contour may be smooth to irregular, with nuclear grooving frequently observed. The nuclei are uniform, and nuclear pleomorphism is rare. Papillary groups without a central fibrovascular core and single cells may be observed. The cytoplasm may contain golden brown pigment, and granularity or vacuoles may be present. Innumerable lipid-laden or foamy macrophages are present in close association with the cell groups and scattered throughout the smear. Psammoma bodies are noted in about 10% of cases.

The differential diagnosis of papillary RCC includes papillary TCC of the renal pelvis and tumors from the breast, ovary, endometrium, thyroid and mesothelioma.

The pitfalls in diagnosis of RCC are as follows:

1. FNA of normal kidney may be confused with well-differentiated nuclear grade I RCC (see Figs. 28–3 and 28–12). This may occur if RCC is diagnosed from scanty or marginal material when just a few tissue fragments are aspirated. Normal renal parenchyma is characterized by a variegated pattern of proximal and distal convoluted tubules that differ

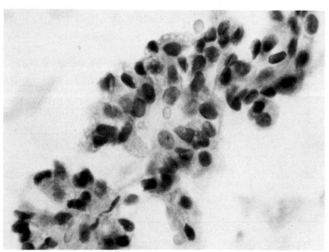

FIGURE 28–15. Papillary renal cell carcinoma aspiration cytology demonstrating a papillary frond with overlapping cuboidal cells with vacuolated cytoplasm and uniform grooved nuclei (Papanicolaou stain; ×425).

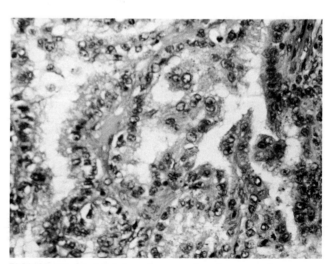

FIGURE 28–16. Histology from **nephrectomy specimen** corresponding to Figure 28–15 that shows well-developed papillary projections containing vacuolated cells with regular vesicular nuclei (hematoxylin and eosin; ×265).

in cytoplasmic texture and nucleocytoplasmic ratio and occur as small, honeycomb sheets of epithelium, frequently admixed with glomeruli. Well-differentiated RCC displays fine vacuoles, best seen on the Diff-Quik stain, and may occur as large sheets of epithelium, a feature not seen in normal renal tissue. The nuclear features of RCC grade I and proximal tubular epithelium may be identical. In one series, 14 of 301 aspirates reported as well-differentiated RCCs were false-positives.[54]

2. Histiocytes of XPN with foamy cytoplasm may be mistaken for single cells of RCC.

3. The cells from an oncocytic RCC or granular RCC may be confused with an oncocytoma. Careful screening of the smears may demonstrate a mixture of clear and granular or oncocytic cells, which will occur in RCC but not in oncocytomas.

4. Hepatocytes may be confused with oncocytes or oncocytic or granular cell RCC. Hepatocytes frequently contain golden brown intracytoplasmic pigment and lie singly or in flat sheets and do not show the overlapping and clustering seen in RCC.

5. Adrenal cortical cells may be confused with well-differentiated RCC because both may appear as clusters of overlapping naked nuclei in a vacuolated background. The former lack the prominent basement membrane material of RCC and may have intranuclear vacuoles.

6. Adenocarcinomas metastatic to or directly invading the kidney may be confused with RCC. These include adrenocortical carcinoma, hepatoma and bronchogenic adenocarcinoma. Adrenocortical carcinomas have characteristic radiologic, clinical and ultrastructural findings (see later) that will allow differentiation from RCC. A mucin stain is very helpful in differentiating metastases to the kidney from renal primary tumors; it may indicate TCC with a mucinous component because RCC is almost always mucin negative. Similarly, tumor cells expressing carcinoembryonic antigen should be considered metastatic to the kidney or derived from TCC because RCC is characteristically negative for carcinoembryonic antigen.

7. Papillary renal cell carcinoma may be misdiagnosed as TCC. The cells of high-grade TCC are distinctive, with higher-grade lesions having a spindle appearance, with dense smooth cytoplasm and hyperchromatic large nuclei. Papillary RCC has uniform cells that may have vacuolated cytoplasm, bland nuclei and fine, powdery chromatin in a background of histiocytes and necrosis.

Sarcomatoid Renal Cell Carcinoma

This is a rare, highly aggressive neoplasm, composing just over 1% of renal parenchymal tumors. To qualify for inclusion in this category, by histology a recognizable RCC component as well as a definite sarcomatoid component must be present. The two components may abut directly upon or blend with each other.[99] Three morphologic appearances of the sarcomatoid compo-

nent are described: malignant fibrous histiocytoma (MFH), fibrosarcoma and unclassified sarcoma. In the 42 patients reported by Ro and coworkers,[99] clinicopathologic stage was a most significant prognostic factor, with the median survival reported as 6.8 months.

Cytology. This carcinoma appears as clusters or single cells with either clear or granular cytoplasm and is of variable nuclear grade, with the cytologic appearance of RCC admixed with cells cytologically consistent with sarcoma. The sarcomatoid cells are large and spindled and frequently occur in large aggregates or dense, tightly coherent fragments (Fig. 28-17). The nuclear features of the sarcoma cells are always high grade; the cells are hyperchromatic with prominent nucleoli and often have multinucleated, pleomorphic forms. Osteoclastic giant cells may be present. Immunocytochemistry stains may show the sarcomatoid cells to be keratin and epithelial membrane antigen (EMA) negative and vimentin positive. In most cases, however, the sarcomatoid cells will be keratin or EMA positive. The smooth muscle actin stain may be positive in these spindle cells.

There are some diagnostic pitfalls. The diagnosis of sarcomatoid RCC by FNA may be overlooked if just the sarcomatoid component is aspirated, resulting in a diagnosis of a sarcoma. Similarly, if the carcinomatous component is the only component aspirated, then a diagnosis of RCC will be made. There also may be difficulty in differentiating sarcomatoid RCC from high-grade RCC. A diagnosis of a high-grade RCC (nuclear grade IV) is made in the presence of a pleomorphic epithelial component without a spindle cell component (see section on renal cell carcinoma).

Use of cell blocks to further elucidate the architectural features and the periodic acid–Schiff stain (with and without diastase) to demonstrate glycogen may aid in discerning a small RCC component on FNA. Additionally, examination of cells ultrastructurally and by

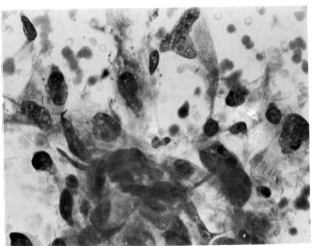

FIGURE 28–17. Aspirate of **sarcomatoid renal cell carcinoma** (RCC) showing large aggregate of highly pleomorphic, large spindle cells. In other areas of the smear a more typical epithelial RCC component was present (not shown) (Papanicolaou stain; ×425).

immunohistochemistry may assist in demonstrating two components.

Immunocytochemistry in RCC

The use of immunocytochemistry may be helpful in differentiating between tumors metastatic to the kidney and high-grade RCC and can be performed on the aspirated specimen. The pattern of antigenic expression in RCC will depend on the specificity of the antibodies selected, the differences in technique, such as prior enzyme digestion, and the differentiation of the tumor.[114] In one series, using a panel that included antibodies against keratins 10, 13, 14, 15, 16 and 19 (AE1) and keratins 8, 18 and 19 (CAM5.2), 87% of RCCs tested demonstrated expression of keratins, with greater reactivity being demonstrated with CAM5.2.[76] RCC has been shown to coexpress keratin and vimentin and may express EMA in the absence of keratin staining.[97] Adrenocortical carcinomas, on the other hand, have been reported to be uniformly nonreactive with EMA and keratins AE1 and AE3. RCCs generally do not express S-100 protein or react with leukocyte-common antigen (LCA), allowing differentiation from metastatic melanoma and lymphoma. Antibodies that are markers of proliferation, such as Ki-67, or cyclin, may have potential for use in differentiating normal renal parenchyma from well-differentiated RCC. A monoclonal antibody that can differentiate well-differentiated and moderately differentiated RCC from normal tissue has been described.[103] The reader is referred to Chapter 38, Immunocytochemistry, for applications and illustrations of this topic.

Tumors of the Renal Pelvis

The epithelial malignant tumors of the pelvis are TCC, which occurs most commonly, followed in frequency by squamous cell carcinoma, adenocarcinoma and undifferentiated carcinoma, the last two occurring only rarely. TCC may show squamous or glandular differentiation or mixed squamous and glandular differentiation. The benign epithelial tumors are papilloma and inverted papilloma, the latter occurring rarely, the likelihood of preoperative diagnosis being low.

The diagnostic efficacy of voided urine cytology in tumorous lesions of the renal pelvis and ureters has been disappointingly low, averaging only 38% of cases,[38] and has been attributed to the presence of ureteral or uteropelvic obstruction and the limitations of cytomorphology in the diagnosis of low-grade urothelial neoplasms. Cytodiagnostic accuracy is increased in specimens collected by ureteral catheter and lavage, with the greatest accuracy reported for renal pelvic brushings.[21] FNA of the renal pelvis is indicated when a mass lesion is detected by radiographic studies and urinary tract cytology is negative. The success rate of FNA of TCC of the renal pelvis has been reported to be 85%.[21]

Transitional Cell Carcinoma. The incidence of TCC has been reported to be 7% of all renal neoplasms, occurring predominantly in men, with a peak incidence in the 7th decade. TCC of the renal pelvis has been observed to occur with increased frequency in workers exposed to industrial dyes that contain alpha- and beta-naphthylamine and benzidine.[95] A relatively high frequency of TCC of the upper urinary tract and bladder has been reported in patients suffering from Balkan nephropathy, an endemic chronic renal disease of unknown etiology.

There is a significant association of TCC of the renal pelvis with synchronous or metachronous urothelial tumors of other sites.[27, 95]

The most common presentation is painless hematuria, with or without flank pain, with a palpable mass noted in only about 10% of cases. Asymptomatic tumors may be discovered during work-up for lower urinary tract neoplasms.

The hallmark of TCC on radiology is an ill-defined mass with preservation of the kidney architecture, which may be accompanied by a filling defect in the renal pelvis, by narrowing of the infundibulum or by hydronephrosis. Lithiasis may occur in 10% of patients.

Staging of TCC of the renal pelvis is similar to that proposed by Jewett and coauthors[95] for the bladder.

Survival of patients is correlated with the stage of disease and tumor grade, with grade I, Stage A tumors being associated with 100% 5-year survival. Stage C tumors are usually of higher grade and associated with a poor prognosis. Overall 5-year survival for all stages ranges from 14 to 57%.[84, 95]

Metastases are observed most frequently in the lungs, liver, regional lymph nodes and bone.

The majority of the tumors are exophytic and papillary, followed by a combination of exophytic and infiltrative growth patterns or, less commonly, a predominantly infiltrative growth pattern. TCC can invade into the renal parenchyma or through the underlying renal pelvic wall into the retroperitoneum. A correlation between the tumor grade and stage of the tumor has been observed, with most low-grade tumors showing no or only minimal invasion, whereas poorly differentiated or high-grade tumors may be widespread when first diagnosed.[84, 95]

Cytology. The cytologic appearance of TCC of the renal pelvis is identical to that described in the bladder, and it is graded in a similar fashion. Exophytic lesions are more commonly associated with low-grade neoplasms, whereas the flat or infiltrative tumors show features of high-grade TCC or carcinoma *in situ*. Review of the tumors diagnosed as TCC of the kidney by FNA at the MD Anderson Cancer Center has shown a predominance of moderately and poorly differentiated tumors, with only a single case of well-differentiated (grade I) TCC being recorded (unpublished data). We use a cytologic grading system based on the World Health Organization histologic grading system of urinary bladder tumors,[79] with grade I signifying the least anaplastic, grade III the most anaplastic and grade II an intermediate stage. Papilloma and TCC grade I are indistinguishable on cytology.

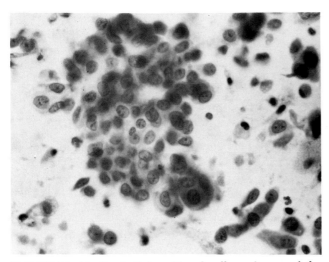

FIGURE 28–18. Grade II transitional cell carcinoma of the renal pelvis. Fine needle aspiration cytology showing cells with intermediate nuclear features arranged in a loose papillary structure, as well as single cells with cytoplasmic tails (Papanicolaou stain; ×265).

Grade I TCC is composed of aggregates of cells and single cells that are columnar or polygonal with minimal nuclear atypia and may be virtually indistinguishable from normal urothelium. The cytoplasm is neither keratinized nor vacuolated but is instead moderately dense and amphophilic.

Grade II TCC is composed of cells with features intermediate between grades I and III. Cells with elongations or cytoplasmic "tails," which are said to be characteristic of TCC, may be seen.[35] The nuclei are more hyperchromatic and round or oval in shape. Papillary structures with or without central fibrovascular cores may be seen (Fig. 28–18).

Grade III TCC is composed of large columnar or polygonal cells with well-defined cell borders and dense cytoplasm without keratinization or vacuolation. The nuclei are large and hyperchromatic, with coarse chromatin and irregular nuclei and high nucleocytoplasmic ratios. Bizarre multinucleated forms, spindle cells and cells with prominent nucleoli may be seen.

Focal squamous differentiation or metaplasia is reported in over 20% of TCC of the upper urinary tract and usually occurs in the higher-grade tumors.[102] Glandular metaplasia, which may produce mucin, has similarly been reported in up to 24% of TCC of the upper urinary tract.[12] The terms squamous carcinoma and adenocarcinoma should be reserved solely for those tumors that are composed exclusively of epidermoid or glandular elements throughout.

The pitfalls in diagnosis are as follows:

1. High-grade TCC with spindle cells may be confused with sarcomatoid RCC. The latter may demonstrate a two-component pattern with areas of recognizable RCC.
2. TCC with either glandular or squamous differentiation may be confused with tumors metastatic to the

kidney, such as bronchogenic carcinomas, and may be impossible to distinguish cytologically.
3. Distinction from RCC or its papillary variant is based on the distinctive nuclear and cytoplasmic features of each entity as well as the characteristic foamy histiocytes, psammoma bodies and hemosiderin pigment found in papillary RCC (see earlier).
4. Distinction from high-grade RCC may be difficult and is based on the presence of focal areas of RCC that may be better differentiated, with clear cell features, lower nucleocytoplasmic ratios and fewer hyperchromatic nuclei. Special stains for mucin and carcinoembryonic antigen are helpful because RCC does not express either, whereas TCC may be positive for both. Occasionally, TCC can coexist with RCC in the same kidney.
5. Reactive urothelial cells in the presence of a filling defect of the renal pelvis due to a blood clot or kidney stones may be overdiagnosed as low-grade TCC. Extreme caution should be exercised in the presence of a specimen containing only a few urothelial cells or cells with minimal atypia, with a request for a surgical biopsy or frozen section prior to definitive therapy.

Squamous Cell Carcinoma. Squamous cell carcinoma is the second most frequent epithelial malignancy of the renal pelvis. It affects both sexes equally and occurs most commonly in the 6th and 7th decades. Both kidneys are equally affected. Associated renal calculi have been observed in up to 57% of reported cases.[95] The tumors are mostly flat and infiltrative. At the time of diagnosis, most patients have invasive disease. The prognosis is generally poor, with a median survival of 5 months.

FNA reveals irregular clusters of malignant squamous cells.

Adenocarcinoma. This is an extremely rare neoplasm, and lithiasis is observed in a high percentage of cases. Chronic inflammation and glandular metaplasia may be associated signs. Histologically, the pattern may be papillary or composed of signet-ring cells. Many tumors bear a striking resemblance to colonic adenocarcinomas. Mucin production may vary from scant to abundant.

Very few reports on the cytology of this entity exist.[82] The gross appearance of the aspirate may be a yellow-white semitransparent mucinous substance. Single or clustered malignant glandular cells may be present.

Adenosquamous Carcinoma. FNA findings of mixed adenosquamous carcinoma of the renal pelvis metastatic to the psoas area indicated by the presence of malignant squamous and mucus-secreting glandular cells.[128]

Undifferentiated Carcinoma. Histologically, this extremely rare tumor resembles small-cell undifferentiated carcinoma of the lung, being composed of solid sheets of small oval cells with hyperchromatic nuclei. It is anticipated that FNA of this entity will reveal cells with cytologic features similar to those described for undifferentiated small-cell carcinoma.

Metastases to the Kidney

Metastases to the kidney occur approximately two to three times as frequently as in RCC. The most common primary sources of renal metastases are breast, lung, intestine, opposite kidney and stomach. Metastatic tumors are often multifocal and bilateral. Knowledge of the clinical history and comparison with the primary tumor will usually confirm the diagnosis of metastases; however, distinction from primary RCC or high-grade TCC may be problematic.

Lymphoma of the Kidney

Lymphoma presents as a solitary mass in the kidney; however, most lymphomatous renal masses represent extensions from adjacent sites of disease or involvement because of generalized disease. Typically these patients present with abdominal or flank pain and by intravenous pyelogram present with a renal mass suggestive of RCC. CT findings are inconsistent with conventional RCC and demonstrate unencapsulated infiltrative solid masses that are hypovascular on angiography. Recognition of lymphoma by FNA in conjunction with marker studies that confirm a monoclonal B cell population is highly successful and avoids the need for nephrectomy to make the diagnosis. Of five cases diagnosed at the MD Anderson Cancer Center,[89] three were large-cell lymphomas, one was a small cleaved cell lymphoma and one a small noncleaved cell (Burkitt's) lymphoma. The differential diagnosis on FNA includes metastatic poorly differentiated carcinoma and Wilms' tumor. The presence of a monotonous population of small, intermediate or large cells with inconspicuous cytoplasm that lie singly associated with lymphoglandular bodies is typical of lymphoma. Papanicolaou smears may be destained and stained for LCA or keratin to confirm lymphoma and rule out carcinoma. Wilms' tumor is characteristically a multicomponent tumor (see section on Wilms' tumor).

Primary Sarcoma of the Kidney

Primary sarcomas of the kidney are extremely rare in adults. The most common type is leiomyosarcoma, followed by MFH, hemangiopericytoma, fibrosarcoma and unclassified sarcomas.[42] These tumors generally have a poor prognosis, with a mean survival time of 23 months after diagnosis. FNA cytology of renal sarcoma will reflect the underlying histology. The typical cytologic features of these sarcomas are the same as those described for other body sites. The use of immunocytochemistry such as keratin, vimentin and smooth muscle studies supplemented by ultrastructural studies will further confirm the histogenesis of the tumor.

Differentiation of renal sarcomas from RCC may be difficult if only the sarcomatoid component of RCC is aspirated. The presence of positive staining for keratin in the spindle cells as well as a recognizable epithelial component favors the diagnosis of sarcomatoid RCC.

Pediatric Neoplastic Tumors

Wilms' Tumor

This important pediatric neoplasm described in the late 19th century by a German surgeon, Max Wilms, composes 6% of all pediatric cancers and represents a complex mixture of stromal and epithelial embryonal tissues.

The histologic appearance of Wilms' tumor, with its mixture of epithelial, stromal and blastemic elements, suggests its derivation from metanephric blastema that undergoes malignant transformation before or after birth. Wilms' tumor is associated with the presence of multicentric or bilateral precursor lesions that have been termed *persistent nodular blastema* or nephrogenic rests[8] or nephroblastomatosis.

The incidence of Wilms' tumor in the United States is reported as 450 cases annually. It occurs most frequently in the 1- to 5-year-old age group; however, a small percentage of cases occur in older children up to the age of 10, and 3% of cases occur in children older than 10.[94] There are over 100 case reports in the literature describing the presence of Wilms' tumor in adults.[94] The tumor presents most frequently as a unilateral mass; however, in 2 to 14% of cases it may occur bilaterally. There is an association between some cases of Wilms' tumor and abnormalities in the short arm of chromosome 11.

The most frequent clinical presentation is that of a unilateral mass, followed by pain and hematuria. Occasionally, children may present with an acute surgical abdomen secondary to massive intratumoral hemorrhage, or they may present with metastases.

By CT, Wilms' tumor shows a well-defined margin with caliceal distortion and abnormal tumor vessels. Occasionally, calcification is present. FNA specimens are usually obtained by CT scan with the patient under general anesthesia.[126] The differential diagnosis by radiology includes neuroblastoma, mesoblastic nephroma and polycystic renal disease. The last condition, however, can be differentiated by ultrasound.

In up to 90% of cases the tumors are greater than 5 cm in diameter, with sizes of more than 10 cm being attained in a third to a half of the cases. Grossly, Wilms' tumor is pseudoencapsulated, enclosing a solid, soft to firm, gray-white tumor mass. Hemorrhage, necrosis and cyst formation can occur but are usually not prominent.

Histology. The histologic appearance of Wilms' tumor is that of a triphasic embryonal neoplasm with the following components: (1) an epithelial component in which the cells may differentiate towards tubular or glomerulus-like structures; (2) a stromal component composed of spindle cells that are usually myxoid or fibroblastic, with the additional presence of smooth or skeletal muscle, fat or cartilage; rarely, Wilms' tumor may be composed of fetal striated muscle (rhabdomyomatous Wilms' tumor); and (3) a blastemic component composed of undifferentiated, densely packed cells that are small with scanty cytoplasm. The blastemic component is seen to be admixed with the spindle stromal component.

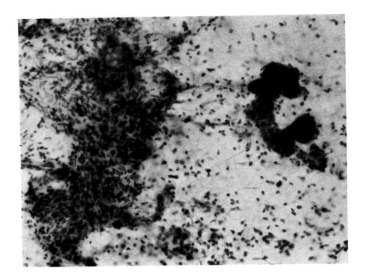

FIGURE 28–19. Wilms' tumor aspiration cytology showing a triphasic pattern composed of a fragment of stromal cells, epithelial structures and intervening blastemic cells (Papanicolaou stain; ×165).

As a result of the studies of tumors accumulated by the National Wilms' Tumor Study Group (NWTS),[7–9] histopathologic criteria have been developed that correlate with an unfavorable outcome for Wilms' tumor and include enlargement of nucleoli, hyperchromasia and multipolar mitotic figures within the stromal, epithelial or blastemic cells.

Two distinctive monophasic tumor subtypes (which are no longer regarded as subtypes of Wilms' tumor but instead as distinct entities) were identified by the first NWTS that, like anaplastic Wilms' tumor, are associated with an unfavorable outcome.[9] These will be discussed under separate headings and are the clear cell sarcoma of kidney (CCSK) and the malignant rhabdoid tumor of kidney (MRTK).

Favorable prognostic factors are principally histologic differentiation, lower stage and age less than 2 years. With improved surgical techniques and adjuvant radiation and chemotherapy the survival rate is currently 85%, compared with a 15% survival rate reported in 1920. FNA has been used preoperatively together with ultrastructural studies to diagnose Wilms' tumor.[3, 17] This is followed by administration of multimodal chemotherapy and x-ray treatment prior to nephrectomy. This approach is particularly useful in patients with bulky disease or extension of tumor into the renal vein or inferior vena cava and facilitates definitive surgical procedures such as subsequent nephrectomy. A case of bilateral rupture of tumor in a patient following FNA was reported[45]; however, the child was alive and free of disease 58 months postbiopsy.

Cytology. The cytologic pattern on FNA reflects the trilinear cellular components described under histology (Figs. 28–19 and 28–20).

1. *Epithelial cells.* These are cells with nuclei that are slightly larger than or the same size as the primitive blastemic cells; however, they are easily recognized by their increased cytoplasmic content and formation into primitive tubular structures or abortive glomerulus-like structures. The epithelial cell clusters are bounded by a basal lamina that stains cyanophilic on the Papanicolaou stain.
2. *Stromal cells.* These are easily distinguished as being arranged into loose sheets of spindle cells that lie in a loose, collagenous matrix.
3. *Blastemal cells.* These compose the remainder of the cells and have small, dark, round or ovoid nuclei with finely granular chromatin, absent to

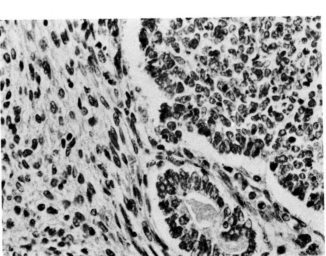

FIGURE 28–20. Corresponding **cell block** prepared from fine needle aspiration showing small undifferentiated blastemic cells, a well-developed epithelial tubular structure, and loose stromal cells (hematoxylin and eosin; ×265).

inconspicuous nucleoli and extremely scant cytoplasm.[1] The blastemic cells generally do not mold to each other and tend to lie haphazardly. A smearing artifact due to chromatin fragility is frequently present.

Electron-microscopic studies may be performed on aspirates and can demonstrate the different cellular components.[3] Clusters of epithelial cells are noted to be separated from the surrounding stroma by well-formed basal lamina. Occasional tubular lumina with projecting microvilli may be present.

Differential diagnosis of Wilms' tumor includes all the blue cell tumors of childhood, namely, embryonal rhabdomyosarcoma, Ewing's sarcoma, lymphoma and neuroblastoma. Embryonal rhabdomyosarcoma may be differentiated by the absence of a bi- or trilinear component as well as by the presence of rhabdomyoblasts with excentric nuclei and eosinophilic cytoplasm. Multinucleated giant cells may be present in rhabdomyosarcoma. Embryonal rhabdomyosarcoma cells are positive for desmin and negative for keratin. Extra-skeletal Ewing's sarcoma should be differentiated by the demonstration of abundant intracellular glycogen and a uniform cell population. Neuroblastoma, when better differentiated, will usually show rosettes as well as a neurofibrillary background and stain positively for neuron-specific antigen (NSE). On electron microscopy, dense core granules, neurofilaments and microtubules will be seen (see Fig. 28–32). The distinction from lymphoma is made based on the characteristic lymphomas of childhood, either large-cell lymphomas or small noncleaved cell (Burkitt's) lymphoma, both of which characteristically have prominent nucleoli and vacuolated cytoplasm—features not noted in the blastemic cells of Wilms' tumor. Furthermore, lymphomas show lymphoglandular bodies in the background, whereas small noncleaved cell lymphomas demonstrate tingible-body macrophages. Lymphomas also stain positive for LCA.

Other conditions with distinct clinical and pathobiologic features that need to be distinguished from Wilms' tumor include congenital mesoblastic nephroma and benign multilocular cystic nephroma as well as two distinctive malignant tumors of childhood, the rhabdoid tumor and clear cell sarcoma.

The pitfalls in the diagnosis of Wilms' tumor are as follows:

1. It may not be possible to detect anaplastic foci on a needle aspirate or a small needle biopsy.
2. Intrarenal neurogenic tumors or neuroblastomas are frequently misdiagnosed as Wilms' tumor. Neuroblastic pseudorosettes as well as the rosettes of peripheral neuroepithelial tumors of the kidney may resemble the embryonic tubular patterns common to Wilms' tumor[7]; however, rosettes usually lack a basal lamina and have stroma composed of neurofibrillary tissue. NSE is helpful in distinguishing these two entities.
3. Ganglion cells have been reported to be present in Wilms' tumor.[7] The presence of ganglion cells in Wilms' tumor may be confused with a ganglioneuroblastoma; however, ganglioneuroblastomas have morphologic features quite distinct from Wilms' tumor. In ganglioneuroblastoma, neuroblasts may form rosettes and stain positively for NSE.

Malignant Rhabdoid Tumor of the Kidney

This tumor was first described by Beckwith and Palmer in 1978[9] as an unfavorable prognostic variant of Wilms' tumor and termed a *rhabdomyosarcomatoid variant* of Wilms' tumor owing to its light-microscopic resemblance to a tumor of myogenic origin. Subsequent ultrastructural studies revealed no myogenic differentiation; instead, rather characteristic whorls of filamentous inclusions were demonstrated. The tumor was thus termed a rhabdoid tumor. The tumor also occurs in children in extrarenal sites[32, 132] as well as in the soft tissue of older patients. The histogenesis is unknown, but derivation from a pluripotential stem cell capable of both mesenchymal and epithelial differentiation has been suggested.[112, 123]

There is an association with MRTK and malignant tumors of the central nervous system. In the third NWTS, 2% of all cases represented MRTK.[8] No difference in incidence between the two sexes has been detected. MRTK is a highly aggressive tumor of childhood, with a mortality rate exceeding 80% even after aggressive adjuvant therapy.

The mean age of infants affected with MRTK is 13 months, with the reported age range being from 3 to 42 months. Occasional cases are associated with elevated levels of parathyroid hormone as well as hypercalcemia. The patients present most commonly with an abdominal mass; in patients with both renal and intracranial tumors, obstructive hydrocephalus may be the presenting sign. Metastases appear shortly after diagnoses and most commonly occur intra-abdominally or in intra-abdominal lymph nodes and lungs. FNA may be used to diagnose both the primary renal tumor as well as its metastases.[129]

MRTK appears as a poorly lobulated, nonencapsulated infiltrative mass and lacks the pseudoencapsulation or lobulation characteristic of classic Wilms' tumor. It is generally not a large tumor at the time of diagnosis.

Histologically the tumor is composed of a monotonous population of round to oval cells that grow in a diffuse pattern. Large hyaline globular cytoplasmic inclusions may be noted in some of the cells. The cells have abundant pink cytoplasm. The nucleus is vesicular with prominent nucleoli.

Cytology. The neoplastic cells are closely associated in sheets and clusters or lie singly and present as a monotonous population of oval to round cells, with centrally to excentrically placed large vesicular nuclei with finely granular chromatin. Nucleoli may vary from one to two in number and may be large and prominent or small and inconspicuous. The cytoplasm stains cyanophilic, and in some cells a cytoplasmic clearing may be appreciated adjacent to the nuclei, imparting a

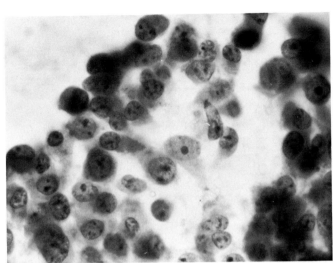

FIGURE 28–21. Rhabdoid tumor aspiration cytology showing a monomorphous population of round-to-oval cells with excentric nuclei and prominent nucleoli. A few cells show a perinuclear cytoplasmic clearing (Papanicolaou stain; ×425).

distinct plasmacytoid appearance (Fig. 28–21). The cytoplasm is not always well preserved, and naked nuclei may be present. Mitoses are frequently noted.

On ultrastructural studies the tumor cells are characterized by relatively abundant cytoplasm within which whorls of 7- to 10-nm–thick intermediate filaments tend to cluster in a paranuclear position (Fig. 28–22). Basement membrane material is not present, nor are Z bands or thick and thin filaments. Some tumor cells may present with condensed filaments resembling tonofilaments.

Immunohistochemistry demonstrates most MRTKs to have concomitant mesenchymal and epithelial markers. Vimentin is usually present on staining and cytokeratin is reported to be present in approximately one half of the tumors. Although most investigators have failed to demonstrate myoglobin or desmin, positive staining for desmin and myoglobin has been reported.[123]

The pitfalls in diagnosis are as follows:

1. Because of the striking resemblance of the cells of MRTKs to rhabdomyoblasts, MRTK can be confused with a rhabdomyosarcoma or a rhabdomyosarcomatoid variant of Wilms' tumor. Malignant rhabdoid tumors lack the strap cells and prominent cytoplasmic spindling of embryonal rhabdomyosarcoma. MRTK generally does not stain for desmin or myoglobin, and ultrastructurally the characteristic myofilaments are absent. Additionally, MRTK will stain for cytokeratin and vimentin, whereas these will be absent in rhabdomyosarcoma.

2. Differentiation from classic Wilms' tumor should not be a problem because of the monotonous distinctive cells of MRTK and the two- or three-component cellular composition of Wilms' tumor.

Clear Cell Sarcoma of the Kidney

Clear cell sarcoma of the kidney (CCSK) is a rare tumor composing approximately 4% of all renal tumors. This is a distinctive tumor both histologically and cytologically with a strong tendency for metastases to the bones. Recognition of this distinctive subtype of tumor is important because of its aggressive clinical behavior and poor prognosis. FNA has been used successfully to diagnose this tumor.[4]

The tumors mostly manifest as an abdominal mass or with hematuria. CCSK affects both sexes equally, occurring in infants and children at a mean age of 3

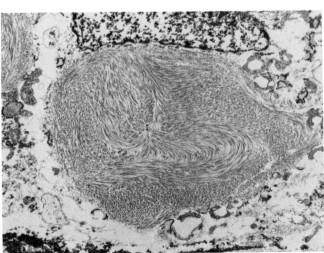

FIGURE 28–22. Ultrastructure of **rhabdoid tumor** from a needle aspirate showing the high magnification view of paranuclear cytoplasm demonstrating characteristic whorls of thick intermediate filaments (×20,379). (Courtesy of Dr. Bruce MacKay, MD Anderson Cancer Center, Houston, Texas.)

years (age range of 7 months to 6 years). The tumors are staged according to the third NWTS. Roughly half of the patients present with Stage I disease, with the remaining patients presenting with spread of disease beyond the kidney. Bone metastases may precede other metastatic sites, with the most frequently affected bones being the skull, spine, ribs and long bones. Other metastatic sites include the lungs and liver.

The gross appearance of CCSK may show a well-demarcated, uniformly lobular gray-white tumor or be variegated with necrotic areas. Some tumors may appear mucinous.

Histologically CCSK is hypercellular with haphazardly arranged cells that have ill-defined clear cytoplasm. Branching fascicles of tightly packed spindle cells may often divide the tumor into nests. Other histologic patterns include an epithelioid-trabecular pattern and a fibrotic hyalinized pattern wherein the stroma is composed of broad bands of dense collagen.[113]

Cytology. The cells occur singly or in small clusters and show variation in shape from polygonal to stellate and spindle shaped. The nuclei are uniform, being round or ovoid. The chromatin pattern is very fine with occasional small nucleoli. Mucoid material is noted in the background and between the cells and stains light pink to deep purple on the Diff-Quik stain. The cytoplasm may show prominent vacuolation, and there may be intranuclear cytoplasmic vacuoles (Fig. 28–23).

Ultrastructural studies reveal cells with slender processes, with an occasional single cilia being noted. The cytoplasm contains a moderate number of organelles. Occasional clusters of collagen are present in the stroma.[4]

This tumor can be differentiated from Wilms' tumor by the presence of a monomorphous cell population devoid of all metanephric elements. Other childhood sarcomas such as rhabdoid tumor and rhabdomyosarcoma can be differentiated based on their characteristic cytologic, ultrastructural and immunocytochemical profiles.

Diagnosis of Renal Allograft Rejection by FNA

FNA has been used to assess rejection of renal transplants by examining the composition of the cellular infiltrates so obtained.[46, 63, 125] Pasternak[92] suggested that the FNA biopsy could be used to analyze the cellular infiltrate for signs of rejection and that serial FNAs could be used to monitor rejection. The field of FNA of renal transplantation has evolved to include an international workshop on renal transplant cytology. It has been shown that FNA is a simple and safe technique to perform in this setting.

Because of the contamination of the cells by peripheral blood, a *corrected increment* is utilized to adjust the cell count.[46] Smears are read by performing a differential count on 200 white cells from the FNA, and the differential of the white cell count on the

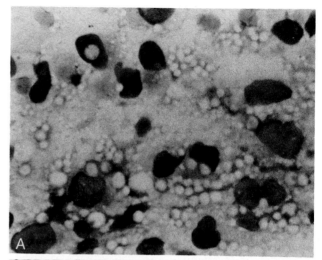

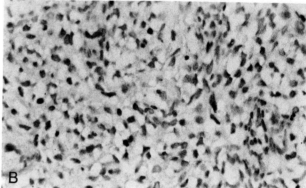

FIGURE 28–23. *A,* Aspiration cytology of **clear cell sarcoma** of the kidney showing round-to-ovoid nuclei with smooth fine chromatin in a background of vacuolated cytoplasm. Note the prominent intranuclear cytoplasm vacuoles (Diff-Quik; ×425). *B,* Corresponding cell block of aspirate of **clear cell sarcoma** of the kidney showing hypercellular tightly packed spindle cells with clear cytoplasm (×265).

peripheral blood is subtracted (corrected increment). It has been shown that when taken at an early post-transplantation period, FNA has a similar diagnostic value to that of core renal biopsy (CRB). FNA has been shown to be complimentary to conventional renal biopsy; however, it cannot evaluate morphologic changes such as fibrosis or vascular rejection. It also cannot accurately assess the intensity of the inflammatory reaction in comparison to histologic criteria. The advantage of FNA over CRB is rapid institution of antirejection therapy.

Deterioration in renal function following transplantation may be due to rejection, drug toxicity, vascular or urinary obstruction or infection. Greater specificity in diagnosing rejection may be obtained by using FNA in conjunction with monoclonal antibodies.[16, 39] Bishop and coworkers[14] have shown that the best indicators for rejection are the presence of T lymphoblasts, (as identified by the T 11 monoclonal antibody), the presence of large, mononuclear cells that strongly express HLA-DR antigens and the presence of renal tubular cells that strongly express the HLA-DR antigen. Using the immunocytochemistry techniques in conjunction with conventional cytology improves the assessment of rejection.

ADRENAL

With improved imaging techniques, increasing numbers of both benign and malignant adrenal lesions are being discovered, either incidentally or as part of the work-up for metastatic disease. Pathologic confirmation of an adrenal lesion is of primary importance because of the high frequency of incidental benign adrenal nodules in the general population. In general, FNA is used (1) to determine the origin of and characterize both cystic and solid adrenal masses, (2) to assist in preoperative staging in patients who have malignant disease because discovery of an adrenal metastasis may radically alter the initial therapy for certain primary tumors, (3) to determine postsurgical adrenal metastases and (4) to investigate further a clinical condition that might be related to the adrenals, e.g., an infectious etiology for adrenal insufficiency.

Imaging Techniques

Radiology in conjunction with FNA cytology plays an important role in the work-up of patients for possible adrenal gland abnormalities.[13, 55, 62, 91, 107]

Adrenal scintigraphy using I^{131}-labeled 19-iodocholesterol has been used to lateralize corticosteroid- or aldosterone-producing adenomas. Using this technique, it is possible to differentiate the cause of Cushing's syndrome as hyperplasia, carcinoma or adenoma. For the diagnosis and localization of pheochromocytoma, I^{131}-labeled metaiodobenzylguanidine has been used.[107]

Gray-scale ultrasonography is helpful in determining whether an adrenal mass is cystic or solid; however, tumors smaller than 2.5 cm can be missed.

The most useful imaging procedure is CT, which is capable of resolving tumors as small as 0.5 cm in diameter.[107] Anatomically on cross-sectional CT images, the right adrenal is located lateral to the right diaphragmatic crus, medial to the right lobe of the liver and immediately posterior to the inferior vena cava. The left adrenal gland is lateral to the left diaphragmatic crus and posterolateral to the aorta. The superior portion of the left gland is posterior to the lesser omental sac, and inferiorly the gland lies posterior to the pancreas with the splenic vessels running between them (Fig. 28–24).

The performance of FNA of the adrenal gland requires a skilled operator, especially if the lesion is small. The procedure may be performed with the patient lying either in the prone or lateral position using 18- to 22-gauge fine needles. Attention to correct placement of the needle in the mass with CT verification is essential if one is to avoid a false-negative diagnosis, such as in the case of a small metastatic lesion. Similarly, a false-positive diagnosis of an adenoma may occur if the aspirating needle obtains normal

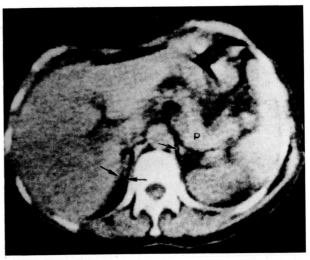

FIGURE 28–24. Computed tomographic scan demonstrating **adrenal glands** (arrows). Right adrenal has an inverted Y shape and is situated behind the liver. Left adrenal is wedge shaped and lies behind the pancreas (P) in the perirenal fat.

adrenal tissue adjacent to a small malignant lesion because the cytology of an adenoma may be identical to that of normal adrenal cortex. To ensure representation of the suspected lesion, it is recommended that immediate cytologic assessment of direct smears be performed. Tissue should be smeared very gently because adrenal cortical cells possess extremely fragile cytoplasm. Depending on the initial impression, additional tissue may be obtained for cell block, immunohistochemistry or other special stains and ultrastructural studies. In some cases, FNA of a right adrenal mass performed from a lateral approach may traverse the liver and result in the aspiration of benign hepatocytes, which should not be confused with adrenal cortical cells.

FNA of the adrenal is generally associated with relatively few complications, the notable exception being the inadvertent needling of catecholamine-producing adrenal tumors. Pneumothorax may be a complication if an approach through the posterior lung sulci is used. FNA may be potentially fatal in patients with pheochromocytomas who do not have clinically recognized paroxysmal hypertensive episodes. Death from extensive intra-abdominal hemorrhage and complications of intra-abdominal bleeding following FNA have been reported.[75] To avoid these complications, screening for elevated levels of urine and serum catecholamines and their products prior to FNA has been advocated in patients with incidental adrenal nodules who do not have a known malignancy or clinical symptoms of steroid hypersecretion.

Anatomy and Histology

The adrenal glands are paired retroperitoneal organs situated within the confines of the perirenal fat inside Gerota's fascia. They lie superior and posterior to the renal vessels. Each gland is 2 to 4 cm long, 2 to 2.5

cm wide and 1.0 cm or less thick. The right adrenal is pyramidal in shape, whereas the left one is crescent shaped. The weight of the normal adrenal gland in a surgical patient is about 4 g. It is essential for the cytopathologist interpreting FNA of the adrenal to obtain the dimensions of the adrenal gland and to be familiar with the normal anatomy on CT. For cytologic interpretation the weight of the gland is less important than the CT-derived dimensions. Each gland is subdivided into head, body and tail, with the head being the larger end, positioned medially in the body. Three separate arteries arising from the inferior phrenic artery, aorta and renal artery supply each gland. The left adrenal vein drains into the renal vein, and the right adrenal vein drains into the inferior vena cava.

The definitive adrenal cortex is composed of three layers, namely, the zona glomerulosa, zona fasciculata and zona reticularis. The outer yellow zone of the cortex corresponds to the zona glomerulosa and zona fasciculata, and the inner brown zone corresponds to the zona reticularis. The adrenal medulla is pale gray in color and sharply differentiated from the cortex and forms approximately one tenth of the mass of the whole gland.

The zona glomerulosa is the outermost layer just beneath the capsule of the adrenal gland and is a narrow zone composed of small polyhedral cells with compact nuclei and clear, lipid-rich cytoplasm. The cells are arranged in small clusters or glomeruli. The cells of this zone are associated with the production of aldosterone, a mineralocorticoid. The zona fasciculata, the widest of the three zones, contains clear cells arranged radially into distinctive columns that possess abundant lipid-laden cytoplasm. The cells of this zone are associated with the production of glucocorticoids, chiefly cortisol. The cells of the zona reticularis, the innermost zone, are compact and acidophilic and demonstrate lipofuscin granules and absence of lipid. The cells of this zone are associated with the secretion of sex steroids, androgens and estrogens.

The ultrastructural appearance of the cortical cells differs according to the zona examined; however, common to each layer are abundant smooth endoplasmic reticulum and numerous mitochondria with tubulovesicular, tubulolamellar or stacked mitochondrial cristae.

The adrenal medulla is composed of pheochromocytes, which are elongated cells arranged in groups set in a rich network of vascular spaces and sympathetic fibers.[131] The pheochromocytes contain eosinophilic cytoplasm and chromaffin granules. Other cells in the medulla are sympathetic ganglia cells derived from the neuroblasts and small round cells. The sympathetic fibers synapse with the pheochromocytes.

Ultrastructural studies of the medulla show the characteristic catecholamine-containing, membrane-bound secretory granules of the pheochromocytes. Norepinephrine granules have an excentrically located core with surrounding halo; epinephrine granules possess a granular dense core with an inconspicuous perimembraneous clearing.

Cytology of the Normal Adrenal Gland

On FNA the cytology of normal adrenal cortical parenchymal cells are characterized by small aggregates and cords of regular polyhedral cells that stain palely to intensely cyanophilic. The cytoplasm is delicate and foamy and frequently the borders are frayed. Cells from the zona fasciculata demonstrate either single, prominent or multiple finely dispersed lipid inclusions that are noted as clear vacuoles following the extraction of lipid by alcohol fixation. The cells derived from the zona reticularis are characterized by densely compact cyanophilic cytoplasm, with fine, golden brown, granular lipofuscin pigment and the absence of lipid. In both types of cells the nuclei are small and round and occupy less than one third of the area of the cell and may be centrally or excentrically located. The nuclear chromatin is fine, and nucleoli are single, small and inconspicuous (Fig. 28–25). Intranuclear intracytoplasmic inclusions consisting of round, clear areas may be conspicuous. Occasionally small, spindle-shaped stromal cells are noted.[56]

Cytology of Benign Entities

Adrenal Cysts

Adrenal cysts are rare lesions, usually incidentally discovered in the 3rd to 5th decade. Endothelial cysts are the most common type, followed by pseudocysts secondary to hemorrhage in normal or neoplastic adrenal tissue. Other rarer cysts may be secondary to degeneration in adrenal adenoma or parasitic cysts often of echinococcal origin. Endothelial cysts may be either lymphangiomatous or angiomatous.[131] The ma-

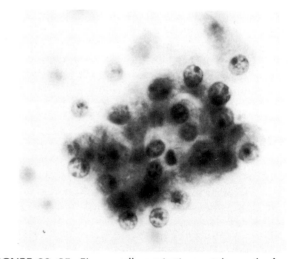

FIGURE 28–25. Fine needle aspiration cytology of **adrenal cortex** showing a cluster of cells derived from the zona fasiculata. Note the uniform round nuclei, inconspicious nucleoli and abundant vacuolated cytoplasm (Papanicolaou stain; ×425).

jority of adrenal cysts are asymptomatic owing to their small size. Larger cysts may cause vague gastrointestinal symptoms related to compression of bowel contents and liver. Plain films of the abdomen may demonstrate peripheral eggshell-type calcification, whereas ultrasound will prove the cystic nature of the mass.[58] Percutaneous FNA can be therapeutic by decompressing the mass.[104] Cyst contents may be bloody, clear or turbid, with few epithelial cells, many leukocytes or hemosiderin-laden macrophages.[56] The treatment of adrenal cysts is primarily conservative, with aspiration of cyst contents followed by cytologic examination. Surgery is indicated if there is malignant cytology or an irregular cyst lining after contrast medium is injected.

Adrenal Myelolipoma

Adrenal myelolipoma is a rare benign tumor of late, middle or old age, ranging in size from microscopic to massive. These tumors are reported in 0.8% of autopsies. These lesions are thought to arise by a metaplasia of adrenocortical cells or from differentiation of previously uncommitted mesenchymal stromal cells into a mixture of mature adipose tissue and hematopoietic cells. The tumors are usually nonfunctioning and asymptomatic and are discovered incidentally. Several tumors have been associated with virilization and Cushing's disease.

Radiologically they reflect their histologic composition of varying proportions of fat and bone marrow and are extremely echogenic on ultrasound and show fatty density on CT.

FNA demonstrates mature adipose tissue, immature hematopoietic cells of myeloid and erythroid origin, lymphocytes and megakaryocytes. Special stains such as naphthol AS-D chloroacetate esterase may be performed on a cell block to demonstrate the immature myeloid element (Fig. 28–26).

The differential diagnosis of a suprarenal fatty mass includes renal angiomyolipoma extending from the kidney, retroperitoneal lipoma and liposarcoma. Identification of the hematopoietic cells mixed in various proportions and mature adipose tissue differentiates myelolipoma from these other entities.

Adrenal Hyperplasia

Adrenal hyperplasia may be functional or nonfunctional. Adrenal hyperplasia may be associated with hypercortisolism or Cushing's syndrome, which is caused by adrenocortical hyperplasia in the absence of pituitary disease. Hypercortisolism caused by an adrenocorticotropic hormone producing pituitary adenoma is known as Cushing's disease and is the most common cause of adrenocortical hyperplasia.[131] Other causes of hypercortisolism are adrenal adenoma and adrenal carcinoma. The diagnosis for the most part is clinical and biochemical.

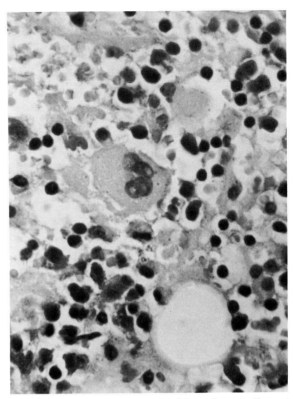

FIGURE 28–26. Cell block prepared from fine needle aspiration of **adrenal myelolipoma** showing mature adipose tissue, immature myeloid and erythroid cells and a megakaryocyte (×425).

By CT the adrenal glands may appear normal or show generalized enlargement without change in shape.

FNA cytology of adrenal hyperplasia reveals whorls of lipid-containing clear cells with small uniform nuclei and cell margins resembling cells of the zona fasciculata. Corresponding cell blocks or core biopsies will show lipid-filled adrenal cells arranged in an alveolar pattern with small homogeneous nuclei.[56]

Adrenal Adenoma

Adrenal adenomas may be functional or nonfunctional. There is a high frequency of incidental benign (nonfunctioning) adrenal nodules in the general population associated with advancing age,[22, 26] diabetes,[48] hypertension[101] and various malignancies, such as RCC. The prevalence of benign nonfunctioning nodules ranges from 8 to 64.5%, which includes both microscopic and grossly visible nodules. The frequency of CT detection of adrenal nodules is estimated to be 0.6%.[37] On CT a functioning adrenal nodule may be associated with atrophy of the contralateral adrenal. Nonfunctioning nodules are generally small with a mean diameter of 2.5 cm (range of 0.5 to 3 cm) and usually involve only one limb of the adrenal gland, with the uninvolved portion of the ipsilateral and the contralateral gland appearing intact. Radiologically they cannot be distinguished from small metastatic lesions.[57] It is most important to differentiate adrenal adenomas from malignant tumors metastatic to the adrenal in view of the therapeutic and prognostic implications. There is close similarity in the clinical and radiologic features of patients with adenomas and metastases to the adrenal in terms of the presenting extra-adrenal neoplasm, mean age, sex, number of adrenal lesions and incidence of bilaterality.[57] At the MD Anderson Cancer Center, the most frequent indication for adrenal FNA is to distinguish between a benign adrenal nodule and a metastasis.

Histology. Adrenal adenomas are usually unencapsulated lesions, better demarcated on low-power scanning, and are composed of aggregates of mainly clear cells lying in an alveolar arrangement; however, occasional masses of more compact cells with eosinophilic cytoplasm may be present. Functioning adenomas that secrete aldosterone appear grossly as small canary-yellow nodules. Pigmented or black adenomas are composed of cortical cells filled with lipofuscin granules that give the adenomas a black appearance.[100]

Cytology. FNA of adrenal adenomas is characterized by two distinct patterns. The first pattern is a hypercellular smear composed of numerous small, round, homogeneous, naked nuclei lying scattered or in aggregates set in a pink granular or bubbly background composed of shattered vacuolated cytoplasm. The nuclei are evenly spaced and occur in an alveolar pattern owing to overlapping of the nuclei or lie in curvilinear arrays (Fig. 28–27). Careful searching reveals cells with intact, lipid-laden cytoplasm. Scattered small spindle cells representing stromal cells may be seen. The second pattern is a less cellular smear composed of discrete aggregates of cells with better preserved vacuolated cytoplasm and small inconspicuous nuclei. In both patterns, the nuclei are round, having fine, even, smooth chromatin, inconspicuous nucleoli and rare intranuclear vacuoles. Nuclear pseudomolding caused by the supraimposition of adjacent nuclei in different focal planes may be noted. Nuclear atypia is unusual but if present is focal and minimal and consists of an occasional enlarged nucleus. Nucleoli are small and inconspicuous. Mitosis and necrosis are absent. FNA of black adenomas reveals cells with features consistent with cells from the zona reticularis, with compact cytoplasm and lipofuscin granules.

The pitfalls in diagnosis are as follows:

1. Care should be taken not to interpret hepatocytes as adrenocortical adenoma cells. Hepatocytes are generally large, polygonal cells with well-defined cell borders and may contain bile pigment.
2. It may be difficult to distinguish metastatic undifferentiated small-cell (oat-cell) carcinoma[72] from an adrenal adenoma because both are characterized by many small, naked nuclei lying singly and in clusters with some degree of nuclear molding (Fig. 28–28). Oat-cell carcinoma shows far more nuclear pleomorphism, more coarsely granular chromatin, nuclear debris and occasional large, irregular nucleoli. Absence of the vacuolated cytoplasmic background and lack of single cells with vacuolated cytoplasm

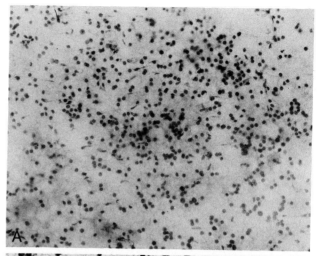

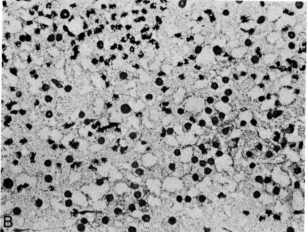

FIGURE 28–27. *A,* Fine needle aspiration of **adrenal adenoma** demonstrating numerous stripped nuclei arranged in an alveolar pattern (Papanicolaou stain; ×165). *B,* Fine needle aspiration smear from the same case as Figure 28–27*A* demonstrating similar alveolar arrangement of small round homogeneous nuclei with intranuclear vacuoles lying in a vacuolated cytoplasmic background best demonstrated on this air-dried smear (Diff-Quik; ×165).

together with lack of an organized aveolar architecture serve as additional distinguishing criteria.[77]

3. Confusion with other small, round tumors such as neuroblastoma and other small-cell anaplastic carcinomas may occur. Electron microscopy and special stains may further help to differentiate these conditions, apart from the previously described morphologic characteristics of adrenocortical adenomas.
4. Differentiation from adrenocortical carcinomas may be difficult on the basis of cytology alone; however, small size (less 3.5 cm) and only minimal focal atypia without necrosis and mitosis favor a diagnosis of adenoma.[56] Although only a very small number of adrenocortical carcinomas are under 6 cm in diameter, regardless of the size of tumor, diffuse cytologic atypia, necrosis and mitosis suggest a diagnosis of adrenal carcinoma. Additionally, any virilizing, feminizing or glucocorticoid-secreting ad-

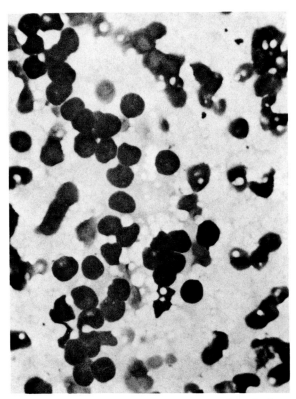

FIGURE 28–28. Fine needle aspiration of an **adrenal adenoma** mimicking oat-cell carcinoma. Note pseudomolding of nuclei, regular round nuclear profiles and smooth chromatin. The stripped nuclei lie in a vacuolated background (Diff-Quik; ×425). (Courtesy of Dr. Alonzo Ashton, Humana Sunrise Hospital, Las Vegas, Nevada.)

renal mass causing abdominal pain, fever or weight loss and failing to become suppressed with high-dose dexamethasone therapy should be suspected of malignancy.[56]

Adrenocortical Carcinoma

Adrenocortical carcinomas are extremely uncommon tumors, with an incidence of 75 to 115 new cases each year in the United States.[18] The average age of the patient is 40 to 50 years; however, the neoplasm can occur any time from early childhood to old age. Adrenocortical carcinomas are classified as either functional or nonfunctional. Hormonal excess produces classic clinical signs such as hypercortisolemia (which occurs in 50% of cases), virilization (20%) or a combination of these (10 to 15%). Between 10 and 15% of tumors are nonfunctional. Levels of precursor steroids may be elevated in clinically "nonfunctional" carcinomas. An adrenocortical carcinoma may present either as a functional tumor that is not suppressed by high-dose dexamethasone therapy or as an intra-abdominal mass. Most carcinomas present as large, advanced masses with an average size at presentation of 16 cm (range of 6 to 40 cm), and the majority of patients have extra-adrenal spread at the time of presentation. Sites of metastases include lungs, liver, lymph nodes, bone,

pancreas and diaphragm. The tumor has a poor prognosis, with an overall median survival reported as 14 months.[25]

Size is one of the most important criteria for assessing malignancy by radiography in primary adrenal masses. Most carcinomas are over 6 cm in diameter. Smaller carcinomas cannot be reliably determined by imaging techniques.

Grossly, carcinomas are frequently necrotic, hemorrhagic and variegated in color. Carcinomas show architectural disarray, including sheet-like growth and marked increase in vascularity. Most tumors show moderate to marked pleomorphism, microscopic foci of necrosis, hemorrhage and calcification. Increased mitotic activity is seen. Capsular and vascular invasion are frequently noted. Small size, in spite of malignant histopathologic features, is most predictive of favorable outcome.[51, 122, 133]

Cytology. The cytologic appearance may range from well-differentiated to highly anaplastic tumors; however, common to all tumors is the presence of hypercellularity, retention of cytoplasm and loss of cohesion of cells. Cells may lie singly or aggregated into densely grouped sheets. Well-differentiated tumors have lipid-laden cells, but the nuclei are enlarged and hyperchro-

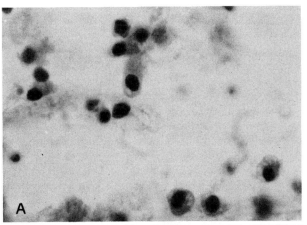

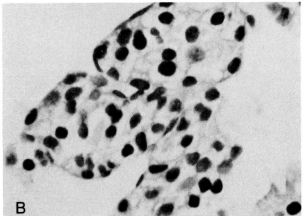

FIGURE 28–29. *A*, Fine needle aspiration cytology demonstrating cells of **well-differentiated adrenocortical carcinoma** (Papanicolaou stain; ×425). *B*, Cell block prepared from fine needle aspirate in *A* showing **well-differentiated adrenocortical carcinoma** (hematoxylin and eosin; ×425).

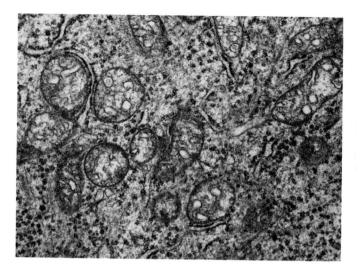

FIGURE 28–30. Ultrastructure of **adrenocortical carcinoma** demonstrating abundant smooth and rough endoplasmic reticulum and mitochondria with tubulovesicular cristae. These features are typical of steroid-secreting tumors (×27,000). (Courtesy of Dr. Bruce MacKay, MD Anderson Cancer Center, Houston, Texas.)

matic and occasional mitoses may be observed (Fig. 28–29). Tumors that are moderately differentiated may show smaller amounts of lipid, with granular cytoplasm and flocculent spheric cytoplasmic aggregates. Poorly differentiated carcinomas exhibit extreme cellular pleomorphism with multinucleated bizarre cells varying from spindle shaped to polyhedral in shape. Nucleoli are prominent and large. Giant cells may be seen.

The pitfalls in diagnosis are as follows:

1. The cells of adrenocortical carcinoma may be indistinguishable morphologically from RCC and pheochromocytoma.[66] Ultrastructually, the cells of adrenocortical carcinoma reveal mitochondria with tubular or vesicular cristae, abundant smooth endoplasmic reticulum and laminar stacks of rough endoplasmic reticulum (Fig. 28–30). These features are not usually seen in either of the other two tumors. In addition, adrenocortical carcinoma is frequently functional.
2. It may be difficult to differentiate well-differentiated adrenocortical carcinoma from an adrenal adenoma; however, this distinction is usually made based on size and degree of nuclear atypia (see earlier).
3. Distinguishing adrenocortical carcinoma from a metastatic poorly differentiated adenocarcinoma may be impossible; however, ultrastructural evidence of features typical of steroid-secreting tumors and evidence of mucin production are helpful diagnostic aids.

Tumors Metatastic to the Adrenal Gland

The adrenal gland is a favored site for metastases, most frequently breast carcinoma, lung carcinoma, lymphoma and melanoma. In two autopsy series the overall incidence of gross and microscopic metastases to the adrenal gland from all sites was found to be 26%.[1, 108] An incidence of adrenal metastases from breast and lung cancer has been reported to be 54% and 36%, respectively. The most important differential diagnosis in small metastatic lesions is a benign adrenal

nodule. The mean size of radiographically detected adrenal metastases in one series was 7.8 cm; however, very small metastases are frequent, and many may be indistinguishable from a benign nodule.[57] Of 16 incidental adrenal nodules in patients with a variety of primary extra-adrenal neoplasms, FNA revealed benign adenomas in seven patients and adrenal metastases in nine.[57] The biologic significance of metastases to the adrenal gland correlates with aggressive behavior, widespread dissemination of the primary tumor and early demise of the patient.

The cytologic diagnosis of metastases to the adrenal is usually straightforward. The clinical history together with close correlation with previous cytologic or histologic accessions, appropriate additional histochemistry stains and ultrastructural examination are helpful.

Tumors of the Medulla

Pheochromocytomas

Pheochromocytomas are tumors of the chromaffin cells of the medulla that are usually symptomatic owing to hypersecretion of catecholamines, resulting in paroxysmal hypertension, sweating and palpations. Up to 20% of tumors may be nonfunctional. Increased levels of urinary or plasma vanillylmandelic acid and catecholamines may occur in 90% of cases. The diagnosis of pheochromocytoma is usually a clinical and biochemical one, followed by surgical excision without the need for preoperative FNA. Up to 20% of tumors, however, may be nonfunctional, and in some cases, biochemical findings may be equivocal.[75] FNA may be used in this situation to obtain the diagnosis; however, the procedure may be fraught with danger, with the potential for producing uncontrollable bleeding and hypertensive crises.[75] Of all pheochromocytomas, 10% are malignant, 10% are bilateral and 10% are extra-adrenal. Pheochromocytomas may be sporadic or may compose part of the multiple endocrine neoplasia (MEN) syndrome. The MEN II syndrome comprises pheochromocytoma, together with medullary carcinoma of the thyroid and parathyroid adenoma. The Sipple syndrome consists of medullary carcinoma of the thyroid and pheochromocytoma. Both of these are familial, with a high incidence of bilateral pheochromocytoma as well as adrenal medullary hyperplasia.

The average pheochromocytoma weighs about 100 g and is a solid ovoid tumor. Microscopically the cells are pleomorphic and are arranged in sheets or clusters and nests, or *zellballen*, surrounded by vascular channels within fibrous septa (Fig. 28–31 *A*). The diagnosis of malignancy is based on invasion of the tumor into adjacent structures or metastases. Few cytologic descriptions of FNA of pheochromocytoma exist.[81, 118]

Cytology. The smears are hypercellular with cells lying singly or in loose groups or pseudorosettes. Three types of cells have been described.[118] The first type are small to moderate-sized polygonal cells with finely granular cytoplasm, uniform round to oval nuclei with granular chromatin and prominent chromocenters. These cells are the prototypic cells of neuroendocrine tumors. The second type are spindle cells with abundant cytoplasm and elongated nuclei with coarse granular chromatin (Fig. 28–31*B*). Finally, large, myoid-like cells with excentric, large nuclei, prominent nucleoli and abundant pale, finely granular cytoplasm

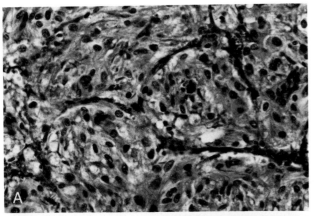
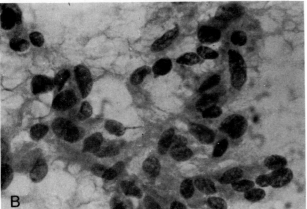

FIGURE 28–31. *A*, Histologic section of **pheochromocytoma** demonstrating pleomorphic cells arranged in zellballen with surrounding fibrovascular channels (hematoxylin and eosin; ×165). *B*, Corresponding fine needle aspiration cytology demonstrating spindle cells with abundant cytoplasm and coarse granular chromatin (Papanicolaou stain; ×425).

have been described. The smears may be composed of a mixture of these cell types, or one cell type may predominate. Recognition of the characteristic polygonal cells will help to make the diagnosis.

We have aspirated one case of pheochromocytoma that demonstrated a ganglioneuromatous component in which large ganglion cells with excentric nuclei with prominent nucleoli were dispersed in a dense neurofibrillary matrix in addition to the pheochromocytes.

Immunochemistry to demonstrate the presence of chromogranin, a constituent of the secretory granules, is supportive evidence of pheochromocytoma. Similarly a Grimelius stain will be positive. Ultrastructurally the pheochromocytoma displays distinctive granules corresponding to norepinephrine and epinephrine.

The differential diagnosis may include adrenocortical carcinoma or metastatic melanoma. Pheochromocytomas may contain melanin, in which case a positive Grimelius stain may lead to an erroneous conclusion of melanoma.

Neuroblastoma, Ganglioneuroblastoma and Ganglioneuroma

Neuroblastoma, ganglioneuroblastoma and ganglioneuroma are tumors derived from the nonchromaffin cells of the sympathetic nervous system of the medulla. Because they are capable of the synthesis and metabolism of catecholamines, elevations in urinary and plasma levels of catecholamines and their metabolites are useful tumor markers. These tumors constitute a spectrum representing progressive stages in the maturation of neuroblasts to mature ganglion cells. Neuroblastoma is a highly malignant tumor of childhood composed of cells that resemble primitive neuroblasts. Apart from tumors of the central nervous system, it is the most common solid tumor in infancy and childhood and occurs most frequently in the first 4 years of life, with a peak incidence in the first 2 years. Metastatic disease to the lymph nodes, bones and liver is frequently present when the patient first presents. Neuroblastoma is the most frequent congenital malignant tumor. It may also occur extra-adrenally in relationship to sympathetic nerve trunks. Prognosis depends on age and stage, with better prognoses recorded for children who are less than 1 year of age and who have low-stage disease. A special category, Stage IVS, occurs in patients with metastases confined to liver, skin or marrow without skeletal involvement and is associated with a good prognosis and the likelihood of spontaneous regression.

The most poorly differentiated tumors histologically occur as cellular neoplasms composed of uniform small, round cells that resemble neuroblasts with hyperchromatic, dense nuclei and scanty cytoplasm. Rosette formation and the presence of a fibrillary matrix that ultrastructurally corresponds to neural cell processes are helpful as early signs of neurodifferentiation. Features suggesting maturation of tumor cells include enlarged and vesicular nuclei with large nucleoli, more

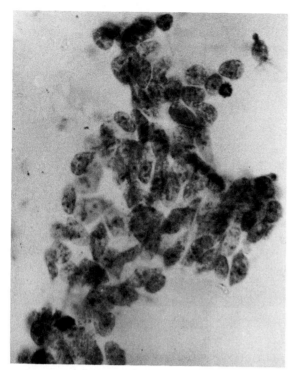

FIGURE 28–32. Fine needle aspiration cytology of **neuroblastoma** demonstrating an aggregate of small round-to-oval cells with high nucleocytoplasmic ratio and coarsely granular chromatin, characteristic of poorly differentiated neuroblastoma (Papanicolaou stain; ×665).

abundant cytoplasm and large amounts of fibrillary matrix material.

Ganglioneuroblastomas are composed of ganglion cells and differentiating neuroblasts, whereas ganglioneuromas consist of differentiated ganglion cells dispersed among nerve bundles and Schwann and fibrous cells.

Cytology. The cells are small and round, with dense, hyperchromatic nuclei and coarsely clumped chromatin with extremely scanty cytoplasm (Fig. 28–32). The Papanicolaou stain reveals the background fibrillary

matrix to stain cyanophilic. The cells may be single or clustered. Ultrastructural studies show sheets of closely opposed small cells with abundant dendritic processes containing microtubules and small, dense, core membrane–bound secretory granules[109] (Fig. 28–33). Cytologically neuroblastomas show features very similar to those described under histology. Signs of differentiation include enlargement and variations in size of nucleoli and vesicular nucleus and increasing prominence of cytoplasmic processes. Ganglion cells may be mature or immature and are noted dispersed with nerve fibers.

Differential diagnosis may include lymphoma, Ewing's sarcoma and rhabdomyosarcoma[124] and, in an adult, undifferentiated small-cell carcinoma. The differentiating characteristics of these small blue cell tumors have been discussed (see section on Wilms' tumor).

RETROPERITONEUM

FNA has revolutionized the evaluation of lesions in the retroperitoneum, which were formerly delineated radiologically and followed by exploratory laparotomy.

Over a 3-year period at the MD Anderson Cancer Center, during which 6797 FNAs were performed, 4.6% represented aspirates from retroperitoneal masses. The most frequent malignant diagnoses in descending order of frequency were metastatic carcinoma, lymphoma, sarcomas, germ cell tumor and other miscellaneous neoplasms. Non-neoplastic lesions accounted for just 3% of the diagnoses (Table 28–2). There were a significant percentage of nondiagnostic or inadequate aspirations, most likely reflecting the technical difficulty of procuring tissue from certain sites or the intrinsic nature of certain lesions.

Imaging Techniques

Transperitoneal percutaneous retroperitoneal lymph node aspiration biopsies are obtained under fluoros-

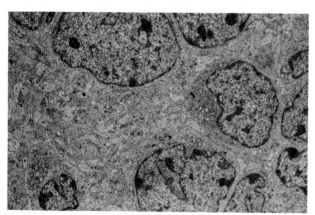

FIGURE 28–33. Ultrastructure of **neuroblastoma** demonstrating small cells with abundant dendritic processes containing microtubules and dense core neurosecretory granules (×4800). (Courtesy of Dr. Bruce MacKay, MD Anderson Cancer Center, Houston, Texas.)

TABLE 28–2. Cytologic Diagnosis of 314 Retroperitoneal Masses by FNA Performed at the MD Anderson Cancer Center*

Diagnosis	Number	%
Metastatic carcinoma (cervix, endometrium, ovary, prostate, bladder)	101	32
Lymphoma	87	28
Sarcoma	17	5
Germ cell tumor	7	2
Other neoplasms (melanoma, ovarian stromal tumor)	6	2
Miscellaneous non-neoplastic lesions (inflammatory, cyst, lymphocele)	10	3
Negative for malignancy	28	9
Inadequate or nondiagnostic	58	19
Total	314	100

*Representing 4.6% of a series of 6797 FNA (1758 deep, 5039 superficial) obtained at the MD Anderson Cancer Center from October 1986 to June 1989.

copy guidance following opacification by bilateral lymphangiography.[40, 136] Lymph nodes involved by carcinomas demonstrate a filling defect following lymphangiography, from which area a biopsy is taken. A more diffuse involvement of a lymph node is seen in lymphoma, and the site of biopsy is not as critical.[136] CT and ultrasound are also well-established modalities used for guiding FNA biopsies of retroperitoneal masses. A flexible 23-gauge needle available in 15- and 20-cm lengths is used.[136] An anterior transperitoneal approach is suitable for biopsy of the periaortic and pelvic lymph nodes, whereas paraspinal masses lateral or posterior to the great vessels are biopsied with the patient in the prone position. Very few complications are reported from large series. Needle passage through bowel or vessels does not pose a greater risk of complications.[136]

For evaluation of carcinomas and sarcoma, smears are prepared in standard fashion and tissue is triaged for cell block and special studies as necessary. FNA tissue from lymphadenopathy caused by lymphoproliferative disorders requires special handling. After determining adequacy, the specimen remaining in the needle is flushed into a preservative medium, from which Cytospin preparations can be prepared for immunohistochemical testing for immunologic classification. Cell lineage is determined using a battery of lymphocyte surface markers for detection of B cell and T cell subsets.[19] Additional cells may be obtained for nucleic acid flow cytometry, cytogenetics and immunoglobulin and T cell receptor gene rearrangements. Together, these studies require a minimum of 10 million cells, which is achievable by performing multiple separate needle passes. Each needle pass will usually yield a cell count of 1 to 2 million cells/ml of preservative fluid.[19]

Anatomy

The retroperitoneal space is mesodermally derived and is the region between the posterior layer of the parietal peritoneum and the muscles of the posterior wall of the abdominal cavity. It extends from the diaphragm superiorly through to the pelvic peritoneal attachments inferiorly and encompasses the lumbar and iliac regions. The anterior extent of the space is limited to the posterior layer of the parietal peritoneum and the mesentery of the small bowel and the colon. The major structures within this area include the abdominal aorta, inferior vena cava, kidneys, ureters and adrenal glands and the sympathetic trunks, celiac and sacral plexus of nerves. The space is filled with fibrous tissue, fat, fascia, loose areolar connective tissue, blood and lymphatic vessels and lymph nodes and nerves.[15, 52]

A primary retroperitoneal tumor is generally considered to be one that originates independently within the retroperitoneal space without primary anatomic connection to any of the retroperitoneal organs.[15] Tumors of the retroperitoneum may be broadly classified as being of mesodermal or neurogenous origin, as arising from tissue remnants and heterotopic tissue or as involving lymph nodes, both primary lymphomas or metastases (Table 28–3).[15]

TABLE 28–3. Tumors of the Retroperitoneum

Tissue	Benign	Malignant
Mesodermally Derived		
Adipose	Lipoma	Liposarcoma
Smooth muscle	Leiomyoma	Leiomyosarcoma
Connective	Fibroma	Fibrosarcoma
Lymphatics	Lymphangioma	Lymphangiosarcoma
Blood vessels	Hemangioma	Angiosarcoma
	Hemangiopericytoma	Hemangiopericytoma
Primitive mesenchyma	Myxoma	Myxosarcoma
	Mesenchymoma	
Histiocytes	Xanthogranuloma	Xanthosarcoma
Neurogenous		
Nerve sheath	Neurofibroma	Neurogenic sarcoma
	Neurilemoma	Malignant schwannoma
Sympathetic nervous system	Ganglioneuroma	Neuroblastoma
Extra-adrenal	Non-chromaffin paraganglioma	Pheochromocytoma
Paraganglion system	Paraganglioma	
	Pheochromocytoma	
Arising from Tissue Remnants and Heterotopic Tissue		
Embryonic	Teratoma	Seminoma
		Embryonal carcinoma
		Teratoma
		Endodermal sinus tumor
		Chordoma
Renal blastema		Wilms' tumor
Heterotopic adrenal tissue		Adrenocortical carcinoma
Lymph Nodes		
		Lymphoma
		Metastatic neoplasms

Neoplastic Lesions

It is beyond the scope of this chapter to detail the multitude of tumors in the retroperitoneum. Some are extremely rare and have not been described by FNA.

Benign Tumors and Masses

There is a limited but growing experience with FNAs from these sites. FNA of a retroperitoneal cystic schwannoma demonstrated numerous single spindle-shaped cells with thin wavy cytoplasm and cigar-shaped nuclei.[80] The presence of isolated cells and clusters of Schwann cells arranged in an organoid pattern of Verocay bodies is characteristic of schwannoma. Deep-seated retroperitoneal lipomas are rare and, in fact, distinction of large lipomas of the retroperitoneum from well-differentiated liposarcomas may be exceedingly difficult. It is likely that most of the huge retroperitoneal lipomas previously described represent well-differentiated liposarcomas. Other miscellaneous benign conditions that can be diagnosed by FNA include abscesses, cysts, hematoma and infectious granulomatous processes such as tuberculoma.

Retroperitoneal Sarcomas

Retroperitoneal sarcomas compose 13% of all sarcomas.[52] The most common sarcomas reported in this site are liposarcoma, leiomyosarcoma, fibrosarcoma, MFH, neurogenic sarcomas and other unclassified sarcomas.[52] Preoperative diagnosis by FNA of soft tissue lesions may be of value in the preoperative evaluation of the patient and in the choice of operation; however, definitive classification should be based on the surgical resection.[78] Reports of the accuracy of cytology in retroperitoneal sarcomas are limited to a few cases or single case reports.

Liposarcoma

The retroperitoneum is the second most common location for this tumor, which may reach a very large size. Because of the difficulty in completely excising these tumors, there is a high rate of local recurrence. Owing to local compression effects, massive recurrence may be fatal. The Armed Forces Institute of Pathology classification[35] divides liposarcoma into four categories: (1) myxoid liposarcoma, (2) round cell liposarcoma, (3) well-differentiated liposarcoma and (4) pleomorphic liposarcoma.

Myxoid liposarcoma is the most common type of liposarcoma and is characterized histologically by proliferating lipoblasts in various stages of differentiation, a delicate plexiform capillary pattern and a myxoid matrix. On cytology the tumor cells appear small and uniform with indistinct cytoplasmic borders. The myxoid background, which stains metachromatically blue-red with the Diff-Quik stain, contains numerous delicate plexiform capillaries composed of small branching aggregates of endothelial cells.[130] A few small multivacuolated lipoblasts may be found, which are characterized by an excentric scalloped hyperchromatic nucleus with surrounding fat vacuoles (Fig. 28–34).[2]

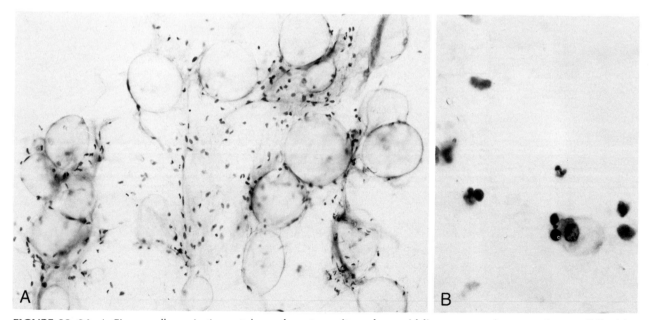

FIGURE 28–34. *A*, Fine needle aspiration cytology of a **retroperitoneal myxoid liposarcoma** demonstrating small lipoblasts and mature adipocytes set in a myxoid background containing a few plexiform capillaries (Papanicolaou stain; ×110). *B*, High magnification demonstrating an occasional lipoblast characterized by an excentric hyperchromatic nucleus with surrounding fat vacuoles (Papanicolaou stain; ×425).

Round cell liposarcomas are closely related to myxoid liposarcomas and tend to be more aggressive.[34] Cytologically there are excessive numbers of uniform small, round cells with vesicular nuclei that may be confused with other small round cell neoplasms. The presence of an occasional vacuolated lipoblast as well as ultrastructural examination for lipid confirms the diagnosis.

Well-differentiated liposarcomas closely simulate lipomas histologically except for the presence of a few lipoblasts, cells with hyperchromatic nuclei or lipocytes showing greater variability in size compared with normal. Dedifferentiated liposarcomas are recognized by the coexistence of a well-differentiated liposarcomatous component with a dedifferentiated cellular component that resembles pleomorphic MFH.[36] By histology, well-differentiated liposarcoma may have a fibrosclerotic and spindle cell component together with focal atypical pleomorphic nuclei.

Pleomorphic liposarcoma resembles MFH cytologically but can be diagnosed based on the demonstration of lipoblasts in smears. Lipoblasts may resemble signet-ring cells or may be large, vacuolated cells with hyperchromatic scalloped nuclei.[130]

The differential diagnosis of liposarcoma, depending on the subtype, includes myxoid fibrosarcoma, MFH of myxoid type and high-grade MFH, extraskeletal myxoid chondrosarcoma and chordoma.[2]

Leiomyosarcoma

Leiomyosarcoma is second in frequency to liposarcoma and frequently arises from the uterus and grows retroperitoneally. The smears are characterized by single cells and clusters of cells with abundant eosinophilic cytoplasm and indistinct cell borders. The nuclei are predominantly cigar shaped with finely granular chromatin and indistinct nucleoli. The cytoplasm is usually abundant and syncytial. Leiomyosarcomas also occur intra-abdominally in the mesentery. The differential diagnosis includes neurogenic sarcoma, whereas the high-grade tumors may resemble MFH. Smooth muscle actin is detected by immunohistochemistry. Ultrastructural studies of differentiated leiomyosarcomas shows thin myofilaments with dense bodies.

Malignant Fibrous Histocytoma

MFH is the most common sarcoma of late life, occurring predominantly in the muscles of the extremities, followed by the retroperitoneum. Pleomorphic, myxoid, giant-cell, inflammatory and angiomatoid subtypes have been described.[34] Inflammatory MFHs occur most commonly in the retroperitoneum and are composed of sheets of histiocytic and inflammatory cells. The histiocytes appear to be xanthomatous because of prominent cytoplasmic lipid. These tumors are most often confused with lymphocytic depleted Hodgkin's disease. Histologically most MFHs are cellular, with a mixture of storiform and pleomorphic areas. FNA of

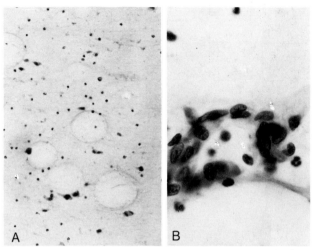

FIGURE 28–35. *A,* Fine needle aspiration cytology of a **low grade myxoid malignant fibrous histiocytoma** showing the myxoid background containing scattered fibroblast- and histiocyte-like cells (Papanicolaou stain; ×110). *B,* High magnification of Figure 28–37A demonstrating an aggregate of spindle cells with hyperchromatic nuclei (Papanicolaou stain; ×265).

low-grade myxoid MFH is composed of a mixture of fibroblast- and histiocyte-like cells in a myxoid background (Fig. 28–35). High-grade MFH shows marked nuclear atypia occurring in a mixture of fibroblast- and histiocyte-like cells with multinucleated giant cells. This may be impossible to differentiate from pleomorphic liposarcoma.

Round Cell Sarcomas

In the retroperitoneum the differential diagnosis of a small round cell tumor includes embryonal rhabdomyosarcoma, extra-skeletal Ewing's sarcoma, neuroblastoma and small-cell undifferentiated carcinoma and lymphoma. For a discussion of their differentiating features see the section on Wilms' tumor.

Embryonal Rhabdomyosarcomas

These are tumors of childhood and adolescence and occur most frequently in the head and neck region, followed by the urogenital tract and the retroperitoneum.[116] By FNA the cells may be small and round or more oval and spindled in a myxoid background. Rhabdomyoblasts, which are cells showing an excentric nucleus and more abundant eosinophilic cytoplasm, may be found (Fig. 28–36). These may be tadpole or racket shaped. Immunoperoxidase stains for desmin and myoglobin are usually positive, the more sensitive stain being desmin, which may demonstrate positive staining even in the most poorly differentiated tumors. By ultrastructural studies, identification of myofilaments and Z band material is confirmatory but may be difficult to demonstrate.

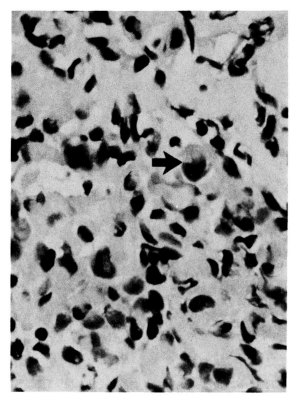

FIGURE 28–36. Fine needle aspiration cytology of **embryonal rhabdomyosarcoma** demonstrating small oval-to-spindle cells set in a myxoid background. Occasional rhabdomyoblasts (arrow) characterized by excentric nuclei and more abundant eosinophilic cytoplasm are present (Papanicolaou stain; ×265).

Lymphoma

One of the most frequent indications for FNA of retroperitoneal masses is for the evaluation of lymphoma. The indications for FNA of lymphoma in this site include establishing an initial diagnosis of lymphoma prior to excisional biopsy, diagnosis of lymphadenopathy in patients with a history of more than one neoplasm, pathologic diagnosis in patients who are poor candidates for excisional biopsy, evaluation of a residual or recurrent mass following either radiation or chemotherapy, staging of lymphoma, evaluation of other lesions (neoplastic or infectious) that may occur in the course of the disease and acquisition of tissue for immunologic markers. For optimal cytologic diagnosis morphology should be supplemented with immunocytochemistry.[19] In a study involving FNA of 238 cases of intra-abdominal and retroperitoneal lymphoma, non-Hodgkin's lymphoma composed 82% of cases, followed by Hodgkin's lymphoma (Table 28–4).[19] The sensitivity of FNA of retroperitoneal lymphomas may not reach the sensitivity of FNAs of lymphomas in superficial sites because of the technical difficulties intrinsic to aspirating in these sites. Some of the pitfalls in FNA of lymphoma include difficulty in interpreting low- and intermediate-grade lymphomas without benefit of immunocytochemistry studies, in which differentiation from reactive processes may be difficult, and poor yield of cells, such as in nodular sclerosing Hodgkin's disease. Lymph nodes showing lymphangiogram effect may be falsely classified as negative if marker studies are not performed. The cytology of lymphangiogram effect is characterized by a polymorphous lymphocytic population with large multinucleated giant cells and histiocytes (Fig. 28–37). Other tumors to be considered in the differential diagnosis of lymphoma include small round blue cell tumors (see earlier) and poorly differentiated carcinoma. For a detailed cytologic description of the various subtypes of non-Hodgkin's and Hodgkin's lymphoma see Chapter 26, Lymph Nodes.

Metatastic Tumors

FNA is frequently utilized in the staging of metastatic disease and may obviate the need for exploratory

TABLE 28–4. Diagnosis of 238 Intra-abdominal or Retroperitoneal Masses Using a Combined Morphologic and Immunochemical Approach

Diagnosis	%	Marker Studies
Lymphoma or consistent with lymphoma	54	
Non-Hodgkin's lymphoma*	82	Monotypic kappa (42%)
		Monotypic lambda (36%)
Immunoblastic	2	T cell lymphoma (1%)
Small noncleaved cell lymphoma	5	No staining for lambda, kappa or Leu-4 (6%)
Lymphoblastic lymphoma	1	
Large-cell lymphoma	47	
Mixed cell lymphoma	11	
Small cleaved cell lymphoma	30	
Small lymphocytic (well-differentiated lymphocytic) lymphoma	4	
Hodgkin's lymphoma	12	
Lymphoma, not classified	6	
Carcinoma	2	
Inconclusive (malignant versus reactive)	11	
Negative for malignancy	12	
Nondiagnostic	22	

*Classified according to the Working Formulation for non-Hodgkin's lymphoma.
(Adapted from Cafferty LL, Katz RL, Ordonez NG, Cabanillas FR: Fine needle aspiration diagnosis of intra-abdominal and retroperitoneal lymphomas by a morphologic and immunocytochemical approach. Cancer 65:72–77, 1990.)

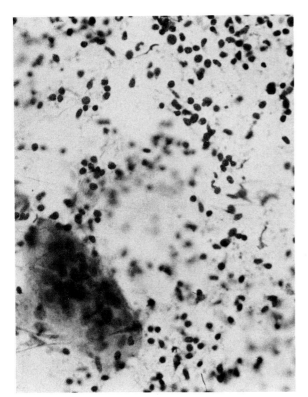

FIGURE 28–37. Fine needle aspiration of a lymph node demonstrating **lymphangiogram effect.** Note the polymorphous lymphocytic population and large multinucleated giant cells (Papanicolaou stain; × 165).

laparotomy. The most frequent carcinomas diagnosed in the retroperitoneum are those arising in pelvic organs, namely, prostate, testes, urinary bladder, cervix and endometrium. These tumors metastasize to pelvic and para-aortic regional lymph nodes in a sequential manner. Tumors from other primary sites that may involve retroperitoneal nodes and present as masses include ovaries, kidneys, adrenals, stomach, colon, pancreas, lungs, breasts and melanoma.[116]

Cytology. The diagnosis of metastatic carcinoma is usually straightforward, relying on the presence of "alien" cells, which are cells not normally indigenous to normal lymph node constituents. Comparing with prior histologies and obtaining the correct clinical history are of paramount importance. The usual types cells that develop into carcinomas are squamous cells from the uterine cervix, vagina and lung. Adenocarcinomas may derive from the gastrointestinal tract, prostate, uterus, ovaries, breast or lung tissue. Their cytologic appearance is similar to that described for their primary locations.

Germ Cell Tumors

Germ cell tumors are usually encountered in the retroperitoneum as metastases from primary germ cell tumors of the testes and ovaries (Fig. 28–38). Rarely, germ cell tumors in the retroperitoneum can occur as primary (extragonadal) germ cell tumors. The most

common malignant germ cell tumor is seminoma. Other germ cell tumors include embryonal carcinoma, endodermal sinus tumor (EST), choriocarcinoma and teratoma. Malignant germ cell tumors composed of a mixture of histologic patterns can occur.

Cytology. FNA of seminoma discloses single cells and loose groups of cells with highly vacuolated cytoplasm and a single large central nucleus with a prominent eosinophilic nucleolus. Differentiation from large-cell lymphoma can be problematic; however, seminoma may be admixed with mature lymphocytes and stain positively for placental alkaline phosphatase and negatively for LCA. On FNA, embryonal carcinomas are composed of syncytial groups of cells with anaplastic primitive nuclear features including prominent nucleoli, resembling poorly differentiated adenocarcinoma. Distinction between embryonal carcinoma and EST tumor is difficult.[116] Immunoperoxidase staining in these tumors is positive for alpha-fetoprotein. Occasionally, the malignant giant cells of a choriocarcinoma may be seen mixed with other germ cell elements and will stain positively with beta-human chorionic gonadotropin.

In children the majority of germ cell–derived neoplasms are composed exclusively or partially of teratomatous components. Teratomas are derived from all three germ cell layers. Common locations for teratomas in children include ovaries, retroperitoneum, stomach,

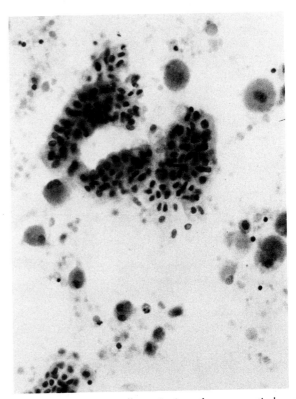

FIGURE 28–38. Fine needle aspiration of a para-aortic lymph node demonstrating a fragment of mature glandular epithelium in a background of histiocytes, consistent with **mature teratoma.** This patient had a history of a mixed germ cell tumor of the testis and had received chemotherapy (Papanicolaou stain; × 165).

TABLE 28–5. Accuracy of FNA Biopsy of Renal Masses Based on a Review of 922 Cases

Authors	Number of Cases		Sensitivity	Specificity	Accuracy	PV Positive	PV Negative
Droese and coworkers[28]	17		70	100	NS	99	75
Porter and coworkers[98]	28		68	NS	66	NS	NS
Juul and coworkers[54]	301		NS	NS	82	93	71
Pilotti and coworkers[96]	132		93	96	NS	93	NS
Nosher and coworkers[85]	17		NS	NS	95	NS	NS
Jeans and coworkers[53]	87*		NS	NS	99	NS	NS
Sundaram and coworkers[120]	20		NS	NS	100	NS	NS
Orell and coworkers[88]	69		NS	NS	90	NS	NS
Suen and coworkers[117]	96		88	NS	92	100	NS
Dekmezian and coworkers[23]	155†		75	100	NS	100	NS
Total	922	Average	79	99	89	99	73

*Predominantly cysts or hypernephrosis.
†Predominantly neoplasms.
PV = predictive value; NS = not stated.

liver and kidneys. Teratomas may be composed of mature or immature components. Retroperitoneal teratomas not associated with an organ account for 2 to 4% of germ cell neoplasms in childhood. The majority of teratomas are microscopically benign by virtue of the exclusive presence of mature somatic tissue. Between 10 and 15% are composed of a mixture of embryonic or fetal elements or immature structures and have an indeterminate biologic behavior.

Diagnostic Accuracy of FNA in Kidney, Adrenal and Retroperitoneum

In a review of ten series encompassing 922 renal aspirates (Table 28–5), the overall sensitivity rate for malignancy was 79%, the specificity was 99% and the overall accuracy was 89%. The predictive value for a positive result was 99%, and the predictive value for a negative result was 73%. There are few studies that have addressed the accuracy of FNA of the adrenal gland. In one study of asymptomatic and incidental masses in 22 patients with adrenal lesions,[56] the overall sensitivity of FNA in detecting the presence of malignancy was 85%, and the number of patients correctly classified for all adrenal masses was 90%. The test was 100% specific for malignant lesions. Two other FNA adrenal studies were associated with accuracies of between 80 and 90% and 93%,[47] respectively.

The reported accuracy of FNA of retroperitoneal lesions has ranged from a low of 53%[93] to a high of 96%.[116] Whereas the sensitivity of FNA of retroperitoneal lymph nodes involved by metastatic carcinoma is high, the sensitivity in the diagnosis of intra-abdominal and retroperitoneal lymphomas is lower. In a large series evaluating FNA of lymphoma in this site, the sensitivity was 66%, the predictive value of a positive result was 100% and the predictive value of a negative result was 42%.[19] The reasons for the last results were the high incidence of nondiagnostic or false-negative FNA specimens due to errors in sampling, the influence of previous radiation or chemotherapy on the recovery of cells and the presence of sclerosing lymphomas. In this situation, open biopsy is mandatory if clinical suspicion is high.

References

1. Abrams HL, Spiro R, Goldstein N: Metastases in carcinoma. Analysis of 1000 autopsied cases. J Urol 81:711–719, 1959.
2. Akerman M, Rydholm A: Aspiration cytology of lipomatous tumors: A 10 year experience at an orthopedic oncology center. Diagn Cytopathol 3:295–301, 1987.
3. Akhtar M, Ashraf A, Sabbah R, Bakry M, Bash NE: Fine-needle aspiration biopsy diagnosis of round cell malignant tumors of childhood. Cancer 55:1805–1817, 1985.
4. Akhtar M, Ashraf AA, Sackey K, Burgess A: Fine-needle aspiration biopsy of clear cell sarcoma of the kidney: Light and electron microscopic features. Diagn Cytopathol 5:181–187, 1989.
5. Amendola MA, Bree BL, Pollack HM, Francis IR, Glazer GM, Jafri SZ, Tomaszewski JE: Small renal cell carcinomas: Resolving a diagnostic dilemma. Radiology 166:637–641, 1988.
6. Barsky SH: Normal histology of the genitourinary tract. In Surgical Pathology of Urologic Diseases. Edited by N Javadpour, SH Barsky. Baltimore, Williams & Wilkins, pp 16–26, 1987.
7. Beckwith JB: Wilms' tumor and other renal tumors of childhood: A selective review from the National Wilms' Tumor Study Pathology Center. Hum Pathol 14:481–492, 1985.
8. Beckwith JB: Wilms' tumor and other renal tumors of childhood: An update. J Urol 136:320–324, 1986.
9. Beckwith JB, Palmer NF: Histopathology and prognosis of Wilms' tumors. Results from the first National Wilms' Tumor Study. Cancer 41:1937, 1978.
10. Bell ET: Renal Disease, 2nd ed. Philadelphia, Lea & Febiger, p 435, 1950.
11. Bennington JL: Tumors of the kidney. In Surgical Pathology of Urologic Diseases. Edited by N Javadpour, SH Barsky. Baltimore, Williams & Wilkins, pp 106–137, 1987.
12. Bennington JL, Benning JL: Tumors of the kidney, renal pelvis, and ureter. In Atlas of Tumor Pathology. Washington, DC, Washington Armed Forces Institute of Pathology, pp 163–166, 1975.
13. Berkman WA, Bernardino ME, Sewell CW, Price RB, Sones PJ: The computed tomography–guided adrenal biopsy. An alternative to surgery in adrenal mass diagnosis. Cancer 53:2098–2103, 1984.
14. Bishop GA, Waugh J, Horvath JS, Johnson JR, Hall BM, Philips J, Duggin GG, Sheil AG, Tiller DJ: Diagnosis of renal allograft rejection by analysis of fine-needle aspiration biopsy specimens with immunostains and simple cytology. Lancet 2:645–650, 1986.
15. Bosniak MA, Siegelman SS, Evans JA: The Adrenal Retroperitoneum and Lower Urinary Tract. Chicago, Year Book Medical Publishers, pp 232–237, 1976.
16. Boudreaux D, Waisman J, Skinner DG, Low R: Giant adrenal myelolipoma and testicular interstitial cell tumor in a man with congenital 21-hydroxylase deficiency. Am J Surg Pathol 3:109–123, 1979.

17. Bray GL, Pendergrass TW, Schaller RT, Kiviat N, Beckwith JB: Preoperative chemotherapy in the treatment of Wilms' tumor diagnosed with the aid of fine needle aspiration biopsy. Am J Pediat Hematol Oncol 8:75–78, 1986.

18. Brennan MF: Adrenocortical carcinoma. Cancer 37:348, 1987.

19. Cafferty LL, Katz RL, Ordonez NG, Cabanillas FR: Fine needle aspiration diagnosis of intra-abdominal and retroperitoneal lymphomas by a morphologic and immunocytochemical approach. Cancer 65:72–77, 1990.

20. Cajulis R, Katz R, Dekmezian R, El-Naggar A, Ro J: Fine needle aspiration biopsy of renal cell carcinoma: Cytologic parameters, its concordance with histology and flow cytometric (FCM) data. Abstract submitted to International Academy of Pathology, March 1990.

21. Clayman RV: Cancer of the Upper Urinary Tract. *In* Principles and Management of Urologic Cancer, 2nd ed. Edited by N Javadpour, SH Barsky. Baltimore, Williams & Wilkins, pp 544–559, 1983.

22. Commons RR, Callaway CP: Adenomas of the adrenal cortex. Arch Intern Med 81:37–41, 1948.

23. Dekmezian R, Sneige N, Katz RL: Fine needle aspiration cytology of kidney masses. Submitted for publication, 1990.

24. Dekmezian R: Papillary carcinoma of the kidney: Fine needle aspiration of eight cases. (In press.) Diagn Cytopathol, 1990.

25. Didolkar MS, Bescher RA, Elias EG, Moore RH: Natural history of adrenal cortical carcinoma: A clinicopathologic study of 42 patients. Cancer 47:2153–2161, 1981.

26. Dobbie JW: Adrenocortical nodular hyperplasia: The ageing adrenal. J Pathol 99:1–18, 1969.

27. Donnelly JD, Koontz WW: Carcinoma of the renal pelvis: A ten year review. South Med J 68:943–946, 1975.

28. Droese M, Altmannsberger M, Kehl A, Lankisch PG, Weiss R, Weber K, Osborn M: Ultrasound-guided percutaneous fine needle aspiration biopsy of abdominal and retroperitoneal masses: Accuracy of cytology in the diagnosis of malignancy, cytologic tumor typing and use of antibodies to intermediate filaments in selected cases. Acta Cytol 28:368–384, 1984.

29. Dunnill MS, Millard PR, Oliver D: Acquired cystic disease of the kidneys: A hazard of long-term intermittent maintenance haemodialysis. J Clin Pathol 30:868, 1977.

30. Flint A, Cookingham C: Cytologic diagnosis of the papillary variant of renal-cell carcinoma. Acta Cytol 31:325–329, 1987.

31. Franzen S, Brehmer-Anderson E: Cytologic diagnosis of renal cell carcinoma. *In* Renal Tumors: Proceedings of the First International Symposium on Kidney Tumors. New York, Alan R Liss, pp 425–432, 1982.

32. Frierson HF, Mills SE, Innes DJ: Malignant rhabdoid tumor of the pelvis. Cancer 55:1963–1967, 1985.

33. Fuhrman SA, Lasky LC, Limas C: Prognostic significance of morphologic parameters in renal cell carinoma. Am J Surg Pathol 6:655–663, 1982.

34. Enzinger FM, Weiss SW: Malignant fibrohistiocytic tumors. *In* Soft Tissue Tumors. St Louis, CV Mosby, pp 166–199, 1983.

35. Enzinger FM, Weiss SW: Liposarcoma. Tumors. *In* Soft Tissue Tumors. St Louis, CV Mosby, pp 166–199, 1983.

36. Gibson TE: Interrelationship of renal cysts and tumors. Report of three cases. J Urol 71:241, 1954.

37. Glazer HS, Weyman PJ, Sagel SS, Levitt RG, McClennan BL: Nonfunctioning adrenal masses: Incidental discovery on computed tomography. AJR 139:81–85, 1982.

38. Glentoj A, Partoft S: Ultrasound-guided percutaneous aspiration of renal angiomyolipoma. Report of two cases diagnosed by cytology. Acta Cytol 28:265–268, 1984.

39. Goldberg J, Rial M, Casadei D, Vila N, Najun Zarazaga C, Mainetti L: HLA-DR expression in fine-needle aspiration biopsy cell samples as a marker of rejection in kidney grafts. Transplant Proc 20:612–613, 1988.

40. Gothlin JH, Rupp N, Rothenberger KH, MacIntosh PK: Percutaneous biopsy of retroperitoneal lymph nodes. A multicentric study. Eur J Radiol 1:46–50, 1981.

41. Grignon DJ, Ayala AG, El-Naggar A, Wishnow KI, Ro JY, Swanson DA, McLemore D, Giacco GG, Guinee VF: Renal cell carcinoma: A clinicopathologic and DNA flow-cytometric analysis of 103 cases. Mod Pathol 2:35A, 1989.

42. Grignon DJ, Ayala AG, Ro JY, El-Naggar A, Papadopoulos NJ: Primary sarcomas of the kidney: A clincopathologic and DNA flow cytometric study of 17 cases. Cancer 65:1611–1618, 1990.

43. Hamperl H: Zur normalen und pathologischen histologie menslicher speicheldusen. Z Mikrosk Anat Forsch 27:1–55, 1931.

44. Hamperl H: Benign and malignant oncocytoma. Cancer 15:1019–1027, 1962.

45. Hanash KA: Recent advances in the surgical treatment of bilateral Wilms' tumor. *In* Therapeutic Progress in Urological Cancers. New York, Alan R Liss, pp 635–652, 1989.

46. Hayry P, von Willebrand E, Ahonen J, Eklund B, Lautenschlager I: Monitoring of organ allograft rejection by transplantation aspiration cytology. Ann Clin Res 13:264–287, 1981.

47. Heaston DK, Handel DB, Ashton PR, Korobkin M: Narrow gauge needle aspiration of solid adrenal masses. AJR 138:1143–1148, 1982.

48. Hedeland H, Ostberg G, Hokfelt B: On the prevalence of adrenocortical adenomas in an autopsy material in relation to hypertension and diabetes. Acta Med Scand 184:211–214, 1968.

49. Helm CW, Burwood RJ, Harrison NW, Melcher DH: Aspiration cytology of solid renal tumors. J Urol 55:249–253, 1983.

50. Holm HH, Pedersen JF, Kristensen JK, Rasmussen SN, Hancke S, Jensen F: Ultrasonically guided percutaneous puncture. Radiol Clin North Am 13:493–503, 1975.

51. Hough AJ, Hollifield JW, Page DL, Hartmann WH: Prognostic factors in adrenal cortical tumors. A mathematical analysis of clinical and morphologic data. Am J Clin Pathol 72:390–399, 1978.

52. Jaques DP, Coit DG: Soft tissue sarcoma of the retroperitoneum. *In* Surgical Management of Soft Tissue Sarcomas. Edited by MF Brennan, C Skin. pp 157–169, 1986.

53. Jeans WD, Penry JB, Roylance J: Renal puncture. Clin Radiol 23:298–311, 1972.

54. Juul N, Torp-Pedersen S, Gronvall S, Holm HH, Koch F, Larsen S: Ultrasonically guided fine needle aspiration biopsy of renal masses. J Urol 133:579–581, 1985.

55. Karstaedt N, Sagel SS, Stanley RJ, Melson GL, Levitt RG: Computed tomography of the adrenal gland. Radiology 129:723–730, 1978.

56. Katz RL, Patel S, Mackay B, Zornoza J: Fine needle aspiration cytology of the adrenal gland. Acta Cytol 28:269–282, 1984.

57. Katz R, Shirkhoda A: Diagnostic approach to incidental adrenal nodules in the cancer patient. Results of a clinical, radiologic, and fine-needle aspiration study. Cancer 55:1995–2000, 1985.

58. Kearney GP, Mahoney EM: Adrenal cysts. Urol Clin North Am 4:273–283, 1977.

59. Khorsand D: Carcinoma within solitary renal cysts. J Urol 93:440–444, 1963.

60. Kiser GC, Totonchy M, Barry JM: Needle tract seeding after percutaneous renal adenocarcinoma aspiration. J Urol 136:1292–1293, 1986.

61. Klein MJ, Valensi QJ: Proximal tubular adenoma of kidney with so-called oncocytic features. Cancer 38:906–914, 1976.

62. Korobkin M, White EA, Kressel HY, Moss AA, Montagne J-P: Computed tomography in the diagnosis of adrenal disease. AJR 132:231–238, 1979.

63. Kreis HA: Use of fine needle aspiration cytology to diagnose rejection. Transplant Proc 16:1569–1572, 1984.

64. Lang EK: Renal cysts puncture studies. Urol Clin North Am 14:91–102, 1987.

65. Leppaniemi A, Wuokko E, Taavitsainen M, Nordling S, Lehtonen T: Xanthogranulomatous pyelonephritis in a functioning kidney. Ann Chir Gynaecol 76:226–229, 1987.

66. Levin NP: Fine needle aspiration and histology of adrenal cortical carcinoma. A case report. Acta Cytol 25:421–424, 1980.

67. Lieber MM, Tomera KM, Farrow GM: Renal oncocytoma. J Urol 125:481–485, 1981.

68. Lindblom K: Percutaneous puncture of renal cysts and tumors. Acta Radiol 27:66–72, 1946.

69. Linsk JA, Franzen S: Aspiration cytology of metastatic hypernephroma. Acta Cytol 28:250–258, 1984.

70. Lizzas EF, Elyaderani MK, Belis JA: Atypical presentation of xanthogranulomatous pyelonephritis: Diagnosis by ultrasonog-

raphy and fine needle aspiration biopsy. J Urol 132:95–97, 1984.

71. Lockhart JL, Wacksman J, White RV, Older RA, Jackson DC, Johnsrude IS, Glenn JF: Renal cyst puncture and abscess formation. Urology 10:98–99, 1977.

72. Lumb G, Mackenzie DH: The incidence of metastases in adrenal glands and ovaries removed for carcinoma of the breast. Cancer 12:521–526, 1959.

73. Ljungberg B, Stenling R, Roos G: Flow cytometric DNA analysis of renal-cell carcinoma. A study of fine needle aspiration biopsies in comparison with multiple surgical samples. Analyt Quant Cytol 9:505–508, 1987.

74. Mancilla-Jimenez R, Stanley RJ, Blath RA: Papillary renal cell carcinoma: A carcinoma: A clinical, radiologic, and pathologic study of 34 cases. Cancer 38:2469–2480, 1976.

75. McCorkell SJ, Niles NL: Fine needle aspiration of catecholamine-producing adrenal masses: A possible fatal mistake. AJR 145:113–114, 1985.

76. Medeiros LJ, Michie SA, Johnson DE, Warnke RA, Weiss LM: An immunoperoxidase study of renal cell carcinomas: Correlation with nuclear grade, cell type, and histologic pattern. Hum Pathol 19:980–987, 1988.

77. Min KW, Song J, Boesenberg M, Acebey J: Adrenal cortical nodule mimicking small round cell malignancy on fine needle aspiration. Acta Cytol 32:543–546, 1988.

78. Miralles TG, Gosalbez F, Menendez P, Astudilla A, Torre C, Buesa J: Fine needle aspiration cytology of soft-tissue lesions. Acta Cytol 30:671–678, 1986.

79. Mostofi FK, Sobin LH, Torloni H: Histological typing of urinary bladder tumors. In International Histological Classification of Tumours, No. 10. Geneva, World Health Organization, 1973.

80. Neifer R, Nguyen G-K: Aspiration cytology of solitary schwannoma. Acta Cytol 29:12–14, 1983.

81. Nguyen G-K: Cytopathologic aspects of adrenal pheochromocytoma in a fine needle aspiration biopsy. A case report. Acta Cytol 26:354–358, 1982.

82. Nguyen G-K: Percutaneous fine-needle biopsy cytology of the kidney and adrenal. Pathol Annu 1:115–134, 1987.

83. Nguyen G-K: Aspiration biopsy cytology of renal angiomyolipoma. Acta Cytol 28:261–268, 1984.

84. Nocks BN, Heney NM, Daly JJ, Perrona TA, Griffin PP, Prout GR: Transitional cell carcinoma of renal pelvis. Urology 19:472–477, 1982.

85. Nosher JL, Amorosa JK, Leiman S, Plafker J: Fine needle aspiration of the kidney and adrenal gland. J Urol 128:895–899, 1982.

86. Nurmi M, Tyrkko J, Puntala P, Sotarauta M, Antila L: Reliability of aspiration biopsy cytology in the grading of renal adenocarcinoma. Scand J Urol Nephrol 18:151–156, 1984.

87. Orell SR, Sterrett GF, Whitaker D: Manual and Atlas of Fine Aspiration Cytology. New York, Churchill Livingstone, pp 164, 1986.

88. Orell SR, Langlois SLP, Marshall VR: Fine needle aspiration cytology in the diagnosis of solid renal and adrenal masses. Scand J Urol Nephrol 19:211–216, 1985.

89. Osborne BM, Brenner M, Weltzer S, Butler JJ: Malignant Lymphomas presenting as a renal mass: Four cases. Am J Surg Pathol 11:375–382, 1987.

90. Osathanondh V, Potter EL: Pathogenesis of polycystic kidneys. Historical survey. Arch Pathol 77:459, 1964.

91. Pagani JJ: Non-small cell lung carcinoma adrenal metastases. Computed tomography and percutaneous needle biopsy in their diagnosis. Cancer 53:1058–1060, 1984.

92. Pasternak A: Fine-needle aspiration biopsy of human renal homografts. Lancet 2:82, 1968.

93. Pereiras RV, Meiers W, Kunhardt B, Troner M, Hutson D, Barkin JS, Viamonte M: Fluoroscopically guided thin needle aspiration biopsy of the abdomen and retroperitoneum. AJR 131:197–202, 1978.

94. Petersen RO: Kidney. In Urologic Pathology. Philadelphia, JB Lippincott, pp 1–179, 1986.

95. Petersen RO: Renal pelvis. In Urologic Pathology. Philadelphia, JB Lippincott, pp 181–228, 1986.

96. Pilotti S, Rilke F, Alasio L, Garbagnati F: The role of fine needle aspiration in the assessment of renal masses. Acta Cytol 32:1–10, 1988.

97. Pinkus GS, Etheridge CL, O'Connor EM: Are keratin proteins a better tumor marker than epithelial membrane antigen? A comparative immunohistochemical study of various paraffin-embedded neoplasms using monoclonal and polyclonal antibodies. Am J Clin Pathol 85:269–277, 1986.

98. Porter B, Karp W, Forsberg L: Percutaneous cytodiagnosis of abdominal masses by ultrasound guided fine needle aspiration biopsy. Acta Radiol [Diagn] 22:663–668, 1981.

99. Ro JY, Ayala AG, Sella A, Samuels ML, Swanson DA: Sarcomatoid renal cell carcinoma: clinicopathologic. A study of 42 cases. Cancer 59:516–526, 1987.

100. Robinson MJ, Pardo V, Rywlin AM: Pigmented nodules (black adenomas) of the adrenal. An autopsy study of incidence, morphology, and function. Hum Pathol 3:317–325, 1972.

101. Russell RP, Masi AT, Richter ED: Adrenal cortical adenomas and hypertension. A clinical pathologic analysis of 690 cases with matched controls and a review of the literature. Medicine 51:211–225, 1972.

102. Sarnecki CT: Urinary cytology in 1400 patients. J Urol 106:761–764, 1971.

103. Scharfe M, Yokoyama M, Alken P, Jacobi GH, Hohenfellner R: Immunoperoxidase staining of the fine-needle aspiration biopsies of renal cell carcinoma using tumor-specific monoclonal antibody. J Urol 13:331–333, 1987.

104. Scheible W, Coel M, Siemers PT, Siegel H: Percutaneous aspiration of adrenal cysts. AJR 128:1013–1016, 1977.

105. Sease WC, Elyaderani MK, Belis JA: Ultrasonography and needle aspiration in diagnosis of xanthogranulomatous pyelonephritis. Urology 24:231–235, 1987.

106. Sherwood T, Trott PA: Needling renal cysts and tumours: Cytology and radiology. Br Med J 3:755–758, 1975.

107. Shirkhoda A: Current diagnostic approach to adrenal abnormalities. J Comput Tomogr 8:277–285, 1984.

108. Siekavizza JL, Bernardino ME, Samaan NA: Suprarenal mass and its differential diagnosis. Urology 18:625–632, 1981.

109. Silverman JF, Dabbs DJ, Ganick DJ, Holbrook CT, Geisinger KR: Fine needle aspiration cytology of neuroblastoma, including peripheral neuroectodermal tumor, with immunocytochemical and ultrastructural confirmation. Acta Cytol 32:367–376, 1988.

110. Skinner DG, Colvin RB, Vermillion CD, Pfister RC, Leadbetter WF: Renal cell carcinoma. A clinical and pathologic study of 309 cases. Cancer 28:1165–1177, 1971.

111. Sneige N, Dekmezian R, Zaatari GS: Liesegang-like rings in fine needle aspirates of renal/perirenal hemorrhagic cysts. Acta Cytol 32:547–551, 1988.

112. Sotelo-Avila C, Gonzalez-Crussi F, deMello MD, Vogler C, Gooch WM, Gale G, Pena R: Renal and extrarenal rhabdoid tumors in children: A clinicopathologic study of 14 patients. Semin Diagn Pathol 3:151–163, 1986.

113. Sotelo-Avila C, Gonzalez-Crussi F, Sadowinski S, Gooch WM, Pena R: Clear cell sarcoma of the kidney: A clinicopathologic study of 21 patients with long-term follow-up evaluation. Hum Pathol 16:1219–1230, 1986.

114. Spagnolo DV, Michie SA, Crabtree GS, Warnke RA, Rouse RV: Monoclonal anti-keratin (AE1) reactivity in routinely processed tissue from 166 human neoplasms. Am J Clin Pathol 84:697–704, 1985.

115. Steg A: Does percutaneous puncture still have a role to play in the diagnosis of renal tumors? In Renal Tumors. Edited by R Kuss. New York, Alan R Liss, pp 417–423, 1981.

116. Suen KC: Retroperitoneum. In Guides to Clinical Aspiration Biopsy, Retroperitoneum and Intestine. Edited by S Tilde, S Kline. New York, Igaku-Shoin, pp 23–100, 1987.

117. Suen KC: Kidneys and urinary tract. In Guides to Clinical Aspiration Biopsy, Retroperitoneum and Intestine. Edited by S Tilde, S Kline. New York, Igaku-Shoin, pp 131–163, 1987.

118. Suen KC: Adrenals. In Guides to Clinical Aspiration Biopsy, Retroperitoneum and Intestine. Edited by S Tilde, S Kline. New York, Igaku-Shoin, pp 165–189, 1987.

119. Sun CN, Bissada NK, White HJ, Redman JF: Spectrum of ultrastructural patterns of renal cell adenocarcinoma. Urology 9:195–200, 1977.

120. Sundaram M, Wolverson MK, Heiberg E, Pilla T, Vas WG, Shields JB: Utility of CT-guided abdominal aspiration procedures. AJR 139: 1111–1115, 1982.
121. Tachibana V, Kamata S, Sihara K, Sekiene H, Goto S, Fukui I, Kitahara S, Oshima H, Yoshida K, Negishi T: Cytology of percutaneous aspiration biopsy of renal angiomyolipoma: A study of 4 cases. Acta Urol Jpn 33:1873–1878, 1987.
122. Tang CK, Gray GF: Adrenocortical neoplasms. Prognosis and morphology. J Urol 5:691–695, 1975.
123. Tsokos M, Triche TJ: Malignant rhabdoid tumor of the kidney and soft tissues. Arch Pathol Lab Med 113, 1989.
124. Triche TJ, Askin FB: Neuroblastoma and the differential diagnosis of small-, round, and blue cell tumors. Hum Pathol 14:569–595, 1983.
125. Ubhi CS, Irving HC, Guillou PJ, Giles GR: A new technique for renal allograft biopsy. Br J Radiol 60:599–600, 1987.
126. Valkov J, Bojikin B: Fine-needle aspiration biopsy of abdominal and retroperitoneal tumors in infants and children. Diagn Cytopathol 3:129–133, 1987.
127. Von Schreeb T, Franzen S, Ljungqvist A: Renal adenocarcinoma: Evaluation of malignancy on a cytologic basis. A comparative cytologic and histologic study. Scand J Urol Nephrol 1:265–269, 1967.
128. Wahl RW: Fine needle aspiration study of metastatic mixed adenosquamous carcinoma of the renal pelvis. A case report. Acta Cytol 29:580–583, 1985.
129. Wakely JE Jr, Giacomantonio M: Fine needle aspiration cytology of metastatic malignant rhabdoid tumor. Acta Cytol 30:533–537, 1986.
130. Walaas L, Kindblom L-G: Lipomatous tumors: A correlative cytologic and histologic study of 27 tumors examined by fine needle aspiration cytology. Hum Pathol 16:6–18, 1985.
131. Warner NE, Strauss FH: The adrenal. In Principles and Practice of Surgical Pathology, Vol 2. Edited by J Silverberg. New York, John Wiley & Sons, p 1467, 1988.
132. Weeks DA, Beckwith B, Mierau GW: Rhabdoid tumor. An entity or a phenotype? Arch Pathol Lab Med 113:113–120, 1989.
133. Weiss LM: Comparative histologic study of 43 metastasizing and nonmetastasizing adrenocortical tumors. Am J Surg Pathol 8:163–169, 1984.
134. Whitmore ER: Hypernephroid tumors of the kidney. South Med J 29:1051–1062, 1936.
135. Zajicek J: Aspiration biopsy cytology. II. Cytology of infradiaphragmatic organs. In Monographs in Clinical Cytology. Basel, S Karger, pp 1–37, 1987.
136. Zornoza J, Wallace S, Goldstein HM, Lukeman M, Jing B-S: Transperitoneal percutaneous retroperitoneal lymph node aspiration biopsy. Radiology 122:111–115, 1977.

29

Prostate

Lambert Skoog
Edneia Miyki Tani
Torsten Löwhagen

In men over 50 years of age, prostatic carcinoma is the most common cancer in Western countries. It often runs a devious clinical course. Some patients might be untreated, whereas others need all the treatment modalities in the oncologist's armamentarium. The unequivocal diagnosis of prostatic carcinoma can be made only by morphologic evaluation, which is done by light microscopy of histologic or cytologic material. The concept of a transperineal fine needle aspiration (FNA) biopsy of the prostate was introduced by Ferguson in 1930.[16] In spite of promising results, the technique did not gain wide acceptance. Thirty years later the idea was revitalized by Franzén and colleagues,[18] who introduced a device that facilitates transrectal FNA biopsy. Today this technique is a standard procedure at many institutions and has been shown to be reliable and cost-effective with excellent patient acceptance. Fine needle aspiration is used not only as a method for detecting prostatic carcinoma but also for tumor grading, which is of utmost importance in deciding therapy.

DIAGNOSTIC PROCEDURES

The diagnostic workup of prostate disease can be subdivided into noninvasive and invasive procedures. A conclusive diagnosis of prostatic carcinoma can be made only by morphologic evaluation. Obviously, this requires an invasive procedure, such as surgical biopsy, cutting needle biopsy or FNA biopsy. The noninvasive procedures, rectal palpation, ultrasonography, computed tomographic (CT)–scan and enzyme marker tests can at best provide circumstantial evidence for a malignant process in the prostate gland. Rectal palpation and ultrasonography are, however, important methods in screening patients for prostatic disease. In addition they are valuable adjuncts in the staging of patients with carcinomas of the prostate.

Rectal Examination

This examination of the prostate is crucial. The peripheral zone is readily accessible for digital evaluation. A carcinoma usually appears as an induration or an enlargement or both. A variety of conditions, such as infections, granulomatous prostatitis and benign hyperplasia, can however be confused with carcinoma on digital examination. The accuracy of rectal evaluation obviously depends on the experience of the examiner. Esposti[14] and Guinan and associates[21] have reported excellent performance for the palpatory detection of carcinoma. In fact, Guinan's group reported it to be the most efficient of ten screening tests for prostatic carcinoma.

Transrectal Ultrasound (US)

This method has been used lately as an adjunct to digital evaluation. It appears to have an excellent sensitivity in detecting small lesions, although the specificity seems lower. Studies comparing US and rectal palpation indicate that US has a higher detection rate of carcinoma.[27, 36] This difference was mostly pronounced for small operable cancers. However, others report that the specificity of transrectal US seems lower than digital examination.[2] Further technical refinements in transrectal US can be expected, and the method already seems to be an indispensable procedure in the clinical workup of a patient who is undergoing evaluation of the prostate.

Additional Noninvasive Screening Tests

Other tests for prostatic carcinoma, such as marker enzymes and cytology after prostate massage, all have a sensitivity that is far too low to warrant their use in the routine search for a localized prostatic carcinoma.[21]

Thus, in summary, both rectal palpation and transrectal US are efficient methods for detecting prostatic carcinoma, but the actual diagnosis can be made only by evaluation of histologic or cytologic material, obtained by invasive procedures, such as core needle biopsy and FNA biopsy.

Core (Cutting) Needle Biopsy

This method, either transperineal or transrectal, is the most common one to obtain tissue for histologic evaluation. Provided the biopsy is representative, it should result in a conclusive diagnosis. In this respect its value is undisputable. Poor patient acceptance together with the risk of infection (transrectal route) make the procedure less suitable in screening for prostatic carcinoma.[30] If the core needle biopsy is guided by US, the efficiency increases and even small lesions can be evaluated.[26]

A spring-triggered device has been constructed to improve the core needle biopsy technique.[29] The instrument automatically moves the two different parts, the cannula and the obturator, of the core biopsy needle. Prostate biopsy can be performed with this instrument via the transrectal route under ultrasonic guidance. The procedure has a very low failure rate. Complications include urosepsis and bleeding.

Fine Needle Aspiration Biopsy

This is an inexpensive technique with excellent patient acceptance. In Europe it has been used for both detecting prostatic carcinoma and providing a final diagnosis, including tumor grading.[13, 31, 41] Thus, there does not seem to be any qualitative difference between the FNA and core biopsy procedures in terms of

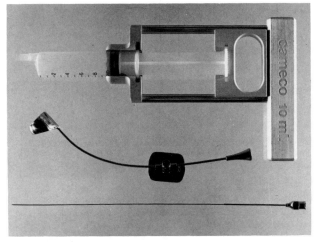

FIGURE 29–1. Material for transrectal aspiration biopsy of the prostate: syringe and the Franzén instruments (needle guide, syringe holder and needle).

contributed morphologic information. Fine needle aspiration biopsy can also be guided by US to increase efficiency.[27]

Technique

The instruments for transrectal FNA biopsy according to the Franzén procedure are presented in Figure 29–1. The holder is designed to fit disposable syringes and to be operated by one hand. The curved needle guide has a ring-like holder at the distal end for insertion of the index finger. The adjustable plate will allow a firm fixation of the guide in the palm during the aspiration procedure. The needle is a 22-gauge 20-cm long, flexible, nondisposable needle. In addition to the instruments depicted in Figure 29–1, gloves and finger cots are required (Fig. 29–2).

For rectal examination and the following biopsy, the

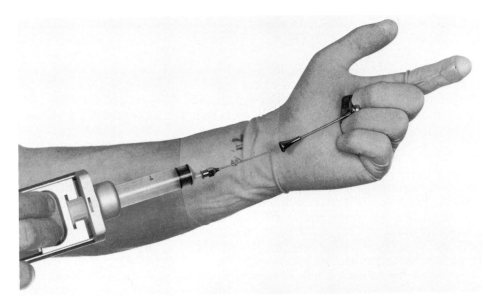

FIGURE 29–2. Franzén instruments positioned before aspiration.

patient should preferably be in the dorsal lithotomy position. He could also be standing and bending forwards or placed in the knee-chest position. Local anesthesia and bowel preparation are not required.

A careful digital examination of the prostate allows identification of areas for biopsy. The needle guide is then mounted on the freshly gloved left index finger (for right-handed persons). The finger cot is utilized to cover the distal part of the guide (see Fig. 29–2). This prevents fecal material from entering the needle when introduced into the rectum. In addition the cot will help to keep the guide in position.

After lubrication the index finger and the guide are inserted into the rectum. The target site is located with the index finger, and the tip of the guide is then pressed firmly against the area. Care should be taken to hold the needle guide parallel to the finger. A deviation from this direction could result in a nonrepresentative biopsy. The needle, attached to the syringe, is then inserted into the guide. The needle tip is pushed into the target. It is important to estimate the depth of the biopsy to avoid sampling from outside the target. Full suction is applied, and the needle is quickly moved back and forth several times with a rotating motion. The negative pressure is released with the needle tip still in the target area. After its withdrawal from the prostate, the needle is detached from the syringe and the aspirate is pressed out on slides. Smears are prepared and air dried or fixed in ethanol.

Patients with acute prostatitis or rheumatism should not be subject to FNA biopsy owing to the risk of septicemia.[15] Patients without these disorders rarely develop septicemia after transrectal FNA biopsy.[15] However, it is still an alarming, life-threatening disease and the patient should be informed about this remote risk. Preferably, written instructions should be given to all patients who undergo prostate FNA biopsy. At some clinics prophylactic antibiotics are prescribed, a policy that always seems to be followed when core needle biopsy is performed. Bleeding from the rectum or penis can occur, but it is quickly self-limiting and requires no treatment.

ANATOMY AND HISTOLOGY

The prostate is a secretory gland that develops during puberty under the influence of testicular androgen. The gland, which encircles the proximal urethra, measures approximately 3 × 3 × 4 cm in an adult man. It is a retroperitoneal organ, separated from the anterior part of the rectum only by the thin septum rectoprostaticum, which makes it accessible to rectal palpation.

Histologically, the gland is a compound tubuloalveolar plexus with a supportive fibromuscular stroma. The acini are lined by a basal myoepithelial cell layer that is covered by a secretory epithelium. The secretory granulae contain acid phosphatase, an enzyme of importance in serum screening tests for prostatic carcinoma.[17] Microscopically, the prostate can be subdivided into a central, a peripheral and a transitional zone as described by McNeal.[33] The central zone rep-

resents about one fourth of the total mass and is composed of large acini. This part of the prostate never seems to be the primary site of prostatic disease. In contrast, the small transitional zone in the upper periurethral part of the gland is the site of the most common prostatic disease—nodular prostatic hyperplasia.[34] This zone seldom is the site of primary malignant changes. The peripheral zone, which is composed of small acini, is the major part of the lateral-caudal part of the gland and constitutes approximately two thirds of the gland. An overwhelming number of the prostatic carcinomas arise in this part of the prostate.[34]

NORMAL GLAND, BENIGN LESIONS

Normal Prostate

The normal prostate gland is firm, but not hard, and has a smooth, well-delineated outer surface on digital examination. Fine needle aspiration biopsy is seldom performed from a palpatory normal gland, except in a patient with metastatic adenocarcinoma of unknown origin.

Cytology

Epithelial cells in monolayers dominate the smears. The cells are uniform with distinct, polygonal outlines and small, round nuclei, sometimes demonstrating a small, indistinct nucleolus (Fig. 29–3). The pale cytoplasm sometimes contains eosinophilic granules in May-Grünwald-Giemsa. A few free-lying nuclei might be found. Stromal cells are very rare.

Nodular Hyperplasia

This condition is so common in men over 50 that it probably does not represent a disease but a normal aging process. It starts in the transitional zone by the formation of discrete nodules of hyperplastic glandular epithelium, accompanied by fibromuscular hyperplasia. These nodules might in some cases compress the urethra leading to urinary tract obstruction of clinical importance. The symtoms include difficulties in starting and stopping the urinary flow, nocturia, urinary retention and dribbling. Acute urinary retention, requiring emergency action, can occur. On digital examination the prostate is diffusely enlarged, often with nodules of varying size. The consistency can vary from soft to boggy to firm.

The microscopic pattern is determined by the predominant proliferative component. Glandular hyperplasia, which is most common, results in cystically dilated glands of varying size. The two-layered epithelium forms prominent papillary folds. The glands are filled with secretion and corpora amylacea. Fibromuscular hyperplasia produces solid strands and areas with few glandular elements. The condition is referred to as fibromyomatous hyperplasia.

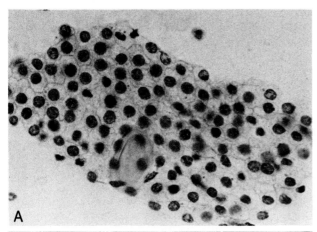

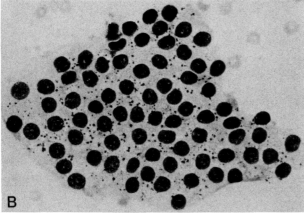

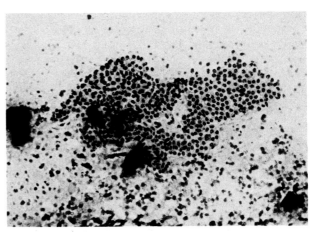

FIGURE 29–4. Benign prostatic hyperplasia. Large sheet of benign epithelial cells and concrements in a proteinaceous background (May-Grünwald-Giemsa stain; ×50).

FIGURE 29–3. Benign prostatic glandular cells. *A*, Flat sheet of epithelial cells with sharp cellular borders and arranged in a honeycomb pattern. Round central nuclei with fine chromatin and without nucleoli. A corpora amylacea is seen with concentrically laminated structure (Papanicolaou stain; ×200). *B*, A sheet of monolayered epithelial cells with cytoplasmic granules (May-Grünwald-Giemsa stain; ×200).

Cytology

The aspirate usually consists of some protein-rich fluid. The amount of epithelium obtained probably relates to the proportion of fibromuscular hyperplasia. The smears are often cellular with sheets of monolayered uniform cells (Fig. 29–4). Cytoplasmic granules are often found and confirm the benign impression. Additional findings include concrement, corpora amylacea, squamous cells and inflammatory cells (see Fig. 29–4). Occasionally, cells from the seminal vesicles or rectal mucosa contaminate the smears. This contamination might present diagnostic difficulties, which are discussed subsequently.

Prostatitis

The acute, chronic and granulomatous variants are described.

Acute prostatitis usually occurs with fever and intense pain. It usually follows surgical manipulation of

the urethra or the prostate but can result from hematogenous spread of distant foci. Bacteria as well as fungi might be the causative agents. The clinical suspicion of an acute infection in the prostate should discourage FNA biopsy attempts because of the risk of septicemia.

Granulocytes and cellular debris are found together with macrophages. Epithelial cells, when present, show degenerative changes (Fig. 29–5).

Chronic prostatitis can be bacterial or nonbacterial. Irrespective of cause the clinical symptoms are vague, including dysuria and low back discomfort. Rectal palpation discloses a slightly enlarged, firm, sometimes irregular prostate, which mimics carcinoma.

Cytologically, the entire spectrum of inflammatory cells can be seen together with histiocytes. The epithelium often exhibits degenerative changes, but reactive alterations can cause diagnostic concern. The presence of inflammatory cells and lack of clear-cut malignant

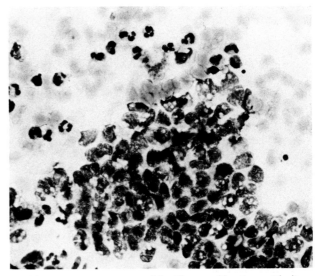

FIGURE 29–5. Acute prostatitis. Cluster of benign epithelium showing degenerative changes and granulocytes (May-Grünwald-Giemsa stain; ×132).

epithelial features should prevent the overdiagnosis of carcinoma. A recommendation of a repeat biopsy seems advisable in this situation.

Granulomatous prostatitis often results from acute or chronic prostatitis. At present, it seems that granulomatous prostatitis is a nonspecific reaction to retention of secretory and inflammatory products. A second type of granulomatous prostatitis is that of tuberculosis. Irrespective of cause, rectal examination reveals an irregular, hard prostate gland giving a strong clinical suspicion of prostatic carcinoma.

Inflammatory cells, including neutrophils, eosinophils, lymphocytes and plasma cells, are observed. Histiocytes containing cellular debris as well as multinuclear giant cells can also be found. Epithelioid cells are required for a conclusive diagnosis (Fig. 29–6).

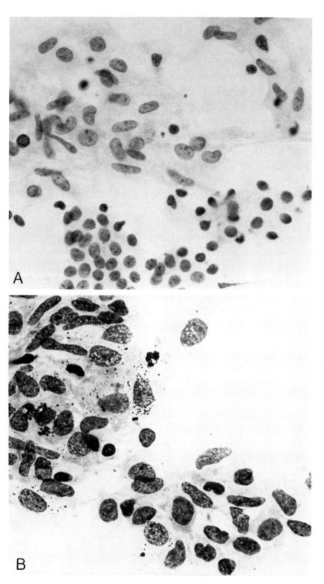

FIGURE 29–6. Granulomatous prostatitis. *A,* Epithelioid histiocytes with elongated or reniform nuclei and epithelial cells with round regular nuclei (Papanicolaou stain; ×160) *B,* Cluster of histiocytes, epithelioid cells and lymphocytes (May-Grünwald-Giemsa stain; ×160).

Epithelial cells often show pronounced reactive changes, including hyperchromasia, prominent nucleoli and crowding. These epithelial changes can in the extreme case be suggestive of carcinoma.[41] The inflammatory components in the smear should, however, alert the cytologist to avoid an overdiagnosis of carcinoma.

Squamous Metaplasia

Focal or extensive squamous metaplasia is a rare condition. It occurs after infarcts, local surgery, estrogen therapy or long-term catheter use.

The smears contain squamous cells without cytologic abnormalities. Inflammatory cells are also present.

MALIGNANT LESIONS

Adenocarcinomas

An overwhelming number of the prostate carcinomas arise in the acini in the peripheral zone and are acinar carcinomas. The incidence of clinical prostatic carcinoma shows a marked racial and age difference. Among Chinese in Hong Kong the incidence is 1 per 100,000; the corresponding figure for African-Americans in the United States is 95 per 100,000.[7, 38] In addition, the age-adjusted incidence increases 100-fold in men between 50 and 75 years.[22]

Latent carcinoma of the prostate is much more prevalent and figures as high as 30% have been reported.[20] The clinical long-term significance of latent carcinomas has not been fully established. However, from the aforementioned figures it can be assumed that only a fraction of the latent carcinomas progress to clinical disease.[9, 24]

Localized prostatic carcinomas rarely cause symtoms and are accidental findings of hard nodules by rectal examination. Larger tumors may produce symptoms indistinguishable from those of benign hyperplasia. The palpatory finding is that of a firm-to-stone hard enlargement, sometimes with overgrowth on surrounding structures. Pain indicates advanced local growth with perineural infiltration. In generalized disease, bone pain and pathologic fractures dominate, but the clinical picture seems immense in variability.

Most malignant lesions are adenocarcinomas. The diagnosis and tumor grading rest on cellular anaplasia, invasion and architectural pattern. Well-differentiated carcinomas exhibit monomorphous epithelia with slightly enlarged nuclei and small nucleoli. The glands are small and lined by one or several layers of neoplastic epithelium, occasionally forming a cribriform pattern. In moderately well-differentiated carcinomas the glands are lined by a multilayered crowded epithelium with distinctly atypical nuclei. Stromal and perineural invasion are readily detectable. In poorly differentiated carcinomas the tumor cells grow essentially without a glandular pattern in sheets, cords and nests. Cellular polymorphism is marked as is nuclear atypia.

A rare variant is the undifferentiated carcinoma, which is composed of small undifferentiated cells with round nuclei and prominent nucleoli. The growth pattern is diffuse. Other uncommon malignant tumors of the prostate are the adenoid cystic, the endometroid, the squamous and the transitional cell carcinomas.

Cytology

The cytologic diagnosis of prostatic carcinoma rests on cellular characteristics as well as on the formation of secondary structures. An integration of these features not only gives a diagnosis but also allows grading.

Well-differentiated carcinomas (grade I) show a marked cellular cohesiveness (Fig. 29–7). The cells occur in tight clusters with crowding and overlapping and with formation of microacini (Fig. 29–8). The cellular borders are indistinct, sharply contrasting with the honeycomb pattern of benign epithelium. Malignant epithelium in most cases lacks cytoplasmic granules but sometimes shows cytoplasmic vacuoles (Fig. 29–9). The nuclei of well-differentiated carcinomas are slightly irregular and enlarged with little polymorphism. Nucleoli are small and inconstant. A high cellularity is often described as an important feature of any prostatic carcinoma. Obviously, this parameter is dependent on so many factors that it is of little diagnostic value. The cytologic characteristics of well-differentiated carcinoma are summarized in Table 29–1.

Moderately differentiated carcinomas (grade II) also exhibit cellular cohesiveness, but microacini are relatively rare. In addition free-lying cells appear as a constant finding. The cytomorphologic features include easily discernable nuclear polymorphism, hyperchromasia and distinct nucleoli (Fig. 29–10). The cells are fragile with poorly retained cytoplasm, and smeared nuclei are seen. These microscopic features of moderately differentiated carcinoma are summarized in Table 29–1.

Poorly differentiated carcinomas (grade III) show lack of cohesiveness, and the majority of cells are free lying, as seen in Figure 29–11. Clusters vaguely resembling acini can occur but are inconstant features. The cytoplasm, when present, is indistinct, but is most often lost. The nuclear polymorphism is often striking, and nucleoli are large. A variant of poorly differentiated carcinoma yields aspirates with completely dissociated, monotonous, often smeared, relatively small cells (Fig. 29–12). The overall picture is that of an undifferentiated neoplasm, and the term "blastic carcinoma" has been suggested. Metastatic lesions are usually the first presentation of this excessively aggressive variant of prostatic carcinoma. Table 29–1 presents the cytologic characteristics of the poorly differentiated carcinoma.

Dysplasia

Duct-acinar dysplasia is a premalignant lesion in preexisting ducts and acini.[35] It is observed in sections from 41% of glands without cancer and 82% of those with invasive carcinoma. The epithelial cells show dysplastic features, such as nuclear enlargement and hyperchromasia, as well as prominent nucleoli. The dysplastic epithelium forms multilayered, sometimes cribriform, structures in ducts and acini. Such lesions have been interpreted as carcinoma *in situ* of the prostate. They are small and thus not detectable by rectal examination. Their relationship to latent carcinoma remains unclear. The cytologic presentation of duct-acinar dysplasia has not been described. It can, however, be anticipated that smears from such lesions will fulfill all the cytomorphologic criteria for malignancy as described.

Accidental aspiration of a small dysplastic lesion will probably yield cells suggestive of carcinoma in a background of normal prostatic epithelium. In the absence of a palpable tumor further diagnostic workup seems mandatory. Normal US or CT scan should result in followup with repeat biopsies and, at this stage, radical prostatectomy should forcibly be discouraged. In this context, it must be emphasized that (1) the biologic behavior of dysplastic lesions is unknown and (2) such lesions are found in approximately 40% of prostates without detectable invasive carcinomas.

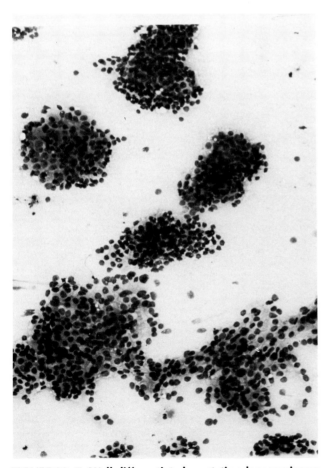

FIGURE 29–7. Well-differentiated prostatic adenocarcinoma (grade I). Cellular smear with clusters of cells with slightly enlarged nuclei showing crowding and overlapping; no cytoplasmic granules (May-Grünwald-Giemsa stain; ×33).

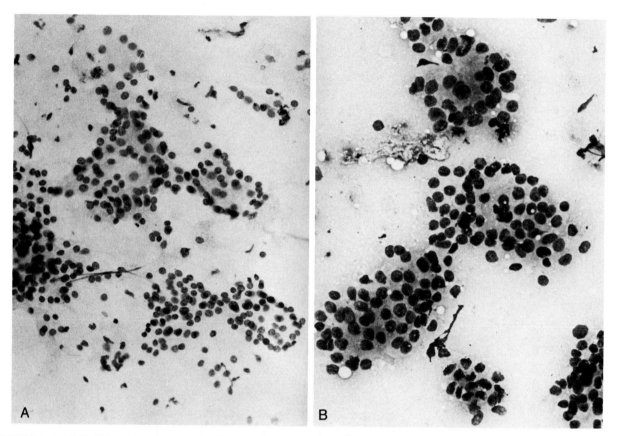

FIGURE 29–8. Well-differentiated prostatic adenocarcinoma (grade I) showing microacinar formations. *A*, Papanicolaou stain; ×66. *B*, May-Grünwald-Giemsa stain; ×66.

TABLE 29–1. Fine Needle Aspiration Cytology of the Prostate

	Normal Hyperplastic Prostate	Prostatic Carcinoma Differentiation		
		Well	*Moderately*	*Poorly*
Cell Pattern				
Monolayers	+ + +	–	–	–
Multilayers/solid clusters	–	+ + +	+ +	(+)
Microglandular	–	+ + +	+ +	(+)
Cell dispersal	–	(+)	(+)+	+ + +
Cell Features				
Defined cell borders	+ + +	(+)	–	–
Cytoplasmic granules	+ + +	–	–	–
Vacuolated cytoplasm	–	+(+)	(+)	–
Nuclear polymorphism	–	+	+ +	+ → + + +
Nucleoli	(+)	+	+	+ +
Periodic acid–Schiff positivity	+ +	+ +	+	(+)

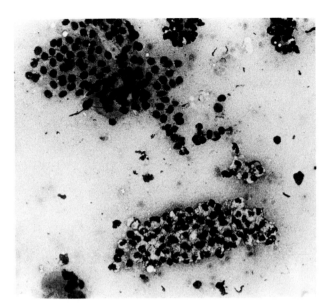

FIGURE 29–9. Well-differentiated prostatic adenocarcinoma (grade I) with vacuolated cytoplasm. Note the contrasting benign epithelium (May-Grünwald-Giemsa stain; ×66).

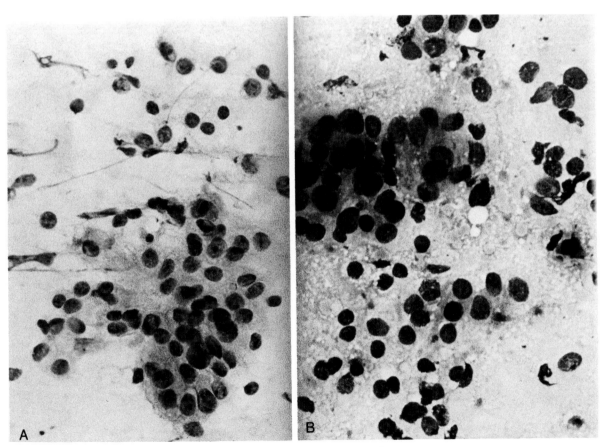

FIGURE 29–10. Moderately well-differentiated prostatic adenocarcinoma (grade II). *A*, Cell clusters and dispersed single cells with enlarged nuclei and prominent nucleoli (Papanicolaou stain; ×80). *B*, Cell clusters and dispersed single cells with enlarged hyperchromatic nuclei (May-Grünwald-Giemsa stain; ×80).

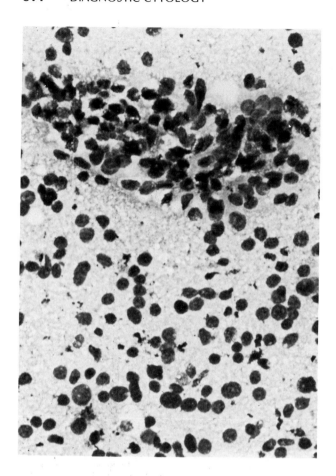

FIGURE 29–11. Poorly differentiated prostatic adenocarcinoma (grade III). Dispersed single cells and a few loose clusters (May-Grünwald-Giemsa stain; ×80).

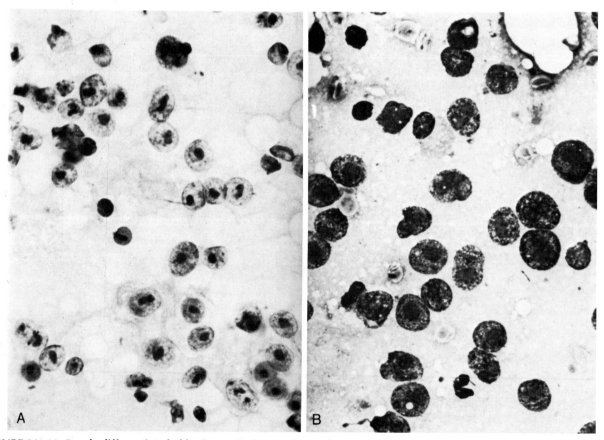

FIGURE 29–12. Poorly differentiated "blastic type" of prostatic carcinoma (grade III). Dispersed monomorphous naked nuclei with large distinct nucleoli. *A*, Papanicolaou stain; ×160. *B*, May-Grünwald-Giemsa stain; ×160.

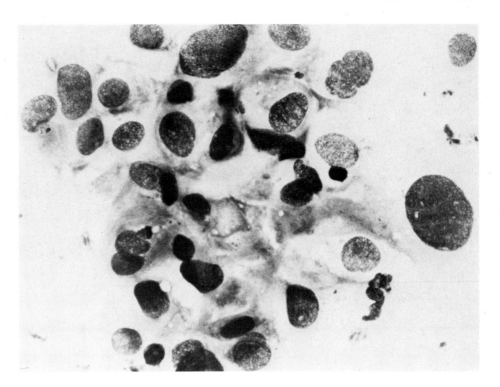

FIGURE 29–13. Transitional cell carcinoma. Cluster of malignant epithelial cells with large polygonal or elongated cytoplasm and polymorphic nuclei (May-Grünwald-Giemsa stain; ×132).

Transitional Cell Carcinomas

These are distinct clinical and morphologic entities.[4, 23] They arise in the periurethral ducts and are thus, in the beginning, confined to the central zone of the prostate. Only when locally advanced is transitional cell carcinoma palpable and then most commonly as a soft midline enlargement. Hematuria and urinary flow obstruction are the most frequent symptoms. The importance in recognizing this tumor lies in the fact that it is not sensitive to hormonal manipulation, but radiation therapy can be effective.[25]

Cytologically, the cells tend to form sheets of varying size, although free cells are common. The individual cell has a distinct, polygonal or elongated, spindle-shaped cytoplasm (Fig. 29–13). The nuclei vary considerably in size and form. Nucleoli are inconstant.

Mucus-producing Carcinomas

These are rare tumors, which should be recognized because they do not respond well to hormonal treatment.[12] Moreover, their biologic aggressiveness seems to be higher than what can be anticipated from tumor grading. Cytologically, the smears are grossly mucinous and contain relatively few cells. The cells are either of the columnar or signet-ring type. The cells show a positive immunoreactivity for prostate-specific antigen, which excludes a secondary carcinoma from the gastrointestinal tract.

Rare Malignant Tumors

Carcinosarcomas, leiomyosarcomas, lymphomas and rhabdomyosarcomas are all extremely rare. Their cytologic presentation is similar to that which occurs in more prevalent sites.

Secondary Tumors

Secondary tumors or direct overgrowth on the prostate from tumors in surrounding organs are relatively rare. Most commonly, bladder carcinomas invade the gland. The clinical symptoms as well as the cytologic features most often allow the identification of such tumors (Fig. 29–14). Metastatic spread to the prostate is seldom seen and can have its primary site in most organs, although lung appears to be most frequent.

EFFECTS OF THERAPY

Fine needle aspiration cytology offers the possibility to evaluate treatment response. Radiation therapy or hormonal manipulation will, when effective, result in a tumor reduction. Simultaneously, the cells of the normal prostate will regress. A firm and small gland is the result. Aspiration biopsy can be painful in contrast to the pretreated gland.

Radiation results in smears with small cells forming compact clusters. Occasional large polymorphic cells

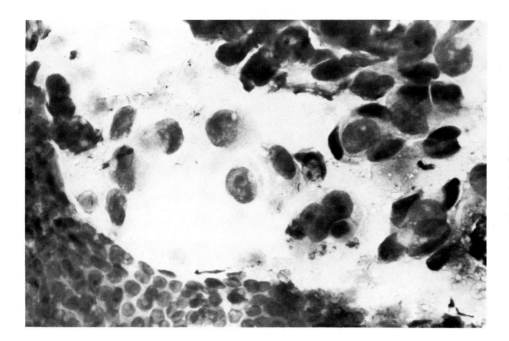

FIGURE 29–14. Bladder carcinoma invading the prostate. Large malignant urothelial cells contrasting the benign regular prostatic epithelium (May-Grünwald-Giemsa stain; ×132).

often with vacuolated nuclei and large basophilic cytoplasm are seen. It is not known whether they represent normal epithelial cells with radiation-induced atypia or degenerated tumor cells (Fig. 29–15). They may cause concern, but the overall picture is that of atrophy. Treatment failure is predicted by the presence of cells with the common malignant changes.

Hormonal manipulation also leads to atrophy and scanty aspirates. The smears have only atrophic epithelial cells. Large cells are not found in a patient with

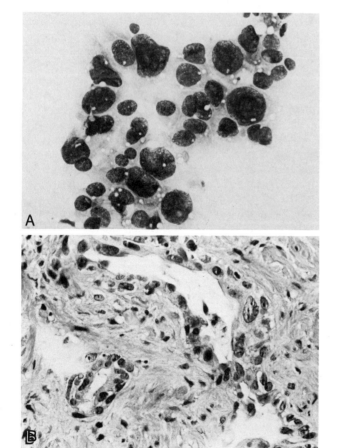

FIGURE 29–15. The effect of radiation therapy. *A*, Aspirate showing cluster of polymorphic cells with vacuolated nuclei and cytoplasm (May-Grünwald-Giemsa stain; ×132). *B*, Tissue section from the same case showing prostatic glands lined by atypical epithelium with polymorphic nuclei (hematoxylin and eosin; ×132).

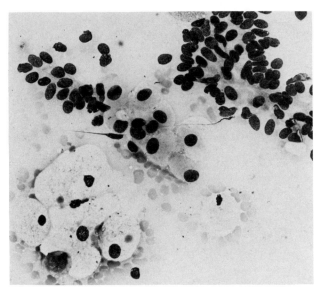

FIGURE 29–16. The effect of hormonal therapy. Presence of metaplastic squamous cells with large polygonal clear cytoplasm and atrophic prostatic epithelial cells (May-Grünwald-Giemsa stain; ×100).

favorable response. Estrogen therapy will after several weeks produce squamous cells, rich in glycogen, as shown in Figure 29–16.[42, 44]

SPECIAL TECHNIQUES

Immunocytochemistry

Prostate specific antigen (PSA) is expressed in the epithelial cells of the normal prostate. It is not found in other normal tissues.[39] Monoclonal antibodies against PSA are commercially available. The antigen is stabile and can be detected in air-dried smears, Papanicolau-stained smears and Cytospin preparations. A majority of prostatic carcinomas express the antigen, both in primary and metastatic tumors. However, we have observed that poorly differentiated tumors express only low levels of the antigen, which thus can be almost impossible to detect. In clinical practice, PSA can aid cytomorphology in identifying prostatic carcinoma as the origin of metastatic adenocarcinoma.

Case. A 69-year-old previously healthy man presented with a well-circumscribed tumor in the groin. Fine needle aspiration smears revealed a moderately well-differentiated carcinoma (Fig. 29–17). The prostate gland appeared normal on rectal examination. A repeat biopsy from the groin tumor was performed, and the cells were evaluated for presence of PSA. A distinct positivity was found, indicating a metastatic prostatic carcinoma (Fig. 29–18). Blind biopsies from the prostate yielded smears with a moderately differentiated prostatic carcinoma (Fig. 29–19).

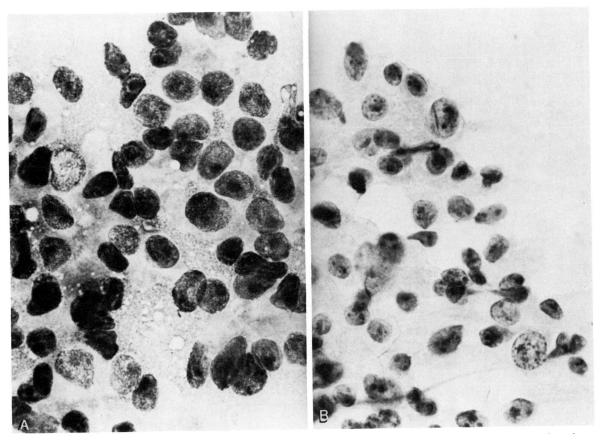

FIGURE 29–17. Aspirate from tumor in the groin. Malignant epithelial cells in a glandular arrangement with polymorphic hyperchromatic nuclei and prominent nucleoli. *A,* May-Grünwald-Giemsa stain; ×132. *B,* Papanicolaou stain; ×132.

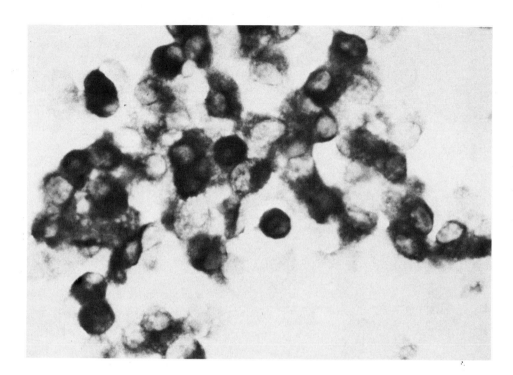

FIGURE 29–18. The **prostatic-specific antigen** visualized by immunocytochemistry in metastatic cells aspirated from a groin tumor (alkaline phosphatase; ×200).

FIGURE 29–19. Prostate aspirate from same patient as in Figures 29–17 and 29–18 revealing a **moderately well-differentiated adenocarcinoma** (grade II) (May-Grünwald-Giemsa stain; ×200).

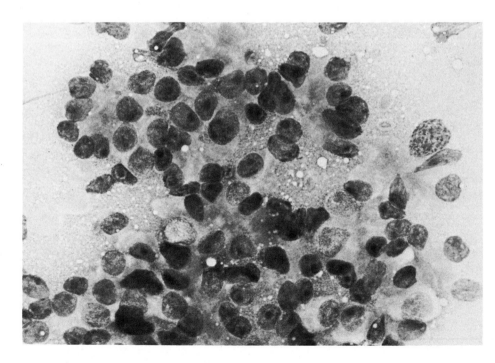

The use of PSA in identifying metastatic prostatic carcinoma is not a futile exercise. On the contrary, it offers the possibility of an effective palliative hormonal treatment.

DNA Analysis

Measurements of tumor cell DNA have been used to predict prognosis in several neoplastic lesions.[3] Fine needle aspiration material from the prostate seems ideal for both single-cell analysis and flow cytometry. Retrospective analysis, using the single-cell technique, showed that patients with diploid tumor cells had a longer disease-free survival as compared with those with aneuploid tumor cells.[45] The predictive capacity of cytophotometric DNA analysis seemed better than that of conventional cytologic grading. Similar results have been reported by Böcking and associates.[8]

Flow cytometric analysis of prostatic carcinoma cells, obtained by FNA, has shown a relationship of ploidy to tumor stage and grade.[40] Thus, small well-differentiated carcinomas were in a majority of the cases diploid. In contrast, aneuploid tumors were cytologically and poorly differentiated and clinically advanced.

These results indicate that the DNA analysis has the potential of aiding cytologic grading, to better predict the clinical course of prostatic carcinoma. It is of importance to underline that DNA analysis is *not* a diagnostic procedure. An euploid or aneuploid DNA pattern has no relevance in the morphologic diagnostic situation. This fact is clear from the following examples. The undifferentiated blastic prostatic carcinoma, which has a diploid DNA content, is excessively aggressive. In contrast, benign vesicular epithelium can have an aneuploid DNA pattern.

The definite clinical value of DNA analysis can be decided only when prospective studies on unselected case material are presented. In this context the importance of a careful cytomorphologic control of the material subject to DNA analysis cannot be overemphasized.

DIAGNOSTIC ACCURACY

A high degree of specificity and sensitivity is an ultimate requirement for a method that is used as a final diagnostic procedure. When discussing the accuracy of such a procedure, one has to assume that all steps involved are performed with a maximum of professional skill. Fine needle aspiration cytology is no exception in this respect. Several studies have been presented on the accuracy of FNA cytology in the diagnosis of prostatic carcinoma. Only those comparing two different morphologic procedures seem relevant. Moreover, the tissue analyzed should be obtained from the same area of the gland. Thus, comparisons between FNA cytology from the peripheral parts and histology on transurethral resection material do not seem valid.

Table 29–2 summarizes studies comparing FNA cytology with histologic diagnoses on core (cutting) biopsy material. It can be seen from this table, which comprises 1162 cases, that a good correlation exists between the two procedures.[5, 6, 11, 30] For FNA cytology, the specificity varies between 96 and 97.8%, whereas the sensitivity varies between 94 and 98%. For core biopsy diagnosis the corresponding figures are difficult to obtain, because this diagnosis is, in most cases, accepted as an end diagnosis. However, published figures for sensitivity and specificity are 76 to 92.2% and 99.3 to 100%, respectively. The figures indicate that both procedures have a low incidence of biopsy failure, including poor yield and biopsy from nonneoplastic areas, as reflected in high figures for sensitivity. Obviously, repeat biopsies in clinically suspect cases should diminish the false-negative diagnoses due to nonrepresentative biopsies. It also seems likely that FNA biopsies, guided by transrectal US, will increase the frequency of representative biopsies to close to 100%.

Misinterpretation of smears, leading to a false-negative diagnosis, is another cause of low sensitivity. The influence of this factor decreases considerably with experience.

The specificity of either cytologic or histologic evaluation is extremely high (see Table 29–2). Overdiagnosis of prostatic carcinoma has been reported for aspiration biopsy material.[41] Evaluation of histologic material is not unique in this respect but can also result in an accidental overdiagnosis.

False-positive FNA cytology has been reported to occur. A definite learning curve seems to be involved. In experienced hands, false-positive cytology seems almost nonexistent. However, smears from some normal structures, as well as some disorders, may mimic carcinoma. Cells from the rectum and seminal vesicles can be misinterpreted. Rectal cells may have distinct nucleoli, appear larger than the normal prostatic epithelium and form acinar structures (Fig. 29–20). How-

TABLE 29–2. Sensitivity and Specificity of Fine Needle Aspiration Biopsy (FNAB) and Core Biopsy

Study	Number of Biopsies	FNAB		Core Biopsy	
		Sensitivity*	*Specificity**	*Sensitivity**	*Specificity†*
Beekhuis-Brussee et al (1988)	826	96.5	97.8	92.2	99.3
Bodner et al (1987)	158	94	96	—	—
Ljung et al (1986)	103	95	97	76	100
Chodak et al (1986)	75	98	Not given	81	Not given

*Compared with the histologic diagnosis.
†Compared with the final diagnosis.

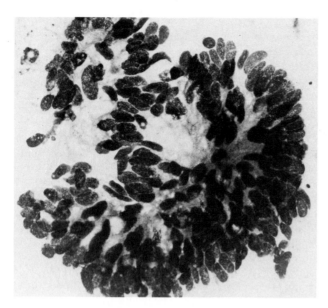

FIGURE 29–20. Rectal mucosa. A cluster of columnar epithelial cells with oval or elongated nuclei in palisade arrangement forming a glandular structure (May-Grünwald-Giemsa stain; ×132).

ever, the presence of fecal material, mucus and palisading of regular columnar cells are features that should prevent an overdiagnosis of carcinoma.

Aspirates from the seminal vesicles may produce a challenging cytologic picture. The cells vary markedly in size and often have distinct nucleoli. The impression of malignancy should, however, be neutralized by the finding of sperms, cytoplasmic vacuoles and typical basophilic cytoplasmic granules (Fig. 29–21). Another helpful feature is that the seminal vesicle cells rarely are smeared, contrasting with poorly differentiated carcinomas.

Prostatitis of unspecific type and the granulomatous variant can contain epithelia with marked reactive changes, which have been mistaken for carcinoma.[32, 41] The presence of different inflammatory cells should, however, alert the cytologist. Occasionally, a conclusive diagnosis cannot be given and a repeat biopsy should be recommended. In this diagnostic dilemma further stress is added by the knowledge that 14% of the patients with prostatitis also have carcinoma.[32]

Grading of prostatic carcinoma on histologic material gives essential prognostic information.[19, 37] Esposti[13] reported a significant correlation between tumor grading on FNA material and survival. The same investigator also found a high correlation between grading high, moderate and poorly differentiated on FNA smears and sections from TUR material. Similarily, high correlation has been reported by Maksem and Johenning.[31] Somewhat less favorable correlations were, however, reported by others.[1, 10, 28, 43] Most studies do not allow a direct comparison, however, because the FNA and histologic biopsy materials were not obtained from the same area of the prostate. It seems prudent to assume that a correlation for true parallel aspiration and core biopsies should be high, if grading on both types of material takes both cytologic features and cellular patterns into account.

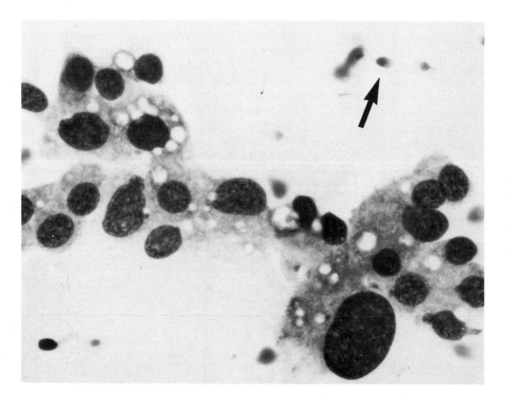

FIGURE 29–21. Seminal vesicle aspirate. Cluster of cells with marked variation in size. Note the cytoplasmic vacuoles and pigment; few spermatozoa in the background (arrow). (May-Grünwald-Giemsa stain; ×200).

References

1. Anandan N, Rowell MJ, MacKenzie E, Johnson DH, Gingell JC: Role of Franzén needle aspiration biopsy in carcinoma of the prostate. J Royal Soc Med 76:828–830, 1983.
2. Andriole GL, Kavoussi LR, Torrence RJ, Lepor H, Catalona WJ: Transrectal ultrasonography in the diagnosis and staging of carcinoma of the prostate. J Urol 140:758–760, 1988.
3. Auer G, Kronenwett M, von Rosen A: DNA measurement: Its value for diagnosis and prognosis. *In* New Frontiers in Cytology. Edited by K Goerttler, GE Feichter, S Witte. Berlin, Springer Verlag, 1988.
4. Bates RH Jr: Transitional cell carcinoma of the prostate. J Urol 101:206–207, 1969.
5. Beekhuis-Brussee JAM, Lycklama a Nijeholt AAB, Bruins JL, Kramer AEJL, Eulderink F, van Krieken HJHM, van Steenis GL, Arentz PW: Comparison between fine-needle aspiration cytology and core biopsy histology in prostatic carcinoma. *In* New Frontiers in Cytology. Edited by K Goerttler, GE Feichter, S Witte. Berlin, Springer Verlag, 1988.
6. Bodner DR, Hampel N, Maksem JA, Suarez M, Resnick MI: Aspiration biopsy of the prostate. World J Urol 5:62–64, 1987.
7. Breslow N, Chan CW, Dhom G, Drury AB, Franks LM, Gellei B, Lee YS, Lundberg S, Sparke B, Sternby NH, Tulinius H: Latent carcinoma of prostate at autopsy in seven areas. Int J Cancer 20: 680–688, 1977.
8. Böcking A, Chatelain R, Orthen U, Gien G, Kalckreuth G, Jocham D, Nohltman D: DNA-grading of prostatic carcinoma: prognostic validity and reproducibility. Anticancer Res 8:129–136, 1988.
9. Cantrell BB: Pathologic factors that influence prognosis in Stage A prostatic cancer: the influence of extent versus grade. J Urol 125:516, 1981.
10. Carter HB, Riehle RA Jr, Koizumi JH, Amberson J, Vaughan ED Jr: Fine needle aspiration of the abnormal prostate: a cytohistological correlation. J Urol 135:294–298, 1986.
11. Chodak GW, Steinberg GD, Bibbo M, Wied G, Straus FS, Vogelzang NJ, Schoenberg HW: The role of transrectal aspiration biopsy in the diagnosis of prostatic cancer. J Urol 135:299–302, 1986.
12. Epstein JI, Lieberman PH: Mucinous adenocarcinoma of the prostate gland. Am J Surg Pathol 9:299–308, 1985.
13. Esposti PL: Cytologic malignancy grading of prostatic carcinoma by transrectal aspiration biopsy. Scand J Urol Nephrol 5:199–209, 1971.
14. Esposti PL: Aspiration biopsy cytology in the diagnosis and management of prostatic carcinoma (Thesis). Stockholm, Stähl och Accidens Tryck, 1974.
15. Esposti PL, Elman A, Norlén H: Complications of transrectal aspiration biopsy of the prostate. Scand J Urol Nephrol 9:208, 1975.
16. Ferguson RS: Prostatic neoplasms: their diagnosis by needle puncture and aspiration. Am J Surg 9:507–511, 1930.
17. Fisher ER, Jeffrey W: Ultrastructure of human normal and neoplastic prostate; with comments relative to prostatic effects of hormonal stimulation in the rabbit. Am J Clin Pathol 44:119, 1965.
18. Franzén S, Giertz G, Zajicek J: Cytological diagnosis of prostatic tumors by transrectal aspiration biopsy: a preliminary report. Br J Urol 32:193–196, 1960.
19. Gleason DF, Mellinger GT: Veterans Administration Cooperative Urological Research Group: Prediction of prognosis for prostatic adenocarcinoma by combined histological grading and clinical staging. J Urol 111:58–64, 1974.
20. Guileyardo JM: Prevalence of latent prostate carcinoma in two U.S. populations. J Natl Cancer Inst 65:311, 1980.
21. Guinan P, Bush I, Ray V, Vieth R, Ras R, Bhatti R: The accuracy of the rectal examination in the diagnosis of prostate carcinoma. N Engl J Med 303:499–503, 1980.
22. Hutchinson GB: Incidence and etiology of prostatic cancer. Urology 17(Suppl 3):4, 1981.
23. Johnson DE, Hogan JM, Ayala AG: Transitional-cell carcinoma of the prostate. Cancer 29:287–293, 1972.
24. Klein LA: Prostatic carcinoma. N Engl J Med 300:824, 1979.
25. Kopelson G, Harisiadis L, Romas NA, Veenema RJ, Tannenbaum M: Periurethral prostatic duct carcinoma: Clinical features and treatment results. Cancer 42:2894–2902, 1978.
26. Lee F, Littrup PJ, McLeary RD, Kumusaka GH, Borlaza GS, McHugh TA, Soiderer MH, Roi LD: Needle aspiration and core biopsy of prostate cancer: comparative evaluation with biplanar transrectal US guidance. Radiology 163:515–520, 1987.
27. Lee F, Littrup PJ, Torp-Pedersen ST, Mettlin C, McHugh TA, Gray JM, Kumusaka GH, McLeary RD: Prostate cancer: comparison of transrectal US and digital rectal examination for screening. Radiology. 168:389–394, 1988.
28. Lin BPC, Davies WEL, Harmata PA: Prostatic aspiration cytology. Pathology 11:607–614, 1979.
29. Lindgren PG: Percutaneous needle biopsy. Acta Radiol. 23:653–656, 1982.
30. Ljung BM, Cherrie R, Kaufman JJ: Fine needle aspiration biopsy of the prostate gland: A study of 103 cases with histological follow-up. J Urol 135:955–958, 1986.
31. Maksem JA, Johenning PW: Is cytology capable of adequately grading prostate carcinoma? Matched series of 50 cases comparing cytologic and histologic pattern diagnoses. Urology 31:437–444, 1988.
32. Maksem JA, Johenning PW, Galang CF: Prostatitis and aspiration biopsy cytology of prostate. Urology 32:263–268, 1988.
33. McNeal JE: Zonal anatomy of the prostate. Prostate 2:35–49, 1981.
34. McNeal J: Normal and pathologic anatomy of prostate. Urology 17:(Suppl 3):11, 1981.
35. McNeal JE: Significance of duct-acinar dysplasia in prostate carcinogenesis. Prostate 13:91–102, 1988.
36. Naito S, Kimiya K, Hasegawa Y, Kumazawa J: Digital examination and transrectal ultrasonography in the diagnoses of prostatic cancer. Eur Urol 14:356–359, 1988.
37. Perez CA: Carcinoma of the prostate, a vexing biological and clinical enigma. Int J Radiat Oncol Biol Phys 9:1427–1438, 1983.
38. Perez CA, Fair WR, Ihde DC, Labrie F: Cancer of the prostate. *In* Cancer—Principles and Practice of Oncology, 2nd ed. Edited by VT DeVita, S Nellman, SA Rosenberg. Philadelphia, JB Lippincott, pp 929–964, 1985.
39. Taylor CR: Immunomicroscopy: A Diagnostic Tool for the Surgical Pathologist. Philadelphia, WB Saunders, 1982, pp 260–266.
40. Tribukait B: Flow cytometry in assessing the clinical aggressiveness of genitourinary neoplasms. World J Urol 5:108–122, 1987.
41. Willems JS, Löwhagen T: Transrectal fine-needle aspiration biopsy for cytologic diagnosis and grading of prostate carcinoma. Prostate 2:381–395, 1981.
42. Williams JP, Still BM, Pugh RCB: The diagnosis of prostatic cancer. Cytological and biomechanical studies using the Franzén biopsy needle. Br J Urol 39:549, 1967.
43. Voeth C, Droese M, Steuer G: Erfahrungen mit dem Zytologischen Grading beim Prostatakarzinom. Urologe [A] 17:367–370, 1978.
44. Zajicek J: Aspiration Biopsy Cytology. II. Cytology of Infradiaphragmatic Organs. *In* Monographs on Clinical Cytology. Edited by GL Wied. Basel, S. Karger, 1979, pp 129–166.
45. Zetterberg A, Esposti PL: Prognostic significance of nuclear DNA levels in prostatic carcinoma. Scand J Urol Nephrol (Suppl)55:53–58, 1980.

30

Liver and Pancreas

Liang-Che Tao

Liver

Cancer growth in the liver is a frequent finding at laparotomy or autopsy. In our series of 1383 cases of aspiration biopsy of the liver, 1037 (75%) were metastatic cancers. Because positive findings for hepatic malignancy imply a grave prognosis and may alter clinical management, biopsy confirmation is often required. For patients with a metastatic liver cancer, confirmation of hepatic metastases may obviate the need for extensive diagnostic procedures or surgery.

For patients with a solitary or localized hepatocellular carcinoma without evidence of lymph node or distant spread, the only definitive treatment is surgical excision when this is technically possible. In fact, there is a tendency for hepatocellular carcinoma to remain localized without distant metastases. In the literature, Anthony[2] reported that 42% of hepatocellular carcinomas in a series of 126 cases were confined to the liver at the time of autopsy. Craig and coworkers[18] reported that a subtype of hepatocellular carcinoma designated *fibrolamellar carcinoma* had a better prognosis with surgical resection. Therefore, the differentiation of primary liver cancer from metastatic tumors and the early recognition of hepatocellular carcinoma are of special importance in our clinical practice in view of the relatively favorable prognosis with resection. This is crucial to the welfare of the patient. With the introduction of an ever-increasing number of sophisticated imaging techniques, the early detection of liver cancer is now possible. In our series, the smallest cancerous lesion of the liver diagnosed by guided fine needle aspiration biopsy was 7 mm. The development of immunocytochemical technique further enhances diagnostic accuracy in the typing of hepatic cancers.

Guided fine needle aspiration biopsy is increasingly being recognized as an excellent diagnostic method for detecting hepatic malignancy.[10, 11, 31, 43, 52, 54, 62, 63] One of the major advantages of fine needle aspiration biopsy is that it can be used to detect malignancy anywhere in the liver, e.g., in the left lobe or in the area of the porta hepatis, where the use of a large-bore needle may be too risky. Another advantage is that we can obtain multiple samples using the fine needle aspiration biopsy technique on the basis of findings visualized by imaging techniques. The chances of obtaining a representative sample are greatly increased. Therefore, for any mass or masses in the liver suspected to be malignant, guided fine needle aspiration biopsy is the method of choice.[8, 15, 31, 44, 56, 57, 62, 65]

IMAGING TECHNIQUES

Prior to aspiration biopsy the lesion or lesions in the liver must be localized by one of the imaging techniques. A number of imaging modalities, including angiography,[118] radioisotopic scan,[31] ultrasonography[10, 17, 56, 57] and computed tomography,[17, 126, 137] have been used for localizing hepatic mass lesions. Selective angiography of the celiac artery may reveal an abnormal configuration of blood vessels and of the blood supply (e.g., hypervascularity in hepatocellular carcinoma). For lesions, especially small lesions causing no blood vessel abnormality, angiography cannot be used for localization. Radioisotopic scan of the liver may demonstrate focal areas or diffuse zones of diminished uptake of radionuclide. However, the radioisotopic liver scan cannot distinguish a solid mass from a cystic lesion, and the lesion for aspiration biopsy has to be large enough to be visualized in two projections.

Ultrasonography and computed tomography have largely replaced all other techniques in the assessment of hepatic lesions because of their sensitivity in detecting small lesions. Ultrasonography can display two-dimensional anatomic cross sections of the abdomen. Special biopsy transducers designed for use with percutaneous aspiration biopsy are currently becoming available. Ultrasonography also has the advantage of greater scanning flexibility, speed, the relatively low cost of the equipment and the absence of radiation exposure. Computed tomography also offers a two-dimensional anatomic display of the human body. It can automatically calculate the optimal distance to the lesion and the angle of needle entry and then display them on the monitor. The position of the needle tip in relation to the lesion can be readily verified prior to aspiration. However, it is expensive to use, and the technique carries with it some exposure to radiation.

NORMAL LIVER

Histology

Normal liver is made up of lobules of hepatic parenchyma. Each lobule contains a central efferent vein, the centrilobular vein and peripheral portal triads. Each portal triad consists of connective tissue in which are embedded a branch of portal vein, arterioles and interlobular bile ducts in addition to lymphatics and nerves. Portal triads may contain a small number of lymphocytes. Interlobular bile ducts drain into larger ones as septal or trabecular ducts. The hepatic parenchyma consists of hepatocytes that form interconnecting plates separated from each other by sinusoids. The sinusoids drain into the centrilobular vein and are lined by an incomplete layer of flattened endothelial cells together with Kupffer cells, which are more numerous near the portal triads. Between the liver cells are the bile canaliculi, which empty into the bile ducts.

Cytology

Aspirates from the normal liver contain hepatocytes, bile duct epithelial cells, sinusoidal endothelial cells and Kupffer cells as well as a few mononuclear cells and fibroblasts. The polygonal hepatocytes occur as monolayered sheets, in cohesive groupings and as solitary cells in aspirate preparations. They have abundant, granular, well-defined cytoplasm and one or two centrally located nuclei with frequent conspicuous nucleoli (Fig. 30–1). There are considerable variations in nuclear size among different individuals. In older people the nuclei of hepatocytes tend to increase in size with age and there is often some variation in nuclear size. Prominent nucleoli may be noted (Fig. 30–2). Intracytoplasmic lipofuscin also becomes more abundant in older people. Hepatocytes may contain fat vacuoles even in the absence of obesity, diabetes or excess alcohol intake. Hepatocytes may appear as stripped nuclei if there is a delay in fixation of aspirated material. This is a pitfall in the interpretation of aspirate specimens because stripped, small-sized nuclei may mimic small-cell anaplastic carcinoma and those

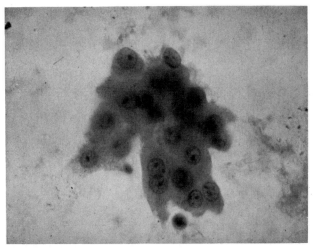

FIGURE 30–1. Normal hepatocytes: liver cells that have one or two centrally located nuclei and an abundance of well-defined cytoplasm. Aspirate preparation (Papanicolaou stain; ×800).

stripped, large-sized nuclei with prominent nucleoli mimic poorly differentiated carcinoma (Fig. 30–3).

Bile ducts in the smallest portal triads are referred to as interlobular ducts, and larger ones, as septal or trabecular ducts. In aspirate preparations, epithelial cells of interlobular bile ducts are often in sheet arrangements. They have relatively scanty, poorly defined cytoplasm and round nuclei without recognizable nucleoli (Fig. 30–4). Tall columnar epithelial cells of the larger bile ducts are usually in cohesive groupings or in palisading arrangements. They have moderate amounts of well-defined cytoplasm and ovoid nuclei (Fig. 30–5).

Hepatocytes are arranged in interconnecting plates that are normally one cell thick and separated from each other by the sinusoids. In aspirate preparations, the sinusoidal endothelial cells are usually seen at the edge of cohesive groupings of hepatocytes and appear as lining cells with spindle-shaped nuclei in a lengthwise

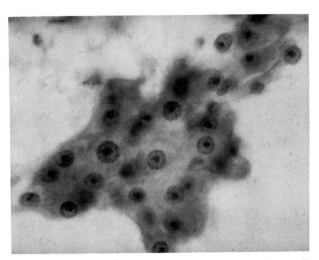

FIGURE 30–2. Hepatocytes in an elderly person: liver cells that have variation in nuclear size and prominent nucleoli. Aspirate preparation (Papanicolaou stain; ×800).

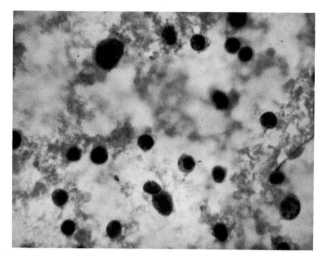

FIGURE 30–3. Hepatocytes stripped of cytoplasm: numerous solitary nuclei of the liver cells stripped of cytoplasm mimicking poorly differentiated carcinoma. Aspirate preparation (Papanicolaou stain; ×800).

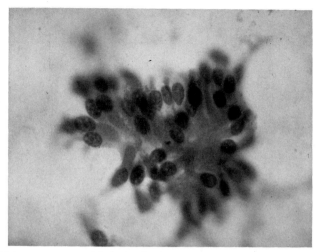

FIGURE 30–5. Epithelial cells from a large, septal bile duct: tall columnar ductal epithelial cells that have ovoid nuclei with indistinct nucleoli, in a palisading arrangement. Aspirate preparation (Papanicolaou stain; ×800).

arrangement. They have relatively scanty cytoplasm (Fig. 30–6).

Kupffer cells are the principal hepatic phagocytes. In tissue sections, they are more numerous near the portal triads and can be distinguished from endothelial cells by their positive staining with periodic acid–Schiff (PAS) after amylase digestion. In aspirate preparations, Kupffer cells have ovoid, elongated or spindle-shaped nuclei and scanty but well-defined cytoplasm. They are often attached to hepatocytes but not as lining cells. They may lie singly and can be distinguished from fibroblasts by their well-defined cytoplasm (Fig. 30–7). When the cytoplasm of Kupffer cells contains phagocytosed material, the cells have a rounded appearance and their nuclei are in excentric positions.

BENIGN DISORDERS

With the increasing use of transabdominal fine needle aspiration biopsy, pathologists are being introduced to a variety of benign hepatic lesions that have not previously been routinely diagnosed by cytologic means.[51] This procedure can be performed on an outpatient basis and thus may spare patients unnecessary hospitalization and operations. Although not all benign disorders of the liver can be diagnosed by cytologic techniques, aspiration biopsy is useful for the diagnosis of diseases in which morphologic changes of hepatocytes and other cytologic appearances are specific enough to be detected by light microscopy.

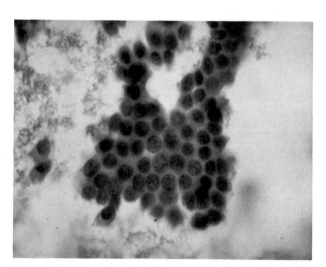

FIGURE 30–4. Epithelial cells from a small, interlobular bile duct: ductal epithelial cells that have round or ovoid nuclei with indistinct nucleoli, and relatively scanty cytoplasm, in a sheet arrangement. Aspirate preparation (Papanicolaou stain; ×800).

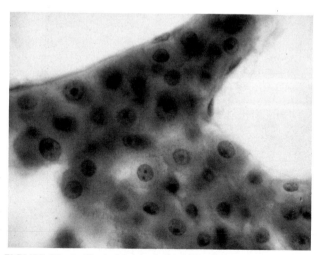

FIGURE 30–6. Sinusoidal endothelial cells: sinusoidal endothelial cells that have spindle-shaped nuclei and small amounts of cytoplasm lining a cohesive grouping of hepatocytes. Aspirate preparation (Papanicolaou stain; ×800).

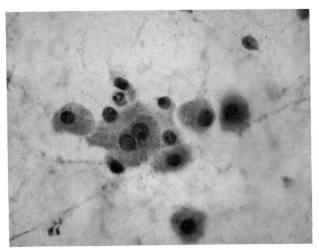

FIGURE 30–7. Kupffer cells: a few Kupffer cells that have ovoid or elongated nuclei and small amounts of cytoplasm. Note that they are attached to hepatocytes. Aspirate preparation (Papanicolaou stain; ×800).

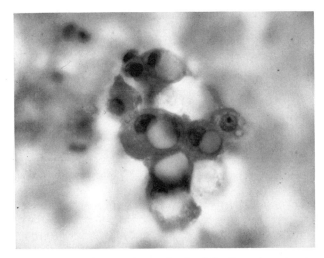

FIGURE 30–8. Fatty metamorphosis of the liver: hepatocytes that contain a single large, intracytoplasmic, clear vacuole or two or more small vacuoles. Note that the large vacuoles displace the nuclei to the periphery of the cells and distend the cells. Aspirate preparation (Papanicolaou stain; ×800).

Fatty Metamorphosis

The accumulation of neutral triglycerides in hepatocytes is one of the most common pathologic changes in the liver. Major causes of fatty metamorphosis of the liver include excess alcohol intake, obesity, malnutrition, diabetes mellitus and debilitating systemic diseases, e.g., leukemias. Excess alcohol intake is by far the most common cause of fatty liver in North America. Fatty changes in alcoholics range from vacuolation of a few liver cells to severe involvement of the whole liver. In severe cases, the liver is enlarged and liver function tests are mildly abnormal.

Cytology

The cytoplasm of hepatocytes contains a single, large, clear vacuole or, less frequently, multiple, small vacuoles of variable sizes. The large vacuoles displace the nuclei to the periphery of the cells and also distend the cells (Fig. 30–8). In the cases of advanced fatty metamorphosis, groupings of liver cells with fatty changes may appear as small fragments of adipose tissue in aspirate preparations. The presence of occasional large, round nuclei in some cells clearly distinguishes liver cell fragments from adipose tissue. It is not possible to tell whether the fatty metamorphosis is due to alcoholism or to other causes on purely cytomorphologic grounds.

Diabetes Mellitus

In diabetes mellitus there is often a combination of prominent nuclear vacuolation and swelling in periportal hepatocytes. Fatty metamorphosis is also a common finding. In most diabetics there is no hepatic fibrosis or inflammation.

Cytology

In aspirate preparations, the hepatocytes appear swollen and have nuclear vacuolation and swelling. The nuclear vacuolation is the result of deposition of glycogen within the nuclei that is dissolved out during processing (Fig. 30–9). Hepatocytes with vacuolated nuclei may also be encountered in aspirate preparations of the liver from normal elderly people. They are not swollen and are seen in only a small number of cells, whereas in cases of diabetes mellitus, nuclear vacuolation is often a common finding and is seen in many hepatocytes. Nuclear vacuolation is different from the intranuclear holes seen in some epithelial cells or

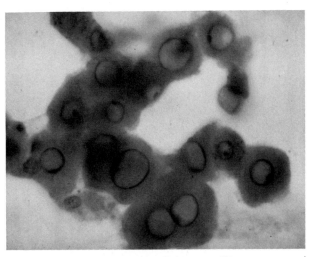

FIGURE 30–9. Hepatocytes in diabetes mellitus: many swollen liver cells that have vacuolated nuclei resulting from the removal of glycogen during processing. Note that the vacuolated nuclei also appear swollen. Aspirate preparation (Papanicolaou stain; ×800).

neoplastic cells that results from invagination of the cytoplasm into the nuclei. In cases of diabetes, the whole nuclei appear vacuolated with well-defined nuclear membranes, whereas intranuclear holes only partially occupy the nuclei.

Cirrhosis

Cirrhosis is a chronic, diffuse process characterized by extensive interstitial fibrosis and the conversion of normal liver architecture into structurally abnormal nodules.[4] Grossly, the nodular pattern may be micronodular or macronodular. In the micronodular category, the nodules of a cirrhotic liver are of the same size, not larger than 0.3 mm in their greatest dimension. In the macronodular category, the nodules are much more variable in size, and many measure more than 1 cm in the greatest dimension. A macronodular, heavily fibrotic liver is typical of the late stage of cirrhosis, whatever its etiology. Microscopically, rounded nodules are well demarcated and separated by dense fibrous septa. The regenerative nodules are composed of hepatocytes exhibiting marked variations in size and shape. Binucleation is a common finding. Focal areas of necrosis may be seen. Bile ductular proliferation and a mixed inflammatory infiltrate occur in some nodules. However, in an inactive cirrhosis, inflammatory infiltration is mild, ductular proliferation is inconspicuous and there is little or no necrosis of hepatocytes. Variation in activity from one part of a cirrhotic liver to another is common.

Cytology

A combination of regenerative changes, fibrosis, degenerative changes and fatty metamorphosis is seen. Regenerative changes are represented by pleomor-

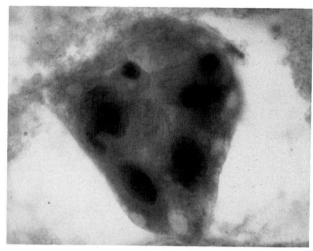

FIGURE 30–11. Liver cell dysplasia in cirrhosis of the liver: large hepatocytes that have marked variations in nuclear size and shape and prominent nucleoli. Aspirate preparation (Papanicolaou stain; × 800).

phism of hepatocytes and an increase in the number of mitotic figures and binucleated hepatocytes. The nuclei of hepatocytes often show variation in size and have prominent nucleoli (Fig. 30–10). In occasional cases, pleomorphism of hepatocytes is very prominent, and multinucleated hepatocytes are present (Figs. 30–11 and 30–12). The hepatocytes are enlarged. Their nuclei are irregular, with prominent nucleoli and marked variations in size. This is designated liver cell dysplasia and is a potential pitfall in the interpretation of liver aspirates because it may be mistaken for hepatocellular carcinoma by inexperienced examiners.[9] However, the overall cytologic findings in aspirate preparations from liver cell dysplasia are different from those seen in hepatocellular carcinoma (see section on Hepatocellular Carcinoma). Anthony and coworkers[3] found a relationship between liver cell dysplasia and hepatocellular carcinoma in an African population.

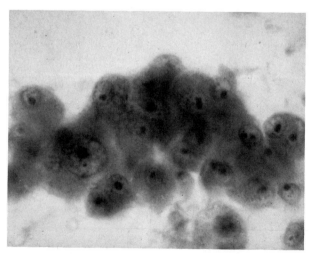

FIGURE 30–10. Pleomorphism of hepatocytes in cirrhosis of the liver: liver cells that have nuclei showing variation in size and prominent nucleoli in cohesive groupings. Aspirate preparation (Papanicolaou stain; × 800).

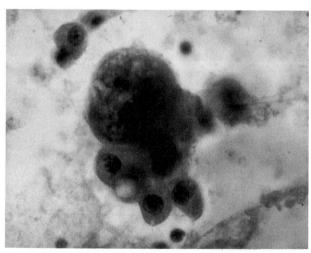

FIGURE 30–12. Liver cell dysplasia in cirrhosis of the liver: a hepatocyte that has several hyperchromatic nuclei. Aspirate preparation (Papanicolaou stain; × 800).

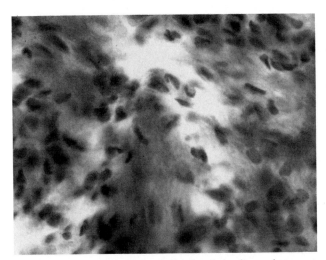

FIGURE 30–13. Fibrosis in cirrhosis of the liver: fragments of fibrous tissue that contain spindle-shaped nuclei in a disorderly arrangement. Aspirate preparation (Papanicolaou stain; ×800).

Liver cell dysplasia may persist for many years, and its presence does not prove the existence of hepatocellular carcinoma in the liver.

Degenerative changes are represented by necrosis of hepatocytes appearing as ghost cells in aspirate preparations. Fibroblasts are present in variable numbers and are intermingled with hepatocytes. Oftentimes, hepatocytes are seen embedded in fragments of fibrous tissue (Figs. 30–13 and 30–14). Fatty changes of hepatocytes is a common finding. Neutrophils and lymphocytes are present in variable amounts in different specimens. Because of variations in activity among different parts of a cirrhotic liver, the cytologic findings in various samples from the same liver may be quite different.

Viral Hepatitis

Viral hepatitis is a necrotizing, inflammatory, regenerative disease of liver parenchymal cells. Etiologically, type A, type B and type non-A, non-B viral hepatitis have been identified; however, they cannot be reliably distinguished from each other on cytohistologic grounds alone.[32, 33] Type A hepatitis is essentially a self-limited illness, and the chronic carrier state has not been shown to exist. However, over 10% of the patients with hepatitis B develop significant symptoms, including acute fulminant illness and a variety of chronic disease states. The viral agents responsible for non-A, non-B hepatitis also have the ability to cause chronic hepatic disease.[32] Hepatitis B virus infection has been found to be a major risk factor in hepatic carcinogenesis in the Orient. In Taiwan, the incidence of hepatocellular carcinoma in hepatitis B surface antigen (HBsAg)-positive patients is 1158 per 100,000, compared with five per 100,000 in HBsAg-negative patients.[7] Reports from Taiwan show that 80% of patients with hepatocellular carcinoma have a chronic form of hepatitis B.[67]

Cytology

A combination of degenerative, inflammatory and regenerative changes is seen. The degenerative changes are represented by ballooning degeneration of hepatocytes and isolated liver cell necrosis in the form of acidophilic bodies. The affected hepatocytes are enlarged and appear swollen, and their cytoplasm is lightly stained (Fig. 30–15). The acidophilic bodies are degenerative hepatocytes that undergo shrinkage and karyopyknosis, with eventual loss of the nucleus (Fig. 30–16). The acidophilic bodies in aspirate preparations prepared with Papanicolaou stain appear either bluish green or eosinophilic. The inflammatory changes in viral hepatitis include mononuclear infiltrate (mainly lymphocytes) and hyperplasia of Kupffer cells. Kupffer cells in noncohesive groupings may be seen. They often stain intensely with PAS after amylase digestion. The regenerative changes include pleomorphism of hepa-

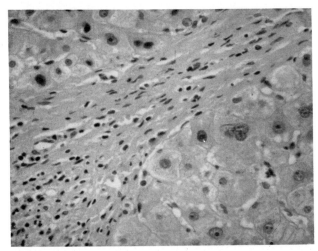

FIGURE 30–14. Cirrhosis of the liver. Histologic section (hematoxylin and eosin; ×200).

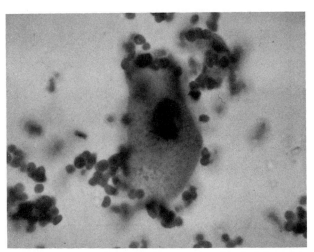

FIGURE 30–15. Ballooning degeneration in viral hepatitis: an enlarged hepatocyte that has swollen and granular cytoplasm and a large, centrally located, round nucleus. Aspirate preparation (Papanicolaou stain; ×800).

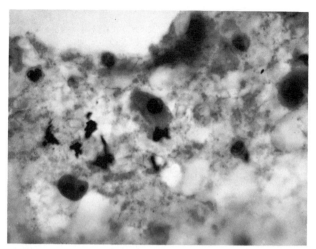

FIGURE 30–16. Acidophilic body in viral hepatitis: a small, acidophilic body (left lower corner) that has dense, well-defined cytoplasm and a small, centrally located, pyknotic nucleus. Aspirate preparation (Papanicolaou stain; ×800).

tocytes, increased mitotic activity and an increase in the number of binucleated hepatocytes. These pleomorphic hepatocytes, unlike those seen in cirrhotic liver, may also undergo ballooning degeneration (Fig. 30–17). In some cases, there is an increase in hemosiderin deposits in Kupffer cells and hepatocytes (Fig. 30–18).

Alcoholic Hepatitis

Ethyl alcohol is a liver toxin and its effects on the liver depend on the duration and level of excess intake.[38] The essential changes of alcoholic hepatitis are liver cell damage and inflammation. Fibrosis is seen in later stages. Fatty change is usually present. In its early stages the changes are seen near centrilobular veins. Later, periportal areas are also affected.

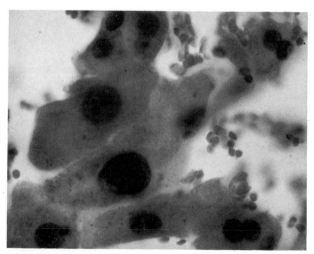

FIGURE 30–17. Pleomorphism of hepatocytes in viral hepatitis: pleomorphic liver cells that show ballooning degeneration and frequent binucleation. Aspirate preparation (Papanicolaou stain; ×800).

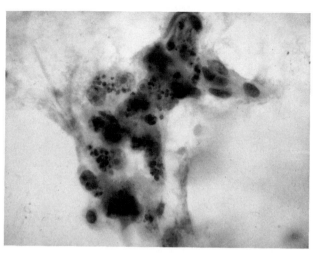

FIGURE 30–18. Hemosiderin deposition in viral hepatitis: hepatocytes and Kupffer cells that have coarsely granular hemosiderin pigment in their cytoplasm. Aspirate preparation (Papanicolaou stain; ×800).

Cytology

A combination of degenerative, inflammatory and fatty changes is seen. The degenerative change is represented by the presence of Mallory's bodies (alcoholic hyalin) in the cytoplasm of hepatocytes. They appear as round or elongated acidophilic clumps located in a perinuclear position (Fig. 30–19). The inflammatory change consists of polymorphonuclear inflammation, and neutrophils are seen surrounding the degenerated liver cells or within damaged liver cells. Fatty changes of the hepatocytes are a common finding.

There are some overlappings of cytomorphologic features seen in aspirate preparations from cirrhosis, viral hepatitis and alcoholic hepatitis. However, their overall cytologic findings are different. In aspirate preparations, the differentiation among alcoholic hepatitis, cirrhosis and viral hepatitis is possible on purely

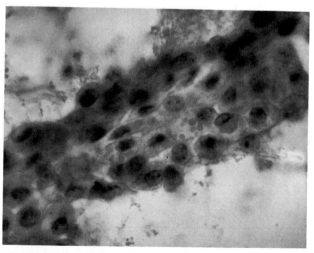

FIGURE 30–19. Mallory bodies in alcoholic hepatitis: some hepatocytes that contain Mallory bodies appearing as intracytoplasmic, round, acidophilic clumps. Aspirate preparation (Papanicolaou stain; ×800).

TABLE 30–1. Comparison of Cytologic Findings in Cirrhosis, Viral Hepatitis and Alcoholic Hepatitis

	Regenerative Changes	Fibrous Stroma	Degenerative Changes	Fatty Changes	Inflammatory Changes
Cirrhosis	+	+	+ (necrosis)	+	+ (mixed inflammatory cells)
Viral hepatitis	+	−	+ (ballooning degeneration and acidophilic bodies)	− +	+ (lymphocytes)
Alcoholic hepatitis	−	−	+ (Mallory's bodies)		+ (polymorphs)

cytomorphologic grounds. The differences in overall cytologic findings among these three conditions are summarized in Table 30–1.

Cholestasis

Cholestasis implies defective excretion of bile by the liver, with reduced amounts of bile reaching the duodenum. It is seen in any variety of jaundice and is a component of many liver diseases, including those primarily involving the biliary tree and those affecting liver cells. However, much of the bilirubin present is removed in routine tissue processing and therefore intracytoplasmic bile granules are not readily appreciated after tissue processing but can be seen in aspirate preparations. Bile plugs that are most commonly associated with mechanical obstruction of the biliary tree are usually recognizable after tissue processing. In histologic sections, centrilobular cholestasis with little or no portal inflammation suggests drug cholestasis or other forms of intrahepatic cholestasis. Portal edema, acute interlobular inflammation and duct proliferation in the absence of widespread liver cell damage are indicative of large bile duct obstruction.

Cytology

Bile pigment that varies greatly in color and texture is present. Intracytoplasmic bile granules are usually yellow or green in color (as a result of oxidation of bilirubin to biliverdin) and vary considerably in size and density. For intrahepatic cholestasis, bile pigments are usually found in the form of granules or clumps within hepatocytes and Kupffer cells. A few bile plugs or thrombi in undilated or minimally dilated canaliculi may be seen, but there is no proliferation of bile ducts and no ductal epithelial hyperplasia.

For cholestasis resulting from obstruction to major bile ducts within or outside the liver, bile is seen in the form of prominent bile plugs or thrombi in the dilated canaliculi between hepatocytes (Fig. 30–20). Owing to proliferation of small bile ducts and bile duct epithelial hyperplasia, large sheets and cohesive groupings of ductal cells are sometimes seen in aspirate preparations. The affected ductal cells may be in slightly disorderly arrangements and show atypical changes. Their nuclei may vary in size and shape.

Clonorchiasis

The liver fluke, *Clonorchis sinensis*, is found in the Far East, and clonorchiasis is seen only in immigrants in North America. The patients contract the infection by ingestion of improperly cooked fish containing immature worms (metacercaria). Clonorchiasis may cause clinical symptoms several years after the patient has left an endemic area.[29] The parasites mature in the upper intestinal tract and then invade the biliary tree and the liver. They induce a localized inflammatory reaction and hyperplasia of the bile duct epithelium that may eventually cause biliary obstruction and rarely cause cholangiocarcinoma. The adult worms reach 2 cm in length and produce eggs in the bile ducts.

Cytology

The cytologic diagnosis is based on finding ova in aspirate preparations from the lesions (Fig. 30–21). Other cytologic findings include abundant mixed in-

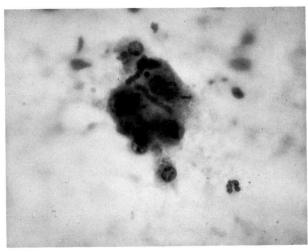

FIGURE 30–20. Cholestasis in large bile duct obstruction: bile plugs or thrombi in dilated canaculi between hepatocytes. Aspirate preparation (Papanicolaou stain; ×800).

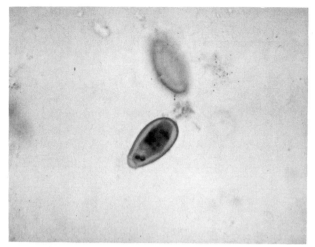

FIGURE 30–21. Clonorchiasis of the liver: an egg produced by a liver fluke, *Clonorchis sinensis*, that contains an immature worm. Aspirate preparation (Papanicolaou stain; ×800).

flammatory cells and bile duct epithelial cells that often show atypia. A large number of eosinophils and Charcot-Leyden crystals may be seen. In the case of *Clonorchis*-induced cholangiocarcinoma, the cytologic findings are essentially the same as those for other cholangiocarcinomas and are discussed in the section on Cholangiocarcinoma in this chapter.

NON-NEOPLASTIC MASS LESIONS

With the increasing use of modern imaging techniques in our clinical practice, many benign, asymptomatic nodules or masses that previously would not be detected are now frequently presented for diagnosis. In many cases of benign lesions of the liver, there are often serious diagnostic problems if no previous radiographs are available for comparison. Most such lesions are presumed to be malignant until proved otherwise. The usefulness of fine needle aspiration biopsy has been increasingly recognized in our clinical practice. This procedure can spare patients unnecessary hospitalization and operations.

Focal Nodular Hyperplasia

Cases of focal nodular hyperplasia of the liver are not rare, but they are often undetected because the lesions in most cases are asymptomatic. The lesions are usually solitary but may be multiple. They are well circumscribed but not encapsulated. They measure 1 to 8 cm in diameter and grow slowly and do not become malignant. The nodules are composed of liver parenchyma intersected by fibrous septa, which often radiate from a central scar. The normal-appearing liver cells are arranged in small pseudolobules. Bile ducts are present. Focal nodular hyperplasia can occur in any age group; most cases, however, are seen during the 3rd to 5th decades of life. Women constitute 85% of the patients with focal nodular hyperplasia. A possible relationship to oral contraceptives has been postulated in many reports.[13, 27, 36]

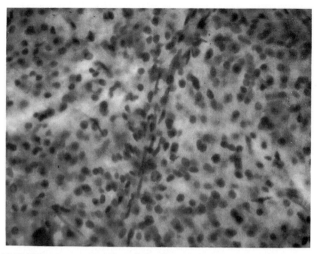

FIGURE 30–22. Focal nodular hyperplasia of the liver: parallel rows of fibrocytes that traverse a fragment of liver parenchyma. Aspirate preparation (Papanicolaou stain; ×800).

Cytology

Normal hepatocytes that are intermingled with numerous fibroblasts or embedded in fragments of fibrous tissue, mimicking cirrhosis, are present. However, in the case of focal nodular hyperplasia, there are no pleomorphism of hepatocytes, no mitotic figures and no necrotic hepatocytes such as those seen in aspirates from the cirrhotic liver. Fatty changes in hepatocytes may be seen. In some instances, the fibrous element is underrepresented in aspirate preparations, and the diagnosis of focal nodular hyperplasia in such cases is difficult on purely cytomorphologic grounds. However, parallel rows of fibrocytes that traverse large fragments of liver parenchyma can usually be found after careful searching and this finding is helpful in establishing the diagnosis (Figs. 30–22 and 30–23).

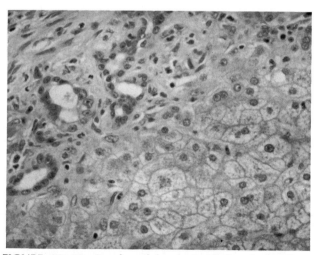

FIGURE 30–23. Focal nodular hyperplasia of the liver: masses of normal-appearing liver cells intersected by fibrous septa that contain bile ducts. Histologic section (hematoxylin and eosin; ×200).

Hydatid Disease

In North America, hydatid disease is caused by ova of the tapeworm *Echinococcus granulosus*, a parasite of dogs and wolves. The ova are passed free in a dog's or wolf's feces and develop into six-hooked embryos in the duodenum when swallowed by a human host. The embryos enter the venules and are filtered by the liver, developing into hydatid cysts that bear numerous scoleces provided with hooklets, which represent the future heads of adult tapeworms.

Cytology

The fluid aspirated from a hydatid cyst is usually clear and contains debris, a few inflammatory cells and numerous scoleces (Fig. 30–24). In old cysts, the scoleces may be difficult to find in aspirate preparations, but the hooklets in a ring-like arrangement often remain. The finding of hooklets is diagnostic of hydatid disease.

Pyogenic Abscess

Most abscesses of the liver are of a bacterial, pyogenic origin. The symptoms may be rather subtle. Pyogenic abscesses are caused by bacterial infections through ascension of the biliary tract (in cases of acute cholangitis), through the portal vein (in cases of pylephlebitis, often a complication of acute appendicitis), by means of an hepatic artery (in cases of septicemia), by direct extension (in cases of subphrenic abscess) or following trauma. They may be single or multiple. Suppurative abdominal disease with or without pylephlebitis may result in septic emboli, giving rise to liver abscesses. These most often occur in the right lobe when the suppurative disorder is drained by the right superior mesenteric vein, whereas disease in the left

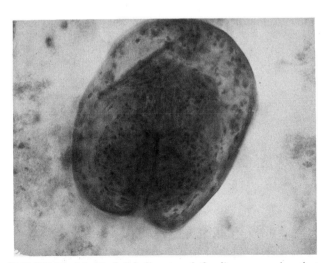

FIGURE 30–24. Hydatid disease of the liver: a scolex that has many hooklets. Aspirate preparation (Papanicolaou stain; × 400).

side of the abdomen may cause suppuration in one or both sides. Occasionally, abscesses of the liver are caused by *Actinomyces israelii*.

Cytology

Aspirate preparations from a pyogenic abscess contain a heavy neutrophilic inflammatory exudate and nuclear debris. Necrotic hepatocytes are usually not seen. The aspirate is purulent-looking and foul-smelling. Material aspirated from a actinomycotic abscess contains numerous neutrophils and phagocytic macrophages. Reactive fibroblasts are abundant. The organisms in the lesions occur as colonies (granules), which are composed of delicate, branching, intertwined, gram-positive filaments with granular, basophilic centers.

Amebic Abscess

Amebic abscesses are a result of amebic infection, caused by *Entamoeba histolytica* protozoa. In about 40% of the cases of amebic colitis, the protozoa enter the circulation and are filtered in the liver, producing solitary or multiple abscesses. The abscesses may vary greatly in size and are often located in the superoposterior portion of the right lobe. The abscess cavity is filled with a chocolate-colored pasty material.

Cytology

Aspirate preparations contain abundant necrotic cellular debris, degenerating hepatocytes and mixed inflammatory cells. Amebae can only be found in the material aspirated from the wall of the abscess. The necrotic material aspirated from the abscess is always negative for parasites. In one of our patients with an amebic abscess of the liver, the aspirate was negative for parasites, but in her cervicovaginal smear, amebae were noted (Fig. 30–25). Protozoa in cytology preparations, if any, are readily identified. They have small, vesicular nuclei and vacuolated cytoplasm that usually contains some phagocytosed red blood cells. The cytologic findings of the aspirate from an abscess plus the gross appearance of the aspirated material are certainly consistent with an amebic abscess. In the diagnosis of amebic abscess, the indirect hemagglutination test is highly sensitive and can be used to confirm the cytologic diagnosis.

Granulomas

The causes of granulomas of the liver include infectious diseases (e.g., tuberculosis, schistosomiasis, brucellosis and histoplasmosis), drug sensitivity, foreign body reaction (e.g., intravenous talc granulomatosis) and sarcoidosis.[35, 47] Tuberculous and sarcoid granulomas are the most frequently seen. Intravenous talc

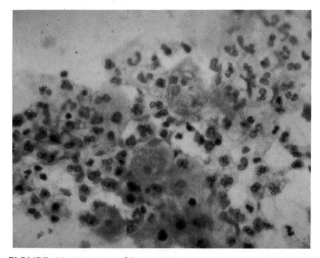

FIGURE 30–25. Amoebic vaginitis: several protozoa, *Entamoeba histolytica*, that have small vesicular nuclei and vacuolated cytoplasm containing phagocytosed red blood cells. Cervicovaginal smear (Papanicolaou stain; × 800).

granulomatosis is seen in narcotic addicts and is caused by intravenous injection of drugs that contain talc. There are two ways by which a narcotic addict may inadvertently inject talc into his or her body: (1) Heroin bought from a "street pusher" may be diluted with a substance that appears similar to the drug. Talc is often used. (2) Intravenous injection of crushed tablets that are intended only for oral administration is not an uncommon practice among narcotic addicts. Talc may be used as a filler substance.[64] The talc crystals lodge in the parenchyma of the lungs and liver and cause granulomatosis.

Cytology

Aspirates from the tuberculous lesions often contain caseous necrosis, epithelioid cells, lymphocytes, other mononuclear cells and Langhans' giant cells. The lesions of sarcoidosis contain epithelioid cells, a few lymphocytes and occasional multinucleated giant cells. No necrosis is seen. Granulomas following drug use are noncaseous and characterized by epithelioid cell reaction with giant cells and eosinophils. Infectious granulomas are often associated with systemic granulomatosis, and the cytologic diagnosis is based on finding organisms or ova. In the cases of intravenous talc granulomatosis, aspirate preparations contain strongly birefringent, plate-like crystals within foreign body giant cells and mononuclear macrophages when examined under polarized light. The crystals are composed of hydrous magnesium silicate.

BENIGN TUMORS

Common benign tumors of the liver include bile duct adenomas, liver cell adenomas and cavernous hemangiomas. With the increasing use of imaging techniques

in our clinical practice, more benign tumors are detected and presented for diagnosis.

Bile Duct Adenoma

Bile duct adenomas are small, firm nodules, rarely over 1 cm in diameter and usually located beneath Glisson's capsule. They are composed of small well-formed bile ducts embedded in a mature fibrous stroma. They are usually solitary but when multiple may mimic metastatic carcinoma.[14]

Cytology

Many cohesive clusters of bile duct epithelial cells, usually columnar in type, are seen (Fig. 30–26). Ductal cells do not show atypia. No cholestasis is noted. Hepatocytes are not seen. Fibroblasts or fragments of fibrous tissue or both may be seen in variable numbers but are usually underrepresented in aspirate preparations compared with the fibrous element seen in tissue sections because they are difficult to aspirate.

Liver Cell Adenoma

Liver cell adenomas were relatively rare until the use of oral contraceptives. Since the first report of liver cell adenomas associated with the use of oral contraceptives in 1973, many similar cases have been published.[6, 25, 36] They almost exclusively occur in women over 30 years of age who have been taking oral contraceptives for longer than 5 years. Estrogen is believed to be responsible. The adenomas are usually solitary, circumscribed and encapsulated, but 10% of cases are multiple. Some adenomas have regressed after withdrawal of the oral contraceptives, but the tumor develops again in 25% of women who resume oral contraceptive use after resection of an adeno-

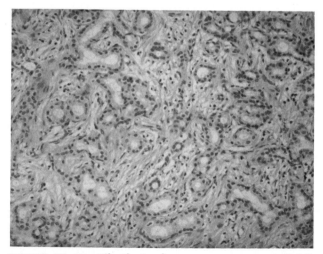

FIGURE 30–26. Bile duct adenoma: numerous small bile ducts surrounded by fibrous stroma. Histologic section (hematoxylin and eosin; × 200).

ma.[22, 36] Malignant transformation has been reported in rare instances.[20] The tumors are composed of liver parenchyma without portal triads or bile ducts. There are abundant small arteries within the tumor, and areas of hemorrhage and necrosis are often present.

Cytology

Aspirate preparations contain numerous closely packed, three-dimensional groupings of hepatocytes and fragments of liver parenchyma. The cytoplasm of these liver cells is frequently rather pale because of increased glycogen deposition (Figs. 30–27 and 30–28). No bile duct epithelial cells or fibroblasts are present. The hepatocytes are normal looking. Mitoses are not seen. Necrotic hepatocytes may be noted. The cytologic findings are not diagnostic of liver cell adenoma on purely cytomorphologic grounds. However, if the operator of aspiration biopsy makes certain that the needle tip is in the lesion and its position has been checked by an imaging technique, the previously mentioned cytologic findings coupled with clinical history are in keeping with a liver cell adenoma.

Cavernous Hemangioma

Cavernous hemangiomas are common incidental findings at autopsy or operation and are often seen in multiparous women, possibly as a result of an increase of circulating estrogenic hormones during pregnancy. They appear as circumscribed, dark red nodules measuring from a few millimeters to several centimeters in diameter. The patients are usually asymptomatic. The lesions are composed of endothelium-lined channels supported by a fibrous stroma.

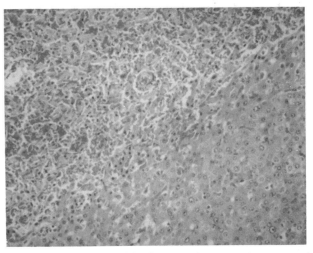

FIGURE 30–28. Liver cell adenoma: the tumor is composed of normal-appearing hepatocytes. No portal triads or bile ducts are present. Note areas of hemorrhage and necrosis. Histologic section (hematoxylin and eosin; ×200).

Cytology

The aspirates from such lesions are invariably very bloody, and aspirate preparations contain scattered noncohesive groupings of stromal cells with elongated nuclei and poorly defined cytoplasm (Figs. 30–29 and 30–30). Rare endothelial cells may be seen, but they are usually hard to find in aspirate preparations because there is no proliferation of endothelial cells in such lesions. As in the diagnosis of liver cell adenoma, only if the operator of aspiration biopsy makes certain that the needle tip is in the lesion and has been checked by an imaging technique can the previously mentioned cytologic findings coupled with radiographic and clinical presentations be considered to be consistent with cavernous hemangioma.

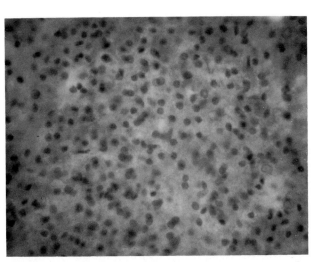

FIGURE 30–27. Liver cell adenoma: a large fragment that contains numerous normal-appearing hepatocytes with relatively pale cytoplasm and uniform, round nuclei. Aspirate preparation (Papanicolaou stain; ×80).

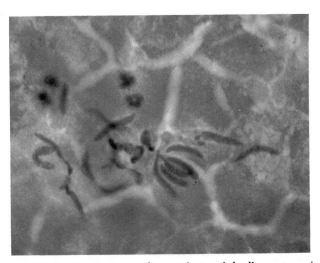

FIGURE 30–29. Cavernous hemangioma of the liver: stromal cells, in loose groupings, appearing as stripped, spindle-shaped nuclei in the absence of endothelial or liver cells on an extremely bloody background. Aspirate preparation (Papanicolaou stain; ×800).

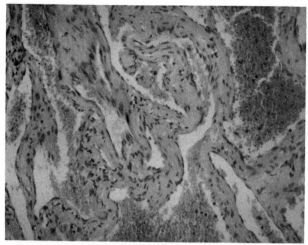

FIGURE 30–30. Cavernous hemangioma of the liver. Histologic section (hematoxylin and eosin; ×80).

PRIMARY MALIGNANT TUMORS

In our series of 1383 cases of aspiration biopsy of the liver, 1037 (75%) were metastatic cancers and 111 (8%), primary liver cancers. Of these 111 primary liver cancers, 83 cases were hepatocellular carcinoma, 19 cases were cholangiocarcinoma, two cases were angiocarcinoma, four cases were malignant lymphoma, two cases were leiomyosarcoma and one case was fibrosarcoma. Cytologic features of primary malignant lymphoma, leiomyosarcoma and fibrosarcoma of the liver seen in aspirate preparations are essentially the same as those in other sites and will not be discussed in this chapter.

Hepatocellular Carcinoma

Hepatocellular carcinoma has a relatively low incidence in western Europe and North America, accounting for 1.2 to 2.5% of all malignancies.[5] However, in the Orient and Africa, hepatocellular carcinoma is one of the most common malignant tumors. In Taiwan, 20% of the deaths from malignancy are from hepatocellular carcinoma.[70] Hepatocellular carcinoma also has a high incidence in all African countries south of the Sahara.[30]

There has been great interest in etiologically related factors in hepatic carcinogenesis during the 1980s. Hepatitis B virus infection has been identified as a major risk factor in the Orient. Reports from Taiwan show that 80% of patients with hepatocellular carcinoma have a chronic form of hepatitis B,[67] and the tumor develops in HBsAg carriers.[7] The incorporation of hepatitis B viral DNA into the DNA of neoplastic cells of hepatocellular carcinoma has been detected.[45, 55] Such hepatitis B viral DNA incorporated into the DNA of neoplastic cells of hepatocellular carcinoma has been observed in patients with hepatocellular carcinoma but with no serologic evidence of past or current hepatitis B infection.[12]

Hepatocellular carcinoma is less likely to develop in patients with alcoholic cirrhosis of the liver. In the United States, only about 4% of patients with alcoholic cirrhosis develop hepatocellular carcinoma. Because alcoholic cirrhosis is much more common in the West than in the Orient, it plays an important role in the etiology of hepatocellular carcinoma in North America.

In some African countries, the ingestion of aflatoxins, metabolic products of the growth of *Aspergillus flavus*, may be involved in the etiology of hepatocellular carcinoma.[48] Studies show that aflatoxin B1, the most toxic of the aflatoxins, is highly carcinogenic for some animal species. In Mozambique, the incidence of hepatocellular carcinoma is the highest in the world and the *per capita* intake of aflatoxins is also the highest.[68]

Grossly, hepatocellular carcinoma may present as a solitary mass, as multiple nodules or as diffuse liver involvement. Hepatocellular carcinoma may permeate the liver through the portal venous system. The growth of carcinoma in the branches of the portal vein may lead to a tumor thrombus of the portal trunk and sudden increase of portal hypertension. Metastases to regional lymph nodes and distant spread may also occur. However, there is a tendency for hepatocellular carcinomas to remain localized in the liver without metastases. With the improved imaging techniques combined with the use of aspiration biopsy, this combination may provide us time to establish the diagnosis before it is too late for surgical excision.

Morphologic differences among different cases of hepatocellular carcinoma are well recognized in histologic sections. As can be expected, aspirate preparations of the tumors from different patients exhibit various cytomorphologic appearances. Many histologic patterns of hepatocellular carcinoma have been described in the literature.[26] They often cannot be appreciated and distinguished from one another in aspirate preparations. The increasing utilization of transabdominal fine needle aspiration biopsy prompts the description of such cytomorphologic features and cytologic diagnostic criteria of different cytologic types of hepatocellular carcinoma, which are helpful in accurately diagnosing this tumor and differentiating it from secondary cancers.

Cytology

On the basis of cytomorphologic features of hepatocellular carcinoma observed in aspirate preparations in correlation with histopathology, the tumors can be classified into three types: well-differentiated cell type, pleomorphic large-cell type and poorly differentiated cell type.[63] In our series of 1383 cases of aspiration biopsy of the liver, 83 were diagnosed as hepatocellular carcinoma, including 44 of the well-differentiated cell type (two cases of clear cell variant), 21 of the pleomorphic large-cell type (four cases of fibrolamellar variant) and 18 of the poorly differentiated cell type.

Histologically, hepatocellular carcinoma of the well-differentiated cell type usually shows a trabecular

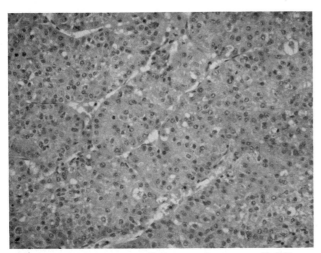

FIGURE 30–31. Hepatocellular carcinoma, well-differentiated cell type: the tumor has a trabecular growth pattern. Trabeculae or plates of tumor cells are separated by sinusoids. Histologic section (hematoxylin and eosin; ×200).

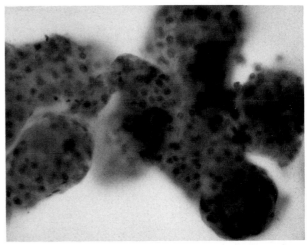

FIGURE 30–33. Hepatocellular carcinoma, well-differentiated cell type: tumor cells that are arranged in papillae and cell balls. Aspirate preparation (Papanicolaou stain; ×200).

growth pattern. Trabeculae or plates of neoplastic cells are separated by sinusoids (Fig. 30–31). Reticulin stain reveals that reticulin is often scanty or absent. The neoplastic cells resemble normal hepatocytes except that their nucleocytoplasmic ratio is higher than that of normal hepatocytes. In hepatocellular carcinomas of the clear cell variant, the tumor cells often contain abundant glycogen and fat. Their cytoplasm appears pale or contains vacuoles in histologic sections. In some areas, the tumor shows a glandular pattern.

The cytomorphologic features of these three types of hepatocellular carcinoma are summarized as follows.

Well-Differentiated Cell Type. The aspirate preparations are usually highly cellular and contain solitary tumor cells and tumor cells in loose groupings as well as many fragments of neoplastic tissue and tightly packed, cohesive cell clusters. The neoplastic cells are often arranged in a trabecular fashion or in thick cords,

papillae or cell balls (Figs. 30–32 and 30–33). They are relatively small cells and have regular, uniform, centrally located round nuclei, with a finely granular chromatin pattern. The cytoplasm is less abundant than that of benign hepatocytes seen in the same specimen, and nucleoli are usually inconspicuous or indistinct (Fig. 30–34). It is not uncommon to find that some cohesive cell clusters are lined by sinusoid endothelial cells with elongated nuclei in a lengthwise arrangement (Fig. 30–35). In some neoplastic cells, intracytoplasmic bile may be found. It stains yellow or green with Papanicolaou stain and appears coarsely granular. Bile thrombi within canaliculi between neoplastic cells are rare. Mitotic figures and multinucleated neoplastic cells are uncommon. Intracytoplasmic hyaline globules may be seen in some cases. They are gray or tan but lightly stained and are surrounded by a clear halo. They are usually single but may be multiple. They are round

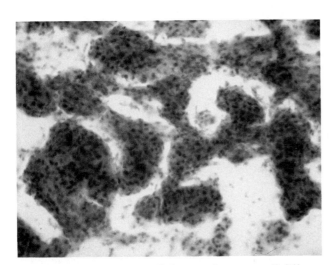

FIGURE 30–32. Hepatocellular carcinoma, well-differentiated cell type: tumor cells in trabecular arrangements. Aspirate preparation (Papanicolaou stain; ×80).

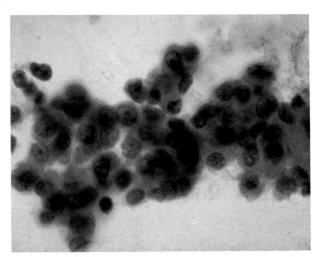

FIGURE 30–34. Hepatocellular carcinoma, well-differentiated cell type: tumor cells that have uniform, regular, centrally located, round nuclei with a finely granular chromatin pattern. Aspirate preparation (Papanicolaou stain; ×800).

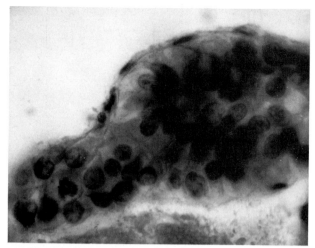

FIGURE 30–35. Hepatocellular carcinoma, well-differentiated cell type: tumor cells in a thick cord arrangement lined by sinusoidal endothelial cells with elongated nuclei. Aspirate preparation (Papanicolaou stain; ×800).

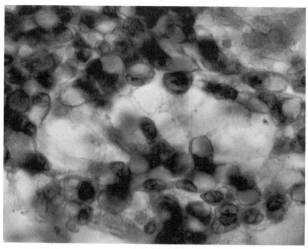

FIGURE 30–37. Hepatocellular carcinoma, well-differentiated cell type, clear cell variant: tumor cells that have vacuolated cytoplasm, in a cohesive grouping with a honeycomb pattern. Aspirate preparation (Papanicolaou stain; ×800).

and fairly large but never distort either the nucleus or the cytoplasmic membrane (Fig. 30–36). Ultrastructurally, they are nonmembrane bound and composed of a mixture of filamentous and finely granular material. They are PAS positive after amylase digestion and usually show negative immunostaining reaction for alpha-fetoprotein or keratin. Intracytoplasmic hyaline globules have also been reported in tumors of the lung, breast, ovary and adrenal.[17]

The aspirate preparations from well-differentiated hepatocellular carcinomas of the clear cell variant contain many tumor cells that have vacuolated cytoplasm in cohesive groupings, some of them with a honeycomb pattern (Fig. 30–37). A special stain (PAS stain with and without amylase digestion) shows that most of these intracytoplasmic vacuoles seen in aspirate

preparations result from a heavy deposition of glycogen that is dissolved out during processing. Intracytoplasmic lipid vacuoles are also present in some areas, and they are indistinguishable from vacuoles resulting from the removal of glycogen. The cytoplasm of tumor cells contains a single large, clear vacuole or, less frequently, multiple small vacuoles of variable size. The large vacuoles displace the nuclei to the periphery of the cells and also distend the cells. The tumor cells have round or ovoid nuclei, centrally or excentrically located, and conspicuous nucleoli. Intracytoplasmic hyaline globules (PAS positive after amylase digestion) are not an uncommon finding.

Pleomorphic Large-Cell Type. Histologic sections of some hepatocellular carcinomas of the pleomorphic large-cell type match the histologic pattern of primary

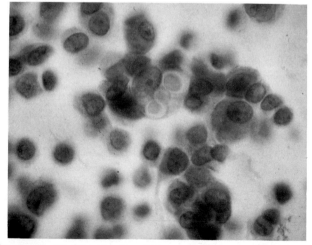

FIGURE 30–36. Hepatocellular carcinoma, well-differentiated cell type: a tumor cell that has three large, intracytoplasmic, round hyaline globules surrounded by prominent clear halos. Aspirate preparation (Papanicolaou stain; ×800).

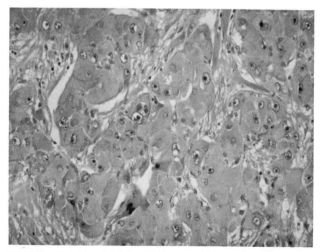

FIGURE 30–38. Hepatocellular carcinoma, pleomorphic large cell type, fibrolamellar variant: nodules of large pleomorphic tumor cells divided by laminated, fibrous stroma. Histologic section (hematoxylin and eosin; ×400).

liver cancer designated as fibrolamellar carcinoma. The pleomorphic, large, often multinucleated neoplastic cells are divided into thin columns or large nodules by fibrous stroma that is composed of many thin hyalinized bands in layers, suggesting a laminated composition (Fig. 30–38). Because the fibrous bands seen in histologic sections are underrepresented in aspirate preparations, the cytologic diagnosis of hepatocellular carcinoma of the fibrolamellar variant is possible only when there are parallel rows of fibrocytes intermingled with tumor cells.[61] However, other hepatocellular carcinomas of the pleomorphic large-cell type do not match the histologic pattern of fibrolamellar carcinoma. In these tumors, the laminated fibrous bands surrounding the tumor cells are not seen in histologic sections. In aspirate preparations from both conditions, tumor cells are large, multinucleation is common and the sinusoids with endothelial linings that are seen in the well-differentiated cell type are not present. Thus, hepatocellular carcinomas of the pleomorphic large-cell type, fibrolamellar variant, are often indistinguishable from other hepatocellular carcinomas of the pleomorphic large-cell type (nonfibrolamellar variant) in aspirate preparations because fibrous stroma in the fibrolamellar variant is often underrepresented or not present in aspirates.

Cytology. Aspirate preparations show that neoplastic cells are present in small, loose groupings or lie singly. They are variable in size and shape but are often large, and some of them giant. The cytoplasm is abundant and well defined. The nuclei also have variations in size and shape and tend to be excentric in position (Fig. 30–39). Nucleoli are prominent in many cells. Multinucleated neoplastic cells are a common finding and may contain more than ten nuclei (Fig. 30–40). Bile production by the tumor cells, either mononuclear or multinucleated, is a frequent finding. Sinusoidal endothelial lining cells, such as those seen in the well-differentiated cell type, are not present. In

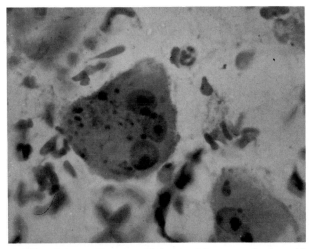

FIGURE 30–40. Hepatocellular carcinoma, pleomorphic large cell type: a tumor cell that has three nuclei with prominent nucleoli and contains an abundance of granular bile pigment. Aspirate preparation (Papanicolaou stain; ×800).

some tumors (the fibrolamellar variant), parallel rows of elongated, benign-looking fibrocytes are seen intermingled with tumor cells and dividing-tumor cells into nests.[61] However, in aspirate preparations, the fibrous stroma is usually underrepresented compared with the neoplastic hepatocytes seen in histologic sections because the fibrous tissue is more difficult to aspirate than are the neoplastic hepatocytes. In two of the four cases of fibrolamellar variant in our series, no fibrocytes were seen in the aspirate preparations. Intracytoplasmic hyaline globules may occasionally be seen. In rare cases of this type, mucin-secreting activity may be seen in some neoplastic cells in which the cytoplasm appears vacuolated and shows positive reaction with mucicarmine stain.[63] In our series, four such cases were identified (Figs. 30–41 and 30–42).

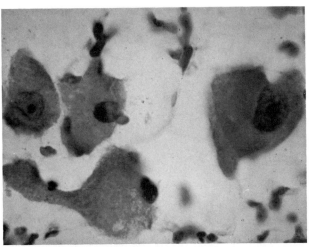

FIGURE 30–39. Hepatocellular carcinoma, pleomorphic large cell type: solitary tumor cells that have large amounts of cytoplasm and excentrically placed nuclei that are variable in size and shape. Aspirate preparation (Papanicolaou stain; ×800).

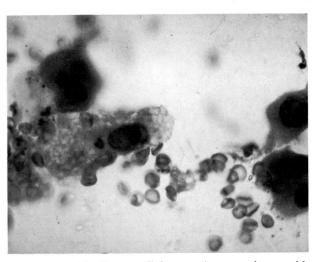

FIGURE 30–41. Hepatocellular carcinoma, pleomorphic large cell type: a solitary tumor cell that has vacuolated cytoplasm indicative of mucin-secreting activity. Aspirate preparation (Papanicolaou stain; ×800).

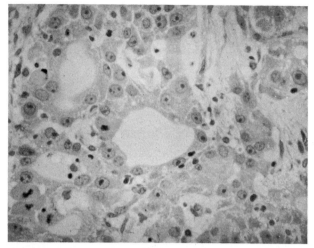

FIGURE 30–42. Hepatocellular carcinoma, pleomorphic large cell type: the tumor has a glandular growth pattern in some areas. Intracellular and extracellular mucin (mucicarmine-positive) is evident. Histologic section (hematoxylin and eosin; ×400).

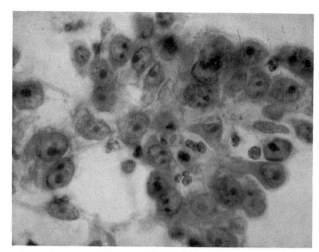

FIGURE 30–44. Hepatocellular carcinoma, poorly differentiated cell type: tumor cells that have large, round or ovoid nuclei and prominent nucleoli, in loose groupings. Aspirate preparation (Papanicolaou stain; ×800).

Poorly Differentiated Cell Type. Histologically, hepatocellular carcinoma of this type shows masses of bizarre-appearing neoplastic cells without a definite cellular arrangement (Fig. 30–43). Occasional sinusoids with endothelial linings may be seen. Multinucleation is unusual, and bile production by neoplastic cells is rare.

Cytology. Aspirate preparations contain a few cohesive cell clusters but many solitary cells and loose groupings of neoplastic cells. The tumor cells appear bizarre and contain large, round or ovoid nuclei with prominent nucleoli. The nuclei are either centrally located or eccentric in position. Binucleation may be seen, but multinucleation is unusual (Figs. 30–44 and 30–45). The cytoplasm is relatively scanty, and thus the nucleocytoplasmic ratio appears high. Bile produc-

tion is rare in this type. Occasional intracytoplasmic hyaline globules may be seen. They are relatively large and surrounded by a clear halo. Cytomorphologically, neoplastic cells of this type somewhat resemble atypical hepatocytes in cirrhotic liver, but their nucleocytoplasmic ratio is much higher than that of the latter.

Cytomorphologic features of hepatocellular carcinomas of these three types are distinctly different and are summarized and compared in Table 30–2. Their cytomorphologic characteristics appear quite different from those of most metastatic cancers. The immunostaining for alpha-fetoprotein, polyclonal carcinoembryonic antigen and alpha-1-antitrypsin is also helpful in establishing the definitive diagnoses in some problem cases.

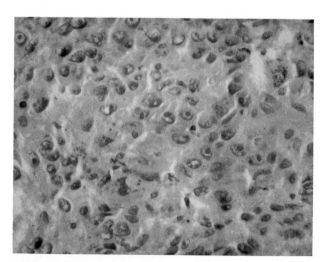

FIGURE 30–43. Hepatocellular carcinoma, poorly differentiated cell type: masses of bizarre-appearing tumor cells without a definite cellular arrangement. Histologic section (hematoxylin and eosin; ×400).

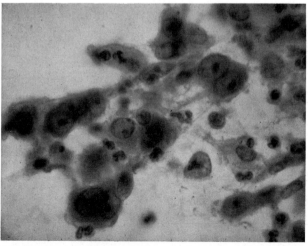

FIGURE 30–45. Hepatocellular carcinoma, poorly differentiated cell type: several binucleated tumor cells that have relatively scanty cytoplasm and large nuclei. Aspirate preparation (Papanicolaou stain; ×800).

TABLE 30–2. Comparison of Cytomorphologic Features of Different Types of Hepatocellular Carcinoma

	Well-Differentiated Cell Type	Pleomorphic Large-Cell Type	Poorly Differentiated Cell Type
Cellular Arrangement			
General cytologic pattern	Many tissue fragments and cohesive groupings	Loose groupings and solitary cells	Cohesive groupings, loose groupings and solitary cells
Sinusoidal endothelial lining	Common findings	Absent	Occasionally seen
Cells			
Average size	Relatively small	Large	Relatively large
Nucleocytoplasmic ratio	Intermediate	Low	High
Cohesion between cells	Good	Poor	Relatively poor
Nuclei			
Shape	Round (mostly) or ovoid	Variable	Round or ovoid
Location	Central	Peripheral	Central or peripheral
Size	Small	Variable	Large
Prominent nucleoli	Unusual	Relatively common	Frequent
Multinucleation	Occasional	Frequent	Unusual
Cytoplasm			
Abundance	Less abundant	Abundant	Scanty
Bile production	Common	Frequent	Rare
Hyaline globules	Uncommon	Rare	Occasional

Cholangiocarcinoma

Cholangiocarcinomas may arise anywhere between the papilla of Vater and the small branches of the bile ducts within the liver but originate most often from the large hilar bile ducts at the bifurcation of the common hepatic duct or from the extrahepatic bile ducts. Intrahepatic cholangiocarcinoma is much less common than hepatocellular carcinoma. Cholangiocarcinoma is known to follow *Clonorchis sinensis* infestation, hemochromatosis and Thorotrast injection, and occasionally the tumor arises in patients with chronic ulcerative colitis.[1] Histologically, cholangiocarcinoma is an adenocarcinoma of the cuboid or columnar cell type. There is much more fibrous stroma than in hepatocellular carcinoma, and the tumor is much less vascular. Mucin is usually demonstrable but rarely abundant. Cholangiocarcinomas with prominent secretory activity are only occasionally encountered in our daily work.

Cytology

Aspirate preparations show that neoplastic cells occur in cohesive groupings without a definite cellular arrangement and, only occasionally, in sheet arrangements. They are relatively small and have ovoid nuclei and small amounts of cytoplasm, resembling atypical bile duct epithelial cells (Fig. 30–46). The variations in nuclear size and prominent nucleoli are noted in some cells. The cytoplasm may appear vacuolated in some cells, indicative of mucin secretion. In our series, most cholangiocarcinomas were nonsecretory or minimally secretory. Only two tumors showed prominent secretory activity and contained numerous neoplastic cells that had vacuolated cytoplasm (Fig. 30–47). Cy-

tomorphologically, cholangiocarcinomas are indistinguishable from adenocarcinomas of the pancreas arising from the pancreatic duct. Findings of imaging techniques, particularly percutaneous transhepatic cholangiography, are helpful in the determination of tumor origin.

Angiosarcoma

Angiosarcomas of the liver are uncommon and highly malignant tumors. They have been associated with injection of Thorotrast,[71] industrial exposure to vinyl chloride[66] and previous arsenic treatment.[37] A relationship to steroid hormones,[24] copper sulfate in

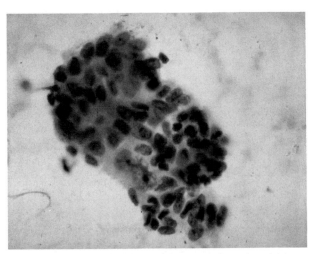

FIGURE 30–46. Cholangiocarcinoma, nonsecretory type: tumor cells that have small ovoid nuclei, in a sheet arrangement, resembling atypical duct epithelium. Aspirate preparation (Papanicolaou stain; × 800).

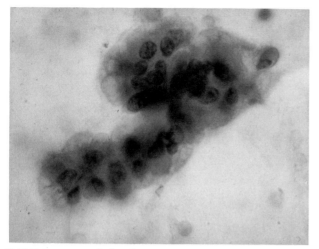

FIGURE 30–47. Cholangiocarcinoma, secretory type: tumor cells that have abundant, vacuolated cytoplasm and relatively small ovoid nuclei, in cohesive groupings. Aspirate preparation (Papanicolaou stain; ×800).

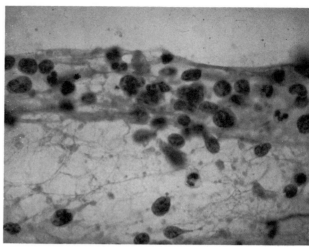

FIGURE 30–49. Angiosarcoma of the liver: solitary tumor cells that have round or ovoid nuclei and no recognizable cytoplasm. Aspirate preparation (Papanicolaou stain; ×800).

vineyard sprayers[51] and phenelzine[19] has also been suggested. The majority of patients (85%) are in their 6th or 7th decade of life. About one third of cases are associated with cirrhosis.[43] The tumors form multiple or, less often, solitary hemorrhagic masses. Both open and percutaneous large-bore needle biopsies for histologic diagnosis are associated with significant intra-abdominal bleeding in 16% of the cases and death in 5%.[40] Fine needle aspiration biopsy of the tumor is expected to greatly reduce this hazard. Histologically, the tumor may show cavernous or solid growth patterns. Irregular vascular spaces lined with neoplastic cells with round, ovoid or elongated nuclei are noted (Fig. 30–48). Thrombosis and infarction are common.

Cytology

Aspirate preparations show that neoplastic cells occur in loose groupings or lie singly. Some of them have round or ovoid nuclei and no recognizable cytoplasm. Other cells appear spindle shaped and have elongated nuclei (Figs. 30–49 and 30–50). Occasionally, large, bizarre-appearing neoplastic cells with intracytoplasmic hemosiderin pigment may be seen. These could be malignant Kupffer cells.[48] The smears are usually bloody, and necrotic cellular debris may be present on the background. Factor VIII is detected in the cytoplasm of some neoplastic cells by means of immunoperoxidase staining, indicative of endothelial origin.

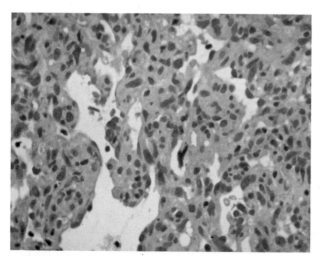

FIGURE 30–48. Angiosarcoma of the liver: some irregular spaces lined by tumor cells that have round, ovoid or elongated nuclei. Histologic section (hematoxylin and eosin; ×400).

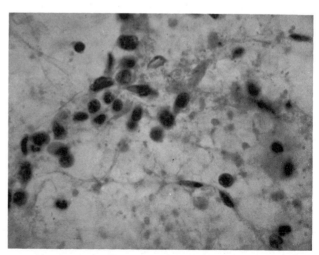

FIGURE 30–50. Angiosarcoma of the liver: some tumor cells that have spindle-shaped nuclei, intermixed with other tumor cells that have round or ovoid nuclei. Aspirate preparation (Papanicolaou stain; ×800).

TUMORS METASTATIC TO THE LIVER

The liver frequently harbors metastatic growths. Approximately 83% of the cases of fine needle aspiration biopsy of the liver in our series were malignant tumors. Among them, 90% were cancers metastatic to the liver. The cancer cells may reach the liver through the portal vein, hepatic artery or hilar lymphatics or by direct extension. Practically all malignant cells grow well in liver parenchyma, and metastatic carcinomas usually grow rapidly in the liver, with patients rarely living more than a year after the establishment of the diagnosis.[34] Primary malignant tumors of the gallbladder, extrahepatic bile ducts, pancreas and stomach frequently involve the liver by direct extension. Distant metastases from carcinomas of the large bowel, kidney, pancreas, stomach, lung and breast appear with appalling frequency. Sarcomas may also metastasize to the liver. Metastasis to the liver occurs in 38% of all cancers—41% of lung cancers, 56% of colon cancers, 70% of pancreatic cancers, 53% of breast cancers and 44% of gastric cancers.[21]

Once implanted in the liver, the cancer cells may form small or large nodules or grow diffusely throughout the liver. In about 10% of the cases metastatic nodules are solitary. Many benign lesions and primary liver tumors may have a gross appearance and roentgenographic features indistinguishable from those of metastatic cancers. Therefore, it is imperative that a microscopic confirmation be obtained in every patient in whom a liver mass or masses are detected by means of imaging techniques. The presence of liver metastases virtually precludes the possibility of curative surgery at the site of the primary cancer. Transabdominal fine needle aspiration biopsy is of great value in patients who are scheduled to undergo operative resection of a primary cancer if ultrasonography or computed tomography demonstrates a lesion or lesions in the liver. The cytomorphologic features of malignant tumors metastatic to the liver seen in aspirate preparations are essentially the same as those of the primary tumors from other organs and will not be discussed in this chapter.

DIAGNOSTIC ACCURACY

An operator capable of obtaining an adequate amount of the target tissue is essential for a successful biopsy. In the 1970s, most aspiration biopsies of the liver in our series were performed under the guidance of radioisotopic scanning or angiography and under fluoroscopic control. Because the position of the needle tip could not be documented before aspiration, the needle sometimes missed the target lesion. According to our results, the chance that a single puncture would yield a representative sample was 72.3%.[62] However, for three punctures with slight modification in the angle of approach, the chances increased to 94% in experienced hands. As a result of improved imaging techniques that can display sectional images, the position of the needle tip in relation to the lesion can now be readily verified prior to aspiration, ensuring the acquisition of the target tissue. With the exception of a few cases due to sampling errors, the aspiration biopsy under the guidance of ultrasonography and computed tomography performed by experienced operators is usually representative. The smallest intrahepatic lesion successfully aspirated in our series was 7 mm in greatest dimension.

The interpretation of aspiration biopsy specimens of hepatic lesions is like morphologic diagnosis in other branches of anatomic pathology, in which subjective recognition of morphologic features and past experience have a major role in diagnostic accuracy. From the literature, the sensitivity for diagnosis of hepatic malignancy ranges from 92 to 96%.[31, 46, 49, 57, 58, 72] False-positive results have also been reported[31, 49, 58] and usually occur in an early stage when the technique is first adopted. False-positive results are more often a reflection of the lack of experience of the examiner. They can be almost completely eliminated with increased experience.

Pancreas

The pancreas is relatively inaccessible to conventional methods of study and is difficult to investigate because of its anatomic location. Clinically, carcinomas of the pancreas are sometimes very difficult to diagnose with certainty, even during laparotomy. The gross appearance of chronic pancreatitis may look similar to that of carcinoma of the pancreas. Cote and coauthors[88] found that the intraoperative wedge biopsy failed to reveal carcinoma in 54% of the patients with carcinoma of the pancreas, and the Vim-Silverman needle missed the diagnosis in 32%.[13] Moreover, wedge biopsy or large-bore needle biopsy often lead to serious complications, e.g., hemorrhage, fistula formation, pancreatitis, pseudocyst and even death. The complication rate has been reported to vary from 3.0 to 20%.[91, 109, 115, 117]

With the introduction of modern imaging techniques, percutaneous fine needle aspiration biopsy is rapidly gaining recognition as an excellent method in obtaining a pathologic diagnosis among patients with malignant lesions in the pancreas.[74–76, 82, 85, 93–101, 112, 119, 121, 124, 127] In our series of 584 cases of aspiration biopsy of the pancreas, the diagnostic rate of carcinomas of the pancreas by guided fine needle aspiration biopsy method has increased from 82% in the 1970s to 94%, and complications following aspiration biopsy were unusual. Therefore, the accuracy and safety of guided aspiration biopsy of the pancreas are superior to those of wedge biopsy or large-bore needle biopsy.

IMAGING TECHNIQUES

The major problem in the diagnosis of carcinoma of the pancreas arises from the difficulty in obtaining representative material, which in turn relies on the techniques used to localize the lesions. Material is obtained by biopsy during selective angiography of the celiac artery with test injections of contrast medium under fluoroscopic control,[125, 126] using endoscopic retrograde cholangiopancreatography (ERCP),[107] during ultrasonography using a special biopsy transducer[87, 103, 135] and with computed tomography to image the position of the biopsy needle.[87, 137]

Selective angiography of the celiac artery may reveal an encasement of a blood vessel by a tumor growth (e.g., encasement of the splenic artery by carcinoma of the pancreas). Endoscopic retrograde cholangiopancreatography permits the visualization of the pancreatic duct. It may reveal small carcinomas of the pancreas because obstruction of the pancreatic duct is often an early change of cancerous growths arising from the ductal epithelium. However, it is not a good localizing method because the site of obstruction is sometimes a result of focal edema, fibrosis or inflammation that may coexist with a malignant tumor. Material aspirated from the site of obstruction may not contain tumor cells.

Improved ultrasonography with a special biopsy transducer has become a preferred method for localization and aspiration biopsy of pancreatic mass lesions in many hospitals because of its ease and accuracy in obtaining representative samples. Computed tomography is also often used, especially if the first attempt under the guidance of ultrasound is unsuccessful.

NORMAL PANCREAS

Histology

The pancreas is composed of exocrine and endocrine portions. The exocrine portion consists of serous acini and ducts. The acini are arranged into many small lobules and produce digestive enzymes that are drained into the duodenum through the pancreatic duct system. The acinar cells have round nuclei and abundant granular cytoplasm. The intralobular ducts are lined by a flattened epithelium, and the epithelium of the interlobular ducts consists of cuboid cells. The main ducts are lined by columnar epithelial cells with interspersed goblet cells. The endocrine portion consists of numerous islets of Langerhans. The islets are dispersed in the pancreas and are more concentrated in the body and tail. The islet cells are arranged in cords, separated by capillaries. They may be classified into at least six types on the basis of the hormones produced, namely, alpha cells (glucagon), beta cells (insulin), delta cells (somatostatin), pancreatic polypeptide cells (pancreatic polypeptide), enterochromaffin cells (5-hydroxytryptamine) and P cells (unknown function). They can be identified by electron microscopy or immunohistochemical study. They are, however, indistinguishable under light microscopy.

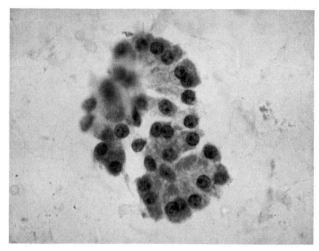

FIGURE 30–51. Normal pancreatic acinar cells: acinar cells that have excentrically placed, round nuclei and an abundance of granular cytoplasm, in small groupings. Aspirate preparation (Papanicolaou stain; × 800).

Cytology

Aspirate preparations from a normal pancreas usually contain acinar cells, islet cells, ductal cells, endothelial cells and mesothelial cells (often seen in aspirates from lesions in the body of the pancreas). If the lesion is in the head of the pancreas, the aspirate may contain some hepatocytes.

In aspirate preparations, acinar cells are present in small clusters with good intercellular cohesion. The nuclei are round or ovoid and have uniformly distributed, finely granular chromatin. They are often excentrically placed and are uniform and regular but may show slight variation in size. The nuclear membranes are smooth and thin. Nucleoli are small but may be conspicuous in some cells. The cytoplasm is abundant and appears granular (Fig. 30–51).

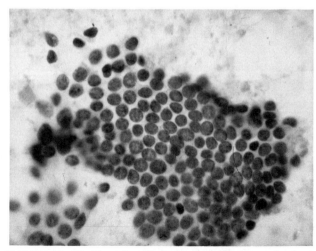

FIGURE 30–52. Ductal cells from a small pancreatic duct: ductal cells that have round nuclei with indistinct nucleoli and relatively scanty, poorly defined cytoplasm, in a sheet arrangement. Aspirate preparation (Papanicolaou stain; × 800).

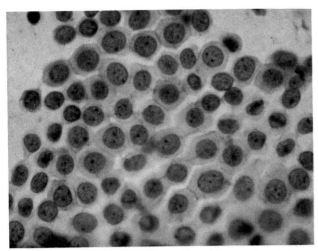

FIGURE 30–53. Mesothelial cells from the peritoneum: mesothelial cells that have large, round or ovoid nuclei, in a sheet arrangement with slits between the cells. Aspirate preparation (Papanicolaou stain; ×800).

Islet cells are an infrequent finding and often not identifiable in aspirate preparations. Special stains may be helpful in their identification. They lie singly or occur in small, loose groupings. The nuclei are usually round, with a finely granular chromatin pattern. The cytoplasm is scanty and often not recognizable in aspirate preparations. Nucleoli are indistinct. The cytologic features of the nuclei of islet cells are similar to those of the nuclei of acinar cells; therefore, islet cells are indistinguishable from acinar cells when stripped of cytoplasm in poorly fixed aspirate preparations.

Epithelial cells of the small pancreatic ducts are often in sheet arrangements in aspirate preparations. They have relatively scanty, poorly defined cytoplasm and round nuclei with indistinct nucleoli (Fig. 30–52). The chromatin pattern of the nuclei is slightly coarsely granular but evenly distributed. Columnar epithelial cells of the larger pancreatic ducts are an infrequent finding in aspirate preparations. They occur in cohesive groupings or in palisading arrangements or lie singly. They have moderate amounts of well-defined cytoplasm and ovoid nuclei. Some of them show vacuolated or foamy cytoplasm, indicative of secretory activity.

In aspirate preparations, mesothelial cells are often seen in aspirates from lesions in the body of the pancreas, which is covered by mesothelial lining. They have round or ovoid nuclei and are in sheet arrangements, often with slits between cells (Fig. 30–53). Endothelial cells from small blood vessels may also be noted. They have ovoid nuclei and abundant cytoplasm. They are also in sheet arrangements like mesothelial cells, but the endothelial sheets usually contain fewer cells. Unlike mesothelial cells, there are no slits between cells.

PANCREATITIS

Inflammation of the pancreas comprises a spectrum of disorders that range from acute hemorrhagic pan-

creatitis, a prostrating disease, to chronic relapsing pancreatitis with eventual pancreatic insufficiency. A late complication of acute pancreatitis is the development of a pseudocyst or an abscess.

Acute Pancreatitis

Acute pancreatitis occurs in adults between 40 and 70 years of age and often follows a heavy meal or an alcoholic debauch. It is a debilitating illness with an abrupt onset. Early in the disease, pancreatic enzymes, such as amylase and lipase, are liberated into the blood stream. The pathogenesis of acute pancreatitis is still not clear. The pancreas appears swollen and edematous. The injury to acinar cells causes release and activation of the digestive enzymes, resulting in necrosis and inflammation of the pancreas and the surrounding tissues. The pancreas contains patches of coagulative necrosis rimmed by heavy neutrophilic infiltrates. Foci of fat necrosis in the peripancreatic tissue, mesentery and omentum may appear as small, ovoid, yellow-white nodules and are due to the formation of calcium soaps through the mechanism of saponification. These foci may be detected by imaging techniques.

Cytology

Aspirate preparations contain tightly packed clusters of necrotic acinar cells with pyknotic nuclei (Fig. 30–54). On the background, finely and coarsely granular necrotic debris is usually present and intermingled with numerous neutrophils. Necrotic ductal cells showing karyorrhexis or appearing as ghost cells are sometimes noted (Fig. 30–55). Degenerating fat cells, lipid droplets and lipid-laden macrophages with foamy or vacuolated cytoplasm are also noted (Figs. 30–56 and 30–57).[105] The von Kossa stain may demonstrate some granular deposition of calcium salts within the necrotic debris. The formation of calcium salts is an indication

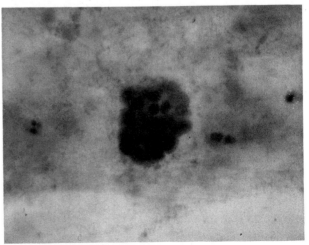

FIGURE 30–54. Necrosis in acute pancreatitis: necrotic acinar cells that have pyknotic nuclei, in a closely packed cluster, on a background of finely and coarsely granular, necrotic debris. Aspirate preparation (Papanicolaou stain; ×400).

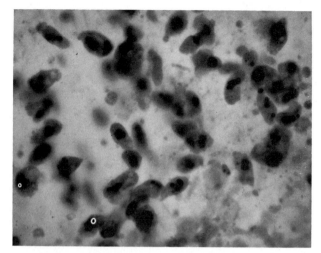

FIGURE 30–55. Necrosis in acute pancreatitis: necrotic ductal cells that undergo karyorrhexis as solitary cells. Aspirate preparation (Papanicolaou stain; ×800).

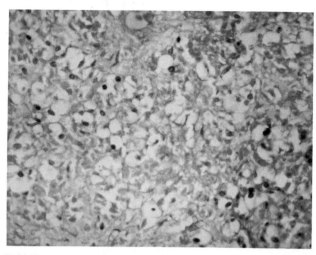

FIGURE 30–57. Acute pancreatitis: necrosis of fat cells and acinar tissue. Histologic section (hematoxylin and eosin; ×200).

of fat necrosis. Irritated mesothelial cells may be seen if the material is aspirated from the body of the pancreas. These cells have slightly enlarged, ovoid nuclei and small nucleoli and occur in groupings with overlapping of cells or in disorderly arrangements. Occasional slits between cells are seen.

Chronic Pancreatitis

In approximately one third of all patients who survive episodes of acute pancreatitis, the disease progresses to chronic pancreatitis. The pancreas is firm and nodular, with areas of dense fibrosis, loss of acinar and islet tissues and infiltration of lymphocytes and plasma cells. Proliferation of ducts and hyperplasia of

ductal epithelial cells with some atypia are noted. Areas of calcification in the interstitial tissue and pancreatic ducts are present. The destruction of the pancreas eventually results in pancreatic insufficiency (Fig. 30–58).

Cytology

The aspirates contain many lymphocytes and plasma cells, fewer acinar cells and more ductal cells. If the material is aspirated from areas of dense fibrosis, the aspirates are often scantily cellular. Fibrocytes and fragments of fibrous tissue are usually present. Atypical acinar cells may be seen. Their nuclei have conspicuous nucleoli and some variation in nuclear size (Fig. 30–59). The cytoplasm of atypical acinar cells may appear vacuolated in some cell clusters. Although atypical ductal cells tend to be in sheet arrangements, overlapping of cells and cells in disorderly arrangements are sometimes noted, mimicking adenocarcinoma (Fig. 30–60). The nuclei of atypical ductal cells are larger than those of normal ones and have variations in nuclear size and shape (Fig. 30–61). Conspicuous nucleoli may be seen. The cytoplasm of atypical ductal cells may appear vacuolated in some cell clusters. Endothelial cells from the small blood vessels in the inflamed tissue or granulation tissue appear somewhat pleomorphic. Their nuclei have some variations in size and shape. Mesothelial cells overlying the inflamed tissue also appear atypical and are seen in aspirated material from the body of the pancreas, which is covered with mesothelial lining. Their nuclei have a slightly coarse chromatin pattern and small or conspicuous nucleoli. The usual sheet arrangements of mesothelial cells are often distorted, with overlapping of cells (see Fig. 30–58). The cytologic differentiation between chronic pancreatitis and adenocarcinoma of the pancreas is summarized in Table 30–3.

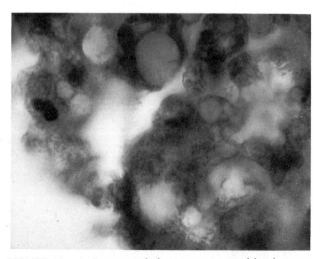

FIGURE 30–56. Fat necrosis in acute pancreatitis: degenerated fat cells and lipid droplets intermixed with lipid-laden macrophages. Aspirate preparation (Papanicolaou stain; ×800).

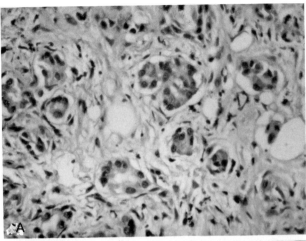

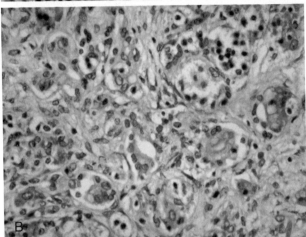

FIGURE 30–58. Chronic pancreatitis. *A,* Loss of acinar cells, fibrosis and infiltration of chronic inflammatory cells. *B,* Atypical acinar and ductal cells that have vacuolated cytoplasm. Histologic section (hematoxylin and eosin; ×200).

Pseudocyst

Pseudocysts of the pancreas are closely related to acute pancreatitis, operative trauma or reflux of bile into the pancreatic duct. They develop as a result of blockage of ducts and leakage of pancreatic juice from the injured pancreatic tissue, which leads to an accumulation of secretion and cyst formation, usually unilocular. The fluid within them has a high amylase content. The cyst gradually increases in size and spreads into the lesser peritoneal cavity. Bile is found in the cavity of the cystic lesion in some cases. Late complications such as hemorrhage have occurred. The splenic artery is the most common source of intracystic hemorrhage, which can be massive and result in sudden death.

Cytology

The aspiration of fluid from a pancreatic pseudocyst may have not only diagnostic but also therapeutic significance. In fact, pseudocysts of the pancreas may

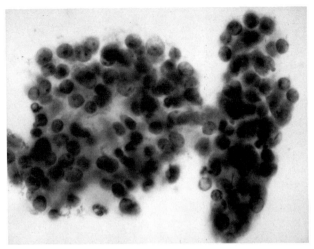

FIGURE 30–59. Atypical acinar cells in chronic pancreatitis: atypical acinar cells that have round nuclei with small nucleoli and variation in nuclear size. Aspirate preparation (Papanicolaou stain; ×800).

disappear after percutaneous aspiration of the fluid, obviating further management. In aspirate preparations prepared by filtration or centrifugation technique, there are varying amounts of mixed inflammatory cells and coarsely granular necrotic debris. Fibroblasts and small fragments of fibrous tissue may be present. Irritated mesothelial cells are usually seen. Some of them are highly atypical. They may be gigantic and have giant nuclei and large nucleoli, mimicking malignancy. However, the nucleocytoplasmic ratio of these cells remains low (Fig. 30–62). In some cases, bile and bile-laden macrophages are abundant (Fig. 30–63).

CYSTADENOMAS

Cystadenomas are uncommon, slow-growing tumors. They occur predominantly in women and usually arise

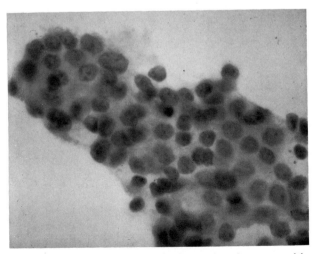

FIGURE 30–60. Atypical ductal cells in chronic pancreatitis: atypical ductal cells in disorderly arrangements mimicking adenocarcinoma. Aspirate preparation (Papanicolaou stain; ×800).

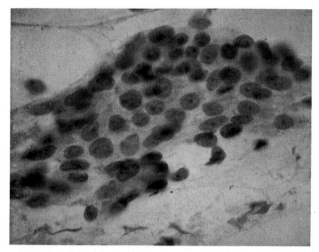

FIGURE 30–61. Atypical ductal cells in chronic pancreatitis: atypical ductal cells that have enlarged nuclei with small nucleoli and variations in size and shape. Aspirate preparation (Papanicolaou stain; ×800).

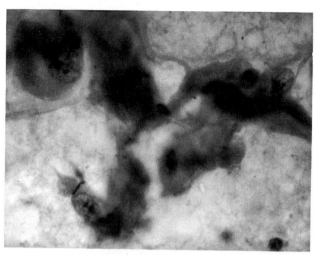

FIGURE 30–62. Irritated mesothelial cells in pseudocyst of the pancreas: atypical mesothelial cells that have large, ovoid nuclei with conspicuous nucleoli and an abundance of cytoplasm. Aspirate preparation (Papanicolaou stain; ×800).

in the body and tail of the pancreas. They can be divided into two distinct groups: serous (microcystic or glycogen-rich) cystadenomas and mucinous cystic tumors.

Serous Cystadenoma

Serous (microcystic or glycogen-rich) cystadenomas are invariably benign tumors, usually large. The patients are usually elderly, and the disease is either discovered incidentally or manifests as an abdominal mass with local discomfort or pain. The tumors are composed of innumerable small cavities and fewer larger cysts containing clear fluids. The cavities of the cysts are lined by cuboid or columnar epithelial cells containing abundant glycogen. Ultrastructural studies have shown that features of the neoplastic epithelial cells are comparable with those of normal centroacinar cells.

Cytology

The aspirates consist of clear fluid. In the cytologic preparations made from the sediment of the fluid or by filtration technique, there are numerous duct epithelial cells. They lie singly or occur in cohesive groupings, in either sheets or palisades. The epithelial cells are either columnar or cuboid in shape. They have moderate amounts of cytoplasm and round or ovoid nuclei. Nucleoli are indistinct (Fig. 30–64). A few foamy macrophages may be present. Other cellular components are rarely seen in the aspirate preparations from serous cystadenomas.

Mucinous Cystic Tumors

Mucinous cystic tumors are seen in a younger age group. The tumors are usually multiloculated or, rarely, uniloculated. The cavities contain mucous material and are lined by tall, mucin-producing epithelial cells. The clinical presentation is similar to that of the serous cystadenomas. Although benign and malignant varieties exist, the distinction between benign and malignant tumors is not always clear-cut and requires an extensive sampling of the specimen. Therefore, all of these mucinous tumors should be regarded as potentially malignant.[82] There have been well-documented cases of "mucinous cystadenoma" recurring as cystadenocarcinoma. Thus, total excision of the tumors is strongly recommended.

TABLE 30–3. Cytologic Differentiation Between Chronic Pancreatitis and Well-Differentiated Adenocarcinoma of the Pancreas

	Chronic Pancreatitis	Well-Differentiated Adenocarcinoma of the Pancreas
Abnormal Ductal Cells	Few groups, vacuolated cells in some groups	Many groups, vacuolated cells intermingled with nonsecretory cells
Cellular Arrangement	Relatively regular, loose, monolayer	Irregular, tight, three-dimensional arrangement; occasional monolayer
Variation in Nuclear Size	Slight	Apparent in some groups

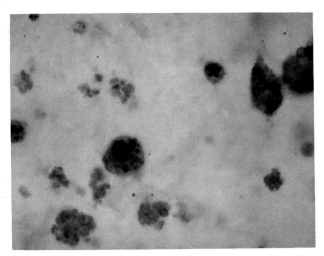

FIGURE 30–63. Bile-laden macrophages in pseudocyst of the pancreas: several macrophages that contain yellow, granular bile pigment. Aspirate preparation (Papanicolaou stain; ×800).

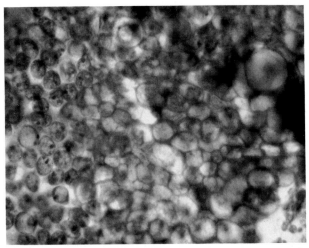

FIGURE 30–65. Mucinous cystic tumor of the pancreas: tumor cells that have vacuolated cytoplasm, in a sheet arrangement with a honeycomb pattern. Aspirate preparation (Papanicolaou stain; ×800).

Cytology

The aspirates are usually highly cellular. The cytologic preparations made from aspirated mucous material show numerous epithelial cells with vacuolated cytoplasm, resembling benign cells from the endocervix.[88] The tumor cells occur in sheet arrangements with a honeycomb pattern (Fig. 30–65) or lie singly, often appearing as goblet cells. The nuclei are round and may have small nucleoli. Atypical epithelial cells are a common finding. They are larger, and the nucleocytoplasmic ratio is higher. Their nuclei often show variations in size and have conspicuous nucleoli and finely granular or slightly coarse chromatin (Fig. 30–66). In some cases, atypical epithelial cells showing malignant transformation are noticed. These highly abnormal cells that have large nuclei with variations in

size and shape and slightly coarse chromatin occur in disorderly arrangements (Fig. 30–67).[103]

CARCINOMAS

Carcinomas of the pancreas rank fourth in frequency among cancer deaths in North America, and their incidence is increasing. Adenocarcinomas arising from the pancreatic ducts compose 80 to 90% of all cases of malignant neoplasms of the pancreas. They occur in the head of the pancreas in about two thirds of the patients and in the body and tail in the other third. Most patients are in their 5th to 7th decade of life. Carcinomas of the head of the pancreas usually cause

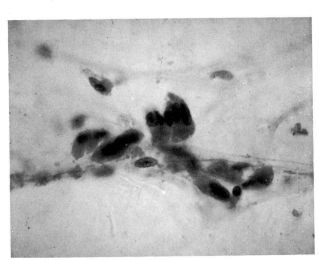

FIGURE 30–64. Serous cystadenoma of the pancreas: columnar tumor cells that have ovoid nuclei, in palisading arrangements. Aspirate preparation (Papanicolaou stain; ×800).

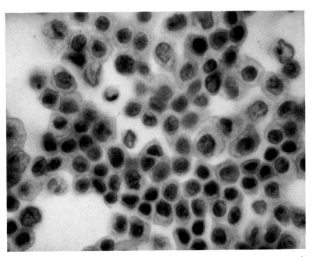

FIGURE 30–66. Atypical epithelial cells in a mucinous cystic tumor of the pancreas: tumor cells that have large, round nuclei with a finely granular chromatin pattern and variation in nuclear size. Aspirate preparation (Papanicolaou stain; ×800).

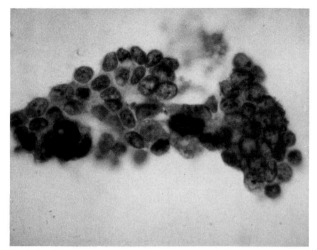

FIGURE 30–67. Malignant transformation in a mucinous cystic tumor of the pancreas: tumor cells that have variations in nuclear size and shape and a slightly coarse granular chromatin pattern, in disorderly arrangements. Aspirate preparation (Papanicolaou stain; ×800).

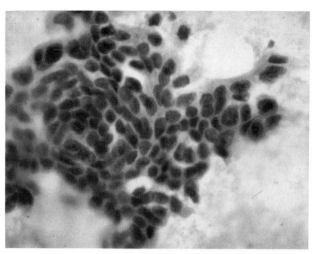

FIGURE 30–69. Well-differentiated adenocarcinoma of the pancreas: tumor cells that have variations in nuclear size and shape, in a monolayer arrangement. Aspirate preparation (Papanicolaou stain; ×800).

progressive jaundice associated with pain, resulting from neoplastic invasion of the wall of the common bile duct. Carcinomas of the body and tail of the pancreas are, on average, larger than those of the head at the time of diagnosis because the tumors rarely produce early symptoms. More than 90% of the patients die within 1 year of diagnosis. Histologic examinations show that carcinomas of the pancreas are often well-differentiated adenocarcinomas. However, the degree of differentiation may vary from neoplasms with well-defined ductal structures to those with anaplastic undifferentiated cells in other tumors. Papillary adenocarcinoma, pleomorphic giant cell carcinoma, adenosquamous carcinoma and cystadenocarcinoma also occur and are uncommon malignant neoplasms of the pancreas. As can be expected, aspirate preparations

from carcinomas of the pancreas from different patients may exhibit various cytomorphologic patterns and features, as discussed in the following sections.

Well-Differentiated Adenocarcinoma

The aspirates from adenocarcinomas of the pancreas of the well-differentiated type are usually cellular. Tumor cells occur in cohesive groupings. They tend to form large, tightly packed cell clusters and flat sheets (Figs. 30–68 and 30–69). Their nuclei are larger than those of normal ductal cells, are round or ovoid with slightly coarse chromatin and have conspicuous nucleoli in some tumor cells (Fig. 30–70). The variation

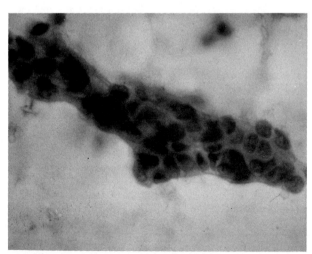

FIGURE 30–68. Well-differentiated adenocarcinoma of the pancreas: tumor cells that have medium-sized, ovoid nuclei, in a tightly packed, cohesive cluster. Aspirate preparation (Papanicolaou stain; ×800).

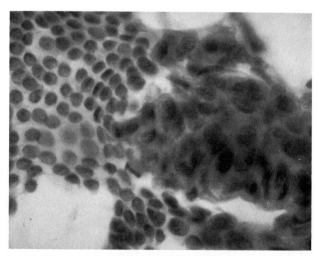

FIGURE 30–70. Well-differentiated adenocarcinoma of the pancreas: tumor cells (right) that have larger nuclei in a three-dimensional grouping as compared with normal ductal cells (left) that have uniform nuclei, in a sheet arrangement. Aspirate preparation (Papanicolaou stain; ×800).

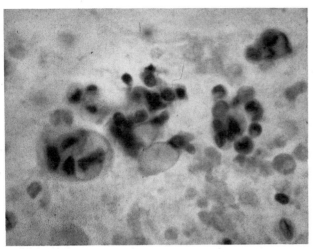

FIGURE 30–71. Well-differentiated adenocarcinoma of the pancreas: tumor cells that have an abundance of vacuolated cytoplasm indicative of mucin secretion. Aspirate preparation (Papanicolaou stain; ×800).

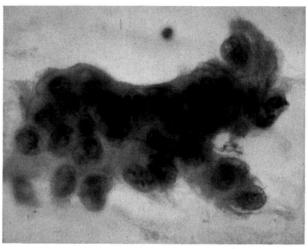

FIGURE 30–73. Moderately differentiated adenocarcinoma of the pancreas: tumor cells that have large, pleomorphic nuclei and moderate amounts of cytoplasm, in a cohesive grouping. Aspirate preparation (Papanicolaou stain; ×800).

in nuclear size is noted in some clusters, and uniformity of nuclei is seen in other groups. The cytoplasm is relatively scanty in nonsecretory tumor cells but may be abundant and appear vacuolated in some tumor cells, indicative of mucin secretion (Figs. 30–71 and 30–72). In our series, carcinomas of the pancreas with prominent secretory activity were uncommon. On some occasions, it may be difficult to differentiate the atypical ductal cells of chronic pancreatitis from the neoplastic cells of well-differentiated carcinoma in aspirate preparations. The individual cells of these two conditions may look alike in the smears. However, the findings of three-dimensional, tightly packed cell clusters with irregularity in cell arrangement and more apparent difference in degree of cellular atypia within the same cell clusters are indicative of adenocarcinoma (see Table 30–3).

Moderately Differentiated Adenocarcinoma

The cytologic diagnosis of adenocarcinomas of the pancreas of the moderately differentiated type is easy and straightforward because the tumor cells are frankly malignant. Large tumor cells occur in cohesive clusters or noncohesive groupings or lie singly. They are bizarre looking, with pleomorphism and irregularity of the nuclei. The nuclei vary in size and shape and have a coarse chromatin pattern and frequent prominent nucleoli. The amount of cytoplasm is variable, from scanty to abundant. Mucin-secreting cells are rare, and mitotic figures are common (Figs. 30–73 and 30–74).

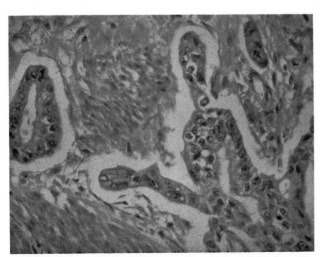

FIGURE 30–72. Well-differentiated adenocarcinoma of the pancreas. Histologic section (hematoxylin and eosin; ×200).

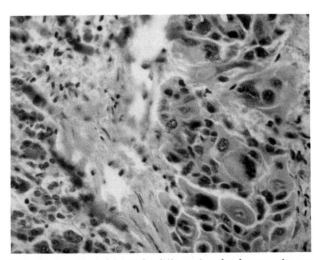

FIGURE 30–74. Moderately differentiated adenocarcinoma of the pancreas. Histologic section (hematoxylin and eosin; ×200).

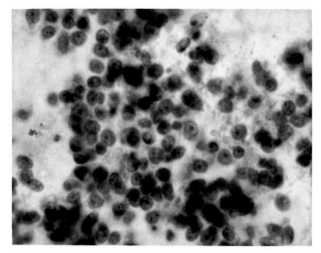

FIGURE 30–75. Poorly differentiated adenocarcinoma of the pancreas: tumor cells that have small or medium-sized nuclei, in loose groupings and as solitary cells. Aspirate preparation (Papanicolaou stain; ×800).

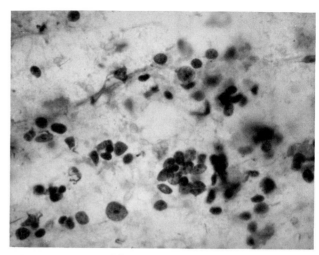

FIGURE 30–77. Undifferentiated small-cell carcinoma of the pancreas: solitary tumor cells that have small, irregularly shaped nuclei and little recognizable cytoplasm. Aspirate preparation (Papanicolaou stain; ×800).

Poorly Differentiated Adenocarcinoma

Poorly differentiated adenocarcinomas of the pancreas are uncommon. In aspirate preparations, tumor cells occur in noncohesive groupings or lie singly (Fig. 30–75). The nuclei are relatively small, tend to be round and have prominent nucleoli and coarsely granular chromatin. The cytoplasm is scanty and poorly defined. At first glance, dispersed neoplastic cells with round nuclei and prominent nucleoli resemble malignant lymphoma of the immunoblastic type. Immunoperoxidase techniques are helpful in the differential diagnosis. Immunostainings for epithelial markers (e.g., cytokeratin, carcinoembryonic antigen) are positive in the cytoplasm of some tumor cells, and immunostainings for lymphoid markers (e.g., common leukocytic antigen) are negative in tumor cells from these tumors (Fig. 30–76).

Undifferentiated Small-Cell Carcinoma

Undifferentiated small-cell carcinomas of the pancreas are rare and highly aggressive. They probably arise from Kulchitsky's cells, which are normally present in this organ in connection with the exocrine ducts.

Cytology

In aspirate preparations, tumor cells are small and occur singly or in loose groupings. The nuclei are irregular and small. The cytoplasm is very scanty and poorly defined. The tumor cells often appear as stripped nuclei in aspirate preparations. Chromatin is usually heavily stained, and nucleoli are indistinct (Figs. 30–77 and 30–78). Nuclear molding may be seen. Cytomorphologically, undifferentiated small-cell

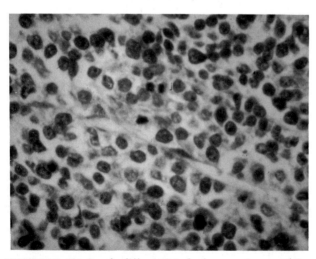

FIGURE 30–76. Poorly differentiated adenocarcinoma of the pancreas. Histologic section (hematoxylin and eosin; ×400).

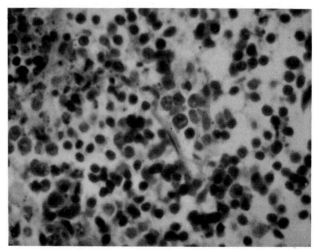

FIGURE 30–78. Undifferentiated small-cell carcinoma of the pancreas. Histologic section (hematoxylin and eosin; ×400).

carcinoma of the pancreas is indistinguishable from small-cell anaplastic carcinoma of the lung, even at the electron-microscopic level.[132]

Papillary Adenocarcinoma

Papillary adenocarcinomas of the pancreas are low-grade malignant tumors and may be solid or partially cystic. They are mostly found in young females. The prognosis is remarkably good following surgical excision.[113] Histologic examinations show that the tumors are extremely cellular and exhibit prominent papillae, which are covered by several layers of tumor cells and have a fibrovascular core.

Cytology

Aspirate preparations contain papillary fragments of neoplastic tissue with branchings and smooth, common cell borders, often in large numbers (Fig. 30–79). Tumor cells are highly cohesive, and dispersed tumor cells are infrequent. The nuclei are round or ovoid and relatively uniform and regular. They appear crowded and frequently molded. Nucleoli are usually inconspicuous but may be prominent in some tumor cells. Tumor cells have moderate amounts of nonsecretory cytoplasm (Figs. 30–80 and 30–81).[80, 84, 95]

Pleomorphic Giant Cell Carcinoma

Pleomorphic giant cell carcinomas of the pancreas are rare, highly malignant tumors, characterized by the presence of a large number of bizarre, mononuclear or multinucleated giant tumor cells. Many terms describing this pathologic entity, including pleomorphic adenocarcinoma, pleomorphic carcinoma, giant cell

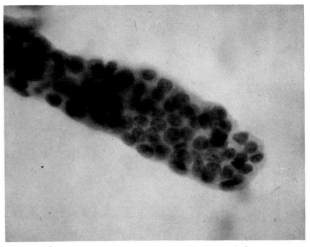

FIGURE 30–80. Papillary adenocarcinoma of the pancreas: tumor cells that have regular, round or ovoid nuclei, in a papillary arrangement. Aspirate preparation (Papanicolaou stain; ×800).

carcinoma and sarcomatoid carcinoma, have been used in the literature. Metastases invariably develop, and hematogenous spread is common. In some tumors, benign-looking osteoclast-like giant cells[118, 142] intermingled with bizarre, giant tumor cells against a background of a sarcomatoid growth pattern are noted.[121] Initially, the prognosis for these tumors containing osteoclast-like giant cells was thought to be better than that of adenocarcinoma of the pancreas, but several reports have attested to negligible patient salvage.[89, 138] However, other authors believe that those tumors composed of osteoclast-like giant cells and relatively uniform spindle cells of mesenchymal appearance without bizarre giant cells (designated as giant cell tumor of the pancreas) have a better prognosis and should be classified separately from pleomorphic giant cell carcinomas.[132] Whether these osteoclast-like giant cells are a mesenchymal response to the tumor or whether

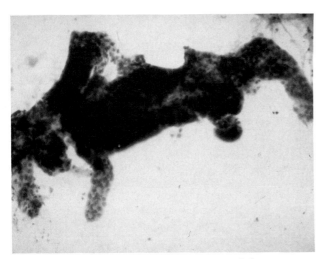

FIGURE 30–79. Papillary adenocarcinoma of the pancreas: a papillary fragment that contains closely packed tumor cells and has smooth, common cell borders. Aspirate preparation (Papanicolaou stain; ×80).

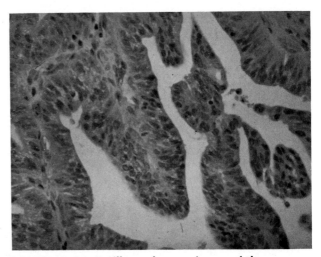

FIGURE 30–81. Papillary adenocarcinoma of the pancreas. Histologic section (hematoxylin and eosin; ×200).

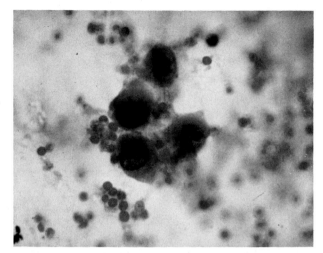

FIGURE 30–82. Pleomorphic giant cell carcinoma of the pancreas: solitary tumor cells that have large nuclei with coarsely granular chromatin and prominent nucleoli. Aspirate preparation (Papanicolaou stain; ×800).

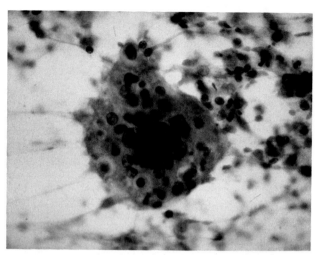

FIGURE 30–84. Pleomorphic giant cell carcinoma of the pancreas: a giant cell that has numerous uniformly small nuclei and an abundance of cytoplasm resembling an osteoclast. Aspirate preparation (Papanicolaou stain; ×800).

they are part of the epithelial components of the tumor is still not clear. Electron-microscopic and immunohistochemical studies suggest an epithelial origin of the osteoclast-like giant cells.[118, 128, 139]

Cytology

The aspirates from some tumors (without osteoclast-like giant cells) contain numerous, dispersed giant tumor cells. Some of them are mononuclear and have bizarre, hyperchromatic nuclei and prominent nucleoli (Fig. 30–82). Other tumor cells are multinucleated and have several pleomorphic nuclei (Fig. 30–83). The aspirates from other tumors contain some benign-looking, osteoclast-like giant cells in addition to bizarre giant tumor cells. The nuclei of osteoclast-like giant

cells are uniformly small and regular (Fig. 30–84). On the background there are relatively uniform spindle cells of mesenchymal appearance.

Adenosquamous Carcinoma

Adenosquamous carcinomas may be seen in many organs. The pancreas is one of the more common sites for the occurrence of adenosquamous carcinoma. Adenosquamous carcinomas constitute about 3 to 4% of exocrine pancreatic neoplasms. They probably arise from squamous metaplasis of the terminal ducts.[83, 129] Pure squamous cell carcinomas of the pancreas are very rare. The aspirates of adenosquamous carcinomas show a dual population: adenocarcinoma cells with evidence of secretory activity and squamous carcinoma cells showing keratinization.[114, 144]

Cystadenocarcinoma

Cystadenocarcinomas have a better prognosis than do noncystic adenocarcinomas. Their documented slow growth rate and prolonged localization within the pancreas contribute to a generally good prognosis.[83, 86] With appropriate surgical resection, these tumors constitute one of the few curable neoplasms of the pancreas.[86] Because the tumors occur mainly in the body and tail of the pancreas, symptoms are late; thus, the tumors often reach a large size. They may be multilocular or unilocular and mucinous or serous. It is possible that some mucinous cystadenocarcinomas derive from benign precursors.

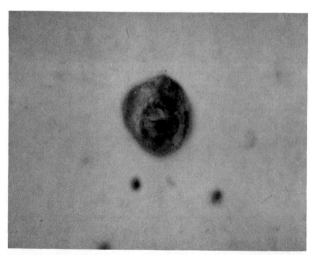

FIGURE 30–83. Pleomorphic giant cell carcinoma of the pancreas: a giant tumor cell that has several pleomorphic nuclei and prominent nucleoli. Aspirate preparation (Papanicolaou stain; ×800).

Cytology

Aspirate preparations from some tumors of the mucinous type contain scattered vacuolated or signet-

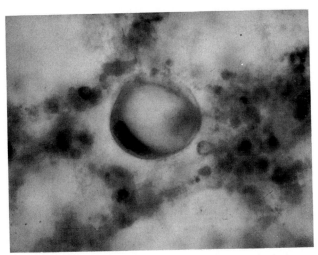

FIGURE 30–85. Cystadenocarcinoma of the pancreas, mucinous type: a tumor cell that has a single, large intracytoplasmic vacuole appearing as a signet ring, on a mucinous background. Aspirate preparation (Papanicolaou stain; ×800).

ring type tumor cells on a mucinous background (Fig. 30–85). The aspirates from such tumors are scantily cellular, and tumor cells are present in small groupings. The large, intracytoplasmic vacuoles displace the nuclei to the periphery of the cells. In other tumors, the aspirates are highly cellular, and groups of benign-looking duct epithelial cells with nuclei in a palisading arrangement are noted in addition to groups of recognizable malignant cells, indicative of malignant transformation from a benign precursor.[140, 141] The aspirates from tumors of the serous type do not have a mucinous background, nor signet-ring type cells. Tumor cells occur in cohesive groupings (Fig. 30–86). They have an abundance of cytoplasm and large round or ovoid nuclei with conspicuous nucleoli.

Ampullary Carcinoma

Carcinomas are much less frequent in the periampullary region than in the pancreas. Because obstruction of the bile duct by the tumor causes early onset of jaundice, ampullary carcinomas are often discovered at an early stage of the disease and are usually much more curable than carcinomas of the head of the pancreas. Most ampullary carcinomas are adenocarcinomas, many of them having a superficial papillary component.[145]

Cytology

In aspirate preparations, the cytologic features are those of well-differentiated adenocarcinoma of the pancreas arising from the pancreatic ducts (Fig. 30–87).[90] The differential diagnosis can be based only on clinical and radiographic findings. In advanced disease with the invasion of adjacent structures and the head of the pancreas, it is often impossible to ascertain the source of the adenocarcinoma.

ISLET CELL LESIONS

Islet cell tumors make up a small fraction (less than 5%) of all pancreatic neoplasms and most commonly are located in the body or tail of the pancreas, where a greater islet concentration is normally present. They are neoplasms of the neuroendocrine system of which the cells are derived, from the neural crest, tube and ridge. Because the cytomorphologic appearances of endocrine tumors are generally not a good indicator for differentiating between benign and malignant lesions, islet cell tumors composed of cells with uniform and regular nuclei do not necessarily indicate a benign lesion, and the presence of nuclear aberration and mitotic figures cannot be used as a criterion for malignancy. Therefore, *islet cell tumor* is the proper termi-

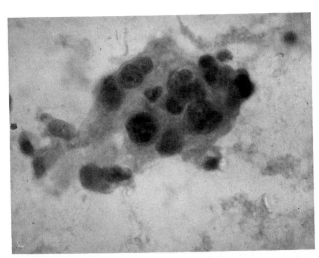

FIGURE 30–86. Cystadenocarcinoma of the pancreas, serous type: tumor cells that have large, round or ovoid nuclei and an abundance of cytoplasm, in a cohesive grouping. Aspirate preparation (Papanicolaou stain; ×800).

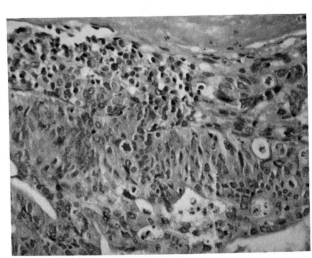

FIGURE 30–87. Ampullary carcinoma. Histologic section (hematoxylin and eosin; ×200).

nology in the cytologic diagnosis of neoplastic lesions of islet cell origin. Moreover, islet cell tumor and islet cell hyperplasia are sometimes indistinguishable on purely cytomorphologic grounds.

Islet Cell Tumor

Islet cell tumors are slow-growing tumors. They may arise from islet cells of any type and may be hormonally active or inactive. Studies of these tumors with immunocytochemical techniques have shown that the majority of them have more than one cell type and that the predominant cell type determines the clinical syndrome. Most tumors are solitary, but they may be multiple. Most tumors occur in adults. Depending on the type of hormones produced, islet cell tumors may be associated with a variety of clinical disorders, such as hyperinsulinism (beta cell tumor), glucagonoma syndrome (alpha cell tumor), Zollinger-Ellison syndrome (ulcerogenic islet cell tumor) and a cholera-like syndrome (diarrheogenic islet cell tumor). Insulin-producing beta cell tumors constitute the most common variety of functioning islet cell tumors. Histologic examinations show that tumor cells resemble normal islet cells. They may be arranged in solid nests, ribbons or festoons and are separated by highly vascular stroma. The only histomorphologic features that show some correlation with metastatic spread are stromal invasion and tumor thrombi in the blood vessels.

Cytology

The aspirates from islet cell tumors are usually highly cellular. In aspirate preparations, tumor cells occur in noncohesive groupings and occasionally in cohesive groupings or lie singly (Fig. 30–88). The tumor cells are generally small. Their nuclei tend to be round and relatively uniform and regular. Nucleoli are inconspicuous, and chromatin is fine and evenly distributed. The cytoplasm is scanty and poorly defined (Fig. 30–89). At first glance, tumor cells from islet cell tumors may look like those from well-differentiated adenocarcinomas of the pancreas, and the former is often mistaken by inexperienced examiners for the latter. However, it is important for us to distinguish this tumor from adenocarcinoma of the pancreas preoperatively because surgical approaches for these two conditions are different. From our experience, the cytologic differentiation between these two conditions is possible and reliable on purely cytomorphologic grounds, although it may be difficult for untrained observers to differentiate. The cytologic differentiation between islet cell tumors and well-differentiated adenocarcinoma of the pancreas is summarized in Table 30–4. The cytomorphologic diagnosis can be readily confirmed by special stains. Immunostaining for neuron-specific enolase or chromogranin is positive in the cytoplasm of some tumor cells from islet cell tumors and negative for tumor cells from adenocarcinomas.[78, 136] The tumor cells from neuroendocrine tumors may also show intracytoplasmic, Grimelius-positive

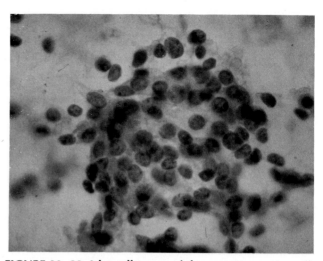

FIGURE 30–88. Islet cell tumor of the pancreas: tumor cells that have round nuclei and little recognizable cytoplasm, in noncohesive groupings and as solitary cells. Aspirate preparation (Papanicolaou stain; ×800).

granules. These findings are helpful in the differential diagnosis.[77, 79, 116, 142, 143]

Islet Cell Hyperplasia

Islet cell hyperplasia of the pancreas, like islet cell tumors, may also present as nodular lesions and may be hormonally active or inactive. The nodules are usually smaller. They are not neoplastic and are always benign. Histologic examinations show that islet cell hyperplasia consists of numerous large islets separated by fibrous stroma. Islets are not fused, and islet cells are not arranged in solid masses.

Cytology

In aspirate preparations, it is not always possible to distinguish islet cell hyperplasia from islet cell tumor.

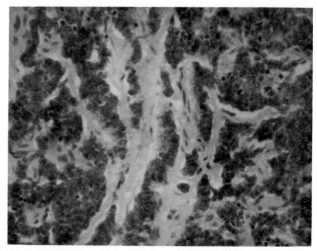

FIGURE 30–89. Islet cell tumor of the pancreas. Histologic section (hematoxylin and eosin; ×200).

TABLE 30–4. Cytologic Differentiation Between Islet Cell Tumors and Well-Differentiated Adenocarcinomas of the Pancreas

	Islet Cell Tumors	Well-Differentiated Adenocarcinomas of the Pancreas
Cellular Arrangement	Three-dimensional groupings, noncohesive	Three-dimensional cohesive groupings, irregular and tight
Nuclei	Tend to be round, relatively uniform and regular; inconspicuous nucleoli	Ovoid, more irregular; prominent nucleoli in some cells
Cytoplasm (Secretory Activity)	Scanty, poorly defined, nonvacuolated	Variable amount, well defined, some vacuolated cells

Cytomorphologic features of these two conditions are similar. However, aspirates from islet cell hyperplasia are usually scantily cellular and contain islet cells in small, noncohesive groupings (Fig. 30–90), whereas aspirates from islet cell tumors are usually highly cellular, and tumor cells are arranged in much larger noncohesive and cohesive groupings. In our practical work, if the specimen is highly cellular and consists of tumor cells in large groupings, islet cell hyperplasia can be readily excluded. If the specimen is scantily cellular and the abnormal islet cells are present in small, noncohesive groupings, islet cell hyperplasia cannot be distinguished from islet cell tumor on purely cytomorphologic grounds.

Islet Cell Carcinoma

Islet cell carcinomas are also slow-growing tumors that may be hormonally active or inactive. Metastases are restricted to peripancreatic lymph nodes and the liver in the majority of cases. About 10% of insulin-producing beta cell tumors are malignant, and approximately 60% of solitary ulcerogenic islet cell tumors are malignant. The large majority of clinically active glucagon-producing alpha cell tumors are malignant. Tumors associated with multihormone production that can be detected by serum determinations are often malignant.

Cytology

In general, cytomorphologic criteria of tumor cells of islet cell origin are not good indicators for the differentiation between benign tumors and carcinomas.[108, 122, 123] In our practical work, islet cell carcinomas cannot be identified as malignant tumors by aspiration biopsy technique in some cases. However, in other cases in our series, the overall cytologic findings were highly suggestive of malignancy, and all of these tumors were confirmed to be malignant in the follow-ups. The cytologic indications of malignancy include (1) tumor cells that show a significant increase in average nuclear size and also variation in nuclear size (Fig. 30–91), (2) tumor cells that are larger and have moderate amounts of well-defined cytoplasm and excentrically located nuclei, (3) the presence of multinucleated tumor cells, (4) the presence of mitotic figures and (5) the presence of necrotic tumor debris. From our experience, any islet cell tumor showing more than four of these five cytologic features is likely a malignant one (Fig. 30–92).

DIAGNOSTIC ACCURACY

The pancreas is considered to be one of the most difficult sites from which to obtain representative ma-

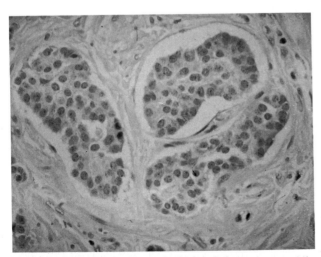

FIGURE 30–90. Islet cell hyperplasia of the pancreas. Histologic section (hematoxylin and eosin; × 200).

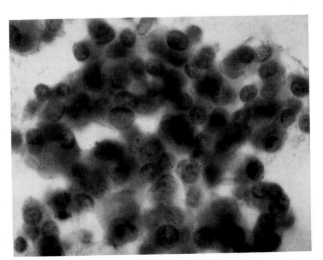

FIGURE 30–91. Islet cell carcinoma of the pancreas: tumor cells that have large, round nuclei and variation in nuclear size, in noncohesive groupings. Aspirate preparation (Papanicolaou stain; × 800).

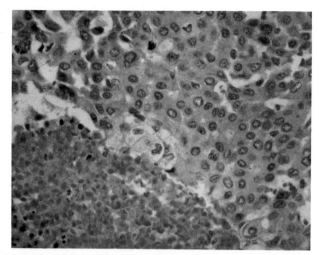

FIGURE 30–92. Islet cell carcinoma of the pancreas. Histologic section (hematoxylin and eosin; × 200).

terial by means of percutaneous fine needle aspiration biopsy technique because of its anatomic location. In the 1970s when most aspiration biopsies of the pancreas in our series were performed under the guidance of ERCP or angiography and under fluoroscopic control, the accuracy rate of needling (usually three passes) in obtaining representative samples was only around 80%. Ultrasonography and computed tomography have largely replaced ERCP and angiography in the diagnosis of pancreatic lesions by aspiration biopsy technique. Computed tomography is particularly useful as a guide to aspiration of small pancreatic lesions. Because the position of the needle tip in relation to the lesion can be readily verified prior to aspiration, the accuracy rate of needling to obtain a representative sample increased to 94% in our series. In the literature, the sensitivity for diagnosis of pancreatic carcinoma ranges from 61 to 91% by percutaneous aspiration biopsy technique[93, 100, 102–104, 119, 121, 133, 140] and from 72 to 96% by intraoperative aspiration biopsy technique.[81, 96, 97, 111]

The cytomorphologic interpretation of aspiration biopsy specimens of the pancreatic lesions is usually straightforward in experienced hands, and the specificity for diagnosis of pancreatic carcinoma should approach 100%. There have been no reports of false-positive diagnoses by aspiration biopsy technique.

References

Liver

1. Akwari OE, VanHeerden JA, Foulk WT, Baggenstoss AH: Cancer of the bile ducts associated with ulcerative colitis. Ann Surg 181:303–309, 1975.
2. Anthony P: Tumors of the liver. *In* Recent Advances in Histopathology. Edited by PP Anthony, W Woolf. Edinburgh, Churchill Livingstone, pp 213–233, 1978.
3. Anthony PP, Vogel CL, Barker LF: Liver cell dysplasia: A premalignant condition. J Clin Pathol 26:217–223, 1973.
4. Anthony PP, Vogel CL, Nayak NC, Poulsen HE, Scheuer PJ,

Sobin LH: The morphology of cirrhosis. J Clin Pathol 31:395–414, 1978.
5. Aoki K: Cancer of the liver: International mortality trends. World Health Stat Rep 31:28–50, 1978.
6. Baum JK, Holtz F, Bookstein JJ, Klein EW: Possible association between benign hepatomas and oral contraceptives. Lancet 2:926–929, 1973.
7. Beasley RP, Hwang LY, Lin CC, Chien CS: Hepatocellular carcinoma and hepatitis B virus. Lancet 2:1129–1133, 1981.
8. Bell DA, Carr CP, Szyfelbein WM: Fine needle aspiration cytology of focal liver lesions: Results obtained with examination of both cytologic and histologic preparations. Acta Cytol 30:397–402, 1986.
9. Berman JJ, McNeill RE: Cirrhosis with atypia: A potential pitfall in the interpretation of liver aspirates. Acta Cytol 32:11–14, 1988.
10. Bognel C, Rougier P, Leclere J, Duvillard P, Charpentier P, Prade M: Fine needle aspiration of the liver and pancreas with ultrasound guidance. Acta Cytol 32:22–26, 1988.
11. Braun B, Dormeyer HH: Ultrasonically guided fine-needle aspiration biopsy of hepatic and pancreatic space-occupying lesions and percutaneous abscess drainage. Klin Wochenschr 59:702–712, 1981.
12. Brechot C, Hadchouel M, Scotto J: Evidence that hepatitis B virus has a role in liver-cell carcinoma in alcoholic liver disease. N Engl J Med 306:1384–1387, 1982.
13. Casarella WJ, Knowles DM, Wolff M, Johnson PM: Focal nodular hyperplasia and liver cell adenoma: Radiologic and pathologic differentiation. AJR 13:393–402, 1978.
14. Cho C, Rullis I, Rogers LS: Bile duct adenomas as liver nodules. Arch Surg 113:272–274, 1978.
15. Civardi G, Fornari F, Cavanna L: Ultrasonically guided fine needle aspiration biopsy: A useful technique for the diagnosis of abdominal malignancies. Eur J Cancer Clin Oncol 22:225–227, 1986.
16. Cohen C: Intracytoplasmic hyaline globules in hepatocellular carcinoma. Cancer 37:1754–1758, 1976.
17. Cooperberg PL, Hutchinson D, Li D: Percutaneous fine needle aspiration biopsy under ultrasound and computed tomographic control. Br Col Med J 23:537–541, 1981.
18. Craig JR, Peters RL, Edmondson HA, Omata M: Fibrolamellar carcinoma of the liver. A tumor of adolescents and young adults with distinctive clinicopathologic features. Cancer 46:372–379, 1980.
19. Daneshmend TK, Scott GL, Bradfield JWB: Angiosarcoma of liver associated with phenelzine. Br Med J 1:1679, 1979.
20. Davis M, Portmann B, Searle M, Wright R, Williams R: Histological evidence of carcinoma in a hepatic tumor associated with oral contraceptives. Br Med J 4:496–498, 1975.
21. Edmondson HA, Peters RL: Tumors of the liver. *In* Diseases of the Liver. Edited by L Schiff, R Engene. Philadelphia, JB Lippincott, pp 1101–1157, 1982.
22. Edmondson HA, Reynolds TB, Henderson B, Benton B: Regression of liver cell adenomas associated with oral contraceptives. Ann Intern Med 86:180–182, 1977.
23. Ekelund P, Wasastjerna C: Cytological identification of primary hepatic carcinoma cells. Acta Med Scand 189:373–375, 1971.
24. Falk H, Thomas LB, Popper H, Ishak KG: Hepatic angiosarcoma associated with androgenic-anabolic steroids. Lancet 2:1120–1123, 1979.
25. Fechner RE: Benign hepatic lesions and orally administered contraceptives. Hum Pathol 8:255–268, 1977.
26. Frias-Hidvegi D: Liver and pancreas. *In* Guides to Clinical Aspiration Biopsy. Edited by TS Kline. New York, Igaku-Shoin, 1988.
27. Gold JH, Guzman IJ, Rosai J: Benign tumors of the liver. Am J Clin Pathol 70:6–17, 1978.
28. Gupta SK, Das DK, Rajwanslin A, Bhusnurmath SR: Cytology of hepatocellular carcinoma. Diagn Cytopathol 2:291–294, 1986.
29. Hartley JPR, Douglas AP: A case of clonorchiasis in England. Br Med J 3:575, 1975.
30. Higginson J: The epidemiology of primary carcinoma of the liver. *In* Tumors of the Liver. Edited by GT Pack, AH Islami.

Recent Results in Cancer Research, vol 26. New York, Springer-Verlag, 1970.

31. Ho CS, McLaughlin MJ, Tao LC, Blendis L, Evans WK: Guided percutaneous fine-needle aspiration biopsy of the liver. Cancer 47:1781–1785, 1981.

32. Iwarson S, Lindberg J, Lundin P: Progression of hepatitis non-A, non-B to chronic active hepatitis. J Clin Pathol 32:351–355, 1979.

33. Iwarson S, Lundin P, Hermodsson S: Liver morphology in acute viral hepatitis related to the hepatitis B antigen. J Clin Pathol 25:850–855, 1972.

34. Jaffe BM: Factors influencing survival in patients with untreated hepatic metastases. Surg Gynecol Obstet 127:1–6, 1968.

35. Klatskin G: Hepatic granulomata: Problems in interpretation. Ann NY Acad Sci 278:427–432, 1976.

36. Klatskin G: Hepatic tumors: Possible relationship to use of oral contraceptives. Gastroenterology 73:386–394, 1977.

37. Lander JJ, Stanley RJ, Sumner HW, Boswell DC, Aach RD: Angiosarcoma of the liver associated with Fowler's solution (potassium arsenite). Gastroenterology 68:1582–1586, 1975.

38. Lelbach WK: Epidemiology of alcoholic liver disease. *In* Progress in Liver Diseases. Edited by H Popper, F Schaffner. New York, Grune & Stratton, pp 494–515, 1976.

39. Lingao AL, Domingo ED, Nishioka K: Hepatitis B virus profile of hepatocellular carcinoma in the Philippines. Cancer 48:1590–1595, 1981.

40. Locker GY, Doroshow JH, Zwelling LA, Chabner BA: The clinical features of hepatic angiosarcoma: A report of four cases and a review of the English literature. Medicine 58:48–64, 1979.

41. Ludwig J, Hoffman HN II: Hemangiosarcoma of the liver: Spectrum of morphologic changes and clinical findings. Mayo Clin Proc 50:255–263, 1975.

42. Lundqvist A: Fine-needle aspiration biopsy for cytodiagnosis of malignant tumor in the liver. Acta Med Scand 188:465–470, 1970.

43. Lundqvist A: Fine-needle aspiration biopsy of the liver. Acta Med Scand [Suppl] 520:1–28, 1971.

44. Lutz H, Weidenhiller S, Rettenmaier G: Ultrasonically-guided fine-needle aspiration biopsy of the liver. Schweiz Med Wochenschr 103:1030–1033, 1973.

45. Marion PL, Salazar FH, Alexander JJ, Robinson WS: State of hepatitis B viral DNA in a human hepatoma cell line. J Virol 33:795–806, 1980.

46. Montali G, Solbiati L, Croce F, Icrace T, Ravetto C: Fine-needle aspiration biopsy of liver focal lesions ultrasonically guided with a real-time probe. Report on 126 cases. Br J Radiol 55:717–723, 1982.

47. Neville E, Piyasena KHG, James DG: Granulomas of the liver. Postgrad Med J 51:361–365, 1975.

48. Nguyen GK, McHattie JD, Jeannot A: Cytomorphologic aspects of hepatic angiosarcoma: Fine-needle aspiration biopsy of a case. Acta Cytol 26:527–531, 1982.

49. Pagani JJ: Biopsy of focal hepatic lesions. Comparison of 18 and 22 gauge needles. Radiology 147:673–675, 1983.

50. Peers FG, Linsell CA: Dietary aflatoxins and liver cancer: A population based study in Kenya. Br J Cancer 27:473–484, 1973.

51. Perry MD, Johnston WW: Needle biopsy of the liver for the diagnosis of nonneoplastic liver diseases. Acta Cytol 29:385–390, 1985.

52. Pilotti S, Rilke F, Claren R, Milella M, Lombardi L: Conclusive diagnosis of hepatic and pancreatic malignancies by fine needle aspiration. Acta Cytol 32:27–38, 1988.

53. Pimentel JC, Menezes AP: Liver diseases in vineyard sprayers. Gastroenterology 72:275–283, 1977.

54. Pinto MM, Avila NA, Heller CI, Criscuolo EM: Fine-needle aspiration of the liver. Acta Cytol 32:15–21, 1988.

55. Prince AM: Hepatitis B virus and hepatocellular carcinoma: Molecular biology provides further evidence for an etiologic association. Hepatology 1:73–75, 1981.

56. Rasmussen SN, Holm HH, Kristensen JK, Barlebo H: Ultrasonically-guided liver biopsy. Br Med J 2:500–502, 1972.

57. Rosenblatt R, Kutcher R, Moussouris HF, Schrieber K, Koss LG: Sonographically guided fine-needle aspiration of liver lesions. JAMA 248:1639–1641, 1982.

58. Schwerk WB, Schmitz-Moormann P: Ultrasonically guided fine-needle biopsies in neoplastic liver disease. Cancer 48:1469–1477, 1981.

59. Soderstrom N: Fine-Needle Aspiration Biopsy. New York, Grune & Stratton, 1966.

60. Suen KC: Diagnosis of primary hepatic neoplasms by fine-needle aspiration cytology. Diagn Cytopathol 2:99–109, 1986.

61. Suen KC, Magee JF, Halparin LS, Chen NH, Greene C: Fine-needle aspiration cytology of fibrolamellar hepatocellular carcinoma. Acta Cytol 29:867–872, 1985.

62. Tao LC, Donat EE, Ho CS, McLoughlin MJ: Percutaneous fine-needle aspiration of the liver: Cytodiagnosis of hepatic cancer. Acta Cytol 23:287–291, 1979.

63. Tao LC, Ho CS, McLoughlin MJ, Evans WK, Donat EE: Cytologic diagnosis of hepatocellular carcinoma by fine-needle aspiration biopsy. Cancer 53:547–552, 1984.

64. Tao LC, Morgan RC, Donat EE: Cytologic diagnosis of intravenous talc granulomatosis by fine needle aspiration biopsy. Acta Cytol 28:737–739, 1984.

65. Tatsuta M, Yamamoto R, Kasugai H: Cytohistologic diagnosis of neoplasms of the liver by ultrasonically guided fine-needle aspiration biopsy. Cancer 54:1682–1686, 1984.

66. Thomas LB, Popper H, Berk PD, Selikoff I, Falk H: Vinyl-chloride–induced liver disease. From idiopathic portal hypertension (Banti's syndrome) to angiosarcomas. N Engl Med J 292:17–22, 1975.

67. Tong MJ, Sun SC, Schaeffer BT: Hepatitis-associated antigen and hepatocellular carcinoma in Taiwan. Ann Intern Med 75:687–691, 1971.

68. VanRensburg SJ, Van der Watt JJ, Purchase IF: Primary liver cancer and aflatoxin intake in a high cancer area. S Afr Med J 48:2508A–2508D, 1974.

69. Wasastjerna C: Liver. *In* Aspiration Biopsy Cytology. II. Cytology of Infradiaphragmatic Organs. J Zajicek. *In* Monographs in Clinical Cytology, vol 7. Edited by GL Wied. Basel, S Karger, pp 167–193, 1979.

70. Weinberg AG, Mize CE, Worthen HG: The occurrence of hepatoma in the chronic form of hereditary tyrosinemia. J Pediatr 88:434–438, 1976.

71. Weinberg CD, Ranchod M: Thorotrast-induced hepatic cholangiocarcinoma and angiosarcoma. Hum Pathol 10:108–112, 1979.

72. Whitlach S, Nuñez C, Pitlik DA: Fine needle aspiration biopsy of the liver. A study of 102 consecutive cases. Acta Cytol 28:719–725, 1984.

Pancreas

73. Al-Kaisi N, Siegler EE: Fine needle aspiration cytology of the pancreas. Acta Cytol 33:145–152, 1989.

74. Alpern GA, Dekker A: Fine-needle aspiration cytology of the pancreas. Acta Cytol 29:873–878, 1985.

75. An-Foraker SH, Fong-Mui KK: Cytodiagnosis of lesions of the pancreas and related areas. Acta Cytol 26:814–822, 1982.

76. Arnesjo B, Stormby N, Akerman M: Cytodiagnosis of pancreatic lesions by means of fine-needle biopsy during operation. Acta Chir Scand 138:363–369, 1972.

77. Ascoli V, Newman GA, Kline TS: Grimelius stain for cytodiagnosis of carcinoid tumor. Diagn Cytopathol 2:157–159, 1986.

78. Banner BF, Myrent KL, Memoli VA, Gould VE: Neuroendocrine carcinoma of the pancreas diagnosed by aspiration cytology. Acta Cytol 29:442–448, 1985.

79. Bell DA: Cytologic features of islet-cell tumors. Acta Cytol 31:485–492, 1987.

80. Bondeson L, Bondeson A, Genell S, Lindholm K, Thorstenson S: Aspiration cytology of a rare solid and papillary epithelial neoplasm of the pancreas. Acta Cytol 28:605–609, 1984.

81. Bourdeou D, Sylvestre J, Lévesque HP: Computerized axial tomography and fine-needle biopsy in surgery of the pancreas. Can J Surg 22:29–33, 1979.

82. Bret PM, Nicolet V: Percutaneous fine-needle aspiration biopsy of the pancreas. Diagn Cytopathol 2:221–227, 1986.

83. Chen J, Baithun ST: Morphological study of 391 cases of exocrine pancreatic tumors with special reference to the classification of exocrine pancreatic carcinoma. J Pathol 146:17–29, 1985.

84. Chen KTK, Workman RD, Efird TA, Cheng AC: Fine-needle aspiration cytology diagnostic of papillary tumor of the pancreas. Acta Cytol 30:523–527, 1986.

85. Clouse ME, Gregg JA, McDonald DG, Seg OA: Percutaneous fine-needle aspiration biopsy of pancreatic carcinoma. Gastrointest Radiol 123:319–322, 1977.

86. Compagno J, Oertel JE: Microcystic neoplasm of the pancreas with overt and latent malignancy (cystadenocarcinoma and adenoma): A clinicopathologic study of 41 cases. Am J Clin Pathol 69:573–580, 1978.

87. Cooperberg PL, Hutchinson D, Li D: Percutaneous fine needle aspiration biopsy under ultrasound and computed tomographic control. Br Col Med J 23:537–541, 1981.

88. Cote J, Dockerty MB, Priestley JT: An evaluation of pancreatic biopsy with the Vim-Silverman needle. Arch Surg 79:588–596, 1959.

89. Cubilla AL, Fitzgerald PJ: Classification of pancreatic cancer (nonendocrine). Mayo Clin Proc 54:449–458, 1979.

90. Dekker A, Lloyd JC: Fine-needle aspiration biopsy in-ampullary and pancreatic carcinoma. Arch Surg 114:595–596, 1976.

91. Dencker H: Evaluation of operative biopsy of periampullary tumors. Acta Chir Scand 138:190–194, 1972.

92. Emmert GM, Bewtra C: Fine-needle aspiration biopsy of mucinous cystic neoplasm of the pancreas: A case study. Diagn Cytopathol 2:69–71, 1986.

93. Evander A, Ihse I, Lunderquist A, Tylen U, Akerman M: Percutaneous cytodiagnosis of carcinoma of the pancreas and bile duct. Ann Surg 188:90–92, 1978.

94. Fekete PS, Nurez C, Pitlik DA: Fine-needle aspiration biopsy of the pancreas: A study of 61 cases. Diagn Cytopathol 2:301–306, 1986.

95. Foote A, Simpson JS, Stewart RJ: Diagnosis of the rare solid and papillary epithelial neoplasm of the pancreas by fine needle aspiration cytology. Light and eletron microscopic study of a case. Acta Cytol 30:519–527, 1986.

96. Forsgren L, Orell S: Aspiration cytology in carcinoma of the pancreas. Surgery 73:38–42, 1973.

97. Frederiksen P, Thommesen P, Skjolborg H: Fine needle aspiration of the pancreas. Scand J Gastroenterol 11:785–791, 1976.

98. Frias-Hidvegi D: Liver and pancreas. In Guides to Clinical Aspiration Biopsy. Edited by TS Kline. New York, Igaku-Shoin, 1988.

99. Goldman MI, Naib ZM, Galambos JT, Rude JC, Oen KT, Bradley EL, Salam A, Gonzales AC: Preoperative diagnosis of pancreatic carcinoma by percutaneous aspiration biopsy. Am J Dig Dis 22:1076–1082, 1977.

100. Goldstein HM, Zornoza J: Percutaneous transperitoneal aspiration biopsy of pancreatic masses. Am J Dig Dis 23:840–843, 1978.

101. Haaga JR, Alfidi RJ: Precise biopsy localization by computed tomography. Radiology 118:603–607, 1976.

102. Hall-Craggs MA, Lees WR: Fine-needle aspiration biopsy: Pancreatic and biliary tumors. AJR 147:399–403, 1986.

103. Hancke S, Holm HH, Kock R: Ultrasonically guided percutaneous fine-needle biopsy of the pancreas. Surg Gynecol Obstet 140:361–364, 1975.

104. Harter LP, Moss AA, Goldberg HI, Gross BH: CT-guided fine-needle aspirations for diagnosis of benign and malignant diseases. AJR 140:363–367, 1983.

105. Hastrup J, Thommesen P, Frederiksen P: Pancreatitis and pancreatic carcinoma diagnosed by preoperative fine needle aspiration biopsy. Acta Cytol 21:731–734, 1978.

106. Hidvegi DF, Nieman HL, DeMay RM, Janes W: Percutaneous transperitoneal aspiration of pancreas guided by ultrasound: Morphologic and cytochemical appearance of normal and malignant cells. Acta Cytol 23:181–184, 1979.

107. Ho CS, McLoughlin MJ, McHattie J, Tao LC: Percutaneous fine-needle aspiration of the pancreas following endoscopic retrograde cholangiopancreatography. Radiology 125:351–353, 1977.

108. Hsiu JG, D'Amato NA, Sperling MH: Malignant islet-cell tumor of the pancreas diagnosed by fine needle aspiration biopsy: A case report. Acta Cytol 29:576–579, 1985.

109. Isaacson R, Weiland LH, McIlrath DC: Biopsy of the pancreas. Arch Surg 109:227–230, 1974.

110. Jones EC, Suen KC, Grant DR, Chen NH: Fine-needle aspiration cytology of neoplastic cysts of the pancreas. Diagn Cytopathol 3:238–243, 1987.

111. Kline TS, Neal HS: Needle aspiration biopsy: A critical appraisal. JAMA 239:36–39, 1978.

112. Kolin MD, Bernacki EG Jr, Schwab R: Diagnosis of pancreatic lesions by percutaneous aspiration biopsy. Acta Cytol 25:675–677, 1981.

113. Kuo TT, Su IJ, Chien CH: Solid and papillary neoplasm of the pancreas: Report of three cases from Taiwan. Cancer 54:1469–1474, 1984.

114. Leiman G, Markowitz S, Svensson LG: Intraoperative cytodiagnosis of pancreatic adenosquamous carcinoma: A case report. Diagn Cytopathol 2:72–75, 1986.

115. Lightwood R, Reber HA, Way LW: The risk and accuracy of pancreatic biopsy. Am J Surg 132:189–194, 1976.

116. Lozowski W, Hajdu SI, Melamed MR: Cytomorphology of carcinoid tumors. Acta Cytol 23:360–365, 1979.

117. Lund F: Carcinomas of the pancreas. Biopsy or not? Acta Chir Scand 135:515–517, 1969.

118. Manci EA, Gardner LL, Pollock WJ, Dowling EA: Osteoclastic giant cell tumor of the pancreas: Aspiration cytology, light microscopy, and ultrastructure with review of the literature. Diagn Cytopathol 1:105–110, 1985.

119. McLoughlin MJ, Ho CS, Langer B, McHattie J, Tao LC: Fine-needle aspiration biopsy of malignant lesions in and around the pancreas. Cancer 41:2413–2419, 1978.

120. Mitchell ML, Carney CN: Cytologic criteria for diagnosis of pancreatic carcinoma. Am J Clin Pathol 83:171–176, 1985.

121. Mitty HA, Effremidis CS, Jeh HC: Impact of fine-needle biopsy on management of patients with carcinoma of the pancreas. AJR 137:1119–1121, 1981.

122. Nguyen G: Cytology of hyperplastic endocrine cells of the pancreas in fine-needle aspiration biopsy. Acta Cytol 28:499–502, 1984.

123. Nguyen G: Hyperplastic and neoplastic endocrine cells of the pancreas in aspiration biopsy. Diagn Cytopathol 2:204–211, 1986.

124. Nosher JL, Plafker J: Percutaneous aspiration biopsy of abdominal and retroperitoneal tumors. J Med Soc 76:741–744, 1979.

125. Oscarson J, Stormby N, Sundgren R: Selective angiography in fine-needle aspiration: Cytodiagnosis of gastric and pancreatic tumors. Acta Radiol [Diagn] 12:737–749, 1972.

126. Pereiras RV, Meiers A, Kunhardt B, Troner M, Huttson D: Fluoroscopically guided thin needle aspiration biopsy of the abdominen and retroperitoneum. AJR 131:197–202, 1978.

127. Pinto MM, Avila NA, Criscuolo EM: Fine needle aspiration of the pancreas: A five-year experience. Acta Cytol 32:39–42, 1988.

128. Pinto MM, Monteiro NL, Tizol DM: Fine needle aspiration of pleomorphic giant-cell carcinoma of the pancreas: Case report with ultrastructural observations. Acta Cytol 30:430–434, 1986.

129. Pour PM, Sayed S, Sayed G: Hyperplastic, preneoplastic and neoplastic lesions found in 83 human pancreas. Am J Clin Pathol 77:137–152, 1982.

130. Pyk TIE, Raaschon-Nielsen T, Seligson U: Percutaneous fine-needle aspiration biopsy during endoscopic retrograde cholangiopancreatography. Scand J Gastroenterol 13:657–662, 1978.

131. Reyes CV, Wang T: Undifferentiated small cell carcinoma of the pancreas. Cancer 47:2500–2502, 1981.

132. Rosai J: Ackerman's Surgical Pathology. St Louis, CV Mosby, 1989.

133. Schwerk WB, Dürr HK, Schmitz-Moormann P: Ultrasound-guided fine-needle bipsies in pancreatic and hepatic neoplasms. Gastrointest Radiol 8:219–225, 1983.

134. Schwerk WB, Schmitz-Moormann P: Percutaneous transperitoneal aspiration biopsy of the pancreatic masses under ultrasonic guidance. Dtsch Med Wochenschr 105:1019–1023, 1980.

135. Smith EH, Bartrum RJ Jr, Chang YC, D'Orsi CJ, Lokrich J, Abbruzzese A, Dantono J: Percutaneous aspiration biopsy of the pancreas under ultrasonic guidance. N Engl J Med 292:825–828, 1975.

136. Sneige N, Ordorez NG, Veanattukalathil S, Samaan WS: Fine-needle aspiration cytology in pancreatic endocrine tumors. Diagn Cytopathol 3:35–40, 1987.

137. Sundram M, Wolverson MK, Neiberg E, Pilla T, Vas WG: Utility of CT-guided abdominal aspiration procedures. AJR 139:1111–1115, 1982.

138. Tao LC, Ho CS, McLoughlin MJ, McHattie JD: Percutaneous fine-needle aspiration biopsy of the pancreas: Cytodiagnosis of pancreatic carcinoma. Acta Cytol 22:215–220, 1978.

139. Trepeta RW, Mathur B, Lagin S, LiVolsi VA: Giant cell tumor ("osteoclastoma") of the pancreas: A tumor of epithelial origin. Cancer 48:2022–2028, 1981.

140. Tylen U, Arnesjo B, Lindberg LG, Lunderquist A, Akerman M: Percutaneous biopsy of carcinoma of the pancreas guided by angiography. Surg Gynecol Obstet 142:737–739, 1976.

141. Vellet D, Leiman G, Mair S, Bilchik A: Fine needle aspiration cytology of mucinous cystadenocarcinoma of the pancreas: Further observations. Acta Cytol 32:43–48, 1988.

142. Walts AE: Osteoclast-type giant cell tumor of the pancreas. Acta Cytol 27:500–504, 1983.

143. Wilander E, Norheim I, Oberg K: Application of silver stains to cytologic specimens of neuroendocrine tumors metastatic to the liver. Acta Cytol 29:1053–1057, 1985.

144. Wilcznski SP, Valente PT, Atkinson BF: Cytodiagnosis of adenosquamous carcinoma of the pancreas: Use of intraoperative fine needle aspiration. Acta Cytol 28:733–736, 1984.

145. Wise L, Pizzimbono C, Dehner LP: Periampullary cancer: A clinicopathologic study of sixty-two patients. Am J Surg 131:141–148, 1976.

31

Effects of Therapy on Cytologic Specimens

Jami L. Walloch
Hi Young Hong
Lisa M. Bibb

Therapeutic modalities in modern medicine are almost as varied as the diseases that they are designed to manage. Therapy falls into four general categories: (1) chemotherapy, (2) immunotherapy, (3) radiation therapy and (4) mechanical therapy. These methods usually have a localized effect on the disease process. In addition they may affect adjacent or distant normal tissues. The changes that many therapies exert on uninvolved normal tissues may mimic malignant transformation. The objectives of this chapter are to present the cytologic changes induced by each category of therapy and, through examples, to discuss the cytologic diagnosis.

RADIATION

Ionizing radiation, electromagnetic or particulate, induces the ejection of electrons during absorption with the production of energy. Electromagnetic radiation, roentgen and gamma radiation, excites electrons, which then generate ion pairs and free radicals. Free radicals interact at the subcellular level causing damage to molecules, which may be reversible or irreversible. Oxygen enhances the reaction of free radicals by peroxidation of the molecules. Deoxyribonucleic acid (DNA) is an important target molecule affected by ionizing radiation. Damage to DNA results in chromosomal breakage or rearrangement. The affected cells may function normally until the next cell division

when abnormal mitosis leads to cell death or abnormal daughter cells.

Nuclear DNA content is an important factor determining radiosensitivity of cells. Cells in the proliferative phase (S, G_2 or M) of the cell cycle are more susceptible to radiation. If structural cytoskeleton macromolecules are affected, the damage to cell membranes could lead to lysis of cells.

Frankl and Amreich[29] reported serial histologic changes of carcinoma of the cervix during radium and x-ray treatment. They observed enlargement, vacuolization and hyalinization of the carcinoma cells. Donaldson and Canti[22] studied immediate and late changes of cervical carcinoma treated with radium by means of serial biopsies. Immediate changes were increased normal and abnormal mitotic figures, necrosis and cellular enlargement. Late changes that occurred after the seventh day consisted of absence of mitosis, karyorrhexis and fibrosis. Graham[33] first introduced a vaginal smear method to study the effects of radiation on cervical malignancy and suggested that vaginal smears were superior to biopsy. Vaginal smears were simpler to perform, and wider areas of the cervix and vagina could be sampled.

General Cellular Changes

Radiation cell changes are divided into two phases: acute and chronic. Acute changes occur within 6 months of irradiation and consist of cellular and nuclear enlargement, vacuolization of the cytoplasm, wrinkling and chromatin condensation of the nuclei, abnormal mitoses and multinucleated or bizarre-shaped cells. Acute changes are rarely observed after the first 6 months following irradiation. In most instances, however, radiation changes may persist for many years. Malignant cells show radiation changes similar to those found in benign cells. Nuclear enlargement may be more pronounced than cytoplasmic swelling, which leads to a higher nucleocytoplasmic ratio. Because malignant cells are more sensitive to radiation than benign cells, they usually disappear within 1 month after termination of radiotherapy.[42]

Chronic radiation changes include cellular enlargement and aberrant basal cells. Epithelial atrophy is commonly encountered. Nuclear and cytoplasmic vacuolization and multinucleated forms are usually less evident.[53]

Radiated cells show cytochemical changes, which may be partly due to destruction of cytoplasmic organelles with release of cytoplasmic enzymes. An increase in nucleolar and cytoplasmic ribonucleic acid (RNA) synthesis occurs followed by a decrease in DNA synthesis.[46] This change is followed by the progressive loss of RNA, as the cells are successfully irradiated. Large glycogen deposits, increased intracellular potassium concentration and disappearance of alkaline phosphatase are observed.

Ultrastructural changes in radiated cells consist of alterations in epithelial and stromal cells. Epithelial cells show alterations in nuclear and cytoplasmic organelles. The nuclear changes that usually precede the cytoplasmic alterations include abnormal clearing of chromatin with a peripheral rim of chromatin-like material along the nuclear envelope.[82] The cytoplasmic changes include a greater number of lysosomes, an accumulation of lipid droplets, a dilatation of endoplasmic reticulum, disrupted cristae in mitochondria, increased fibrils and a disruption of cytoplasmic membranes.[3, 82] In the stroma, active fibroblasts with abundant endoplasmic reticulum and Golgi apparatus are increased.

Female Genital Tract

Acute Radiation Changes

The most frequent changes found in benign cervical and vaginal cells include marked nuclear and cellular enlargement, vacuolization of the cytoplasm, degenerative nuclei and the appearance of bizarre cell shapes, such as tadpole-shaped cells. These changes are found in all layers of the ectocervical and vaginal squamous epithelium and endocervical cells. Cellular enlargement is proportional to nuclear increase except in superficial cells, thus the nucleocytoplasmic ratio is maintained. Vacuolization is first found in parabasal cells followed by intermediate and superficial cells. The vacuoles vary in size from fine multiple vacuoles to a large single vacuole displacing the nucleus to one side.

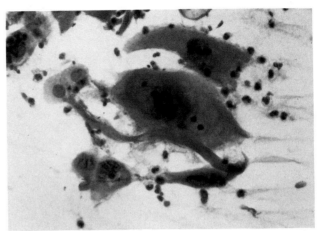

FIGURE 31–1. Acute radiation changes in the uterine cervix. The cells are markedly enlarged with bizarre shapes, vacuolated cytoplasm, phagocytosis of neutrophils and pleomorphic hyperchromatic nuclei with nucleoli. Cervicovaginal smear (Papanicolaou stain; ×400).

The nuclei may also contain vacuoles. Other cytoplasmic changes include alteration in staining characteristics, amphophilia and invasion or phagocytosis of neutrophils. Nuclear changes consist of size increase, wrinkling, multinucleation, pyknosis and karyorrhexis. Hyperchromasia may be present; however, chromatin distribution usually is homogeneous and finely granular. The smear background contains a heavy infiltration of neutrophils, leukocytes, histiocytes and other inflammatory cells (Fig. 31–1).

Malignant cells undergo the same changes as benign epithelial cells. Nuclear enlargement may be greater than that of the cytoplasm maintaining an altered nucleocytoplasmic ratio. It may be difficult to separate malignant cells from benign cells after irradiation.

Chronic Radiation Changes

Persistent radiation changes can be found for several years after radiation therapy. The smear often has an atrophic pattern with a predominance of basal and parabasal cells (Fig. 31–2). The epithelial cells still demonstrate nuclear and cytoplasmic enlargement. The nuclei are hyperchromatic; however, the chromatin is homogeneous without clumping. Aberrant basal cells are frequently found. Multinucleated epithelial cells may be present. Kaufman[48] described a net-like background of amorphous acellular pink material as a characteristic late radiation effect. Although the background is usually clean, a foreign body giant cell reaction and fibroblasts may be encountered.

Prediction of Prognosis and Recurrence

Periodic cytologic examination after radiation therapy is important for the assessment of the effectiveness of treatment and for the detection of persistent or

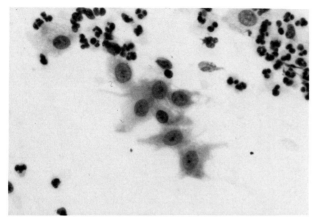

FIGURE 31–2. Chronic radiation changes in the uterine cervix. The smear is atrophic with aberrant parabasal and basal cells. Cervicovaginal smear (Papanicolaou stain; ×400). (Courtesy of Dr. Marluce Bibbo, Chicago, Illinois.)

recurrent tumor. Features that may be related to prognosis include radiation response, host inflammatory reaction, high karyopyknotic index and presence of malignant cells.

Radiation response (RR) was described by Graham and Graham in 1955.[35] It is the percentage of benign squamous cells showing radiation effect in a vaginal smear. The cytologic features of radiation effect include cytoplasmic vacuolization, cellular enlargement, degenerative nuclear changes and multinucleation. If more than 75% of benign cells show radiation changes, the radiation reaction is considered good. An RR of 60% or less indicates a poor response. Although the two groups studied had a significant difference in 5-year survival, these results have not been reproduced by other investigators. Thus, the reliability of RR as a prognostic indicator is controversial.

The inflammatory response consists of large numbers of neutrophils that usually appear during or immediately after radiation and histiocytes with phagocytized red blood cells or debris. Lymphocytes are seen in variable numbers. Giant histiocytes start to appear 25 days after radiation.[40] If degenerating leukocytes and hemolyzed red blood cells persist, it is considered as a poor host response, which may lead to the formation of fistulas, sinuses or deep abscesses.[42]

Postirradiation dysplasia is the appearance of abnormal cellular changes in benign epithelial cells after radiotherapy. The abnormal cells are characterized by cytoplasmic and nuclear enlargement with an altered nucleocytoplasmic ratio, oval-to-irregular shaped hyperchromatic nuclei with finely to coarsely granular chromatin and eosinophilic or amphophilic staining of the cytoplasm.[71] Wentz and Reagan[91] reported 84 patients with postirradiation dysplasia that occurred from 9 months to 12 years after the initial diagnosis of carcinoma. Of all patients with recurrent carcinoma, 80.8% developed postirradiation dysplasia within 3 years after the initial diagnosis of carcinoma (Fig. 31–3). The 5-year survival rate for the patients with a less than 3-year latent period of postirradiation dysplasia was

33.8% as compared with 100% 5-year survival rate for the patients with a greater than 3-year latent period. Postirradiation dysplasia within 3 years after treatment for cervical carcinoma indicated a poor prognosis. Patten[70] later claimed that postradiation dysplasia is a malignancy-associated change. However, the significance of postirradiation dysplasia has been debated by several workers.[34, 62] At present, the prognostic significance of postirradiation dysplasia is controversial.

Karyopyknotic index (cornification index) is the ratio of superficial cells showing karyopyknosis to all squamous cells in the smear, expressed as a percentage. A high karyopyknotic index indicates estrogen effect and is related to the presence of malignancy.[37, 89]

Although some disagreement exists on the significance of malignant cells in a postirradiation smear, it is generally considered as a poor response to the therapy. Graham and Graham[35] demonstrated no significant correlation between the presence of cancer cells in the smear at the end of treatment and the survival of the patients. McLennan and McLennan[62] and Gupta and associates[37] reported that the presence of malignant cells at any time after completion of therapy indicated poor response or recurrence. Gupta and colleagues[40] later stated that cancer cells in the first postradiation smear were not significant in prognosis, but if present after 4 months, they indicated a relatively poor prognosis. In cases of persistent cancer, the malignant cells exhibit little or no radiation effect. If malignant cells appear in a postirradiation smear, a thorough colposcopy and biopsies should be carried out to identify persisting or recurrent lesions.

Oral Mucosa

Oral mucosal changes occur when the radiation therapy is part of the therapeutic regimen in head and neck malignancies. The radiation changes of the oral squamous cells are similar to those seen in the uterine cervix. Nuclear and cytoplasmic enlargement, cyto-

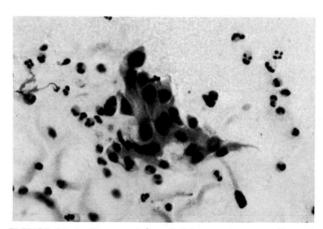

FIGURE 31–3. Recurrent keratinizing squamous cell carcinoma after radiation therapy. Cervicovaginal smear (Papanicolaou stain; ×400). (Courtesy of Dr. Marluce Bibbo, Chicago, Illinois.)

plasmic vacuolization, multinucleation and increased cytoplasmic eosinophilia are the common findings. Cytoplasmic granules, which may represent RNA accumulation,[74] and perinuclear halo formation are also described. Silverman and Sheline[83] reported that the RR of oral squamous cells did not correlate with the local recurrence rate. The presence of malignant cells usually indicates persistent or recurrent lesions. Negative cytology findings do not necessarily rule out underlying submucosal malignant recurrence, because the surface may be reepithelialized with benign mucosa.

Lower Respiratory Tract

Irradiation of the chest for chest wall, lung or mediastinal malignancies may cause acute and chronic injuries to the lung. In the acute stage, bronchial epithelium undergoes marked nuclear and cytoplasmic enlargement with the formation of bizarre giant cells. Nuclei may show granular-to-coarse chromatin and prominent nucleoli. The benign nature of these cells can be reassured by finding cilia. Acute radiation pneumonitis may superimpose an inflammatory process on the epithelial cellular changes.

Chronic radiation changes consist of interstitial fibrosis, chronic inflammation and squamous metaplasia of bronchial lining cells. Columnar cells and metaplas-tic squamous cells may show significant atypia, which may be difficult to differentiate from malignancy. Metaplastic squamous cells can show all the features of malignancy including high nucleocytoplasmic ratio, hyperchromasia, irregular clumping of chromatin and prominent nucleoli (Fig. 31–4). Obtaining the patient's history of irradiation is of critical importance to avoid making a diagnosis of malignancy based on only a few highly atypical cells. The chronic radiation changes are similar to the chemotherapeutic changes found with bleomycin, busulfan and other pulmonary toxic antineoplastic drugs.

Urinary Tract

The urinary bladder is affected when irradiation is given for urinary bladder cancer and other pelvic malignancies. Radiation changes of the urothelium occur relatively early, as soon as the second day of treatment.[44] Benign urothelial cells show pronounced cellular enlargement accompanied by nuclear swelling and cytoplasmic vacuolization. Other nuclear changes include hyperchromasia, irregular shapes, pyknosis, karyorrhexis and multinucleation (Fig. 31–5). Cytoplasmic vacuolization and multinucleation are not specific for radiation effect. They can be found in nonirradiated bladder epithelium secondary to chronic cystitis or calculi. Recognition of unaffected high-grade

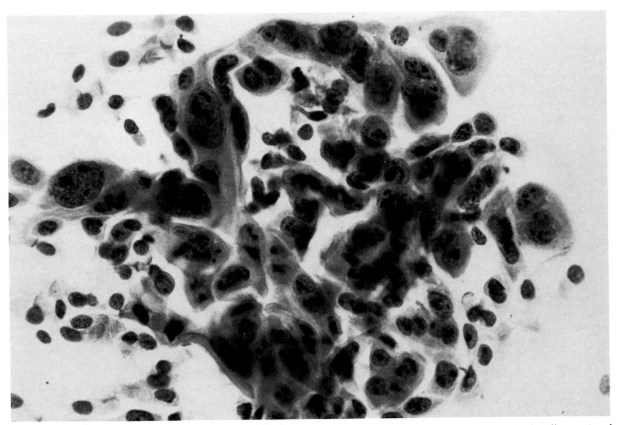

FIGURE 31–4. Chronic radiation change in the lung. The smear contains a loose aggregate of bronchial cells ranging from minimally reactive columnar cells with cilia to large cells with pleomorphic nuclei, coarse chromatin, irregular nuclear membranes, multiple nuclei and an increased nucleocytoplasmic ratio. Bronchial brush (Papanicolaou stain; ×400).

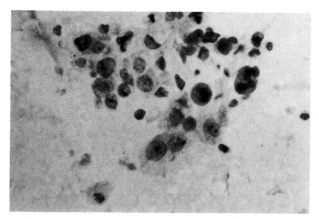

FIGURE 31–5. Radiation change in the urinary bladder. The affected urothelial cells have vacuolated cytoplasm, nuclear enlargement, finely granular chromatin and small nucleoli. Catheterized urine (Papanicolaou stain; ×400). (Courtesy of Dr. Marluce Bibbo, Chicago, Illinois.)

malignant cells is often not very difficult in urine cytology. They maintain a high nucleocytoplasmic ratio with hyperchromatic nuclei having prominent irregular nucleoli. Irradiated urothelial cells may mimic squamous cell carcinoma causing a diagnostic problem when the radiation therapy is given for carcinoma of the cervix.[53]

Urine cytology is a useful method for the follow-up of patients with irradiated bladder cancer. Esposti and associates[26] reported 89% accuracy in detecting persistent or recurrent carcinoma. Only one patient among 25 with radioresistant tumor had negative cytology findings. Among 54 patients with recurrences, urine cytology revealed frankly malignant cells in 46 cases. Of patients with recurrence, 17 had positive urine cytology findings 3 to 24 months preceding the clinical recognition of recurrence.

As a complication of radiotherapy, malignant neoplasms can develop in the urinary bladder. Transitional cell carcinoma, squamous cell carcinoma and sarcoma have been reported.[25]

Breast

Radiation-induced change to the breast cytology is a somewhat newly recognized problem because of the greater tendency to treat small localized breast cancer conservatively with lumpectomy or quadrantectomy combined with radiation.

Schnitt and coworkers[80] studied the radiation effect on breast tissue in 30 patients with breast cancer. Epithelial atypia in the terminal duct lobular unit associated with lobular sclerosis and atrophy was the characteristic finding. Epithelial atypia in large ducts, stromal changes and vascular changes were less frequent. The atypical epithelial cells still maintained polarity and cohesion without evidence of cellular pleomorphism or proliferation. These changes could easily be distinguished from malignancy.

Cytology

Interpretation of the needle aspiration biopsy of a recurrent breast mass after irradiation may be more intriguing. Normal breast ductal and lobular epithelia may have discohesion and severe atypia with large, pleomorphic, hyperchromatic nuclei and only rare bipolar naked nuclei making a distinction from malignant change difficult.[10] These cytologic features markedly contrast the histologic epithelial changes described by Schnitt.[80] A clue that the changes may be radiation induced is the hypocellularity of the smears due to the fibrosis. The presence of myoepithelial cells or bipolar naked nuclei or the transition between normal and highly atypical cells within an aggregate of cells may indicate the benignity of the lesion.[52]

Prostate

Irradiation is an accepted mode of treatment for locally advanced, Stage C, prostatic adenocarcinoma. Follow-up of patients with irradiated prostate to evaluate radiation injury and persistence of malignancy by aspiration biopsy has been poorly studied.

Bostwick and colleagues[12] studied histologic features of normal and neoplastic prostate tissue after radiotherapy. The radiation injury changes included atrophy and squamous metaplasia of the non-neoplastic glands, with or without atypia; stromal fibrosis and arterial stenosis. The neoplastic glands were unaffected without architectural alteration or dedifferentiation. Cytologic changes in the neoplastic glands were not useful criteria in differentiating them from non-neoplastic glands with radiation-induce atypia.

Cytology

Aspiration biopsy of the irradiated prostate usually yields a hypocellular specimen because of fibrosis that occurs within a few days after radiotherapy.[85] Cytologic changes found in normal and neoplastic glandular epithelium consist of cellular and nuclear enlargement, cytoplasmic vacuolization and bizarre giant nuclear forms (Fig. 31–6). Squamous metaplasia may develop. Degenerative nuclear changes, such as karyorrhexis, karyolysis or pyknosis, are also found in the malignant cells. Nucleoli in the malignant cells may shrink and may no longer be prominent. No definite criteria exist for the viability of malignant cells. The presence of well-preserved eosinophilic nucleoli and cellular dyshesion suggests a viable neoplasm.[50]

The significance of persistent malignant cells and the value of post-therapy biopsy to assess the tumor response is controversial because of poor correlation between the biopsy results and patient survival. Persistent positive biopsy findings 12 to 18 months post-therapy may indicate residual viable neoplasm.[12] Biopsy conversion from malignant to benign can occur as late as 1 to 2 years following radiation.[18, 55] After

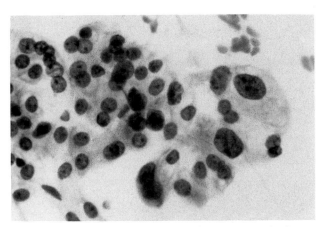

FIGURE 31–6. Radiation change in the prostate. The benign prostatic glandular cells have nuclear atypia and loss of polarity. Distinguishing these changes from malignancy may be difficult. Fine needle aspiration biopsy of prostate (Papanicolaou stain; ×400). (Courtesy of Dr. Marluce Bibbo, Chicago, Illinois.)

2.5 years, 20% of prostate biopsy samples will contain malignant cells. A direct correlation with prognosis is difficult to assess because of problems in evaluating the viability and metastatic potential of the residual malignant cells.[12] Serial rectal examination and biopsy, TruCut or fine needle aspiration, still remain the accepted method of following a patient with irradiated prostate carcinoma.

Thyroid

Internal radiation by administering [131]iodine is used for the treatment of Graves' disease and, in some cases, of functioning thyroid carcinomas. [131]Iodine mostly emits beta rays, which centrifugally spread approximately 2 mm, thus sparing structures adjacent to the thyroid. The effect of radioactive iodine on the thyroid depends on the dose of radioiodine per gram of thyroid tissue, duration and sensitivity of the cells to radiation.

Histologic changes are acute and chronic. Acute changes include cytoplasmic oxyphilia, stromal edema and nuclear pyknosis. Acute inflammation or necrosis is rarely found in therapeutic doses. By the third week, the stromal edema has been replaced by interstitial fibrosis with a decrease in follicle size. Chronic changes, after 6 weeks, include interstitial fibrosis, cytoplasmic swelling and oxyphilia resembling Hürthle cells, nuclear atypia with hyperchromasia and bizarre giant forms, small follicles and vascular alterations. The nuclear changes are most prominent in the oxyphilic cells and may be indistinguishable from malignancy.[21] A lymphocyte infiltrate and multinucleated histiocytes with the oxyphilic cells may mimic Hashimoto's thyroiditis.[19] Although Vickery[88] reported a 39% incidence of Hashimoto's thyroiditis in the irradiated glands, it is a relatively uncommon finding in other series. Regenerative or adenomatous nodules in the long-term postirradiation period may develop.

Cytology

Cytologic features of the irradiated thyroid consist of nuclear enlargement with bizarre nuclear forms, clumping of chromatin, cytoplasmic swelling or eosinophilic granularity and naked nuclei. Intranuclear inclusions and blue-black cytoplasmic pigment granules in the follicular cells have been described by Kini.[49] These features may be indistinguishable from malignancy, and a history of [131]iodine therapy is needed for clarification. In the chronic stage, aspiration biopsy may yield scant cellularity owing to fibrosis and follicular atrophy.

ANTINEOPLASTIC CHEMOTHERAPY

Bleomycin

Bleomycin is an antineoplastic and antimicrobial polypeptide antibiotic isolate from the fungus *Streptomyces verticullus*. Briefly, the mechanism of action is the binding of bleomycin to guanine bases in DNA with the hydrolyzation of Fe^{+2} (ferrous iron) to Fe^{+3} (ferric iron). The liberated electron is accepted by oxygen to form superoxides and hydroxyl radicals. These active oxygen intermediates attack DNA bases leading to single- and double-stranded DNA breaks and deletions.[15] The primary toxicity of bleomycin is a subacute or chronic pneumonitis with progression to interstitial pneumonitis.

Chest radiography shows bibasilar pulmonary infiltrates that must be differentiated from metastatic tumor, infectious processes, such as *Pneumocystis carinii* and cytomegalovirus, and radiation injury. Diagnosis is often made by open lung biopsy. Less aggressive diagnostic methods include sputum, bronchial and fine needle aspiration cytology.[30]

The incidence of fatal bleomycin toxicity is about 1 to 2%. An additional 2 to 3% of patients experience nonlethal pulmonary fibrosis. Toxicity usually does not occur below the cumulative dosage of 400 units. McLeod and associates[63] reported that a case occurred after a dose of only 60 units, suggesting that a true threshold does not exist. Other factors may be synergistic and increase the incidence of bleomycin-induced pulmonary toxicity. These include age (older than 70 years), prior radiation therapy, combination chemotherapy in non-Hodgkin's lymphomas and high pO_2 during anesthesia.[30]

The histologic and ultrastructural changes in bleomycin-induced pulmonary toxicity have been well-documented in animal models.[1, 6, 60] The earliest changes are endothelial and perivascular edema of pulmonary vessels. Ultrastructural studies show subendothelial blebbing with intracytoplasmic edema. These progress to interstitial edema. Alveolar epithelium reveals type I pneumocyte necrosis with a proliferation and desquamation of type II pneumocytes. The type II pneumocytes have bizarre elongated cytoplasmic shapes, nuclear pleomorphism, hyperchromasia, occasional mitotic figures and metaplastic change to squamous

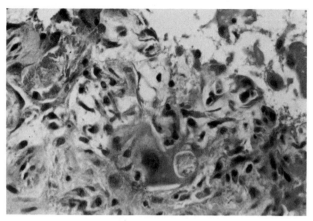

FIGURE 31–7. Bleomycin toxicity in the lung. The pulmonary parenchyma has marked interstitial fibrosis with a proliferation of atypical type II alveolar pneumocytes. Open lung biopsy (hematoxylin and eosin; ×200).

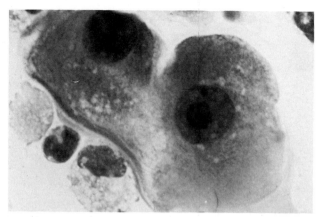

FIGURE 31–8. Bleomycin toxicity in the lung. The smear contains large atypical type II alveolar pneumocytes with fine cytoplasmic vacuoles, large nuclei with smooth membranes and macronucleoli. Fine needle aspiration biopsy of lung (Diff-quik stain; ×1000).

epithelium. Intra-alveolar fibrin deposition due to vascular leakage also occurs. The interstitium develops septal fibrosis with collagen/elastin fiber deposition and smooth muscle proliferation. End stage bibasilar fibrosis develops leading to a sequela of "honeycomb" lung (Fig. 31–7).

Cytology

Sputum, bronchial and fine needle aspiration biopsy cytology may have distinctly different findings in bleomycin-induced pulmonary toxicity. In the sputum of treated patients as compared with matched controls, Bedrossian and Corey[5] reported increased ciliocytophoria (30 to 56.2%) and increased low-grade dysplasia (10 to 37.5%) in the treated group. No significant difference in inflammation or atypical columnar cells was found. In addition, 40% of the treated patients had abnormalities of the squamous cells in the oral cavity. The low-grade dysplastic cells varied in size and shape and had amphophilic cytoplasm and irregular hyperchromatic nuclei. The abnormalities occurred as early as 12 weeks after the start of therapy.

Bronchial cytology contains a majority of normal bronchial cells and occasional scattered large abnormal columnar cells with bizarre large nuclei. The chromatin is clumped and prominent large eosinophilic nucleoli are also found. Despite these malignant features, the cells maintain their delicate translucent, basophilic cytoplasm and well-defined cilia as evidence of their benign nature.[90]

Fine needle aspirates are low to moderately cellular depending on the degree of fibrosis. Scattered lymphocytes and plasma cells are in the background. Atypical epithelial cells form cohesive two-dimensional sheets with a few scattered single cells. The cells are large, polygonal and pleomorphic with well-defined cell membranes. The cytoplasm is dense (squamoid). Perinuclear microvacuoles are also found. Minimal cellular overlap is seen. The cohesive clusters resemble a reparative epithelial arrangement. The nuclei are cen-

tral or excentric with a smooth membrane, coarsely granular chromatin and single or multiple macronucleoli. The cytologic appearance mimics malignant change (Fig. 31–8). The clinical history is essential to verify a benign reactive process. The cellular changes observed in bleomycin-induced pulmonary toxicity are similar to radiation-induced changes.

No effective therapy is available in bleomycin-induced pulmonary fibrosis. The drug-induced toxic pulmonary changes and subsequent end stage fibrosis are not unique to bleomycin and may be found in other cases involving antineoplastic drugs (Table 31–1) (Fig. 31–9).

Busulfan

Busulfan is an alkylating agent that binds to nucleophilic sites of DNA bases. This activity leads to the misreading of the DNA codes, single-strand breaks and crosslinking of DNA. The cytotoxic activity occurs throughout the cell cycle but is exaggerated during the proliferative S-phase.[15]

Busulfan in 1961 was the first chemotherapeutic drug to be associated with pulmonary toxicity.[78] The chest

TABLE 31–1. Drug-Induced Interstitial Pulmonary Fibrosis

Chemotherapy Agent	Pulmonary Toxicity
Bleomycin	Pulmonary fibrosis
Mitomycin-C	Pulmonary fibrosis with lymphocytes and eosinophils
Bischloroethylnitrosourea	Pulmonary fibrosis
Busulfan	Pulmonary fibrosis and possibly dystrophic pulmonary calcification and ossification
Cyclophosphamide	Pulmonary fibrosis
Chlorambucil	Pulmonary fibrosis
Melphalan	Pulmonary fibrosis
Methotrexate	Pulmonary fibrosis with eosinophils and occasional nodular aggregates of multinucleated giant cells

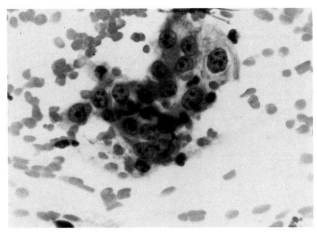

FIGURE 31–9. Methotrexate toxicity in the lung. The smear contains atypical reactive bronchial cells with enlarged nuclei and prominent nucleoli. Bronchial brush (Papanicolaou stain; ×400).

radiograph usually reveals a diffuse linear infiltrate, although normal radiographs or alveolar infiltrate findings have also been reported.[30]

The incidence of clinical pulmonary toxicity clinically has been reported at 4% with atypical histologic changes reported as high as 12%.

The histologic and ultrastructural changes in the lung due to the busulfan toxicity are similar to those reported in bleomycin. Dystrophic calcification and pulmonary ossification have been reported in a few cases.[30] Kyung-Whan and Gyorkey[56] reported a case of bronchioloalveolar carcinoma, diffuse interstitial fibrosis and atypical alveolar pneumocyte hyperplasia occurring in a patient after long-term busulfan therapy suggesting a possible carcinogenic role.

Cytology

The pulmonary cytologic changes are similar to those reported in bleomycin toxicity.

The cytomegalic changes are not limited to the lung and have been described in the pancreas, liver, adrenal gland, kidney, urinary bladder, esophagus, pituitary gland, skin, breast and uterine cervix in autopsy series.[41, 54, 69] The epithelial cells are markedly enlarged with cytoplasmic vacuoles and display an increased nucleocytoplasmic ratio. The nuclei are markedly pleomorphic with irregular elongated and multilobulated forms measuring up to 50μ in diameter. Coarsely granular chromatin and nucleoli are found. Mitotic figures are not observed.[41]

The uterine cervix shows a decreased estrogen effect with a preponderance of parabasal and intermediate cells.[90] The stratified squamous epithelium contains a large number of scattered cytomegalic cells mainly located in the upper layers.[69] In some areas, the full thickness is involved with abnormal cells and resembles carcinoma *in situ* except for the abundant cytoplasm, thinning of the epithelium and lack of mitotic figures. The cervicovaginal smear may have the cellular

changes of a high-grade dysplasia or carcinoma *in situ* (Fig. 31–10).[54, 90] Similar cells from the urinary transitional mucosa may be observed in urine cytology.[54]

Thiotepa

Thiotepa (triethylenethiophosphoramide) is a polyfunctional alkylating drug instilled intravesically in the treatment of superficial bladder cancers and carcinoma *in situ*. Mouse models with normal bladder urothelium treated with thiotepa show mild lymphocytic infiltrates. No atypical changes of the bladder urothelium are found.[66] In mouse models with chemically induced urothelial neoplasms, toxic effects include cellular degeneration with cytoplasmic vacuolization and exfoliation. Nuclear changes are rare. Neither multinucleation nor mitoses are found.[67] In normal dog urothelium treated with thiotepa at weekly intervals, the initial changes include hypercellularity and cytoplasmic vacuolization (at weeks 2 to 3). These are followed by nuclear and nucleolar enlargement and multinucleation (at weeks 3 to 5). The nuclei degenerate, becoming pyknotic and karyorrhectic (at weeks 5 to 10). At autopsy (at 10 weeks), the urothelium is hyperplastic, and individual cells have nuclear enlargement and multiple nucleoli.[77]

Cytology

In humans, thiotepa-related changes are similar to reactive changes and differ from neoplastic changes. The nuclei become slightly to markedly enlarged without a significant increase in chromatin. Mild-to-moderate hyperchromasia may exist in rare cells, but the nuclei are smudged lacking sharply defined chromatin detail. The nuclei are round to oval with smooth membranes. Cellular degeneration may cause the nuclear membrane to wrinkle. Large multinucleated cells may be present. The cytoplasm has degenerated vac-

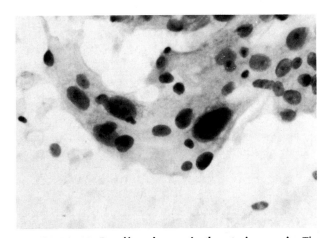

FIGURE 31–10. Busulfan changes in the uterine cervix. The squamous cell changes resemble a high-grade dysplasia. Cervicovaginal smear (Papanicolaou stain; ×400). (Courtesy of Dr. Marluce Bibbo, Chicago, Illinois.)

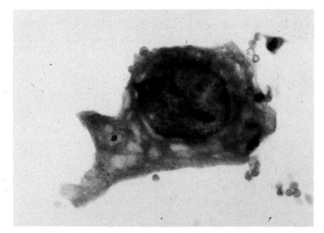

FIGURE 31–11. Thiotepa changes in the urinary bladder. The smear contains markedly enlarged superficial umbrella cells with cytoplasmic vacuoles, neutrophil phagocytosis and irregular frayed cytoplasmic membranes. The nucleus is gigantic with smudged chromatin and macronucleoli. Catheterized urine (Papanicolaou stain; × 400).

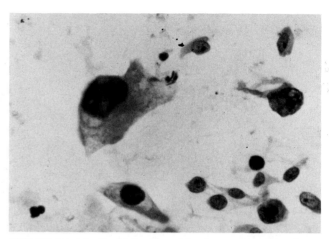

FIGURE 31–12. Cyclophosphamide changes in the urinary bladder. The smear contains enlarged urothelial cells with cytoplasmic vacuoles, frayed cytoplasmic membranes and large hyperchromatic nuclei with distorted membranes. Catheterized urine (Papanicolaou stain; × 400). (Courtesy of Dr. Marluce Bibbo, Chicago, Illinois.)

uoles and frayed borders. The changes are most prominent in the large superficial umbrella cells (Fig. 31–11). Similar changes may be found after radiation therapy or after use of other alkylating drugs, such as mitomycin C. The changes are easily distinguishable from neoplastic changes and do not obscure the presence of occult neoplasia.[24, 65]

Cyclophosphamide

Cyclophosphamide is an alkylating drug activated in a multistep process to the metabolite phosphoramide mustard, the active compound. A side product of the reaction is acrolein, a weakly cytotoxic compound responsible for the common side effect of hemorrhagic cystitis.[15] The presenting signs and symptoms of toxicity include urinary frequency, hematuria and sterile cystitis. In animal models, extensive urothelial ulceration occurs 1 day after initiating therapy. The ulcerated areas contain necrotic epithelium with an associated bloody inflammatory exudate. The mucosa in the intact areas is thinned. The urothelial cells show atypia and karyorrhexis. Surface reepithelialization starts by the fourth day. By day 8, the ulcerated area is covered with an attenuated regenerating mucosa. After 12 to 13 days the normal mucosa is intact, and the only evidence of an insult is hemosiderin-laden histiocytes within the submucosa.[75]

Cytology

The urothelial changes in humans are radiomimetic and similar to thiotepa-induced changes. The nuclei are enlarged and excentric, with a slightly irregular outline. The chromatin is coarsely granular. Occasional large chromocenters and nucleoli with distorted irreg-

ular borders are found. Late changes include nuclear pyknosis with chromatin smudging. Occasional multinucleated cells are found. The cytoplasm is also enlarged with degenerative vacuoles, frayed borders, phagocytosis of foreign debris and neutrophil infiltration (Fig. 31–12). The background often contains numerous erythrocytes, cellular debris and neutrophils.[28]

ANTINEOPLASTIC IMMUNOTHERAPY

BCG

Bacillus Calmette-Guérin (BCG) is a preparation of attenuated bovine tubercle bacillus first used as a vaccine against tuberculosis in 1921. Antineoplastic effects of BCG were first suggested when guinea pigs infected with viable organisms were found to be resistant to the development of neoplasms.[96] Requirements for a therapeutic effect include (1) a small tumor load, (2) an ability by the host to mount an immune response to mycobacterial antigens, (3) an adequate amount of inoculate of viable organisms and (4) an administration of the inoculate in close proximity to the neoplasm. The mechanism of action is not well understood. Interactions among macrophage activation, interferon production, stimulation of cell suppressor activity and enhancement of natural killer cell cytotoxicity are postulated.[23] The antineoplastic effect may be direct cytotoxicity or, more likely, a bystander phenomenon due to the generalized inflammatory response. Intravesical BCG immunotherapy has become an effective method in tumor cytoreduction in patients with superficial bladder cancers.[86] Post-therapy urine cytology and fine needle aspiration biopsy findings of the prostate may show the effects of this therapy.

Prostate

Grossly, the prostate is enlarged, indurated and distorted. By rectal examination, the prostate is indistinguishable from a malignant prostate.

The histology on core needle biopsy or transurethral resection specimen contains multiple small noncaseating to large caseating granulomas. The adjacent prostatic tissue is markedly inflamed. Atypical squamous metaplasia is most prominent adjacent to the caseating lesions.[86] The incidence of developing prostatic granulomata after BCG therapy is close to 100%. The interval between therapy and granuloma appearance is as short as 3 months.

Cytology. The fine needle aspiration of the prostate is very cellular with a necrotic background. The inflammatory cellular components include histiocytes, lymphocytes, multinucleated giant cells, neutrophils and epithelioid histiocytes. Atypical squamous metaplasia contains small groups of dyskaryotic squamous cells with pleomorphic nuclei having irregular membranes and clumped and unevenly distributed chromatin. Enlarged often multiple nucleoli are found. The benign prostatic epithelial cells are in cohesive monolayered sheets. The Ziehl-Neelsen stain for acid fast bacilli is positive in many cases.

Urinary Bladder

The histology of cystoscopic biopsies shows a denuded mucosal surface with a markedly edematous and inflamed lamina propria. Within the lamina propria and submucosa are granulomas ranging from small noncaseating to large caseating processes. The Ziel-Neelsen stain is often positive for acid fast bacilli.

Cytology. Urine cytology shows the effects of the marked localized inflammatory response. The hypercellular specimen contains abundant mixed inflammatory cells including neutrophils, lymphocytes and histiocytes. Necrotic cellular debris is also found. Sloughed groups and single urothelial cells have degenerative changes as found in chronic cystitis. The cells are slightly enlarged with a mildly increased nucleocytoplasmic ratio. The cytoplasm has degenerative vacuoles. The enlarged nuclei have vesicular to smudged chromatin and small nucleoli (Fig. 31–13). Distinction between sloughed neoplastic cells and inflammatory urothelial cell changes may be difficult. Epithelioid histiocytes and multinucleated giant cells are rarely found.

TRANSPLANT IMMUNOSUPPRESSIVE THERAPY

Immunotoxicity and Neoplasia After Transplant Immunosuppressive Therapy

Several epidemiologic studies have shown an increased incidence of certain neoplasms after organ transplantation.[73] The neoplasms include skin cancer, non-Hodgkin's lymphoma, uterine cervix *in situ* carcinoma, Kaposi's sarcoma, vulvar and anal carcinoma and liver cancer. The etiology for neoplastic transformation is postulated to be immunosuppressive therapy[73, 92] associated with an Epstein-Barr virus infection.[43] In allograft transplantation of kidney, heart, liver, heart-lung, pancreas and bone marrow, host immunosuppression is necessary to prevent rejection. Single or combination drug therapy is used for immunosuppression. Cyclosporin A has been implicated alone or in combination with other drugs as the most carcinogenic immunosuppressive drug.[92]

Cyclosporine

Cyclosporin A is a fungal metabolite and a powerful immunosuppressant in all species tested. It is relatively specific for T lymphocytes and is postulated to act by inhibiting the expression of antigen-induced signals from T cells necessary for the subsequent recruitment, proliferation and maturation of T cell–dependent immune responses.[20, 95]

The therapy-induced neoplasms that are most likely to be diagnosed by cytology findings include malignant lymphomas by fine needle aspiration biopsy and intraepithelial neoplasia of the uterine cervix by cervicovaginal smear.

Lymphomas and Lymphoproliferative Disorders. The incidence of lymphomas and lymphoproliferative disorders ranges from 0.4% in 5550 transplant patients[72] to 5.3% in 132 transplant patients.[92] The lesions may be polyclonal polymorphic B-cell hyperplasia (PBCH) or monoclonal/oligoclonal polymorphic B-cell lymphoma (PBCL).[16, 43] The site of origin may be nodal or extranodal including the gastrointestinal tract, liver, spleen, lungs or central nervous system. In

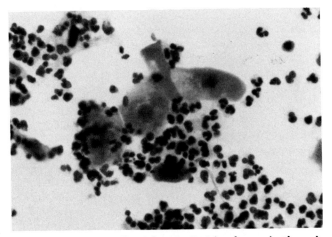

FIGURE 31–13. Bacille Calmette-Guérin change in the urinary bladder. The smear contains enlarged degenerated urothelial cells and marked acute inflammation. This pattern resembles chronic cystitis. Catheterized urine (Papanicolaou stain; ×400).

PBCH, the presenting symptomatology is often an infectious mononucleosis-like illness; PBCH is usually widely disseminated.

Lymphoproliferative Disorder. The lymph node histology consists of a polymorphic, diffuse, B-cell proliferation of follicular center cells (small cleaved and large noncleaved) and "post-follicular" lymphocytes with varying degrees of plasmacytic differentiation (plasmacytoid lymphocytes, plasma cells and immunoblasts). The immunoblastic lymphocytes do not show nuclear atypia.[43]

Cytology. Fine needle aspiration contains a cellular polymorphic population of lymphocytes (large noncleaved and small cleaved), plasmacytoid lymphocytes, plasma cells and immunoblasts without significant atypia. Tingible-body macrophages are also found. The polymorphic pattern of the aspirate suggests a benign process with a follicular center and parafollicular hyperplasia (Fig. 31–14). The immunoblasts, although increased in number, are not sufficient to suggest outright malignancy.[43] Immunophenotyping and gene rearrangement studies reveal a polyclonal B-cell population. This lymphoproliferative disorder may progress to a polymorphic B-cell lymphoma. Even though the process is polyclonal, it is progressive, frequently leading to the patient's demise. The therapeutic regimens include an antiviral agent "acyclovir" and a decrease, cessation or change in immunosuppressive therapy. Hanto[43] reported a good response with this therapy.

Lymphoma. In PBCL, the process appears with localized solid tumor masses. In contrast to PBCH, typical signs or symptoms of infection are not present. The PBCL shows a diffusely replaced lymph node with large atypical immunoblasts and areas of necrosis (Fig. 31–15). The polymorphic B-cell hyperplasia features are minimized.[43]

Cytology. Fine needle aspirate contains a monomorphic population of large atypical immunoblasts. The cells have an intermediate amount of excentric

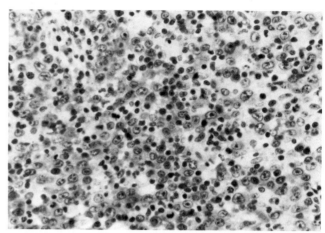

FIGURE 31–15. Cyclosporine (Cyclosporin A)-induced polymorphic B-cell (immunoblastic) lymphoma. The lymph node is diffusely effaced with abundant immunoblasts admixed with scattered plasma cells and plasmacytoid lymphocytes. Lymph node biopsy (hematoxylin and eosin; ×100).

cytoplasm often containing small vacuoles. The nuclei are large and noncleaved, with vesicular chromatin and prominent single or multiple central nucleoli. Admixed with the immunoblasts are a minor population of small lymphocytes and plasma cells.[43] Immunophenotyping and gene rearrangement studies reveal a monoclonal or oligoclonal B-cell population.[16, 43] The therapy of choice is cessation or change of the immunosuppressive therapy with aggressive antineoplastic chemotherapy, radiation therapy or both. In general, antiviral therapy is not effective in PBCL.[43]

Uterine Cervix. Cervical neoplasia shows a 14-fold increase in the immunosuppressed population compared with the general population.[76] The predominant lesion is intraepithelial. Rarely have invasive neoplasms been found. The cytologic features of the immunosuppression-induced dysplasia or cancer are identical to those of the cervical neoplasia of the general population. A recommendation is made for women to have a baseline cervicovaginal smear prior to immunosuppressive therapy and at regular intervals thereafter to monitor for early dysplastic changes. Most neoplasms respond to conventional cancer therapy. High-grade malignancies may necessitate a reduction or cessation of immunosuppressive therapy.[76]

Evaluation of Allograft Transplant Rejection and Immunosuppressive Toxicity

Fine Needle Aspiration of Renal Allograft

Since the advent of renal allograft transplantation, core needle biopsy has been the standard in evaluating host rejection, immunotherapy toxicity and renal function. Fine needle aspiration biopsy has also become an accepted method for monitoring renal transplant pa-

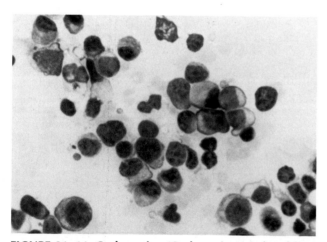

FIGURE 31–14. Cyclosporine (Cyclosporin A)-induced lymphoproliferative disorder. The smear contains polymorphic mononuclear cells including immunoblasts, plasma cells and plasmacytoid lymphocytes. Fine needle aspiration biopsy of lymph node (Diff-quik stain; ×400).

tients.[93] Fine needle aspiration is a less morbid procedure, allowing for more frequent sampling of the allograft with less risk for complications. Fine needle aspiration and core needle biopsy correlate well in evaluating host rejection.[11, 13] Complications during the immediate post-transplant period that can be differentiated by fine needle aspiration biopsy include acute tubular necrosis, cyclosporine toxicity, acute cellular rejection and graft necrosis.[58] These diagnoses can be differentiated by evaluation of the subpopulations of the inflammatory cells using standard cytologic stains, such as May-Grünwald-Giemsa,[93] and by evaluation of the lymphocyte subpopulations (T cell and B cell) and renal tubular HLA-DR antigen expression, using immunocytochemistry, immunogold-immuno silver markers and flow cytometry immunophenotyping.[9, 58, 93] Other studies amenable to fine needle aspiration material include DNA *in situ* hybridization for viral infections (cytomegalovirus, Epstein-Barr virus and herpes virus) and electron microscopy to detect changes at the subcellular level. Although fine needle aspiration can duplicate core needle biopsy results with less morbidity, a core needle biopsy is necessary to evaluate vascular changes in chronic rejection.[58]

Urine Cytology of Renal Allograft

Another method for evaluating renal transplant function is urine cytology. Sandoz[79] correlated lymphocyturia or a sharp increase in preexisting lymphocyturia as a marker for immunologic rejection: 400 cells per case are counted in three groups, lymphocytes, neutrophils and nonsquamous epithelial cells. If the lymphocytes constitute greater than 20% and the neutrophils less than 55% of the cells, this correlates with immunologic rejection. In a series of 24 cases, the sensitivity was 77% and the specificity was 91%. Kline and Craighead[51] recognized two epithelial cell populations in transplant patients' urine. Type I cells are small (7 to 9 μ in diameter) and are clustered in groups of 5 to 20. The cells have scant cytoplasm and variably sized hyperchromatic nuclei. Their origin is postulated to be renal tubular cells exfoliated secondary to ischemia. They are present immediately after transplantation, 2 weeks prior to death and during episodes of threatened rejection. Type II cells are larger (10 to 80 μ in diameter) and are scattered individually in the urine sediment. They have irregular cell margins, enlarged nuclei and clumped chromatin. The origin of these cells is unknown. They are found in the urine of all renal transplant patients at nonspecific times post-transplant and are not associated with the perioperative period, threatened rejection or death. Type II cells are postulated to represent cellular changes due to the immunosuppressive drugs.

Cyclosporin A toxicity may also be evaluated by exfoliative urine cytology. Ashton and colleagues[4] described a sterile leukocyturia (> 1000 neutrophils/10 high-power fields), which occurs in a higher frequency in cyclosporine-treated patients (93%) compared with azathioprine-treated patients (62%). Cortesini[17] char-

acterized cyclosporin A toxicity by finding proximal renal tubular cells containing prominent intracytoplasmic eosinophilic granules. In the late phase, damaged renal epithelial cell fragments, necrotic cellular debris and degenerated tubular cells are found. Winkleman[94] confirmed the finding of the abnormal renal tubular cells and found their number to be dose dependent. Urine cytology may be advantageous in the evaluation of immunologic rejection and cyclosporin A toxicity compared with renal fine needle aspiration biopsy because of its less invasive nature. Fine needle aspiration biopsy is a more objective method and correlates better with core needle biopsy. Both cytologic methods are complementary in the evaluation of renal allograft function.

THYROID-SUPPRESSIVE THERAPY

Carbimazole

Carbimazole and methimazole are thyroid-suppressive agents that have a cytostatic effect in hyperthyroidism. The cytologic changes induced by these drugs may mimic malignancy. Clinical history of their usage is important when interpreting a fine needle aspirate of the thyroid.

The histologic changes in carbimazole-treated thyroid glands include the increased number of unopened acini, the pseudostratification of the follicular epithelium and the presence of papillae and pseudopapillae. The follicular cells display anisonucleosis and moderate pleomorphism. Atypical mitoses may be found. The cytoplasm is abundant and oxyphilic.

Cytology

Smejkal and coworkers[84] observed cytologic changes due to these drugs in two thirds of treated patients. The smears were cellular, displaying a striking anisonucleosis with large irregular nuclei measuring up to 30 μ in diameter. Toluidine blue staining is useful in distinguishing the small ring-shaped benign nucleoli in the treated atypical follicular cells from the large compact nucleoli found in malignant follicular cells. The large nuclei are postulated to be polyploid due to inhibition of nuclear division.

MECHANICAL THERAPY

Electrocautery of the Uterine Cervix

Electrocautery is a therapy causing coagulative "thermal" tissue necrosis by means of a biterminal, high frequency, electrical current. In the uterine cervix, it is used to treat benign processes, such as erosions, cervicitis, and preneoplastic and neoplastic lesions. Electrocautery is postulated to cause a host immune response with activation of lymphocytes that are stimulated against the epithelial cells in the lesion. Clinical information including the types of therapy and the dates of the procedures are essential in evaluation of post-therapy smears. Bukovsky and Zidovsky[14] reported abnormal cells in 42% of the cervicovaginal smears of patients treated by electrocautery for benign cervical lesions. The abnormal cells were found in the first 8 weeks after the therapy and persisted for up to 20 weeks.

Acute Phase

Early cytologic features include a necrosis resembling "tumor diathesis" and a marked inflammatory response composed of neutrophils and lymphocytes. In neoplastic lesions, a repeat cervicovaginal smear is recommended 4 to 6 weeks after therapy. This interval allows the necrotic inflammatory background to clear and not obscure persistent neoplastic cells. The abnormal, non-neoplastic cells are mostly atypical parabasal and intermediate cells with enlarged coarsely granular nuclear chromatin. Prominent nucleoli, often multiple, are found. These cells have fairly abundant, usually cyanophilic cytoplasm. The nucleocytoplasmic ratio remains close to normal.

Abnormal endocervical cells are also found. These cells usually occur in aggregates. They are enlarged with variable nuclear sizes. The nucleocytoplasmic ratio is sometimes markedly increased. The endocervical cells have coarse chromatin often condensed at the nuclear membrane. Koss[53] has described characteristic "beading" of the chromatin in these cells. The nucleoli are enlarged; one or more cytoplasmic vacuoles are found.

Early Healing

Bukovsky and Zidovsky[14] have reported two cytologic phenomena that occur during the healing process after electrocautery. These are the "contact-developed lucid cell" and the "regression field." Contact-developed lucid cells are first observed approximately at the fourth week. They are round cells with pale, translucent cytoplasm and finely granular, homogeneous chromatin. The early forms resemble large lymphoid cells with narrow rims of cytoplasm. A larger cell with abundant translucent cytoplasm and a thickened cytoplasmic membrane is also found. These cells have one to two prominent nucleoli. Contact-developed lucid cells are never observed alone but rather are firmly attached to an abnormal target cell nucleus in a "cell-in-a-cell" pattern. As many as 12 contact-developed lucid cells may be adherent to one target cell. The target cells, epithelial cells stimulating the host immune response, have degenerative cytoplasmic changes with nuclear shrinking and wrinkling. The nucleus of the target cell assumes a crescent shape. In the later stages of the immune response, the contact-developed lucid cell resembles a cystic inclusion within the target cell.

The second healing phenomenon, the regression field, peaks approximately at the eighth week. The

smear background is granular. This appearance is secondary to cytoplasmic debris from destruction of abnormal cells. This background mimics the tumor diathesis found in smears with invasive carcinoma. Within the regression field, intact and degenerated abnormal cells are found. Normal cells are not affected. Dark round bodies the size of red blood cells, representing killer lymphocytes, are found either within or adherent to target cells. The nuclei of the target cells are heavily damaged and may even be lysed or ejected from the cell. A yellow-staining "ghost" vacuole remains.

Repair

The reparative process starts with a single layer of reparative epithelium covering the ulcerated coagulative area 1 week after the therapy is completed. By the third to eighth week, the treated area is covered by a mature stratified squamous epithelium. The reparative process is postulated to start from the columnar or squamous cells adjacent to the treated area rather than from the reserve cells at the ulcer base. The cytologic features of epithelial repair in electrocautery damage are similar to repair due to other causes of cervical mucosal disruption and are discussed under Cryotherapy.[8, 32]

Cryotherapy

Cryotherapy (freezing) has been used since 1966 in the treatment of chronic cervicitis and premalignant lesions of the uterine cervix. The precise mechanism of cellular injury following this form of therapy is unclear. It may be due to the formation of extracellular and intracellular ice crystals.[45] As in other uterine cervix ablative therapies, a clinical history regarding cryotherapy is needed to evaluate the cervicovaginal smear. Freeze-associated cytologic changes may simulate neoplasia. Interpretation of smears prior to 6 weeks following cryotherapy or until complete healing has occurred is not advised. Cancer cells may persist in smears for several weeks following cryotherapy. A false-positive smear is avoided if it is taken after 6 weeks.

Cytology

The acute cytologic findings include granular necrosis and a marked inflammatory exudate composed of neutrophils and lymphocytes similar to electrocautery acute changes. Marked cellular and nuclear enlargement is not a feature of cryotherapy as in electrocautery.[31] Hasegawa[45] reported two categories of atypical cells found in 19% of cervicovaginal smears up to the fourth week following cryotherapy. The first category of atypical cells has features identical to "tissue repair." The cells occur in large sheets, small aggregates and, rarely, as isolated cells. Within the tissue aggregates, the cells display indistinct cell borders with maintenance of nuclear polarity. The single cells demonstrate abundant cytoplasm with irregular borders and occasional small vacuoles. The nuclei are oval with a finely granular chromatin, smooth membranes and perinuclear halos. There may be moderate anisonucleosis. Prominent macronucleoli, some with irregular borders, and multiple nucleoli are found. The postulated origin of the cells may be from basal cell hyperplasia or atypical reserve cell hyperplasia. Bibbo and associates[8] also reported these reparative cell changes, remarking on the cyanophilic cytoplasm with long, ribbon-like extensions and mitotic figures. The second atypical cell type occurs in aggregates and syncytia with small uniform nuclei having finely granular chromatin and chromocenters. These cells are postulated to arise from reserve cell hyperplasia or immature squamous metaplasia. Both atypical cell types regress or are no longer observed in smears 5 to 6 weeks after cryotherapy.[45]

Gondos and colleagues[31] reported degenerative nuclear changes characterized by karyorrhexis involving intermediate and parabasal cells. The changes are extensive from 2 to 4 weeks following cryotherapy. Cytoplasmic vacuoles in parabasal cells with occasional indentation of the nucleus and nuclear folds are also found. The vacuoles may be single or multiple, appear to be membrane-bound and are filled with pale eosinophilic material. The karyorrhexis and cytoplasmic vacuolization persist up to 6 months after cryotherapy and are present in cervicovaginal smears despite a grossly normal cervix on clinical examination.

Early postcryotherapy reparative cells are polyploid with a significant proliferative activity by quantitative DNA analysis. After 6 to 8 weeks, when the reparative process is completed, the nuclear DNA reverts to diploid.[8, 87]

Laser Therapy

Carbon-dioxide laser tissue vaporization was first introduced as a treatment modality for uterine cervical dysplasia and carcinoma *in situ* in England in 1977.[68] A colposcopically guided laser can be focused on any area of the cervix, in various directions and to any tissue depth. Virtually no bleeding or tissue necrosis occurs with this form of therapy as compared with electrocautery and cryotherapy. The laser produces intense focused heat in the tissue inactivating cellular components, including DNA and RNA. This effect interrupts the cellular replication process. Cytology, histology and scanning electron microscopy reveal the greatest thermal damage occurs in the superficial epithelial layers where the water content is low.[7] The energy is rapidly dissipated in the superficial cells causing less destruction to the parabasal, basal and stromal cells, which have a higher water content. Adjacent tissue necrosis is consequently minimal to absent with resultant minimal scar formation and rapid healing.

Several histologic studies have delineated the sequence of events following laser therapy.[2, 7, 81] The

ulcer formation and epithelial repair are similar to those following electrocautery and cryotherapy, except the healing time is shortened to 2 to 4 weeks from 6 to 8 weeks. Ultrastructural studies have confirmed the origin of the regenerative epithelium to be the lateral epithelial edges of the ulcer and not the reserve or stromal cells at the base of the ulcer.[2, 81]

Colposcopy confirms this sequence of events. At 1 week, the treated area is charred or red with little evidence of reepithelialization. At 2 weeks, a thin layer of epithelium spreads over the ulcer. By 4 weeks, a nearly full-thickness squamous epithelium covers the ulcerated area and has the appearance of native squamous epithelium. The Schiller test finding at this site is positive. At 6 weeks, the epithelium is mature and the Schiller test finding reverts to negative. The ulcerated site is now unrecognizable. The original squamocolumnar junction is maintained.[68]

Cytology

The sequence of events follows an epithelial reparative process previously described under Cryotherapy. After 1 day, a marked acute inflammatory infiltrate is found. Typical squamous cells are absent. Elongated distorted squamous cells and markedly lengthened columnar cells are found. The cellular changes are postulated to be due to dehydration resulting from the thermal insult. By the seventh to tenth day, the reparative epithelial process has begun and the inflammatory exudate has changed to histiocytes and multinucleated giant cells. By day 21, the normal intermediate and superficial squamous cells are found and the inflammatory exudate is absent.[7, 47]

Intrauterine Devices

The exact mechanism of action of the intrauterine device (IUD) accounting for its contraceptive property is not known. The IUD initiates an inflammatory response on the surface of the endometrium, which may inhibit implantation of the fertilized ovum. The use of an IUD is often associated with an exfoliation of atypical cells that may be mistaken for endometrial adenocarcinoma, endometrial hyperplasia or squamous cell carcinoma. History of IUD use, especially in a reproductive-age woman, should always be considered in the interpretation and reporting of this type of atypia.

The uterine cervix shows chronic cervicitis with varying degrees of squamous metaplasia. No distinct atypia is identified. The endometrial tissue has chronic endometritis with endocervical and squamous metaplasia. Hyperchromasia and cellular atypia of a reparative type are found in the endometrium.[36]

Cytology

The cytologic changes are also described in Chapter 8, Inflammation and Viral Microbiology Infections.

The inflammatory response found in cervicovaginal smears of women wearing IUDs varies, depending on the length of time the IUDs have been in place.[39] The initial inflammatory response is acute with many neutrophils. By the third day, macrophages are recognized. They are abundant by the seventh day. The macrophage population increases in proportion to the duration of IUD usage. It is postulated that macrophage proliferation and accumulation may be the primary effect of the IUD. Erosions of the endometrium and underlying stroma by the IUD probably cause shedding of histiocytes and endometrial cells.[36] Occasional foreign body giant cells are found from the third day on (Fig. 31–16). Plasma cells and lymphocytes also increase. Neutrophils are almost completely absent by the fourth week. Phagocytosed foreign material, including hemosiderin and degenerated spermatozoa, may be found. Atypical glandular cells appear at approximately day 10. Between 12 weeks and up to 7 years, macrophages and giant cells remain conspicuous. Fragments of refractile foreign material from the IUD are found surrounded by macrophages or embedded within endometrial cells. Atypical epithelial repair is found and may be caused by the large number of inflammatory cells that migrate from the uterus or from the ulceration at the site of cervical contact with the carrier thread.

Three types of atypical epithelial cells, squamous, glandular and indeterminant, have been described.[36] The squamous atypia is metaplastic with macronucleoli.

Several reports have described the atypical changes found in glandular cells of endocervical[27, 36] and endometrial[27] origin. The atypical glandular cells usually occur in clusters containing from 3 to 15 and up to 30 cells. An occasional single atypical columnar cell may be found. The glandular cells have a variable amount of cytoplasm. Some have dense scanty cytoplasm with distinct cell borders. The nuclei are en-

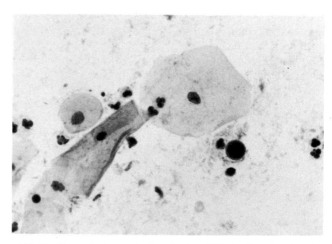

FIGURE 31–17. Intrauterine-device (IUD) changes in the uterine cervix. The smear contains an indeterminant cell resembling carcinoma *in situ*. Note the paucity of other cells suggesting dysplasia. Cervicovaginal smear (Papanicolaou stain; ×400).

larged with moderate variation in size and shape. The chromatin is coarsely granular and clumped. The nucleocytoplasmic ratio is high. The nucleus contains single-to-multiple round nucleoli. The cytoplasm has many large vacuoles pushing the nucleus aside. These cytologic changes cause the atypical columnar cells to strongly mimic adenocarcinoma of either endocervical or endometrial origin.

The third atypical epithelial cell type is the so-called indeterminant cell. These cells fit into no definite morphologic cell type, although they are postulated to be endometrial in origin. The cells resemble the cells shed from carcinoma *in situ* (Fig. 31–17). Most are single and enlarged with a high nucleocytoplasmic ratio and scant cytoplasm. The nuclei have hyperchromatic granular chromatin with irregular nuclear membranes. Unlike carcinoma *in situ*, the cells are usually bi- or trinucleated and contain nucleoli. The nucleoli may be inconspicuous and multiple. An additional cytologic feature separating these atypical indeterminant cells from those of carcinoma *in situ* is the homogeneity of the cell population. In carcinoma *in situ*, cells displaying a full spectrum of dysplastic changes, from mild to severe, are found. Gupta and colleagues[36] observed this cytologic atypia to revert to normal 1 to 13 months after removal of the IUD.

Actinomyces and Intrauterine Devices

Another feature associated with IUD is the presence of *Actinomyces* species in the cervicovaginal smears. The incidence of *Actinomyces* in IUD users varies from 7 to 44%. The type of IUD (metal or plastic) does not influence the presence of *Actinomyces*.[61] The use of an IUD for greater than 2 years promotes the overgrowth of *Actinomyces* in the vagina. The predominant species isolated in such cases is *A. israelii*.[59, 61]

Actinomyces is a rare inhabitant of the normal female

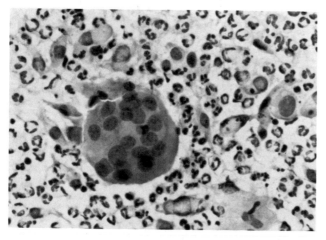

FIGURE 31–16. Intrauterine-device (IUD) changes in the uterine cervix. The smear contains a marked inflammatory exudate with neutrophils, histiocytes and multinucleated giant cells. Cervicovaginal smear (Papanicolaou stain; ×400). (Courtesy of Dr. Marluce Bibbo, Chicago, Illinois.)

genital tract. Most women with smears positive for *Actinomyces* are asymptomatic. However, many case reports implicate IUD-related *Actinomyces* as a cause of pelvic inflammatory disease. Actinomycosis has been reported in 17 to 30% of IUD users with pelvic inflammatory disease. *Actinomyces* may cause cervicitis and endometritis and result in permanent damage to the fallopian tubes with complications of salpingo-oophoritis, tubo-ovarian abscesses, infertility or ectopic pregnancy.

Cytology

All cervicovaginal smears show moderate or marked chronic inflammation with histiocytes. The organisms are small and irregular masses, which stain blue, purple, brown or black with the Papanicolaou stain. In the center of the masses is a haphazard arrangement of filaments. Delicate, branching and sometimes beaded filamentous hyphae radiate to the periphery of the masses, extending in parallel rays, giving a fern-like pattern. The hyphae branch at acute angles. The tips of most of the filaments are slightly blunted or clubbed. Occasionally, the organisms may form a central denser eosinophilic core, which may consist of IUD-associated material (fragments of IUD or calcium carbonate crystals). Typical "sulfur granules" are infrequent. The granules are thick and have a central homogeneous core from which the organism's filaments radiate. A heavy neutrophil and histiocytic infiltrate is found along the periphery. An occasional foreign body type giant cell is observed.[38]

Transurethral Resection and Core Needle Biopsy of the Prostate

Transurethral resection of the prostate (TURP) is an endoscopic surgical procedure commonly employed to relieve urethral obstruction secondary to enlargement of the prostatic periurethral transition zone. A transurethral endoscopically placed tungsten wire loop passes an electrical current and cuts fragments of periurethral prostatic tissue to relieve the obstruction. Another surgical procedure employed to evaluate transrectally palpable nodules in the peripheral zone of the prostate is the core needle biopsy. The procedure may be performed transperineally or transrectally with a TruCut or Biopty gun needle. Subsequent fine needle aspiration, TURP or core needle biopsy may detect changes due to the previous surgical intervention.

Core needle biopsies and TURP may induce the formation of large well-circumscribed granulomas with necrotic or collagenous centers, palisading epithelioid histiocytes, occasional multinucleated giant cells and a dense mantle of inflammatory cells. The granulomas are associated with acini, ducts or vessels.[64] The granulomas may resemble rheumatoid nodules.[57]

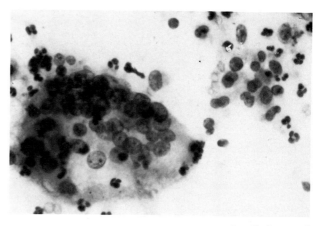

FIGURE 31–18. Transurethral resection–induced changes in the prostate. The smear contains a multinucleated giant cell and neutrophils from granulomatous prostatitis. Fine needle aspiration biopsy of prostate (Papanicolaou stain; ×400). (Courtesy of Dr. Marluce Bibbo, Chicago, Illinois.)

Cytology

The findings of fine needle aspiration of the prostate are similar to those of BCG therapy changes except the atypical squamous metaplasia is less frequent. The aspirate is often cellular with neutrophils, lymphocytes, histiocytes, eosinophils, occasional epithelioid histiocytes and multinucleated giant cells (Fig. 31–18). Necrosis can be found in the background. The benign prostatic epithelial cells may show atypical reactive changes including disturbed polarity within the monolayered sheets, few microacini and small nucleoli. Overt malignant changes are not found. Findings using special stains for microorganisms are negative.

The etiology of the granuloma formation is unknown. A hypersensitivity reaction to heat coagulation necrosis of the collagen or impaired healing may initiate the process.[64]

References

1. Adamson IYR, Bowden DH: The pathogenesis of bleomycin-induced pulmonary fibrosis in mice. Am J Pathol 77:185–190, 1974.
2. Allen JM, Stein DS, Shingleton HM: Regeneration of cervical epithelium after laser vaporization. Obstet Gynecol 62(6):700–706, 1983.
3. Antonakopoulos GN, Hicks RM, Berry RJ: The subcellular basis of damage to the human urinary bladder induced by irradiation. J Pathol 143:103–116, 1984.
4. Ashton A, Alexander DP, DeBellis C, Schumann GB: Leukocyturia in cyclosporine-treated renal allograft recipients. Am J Clin Pathol 89(1):113–117, 1988.
5. Bedrossian CWM, Corey BJ: Abnormal sputum cytopathology during chemotherapy with bleomycin. Acta Cytol 22(4):202–207, 1978.
6. Bedrossian CWM, Luna MA, Mackay B, Lichtiger B: Ultrastructure of pulmonary bleomycin toxicity. Cancer 32:44–51, 1973.
7. Bellina JH, Seto YJ: Pathological and physical investigations into CO_2 laser-tissue interactions with specific emphasis on

cervical intraepithelial neoplasm. Lasers Surg Med 1:47–69, 1980.

8. Bibbo M, Keebler CM, Weid GL: The cytologic diagnosis of tissue repair in the female genital tract. Acta Cytol 15:133–137, 1971.

9. Bishop GA, Waugh J, Horbath JS, Johnson JR, Hall BM, Philips J, Duggin GG, Sheil AGR, Tiller DJ: Diagnosis of renal allograft rejection by analysis of fine-needle aspiration biopsy specimens with immunostains and simple cytology. Lancet 2:645–649, 1986.

10. Bondeson L: Aspiration cytology of radiation-induced changes of normal breast epithelium. Acta Cytol 31:309–310, 1987.

11. Boshkos C, Steinmuller DR, Novick AC, Streem S, Cunningham RJ, Fishleder A, Dlugosz, B: Correlation of fine-needle aspirate biopsies with core biopsies after renal transplantation. Transplant Proc 20(4):592–594, 1988.

12. Bostwick DG, Egbert BM, Fajardo LF: Radiation injury of the normal and neoplastic prostate. Am J Surg Pathol 6:541–551, 1982.

13. Brown S, Horsburgh T, Veitch PS, Bell PRF: Comparison of fine needle aspiration biopsy and Tru-Cut biopsy performed under ultrasound guidance. Transplant Proc 20(4):595–596, 1988.

14. Bukovsky A, Zidovsky J: Cytologic phenomena accompanying uterine cervix electrocoagulation. Acta Cytol 29(3):353–362, 1985.

15. Chabner BA, Myers CE: Clinical pharmacology of cancer chemotherapy. *In* Cancer: Principles and Practice of Oncology, 3rd ed. Edited by VT Devita, S Hellman, SA Rosenberg. Philadelphia, JB Lippincott, 1989.

16. Cleary ML, Sklar J: Lymphoproliferative disorders in cardiac transplant recipients are multiclonal lymphomas. Lancet 2:489–493, 1984.

17. Cortesini R, Stella F, Molajoni ER, Lemeni AR, Rossi M, Pretagostini R, Alfani D: Urinary exfoliative cytology in kidney allographs under cyclosporine therapy. Transplant Proc 16(5):1200–1201, 1984.

18. Cox JD, Stoffel TJ: The significance of needle biopsy after irradiation for stage C adenocarcinoma of the prostate. Cancer 40:156–160, 1977.

19. Dailey ME, Lindsay S, Miller ER: Histologic lesions in the thyroid glands of patients receiving radioiodine for hyperthyroidism. J Clin Endocrinol Metab 13:1513–1529, 1953.

20. Demetris AJ, Nalesnik MA, Kunz HW, Gill TJ III, Shinozuka H: Sequential analyses of the development of lymphoproliferative disorders in rats receiving cyclosporine. Transplantation 38(3):239–246, 1984.

21. Dobyns BM, Vickery AL, Maloof F, Chapman EM: Functional and histologic effects of therapeutic doses of radioactive iodine on the thyroid of man. J Clin Endocrinol Metab 13:548–567, 1953.

22. Donaldson M, Canti RG: Fifty cases of carcinoma of the cervix treated with radium. Br Med J 2:12–16, 1923.

23. Droller MJ: Immunotherapy in genitourinary neoplasia. Urol Clin North Am 11(4):643–657, 1984.

24. Droller MJ, Erozan YS: Thiotepa effects on urinary cytology in the interpretation of transitional cell cancer. J Urol 134(4):671–674, 1985.

25. Duncan RE, Bennett DW, Evans AT, Aron BS, Schellhas HF: Radiation-induced bladder tumors. J Urol 118:43–45, 1977.

26. Esposti PL, Edsmyr F, Moberger G, Wadstrom L, Zajicek J: Cytologic diagnosis in bladder carcinoma treated by supervoltage irradiation. Scand J Urol Nephrol 3:201–203, 1969.

27. Fornari ML: Cellular changes in the glandular epithelium of patients using IUCD—A source of cytologic error. Acta Cytol 18(4):341–343, 1974.

28. Forni AM, Koss LG, Geller W: Cytological study of the effect of cyclophosphamide on the epithelium of the urinary bladder in man. Cancer 17:1348–1355, 1964.

29. Frankl O, Amreich I.: The histological changes incident to radium and X-ray treatment of uterine carcinoma. Surg Gynecol Obstet 33:162–163, 1921.

30. Ginsberg SJ, Comis RL: The pulmonary toxicity of antineoplastic agents. Semin Oncol 9(1):34–51, 1982.

31. Gondos B, Smith LR, Townsend DE: Cytologic changes in

cervical epithelium following cryosurgery. Acta Cytol 14(7):386–389, 1970.

32. Gonzalez-Merlo J, Ausin J, Lejarcegui JA, Marquez M: Regeneration of the ectocervical epithelium after its destruction by electrocauterization. Acta Cytol 17(4):366–371, 1973.

33. Graham RM: The effect of radiation on vaginal cells in cervical carcinoma. Surg Gynecol Obstet 84:153–165, 1947.

34. Graham RM: The Cytologic Diagnosis of Cancer. Philadelphia, WB Saunders, 1972.

35. Graham RM, Graham JB: Cytological prognosis in cancer of the uterine cervix treated radiologically. Cancer 8:59–70, 1955.

36. Gupta PK, Burroughs F, Luff RD, Frost JK, Erozan, YS: Epithelial atypia associated with intrauterine contraceptive devices (IUD). Acta Cytol 22:286–291, 1978.

37. Gupta S, Gupta YN, Sanyal B: Radiation changes in vaginal and cervical cytology in carcinoma of the cervix uteri. J Surg Oncol 19:71–73, 1982.

38. Gupta PK, Hollander DH, Frost JK: *Actinomyces* in cervicovaginal smears: An association with IUD usage. Acta Cytol 20(4):295–297, 1976.

39. Gupta PK, Malkani PK, Bhasin K: Cellular response in the uterine cavity after IUD insertion and structural changes of the IUD. Contraception 4:375–384, 1971.

40. Gupta S, Mukherjee K, Gupta YN, Kumar M: Sequential radiation changes in cytology of vaginal smears in carcinoma of cervix uteri during radiotherapy. Int J Gynecol Obstet 25:303–308, 1987.

41. Gureli N, Denham SW, Root SW: Cytologic dysplasia related to busulfan (Myleran) therapy. Obstet Gynecol 21:466–470, 1963.

42. von Haam E: Radiation cell changes. *In* Compendium on Diagnostic Cytology, 6th ed. Edited by GL Wied, CM Keebler, LG Koss, JW Reagan. Chicago, University of Chicago Press, 1988.

43. Hanto DW, Gajl-Peczalska KJ, Frizzera G, Arthur DC, Balfour HH, McClain K, Simmons RL, Najarian JS: Epstein-Barr virus (EBV)–induced polyclonal and monoclonal B-cell lymphoproliferative diseases occurring after renal transplantation. Ann Surg 198(3):356–369, 1983.

44. Haour P: Comparison of radiation cell changes in exfoliated vaginal cells and in exfoliated cells from the urinary tract (urocytogram). Acta Cytol 3:449–450, 1959.

45. Hasegawa T, Tsutsui F, Kurihara S: Cytomorphologic study on the atypical cells following cryosurgery for the treatment of chronic cervicitis. Acta Cytol 19(6):533–537, 1975.

46. Herovici C: Cytochemistry of irradiated cells. Acta Cytol 3:360–361, 1959.

47. Holmquist ND, Bellina JH, Danos ML: Vaginal and cervical cytologic changes following laser treatment. Acta Cytol 20(4):290–294, 1976.

48. Kaufman RH, Topek NH, Wall JA: Late irradiation changes in vaginal cytology. Am J Obstet Gynecol 81:859–866, 1961.

49. Kini SR: Guides to Clinical Aspiration Biopsy: Thyroid. Tokyo, Igaku-Shoin, 1987.

50. Kline TS: Guides to Clinical Aspiration Biopsy: Prostate. Tokyo, Igaku-Shoin, 1985.

51. Kline TS, Craighead JE: Renal homotransplantation. The cytology of the urine sediment. Am J Clin Pathol 47(6):802–806, 1967.

52. Kline TS, Kline IK: Guides to Clinical Aspiration Biopsy: Breast. Tokyo Igaku-Shoin, 1989.

53. Koss LG: Diagnostic Cytology and Its Histopathologic Bases. Philadelphia, JB Lippincott, 1979.

54. Koss LG, Melamed MR, Mayer K: The effect of busulfan on human epithelia. Am J Clin Pathol 44(4):385–397, 1965.

55. Kurth KH, Altwein JE, Skoluda D, Hohenfellner R: Followup of irradiated prostatic carcinoma by aspiration biopsy. J Urol 117:615–617, 1977.

56. Kyung-Whan M, Gyorkey F: Interstitial pulmonary fibrosis, atypical epithelial changes and bronchiolar cell carcinoma following busulfan therapy. Cancer 22(5):1027–1032, 1968.

57. Lee G, Shepherd N: Necrotizing granulomata in prostatic resection specimens—a sequel to previous operations. J Clin Pathol 36:1067–1070, 1983.

58. Loveras J, Hayry P: Fourth International Workshop on Transplant Aspiration Cytology. Transplant Proc 20(4):567–569, 1988.

59. Luff RD, Gupta PK, Spence MR, Frost JK: Pelvic actinomycosis and the intrauterine contraceptive device. A cytohistomorphologic study. Am J Clin Pathol 69:581–586, 1978.

60. Luna MA, Bedrossian CWM, Lichtiger B, Salem PA: Interstitial pneumonitis associated with bleomycin therapy. Am J Clin Pathol 58:501–510, 1972.

61. Mali B, Joshi JV, Wagle U, Hazari K, Shah R, Chadha U, Gokral J, Bhave G: *Actinomyces* in cervical smears of women using intrauterine contraceptive devices. Acta Cytol 30(4):367–371, 1986.

62. Mc Lennan MT, Mc Lennan CE: Significance of cervicovaginal cytology after radiation therapy for cervical carcinoma. Am J Obstet Gynecol 121:96–100, 1975.

63. McLeod BF, Lawrence HJ, Smith DW, Vogt PJ, Gandara DR: Fatal bleomycin toxicity from a low cumulative dose in a patient with renal insufficiency. Cancer 60(11):2617–2620, 1987.

64. Mies C, Balogh K, Stadecker M: Palisading prostate granulomas following surgery. Am J Surg Pathol 8(3):217–221, 1984.

65. Murphy WM, Soloway MS, Finebaum PJ: Pathological changes associated with topical chemotherapy for superficial bladder cancer. J Urol 126:461–464, 1981.

66. Murphy WM, Soloway MS, Lin CJ: Morphologic effects of thio-TEPA on mouse urothelium. Acta Cytol 21(5):701–704, 1977.

67. Murphy WM, Soloway MS, Lin CJ: Morphologic effects of thio-TEPA on mammalian urothelium. Changes in abnormal cells. Acta Cytol 22(6):550–554, 1978.

68. Mylotte MJ, Allen JM, Jordan JA: Regeneration of cervical epithelium following laser destruction of intraepithelial neoplasia. Obstet Gynecol Surv 34:859–860, 1979.

69. Nelson BM, Andrews GA: Breast cancer and cytologic dysplasia in many organs after busulfan (Myleran). Am J Clin Pathol 42(1):37–44, 1964.

70. Patten SF: Postradiation dysplasia of the uterine cervix: cytopathology and clinical significance. *In* Compendium on Diagnostic Cytology, 6th ed. Edited by GL Wied, CM Keebler, LG Koss, JW Reagan. Chicago, University of Chicago Press, 1988.

71. Patten SF, Reagan JW, Obenauf M, Ballard LA: Postirradiation dysplasia of uterine cervix and vagina: an analytical study of the cells. Cancer 16:173–182, 1963.

72. Penn I: Cyclosporine and oncogenesis. Mt Sinai J Med 54(6):460–464, 1987.

73. Penn I, Brunson ME: Cancers after cyclosporine therapy. Transplant Proc 20:885–892, 1988.

74. Peters H: Cytologic smears from the mouth; cellular changes in disease and after radiation. Am J Clin Pathol 29:219–225, 1958.

75. Philips FS, Sternberg SS, Cronin AP, Vidal, PM: Cyclophosphamide and urinary bladder toxicity. Cancer Res 21:1577–1589, 1961.

76. Porreco R, Penn I, Droegemueller W, Greer B, Makowski E: Gynecologic malignancies in immunosuppressed organ homograft recipients. Obstet Gynecol 45(4):359–364, 1975.

77. Rasmussen K, Peterson BL, Jacobo E, Penick GD, Sall J: Cytologic effects of thiotepa and adriamycin on normal canine urothelium. Acta Cytol 24(3):237–243, 1980.

78. Rosenow EC III: The spectrum of drug-induced pulmonary disease. Ann Int Med 77:977–991, 1972.

79. Sandoz PF, Bielmann D, Mihatsch M, Thiel G: Value of urinary sediment in the diagnosis of interstitial rejection in renal transplants. Transplantation 41(3):343–348, 1986.

80. Schnitt SJ, Connolly JL, Harris JR, Cohen RB: Radiation-induced changes in the breast. Hum Pathol 15:545–550, 1984.

81. Sharp GLM, Cordiner JW, Murray EL, More IAR: Healing of cervical epithelium after laser ablation of cervical intraepithelial neoplasia. Clin Pathol 37:611–615, 1984.

82. Silverman S: Ultrastructure observations of radiation response in oral exfoliative cytology. Acta Cytol 13:292–301, 1969.

83. Silverman S, Sheline GE: Effects of radiation on exfoliated normal and malignant oral cells. Cancer 14:587–596, 1961.

84. Smejkal V, Smejkalova E, Rosa M, Zeman V, Smetana K: Cytologic changes simulating malignancy in thyrotoxic goiters treated with carbimazole. Acta Cytol 29(2):173–178, 1985.

85. Spieler P, Gloor F, Egle N, Bandhauer K: Cytological findings in transrectal aspiration biopsy on hormone- and radio-treated carcinoma of the prostate. Virchows Arch 372(2):149–159, 1976.

86. Stilmant M, Siroky MB, Johnson KB: Fine needle aspiration cytology of granulomatous prostatitis induced by BCG immunotherapy of bladder cancer. Acta Cytol 29(6):961–966, 1985.

87. Tenjin Y, Yamamoto K, Sugishita T, Igarashi Y: Basic studies on repair, especially histology, cytology, and microspectrophotometry of DNA contents. Acta Cytol 23(3):245–251, 1979.

88. Vickery AL Jr: Thyroid alterations due to irradiation. *In* The Thyroid. International Academy of Pathology Monograph no.5. Edited by BJ Hazard, DE Smith. Baltimore, Williams & Wilkins, 1964.

89. Wachtel E: A simple cytological test for cancer cure. Br Med J 1:20–22, 1958.

90. Ward HN, Konikov N, Reinhard EH: Cytologic dysplasia occurring after busulfan (Myleran) therapy. Ann of Int Med 63:654–660, 1965.

91. Wentz WB, Reagan JW: Clinical significance of postirradiation dysplasia of the uterine cervix. Am J Obstet Gynecol 106:812–817, 1970.

92. Wilkinson AH, Smith JL, Hunsicker LG, Tobacman J, Kapelanski DP, Johnson M, Wright FH, Behrendt DM, Corry RJ: Increased frequency of posttransplant lymphomas in patients treated with cyclosporine, azathioprine, and prednisone. Transplantation 47(2):293–296, 1989.

93. von Willebrand E: Long-term experience with fine needle aspiration in kidney transplant patients. Transplant Proc 21(4):3568–3570, 1989.

94. Winkelmann M, Burrig KF, Koldovsky U, Witkowski M, Grabensee B, Pfitzer P: Cyclosporin A—altered renal tubular cells in urinary cytology. Lancet 2:667, 1985.

95. Wish JB: Immunologic effects of cyclosporine. Transplant Proc 28:15–18, 1986.

96. Zbar B, Rapp HJ: Immunotherapy of guinea pig cancer with BCG. Cancer 34:1532–1540, 1974.

PART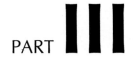

Special Techniques in Cytology

32

Cytopreparatory Techniques

Catherine M. Keebler

Diagnostic cytologic criteria are based on cell samples prepared in a variety of ways. The methods of fixation and sample preparation vary from laboratory to laboratory. Many of the methods are similar in their basic concepts and goals: to reduce artificial cell changes while producing an optimal diagnostic cell sample.[3–6, 9, 10, 12, 20–22, 25, 30, 35–42, 44, 46, 48–50, 55, 57–59, 65, 68, 70, 72, 76, 77, 81]

Collection methods are discussed within each body site section, if warranted.

FIXATION

General Comments on Fixation Procedures

The purpose of the cytologic fixative is to maintain as closely as possible the cytomorphologic characteristics and the diagnostically essential cytochemical elements of the cell.[23] An appropriate fixative for cytodiagnostic purposes should
1. Penetrate cells rapidly
2. Minimize cell shrinkage
3. Maintain morphologic integrity
4. Inactivate autolytic enzymes
5. Replace cellular water
6. Allow permeability of dyes across cell boundaries
7. Permit cell adhesion to a glass surface
8. Be matched to the subsequent staining method used
9. Be bacteriocidal
10. Be reproducible
11. Represent a permanent cellular record.

Historically, Papanicolaou,[63] like Reider[66] before him, utilized ether and 95% ethanol (1:1) as the cytologic fixative of choice. Currently, 95% ethanol, 80% isopropanol, 100% methanol, 95% denatured alcohol and various commercially available spray fixatives have replaced ether and ethanol as the fixative of

choice. The fixative most commonly used today is 95% ethanol. Laboratories not eligible for tax-free alcohol seek equivalent, often less-expensive alternatives. Using the previously mentioned substitutes, there appears to be a minimal amount of cell alteration compared with the original alcohol and ether fixation. Some artifacts are present, as with any fixative, but most cytologists are familiar with those artifacts resulting from the variety of alcohol-based fixatives.

Fixation methods fall into one of three categories.
1. *Wet fixation,* i.e., the immediate submersion of wet cell samples into a fixative solution. The cell samples remain in the fixative solution until arrival in the laboratory, where they are numbered and stained. The cells are not exposed to air.
2. *Wet fixation with subsequent air drying,* i.e., immediately submersing cell samples into a fixation solution, removing from the fixative after a specified time period, allowing to air dry and placing in a container for transportation to the laboratory. Upon arrival in the laboratory the smear is placed in 95% ethanol or its equivalent prior to staining.
3. *Spray fixation,* i.e., the immediate fixation of the wet cell sample with a spray fixative. The spray-fixed cell sample is allowed to dry in the air and is then placed in a container for transportation to the laboratory. Upon arrival in the laboratory the sample is placed into two separate rinses of 95% ethanol to remove the polyethylene glycols (Carbowax) and to complete fixation prior to staining.

The following is a list of alcohol fixatives that are equivalent.
1. 95% ethanol (fast acting, nontoxic and reliable; some distortion due to shrinkage)
2. 80% isopropanol
3. 80% propanol
4. 100% methanol (toxic and cannot be used with Millipore filters; useful mainly for air-dried samples)
5. 95% denatured alcohol (90 parts 95% ethanol, five parts absolute methanol, five parts absolute isopropanol)

6. Reagent-grade alcohol (absolute methanol, 80% isopropanol, 90% acetone)
7. Proprietary-grade alcohol (one part each ethyl acetate, methylisobutylketone and aviation gasoline and 100 parts ethanol).

Immediate Fixation

Whatever the fixative used, be it 95% ethanol, its equivalent or a spray fixative, *immediate fixation while the sample is still wet* is necessary to preserve the cellular features needed for cytomorphologic interpretation because even minimal air drying of the sample alters cellular features. In addition to written instructions, consultative contacts between laboratory and clinical staff usually improve the quality of the cell sample.

Thickness of the Cell Sample (Monolayer Versus Multilayer Specimens)

Fixatives must penetrate the cell surface. The optimal sample for fixation and staining is the monolayer smear. A cellular monolayer is easy to fix, stain, coverslip and screen. However, preparation of true monolayer samples can be performed only on material submitted to the laboratory as a cellular suspension and usually requires sophisticated instrumentation.[1] Gynecologic samples are usually submitted as prefixed smears rather than cellular suspensions and therefore do not lend themselves to monolayer preparations. The gynecologist who takes the sample is advised to prepare thin smears because thick samples prevent rapid penetration of the fixative, result in uneven staining of the cell sample and, in some cases, may cause difficulty in the adequate visualization of the cells. Using the Bethesda system[8] for reporting gynecologic cell diagnoses, smears that are improperly fixed or prepared are identified as unsatisfactory.

Usage of Lubricants Prior to Preparation of the Cell Sample

Usage of lubricants prior to taking the gynecologic cell sample should be avoided. Cells coated by lubricant may be difficult to interpret, and such specimens should be identified as "less than optimal" or "unsatisfactory," depending on the degree of cellular distortion.

Adherence of Cells to Glass Slide

The degree of cellular adherence to the glass slide depends on the body site from which the specimen is derived and on the condition of a given body site. For example, cells from voided urine adhere less well to a glass slide than cells from a sputum sample, and cells from a normal uterine cervix usually adhere better to a glass slide than cells from a patient with an inflammatory, watery discharge. In the last case, spray fixation may yield better results than placing the sample in 95% ethanol. Mayer's albumin, polylysine hydrobromide in a 0.1% aqueous solution, may be added to fluid samples prior to centrifugation or placed on a glass slide to help cells adhere to the slide. For fine needle aspirates it is suggested by some to first place the fixative onto the glass slide and then the cells in order to achieve optimal cellular fixation.

Spray Fixation

Spray fixatives usually consist of an alcohol base and a waxy substance (Carbowax)[32, 43] that provides a thin protective coating for cells. When received in the laboratory, the spray-fixed slides are placed in two separate rinses of 95% ethanol to (1) remove the Carbowax, (2) complete fixation and (3) begin step 1 of the Papanicolaou staining procedure. The slides remain in the first ethanol rinse for approximately 30 minutes. One may see opaque, waxy like particles float to the surface of the solution. This first 95% ethanol rinse is discarded after each use. The samples are then placed into the second freshly prepared 95% ethanol rinse for 10 to 15 minutes. The use of these two ethanol rinses is usually enough to dissolve the waxy substance, except in hot and humid environments, where it may be necessary to add a third ethanol rinse.

Some manufacturers of spray fixatives recommend removal of Carbowax with water. We have found 95% ethanol to be more effective and less time consuming than water rinses. After the ethanol rinses, the cells appear to be better prepared for the uptake of dyes than with water rinses alone. If the Carbowax has not been removed completely, it will be carried into the staining solutions. If that happens, nuclei will appear foggy and lack detail, and the cytoplasm will appear pale blue.

Alcohol-based, nonaerosol spray fixatives are preferred. One spray container can fix approximately 700 to 1000 cell samples. It is suggested that one use a commercially prepared fixative designed specifically for cytologic use instead of alcohol-based hair sprays, as was done in the past. One of the reasons for this recommendation is that companies producing hair sprays may alter their formulas, replacing chemicals with available substitutes that may alter the quality of cell preservation.

The holes of the spray nozzle sometimes become clogged. It is advisable at the beginning of each day to test the spray emitted from the nozzle to ensure that the spray is evenly distributed. Nonaerosol sprays are more likely to exhibit an uneven spray than aerosol sprays. Nonaerosol spray fixatives can be held closer to the specimen than aerosol sprays. For some products, 3 to 6 inches is recommended, whereas for others, 6 to 10 inches is still the best distance. One should try to obtain an even spray across the entire slide and avoid spraying the labeled or frosted portion of the slide where a heavy coating of waxy residue will make it difficult to number or label the slide. It may be necessary to scrape off the waxy coating on the frosted end of the slide prior to numbering the slide so that identification of the slide will be readable.

Bloody Cell Samples

The presence of erythrocytes that partially or completely obscure the epithelial cells should be reported in the quality report of the slide according to the Bethesda system as either less than optimal or unsatisfactory. Boschann[14] recommends placing a drop of acetic acid in 95% ethanol in a Coplin jar both to fix cells and to lyse red blood cells. Some laboratories use Carnoy's fixative. Others prefer Clarke's fixative or a modification of either Carnoy's or Clarke's fixative.

There are different methods suggested for fixation and treatment of bloody cell samples. Some recommend fixing the sample first and then placing the slide into a lysing solution, whereas others place the sample directly into the lysing medium. It is important in either approach to rinse the sample thoroughly following the lysing solution and prior to the staining procedure. Whichever fixation and lysing method is applied to bloody samples, the solutions should be discarded after each use.

Because cells may shrink or round up when lysing media are used, it is important to reduce the staining times in hematoxylin and EA.

The following are methods for lysing red blood cells.

Lysing Fixatives

1. Carnoy's (always prepare fresh) (absolute ethanol, chloroform, glacial acetic acid [6:3:1])
2. Modified Carnoy's
   95% ethanol, chloroform, glacial acetic acid (7:2.5:0.5)
   95% ethanol, chloroform, glacial acetic acid (6:3:1)
   95% ethanol, glacial acetic acid (6:1)
   Its shelf life is not known, but it does turn into hydrochloric acid at some point in time. This is the reason why it should be mixed fresh each time it is used and discarded after each use.
   Carnoy's fixative is an excellent nuclear fixative as well as a preservative of glycogen.
3. Clarke's (absolute ethanol, glacial acetic acid [3:1])
4. 1 drop hydrochloric acid:500 ml 95% ethanol
5. 10% glacial acetic acid (this is followed by placing the slide in 95% ethanol)
6. 2 M urea (120 g powdered urea per liter of distilled water).

Lysing Fixative Procedures

Procedure 1
1. Fix in 95% ethanol for 15 to 20 minutes.
2. Place in Carnoy's fixative for 10 minutes or less.
3. Immerse in 95% ethanol.

Procedure 2
1. Place in Carnoy's fixative for 3 to 5 minutes until material on slide becomes colorless.
2. Transfer to 95% ethanol or its equivalent.

Procedure 3
1. Fix in 95% ethanol for 5 minutes.
2. Immerse in 2 M urea solution for 30 seconds.

Procedure 4
1. Fix in 95% ethanol for 15 to 20 minutes.
2. Place in 2 M urea solution for up to 1 minute.

Procedure 5
1. Place in Clarke's fixative for 10 to 15 minutes.
2. Rinse in 95% ethanol.

Monitoring Procedure

The quality of fixation should be monitored by laboratory personnel and reported to the clinician. Inadequately or poorly fixed specimens should be reported to the clinician. Accreditation bodies require (1) monitoring of each occurrence, (2) documenting of each incident, (3) maintaining a record of each event and (4) taking corrective action to solve the problem.

Fine Needle Aspirates: Fixation and No Fixation

There are many instances in which both a fixed and an unfixed cell sample are required to provide an adequate cytologic evaluation, especially for fine needle aspirates and body fluids.

The air-dried sample is stained with methods other than the Papanicolaou procedure such as Wright-Giemsa,[48] Diff-Quik,[21] May-Grünwald-Giemsa[48] and so on. The air-dried slide is immersed in a methanol fixative upon arrival in the laboratory, where it remains until it is stained.

For fine needle aspirates, Boccato[11] has recommended a polyvalent fixative to allow the performance of some immunocytochemical reactions by the Papanicolaou method. However, restaining of Papanicolaou stained samples fixed in 95% ethanol may be satisfactory for some immunostaining procedures. The reader is referred to Chapter 38, Immunocytochemistry, for detailed procedures.

Collecting Nongynecologic Specimens in Alcohol-Based Solutions

Fresh, unfixed cell samples are preferred. If fresh specimens cannot be brought directly to the laboratory, the samples may be refrigerated. Prefixation, with the exception of sputum samples, is not recommended. Alcohol (1) coagulates protein and, unless removed from the cells, hinders their visibility, (2) interferes with the adherence of cells to glass slides so that one must add an adhesive substance to the slide (the adhesive substance increases the uptake of background dye), (3) "rounds up" cells (stains cannot penetrate cell when they are balled up as well as when they lie on a flat surface) and (4) limits the choice of preparatory methods that can be used for a particular cell sample.

Table 32–1 shows collecting fixatives or preservative solutions for cell samples collected from various body sites that are used in some laboratories.

STAINING

Staining Techniques Based on the Papanicolaou Method

The polychrome Papanicolaou staining method has gained worldwide acceptance for cytologic samples.[63, 64, 78] The staining method and its modifications consists of a nuclear stain and two counterstains. Hydration prepares the cell sample for the uptake of the nuclear dye; dehydration prepares the cell sample for the uptake of counterstains. Dehydration and clearing solutions result in cellular transparency and prepare the cell samples for the final step: mounting and coverslipping.

Papanicolaou defined a good staining method as one in which nuclear detail was defined, transparency of cytoplasm was assured when cells overlapped and cell types could be differentiated from one another. One might add to this list the stability of the stain over a period of time, stability of color and reproducibility of results.

Modifications of the technique vary from laboratory to laboratory. Visually as well as analytically there are differences. There are also differences in solutions and staining times depending on whether one stains slides or cellulose filters. Of importance to the Papanicolaou staining method is the length of time in the hematoxylin and EA dyes. When adjusting staining times one begins by doubling or halving the time in the dyes to see if time changes result in a color change. One then can fine-tune the time changes until one achieves the results desired.

Whichever modification of the Papanicolaou method is used, it is advisable to standardize as much as possible the staining method employed to achieve reproducible results.

There are several factors that affect the Papanicolaou staining reaction.[24, 33] Some of these are
1. The type of fixative used
2. The type of hematoxylin formula selected
3. Formulas of the counterstains
4. Length of staining times
5. Number of slides stained in each particular dye
6. pH and chemical content of tap water used (such as excessive amount of chlorine)
7. Temperature of the water
8. pH of the solution and dyes
9. Age of the dyes used
10. Presence of dye particles in unfiltered solutions
11. Inconsistency of the staining technique

TABLE 32–1. Cell Samples and Preservative Collection Fluids

Sample Type	Preservative Collection Fluid (only if necessary, except for sputum samples)
Sputum or viscous samples, i.e., some bronchial or tracheal specimens, some synovial fluids, etc.	2% Carbowax in 50% ethanol (1:1)* 50% ethanol (1:1) 70% ethanol (1:1)
Bronchial washings	2% Carbowax in 50% ethanol (1:1) 50% ethanol (1:1) 70% ethanol (1:1)
Pleural, peritoneal, cul-de-sac, pericardial fluids	50% ethanol (1:1)
Urine	70% ethanol (two parts urine: one part alcohol) 2% Carbowax in 70% ethanol (1:1) Esposti's fixative (add 10 ml of fixative to urine sample)[26, 27] 5% glacial acetic acid 50 ml distilled water 225 ml 95% methanol 225 ml
Gastric washings	95% ethanol (if Ringer's solution or saline used)
Esophageal washings	2% Carbowax in 50% ethanol (1:1)
Fine needle aspirate fluids	Boccato[11] polyvalent fixative:† Hydrogen peroxide–methanol solution 3% hydrogen peroxide 10 ml Absolute methanol 90 ml
Cerebrospinal fluid	None recommended

*Saccomanno's preservative[32, 43, 69, 70]
  Distilled water   454 ml
  95% ethanol   526 ml
  Melted Carbowax   20 ml
Place distilled water into 1000-ml cylinder, add ethanol, pour 20 ml melted Carbowax 1540 into graduated 1-liter cylinder containing the distilled water and 95% ethanol.

1. Polyethylene glycol 2% in 50% ethanol or isopropanol. Shake well to permit preservative to rapidly reach cells surrounded by mucus. Red blood cells are lysed. Never use absolute alcohol for preparation of Saccomanno fixative because it may contain dehydrating agents that cause mucus to harden and become rubbery and difficult to blend.

2. Carbowax 2% solution: Add 2 ml melted Carbowax 1540 to 98 ml of 50% ethanol. Mix Carbowax and ethanol on magnetic stirrer for 30 minutes. Once in solution Carbowax does not harden. Melted Carbowax may be kept in solution in a 56°C oven for ready availability. Glassware must be kept warm to prevent hardening of wax on the surface. This can cause inaccurate measurement.

Carbowax 1540 is a water soluble wax at room temperature, with a melting range of 43° to 46°C. It can be mixed with ethanol. Place straight-sided gallon can with cap removed in an 80° to 100°C hot-air oven for several hours. Check frequently to ensure that expanding Carbowax does not overflow container. Wear insulated gloves when handling hot container. Support top, sides, bottom of container. Do not lift by handle: It can snap off.

†Allows performance of some immunocytochemical reactions by the PAP method.[11]
1. Kappa or lambda chains or both in lymphoma
2. Calcitonin in medullary carcinomas of the thyroid
3. Myoglobin in rhabdomyosarcomas
4. Prostate-specific antigen in bone metastases from prostatic carcinoma
For further information concerning immunocytochemical reactions, the reader is referred to Chapter 38, Immunocytochemistry.

12. Possible contamination of dehydrating solutions
13. Type of staining method employed (regressive or progressive)
14. Quality of preparation of the cell sample by the clinician (thick or thin, air dried or well fixed)
15. pH of the specimen
16. Presence or absence of inflammatory cell changes.

There are two ways the Papanicolaou method is applied: progressively or regressively. A simplified diagram of the two methods is depicted in Table 32–2.

The Progressive Method

In the progressive method the nucleus is stained with hematoxylin to the intensity desired. The "blueing" agent, following the hematoxylin, sets the nuclear dye in place. The cytoplasm is barely tinted. Ammonium hydroxide, lithium carbonate and Scott's tap water substitute (STWS) are the most commonly used blueing agents. Tap water may serve as a blueing agent if the pH is higher than 8.

The Regressive Method

Using the regressive method one deliberately overstains the nucleus with a nonacidified hematoxylin. The excess stain is removed with a diluted hydrochloric acid solution. The decolorizing acid is then removed by a bath or running tap water. Timing in the acid bath is essential for the final appearance of the nuclear pattern. More often than not, hypochromasia rather than hyperchromasia is the result. The cytoplasm as well as the nucleus is decolorized by the diluted hydrochloric acid. If the acid bath is inadequate, there will be less contrast between chromatin and parachromatin and uptake of the counterstains will be lessened.

General Comments

The Papanicolaou method and its various modifications are not exactly stoichiometric as is the Feulgen staining reaction,[7] although linearities between these two reactions exist. In 1973, Bahr and coauthors wrote that "in view of the fact that the Papanicolaou stain is not considered quantitative" the correlation between the Feulgen-stained and Papanicolaou-stained material was unexpectedly high, with relation to total extinction values at 540 nm.

Even when the same formulas are selected for use in a particular laboratory the hydrating and dehydrating solutions may vary. When the regressive method is selected, there will be a variety of formulas used to obtain the diluted hydrochloric acid rinses to remove the excess hematoxylin. If the progressive method is

TABLE 32–2. Common Steps and Procedures in the Papanicolaou Staining Method

Common Steps and Procedures	Papanicolaou Staining Method		
	Progressive		Regressive
Selection of Method	Progressive		Regressive
Fixation		95% ethyl alcohol or equivalent	
Rinses to remove Carbowax		95% ethyl alcohol for spray-fixed slides	
Hydration		Water	
Nuclear stain (DNA related)	Stain to desired intensity	Hematoxylin	Overstain
Rinse		Water	
Blueing or removal of hematoxylin	Ammonium hydroxide or lithium carbonate or Scott's tap water substitute (pH 8.02) or 0.5% sodium acetate (pH 7.13) 1.0% potassium acetate (pH 7.45) 0.1% sodium bicarbonate (pH 8.05)		Dilute hydrochloric acid 0.05%, 0.5% or 5%
Rinse to prevent precipitation of salts on slide or stop of acid		Water	
Dehydration		95% ethyl alcohol	
Cytoplasmic stain		OG	
Rinse		95% ethyl alcohol	
Cytoplasmic and nucleolar stain (RNA related)		EA polychrome	
Rinse		95% ethyl alcohol	
Dehydration		Absolute ethyl alcohol	
Clearing		Absolute ethyl alcohol xylene	
Mounting		Mounting medium	

selected, there are often a variety of both the blueing solutions selected and the formulas to make up the solutions. There are also differences in the selection of staining times for each solution and in the use of tap water or distilled water. Whether these specifications were selected for a particular purpose or by chance is not always clear. Some of the variations of the staining procedures for gynecologic samples are illustrated in Tables 32–3 and 32–4.

The Nuclear Stain: Hematoxylin

Discovered in 1840 and first used by Bohmer in 1865, hematoxylin is the nuclear dye in the Papanicolaou procedure. Hematoxylin is, however, one of the most difficult dyes to control and standardize. Luna and Gaffney,[52] in a study of nine commercially available hematoxylins used for hematoxylin and eosin (H&E) staining, concluded "most H&E staining defi-

TABLE 32–3. Progressive Staining Method: Gynecologic Staining Procedures

Steps	Johns Hopkins University[34]	Case Western Reserve University[74]	UCLA Medical Center[67]	University of Chicago Hospitals
Fixation	95% ethyl alcohol	80% isopropanol—30 minutes or spray fixation	95% ethyl alcohol	95% ethyl alcohol or spray fixation
Preparation to remove Carbowax if spray fixed		95% isopropanol—30 minutes to 1 hour		95% ethyl alcohol—30 minutes 95% ethyl alcohol—10 minutes
Hydration	Tap water (×2)—ten dips each	80% ethyl alcohol (if alcohol-fixed) 80%, 70%, 50% ethyl alcohol—ten dips each Distilled water—12 dips	70% ethyl alcohol—ten dips Distilled water—ten dips	Tap water—until glassy look disappears
Nuclear stain (DNA specific)	Gill's half-oxidized hematoxylin—2 minutes	Harris hematoxylin with acetic acid—2–4 minutes (used full strength and filtered weekly)	Mayer's hematoxylin—4 minutes	Gill's half-oxidized hematoxylin—4 minutes
Rinse	Tap water (×2)—ten dips each	Distilled water—five dips Tap water—ten dips	Tap water—15 minutes (stream of gently running water)	Running tap water—until clear
Blueing agent	Scott's tap water substitute—1 minute (10 g magnesium sulfate, anhydrous MqSO₄, 2 g sodium bicarbonate, 1000 ml tap water)	0.5% aqueous ammonium hydroxide—30 seconds (5 ml ammonium hydroxide in 1000 ml distilled water)		Scott's tap water substitute—1 minute
Rinse	Tap water (×2)—ten dips	Running tap water—5 minutes Distilled water—ten dips		Tap water—40–50 dips
Dehydration	95% ethyl alcohol (×2)—ten dips each	50%, 70%, 80%, 95% ethyl alcohol—ten dips each	70%, 95% ethyl alcohol—ten dips each	95% ethyl alcohol (×2)—ten dips each
Cytoplasmic stain	Modified OG-6—15 seconds to 1½ minutes	OG-6—2 minutes	OG—1 minute	Modified OG—1 minute
Rinse	95% ethyl alcohol (×2)—ten dips each	95% ethyl alcohol—three dips each	95% ethyl alcohol (×2)—ten dips each	95% ethyl alcohol (×3)—ten dips each
Cytoplasmic and nucleolar stain (RNA specific)	Modified EA—10 minutes	EA 65—4–6 minutes	EA—1½ minutes	Modified EA—10 minutes
Rinse	95% ethyl alcohol (×3)—20 dips each	95% ethyl alcohol (×2)—three dips each	95% ethyl alcohol (×2)—ten dips each	95% ethyl alcohol (×3)—20 dips each
Dehydration	Absolute ethyl alcohol (×3)—ten dips each	Absolute ethyl alcohol five dips (slowly) Absolute ethyl alcohol—three dips	Absolute ethyl alcohol (×2)—ten dips each	Absolute ethyl alcohol (×4)—ten dips each
Clearing	Xylene (×3)—ten dips each	Absolute ethyl alcohol and xylene (1:1)—five dips (slowly) Xylene (×3)—five dips each	Absolute ethyl alcohol and xylene (1:1)—1 minute Xylene (×3)—ten dips each	Xylene (×3)—ten dips each
Mounting	Permount	Permount	Permount	Preservaslide

TABLE 32–4. Regressive Staining Method: Gynecologic Staining Procedures

Steps	Papanicolaou Laboratory[78]	University of Michigan[72]	University of Rochester[21]	Memorial Sloan-Kettering Cancer Center[28]
Fixation	95% ethyl alcohol	95% ethyl alcohol	95% ethyl alcohol	95% ethyl alcohol
Preparation	If spray-fixed, place in water for 10 minutes			80% ethyl alcohol—until slides are labeled
Hydration	80%, 70%, 50% ethyl alcohol–six to eight dips each Distilled water—six to eight dips each	50% ethyl alcohol—ten dips Distilled water—ten dips	95%, 80%, 70%, 50% ethyl alcohol—ten dips each Running tap water—1 minute or until beading disappears	70%, 50% ethyl alcohol—five dips each Distilled water—five dips
Nuclear stain (DNA specific)	Harris hematoxylin (no acetic acid)—6 minutes: run pilot slides to determine times for each batch	Harris hematoxylin—1–3 minutes	Harris hematoxylin—4–6 minutes (depending on desired nuclear stain intensity and dye lot strength)	Harris hematoxylin (without acetic acid)—6 minutes
Rinse	Distilled water ($\times 2$)	Running tap water—rinse well	Running tap water—1 minute or until water runs clear	Distilled water—five dips
Removal of hematoxylin	0.25% HCl—six dips	0.5% HCl—five dips	0.25% HCl—4–5 quick dips	0.5% HCl aqueous solution—3–5 dips slowly (number of dips depends on strength of hematoxylin)
Rinse	Running tap water (lukewarm)—6 minutes	Running tap water—4 minutes	Running tap water—30 seconds	Running tap water—6 minutes
Blueing agent		Dilute lithium carbonate (20 drops saturated aqueous Li_2CO_3 per 100 ml water) 2 minutes, then visual check		
Rinse		Running tap water—30 seconds		
Dehydration	50%, 70%, 80%, 95% ethyl alcohol 6–8 dips each	50%, 96% ethyl alcohol—ten dips each	50%, 70%, 80%, 95% ethyl alcohol—ten dips each	50%, 70%, 80%, 95% ethyl alcohol—five dips each
Cytoplasmic stain	OG-6—1.5 minutes	OG-6—1 minute	OG-6—1.25 minutes	OG-6—3 minutes
Rinse	95% ethyl alcohol ($\times 2$)—rinse gently; do not allow to stand in alcohol or cells will be discolored	96% ethyl alcohol ($\times 2$)—ten dips each	95% ethyl alcohol ($\times 2$)—ten dips each	95% ethyl alcohol ($\times 2$)—five dips each (slowly)
Cytoplasmic and nucleolar stain (RNA specific)	EA 36 (EA 50 or EA 65)—1.5 minutes	EA 65—2 minutes	EA 65—4–6 minutes (intensity depends on dye lot)	EA 50—3 minutes (drain carrier on paper towel)
Rinse	95% ethyl alcohol ($\times 3$)—Rinse gently but thoroughly	96% ethyl alcohol ($\times 2$)—ten dips each	95% ethyl alcohol ($\times 2$)—ten dips each	95% ethyl alcohol ($\times 3$)—five dips each (slowly)
Dehydration	Absolute ethyl alcohol ($\times 2$)—six to eight dips each	Absolute ethyl alcohol—ten dips Absolute ethyl alcohol—1 minute	Absolute ethyl alcohol ($\times 2$)—ten dips each	Absolute ethyl alcohol ($\times 2$)—five dips each (slowly)
Clearing	Absolute ethyl alcohol and xylene—six to eight dips each Xylene ($\times 4$)—six to eight dips each	Xylene—1 minute	Absolute ethyl alcohol and xylene (1:1)—ten dips Xylene ($\times 3$)—ten dips each	Absolute ethyl alcohol and xylene (1:1)—five dips
Mounting	Permount	Permount	Permount	Histoclear ($\times 7$)—five dips each (slowly)

ciencies seen on stained slides are not due to the hematoxylin used, but to the quality of fixation and the way the hematoxylin solutions were used.''

A variety of hematoxylin formulas have been utilized over the years. Harris hematoxylin is usually combined with regressive staining methods, whereas Mayer's, Delafield's, Gill-Baker-Mayer and Gill's[29] half-oxidized hematoxylin usually are used with a progressive staining method. Mayer's hematoxylin is said to have a short useful life in solution (2 to 3 months) and tends to fade with time in storage.

Lillie,[51] in 1974, reported on the variability of hematoxylin samples submitted to the Biological Stain Commission for certification since the reported hematoxylin shortage in 1973. The shortage of hematoxylin resulted in a lower-quality product. Some post-1973 samples do not dissolve well in alcohol and formulas such as Gill's may be more appropriate. Water should be added to the alcohol to help dissolve the hematoxylin: 90% alcohol is suggested. Some batches require two or three times more hematoxylin than was previously required to produce the same results. It is advisable to check the batch number and color index (CI) printed on the hematoxylin bottle and include this information in the laboratory procedure book so one can be assured the same ingredients are used to make up each batch of hematoxylin. Differences in hematoxylin may be due to differences in the soil where it is grown. A listing from the Biological Stain Commission shows code names for current batches of dye and compares them with batches in use prior to 1973 (Table 32–5).

It is important to date hematoxylin when it is received in the laboratory because the dye may oxidize over time, especially in moist climates. The lighter the crystals, the less oxidized the hematoxylin; the darker the crystals, the more hematein (or oxidized hematoxylin) is present. Lillie[51] stated that overoxidation is one of the main causes of a poor hematoxylin stain.

The information provided by the manufacturer may not indicate the actual shelf life of dyes. It is best to date the bottle when it is received and record the date when it is opened. For stock and working solutions the date when it was made and date when it was first used may help the laboratory establish a beginning to the quality control of items so marked.

TABLE 32–5. Hematoxylin Certified by the Biological Stain Commission

Company Code	Prior to 1973 Numbers	Since 1973 Numbers
CH	1 through 43	44 and greater
EH	1 through 30	33 and greater
LH	1 through 38	39 and greater
AbH		1 and greater
AcH		1 and greater
BaH		1 and greater
BcH		1 and greater
CcH		1 and greater
LeH		1 and greater
TH		1 and greater
ZH		3 and greater

TABLE 32–6. Comparison of Cytologic Findings for Progressive and Regressive Staining Methods by Soost and Coworkers[75]

Progressive	Regressive
Finely distributed chromatin structure	Uniformly stained, dark nuclei
Accentuated hyperchromasia	Significantly higher nuclear areas found
Moderate staining of nuclear envelope	Accentuated textural features as well as contrast between nucleus and cytoplasm
Accentuated polychromasia	
One peak of nuclear absorption at 540 nm	Two peaks of nuclear absorption at 530 and 590 nm

Certain components in hematoxylin formulas help transform hematoxylin into a useable nuclear dye. These are (1) an oxidizing agent, (2) a mordant, (3) a solvent and (4) a substance used for acidification.

The oxidizing agent is used to begin the ripening process that helps to transform hematoxylin to hematein, the active coloring agent. The oxidizing agents most often used are sodium iodate and mercuric oxide. The mercuric oxide used to oxidize and ripen the Harris hematoxylin and the chloral hydrate added as a preservative, as recommended by Mayer, are toxic chemicals and, if possible, should be avoided.

The mordant is a substance that is responsible for the induction of color in the dye. Aluminum sulfate or alum supplies positively charged ions that act as a bridge to chemically unite the negatively charged hematein to the negatively charged phosphoric acid on the DNA chain.

The solvent in hematoxylin is the substance that dissolves hematein into solution. Ethylene glycol is used in certain formulas for this purpose. The solvent acts as a leveling agent and helps reduce the rate of oxidation.

Acidification, the final component, ensures selectivity to nuclear material and aids in preventing oxidation of the dye. It does so by stabilizing the aluminum-hematein complex. Glacial acetic acid or citric acid is used for this purpose.

Soost and coauthors[75] in a controlled study used Harris hematoxylin both progressively and regressively. Their findings are shown in Table 32–6.

Soost and coauthors concluded that the progressive method is better for cell measurement and fits the requirements for automated systems and there is better correlation of visually described chromatin patterns with quantitative data. Soost and coauthors also reported that the total amount of stain (total extinction values) in the nucleus does increase significantly with the length of time in the staining solution. The total amount of stain bound in the nucleus is not materially different for cells lying singly or in clusters. It was also noted that stained samples stored for 6 months led to optical extinction and readings approximately 6% lower than the original measurements. For the given precision of the technique, this difference is statistically significant.

Wiseman[84] presented the findings on a comparative study. Six different formulations of hematoxylin were used; five with the progressive staining method and the sixth with a regressive staining method. The half-oxidized formulas were made with varying amounts of hematoxylin, and the oxidizing agent was sodium iodate. Initial studies were planned to determine if such variations could be detected by computerized measurements of the extinction values of buccal cell nuclei prepared with a monolayer technique. A ratio of 2.0 g of hematoxylin dye to 0.2 g of sodium iodate, as recommended by Gill,[29] provided the most condensed range of total extinction measurements. These values were then compared with extinction values obtained using the Harris hematoxylin formula with the regressive staining method. The half-oxidized hematoxylin yielded the most condensed range of total extinction values.

At the University of Chicago, the progressive staining method with Gill's half-oxidized hematoxylin formula is used. The formula is easy to prepare, is stable in solution and is cost effective. No scum (the actual coloring agent) forms on the surface of the hematoxylin solution, and it can be used immediately after preparation. Once the staining times have been standardized little or no alteration is required. In a laboratory with a volume of approximately 40,000 gynecologic slides per year, the hematoxylin solution is changed every 6 weeks or after every 2000 slides, whichever comes first.[33, 34]

Hematoxylin Formulas

Table 32–7 contains the ingredients to make 1 liter or more of hematoxylin solution. It should be noted, however, that in some procedures the solution is further diluted when in actual use. Some laboratories use the stock solution exclusively, whereas others may use a diluted stock solution for daily work.

Papanicolaou Counterstains: Orange G and EA

The Biological Stain Commission certifies most synthetic biologic dyes. In preparing the counterstains orange G (OG) and EA, it is important to check the dye content on the outside label. OG usually contains 80% dye content, light green, 65%, eosin Y, 80% and Bismarck brown Y, 45%. Information from the Biological Stain Commission reveals that current dye contents for these dyes are quite different: OG contains 89% dye, light green, 71% and eosin, 92 to 94%. To compensate for variations in dye content, one divides the desired amount of total dye content required by the actual percentage of dye content listed on the label. Published staining procedures usually do not contain this information and therefore, in attempting to reproduce a staining procedure, it is necessary to obtain this information directly from its original source.

TABLE 32–7. Formulas for Alum Hematoxylin*

Ingredients	Gill[29], Half-Oxidized	Harris	Mayer† (UCLA)	Harris‡ (Case Western Reserve University)
Hematoxylin CI 75290	2 g§	5 g	1 g (powder)	8 g
Absolute methanol	—	50 ml	—	80 ml
Distilled water	730 ml	1000 ml	1000 ml	1680 ml
Ethylene glycol	250 ml	—	—	—
Chemical ripening agent	Sodium iodate (NaIO₃) 0.2 g	Mercuric oxide (HgO) 2.5 g	Sodium iodate (NaIO₃) 0.2 g	Sodium iodate 550 mg (0.55 g)
Aluminum ammonium sulfate (alum)	23.5 g (or 17.6 g aluminum sulfate)	100 g	50 g	160 g
Glacial acetic acid	20 ml (or 1 g citric acid)	None (or 40 ml)	None (40 ml or 1 g citric acid)	20 ml
Preservative	—	—	50 g chloral hydrate	—
Stated life	Over 1 year	Months to years	2–3 months	—

*Hematoxylin dated after 1973 is to be mixed with 90% ethanol to help it dissolve.
†Mayer's instructions[67]
1. Dissolve the hematoxylin in the distilled water, which has been heated to 55° to 60°C, and rotate until all stain is in solution. (Mixture will look like orange tea in color. If color is incorrect, check purity of the distilled water.)
2. Add the alum. (The mixture turns to a deep red wine color. The mixture appears to be opaque.)
3. Add chloral hydrate. (The mixture appears to run down the sides of the flask as one rotates the solution.) Be sure to observe whether the crystals are in solution before adding the next ingredient.
4. Allow the solution to stand overnight before use. Pour the hematoxylin into dark brown stock solution bottles. As a stock solution, this stain is stable indefinitely. As a working solution, it can be stable up to 2 months if the length of staining time is increased after prolonged use.
‡Harris hematoxylin instructions[74]
Use magnetic mixer for the following.
1. Dissolve aluminum ammonium sulfate in distilled water without the aid of heat for about 1 hour.
2. Add hematoxylin to sulfate solution.
3. Add absolute alcohol to solution.
4. Slowly add sodium iodate while stirring.
5. Let solution stand for 30 minutes.
6. Add 20 ml acetic acid in 80 ml distilled water to final solution.
Note: Hematoxylin is variable in the presence of blood. Check microscopically for depth of nuclear staining.
§2.0 g anhydrous hematoxylin or 2.36 g crystalline form.

Orange G

OG is an acidic dye. It stains keratin a bright and intense orange. The granules in eosinophilic, superficial cells (possibly those containing eleidin) are also stained. Because keratin, not normally present in squamous epithelial cells, may be found in the presence of keratinizing squamous cancers, the presence of intense orangeophilia is of importance to the diagnostician.

In the modified OG formula, the dye content is quantitatively controlled. OG is slightly soluble in 95% ethanol and even more soluble in water. In the modified formulas the OG content is reduced to a level of its solubility in 95% ethanol. When glacial acetic acid is added to the formula the solution stains rapidly and intensely. Positive hydrogen ions are added to the amino acids of cellular proteins, shifting the balance of charges to the acidic side of the proteins' isoelectric point and thus increasing the bonding sites to which the negatively charged OG can attach. The staining time must be limited or the subsequent uptake of eosin Y will be inhibited. The addition of phosphotungstic acid, a mordant that strongly binds to proteins, helps intensify the color achieved. Following is an example of how to calculate the amount of dye needed for a particular formula.

Preparation of Orange G Stain

Amount of dye required ÷ percent of dye content =

Actual amount of dye to be used to yield appropriate amount of dye needed
Examples:

OG 10 g (CI 16230) ÷ 89% or 0.89 = 11.2 g
OG 10 g (CI 16230) ÷ 80% or 0.80 = 12.5 g

The higher the dye content, the less dye will be required to obtain the required 100% dye content.

Modified Orange G Stain

Stock Solution. Prepare an OG (CI 16230) aqueous *stock* solution, 10% total dye content. The dye content contained in the OG container is 80%.

10 g ÷ 80% or 0.80 = 12.5 g; therefore, dissolve 12.5 g OG-6 in up to 100 ml of distilled water heated to 70° to 80°C.

Working OG solution[33]

OG, 10% aqueous solution	20 ml	or	20 ml
Phosphotungstic acid	0.15 g		—
95% ethyl alcohol	980 ml		970 ml
Glacial acetic acid (optional)	—		10 ml

1. Combine ingredients.
2. Filter prior to usage.

The solution can be used immediately upon preparation and should be filtered after each use. The working solution can be replenished daily to maintain satisfactory results. It is usually discarded after staining 40 baskets of 50 slides each.

EA

EA is a polychrome stain. It is a combination of light green SF yellowish, eosin Y and, in some cases, Bismarck brown Y.

Light green SF yellowish is an acid dye. It stains the cytoplasm of metabolically active cells, intermediate squamous cells, parabasal and columnar cells, histiocytes, leukocytes, large- and small-cell undifferentiated carcinoma cells and cells deriving from adenocarcinoma a green color. It binds well to basic protein side chains. It is the most light-sensitive of the dyes used in the Papanicolaou method.

Eosin Y is an acid dye. Various bromine atoms may or may not be present. When all four bromine atoms are present, it is at its deepest red; at lower bromine content, the stain is yellowish. Eosin Y mainly stains the cytoplasm of superficial squamous cells, nucleoli, erythrocytes and cilia.

The modified EA allows eosin and light green to stain the cytoplasm differentially. The addition of fast green to the formula is an individual choice. When the green color fades from the blue-green stained cytoplasm one has a clue that the EA is exhausted and should be changed. This may occur prior to the 6-week scheduled time period for changing the dye solutions. The dye should be filtered daily and stored in a dark, well-sealed bottle when not in use. Some laboratories make special opaque covers to sit over the dishes containing the dyes so light reaches the dyes as little as possible.

EA has three separate formulations: 36, 50 and 65. EA 36 was originally formulated for staining gynecologic smears but may be used for other cell samples. The original formula was modified in 1954. EA 65 is a modification of EA 36 and was developed for staining thicker cell samples. EA 50 is a commercially prepared solution; it is supposed to be similar to EA 36 but its formula may vary from one manufacturer to another.

Modified EA is a result of experimentation by Gill.[33, 34] Bismarck brown Y has been eliminated from the Gill formula and its presence in the original formulation is debated. It is known that Bismarck brown Y precipitates phosphotungstic acid, the ingredient responsible for differential staining by light green and eosin.[38] Modified EA may be used for both gynecologic and nongynecologic samples.

To the modified EA solution we have added fast green dye to increase the concentration of cytoplasmic green dye.[48] Its lower solubility in alcohol makes it less prone to being washed away from cells.

Modified EA

Stock Solutions. There are two stock solutions contained in the modified EA dye: (1) a 3% total dye content of light green SF yellowish (CI 42095) and (2) a 20% TDC aqueous solution of eosin Y (CI 45380). Dissolve corrected weights of each dye in 70° to 80°C distilled water up to 100 ml each. The University of Chicago Hospitals adds fast green to that formulation.

The following are two stock solutions.

1. *Light green, 3% aqueous solution.* Dissolve 5.0 g of light green dye (CI 42095–1B211) into 100 ml of distilled water that has been heated to 70° to 80°C.

Dissolve 0.3 g of fast green dye into that solution while it is still warm. Fast green is added to increase the concentration of green dye. Its lower solubility in alcohol makes it less prone to being washed from cells.

Allow to cool in brown-colored bottle and store.

2. *Eosin, 20% (total dye content) aqueous solution of eosin Y (CI 45380).* Dissolve 25.0 g of eosin Y (CI 45380) in 100 ml of distilled water that has been heated to 70° to 80°C.

Allow to cool in brown-colored bottle and store.

Working EA Solution

95% ethanol	700.0 ml
Absolute methanol	250.0 ml
Glacial acetic acid	20.0 ml
Light green stock (3% aqueous solution)	10.0 ml
Eosin stock (20% aqueous solution)	20.0 ml
Phosphotungstic acid	4.0 g

Point of Emphasis

Dipping cellulose filters rapidly strips dyes, particularly light green, from cells but slowly extracts it from the filter background. Letting the filter sit undisturbed in the alcohols following EA reverses events. Cells retain their green color and the filters lose their green color.

Avoiding Staining Problems

Helpful Hints in Staining Slides with the Papanicolaou Method

1. When transferring slides from water to hematoxylin the glassy droplets of water on the slide must have disappeared prior to placement in hematoxylin. This step may take as long as 30 minutes and depends on the thickness of the cell sample. If the glassy appearance does not disappear from the slide, the hematoxylin dye will not penetrate the nucleus and the cells may show a hazy appearance. Discard the water rinse after each use.

2. If STWS, a salt solution, is used as a blueing agent the salt solution must be removed from the slide or a filmy white coating will appear on the underside of the slide after coverslipping. The salt solution is usually removed in two separate tap water rinses. Discard the water rinses following STWS after each use.

3. Cells require gentle dipping to avoid cell loss during the staining process. A dip is described as a complete submersion of the slides in a solution

and then complete lifting of the slides out of solution. This is performed in a continuous and regular movement. It is suggested that one not allow the slides to hit the bottom of the staining dish. It is here where cells that have floated off from other slides may be present. A dip usually takes a second.

4. It may take ten dips to have one solution replace another.

5. It is recommended that slides not be permitted to sit in the alcohol solutions following the OG and EA dyes. The stains that have penetrated the cells will be washed out of the cells if slides are allowed to sit for any length of time. In other words, all the work you have done will be erased by letting the solutions sit in high concentrations of alcohol for longer than necessary.

6. Ethanol rinse solutions following the dyes are rotated as the ethanol nearest the dye becomes discolored. The highly colored alcohol is discarded and the cleaner alcohols are moved closer to the dye. The final rinse is usually the cleanest rinse.

7. Xylene is filtered each day.

8. Xylene is discarded in a special disposable bottle as soon as it either becomes pinkish in color, contains small bubbles (water contamination) or becomes milky in color. Xylene cannot be discarded in the sink. Each laboratory is required to follow specific regulations for disposal of xylene and other hazardous solutions and chemicals.

9. Slides should be well drained between each solution so that they do not contaminate the next solution.

10. The level of solutions should be maintained during the entire staining procedure. It is suggested that the level of the solutions following the EA dye should be higher than the other solutions in order to achieve complete dehydration prior to placement in the clearing solutions.

11. If the pH of tap water following the hematoxylin is not sufficiently alkaline (pH 7.4), then the staining results will vary from one laboratory setting to another. The pH of water may change with the seasons.

12. On a daily basis, dyes are added from the working solutions to maintain the appropriate dye level of the staining solutions. In some institutions dyes may be added from the stock solutions.

13. The pH of EA is supposed to be between 4.5 and 5 to achieve maximum results.

14. Staining times are to be recorded each day, along with a notation of any changes made and the initials of the recorder.

15. Solutions should be kept covered when not in use and all stains transferred to airtight dark brown containers when not in use.

COVERSLIPPING

General Comments

Coverslipping is performed under a well-ventilated fume hood to avoid inhaling toxic vapors. It is suggested that safety glasses be worn during coverslipping unless the xylene can be handled so that there is a physical separation between the worker and the xylene solution.

An instrument such as forceps may be used to remove slides from xylene to avoid irritation and drying of skin.

A No. 1 thinness coverglass, optimal size 24 × 60, is the coverslip of choice, both to cover all cells present on the glass slide and because of its optical properties. The optimal refractive index of a glass slide is 1.515 ± 0.015, with a thickness range of 0.96 to 1.06 mm; this is best matched to a No. 1 thinness coverglass.

If photography is to be performed the selection of coverglass and coverslip is critical and a No. 1 thinness coverslip is essential.

Liquid Mounting Solutions

Liquid substitute mounting solutions (1) are likely to produce potentially toxic vapors, (2) produce an irregular layer of mounting medium over the cells, (3) produce a wavy layer that may be difficult to screen, (4) have a lower refractive index than that of cells, (5) may increase fading and (6) when dry, will allow the surface to scratch and crack with age.

Prevention of Fading

Some laboratories add an antioxidant to the mounting medium to prevent eosin from fading over time. Butylated hydroxytoluene is such a substance.

In a 1% concentration, 2,6-di-tert-butyl-p-cresol helps preserve Romanowsky-type blood stains but does not affect the preservation of hematoxylin, OG, eosin Y or light green SF yellowish.[35]

Filters

To mount cellulose filter preparations properly, the mounting medium must replace the xylene contained within the pores of the filter. If the mounting medium does not replace the xylene, then the filter will dry out as the xylene evaporates. Dehydration and clearing solutions also help prepare the filter for coverslipping. The final dehydration solutions should cover the slides and the filter holder to avoid improper dehydration of the filter.

A medium with a refractive index as close to the filter type as possible will produce the necessary transparency and visibility of cells when viewed under the microscope.

Procedure for Coverslipping Cellulose Filters

Precaution: Coverslipping is performed under a fume hood or in a well-ventilated area.

1. Match filter number with identification number on glass slide.
2. Apply mounting medium in one thick strip on glass slide surface.
3. Remove filter from filter holder in xylene.
4. Place filter on paper toweling, cell side up, to absorb some of excess xylene.
5. Center filter cell side up on glass slide directly on top of mounting medium.
6. Take a clean applicator stick.
7. Place in middle of filter.
8. Roll smooth applicator stick firmly along top of filter from center of filter to each end to remove excess xylene.
9. Apply ample amount of mounting medium on top of filter.
10. Turn slide slightly sideways.
11. Apply coverslip as mounting medium and coverslip meet.
12. Place slide in horizontal position.
13. Take clean applicator stick and apply some pressure to top of coverslip to help mounting medium to spread evenly across filter, allowing for complete and ample coverage.
14. Check to see that there are no air bubbles.
15. Place on rack covered by filter paper in drying oven set at 80°F.
16. Allow filter to dry in oven for a few hours before microscopic evaluation is made so that cells can be marked without moving the coverslip. We have noted that the cells need to "settle" into the mounting medium before giving their characteristic cellular pattern. If Eukitt mounting medium is used, this step may not be necessary.
17. Allow filters to dry in horizontal position for 3 months before filing.

Procedure for Coverslipping Polycarbonate Filters

Rinse in xylene rapidly to avoid curling of the filter and then follow steps 1 to 17, just described.

If dissolving the filter is desired to avoid visualizing the holes under the microscope, perform the following steps.

1. Place filter cell side down onto a coverslip.
2. Quickly flatten filter to coverslip and drain all xylene off, using absorbant tissue and very gentle finger pressure.
3. Immediately tilt coverslip onto absorbent paper towel and flood with anhydrous chloroform, allowing excess to flow onto towel.
4. Place coverslip on gauze bed and flood again with chloroform.
5. Cover with glass Petri dish and allow chloroform to evaporate completely.
6. Dip labeled slide and coverslip in xylene, add mounting medium to slide and place coverslip in position.

Procedure for Coverslipping Slides

1. Remove slide from xylene and let excess drain off slide.
2. Apply mounting medium (amount depends on thickness of sample).
3. Tilt slide with mounting medium toward you as you place coverslip to meet mounting medium.
4. Check to see there are no air bubbles.
5. Place in horizontal position on drying oven rack covered with filter paper.
6. Place in oven set at 26.7°C overnight.

DESTAINING PROCEDURES

Destaining the Cell Sample

Destaining and restaining a slide with the Papanicolaou method can be performed on most samples but will produce optimal results only when the original cell sample was properly fixed.

There are several methods of removing the coverslip. Once this is achieved the next step is the removal of the mounting medium, which may take several hours' immersion in xylene. The older the slide, the more time this step will take. Time will vary depending on the amount and type of mounting medium used.

The next step is the removal of the nuclear dye. It is usually necessary to place the slide in a dilute hydrochloric acid, either an aqueous or alcohol-based solution. The removal of hematoxylin may take from 5 to 20 minutes or longer depending on the thickness of the cell sample. The slide is then rinsed gently in running tap water for 10 to 15 minutes.

Destaining Procedure

Step 1. Removing Coverslip

Method 1

1. Place slide in xylene until coverslip falls away from slide. Pressure is not used to remove coverslip. (This step may take hours or even days depending on age of slide and mounting medium utilized.)
2. Place slide in clean xylene solution until mounting medium is removed.
3. Proceed to destaining procedures.

Method 2

1. Place slide in freezer, coverslip side directly on ice.
2. Wait for 10 to 15 minutes or until frosted area appears along periphery of slide. (This step may take hours depending on age of slide and mounting medium used. Usually the older the slide, the shorter the time period.)
3. Put on gloves and safety glasses.
4. Insert razor blade between coverslip and cell material. Coverslip, if properly frosted, will flip away from slide material.
5. Place slide in xylene until mounting medium is removed.
6. Proceed to destaining procedure.

Step 2. Destaining Procedure

Two procedures are listed, one from the University of Chicago (Procedure 1) and one from Case Western Reserve University (Procedure 2).[23]

Procedure 1
---

1. Rinse in xylene.
2. Rinse in absolute ethanol (×3)—ten dips each.
3. Rinse in 95% ethanol (×2)—ten dips each.
4. Rinse in tap water.
5. Soak in acid-alcohol solution* for 3 to 5 minutes or until slide appears colorless.
6. Run under water for 5 to 10 minutes to remove all traces of acid.
7. Restain with Papanicolaou staining method.

Procedure 2
---

1. Rinse in absolute ethanol with xylene.
2. Rinse in absolute ethanol (×2).
3. Rinse in 95% (×4), 80%, 70%, 50% ethanol.
4. Rinse in distilled water.
5. Place slides in 1% HCl for 1 to 20 minutes to remove "hematoxylin" (actually hematein). The length of time will vary depending on the thickness of the material.
6. Wash slides under gently running tap water for 10 minutes to remove all traces of acid.
7. The slides are now ready to restain.

Note: The same procedure can be used to remove golden brown artifact "corn flakes."

---

*10.0 ml HCl (5N) concentrate reagent grade and 1000 ml 70% ethanol.

CROSS-CONTAMINATION CONTROL

The use of a separatory funnel permits solutions to be filtered so that they are cell-free without losing staining constituents.[31] This is especially important to know if using the Harris hematoxylin because other methods of filtration may result in weakening the staining solution.

Cross-contamination is controlled more stringently with the separatory funnel system. The filter type is different for different solutions. Filters need replacement when filtration becomes labored after several filtrations. Filtration may be slow to start if the pores are wet. Wet pores may require substantial vacuuming to break loose the liquid held in the pores. Once the pores are opened, filtration proceeds smoothly. In other words, slow-starting filtration may mimic an overloaded filter that needs replacement.

With the separatory filter system, cross-contamination can be reduced virtually to zero. Storage of stains prevents evaporation of dyes. Spills are avoided because one vacuums up the dye into the stain storage unit. Soiled laboratory coats and hands can also be avoided if the tube for vacuuming up the solution is long enough to be placed into the base of the staining dish containing the dye.

Three functions of the separatory funnel filtering procedure are (1) convenient and absolute removal of cells and debris from suspension in any solution, (2) airtight storage of filtered solution until ready for use

TABLE 32–8. Macroscopic Differences in Body Fluids

				Type				
	Serous	*Chylous*	*Pseudo-chylous*	*Cirrhotic*	*Eosinophilic*	*Inflammatory*	*Infectious*	*Hemorrhagic*
Gross appearance	Watery, clear	Milky, white	Milky, green	Watery, brown	Watery, smooth	Yellowish white	Greenish with odor	Brownish or opaque, deep red
Microscopic findings	Hypocellular	Fat-filled cells	Foamy cells	Atypical cells	Eosinophils	Polys, lymphocytes	Lymphocytes	Malignant cells
Possible significance	Transudate	Lymph retention	Cholesterol crystals	Transudate, bilirubin	Allergic process	Collagen disease	Tuberculosis	Mesothelioma, carcinoma

and (3) simple and mess-free drainage of the cell-free and debris-free solution into a clean staining disk. The potential pitfalls are (1) using the wrong separatory funnels and (2) forgetting to close the stopcock when filtering.

Floaters can be avoided by

1. Using the separatory funnel system
2. Changing alcohols twice daily
3. Discarding water rinses after each use
4. Replacing blueing and differentiation solutions frequently during the day
5. Utilizing the toluidine blue technique to determine if a given fluid or specimen is positive (procedure discussed in next section)
6. Staining known positive cases separately in disposable tubes or Coplin jars or staining last and then discarding all solutions.

NONGYNECOLOGIC SAMPLE PREPARATION

Pleural, Peritoneal and Pericardial Fluid Preparation

Transudates and Exudates

Transudates and exudates are formed within the mesothelial-lined body cavities. The classification as an exudate or transudate is made on the basis of the specific gravity, protein content and other biochemical parameters of the body fluid itself. Transudates have a lower protein content and a lower specific gravity than do exudates. Transudates are usually clear. Exudates are usually cloudy. Exudates are usually rich in fibrin and protein and may coagulate upon staining; transudates do not coagulate. Cells from an exudate will usually adhere better to a glass slide surface than cells from a transudate. Some exudates may contain fat (chyle) and will appear milky white in color and

consistency. Chylous fluids may occur when there is perforation or obstruction of the thoracic duct by trauma, malignant neoplasm, tuberculosis or filariasis. There are also fluids that appear to be chylous but may contain foamy cells due to the presence of fine fat droplets or albuminous material (pseudochyle), but these are not true chylous fluids. Biochemical studies may be required to distinguish between these two fluids.

There is also the rare gelatinous fluid, deriving from the patient with pseudomyxoma peritonei. It does not lend itself to the routine fluid preparation and requires special handling.

In addition to the cell diagnostic examination of transudates and exudates, the evaluation of peritoneal washings in staging of ovarian malignancies and follow-up studies on treated patients have expanded the usefulness of fluid cytology.

Effusions may result from a variety of causes: collagen vascular diseases, circulatory disorders, neoplasms and infections. It is the last that is of special concern to preparatory personnel. Because information regarding potentially infectious material is not given to laboratory personnel in every case, all samples are handled as if they were infectious.[60] Tuberculosis, viral infections, parasites such as *Strongyloides stercoralis* (infrequently observed in peritoneal fluids) and the currently high prevalence of samples taken from patients with immunosuppressed conditions, with the finding of opportunistic pathogens such as the parasite *Pneumocystis carinii*, may be expected findings.

The importance of noting the macroscopic differences in body fluids is emphasized. Notations are made on the requisition form and available to the evaluator of the sample. Clinical history is correlated with the gross findings of the fluid itself. A record of the amount of fluid, its gross appearance and any special problems related to the preparation of the fluid are noted on the requisition form (Tables 32–8 and 32–9).

TABLE 32–9. Transudates and Exudates

	Gross Appearance	Coagulation Factor	Bacteriologic Yield	Cellularity
Exudate	Cloudy	Coagulates on standing	May yield bacterial growth	Highly cellular, predominantly inflammatory
Transudate	Clear	Does not coagulate	Usually sterile	Sparse, predominantly mesothelial

If the patient has a history of malignancy, the previous histologic samples may be obtained so that the newly prepared cell sample and the previous histologic sections are available for comparative assessments.

Cytopreparation

The method of cytopreparation may be selected on the basis of the physical properties of the specimen and patient history. The cytotechnologist needs pertinent clinical information on hand to correlate with the cell findings. The variety and types of cell samples required for routine cytodiagnostic purposes, immunologic studies (see Chapter 38, Immunocytochemistry), microbiologic evaluation and special stains may be prepared in advance of the actual cytologic evaluation. The preparatory method may be based on the results of the toluidine blue test. For example, if the toluidine blue-stained specimen appears to be from a lymphoma, air-dried samples stained with Diff-Quik,[21] in addition to routine Papanicoloau stained samples, will be prepared. The following options are available.

1. If the cell sample is low in volume, clear in appearance and contains few cells, then the method of choice may be a filter preparation (see procedure 1).
2. If the cell sample is cloudy, has a cell button after initial centrifugation and is cellular with the toluidine blue test, the following may be performed: direct smears from the sediment, cytocentrifugation procedure (see procedure 2)[13, 38] or filter preparation. Direct smears are both fixed and air dried to permit both Diff-Quik and Papanicolaou staining.
3. If the cell sample is bloody and a cell button is not visualized after initial centrifugation, the saponin method (see procedure 3) combined with a filter preparation, direct smears or cytocentrifugation may be performed.
4. If the cell sample is mucoid, direct smears or the Saccomanno concentration method may be utilized.[70]
5. All sample types may be prepared by filtration methods, but not all cell samples will produce a good yield of cells by the direct smear method.

General Preparation Procedure for Direct Smears, Filter Preparations and Cytospin 2 Samples

1. Turn on germ-free hood half an hour before work is to begin.
2. Check pressure gauge on vacuum pump.
3. Put on gown and gloves.
4. Remove specimens from refrigerator and place in hood. *Note:* Specimens are easier to prepare when at room temperature.
5. Organize work area.
6. Wipe outside of all specimen containers with 70% isopropanol or 10% Clorox solution.
7. Wipe all requisition forms with decontamination solution.
8. Match specimens to requisition forms. If there are any discrepancies, contact physician requesting test.
9. Assign a laboratory number to each case.
10. List cases on log sheet.
11. Label specimen container, requisition form, slides, test tubes and Petri dish with laboratory number, patient identification and type of sample.
12. Label filters with laboratory number and patient identification. Use a permanent marker pen that is insoluble in staining solution.
13. Pre-expand labeled Millipore filters in labeled Petri dish containing 95% ethanol for 10 to 15 seconds. Pre-expand Nuclepore filters in a Petri dish containing a physiologic solution for 10 to 15 seconds (a balanced salt solution, *not* normal saline solution). *Note:* Pre-expansion reduces wrinkling, waviness and pleating of filter during cell preparation.
14. Place specimen containers in hood.
15. Place Petri dishes with pre-expanded filters in hood.
16. Mix specimen thoroughly in collection container so that aliquots will contain equivalent cellular contents.
17. Place well-mixed fluid sample into two separate, capped and labeled disposable plastic test tubes (amount in each test tube depends on total fluid received). Two 50-ml aliquots are usually adequate if specimen has been well mixed. Two conic 15-ml test tubes may be used for smaller samples.
18. Centrifuge sample in 50-ml plastic test tubes for 10 minutes at 2500 rpm.
19. Carefully decant one test tube. Save and refrigerate second test tube.
20. Place one drop of toluidine blue onto glass slide.
21. Place one drop of sediment onto glass slide with disposable pipette.
22. Mix drops together with clean applicator stick.
23. Cover with 24 × 24 thinness No. 1 coverslip.
24. Wait 1 minute.
25. Observe under microscope with 10× objective.
26. Estimate the number of cells. Cellularity is determined by cell population per microscopic field. *Note:* The microscope used to examine toluidine blue samples should be in the cytopreparatory laboratory. It requires decontamination similiar to that used for other equipment used in cell preparation.
27. Decide what type of preparation should be made based on cellularity of sample, type of cells observed and clinical history. Direct smears may be made at this time. Make one air dried and three 95% ethanol-fixed slides—the air-dried slide for Diff-Quik stain[21] and the wet-fixed slides for Papanicolaou stain. For cellulose filter preparation proceed to step 28.

The Cytospin 2 procedure is described later in this chapter.

Procedure 1: Cellulose Filter Preparation

28. Reconstitute cell button by mixing 10 to 20 ml of Hank's solution (Table 32–10) with sediment on a Vortex mixer.
29. Moisten wire mesh grid with physiologic salt solution.
30. Remove pre-expanded filter from Petri dish. Turn on vacuum pump and check pressure. *Note:* Do not exceed red line on gauge.
31. Place premoistened, pre-expanded membrane filter on grid, labeled side up. *Note:* For those who have difficulty with placement of filter on grid when using the rectangular style of filter, place filter directly on underside of rectangular side of funnel with label facing upwards, then place funnel with filter already in place on grid.
32. Secure filter funnel to the grid.
33. Add 15 to 20 ml of Hank's solution to funnel. *Note:* Normal saline solution should not be used because it irreversibly damages cytomorphology of cells exposed to it.
34. Draw small amount of solution through filter to secure filter in place.
35. Add sample from sediment according to estimated cell content with disposable pipette to try to obtain even distribution of cells across the filter. Experience with this part of the procedure will help to not overload filter. *Note:* Filter *must* be covered by fluid medium at all times. *Never* permit filter to air dry.
36. Turn on vacuum.
37. Check pressure gauge on vacuum pump. For Millipore filters negative pressure may reach 100 mm Hg without damaging cells. *Note:* Nuclepore filter does not require vacuum pressure.
38. Check dripping through vacuum.
39. Stop vacuum as soon as filter flow slows down.
40. Watch surface of filter to see that filter is always covered by fluid. *Note:* Surface of filter can be observed at all times by building a movable mirror above filter apparatus within germ-free hood.
41. Add 95% ethanol to reservoir to fix cells on filter. *Note:* Adding 95% ethanol to physiologic solution will yield 50% solution. Red blood cells usually lyse. This action is visible when red-covered filter turns white.
42. Allow fixative to remain over cells for 1 minute.
43. Begin vacuum again and pull most of fixative through filter. A small amount of fixative fluid should cover cells.
44. Stop vacuum. *Note:* If filter appears reddish, adding 95% ethanol to Hank's solution (1:1) will lyse red blood cells. Filter will change color from red to white. If this does not occur, filter may be overloaded with red blood cells and sample may have to be prepared from scratch.
45. Lift funnel and transfer to disinfectant solution.
46. Remove filter from grip with forceps and quickly place, cell side up, in a Petri dish containing 95% ethanol.
47. Add 70% isopropanol to grid and allow vacuum to pull isopropanol solution through grid.
48. Decontaminate surface areas and microscope and all permanent equipment with 70% isopropanol or 10% Clorox solution for 15 to 20 minutes.

Procedure 2: Cytospin 2 Cell Preparation

1. Turn on germ-free hood half an hour before work is to begin.
2. Check pressure gauge on vacuum pump.
3. Put on gown and gloves.
4. Remove specimens from refrigerator and place in hood. *Note:* Specimens are easier to prepare when at room temperature.
5. Organize work area.
6. Wipe outside of all specimen containers with 70% isopropanol or 10% Clorox solution.
7. Wipe all requisition forms with decontamination solution.
8. Match specimens to requisition forms. If there are any discrepancies contact physician requesting test.
9. Assign a laboratory number to each case.
10. List cases on log sheet.
11. Number slides.
12. Place labeled slide, filter card, sample chamber and slide clip into cytospin head.

TABLE 32–10. Properties of Salt Solutions Used in Cytopreparatory Techniques

| Solution | Properties | | | | |
	pH	Buffered	Isosomotic	Inorganic Ion Compound	Energy Source
Normal saline	6.0	No	Yes	Unbalanced	None
Polysal	6.0	No	Yes	Balanced	None
Hank's balanced salt solution*	7.4	Yes	Yes	Balanced	Glucose

*Preferred over other saline solutions in the preparation of fresh body fluids because it is physiologic.
Procedure to make Hank's balanced salt solution:
1. Stir powdered Hank's balanced salt solution medium into 950 ml deionized, distilled water at room temperature.
2. Rinse out package to remove all traces of powder.
3. Add 0.35 gms of $NaHCO_3$ per 1 liter medium.
4. Add 50.0 ml deionized, distilled water to bring volume to 1 liter.

13. Place well-mixed fluid sample into two separate, capped and labeled disposable plastic test tubes (amount in each test tube depends on total fluid received). Two 50-ml aliquots are usually adequate if specimen has been well mixed. Two conic 15 ml-test tubes may be used for smaller samples.

14. Centrifuge sample in 50-ml plastic test tubes for 10 minutes at 2500 rpm. Urine samples centrifuge for 10 minutes at 2000 rpm.

For Samples with a Cell Button

15. Pour off supernatant in disposable plastic container.
16. Resuspend button in 10 ml of Hank's balanced salt solution (BSS).
17. Take one drop of toluidine blue.
18. Mix with one drop of resuspended fluid on a glass slide.
19. Examine under microscope to determine how many drops of fluid should be added to chamber or determine amount of drops to be added to chamber by the following scheme:
    Four drops for body fluids and bronchial washings
    Two drops for urine samples
    Four to six drops for acquired immunodeficiency syndrome cases when filter will not be made or for patients with Creutzfeldt-Jakob disease.
20. Resuspend button with 30 ml of Hank's solution.
21. Place test tube on Vortex mixer to complete suspension of button in Hank's solution.
22. Add one drop of Saccomanno preservative to cytocentrifuge chamber if slide is to be Papanicolaou-stained. If slide is to be air dried, only add cell sample.
23. Spin specimen for 4 minutes at 600 rpm or if cerebrospinal fluid (CSF) for 5 minutes at 500 rpm.
24. Remove slides with care.
25. Place filters and disposable cytofunnel chambers directly into red bag.
26. Place chambers and slide clips into disinfectant.
27. Place slides for Papanicolaou stain into 95% ethanol or fix with spray fixative. The latter may help cells adhere to glass slide surface.
28. Allow air-dried sample to continue to air dry prior to staining with Diff-quik.
29. Remove equipment from disinfectant after 15 to 20 minutes.
30. Rinse well and dry thoroughly.

For Samples with No Cell Button

15. Invert test tube to drain off supernatant.
16. Take sample from base of test tube and mix with Hank's solution.
17. Mix on Vortex mixer to resuspend cells.
18. Add preservative to each cytocentrifuge chamber.
19. Add a few drops of resuspended specimen to chamber.
20. Spin specimen for 4 minutes at 600 rpm or if CSF for 5 minutes at 500 rpm.
21. Remove slides with care.
22. Place filters and disposable cytofunnel chambers directly into red bag.
23. Place chambers and slide clips into disinfectant.
24. Place slides for Papanicolaou stain into 95% ethanol or fix with spray fixative. The latter may help cells adhere to glass slide surface.

25. Allow air-dried sample to continue to air dry.
26. Remove equipment from disinfectant after 15 to 20 minutes.
27. Rinse well and dry thoroughly.

Procedure 3: Preparation of Bloody Cell Samples: Saponin Methods[39]

Saponin, an enzyme that lyses red blood cells, may be helpful in the preparation of bloody cell samples. The saponin procedure will hemolyze red blood cells while cells are in suspension. It has been suggested that this technique should be applied to all cell samples in which erythrocytes are visualized after initial centrifugation.

When the procedure is performed properly the supernatant will be colored red and the cell button will be white, just the opposite of what one normally obtains with centrifugation. The saponin selectively lyses the red blood cells, and the remaining red blood cell ghosts remain in suspension. One must be cautious in the application of saponin because an excess may destroy the cellular component of the cell sample. Time is critical and the action of saponin must be stopped after 1 minute by the action of the calcium ions in the calcium gluconate solution. Damage to all cell types may be seen in the uneven cytoplasmic borders. Saponin solution is prepared under a protective hood to avoid inhalation of saponin powder.

Saponin Solution

- 1.0 g saponin
- 0.2 g *p*-hydroxybenzoic acid sodium salt
- 100 ml distilled water

1. Mix thoroughly
2. Filter through 8-μm membrane filter

Calcium Gluconate Solution

- 3.0 calcium gluconate
- 0.02 g *p*-hydroxybenzoic acid sodium salt
- 100 ml distilled water

1. Mix thoroughly
2. Filter through 8-μm membrane filter
Note: Fungi grow rapidly in this medium.

Saponin Methods

Method 1[50]

---

1. Centrifuge specimen at 3000 rpm for 10 minutes.
2. Discard supernatant.
3. Resuspend sediment in 30 ml BSS.
4. Add five drops saponin solution.
5. Agitate gently for 1 minute.
6. Add 15 drops calcium gluconate solution to stop action of saponin enzyme.
7. Mix well.
8. Centrifuge at 2000 rpm.
9. If sediment is still bloody, repeat procedure. If no sediment is visible, prepare membrane filter.
10. Prepare direct smears if sediment is visible.
11. Spray fix.
12. Stain.

Method 2[38]

1. Centrifuge specimen at 3000 rpm for 10 minutes.
2. Discard supernatant.
3. Add 25 ml Hank's BSS to button.
4. Mix well on Vortex.
5. Add Hank's solution to 45 ml level and mix.
6. Add 2 ml 1% saponin.
7. Mix by inversion.
8. Wait 1 minute.
9. Add 3 ml 3% calcium gluconate.
10. Mix by inversion.
11. Centrifuge at 3000 rpm for 10 minutes.
12. Prepare smears on cytospin samples or filters.
13. Fix.
14. Stain.

Centrifugation

Centrifugation of cell samples is variable among authors. Cell fractionation experiments show that whole cells sediment optimally at 600 × gravity in 10 minutes. To determine what speed will produce 600 × gravity in your centrifuge, do the following: (1) Measure radius (in cm) of rotating head of centrifuge (from center to bottom of test tube holder). (2) Locate G 600 and relate centrifugal force G to revolutions per minute to radius of centrifuge head (in cm). (3) Place a line that will intercept 600 G and known radius of centrifuge. Adequacy of sedimentation can be verified by passing supernatant through a cellulose filter, staining the filter and examining it for cells. Finding a few cells is acceptable. From Tables 32–11 and 32–12, one can see the variability among laboratories.

Supravital Staining

Supravital staining of a drop of sediment with a drop of staining solution in a fresh, unfixed cell sample can provide information in the cytopreparatory laboratory that can help the cytotechnologist to

1. Avoid contamination of staining solutions if malignant tumor cells are apparent
2. Anticipate the need for special stains when there may be a potential differential diagnostic problem
3. Observe the presence of crystals and casts in urine samples that are lost in ethanol fixation
4. Decide what type of preparation will be performed: filter, direct smears or cytocentrifugation

5. Determine how many drops of sediment should be used to prepare a filter or cytospin sample
6. Determine the necessity of lysing red blood cells in a sample that was not thought to contain many red blood cells until microscopically examined
7. Prepare extra slides for educational purposes.

Toluidine blue provides good nuclear detail, with easily visualized three-dimensional formations and prominent vacuoles. The working solution keeps well under refrigeration and does not require frequent filtration (Table 32–13).[56] Thionin is also an excellent nuclear stain. It does require frequent filtration to remove the crystals that may obscure microscopic observation. Methylene blue is used to stain urinary sediment to visualize malignant tumor cells. Methyl green and pyronine stain exhibit brilliant colors: blue-green nuclear chromatin and red cytoplasm. The stain can be erratic and modifications may be necessary. There are also other supravital stains that have been used to distinguish histiocytes and leukocytes from mesothelial cells and malignant cells in body fluids.[47]

These methods require the cytotechnologist to feel comfortable with the visual patterns observed with these stains. If one elects to show the slide for a second opinion, then the coverslip may be sealed with clear fingernail polish or petroleum jelly. The sample will be preserved for a few hours. Another method to maintain the sample for additional viewing is to place the slide in a covered Petri dish containing a moistened gauze pad. The sample will not dry out for a few hours.

McCormack[56] originally suggested the following:

1. Add 10 ml toluidine blue solution to 10 ml of equine serum.
2. Centrifuge mixture to remove sediment.
3. Decant the supernatant (this is the staining fluid).
4. Add a few thymol crystals to staining fluid.
5. Store in dropper bottle in refrigerator. Write date on bottle (it is stable for several months).

Toluidine Blue Procedure

1. Place small drop of sediment on a slide.
2. Put a drop of toluidine blue near the cell sample on slide.
3. Mix the two drops together.
4. Coverslip.
5. Evaluate microscopically.

TABLE 32–11. Centrifugation Times for Various Types of Cell Samples

Cell Samples	RPM	Time	Place or Author
Body fluids	1500	5 minutes	Johns Hopkins[37, 38] (for cells exposed to alcohol)
	3000	10 minutes	Johns Hopkins (for fresh fluids)
	2500	5 minutes	University of Illinois (50-ml round-bottom test tube)
	2500	10 minutes	University of Chicago
Cerebrospinal fluids	2000	5 minutes	Naylor[61] (conic tube)
	1500	4 minutes	Whitmore and coworkers[83]
Urine	2500	10 minutes	University of Chicago
	2000	10 minutes	Kini and Smith[50]
Sputum (with Carbowax preservative)	1500	5 minutes	Saccomanno[3, 70]

TABLE 32–12. Cytospin Centrifugation Times for Various Types of Cell Samples

Cell Samples	RPM	Time	Place or Author
Body fluids	600	4 minutes	University of Chicago
	1000	2.5 minutes	Cytospin 1[5]
	1000	6 minutes	Cytospin 2 book (samples up to 0.5 ml; avoid in excess of 1000 rpm)
Cerebrospinal fluids	500	5 minutes	University of Chicago
	800	6 minutes	Gill[38]
	825	5 minutes	Rosenthal[68]
	1200	1 minute	Tutuarima and coworkers[81]
	1500	5–7 minutes	Bigner and coworkers[10]

Smith and Naylor[71] recommend obtaining the sample from the topmost layer of sediment.

The described procedure has been used mostly with body fluids, but the same procedure may be used to provide a rapid evaluation of fine needle aspirates.

Toluidine Blue Procedure for Fine Needle Aspirates

1. Put on disposable gloves to handle patient samples.
2. Express a drop of the aspirate in center of slide.
3. Place a drop of toluidine blue stain next to cell sample.
4. Mix the two drops together with wooden applicator stick.
5. Discard applicator stick in designated red bag.
6. Place a small 24 × 30 mm coverslip over specimen.
7. Let sample sit for a minute.
8. Place sample under microscope.
9. Evaluate sample.
10. Discard sample. If you decide to keep the sample, drop the slide with the coverslip into 95% ethanol to fix for permanent record.
11. Decontaminate microscope stage, objectives and oculars and fine adjustment with 70% isopropanol if microscope is used by others not handling fresh samples.
12. Remove and discard gloves in designated red bag.

Staining of Body Fluids on Millipore Filters

The staining procedure is as follows for the Millipore filter preparations.

Procedure
1. 95% ethanol — Fixation
2. Tap water (×2) — Ten dips each
3. Gill's half-oxidized hematoxylin — 45 seconds to 1 minute
4. Tap water (×2) — Ten dips each
5. 0.05% HCl — 30 seconds or until filter turns buttercup yellow
6. Tap water (×2) — Ten dips each; filter will turn blue
7. Scott's solution — 1 minute
8. Tap water (×2) — Ten dips each
9. 95% ethanol (×2) — Ten dips each
10. Modified OG-6 — 2 minutes

11. 95% ethanol (×2) — 1 minute each
12. Modified EA — 10 minutes (Dipping cellulose filters rapidly strips dyes, particularly light green, from cells but slowly extracts it from the filter background. Letting the filter sit undisturbed in the alcohols following EA reverses events. Cells retain their green color and the filters lose their green color.)
13. 95% ethanol — 4 minutes
14. 95% ethanol — 2 minutes
15. 95% ethanol — 1 minute
16. Absolute 2 and propanol (×2) — 1 minute each
17. Xylene (×3) — 1 minute each
18. Xylene until coverslipped

Staining of Body Fluids for Slides

1. 95% ethanol — Fixation
2. Tap water (×2) — Ten dips each
3. Gill's half-oxidized hematoxylin — 1 minute
4. Tap water (×2) — Ten dips each
5. Scott's solution — 1 minute
6. Tap water (×2) — Ten dips each
7. 95% ethanol — Ten dips each
8. Modified OG-6 — 2 minutes
9. 95% ethanol (×3) — Ten dips each
10. Absolute ethanol (×2) — Ten dips each
11. Xylene (×2) — Ten dips each
12. Xylene until coverslipped

CEREBROSPINAL FLUID PREPARATION

The preparation and staining of CSF is performed separately from other fluid samples. The method we use is a filtration method in which the entire cell sample is utilized for diagnostic purposes.

There are a variety of cytopreparatory methods in current use: cellulose and polycarbonate filter methods, centrifugation and direct smears and cytocentrifuga-

TABLE 32–13. Toluidine Blue: Stock Solutions

Ingredients	University of Rochester	University of Chicago	McCormack and Coworkers[58]
Toluidine blue	0.50 g	0.50 g (Cl#52040)	1 g*
95% ethyl alcohol	20 ml	20 ml	20 ml
Distilled water	30 ml	80 ml	80 ml

*Mortar the dry stain with the alcohol and add the water slowly.

tion. If the direct smear method is used, the addition of an adhesive solution on the glass slide such as polylysine, dextran or Mayer's albumin is suggested so that cells will adhere more readily to the glass surface. Prefixation with alcohol is not recommended for CSF because alcohol may precipitate any protein present in the fluid sample.

Staining of CSF is performed separately so that cross-contamination from other specimen types does not occur. If all CSF fluids prepared in a single day are microscopically monitored by the cytopreparatory individual, cross-contamination within the samples themselves can be recognized.

Preparation of Clear Cerebrospinal Fluids of Less than 5 ml in Volume

Equipment

All preparatory equipment for CSF as well as the staining solutions are kept separate from all other fluids. The equipment is marked so that it will not be confused with the body fluid preparatory equipment.

Procedure

1. Make a permanent marking along the filter margin. *Note:* Select numbers or letters that cannot be misinterpreted when viewed backwards. Write the information twice if the filter is to be cut in half. Berol All-Rite and Plymouth ball-point pens work well and are indelible.
2. Label slides and test tubes.
3. Pre-expand cellulose filter in 95% ethanol for 10 to 15 seconds. *Note:* Pre-expansion of filter helps reduce pleating or wrinkling during preparation.
4. Moisten grid of filter apparatus with Hank's solution.
5. Place premoistened, pre-expanded membrane filter on grid with label side up.
6. Place funnel carefully in position guiding with fingers.
7. Add 20 ml of Hank's solution to funnel. *Note:* When adding solutions to the filter on the grid let the fluid run along the sides of the funnel.
8. Begin vacuuming, allowing some of the Hank's solution to go through the filter. *Note:* The filter will flatten out on the grid. Pleating or wrinkling of the filter is avoided. The filter apparatus is now ready for the clamp to be applied.

9. Stop vacuum.
10. Add specimen to Hank's solution in funnel. *Note:* The cells will be washed of proteinaceous material as Hank's solution is pulled through the filter and over the cells.
11. Begin vacuuming slowly. *Note:* Vacuuming to 100 mg of Hg has not been shown to cause cellular damage or distortion to cellulose filters. The filter must be covered by a fluid medium at all times.
12. Add more Hank's solution from rinse bottle to sides of reservoir to retrieve any cells clinging to sides of funnel.
13. After Hank's solution has almost disappeared, stop vacuum.
14. Add 95% ethanol to reservoir to fix cells on the filter itself (1:1).
15. Allow fixative to remain on cells for 1 minute.
16. Begin vacuuming again and pull most of the fixative through filter. A small amount of fixative should cover cells on the filter.
17. Stop vacuum.
18. Remove filter from apparatus and quickly place filter, cell side up, in Petri dish containing 95% ethanol.
19. Remove clamp, lift funnel and transfer to disinfectant solution along with grid.
20. Place all equipment in disinfectant.

Staining of Cerebrospinal Fluids on Millipore Filter

The staining procedure is as follows for the Millipore filter preparations.

Procedure

1. 95% ethanol	15 minutes
2. Tap water	Ten dips
3. Gill's half-oxidized hematoxylin	Less than 1 minute
4. Tap water (×2)	Ten dips each
5. 0.05% HCl	30 seconds (time may vary until filter turns buttercup yellow)
6. Tap water (×2)	Ten dips each
7. Scott's solution	1 minute (filter turns pale blue)
8. Tap water (×2)	Ten dips each
9. 95% ethanol (×2)	Ten dips each
10. 95% ethanol	1 minute
11. Modified EA	Ten minutes
12. 95% ethanol (×2)	20 dips each

13. Absolute 2-pro-   1 minute each
    panol (×2)
14. Xylene   1 minute (filter becomes
        translucent)
15. Xylene   1 minute
16. Xylene until cov-
    erslipped

Precautions for preparation of samples from patients with Creutzfeldt-Jakob disease include using disposable equipment whenever possible. For the staining setup, we use 50-ml plastic test tubes that are discarded after use.

Reusable items shall be immersed for 2 hours in 5% sodium hypochlorite (undiluted household bleach) or autoclaved at 121°C for 1 hour before being cleaned or discarded. Surfaces contaminated with body fluids during processing of samples should be disinfected for 2 hours with 5% sodium hypochlorite before routine cleaning. The prepared slides are discarded after the case has been signed out.

PREPARATION OF GENITOURINARY TRACT AND OTHER WATERY SAMPLES

Urinary tract samples contain cells that are suspended in an unfriendly environment and may already be degenerated prior to leaving the body, according to Harris and coworkers.[44, 46] Crabtree and Murphy[19] wrote, "Most of the morphologic changes recognized as degenerative occur prior to voiding." Cell preservation is in further jeopardy once the specimen has left the body. Variations in cellularity and cell preservation may also be reflected in a variety of urologic diseases. Early-morning and 24-hour samples are not recommended for cytologic evaluation.

Holmquist[47] states that a urine sample can sit out at room temperature if prepared the same day that it was obtained; if left out overnight or over a weekend, however, the specimen should be refrigerated. If a longer delay is anticipated, it is then and only then that 70% ethanol (two parts urine to one part alcohol) may be added to the urine sample. Although refrigeration of the cell sample may retard cell degeneration, the addition of an ethanol fixative may not.

Urine sample preparation is difficult to perform on cool or cold samples. Salts crystallize in cold urine samples and may cause the filter to clog. Salts will dissolve in solution if the urine is brought to room or body temperature prior to preparation. It is advisable to let the urine sample reach room temperature prior to processing the sample.

If the sample is collected in an alcohol fixative it is difficult for the cells to attach themselves to the surface of a clean glass slide. Cells collected in alcohol tend to round up and harden, and nuclear pyknosis frequently occurs. The use of albumin as a cohesive agent (in the sample or on the slides) does not improve the results.[9] If the specimen has been fixed in a suspension it should be centrifuged, the supernatant poured off and the sediment resuspended, preferably in a balanced salt solution before further processing. Alcohol added to urine samples also causes protein coagulation in the supernatant. The coagulated protein may clog the pores of filter preparations unless the cells are washed clear of the protein. There will also be a background of densely stained protein that may obscure epithelial cells; if the protein is not washed from them, then the cells will not take up the dyes properly in the staining process.

Holmquist[47] states that all urine samples should be centrifuged and rinsed once with a salt solution. If the specimen is bloody or contains ample sediment, then more than one rinse may be necessary to help uptake of dyes in the staining process. A 0.9% isotonic and isosmotic solution is recommended in the preparation of Millipore filters in the handling of urine samples in particular and body fluids in general.

Centrifugation of genitourinary tract samples prior to filtration is the usual procedure. One may also allow the urine to form a sediment at room temperature. In the latter case, cells obtained from the bottom of the container are usually adequate in number to obtain a diagnostic cell sample, provided it is placed into a conic container for cytospin preparation or applied to a membrane filter.[3]

Centrifugation and direct smears used to be the most common methods. Because urine samples have a tendency to become detached from glass slides during fixation and staining, a coating agent such as albumin 0.1% polylysine hydrobromide or frosted Dakin slides were used. Bales[2] and Bales and Durfee[3] describe a technique for handling a high volume of urine samples. The technique is semiautomated, and rapid preparation of urine samples can be performed by personnel with limited experience. Samples are coated with 2% Carbowax in 70% ethanol. This method also proved to be excellent in preserving casts, crystals and blood cells.

The first voided urine is thought by some to have poorer cellular preservation because of prolonged exposure of cells to urine. However, Pearson and coauthors[65] show that if the pH is low, exposure of cells to unfixed urine for as long as 72 hours causes little loss of preservation.

The addition of a fixative to specimens that have a higher pH or that must undergo prolonged storage before preparation can improve the preservation of cellular detail.

No relationship could be distinguished between the number of cells in the original sample and the variation in cell counts in the material prepared with various techniques: air drying, wet fixing and Millipore filtering.[9]

Staining of urine samples is the same as staining of other body fluids.

MUCOID SAMPLE PREPARATION

Respiratory Tract Specimen Preparation and Other Mucoid Samples

Methods of processing mucoid specimens such as sputum, bronchial washings, bronchoalveolar lavages and tracheal aspirates vary from laboratory to laboratory.[35, 36, 50, 54, 57, 60] Some laboratories use the "pick and smear" method and some use the Saccomanno method, which is designed to homogenize the sample prior to spreading the material onto a glass slide. Others collect the sample in an alcohol solution. The goal of each method is to obtain the best diagnostic sample for screening and diagnosis.

Unfixed Respiratory Tract Samples

1. Turn on light and power in germ-free hood half an hour before beginning procedure.
2. Put on protective clothing, gloves and gown.
3. Place specimen under germ-free hood. *Note:* If specimen has been refrigerated, bring to room temperature.
4. Label four slides with patient identification and laboratory acquisition number.
5. Label collection cup with acquisition number and patient name.
6. Examine specimen carefully. *Note:* This may require that the specimen be transferred to a Petri dish placed on a dark background to visualize suspicious areas.
7. Look for fresh or old blood-tinged areas, discolored portions of sample and tissue fragments.
8. Transfer suspect areas with a disposable instrument or applicator sticks to a glass slide. Spread material across surface of glass slide.
9. Take a second glass slide.
10. Crush specimen firmly but gently between the two slides until an even distribution of material is obtained. *Note:* If the slides do not pull apart cleanly, continue working with the sample until successful. A drop of Hank's solution or tap or distilled water on the sample will help soften the material and at the same time prevent the material from air drying during the smearing process.
11. Fix slides in 95% ethanol for 15 to 30 minutes.

Respiratory Tract Samples Collected in a Preservative

Specimens collected in 50% or 70% ethanol yield a hardened specimen owing to coagulation of mucoproteins. Erythrocytes hemolyze when collected in alcoholic preservative. The fixative is one part specimen and one part preservative. The alcohol collecting solutions kill cells, stop autolysis and prevent growth of microorganisms. The negative side of alcoholic preservation is that cells shrink and harden and no longer adhere to a glass surface and it is difficult to achieve a monolayer of cells. It may be necessary to albuminize slides well in advance of their use or both the cells and the albumin may fall away from the glass slide when placed in 95% ethanol fixative. The slide's surface must be sticky to the touch. The prealbuminized slides may be kept in a covered box prior to use.

Steps 1 to 7 are the same as for unfixed respiratory tract samples except that the slides for alcohol-preserved sputum cells are albuminized in advance.

8. Place the second slide over the selected material and, with a firm grinding or rotating motion, break up the material. To avoid air drying of specimens, moisten sample with a few drops of tap or distilled water or Hank's solution.
9. Place a drop of Hank's solution or tap or distilled water on sample to help soften the material and at the same time not allow the material to air dry.
10. Continue to work with sample until there is an even distribution of the sample on the glass slide. Well-prepared slides will come apart easily.
11. Pull slides apart.
12. Fix slides in 95% ethanol for at least 30 minutes.
13. Remove slides from fixative.
14. Immerse in water (tap or distilled) for 15 to 20 minutes.
15. Drain well prior to staining. Air drying will reduce the risk of cell loss.

Respiratory Samples in Carbowax and Alcohol Solution

Unfixed samples may have Carbowax or alcohol preservative added to the specimen upon receipt in the laboratory, or the preservative may be used as a collection fluid. A Carbowax solution or 50% ethanol (1:1) is added to the specimen. The specimen and preservative should be well mixed and allowed to sit for 1 hour.

With the Carbowax or alcohol prefixation and the concentration technique of Saccomanno,[70] a representative sample of the entire sputum sample is obtained. Experience in the selection of suspect areas is not required. For some, handling sputum in this manner is more acceptable than the pick and smear method. Saccomanno[70] states that false-negative rates were 12% with the concentration method and 46% with direct cough and direct smear.

A word of caution is necessary. When using the Saccomanno sputum preparation technique: The blender produces potentially infectious aerosols. The blender should be one made for laboratory use only and not a kitchen model. The cap should prevent leakage. It is recommended that the blender cap not be opened for at least 1 hour after the blending operation has been completed because it may take that long for the infectious aerosols to settle within the blender jar. If the laboratory is equipped with a germ-free hood, the 1 hour wait may not be necessary; however, the area where the blender sits should be in the middle of the hood so that the aerosol sprays will be carried away from the operator.

The blender is placed in a negative pressure cabinet that has an airflow velocity across the face of the cabinet of at least 75 linear feet per minute.[45]

The blender is decontaminated after each use by filling the container with household bleach, blending and then rinsing well with water. Saccomanno adds 3 mg of rifampin to each bottle of fixative and a similar amount to the specimen upon receipt in the laboratory.[3] The sample is then allowed to sit for 24 hours before preparation is begun.

The use of the Saccomanno method yields
1. A representative sample
2. A reduction in mucus in smears
3. A concentration of cells from the entire specimen versus the selection of cells by an experienced technologist.

Ferruginous Bodies

Sputum samples processed by the three described methods may not be optimal to detect ferruginous bodies.[73] The Saccomanno technique is not as sensitive as the pick and smear method when staining for iron. Membrane filtration may yield a better detection rate for this purpose. Bronchial washings may yield better results than either sputum samples or bronchoalveolar lavage. Specimens from patients with a history of asbestos exposure might be prepared for Prussian blue staining to improve the detection rate of ferruginous bodies.[18, 21, 62, 71, 82]

Pneumocystis carinii

Detection of *P. carinii* in bronchial wash samples stained with the Diff-Quik method is fairly reliable and rapid. The routine Papanicolaou stain[53, 80] may be less sensitive for the washings but is improved in bronchoalveolar lavage specimens.[20] Sensitivity is increased with the use of Grocott-Gomori methenamine-silver stain[16, 17] and cresyl echt (fast violet) in addition to the Diff-Quik stain.[15] The Gram-Weigert stain is also good. The Diff-Quik method is easy and rapid and has a reported sensitivity of 76%.[15, 79]

Procedure for the Saccomanno Concentration Method

Specimen Identification Procedure

1. Check forms with specimen to determine if both match and are identified properly.
2. Write in laboratory acquisition number on form; at the same time, label specimen both on side and top of container with adhesive (this taped label is to be placed on blender cup).
3. Log in all samples.
4. Describe sample (amount and consistency) and indicate gross picture on yellow form on lower left side.
5. Wipe outside of sample containers with 70% isopropanol.
6. Label all slides with patient identification number and name. Check twice to see that number on form matches number on slide.
7. Label two 15-ml test tubes with proper number; place in rack.
8. Take all samples to germ-free hood.

Procedure for Concentration Method

1. Turn on light and power in germ-free hood half an hour before use.
2. Add 2% Carbowax-50% ethanol fixative to double amount of specimen. If specimen is scant, add enough Carbowax to equal 30 ml.
3. Agitate or mix with tongue blade the specimen container with the Carbowax fixative. Specimens should fix for up to 1 hour in 2% Carbowax-50% ethanol fixative under the hood.
4. Remove labeled identification tape from cap of sputum sample and place on side of blender cup.
5. Under hood, open sample and pour total amount into blender cup.

Time to be blended varies with sample:

Watery	2 seconds on low power 6 seconds on high power	Check sample
Semimucoid	2 seconds on low power 8 seconds on high power	Check sample
Mucoid	2 seconds on low power 10 to 30 seconds on high power	Check sample

6. Pour entire sample into two 15-ml capped test tubes. Check to see that material in each test tube contains an equal amount of sample prior to centrifugation. Wipe outside of tubes with 70% isopropanol.
7. Take test tubes to centrifuge.
8. Place each sample tube directly across from its twin.
9. Centrifuge at 1500 rpm for 5 minutes.
10. Return to hood to clean blender cups with 70% isopropanol. (To clean blender cup, blend full-strength household bleach in blender cup for 20 seconds.)
11. Rinse cup well with hot water and wash with germicidal soap.
12. Remove 15-ml tubes from centrifuge and place in rack; return to hood with tubes, disposable pipettes, glass slides and paper towels.
13. Pour off supernatant from one tube of each specimen into discard container, leaving about 2 ml of supernatant in tube to cover sediment. Watch button at all times while pouring to make sure it is not poured off with supernatant.
14. Resuspend remaining supernatant and sediment by placing test tube on Vortex mixer for a few seconds.
15. Pipette the mixture onto four slides using one to three drops on each slide, depending on thickness of sediment. Using two slide smear technique, make a *monolayer* by spreading drops between

two slides. Work with sample until a smooth layer of sample is attained.

16. With a disposable glass pipette, place a few drops of cell concentrate directly on glass slide; cover with another slide and gently pull the two apart. This method distributes the cells in a monolayer over the two slides. Leave slides under hood until dry. When dry, rack up slides and stain according to posted procedure.

17. Refrigerate and save any remaining specimen until case has been signed out.

Staining for Sputum Samples

1. 95% ethanol	Fixation
2. 95% ethanol	Removal of Carbowax
3. Tap water (×2)	Ten dips each
4. Gill's half-oxidized hematoxylin	1 minute
5. Tap water (×2)	Ten dips each
6. Scott's tap water substitute	2 minutes
7. Tap water (×2)	Ten dips each
8. 95% ethanol	Ten dips each
9. Modified OG	2 minutes
10. 95% ethanol (×2)	Ten dips each
11. Modified EA	Ten minutes
12. 95% ethanol (×3)	Ten dips each
13. Absolute ethanol (×2)	Ten dips each
14. Xylene (×2)	Ten dips each
15. Xylene until coverslipped	

OTHER FACTORS RELATED TO CYTOPREPARATION

Time for cytopreparation is usually limited and decisions related to preparatory techniques may relate to the daily workload and the available staff. Most laboratories provide results within a 24-hour period. The volume of stat requests also influences the selected preparatory methods in a given setting.

Laboratories in which the cytotechnologist does not prepare the cell sample may best be served by the design of a strict protocol in which all possibilities are covered and a variety of sample preparations can be prepared at one time; many of the preparations may not be required but would be available if necessary. This system requires availability of ample staff.

The human factor also plays a role in the preparatory laboratory. Procedures change over time. Short cuts or modifications are made by those preparing cell samples. It is advisable to observe or monitor preparation performed by various staff members on a regular basis to compare the written procedures with what is actually being done. Some modifications may save time and be equivalent to the written procedure; others are not. In any event, the written procedure should reflect what is actually being done by laboratory personnel.

INFECTION CONTROL

At the University of Chicago Hospitals, the Committee on Infections and Epidemiology works with each department to develop and write up infection-control policies and procedures. These policies and procedures are reviewed and updated annually. Each department is then responsible for in-service education programs for their staff. Guidelines are in accordance with those issued by the Centers for Disease Control.

The state of Illinois also has a set "Rules and Regulations for the Control of Communicable Diseases," concerning the reporting of communicable disease cases. It is suggested that readers make themselves aware of federal, state and local regulations.

Cytopathology laboratories that perform diagnostic tests on biologic specimens that may contain infectious agents must take precautions to minimize the risk to laboratory personnel. Red bags placed at appropriate places in the cytopreparatory laboratory help separate contaminated articles for incineration, and color-coded, red-marked areas may alert laboratory workers to exert more caution in the day-to-day processing of cell samples.

References

1. Bahr GF, Bartels PH, Bibbo M, de Nicolas M, Wied GL: Evaluation of the Papanicolaou stain for computer assisted cellular pattern recognition. Acta Cytol 17:106–112, 1973.
2. Bales CE: Tech sample No. CY-1. Preparation of scant cellular samples. Am Soc Clin Pathol 1:1–4, 1985.
3. Bales CE, Durfee GR: Cytologic techniques. *In* LG Koss: Diagnostic Cytopathology and Its Histologic Bases, 3rd ed. Philadelphia, JB Lippincott, pp 1187–1266, 1979.
4. Barrett DL: Cytocentrifuge technique. *In* Compendium on Cytopreparatory Techniques, 4th ed. Edited by CM Keebler, JW Reagan, GL Wied. Chicago, Tutorials of Cytology, pp 80–83, 1976.
5. Barrett DL, King EB: Comparison of cellular recovery rates and morphological detail using membrane filter and cytocentrifuge techniques. Acta Cytol 20:174–180, 1976.
6. Barrett DL: Sources of cell loss using membrane filter and cytocentrifuge preparatory techniques. Cytotechnol Bull 12:7–8, 1975.
7. Bartels PH, Bahr GF, Bibbo M, Richards DL, Sonek MG, Wied GL: Analysis of variance of the Papanicolaou staining reaction. Acta Cytol 18:522–531, 1974.
8. Bethesda system for reporting cervical/vaginal cytological diagnosis. JAMA 262:931–934, 1989.
9. Beyer-Boon ME, Voorn-Den Hollander MJA: Cell yield obtained with various cytopreparatory techniques for urinary cytology. Acta Cytol 22:589–594, 1978.
10. Bigner SH, Johnston WW: Cytopreparation. *In* Cytopathology of the Central Nervous System. Edited by WW Johnston. New York, Masson Publishing, pp 5–15, 1983.
11. Boccato P: Polyvalent fixative for staining of fine needle aspirates. Acta Cytol 29:647–648, 1985.
12. Bonfiglio TA: Cytopathologic intepretation of transthoracic biopsies. *In* Masson Monographs in Diagnostic Cytopathology. Edited by WW Johnston. New York, Masson Publishing, pp 187–194, 1983.
13. Boon ME, Wickel AF, Davoren RAM: Role of the air bubble in increasing cell recovery using cytospin I and II. Acta Cytol 27:699–702, 1983.
14. Boschann HW: Personal communication.
15. Chandra P, Delaney MD, Tuazon CU: Role of special stains in

the diagnosis of *Pneumocystis carinii* infection from bronchial washing specimens in patients with acquired immune deficiency syndrome. Acta Cytol 32:105–108, 1988.

16. Churukian CJ: Manual of Special Stains. Rochester NY, Department of Pathology, University of Rochester, 1979.

17. Churukian CJ, Schenk EA: Rapid Grocott's methenamine-silver nitrate method for fungi and *Pneumocystis carinii*. Am J Clin Pathol 68:427–428, 1977.

18. Clark G: Staining Procedures, 4th ed. Published for the Biological Stain Commission. Baltimore, Williams & Wilkins, pp 1–2, 23–34, 439, 468, 1981.

19. Crabtree WN, Murphy WM: The value of ethanol as a fixative in urinary cytology. Acta Cytol 24:452–455, 1980.

20. Crabtree WN, Stine CR: The polycarbonate disc versus the cellulose membrane filter in urinary cytology. Acta Cytol 27:577, 1983.

21. Danos ML, Keebler CK: Cytopreparatory techniques. *In* A Manual of Cytotechnology, 4th ed. Edited by CM Keebler, JW Reagan. Chicago, American Society of Clinical Pathologists, pp 262–317, 1975.

22. Danos-Holmquist ML: Preparation of Urine Samples. Cytotechnology Tech Sample No. CY-2. Chicago, American Society of Clinical Pathologists, pp 1–9, 1984.

23. Danos ML: Fixatives for cytologic use. *In* Compendium on Cytopreparatory Techniques, 3rd ed. Edited by CM Keebler, JW Reagan, GL Wied. Chicago, Tutorials of Cytology, pp 6–8, 1974.

24. Danos ML: On understanding the Papanicolaou stain. Cytotechnol Bull 7:1–2, 1972.

25. Dekker A, Bupp PA: Cytology of serous effusions: A comparative study of two slightly different preparative methods. Acta Cytol 20:394–399, 1976.

26. Esposti PL, Moberger G, Zajicek J: The cytologic diagnosis of transitional cell tumors of the urinary bladder and its histologic basis. Acta Cytol 14:145–155, 1970.

27. Esposti PL, Zajicek J: Grading of transitional cell neoplasms of the urinary bladder from smears of bladder washings. A critical review of 326 tumors. Acta Cytol 16:529–537, 1972.

28. Gatscha RM: Personal communication.

29. Gill GW, Frost JK, Miller KA: A new formula for a half-oxidized hematoxylin solution that neither overstains nor requires differentiation. Acta Cytol 18:300–311, 1974.

30. Gill GW: Comparative filter techniques. Acta Cytol 19:207–209, 1975.

31. Gill GW: A cross contamination control and stain storage system. Cytotechnol Bull 12:12–13, 1975.

32. Gill GW: Carbowax in fixatives. Cytotechnol Bull 10:19–20, 1973.

33. Gill GW: The Papanicolaou Stain: Material and Methods. (Booklet for the film "The Papanicolaou Stain: Materials and Methods.") Bethesda, Health & Education Resources, pp 1–8, 1975.

34. Gill GW: Controlling the Papanicolaou Stain. Cytotechnology Check Sample No. C-66. Chicago, American Society of Clinical Pathologists, 1979.

35. Gill GW: Collection and Preparation of Bronchoscopy Specimens. (Booklet for the film "Pulmonary Cytology-I: Collection and Preparation of Sputum Specimens.") Bethesda, Health & Education Resources, pp 1–26, 1978.

36. Gill GW: Collection and Preparation of Bronchoscopy Specimens. (Booklet for the film "Pulmonary Cytology-II: Collection and Preparation of Bronchoscopy Specimens.") Bethesda, Health & Education Resources, pp 1–26, 1978.

37. Gill GW: Cytopreparation with Micro Slides and Membrane Filters. (Booklet for the film "Cytopreparation with Micro Slides and Cytopreparation with Membrane Filters.") Bethesda, Health & Education Resources, pp 1–6, 1976.

38. Gill GW: Techniques, tips and troubleshooting for cell suspensions in cytology, hematology and all disciplines. *In* The Shandon Cytospin 2 in Diagnostic Cytology: Techniques, Tips and Troubleshooting. Sewickley, Pennsylvania, Shandon Southern Instruments, pp 1–174, 1982.

39. Gill GW: Saponizing bloody cytologic specimens. *In* The Shandon Cytospin 2 in Diagnostic Cytology: Techniques, Tips and Troubleshooting. Sewickley, Pennsylvania, Shandon Southern Instruments, pp 44–46, 1982.

40. Gill GW: Exfoliative Cytology. Application Report No. 24. Bedford, Massachusetts, Millipore Corporation, 1969.

41. Gondos B, King EB: Cerebrospinal fluid cytology: Diagnostic accuracy and comparison of different techniques. Acta Cytol 20:542–547, 1976.

42. Graham RM: Advantages and disadvantages of fixation methods other than alcohol-ether. Acta Cytol 1:66, 1951.

43. Hajdu SI: A note on the history of Carbowax. Acta Cytol 27:204–206, 1983.

44. Harris MJ, Schwinn CP, Morrow JW, Gray RL, Browell BM: Exfoliative cytology of the urinary bladder irrigation specimen. Acta Cytol 15:385–399, 1971.

45. Harris MJ: Sputum fixatives. Acta Cytol 21:493, 1977.

46. Harris MJ, Keebler CM, Schwinn CP: Cytopreparatory Techniques in Urinary Cytology. Cytotechnology Check Sample No. 31. American Society of Clinical Pathologists, pp 1–13, 1976.

47. Holmquist ND: Diagnostic Cytology of the Urinary Tract. Basel, S Karger, p 72, 1977.

48. Keebler CM, Reagan JW, Wied GL: Compendium on Cytopreparatory Techniques, 4th ed. Chicago, Tutorials of Cytology, 1976.

49. Kini SR: Guides to clinical aspiration biopsy. *In* Thyroid. Edited by TS Kline. New York, Igaku-Shoin, pp 22–28, 1987.

50. Kini SR, Smith MI: Diagnostic Cytology by Membrane Filter Application. Bulletin 100. Ann Arbor, Gelman Science, 1978.

51. Lillie RD: The Hematoxylin Shortage and the Availability of Synthetic Substitutes. American Society of Medical Technology, p 40, 1974.

52. Luna LG, Gaffney E: Evaluation of commercial hematoxylin for H & E staining. Histology 18:34–35, 1988.

53. Markowitz S, Leiman G: Cytologic detection of *Pneumocystis carinii* by ultraviolet light examination of Papanicolaou-stained sputum specimens. Acta Cytol 30:79–80, 1986.

54. Marsan C, Pasteur X, Alepee B, Laurent JL, Accard JL, Cava E, Eloit P, Maoret JJ: Automatic cytopathologic diagnosis of bronchial carcinoma. I. Cytocentrifugation of bronchial brushings for image analysis. Acta Cytol 26:545–550, 1982.

55. Maswah S, Devlin D, Dekker A: A comparative cytologic study of 100 urine specimens processed by the slide centrifuge and membrane filter techniques. Acta Cytol 22:431–434, 1978.

56. McCormack LJ, Hazard JB, Belovich D, Gardner WJ: Identification of neoplastic cells in cerebrospinal fluids by wet-film method. Cancer 10:1293–1299, 1957.

57. Miller FK: Preparation of sputum specimens. *In* A Manual of Cytotechnology, 4th ed. Edited by CM Keebler, JW Reagan. Chicago, American Society of Clinical Pathologists, pp 289–290, 1975.

58. Miller FK: Cytopreparatory methods—Collection, smearing and reporting. *In* Compendium on Cytopreparatory Techniques, 4th ed. Edited by CM Keebler, JW Reagan, GL Wied. Chicago, Tutorials of Cytology, pp 59–69, 1976.

59. Miller F, Woolner LB: Specimen preparation for material from the respiratory tract. *In* Compendium on Diagnostic Cytology, 3rd ed. Edited by LG Koss, JW Reagan, GL Wied. Chicago, Tutorials of Cytology, pp 254–261, 1974.

60. Mitchell PD: Sputum fixatives. Acta Cytol 21:493–494, 1977.

61. Naylor B: An exfoliative cytologic study of intracranial fluids. Acta Cytol 8:141, 1964.

62. Naylor B: Regarding cyanophilic bodies, toxoplasma cysts and ferruginous bodies. Acta Cytol 21:490–491, 1977.

63. Papanicolaou GN: A new procedure for staining vaginal smears. Science 95:438–439, 1942.

64. Papanicolaou GN: Atlas of Exfoliative Cytology. Cambridge, Harvard University Press, 1954.

65. Pearson JC, Kromhout L, King EB: Evaluation of collection and preservation techniques for urinary cytology. Acta Cytol 25:327–333, 1981.

66. Reider H: Zur Diagnose der Neubildungen bei klinisch-mikroskopischin Untersuchungen von Transsudatan. Dsch Arch Klin Med 54:150–544, 1985.

67. Rosenthal DL: Personal communication.

68. Rosenthal DL: Cytology of the central nervous system. *In* Monographs in Clinical Cytology. Edited by GL Wied. New York, S Karger, pp 171–178, 1984.

69. Saccomanno G: Sputum fixatives. Acta Cytol 21:495, 1977.
70. Saccomanno G, Saunders RP, Ellis H, Archer VE, Wood BG, Beehler PA: Concentration of carcinoma or atypical cells in sputum. Acta Cytol 7:305–310, 1963.
71. Smith MJ, Naylor B: Digestion technique for detecting ferruginous (or "asbestos") bodies in lung and sputum. *In* Compendium on Cytopreparatory Techniques. Edited by CM Keebler, JW Reagan, GL Wied. Chicago, Tutorials of Cytology, pp 79–81, 1970.
72. Smith MJ, Naylor B: Techniques of Cytopathology: Laboratory Manual. Ann Arbor, Department of Pathology, University of Michigan, pp 8–10, 1970.
73. Smith MJ, Naylor B: A method for extracting ferruginous bodies from sputum and pulmonary tissue. Am J Clin Pathol 58:250–254, 1972.
74. Somrak T: Personal communication.
75. Soost HJ, Falter EW, Otto K: Comparison of two Papanicolaou staining procedures for automated prescreening. Anal Quant Cytol 1:37–42, 1979.
76. Spriggs AI: The Cytology of Effusions in Pleural, Pericardial and Peritoneal Cavities, 2nd ed. London, Heineman, pp 22–26, 1972.
77. Spriggs AI, Boddington MM: The Cytology of Effusions and of Cerebrospinal Fluid, 2nd ed. New York, Grune & Stratton, pp 51–57, 1968.
78. Street CM: Papanicolaou techniques in exfoliative cytology. *In* Laboratory Technique in Biology and Medicine, 3rd ed. Edited by EV Cowdry. Baltimore, Williams & Wilkins, pp 253–259, 1952.
79. Street CM: Personal communication.
80. Tsieh S, Quintus C, Tanenbaum B: Morphologic criteria for the identification of *Pneumocystis carinii* in Papanicolaou-stained preparations. Acta Cytol 30:80–81, 1986.
81. Tutuarima JA, Hesche EA, Sylva-Steenland RMR, Wander-Helm HJ: A cytopreparatory method for cerebrospinal fluid in which the cell yield is high and the fluid is saved for chemical analysis. Acta Cytol 2:425–427, 1988.
82. Wheeler TM, Johnson EH, Coughlin D, Greenberg SD: The sensitivity of detection of asbestos bodies in sputum and bronchial washings. Acta Cytol 32:647–650, 1988.
83. Whitmore EL, Hochberg F, Wolfson L, Royalty J, Taft P: Quantitative cytocentrifugation in the evaluation of cerebrospinal fluid. Acta Cytol 26:847–850, 1982.
84. Wiseman C: DNA assessments of various modifications of Papanicolaou stained samples. Presented at the Illinois Society of Cytology Annual Spring Meeting, 1982.

33

Light Optical Microscopy

Peter H. Bartels

The light optical microscope is essential to the diagnostic assessment of clinical samples in cytopathology and histopathology. Optical instruments, such as telescopes and microscopes, present the observer with images of objects under greatly increased viewing angles, i.e., magnified, so that they appear to be nearer to the eye and finer detail can be discerned. One does not see the object itself but an image of the object. What we can learn about the object thus depends entirely on the quality of the image, and this is crucially dependent on the performance of the microscope objective.

Light optical microscopy offers a multitude of imaging modalities. Each is optimized either to bring out particular properties of the microscopic object or to allow the observation of specific processes.

We distinguish two basic types of objects: (1) objects that absorb light—their structures appear in different gray tones or in different colors—and (2) objects in which structures are optically revealed merely by differences in refractive index. Such objects have no natural contrast. They appear transparent, much like a piece of clear glass submerged in water.

Absorbing objects diminish the amount of light that transilluminates them. They are therefore called amplitude objects. Clear objects, which differ only in their refractive properties, affect the speed of propagation of the transilluminating light as it traverses the object. The wavefronts are distorted and emerge from the object delayed relative to portions of the wavefronts passing through the free background. Such deformations of the wavefront are called phase shifts. The objects causing them are called phase objects.

The vast majority of objects in clinical samples are pure phase objects, such as live cells or fresh unstained sections. Human eyes, photographic emulsions and electronic imaging devices such as video tubes, are all amplitude detectors. They detect only differences in image brightness. For phase objects to be viewed, it is necessary to generate image contrast. The rationale behind most of the different imaging modes in light optical microscopy is to generate contrast.

In **ordinary transmitted light microscopy,** objects are stained with multicolored dyes to generate contrast. In **fluorescence microscopy,** fluorophors are used to stain specific object structures. These are then seen selectively, shining with high luminosity in stark contrast against a completely dark background. In **dark field microscopy,** indirect highly oblique lighting is employed to show object contours brightly outlined against a dark background.

In **phase contrast microscopy,** the imparted phase differences are optically converted to differences in amplitude and the object appears in light/dark contrast.

Interference contrast methods take the conversion of phase differences into differences of image brightness one step further. They offer a quantitative image, in which image brightness at each point is proportional to the amount of phase difference. Other interference contrast methods generate dual images, very slightly displaced relative to each other, so that objects with phase structures appear in stark relief as if embossed. This imaging mode is also known as differential interference contrast or DIC imaging.

Polarization optics exploits natural birefringence properties of biologic objects to present images of high contrast. Polarization optics are also used in optical configurations to produce interference contrast.

Video-enhanced contrast microscopy uses both optical methods to generate contrast and video technology to enhance such contrast, to make the object's structures with extremely small phase differences visible.

In **confocal microscopy,** images are scanned, point by point, under conditions that allow greatly enhanced depth discrimination. This permits extremely thin optical sectioning of objects, and the observation of fine structures well inside a large cell or within a thick layer of tissue without being affected by degrading effects caused by the overlying material. Optical sectioning is also used to create three-dimensional reconstructions of cells and tissues. In addition, confocal microscopes image small phase differences in varying brightness.

In **micromorphometry** and in **image analysis,** images are digitized and quantitative measurements are performed.

Many of these imaging modes are finding widespread application in research and, increasingly, in diagnostic assessment of clinical samples.

An extensive literature exists on light optical microscopy. An excellent introduction to the optics of the light microscope is provided by Inoue.[11] The theory of light optical microscopy is presented in the classic text by Michel.[14] Fluorescence microscopy and the multitude of techniques based on its principles are exhaustively described in the monographs by Taylor and associates[19, 20, 21] and by Thaer and Sernetz.[22] Phase contrast microscopy is treated by Bennett and associates.[5] Wolter[24] provides a superb and exhaustive discussion of the microscopy of phase structures. For the light optical microscopy of biologic materials under polarized light, a number of specialized texts are available—the well-known text by Bennett[6] and a particularly well-written chapter by Schmidt.[18] Application of polarization optical methods to histopathology is the exclusive subject of a text by Scheuner and Hutschenreiter.[17] Inoue discusses very high sensitivity polarizing microscopy.[10] For interference microscopy the most comprehensive discussion of light optical instrumentation is given by Krug and colleagues.[13] There is also the text by Hale[9] and the rigorous discussion of the optics involved by Francon.[8] Video-enhanced microscopy is discussed by Inoue[11] and by Allen and coworkers.[1, 2, 3] Confocal microscopy is the subject of a text by Wilson and Sheppard[23] and of the excellent monograph edited by Pawley.[16] Digital image analysis in the cytopathologic and histopathologic laboratory is the subject of texts by Baak and Oort,[4] Oberholzer[15] and Burger and associates.[7]

It is the goal of this chapter to present those principles of light optical microscopy whose understanding is essential to attain effective use of the instrument.

IMAGE FORMATION

In all imaging modalities, it is the performance of the objective that determines the information contents of the image. It may therefore be helpful to begin with a discussion of image formation in a light optical microscope. To facilitate an understanding of the processes involved in image formation, and of the factors ultimately limiting performance, idealized model objects are useful. For the imaging of an object point into an image point we consider a very small, round, back-illuminated object, such as a tiny pinhole in a metallized slide. For the discussion of image resolution and diffraction limited imaging, we consider model objects, such as gratings, i.e., arrays of parallel, opaque and fully transparent stripes, each grating with a different spacing of the stripes.

The imaging of an object point into an image point

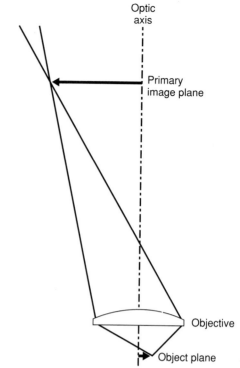

FIGURE 33–1. Object point imaged into image point; **geometric optics** representation.

by an objective is shown in Figure 33–1. The process is illustrated by drawing straight lines, or rays, to show the resulting magnification and how the rays emanating from the object point come to a sharp focus at the image point. This representation by **geometric optics** is eminently useful for the design of optical systems. Light paths are indicated by straight lines that bend at sharply defined angles when refracted by an optical element and which intersect to form a mathematically fine image point.

Geometric optics are, however, a simplified abstraction, which provides valid predictions only under conditions in which light interacts with relatively large objects. Geometric optics ignores the wave nature of light.

In reality, light propagates in the form of electromagnetic waves. The wavefield has a distinct structure, defined by the frequency of the radiation, the amplitude of the electromagnetic field and the divergence of the wavefronts. The imaging of a luminous object point into an image point is therefore better represented by the process shown in Figure 33–2, where the focus is seen as the point of greatest constriction of the wavefield.

Geometric optics with its rays and extremely sharp focus ignores the inherent structure of the imaging medium. It assumes the wavelength to be zero. Thus, all objects are large when compared with this inherent structure, and **resolution** is infinite in geometric optics. In the real world, light waves interact with objects. When the objects are comparable in dimension to the wavelength of light, the predictions derived from geo-

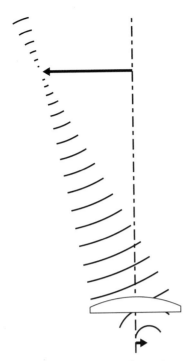

FIGURE 33–2. Object point imaged into image point; **converging wavefronts** shown.

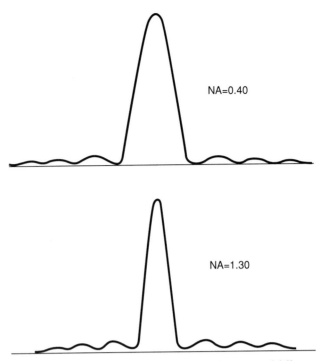

FIGURE 33–4. Point spread functions of objectives of different numerical apertures (N.A.).

metric optics are no longer valid. To describe the interaction of light with small objects, one has to consider **diffraction theory.** Most certainly this is the case when one discusses the limit of resolution of a light optical microscope.

The image of the small, back-illuminated pinhole is not simply a sharply delineated small round spot. Instead, the image consists of a **diffraction pattern,** with a central bright maximum, surrounded by a series of alternating dark and bright rings, decreasing rapidly in brightness, as seen in Figure 33–3. The diameter of the central maximum is determined by the objective, specifically by the numerical aperture of the objective and by the wavelength of light. The diameter of the central maximum is independent of how small the pinhole in the object plane is. This is as small a point as the particular objective will image. The diffraction pattern is also known as the **point spread function** (PSF) of the objective. The higher the numerical aperture of an objective, the smaller is the half-inten-

sity diameter of the PSF, as is shown in Figure 33–4. If the PSF is as sharply defined as the objective's design specifications allow, and if it is not broadened by optical system aberrations, one speaks of **diffraction-limited imaging.**

Clearly, the PSF sets a limit to how closely spaced two points could be in the object plane and still be discerned as two separate points.

Convention has set this limit of resolution to the distance from the maximum of the PSF to the location of the first dark ring. If the maximum of one point's diffraction pattern is not closer than this distance to another point's maximum of the diffraction pattern, the dip in image intensity is considered to offer sufficient contrast for the human eye to discern two points. This limit is also known as the Rayleigh limit (Fig. 33–5), and it is calculated as

d = 1.22 × wavelength / 2 × Numerical Aperture

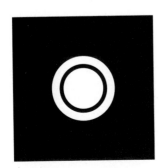

FIGURE 33–3. Diffraction pattern or "Airy disk."

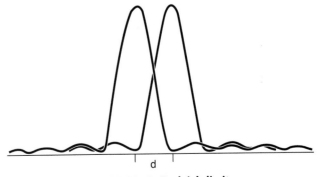

FIGURE 33–5. Rayleigh limit.

To give a numeric example, an objective with a numerical aperture (N.A.) of 1.40 and illuminating light of a wavelength of 560 nm would have a Rayleigh limit of $1.22 \times 0.56 / 2 \times 1.4 = 0.24\,\mu = d$. Applied to the resolution of a set of alternating opaque and fully transparent stripes, the distance d translates into line pairs/mm. To sample the image information fully, the Nyquist theorem requires that sample spacing provide two sampling spots for the highest spatial frequency, hence, the line pair. The spatial frequency where contrast has decreased so that the line structure can no longer be seen, and where the area simply appears uniformly gray, is called the **spatial cut-off frequency of the objective.** For the objective considered in the numeric example here, this would be at 4166 line pairs/mm.

The ability of the objective to render object contrast in the image, as a function of spatial frequency, is defined by the **contrast transfer function.** At low spatial frequencies (when opaque and transparent stripes are wide and the number of line pairs/mm is modest), contrast may be fully preserved in the image, at 100%. As the spatial frequency of the grating increases to more line/mm, image contrast will decrease gradually until, at the Rayleigh limit, the human eye can just discern stripes (Fig. 33–6).

When the object contrast is described by a square wave function (black and transparent stripes), one speaks of the contrast transfer function. When object contrast follows a sinusoidal curve, one speaks of the modulation transfer function (MTF) and the modulation of object contrast in the image.

Gratings of different spatial frequencies are, in fact, the model underlying the mathematic considerations that enter into the analysis of diffraction-limited imaging. Objects in general, be they cells or tissue sections, are composed of structural details falling into a wide range of spatial frequencies. Object structures diffract light, as discussed subsequently in more detail, and may be modeled as a superposition of diffracting gratings spanning the full range of spatial frequencies. Gratings of different spatial frequencies thus may serve for a discussion of the processes involved in the imaging of objects in light optical microscopy.

The equation defining the smallest detail that a microscope objective can resolve, or the highest spatial frequency for which the image still offers acceptable contrast, contains two quantities: the wavelength of light and the N.A. of the objective. To understand how these two entities are involved, we have to examine the phenomenon of diffraction.

Figure 33–7 shows how a plane wavefront coming from below encounters a very small object. The direct illuminating wavefront interacts with the object's structure. This results in "kicking off" a wavelet, also called an elementary wave, an object wave or a **diffracted wave.** A wavelet has the object structure as its point of origin and it spreads forward with a spheric, diverging wavefront. Let us assume that there is another tiny object close by. Its interaction with the same wavefront also produces an object wave. The two object waves have in common that they were generated by the same wavefront; thus, they retain a fixed mutual relationship. They are **in phase,** they are **coherent** and, there-

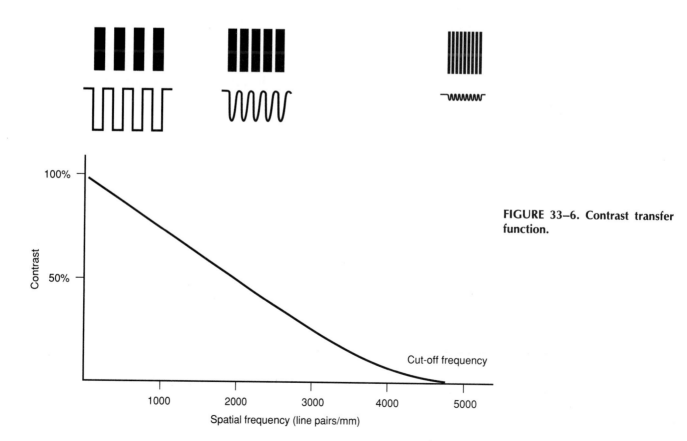

FIGURE 33–6. Contrast transfer function.

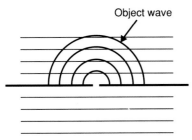

Object wave

FIGURE 33–7. Plane wavefronts transilluminating an object; an object structure giving rise to a diffracted wavelet.

fore, their electromagnetic wavefields can interact. This interaction takes the form of **interference.** The strength or the amplitude of each of the two wavefields at a given point may add up, leading to **constructive interference.** Under slightly different conditions, the two wavefields may counteract each other and cancel out, in a process called **destructive interference.**

It is instructive to draw this to scale. In Figure 33–8, two object points giving rise to diffraction are shown. They have a distance from each other that is of the same order of magnitude as the wavelength.

The semicircles represent the spheric wavefronts of the two object waves. We assume that they are drawn on the wavecrest, i.e., at the point of greatest amplitude of the wavefield. Where wavecrest falls upon wavecrest, constructive interference will occur. The two wavelets will reinforce each other. As we see in Figure 33–8, such reinforcement occurs in certain directions only. These directions are called the **orders of diffraction.** Conditions for constructive interference exist in direction of propagation of the original illuminating wavefront; this is called the zero order. Higher orders are also possible. The first order appears under an angle closest to the zero order. There is symmetry about the direction of the original illuminating wavefront. Thus, there is a +I. order, and a −I. order. At higher angles, one can observe the +II. order and the −II. order, a +III. order and a −III. order and so forth, as shown in Figure 33–8.

If there were no object structure there would, of course, not be any diffracted light. The information about the object is, so to speak, entrusted to the diffracted wavelets to carry forward and form an image. To be able to do so, clearly, the diffracted light must enter the objective. Here is where we begin to understand the role of the N.A. of the objective. The N.A. of the objective measures the angle of acceptance for light, as illustrated in Figure 33–9.

Light diffracted under a very high angle, e.g., for the higher orders, at an angle beyond the angle of acceptance of the objective, simply cannot contribute to the formation of an image. It is lost, as is the information it carries. Although contribution of light of the higher orders to the formation of the image certainly is helpful, it has been established that sufficient information to image the object is retained if at least light diffracted into the first order enters the objective.

To examine the relationship among N.A., diffraction of light by the object structures and attainable resolution, we consider Figure 33–10. Here, the same situation as in Figure 33–8 is depicted. However, the two diffracting object points are much closer together. One can see that the directions under which conditions for constructive interference occur now appear under a much greater angle. Let it be assumed that the first order of diffracted light in this case still enters the objective aperture, i.e., the dimension of the object structure is still above the spatial cut-off frequency. For two object points any closer, the angle of diffraction for the first order would be so high that the diffracted light by-passes the objective aperture. One has reached the limit of resolution. Actually, this is not quite true. It has also been shown that it is not necessary to have diffracted light from both the −I. order and the +I. order to image the object. The contribution of one of the two is sufficient. If one illuminated the object with a plane wavefront under a high angle to begin with, so that the zero order barely entered the aperture on one side, one would have the full angle of the objective aperture open to accept the

FIGURE 33–8. Diffraction into different orders.

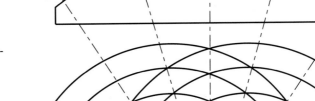

0.

−I.   +I.

Order

−II.   +II.

−III.   +III.

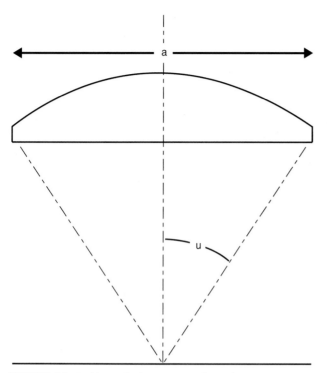

FIGURE 33–9. Numerical aperture of an objective—**acceptance angle u.**

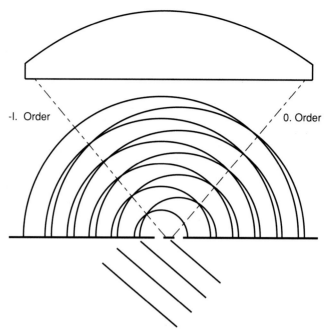

FIGURE 33–11. Object structure of a smaller dimension, illuminated under high aperture, such that at least one of the first orders still enters the objective's aperture.

first order of light diffracted by object points twice as close as shown in Figure 33–10. This illumination is shown in Figure 33–11. It explains why, for the full resolution, objective and condensor aperture should match, and the aperture stop in the condensor should be fully opened. Only then can the object be illuminated with parallel light under such a high angle of incidence.

What remains to be shown is the role of the wavelength of the illuminating light on resolution. A scale drawing of two diffracting object points is helpful. In Figure 33–12, the situation is shown for two object points spaced such that the first order of diffraction, for red light of 650 nm wavelength, appears under a certain angle. In Figure 33–13 the same point spacing

is given, but now the wavelength of the illuminating light is much shorter—blue light of 400 nm wavelength.

Blue light is diffracted at a lesser angle than red light. Therefore, for even smaller structures than shown here where the first order of diffraction for red light already misses the aperture of the objective, the first order of diffraction for blue light still contributes to the image. Blue light can therefore resolve finer detail. The PSF is smaller, and the system has a higher spatial cut-off frequency for shorter wavelengths. The discussion up to here has concerned itself with the process of diffraction, the role of the wavelength of light in its relation to the dimension of object structures and the role of the N.A. of the objective. What has not yet been addressed is the formation of the image.

We are using a model object to discuss the underlying processes—a grating with opaque and transparent parallel stripes of a spatial frequency that even some of the higher orders of diffraction can enter the aper-

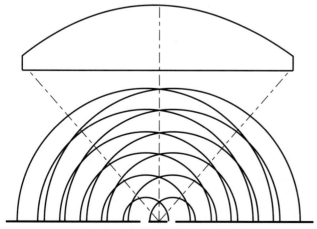

FIGURE 33–10. Object structure of a dimension such that first order of diffraction still just enters aperture of the objective.

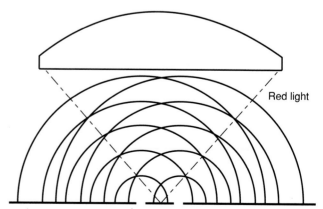

FIGURE 33–12. Object structure of a dimension that for illumination in red light first order still just enters objective.

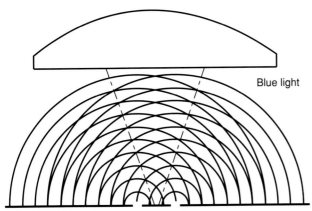

FIGURE 33–13. Illumination in blue light of the same structure as in Figure 33–12 still admits the second order. In blue light, object structures of even higher spatial frequency could be resolved.

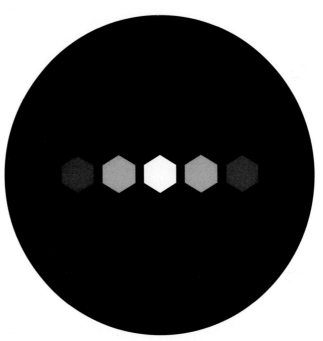

FIGURE 33–15. Appearance of **back focal plane** of the objective. Aperture stop almost closed, and a grating is used as object, e.g., a stage micrometer. The different orders of diffraction each form an image of the source and of the aperture stop. From here, light of the different orders spreads into the interference space towards the primary image plane.

ture of the objective. Also, for the following discussion, we assume that the aperture stop has been closed almost completely. Light diffracted by the specimen, and, of course, the direct light (the zero order), enters the objective as parallel beams—under different angles, but as parallel beams—each with straight wavefronts. The objective thus will focus these beams in its back focal plane (see Fig. 33–14). There, a small image of the source and of the nearly closed aperture stop is formed on axis, flanked by fainter side images of the + − I. order, and the + −II. order of the diffracted light. They all lie on one diameter of the back focal

plane of the objective, spread out in the direction of the diffraction grating serving as object (Fig. 33–15).

Wavefronts propagating in the space between object and objective, under different angles with respect to the optic axis, come to focus in the back focal plane of the objective in different locations. The greater the angle to the optic axis in the object space, the more towards the periphery in the back focal plane will they come to focus.

Because, as we have seen, structures of higher spatial frequencies give rise to diffracted light whose first orders form a large angle with the optic axis, the high frequency information about the object, the information about the finest object structures, appears at the periphery in the back focal plane of the objective.

The higher the N.A. of the objective the more of the high frequency detail of the object can contribute to the image. If one closes the aperture stop in the condensor—which is in the plane that is conjugated and imaged into the back focal plane of the objective—diffraction from some of the higher spatial frequency components in the object never even enters the objective.

From the back focal plane the light from all of these source images spreads out into the space behind the back focal plane, with all of the wavefields permeating each other. However, the diffracted light and the direct light are coherent and can interfere. This is precisely what happens throughout this space, which therefore is also referred to as the **interference space.** The interference leads to a distinctive distribution of brightness and darkness throughout the interference space. However, we are interested only in the distribution of

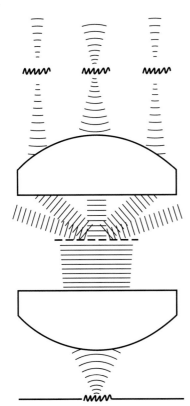

FIGURE 33–14. Diffracted orders coming to focus in the back focal plane of the objective, forming images of the filament and aperture stop.

brightness and darkness—and of color— in a very specific plane in that space. This is the plane at right angles to the optic axis, which is conjugated to the object. It is the plane where all the rays, as traced by geometric optics from the object and through the objective, come to focus. This is the image of the object plane. The distribution of brightness and darkness and of color is the result of the multitudinous interference processes between the direct and the diffracted light. We hope that the image reflects, in its visual appearance, in its morphometric properties and photometric values, the physical characteristics of the object.

KOEHLER ILLUMINATION

Any light optical microscope is made of five distinctive functional components: (1) the light source and the optics to transilluminate the specimen, (2) the microscope objective, (3) the ocular (and, if applicable, a projective lens system), (4) the field diaphragm or **bright field stop** and (5) the aperture stop in the condensor.

The field diaphragm is an adjustable stop. It is usually mounted close to the collector lens in front of the light source. It is the role of the **field stop** to provide a clear delineation of the illuminated area of the specimen, to limit it to the area that the objective actually shows. It thus **prevents stray light** originating in object areas not even in the field of view from entering the objective and lowering image contrast.

The aperture stop also is an adjustable iris diaphragm. It is, in most microscopes, firmly built into the substage condensor. The **aperture stop** is one of the most crucial controls of a light optical microscope. It allows the user to control **image contrast,** and with that, the **attainable resolution.** For a specimen of ideal contrast, prepared with a coverglass of correct thickness and not an excessive layer of mounting medium, the aperture stop could be left all the way open. Most average specimens, however, have deficiencies—low contrast staining, too thick a layer of mounting medium and coverglass of incorrect thickness. These cause problems for observation under high-dry objectives. The most serious problem is spherical aberration in the image (not to be confused with image curvature). Spherical aberration causes a milky image from center to periphery. This can be reduced by closing the aperture stop in the condensor, by about a third, but one should be aware that this is a necessary compromise. The gain in contrast, after removal of the spherical aberration, has to be paid for by a loss of resolution.

To attain high quality imaging, proper alignment of all components is essential. The almost universally accepted optical alignment is known as **Koehler illumination.** It provides several advantages.

In Koehler[12] illumination the field of view is uniformly illuminated. It is possible to exert independent control over the area of the illuminated field—by adjusting the field stop—and over image contrast, and

effective N.A., by adjusting the aperture stop. In Koehler illumination, the specimen is transilluminated by parallel beams. This provides conditions under which both lateral and axial resolution are maximized.

In a microscope set up for Koehler illumination there exist two simultaneous beam paths. The first provides for the illumination; it is referred to as the **direct light** beam path, and it is shown in Figure 33–16. Light from the filament of the **source** is collected

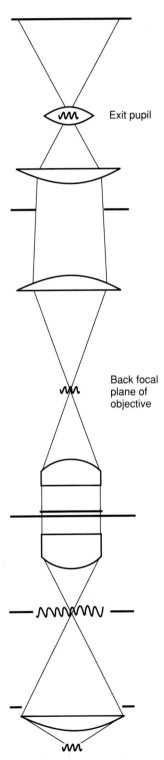

Exit pupil

Back focal plane of objective

FIGURE 33–16. Koehler illumination, **direct light beam path.**

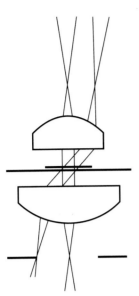

FIGURE 33–17. Transillumination of object by **beams of parallel light.** Points at the periphery of the aperture stop give rise to parallel beams transilluminating the object under the highest aperture.

by a collector lens, which projects an enlarged image of the filament into the plane of the **aperture stop.** This image of the source, in the aperture stop plane, becomes effectively the light source. The aperture stop is mounted in the front focal plane of the condensor. Therefore, the light emerging from the condensor and transilluminating the object is parallel. The parallel beam in the direction of the optic axis originates at the center of the aperture stop. For points off axis, the beams emerging from the condensor and traversing the specimen are also parallel beams even though they form an angle with the optic axis (Fig. 33–17).

Geometric optics tells us that any beam entering an objective as a parallel beam comes to focus at the **objective's back focal plane.** There, an image of the aperture stop, and of the filament, is formed. From the back focal plane of the objective the direct light diverges. Its divergence is slightly reduced by the bottom lens of the ocular, the so-called field lens. The direct light proceeds to illuminate the plane of the primary image uniformly. That is the plane in which the ocular has its round, fixed stop. Leaving the ocular, the direct light converges once more, in a plane a few millimeters above the ocular, in the so-called **exit pupil of the microscope.** This plane is also conjugate to the light source, the aperture stop and the back focal plane of the objective. The exit pupil of microscope is where the pupil of the observer's eye should be, so that the exit pupil of one system—the microscope—and the entrance pupil of the next—the eye—coincide. When the pupils do not coincide, vignetting occurs, i.e., one will see only the center of the field.

The second beam path is associated with the formation of the image, imparting structure on the uniformly bright background provided by the direct light. This second beam path is often referred to as the beam

path of the diffracted light, or as the **image-forming beam path,** as seen in Figure 33–18.

Light is diffracted by the object and spreads into a wide cone. The object plane is focused by the objective into the primary, or **intermediary image** plane, located inside the ocular. It is in the front focal plane of the ocular's eye lens. The beams thus leave the ocular as parallel beams; to the observer, they seem to come from infinity. Because the object seems to be at infinity the eye is adapted to infinity and relaxed. The lens in the observer's eye focuses the beam onto the retina, forming a **retinal image** of the object.

A second component to the image-forming beam path exists. The condensor projects an image of the **field stop** sharply into the object plane. It appears in sharp focus together with the object.

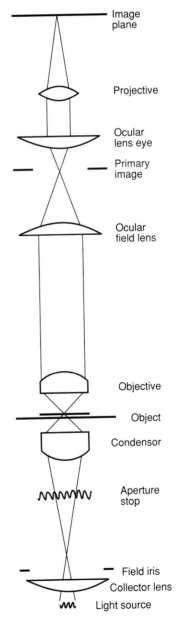

FIGURE 33–18. Koehler illumination, **image-forming beam path.**

Thus, in Koehler illumination, two sets of conjugated planes are present. In the direct beam path, the source filament, the aperture stop, the back focal plane of the objective and the exit pupil of the microscope appear in simultaneous focus. In the image-forming beam path, the field stop, the object, the primary image and the final image are in simultaneous focus. This final image may be projected onto the retina, a film plane or the face plate of a video tube.

It is not difficult to check whether a microscope is properly adjusted for Koehler illumination. The object is brought into focus. The field stop is closed down. The condensor is focused until the image of the field stop in the object plane is sharp. This focusing is done with the condensor's rack and pinion. One should not touch the fine focus of the objective during this adjustment. As one sees the edges of the field stop in sharp focus, one can also see whether the condensor is centered. If not, the centering screws in the condensor mount are adjusted until, as one opens the field diaphragm, it disappears symmetrically around the field's perimeter. Because the aperture stop is rigidly mounted in the condensor, one automatically has it in its proper position. The microscope is now set to Koehler illumination. This procedure assumes that the source filament had already been centered and focused. This can be checked in two ways. One may remove an ocular and look down into the tube, towards the back focal plane of the objective. One will see an image of the aperture stop and can observe its closing. One should also see a small image of the source filament there and whether it is centered. Unfortunately, many microscopes have built-in diffusing glass surfaces in the illuminating beam path close to the source, making it difficult to see the filament.

One may also close the aperture stop and observe the leaves of this iris from below, with a small mirror, to see the projected image of the filament.

References

1. Allen RD, Allen NS: Video-enhanced microscopy with a computer frame memory. J Microsc 129:3–17, 1983.
2. Allen RD, Allen NS, Travis JL: Video-enhanced contrast, differential contrast (AVEC-DIC) microscopy. Cell Motil 1:291–302, 1981.
3. Allen RD, Travis JL, Allen NS, Yilmaz H: Video-enhanced contrast-polarization (AVEC-POL) microscopy. Cell Motil 1:275–289, 1981.
4. Baak JPA, Oort J: Morphometry in Diagnostic Pathology. Berlin, Springer-Verlag, 1983.
5. Bennet AHB, Jupnik H, Osterberg H, Richards OW: Phase Microscopy. New York, John Wiley & Sons, 1951.
6. Bennett HS: The microscopical investigation of biologic materials with polarized light. *In* Handbook of Microscopical Technique. Edited by CE McClung. New York, Harper & Row, 1950.
7. Burger G, Oberholzer M, Goessner W: Morphometrie in der Zyto-und Histopathologie. Berlin, Springer-Verlag, 1988.
8. Francon M: Interferences, diffraction et polarisation. *In* Handbuch der Physik. Edited by S Fluegge. Berlin, Springer-Verlag, 1956.
9. Hale AJ: The Interference Microscope in Biological Research. Edinburgh, ES Livingstone, 1958.
10. Inoue S: Polarizing microscope: Design for maximum sensitivity. *In* Encyclopedia of Microscopy. Edited by GL Clarke. New York, Reinhold, 1961.
11. Inoue S: Videomicroscopy. New York, Plenum Press, 1986.
12. Koehler A: Ein neues Beleuchtungsverfahren fuer mikrophotographische Zwecke. Z Wiss Mikr 10:433–440, 1983.
13. Krug W, Rienitz J, Schulz G: Beitraege zur Interferenzmikroskopie. Berlin, Akademie Verlag, 1961.
14. Michel K: Grundzuege der Theorie des Mikroskops. Stuttgart, Wiss Verlagsgesellschaft, 1981.
15. Oberholzer M: Morphometrie in der klinischen Pathologie. Berlin, Springer-Verlag, 1983.
16. Pawley J: Handbook of Biological Confocal Microscopy. Madison, Wisconsin, IMR Press, 1989.
17. Scheuner C, Hutschenreiter J: Polarisationsmikroskopie in der Histophysik. Leipzig, Georg Thieme Verlag, 1972.
18. Schmidt WJ: Instrumente und Methoden zur mikroskopischen Untersuchung optisch anisotroper Materialien mit Ausschluss der Kristalle. *In* Handbuch der Mikroskopie in der Technik, vol 1. Edited by H Freund. Frankfurt, Umschau Verlag, 1957.
19. Taylor DL, Waggoner AS, Lanni F, Murphy RF, Birge R: Application of Fluorescence in the Biological Sciences. New York, Alan R. Liss, 1986.
20. Taylor DL, Wang YL: Methods in Cell Biology. Quantitative Fluorescence Microscopy, Imaging and Spectroscopy, vol 29, part A. San Diego, Academic Press, 1989.
21. Taylor DL, Wang YL: Methods in Cell Biology. Fluorescence Microscopy of Living Cells in Culture, vol 30, part B. San Diego, Academic Press, 1989.
22. Thaer A, Sernetz M: Fluorescence Techniques in Cell Biology. New York, Springer-Verlag, 1973.
23. Wilson T, Sheppard C: Theory and Practice of Scanning Optical Microscopy. New York, Academic Press, 1984.
24. Wolter H: Schlieren-, Phasenkontrast- und Lichtschnittverfahren. *In* Handbuch der Physik, volume XXIV. Edited by S Fluegge. Berlin, Springer-Verlag, 1956.

34

Electron Microscopy

Denise Frias Hidvegi
A. Marion Gurley

The concepts of surface and intracellular ultrastructure and organization have been developed as a result of studies done with the aid of scanning (Fig. 34–1) and transmission (Fig. 34–2) electron microscopy, respectively. Microscopes using electron beams instead of light for definition of cellular images can be of two types: transmission electron microscopy (TEM) and scanning electron microscopy (SEM).

TRANSMISSION ELECTRON MICROSCOPY

The TEM uses an electron beam in a high vacuum environment that acts upon biologic specimens that have been turned opaque by staining them with heavy metals, such as osmium or uranium. This technique enables the visualization of the relationships among cells, cytoplasmic structures and intranuclear structures as well as morphologic features related to the nuclear envelope and cell membranes.

Because these pictures are static they do not evaluate cell function. Only by utilizing a more sophisticated technique, immunoelectron microscopy, can some facets of cell function be characterized. This technique has been used to evaluate, sometimes quantitatively, the distribution of certain antigenic determinants, within cytoplasmic and nuclear structures, by labeling antibodies with colloidal gold. The advantage of this method is that molecules (usually proteins) that are too small to be seen by conventional TEM are localized using the larger colloidal gold structures, which are visualized with TEM without difficulty (Fig. 34–3).

The intracytoplasmic and nuclear structures present in normal cells are also present to varying degrees in their malignant counterparts, and therefore the differentiation between benign and malignant cells cannot usually be made by TEM. The main use of TEM is to detect the presence of cell markers that indicate the origin of the tumor. Several intracytoplasmic structures, such as desmosomes, tonofilaments, intracytoplasmic lumina, neurosecretory granules and zymogen granules, can aid in identifying the precise origin of the neoplasm (Table 34–1).

Non-neoplastic processes, such as abnormal structure of the cilia of the respiratory passages, may cause abnormal motility of the cilia producing serious respiratory illness as in Kartagener's syndrome.[1, 30] In addition, the understanding of several medical diseases, such as amyloidosis, numerous renal diseases, Alzheimer's disease and some storage disorders, has been improved with TEM.

On April 7, 1931, the first electron microscope (EM), as we know it today, was built by Max Knoll and Ernst Riiska at the Technical University of Berlin.[33] This was the first time that two electromagnetic lenses were employed in series to create a magnified image.

Several aspects in the development of this technology were equally important and took place in a span of slightly over 50 years, following the initial design and construction of the instrument. Refinement of techniques for the preparation of biologic specimens, such as overcoming destruction of the specimens due to the heat generated by high-voltage sources, was a major initial step. Numerous scientists worked on perfecting the preparation of specimens, but the pioneer work of Ladislas Marton, initiated at the Free University of Brussels, accurately identified the problems of specimen preparation and some basic aspects of the solutions to these problems. His work suggested that biologic specimens could be spared from heat damage in two major ways: cooling the specimens and impregnating the material with a supporting medium.

Subsequently, osmium fixation with simultaneous staining became a part of the technique and is still used today with the later modification of Palade. This worker introduced buffering of osmium tetroxide solutions at pH 7.3 to 7.5 with acetate veronal, following

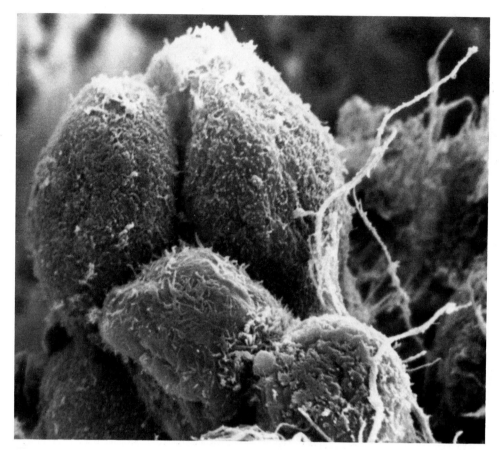

FIGURE 34–1. Adenocarcinoma in an ascitic fluid. The specimen was centrifuged and fixed in glutaraldehyde. The pellet was then dehydrated, dried at critical point and broken into several pieces. The pieces were coated in gold and examined with a scanning electron microscope. Note the fibrin in the background, and in which the cells were embedded, necessitating the fracturing of the pellet to reveal the cells (×2200).

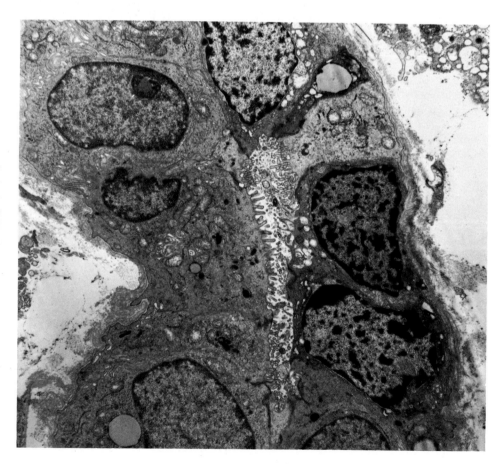

FIGURE 34–2. Adenocarcinoma of pancreas tissue fragments was harvested by scraping the surgical specimen. The material was immediately fixed in glutaraldehyde and then processed for transmission electron microscopy (uranyl acetate and lead citrate; ×3000).

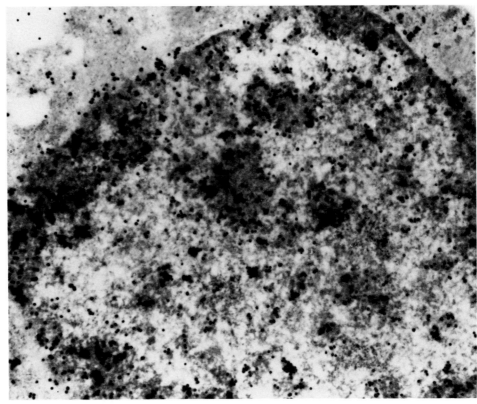

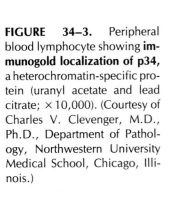

FIGURE 34–3. Peripheral blood lymphocyte showing **immunogold localization of p34,** a heterochromatin-specific protein (uranyl acetate and lead citrate; ×10,000). (Courtesy of Charles V. Clevenger, M.D., Ph.D., Department of Pathology, Northwestern University Medical School, Chicago, Illinois.)

TABLE 34–1. Selected Ultrastructural Features: Their Occurrence and Diagnostic Significance

I. Extracellular features
  A. Amyloid
    Medullary carcinoma of the thyroid
  B. External lamina
    1. Epithelial cells
    2. Carcinomas
    3. Endothelial cells
    4. Vascular tumors
    5. Schwannoma, lamina thrown into big folds
    6. Fibroblasts (Fig. 34–21)
  C. Luse bodies
    Schwannoma
  D. Reduplicated basement membrane
    Adenoid cystic carcinoma

II. Cell surface features
  A. Pseudopods
    1. Leukocytes (Figs. 34–5 and 34–14)
    2. Glomerular epithelial cells
  B. Filopodia
    1. Synovial cells
    2. Endothelial cells
  C. Interdigitations
    1. Schwann cells
    2. Schwannoma
    3. Meningial cells
    4. Meningioma
  D. Microvilli
    1. Glandular epithelium
    2. Adenocarcinoma—Figs. 34–2 and 34–17. Glycocalyx/
       glycocalyceal bodies/rootlets: well-differentiated adeno-
       carcinoma, most common in primary tumors of the colon,
       appendix and rectum but, occasionally, seen in other
       adenocarcinomas (gastric, gallbladder, pancreas, bron-
       choalveolar, mucinous cancer of ovary, endocervical).
    3. Mesothelial cells (Fig. 34–4)
    4. Mesothelioma
  E. Cilia
    Specialized glandular epithelium. In almost all instances,
    adenocarcinomas arising from these cells lose this feature
    of differentiation.
    1. Epithelium of the upper airways
    2. Bronchial epithelium
    3. Epithelium of the small bowel
    4. Endocervical epithelium
    5. Epithelium of the epididymis
  F. Junctions
    1. Desmosomes
       a. Squamous epithelium
       b. Squamous cell carcinoma (Fig. 34–18)
       c. Meningeal cells
       d. Meningioma
       e. Synovial cells
       f. Synovial sarcomas
    2. Tight junctions
       a. Glandular epithelium
       b. Adenocarcinoma
       c. Endothelial cells
       d. Vascular tumors (Fig. 34–25)
    3. Intermediate junctions
       a. Glandular epithelium
       b. Adenocarcinoma
       c. Smooth muscle cells (Fig. 34–24D)
    4. Gap junctions
       a. Squamous epithelium
       b. Squamous cell carcinoma (Fig. 34–18)
  G. Bile canaliculi
    1. Hepatocytes
    2. Hepatocellular carcinoma (Figs. 34–6 to 34–8)
  H. Pinocytotic vesicles
    1. Endothelial cells
    2. Vascular tumors (Fig. 34–25)

III. Cytoplasmic features
  A. Abundance of common structures
    1. Mitochondria
       a. Parathyroid (oxyphil cells)
       b. Thyroid (Hürthle cells)
         (1) Thyroiditis
         (2) Hürthle cell neoplasm
         (3) Hürthle cell change in follicular neoplasms
       c. Salivary gland (Oncocytes)
         (1) Oncocytoma
         (2) Warthin's tumor
       d. Liver
         Oncocytes in fibrolamellar hepatocellular carcinoma
       e. Pancreas
         Oncocytes in oncocytic neuroendocrine tumor of the
         pancreas
       f. Kidney
         Oncocytes in oncocytoma
       g. Pituitary
         Null cell adenoma
    2. Golgi apparatus
       a. Plasma cells
       b. Plasmacytoma
       c. Hepatocellular carcinoma
    3. Smooth endoplasmic reticulum
       Steroid-producing cells and their tumors
    4. Rough endoplasmic reticulum
       a. Hepatocytes
       b. Well-differentiated hepatocellular carcinoma
       c. Pancreatic acinar cells (Fig. 34–13)
       d. Plasma cells
       e. Osteoblasts
       f. Fibroblasts (Fig. 34–21)
       g. In stacked cisternae
          Steroid-producing cells and their tumors
       h. Accompanied by pleomorphic granules
          Juxtaglomerular tumors
    5. Lysosomes
       a. Tumors
         (1) Granular cell myoblastoma/schwannoma
         (2) Steroid-producing tumors as residual bodies
       b. Storage diseases
         (1) Gaucher's disease, contain 30 to 60 nm tubules
             (Figs. 34–30 and 34–31)
         (2) Fabry's disease, contain zebra bodies
         (3) Pompe's disease, contain glycogen
  B. Presence of specialized structures
    1. Filaments
       a. Thin filaments with focal densities and orderly ar-
          rangement
         (1) Myoepithelial cell
         (2) Myoepithelioma
         (3) Myofibroblast
         (4) Myofibroblastoma
         (5) Smooth muscle cell
         (6) Leiomyoma
         (7) Leiomyosarcoma (Fig. 34–23)
       b. Intermediate filaments (cytoskeletal proteins) (Fig.
          34–24C)
         (1) nonspecific morphology
            (a) Chondrocytes
            (b) Chondroid tumors
            (c) Astrocytes
            (d) Astrocytoma
            (e) Neurons
            (f) Neuroblastoma
            (g) Ganglioneuroma
         (2) Tonofilaments
            (a) Squamous epithelium (Fig. 34–24B)
            (b) Squamous cell carcinoma (Fig. 34–18)
            (c) Meningeal cells
            (d) Meningioma

TABLE 34–1. Selected Ultrastructural Features: Their Occurrence and Diagnostic Significance *Continued*

(3) Paranuclear whorls
  (a) Neuroendocrine tumors
(4) Neurofilament
  Neuroblastoma
(5) Mallory bodies
  (a) Alcoholic hepatitis
  (b) Hepatocellular carcinoma
  c. Thick filaments (myosin/Z lines)
  (1) Skeletal muscle cells (Fig. 34–24A)
  (2) Rhabdomyoma
  (3) Rhabdomyosarcoma (may also see A and I bands)
2. Discrete bodies, cytoplasmic
  a. Weibel-Palade bodies
  (1) Endothelial cells
  (2) Vascular tumors (Fig. 34–25)
  b. Zymogen granules
  (1) Chief cells of stomach
  (2) Acinar cells (Fig. 34–13)
  (3) Acinic cell carcinoma
  c. Neurosecretory granules
  (1) In large numbers
  (a) Medullary carcinoma of thyroid
  (b) Pancreatic islet cells (Fig. 34–12)
  (c) Neuroendocrine tumors
  (d) Pituitary adenoma
  (2) In small numbers
  (a) Small cell carcinoma
  (b) Neuroblastoma
  (c) Sparsely granulated prolactinoma (misplaced exocytosis)
  d. Norepinephrine granules
  (1) Adrenal medulla cells
  (2) Pheochromocytoma
  e. Beta granules
  (1) Beta islet cells
  (2) Insulinoma
  f. Birbeck bodies
  (1) Interdigitating histiocyte
  (2) Histiocytosis X
  g. Electron dense scrolled bodies
  (1) Mast cells
  (2) Mastocytosis
  h. Melanosomes
  (1) Melanocytes
  (2) Nevi
  (3) Melanoma (Fig. 34–19)
  (4) Melanotic schwannoma
  (5) Clear cell sarcoma
  i. Annulate lamellae
  (1) Germ cells and fetal cells
  (2) Germ cell tumors
  (3) Occasionally seen in many other different tumors
  j. Rod-like microtubules in rough endoplasmic reticulum
  Melanoma
  k. Mitochondria with tubulovesicular cristae. Steroid-

producing cells and their tumors
  l. Myelinoid bodies*
  (1) Type 2 pneumocytes
  (2) Bronchioloalveolar carcinoma
  m. Neurotubules
  Neuroblastoma
  n. Ribosomal-lamellar
  (1) Lymphoma
  (2) Leukemia, especially hairy cell leukemia
  o. Crystals, with 10 nm periodicity
  Alveolar soft part sarcoma
3. Abundance of intracytoplasmic substances
  a. Glycogen
  (1) Cytoplasmic
  (a) Hepatocytes
  (b) Ewing's tumor
  (c) Rhabdomyosarcoma
  (d) Renal cell adenocarcinoma
  (2) In vacuoles
  Sugar tumor of the lung
  b. Lipid
  (1) Adipocytes
  (2) Lipoma/liposarcoma (Fig. 34–20B)
  (3) Fatty change of the liver
  (4) Steroid-producing cells and their tumors (lipid is both cytoplasmic and mitochondrial)
  (5) Renal cell adenocarcinoma

IV. Nuclear features
  A. True inclusions
  1. Viral infections (most viruses that are assembled in the nucleus are DNA viruses, except measles virus, which is assembled partially in the nucleus and partially in the cytoplasm of the infected cell)
  a. Adenovirus (appears as spheric electron-dense particles in crystalline array, similar to Fig. 34–34)
  b. Herpes virus
  Core and capsid arrangement
  c. Measles virus
  Aggregates of viral microtubules
  2. Heavy metals
  a. Lead
  Feathery border
  b. Bismuth
  Sharp border
  B. Pseudoinclusions (common in papillary carcinoma of thyroid, Fig. 34–15; occasionally seen in a wide variety of other tumors)
  1. Melanoma
  2. Hepatocellular carcinoma
  C. Nuclear pockets
  Leukemia/lymphoma
  D. Nuclear fibrous lamina (thick (200 nm) in *Amoeba proteus;* up to 110 nm in reparative human cells, e.g., myofibroblasts in rheumatoid arthritis)

*May also occur artifactually, owing to formalin fixation, in cells that have phagocytosed red blood cells and because of some medications, e.g., chloroquine and amiodarone.

his discovery that excess acidity produced morphologic damage to the cell, at the ultrastructural level.[33]

In the early 1960s, the introduction of glutaraldehyde fixation greatly improved the penetration of fixative into the cells, providing much better preservation. Subsequently, the utilization of epoxy resins and sophisticated microtomes contributed to the ability to cut ultrathin sections.

Finally, an electron beam generated with a high voltage power source, 1 to 2 million volts, was developed. The heightened voltage produced images of

greater quality because the higher energy electrons have a short wavelength and, therefore, resulted in much better resolution.

SCANNING ELECTRON MICROSCOPY

Von Ardenne built the first scanning electron microscope in 1938. The function of the scanning electron microscope is based on the action of a very fine electron

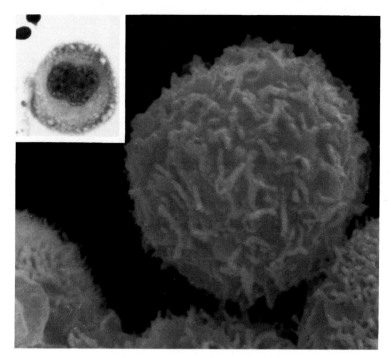

FIGURE 34–4. Mesothelial cells in a pleural fluid as seen by scanning electron microscopy (SEM). The fluid was centrifuged, fixed in glutaraldehyde, post fixed in osmium tetroxide, dried at critical point, coated in gold and examined with SEM (gold coating; ×2500). *Inset,* Light microscopic appearance of mesothelial cells (Papanicolaou stain; ×1300).

beam that scans the specimen in a television-type raster.[33] The electrons are scattered by the metal-coated specimen and collected by the scintillation crystal. The signal is then amplified by a photomultiplier and displayed on a cathode-ray tube. The extremely fine electron beam produces an excellent depth of focus, yielding impressive three-dimensional pictures.[33]

This technique provides information about the cell surface only. Several investigators have suggested that if employed selectively, and in light of clinical information and cytologic findings, SEM can be useful in the distinction between (1) atypical mesothelial cells (Fig. 34–4) and adenocarcinoma (Fig. 34–1) cells,[5, 15, 17, 28] (2) benign and malignant transitional cells[7, 8, 11, 16, 21, 24, 32, 38] and (3) benign lymphocytes (Fig. 34–5) and malignant lymphomas.[13, 14] Interpretation in this regard should be done with extreme care, as to assess the use of this technique, considering the degree of controversy in this area among various well-regarded workers.

By combining SEM with autoradiographic techniques, the possibility exists of demonstrating molecules that are synthesized by the cell, as well as cell surface receptors and antigens, using direct and indirect labeling techniques.[22]

METHODS

Cell Collection

Specimens to be submitted for EM may come from a variety of sources, and some cell types require particular collection and preparation techniques.

Aspiration

Fine needle aspirates are obtained from peripheral and deep organs, the latter with a variety of radiologic guidances.[31] Numerous techniques have been advocated, but they are basically modifications of a standard method.[20, 26, 30] The material obtained is a combination of small fragments and isolated cells mixed with fluid

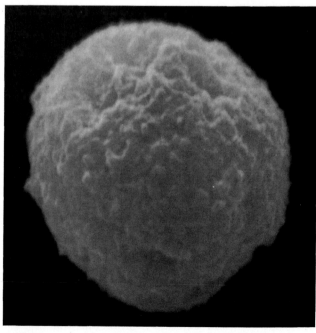

FIGURE 34–5. Lymphocyte in a pleural fluid as seen by scanning electron microscopy (gold coating; ×5000).

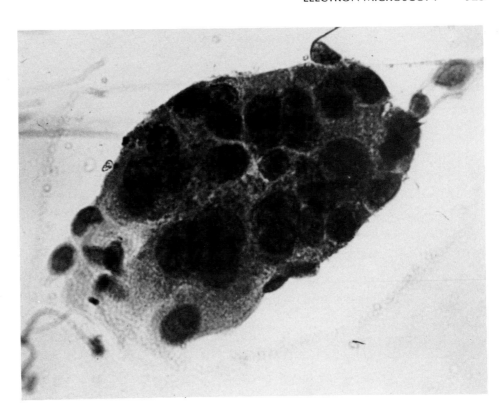

FIGURE 34–6. Fine needle aspiration of hepatic mass. A cluster of **poorly differentiated carcinoma cells** is shown (Papanicolaou stain; ×1300).

and red blood cells. These microbiopsies and single cells are adequate for studies with SEM and TEM. Some laboratories may do EM mostly in aspirates and in these instances the syringe can be rinsed with buffer. Most commonly, however, the specimen remaining in the tube after expulsion to the glass slides, is diluted with saline solution. In this instance, when a problem of interpretation by light microscopy arises, and there is a need for further studies by EM, the saline/cell solution is centrifuged and the pellet fixed with glutaraldehyde. In spite of degenerative changes, useful information can be obtained (Figs. 34–6, 34–7 and 34–8).

Exfoliated Cells—Serosal Cavities, Urinary Bladder and Spinal Fluid

Exfoliated cells, depending on the body site, may show some degree of degeneration and may be accompanied by mucus or fibrin strands, rendering the specimens technically difficult to prepare for EM studies.

Cells that float in fluids are suitable for EM even when not absolutely fresh.[4] Refrigeration at 4°C will maintain their preservation for up to 48 hours.[4] This time facilitates the cytopathologist's work when a diagnostic problem is encountered on light microscopic analysis of the cells. Although most cells found in pleuroperitoneal and pericardial effusions can be identified by TEM and SEM,[25] the diagnosis of malignancy is facilitated if the cell type identified is foreign to the environment, most commonly cells of adenocarcinoma showing glandular differentiation. Some non-neoplastic

diseases can be assessed only by light microscopy with support from TEM studies. In these cases SEM is of little value. For example, in systemic lupus erythematosus (SLE) or in drug-induced SLE-like syndromes, the characteristic cells in the effusions are polymorphonuclear leukocytes (PMLs) or histiocytes with a cytoplasmic inclusion, representing the depolymerized DNA of a lymphocyte nucleus. This depolymerization is due to the presence of anti-DNA antibodies. The cytoplasmic inclusion can be seen by light microscopy and TEM (Figs. 34–9 and 34–10) but not by SEM, which reveals only the surface features of cells. In this case, they are no different than histiocytes without the inclusion (Fig. 34–9, inset).

Cells from urine are usually well preserved except if overwhelming infection by bacterial or viral organisms is present. The red cytoplasmic inclusions commonly seen in degenerated cells do not represent viral particles. Transmission electron microscopy demonstrates that they are of a homogeneous nature without viral particles or crystalline arrays, which indicates their nonviral nature (Fig. 34–11). Spinal fluids must be refrigerated to assure preservation of cells, especially if they are of lymphoid origin.

Cyst Fluid

Fluids from cystic cavities are less well preserved than those from serosal spaces. However, despite degeneration, some useful information can be obtained from cells originating in specimens of cystic cavities. Cells obtained from cystic cavities may be from a true

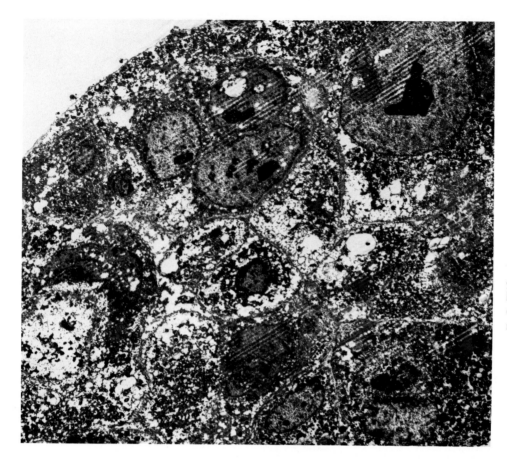

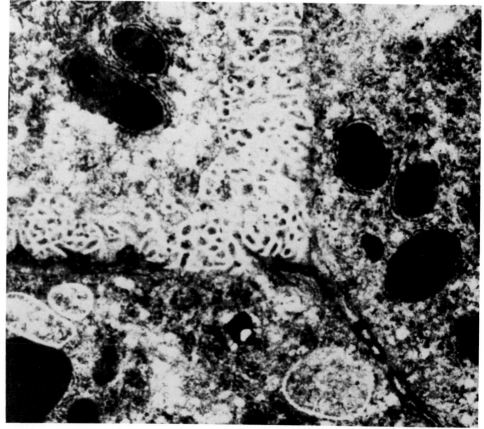

FIGURE 34–7. Transmission electron microscopy (TEM) of the aspirate shown in Figure 34–6. After preparing the slides, the needle was rinsed with saline. The rinse was then centrifuged, the pellet fixed in 2% glutaraldehyde and processed for TEM. The participation of malignant cells in the formation of a bile canaliculus establishes the diagnosis of **hepatocellular carcinoma** (uranyl acetate and lead citrate; ×960).

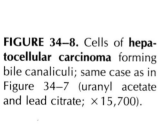

FIGURE 34–8. Cells of **hepatocellular carcinoma** forming bile canaliculi; same case as in Figure 34–7 (uranyl acetate and lead citrate; ×15,700).

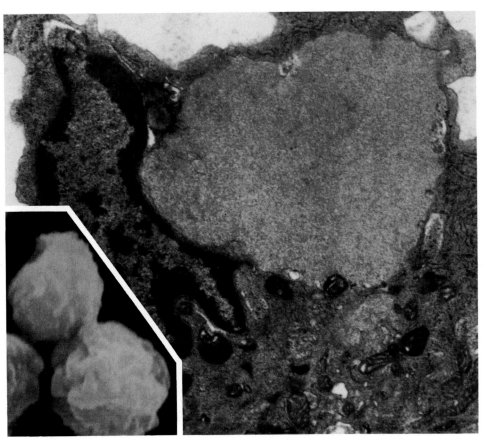

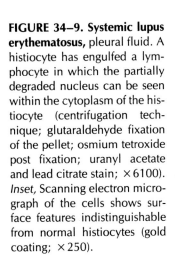

FIGURE 34–9. Systemic lupus erythematosus, pleural fluid. A histiocyte has engulfed a lymphocyte in which the partially degraded nucleus can be seen within the cytoplasm of the histiocyte (centrifugation technique; glutaraldehyde fixation of the pellet; osmium tetroxide post fixation; uranyl acetate and lead citrate stain; ×6100). *Inset,* Scanning electron micrograph of the cells shows surface features indistinguishable from normal histiocytes (gold coating; ×250).

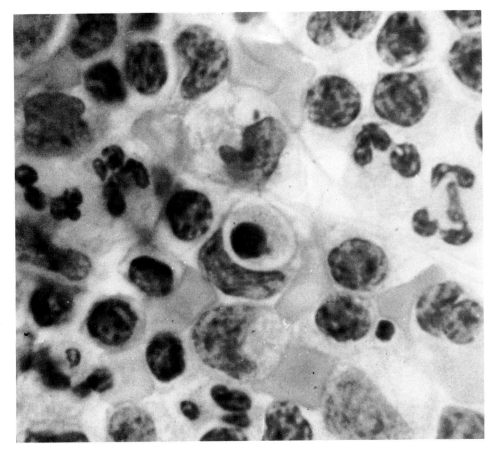

FIGURE 34–10. Systemic lupus erythematosus, pleural fluid. In the center is a histiocyte that has engulfed a lymphocyte. The chromatin of the lymphocyte is homogeneous (Papanicolaou stain; ×1300).

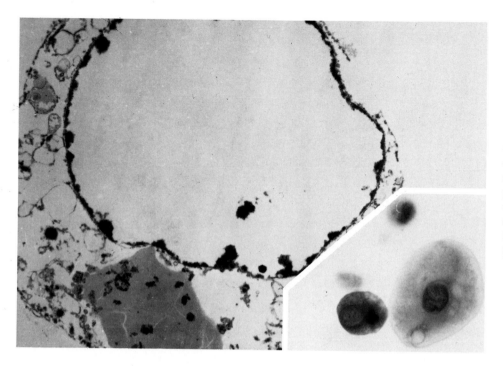

FIGURE 34–11. Urinary sediment degenerated transitional cell as seen by transmission electron microscopy. The cytoplasmic inclusion is homogeneous, without evidence of viral structures (uranyl acetate and lead citrate; ×4000). *Inset,* Papanicolaou stain; ×1300.

cystic cavity or from areas of hemorrhage and necrosis of rapidly growing solid neoplasms.

Differentiation between histiocytes and epithelial cells is not always possible by light microscopy. In this case, TEM can be of great assistance in making this distinction, despite the marked degenerative changes frequently seen in epithelial cells when they float in the cystic fluid for long periods of time. Occasionally, the epithelial cells encountered in true cystic lesions show a remarkable degree of preservation, helping in the differential diagnosis between the two cell types.

Abrasion

This method involves scrapes or brushings from the endocervix, bronchus, esophagus, stomach, colon and so forth.

The mucus that is often present in these specimens must be removed, prior to fixation for SEM studies, by saline washings of the specimens or by mechanical methods.[4] Otherwise, they obstruct partially or totally the cell surface rendering them inadequate for SEM studies. The cells are usually well preserved and suitable for TEM ultrastructural studies.

Scraping of Surgical Specimens

Scraping of the tissue surface of biopsies, during frozen section or at autopsy, can be done with excellent results. Surgical material often produces better results as preservation is usually superior. This technique is especially advantageous when very small biopsy specimens are available and EM studies are necessary. The scrape is done with a surgical blade and the small

particles of cell aggregates are placed directly into glutaraldehyde (Figs. 34–12 and 34–13). The material is further prepared using the same technique as for aspirates.

Retrieval of Cells from Slide Surface

Most frequently, this technique is employed when all the material is smeared on the glass slides and, after an attempt to diagnose by light microscopy, the need for ultrastructural studies arises.

Several modifications of a basic method by Coleman and associates[10] have been described, but most of the steps are almost the same in the various methods advocated in the literature.[4, 10, 23]

For precise identification of the cellular material to be studied, the cells are marked with a diamond pen on the undersurface of the slide and photographed. The slides are immersed in xylene and the coverslip gently removed. The xylene is removed by immersing the slides in descending grades of ethyl alcohol[4] and aqueous solution, and finally they are fixed in 2% glutaraldehyde. A capsule is filled with a monomer mixture of resin and its tip is placed over the cellular material to be examined. Where polymerization of the resin occurs, the undersurface of the slide is cooled with dry ice, and the capsule with the cells embedded in the resin is separated from the slide.

The tip of the resin cone is sectioned with the microtome, and a slice of the resin containing the cells is placed in a receiving grid to be studied by TEM (Figs. 34–14 and 34–15).

Cells attached to slide surfaces can also be studied by the SEM method. The slide can be cut in smaller pieces with the aid of a diamond pen, containing the

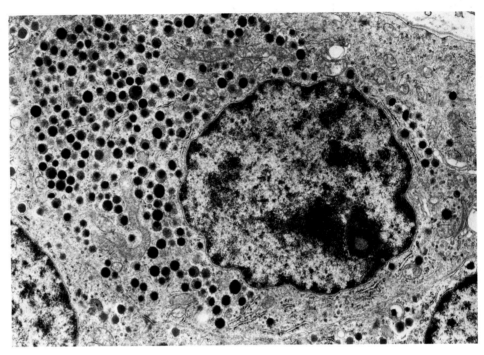

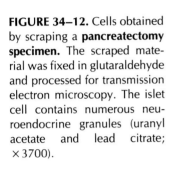

FIGURE 34–12. Cells obtained by scraping a **pancreatectomy specimen.** The scraped material was fixed in glutaraldehyde and processed for transmission electron microscopy. The islet cell contains numerous neuroendocrine granules (uranyl acetate and lead citrate; ×3700).

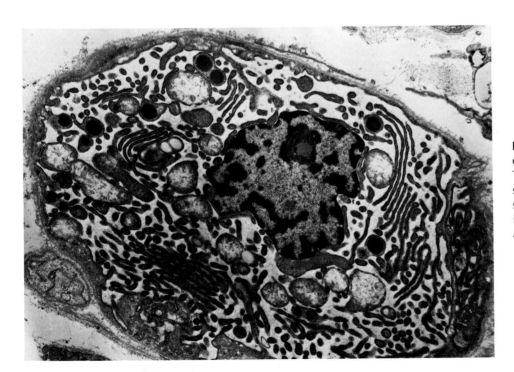

FIGURE 34–13. An **acinar cell** containing zymogen granules. The material was obtained by scraping a pancreatectomy specimen and processing it as in Figure 34–12 (uranyl acetate and lead citrate; ×7800).

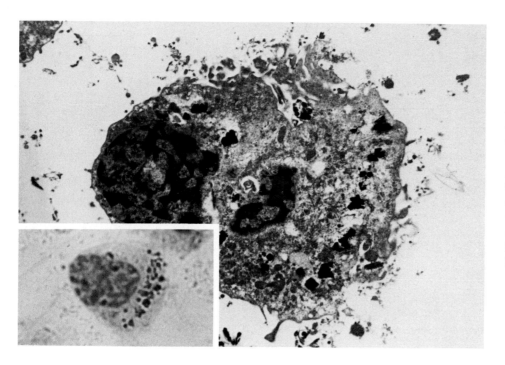

FIGURE 34–14. Kupffer cell from a rat following the injection of carmine into the caudal vein. After examination and photography of the smear *(inset),* the cell was removed from the slide as outlined in the text and stained (uranyl acetate and lead citrate; ×3200). *Inset,* Note the cell with particulate material in its cytoplasm (Papanicolaou stained smear; ×1300)

FIGURE 34–15. Fine needle aspiration of thyroid, **papillary carcinoma.** Smears were fixed in paraformaldehyde and glutaraldehyde and stained by a modified Papanicolaou stain, omitting xylene. After cytologic examination, the same cells were removed from the slide as described in the text and processed for transmission electron microscopy (uranyl acetate and lead citrate; ×3433. *Inset,* Papanicolaou stain; ×1100).

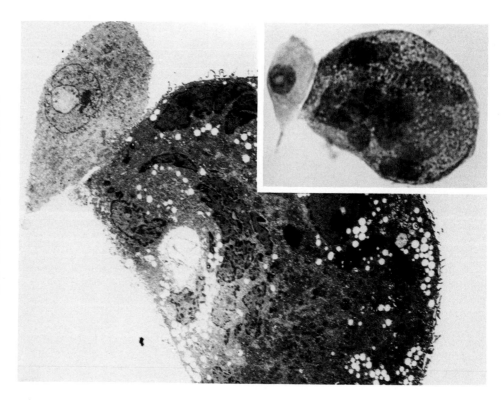

cells to be analyzed. The steps for preparation are identical to the ones used for TEM except that after dehydration the fragment of glass containing the cells is critical-point dried and coated with gold or palladium directly on the original slide.

For cells harvested from slide surfaces that have not been fixed in 95% ethyl alcohol, a more refined technique can be employed with excellent preservation of cellular detail.[23] During this procedure, air drying must be prevented.[10] The cellular material on the slide surface is fixed rapidly in 2% paraformaldehyde and 2.5% glutaraldehyde in 0.1 m sodium cacodylate buffer (pH 7.4) for 2 hours at 4°C.[26] This fixation transforms protein into stable gels with much distortion of the final state.[10] The cells are immersed overnight in cacodylate buffer to remove the excess of glutaraldehyde, to avoid reaction with OsO$_4$ during postfixation. The cells are stained by modification of the Papanicolaou technique, omitting xylene to avoid extraction of lipids from the cytoplasm, which induces pronounced degenerative changes. Also, reduced osmium is soluble in xylene, which would prevent adequate staining.[2] Lactate Ringer's solution is utilized as a washing medium, which prevents changes in osmotic pressure,[18, 19, 35] precluding cellular swelling.[42] Glycerol is utilized as a temporary mounting medium for simple removal of the coverslip to avoid damage of the cells (see Figs. 34–14, inset, and 34–15, inset).

Preparation Techniques

Several preparation techniques can be employed to harvest cells for TEM and SEM, including centrifugation and filter preparation.

Centrifugation

The cells from aspirates, fluids and cyst fluids are suspended in saline or buffer and centrifuged at 2000 revolutions/minute (RPM) for 5 minutes. Bloody specimens produce a coat of nucleated cells on top of the red blood cells, and this detail should be observed when cutting the cell blocks after fixation. For TEM after carefully pipetting the supernatant fluid, the pellet is fixed with glutaraldehyde for 1 hour, after which time it is removed and diced into 1- to 2-mm cubes.

After being processed as in the original EM procedures and embedded in resin, thick sections (1 to 2 μ) are cut with the microtome, placed on a glass slide surface and stained with toluidine blue. The thick sections are assessed by light microscopy and a field containing the pertinent cells is chosen. By trimming the block around the field containing diagnostic cells, a small portion of the block can be cut in thin section (75 nm) and placed on grids to be stained with osmium and studied by TEM.

For SEM after the supernatant is discarded some cells are pipetted from the uppermost layer smeared on the slide and prepared as described for smears.

Filter

Fluids containing cells and aspirates suspended in saline solution can be passed through filters and analyzed by TEM and SEM. Nucleopore filters (13 μ in diameter: Nucleopore Corporation, 7035 Commerce Circle, Pleasanton, CA 94566) give superior results and are the best choice.[4]

The fluid is passed through the filter, followed by glutaraldehyde for fixation and postfixed with OsO$_4$. The specimen is then further dehydrated to absolute alcohol[4] and cut in two halves for TEM and SEM.

For embedding, the filters can be cut in smaller portions before placing them in the embedding molds containing the epoxy resin. After embedding, the molds are trimmed, thick sections are cut, stained and analyzed and finally thin sections are produced to be examined by TEM

Beals[4] has written a detailed account of all the steps of filter preparation for SEM and TEM and helpful hints regarding their preparation.

Fixation

Alcohol

For EM 95% ethanol gives adequate results; however, some degree of degeneration can be seen in the photographic material (see Figs. 34–6, 34–7 and 34–8).

Usually, the specimen has been smeared and stained by the Papanicolaou technique and then retrieved from the slides. During the Papanicolaou staining the xylene dissolves lipid material from the cells, including the components of the cell membrane.[4] When the coverslip is removed, in the xylene bath, for cell retrieval, the damage is already done; no extra care should be taken to avoid further degeneration.[4] Despite the drawbacks of specimens fixed in 95% alcohol and retrieved from slides, the material is still adequate for diagnostic purposes.

Glutaraldehyde

Cells smeared on slides from various sources, such as tissue imprints, centrifuged fluids and filter preparations, can be fixed in glutaraldehyde with excellent results. The quality of the material is excellent and the preservation of the cells is very good, even when the cells are retrieved from the slide surface (Fig. 34–15).

Cellular material, smeared on glass slides and stained by the Papanicolaou technique, following fixation with glutaraldehyde instead of 95% ethyl alcohol, loses some of the staining qualities demonstrated by fixation with 95% ethyl alcohol by light microscopy. The stain of the cytoplasm and nuclei is of a flat uniform bluish color. However, the preservation of the smear is excellent for electron microscopy studies and more than adequate for diagnostic purposes.[23]

INTERPRETATION

Examination of specimens by TEM should be approached in a systematic fashion. Features to be assessed include the presence of extracellular material, the relationship of cells to each other, the presence and nature of intercellular junctions, the presence and type of cytoplasmic structures and the presence of specific nuclear structures. Table 34–1 lists, in such a systematic fashion, the most commonly encountered ultrastructural features and their diagnostic significance. When the features are illustrated in this chapter, the figure numbers are also indicated in Table 34–1.

Histogenesis of Tumors

Epithelial Cells

Epithelial cells usually have ultrastructural characteristics that can identify them as such. Commonly, adenocarcinomas may have mucin production (Fig. 34–16) or intracytoplasmic lumina containing mucin droplets (Fig. 34–17). Benign glandular epithelium shows lumen formation between two or more epithelial cells, creating a ductule or duct. In malignant epithelium, this higher degree of organization is commonly lacking and many adenocarcinomas contain cells with lumina completely formed within the cytoplasm of a single cell.

More specialized structures may resolve diagnostic dilemmas. For example, in Figure 34–6 a cluster of poorly differentiated cells from a fine needle aspiration (FNA) of liver is shown. In this case TEM was performed and demonstrated the participation of malig-nant cells in the formation of bile canaliculi (Figs. 34–7 and 34–8), establishing the diagnosis of hepatocellular carcinoma. However, two other ultrastructural features, desmosomes and tight junctions (Fig. 34–18), represent the most commonly seen indicators of epithelial differentiation. Although desmosomes are specific for epithelial differentiation, tight junctions may also be seen in some nonepithelial tumors.

The cytoskeleton of epithelial cells is composed of cytokeratins. Cytokeratins belong to a family of proteins known as intermediate filaments, which can be seen by TEM and are 10 to 15 nm in diameter.[36] Most commonly, they are of nonspecific morphology and therefore can be identified only biochemically, by immunocytochemistry. However, when they participate in the formation of specialized structures, such as tonofilaments, they can be identified by TEM (Fig. 34–18, inset).

Some tumor cells contain specific intracytoplasmic structures as seen in their benign counterparts such as neurosecretory granules (Fig. 34–12), zymogen granules (Fig. 34–13) and melanosomes (Fig. 34–19). The presence of such structures establishes the diagnoses of neuroendocrine tumor, acinic cell carcinoma and melanoma, respectively. When the diagnosis of neuroendocrine tumor is made, further classification requires correlation with the site of the tumor, hormone production and the clinical history. Depending on the degree of differentiation of the tumor, these specific cell markers may or may not be present. Another drawback is the material that may be limited in cytologic samples.

Some of these features are specific for a cell type and others overlap with a variety of cells of different histogenesis.

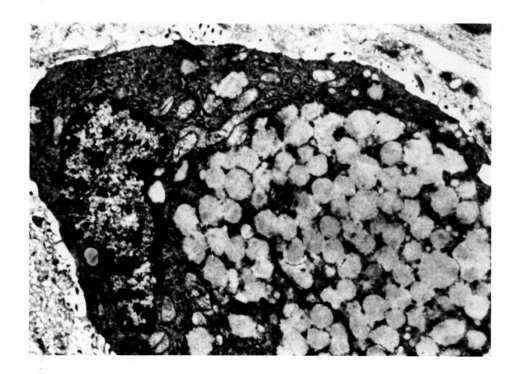

FIGURE 34–16. Mucus-producing adenocarcinoma as seen with transmission electron microscopy. Notice the many cytoplasmic droplets (uranyl acetate and lead citrate; ×7800).

FIGURE 34–17. Adenocarcinoma, pleural fluid. Within the cell is an intracytoplasmic lumen lined by microvilli, which contains a drop of mucus (centrifugation, fixation of the pellet with glutaraldehyde, post fixed with osmium tetroxide, uranyl acetate and lead citrate stain; ×15,600). *Inset,* The corresponding cytologic appearance. Two cells with intracytoplasmic lumina, each containing a drop of mucin (cytocentrifugation, Papanicolaou stain; ×1300).

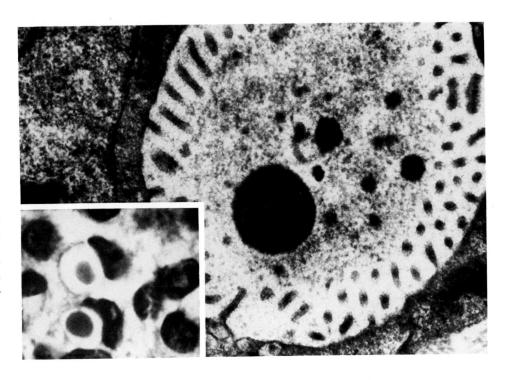

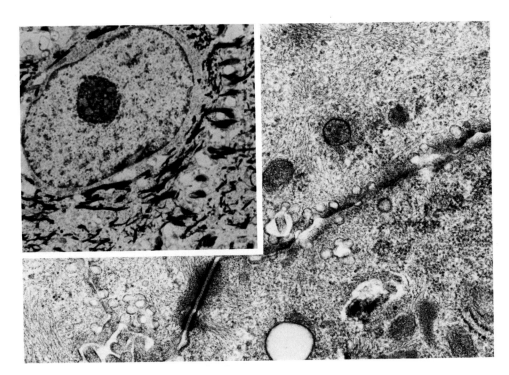

FIGURE 34–18. Squamous carcinoma showing desmosomes (×43,100). *Inset,* numerous tonofilaments are apparent (uranyl acetate and lead citrate).

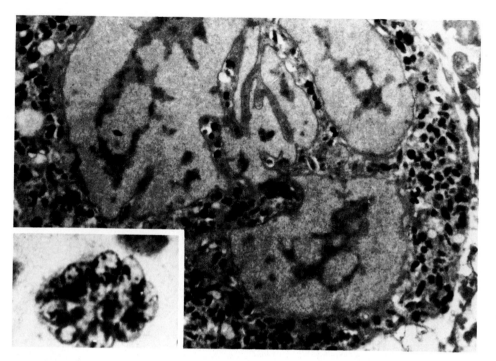

FIGURE 34–19. Malignant melanoma. Material from cerebral metastasis at autopsy. Transmission electron microscopy shows a lobulated nucleus and numerous melanosomes (glutaraldehyde fixation, osmium tetroxide, post fixation, uranyl acetate and lead citrate stain; ×5000). *Inset,* Cytologic appearance of a cell from the same case. Note the corresponding nuclear lobulations (Papanicolaou stain; ×1300). (Reproduced with permission from Hidvegi D, Koizume J, Sorensen K: Pale nodular nuclei not diagnostic of adenocarcinoma of the pancreas. Acta Cytol 26:167, 1982.)

Mesenchymal Cells

Mesenchymal cells may have specific markers in benign and malignant states, which can identify their histogenesis. Because of the intracytoplasmic location of these structures, SEM is not helpful in their identification and it is only by TEM that they can be seen.

The most important role of TEM is in establishing the histogenesis of the tumor and it is of little help in distinguishing between benign and malignant counterparts.

In malignant neoplasms of mesenchymal origin, these specific cell markers may or may not be present, depending on the degree of differentiation. In addition, because of sampling limitations, it is not always possible to successfully establish the nature of the tumor by TEM.[39]

The most frequently encountered mesenchymal tumors in cytology are liposarcomas, leiomyosarcomas and fibrosarcomas. For example, myxoid liposarcoma shows a myxoid background, with rich capillary network, fusiform mesenchymal cells and occasional lipoblasts (Fig. 34–20A). Lipoblasts, the characteristic cell of this tumor, are round cells with abundant cytoplasm that contain droplets of lipid that indent the nucleus (Fig. 34–20A, inset). Transmission electron microscopy studies confirm that the vacuolated cell is in fact a lipoblast and discloses two cell types, one with a centrally placed nucleus and the other with an excentrically placed nucleus, each with identical cytoplasmic features (Fig. 34–20A inset and Fig. 34–20B). Fibrosarcomas, when well differentiated, are difficult to distinguish from their benign counterparts in FNA. The basic cell type, the fibroblast, is an elongated cell

with a bipolar nucleus, which has pencil-shaped ends. Ultrastructurally, the spindle-shaped cell is surrounded by a basal lamina. The cell membrane contains pinocytotic vesicles. The cytoplasm is rich in rough endoplasmic reticulum, mitochondria and filaments. The nucleus, which is elongated, possesses a marginal zone of heterochromatin (Fig. 34–21).

As in fibrosarcoma, tumors of smooth muscle origin present the problem of differentiating between benign and malignant forms in FNA specimens. This same difficulty is also frequently encountered in the tissue. The cells of leiomyosarcoma are also spindle shaped. However, their bipolar nuclei have rounded ends in contrast to fibrosarcomas (Fig. 34–22). Transmission electron microscopy discloses an elongated cell invested with basal lamina with numerous pinocytotic vesicles. The cytoplasm contains myofilaments, and the cylindrically shaped nucleus is often "clefted," especially in contracted cells (Fig. 34–23).

Very few intracytoplasmic structures, when present, identify without question the histogenesis of a mesenchymal tumor. Two examples are Z bands, seen in rhabdomyosarcoma (Fig. 34–24), and Weibel-Palade bodies, seen in vascular tumors (Fig. 34–25).[34, 41]

Frequently, rather than the presence of a single feature, it is the presence of a combination of ultrastructural features that determines the histogenesis. In the majority of cases, the features demonstrated by TEM need to be interpreted in relation to the light microscopic appearances, the site of the tumor and the age of the patient. Chordoma, a neoplasm arising from notochord remnants, is characterized by the presence of physaliferous cells within a myxoid background. The physaliferous cell contains numerous cytoplasmic

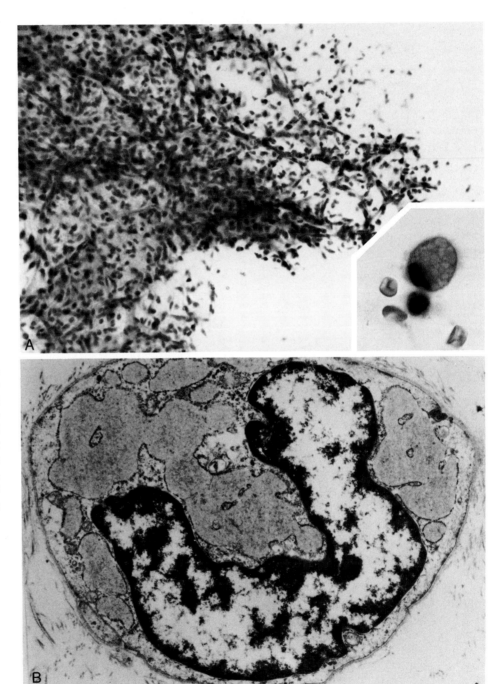

FIGURE 34–20. *A,* **Myxoid liposarcoma.** Low power appearance of smear prepared from the scrape of a surgical specimen. Notice the characteristic chickenwire like appearance of the blood vessels (Papanicolaou stain; ×260). *Inset,* A single, multivacuolated lipoblast. The vacuoles indent the nucleus (Papanicolaou stain; ×1300). *B,* Transmission electron microscopy view of a **lipoblast.** The lipid vacuoles, indenting the nucleus, are apparent (uranyl acetate and lead citrate; ×1500). (Reproduced with permission from Trump BF, Jones RT: Diagnostic Electron Microscopy, vol. 3. New York, Churchill Livingstone, 1980.)

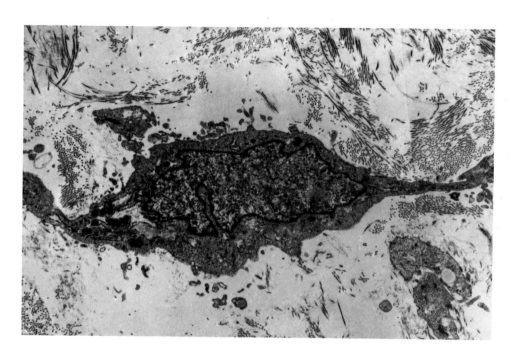

FIGURE 34–21. Fibroblast. A spindle-shaped cell with rough endoplasmic reticulum and pinocytotic vesicles (uranyl acetate and lead citrate; ×7800).

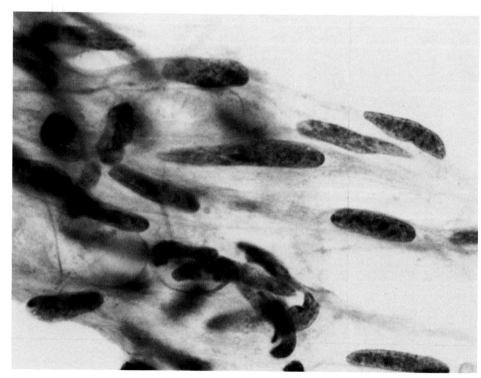

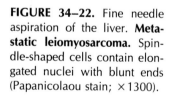

FIGURE 34–22. Fine needle aspiration of the liver. **Metastatic leiomyosarcoma.** Spindle-shaped cells contain elongated nuclei with blunt ends (Papanicolaou stain; ×1300).

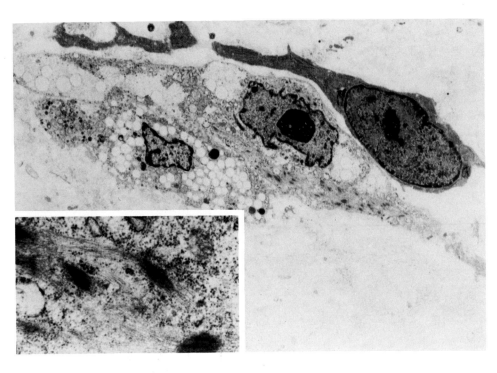

FIGURE 34–23. Leiomyosarcoma, material prepared from scrapings. Spindle-shaped cell with numerous cytoplasmic filaments (×3600). *Inset,* The filaments, which are parallel in arrangement, show focal condensations. In addition a moderate amount of glycogen is present (glutaraldehyde fixation, osmium post fixation, uranyl acetate and lead citrate; ×15,700). (Reproduced with permission from Trump BF, Jones RT: Diagnostic Electron Microscopy, vol. 3. New York, Churchill Livingstone, 1980.)

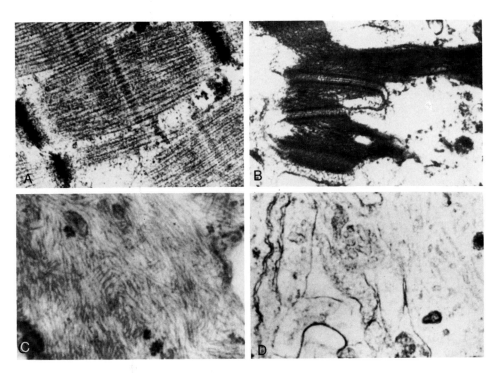

FIGURE 34–24. Various **cytoplasmic filaments.** *A,* Thick filaments with Z lines and A and I bands. *B,* Intermediate filaments forming tonofilaments that insert into desmosomes. *C,* Intermediate filaments of a nonspecific morphology. *D,* Gap junction (uranyl acetate and lead citrate).

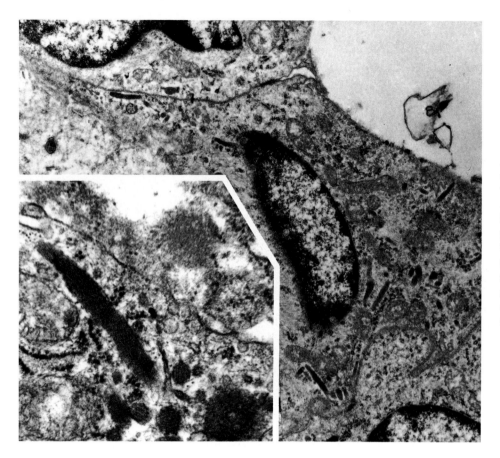

FIGURE 34–25. Cells lining a vascular lumen have tight junctions, pinocytotic vesicles and an intracytoplasmic structure (Weibel-Palade bodies). *Inset,* A closer view of the Weibel-Palade body shows the parallel arrangement of the internal structure. In this view, some are cut in cross section and others are cut longitudinally (glutaraldehyde fixation, osmium tetroxide post fixation, uranyl acetate and lead citrate; ×22,000).

vacuoles that can be appreciated on TEM along with desmosomes and intermediate filaments (Figs. 34–26 and 34–27).

Lymphoreticular Cells

The lymphoreticular system is composed of lymph nodes, bone marrow, spleen and dispersed aggregates of lymphocytes in other body sites.

The main cellular components of lymph nodes and spleen are lymphocytes in varying stages of maturation, reticulum cells and macrophages. The variability of maturation is dependent on the presence in these organs of the organized structure composed of immature cells in the germinal center that are surrounded by a mantle of mature lymphocytes. When those lymphoid follicles are aspirated, a pleomorphic population of immature and mature cells is obtained. The bone marrow contains, in addition, the precursors of the erythrocytic series, the granulocytic series and megakaryocytes.

Scanning electron microscopy has been used in some instances to differentiate between benign and malignant lymphocytes by the appearance of their surface.[13] This is a very controversial matter and for practical purposes, currently, the only malignant cell type recognized by this technique is the hairy cell leukemia (Fig. 34–28).[12] However, even benign cells may have

a striking resemblance to those neoplastic cells (Fig. 34–29).

Transmission electron microscopy rarely has application in diagnostic problems of lymphoreticular neoplasms. Benign and malignant lymphocytes appear to a certain extent morphologically similar by TEM, and monoclonality of the cells can best be evaluated by immunophenotyping using either flow cytometry or immunohistochemistry.

Occasionally, TEM is used in cytologic specimens to differentiate between a high-grade lymphoma and an undifferentiated epithelial malignant neoplasm. Also, in rare instances, when the specimen has been stained only by the Papanicolaou technique, some difficulties arise in differentiating between a lymphoma and a plasmacytoma, especially when this latter tumor is in an unusual location. However, if air-dried specimens stained by Giemsa are available, the differentiation is obvious, and no ultrastructural studies are necessary to elucidate the cell type.

Histiocytes can be transformed in benign conditions, such as in storage diseases (Figs. 34–30 and 34–31) and in benign soft tissue tumors, involving the proliferation of histiocytic cells, and in malignant conditions, such as in malignant histiocytosis, and as components of solid sarcomatous lesions, such as in malignant fibrous histiocytomas. Their morphologic appearance, especially in neoplastic processes, can be deceiving. Transmission electron microscopy assistance in these

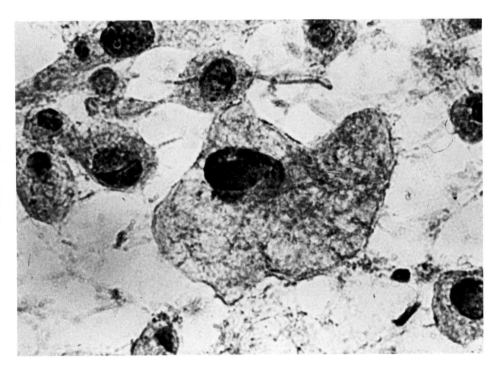

FIGURE 34–26. Fine needle aspiration of a sacral mass, **chordoma.** Several physaliferous cells are shown. They have abundant, vacuolated cytoplasm (Papanicolaou stain; ×1300).

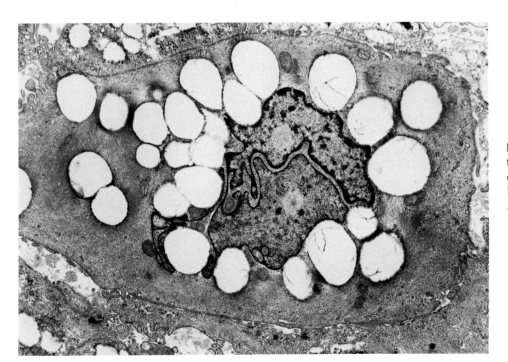

FIGURE 34–27. Chordoma, transmission electron microscopy. The physaliferous cell has vacuoles, cytoplasmic filaments and a single, small desmosome (uranyl acetate and lead citrate; ×15,100).

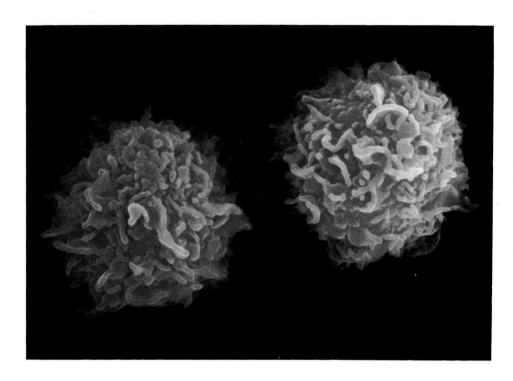

FIGURE 34–28. Hairy cell leukemia. Scanning electron microscopy demonstrates the classic cytoplasmic projections in the circulating leukemic cells (×5000). (Courtesy of Haim Gamliel, Ph.D., Department of Medicine, University of Chicago, Chicago, Illinois.)

FIGURE 34–29. Cultured human fibroblasts. Scanning electron microscopy is utilized to study cell motility. Cells are plated onto coverslips and allowed to attach to them for various lengths of time (10, 30, 50 and 70 minutes). The specimens are then dried at critical point and coated with gold before being examined with the scanning electron microscope. (Courtesy of Martin Zand, graduate student, Department of Anatomy and Cell Biology, Northwestern University Medical School, Chicago, Illinois.)

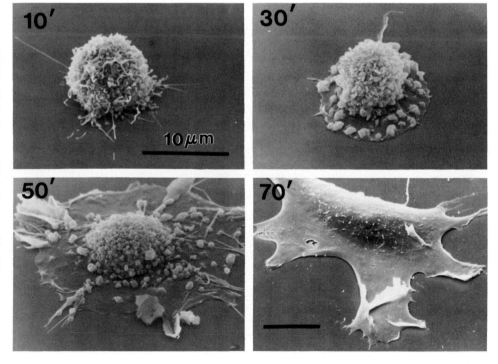

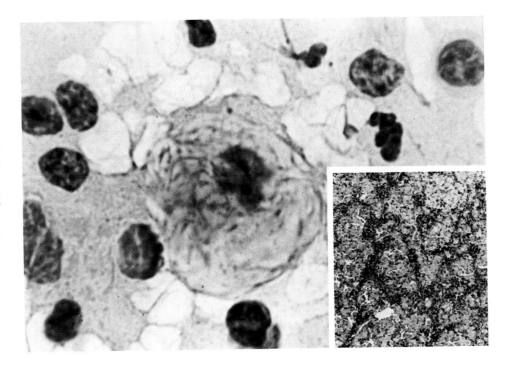

FIGURE 34–30. Gaucher's disease. A Gaucher's cell with abundant delicate cytoplasm (Giemsa stain; ×1300). *Inset,* Gaucher's disease, lymph node. Extensive infiltration of histiocytes with abundant delicate cytoplasm is shown (hematoxylin and eosin; ×260).

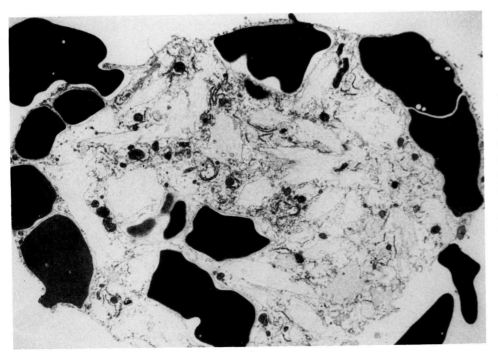

FIGURE 34–31. Gaucher's cells, transmission electron microscopy. Microtubules are contained within lysosomes (uranyl acetate and lead citrate; ×3250). (Courtesy of Zelma V. Molnar, M.D., Ph.D., Department of Pathology, Hines Veteran Administration Hospital, Loyola University, Maywood, Illinois.)

instances, especially in malignant fibrous histiocytomas, can be of great help to elucidate their nature.

Infectious Agents

The EM can be employed to study microorganisms, particularly bacteria and viruses. Its use is especially important in the detection of tumor-specific viral particles.[6] For diagnostic purposes, EM is indicated to confirm the findings encountered with light microscopy.[6]

The same methods for studying morphologic features of cells are used to study microorganisms. However, several modifications are advocated as being improvements for studying microbiologic specimens.[6]

Viruses

Cells from various sources can be examined to establish the presence of viral infection by TEM. Cells transformed by viruses can be studied by SEM, but their morphologic changes are not indicative of viral infections.

Some viral groups, such as pox viruses and herpes viruses, can be recognized by characteristic structure, by light microscopy and by TEM. Helpful ultrastructural features include size and the appearance of their cores (nucleocapsids) and of their envelopes.

Inclusions, depending on the virus, can be encountered in the cytoplasm or in the nucleus. For instance, most DNA viruses, e.g. the herpes-cytomegalic, polyoma and papilloma groups, are present in the nucleus, whereas most RNA viruses, e.g., the pox virus, are associated with intracytoplasmic inclusions, such as variola, vaccinia, cowpox and molluscum contagiosum (Figs. 34–32 and 34–33).

In cytomegalovirus, inclusions are found both in the nucleus and in the cytoplasm. Taking into account the gross and clinical findings, it is not difficult to diagnose viral changes in most cytology samples. However, some cells infected by viral particles such as papillomavirus, show only cytopathic changes and no inclusions by light microscopy. In other instances, the changes are very subtle and only by TEM can the presence of viral particles be supported.

Another virus commonly encountered in urine samples in hospital practices is polyoma virus. The polyoma virus belongs to the papovirus family and can be identified in the urinary sediments of patients with a variety of immunosuppressive states, such as renal and liver transplantations,[27] and in patients undergoing allogenic bone marrow transplantations in the treatment of various malignancies. The same virus is sometimes seen in the cervicovaginal smears of patients without immunosuppression.[10] Within the inclusion, the virus characteristically exists in the nonencapsulated state and can be demonstrated by TEM (Fig. 34–34).[10, 27] The morphology of most viruses is well maintained even with cell destruction and pronounced degenerative changes in cytologic material (Fig. 34–34).

Immunoelectron microscopy can also be utilized based on the principle that very small particles can be labeled with specific antisera, using ferritin or enzyme-conjugated antibodies, and then visualized by TEM.

Bacteria

Ultrastructural analysis of bacteria in cytology samples is of limited clinical utility. This type of work is

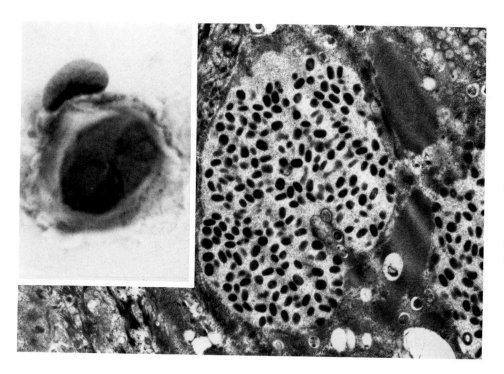

FIGURE 34–32. Molluscum contagiosum. Transmission electron microscopy prepared from material obtained by scraping the skin lesion. Notice the numerous viral structures contained with the cytoplasmic inclusion (uranyl acetate and lead citrate; ×20,300). *Inset,* An infected cell as seen in cytologic material. Note the large cytoplasmic inclusion (Papanicolaou stain; ×1300).

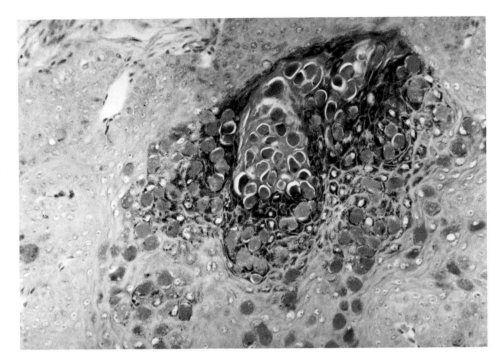

FIGURE 34–33. Molluscum contagiosum tissue (hematoxylin and eosin; ×250).

performed mainly by investigators who use microorganisms grown *in vitro*.

Protozoa

With the present cytologic and cytochemical techniques it is not necessary to perform EM studies to identify most protozoans.

The most frequent pathogenic protozoan is *Pneumocystis carinii*, frequently encountered in immunocompromised patients. *P. carinii* is a protozoan with a two-stage life cycle, the cysts and trophozoites. The cysts are thick walled and contain four to eight sporozoites. This entire structure is seen only in specimens stained by Giemsa (Fig. 34–35A) and by TEM (Fig. 34–35B).

By Papanicolaou, the cysts are viewed as negatively stained forms surrounded by cyanophilic foamy material (Fig. 34–35C).[9]

By silver stain the cysts are seen as half moons, some with longitudinal clefts, or the cysts may show a darker spot in the lighter-stained cyst walls, which has been termed "intracystic body" or "bull's eye" (Fig.

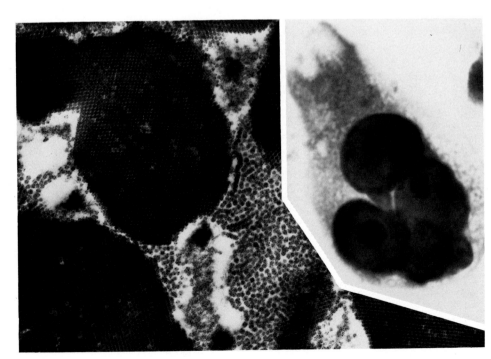

FIGURE 34–34. Polyoma virus. Urinary sediment from a bone marrow transplant patient. Transmission electron microscopy reveals the presence of viral particles (uranyl acetate and lead citrate; ×20,300).

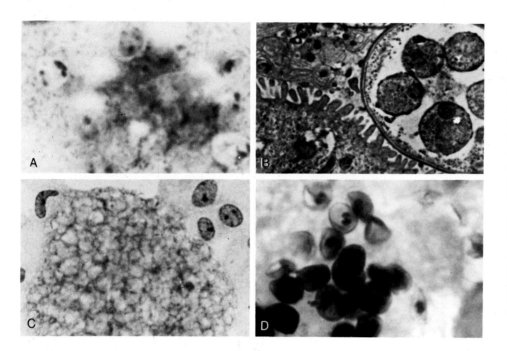

FIGURE 34–35. *A,* Bronchial brushings, ***Pneumocystis carinii.*** The cystic forms are evident, containing several sporozoites (Giemsa stain; ×1300). *B,* Electron microscopic view of *P. carinii.* A single cyst contains five trophozoites and is seen adjacent to the microvilli of the respiratory epithelial cell (uranyl acetate and lead citrate; ×9600). *C,* ***P. carinii* infection,** bronchial brushings. Note the fluffy material that forms a negative image of the organism (Papanicolaou stain; ×1300). *D,* ***P. carinii*** cysts showing collapsed walls and bull's eye formation (silver stain; ×1300).

FIGURE 34–36. Budding organism *(Cryptococcus neoformans)* demonstrating a thinner cell wall in the bud portion. Capsular material with fibrils is also shown (culture; ×10,000). *Inset,* Microfibrils in the capsule of *C. neoformans.* Some are long and coiled (autopsy brain specimens fixed in formalin; ×6300). (Reproduced with permission from Trump BF, Jones RT: Diagnostic Electron Microscopy, vol. 3. New York, Churchill Livingstone, 1980.)

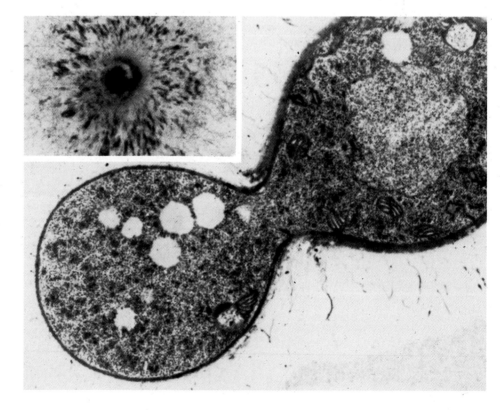

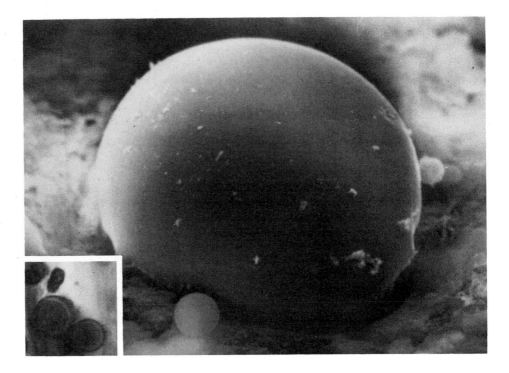

FIGURE 34–37. *Blastomyces dermatitidis,* scanning electron microscopy. The organism has a smooth surface (gold coating; ×1250). *Inset, B. dermatitidis,* budding organism (Papanicolaou technique; ×1250).

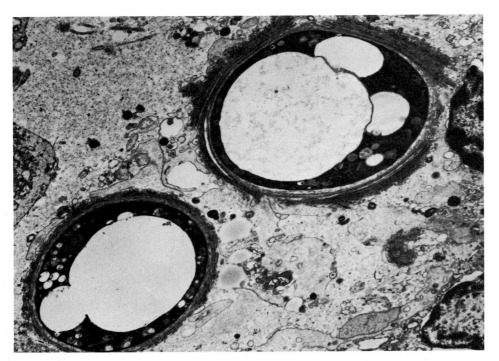

FIGURE 34–38. *Blastomyces dermatitidis.* The organisms as seen by transmission electron microscopy (uranyl acetate and lead citrate; ×3000).

34–35D). It has been demonstrated by TEM that this finding corresponds to a localized thickening of the cyst wall and is not related to sporozoites or cellular organelles.[40] The cysts' vegetative replicating states are the intracystic sporozoites that excyst as trophozoites and cannot be seen in their free stages in cytologic specimens.

The foamy material observed in samples from lungs is composed of fragments of cystic membranes, degenerated organisms or collapsed cysts as demonstrated by TEM.

Sueishi and associates,[37] using scanning EM, encountered two main structures: the thick-walled cyst that shows a smooth-surfaced wall and a structure that shows a rough surface and probably represents a trophozoite.

Fungi

Several species of fungi can be demonstrated with cytologic and cytochemical methods without the aid of EM. These microorganisms as seen by EM show remarkable preservation, regardless of the degenerative changes of the epithelial cells, probably due to the rigidity of their cell walls. In some species, such as *Cryptococcus,* an outer layer represents a thick capsule formed by intertwined microfibrils radiating from the capsule (Fig. 34–36). This layer is composed of mucopolysaccharides and can be stained with mucicarmine and seen as a thick red capsule.

It has been postulated that the thickness of the capsule is related to aging and degree of degeneration of the organism.[6]

New organisms supposedly have scarce fibrillary components,[6] whereas older more degenerated organisms have more abundant fibrillary components. Fungi are for the most part mononuclear, but multinucleation may occur as in *Blastomyces dermatitidis.* This is a biphasic fungus, identified in cytologic samples without difficulty. The attachment of daughter cells is broad based in contrast to the narrow-based attachment of *Cryptococcus* species. This fungus can be identified simply in cytologic specimens (Fig. 34–37, inset). Electron microscopy techniques only emphasize the smooth surface of the yeast by SEM (Fig. 34–37) and the budding effect of plasma membrane prior to the entrance of cell wall involvement in this process (Fig. 34–38).

References

1. Afzelius BA, Mossberg B: Immotile cilia. Thorax 35:401–404, 1980.
2. Baker JR: Principles of Biological Microtechnique: A Study of Fixation and Dyeing. New York, John Wiley & Sons, 1958.
3. Bauer KD, Clevenger CN, Endow RK, Murad T, Epstein AL, Scarpelli DG: Simultaneous nuclear antigen and DNA content quantitation using paraffin-embedded colonic tissue and multi-parameter flow cytometry. Cancer Res 46:2428–2434, 1986.
4. Beals TF: Cytology and electron microscopy. *In* Diagnostic Electron Microscopy. Edited by BF Trump and RT Jones. New York, John Wiley & Sons, 1980.
5. Berliner JA, Janssen M, McLatchie C: The use of scanning electron microscopy in the diagnosis of malignancy in human serous effusions. *In* Scanning Electron Microscopy 1978/2. Edited by O Johari and RP Becker. Chicago, Scanning Electron Microscopy, Inc., 1978.
6. Burns WA: Microorganisms. *In* Diagnostic Electron Microscopy. Edited by BF Trump and RT Jones. New York, John Wiley & Sons, 1980.
7. Carter HW: The role of scanning electron microscopy in pathology: A pathologist's viewpoint. *In* Scanning Electron Microscopy 1977/2. Edited by O Johari and RP Becker. Chicago, Int. Research Institute, 1977.
8. Carter H, Tannenbaum S, Tannenbaum M: Correlative light microscopic cytology and ultrastructural membrane pathology. Acta Cytol 22:603, 1978.
9. Chandra P, Delaney MD, Carmelita UT: Role of special stains in the diagnosis of *Pneumocystis carinii* infection from bronchial washings in patients with the acquired immune deficiency syndrome. Acta Cytol 32:105–108, 1988.
10. Coleman DV, Russell WJI, Hodgson J, Tun PE, Mowbray JR: Human papovavirus in Papanicolaou smears of urinary sediment detected by transmission electron microscopy. J Clin Pathol 30:1015–1020, 1977.
11. Croff WA: Scanning electron microscopy of exfoliated malignant and nonmalignant human urothelial cells. Scand J Urol Nephrol 13:31–42, 1979.
12. Domagala W: The hairy cell. Hum Pathol 6:760–761, 1975.
13. Domagala W, Koss LG: Configuration of surfaces of human cancer cells in effusions: A scanning electron microscopic study of microvilli. Virchows Arch IV [Cell Pathol] 26:27–42, 1977.
14. Domagala W, Koss LG: Configuration of surfaces of cells in effusions by scanning electron microscopy. *In* Advances in Clinical Cytology. Edited by LG Koss and DV Coleman. London, Butterworths, 1981.
15. Domagala W, Woyke S: Transmission and scanning electron microscopic studies of cells in effusions. Acta Cytol 19:214–224,1975.
16. Gilchrist KW, Benson RC Jr, Albrecht RM, Kutchera AR, Inhorn SL: Scanning microscopy of urinary cells: Requirement for direct correlation with cytology. Lab Invest 42:120, 1980.
17. Gondos B, Lai C, King EB: Distinction between atypical mesothelial cells and malignant cells by scanning electron microscopy. Acta Cytol 23:321–326, 1979.
18. Greenberg DM: The interaction between the alkali earth cations, particularly calcium and proteins. Adv Protein Chem I:121–151, 1944.
19. Hayat MA: Principles and Techniques of Electron Microscopy: Biological Applications. New York, Van Nostrand Reinhold, 1970.
20. Hidvegi DF, Hultgren SJ: Origin of giant cells from papillary carcinoma of thyroid: Immunologic, enzymatic and ultrastructural aspects of cytopreparations. Acta Cytol 26:742, 1982.
21. Hodges GM: Normal and neoplastic urothelium of human bladder *in vivo* and *in vitro*: An assessment of SEM studies. *In* Scanning Electron Microscopy 1978/2. Chicago, Scanning Electron Microscopy, Inc., 1978.
22. Hodges GM, Muir MD: Autoradiography of biological tissues in the scanning electron microscope. Nature 247:383–385, 1974.
23. Hultgren S, Hidvegi DF: Improved transmission electron microscopy for the study of cytologic material. Acta Cytol 29:179–183, 1985.
24. Jacobs JB, Cohen SM, Arai M, Friedell GH: SEM on bladder cells. Acta Cytol 21:3–4, 1977.
25. Kaneshima S, Kiyasu Y, Kudo H, Koga S, Tanaka K: An application of scanning electron microscopy to cytodiagnosis of pleural and peritoneal fluids. Comparative observation of the same cells by light and microscopy and scanning electron microscopy. Acta Cytol 22:490–499, 1978.
26. Karnovsky MJ: A formaldehyde-glutaraldehyde fixative of high osmolarity for use in electron microscopy. J Cell Biol 27:127A, 1965.
27. Koss LG: Diagnostic Cytology and Its Histopathologic Bases, 3rd ed. Philadelphia, JB Lippincott, 1979.
28. Koss LG, Domagala W: Configuration of surfaces of human

cancer cells in effusions: A review. *In* Scanning Electron Microscopy 1980/3. Edited by Johari O and Becker RP. Chicago, Scanning Electron Microscopy, Inc., 1980.

29. Melamed MR, Wolinska WH: On the significance of intracytoplasmic inclusions in the urinary sediment. Am J Pathol 38:711, 1961.

30. Moreau MF, Chretien MF, Dubin J, Rebel A, Malkani K: Transposed ciliary microtubules in Kartagener's syndrome: A case report with electron microscopy of bronchial and nasal brushings. Acta Cytol 29:248–253, 1985.

31. Neiman LH: Radiologic observations and techniques. *In* Liver and Pancreas. Guides to Clinical Aspiration Biopsy. Edited by DF Hidvegi. Tokyo, Igaku-Shoin, 1988.

32. Nelson CE: Surface characteristics of malignant human bladder epithelium studied with scanning electron microscopy. Scand J Urol Nephrol 12:31–42, 1979.

33. Peven DR, Gruhn JD: The development of electron microscopy. Arch Pathol Lab Med 109:683–691, 1985.

34. Rosai J, Sumner HW, Kostianovski M, Perez-Mesa C: Angiosarcoma of the skin: A clinicopathologic and fine structural study. Hum Pathol 7:83–109, 1976.

35. Roth LE, Jenkins RA, Johnson CW, Robinson RW: Additional stabilizing conditions for electron microscopy of the mitotic apparatus of giant amoeba. J Cell Biol 19:62A, 1963.

36. Steiner PM, Roop DR: Molecular and cellular biology of intermediate filaments. Ann Rev Biochem 57:593–625, 1988.

37. Sueishi K, Hisano S, Sumiyoshi A, Tanaka K: Scanning and transmission electron microscopic study of human pulmonary pneumocystosis. Chest 72:213–216, 1977.

38. Tannenbaum M, Tannenbaum S, Carter HW: SEM, BEI and TEM ultrastructural characteristics of normal, preneoplastic, plastic and neoplastic human transitional epithelium. Scan Electr Micros 2:949–958, 1978.

39. Taxy JB, Battifora H: The electron microscope in the study and diagnosis of soft tissue tumors. *In* Diagnostic Electron Microscopy. Edited by BF Trump and RT Jones. New York, John Wiley & Sons, 1980.

40. Watts JC, Chandler FW: *Pneumocystis carinii* pneumonitis: The nature and significance of the methenamine silver positive "intracystic bodies." Am J Surg Pathol 9:744–745, 1985.

41. Weibel ER, Palade GE: New cytoplasmic components in arterial endothelia. J Cell Biol 23:101, 1964.

42. Wood RL, Luft JH: The influence of buffer systems on fixation with osmium tetroxide. J Ultrastruct Res 12:22–45, 1965.

35

Morphometry

Paul J. van Diest
Jan P. A. Baak

The field of cytopathology has made tremendous progress over the last century. Screening programs for breast and cervical cancers have increased the role of cytopathologists in diagnosis and clinical follow-up. The criteria used for making a diagnosis, although subjective, can in most cases be quantified (Table 35–1). However, the cytopathologist sometimes finds the distinction between reactive and malignant cells can be extremely difficult because subjective assessment of size is less accurate and reproducible than overall pattern recognition. In these situations, the objective measurement of quantitative parameters can be of use (Fig. 35–1).

Because quantitative parameters are *objective* and *reproducible,* they may be important aids in the making of a cytopathologic diagnosis. This is further exemplified in Applications of Morphometry in Cytopathology in this chapter.

Formally, the word morphometry means measurement of form (Greek μορφοσ = form), but in this chapter we use the definition by Baak:[5] *Morphometry is the quantitative description of geometric features of structures with any dimension.* This is a more restricted definition of morphometry than that of Weibel,[56] who

includes stereology in the definition of morphometry. For an elaborate discussion on definitions, we refer to Baak.[5] The term planimetry is employed to denote measurement of geometric features of structures in a two-dimensional image, although these structures themselves originally may not be two-dimensional. For example, cells and nuclei in a cytologic specimen appear as flat (two-dimensional) images if the magni-

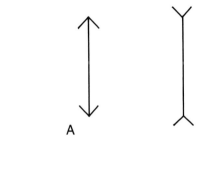

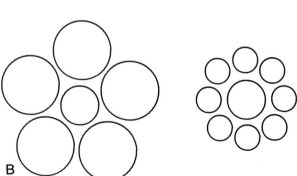

FIGURE 35–1. Misleading factors when estimating size. *A,* Both lines have the same length, although the right line seems longer because of the differently positioned arrowheads. *B,* The inner circles have exactly the same size, although the left inner circle seems smaller because of the large surrounding circles.

TABLE 35–1. Subjective Cytologic Criteria That May Be Quantified

Subjective Criteria	Objective Quantitative Parameters
Enlarged cells, nuclei, nucleoli	Increased cytoplasmic area Increased nuclear area Increased nucleolar area
Anisokaryosis	Increased SD of nuclear area
Pleomorphism	Altered shape factors
Disturbed nucleocytoplasmic equilibrium	Altered nucleocytoplasmic area ratio
Disturbed chromatin pattern	Altered nuclear texture parameters
Decreased cellular cohesion	Small cluster size, few elements per cluster

fication factor is not too high. Yet they have a certain thickness, which becomes more apparent at higher magnification; but, if the nuclear and cytoplasmic (=cell) area is measured, this thickness is usually irrelevant. Although the term planimetry formally would be more correct, studies of this type are often called morphometric studies. This practice is of course perfectly in order, and in this chapter morphometry and planimetry are therefore both utilized.

Stereologic techniques have found limited applications in cytopathology and are therefore not discussed in this chapter. For more details on stereology, we refer to the books of Baak and Oort,[7] Baak,[5] Aherne and Dunnill[3] and Burger, Oberholzer and Gössner.[19] Most quantitative studies in cytopathology employ planimetric techniques. For this reason, we further limit the scope of this chapter to planimetric techniques.

INTERACTIVE VERSUS AUTOMATED ANALYSIS

Interactive as well as fully automated equipment is available for morphometric assessments. For routine laboratory use, a well-developed digitizing interactive (graphic tablet or video overlay) system can be as good or even better than an automated image analysis system. Digitizing interactive systems utilize reliable, well-established and relatively inexpensive technology. Moreover, the resolution of a graphic tablet is usually 0.1 mm, yielding a theoretic picture element array on the pad of around 2800 × 2800 pixels. This exceeds the resolution of most digital image analysis systems currently available. In practice, this means that under certain conditions a high sampling rate (pixels/micron) can be achieved, even at low magnification. The implication for routine use is that the error due to approximations made in the digitization of the contours of traced objects can be kept low.

In contrast, quantitation of objects with automated image processing systems must be performed at a higher magnification to achieve a similar resolution. Because of low spectral contrast between foreground and background in ordinary microscopic specimens and hence segmentation problems, many images require user delineation of object boundaries—a task best suited to an interactive (graphic tablet) system rather than a digital image processing and analysis system. However, the theoretic 2800 × 2800 (or 0.1 mm) resolution of a graphic tablet is generally too optimistic a view, as the tablet resolution is not the only factor that determines the final resolution of the measurement. Even more important factors affecting the final drawing resolution are the processing speed of the computer and the manual tracing speed. The *processing speed* is the maximum number of coordinates that can be processed per second by the microcomputer to which the tablet or mouse is linked. The processing speed of an 80286/80287 machine is approximately 30 compared with 50 on an 80386/80387 processor-based computer. The *optimal manual tracing speed* is usually 7.5 to 20 mm per second (average: 15 mm per second).[31] This factor reduces the true drawing resolution considerably to approximately 0.25 mm when using a 286 machine and drawing at 7 mm per second which is fairly slow, and 0.67 mm when drawing at a much more usual speed of 20 mm per second. Similarly, the resolution on a 386 machine will be 0.15 to 0.5 mm. Thus, resolution of a digitizing graphic tablet system in practice is approximately between 580 × 580 picture points (on 286/287 processor-based systems) and 930 × 930 picture points (on 386/387 machines). Because the weakest link in the chain of resolution of interactive systems is the processing speed of the computer, approximately the same resolution can be obtained with video overlay systems that use an ordinary computer mouse instead of a graphic tablet, in spite of the fact that the mouse resolution is theoretically lower. Provided that the same magnification is used, this still may be better than the resolution of most digital image processing and analysis systems, which at present usually have a standard resolution of 512 × 512 picture points, although higher resolutions up to 1024 × 1024 are expected within 2 years.

Thus, at the present state of development, for routine quantitative pathology interactive graphic tablet and video overlay systems are in no way inferior to automated digital image cytometers and provide an inexpensive and simple entry to quantitative pathology.

Automated image processors are discussed in Chapter 36, Cell Image Analysis. The scope of this chapter is limited to interactive planimetric techniques.

EQUIPMENT FOR INTERACTIVE MORPHOMETRY

Computerized planimetry systems are available in several configurations. They may consist of a microcomputer connected to a digitizing tablet (an electromagnetic sensitive plate, usually approximately 30 × 30 cm) with a cursor, often employed in combination with a microscope equipped with a drawing tube. Video overlay systems using a camera mounted on top of the microscope are also available. Some video overlay systems utilize a computer mouse instead of a graphic tablet with a cursor, both yielding approximately the same resolution.

The movements of the cursor over the surface of the digitizing tablet or the movements of the computer mouse as an image are traced and generate X, Y-coordinate data. These are translated by the attached computer into measurement data, such as lengths, areas and counts, as well as derived parameters (e.g., shape factors), usually with a resolution of ± 0.1 to 0.7 mm, depending on the tracing speed, of the actual measured line. The price of a basic unit varies between $3000 and $25,000. The difference in price does not however always reflect a difference in performance. The net working time required for one sample is usually between 10 and 30 minutes.

Video Overlay or Drawing Tube?

Points to be considered in the choice between a *video overlay and a drawing tube* (camera lucida or drawing mirror) system are price, resolution and image quality, ease of use and other possibilities. The price of video overlay and drawing tube systems is about the same. With a 1.2-to 2.0-fold magnification objective in front of the camera, a fairly common feature of many cameras, video overlay/interactive mouse-based tools, in practice, can have a resolution comparable to standard digitizing interactive graphic tablet systems. In drawing tube systems, the real microscopic image is employed, which is familiar and flicker free, and has the resolution of the human retina (3000×3000 pixels). The same demands have to be made on video overlay systems, and noninterlaced 60 Hertz NTSC video boards, which provide high quality flicker-free images on the computer screen with enhanced graphics adaptor (EGA) resolution, have become available. Interaction between image and tracing can initially be difficult in drawing tube systems, and no control exists over the precise match between tracing and object. Video overlay facilities do allow such visual control. In addition, video overlay systems provide slide demonstration facilities and some allow stereologic analysis by overlay of graticles on the microscopic images. Although video overlay systems provide more facilities, especially in histopathology, a drawing tube system may also be adequate for cytomorphometric applications. The choice can be made only as based on personal experience using trial equipment.

Parameters

The available parameters vary considerably among various systems. Some parameters that are available in general are discussed hereafter. Planimetric parameters can be divided into four groups: simple parameters, shape factors, two-phase parameters and contextual parameters. These groups are also discussed subsequently.

Simple Parameters

Area is the total area of the object included by a smoothed curve through the contour points.

Diameter or *size* is the diameter of a circle with the same area as the traced object diameter = $2*\sqrt{(area/\pi)}$.

Perimeter is the length of the contour of the object. It is best calculated with Freeman codes:

$$Perimeter = 0.98*N_e + 1.406*N_o - 0.091*N_c$$

Where N_e = number of even Freeman codes; N_o = number of odd Freeman codes and N_c = number of angles.

Shortest axis is the shortest axis of an ellipse having the same area as the traced object fitted on the traced object.

Longest axis is the longest axis of an ellipse having the same area as the traced object fitted on the traced object.

Feret X is the length of the projection of the traced object on the x-axis.

Feret Y is the length of the projection of the traced object on the y-axis.

Shape Factors

Shape factors describe the irregularity of the traced object. Several shape factors are frequently implemented in morphometric equipment

Axis ratio (form EU) = (longest axis)/(shortest axis)
Form AR = $1/4*\pi*$(longest axis)*(shortest axis)
Form PE = $(4*\pi*area)/((perimeter)^2)$
Nuclear contour index = perimeter/(area)
Contour ratio = $(perimeter)^2/(4*\pi*area)$
Nuclear roundness = perimeter/$2*\pi$

Two-phase Parameters

Nucleocytoplasmic (NC) ratio is calculated by dividing the nuclear area by the cytoplasmic area. If several nuclei are present within one cell, the mean of the areas of the nuclei is usually used.

Nuclear/nucleolar (NN) ratio is calculated by dividing the nuclear area by the nucleolar area. If several nucleoli are present within one nucleus, the mean of the areas of the nucleoli is usually used.

Area difference is calculated by subtracting the (total) area of the second phase from the area of the first phase.

Excentricity of the second phase within the first phase is calculated with the formula:

$$Exc = \sqrt{((Cmassx_1 - Cmassx_2)^2 + (Cmassy_1 - Cmassy_2)^2)/D_1}$$

Where $Cmassx_1/Cmassx_2$ are the x coordinates of the centroids of the first and second phase, respectively. $Cmassy_1/Cmassy_2$ are the y coordinates of the centroids of the first and second phase, respectively. D_1 is the diameter of the first phase.

If several objects are present in the second phase, usually the mean of the excentricity of the different objects within the second phase is employed.

Contextual Parameters

Cluster area is calculated with the usual area algorithm, although in general a lower magnification is used.

The number of *elements per cluster* is calculated by either tracing all elements per cluster or, after tracing the cluster, clicking the cursor button as many times as elements are present in the cluster. With the clicking method, an indirect measure of mean cytoplasmic area may be calculated.

Cluster shape is calculated with the usual shape algorithms, although in general a lower magnification is used.

Distance between clusters is calculated from cluster centroid to cluster centroid.

RELIABILITY OF MORPHOMETRIC ASSESSMENTS

As explained in the beginning of this chapter, important arguments for the employment of morphometric techniques are their objectivity and reproducibility, or, in other words, their reliability. However, repeated measurements of one object or of samples drawn from one population usually do not yield identical results but rather a distribution of measurement data within a certain interval. Thus, morphometric assessments are subject to measurement errors that should be controlled as much as possible to guarantee the reliability of measurements in diagnostic cytopathology.

In the next discussions, we first present the terminology used to describe measurement errors. Secondly, factors that can influence the results of quantitative assessments in cytopathology are dealt with. Practical guidelines are given, which can help to improve the reproducibility of interactive planimetry.

Terminology of Measurement Errors

Measurement errors usually consist of two components called stochastic and systematic errors. *Stochastic measurement errors* are caused by random influences on the measurement process. A consistent factor deflecting measurement results in a certain direction causes *systematic* measurement errors. Unfortunately, in the terminology of measurement errors (reproducibility, precision, accuracy), the same words are often loosely used to express different ideas and vice versa. In order to give a clear understanding of what is meant, we will put forward some basic definitions as adapted from Baak.[5]

Reproducibility denotes the degree of concordance in measurement results obtained from repeated assessments of a certain object or samples from one population.

Allowing for some simplification, three important aspects of reproducibility can be distinguished: precision, accuracy and bias. Let us assume, for instance, that a nucleus with the true area T has been measured *n* times; in other words, a sample of *n* measurements has been taken. Subsequently, the sample mean *x* has been calculated to obtain a representation of the average measurement result, which is an estimation of the unknown true area T. A frequency distribution of all measurements may then look like the hypothetic distribution illustrated in Figure 35–2. Neither do the individual nuclear area measurements all equal the sample mean *x* nor does *x* equal the true area T. Figure 35–2 thus provides a graphic explanation of the terms precision, accuracy and bias as defined next.

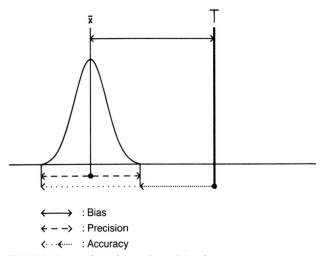

FIGURE 35–2. The relationship of the **three aspects of reproducibility:** precision, accuracy and bias. (Reproduced with permission from Baak JPA: Manual of Quantitative Pathology. Berlin, Springer-Verlag, in press.)

Precision expresses the closeness of the measurement results around the sample mean, x.

Accuracy indicates the closeness of the measurement data to the true value T.

Bias, in contrast to the aforementioned stochastic errors, describes the degree of systematic overestimation or underestimation of the true value T by the sample mean, x.

Several statistical parameters are employed to describe precision and accuracy. The *coefficient of variation (CV)* expresses the absolute dispersion of a data distribution as a percentage of the mean statistic (mean). For example, the CV of area measurements can be calculated by (SD/mean) $\times$ 100%. Because the CV is a dimensionless measure of dispersion, it is particularly useful for the comparison of populations in which the mean and the standard deviation both vary. The CV of a certain quantitative feature may describe its biologic variation within a tumor population (e.g., CV of nuclear measurements describes degree of anisokaryosis). The *standard error (SE)* is the SD of a sampling distribution of a certain statistic yielded from different samples that are taken from one population (e.g., from a tumor nucleus population). For instance, the SE of the mean (SEM), which consequently is the SD of the sample means from their grand mean M, can be estimated by dividing the SD of a sample by the square root (sq rt) of the number of sample elements (*n*): SEM = SD/sq rt(*n*). Therefore, the more elements the sample contains, the smaller the SEM becomes. Provided that no measurement bias is present, *n* is large, and the measured feature is approximately normally distributed; a *confidence interval* of M $\pm$ 1.96*SEM indicates that the true mean of the population lies within this interval with a probability of 95%. The borders of such an interval are called the confidence limits. The *coefficient of error (CE)* expresses the SE as a percentage of the mean statistic (mean): CE = (SE/mean)*100%.

Potentially Influencing Factors

Having defined the terminology, we now discuss the factors that can influence morphometric assessments in cytopathology and must therefore be controlled to ensure reliability.
1. Cell processing
2. Definition and segmentation of particles
3. Measuring system parameters
4. Selection methods, sample size and measurement protocols
5. Experience and quality control

Cell Processing

Certain specimen preparation procedures used in cytology may lead to selective loss of particular subsets of cells or nuclei. For example, mechanical cell destruction by the syringe may be considerable.[37] Multinucleated or mitotic cells are especially susceptible to preparation influences because they are more fragile owing to a greater instability or absence of their cellular or nuclear membranes. When preparing imprint slides from tumor material, a subpopulation of particularly loose cells may become detached from the primary tumor. Various studies have been devoted to the influence of specimen sampling procedures on quantitative cytopathologic data, but substantial evidence for a specific influence is lacking. Molengraft and coworkers[42] found no difference, for example, in cellular, nuclear and nucleolar diameters between solitary and clustered cells. However, it is advisable to standardize the specimen sampling procedure for each study as much as possible. Van Diest and associates[30] investigated the mechanical influences of the smear and of preparation techniques on cells and nuclei. Neither method led to an area-dependent distribution (area gradient) of the cells or nuclei on the slide nor induced orientation of the cells or nuclei. Lower measurement CEs were, however, obtained in the smear slides owing to a more uniform distribution of the cells and nuclei over the glass slide.

Beyer-Boon and colleagues[10] have investigated the influence of some routine fixation and staining procedures on quantitative cytopathologic data utilizing smears of urinary bladder scrapes. Table 35–2 summarizes their results.

Compared with the unfixed and unstained cells measured under a phase contrast microscope, none of the cell processing procedures preserved the dimensions of cells and nuclei exactly. Air drying resulted in an increase of 58% and 33% in the nuclear and cellular areas, respectively, and in an increase of 9% in the NC ratio. The other preparation techniques led to a decrease in nuclear and cellular area and the NC ratio. As the staining and mounting of cells appeared to have little effect on these quantitative parameters, these changes must be attributed to the fixation procedures. Air drying and the percentage of alcohol in the fixative are therefore important influencing factors in cytopreparatory procedures and should be standardized as much as possible.

Definition and Segmentation of Particles

At the microscopic level the *definition* and the ease of *segmentation* of particles should be considered. In the definition of particles, certain objects to be measured can be defined unambiguously. Macrophagocytes, for example, are characterized by their large size, small benign-appearing nucleus, foamy cytoplasm and often cytoplasmic inclusions. Even if these characteristics are only partly present, the definition of such particles will usually be clear-cut and their identification will be highly reproducible. However, biologic objects unavoidably show variation in their spatial, densitometric and spectral characteristics. If these variations are considerable, lack of reproducibility may occur, as illustrated by Smeulders and Dorst.[52] They asked several observers to measure the nuclear area of "intermediate cells" in cervical smears. Because a gradual transition occurs and no sharp demarcation between "intermediate cells" and "parabasal and superficial cells" in cervical smears is seen, considerable variation resulted in the morphometric assessments among the observers. A sharp definition of the objects to be measured or not to be measured using strict qualitative criteria, is therefore essential. Also, poor quality slide preparation can cause difficulty in the identification of the objects to be measured. Moreover, poor fixation resulting in "ballooning" and vague outlines and understaining or overstaining hinder the segmentation (discrimination between foreground and background) and should therefore be avoided. Optimizing staining techniques and the quality of slides is therefore of major importance in quantitative cytopathology.

TABLE 35–2. Influence of Several Routine Cytopreparatory Techniques on Quantitative Features of Normal Bladder Cells

Cell Processing Technique	Nuclear Area	Cellular Area	Nucleocytoplasmic Ratio
Air drying, May-Grünwald-Giemsa	95 μm²	277 μm²	0.37
50% ethyl alcohol, Papanicolaou	49 μm²	176 μm²	0.30
96% ethyl alcohol, Papanicolaou	32 μm²	114 μm²	0.29
Spray fixative, Papanicolaou	40 μm²	131 μm²	0.31
No fixation, no staining	60 μm²	208 μm²	0.34

Modified from Beyer-Boon ME, Voorn-Den Hollander MJA, Van der Arentz PW, Cornelisse CJ, Schaberg A, Fox CH: Effect of various routine cytopreparatory techniques on normal urothelial cells and their nuclei. Acta Pathol Microbiol Scand [A]87:63–69, 1979.

Measuring System Parameters

Although nuclear morphometric analysis by means of an interactive digitizing system is highly reproducible in principle, some studies, by Barry and Sharkey[9] and Chan and coworkers,[21] described considerable variation in morphometric assessments, in contrast to the findings of Dardick and Caldwell[25] and our own findings. However, the methodology of the measurements in these studies differed. Therefore, the influence of the following measuring system parameters on the reproducibility was further evaluated at our laboratory: tracing speed, "projected" particle size (total magnification at the digitizing tablet level), orientation and localization on the digitizing tablet, pen-photograph versus cursor-microscope usage and particle shape.[31] The magnification, the tracing tool and the tracing speed were found to be the most important influencing factors.

Figure 35–3 demonstrates the superiority of the cursor-microscope combination in comparison with the pen-photograph setting, which can be explained by the lower influence of manual tremor; a cursor is more stable than a pen, and tracing on a digitizing tablet is smoother than on a photograph. Coefficients of variation decrease with increasing "projected" diameter at the digitizing tablet level. The larger the actual tracing diameter, the less the effect of tremor. From a minimal particle diameter of 15 mm onwards, the CV remains fairly stable and below 1.5%, which is in practice the minimal CV of one observer repeatedly measuring the same object. This finding means that for measurements of average nuclei in cytologic specimens (diameter range of 6 to 12 μm), a total magnification at the digitizing tablet level of 2000× is usually sufficient. With the digitizing tablet system used in this study, it was found that the tracing speed should be kept between 7 and 20 mm per second; higher speeds resulted in increased CVs. However, the optimal trac-

ing speed may vary depending on the processing speed of the computer of the interactive digitizing system. Interestingly, in the study of Barry and Sharkey,[9] the areas of the tracings were small (3 to 6 mm), which may at least in part explain their poor reproducibility.

Black and white photographs have the advantage over live microscopy in that the images are fixed and focusing variations from one observer to another are excluded. However, poorer contrast of photographs leading to less sharp object boundaries may result in a higher measurement imprecision. Furthermore, the plane of focus of a photograph is always a compromise because only a few nuclei are caught at their largest diameter. Measuring from photographs may therefore lead to a systematic underestimation of the mean value when compared with drawing tube or video-overlay measurements, in which each object can be focused individually.

When utilizing a digitizing tablet and drawing tube configuration, the position of the measuring spot on the digitizing tablet may be another important feature. The reason is that an image transmitted from a small lens via a divergent projection beam and cast onto a flat surface is optically overstretched in a radial way. For the digitizing tablet (a flat surface) and drawing tube (equipped with a small lens) system, the same is true. Because the travel of light is reversible, the cursor light spot will make larger movements when outlining objects in the periphery of the field of vision than in the middle. This effect results in overestimation of the area when objects are not measured at the center of the field of vision.[33] However, this effect of overestimating is counteracted by the fact that the light on top of the cursor will become blurred in the periphery of the field of vision because it gets out of focus. This factor hinders accurate tracing and automatically limits the operator to measuring in the center. *Therefore, it is advisable not to measure in the (extreme) periphery of the field of vision.*

Proper calibration of the measurement equipment is obviously essential to obtain reliable measurement results. Calibration has to be performed before *each* measurement session. Linear features, such as perimeter and axis length, as well as most shape factors are less sensitive to inappropriately chosen measuring system parameters than area. Therefore, tuning a measuring system employing area measurements usually yields an adequate precision for other features. When the influence of the described measuring system parameters is taken into account, they can be well adjusted to optimize the performance of the measuring system. With such a regimen the CV of cytopathologic measurements can be kept low and errors due to measuring system parameters can be virtually eliminated.

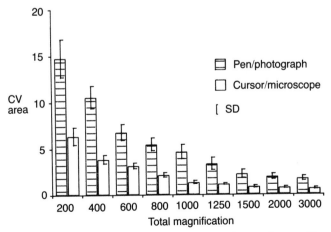

FIGURE 35–3. The **relationship between the total magnification at digitizing tablet level and the coefficient of variation (CV) of area measurements** for the pen/photograph and the cursor/microscope combination. (SD = standard deviation.) (Reproduced with permission from Fleege JC, Baak JPA, Smeulders AWM: Hum Pathol 19:513–517, 1988.)

Selection Methods

Selection is the cornerstone of diagnostic pathology.[22] Likewise, in cytomorphometry, a careful choice of a particular *measurement field* with cells having certain qualitative attributes is often of the utmost importance in achieving an adequate diagnosis or prediction of prognosis and, hence, therapy selection. To accomplish this usually means selecting a field with the most atypical cells.

In choosing a selection method, one has to realize that different biologic variation phenomena may be present within the selected measurement field: (1) *object variation,* which is the variation of a certain quantitative feature from object to object (e.g., pleomorphism, anisokaryosis), and (2) *object clustering,* which denotes the presence of groups each containing objects that show a relatively high similarity for a certain feature within one group but reveal differences for that particular feature among the various groups. Object variation and object clustering have completely different consequences for the choice of the selection method. *The higher the degree of object variation* (and thus the higher the SD of the quantitative feature), the *more objects have to be measured* to achieve a certain level of measurement precision. *The more pronounced the object clustering,* the more care should be taken that *the selection method uniformly covers the whole measurement field.* If a specific orientation (on average, ellipsoid) of objects is present, this has consequences for the selection method to be applied. This phenomenon, however, hardly ever occurs and is not induced by the smear technique.[30] This phenomenon therefore is not considered further.

In the following discussions we present four *selection methods* that have been employed in different publications on cytomorphometry. They are based on the following.

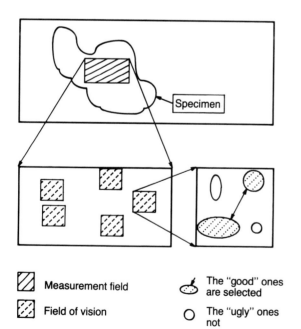

FIGURE 35-4. The "at convenience" method. The hatched nuclei are selected for measurement. This method is dangerous as different preferences among observers for "good" nuclei may result in biased and unpredictable measurement results. (Reproduced with permission from Baak JPA: Manual of Quantitative Pathology. Berlin, Springer-Verlag, in press.)

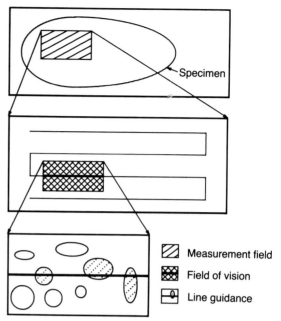

FIGURE 35-5. The line method. The hatched nuclei that touch the line are selected for measurement. This method provides more reproducible results than the "at convenience" method but may cause a systematic overestimation of the nuclear area because larger nuclei have a higher probability of being in contact with the line. (Reproduced with permission from Baak JPA: Manual of Quantitative Pathology. Berlin, Springer-Verlag, in press.)

1. "At convenience" selection
2. Line-guided selection
3. Zone-guided selection
4. Random selection.

"At Convenience" Selection (Fig. 35-4). This means measuring objects "as you like" while scanning through the slide. Within a marked measurement field the observer selects here and there a field of vision and measures one to five or more "good" nuclei or cells in that field. This widely utilized method is generally called "random," but it is obviously not random, and in fact it is strongly liable to undesired observer subjectivity.

Line-guided Selection (Fig. 35-5). Only those objects are allowed to be measured that "touch" one specified line of a grid in the eyepiece of the microscope. By this method reproducibility can be markedly increased.[30, 52] An advantage of this method is that a large area within the measurement field is scanned, which thereby deals better with object clustering. However, this method is open to criticism because larger objects have a higher probability of being in "contact" with the specified crosshair line, which may lead to a systematic overestimation (bias) of the mean area and underestimation of the SD.[30]

Zone-guided Selection (Fig. 35-6). The preference for larger objects as present in the line method can be virtually eliminated by measuring (*all*) objects with centroids that lie within a zone with a specific width, for instance, three to four times the diameter of the largest object.

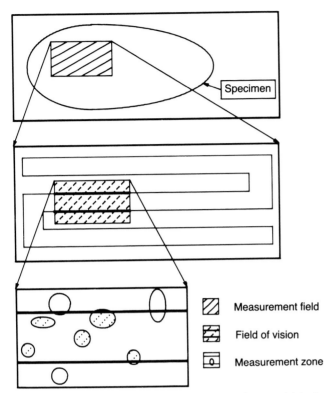

FIGURE 35–6. The zone method. Only nuclei in which the centroid lies within the zone (the hatched ones) are selected for measurement. Overestimation of the mean area in the line method is thereby largely avoided. (Reproduced with permission from Baak JPA: Manual of Quantitative Pathology. Berlin, Springer-Verlag, in press.)

Random Selection (Fig. 35–7). Employment of a random graticule, whether or not combined with an automated scanning stage, offers the possibility of truly random sampling. Only nuclei that are "touched" by one of the random points of the grid are measured. Compared with the aforementioned methods, the random method is theoretically optimal as it excludes all personal influences. Perfect random sampling is, however, often not completely possible, because of the necessity to apply subjective criteria for selection or rejection of a particular object for quantitation. For example, damaged nuclei or nontumor nuclei will be rejected. Therefore, a certain degree of subjectivity in the selection process cannot be excluded and is usually a necessity. To our knowledge, truly random sampling has not been reported in cytopathology. *The zone method, therefore, seems adequate in cytology.*

Sample Size

The determination of *sample size* is an important factor in obtaining reliable measurement results. The most reliable sample consists of all elements of a population. Because many ten thousands of cells may be present in cytologic specimens, it is in practice impossible to measure all elements using semiautomated measuring equipment. Measuring only a small sample is timesaving but may be imprecise. Therefore, a compromise between time spent and reliability has to be sought, and the optimal solution between size and representativeness of a sample must be assessed for each population. A theoretic method of calculation of the required sample size for a desired level of precision was described by DeHoff,[26] using the SD of a small test sample. In nearly normal populations with high variation in the feature of interest, this formula readily leads to relatively large (up to 750) sample sizes when the CE is set to a reasonable low level of $\leq 2\%$.[30] Because such sample sizes defy the patience of the average observer, one should accept a lower precision (i.e., a higher CE) in such cases, thus allowing fewer cells to be measured. This practice is often acceptable as precision is not the ultimate goal in quantitative pathology but must be chosen in balance with the desired discriminatory power needed to distinguish different populations. For many purposes, a CE of 5% may be satisfactory. For area measurements in a population having an SD of 15 μm^2 and a mean nuclear area (x) of 60 μm^2 the sample size (n), calculated according to DeHoff's formula of $n = [(Z*100*SD)/(CE*x)]^2$, is 96 assuming a precision (CE) of 5%, a 95% level of confidence and a standard score of z = 1.96 ($n = [(1.96*100*15)/(5*60)]^2 = 96$).

Measurement Protocols

A measurement protocol should contain clear guidelines describing where, what, how and how much to measure. The following basic points form the skeleton

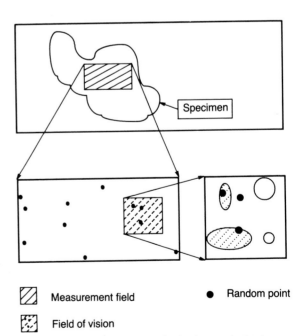

FIGURE 35–7. The random method. The nuclei hit by one of the random graticule points (the hatched ones) are selected for measurement. (Reproduced with permission from Baak JPA: Manual of Quantitative Pathology. Berlin, Springer-Verlag, in press.)

for the formulation of a more detailed and specimen specific measurement protocol:

1. Sharply demarcate a measurement field at a location where the highest nuclear atypicality of tumor cells is found and the least inflammatory or necrotic changes are observed.
2. Within the selected measurement field measure all, according to the definition of the desired objects, well-preserved, nonoverlapping nuclei with clear identifiability of the nuclear membrane, rejecting poorly fixed and understained objects.
3. Tune the measurement system parameters previously described optimally to guarantee a high measurement reproducibility. Furthermore, calibrate the measurement system and frequently check its adjustment; improve the microscopic or video monitor image quality as much as possible and allow the adjusted focus plane to remain unchanged during one measurement.
4. The chosen selection method (see previous discussion) should be maintained for all measurements of a certain experiment or diagnostic goal. Establish the number of objects necessary to attain a certain degree of precision in the assessments.

Of course, other criteria are possible as well, e.g., whichever one correlates best with the prognosis or fits the purpose of the study well.

Experience and Quality Control

The level of *experience* of the operator is an important factor in the interobserver and intraobserver variation of interactive planimetric analysis. Gamel and colleagues[32] pointed to this when testing the reproducibility of nucleolar measurements in ocular melanoma. It was demonstrated that the measurements of an experienced operator were more precise and less biased than those of an inexperienced operator. A person inexperienced in performing nuclear measurements with a digitizing tablet may, for instance, preferentially select larger or smaller nuclei or may systematically trace the outer or inner, depending on the person, boundary of the object instead of its middle, which results in bias and low accuracy, whereas the initially high manual instability leads to unwanted measurement noise (low precision). A thorough training phase should therefore precede diagnostic quantitative measurements to allow the technician to become acquainted with the equipment, the selection procedure and the different measuring techniques. Training programs for interactive planimetric, stereologic and cytometric analysis, which have been developed at our laboratory, have proved to be very useful.

In a diagnostic session, it is of the utmost importance to set up programs for *ongoing quality control* to guarantee the reliability of morphometric measurements in any department. A multicenter quality control program was started in the Netherlands for breast cancer histomorphometry. Test preparation sets have been employed for digitizing tablet, stereologic and mitotic activity index assessments. Prior to the application of these sets as a quality calibration tool in other laboratories, they were extensively measured at our laboratory. Because the true values are normally not known, the mean values of several experienced technicians served as the reference values.

Summary of Guidelines for Reliable Application of Morphometry in Cytopathology

Cell Processing

- As air drying and alcohol fixation give very different results, standardization must be applied as much as possible.

Definition and Segmentation

- Particles (cells, nuclei, nucleoli) should be defined as clearly as possible on the bases of qualitative criteria. The stain should distinguish adequately between foreground and background; the more "black and white" the better. Poorly fixed and understained or overstained slides must be rejected.

Measuring System Parameters

- The diameter of an object on the digitizing tablet level should be at least 15 mm, usually obtained at a $2000\times$ magnification, and the tracing speed should be kept between 7 and 20 mm per second. A cursor-microscope combination is preferable to a pen-photograph combination. Measuring at the periphery of the field of vision should be avoided if a drawing tube system is employed.

Selection Methods, Sample Size, Measurement Protocols

- If variation among objects is large, many objects should be measured to obtain reliable results.
- If clustering is prominent, take care that the selection method used covers the whole measurement field. The zone method for cell selection is adequate for cytologic specimens.
- Establish the optimal sample size with respect to reliability, required discriminatory power and time spent.
- Develop a clear-cut measurement protocol.

Experience and Quality Control

- A thorough training phase should precede diagnostic morphometric assessments.
- Ongoing quality control is of the utmost importance in order to guarantee the reliability of morphometric assessments in time.

APPLICATIONS OF MORPHOMETRY IN CYTOPATHOLOGY

The number of morphometric publications is rapidly increasing, and cytomorphometric studies have been performed on many different tumors from many different sites. It would go far beyond the scope of this chapter to describe them all, so hereafter some applications of morphometry in cytopathology are presented. The decision thresholds given should not be regarded as strict laws, but merely as guidelines, because it is advisable for each laboratory to set its own standards.

For all nuclear measurement applications described, a final magnification of $\times 2000$ is advisable. Measurements may be performed on a graphic tablet system or video-overlay system.

Breast

In breast cancer cytology, quantitative cell analysis has been utilized for the distinction between benign and malignant lesions and because of its ability to provide data to predict the prognosis of an individual patient.

Distinction Between Benign and Malignant Lesions

Cornelisse and associates[23] could improve the cytodiagnosis of suspicious breast smears using the mean nuclear area, the maximum nuclear area and the percentage of nuclei larger than 200 μ^2. Boon and colleagues[17] found the mean nuclear size ($2*(\mathrm{sq}\ \mathrm{rt}(\mathrm{area}/\pi))$) to be the best discriminating feature when measuring the nuclei of 100 abnormal cells, characterized by large nuclei, abnormal nuclear borders and chromatin patterns, in air-dried May-Grünwald-Giemsa (MGG)–stained slides. A mean nuclear size of > 13 was very indicative of malignancy. The SD of the nucleocytoplasmic ratio had some additional value for discriminating benign from malignant cells. However, a complete separation of benign from malignant cases could not be obtained in these studies. Detweiler and associates,[27] in contrast, completely separated benign from malignant smears employing a combination of contextual, textural and geometric features (Table 35–3). The number of cases in this study was limited, however ($n = 18$). Follow-up studies are therefore necessary to further establish objective classification of difficult breast cancer smears utilizing geometric, textural, contextual and densitometric parameters.

Prediction of Prognosis

Prognosis prediction from cytologic specimens could have important advantages because a preoperative indication of a patient's prognosis could guide the therapy strategy, especially in breast cancer screening programs. Several studies have emphasized the importance of quantitative features in this field.

Van Diest and coworkers[28] studied the value of morphometry as an aid to subjective cytoprognostic grading of cytologic breast cancer specimens. Grading has proved its value in several studies[43, 45] but is difficult in some cases, and observers sometimes disagree on the grade. The discriminative power of morphometric features for the three subjective grades in cytologic breast cancer specimens as an auxiliary tool in subjective grading was therefore evaluated. Cytologic specimens from 76 patients with histologically proven invasive breast cancer tumor fixed in methanol/acetone (50/50) at pH 8.1 and stained according to a hypochromic Papanicolaou staining procedure, which delicately outlines the distribution of chromatin and visualizes nucleoli,[44] were independently classified by experienced cytologists in two different centers into three grades of increasing severity in order to select clear cases (unequivocally graded slides) for a training set to develop classification rules based on morphometric criteria. In 22 slides (28.9%), disagreement occurred in grading. Nine cases (11.8%) were equivocally graded 1/2; 13 cases (17.1%) were equivocally graded 2/3. Discrepancy in grading between grades 1 and 3 did not occur. The 54 unequivocally graded slides (72.1%) were considered to be unambiguous cases and were used as a training set to develop classification rules with discriminant analysis based on morphometric features. In the slides, the field with the most atypical cells was selected and 100 nuclei and their nucleoli were measured at a final magnification of $\times 2800$. Many morphometric features showed significant p- values in univariate analysis when comparing different grades. Multivariate discriminant analysis showed that the mean nuclear area and the number of mitoses per slide appeared to be the optimal combination for discrimination between grades 1 and 2 (87.5% correct classifications).

Addition of the mean nuclear shape factor to these two features provided the optimal combination for discrimination between grades 2 and 3 (83.3% correct classifications). The 22 equivocally graded slides were classified employing the described classification rules.

TABLE 35–3. Statistically Significant* High Resolution and Contextual Features for Discrimination Between Benign and Malignant Breast Cancer Smears†

	Benign	Malignant
High Resolution Features		
Area	44.4 ± 14.1	146.2 ± 56.4
Texture (long runs)	57.0 ± 50.8	31.1 ± 14.0
Texture (gray distribution)	12.5 ± 5.1	36.2 ± 13.3
Texture (run distribution)	51.1 ± 36.1	161.7 ± 91.2
Average gray level	92.0 ± 31.9	118.3 ± 24.2
Bending energy	1.9 ± 0.3	3.2 ± 1.2
Integrated darkness	113.1 ± 50.8	315.7 ± 127.3
Contextual Features		
Number of clusters per scene	3.3 ± 3.3	14.3 ± 6.1
Average area of clusters	4478.6 ± 4845.6	645.3 ± 406.1
Average gray level/cluster	131.8 ± 31.9	171.8 ± 18.8
SD of distance between clusters	6.7 ± 3.9	11.3 ± 1.3
SD of polarity of clusters	20.5 ± 21.9	40.6 ± 9.7

*$p < 0.001$, Student's t-test.
†In hematoxylin and eosin–stained aspirates.
(Adapted from Detweiler R, Zahniser DJ, Garcia GC, Hutchinson M: Contextual analysis complements single-cell analysis in the diagnosis of breast cancer in fine needle aspirates. Analyt Quant Cytol Histol 10:10–15, 1988.)

TABLE 35–4. Prognostically Significant Features in Cytologic Breast Cancer Specimens

Nuclear Parameters		P Value	MC Value
Area	Mean	0.01	9.02
	SD	NS	5.86
Perimeter	Mean	0.05	6.22
	SD	0.04	6.32
Short axis	Mean	0.008	9.63
	SD	0.005	10.64
Diameter	Mean	0.03	7.21
	SD	0.05	6.00
Nucleolar Parameters			
Area	Mean	0.05	6.13
	SD	0.006	7.58
Perimeter	Mean	0.009	9.42
	SD	0.04	6.51
Long axis	Mean	0.02	8.33
	SD	NS	4.58
Short axis	Mean	0.01	8.88
	SD	0.03	7.35
Diameter	Mean	0.03	7.30
	SD	NS	5.97
NF		0.004	11.07
Combined Parameters			
% Nuclei without nucleoli		0.005	10.46
% Nuclei with 3 nucleoli		0.04	6.54
% Nuclei with >3 nucleoli		0.004	8.29

MC = Mantel-Cox; SD = standard deviation; NS = not significant; NF = nucleolar frequency; number of nucleoli per 100 nuclei.
(Adapted from van Diest PJ, Mouriquand J, Schipper NW, Baak JPA: Prognostic value of nucleolar morphometric variables in cytological breast cancer specimens. J Clin Pathol 43:157–159, 1990.)

Five of the nine cases that were equivocally graded 1/2 were classified grade 1, and four cases as grade 2. Seven of the 13 cases that were equivocally graded 2/3 were classified grade 2 and 6 cases grade 3. In total, 16 of the 22 equivocally graded cases (72.7%) could be classified with high (≥ 0.60) posterior probability. Therefore, such morphometric grading may be a useful aid in cytoprognostic grading of difficult cases.

In a subsequent study,[29] the prognostic value of nuclear and nucleolar features was studied in a group of 86 patients. Univariate recurrence-free survival analysis according to Kaplan-Meier showed that many features had prognostic value (Table 35–4).

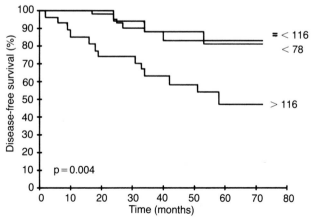

FIGURE 35–8. Survival curves for the **total number of nucleoli per 100 nuclei.**

The total number of nucleoli per 100 nuclei (nucleolar frequency, NF) was the best single prognostic parameter ($p = 0.004$, Mantel-Cox value 11.07). Survival at 6 years was 82% for cases with NF ≤ 78, 83% for cases with NF < 116 and 47% for cases with NF ≥ 116. Figure 35–8 shows the survival curves for this feature. Multivariate survival analysis (Cox regression model) revealed that no other features added further prognostic information to the total number of nucleoli.

Other cytomorphometric studies have also demonstrated the prognostic value of morphometric features. Nuclear parameters, such as area and diameter, have proved to be useful.[55, 59] In the study of Kuenen-Bouwmeester and coworkers[35] on air-dried, MGG–stained aspirates of 73 cases, a multivariate combination of nuclear area variation (the difference between the 90th and 10th percentile of 100 randomly selected carcinoma cells) and lymph node status showed strong prognostic value. Using the following formula, 0.03* range (in μm) + 1.9 (if positive lymph nodes are present), a score < 2.5 indicated a very good prognosis ($n = 15$, 6-year survival 100%), a score > 5.5, a very poor prognosis ($n = 11$, 6-year survival 17%) and a score in between ($n = 45$), an intermediate prognosis.

Cervix

Most quantitative studies of cervical lesions apply automated techniques.[11, 47, 57] This is a very important development because of the possible role of automated quantitative analysis in cervical screening. Automated techniques are beyond the scope of this chapter; hereafter, an example of a study on cervical lesions using interactive techniques is discussed.

Simultaneous condyloma acuminatum and dysplasia of the uterine cervix were studied by Boon and Fox.[12] They compared a group of 50 women with severe dysplasia with a group of 50 women with both severe dysplasia and koilocytosis, utilizing spray fixed, Papanicolaou-stained smears. Morphometric measurements were performed on a minimum of 50 abnormal cells (koilocytic cells with and without nuclear abnormalities in the koilocytic cases and an admixture of slightly and severely dysplastic cells in the classic dysplasia cases) per case.

Table 35–5 clearly shows the differences between the koilocytic cells and the classic dysplastic cells. In a relatively short follow-up period of 3 years, it could not, however, be demonstrated that the patients with dysplasia accompanied by koilocytosis were at higher risk for development of *in situ* or invasive carcinoma.

Lung

In a cytomorphometric study of *large-cell carcinoma* (LCC) of the lung, Burns and associates[20] measured nonoverlapping cells in routinely prepared Papanicolaou-stained slides from sputum material (nine cases) or bronchial washings (one case). Cellular and nuclear

TABLE 35–5. Mean Values (± SD) of Nuclear Area, Cytoplasmic Area and Nucleocytoplasmic Ratio of Cells*

	No. of Cells	Nuclear Area (μm^2)	Cytoplasmic Area (μm^2)	Nucleocytoplasmic Ratio
Normal epithelial cells from negative controls	500	67.2 ± 20.6	2105.2 ± 824.1	0.038 ± 0.018
Classic dysplastic cells	500	92.3 ± 80.9	279.3 ± 233.0	0.358 ± 0.275
Koilocytes	500	115.2 ± 134.8	1752.1 ± 1410.9	0.094 ± 0.503

*Measured in 10 different slides from 10 different patients.
(Adapted from Boon ME, Fox CH: Simultaneous condyloma acuminatum and dysplasia of the uterine cervix. Acta Cytol 25:393–399, 1981.)

areas were found to be significantly larger in adenocarcinoma areas whereas nucleolar areas were greater in LCC, leading to a higher nucleolar/nuclear area ratio in LCC. In a logistic regression, cellular area, nucleolar/nuclear area ratio and cellular and nuclear shape factors appeared to be significant contributors to the discrimination of LCC from adenocarcinoma, with a positive predictive value of 92%. Morphometry may therefore be helpful in the differential cytologic diagnosis of adenocarcinoma and LCC.

A quantitative cytologic study of sputum in *early squamous cell bronchogenic carcinoma* was performed by Saito and associates.[48] Sputum was processed by the Saccomano method, and in each case 50 borderline atypical squamous cells or cancer cells were measured. In *in situ* and early invasive squamous cell carcinomas, the mean nuclear diameters were larger and multinucleated cells and distinct nucleoli were more frequent than in borderline cases. Furthermore, the mean cellular diameters and the number of abnormal cells per slide were smaller, distinct nucleoli were less frequent and acidophilic cytoplasms were more frequent than in frankly invasive squamous cell carcinomas. Table 35–6 summarizes the quantitative results.

They concluded that *in situ* and early invasive squamous cell carcinomas are generally distinguishable cytologically from borderline cases and from frankly invasive squamous cell carcinomas, but the cytologic differentiation between *in situ* and early invasive squamous cell carcinomas is quantitatively insufficient.

In *small-cell lung cancer* (SCLC) cases, Abe and coworkers[1, 2] measured the mean nuclear diameter (range 5.9 to 20.6 μm) in bronchial brushings immediately after the preparation of cytologic smears. The specimens were fixed in 95% alcohol and stained by the Papanicolaou technique. The dimensions of tumor cells were measured with a micrometer, and at least 200 tumor cells were evaluated per patient. No significant correlation was found between subtype or nuclear diameter and survival.

Horan and associates[34] succeeded in making the clinically very relevant *discrimination between bronchial carcinoid tumors and SCLC* with morphometric parameters. Material was collected by transthoracic fine needle aspiration under radiologic guidance, placed onto glass slides, immediately fixed in 95% ethanol and stained with Papanicolaou stain. In each case, the nuclear and cytoplasmic areas of 100 cells were measured from several areas on the slide. All seven bronchial carcinoid cases and four small-cell anaplastic carcinomas (intermediate type) could be discriminated employing mean nuclear and cytoplasmic area (Fig. 35–9). Although the number of cases in this study was small, the results indicate that morphometry may be of help in discriminating carcinoid tumors from SCLC.

Effusions

Morphometry has been utilized to discriminate between benign and malignant cells in pleural and peritoneal effusions and to trace the pleural or peritoneal origin of mesothelial tumors.

Distinction Between Benign and Malignant Cells in Pleural Effusions

Various studies have been undertaken to evaluate the power of quantitative features as an aid in the

TABLE 35–6. Quantitative Cellular Features of Abnormal Cells in Borderline Cases and *In Situ*, Early Invasive and Frankly Invasive Squamous Cell Carcinomas

Lesion	No. of Cases	No. of Abnormal Cells per Slide*	Dissociating Ratio*†	Multinucleated Cells per Abnormal Cells*
Borderline	12	9.1 ± 1.5	0.54 ± 0.05	0.08 ± 0.03
Carcinoma *in situ*	12	10.8 ± 1.6	0.73 ± 0.07	0.15 ± 0.03
Invasive Carcinoma				
Early	20	11.3 ± 1.2	0.76 ± 0.04	0.16 ± 0.02
Frankly	11	21.2 ± 4.1	0.90 ± 0.04	0.10 ± 0.02

*Mean ± SE.
†Number of single abnormal cells and clusters per total number of abnormal cells.
(Adapted from Saito Y, Imai T, Nagamoto N, et al: A quantitative cytologic study of sputum in early squamous cell bronchogenic carcinoma. Analyt Quant Cytol Histol 10:365–379, 1988.)

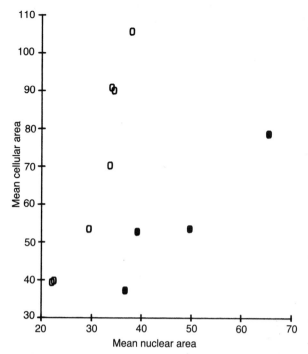

FIGURE 35–9. Scatter diagram of **mean nuclear area and mean cytoplasmic area of bronchial carcinoid tumors** *(open)* and **small-cell lung cancer** *(filled).* (Modified from Horan DC, Bonfiglio TA, Patten SF: Analyt Quant Cytol Histol 4:105–109, 1982.)

sometimes very difficult cytologic differentiation between benign and malignant cells in pleural effusions. Kwee and colleagues[36] were able to correctly classify 85% of the cases within a group of 20 reactive and 40 malignant mesothelial proliferations employing nuclear and cytoplasmic area (Fig. 35–10). The doubtful cases could subjectively be correctly classified considering morula formation and chromatin pattern.

The value of nuclear and cytoplasmic size was confirmed by Marchevsky and associates.[39] Boon and colleagues[18] showed that a size-independent distribution index of cytoplasmic lipid vacuoles can also aid in

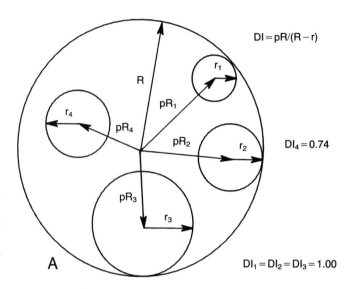

$$DI = pR/(R-r)$$

$$DI_4 = 0.74$$

A

$$DI_1 = DI_2 = DI_3 = 1.00$$

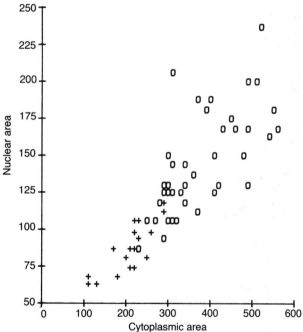

FIGURE 35–10. Scatter diagram of **cases with reactive mesothelial changes** *(plus)* and **primary pleural mesotheliomas** *(open),* with mean cytoplasmic and mean nuclear area. (Modified from Kwee WS, Veldhuizen RW, Alons CA, Morawetz F, Boon ME: Acta Cytol 26:401–406, 1982.) Effusion specimens were centrifuged at 2500 rpm for 10 minutes and air dried. May-Grünwald-Giemsa–stained specimens were prepared. The nuclear and cytoplasmic areas of 50 mesothelial cells were measured at a final magnification of ×2000.

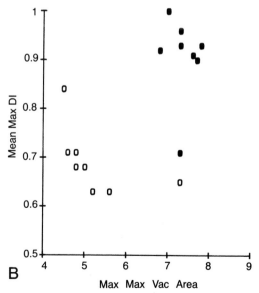

B

FIGURE 35–11. *A,* Calculation of the **distribution index.** *B,* Scatter diagram showing the **separation of the eight benign** *(open)* **from the eight malignant cases** *(filled)* with maximum maximal vacuolar area (abscissa) and mean maximum distribution index (ordinant). For each case, six vacuoles containing cells were considered. (Modified from Boon ME, van Velzen D, Ruinaard C, Veldhuizen PW: Analyt Cytol Histol 6: 221–226, 1984.)

distinguishing between benign and malignant cells in air-dried, oil red O–stained specimens of pleural effusions. Benign mesothelial cells had fewer and smaller lipid vacuoles, which were found predominantly around the nuclei. A complete separation between benign and malignant cases could be obtained with the maximum vacuolar area and the mean maximum distribution index (Fig. 35–11).

Distinction Between Benign and Malignant Cells in Ascitic Effusions

Van Molengraft and associates[42] studied the value of morphometric features for distinction between atypical mesothelial cells and malignant cells in ascitic fluid of eight patients with cirrhosis-related ascites and nine with adenocarcinomas metastatic to the peritoneal cavity. Using methanol:acetic acid (9:1)–fixed, Papanicolaou-stained slides, they measured 750 cells from both the benign and malignant cases. The largest cellular, nuclear and nucleolar diameters of these cells were assessed with the use of an ocular micrometer in the eyepiece of the microscope. The scale of the micrometer was read to the nearest 0.5 μm. Furthermore, the number of nucleoli per measured cell was recorded as well as the percentage of irregular nucleoli. Table 35–7 summarizes their results.

The observed differences were highly significant, and although measuring nuclear diameter with an ocular grid is less reliable than measuring diameter on a graphic tablet or with a video-overlay system, these results indicate the value of morphometric features in the diagnosis of ascitic effusions.

Scott and colleagues[49] confirmed the value of nuclear area in a study on serous effusions of both pleural and peritoneal origin, although much overlap among the benign, suspicious and malignant groups was present, perhaps due to the different cell processing techniques (spray fixation and hematoxylin and eosin staining). These investigators especially pointed to the significance of outlying values, such as largest nuclear area. However, sample sizes of up to 300 cells were necessary to derive reproducible assessments of outlying values, which may be too high for routine interactive applications.

Peritoneal or Pleural Origin of Mesothelial Tumors

Although only 6 to 10% of the mesothelial tumors derive from a primary peritoneal location, transcoelomic metastases may occur. It is therefore important to establish criteria that indicate peritoneal origin of mesothelioma cells in pleural effusions and vice versa. Morphometric criteria are helpful as demonstrated by Boon and associates.[15] They measured nuclear and cytoplasmic features of 50 cells in air-dried, MGG–stained specimens of 64 mesothelioma cases: 40 cases with primary pleural location, 16 with primary peritoneal location and eight with involvement of both pleura and peritoneum. With nuclear area and NC ratio, cells from different origins could be well separated (Fig. 35–12).

Thyroid

The extent of surgery in a case of a thyroid nodule depends in general on the benign or malignant nature of the lesion. Because interpretation of intraoperative frozen sections may be difficult and often requires many slides, a preoperative quantitative cytologic approach as described by Boon and coworkers,[16] may be useful. Employing mean cell size $(2(\sqrt{\text{area}/\pi}))$ and mean nuclear/cytoplasmic size ratio of 50 cells in follicular formation, assessed in air-dried, MGG–stained smears, they could identify all but two of 33 adenomas and carcinomas (Fig. 35–13).

Wright and colleagues[58] described the value of nuclear area in discriminating adenomas from carcinomas in ethanol-fixed Papanicolaou-stained smears. The mean values for nuclear area in follicular adenomas and carcinomas were 50 ± 9.3 and 64.2 ± 8.0 μm^2, respectively. These findings are comparable to the discrimination thresholds found by Boon and colleagues[16] on air-dried specimens, but Luck and colleagues[38] found no discriminative value of nuclear area in air-dried specimens stained with Wright's stain. These results are apparently influenced by differences in tissue processing.

Masuda and associates[40] demonstrated the value of contextual parameters in air-dried, MGG–stained im-

TABLE 35–7. Differences in Mean Values for Several Quantitative Parameters Between Benign and Malignant Cells in Effusions

	Benign Effusions		Malignant Effusions	
	Mean	**SD**	**Mean**	**SD**
Cellular diameter (μm)	12.9	0.9	15.2	1.6
Nuclear diameter (μm)	6.9	0.4	9.5	1.0
Nucleocytoplasmic ratio (%)	54.5	2.4	63.9	4.6
Nucleolar diameter (μm)	1.06	0.12	2.18	0.37
Nucleolar number/cell	1.66	0.19	1.22	0.16
Irregular nucleoli (%)	6.6	4.8	58.8	15.2

Adapted from van Molengraft FJJM, Van't Hot MA, Herman CJ, Vooijs PG: Quantitative light microscopy of atypical mesothelial cells and malignant cells in ascitic fluid. Analyt Quant Cytol 4:217–220, 1982.

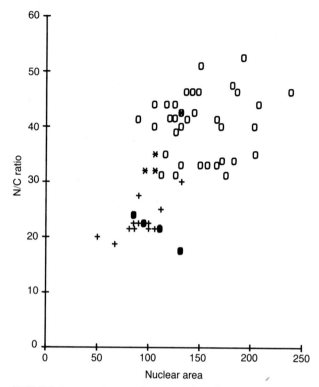

FIGURE 35–12. Scatter diagram of **nuclear area versus nucleocytoplasmic (NC) ratio of mesothelioma cases.** *(Open)*: pleural mesotheliomas. *(Plus)*: peritoneal mesotheliomas. *(Asterisk)*: primary pleural mesothelioma in ascites. *(Filled)*: primary peritoneal mesothelioma in pleural effusion. (Modified from Boon ME, Kwee HS, Alons CL, Morawetz F, Veldhuizen RW: Acta Cytol 26: 103–108, 1982.)

print slides of excised thyroid lesions. Their results indicated that the presence of large cell clusters indicates malignancy; *clusters with a size (2*sq rt(area/π)) above 300 μm were found exclusively in malignant lesions.* It is, however, not clear from their study whether carcinoma cases without large cell clusters occurred.

Non-Hodgkin's Lymphomas

Treatment of patients with B-cell lymphoma varies significantly for different subclassifications. However, Metter and associates[41] have reported that major problems in quantitating cells of different types are inherent in the subjective classification of follicular lymphomas, including major disagreement (small-cell/large-cell discrepancies) in 25 to 37%. Thus, a considerable percentage of patients may be inappropriately treated.

Ball and coworkers[8] studied the value of morphometry for the differential diagnosis of centroblastic and B-immunoblastic subtypes by morphometry on air-dried, MGG–stained imprints of biopsy specimens from 18 cases of centroblastic and nine cases of B-immunoblastic non-Hodgkin's lymphomas (NHL). The nuclear and nucleolar areas of at least 100 cells were measured from photographs (final magnification, ×1200) on a digitizing graphic tablet system. All cells

with a nuclear area < 35 μm² were regarded as normal lymphocytes and thus excluded. Statistically significant differences were present for the mean and SD of nuclear area, the mean nuclear area and the number of nucleoli per nucleus. The best discriminator was the mean nucleolar area. The mean percentage of immunoblasts, defined as cells with a nuclear area > 35 μm² and a mean nucleolar area > 3 μm², was significantly different between the two groups of patients (Fig. 35–14).

Stevens and colleagues[53] further confirmed that morphometric analysis of cytologic preparations can be employed for the diagnosis of follicular NHL. Nodular poorly differentiated, nodular mixed and diffuse and nodular histiocytic NHL could be distinguished by the percentage of cells with nuclei larger than 87 μm² (thresholds, 20 and 50%).

Childhood Acute Lymphoblastic Leukemia

In a morphometric study on 21 children with acute lymphoblastic leukemia (ALL), Tosi and coworkers[54] utilized bone marrow aspirates, which were prepared as follows: a small drop of bone marrow was placed in the middle of a cover glass, and a second cover glass was placed over the first so that they did not cover each other but so that the second cover glass was rotated 45 degrees on the first. The slides were then

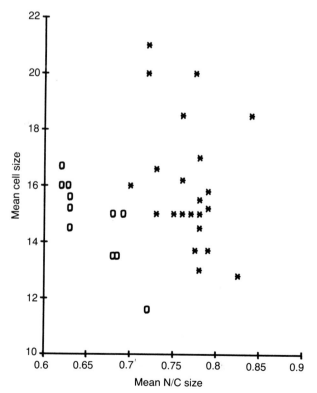

FIGURE 35–13. Scatter diagram of **follicular adenomas** *(open)* **and carcinomas** *(asterisk)*. (Modified from Boon ME, Lowhagen T, Lopes Cardozo PL, Blonk DI, Kurver PHJ, Baak JPA: Analyt Quant Cytol Histol 4: 1–5, 1982.)

Centroblastic Immunoblastic

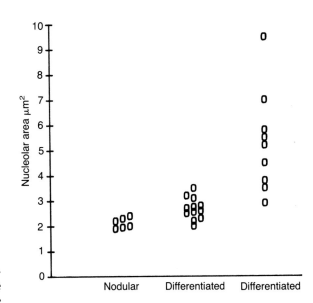

FIGURE 35–14. Mean nucleolar areas and percentage of immunoblasts from each case: six nodular centroblastic, 12 diffuse centroblastic and nine B-immunoblastic lymphoma patients. The percentage immunoblasts is the percentage of cells with nuclear area > 35 μm² and mean nucleolar area > 3 μm² in each patient. (Modified from Ball PJ, van der Valk P, Kurner PHJ, Lindeman J, Meijer CJLM: Cancer 55: 486–492, 1985.)

Centroblastic Immunoblastic

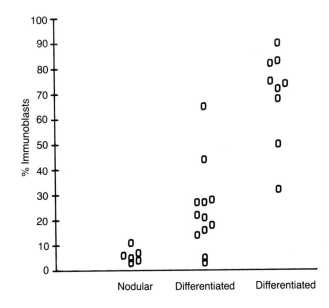

air dried and stained immediately with Romanowsky-Giemsa stain.

Among the prognostic variables, age, sex, white blood cell count and French-American-British (FAB) subtype were used as identifiers for low, medium and high risk. With these criteria, two of the patients were at high risk (therapeutic protocol, AIL 7602), and the others were at medium risk (therapeutic protocol, AIL 7401). (For details of the extensive cytostatic protocols, see reference 4.) Central nervous system prophylaxis with cranial irradiation (2400 rads) was performed on all the children. Differences in classification and treatment did not interfere with the morphometric analysis or prognosis of the two subgroups studied.

The morphometric analyses were performed at a final magnification of ×1250. After a thorough search of the whole slide, the most cellular areas were selected in which 100 blast cells as well as their nuclei were outlined. In each selected field, all lymphoblastic cells with clear profiles were measured. Nonblast cells, such as myeloid cells, erythrocytes, obvious plasma cells and megakaryocytes, were not measured if present.

The results showed that by combining the nuclear/cellular area ratio and the cellular area, a good discrimination between short-term and long-term survivors (survival less and more than 5 years, respectively) could be obtained (Fig. 35–15). Although these results will have to be confirmed in larger material, objective

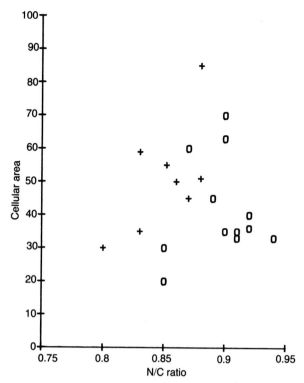

FIGURE 35–15. Scatter diagram of **nuclear/cellular area ratio and cellular area in children with acute lymphoblastic leukemia.** The *(plus)* represent the long-term survivors and the *(open)* the short-term survivors. (Modified from Tosi P, Luzi P, Miracco C, Santopietro R, Baak JPA, Bernardini C, Acquaviva A: Pathol Res Pract 182:416–420, 1987.)

and reproducible morphometric parameters may be of great value in the diagnosis of ALL.

Urinary Bladder

Boon and colleagues[13] studied the morphometric differences between cells in voided urine of patients with grade I and grade II bladders. For all cases, 50 urothelial cells in air-dried and MGG–stained smears were measured. Table 35–8 summarizes the results.

With a cut off point of 0.59 for NC size ratio (values > 0.59 indicating grade II), 20 of the 22 cases were

correctly classified as grades I and II. Only two grade I cases were misclassified as grade II using this threshold.

Van der Poel and colleagues[46] compared cytomorphometry with histomorphometry for grading of bladder tumors employing Papanicolaou-stained centrifuged sediments of urinary bladder washings. They confirmed the value of nuclear area for cytomorphometric grading and showed that in some cases cytomorphometric grading is preferable to histomorphometry.

Stomach

Brush cytology of the gastric mucosa has progressed very much. The accuracy of diagnosis in gastric brush cytology, however, greatly depends on the expertise of the cytologist interpreting the smears. Objective quantitative criteria may therefore be of help to less experienced observers and, in difficult cases, even to very experienced observers. Successful application of morphometry to gastric cytology has been reported by Danno,[24] who showed significant differences in the NC ratio between benign cells and malignant cells. These findings were confirmed by Boon and colleagues[14] who also found the NC ratio to be the best discriminating variable. In their study, smears were prepared from gastric brushes obtained during endoscopy, fixed in 75% ethyl alcohol and stained by the Papanicolaou technique. In each smear, the nuclear and cytoplasmic area of 25 abnormal cells, characterized by enlarged nuclei, abnormal nuclear shapes and abnormal chromatin pattern, were measured at ×1000 magnification. Abnormal cells without visible cytoplasm were also included in the measurement, because they are considered to be poorly differentiated cells that have lost their cytoplasm. The NC ratio of these cells was defined as 1.0. In the cell groupings, only peripherally localized cells with well-spread cytoplasm were measured, thereby excluding the centrally localized cells from measurement. All cases with NC ratios below 0.50 were benign; NC ratios above 0.60 indicated malignancy and an intermediate value should be regarded as doubtful.

TABLE 35–8. Mean Values (± SD) of Air-dried MGG–stained Cells of Voided Urine in Grade I and Grade II Tumors

Parameters (2 sq rt area/π)	Mean ± SD Grade I	Grade II	Probability of Difference (Wilcoxon's Test)
Nuclear perimeter (μm)	40.3 ± 7.69	39.2 ± 7.56	0.67
Cell perimeter (μm)	81.2 ± 21.3	64.1 ± 16.9	0.02
Nuclear area (μm²)	88.2 ± 32.9	89.2 ± 36.0	0.92
Cell area (μm²)	363 ± 208	229 ± 122	0.03
Nuclear size (μm)	10.3 ± 1.94	10.3 ± 1.95	0.97
Cell size (μm)	20.3 ± 5.65	16.1 ± 3.96	0.03
NC area ratio	0.31 ± 0.12	0.34 ± 0.12	0.00
NC size ratio	0.54 ± 0.11	0.66 ± 0.09	0.00

MGG = May-Grünwald-Giemsa; NC = nucleocytoplasmic.
(Adapted from Boon ME, Kiver PHJ, Baak JPA, Ooms ECM: Morphometric differences between urothelial cells in voided urine of patients with grade I and grade II bladder tumours. J Clin Pathol 34:612–615, 1981.)

Endometrium

Equipment has now become available for sampling of cytologic material from the endometrium. Accuracy tests on such sampled material have shown that it may be as reliable as curettements and that cytologic evaluation can be as accurate as histologic evaluation in malignant cases. Skaarland[50] studied the value of morphometry on endometrial cytologic material in 55 cases (35 normal cases and 20 moderately or well-differentiated adenocarcinomas) in which the cytologic sampling had been followed by curettage to establish the histologic diagnosis. The cytologic material obtained with either the Isaacs cell sampler or the Endoscann instrument was smeared on glass slides, fixed in 96% alcohol and stained according to Papanicolaou. Nuclear measurements were performed at a magnification of $\times 400$. In each case, 20 well-preserved nuclei in each of 10 different epithelial structures were measured. The best distinction between normal and malignant cases was obtained with a cutoff value for a nuclear area of 45 μm^2, leading to 17% false-negative and 25% false-positive reports. Although this finding illustrates the value of quantitation in this field, nuclear area as a single parameter is not good enough as a screening method. Further research is therefore necessary to establish quantitative features with additional discriminative value. In this respect it is promising that the SD of nuclear area seemed to improve discrimination. In a subsequent study, Skaarland[51] studied cystic and adenomatous hyperplasia cases in comparison with benign and malignant endometrial conditions. The mean nuclear area in the ten cystic hyperplasias was significantly lower compared with the four adenomatous hyperplasias. Both groups differed from normal endometrium but could not be distinguished from malignant lesions. In the cytologic diagnosis of hyperplastic lesions, nuclear area therefore seems to be of limited value.

References

1. Abe S, Makimura S, Itabashi K, Kawakami Y: Nuclear DNA content, cytomorphologic features and clinical characteristics of small cell carcinoma of the lung. Analyt Quant Cytol Histol 9:495–498, 1987.
2. Abe S, Tsuneta Y, Makimura S, Itabashi K, Nagai T: Nuclear DNA content as an indicator of chemosensitivity in small-cell carcinoma of the lung. Analyt Quant Cytol Histol 9:425–428, 1987.
3. Aherne WA, Dunnill MS: Morphometry. London, Edward Arnold, 1982.
4. AIL (Italian Association Against Leukemia) Study Group: A cooperative study on the therapy of acute lymphoblastic leukaemia. Results of Italian Association Against Leukemia. Haematologica 64:119–147, 1979.
5. Baak JPA: Manual of Quantitative Pathology. Berlin, Springer-Verlag, in press.
6. Baak JPA, van Diest PJ, Ariens ATH, van Beek MWPM, Bellot SM, Fijnheer J, van Gorp LHM, Kwee WS, Los J, Peterse JC, Ruitenberg HM, Schapers RFM, Schipper MEI, Somsen JG: The Multicenter Morphometric Mammary Carcinoma Project. A nationwide study on reproducibility and prognostic value of quantitative features in breast cancer. Pathol Res Pract 185:664–670, 1989.
7. Baak JPA, Oort J: A manual of morphometry in diagnostic pathology. Berlin, Springer-Verlag, 1983.
8. Ball PJ, van der Valk P, Kurver PHJ, Lindeman J, Meijer CJLM: Large cell lymphoma. II. Differential diagnosis of centroblastic and B-immunoblastic subtypes by morphometry on cytologic preparations. Cancer 55:486–492, 1985.
9. Barry JD, Sharkey FE: Observer reproducibility during computer-assisted planimetric measurements of nuclear features. Hum Pathol 16:225–227, 1985.
10. Beyer-Boon ME, Voorn-Den Hollander MJA, van der Arentz PW, Cornelisse CJ, Schaberg A, Fox CH: Effect of various routine cytopreparatory techniques on normal urothelial cells and their nuclei. Acta Pathol Microbiol Scand [A] 87:63–69, 1979.
11. Bibbo M, Bartels PH, Dytch HE, Wied GL: Ploidy patterns in cervical dysplasia. Analyt Quant Cytol Histol 7:213–217, 1985.
12. Boon ME, Fox CH: Simultaneous condyloma acuminatum and dysplasia of the uterine cervix. Acta Cytol 25:393–399, 1981.
13. Boon ME, Kurver PHJ, Baak JPA, Ooms ECM: Morphometric differences between urothelial cells in voided urine of patients with grade I and grade II bladder tumours. J Clin Pathol 34:612–615, 1981.
14. Boon ME, Kurver PHJ, Baak JPA, Thompson HT: The application of morphometry in gastric cytological diagnosis. Virchows Arch [A] 393:159–164, 1981.
15. Boon ME, Kwee HS, Alons CL, Morawetz F, Veldhuizen RW: Discrimination between primary pleural and primary peritoneal mesotheliomas by morphometry and analysis of the vacuolization pattern of the exfoliated mesothelial cells. Acta Cytol 26:103–108, 1982.
16. Boon ME, Lowhagen T, Lopes Cardozo PL, Blonk DI, Kurver PHJ, Baak JPA: Computation of preoperative diagnosis probability for follicular adenoma and carcinoma of the thyroid on aspiration smears. Analyt Quant Cytol Histol 4:1–5, 1982.
17. Boon ME, Trott PA, van Kaam H, Kurver PHJ, Leach A, Baak JPA: Morphometry and cytodiagnosis in breast lesions. Virchows Archiv [A] 396:9–18, 1982.
18. Boon ME, van Velzen D, Ruinaard C, Veldhuizen RW: Analysis of number, size and distribution patterns of lipid vacuoles in benign and malignant mesothelial cells. Analyt Quant Cytol Histol 6:221–226, 1984.
19. Burger G, Oberholzer M, Gössner W: Morphometrie in Zyto- und Histopathologie. Berlin, Springer-Verlag, 1988.
20. Burns TR, Underwood RD, Greenberg SD, Teasdale TA, Cartwright J: Cytomorphometry of large cell carcinoma of the lung. Analyt Quant Cytol Histol 11:48–52, 1989.
21. Chan KW, Chiu KY, Fu KH, Ling JM: Observer variability in microcomputer-assisted morphometric study of nuclear parameters. Pathology 19:407–409, 1987.
22. Collan Y, Torkkeli T, Koswa VM, Pesonen E, Kosunen O, Jantunen E, Mariuzzi GM, Montironi R, Marinelli F, Collina G: Sampling in diagnostic morphometry. Pathol Res Pract 182:401–406, 1987.
23. Cornelisse CJ, Koning HR de, Arentz PW, Raatgever JW, van Heerde P: Quantitative analysis of the nuclear area variation in benign and malignant breast cytology specimens. Analyt Quant Cytol Histol 3:128–134, 1981.
24. Danno M: Statistical criteria for the cytology of gastric cancer. A proposal of distance index. Acta Cytol 20:466–468, 1976.
25. Dardick I, Caldwell D: Reproducibility of morphometric image analysis. Hum Pathol 16:1178, 1985.
26. DeHoff RT: Sampling of material and statistical analysis in quantitative stereology. In Stereology: Proceedings of the Second International Congress for Stereology. Edited by H Elias. Berlin, Springer-Verlag, 1967.
27. Detweiler R, Zahniser DJ, Garcia GL, Hutchinson M: Contextual analysis complements single-cell analysis in the diagnosis of breast cancer in fine needle aspirates. Analyt Quant Cytol Histol 10:10–15, 1988.
28. van Diest PJ, Mouriquand J, Risse EKJ, Schipper NW, Baak JPA: Comparison of light microscopic grading and morphometric features in cytological breast cancer specimens. Pathol Res Pract, in press.
29. van Diest PJ, Mouriquand J, Schipper NW, Baak JPA: Prognostic value of nucleolar morphometric variables in cytological breast cancer specimens. J Clin Pathol 43:157–159, 1990.

30. van Diest PJ, Smeulders AWM, Thunnissen FBJM, Baak JPA: Cytomorphometry: A methodological study on preparation techniques, selection methods and sample size. Analyt Quant Cytol Histol 11:225–231, 1989.

31. Fleege JC, Baak JPA, Smeulders AWM: Analysis of measuring system parameters that influence reproducibility of morphometric assessments with a graphic tablet. Hum Pathol 19:513–517, 1988.

32. Gamel JW, Gleason J, Williams H, Greenberg R: Reproducibility of nucleolar measurements in human intraocular melanoma cells on standard histologic microslides. Analyt Quant Cytol Histol 7:174–177, 1985.

33. Gamel JW, McLean IW: Computerized histopathologic assessment of malignant potential: III. Refinements of measurement and data analysis. Analyt Quant Cytol Histol 6:37–43, 1984.

34. Horan DC, Bonfiglio TA, Patten SF: Fine needle aspiration cytology of bronchial carcinoid tumors. An analytical study of the cells. Analyt Quant Cytol Histol 4:105–109, 1982.

35. Kuenen-Bouwmeester V, Hop WCJ, Blonk DI, Boon ME: Prognostic scoring using morphometry and lymph node status of patients with breast carcinoma. Eur J Cancer Clin Oncol 20:337–345, 1984.

36. Kwee WS, Veldhuizen RW, Alons CA, Morawetz F, Boon ME: Quantitative and qualitative differences between benign and malignant mesothelial cells in pleural fluid. Acta Cytol 26:401–406, 1982.

37. Lopez PA, Cambier MA, Wheeless LL: Syringing as a method of cell dispersal. II. Effect on abnormal cells. Analyt Quant Cytol Histol 3:235–238, 1981.

38. Luck JB, Mumaw VR, Frable WJ: Fine needle biopsy of the thyroid. Differential diagnosis by videoplan image analysis. Acta Cytol 26:793–796, 1982.

39. Marchevsky AM, Hauptman E, Gil J, Watson C: Computerized interactive morphometry as an aid in the diagnosis of pleural effusions. Acta Cytol 31:131–136, 1987.

40. Masuda T, Tezuka F, Konno H, Togashi A, Itoh Y, Sugawara T: Intraoperative imprint cytology of the thyroid gland with computer-assisted morphometric analysis of cell clusters. Analyt Quant Cytol Histol 10:294–298, 1988.

41. Metter GE, Nathwani BN, Burke JS, Winberg CD, Mann RB, Barcos M, Kjeldsberg CR, Whitcomb CC, Dixon DO, Miller TP: Morphological subclassification of follicular lymphoma: Variability of diagnoses among hematopathologists: A collaborative study between the Repository Center and Pathology Panel for Lymphoma Clinical Studies. J Clin Oncol 3:25–38, 1985.

42. van Molengraft FJJM, van't Hot MA, Herman CJ, Vooijs PG: Quantitative light microscopy of atypical mesothelial cells and malignant cells in ascitic fluid. Analyt Quant Cytol Histol 4:217–220, 1982.

43. Mouriquand J, Gozlan-Fior M, Villemain D, Bouchet Y, Sage JC, Mermet MA, Bolla M: Value of cytoprognostic classification in breast carcinomas. J Clin Pathol 39:489–496, 1986.

44. Mouriquand J, Mouriquand C, Petitpas E, Louis J, Mermet MA: Differential nucleolar staining affinity with a modified Papanicolaou staining procedure. Stain Technol 56:215–219, 1981.

45. Mouriquand J, Pasquier D: Fine needle aspiration of breast carcinoma. A preliminary cytoprognostic study. Acta Cytol 24:153–159, 1980.

46. van der Poel HG, Boon ME, Kok LP, Tolboom J, van der Meulen B, Ooms ECM: Can cytomorphometry replace histomorphometry for grading of bladder tumours? Virchows Arch[A]413:249–255, 1988.

47. Rosenthal DL, Philippe A, Hall TL, Harami S, Missirlial N, Suffin SC: Prognosis of moderate dysplasia. Predictive value of selected markers in routinely prepared cervical smears. Analyt Quant Cytol Histol 9:165–168, 1987.

48. Saito Y, Imai T, Nagamoto N, Sato M, Ota S, Kanma K, Takahashi S, Usuda K, Sagawa M, Suda H, Sato H, Hashomoto K, Nakada T, Higashiiwai H: A quantitative cytologic study of sputum in early squamous cell bronchogenic carcinoma. Analyt Quant Cytol Histol 10:365–370, 1988.

49. Scott N, Sutton J, Gray C: Morphometric diagnosis of serous effusions: refinement of differences between benign and malignant cases by use of outlying values and larger sample size. J Clin Pathol 42:607–612, 1989.

50. Skaarland E: Morphometric analysis of nuclei in epithelial structures from normal and neoplastic endometrium: a study using the Isaacs cell sampler and Endoscann instruments. J Clin Pathol 38:496–501, 1985.

51. Skaarland E: Nuclear size and shape of epithelial cells from the endometrium: lack of value as a criterion for differentiation between normal, hyperplastic, and malignant conditions. J Clin Pathol 38:501–506, 1985.

52. Smeulders AWM, Dorst L: Measurements issues in morphometry. Analyt Quant Cytol Histol 7:242–249, 1985.

53. Stevens MW, Crowley KS, Fazzalari NL, Woods AE: Use of morphometry in cytological preparations for diagnosing follicular non-Hodgkin's lymphomas. J Clin Pathol 41:370–377, 1988.

54. Tosi P, Luzi P, Miracco C, Santopietro R, Baak JPA, Bernardini C, Acquaviva A: Morphometry for the prognosis of acute lymphoblastic leukaemia in childhood. Pathol Res Pract 182:416–420, 1987.

55. Wallgren A, Zajicek J: The prognostic value of the aspiration biopsy smear in mammary carcinoma. Acta Cytol 20:479–485, 1976.

56. Weibel ER: Stereological methods. In Practical Methods for Biological Morphometry, vol 1. Edited by ER Weibel. London, Academic Press, 1979.

57. Wied GL, Bibbo M, Dytch HE, Bartels PH: Computer grading of cervical intraepithelial neoplastic lesions. I. Cytologic indices. Analyt Quant Cytol Histol 7:52–60, 1985.

58. Wright RG, Castles H, Mortimer RH: Morphometric analysis of thyroid cell aspirates. J Clin Pathol 40:443–445, 1987.

59. Zajdela A, De LaRiva LS, Ghossein NA: The relation of prognosis to the nuclear diameter of breast cancer cells obtained by cytologic aspiration. Acta Cytol 23:75–80, 1979.

36

Cell Image Analysis

Marluce Bibbo

Peter H. Bartels

Harvey E. Dytch

George L. Wied

Over 50 years ago, Caspersson[39] laid the foundations for quantitative microphotometric methodology and defined the conditions under which exact determinations of cellular constituents, such as DNA and RNA, could be obtained. The scanning microscope was developed about 30 years ago but did not become commercially available until the late 1960s[40] and was very expensive. The somewhat cumbersome determination of DNA contents in cell nuclei, based on ultraviolet (UV) absorbance, was replaced by visible light microphotometry employing a stoichiometric cytochemical procedure, the Feulgen reaction.[55] Over the past two decades, advances in image sensing and recording techniques have all but replaced analogue microphotometry with digital methods. For each spot measurement in the scanned image, the amount of light absorbed (the optical density, OD) is converted to a number. The image is represented as an array of numbers, i.e., a digital image. Microphotometers that record digital images at video rates are now generally available.[119]

Microphotometric applications were augmented by micromorphometric procedures, implemented on videophotometers and supported by personal computers. Videophotometers with special processing boards offer all of the capabilities of mathematic morphology.[103] Computer assessment of digitized cell images has developed into a methodology of great refinement and substantial potential.

The overall goal of cell image analysis is to bring measurement and objectivity to pathology. Cell image analysis aims to determine numeric values for the cellular characteristics used by human diagnosticians, e.g., nucleocytoplasmic (N/C) ratio, nuclear area, staining density, coarseness of the nuclear chromatin, peripheral tendency of the nuclear chromatin, number and size of nucleoli and shape of nuclei. The analysis is continued at the next level by characterizing the cell population of a clinical sample and computing numeric values for such sample properties as the proportional composition of cells of different cell types, the ploidy pattern, the mean atypicality index for abnormal cells, the nuclear polymorphism and the degree of anisonucleosis.

This level of analysis is followed by a characterization of clinical samples falling into different cytodiagnostic categories, such as patients with mild dysplasia or carcinoma *in situ*. It is continued by studies of the sequential development of disease processes, the homogeneity of such processes among patients and the response to treatment.

Cell image analysis has, however, not remained restricted to those diagnostic clues that human observers notice. An important clinical application has evolved with the determination of the ploidy pattern as a diagnostic and prognostic indicator. Based on a cytochemical reaction, the ploidy pattern adds diagnostic information not readily available in visual cytodiagnosis.

Computer analysis of digitized imagery has led to the discovery of computable diagnostic clues too subtle to be noticed by visual inspection. Visually, clearly "normal" cells from patients with malignant lesions have been shown to express micromorphometric characteristics obviously different from cells of the same cell type from patients free of malignant lesions. Here, the discriminatory capabilities of computation expand our ability for diagnostic detection.

Measurements can unequivocally demonstrate differences — for instance, in nuclear area — that for the human eye are simply too small to be noticed. Here, statistical hypothesis testing is employed as a tool for the demonstration of diagnostic clues.

The extraction of diagnostic information, however,

is only the first stage of image analytic assessment. It is followed by classification and diagnostic evaluation, in which measurement results are converted to human diagnostic concepts and judgment. Such diagnostic assessment may now be supplemented by indices of atypia on malignancy or by objectively computed gradings derived from the measured features.

A number of applications of this powerful methodology have reached the stage of practical and daily clinical use, in particular, the recording of DNA ploidy patterns. A rich literature shows a substantial number of other applications in the research and development stage.

A number of publications may serve as introductory texts to the field (see references 12, 15, 22, 37, 38, 52, 91, 98, 103, 105, 113, 115, 116 and 121).

METHODOLOGY

Quantitative measurements, whether of a microphometric, micromorphometric or stereologic nature, demand standardized conditions. These include the sample preparation, the fixation, the staining and the recording of the digitized imagery.

Sample Preparation

Fixation

Fixation may have pronounced effects on a number of important micromorphometric features of cells and tissues.

The chromatin pattern provides a rich source of diagnostically discriminating features, and the nuclear chromatin texture changes in a most sensitive fashion in response to even slight variations in the functional state of the cell. The nature of the changes is different for different types of cell injuries, such as radiation damage, viral infection and chemical toxicity.[94] Morphometry can be utilized to quantitate these changes. However, because fixation may also induce chromatin changes, quantitative micromorphometry requires rigid control and careful choice of fixation conditions.

Ethanol (ethyl alcohol, ETOH) is the alcohol originally recommended as a cytologic fixative; it causes the desired amount of cell contraction to yield optimal information from the nuclear chromatin patterns. The desired effect on nuclear content can be produced by using 95% ethanol alone.[73] Alcohols that have similar effects on cells are 100% methanol, 95% denatured alcohol and 80% propanol and isopropanol.

Immediate submission of freshly obtained cells in a liquid fixative is known as wet fixation. Slides may be wet fixed for 20 to 30 minutes, removed from the alcohol and allowed to dry.

Coating fixatives are substitutes for wet fixation. Coating fixatives can be either aerosols applied by spraying the cell sample or liquids placed onto the slide. They are composed of an alcohol base that fixes the cells and a waxlike substance that forms a thin protective coating over the cells. The coating fixative must be removed from the cell sample before staining. Formalin is the most commonly used fixative for tissues. For more details on cell fixation, see Chapter 32 on Cytopreparatory Techniques.

Cell Preparation

For image analysis, cells or tissues are prepared on microscope slides. They can be placed directly on slides as smears or touch preparations, as tissue sections or as single cell suspensions placed on slides.[4, 16, 67, 10]

Single cell suspensions of cytologic preparations can be obtained with automated devices.[16] The steps involve the depositing of the cellular sample in a collection fluid, the adjustment of the concentration to about 30,000 cells per milliliter, the dispersion of the sample by syringing and the deposition of the cellular content onto microscope slides by centrifugation.

Thick or thin tissue sections (up to 50 μ) from paraffin-embedded specimens are deparaffinized, protease treated and placed on slides.[67]

Staining Procedures

The need for standardization of stains and staining procedures has been widely recognized.[122] Although stoichiometry of staining is desirable, it is not mandatory for reproducibility in micromorphometric or even microphotometric measurements; this does not apply, of course, to quantitative cytochemical determinations. Even for the Feulgen procedure, stoichiometry is obtained only under certain preparatory conditions. Reviews of the extensive early literature in the field have been provided by Hale[65] and Deitch.[45]

The recipe for the Feulgen procedure, one of the most important stoichiometric stains, is given in Table 36–1.

INSTRUMENTATION

Many instruments are commercially available for microphotomery.[98] Instruments are also available that have been developed for research purposes.[97–99]

Hardware

A videomicrophotometer comprises four basic components: a microscope, a video camera, a video digitizer/imaging board and a computer (Fig. 36–1).[99]

Microscope

In converting a laboratory microscope into a microphotometer, a number of requirements should be met. It must be possible to set up the microscope for Koehler illumination to provide as even an illumination as

TABLE 36–1. Feulgen Stain for DNA Analysis

Procedure		Points of Emphasis
1. Xylene	2–3 hours	This wash is designated to remove paraffin coating or other fixative from tissue section.
2. 95% ethanol	20 dips	
3. 95% ethanol	10 dips	
4. 70% ethanol	10 dips	
5. 50% ethanol	10 dips	
6. 30% ethanol	10 dips	
7. Distilled water	10 dips	
8. Distilled water	10 dips	
9. 5N HCl	20 minutes	Hydrolysis
10. Schiff's reagent	1 hour	
11. Sulfurous acid bleach	10 minutes	Bleach solution must be made immediately before use. Must be used in well-covered screw-cap jars.
12. Sulfurous acid bleach	10 minutes	
13. Sulfurous acid bleach	10 minutes	
14. Running tap water	5 minutes	
15. Distilled water	10 dips	
16. Distilled water	10 dips	
17. 30% ethanol	10 dips	
18. 50% ethanol	10 dips	
19. 70% ethanol	10 dips	
20. 95% ethanol	10 dips	
21. 100% ethanol	10 dips	
22. Xylene	10 dips	
23. Xylene	10 dips	
24. Xylene	10 dips	
25. Cover		

Schiff's Reagent (100 mml)

Materials

0.5	gm of Fuchsin
100.0	ml of boiled distilled water
10.0	mg of 1N HCl
2.0	gm of potassium metabisulfite
0.25	gm of neutral activated charcoal

Thermometer
Coarse filter paper
Funnel
2 chemically clean bottles
1 heat resistant flask

Procedure
1. Dissolve fuchsin in distilled water.
2. Shake thoroughly.
3. Cool to 50°C.
4. Filter into chemically clean bottle.
5. Add 1N HCl to filtrate.
6. Add potassium metabisulfite to filtrate.
7. Shake.
8. Close tightly and store for 24 hours in dark. (After this time period, the solution should be straw colored.)
9. Add neutral activated charcoal.
10. Shake for 1 minute.
11. Filter rapidly.
12. Store clear filtrate in chemically clean brown bottle in refrigerator.

Sulfurous Acid Bleach (200 ml); Made Immediately Before Use

Materials

190.0	ml of distilled water
1.00	ml of potassium metabisulfite
10.0	ml of 1N HCl

Procedure
1. Dissolve potassium metabisulfite in distilled water.
2. Stir.
3. Add 1N HCl.
4. Shake thoroughly.
5. Store in tightly covered screw-cap jars.

Reproduced with permission from Deitch AD: Cytophotometry of nucleic acids. *In* Introduction to Quantitative Cytochemistry. Edited by GL Wied. New York, Academic Press, pp 327–354, 1966.

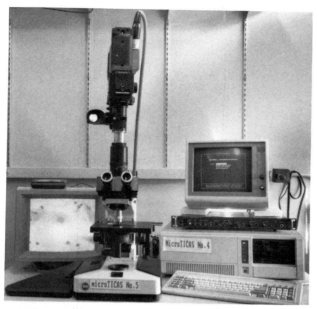

FIGURE 36–1. MicroTICAS image analysis system.

possible and to control stray light.[70] For practical purposes, the condensor should have its aperture iris in its lower focal plane, which is the case for practically all condensors. The condensor should be focusable so that the image of the field iris can be focused into the object plane. The field iris is usually close to the light source and is sometimes built into the base of the microscope stand.

A rather bright light source is needed, preferably with a flat filament and power of 30 to 60 watts. It is essential that the bulb be simple to center exactly. Also, a very well-stabilized power supply is necessary; very small voltage fluctuations — down to the millivolt range — may cause several percentage points of variation in photometric values.

The microscope should have a trinocular tube, so that a video camera can be mounted. Videophotometers are image scanning systems, i.e., the object remains stationary, and the image is scanned as it is projected onto the faceplate of the videotube.

Because the object is stationary, it is not necessary to have a scanning microscope stage. The ordinary mechanical stage of the microscope may serve. However, a number of applications exist in which one may want to map the locations of measured cells.[121] A computer file of locations could drive a scanning stage back to all listed fields. For this, a relatively slow stage, moving at, for example, 200 steps per second, is adequate. It is helpful to have a scanning stage that can cover a 20×20 mm area. The manual reading of micrometers on the mechanical stage, as an alternative, is cumbersome and not recommended. A compromise is mounting small digital readout location indicators on the microscope stage.

Video Camera

It is advisable to seek the optical manufacturer's advice for the mounting of a video camera. The micro-

scope projects the image onto the faceplate of the videotube. The active area in United States–standards cameras is 12.8 x 9.6 mm. As a rule, the ocular would be left in place in the phototube, followed by a relay projective to project the image onto the videotube. This is done for two reasons. First, the relay projective permits the microscope objective to remain at its designed working distance; thus, the images on the video display and in the binocular viewing tubes are parafocal. Second, the image is kept free from spherical aberration, which would result in a milky or hazy image appearance and in contrast loss. This is a serious problem in high-dry objectives. Also, the relay projective allows the "resolution" of the microscope optics to be matched to that of the video system, an important point that is discussed further.

To attain a certain magnification, the focal length required for the relay projective is given by $M_{rel} \times 250$ mm $= f_{rel}$ in mm. Thus, to reach a 0.33:1 demagnification, a focal length of 83.3 mm is needed. However, because the active area on a videotube is relatively small, relay projectives of 20 to 50 mm focal lengths are common. Video camera objectives are rarely suitable as relay projectives because the location of the entrance pupil — where the objective has its "f stop" iris — is deep inside the optics, and the exit pupil of the microscope is too close to the ocular. The exit pupil of the microscope and the entrance pupil of the videosystem cannot be brought to coincidence. This would result in vignetting, i.e., a keyhole effect with only the center of the field visible.

For purposes of matching microscope resolution and videotube sampling geometry,[66] it is customary to include the ocular as part of the relay projection optics and to compute a common magnification. Thus, to attain a total relay projection of 3:1 magnification, with a $10\times$ ocular, a relay lens of 0.33:1 magnification is needed, i.e., of 83.3 mm.

Some optics manufacturers have their objectives corrected so that only a relay projective is needed and no ocular is used. The focal length calculation remains the same.

Optical Requirements for Microphotometers

The two principal uses of microphotometers are microphotometry and micromorphometry. They have somewhat differing optical requirements. In microphotometry, the principal goal is accurate photometry. For this, among other requirements, the condensor's aperture should not exceed 0.3 in value; otherwise, the high aperture oblique rays traverse the specimen in a noticeably longer path than do rays close to the optic axis. In micromorphometry, the primary goal is often the measurement of an area or outline. This requires as fine a sampling capability as possible, for which the condensor aperture should match that of a high aperture objective. The actual photometry in micromorphometry often serves only to establish a threshold for defining an object structure.

It is not advisable to have an adjustable aperture stop in a condenser system used for accurate photometry. The very slightest change in setting has a marked effect on the contrast transfer of the microscope and can make reproducible photometric results such as a ploidy measurement difficult to achieve. For microphotometry, a fixed round stop in the front focal plane of the condenser is a good idea. For micromorphometry, some provision should be made that allows setting the aperture stop as reproducibly as possible.

The choice of objective for either microphotometry or micromorphometry is guided by two considerations: the size of the imaged field and the spatial resolution. The diameter of the field of view (FOV) for a given microscope objective in mm is computed as (FOV number of ocular in mm)/(magnification of objective) × (tube factor of microscope). The FOV number of the ocular is listed by the manufacturer for each ocular. For a typical wide field ocular, it may be 18 mm. The tube factor varies with manufacturers, often it is 1.25. Thus, for a 20:1 objective and an FOV number of the ocular of 18 mm with a tube factor of 1.25, the diameter of the visible field of view is 0.615 mm. The "resolution" is determined by the numeric aperture (N.A.) of the objective, as discussed elsewhere in this text. Generally, the higher the power of the objective, the higher the N.A. and the smaller the diameter of the FOV.

In cell image analysis, one often wishes to record the texture of nuclear chromatin. One is trying to find an objective of as high an N.A. as possible, even if this means recording images of individual cells. In histologic sections, the placement pattern of nuclei is an important feature, and one may have to settle for a large field of view and lower magnification. For these reasons, a 40:1 objective is often chosen as a compromise. However, 40:1 objectives have a high N.A. and are very sensitive to spherical aberration introduced by the specimen, specifically by a coverglass of incorrect thickness, which produces hazy or milky images. The effect is particularly insidious in videophotometry because the observer usually simply adjusts the contrast on the display monitor; however, the image from which the cytometric features are computed has poor contrast. It is therefore advisable to use oil immersion objectives even for the 20:1 high aperture objectives in microphotometry. It is definitely not advisable to use high-dry objectives with an adjustment collar that allows compensation for coverglass thickness in visual microscopy. These systems introduce a change in magnification, and measurements from slide to slide are no longer comparable.

Software

Support software is the single most significant factor that determines the utility of a computer-assisted microphotometry system. The software has to provide a number of functions, such as the operating system, the data acquisition and recording, the image processing and editing, the image analysis and the data evaluation.[50] Beyond these are important general considera-tion.[50] Beyond these are important general considerations that enter into the acquisition or assembly of a software support package.

If the microphotometer is intended as a single-purpose instrument to carry out a well-defined procedure and to be operated as a "turnkey" system, one of the commercial software packages may be an excellent choice. They are usually very carefully "debugged" and provide "help" instructions. A potential user can try them out before a decision is made. They do not require programming personnel and can be placed in operation immediately. Several disadvantages exist. Such systems cannot be modified and usually cannot be used for other procedures unless additional fixed-purpose software modules are obtained.

Because most research applications require a large variety of options, software systems are often assembled from a variety of programs. Programs obtained from software vendors usually do not include the source code, which makes it difficult to integrate the output from one program with the data in other modules in the software package. Also, many commercial programs contain hardware-dependent codes and may no longer work if, for example, the imaging board was upgraded. One should, therefore, insist on the source code for every hardware-dependent subroutine in such software.

In assembling a software package it is important to make its operation simple for the user. The user should never have to remember obscure system's commands or to guess what answer the system expects to a query. A menu with help frames is a good idea. Furthermore, the output from any program should be acceptable as input into any other program.

Choice of Operating System

The choice of operating system is a decision of some consequence. A user may select a general purpose and highly standardized operating system, such as MS-DOS, or a much more versatile, but also more complex, operating system, such as UNIX. A system like MS-DOS can be used even by a novice, without extensive training. Such systems have wide distribution and are inexpensive. A very large number of software packages, different languages and low-cost compilers are available. The disadvantages are that operating systems of this kind usually limit programs to around 640K of memory and offer only a limited number of system commands. Generating a report, for example, from a data base, could be cumbersome.

The more research-oriented operating systems require programming personnel with special experience to utilize the system effectively. They allow programs with memory requirements in the megabyte range. However, the cost of these operating systems also is an order of magnitude greater than that of a general system. Likewise, compilers for different languages, if they are available, are also much more expensive. Because the options and capabilities are complex and powerful, on the one hand, the user is facing a system that requires considerable knowledge to operate. On the other hand, the large memory makes feasible operations that a general operating system would not.

One important consideration for cell image analysis is whether the operating system offers a driver for an imaging board. If it does not, a significant programming effort may be required.

Photometer Calibration

A system's calibration software module offers several service functions.[13, 41, 51, 72] It should allow the user to set up uniform illumination in the field of view, to set up a standardized brightness level and to establish linearity of response.

Uniformity of illumination is usually attained in a two-step procedure. The microscope is first manually set up for Koehler illumination. Next, a service routine on the videophotometer displays on the monitor the image brightness, e.g., in the four corners of the field and at the center. The light source is then centered until a uniform, or at least as symmetric a response as possible, is achieved.

Next, the power supply of the source is adjusted until the video camera reaches full response in a clear field. Finally, the object slide is moved to an empty field and the free background is recorded. Actually, several different empty fields are recorded and averaged to eliminate the effect of blemishes or dust. The average is stored as a photometric reference map for background correction and uniformity of illumination. The procedure should be repeated every time the condenser is recentered or refocused.

The next step is calibration for linearity of response. This involves setting up an empty field at full illumination and recording the response as 100%, utilizing a clear glass insert in the beam path. A series of neutral density filters of known OD are then sequentially inserted, and the recorded response is stored. The software displays the response curve and establishes a "lookup table" to relate the photometric response to the OD.

Cytochemical linearity of response requires a separate calibration that is often neglected. It involves the use of nuclei that contain known amounts of DNA to create a lookup table for the stoichiometry of the Feulgen reaction[87]

DATA COLLECTION

Many cell properties or parameters are readily accessible to image cytometry: size, DNA and protein content, surface antigens, intracellular antigens, motility, N/C ratio, shape and texture.[84]

Image Acquisition

One of the great advantages of image cytometry is its basis in the familiar techniques of light microscopy. The operator, whether a pathologist, clinician or tech-

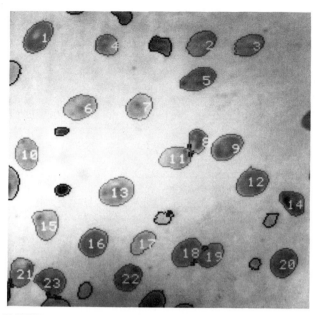

FIGURE 36–2. Scene segmentation in Feulgen-stained tissue. Acceptable nuclei are shown with a black boundary and a number tag whereas rejected nuclei have only a black boundary.

nician, can relate to the material being measured and interact with the system, editing it if necessary.

It is desirable to choose an image board that digitizes at video rates so that the image moves with the slide, in real time, during the search for fields to be recorded. Once a field of interest is located, the image is "frozen" and stored. In most videophotometers, several frames of the image are automatically averaged to reduce noise.

Image acquisition is followed by scene segmentation. In most cytologic scenes, only certain cells in the field are of interest. The software should allow the user to segment these images out, give them separate names and identification numbers and store them for further processing. This interaction may involve a light pen; the observer may use the keyboard to move a cursor or the system may have a "mouse."

In applications such as ploidy determinations, segmentation may involve the automatic processing of the entire field, or selected subfields, trying out a threshold and then displaying the segmentation results as outlines. Overlapping nuclei may then be interactively separated, or identified and processed individually (Fig. 36–2).[51]

Computer Graphics

One important way in which data display can aid the diagnostician is by summarizing the cytometric data from hundreds of cells from a scraping, aspirate or biopsy sample. One type of summary is represented by the nuclear DNA histograms that summarize hundreds of ploidy measurements made in Feulgen-stained tissue sections or Papanicolaou-stained cells,

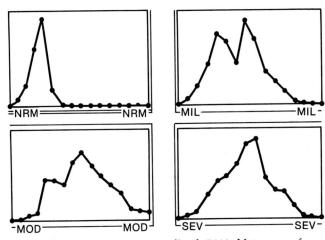

FIGURE 36–3. Average normalized DNA histograms from groups of patients of different diagnostic categories showing intergroup spectral variations. (Reproduced with permission from Dytch HE, Bibbo M, Bartels PH, Wied GL: Analyt Quant Cytol Histol 8:81 to 88, 1986.)

such as the one shown in Figure 36–3. Such displays enable the diagnostician to see clearly the patterns and trends that might not be noticed when the data is presented in numeric form.

Computer graphics may also provide a means of examining cytodiagnostic criteria that are difficult or impossible to visualize otherwise.[50] One example is the use of pseudocolor density mapping to bring out chromatin clumping patterns within dark nuclei. Transparent colored overlays may be employed to highlight nuclei of a given ploidy range, for example, all nuclei exceeding the 5N ploidy level, and computer graphics may be employed to frame cell images in a color tone reflecting an atypicality measure that has been computed. Computer graphics provide a valuable analytic tool to the researcher in automated diagnostic cytometry. Various plotting techniques allow the examination of interrelations between cytometric variables. In addition, there are secondary graphics, which display not the original or processed image, but the computation of mathematic features derived from such images. This image represents a still greater extent of information condensation and abstraction. Although a few of these features have direct graphic analogues, such as the Fourier shape approximations, most do not. Their primary visual representation is in the form of histograms or scatterplots. Displays may involve a single type of information about a single object, such as the histogram of OD values shown in Figure 36–3. They may also display, in a multidimensional way, the relationship between several types of features measured within a group of many related objects.[50]

Analysis

In general, the methodology for the analysis of data obtained by high-resolution cell image analysis is similar, regardless of the particular study involved. An experimental design is set up to test a given hypothesis.

Appropriate cell images are then collected and segmented, and the cytometric features are extracted. The most discriminatory features and feature combinations are then selected by one of a variety of statistical methods, such as discriminant analysis. Analysis of variance and other statistical techniques are utilized to test the initial hypothesis according to the experimental design set up originally.[19, 56]

CLINICAL APPLICATIONS

A variety of clinical applications, involving both individual cells and cells in embedded tissues, are illustrated.

Diagnosis

DNA aneuploidy is unquestionably the most universal marker of malignancy. When present, an abnormal DNA stem line, even in precancerous conditions, implies neoplasia.[18, 31, 61, 100, 111] Many investigations have shown that 80 to 90% of solid tumors are aneuploid.[18] A similar frequency of aneuploidy has been observed in malignant effusions, predominantly those secondary to solid tumors.[68] Figure 36–4 shows an adenocarcinoma metastatic to the pleural cavity with its aneuploid histogram. For comparison, a diploid histogram of reactive mesothelial cells is shown in Figure 36–5.

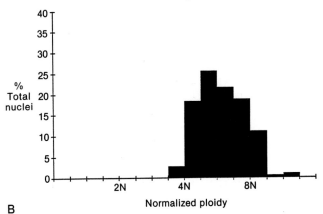

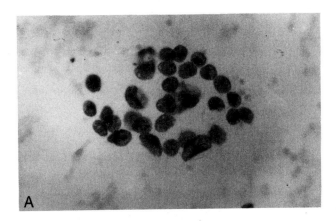

FIGURE 36–4. *A,* **Metastatic adenocarcinoma** to the pleural cavity (Feulgen stain; ×400). *B,* **Aneuploid histogram.**

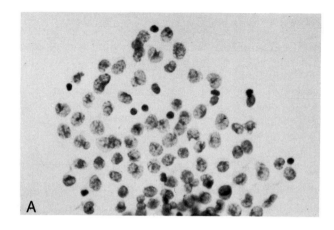

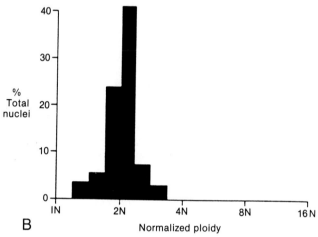

FIGURE 36–5. *A,* **Reactive mesothelial cells** (Feulgen stain; ×400). *B,* **Diploid histogram.**

Prognosis

Quantitative DNA analysis reflects the total chromosomal content of tumor cells. Evidence is accumulating that tumor ploidy reflects the biologic behavior of a large number of tumor types and that patients with tumors with DNA contents in the diploid range have better prognoses than do patients with aneuploid tumors.[32, 59]

Ploidy assessment provides significant information for the management of patients with tumors in almost any organ site. Table 36–2 presents a review of the literature on the prognostic significance of DNA ploidy by image analysis in solid tumors of various organ sites. Ploidy assessment also has predictive value in premalignant atypias.[28, 32, 59, 92] Figure 36–6 shows a cervical intraepithelial neoplasia (CIN) lesion with an aneuploid histogram consistent with a poor prognosis.[31]

Good correlation exists between DNA contents determined by image cytometry and by flow cytometry.[8]

Quality Control

One of the great potentials of rapid high-resolution cytometry is in the area of quality control of cytologic

and histologic diagnoses. Comparison of the results obtained on the histologic and cytologic samples can determine whether the correct site was biopsied.[27] Figure 36–7 shows cytologic and histologic samples consistent with high-grade CIN. The absorption measurements on the histologic material are representative of the detected cytologic atypia, indicating an agreement between the cytologic and histologic sampling.

Response to Therapy

Ploidy assessment can monitor the response to radiation therapy, chemotherapy, laser therapy or surgery, with recurring aneuploidy pointing to a poor response.[32, 92] Figure 36–8 shows smears taken before and after treatment of an invasive carcinoma. Although the post-treatment smear shows only postradiation dysplasia, it retains the aneuploid DNA pattern of the pretreatment smear, indicating a poor therapeutic response.

Tumor Heterogeneity

The phenomenon of tumor heterogeneity has gained increased interest because of its important implications

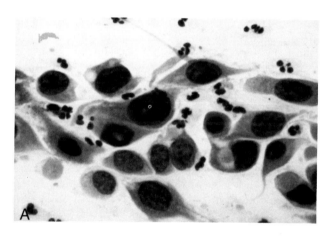

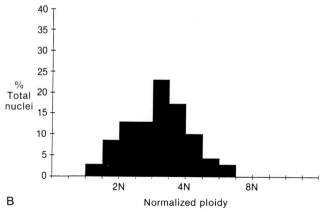

FIGURE 36–6. *A,* **High-grade cervical intraepithelial neoplasia lesion** (Papanicolaou stain; ×400). *B,* **Aneuploid histogram** consistent with a poor prognosis.

TABLE 36–2. DNA Ploidy by Image Analysis—Prognostic Significance Reported in the Literature

Solid Tumor Type	Author, Reference	Survival Advantage of Diploid Tumors	Correlation with Histologic Grade	Other Correlations or Findings
Breast	Atkin and Kay[7]	+	+	
	Auer et al[8-10]	+	+	Stability DNA content, ER expression
	Erhardt and Auer[53]			Same DNA content in invasive and noninvasive tumors
	Izuo et al[71]			Aneuploid benign tumors progress
	Meek[86]			Stability DNA content tumor and metastases
	Stenkvist et al[108]			Aneuploidy and recurrence and variance nuclear area
	Zajicek et al[124]			Diagnostic cytophotometry
Ovary	Atkin and Kay[5, 7]	+	−	Stage
	Bader et al[14]		+	
	Weiss et al[114]	+	−	Borderline malignancy
Cervix	Atkin and Kay[7]			High ploidy squamous tumors have better prognosis.
	Fu et al[61]			Precursor lesions
	Fu et al[60]	+		Stage (adenocarcinoma)
Endometrium	Atkin[6]	+	−	
Colon	Rognum et al[101]	+	−	CEA production
	Suzuki et al[109]	+	−	
	Wolley et al[123]	+	−	
Stomach	Korenaga et al[76, 77]	+	−	Tumor size, lymph node involvement in higher ploidy groups
	Okamura et al[93]			Modes of cancer growth
	Sowa et al[106]	+	−	
Liver	Ezaki et al[54]		−	No correlation between DNA and prognosis
	Kuo et al[81]			Stability DNA content in primary and metastases for hyperdiploid tumors
Lung	Abe et al[1]	+		Indicator of chemosensitivity
	Adams and Dahlgren[3]	+	−	Cytology and histology classification
	Nasiell et al[90]		+	Preneoplastic changes
	Pak et al[95]			Cancer screening
Prostate	Auer and Zetterberg[11]	+		
	Tavares et al[110]	+	+	
	Zetterberg and Esposti[125]	+	+	
	Zetterberg and Esposti[126]	+	+	Hormonal response
Bladder	Bartels et al[21]			Indices of atypia
	Fossa et al[57]	+	+	
	Koss et al[110]			Sample profiles
	Tavares et al[110]	+	+	
Kidney	Baisch et al[17]	+	+	
	Bennington and Mayall[26]	+	+	
	Bibbo et al[33]		+	
Thyroid	Bengtsson et al[25]			Differential diagnosis between benign and malignant lesions
	Cohn et al[43]	+		
	Galera-Davidson et al[62]	+	−	
	Sprenger et al[107]			Differential diagnosis between benign and malignant lesions
Bone	Auer and Zetterberg[11]	+	−	
	Kreicbergs et al[79]	+	−	
	Kreicbergs et al[80]	+	−	

+ = positive correlation
− = no correlation
ER = estrogen receptor; CEA = carcinoembryonic antigen.

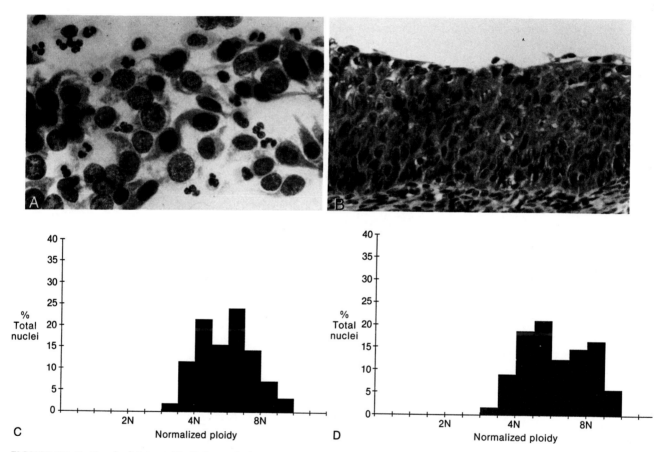

FIGURE 36–7. Cervical intraepithelial neoplasia. *A,* Papanicolaou-stained smear (×400). *B,* Hematoxylin and eosin–stained tissue (×40). *C,* DNA histogram of the absorption measurements of the Papanicolaou-stained smear is similar to *D. D,* DNA histogram of the Feulgen-stained tissue section.

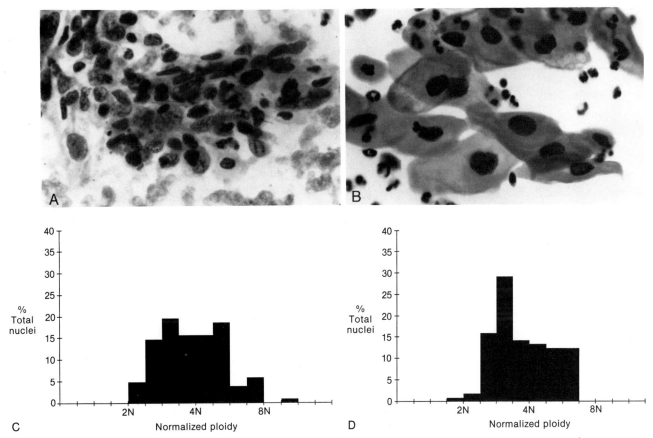

FIGURE 36–8. Invasive squamous carcinoma of the cervix. *A,* Papanicolaou-stained smear prior to treatment shows invasive carcinoma (×400). *B,* Papanicolaou-stained smear following treatment shows postradiation dysplasia (×400). *C,* Histogram of absorption measurements of the smear prior to treatment shows an aneuploid pattern. *D,* Histogram of absorption measurements of the smear showing postradiation dysplasia also has an aneuploid pattern. (Reproduced with permission from Bibbo M, Dytch HE, Bartels PH, Wied GL: Acta Cytol 30:372–378, 1986.)

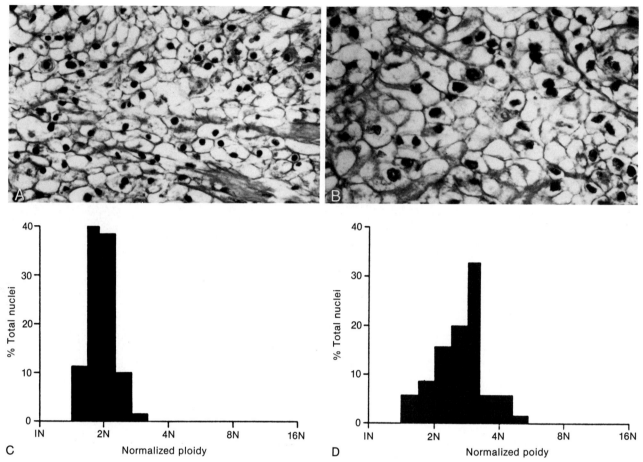

FIGURE 36–9. Renal cell carcinoma. *A*, Sample A and *B*, sample B of the hematoxylin and eosin–stained tissue section (×40). *C*, The DNA histogram of sample A shows a diploid DNA content. *D*, The DNA histogram of sample B shows an aneuploid DNA content, indicating tumor heterogeneity. (Reproduced with permission from Bibbo M, Dytch HE, Bartels PH, Wied GL: Acta Cytol 30:372–378, 1986.)

for the clinical behavior of heterogeneous tumors, including metastatic potential and therapeutic response. Therapy in such cases must be directed against coexisting cell clones, which can be shown by DNA measurements of the tumor cells.[32, 82] In Figure 36–9, DNA analysis of two different areas of a renal cell carcinoma reveals tumor heterogeneity.

Quantitation of Immunologic Staining

For many years, hormone receptor content has been measured by biochemical assays performed on aqueous tissue extracts of fresh-frozen tumor tissue.[42] The development of monoclonal antibodies against human estrogen receptor (ER) and progesterone receptor (PR) has made immunocytochemical detection of both hormone receptors possible.[64] Early prognostic studies suggest that the immunocytochemical ER assay has a predictive value similar to that of older biochemical methods.[46, 85, 96]

By employing a computerized image analysis system, it is possible to reduce the subjectivity inherent in the visual evaluation of immunostains and to offer more

conclusive information about a carcinoma's hormone receptor content and expression of intratumoral heterogeneity, to which the clinical response can be related with greater accuracy than has previously been possible.[36, 44, 58, 75] Three hormone receptor distribution patterns, designated A, B and C, were identified by image analysis among breast tumors. In the type A pattern, tumor cell nuclei are diffusely and uniformly labeled. In type B, both clearly negative as well as distinctly positive cells are present. In type C tumors, a broad range of labeling reactions, from negative to intensely positive, are observed.[44, 75] Figures 36–10 and 36–11 illustrate the A and B staining patterns in breast carcinomas immunostained for hormone receptors. Virtually any antibody that can be localized by immunohistochemical methods can be quantitated utilizing cell image analysis.

Cell Proliferation Rates

Cytokinetic studies using monoclonal antibody Ki-67 produce a direct measurement of proliferative status. This is one of the most powerful markers of

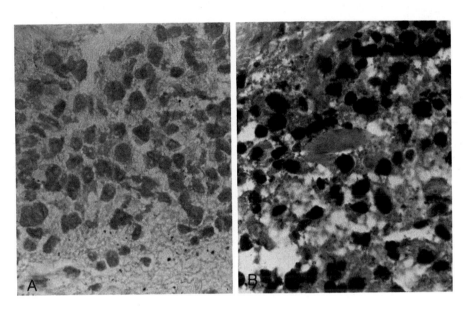

FIGURE 36–10. Invasive ductal breast carcinoma. *A,* Negative control; ×180. *B,* Tumor cells show uniform, strong specific estrogen receptor (ER) labeling (ER immunostain; ×180). *C,* Image analysis graph showing type A staining pattern. (Reproduced with permission from Colley M, Kommoss F, Bibbo M, Dytch HE, Holt J, Wied GL, Franklin WA: Analyt Quant Cytol Histol 11:307–314, 1989.)

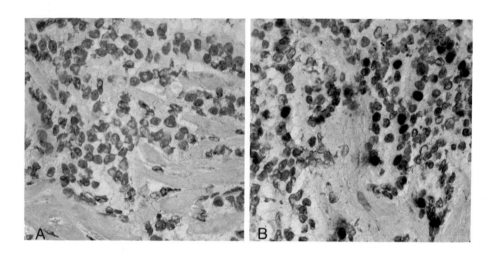

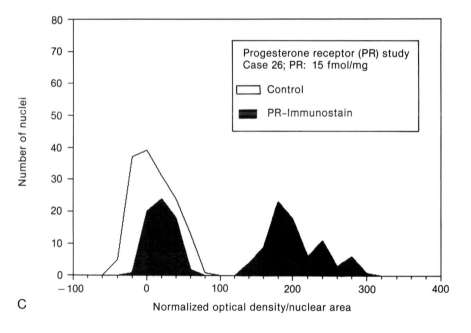

FIGURE 36–11. **Invasive ductal breast carcinoma.** *A*, Negative control, ×180. *B*, Clearly negative as well as strongly progesterone receptor (PR)–positive tumor cells are present (PR immunostain, ×180). *C*, Image analysis graph showing type-B staining pattern. (Reproduced with permission from Kommoss F, Bibbo M, Colley M, Dytch HE, Franklin WA, Holt J, Wied GL: Analyt Quant Cytol Histol 11:298–306, 1989.)

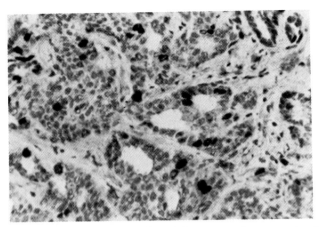

FIGURE 36–12. Invasive ductal breast carcinoma stained with monoclonal antibody Ki-67 (×180). Scattered tumor cell nuclei are densely labeled and are clearly distinguished from unlabeled cells.

abnormality in tissues or cells and is related to tumor grade and aggressiveness. The cells in proliferation are labeled and clearly distinguished from unlabeled cells by Ki-67 immunostaining (Fig. 36–12). For labeling with this monoclonal antibody, cells or tissues must be processed fresh.

Cell image analysis with special software has been employed to assess the cell proliferation rates in various tissues. With appropriate adjustment for image contrast, 1000 cells can be analyzed for Ki-67 content in a few seconds. The system can be used with standard immunoperoxidase substrates and hematoxylin counterstain; optimal combinations of immunoenzymatic substrate colors and counterstains are currently being developed.[48, 58] A close linear correlation exists between Ki-67 counts determined by image analysis and by direct visual counting.

Contextual Karyometry

Contextual karyometry considers the expression of diagnostic clues in nuclei as observed in the context of other nuclei in their vicinity. A good example of this methodology is given by the capabilities offered by the mesoTICAS software system for stratified epithelia.[49] This system computes not only the basic karyometric features, such as total OD for ploidy evaluation, nuclear area, roundness, elongation and shape information, but also the position and orientation of the nuclei, which allows these features to be examined in the context of the epithelial profile as a whole. The depth of each nucleus within the epithelium and the total epithelial height at that point are recorded for stratified epithelium by measuring along a line orthogonal to the stratum germinativum from the center of that nucleus. This practice allows later examination of the relationship of the karyometric features to the relative epithelial depth. The orientation of the major axis of the nucleus to that of the basal layer is computed and used to determine the angle of each nucleus to the stratum germinativum. A measure of nuclear proximity is cal-

culated for each nucleus by determining the distance to its nearest neighbor after the entire field has been segmented. This technique provides measures of nuclear crowding and regularity of internuclear spacing. Figure 36–13 shows the karyometric and histometric features in a typical section of stratified epithelium.

The contextual analysis of nuclei in renal cell carcinomas showed that differences in histologic grade are significantly associated with several histometric variables, including nuclear area, shape, crowding, elongation and mitotic density. A significant relationship between the patient's survival and metastases and the histometric parameters of nuclear elongation, nuclear crowding and mitotic density, as well as tumor grade, was shown. Patients who later died tended to have a high mitotic density, elongated and crowded nuclei and high-grade tumors.[33] Figure 36–14 shows a scatterplot of histologic grades versus nuclear elongation in cases of renal cell carcinoma labeled by follow-up.

The contextual analysis of nuclei in cell clusters in fine needle aspirates of the breast was found by Detweiler and coworkers[47] to considerably improve the accuracy of the classification of samples as benign or malignant. A correct classification as benign or malignant was achieved in 22 of 26 prostatic aspirates and in 15 of 18 mammary aspirates by Hutchinson and associates[69] with contextual analysis.

Chromatin Markers

The computer assessment of digitized images and the statistical evaluation of micromorphometric fea-

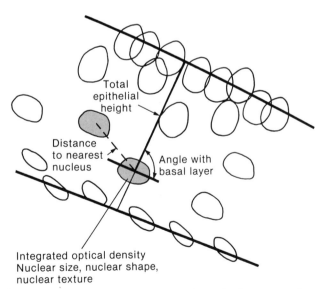

FIGURE 36–13. This diagram schematically summarizes **measurements made by the mesoTICAS system in a typical section of stratified epithelium.** These include features derived from measurements made within the nucleus in isolation (box at the lower left) and those that enable the karyometry to be examined in the context of the section as a whole. (Reproduced with permission from Dytch HE, Bibbo M, Bartels PH, Duls JH, Wied GL: Analyt Quant Cytol Histol 9:69–78, 1987.)

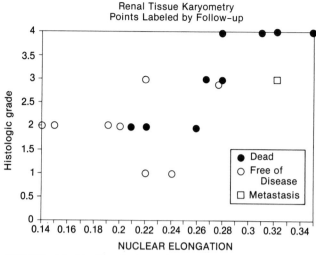

FIGURE 36–14. Renal tissue karyometry. Scatter plot of histologic grade versus elongation, showing, by case, the distribution of renal cell carcinomas labeled by follow-up. (Reproduced with permission from Bibbo M, Galera-Davidson H, Dytch HE, Chaves JG, Lopez-Garrido J, Bartels PH, Wied GL: Analyt Quant Cytol Histol 8: 182–187, 1987.)

tures have been shown to provide a range of measurable clues that render highly discriminating information for diagnosis. Such computed diagnostic clues (certain differences in the nuclear chromatin texture and subtle differences in cellular shape and area) are also referred to as "subvisual clues" because, as a rule, they cannot be perceived consistently and reliably by visual inspection alone. Computed clues constitute new information that has previously not been applied to diagnostic assessment but that offers great potential for finer discrimination and more sensitive and reliable detection of pathologic changes.

Possibly the most intriguing example was the finding of "markers" in normal-appearing intermediate epithelial cells from the ectocervix, thus offering clues for the presence of premalignant and malignant lesions in these cases.[30, 118, 120] Marker features have also been described in foam cells from breast exudates[74] in urothelial cells[104] in glands adjacent to thyroid tumors[29] and in glands adjacent to colonic carcinomas (Fig. 36–15).[34]

Other Applications

Computer image analysis has been employed for a wide variety of other applications. Brenner and colleagues[35] used computer image techniques to quantify components in bone marrow smears and tissues. A method for automated screening for micrometastases of breast cancer in bone marrow smears was described by Mansi and coworkers.[83] Moruzzi and coworkers[88] were able to classify human sperm morphology by computer-assisted analysis. Gamel and McLean[63] conducted extensive studies on the malignant potential of uveal melanomas. In environmental pathology, toxi-

cology and carcinogenesis, studies were conducted by Nair and colleagues[89] on the effects of subtoxic levels of chlordane on rat hepatocytes and by Abmayr and colleagues[2] on the nuclear morphology of hepatocytes after the application of polychlorinated biphenyls.

In tissues, the extraction of diagnostic information has been approached at different levels of complexity and is described by Wied and associates[117] and Bartels.[20]

SUMMARY AND PROSPECTS

Cell image analysis, at this time, is not only a well-established and highly developed methodology, but it is becoming widely utilized and increasingly applied to a wide variety of diagnostic problems in the clinical laboratory.

The analysis of digitized images often provides a more sensitive detection of subtle changes in cells and tissues than does mere visual assessment, thus leading to new insights into the development of pathologic conditions.

Beyond that is a fundamental aspect to this development. Diagnostic practice in pathology is gradually

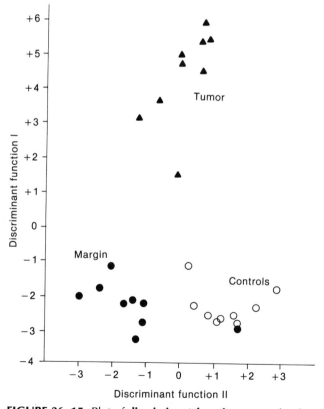

FIGURE 36–15. Plot of **discriminant function scores** for data recorded in the normal-appearing margins of colonic carcinomas in the tumor areas and in controls. Note the clear separation of chromatin markers data recorded in normal-appearing areas from the data in controls. (Reproduced with permission from Bibbo M, Michelassi F, Bartels PH, Dytch HE, Bania C, Lerma E, Montag A: Cancer Research 50:147–151, 1990.)

being moved, by cell analytical methods, to a quantitative basis. This move can be expected to have a far-reaching impact on the standardization, reproducibility and quality of diagnostic procedures. Cell image analytic measurements provide the foundation for data bases, which, combined with long-term patient records, will allow validation and improvement in the ability to render diagnostic and prognostic assessments. High volume, high storage density digital image data bases can make a valuable contribution to the continuing education of practicing cytodiagnosticians.

Cell image analysis plays an important role in preserving and widely distributing human diagnostic expertise in the form of interactive expert systems. Such systems can serve as diagnostic "consultants," providing guidance in data analysis and interpretation. Eventually, in the form of machine-vision systems in which human conceptual diagnostic knowledge is correlated with machine computable data, these systems will allow an encompassing and exhaustive utilization of all of the information offered by a clinical sample.[23, 24, 112, 117]

References

1. Abe S, Tsuneta Y, Makimura S, Itabashi K, Nagai T, Kawakami Y: Nuclear DNA content as an indicator of chemosensitivity in small-cell carcinoma of the lung. Analyt Quant Cytol Histol 9:425–428, 1987.
2. Abmayr W, Deml E, Oesterle D, Gossner W: Nuclear morphology in preoplastic lesions of rat liver. Analyt Quant Cytol 5:275–284, 1983.
3. Adams LR, Dahlgren SE: Cytophotometric measurements of the DNA content of lung tumors. Acta Pathol Microbiol Scand 72:561–574, 1968.
4. Amberson JB, Wersto RP, Agarwal V, Suhrland M, Koss LG: Preparation of paraffin-embedded tissue for flow and image cytometric analysis: An improved and more efficient procedure. Cytometry (Suppl) 2:34, 1988.
5. Atkin NB: Modal DNA value and chromosome number in ovarian neoplasia: A clinical and histopathologic assessment. Cancer 27:1064–1073, 1970.
6. Atkin NB: Prognostic significance of ploidy level in human tumors: I. Carcinoma of the uterus. J Natl Cancer Inst 56:909–910, 1976.
7. Atkin NB, Kay R: Prognostic significance of modal DNA value and other factors in malignant tumors based on 1465 cases. Br J Cancer 40:210–221, 1979.
8. Auer GU, Arrhenius E, Granberg P, Fox CH: Comparison of DNA distributions in primary human breast cancers and their metastases. Eur J Cancer 16:273–278, 1980.
9. Auer GU, Caspersson TO, Gustafsson SA, Humla SA, Ljung BM, Nordenskjold BA, Silfversward C, Wallgren AS: Relationship between nuclear DNA distribution and estrogen receptors in human mammary carcinomas. Analyt Quant Cytol 2:280–284, 1980.
10. Auer G, Caspersson TO, Wallgren AS: DNA content and survival in mammary carcinoma. Analyt Quant Cytol 2:161–165, 1980.
11. Auer GU, Zetterberg A: The prognostic significance of nuclear DNA content in malignant tumors of breast, prostate and cartilage. In Advances in Clinical Cytology, volume 2. Edited by LG Koss, DV Coleman. New York, Masson Publishing USA, pp 123–134, 1984.
12. Baak JPA, Oort J: Morphometry in Diagnostic Pathology. Berlin, SpringerVerlag, 1983.
13. Bacus JW, Grace LJ: Optical microscope system for standardized cell measurements and analyses. Appl Optics 26:3280–3293, 1987.
14. Bader S, Taylor HC, Engle ET: Deoxyribonucleic acid (DNA) content of human ovarian tumors in relation to histological grading. Lab Invest 9:443–459, 1960.
15. Bahr GF, Bartels PH, Wied GL, Koss LG: Automated cytology. In Diagnostic Cytology and Its Histopathologic Bases. Edited by LG Koss. Philadelphia, JB Lippincott, pp 1123–1164 1979.
16. Bahr GF, Bibbo M, Oehme M, Puls JH, Reale FR, Wied GL: An automated device for the production of cell preparations suitable for automatic assessment. Acta Cytol 22:243–249, 1978.
17. Baisch H, Otto U, Konig K, Kloppel G, Kollerman M, Linden WA: DNA content of human kidney carcinoma cells in relation to histological grading. Br J Cancer 45:878–886, 1982.
18. Barlogie B: Perspectives and commentaries: Abnormal cellular DNA content as a marker of neoplasia. Eur J Cancer Clin Oncol 20:1123–1125, 1984.
19. Bartels PH: Numerical evaluation of cytologic data. III. Selection of features for discrimination. Analyt Quant Cytol 1:153–159, 1979.
20. Bartels PH, Bibbo M, Graham A, Paplanus S, Shoemaker RL, Thompson D: Image understanding system for histopathology. Analyt Cell Pathol 1:195–214, 1989.
21. Bartels PH, Koss LG, Sychra JJ, Wied GL: Indices of cell atypia in urinary tract cytology. Acta Cytol 22:3873–91, 1978.
22. Bartels PH, Olson GB: Computer analysis of lymphocyte images. In Methods of Cell Separation, Vol. 3. Edited by N Catsimpoolas. New York, Plenum Press, pp 1–99, 1980.
23. Bartels PH, Weber JE: Expert systems in histopathology: I. Introduction and overview. Analyt Quant Cytol Histol 11:1–7, 1989.
24. Bartels PH, Weber JE: Expert systems in histopathology. II. Knowledge representation and rule-based systems. Analyt Quant Cytol Histol 11:147–153, 1989.
25. Bengtsson A, Malmaeus J, Grimelius L, Johansson H, Ponten J, Rastad J, Akerstroem G: Measurement of nuclear DNA content in thyroid diagnosis. World J Surg 8:481–486, 1984.
26. Bennington JL, Mayall BH: DNA cytometry on four-micrometer sections of paraffin-embedded human renal adenocarcinomas and adenomas. Cytometry 4:31–39, 1983.
27. Bibbo M, Alenghat E, Bahr GR, Bartels PH, Dytch HE, Herbst AL, Keebler CM, Pishotta FT, Wied GL: A quality-control procedure on cervical lesions for the comparison of cytology and histology. J Reprod Med 28:811–822, 1983.
28. Bibbo M, Bartels PH, Dytch HE, Wied GL: Ploidy measurements by high-resolution cytometry. Analyt Quant Cytol Histol 7:81–88, 1985.
29. Bibbo M, Bartels PH, Galera-Davidson H, Dytch HE, Wied GL: Markers for malignancy in the nuclear texture of histologically normal tissue from patients with thyroid tumors. Analyt Quant Cytol Histol 8:168–175, 1986.
30. Bibbo M, Bartels PH, Sychra JJ, Wied GL: Chromatin appearance in intermediate cells from patients with uterine cancer. Acta Cytol 25:23–28, 1981.
31. Bibbo M, Dytch HE, Alenghat E, Bartels PH, Wied GL: DNA ploidy profiles as prognostic indicators in CIN lesions. Am J Clin Pathol 92:261–265, 1989.
32. Bibbo M, Dytch HE, Bartels PH, Wied GL: Clinical applications for an inexpensive, microcomputer-based DNA-cytometry system. Acta Cytol 30:372–378, 1986.
33. Bibbo M, Galera-Davidson H, Dytch HE, Chaves JG, LopezGarrido J, Bartels PH, Wied GL: Karyometry and histometry of renal cell carcinoma. Analyt Quant Cytol Histol 8:182–187, 1987.
34. Bibbo M, Michelassi F, Bartels PH, Dytch HE, Bania C, Lerma-Puertas E, Montag AG: Karyometric marker features in normal-appearing glands adjacent to human colonic adenocarcinoma. Cancer Res 50:147–151, 1990.
35. Brenner JF, Necheles TF, Bonacossa A, Fristensky R, Weintraub BA, Neurath PW: Scene segmentation techniques for the analysis of routine bone marrow smears from acute lymphoblastic leukemia patients. J Histochem Cytochem 25:601–613, 1977.
36. Bur M, Bibbo M, Holt J, Dytch HE, Greene G, Lorincz M, Wied GL, Press M: Computerized image analysis of estrogen

receptor in fine needle aspirations of breast cancer: A preliminary report. Lab Invest 56:9, 1987.

37. Burger G, Oberholzer M, Goessner W: Morphometrie in der Zyto und Histopathologie. Berlin, SpringerVerlag, 1988.

38. Burger G, Ploem JS, Goerttler K: Clinical Cytometry and Histometry. San Diego, Academic Press, 1987.

39. Caspersson TO: Ueber den chemischen Aufbau der Strukturen des Zellkernes. Scand Arch Physiol 73:1–151, 1936.

40. Caspersson TO, Lomakka GM: Scanning microscopic techniques for high resolution quantitative cytochemistry. Ann NY Acad Sci 97:449–462, 1962.

41. Castleman KR: Spatial and photometric resolution and calibration requirements for cell image analysis instruments. Appl Optics 26:3338–3342, 1987.

42. Chamness GC, McGuire WL: Steroid receptor assay methods in human breast cancer. *In* Steroid Receptors in the Management of Cancer, Vol 1. Edited by EB Thompson, EB Lippman. Boca Raton, Florida, CRC Press, pp 3–29, 1979.

43. Cohn K, Baeckdahl M, Forsslund G, Auer G, Lundell G, Lowhagen T, Tallroth E, Willems JS, Zetterberg A, Granberg PO: Prognostic value of nuclear DNA content in papillary thyroid carcinoma. World J Surg 8:474–480, 1984.

44. Colley M, Kommoss F, Bibbo M, Dytch HE, Holt JA, Wied GL, Franklin WA: Assessment of hormone receptors in breast carcinoma by immunocytochemistry and image analysis: II. Estrogen receptors. Analyt Quant Cytol Histol 11:307–314, 1989.

45. Deitch AD: Cytophotometry of nucleic acids. *In* Introduction to Quantitative Cytochemistry. Edited by GL Wied. New York, Academic Press, pp 327–354, 1966.

46. DeSombre ER, Thorpe SM, Rose C, Blough RR, Andersen KW, Rasmussen BB, King WJ: Prognostic usefulness of estrogen receptor immunocytochemical assays for human breast cancer. Cancer Res 46:4256–4264, 1986.

47. Detweiler R, Zahniser DJ, Garcia GL, Hutchinson M: Contextual analysis complements single-cell analysis in the diagnosis of breast cancer in fine needle aspirates. Analyt Quant Cytol Histol 10:10–15, 1988.

48. Doria MI, Dytch HE, Puls JH, Franklin WA, Bibbo M, Wied GL: Computer analysis of cell proliferation rates in sections stained with the monoclonal antibody Ki67. Lab Invest 56:90, 1987.

49. Dytch HE, Bibbo M, Bartels PH, Puls JH, Wied GL: An interactive microcomputer-based system for the quantitative analysis of stratified tissue sections. Analyt Quant Cytol Histol 9:69–78, 1987.

50. Dytch HE, Bibbo M, Bartels PH, Wied GL: Computer graphics in cytologic and pathologic microscopy: Tools for the clinician and researcher. Analyt Quant Cytol Histol 8:81–88, 1986.

51. Dytch HE, Bibbo M, Puls JH, Bartels PH, Wied GL: Software design for an inexpensive, practical microcomputer-based DNA cytometry system. Analyt Quant Cytol Histol 8:8–18, 1986.

52. Eins S: Quantitative and Strukturelle Bildanalyse in der Medizin. Darmstadt, GIT Verlag, 1987.

53. Erhardt K, Auer GU: Mammary carcinoma: Comparison of nuclear DNA content from *in situ* and infiltrative components. Analyt Quant Cytol Histol 9:263–267, 1987.

54. Ezaki T, Kanematsu T, Okamura T, Sonoda T, Sugimachi K: DNA analysis of hepatocellular carcinoma and clinicopathologic implications. Cancer 61:106–109, 1988.

55. Feulgen R, Rossenbeck H: Mikroskopischchemischer Nachweis einer Nukleinsäure vom Typus der Thymonukleinsäure und die darauf beruhende elektive Färbung von Zellkernen in mikroskopischen Präparaten. Z Physiol Chem 125:203–248,1924.

56. Fisher RA: Statistical Methods for Research Workers, 11th ed. Edinburgh, Oliver and Boyd, pp 147–173, 1950.

57. Fossa SD, Kaalhus O, SconKnudsen O: The clinical and histopathological significance of Feulgen DNA-values in transitional cell carcinoma of the human urinary bladder. Eur J Cancer 13:1155–1162, 1977.

58. Franklin WA, Bibbo M, Doria MI, Dytch HE, Toth J, DeSombre E, Wied GL: Quantitation of estrogen receptor content and Ki67 staining in breast carcinoma by the microTICAS image analysis system. Analyt Quant Cytol Histol 9:279–286, 1987.

59. Friedlander ML, Hedley DW, Taylor IW: Clinical and biolog-

ical significance of aneuploidy in human tumors. J Clin Pathol 37:961–974, 1984.

60. Fu YS, Reagan JW, Fu AS, Janiga KE: Adenocarcinoma and mixed carcinoma of the uterine cervix. II. Prognostic value of DNA analysis. Cancer 49:2571–2577, 1982.

61. Fu YS, Reagan JW, Richart RM: Definition of precursors. Gynecol Oncol 12:220–231, 1981.

62. Galera-Davidson H, Bibbo M, Bartels PH, Dytch HE, Puls JH, Wied GL: Correlation between automated DNA ploidy measurements of Huerthle-cell tumors and their histopathologic and clinical features. Analyt Quant Cytol Histol 8:158–167, 1986.

63. Gamel JW, McLean IW: Computerized histopathologic assessment of malignant potential: A method for determining the prognosis of uveal melanomas. Hum Pathol 13:834–837, 1982.

64. Greene GL, Press MF: Immunochemical evaluation of estrogen receptor and progesterone receptor in breast cancer. *In* Immunological Approaches to the Diagnosis and Therapy of Breast Cancer. Edited by RL Ceriani. New York, Plenum Publishing, pp 119–135, 1987.

65. Hale AJ: Feulgen microspectrophotometry and its correlation with other histochemical methods. *In* Introduction to Quantitative Cytochemistry. Edited by GL Wied. New York, Academic Press, pp 183–199, 1966.

66. Hansen E: Modulation transfer function analysis in video microscopy. *In* Video Microscopy. Edited by S Inoue. New York, Plenum Publishing, pp 467–475, 1986.

67. Hedley DW, Friedlander ML, Taylor IW, Rugg CA, Musgrove EA: Method for analysis of cellular DNA content of paraffin-embedded pathological material using flow cytometry. J Histochem Cytochem 31:1333–1335, 1983.

68. Hedley DW, Philips J, Rugg CA, Taylor IW: Measurement of cellular DNA content as an adjunct to diagnostic cytology in malignant effusions. Eur J Cancer Clin Oncol 20:749–752, 1984.

69. Hutchinson ML, Schultz DS, Stephenson RA, Wong KL, Harry T, Zahniser DJ: Computerized microscopic analysis of prostatic fine needle aspirates: Comparison with breast aspirates. Analyt Quant Cytol Histol 11:105–110, 1989.

70. Inoue S: Video Microscopy. New York, Plenum Publishing, 1986.

71. Izuo M, Okagaki T, Richart RM, Lattes R: Nuclear DNA content in hyperplastic lesions of cystic disease of the breast with special reference to malignant alteration. Cancer 28:620–627, 1971.

72. Jarvis LR: A microcomputer system for video image analysis and diagnostic microdensitometry. Analyt Quant Cytol Histol 8:201–209, 1986.

73. Keebler CM, Reagan JW, Wied GL (editors): Compendium on Cytopreparatory Techniques, 4th ed. Chicago, Tutorials of Cytology, 1976.

74. King EB, Kromhout LK, Chew KL, Mayall BH, Petrakis NL, Jensen RH, Young IJ: Analytical studies of foam cells from breast cancer precursors. Cytometry 5:124–130, 1984.

75. Kommoss F, Bibbo M, Colley M, Dytch HE, Franklin WA, Holt J, Wied GL: Assessment of hormone receptors in breast carcinoma by immunocytochemistry and image analysis: I. Progesterone receptors. Analyt Quant Cytol Histol 11:298–306, 1989.

76. Korenaga D, Mori M, Okamura T, Sugimachi K, Enjoji M: DNA ploidy in clinical malignant gastric lesions less than 5 mm in diameter. Cancer 58:2542–2545, 1986.

77. Korenaga D, Okamura T, Saito A, Baba H, Sugimachi K: DNA ploidy is closely linked to tumor invasion, lymph node metastasis, and prognosis in clinical gastric cancer. Cancer 62:309–313, 1988.

78. Koss LG, Bartels PH, Sychra JJ, Wied GL: Diagnostic cytologic sample profiles in patients with bladder cancer using TICAS system. Acta Cytol 22:392–397, 1978.

79. Kreicbergs A, Zetterberg A, Soderberg G: The prognostic significance of nuclear DNA content in chondrosarcoma. Analyt Quant Cytol 2:272–279, 1980.

80. Kreicbergs A, Brostrom LA, Cewrien G, Einhorn S: Cellular DNA content in human osteosarcoma: Aspects on diagnosis and prognosis. Cancer 50:2476–2481, 1982.

81. Kuo SH, Sheu JC, Chen DS, Sung JL, Lin CC, Hsu HC: DNA

clonal heterogeneity of hepatocellular carcinoma demonstrated by Feulgen DNA analysis. Liver 7:359–363, 1987.

82. Ljungberg B, Stenling R, Roos G: DNA content in renal cell carcinoma with reference to tumor heterogeneity. Cancer 56:503–508, 1985.

83. Mansi JL, Mesker WE, McDonnell T, van DrielKulker AMJ, Ploem JS, Coombes RC: Automated screening for micrometastases in bone marrow smears. J Immunol Methods 112:105–111, 1988.

84. Mayall BH: Current capabilities and clinical applications of image cytometry. Cytometry [Suppl] 3:78–84, 1988.

85. McClelland RA, Berger U, Miller LS, Powles TJ, Jensen EV, Coombes RJ: Immunocytochemical assay for estrogen receptor: Relationship to outcome of therapy in patients with advanced breast cancer. Cancer Res 46:4241–4243, 1986.

86. Meek ES: The cellular distribution of deoxyribonucleic acid in primary and secondary growths of human breast cancer. J Pathol Bacteriol 82:167–172, 1962.

87. Mikel UV: Absolute DNA values from Feulgen microspectrophotometric measurements and quantitative electron microscopy. Analyt Quant Cytol Histol 9:13–16, 1987.

88. Moruzzi JF, Wyrobek AJ, Mayall BH, Gledhill BL: Quantification and classification of human sperm morphology by computer-assisted image analysis. Fertil Steril 50:142–152, 1988.

89. Nair KK, Bartels PH, Mahon DC, Olson GB, Oloffs PC: Image analysis of hepatocyte nuclei from chlordane-treated rats. Analyt Quant Cytol 2:285–289, 1980.

90. Nasiell M, Kato H, Auer G, Zetterberg A, Roger V, Karlen L: Cytomorphological grading and Feulgen DNA analysis of metaplastic and neoplastic bronchial cells. Cancer 41:1511–1521, 1978.

91. Oberholzer M: Morphometrie in der Klinischen Pathologie. Berlin, Springer Verlag, 1983.

92. Okagaki T, Meyer AA, Sciarra JJ: Prognosis of irradiated carcinoma of cervix uteri and nuclear DNA in cytologic post-irradiation dysplasia. Cancer 33:647–652, 1974.

93. Okamura T, Korenaga D, Haraguchi M, Tsujitani S, Sugimachi K, Mori M, Enjoji M: Growth mode and DNA ploidy in mucosal carcinomas of the stomach. Cancer 59:1154–1160, 1987.

94. Olson GB, Bartels PH: Assessment of environmental-induced insults upon lymphoid cells by computerized morphometric analysis. *In* Biological Dosimetry. Edited by WG Eisert, MC Mendelsohn. Berlin, Springer-Verlag, pp 203–218, 1982.

95. Pak HY, Ashdjian V, Yokota SB, Teplitz RL: Quantitative DNA determination by image analysis. I. Application to human pulmonary cytology. Analyt Quant Cytol 4:95–98, 1982.

96. Pertschuk LP, Eisenberg KB, Carter AC, Feldman GJ: Immunohistologic localization of estrogen receptors in breast cancer with monoclonal antibodies: Correlation with biochemistry and clinical endocrine response. Cancer 55:1513–1518, 1985.

97. Ploem JS: Imaging systems for DNA measurements and other tumor markers and probes: *In* DNA Measurements and Other Markers and Probes and Diagnostic and Prognostic Factors in Human Solid Tumors. Organ Systems Coordinating Center at Roswell Park Institute Symposium, DuPont Experimental Station, Wilmington, Delaware, 1988.

98. Preston K, Bartels PH: Automated image processing for cells and tissues. *In* Progress in Medical Imaging. Edited by VL Newhouse. New York, Springer-Verlag, pp 11–21, 1988.

99. Puls JH, Bibbo M, Dytch HE, Bartels PH, Wied GL: MicroTICAS: The design of an inexpensive videobased microphotometer/computer system for DNA ploidy studies. Analyt Quant Cytol Histol 8:1–7, 1986.

100. Rigaut JP, Reith A, El Kebir FZ: Karyometry by automated image analysis: Application to precancerous lesions. Pathol Res Pract 179:216–219, 1984.

101. Rognum TO, Thorud E, Elgjo K, Brandtzaeg P, Orjasaeter-Nygaard K: Large-bowel carcinomas with different ploidy related to secretory component: IgA and CEA in epithelium and plasma. Br J Cancer 45:921–934, 1982.

102. Rosenthal DL, Manjikian V: Techniques in the preparation of a monolayer of gynecologic cells for automated cytology: An overview. Analyt Quant Cytol Histol 9:55–59, 1987.

103. Serra J: Image Analysis and Mathematical Morphology. New York, Academic Press, 1982.

104. Sherman AB, Koss LG: Morphometry of benign urothelial cells in the presence of cancer. Analyt Quant Cytol 5:221, 1983.

105. Simon H, Kunze D, Voss K, Herrmann WR: Automatische Bildverarbeitung in Medizin und Biologie. Dresden, T Steinkopff Verlag, 1975.

106. Sowa M, Yoshino H, Kato Y, Nishimura M, Kamino K, Umeyama K: An analysis of the DNA ploidy patterns of gastric cancer. Cancer 62:1325–1330, 1988.

107. Sprenger E, Lowhagen T, Vogt-Schaden M: Differential diagnosis between follicular adenoma and follicular carcinoma of the thyroid by nuclear DNA determination. Acta Cytol 21:528–530, 1977.

108. Stenkvist B, Bengtsson E, Eriksson O, Jarkrans T, Nordin B, Westman-Naeser S: Correlation between cytometric features and mitotic frequency in human breast carcinoma. Cytometry 1:287–291, 1981.

109. Suzuki H, Matsumoto K, Masuda T, Koike H: DNA ploidy of colorectal carcinoma. Correlation with conventional prognostic variables. J Clin Gastroenterol 10:176–178, 1988.

110. Tavares AS, Costa J, De Carvalhi A, Reis M: Tumour ploidy and prognosis in carcinoma of the bladder and prostate. Br J Cancer 20:438–441, 1966.

111. Teodori L, Capurso L, Cordelli E, De Vita R, Koch M, Tarquini M, Pallone F, Mauro F : Cytometrically determined relative DNA content as an indicator of neoplasia in gastric lesions. Cytometry 5:63–70, 1984.

112. Weber JE, Bartels PH, Griswold W, Kuhn W, Paplanus SH. Graham AR: Colonic lesion expert system: Performance evaluation. Analyt Quant Cytol Histol 10:150–159, 1988.

113. Weibel ER: Practical Methods for Biological Morphometry, vol 1. Stereological Methods. New York, Academic Press, 1980.

114. Weiss RR, Richart RM, Okagaki T: DNA content of mucinous tumors of the ovary. Am J Obstet Gynecol 103:409–424, 1969.

115. Wied GL: Introduction to Quantitative Cytochemistry. New York, Academic Press, 1966.

116. Wied GL, Bartels PH, Bahr GF, Oldfield DG: Taxonomic intracellular analytic system (TICAS) for cell identification. Acta Cytol 12:177–210, 1968.

117. Wied GL, Bartels PH, Bibbo M, Dytch HE: Image Analysis and Quantitative Cyto and Histopathology. IAC Technical Report No. 20. Chicago, International Academy of Cytology, 1988.

118. Wied GL, Bartels PH, Bibbo M, Sychra JJ: Cytomorphometric markers for uterine cancer in intermediate cells. Analyt Quant Cytol 2:257–263, 1980.

119. Wied GL, Bartels PH, Dytch HE, Bibbo M: Rapid DNA evaluation in clinical diagnosis. Acta Cytol 27:33–37, 1983.

120. Wied GL, Bartels PH, Dytch HE, Pishotta FT, Yamauchi K, Bibbo M: Diagnostic marker features in dysplastic cells from the uterine cervix. Acta Cytol 26:475–483, 1982.

121. Wied GL, Bibbo M, Bartels PH: Computer analysis of microscopic images: application in cytopathology. In Pathology Annual. Edited by PP Rosen. New York, Appleton-Century-Crofts, 1981, pp 367–409.

122. Wittekind D: Standardization of dyes and stains for automated cell pattern recognition. Analyt Quant Cytol Histol 7:6–30, 1985.

123. Wolley RC, Schreiber K, Koss LG, Karas M, Sherman A: DNA distribution in human colonic carcinomas and its relationship to clinical behavior. J Natl Cancer Inst 69:15–22, 1982.

124. Zajicek J, Caspersson T, Jakobsson P, Kudynowski J, Linsk J, Us-Krasovec M: Cytologic diagnosis of mammary tumors from aspiration biopsy smears: Comparison of cytologic and histopathologic findings in 2,111 lesions and diagnostic use of cytophotometry. Acta Cytol 14:370–376, 1970.

125. Zetterberg A, Esposti PL: Cytophotometric DNA-analysis of aspirated cells from prostatic carcinoma. Acta Cytol 20:46–57, 1976.

126. Zetterberg A, Esposti PL: Prognostic significance of nuclear-DNA levels in prostatic carcinoma. Scand J Urol Nephrol 55:53–59, 1980.

37

Flow Cytometry

Cornelis J. Cornelisse
Hans J. Tanke

Routine cytologic and histologic examinations are indispensable for the diagnosis of premalignant and malignant lesions. Although the clinical value of these examinations is not in doubt, several attempts have been made to improve the cytologic and histologic diagnosis over the past 20 years. These studies are directed towards standardization and improvement of reproducibility and aim to refine the diagnosis with respect to prognostic information. Quantitative analysis of stained cells and tissues has played an important role in this respect. As occurred earlier with respect to the automated classification of white blood cells, parameters such as cell size, nuclear size, stain intensity and nucleocytoplasmic ratio were used to gain additional information to support the diagnosis or even to classify cells and preparations in an automated way.

Simultaneously with these studies considerable progress was made in the field of cytochemistry. Rather than the routine Papanicolaou and Giemsa stains, cytochemical methods aiming at the demonstration of specific cellular macromolecules such as nucleic acids or proteins were introduced; possibilities for demonstrating the latter were significantly increased by the introduction of monoclonal antibodies.

Parallel with the development of cytochemistry, cytometric techniques were developed to derive quantitative information not only about morphologic cellular parameters such as size and shape but also—in combination with cytochemical staining—about the molecular composition of the intact cell. The discipline that aims at quantitative cell analysis is called analytic cytology. Some approaches are based on analysis of microscopic images of cells on glass slides (image cytometry); other methods analyze cells on the basis of interaction with light when they are passed through a focused beam of light (flow cytometry).

As discussed previously, a variety of instruments have been developed based on different principles but with the same purpose: the acquisition of quantitative information from cells in flow. Consequently, various names for this technique have been used, such as flow cytofluorometry, pulse cytophotometry and flow cytophotometry. The commonly accepted name *flow cytometry* will be used throughout this chapter.

A well-known application of flow cytometry is the measuring of nuclear DNA content using fluorescent staining methods for DNA. This technique was introduced relatively early, and its diagnostic and prognostic value in cases of malignancy has been studied since the 1970s. This chapter introduces clinicians and researchers to the method of DNA flow cytometry and summarizes its clinical achievements that have been made so far for malignancies of various origins.

HISTORY OF FLOW CYTOMETRY

Development of flow cytometric equipment started in the 1940s with the construction of systems aiming at the counting of particles in suspension, such as blood cells. In 1941, Kielland[170] described a method for counting blood cells very similar to an earlier procedure of Moldavan.[205] He used an apparatus in which cells in suspension were directed through a capillary tube on a microscope stage. The passage of each cell was registered by a photosensor attached to the ocular. Major problems of these early prototypes were the maintenance of flow in narrow channels, avoidance of obstructions by larger objects (cell aggregates) and proper focusing. A significant improvement was made in 1953 when Crosland-Taylor[59] introduced hydrodynamic focusing for flow cytometry, based on pioneering studies by Reynolds[239] in 1883 on laminar flow. Cells were injected slowly in the middle of a relatively fast flowing sheath fluid, permitting focusing of the cells within a small inner core of a larger channel. Most of the commercially available flow systems nowadays use this principle of hydrodynamic focusing. Besides photoelectric sensing as used by Moldavan, electric sensing was investigated. One of the earliest flow systems is the Coulter[53]-type cell counter. In this apparatus cells are passed through an aperture where the presence of an object results in a detectable change in conductivity between two electrodes, provided that cells and suspension medium differ in conductivity.

Kamentsky and colleagues[167] demonstrated in 1965 that cellular macromolecules can be quantified using flow cytometry and multiparameter spectrophotometry. Shortly thereafter, the use of fluorescence was introduced by various groups. In 1968 and 1969 Dittrich and Göhde[71, 72] described a microscope-based system for the measurement of particles moving in a flow stream parallel to the optical axis of the light microscope and through the focal plane of an objective with a high numeric aperture. Van Dilla and colleagues[296] at the Los Alamos National Laboratory simultaneously developed the so-called orthogonal flow systems. These systems had three orthogonal pathways: fluid stream, excitation pathway (lasers were introduced at this time as excitation light sources) and detection pathway for light (fluorescence emission, scattered light). Although the Dittrich-Göhde flow cytometer has proved to be a relatively inexpensive but sensitive and accurate measuring instrument, the orthogonal systems had a major advantage. The configuration of the latter allowed physical separation of measured particles from the mainstream by means of electrostatic deflection of droplets containing the cells of interest. This principle of cell sorting was first described by Fulwyler.[105] A multiparameter flow cytometer incorporating this principle was described by Bonner and coauthors.[33]

Cell sorting followed by visual examination of the isolated cells using a fluorescence microscope offers a way of checking the measuring data by correlating the measurements with the observed microscopic image. Moreover, sorting of cells (live or dead) or subcellular organelles such as chromosomes on the basis of physical or immunologic properties for biochemical purposes (cloning of DNA) or reconstruction experiments offers a unique and extremely flexible tool in cell biology and experimental medicine.

A very important step in the development of flow cytometric instrumentation has been the introduction of microcomputers for signal handling, manipulation and operation control. Flow cytometers have developed from complicated research instruments into user-friendly laboratory systems. Flow cytometers are increasingly used in clinical laboratories.

PRINCIPLES OF FLOW CYTOMETRY

The principle of flow cytometry is that cells or cellular components in aqueous suspension are passed through a sensing region where optical or electrical signals are generated and measured. Such an analysis may be very fast: The typical analysis rate of commercial instruments is on the order of several thousand objects per second. In many cases cells to be analyzed are stained with fluorescent dyes. The reproducibility of fluorescence measurements is 2% or better, and the detection limit of most commercial instruments is 2000 to 3000 molecules of fluorescein per cell. Information about unstained cells can be derived on the basis of their light scatter properties or electrical resistance (see the following).

Configuration and Hydrodynamic Focusing

Flow cytometers differ in configuration. Among the earliest developed systems are configurations that are similar to microscopes. An example is shown in Figure 37–1. To obtain accurate and reproducible measurements it is necessary to transport the cells in suspension by means of hydrodynamic focusing, a technique by which the speed and the position of the cells are controlled by various coaxial fluid streams. In a high-speed analysis cells may be transported with a speed of 10 m per second (there are even much faster systems) to a region onto which a high-intensity light source, usually a laser or high-pressure arc lamp, is focused to generate light scatter signals and fluorescence emission. Properly oriented photodetectors collect a fraction of the signals and generate electrical signals proportional to the optical signals. These signals are accumulated, analyzed and usually presented as single parameter or multiparameter frequency distributions (histograms). Many flow cytometers are based

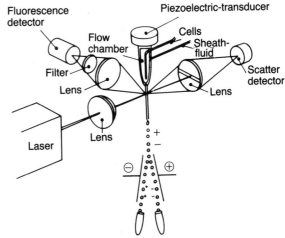

FIGURE 37–1. Schematic representation of a **flow-through chamber,** where the fluid stream with the objects flows parallel to the optical axis. Focusing problems do not occur because each object has to go through the optimal focus plane of the objective. The excitation is performed according to the Köhler illumination principle. This configuration is not suitable for sorting based on deflection of droplets. However, sorting may be accomplished in an adapted flow chamber (not shown here), in which the various fluid pathways after the illumination area can be closed by instantaneously generated gas bubbles (electrolysis), thereby forcing the cells of interest in a defined direction. The speed, however, is much lower than that achievable with sorters based on electrostatic deflection of droplets.

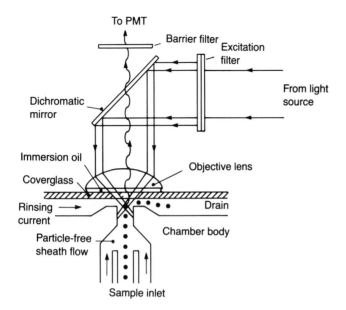

FIGURE 37–2. Schematic representation of a **fluorescence flow cytometer and sorter** with orthogonal axes of cell flow, illumination and emission. Fluorescently stained cells are passed through a focused laser beam, and the generated light scatters. Fluorescence emission signals are sensed, digitized and displayed as frequency distributions. Two sorting windows may be defined for each single parameter or combination of parameters. After the sensing area, the fluid stream breaks up into uniform droplets generated by a piezoelectric transducer. Sorting is accomplished by selectively charging the fluid stream (positively or negatively for the two defined sorting windows) with an electrode, exactly at the moment that the cell of interest is about to pinch off into a droplet. Charged droplets are consequently deflected in an electric field downstream and collected. The example shown allows detection of forward-angle light scatter and one fluorescence parameter. Extensions may include the Coulter sensor or additional photomultipliers for measurements of multicolor fluorescence or for perpendicular light scatter. (PMT = photomultiplier tube.)

on an orthogonal configuration (Fig. 37–2). Orthogonal systems mostly use lasers as light sources. The measuring principle, however, is the same as discussed previously. A major advantage of orthogonal flow cytometers is their ability to sort cells on the basis of electrostatic deflection of droplets that contain these cells (see Principles of Cell Sorting).

Modern flow cytometers are able to derive a large amount of information that is related to physical parameters or, especially if cytochemical staining produces are used, to the chemical composition of the intact cell. Cell characterization may often be based on the interpretation of combined fluorescence, light scatter and electrical resistance signals. The various measuring techniques are therefore briefly discussed. For more details, the reader is referred to specialized books on flow cytometry.[200, 201, 264, 297]

Cell Volume (Electrical Resistance) Measurements

Measurements of biologic objects in suspension were introduced by Coulter[53] in 1949. His idea was to pass cells suspended in a conducting fluid through an orifice that had a small diameter. Across the orifice a constant current was maintained by two electrodes, positioned at either side. Each cell, being a relatively poor conductor owing to its membrane composition, that passed between the electrodes would change the electrical resistance and therefore, according to Ohm's law, generate a voltage pluse, which is easily amplified and measured. As found by Coulter, this signal is proportional to the volume of the cells or particles. A volume distribution curve of objects thus can be derived from a recorded pulse height distribution. Coulter volume measurements obviously require differences in electrical resistance between the suspension medium and the objects. This can easily be achieved for live cells. It

should be realized that cell death or fixation significantly reduces the electrical resistance of cellular membranes. Furthermore, cell volume measurements require an orifice size adapted to the size of the objects to achieve optimal resolution. Coulter volume measurements are widely applied for cell counting purposes in clinical hematology, e.g., counting of leucocytes, erythrocytes and platelets in blood samples. Furthermore, these measurements are very useful to distinguish different cell types in heterogeneous samples on the basis of size and to distinguish live from dead cells based on their difference in electrical resistance. An overview of electrical resistance pulse sizing has been given by Kachel.[162]

Light Scatter Measurements

Measurements of the light scatter properties of cells are used in several flow systems for cell sizing and discrimination among cells with different morphologies. Light scatter signals of irregularly shaped biologic objects are complex and sometimes difficult to interpret. If light, being an electromagnetic wave, is directed onto a cell immersed in a uniform medium, the electrons are slightly displaced relative to the nuclei of the atoms of the cell. This generates dipoles, which oscillate at the frequency of the incident light and reradiate light at the same wavelength as the incident light. The observed scattered light represents the summation of all reradiated waves, taking into account phase relationships. The signal depends on the size and refractive index distribution of the biologic objects, the refractive index of the medium, the wavelength of the incident light and the angle of observation. For theoretic considerations the objects are mostly assumed to be spheric. Approximations for objects larger than the wavelength of the incident light have been made by Rayleigh-Debye. Application of this theory requires that the relative refractive index is close to one and that the phase shift is small.[169] Narrow angle (forward) light scatter signals are proportional to d exp3 for particles with a diameter d between roughly 0.5 and 10 μ.[207] Low-angle light scatter also allows discrimination between live and dead cells. This provides an important application, in particular for membrane immunofluorescence studies, in which nonspecifically stained dead cells may often represent a problem. Light scatter signals measured in a direction perpendicular to the incident light rays are strongly influenced by the regularity of internal cellular compartments. A cell with an irregularly shaped nucleus or cytoplasmic granules or both will generally have a higher perpendicular light scatter than a cell without granules or with a round nucleus. Measurements of forward and perpendicular light scatter signals can be used to distinguish different types of cells in blood and bone marrow.[251] Light scatter signals are predominantly measured using orthogonal laser-based systems. However, microscope-based flow cytometers have been adapted for scatter measurements as well.[271] In comparison with Coulter volume measurements, forward light scatter provides comparable information. Forward angle scatter measurements allow the detection of particles as small as approximately 0.2 μ, depending on their refractive index with standard flow cytometric equipment. The lower detection limit for Coulter volume measurements is in the order of a few μ for most systems. Moreover, light scatter signals do not require a special sensing orifice as is necessary for Coulter volume measurements because in many cases a focused laser light beam is used to generate fluorescence.

Fluorescence Measurements

The amount of cytochemically bound dye can be measured among others on the basis of absorption or fluorescence emission. The latter technique has the advantage that under controlled conditions, a linear relationship between the fluorescence signal and the amount of fluorophore-bound macromolecules exists, rather than the logarithmic relationship that holds for absorption. Practically this implies that no scanning of the object is required to avoid the influence of the distributional error; rather, the single fluorescence signal can be related directly to the amount of fluorophore-bound macromolecules. However, fluorescence is a very complex luminescence phenomenon.[161] For reproducible cytofluorometry, strictly controlled conditions have to be used, and the use of appropriate standards is necessary.

The major advantage of the use of fluorophores for flow cytometry is their sensitivity. Modern flow cytometers allow the specific detection of a few thousand fluorophores per cell and are therefore suitable to demonstrate or quantify low amounts of cellular macromolecules. This has been achieved by combining high power lasers, efficient light-collecting optics and sensitive photodetectors.

Optics: Light Sources, Lenses and Filters

Flexible use of flow cytometers requires the availability of multiple excitation possibilities of various fluorophores, ranging from the near ultraviolet to the green part of the spectrum. In practice this is mostly achieved with lasers (argon, krypton) or with high-pressure vapor lamps (mercury, xenon). In most commercial flow systems sensitive light detectors are positioned in such a way that at least two colors of fluorescence emission can be measured simultaneously with light scatter of electrical resistance signals. The recording of multiple signals is relatively complex. "Crosstalk," i.e., interference between the various detection systems, can only be avoided by use of appropriate lenses and diaphragms as well as by spectral filters that transmit or suppress defined regions of the wavelength spectrum.

Principles of Cell Sorting

Besides analysis several flow cytometers allow the sorting of cells of interest on the basis of the recorded signals. During the analysis procedure generally two populations in the multiparameter histograms may be defined that contain cells with certain defined properties (fluorescence of light scatter intensity). Once cells that fulfill the requirements are passing by, a sorting procedure is started. During the entire measuring procedure, acoustic energy is transferred to the fluid stream, causing the jet to break up into uniform, equally spaced droplets after the laser intersection point. The sorting action indicates that the droplets that contain the cells of interest are charged based on the signals measured. Subsequently, they are deflected from the main stream into an electric field downstream (see Fig. 37–2). This cell-sorting procedure allows the isolation of biologic (live) objects with defined properties on the basis of measurements of light scatter or fluorescence emission for cell culture, biochemical analysis or visual examination under the microscope. The last aspect allows the investigator to visually control the analysis procedure or to examine the cytologic characteristics of sorted subpopulations.[49]

Data Analysis and Presentation

Flow cytometers are able to measure simultaneously several parameters of one object. A typical number of parameters for clinically used instruments is three to five; however, larger experimental systems allow measurements of up to eight parameters. After detection and amplification analog signals are first digitized using proper analog-to-digital converters. AD conversion in flow cytometry must be fast. For example, to record five-parametric data at a speed up to 2000 cells per second, digitizing and storing of a single signal must be performed within 20 microseconds. At higher rates,

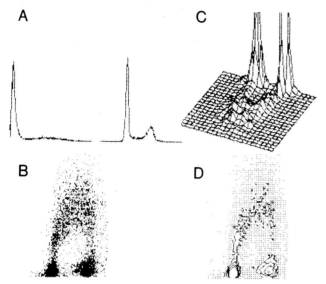

FIGURE 37–3. Examples of univariate and bivariate histograms for **simultaneous analysis of DNA content** (red PI, propidium iodide) (fluorescence) **and incorporated BrdUrd** (green FITC anti-BrdU fluorescence) **in cultured breast tumor cells** in S phase at the moment of incubation with BrdUrd. *A,* Single parameter distributions of BrdUrd-FITC and DNA content, respectively. *B,* Correlated two-parameter data (dot plot). *C,* Pseudo-three-dimensional display of correlated two-parameter data. *D,* Contour map. Projection of the data shown in *(C)* with contour lines set at a defined number of cells. (BrdU = 5′ bromodeoxyuridine.)

such as those used in high-speed cell sorting, the complexity of data acquisition increases.

Digitized data may be displayed directly using *univariate or bivariate frequency distributions (histograms).* Examples are given in Figure 37–3. The display of more than two parameters (multivariate data) becomes very complex. A third parameter may be displayed in the vertical direction. The result is the display of a cube containing dots, each point representing the location of a parameter triplet of a corresponding cell in this cube. Another possibility to simplify visualization of multiparameter flow data is to use color for the third parameter and color intensity for frequency.[275] Multiparameter data are preferably recorded in list mode. This means that the correlated data are digitized and directly stored on disk or tape while the sample is being analyzed. Selection of the most discriminative parameters as well as gated analysis of the data may then be performed later.

Flow cytometric data may contain a wealth of biologically relevant information. Mathematic analysis of the data is often required to extract this information. Most analysis is performed on univariate data, although there is an increasing interest in quantitative analysis of multivariate data (partly explained by the dramatically improved computing facilities for this purpose). Methods in use range from graphic procedures through nonlinear curve-fitting procedures to cluster analysis. This chapter only discusses the general aspects of analysis of flow cytometric data. For more detailed

information on the mathematic procedures the reader is referred to an overview on this subject by Dean.[62]

Analysis of DNA Content Distributions

The mathematic procedures for the analysis of DNA content distributions were originally developed to analyze the growth characteristics of cells in culture, assuming that the cell population was homogeneous and growing asynchronously. On the basis of total DNA content three compartments then can be distinguished: cells in G0 and G1 phase (with a 2C DNA content corresponding to two haploid sets of chromosomes), cells in G2 and M (mitosis) phase (with a 4C DNA content corresponding to four haploid sets of chromosomes) and cells in S (synthesis) phase (with a DNA content of any value between 2C and 4C).

Analysis of DNA distributions, if necessary in combination with measurements of incorporated base analogues (either using radioactive or fluorescent markers, such as tritiated thymidine or bromodeoxyuridine [BrdUrd]), allows the determination of cell kinetic parameters such as total cell cycle time, duration of the G0G1, S and G2M phase and the potential cell doubling time.[15, 16, 63, 97, 113] Using these methods, the mechanism and effect of cytoxic drugs or radiation on the cell cycle characteristics have been studied and quantified. Application of this methodology to the analysis of solid tumors is only allowed if certain criteria are fulfilled.

The first difference with cells *in vitro* is the fact that solid tumors are generally heterogeneous and consist of various cell types such as epithelial, stromal and inflammatory cells. Some of these populations still grow with their own typical characteristics; other cells are end-stage cells that do not cycle. The second difference is caused by the fact that solid tissue is generally more difficult to prepare for flow cytometry than cells in monolayer culture. Even the best preparation technique for solid tissue unavoidably results in a certain percentage of aggregates of two or more cells and also in cell debris. The first problem can be countered by applying DNA analysis only to determine the ploidy of the main tumor cell population (tumor stemline) and omitting the analysis of cell cycle characteristics; this is carried out in the majority of applications. If the tumor is very homogeneous and controlled sampling can be guaranteed, cell cycle analysis can be performed; the interference of nontumor cells with a DNA content falling within the DNA range of the tumor can be corrected for by microscopic investigation of stained sections of the tumor and by counting the percentage of these cells.

A second possibility is to distinguish the various cell types on the basis of their intermediate filament composition using fluoresceinated antibodies as introduced by Ramaekers.[58, 234, 235] Selective measurement of the tumor populations, using two color fluorescence analysis, is not only more accurate but also provides better sensitivity for detecting relatively low amounts of tumor cells (e.g., between 1 and 5%).

The second problem, i.e., the occurrence of cell aggregates and debris, can be solved to a large extent by mathematically correcting the DNA distributions.[25, 55, 118, 255] The presence of cell debris leads to a background signal that is relatively high in the lower channels and low in the higher channels, which can be fitted with an exponential function. Simple subtraction of this curve effectively eliminates the influence of debris. Cell aggregates can dramatically influence cell cycle characteristics because an aggregate of two cells with G0,1 DNA content will be counted as one cell with a DNA content corresponding to the G2M value. In such a case the frequency of aggregates of three and four cells is determined from the histogram (when possible), and the frequency of cell doublets is calculated assuming that the distribution of the aggregates types is Poisson-like. An increasingly used approach is the application of pulse-processing methods, by which single cells with high DNA content are distinguished from cell aggregates on the basis of the length of the fluorescence pulse. Elimination of cell aggregates using pulse processing is becoming a standard feature on most flow cytometers that are used for clinical investigations.

Practical graphic methods for cell cycle analysis have been published by Baisch and coworkers[15] and Ritch and colleagues.[240] More sophisticated procedures for the mathematic analysis of DNA distributions allow curve fitting of multiple cell populations and correction.[74, 195, 257] They are also able to warn the user in many cases if the distribution to be analyzed does not fit certain criteria: For instance, a warning is given if the coefficient of variation (CV) of the analysis is too high for appropriate fitting of the gaussian distribution. Owing to the problems listed, the accurate determination of the percentage of proliferating cells (S, G2M phase) in clinical material may be very difficult. This holds in particular for DNA profiles derived from paraffin-embedded material.[126] However, provided that the correct procedures are used and proper correction methods are carried out, determination of percentage of cells in S and G2M phase in solid tumors may be meaningful. Typical examples of diploid and aneuploid DNA distributions are given in Figure 37–4.

Convention on Nomenclature for DNA Cytometry

In 1984, a Committee on Nomenclature of the Society for Analytical Cytology presented guidelines for the analysis of DNA content by cytometry. These guidelines cover staining of DNA, cytogenetic and cytometric terminology, DNA index, resolution of measurements and cytometric standards.[133] In summary, this committee recommends using the terms normal and abnormal DNA stemline rather than diploid and aneuploid (these latter terms should be reserved for cytogenetic evaluation). If the term aneuploidy is used in cytometry, the prefix DNA should be

added. Thus, DNA aneuploidy refers to an abnormal stemline determined by cytometry. DNA index is the ratio of the mode (or mean) of the relative DNA content of the G0,1 cells of the sample divided by the mode (or mean) of the relative DNA measurements of the diploid G0,1 reference cells. All cytometric measurements should include the coefficient of variation of the G0,1 peak of the cells analyzed. Reference cells should always be used when determining the DNA

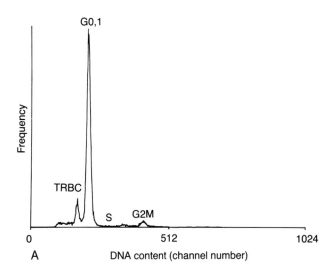

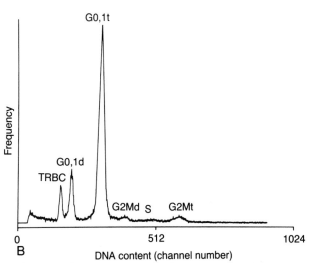

FIGURE 37–4. Flow cytometric DNA content distributions from fresh tumor samples prepared with the Vindelv technique. *A*, DNA-diploid distribution (DNA index = 1.00, CV = 2.9%) from a renal cell carcinoma. TRBC = trout red blood cells used as a ploidy reference. G0,1 = G0,1 peak DNA-diploid cells. S = S-phase compartment. G2M = G2M peak. The small peak in the S-phase compartment represents TRBC doublets. *B*, DNA-aneuploid distribution (DNA-index = 1.52, CV = 3.3%) from a breast carcinoma. G0,1d = G0,1 peak DNA-diploid population. G0,1t = G0,1 peak DNA-aneuploid population. G2Md = G2M peak DNA-diploid population situated within the S-phase compartment of the DNA-aneuploid stemline. G2Mt = G2M peak DNA-aneuploid population. (CV = coefficient of variation.)

index of an unknown population. The ideal reference cells are diploid cells from the same tissue and the same individual. Normal cells from another species (avian or fish erythrocytes) or nonbiologic standards such as fluorescent beads are useful standards for instrument calibration but should not be used in calculating the DNA index.

Although in general we agree with these recommendations, in practice the use of normal human diploid cells as a ploidy reference is not without problems. In clinical laboratories where samples of widely varying tissue types have to be analyzed, it is impossible to keep stocks of all these matched normal cell types for reference purposes. Also, the use of normal peripheral blood leukocytes is not without pitfalls. Artifactual differences in DNA fluorescence may lead to overestimations of DNA aneuploidy when reference leukocytes and test cells are mixed *after* the enzymatic treatment.[142] A workable compromise is to use the admixed benign cell populations that are nearly always present in most tumor types as an internal diploid ploidy reference. In order to find out which of the $G_{0,1}$ peaks represents the diploid cell population, trout red blood cells can be included (before enzymatic and detergent treatment) as an additional reference in one aliquot of the sample.[303] The proportion of normal diploid cells as well of tumor cells in the sample preferably should be estimated in a histologic control section.

The classification of flow cytometric DNA profiles for DNA ploidy determinations in the majority of cases does not present problems. There are several situations in which the interpretation of the results is less straightforward, however. Extra $G_{0,1}$ peaks may occur when preparation procedures have not been carried out properly. Such erroneous results are easily overlooked unless samples of well-characterized standard cell populations are regularly included in the work-up procedure. A second problem is the interpretation of unimodal DNA profiles with an asymmetric or broadened $G_{0,1}$ peak or a shoulder on the $G_{0,1}$ peak. In particular, DNA profiles from deparaffinized tissue samples may present these problems. In our laboratory we routinely classify such cases as "peridiploid," using an (arbitrary) cutoff CV value of 5.5% to discriminate between diploid and peridiploid tumors (Fig. 37–5). A notorious problem is also the interpretation of DNA profiles showing an increased proportion of cells with the normal G2M DNA content.[262] When the tetraploid cell population is accompanied by its own S phase and G2M compartment, there is no problem in classifying such tumors as DNA aneuploid (tetraploid). Problems arise when only an elevated G2M population is visible. For such cases arbitrary cutoff values for the size of the G2M fraction, ranging from 10 to 35% have been used to discriminate between a diploid G2M and a tetraploid $G_{0,1}$ fraction. A possible way out of this dilemma may be offered by the use of a second parameter such as cytokeratins, as has been demonstrated for bladder tumors (see also Data Analysis and Presentation).[90]

A third interpretational problem that is particularly

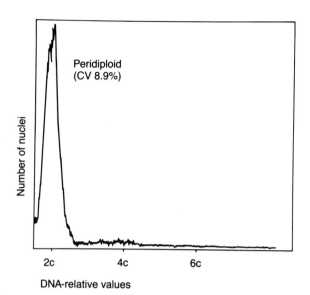

FIGURE 37–5. Example of a **DNA-distribution from a deparaffinized tissue sample of a thyroid carcinoma** showing a broad $G_{0,1}$ peak with a high CV (= 8.9%). Such distributions create interpretational problems because these broad $G_{0,1}$ peaks may conceal the presence of low-aneuploid stem lines and therefore may be classified as "peridiploid." (CV = coefficient of variation.)

associated with the evaluation of DNA profiles from deparaffinized tissue is the discrimination between hypo- and hyperdiploid DNA stemlines. For fresh or frozen tissue samples this problem can be circumvented by the use of ploidy reference cells to mark the position of the diploid peak. For paraffin-embedded samples it may be possible to identify the diploid fraction when the size of the two $G_{0,1}$ peaks differs substantially and can be matched with the estimated proportions of tumor cells and normal cells in histologic control sections.

Autolysis is a potential source of false aneuploid peaks in DNA profiles from paraffin-embedded tissues, as was demonstrated by Alanen and coauthors.[4] Although the DNA indexes of the spurious peaks were usually less than 1.3, the occurrence of this phenomenon calls for caution in the interpretation of tumor samples containing necrotic parts.

SAMPLE PREPARATION AND STAINING FOR FLOW CYTOMETRY

Sampling of the Cells and Preparation

A cell suspension of good quality is a prerequisite for optimal flow cytometric analysis. Such a suspension ideally consists of well-preserved single cells, without too much cell debris or other artifacts such as cell aggregates and clumps. This may be easily achieved for blood cells but is very difficult in the case of solid tissues. Moreover, one general method suitable for all types of tissue cannot be given. As is important for all sampling procedures, care should be taken that the end result is a true reflection of the native sample and that no selective loss of one particular cell type occurs in cases of heterogeneous tissues (and most cases are heterogeneous).

Isolation of cells from solid tissue is generally based on *mechanical disaggregation* of the tissue or on *enzymatic digestion* (often a combination of both). Mechanical disaggregation may consist of a simple cutting of the tissue with razor blades followed by syringing of the smaller pieces to generate more single cells. Adequate precautions should be taken in order to prevent cutting accidents when handling fresh or frozen human tissues. The routine use of protective gloves and forceps for manipulation of tissue samples must be strongly recommended. The minced tissue is then sieved through appropriate nylon mesh filters. Another method consists of scraping cells from a piece of tissue with the edge of a microscopic glass slide. Mechanical disaggregation generally results in sufficient cells for flow analysis. However, the procedure may lead to considerable cell damage. Whether this will influence the flow cytometric analysis strongly depends on the parameters under investigation. For instance, mechanical cell damage generally will affect analysis of membrane antigens more than that of nuclear DNA.

A generalized procedure for *enzymatic digestion* of fresh tissue consists of the following steps. Tissue obtained by surgery is placed in cold culture medium, supplemented with 10% fetal calf serum. The tissue is minced and washed with medium and subsequently incubated in medium containing the digestive enzyme under gentle stirring. The cell suspension is decanted from the tissue fragments, cooled in ice and filtered through appropriate filters to obtain a suspension of single cells. Enzymes that may be used are trypsin, pronase, collagenase and hyaluronidase. The procedures just discussed may be used for fresh or frozen tissue. Since 1983, it has become possible to prepare *formalin-fixed, paraffin-embedded archival material* for flow cytometric analysis of DNA content.[124] The method consists of preparing 40- to 60-μ sections from the tissue blocks, which are subsequently dewaxed in xylene and rehydrated. A nuclear suspension may then be prepared by digesting the sections with pepsin. Most of the connective tissue as well as the cell cytoplasm is digested by this procedure. Because this procedure allows retrospective investigations, it is very useful for prognostic studies of DNA aneuploidy in solid tumors. The following two preparation and staining methods for flow cytometric analysis of nuclear DNA content are given in detail because they are (sometimes slightly adapted to the type of tissue) extensively used for analysis of fresh or paraffin-embedded material. The techniques were originally described by Vindeløv and coauthors[302] and Hedley and associates,[124] respectively.

Fixation and Storage

Fixation of the cells in suspension prior to staining may be necessary, either to guarantee preservation of the cellular components or simply to make membranes permeable for dye accessibility. Two main aspects are important: Some fixatives may induce cell aggregation (for instance, ethanol) and other fixatives will influence the fluorescence properties of fluorochromes (for instance, glutaraldehyde and formaldehyde cause quenching of the nucleic acid dyes ethidium bromide and propidium iodide). Clumping may be kept to a minimum by vigorous stirring of the cell suspension while slowly increasing the ethanol concentration preferably to 70%.

Cytochemical Staining Methods

In the staining of DNA, most dyes are used under so-called equilibrium conditions, i.e., cells are resuspended in dye solution, allowed to take up stain and analyzed by flow cytometry while suspended in dye solution. Among the fluorescent DNA dyes, some show base specificity: Chromomycin and 7–Aminoactinomycin D are specific for GC base pairs, nonintercalating dyes, whereas the nonintercalating bisbenzimidazol dye Hoechst 33258 binds preferentially to AT base pairs. Other dyes such as the phenanthridinium dyes ethidium bromide and propidium iodide intercalate in double-stranded nucleic acid without much base specificity. When used for quantitation, DNA treatment with ribonuclease (RNase) is required because binding to double-stranded RNA will occur as well. An excellent overview of fluorescent probes for DNA has been given by Latt.[181]

Staining for DNA may be combined with protein stains of different fluorescent properties.[57, 276] Optimal separation of the two fluorescence signals is achieved by sequentially exciting the cells in flow at two different wavelengths.[64, 274]

In situ hybridization methods for nucleic acids have been applied to cells in suspension for flow cytometric analysis.[288] With these methods specific base sequences can be demonstrated.[24]

Staining Methods for DNA Analysis of Solid Tumors

Staining of Fresh Material[300–303]

Among various methods developed for staining of nuclear DNA for flow cytometry the technique described by Vindeløv and coworkers[302] is of particular interest. The method is fast, widely applicable for a variety of tissues and results in low coefficients of variation.[300] An important practical aspect is that the procedure can be applied to fresh as well as to frozen tissue. Preparation is based on the trypsinization of unfixed tissue in the presence of a detergent to digest cell cytoplasm and spermine to prevent complete disintegration of the nuclei. A long-term storage step is incorporated in the procedure, involving freezing of the native tissue or cells in a citrate buffer, containing sucrose and dimethyl sulfoxide.[301] Fluorescent DNA staining is performed with propidium iodide after removal of interfering double-stranded RNA with RNase. The conditions for appropriate preparation and staining, e.g., the concentrations of trypsin and spermine as well the storage procedure, are critical; the reader is referred to the original papers by Vindelv. However, because all reagents can be prepared beforehand and kept frozen and because excellent results are obtained, the method is highly recommended for clinical material.

The same authors have developed procedures to determine the DNA index of tumors on the basis of two independent DNA standards, e.g., trout and chicken erythrocytes with approximately 35 and 80% of the total human DNA content, respectively.[303]

Staining of Paraffin-Embedded Material[124]

The blocks of paraffin-embedded material are cut in relatively thick sections. Thickness of these sections may vary from 30 to 50 μ, depending of the size of cell nuclei that have to be isolated. Thinner sectioning results on one hand in improved enzymatic digestion but on the other hand in an increased percentage of cut nuclei, leading to cell debris. The sections are dewaxed in three fractions of xylene and rehydrated by sequentially immersing in 100, 95, 70 and 50% ethanol before washing in distilled water. (*Note:* It is important to remove all of the rest of the paraffin; when necessary, warm xylene may be applied to speed up the procedure.) The rehydrated section are then treated with 1 ml of 0.5% pepsin (Sigma) in 0.9% sodium chloride, adjusted to pH 1.5 with 2 N hydrochloric acid, at 37° C for 30 minutes to prepare suspensions of single nuclei. Optimal incubation conditions (time, enzyme concentration) may be adjusted depending on the cell type. It is recommended that the digestion of the sections be controlled by judging the number of single cells in the supernatant by microscopy. After digestion the cells are washed, counted and stained with 1 μg/mg 4′,6′-diamidino-2-phenylindole for 30 minutes, filtered through nylon mesh filters and analyzed by flow cytometry. A minimum of 100,000 cells is considered necessary for proper flow cytometric analysis, as given by the authors. DAPI stained cells require excitation with ultraviolet light (either from an argon ion laser or from a mercury arc lamp); the blue fluorescence emission is measured through a band pass 450-nm filter (or equivalent).

Hedley[127] has evaluated his method in a large series of samples of various organs and on the basis of more than 100 published papers in the literature. His initial studies indicated an excellent correlation of the DNA index for fresh and paraffin-embedded material (r-0.996), as found in a controlled comparative study. Retrospective analysis of archival material is, however, more problematic owing to variation in preparation and fixation of the material. Improper fixation of the material, resulting in very high coefficients of variation, leads to a significant number of cases that cannot be

properly evaluated (up to 30% depending on the type of tumor). Another limitation of the technique is the fact that no external reference cells such as trout or chicken erythrocytes can be applied to determine the diploid DNA value; in practice DNA scaling is performed using leucocytes or other normal (e.g., stromal) cells from the sample itself. Also, admixtures of large numbers of nonepithelial cells (inflammatory cells) that can mask the presence of cells with aneuploid DNA content present a difficulty because anticytokeratin antibodies that are used on fresh material to identify these cells can generally not be applied on formalin-fixed, paraffin-embedded material. Accurate determination of the percentage of cells in S phase, hampered by significant background signals due to cell debris, may also be very difficult. Considering the difficulties discussed, it is of the utmost importance to use hematoxylin stained reference sections that should be examined microscopically to anticipate occurring problems. When carried out properly flow cytometric analysis of paraffin-embedded material provides clinically useful information.

BIOLOGIC AND CLINICAL SIGNIFICANCE OF DNA ANEUPLOIDY

Biologic Significance of DNA-Aneuploidy

The DNA content of normal, nondividing cells is a tightly controlled cell characteristic representing two haploid (or diploid) sets of 22 autosomes and one pair of sex chromosomes. The genetic information that cells need to grow, divide and fulfill their specific functions in the organism is dispersed over these 23 pairs of chromosomes. Structural as well as numeric chromosomal changes may disrupt the genetic programming of cells and lead to deviant biologic behavior or cell death. More than 40 years before the correct number of chromosomes in human cells was established, Boveri[34] postulated that chromosomal alterations might lead to the development of cancer. This hypothesis was proved correct with the advent of chromosome analysis techniques, the classic example being the t(9;22) chromosome (Philadelphia chromosome) as a specific chromosomal abnormality in chronic myelocytic leukemia.[210–212] Since then, great progress has been made in describing the cytogenetic changes in hematologic malignancies, but knowledge about specific chromosomal aberrations in solid tumors is advancing more slowly.[128, 252] The main reasons for solid tumor cytogenetics lagging behind that of hematologic malignancies are the technical difficulties associated with the culturing of primary solid tumors, the low yield of metaphases and the often very complex karyotypes showing numerous structural and numeric changes.

Because the total nuclear DNA content of cells in the G0,1 phase of the cell cycle is roughly proportional to the average number of chromosomes, DNA cytometry can provide an estimate for the extent of numeric chromosome changes in neoplastic cells. In contrast to karyotype analysis requiring cells in metaphase, all cells in a population are accessible for DNA content measurements. It is obvious that in this way no information on specific structural or numeric chromosome aberrations is obtainable. In spite of the global nature of DNA content information there is growing evidence for a correlation between DNA aneuploidy and biologic aggressiveness of solid tumors. Such correlations were already anticipated in the first publication on DNA content distributions in solid tumors by Leuchtenberger and coworkers.[184]

One of the more simple explanations for the observed associations between DNA ploidy and biologic behavior is that it reflects the degree of disarrangement of the genome of the tumor cell. This could interfere with the proper functioning of normal cellular differentiation programs and of proliferation control. This view is probably too simplistic because it does not discriminate between specific genetic events involved in initiation and tumor progression and genomic changes that are "byproducts" of increased genetic tumor instability without phenotypic effects.

Loss or duplication of chromosomes may affect the dosage of genes whose products have to be maintained at a critical level for the regulation of cell growth. The best-known example of the effect of a deletion of part or all of a chromosome is presented by retinoblastoma. Detection of frequent allelic losses at band 13q14 led to the identification and cloning of the Rb gene, the first human tumor suppressor gene.[39, 104, 182] Similar allelic losses have now been found in a variety of other solid tumors and even at multiple loci in colorectal and breast cancer.[69, 304] It is not clear, however, whether all these loci harbor tumor suppressor genes or whether the observed allele losses reflect increased genetic instability.

DNA aneuploidy and its underlying numeric and structural chromosome abnormalities can be seen as evidence for genome destabilization during tumor development. Although genomic instability is attributed a central role in the clonal evolution of tumors, the mechanisms involved are still poorly understood.[129, 138, 211, 308] An unsolved paradox is how genetically unstable clones ultimately can develop into apparently more stable tumor stemlines that can maintain the same DNA ploidy level in metastases even over many years.[10] Computer modeling experiments by Shackney and coworkers[263] suggest that an essential condition for the establishment of discrete aneuploid peaks in genetically unstable cell populations is the prior development of a growth-promoting structural chromosome abnormality. This very interesting approach may lead to further insights in the development of aneuploidy and genetic evolution of human solid tumors.

Finally, the development of nonradioactive *in situ* hybridization techniques enables the detection of chromosome-specific repetitive DNA sequences in interphase nuclei.[56, 225] These techniques have already successfully been applied in combination with DNA flow cytometry to identify the chromosomes showing numeric aberrations in primary breast and bladder carcinomas.[68, 138]

DNA Aneuploidy in Solid Tumors

Breast Cancer

Breast cancer is the most common type of cancer in women in many western European countries and the United States. About 70% of the patients eventually die from metastatic disease even after disease-free intervals of more than 20 years. Owing to the heterogeneity and complexity of the disease, large numbers of patients and relatively long clinical follow-up periods are required for evaluating prognostic factors. Classic prognostic factors are the number of axillary lymph node metastases, tumor size, nuclear and histologic grade and clinical stage. More recently, steroid hormone receptor levels and amplification of the HER-2/neu oncogene have been attributed prognostic significance.[192, 266]

For more than 3 decades, DNA content measurements have been carried out on benign and malignant breast tumors.[9, 184] At present, breast cancer is the most extensively investigated type of solid tumor by flow cytometry. The first flow cytometric studies date from the early 1980s.[28, 215, 216] These studies were done on limited series of patients and predominantly compared DNA ploidy and S phase fractions with a number of clinicopathologic variables. Because most studies had to be done prospectively on freshly sampled tumor specimens, follow-up periods were too short to evaluate the prognostic effects of aneuploidy and S phase fraction. This situation changed after Hedley and associates[124] introduced their technique for flow cytometric analysis of archival paraffin-embedded tumor specimens enabling retrospective studies on well-documented series of patients with adequate follow-up.

The majority of breast carcinomas contain one or more aneuploid cell populations. The overall percentage of aneuploid tumors reported in the literature ranges from 54 to 92%, but in the majority of studies between 60 and 80% of the tumors are aneuploid (Table 37–1). The occurrence of multiple aneuploid stemlines is reported in about half of the studies at frequencies from 6 to 19%. Many investigators report a typical bimodal distribution of DNA indexes in breast cancer (Fig. 37–6), with most of the values in the near-diploid and hypotetraploid range and scattered values in the hypertetraploid-hexaploid range. The distributions show a minimum in the DNA index range of 1.2 to 1.4. Hypodiploid tumors occur at frequencies below 10%. It must be emphasized, however, that classifying tumors as hypodiploid requires an adequate internal standard with a DNA content sufficiently different from the normal human diploid value. For this reason the identification of hypodiploid tumors in deparaffinized samples is hardly possible unless the proportion of normal diploid cells in the sample can be estimated with high accuracy. Interestingly, canine mammary

TABLE 37–1. Correlation of DNA Ploidy with Clinicopathologic Variables in Breast Cancer

Author	Year	N	A (%)	H	G	E	P	T	N	St	M	SV
Bedrossian et al[28]	1981	43	72	−	+	−			−	−	−	−
Kutre et al[178]	1981	70	56	−		±			−			
Olszewski et al[215]	1981	92	92	+	+							
Bichel et al[29]	1982	46	54		+	+						
Raber et al[229]	1982	80	85			±				−		−
Taylor et al[282]	1983	114	80	−		−	−		−		+	
Cornelisse et al[50]	1984	166	69	+		+			−			
Coulson et al[54]	1984	74	79	−	−	+				−	+	
Ewers et al[84]	1984	638	66					+	−	+	−	+
Fossa et al[93]	1984	66	61		+	−		−		+	−	
Hedley et al[125]	1984	165	68			−			+		−	+
Haag et al[117]	1984	155	54	−	−			−			−	
Jakobsen et al[147]	1984	143	70		+	±	−	±	±		−	
Moran et al[206]	1984	76	89	+	+	+	+		−			
Kute et al[179]	1985	226	54		±	+	+	±	−			
Stuart-Harris et al[280]	1985	42	74									−
Horsfall et al[139]	1986	145	57	+		+	+					
McDivitt et al[191]	1986	168	55	+	+	−	−					
Klintenberg et al[173]	1986	210	58			−						−
Nesland et al[209]	1986	61	57	+	+							
Thorud et al[285]	1986	59	54		+	−		+			+	±
Ucelli et al[294]	1986	54	63						+			
Abandowitz et al[1]	1987	163	68			±					+	
Abe and Ueki[2]	1987	60	37						−	±		
Baildam et al[14]	1987	136	62			+	−					+
Cornelisse et al[52]	1987	565	71			+		+	±	−	−	+
Dowle et al[72]	1987	354	60		+	−		+	−		−	+
Hedley et al[126]	1987	490	68		+	+	−	−	−		+	+
Kallioniemi et al[164]	1987	93	60		+	+		±	±	±	−	+
Kallioniemi et al[165]	1987	308	64	±	+	+	+	−	+	±	±	+
Masters et al[196]	1987	125	79		+							
Meckenstock et al[198]	1987	100	55		+	+	+	±	+			
Owainati et al[222]	1987	280	60		+	+		−			−	
Spyratos et al[269]	1987	106	67		+	±		−				
Dressler et al[75]	1988	1331	57		+				−			
Feichter et al[88]	1988	300	62	+	+	+	+	±	+		−	
Remvikos et al[237]	1988	206	78					−	−			
Roos et al[248]	1988	72	58							−	−	+
Uyterlinde et al[295]	1988	63	67					−	−			−
Beerman et al[27]	1990	690	73					−	+	+	−	+
Clark et al[45]	1989	345	68									+
Stal et al[270]	1989	472	63		+			−	+		−	+

N = number of patients, A = percentage of aneuploid cases, H = histology, G = histologic or nuclear grade, E = estrogen receptor level, P = progesterone receptor level, T = tumor size, N = lymph node involvement, St = clinical stage, M = menopausal status or age, SV = overall or disease-free survival, + = correlation with DNA ploidy, − = no correlation.

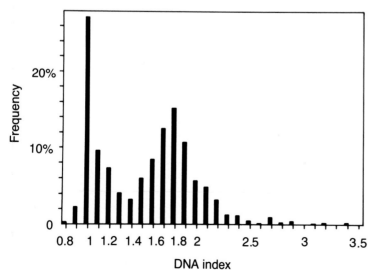

FIGURE 37–6. DNA-index frequency distribution of 839 breast carcinomas measured in my laboratory. Note the typical bimodal clustering of DNA-stem lines in the near-diploid and hypotetraploid region.

tumors show a much higher proportion of hypodiploid stemlines than human mammary cancers.[250]

Prevalence and degree of aneuploidy are correlated with histologic tumor type, although this has been investigated in a limited number of studies only (see Table 37–1). The majority of infiltrating duct carcinomas not otherwise specified are aneuploid. The mean DNA index of this group ranges from 1.5 to 1.6. Special types of infiltrating duct carcinoma show a different pattern of DNA ploidy aberrations. Tubular as well as mucinous carcinomas are mostly (near) diploid, whereas medullary carcinomas are mostly (highly) aneuploid.[50, 89, 139, 163, 191, 206, 215, 287] In the majority of studies, less than 30% of the infiltrating lobular carcinomas are aneuploid. Data on aneuploidy in *in situ* ductal and lobular carcinoma are still scanty and do not permit general conclusions.[49, 163, 237]

In many studies a correlation between DNA ploidy and histologic or nuclear grade or both has been found (see Table 37–1). Well-differentiated tumors are more often diploid than poorly differentiated tumors, and aneuploid tumors show a higher degree of nuclear atypia than diploid tumors. The evaluation of the relationship between DNA ploidy and clinical stage requires a rather large number of patients and such studies are still scanty. A positive correlation was found by Ewers and coworkers,[84] whereas in two other studies no significant differences were found except for a somewhat lower percentage of aneuploid tumors in patients with Stage I disease.[52, 163] In a study from our own group we found a significant correlation between DNA ploidy and tumor, node, metastasis (TNM) stage when tumors were classified as near diploid (DNA index < 1.4), hypotetraploid (1.4 < DNA index < 1.9), tetraploid (1.9 < DNA index < 2.1) or hypertetraploid (DNA index > 2.1).[27] This showed a significant decrease of near diploid stemlines and a concomitant increase in hypotetraploid, tetraploid and hypertetraploid stemlines with increasing stage.

As with stage, no unanimity exists with respect to the correlation between DNA ploidy and tumor size. In several studies the percentage of aneuploid stemlines in T1 tumors was significantly lower than in T2 to T4 tumors.[52, 73, 84] Again, subdivision according to DNA index range showed a strong decrease in the percentage of near diploid and an increase in the percentage of higher aneuploid DNA stemlines (DNA index > 1.4) in T2 to T4 tumors compared with T1 tumors.[27]

The evidence for a correlation between DNA ploidy and the number of positive lymph nodes is rather weak. In the majority of studies no association was found. In some others only extensive lymph node involvement was associated with a higher percentage of aneuploidy.[52, 125, 126] Associations with N stage or with the presence or absence of nodal involvement have been reported by several investigators.[89, 147, 163, 294] In one study we found a strong correlation between hypertetraploidy and lymph node involvement.[27] It is possible, therefore, that stratification according to the degree of aneuploidy may unmask correlations with lymph node involvement not seen with the conventional binary DNA ploidy classification.

A higher prevalence of DNA ploidy in tumors from postmenopausal patients has been reported in several studies.[73, 126, 282, 285] In the majority of studies no correlation with age has been found; however, the relationship between DNA ploidy and age of the patients remains unclear.

There is growing evidence for a correlation between DNA ploidy and presence of steroid hormone receptors. The majority of investigators report that aneuploid tumors more frequently have low or negative estrogen receptor levels than diploid tumors (see Table 37–1). However, the differences are often small and not confirmed in all studies, indicating that the association is rather weak. Data on the correlation between DNA ploidy and progesteron receptor levels is more limited but shows a similar trend (see Table 37–1).

The prognostic value of DNA ploidy measurements in breast cancer is still a matter of controversy. Although in the majority of studies some favorable effect of diploidy on disease-free and overall survival has been found in univariate analyses (see Table 37–1), the question of whether DNA ploidy is an independent prognostic factor in multivariate analyses remains unsettled. Also, the magnitude of the observed prognostic effect differs between the various studies and comparison of the results is complicated by differences in the composition of the series of patients as well as by the use of diverging DNA ploidy classifications.

DNA ploidy was found to be an independent prognostic variable for overall survival by Cornelisse and coworkers[52] and by Kallioniemi and coauthors.[163] We found a significant effect on survival in patients with more advanced stages of disease only, whereas Kallioniemi and colleagues also report an effect in node-negative patients. For the series of 345 node-negative patients studied by Clark and colleagues,[45] DNA ploidy was the only significant prognostic factor for disease-free survival but not for overall survival. In some studies the prognostic effect of aneuploidy on disease-free or overall survival disappeared after allowance was made for established prognostic variables by multivariate analysis.[73, 125, 127] Several investigators have inquired whether classification of tumors according to DNA index range could improve the discrimination between prognostically different groups of patients. Evidence was obtained that indicated that particularly patients with hypertetraploid tumors may form a high-risk group.[26, 45, 163, 173]

Results from ³H thymidine labeling studies have demonstrated the prognostic importance of cell kinetic information in breast cancer.[108, 202, 293] This has prompted a number of groups to investigate the prognostic value of flow cytometric S phase determinations in addition to DNA ploidy (Table 37–2). The heterogeneity of breast cancer samples raises considerable problems for the accurate calculation of S phase fractions, requiring the development of sophisticated software programs.[74] Flow cytometrically determined S phase fractions vary over a wide range (1 to 40%) in breast cancer, with mean or median values between 5 and 15% in the majority of the studies. Good correlations have been found between the S phase fractions

TABLE 37–2. Correlation of S Phase Fraction or Proliferation Index* with DNA Ploidy and Clinicopathologic Variables in Breast Cancer

Authors	Year	NT	NS	An	G	ER	T	N	M	Surv
Bedrossian et al[28]	1981	43	43	−	−	+	−	−	−	
Olszewski et al[216]	1981	90	90		+	+	−		±	
Raber et al[229]	1982	80	80	−	−	+		−		
Haag et al[117]	1984	155	155	+				−		
Moran et al[206]	1984	76	58	+	±	+		−		
Kute et al[179]	1985	226	179	+	+	+	+	−	+	
Klintenberg et al[173]	1986	210	148	+		+				+
McDivitt et al[191]	1986	168	168	+		+	±	−		
Ucelli et al[294]	1986	54	54	+						
Abandowitz et al[294]	1987	163	52			±			±	
Abe and Ueki[2]	1987	60	60	+			+	+		
Hedley et al[126]	1987	490	188	+	+	±		±	±	+
Masters et al[196]	1987	125	86	+	+					
Meckenstock et al[198]	1987	100	41		−	+				
Dressler et al[75]	1988	1331	1084	+		+		+	+	
Feichter et al[88]	1988	300	300	+	+	+	−	−	−	
Kallioniemi et al[165]	1988	308	308	+	+	±	−	−	−	+
Clark et al[45]	1989	345	253	+						+
Stal et al[270]	1989	472	290	+		+	+	−		+

*Proliferation index = S + G$_2$M fraction.

NT = total number of cases, NS = evaluable number of cases for S phase fraction, An = DNA aneuploidy, G = histologic grade, ER = estrogen receptor level, T = tumor size, N = lymph node involvement, M = menopausal status or age, Surv = overall or disease-free survival, + = correlation with S phase fraction, − = no correlation.

and ³H thymidine labeling indexes in breast cancer, although the latter are usually lower.[191, 203] As with types of solid tumors, S phase fractions reported for aneuploid breast cancers are often significantly higher than for diploid tumors (see Table 37–2).[94] In the majority of studies, however, the effect of contaminating normal host cells on the accuracy of S phase determinations in diploid tumors as discussed by Hedley and associates[126] and Dressler and coworkers[75] has not been systematically investigated. In most studies, a correlation is found between S phase fraction and loss of estrogen receptors, but except for histologic grade, correlations with other clinicopathologic variables are less well established (see Table 37–2).

A high S phase fraction (cutoff values ranging from 7 to 10%) was found to be associated with a lower disease-free or overall survival or both in several studies.[45, 126, 165, 270] In the study of Clark and coworkers[45] involving 345 node-negative patients, the prognostic effect on both disease-free and overall survival was limited to patients with diploid tumors only. Multivariate analysis showed the S phase fraction to be the only significant prognostic factor for disease-free or overall survival. However, in Hedley and coworkers'[126] study of 285 patients with node-positive breast cancer, S phase was no longer an independent prognostic factor when allowance was made for its strong correlation with tumor grade in the Cox model.

Several authors have attempted to define classes of DNA profiles that integrate the prognostically important DNA ploidy and S phase fraction differences.[45, 54, 165, 191] These systems have in common the consideration that patients having diploid tumors with low S phase fractions form the most favorable prognostic category. In combination with other established prognostic factors these may well lead to a more objective and rational prognostic stratification of patients with breast cancer. However, in spite of these promising results, more data are needed from long-term follow-up studies before the use of DNA cytometry data for patient management can be justified.[26]

Colorectal Carcinoma

DNA aneuploidy is found in 60 to 80% of the colorectal carcinomas (Table 37–3). Results from two different studies show a very good correlation between DNA indexes measured by flow cytometry and those calculated from the number of chromosomes in karyograms.[224, 238] Several investigators obtained evidence for a considerable intratumor heterogeneity of DNA ploidy by analysis of multiple samples from different tumor sites.[134, 223, 227, 261, 290] Despite the reported heterogeneity of DNA ploidy patterns in colorectal cancer, it appears to be possible to reliably determine DNA ploidy on superficial forceps biopsy specimens in the majority of cases.[261]

There is no unanimity with respect to the correlation between tumor ploidy and stage (see Table 37–3). In the majority of studies there is some trend towards an increased prevalence of DNA aneuploidy in tumors of higher stage (predominantly Dukes' C stage). In none of the studies was an association between tumor ploidy and histologic differentiation found. Two groups reported significant associations with other prognostic variables such as nodal status, growth pattern characteristics and lymphocytic infiltration.[17, 151]

After the first encouraging publication by Wolley and associates[316] showing a strong effect of DNA aneuploidy on survival in a series of 33 patients, results from later studies on larger series of patients indicated a more complex relationship between ploidy and prognosis (see Table 37–3). Tumor ploidy was found to be

TABLE 37–3. DNA Aneuploidy in Colorectal Cancer: Relationship with Differentiation and Clinical Stage

Author	Year	N	A (%)	H	Stage
Rognum et al[245]	1982	85	67		
Wolley et al[316]	1982	33	39		+
Tribukait et al[290]	1983	66	60	−	−
Armitage et al[8]	1985	134	55	−*	−
Banner et al[17]	1985	56	75	−	+
Quirke et al[227]	1985	66	72		
Williams et al[313]	1985	45	69–89		
Durrant et al[76]	1986	50	33		
Finan et al[9]	1986	46	59	−	
Hiddemann et al[134]	1986	88	82	−	+
Kokal et al[174]	1986	133	74	−	+
Melamed et al[199]	1986	33	55		
Rognum et al[246]	1986	100	63		
Schwartz et al[260]	1986	23	43		
Chang et al[40]	1987	30	50		
Bauer et al[22]	1987	120	82		
Emdin et al[80]	1987	37	62	−	+
Goh et al[117]	1987	203	64		
Rognum et al[242]	1987	100	63	−	−
Scott et al[261]	1987	30	52		
Schutte et al[258]	1987	279	62		
Jones et al[160]	1988	123	75	−	+
Wiggers et al[312]	1988	350	42	−*	+
Jass et al[151]	1989	369	72	−*	+

N = number of cases, A = percentage of aneuploid cases, H = degree of histologic differentiation, * = correlation with other pathologic variables such as nodal status, lymphocytic infiltration, growth pattern, + = correlation with DNA aneuploidy, − no correlation.

an independent prognostic factor in the studies of Armitage and coworkers[8] and Kokal and coworkers.[174] In the latter, DNA ploidy was found to be the single most important variable for overall and disease-free survival in patients with primary colorectal cancer but not in patients with liver metastases. In a series of 279 patients investigated by Schutte and colleagues,[258] DNA ploidy and proliferative activity were of prognostic significance only in patients with Dukes' C disease. However, in a later study from the same group on an extended series of 369 patients, the prognostic difference had largely disappeared.[312] S phase fraction

rather than DNA ploidy had prognostic value independent of stage and grade in a series of 120 patients studied by Bauer and associates.[22] DNA ploidy was found to be a weak but independent prognostic factor by Goh and coworkers.[112] In a later study by Jass and associates[151] on a series of 369 patients, DNA ploidy was still a highly significant prognostic variable in univariate survival analysis but no independent prognostic factor in multivariate analysis.[151] In a series of 30 patients with low rectal tumors, all treated by local excision, DNA aneuploidy was associated with local recurrence but not with survival.[40] Finan and coworkers[91] found no evidence for a prognostic effect of DNA ploidy in patients with advanced colorectal cancer (Table 37–4).

Although the data available so far indicate some kind of association between DNA ploidy and tumor aggressiveness in colorectal cancer, there is still little evidence that it could serve as an independent, additional prognostic factor. However, it may prove to be of some use for prognosis assessment on biopsies before surgery or in other situations in which established prognostic variables cannot be or can only be insufficiently evaluated.[17, 151]

Several investigators have reported the occurrence of aneuploid cell populations in colorectal adenomas.[18, 109, 111, 121, 228, 298, 311] The frequency of aneuploid stemlines ranges from less than 10 to over 30%. Aneuploidy tends to be more frequently found in fresh samples than in deparaffinized samples. Aneuploidy correlates more frequently with size than with histologic type or degree of dysplasia. No aneuploidy has been found in adenomas of less than 1 cm.[109, 228, 298] In comparison with colorectal adenocarcinoma, the average DNA index of aneuploid adenomas tends to be lower.[109, 298] A highly significant correlation between DNA ploidy of adenomas and family history of colorectal cancer has been reported by Sciallero and coworkers.[253] No DNA aneuploidy has been found in hyperplastic polyps and other nonadenomatous polyps, but Hammarberg and coauthors[122] report the occurrence of aneuploid stemlines in patients with ulcerative colitis. The occur-

TABLE 37–4. Relation Between DNA Content and Survival in Colorectal Cancer

Author	Year	N	Summary of Results
Wolley et al[316]	1982	33	Aneuploidy associated with poor survival
Armitage et al[8]	1985	134	Aneuploidy associated with worse prognosis, independent of stage and grade
Finan et al[91]	1986	46	No association
Kokal et al[174]	1986	133	Aneuploidy is an independent prognostic factor in primary colorectal cancer, not in metastatic disease
Melamed et al[199]	1986	33	No association
Rognume et al[246]	1987	100	No significant association
Schutte et al[258]	1987	279	Unfavorable prognostic effects of aneuploidy and proliferative activity limited to Dukes' C disease
Bauer et al[22]	1987	120	High S phase fraction associated with worse prognosis, independent of stage and grade
Chang et al[40]	1987	30	Aneuploidy associated with local recurrence, not with survival
Emdin et al[80]	1987	37	Aneuploidy associated with worse survival
Goh et al[112]	1987	203	Aneuploidy weak but independent prognostic factor
Jones et al[160]	1988	123	Aneuploidy associated with worse survival but no independent prognostic factor
Wiggers et al[312]	1988	350	Weak effect in multivariate analysis
Jass et al[151]	1989	369	Aneuploidy associated with worse survival but no independent prognostic factor

N = number of patients.

rence of aneuploidy in colorectal adenomas supports the view that these lesions are neoplastic and may be part of an "adenoma-carcinoma" sequence in the development of colorectal cancer.[61]

Bladder Carcinoma

Analysis of nuclear DNA content in bladder cancer has been used in a number of ways. One has to distinguish the analysis of cytologic specimens encompassing cells in voided urine, bladder washings or fine needle biopsies taken during cystoscopy[84] and the analysis of biopsy material, either fresh, frozen or formaldehyde fixed and embedded in paraffin. The efficacy of flow cytometric analysis of cytologic samples for the detection of malignancies and premalignancies of the bladder is doubtful.

In cases of the analysis of voided urine samples sensitivity is optimal when three samples per patient can be examined, similar to routine cytologic investigations. The low total number of cells collected, the sometimes poor quality of the material and the low frequency of cells with abnormal DNA content hamper successful application of flow cytometry for screening purposes. Moreover, because low-grade tumors are frequently diploid and cytologically negative, no DNA abnormalities are expected in many cases. Samples obtained by bladder washings and fine needle biopsy show a significantly better quality, however. The detection sensitivity of flow cytometric analysis of such material using DNA and RNA analysis provided by acridine orange staining has been found to be more sensitive than conventional cytology.[13]

Mass screening for bladder cancer based on analysis of irrigation specimens is an issue of discussion. However, monitoring of patients with bladder cancer after treatment (surgery or chemotherapy) using flow cytometry of bladder washings has proved to be quite adequate:[70, 171] Flow cytometric evaluation appeared to be more sensitive in detecting recurring tumors than conventional cytology, especially as demonstrated in surgically treated patients with low-stage bladder tumors. It should be stressed that the role of acridine orange staining is important because atypia may be based both on the detection of DNA aneuploidy and on RNA abnormality. An example is the detection of DNA abnormality in atypical papilloma (57%) versus 86% RNA abnormality.[171] Farsund and coworkers[86] demonstrated that flow cytometric DNA analysis of material obtained by cystoscopically controlled sampling using a fine needle may be used to study the effect of local chemotherapy, as reflected in changing ratios of diploid and aneuploid cells.

Flow cytometric DNA analysis of biopsy material mainly aims at further unbiased characterization of histologically proved abnormalities, in many cases with respect to grading and prognosis. In a large series of studies the presence of DNA aneuploidy has been investigated as an objective measure for grading of carcinoma of the bladder.[116] Generally, high-grade (poorly differentiated) tumors are frequently aneuploid, whereas low-grade (well-differentiated) tumors are rarely aneuploid; primary carcinoma in situ is almost exclusively aneuploid. The same correlation has been shown for tumor stage (T staging). Chin and associates[42] found no aneuploidy in T0 tumors; 27% of T1, 71% of T2 and 75% of T3 and T4 were aneuploid. It is remarkable that the frequency of aneuploidy in low-stage (Ta, T1) tumors is similar to the known incidence of subsequent progression of these tumors.

Grade II tumors are roughly half diploid. The meaning of this bimodal distribution of the interesting grade II group has been investigated with respect to prognosis.[30, 70, 130, 214, 292] The prognostic importance of this distinction is clear because it has been shown that the recurrence rate of surgically treated grade II tumors increases with an increasing DNA index,[214] ultimately resulting in a significantly decreased survival rate.[30] In several studies it has been observed that bladder cancers with diploid or tetraploid stemlines have a relatively good prognosis, whereas tumors with stemlines between 1.4 and 2.0, and especially with stemlines higher than 2.0, have a less favorable prognosis.

Although the flow cytometrically derived DNA index provides clinically useful information, the effect on management and therapy is rather minimal. A significant change in therapy regimen is then justified only if a large-scale, randomized prospective study shows that cases with an unfavorable DNA index but that are not candidates for aggressive therapy on the basis of conventional indicators do, indeed, benefit from adjuvant therapy or radical surgery. Such large-scale studies, however, are rare.

Prostate Carcinoma

Histologic grade is the most important prognostic factor in prostate carcinoma.[110] A number of investigators have studied the question of whether DNA ploidy would be of additional prognostic value. As with several other common types of solid tumors, the frequency distribution of DNA indexes found in prostate carcinoma is typically bimodal.[292] In several studies tumor ploidy correlated with histologic grade and clinical stage.[65, 96, 193, 291, 292] The overall percentage of aneuploidy in Tribukait's[292] series of 500 patients ranges from about 20% in T1 to nearly 100% in T4 tumors. However, in a series of 109 patients with clinically localized carcinoma of the prostate analyzed by Ritchie and coworkers,[241] ploidy did not correlate with histologic grade or anatomic extent. Similarly, no correlation was found with histologic grade in a series of 50 patients studied by Lundberg and colleagues.[190] In the majority of studies aneuploidy was associated with an impaired prognosis.[92, 183, 190, 232, 273, 292, 315] Aneuploidy emerged as an independent prognostic factor in three of these studies.[190, 232, 273] In Tribukait's[292] study patients with tetraploid tumors had a significantly higher survival rate than those with nontetraploid aneuploid or multiploid tumors. No relatively favorable prognostic effect of tetraploidy was seen in two other studies, however.[241, 315] Taken together, most of the literature data indicate that DNA ploidy is of prognostic significance in prostate carcinoma and deserves further evaluation in prospective clinical studies.

Some investigators report the occurrence of DNA aneuploidy in benign prostate lesions at frequencies ranging from 2 to 30%.[67, 193, 241, 292] This interesting phenomenon needs to be studied in larger series of histologically well-documented cases before any conclusions can be drawn from these observations.

Renal Cell Carcinoma

Several flow cytometric studies have been published on renal cell carcinoma. The average percentage of aneuploid tumors is about 50%. Evidence for the existence of considerable intratumor DNA ploidy heterogeneity has been reported by Ljungberg and coworkers.[185] In the majority of studies, a positive association has been found between DNA aneuploidy and nuclear or histologic grade or both.[78, 115, 185, 219, 259] Otto and colleagues[221] and Oosterwijk and coworkers[219] report a higher percentage of DNA aneuploid tumors among patients with metastatic disease, but this was not confirmed by Ekfors and associates.[78] In patients with clear cell carcinomas aneuploidy correlates with stage.[231] DNA aneuploidy and tetraploidization have also been reported in renal oncocytomas, which are usually nonmetastasizing tumors with a limited tendency for locally invasive growth.[230] This illustrates once more that the presence of a DNA aneuploid stemline does *not always* indicate malignancy.

Most studies indicate a better survival for patients with DNA diploid renal cell carcinomas,[42, 78, 115, 186,] [219, 221] although it is not clear whether ploidy is an independent prognostic factor.

Ovarian Carcinoma

In epithelial ovarian cancer DNA aneuploidy is related to histologic grade and International Federation of Gynecology and Obstetrics (FIGO) stage (Table 37–5). High-stage and high-grade tumors are mostly aneuploid, whereas tumors of a low grade and stage are predominantly diploid. In several studies a correlation between aneuploidy and high S phase fraction was also found.[82, 88, 143] The DNA index in ovarian carcinoma appears to be a remarkably stable feature in different parts of the same tumor as well as in metastases and seems not to change even after chemotherapy.[32, 100, 150, 243] DNA flow cytometry is therefore a valuable technique for discriminating intragenital metastatic disease from multiple primary tumors.[267]

Evidence is accumulating that DNA ploidy is an important prognostic factor in early as well as in advanced ovarian carcinoma (see Table 37–5). Patients with diploid tumors generally survive for significantly longer periods than those with aneuploid tumors. In several studies, DNA ploidy emerged as one of the strongest independent prognostic variables for advanced ovarian carcinoma in the Cox model.[32, 100, 243] In a later study by Friedlander and colleagues,[103] the favorable prognostic effect of diploidy was limited to patients with FIGO Stage III disease and not seen in patients with FIGO Stage IV disease. Only a weak and statistically insignificant association between ploidy and survival is reported by Erba and associates.[82] There is some evidence that proliferative activity may be of prognostic significance as well.[166, 177, 305] Although the

TABLE 37–5. DNA Aneuploidy in Ovarian Carcinoma: Relationship with Clincopathologic Variables and Survival

Author	Year	N	A%	G	H	St	SV
Friedlander et al[98]	1983	50	40	−		+	
Friedlander et al[100]*	1984	44	5				
Friedlander et al[101]	1984	91	69				+
Erba et al[81]	1985	56	57	+			
Feichter et al[88]	1985	42	40	+		+	
Volm et al[305]	1985	37	81				+
Baak et al[12]†	1987	33	24				+
Blumenfeld et al[32]	1987	84	61				+
Christov and Vassilev[44]	1988	24	67	+			
Iversen and Skaarland[143]	1987	50	52	+	−	+	
Rodenburg et al[243]	1987	74	61	+		+	+
Jakobsen et al[150]	1988	37	54				
Kallioniemi et al[165]	1988	157	58	+	±	+	+
Friedlander et al[103]	1988	128	73				+
Iverson[144]	1988	50	52				+
Erba et al[82]	1989	101	78	+		+	−
Künn et al[177]	1989	111	65		+	−	+
Murray et al[208]	1989	41	60	−	−	−	+
Robey et al[242]	1989	36	94			−	−

*Borderline tumors.

†Only Stage I patients.

N = number of patients, A = percentage of aneuploid cases, G = grade, H = histology, St = stage, SV = survival, + = correlation with DNA aneuploidy, − = no correlation.

results obtained so far suggest that ploidy and probably also S phase fraction may be clinically important variables in epithelial ovarian cancer, results from further prospective studies must be awaited before final conclusions can be drawn.

Borderline ovarian tumors are predominantly diploid, which fits their usually indolent biologic behavior.[101, 143, 177, 310] Of the 44 patients with borderline tumors studied by Friedlander and coworkers,[101] 42 had diploid tumors. During follow-up only the two patients with aneuploid tumors died within 7 months of the initial diagnosis. Brenner tumors form a distinct group of ovarian tumors of epithelial origin, of which the majority show a benign behavior. From the 54 Brenner tumors analyzed by Trebeck and colleagues,[289] all 50 benign tumors were diploid, whereas from the four higher-grade tumors, two were aneuploid.

It can be concluded that DNA content aberrations in ovarian tumors in general appear to correlate quite well with histologic and clinical features of biologic aggressiveness.

Squamous Cell Carcinoma of the Uterine Cervix

In the 1970s many studies concentrated on the application of flow cytometry for the automation of cervical cytology.[132, 204] In spite of large efforts by many groups, problems such as that of "false alarms"[197] have frustrated the development of commercial flow-based prescreening instruments, and this approach was abandoned in the 1980s.

Relatively few studies have appeared on the prognostic value of flow cytometry in squamous cell carcinoma of the uterine cervix. The ploidy distribution in cervical carcinomas shows a similar bimodal clustering of DNA indexes[149, 277] to those of breast and ovarian cancer. The overall percentage of aneuploid cases is in the 60 to 80% range.[60, 119, 149, 277] Some authors report a moderate to high degree of stemline heterogeneity in aneuploid tumors.[77, 277, 278] Evidence was obtained that part of the additional stemlines probably had evolved via polyploidization of the first stemline.[278] The literature on the prognostic effect of tumor ploidy in squamous cell carcinoma of the cervix is conflicting. Jakobsen[146] and Jakobsen and associates[148, 149] report that a DNA index of more than 1.5 correlated with the degree of lymph node involvement and recurrence rate. They stated that the combination of ploidy information with histopathologic grading could contribute to the identification of patients needing more aggressive treatment. However, the prognostic effect of DNA indexes above or below 1.5 was not confirmed by Willen and colleagues,[314] who found a significant correlation between ploidy, histologic malignancy grading score and stage. Similarly, no association between aneuploidy and prognosis was found in some other studies,[60, 77, 279] whereas Rutgers and coauthors[249] report that patients with peridiploid and peritetraploid have a worse prognosis than those with nondiploid and

nontetraploid tumors. A high S phase fraction correlated with early recurrence in one study.[279]

Endometrial Adenocarcinoma

Flow cytometric studies on endometrial adenocarcinoma were performed by several groups.[87, 107, 141, 146, 226] DNA aneuploidy was found to correlate with histologic grade in three studies, but data on the prognostic significance are conflicting.[107, 141, 146, 226]

It can be concluded that there is still insufficient evidence for an important role of DNA flow cytometry in prognosis assessment in squamous carcinoma of the uterine cervix and endometrial adenocarcinoma.

Lung Carcinoma

In comparison with other solid tumors, relatively few flow cytometric studies have been published on lung cancer. The overall prevalence of aneuploidy in lung cancer is quite high. Bimodal DNA index distributions have been reported for small cell carcinoma, squamous cell carcinoma and adenocarcinomas.[299, 306] Squamous cell carcinomas more often have lower DNA indexes than adenocarcinomas.[217, 306] Jones and colleagues[159] found a lower percentage of DNA aneuploid stemlines (49%) in a series of 53 bronchopulmonary carcinoid tumors. Several investigators report a high frequency of multiploidy (20% or more) in small-cell as well as in nonsmall-cell lung cancer.[286, 299, 307] Tirindelli-Danesi and associates[286] found by analysis of multiple-site biopsies that 62% of the surgical specimens showed multiploidy, whereas in nonsurgical samples, e.g., bronchial washings, multiploidy was found in only 25% of the cases. These results indicate that the prevalence of multiploidy may be underestimated by limited sampling.

Aneuploidy and also high S phase fraction were associated with a significantly shorter survival in patients with nonsmall-cell lung cancer in the study of Volm and colleagues.[306] Later, Volm and coworkers[307] published the results of a series of patients with epidermoid carcinoma after a minimal follow-up period of 5 years. This study confirmed the negative effect of aneuploidy on prognosis and showed that tumor ploidy was an independent prognostic factor in the Cox model. Associations between tumor ploidy and prognosis were also found in some other studies[31, 286, 319] but not in those of Bunn and coauthors[38] and ten Velde and colleagues.[284] Therefore, results from further studies must be awaited before there is a sufficient basis to recommend the clinical use of DNA ploidy data in lung cancer such as was done by Zimmerman and colleagues.[319]

Melanoma

The correlation of DNA ploidy with clinicopathologic variables and survival in melanoma patients has been investigated in only a limited number of studies.[21, 37, 120, 265, 268, 309, 318] Most investigators report aneuploidy frequencies in the range of 60 to 80%, but a markedly lower frequency was found by Coon and associates[47] in a study of 167 Stage I patients. Apart from differences in the composition of the patient population, the authors mention the possibility that underdetection of aneuploidy in deparaffinized samples of small tumors may account for this discrepancy. DNA aneuploidy has been described also in patients with congenital melanocytic nevi but not in patients with acquired nevi.[272] As with other solid tumor types, DNA index distributions in melanomas show a bimodal clustering in the near diploid and near tetraploid mode.[21, 120, 318]

There is evidence that aneuploidy increases with tumor thickness.[21, 268, 309] In several studies[37, 47, 265, 268, 309] aneuploidy correlated with a higher recurrence rate and impaired survival, but no difference was found in a series by Zaloudik and coauthors[318] of 50 patients with Stage I nodular melanomas. Although not conclusive, most of the present data indicate a prognostic effect of DNA ploidy in patients with cutaneous melanoma.

Endocrine Tumors

Thyroid Carcinoma. Both the need for additional diagnostic criteria for discriminating benign from malignant thyroid disease as well as for additional prognostic factors have prompted a number of flow cytometric studies on thyroid tumors. Owing to the finding of significant percentages of diploid carcinomas as well as of aneuploid adenomas, the diagnostic value of DNA flow cytometry for now must be considered as limited, although some investigators hold a more optimistic view.[154, 175]

About 75% of the papillary carcinomas were found to be DNA diploid or peridiploid in two different studies in which a relative large number of cases (n = 81 and n = 72, respectively) were analyzed.[153, 254] In the same studies, about 30 to 40% of the follicular carcinomas (n = 36 and n = 42, respectively) were diploid, too. Moreover, several investigators have demonstrated aneuploid cell populations in follicular adenomas.[79, 114, 152, 155, 157, 175, 254] In some of the larger series, about 25% of the cases showed aneuploidy.[152, 254] Greenebaum and associates[114] after histologic revision concluded that the three aneuploid cases in their study represented noninvasive, low-grade follicular carcinomas. However, no evidence of capsule or blood vessel invasion was seen after meticulous serial sectioning of the 18 aneuploid cases in the study of Joensuu and colleagues,[152] and no metastases developed in these patients after a minimal follow-up period of 5 years. These results indicate that aneuploidy occurs relatively frequently in follicular adenomas and does not seem to be associated with increased risk of metastasis if they are surgically removed. The DNA index of thyroid carcinomas is a quite stable tumor property that is maintained in regional lymph node metastases.[155]

A relation between DNA aneuploidy and loss of differentiation characteristics has been reported in two studies.[43, 254] Results from several studies indicate an adverse prognosis for patients with DNA aneuploid tumors.[11, 79, 123] Multiploidy was the only significant prognostic factor for overall survival and second to age for disease-free survival in patients with papillary and follicular thyroid carcinoma studied by Hamming and coauthors.[123] The few data on medullary thyroid carcinomas are conflicting and involve only small series of patients.[256, 281] In conclusion, it appears that DNA flow cytometry has little value for the diagnosis of malignant thyroid disease but may be a prognostic factor in papillary and follicular carcinoma.

Adrenal Tumors

Tumor size is at present the most important diagnostic criterion to discriminate benign from malignant adrenocortical tumors. Although aneuploidy is found in more than 50% of the adrenocortical tumors with histologic and clinical features of malignancy including large tumor size,[6, 35, 172, 283] this is not an uncommon finding in adrenocortical adenomas, either, and thus cannot be taken as a definitive criterion for malignancy.[156, 233] Data on the prognostic significance of DNA aneuploidy in adrenocortical tumors are scanty, but some tentative associations with metastasis formation and survival have been reported.[6, 35, 140, 283]

DNA aneuploidy was also found in 12 out of 16 pheochromocytomas studied by Amberson and coauthors.[7] The frequent presence of aneuploid stemlines in these mostly benign tumors of the adrenal medulla underscores that DNA aneuploidy cannot be taken as definitive proof for malignancy.

Neuroblastoma is a highly malignant neoplasm of the adrenal medulla that is mostly found in children under the age of 5 years. The percentage of DNA aneuploidy reported for these tumors ranges from 20 to 60%, which is lower than that found in most common types of solid tumors.[3, 106, 187, 220] This tumor appears to be a striking exception to the general trend of DNA aneuploidy being associated with clinicopathologic features of higher malignancy and impaired survival reported for many other tumor types. In all four studies aneuploidy rather than diploidy correlated with favorable clinical stage.[3, 106, 187, 220] Clinical follow-up in three of these studies also showed a better response to chemotherapy and better prognosis for patients with aneuploid tumors.[106, 187, 220] DNA diploid tumors also appear to be biochemically more primitive because they secrete relatively higher levels of early catecholamine metabolites than aneuploid tumors.

Results from a cytogenetic study showed that the karyotype of the majority of aneuploid tumors consisted of three nearly complete haploid sets of chromosomes in contrast to that of diploid tumors, which were characterized by extensive structural chromosomal aberrations.[168] It seems, therefore, that two entirely different ploidy evolution mechanisms are operational in the development of neuroblastomas, leading to profound differences in biologic potential.

Bone Tumors

Bone tumors are relatively rare and the diagnosis often requires expert consultation. Therefore, several groups have investigated whether DNA flow cytometry could provide additional criteria for the diagnosis and prognostic grading of malignancy in bone tumors.[5, 23, 131, 135, 176, 188, 194, 317] Bauer and coworkers[23] report flow cytometric DNA measurements on 158 osteosarcomas and 41 benign tumors. All benign tumors were diploid, whereas of the 96 high-grade osteosarcomas, 96% were aneuploid. Four paraosteal sarcomas were diploid. In the diagnostically controversial group of 17 cases, DNA aneuploidy was associated with recurrence or death. These results are in agreement with those from an earlier study from the same group[176] and with those from other investigators all showing that about 90% of the high-grade osteosarcomas are aneuploid.[131, 135, 188, 317] These results indicate that aneuploidy may be a useful parameter in the diagnosis of high-grade osteosarcoma.

SUMMARY AND PROSPECTS

Flow cytometry is a versatile and increasingly user-friendly technique for extracting quantitative information on a variety of parameters from individual cells. To date, the most important application in cytopathology has been the measurement of nuclear DNA content in order to get information on the biologic nature and the proliferative activity of a wide variety of human neoplasms. Other important clinical applications are in hematology and immunology, in which it has become a standard technique for the immunophenotyping of white blood cells. In this chapter, the current status with respect to the value of flow cytometric DNA content measurements for the prognostic grading of different types of solid tumors has been reviewed. Similar reviews have been published by other investigators.[19, 20, 47, 99, 127, 158, 189, 262]

It is now evident that the majority of human solid tumors are DNA aneuploid. In this respect, flow cytometry has contributed significantly to the knowledge about the prevalence of cytogenetic aberrations in solid tumors. Although no information on specific chromosomes can be obtained, it is becoming increasingly clear that the observed DNA index distributions are often nonrandom and may reflect the major mechanisms of ploidy evolution for a certain type of tumor. A well-known example is the typical bimodal DNA index distribution found for breast cancer and several other types of common cancers. Such distributions indicate that tetraploidization and chromosome loss are important events in the development of highly aneuploid tumors that may endow cells with a growth advantage by disturbing the balance between growth-promoting and growth-suppressing genes.[52, 84, 219, 263, 292] The conventional, binary classification of tumors as DNA diploid or DNA aneuploid does not account for differences in the degree of DNA aneuploidy. There is evidence that in this way significant correlations between DNA index range and clinical aggressiveness

may be obscured.[27, 165, 292] Furthermore, DNA diploid tumors may still harbor numeric chromosome aberrations that are not resolvable by DNA flow cytometry.[236] In combination with the fact that DNA diploidy is a more or less operational definition depending on measurement resolution, it can be expected that the DNA index range will become integrated in biologically relevant and more refined DNA ploidy classification systems. However, it is important to realize that tumors with the same DNA index may still harbor different numeric chromosome aberrations and thus may have inherently different biologic potentialities.[236] On the other hand, the probability that two independent tumors in the same patient will have the same (aneuploid) DNA index is rather low and can be estimated from the DNA index frequency distribution for that type of tumor.[260] Because metastases often have the same DNA index as primary tumors, DNA flow cytometry can help to discriminate multiple primary tumors from metastatic disease.[83, 96, 102, 238, 260, 267]

In spite of the evidence for the prognostic value of S phase determinations, the calculation of this parameter as well as its interpretation is far less standardized than DNA ploidy determinations. Because the reliability of this parameter is highly influenced by the heterogeneity of the cell sample, multiparameter analysis using cell-type specific markers such as monoclonal antibodies against intermediate filaments will be needed to more specifically identify the relevant cell populations.[58, 90] Monoclonal antibodies that have been developed to be directed against nuclear proliferation–associated antigens such as PCNA/cyclin offer a new way for the direct identification of cycling cells without the need to label cells *in vivo* or *in vitro* with BrdUrd.[213] Procedures for the simultaneous analysis of cytoplasmic and nuclear antigens with nuclear DNA content have been developed by several groups, and we expect that these gradually will be implemented for the analysis of clinical samples.[46, 66, 180]

DNA flow cytometry is now being implemented as a routine technique in many pathology laboratories, predominantly with the intention to use it for the malignancy grading of tumors. This development seems to be justified by the results of many studies in which correlations between DNA content parameters and various aspects of biologic behavior have been demonstrated. Such associations have been found in ovarian carcinoma, bladder carcinoma, prostate carcinoma, breast carcinoma, renal carcinoma, colorectal carcinoma, lung carcinoma, thyroid carcinoma, bone tumors and melanoma. To date, most of this evidence comes from retrospective studies on paraffin-embedded tissue. In part of the publications no or incomplete information on clinical stage and histologic degree of differentiation is given, which makes it difficult to weigh the observed prognostic effects of DNA ploidy and S phase fraction against the impact of established prognostic factors. The most convincing evidence for an important, independent effect of DNA aneuploidy so far is found in ovarian carcinoma. For melanoma and prostate carcinoma there is similar but less strong evidence. The situation is less clear for common tumors such as breast and colorectal cancer, in which many other prognostic variables have to be considered before conclusions can be drawn. Ultimately, the prognostic value of DNA ploidy has to be evaluated on the basis of the results from prospective studies on well-documented series of patients.

It may take another 5 years before sufficient information is available to establish generally accepted guidelines of how DNA content parameters are to be used in therapy planning and patient management. In the meantime it should be realized that even when such studies show that the prognostic effect of DNA content parameters for certain tumor types can be largely explained by their strong correlation with established prognostic factors such as grade and stage, the objectivity of DNA flow cytometry may help to detect inconsistencies that are associated with the subjectivity and interobserver variability of grading and staging systems.[283]

The large-scale introduction of flow cytometry in clinical laboratories has created an urgent need for quality assurance and standardization. Initiatives to establish standards and quality assurance programs have been taken by several organizations and institutes; also, the manufacturers of flow cytometry instrumentation and reagents have put considerable effort into developing instrumental controls for monitoring performance.[36, 47, 137]

Finally, besides flow cytometry, there is an increased interest in the application of image cytometry in diagnostic cytopathology. Although aiming at the same goal, the assessment of DNA ploidy and proliferative activity, these techniques are intrinsically different in nature. Rather than being competitive, they are to a large extent complementary.[51, 244] The combined use of various cytometric techniques in diagnostic cytopathology is therefore indicated.

References

1. Abandowitz HM, Ow KT, Hardy D, Keightly DD, Sarfaty G, Nash A: Relationship between flow cytometric parameters, steroid receptors, and menopausal status in breast cancers. Oncology 44:24–29, 1987.
2. Abe R, Ueki H: Flow cytometric analysis for assessing the malignant potential of breast cancer. J Surg Oncol 36:259–262, 1987.
3. Abramowsky CR, Taylor SR, Anton AH, Berk AI, Roederer M, Murphy RF: Flow cytometric DNA ploidy analysis and catecholamine secretion profiles in neuroblastoma. Cancer 63:152–1756, 1989.
4. Alanen KA, Joensuu H, Klemi PJ: Autolysis is a potential source of false aneuploid peaks in flow cytometric DNA histograms. Cytometry 10:417–425, 1989.
5. Alho A, Connor JF, Mankin HJ, Schiller AL, Campbell CJ: Assessment of malignancy of cartilage tumors using flow cytometry. J Bone Joint Surg 65:779–785, 1983.
6. Amberson JB, Vaughan D, Gray GF, Naus GJ: Flow cytometric analysis of nuclear DNA from adrenocortical neoplasms. Cancer 59:2091–2095, 1987.
7. Amberson JB, Vaughan ED, Gray GF, Naus GJ: Flow cytometric determination of nuclear DNA content in benign adrenal pheochromocytomas. Urology 30:102–104, 1987.
8. Armitage NC, Robins RA, Evans DF, Turner DR, Baldwin RW, Hardcastle JD: The influence of tumor cell DNA abnor-
malities on survival in colorectal cancer. Br J Surg 72:828–830, 1985.
9. Atkin NB: Modal deoxyribonucleic acid value and survival in carcinoma of the breast. Br Med J 1:271–272, 1972.
10. Auer G, Fallenius A, Erhardt K, Sundelin B: Progression of mammary adenocarcinomas as reflected by nuclear DNA content. Cytometry 5:420–425, 1984.
11. Auer GU, Bäckdahl M, Forsslund GM, Askensten UG: Ploidy levels in nonneoplastic and neoplastic thyroid cells. Anal Quant Cytol Histol 7:97–106, 1985.
12. Baak JP, Wisse-Brekelmans EC, Uyterlinde AM, Schipper NW: Evaluation of the prognostic value of morphometric features and cellular DNA content in FIGO I ovarian cancer patients. Anal Quant Cytol Histol 9:287–290, 1987.
13. Badalament RA, Hermansen DK, Kimmel M, Gay H, Herr H, Fair WR, Whitmore WF, Melamed MR: The sensitivity of bladder wash flow cytometry, bladder wash cytology, and voided cytology in the detection of bladder carcinoma. Cancer 60:1423–1427, 1987.
14. Baildam AD, Zaloudik J, Howell A, Barnes DM, Turnbull L, Swindell R, Moore M, Sellwood RA: DNA analysis by flow cytometry, response to endocrine treatment and prognosis in advanced carcinoma of the breast. Br J Cancer 55:553–559, 1987.
15. Baisch H, Göhde W, Linden WA: Analysis of PCP data to determine the fraction of cells in various phases of the cell cycle. Radiat Environ Biophys 12:31–39, 1975.
16. Baisch H, Beck HP, Christensen IJ, Hartmann NR, Fried J, Dean PN, Gray JW, Jett JH, Johnson DA, White RA, Nicolini C, Zietz S, Watson JV: A comparison of mathematical methods for the analysis of DNA histograms by flow cytometry. Cell Tissue Kinet 15:235–249, 1982.
17. Banner BF, de la Vega T, Roseman DL, Coon JS: Should flow cytometric DNA analysis precede definitive surgery for colon carcinoma? Ann Surg 302:740–744, 1985.
18. Banner BF, Chacho MS, Roseman DL, Coon JS: Multiparameter flow cytometric analysis of colon polyps. Am J Clin Pathol 87:313–318, 1987.
19. Barlogie B, Drewinko B, Schumann J, Göhde W, Dosik G, Latreille J, Johnston DA, Freireich EJ: Cellular DNA content as a marker of neoplasia in man. Am J Med 69:195–203, 1980.
20. Barlogie B: Abnormal cellular DNA content as a marker of neoplasia. Eur J Cancer Clin Oncol 9:1123–1125, 1984.
21. Bartkowiak D, Schumann J, Otto FJ, Lippold A, Drepper H: DNA flow cytometry in the prognosis of primary malignant melanoma. Oncology (in press).
22. Bauer KD, Lincoln ST, Vera-Roman JM, Wallemark CB, Chmiel JS, Madurski ML, Murad T, Scarpelli D: Prognostic implications of proliferative activity and DNA aneuploidy in colonic adenocarcinomas. Lab Invest 57:329–335, 1987.
23. Bauer HC, Kreicsbergs A, Silfversbärd C, Tribukait B: DNA analysis in the differential diagnosis of osteosarcoma. Cancer 61:2432–2540, 1988.
24. Bauman JGJ, van der Ploeg M, van Duijn P: Fluorescent hybridocytochemical procedures: DNA/RNA hybridization in situ. In Investigative Microtechniques in Medicine and Biology. Edited by J Chayen, L Bitensky. New York, Marcel Dekker, pp 41–87, 1984.
25. Beck HP: Evaluation of flow cytometric data of human tumors: Correction procedures for background and cell aggregations. Cell Tissue Kinet 13:173–181, 1980.
26. Beerman H, Kluin PM, van de Velde CJH, Hermans J, Cornelisse CJ: DNA flow cytometry in the prognosis of node-negative breast cancer. N Engl J Med 321:473–474, 1989.
27. Beerman H, Kluin PM, Hermans J, van de Velde CJH, Cornelisse CJ: Prognostic significance of DNA-ploidy in a series of 690 primary breast cancer patients. Int J Cancer 45:34–39, 1990.
28. Bedrossian CWM, Raber M, Barlogie B: Flow cytometry and cytomorphology in primary resectable breast cancer. Anal Quant Cytol 3:112–116, 1981.
29. Bichel P, Poulsen HS, Andersen J: Estrogen receptor content and ploidy of human mammary carcinoma. Cancer 50:1771–1774, 1982.
30. Blomjous CEM, Schipper NW, Baak JPA, Van Galen EM, de

Voogt HJ, Meyer CJLM: Retrospective study of prognostic importance of DNA flow cytometry of urinary bladder carcinoma. J Clin Pathol 41:21–25, 1988.

31. Blöndal T, Pontén J: DNA ploidy in small cell carcinoma of the lung. Anticancer Res 3:47–51, 1983.

32. Blumenfeld D, Braly PS, Ben-Ezra J, Klevecz RR: Tumor DNA content as a prognostic feature in advanced epithelial ovarian carcinoma. Gynecol Oncol 27:389–402, 1987.

33. Bonner WA, Hulett HR, Sweet RG, Herzenberg LA: Fluorescence cell sorting. Rev Sci Instrumen 43:404–409, 1972.

34. Boveri T: Zur Frage der Entstehung Maligner Tumoren. Jena, Gustav Fischer, 1914.

35. Bowlby LS, Debault LE, Abraham SR: Flow cytometric analysis of adrenal cortical tumor DNA. Cancer 58:1499–1505, 1986.

36. Bray RA, Landay AL: Identification and functional characterization of mononuclear cells by flow cytometry. Arch Pathol Lab Med 113:579–590, 1989.

37. Büchner T, Hiddemann W, Wörmann B, Kleinemeier B, Schumann J, Gönde W, Ritter J, Müller KM, von Bassewitz, DB, Roessner A, Grundmann E: Differential pattern of DNA-aneuploidy in human malignancies. Pathol Res Pract 179:310–317, 1985.

38. Bunn PA, Carney DN, Gazdar AF, Whang-Peng J, Matthews MJ: Diagnostic and biological implications of flow cytometric DNA content analysis in lung cancer. Cancer Res 43:5026–5032, 1983.

39. Cavenee WK, Dryja TP, Phillips RA, Benedict WF, Godbout R, Gallie BL, Murphree AL, Strong LC, White RL: Expression of recessive alleles by chromosomal mechanisms in retinoblastoma. Nature 305:779–784, 1983.

40. Chang KJ, Enker WE, Melamed M: Influence of tumor cell DNA ploidy on the natural history of rectal cancer. Am J Surg 153:184–188, 1987.

41. Chin JL, Huben RP, Nava E, Rustum YM, Grevo JM, Pontes JE, Frankfurt OS: Flow cytometric analysis of DNA content in human bladder tumors and irrigation fluids. Cancer 56:1677–1681, 1985.

42. Chin JL, Pontes JE, Frankfurt OS: Flow cytometric deoxyribonucleic acid analysis of primary and metastatic human renal cell carcinoma. J Urol 133:582–585, 1985.

43. Christov K: Flow cytometric DNA measurements in human thyroid tumors. Virchows Arch [Cell Pathol] 51:255–263, 1986.

44. Christov K, Vassilev N: Flow cytometric analysis of DNA and cell proliferation in ovarian tumors. Cancer 61:121–125, 1988.

45. Clark GM, Dressler LG, Owens MA, Pounds G, Oldaker T, McGuire WL: Prediction of relapse or survival in patients with node-negative breast cancer by DNA flow cytometry. N Engl J Med 320:627–633, 1989.

46. Clevenger CV, Bauer KD, Epstein AL: A method for simultaneous nuclear immunofluorescence and DNA content quantitation using monoclonal antibodies and flow cytometry. Cytometry 6:208–214, 1985.

47. Coon JS, Landay AL, Weinstein RS: Biology of disease. Advances in flow cytometry for diagnostic pathology. Lab Invest 57:453–479, 1987.

48. Coon JS, Deitch AD, de Vere White RW, Koss LG, Melamed MR, Reeder JE, Weinstein RS, Wersto RP, Wheeless LL: Check samples for laboratory self-assesment in DNA flow cytometry. Cancer 63:1592–1599, 1989.

49. Cornelisse CJ, Tanke HJ, de Koning H, Brutel de la Rivière G: DNA ploidy analysis and cytologic examination of sorted cell populations from human breast tumors. Anal Quant Cytol 5:173–183, 1983.

50. Cornelisse CJ, de Koning HR, Moolenaar AJ, van de Velde CJH, Ploem JS: Image and flow cytometric analysis of DNA content in breast cancer. Anal Quant Cytol 6:9–18, 1984.

51. Cornelisse CJ, Van Driel-Kulker AM: DNA image cytometry on machine-selected breast cancer cells and a comparison between flow cytometry and scanning cytophotometry. Cytometry 6:471–477, 1985.

52. Cornelisse CJ, van de Velde CJH, Caspers RJC, Moolenaar AJ, Hermans J: DNA ploidy and survival in breast cancer patients. Cytometry 8:225–234, 1987.

53. Coulter WJ: Means for counting particles suspended in a fluid.

US Patent No. 2,656,508. Filed August 27, 1949. Issued October 20, 1953.

54. Coulson PB, Thornthwaite JT, Woolley TW, Sugarbaker EV, Seckinger D: Prognostic indicators including DNA histogram type, receptor content, and staging related to human breast cancer patient survival. Cancer Res 44:4187–4196, 1984.

55. Cremer C, Cremer T, Gray JW: Induction of chromosome damage by ultraviolet light and caffeine: Correlation of cytogenetic evaluation and karyotype. Cytometry 5:287–290, 1982.

56. Cremer T, Landegent J, Bruckner A, Scholl H, Schardin M, Hager H, Devilee P, Pearson P, Van der Ploeg M: Detection of chromosome aberrations in the human interphase nucleus by visualization of specific target DNAs. Hum Genet 74:346–352, 1986.

57. Crissman HA, Oka MS, Steinkamp JA: Rapid staining methods for analysis of deoxyribonucleic acid and protein in mammalian cells. J Histochem Cytochem 24:64–71, 1976.

58. Croonen AM, van der Valk P, Herman CJ, Lindeman J: Cytology, immunopathology and flow cytometry in the diagnosis of pleural and peritoneal effusions. Lab Invest 58:725–732, 1988.

59. Crosland-Taylor PK: A device for counting small particles suspended in a fluid through a tube. Nature 171:37–38, 1953.

60. Davis JR, Aristizibal S, Way DL, Weiner SA, Hicks MJ, Hagaman RM: DNA ploidy, grade and stage in prognosis of uterine cervical cancer. Gynecol Oncol 32:4–7, 1989.

61. Day DW, Morson BC: The adenoma. *In* The Pathogenesis of Colorectal Cancer. Edited by BC Morson. London, WB Saunders, pp 58–71, 1978.

62. Dean PN: Methods of data analysis in flow cytometry. *In* Flow Cytometry: Instrumentation and Data Analysis. Edited by MA van Dilla, PN Dean, OD Laerum, MR Melamed. London, Academic Press, pp 195–221, 1985.

63. Dean PN, Jett JH: Mathematical analysis of DNA distributions derived from flow microfluorometry. J Cell Biol 60:523–527, 1974.

64. Dean PN, Pinkel D: High-resolution dual laser flow cytometry. J Histochem Cytochem 26:622–627, 1978.

65. Dejter SW, Cunningham RE, Noguchi PD, Jones RV, Moul JW, McLeod DG, Lynch JH: Prognostic significance of DNA ploidy in carcinoma of the prostate. Urology 33:361–366, 1989.

66. Dent GA, Leglise MC, Pryzwansky KB, Ross DW: Simultaneous paired analysis by flow cytometry of surface markers, cytoplasmic antigens, or oncogene expression with DNA content. Cytometry 10:192–198, 1989.

67. de Vere White RW, Tesluk H, Deitch AB: The paradox of aneuploidy in the benign and malignant prostate. Cytometry [Suppl] 8 Abstracts Society for Analytical Cytology, Abstract No. 10, 1987.

68. Devilee P, Thierry RF, Kievits T, Kolluri R, Hopman AHN, Willard HF, Pearson PL, Cornelisse CJ: Detection of chromosome aneuploidy in interphase nuclei from human primary breast tumors using chromosome-specific repetitive DNA probes. Cancer Res 48:5825–5830, 1988.

69. Deville P, Van den Broek M, Kuipers-Dijkshoorn NJ, Kolluri R, Meera Khan P, Pearson PL, Cornelisse CJ: At least four different chromosomal regions are involved in loss of heterozygosity in human breast carcinoma. Genomics 5:554–560, 1989.

70. Devonec M, Darzynkiewicz Z, Kostyrka-Claps, Collste L, Whitmore WF, Melamed MR: Flow cytometry of low-stage bladder tumors. Cancer 49:109–118, 1982.

71. Dittrich W, Göhde W: Automatic measuring and counting device for particles in a dispersion. British Patent No. 1,300,585. Filed December 18, 1968 in Germany. Issued December 20, 1972.

72. Dittrich W, Göhde W: Automatic measuring and counting device for particles in a dispersion. British Patent No. 1,305,923. Filed April 18, 1969 in Germany. Issued February 7, 1973.

73. Dowle CS, Owainati A, Robins A, Burns K, Ellis IO, Ellston CW, Blamey RW: Prognostic significance of the DNA content of human breast cancer. Br J Surg 74:133–136, 1987.

74. Dressler LG, Seamer L, Owens MA, Clark GM, McGuire WL: Evaluation of a modeling system for S-phase estimation

in breast cancer by flow cytometry. Cancer Res 47:5294–5302, 1987.

75. Dressler LG, Seamer LC, Owens MA, Clark GM, McGuire WL: DNA flow cytometry and prognostic factors in 1331 frozen breast cancer specimens. Cancer 61:420–427, 1988.

76. Durrant LG, Robins RA, Armitage NC, Brown A, Baldwin RW, Hardcastle JD: Association of antigen expression and DNA ploidy in human colorectal tumors. Cancer Res 46:3543–3549, 1986.

77. Dyson JE, Joslin CA, Rothwell RI, Quirke P, Khoury GG, Bird CC: Flow cytometric evidence for the differential responsiveness of aneuploid and diploid cervix tumors. Radiother Oncol 8:263–272, 1987.

78. Ekfors TO, Lipasti J, Nurmi MJ, Eerola E: Flow cytometric analysis of the DNA profile of renal cell carcinoma. Pathol Res Pract 182:58–62, 1987.

79. el-Naggar AK, Batsakis JG, Luna MA, Hickey RC: Hürthle cell tumors of the thyroid. Acta Otolaryngol Head Neck Surg 114:520–521, 1988.

80. Emdin SO, Stenling R, Roos G: Prognostic value of DNA content in colorectal carcinoma. Cancer 60:1282–1287, 1987.

81. Erba E, Vaghi M, Pepe S, Amato G, Bistolfi M, Ubezio P, Mangioni C, Landoni F, Morasca L: DNA index of ovarian carcinomas from 56 patients: *In vivo in vitro* studies. Br J Cancer 52:565–573, 1985.

82. Erba E, Ubezio P, Pepe S, Vaghi M, Marsoni S, Torri S, Mangioni C, Landoni F, d'Incalci M: Flow cytometric analysis of DNA content in human ovarian cancers. Br J Cancer 60:45–50, 1989.

83. Erhardt K, Auer G: Mammary carcinoma: Comparison of DNA-content in the primary tumor and the corresponding axillary lymph node metastases. Acta Pathol Microbiol Immunol Scand [A], 94:29–34, 1986.

84. Ewers SB, Langström E, Baldetorp B, Killander D: Flow-cytometric DNA analysis in primary breast carcinomas and clinicopathological correlations. Cytometry 5:408–419, 1984.

85. Farsund T, Hostmark JG, Laerum OD: Relation between flow cytometric DNA distribution and pathology in human bladder cancer. Cancer 54:1771–1777, 1984.

86. Farsund T, Laerum OL, Hostmark J, Jordfald G: Local chemotherapy effects in bladder cancer demonstrated by selective sampling and flow cytometry. J Urol 131:22–32, 1984.

87. Feichter GE, Hoffken H, Heep J, Haag D, Heberling D, Brandt H, Rummel H, Goerttler K: DNA flow-cytometric measurements on the normal, atrophic, hyperplastic and neoplastic human endometrium. Virchows Arch [A], 398:53–65, 1982.

88. Feichter GE, Kühn W, Czernobilsky B, Müller A, Heep J, Abel U, Haag D, Kaufmann M, Rummel HH, Kubli F, Goerttler K: DNA flow cytometry of ovarian tumors with correlation to histopathology. Int J Gynecol Pathol 4:336–345, 1985.

89. Feichter GE, Müller A, Kaufmann M, Haag D, Born IA, Abel U, Klinga K, Kubli F, Goerttler K: Correlation of DNA flow cytometric results and other prognostic factors in primary breast cancer. Int J Cancer 41:823–828, 1988.

90. Feitz WFJ, Beck HLM, Smeets AWGB, Debruyne FMJ, Vooijs GP, Herman CJ, Ramaekers FCS: Tissue-specific markers in flow cytometry of urological cancers: Cytokeratins in bladder carcinoma. Int J Cancer 36:349–356, 1985.

91. Finan FJ, Quirke P, Dixon MF, Dyson JED, Giles GR, Bird CC: Is DNA aneuploidy a good prognostic indicator in patients with advanced colorectal cancer? Br J Cancer 54:327–330, 1986.

92. Fordham MV, Burdge AH, Matthes J, Williams G, Cooke T: Prostatic carcinoma cell DNA content measured by flow cytometry and its relation to clinical outcome. Br J Surg 73:400–403, 1986.

93. Fossa SD, Thorud E, Shoaib MC, Pettersen EO, Hoie J, Knudsen, SO: DNA flow cytometry in primary breast carcinoma. Acta Pathol Microbiol Immunol Scand [A], 92:475–480, 1984.

94. Frankfurt OS, Greco WR, Slocum HK, Arbuck SG, Gamarra M, Pavelic ZP, Rustum YM: Proliferative characteristics of primary and metastatic human solid tumors by DNA flow cytometry. Cytometry 5:629–635, 1984.

95. Frankfurt OS, Slocum MK, Rustum YM, Arbuck SG, Pavelic ZP, Petrelli N, Huben RP, Pontes EY, Greco WR: Flow cytometric analysis of DNA aneuploidy in primary and metastatic human solid tumors. Cytometry 5:71–80, 1984.

96. Frankfurt OS, Chin JL, Englander LS, Greco WS, Pontes JE, Rustum YM: Relationship between DNA ploidy, glandular differentiation, and tumor spread in human prostate cancer. Cancer Res 45:1418–1423, 1985.

97. Fried J: Method for the quantitative evaluation of data from flow microfluorometry. Comput Biomed Res 9:263–276, 1976.

98. Friedlander ML, Taylor IW, Russel P, Musgrove EA, Hedley DH, Tattersall MH: Ploidy as prognostic factor in ovarian cancer. Int J Gynecol Pathol 2:55–63, 1983.

99. Friedlander ML, Hedley DW, Taylor IW: Clinical and biological significance of aneuploidy in human tumours. J Clin Pathol 37:961–974, 1984.

100. Friedlander ML, Hedley DW, Taylor IW, Russell P, Coates AS: Influence of cellular DNA content on survival in advanced ovarian cancer. Cancer Res 44:397–400, 1984.

101. Friedlander ML, Russell P, Taylor IW, Hedley DW, Tattersall MH: Flow cytometric analysis of cellular DNA content as an adjunct to the diagnosis of ovarian tumours of borderline malignancy. Pathology 16:301–316, 1984.

102. Friedlander ML, Taylor IW, Russell P, Tattersall MH: Cellular DNA content: A stable feature in epithelial ovarian cancer. Br J Cancer 49:173–179, 1984.

103. Friedlander ML, Hedley DW, Swanson C, Russell P: Prediction of long-term survival by flow cytometric analysis of cellular DNA content in patients with advanced ovarian cancer. J Clin Oncol 6:282–290, 1988.

104. Friend SH, Bernards R, Rogelj S, Weinber RA, Rapaport JM, Albert DM, Dryja TP: A human DNA segment with properties of the gene that predisposes to retinoblastoma and osteosarcoma. Nature 323:643–646, 1986.

105. Fulwyler MJ: Electronic separation of biological cells by volume. Science 150:910–911, 1965.

106. Gansler T, Chatten J, Varello MT, Bunin GR, Atkinson B: Flow cytometric DNA analysis of neuroblastoma. Correlation with histology and clinical outcome. Cancer 58:2453–2458, 1986.

107. Geisinger KR, Homesley HD, Morgan TM, Kute TE, Marshall RB: Endometrial adenocarcinoma. A multiparameter clinicopathologic analysis including the DNA profile and the sex steroid hormone receptors. Cancer 58:1518–1525, 1986.

108. Gentili C, Sanfilippo O, Silvestrini R: Cell proliferation and its relationship to clinical features and relapse in breast cancers. Cancer 48:974–979, 1981.

109. Giaretti W, Sciallero S, Bruno S, Geido E, Aste H, di Vinci A: DNA flow cytometry of endoscopically examined colorectal adenomas and adenocarcinomas. Cytometry 9:238–244, 1988.

110. Gleason DF, Mellinger GT, Veterans Administration Research Group: Prediction of prognosis for prostatic adeno-carcinoma by combined histological grading and clinical staging. J Urol 111:58–64, 1974.

111. Goh HS, Jass JR: DNA content and the adenoma-carcinoma sequence in the colorectum. J Clin Pathol 39:387–392, 1986.

112. Goh HS, Jass JR, Atkin WS, Cuzick J, Northover JMA: Value of flow cytometric determination of ploidy as a guide to prognosis in operable rectal cancer: A multivariate analysis. Inter J Colorect Dis 2:17–21, 1987.

113. Gray JW, Darzynkiewicz Z: Techniques in cell cycle analysis. Clifton, New Jersey: Humana Press, 1987.

114. Greenebaum E, Koss LG, Elequin F, Silver CE: The diagnostic value of flow cytometric DNA measurements in follicular tumors of the thyroid gland. Cancer 56:2011–2018, 1985.

115. Grignon DJ, el-Naggar A, Green LK, Ayala AG, Ro JY, Swanson DA, Troncoso P, McLemore D, Giacco GG, Guinee VF: DNA flow cytometry as a predictor of outcome of Stage I renal cell carcinoma. Cancer 63:1161–1165, 1989.

116. Gustafson H, Tribukait B: Characterization of bladder carcinomas by flow DNA analysis. Eur Urol 11:410–417, 1985.

117. Haag D, Goerttler K, Tschahargane C: The proliferative index (PI) of human breast cancer as obtained by flow cytometry. Pathol Res Pract 178:315–322, 1984.

118. Haag D, Feichter GE, Goerttler K, Kaufmann M: Influence of systematic errors on the evaluation of the S-phase portions

from DNA distributions of solid tumors as shown for 328 breast carcinomas. Cytometry 8:377–385, 1987.

119. Hanselaar AG, Vooijs GP, Oud PS, Pahlplatz MM, Beck JL: DNA ploidy patterns in cervical intraepithelial neoplasia grade III, with and without synchronous invasive squamous cell carcinoma. Cancer 62:2537–2545, 1988.

120. Hansson J, Tribukait B, Lewensohn R, Ringborg U: Flow cytofluorometric DNA analyses of metastases of human malignant melanomas. Anal Quant Cytol 4:99–104, 1982.

121. Hamada S, Namura K, Fujita S: The possibility of nonpolyploid carcinogenesis in the large intestine as inferred from frequencies of DNA aneuploidy of polypoid and crater-shaped carcinomas. Cancer 62:1503–1510, 1988.

122. Hammarberg C, Slezak P, Tribukait B: Early detection of malignancy in ulcerative colitis. Cancer 53:291–295, 1984.

123. Hamming JF, Schelfhout LJ, Cornelisse CJ, van de Velde CJ, Goslings BM: Prognostic value of nuclear DNA content in papillary and follicular thyroid cancer. World J Surg 12:503–508, 1988.

124. Hedley DW, Friedlander ML, Taylor IW, Rugg CA, Musgrove EA: Method for analysis of cellular DNA content of paraffin-embedded pathological material using flow cytometry. J Histochem Cytochem 31:1333–1335, 1983.

125. Hedley DW, Rugg CA, Ng AB, Taylor IW: Influence of cellular DNA content on disease-free survival of Stage II breast cancer patients. Cancer Res 44:5395–5398, 1984.

126. Hedley DW, Rugg CA, Gelber RA: Association of DNA index and S-phase fraction with prognosis of nodes positive for early breast cancer. Cancer Res 47:4729–4735, 1987.

127. Hedley, DW: Flow cytometry using paraffin-embedded tissue: Five years on. Cytometry 10:229–241, 1989.

128. Heim S, Mitelman F: Cancer Cytogenetics. New York: Alan R Liss, 1987.

129. Heim S, Mandahl N, Mitelman F: Genetic convergence and divergence in tumor progression. Cancer Res 48:5911–5916, 1988.

130. Helander K, Kirkhus B, Iversen OE, Johansson SL, Nilsson S, Vaage S, Fjordvang H: Studies on urinary bladder carcinoma by morphometry, flow cytometry, and light microscopic malignancy grading with special reference to grade II tumours. Virchows Arch [A], 408:117–126, 1985.

131. Heliö H, Karaharju E, Nordling S: Flow cytometric determination of DNA content in malignant and benign bone tumours. Cytometry 6:165–171, 1985.

132. Herman CJ, Bunnag B, Cassidy M: Clinical cytology specimens for cancer detection. In Flow cytometry and cell sorting. Edited by MR Melamed, PF Mullaney, ML Mendelsohn. New York: John Wiley, pp 559–572, 1979.

133. Hiddemann W, Schumann J, Andreeff M, Barlogie B, Herman CJ, Leif CR, Mayall BH, Murphy RF, Sandberg AA: Convention on nomenclature for DNA cytometry. Cytometry 5:445–446, 1984.

134. Hiddemann W, von Bassewitz DB, Kleinemeier HJ, Schulte-Brochterbeck E, Hauss J, Lingemann B, Büchner T, Grundmann E: DNA stemline heterogeneity in colorectal cancer. Cancer 58:258–263, 1986.

135. Hiddemann W, Roessner A, Wörman B, Mellin W, Klockenkemper B, Bösing T, Büchner T, Grundmann E: Tumor heterogeneity in osteosarcoma as identified by flow cytometry. Cancer 59:324–328, 1987.

136. Holliday R: Chromosome error propagation and cancer. Trends Genet 5:42–45, 1989.

137. Homburger HA, McCarthy RM, Deodhar S: Assessment of interlaboratory variability in analytical cytology. Arch Pathol Lab Med 113:667–672, 1989.

138. Hopman AHN, Ramaekers FCS, Raap AK, Beck JLM, Devilee P, van der Ploeg M, Vooijs GP: In situ hybridization as a tool to study numerical chromosome aberrations in solid bladder tumors. Histochemistry 89:307–316, 1988.

139. Horsfall DJ, Tilley WD, Orell SR, Marshall VR, Cant EL: Relationship between ploidy and steroid hormone receptors in primary invasive breast cancer. Br J Cancer 53:23–28, 1986.

140. Hosaka Y, Rainwater LM, Grant CS, Young WF, Farrow GM, van Heerden JA, Lieber MM: Adrenocortical carcinoma: Nuclear deoxyribonucleic acid ploidy studied by flow cytometry. Surgery 102:1027–1034, 1987.

141. Iversen OE: Flow cytometric deoxyribonucleic acid index: A prognostic factor in endometrial carcinoma. Am J Obstet Gynecol 155:770–776, 1986.

142. Iversen OE, Laerum OD: Trout and salmon erythrocytes and human leukocytes as internal standards for ploidy control in flow cytometry. Cytometry 8:190–196, 1987.

143. Iversen OE, Skaarland E: Ploidy assessment of benign and malignant ovarian tumors by flow cytometry. A clinicopathologic study. Cancer 60:82–87, 1987.

144. Iversen OE: Prognostic value of the flow cytometric DNA index in human ovarian carcinoma. Cancer 61:971–975, 1988.

145. Iversen OE, Utaaker E, Skaarland E: DNA ploidy and steroid receptors as predictors of disease course in patients with endometrial carcinoma. Acta Obstet Gynecol Scand 67:531–537, 1988.

146. Jakobsen A: Ploidy level and short-time prognosis of early cervical cancer. Radiother Oncol 1:271–275, 1984.

147. Jakobsen A, Poulsen HS, Madsen EL, Petersen SE, Hansen HS: Ploidy level of human breast carcinoma. Acta Radiol 23:103–107, 1984.

148. Jakobsen A, Bichel P, Vaeth M: New prognostic factors in squamous carcinoma of cervix uteri. Am J Clin Oncol 8:39–43, 1985.

149. Jakobsen A, Bichel P, Kristensen GB, Nyland M: Prognostic influence of ploidy level and histopathological differentiation in cervical carcinoma Stage Ib. Eur J Cancer Clin Oncol 24:969–972, 1988.

150. Jakobsen A, Hansen V, Poulsen HS: DNA profile and receptor content of human ovarian cancer. Eur J Gynaecol Oncol 9:461–463, 1988.

151. Jass JR, Mukawa K, Goh HS, Love SB, Capellaro D: Clinical importance of DNA content in rectal cancer measured by flow cytometry. J Clin Pathol 42:254–259, 1989.

152. Joensuu H, Klemi P, Eerola E: DNA aneuploidy in follicular adenomas of the thyroid gland. Am J Pathol 124:373–376, 1986.

153. Joensuu H, Klemi P, Eerola E, Tuominen J: Influence of cellular DNA content on survival in differentiated thyroid cancer. Cancer 58:2462–2467, 1988.

154. Joensuu H, Klemi PJ, Eerola E: Diagnostic value of flow cytometric DNA determination combined with fine needle aspiration biopsy in thyroid tumors. Anal Quant Cytol Histol 9:328–334, 1987.

155. Joensuu J, Klemi P: Comparison of nuclear DNA content in primary and metastatic differentiated thyroid carcinoma. Am J Clin Pathol 89:35–40, 1988.

156. Joensuu J, Klemi J: DNA-aneuploidy in adenomas of endocrine organs. Am J Pathol 132:145–151, 1988.

157. Johannessen JV, Sobrinho-Simoes M, Tangen KO, Lindmo T, Tangen KO: The diagnostic value of flow cytometric DNA measurements in selected disorders of the human thyroid. Am J Clin Pathol 77:20–25, 1982.

158. Johnson TS, Katz RL, Pershouse M: Flow cytometric applications in cytopathology. Anal Quant Cytol Histol 6:423–458, 1988.

159. Jones DJ, Hasleton PS, Moore M: DNA ploidy in bronchopulmonary carcinoid tumours. Thorax 43:195–199, 1988.

160. Jones DJ, Moore M, Schofield PF: Refining the prognostic significance of DNA ploidy status in colorectal cancer: A prospective flow cytometric study. Int J Cancer 41:206–210, 1988.

161. Jovin T: Fluorescence polarization and energy transfer: Theory and application. In Flow Cytometry and Sorting. Edited by MR Melamed, PF Mullaney, ML Mendelsohn. New York, John Wiley, pp 137–165, 1979.

162. Kachel V: Electrical resistance pulse sizing (Coulter sizing). In Flow Cytometry and Sorting. Edited by MR Melamed, PF Mullaney, ML Mendelsohn. New York, John Wiley, pp 61–104, 1979.

163. Kallioniemi OP, Blanco G, Alavaikko M, Hietanen T, Mattila J, Lauslahti K, Koivula T: Tumour DNA ploidy as an independent prognostic factor in breast cancer. Br J Cancer 56:637–642, 1987.

164. Kallioniemi OP, Hietanen T, Mattila J, Lehtinen M, Lauslahti K, Koivula T: Aneuploid DNA content and high S-phase fraction of tumour cells are related to poor prognosis in patients

with primary breast cancer. Eur J Cancer Clin Oncol 23:277–282, 1987.

165. Kallioniemi OP, Blanco G, Alavaikko M, Hietanen T, Mattila J, Lauslahti K, Lehtinen M, Koivula T: Improving the prognostic value of DNA flow cytometry in breast cancer by combining DNA index and S-phase fraction. Cancer 62:2183–2190, 1988.

166. Kallioniemi OP, Punnonen R, Mattila J, Lehtinen M, Koivula T: Prognostic significance of DNA index, multiploidy, and S-phase fraction in ovarian cancer. Cancer 61:334–339, 1988.

167. Kamentsky LA, Melamed MR, Derman H: Spectrophotometer: New instrument for ultrarapid cell analysis. Science 150:630–631, 1965.

168. Kaneko Y, Kanda N, Maseki N, Sakurai M, Tsuchida Y, Takeda T, Okabe I, Sakurai M: Different karyotypic patterns in early and advanced stage neuroblastomas. Cancer Res 47:311–318, 1987.

169. Kerker M: The Scattering of Light and Other Electromagnetic Radiation. New York, Academic Press, 1969.

170. Kielland J: Method and apparatus for counting blood corpuscles. US Patent No. 2,369,577. Filed May 12, 1941. Issued February 13, 1945.

171. Klein FA, Herr HW, Sogani PC, Whitmore WF, Melamed MR: Detection and follow-up of carcinoma of the urinary bladder by flow cytometry. Cancer 50:389–395, 1982.

172. Klein FA, Kay S, Ratliff JE, White FK, Newsome HH: Flow cytometric determinations of ploidy and proliferation patterns of adrenal neoplasms: An adjunct to histological classification. J Urol 134:862–866, 1985.

173. Klintenberg C, Stal O, Nordenskjold B, Wallgren A, Arvidsson S, Skoog L: Proliferative index, cytosol receptor and axillary node status as prognostic predictors in human mammary carcinoma. Breast Cancer Res Treat [Suppl]7:99–106, 1986.

174. Kokal WA, Duda RB, Azumi N, Sheibani K, Kemeny MMM, Terz JJ, Harada R: Tumor DNA content in primary and metastatic colorectal carcinoma. Arch Surg 121:1434–1439, 1986.

175. Kraemer BB, Srigley JR, Batsakis JG, Silva EG, Goepfert H: DNA flow cytometry of thyroid neoplasms. Arch Otolaryngol 111:34–38, 1985.

176. Kreicsbergs A, Silfversward C, Tribukait B: Flow DNA analysis of primary bone tumors. Cancer 53:129–136, 1984.

177. Kühn W, Kaufmann M, Feichter GE, Rummel HH, Schmid H, Herberling D: DNA flow cytometry, clinical and morphological parameters as prognostic factors for advanced malignant and borderline ovarian tumors. Gynecol Oncol 33:360–367, 1989.

178. Kute TE, Muss HB, Anderson D, Crumb K, Miller B, Burns D, Dube LA: Relationship of steroid receptor, cell kinetics, and clinical status in patients with breast cancer. Cancer Res 41:3524–3529, 1981.

179. Kute TE, Muss HB, Hopkins MB, Marshall R, Case D, Kammire L: Relationship of flow cytometry results to clinical and receptor status in human breast cancer. Breast Cancer Res Treat 6:113–121, 1985.

180. Laffin J, Fogleman D, Lehman JM: Correlation of DNA content, p53, T antigen, and V antigen in simian virus 40-infected human diploid cells. Cytometry 10:205–213, 1989.

181. Latt S: Fluorescent probes of DNA microstructure and synthesis. *In* Flow Cytometry and Cell Sorting. Edited by MR Melamed PF Mullaney, ML Mendelsohn. New York, John Wiley, pp 256–273, 1979.

182. Lee WH, Bookstein R, Hong F, Young LH, Shew JY, Lee EY-HP: Human retinoblastoma susceptibility gene: Cloning, identification and sequence. Science 235:1394–1399, 1987.

183. Lee SE, Currin SN, Paulson DF, Walther PJ: Flow cytometric determination of ploidy in prostatic adenocarcinoma: A comparison with seminal vesicle involvement and histopathological grading as a predictor of clinical recurrence. J Urol 140:769–774, 1988.

184. Leuchtenberger C, Leuchtenberger R, Davis AM: A microspectrophotometric study of the deoxyribonucleic acid (DNA) content in cells of normal and malignant human tissue. Am J Pathol 30:65–85, 1954.

185. Ljungberg B, Stenling R, Roos G: DNA content in renal cell carcinoma with reference to tumor heterogeneity. Cancer 56:503–508, 1985.

186. Ljungberg B, Stenling R, Roos G: Prognostic value of deoxyribonucleic acid content in metastatic renal cell carcinoma. J Urol 136:801–804, 1986.

187. Look AT, Hayes FA, Nitschke R, McWilliams NB, Green AA: Cellular DNA content as a predictor of response to chemotherapy in infants with unresectable neuroblastoma. N Engl J Med 311:231–235, 1984.

188. Look AT, Douglass EC, Meyer WH: Clinical importance of near-diploid stemlines in patients with osteosarcoma of an extremity. N Engl J Med 318:1567–1572, 1988.

189. Lovett EJ, Schnitzer B, Keren DF, Flint A, Hudson JL, McClatchey KD: Application of flow cytometry to diagnostic pathology. Lab Invest 50:115–140, 1984.

190. Lundberg S, Carstensen J, Rundquist I: DNA flow cytometry and histopathological grading of paraffin-embedded prostate biopsy specimens in a survival study. Cancer Res 47:1973–1977, 1987.

191. McDivitt RW, Stone KR, Craig RB, Palmer JO, Meyer JS, Bauer WC: A proposed classification of breast cancer based on kinetic information. Cancer 57:269–276, 1986.

192. McGuire WL, Clark GM, Dressler LG, Owens MA: Role of steroid hormone receptors as prognostic factors in primary breast cancer. Natl Cancer Inst Monogr 1:19–23, 1986.

193. McIntire TL, Murphy WM, Coon JS, Chandler RW, Schwartz D, Conway S, Weinstein RS: The prognostic value of DNA ploidy combined with histological substaging for incidental carcinoma of the prostate gland. Am J Clin Pathol 89:370–373, 1988.

194. Mankin HJ, Connor JF, Schiller AL, Perlmutter N, Alho A, McGuire M: Grading of bone tumors by analysis of nuclear DNA content using flow cytometry. J Bone Joint Surg 67:404–413, 1985.

195. Mann RC, Hand RE, Braslawsky GR: Parametric analysis of histograms in flow cytometry. Cytometry 4:75–82, 1983.

196. Masters JRW, Camplejohn RS, Millis RR, Rubens RD: Histological grade, elastosis, DNA ploidy and the response to chemotherapy of breast cancer. Br J Cancer 55:455–457, 1987.

197. Mayall BH: System operating characteristics and cost analysis in automated cytodiagnosis of gynecological specimens. J Histochem Cytochem 27:584–590, 1979.

198. Meckenstock G, Bojar H, Hort W: Differentiated DNA analysis in relation to steroid receptor status, grading, and staging in human breast cancer. Anticancer Res 7:749–745, 1987.

199. Melamed MR, Enker WE, Banner P, Janov AJ, Kessler G, Darzynkiewicz Z: Flow cytometry of colorectal carcinoma with three-year follow-up. Dis Colon Rectum 29:184–186, 1986.

200. Melamed MR, Mullaney PF, Mendelsohn ML: Flow cytometry and cell sorting. New York, John Wiley, pp 317–334, 1979.

201. Melamed MR, Lindmo T, Mendelsohn ML: Flow cytometry and sorting. New York, John Wiley, 1989.

202. Meyer JS, Friedman E, McCrate MM, Bauer WC: Prediction of early course of breast carcinoma by thymidine labeling. Cancer 51:1879–1886, 1983.

203. Meyer JS, Micko S, Craver JL, McDivitt RW: DNA flow cytometry of breast carcinoma after acetic-acid fixation. Cell Tissue Kinet 17:185–197, 1984.

204. Miller RE, Herman CJ: Automated cervical cytology screening: Performance requirements and instrument evaluation. J Histochem Cytochem 27:512–519, 1979.

205. Moldavan A: Photo-electric technique for the counting of microscopical cells. Science 80:188–189, 1934.

206. Moran RE, Black MM, Alpert L, Straus MJ: Correlation of cell-cycle kinetics, hormone receptors, histopathology, and nodal status in human breast cancer. Cancer 54:1568–1590, 1984.

207. Mullaney PF, Dean PN: Cell sizing: A small-angle light-scattering method for sizing particles of low refractive index. Appl Optics 8:2361–2362, 1969.

208. Murray K, Hopwood L, Volk D, Wilson JF: Cytofluorometric analysis of the DNA content in ovarian carcinoma and its relationship to patient survival. Cancer 63:2456–2460, 1989.

209. Nesland JM, Pettersen J, Fossa SD, Hoie J, Johannessen JV: Nuclear DNA content in breast carcinomas with neuroendocrine differentiation. J Pathol 150:181–185, 1986.

210. Nowell PC: The clonal evolution of tumor cell populations. Science 194:23–28, 1976.
211. Nowell PC: Mechanisms of tumor progression. Cancer Res 46:2203–2207, 1986.
212. Nowell PC, Hungerford DA: A minute chromosome in human chronic granulocytic leukemia. Science 132:1497–1499, 1960.
213. Ogata K, Kurki P, Celis JE, Nakamura RM, Tan EM: Monoclonal antibodies to a nuclear protein (PCNA/cyclin) associated with DNA replication. Exp Cell Res 47:475–486, 1987.
214. Oljans PJ, Tanke HJ: Flow cytometric analysis of DNA content in bladder cancer: Prognostic value of the DNA index with respect to early tumour recurrence in G2 tumours. World J Urol 4:205–210, 1986.
215. Olszewski W, Darzynkiewicz Z, Rosen PP, Schwartz M, Melamed MR: Flow cytometry of breast carcinoma. I. Relation of DNA ploidy level to histology and estrogen receptor level. Cancer 48:980–984, 1981.
216. Olszewski W, Darzynkiewicz Z, Rosen PP, Schwartz MK, Melamed MR: Flow cytometry of breast carcinoma. II. Relation of tumor cell cycle distribution to histology and estrogen receptor. Cancer 48:985–988, 1981.
217. Olszewski W, Darzynkiewicz Z, Claps ML, Melamed MR: Flow cytometry of lung carcinoma. Anal Quantit Cytol 4:90–94, 1982.
218. Oosterhuis JW, Castedo SMM, de Jong B, Cornelisse CJ, Dam A, Sleijfer DT, Schraffordt Koops H: Ploidy of primary germ cell tumors of the testis. Lab Invest 60:14–21, 1989.
219. Oosterwijk E, Warnaar SO, Zwartendijk J, van der Velde EA, Fleuren GJ, Cornelisse CJ: Relationship between DNA ploidy, antigen expression and survival in renal cell carcinoma. Int J Cancer 42:703–708, 1988.
220. Oppedal BR, Storm-Mathisen I, Lie SO, Brandtzaeg P: Prognostic factors in neuroblastoma. Cancer 62:772–780, 1988.
221. Otto U, Baisch H, Huland H, Klöppel G: Tumor cell deoxyribonucleic acid content and prognosis in human renal cell carcinoma. J Urol 132:237–239, 1984.
222. Owainati AAR, Robins RA, Hinton C, Ellis IO, Dowle CS, Ferry B, Elston CW, Blamey RW, Baldwin RW: Tumour aneuploidy, prognostic parameters and survival in primary breast cancer. Br J Cancer 55:449–454, 1987.
223. Petersen SE, Bichel P, Lorentzen M: Flow-cytometric demonstration of tumour cell subpopulations with different DNA content in human colo-rectal carcinoma. Eur J Cancer Clin Oncol 15:383–386, 1978.
224. Petersen SE, Friedrich U: A comparison between flow cytometric ploidy investigation and chromosome analysis of 32 human colorectal tumors. Cytometry 7:307–312, 1986.
225. Pinkel D, Gray J, Trask B, van den Engh G, Fuscoe J, van Dekken H: Cytogenetic analysis by in situ hybridization with fluorescently labeled nucleic acid probes. Cold Spring Harbor Symposia on Quantitative Biology, vol. L1, pp 151–157, 1986.
226. Quillamor RM, Furlong JW, Hoschne JA, Wynn RM: Relative prognostic significance of DNA flow cytometry and histologic grading in endometrial carcinoma. Gynecol Obstet Invest 26:332–337, 1988.
227. Quirke P, Dyson JED, Dixon MF, Bird CC, Joslin CAF: Heterogeneity of colorectal adenocarcinomas evaluated by flow cytometry and histopathology. Br J Cancer 51:99–106, 1985.
228. Quirke P, Fozard JBJ, Dixon MF, Dyson JED, Giles GR, Bird CC: DNA aneuploidy in colorectal adenomas. Br J Cancer 53:477–481, 1986.
229. Raber MN, Barlogie B, Latreille J, Bedrossian C, Fritsche H, Blumenschein G: Ploidy, proliferative activity and estrogen receptor content in human breast cancer. Cytometry 3:36–41, 1982.
230. Rainwater LM, Farrow GM, Lieber MM: Flow cytometry of renal oncocytoma: Common occurrence of deoxyribonucleic acid polyploidy and aneuploidy. J Urol 135:1167–1171, 1986.
231. Rainwater LM, Hosaka Y, Farrow GM, Lieber MM: Well-differentiated clear cell carcinoma: Significance of nuclear deoxyribonucleic acid patterns studied by flow cytometry. J Urol 137:15–20, 1987.
232. Rainwater LM, Zincke H: Radical prostatectomy after radiation therapy for cancer of the prostate: Feasibility and prognosis. J Urol 140:1455–1459, 1988.
233. Rainwater LM, Young WF, Farrow GM, Grant CS, van Heerden JA, Lieber MM: Flow cytometric analysis of deoxyribonucleic acid ploidy in benign and malignant aldosterone-producing neoplasms of the adrenal gland. Surg Gynecol Obst 168:491–496, 1989.
234. Ramaekers FCS, Beck HLM, Feitz WFJ, Oud PS, Debruyne FMJ, Vooijs GP, Herman J: Application of antibodies to intermediate filament proteins as tissue-specific probes in the flow cytometric analysis of complex tumors. Anal Quant Cytol Histol 8:271–280, 1986.
235. Ramaekers FCS, Beck H, Vooijs GP, Herman CJ: Flow cytometric analysis of mixed populations using intermediate filament antibodies. Exp Cell Res 153:249–253, 1984.
236. Remvikos Y, Gerbault-Seurreau M, Vielh P, Zafrani B, Magdalénat H, Dutrillaux B: Relevance of DNA ploidy as a measure of genetic deviation: A comparison of flow cytometry and cytogenetics in 25 cases of human breast cancer. Cytometry 612–618, 1988.
237. Remvikos Y, Magdelénat H, Zajdela A: DNA flow cytometry applied to fine needle sampling of human breast cancer. Cancer 61:1629–1634, 1988.
238. Remvikos Y, Muleris M, Vielh P, Salmon RJ, Dutrillaux B: DNA content and genetic evolution of human colorectal adenocarcinoma. Int J Cancer 42:539–543, 1988.
239. Reynolds O: An experimental investigation of the circumstances which determine whether the motion of water shall be direct or sinuous, and the law of resistance in channels. Philos Trans 935, 1883.
240. Ritch PS, Shackney SE, Schuette WH, Talbot TL, Smith CA: A practical graphical method for estimating the fraction of cells in S in DNA histograms from clinical tumor samples containing aneuploid populations. Cytometry 4:66–74, 1983.
241. Ritchie AW, Dorey F, Layfield LJ, Hannah J, Lovrekovich H, de Kernion JB: Relationship of DNA content to conventional prognostic factors in clinically localised carcinoma of the prostate. Br J Urol 62:245–260, 1988.
242. Robey SS, Silva EG, Gershenson DM, McLemore D, el-Naggar A, Ordonez NG: Transitional cell carcinoma in high-grade, high-stage ovarian carcinoma. Cancer 63:839–847, 1989.
243. Rodenburg CJ, Cornelisse CJ, Heintz PA, Hermans J, Fleuren GJ: Tumor ploidy as a major prognostic factor in advanced ovarian cancer. Cancer 59:317–323, 1987.
244. Rodenburg CJ, Ploem-Zaaijer JJ, Cornelisse CJ, Mesker WE, Hermans J, Heintz PAM, Ploem JS, Fleuren GJ: Use of DNA image cytometry in addition to flow cytometry for the study of patients with advanced ovarian cancer. Cancer Res 47:3938–3941, 1987.
245. Rognum TO, Thorud E, Elgjo K, Brandtzeg P, Orjasaeter H, Nygaard K: Large-bowel carcinomas with different ploidy, related to secretory component, IgA, and CEA in epithelium and plasma. Br J Cancer 45:921–934, 1982.
246. Rognum TO, Heier HE, Orjasaeter H, Thorud E, Brandtzaeg P: Comparison of two CEA assays in primary and recurrent large bowel carcinoma with different DNA ploidy pattern. Eur J Cancer Clin Oncol 22:1165–1169, 1986.
247. Rognum TO, Thorud E, Lund E: Survival of large bowel carcinoma patients with different DNA ploidy. Br J Cancer 56:633–636, 1987.
248. Roos G, Arnerlöv C, Emdin S: Retrospective DNA analysis of T3/T4 breast carcinoma using cytophotometry and flow cytometry. Anal Quant Cytol Histol 10:189–194, 1988.
249. Rutgers DH, van der Linden PM, van Peperzeel HA: DNA-flow cytometry of squamous cell carcinomas from the human uterine cervix: The identification of prognostically different subgroups. Radiother Oncol 7:249–258, 1986.
250. Rutteman GR, Cornelisse CJ, Dijkshoorn NJ, Poortman J, Misdorp W: Flow cytometric analysis of DNA ploidy in canine mammary tumors. Cancer Res 48:3411–3417, 1988.
251. Salzman GC, Growell JM, Martin JC: Cell classification by laser light scattering. Identification and separation of unstained leukocytes. Acta Cytol 19:374–377, 1975.
252. Sandberg AA, Turc-Carel C, Gemmill RM: Chromosomes in solid tumors and beyond. Cancer Res 48:1049–1059, 1988.
253. Sciallero S, Bruno S, di Vinci A, Geido E, Aste H, Giaretti W: Flow cytometric DNA ploidy in colorectal adenomas and family history of colorectal cancer. Cancer 61:114–120, 1988.

254. Schelfhout LJDM, Cornelisse CJ, Goslings BM, Hamming JF, Kuipers-Dijkshoorn NJ, van de Velde CJH, Fleuren GJ: Frequency and degree of aneuploidy in malignant neoplasms. Int J Cancer 45:16–20, 1990.

255. Scholz KU: Mathematical evaluation of two-parameter cytometric histograms. Cytometry 2:159–164, 1981.

256. Schröder S, Böcker W, Baisch H, Bürk CG, Arps H, Meiners H, Kastendieck H, Heitz PU, Klöppel G: Prognostic factors in medullary thyroid carcinomas. Cancer 61:806–816, 1988.

257. Schuette WH, Shackney SE, MacCollum MA, Smith CA: High resolution method for the analysis of DNA histograms that is suitable for the detection of multiple aneuploid G1 peaks in clinical samples. Cytometry 3:376–386, 1983.

258. Schutte B, Reynders MM, Wiggers T, Arends JW, Volovics L, Bosman FT, Blijham GH: Retrospective analysis of the prognostic significance of DNA content and proliferative activity in large bowel carcinoma. Cancer Res 47:5494–5496, 1987.

259. Schwabe HW, Adolphs HD, Vogel J: Flow-cytometric studies in renal cell carcinoma. Urol Res 11:121–125, 1983.

260. Schwartz D, Banner BF, Roseman DL, Coon JS: Origin of "primary" colon carcinomas. Cancer 58:2082–2088, 1986.

261. Scott NA, Grande JP, Weiland LH, Pemberton JH, Beart RW, Lieber MM: Flow cytometric DNA patterns from colorectal cancers. Mayo Clin Proc 62:331–337, 1987.

262. Seckinger D, Sugarbaker E, Krankfurt O: DNA content in human cancer. Arch Pathol Lab Med 113:619–626, 1989.

263. Shackney SE, Smith CA, Miller BW, Burholt DR, Murtha K, Giles HR, Ketterer DM, Pollice AA: Model for the genetic evolution of human solid tumors. Cancer Res 49:3344–3354, 1989.

264. Shapiro H: Practical flow cytometry, 2nd ed. New York, Alan R Liss, 1988.

265. Silver HKB, Karim KA, le Riche J, de Jong G, Spinelli J, Worth A, McLean DI: Nuclear DNA, serum sialic acid, and measured depth in malignant melanoma for predicting disease recurrence and survival. Int J Cancer 44:31–34, 1989.

266. Slamon DJ, Clark GM, Wong SG, Levin WJ, Ullrich A, McGuire WL: Human breast cancer: Correlation of relapse and survival with amplification of the HER-2/neu oncogene. Science 235:177–182, 1987.

267. Smit VTHBM, Cornelisse CJ, De Jong D, Dijkshoorn NJ, Peters AAW, Fleuren GJ: Analysis of tumor heterogeneity in a patient with synchronously occurring female genital tract malignancies by DNA flow cytometry, DNA fingerprinting, and immunohistochemistry. Cancer 62:1146–1152, 1988.

268. Sondergaard K, Larsen JK, Moller U, Christensen IJ, Hou-Jensen K: DNA ploidy characteristics of human malignant melanoma analysed by flow cytometry and compared with histology and clinical course. Virchows Arch Cell Pathol, 42:43–52, 1983.

269. Spyratos F, Briffod M, Gentile A, Brunet M, Brault C, Desplaces A: Flow cytometric study of DNA in cytopunctures of benign and malignant breast lesions. Anal Quant Cytol Histol 9:485–494, 1987.

270. Stal O, Wingren S, Carstensen J, Rutqvist LE, Skoog L, Klintenberg C, Nordenskjöld B: Prognostic value of DNA ploidy and S-phase fraction in relation to estrogen receptor content and clinicopathological variables in primary breast. Eur J Cancer Clin Oncol 25:301–309, 1989.

271. Steen HB: Further developments of a microscope-based flow cytometer: Light scatter detection and excitation compensation. Cytometry 1:26–31, 1980.

272. Stenzinger W, Suter L, Schumann J: DNA aneuploidy in congenital melanocytic nevi: Suggestive evidence for premalignant changes. J Invest Dermatol 82:569–572, 1984.

273. Stephenson RA, James BC, Gay H, Fair WR, Whitmore WF, Melamed MR: Flow cytometry of prostate cancer: Relationship of DNA content to survival. Cancer Res 47:2504–2509, 1987.

274. Stöhr M, Eipel H, Goerttler K: Extended applications of flow microfluorometry by means of dual laser excitation. Histochemistry 51:305–313, 1977.

275. Stöhr M, Futterman G: Visualization of multidimensional spectra in flow cytometry. J Histochem Cytochem 27:560–563, 1979.

276. Stöhr M, Vogt-Schaden M, Knobloch M, Vogel R, Futterman G: Evaluation of eight fluorochrome combinations for simultaneous DNA-protein flow analysis. Stain Technol 53:205–215, 1978.

277. Strang P, Stendahl U, Frankendal B, Lindgren A: Flow cytometric DNA patterns in cervical carcinoma. Acta Radiol [Oncol] 25:249–254, 1986.

278. Strang P, Stendahl U, Sorbe B: Polyclonal cervical tumors detected by flow cytometry. Anticancer Res 6:171–175, 1986.

279. Strang P, Eklund G, Stendahl U, Frankendahl B: S-phase rate as a predictor of early recurrence in carcinoma of the uterine cervix. Anticancer Res 7:807–810, 1987.

280. Stuart-Harris R, Hedley DW, Taylor IW, Levene AL, Smith IE: Tumour ploidy, response and survival in patients receiving endocrine therapy for advanced breast cancer. Br J Cancer 51:573–576, 1985.

281. Tangen KO, Lindmo T, Sobrinho-Simoes M, Johannessen JV: A flow cytometric DNA analysis of medullary thyroid carcinoma. Am J Clin Pathol 79:172–177, 1983.

282. Taylor IW, Musgrove EA, Friedlander ML, Foo MS, Hedley DW: The influence of age on the DNA ploidy levels of breast tumours. Eur J Cancer Clin Oncol 19:623–638, 1983.

283. Taylor SR, Roederer M, Murphy RF: Flow cytometric DNA analysis of adrenocortical tumors in children. Cancer 59:2059–2063, 1987.

284. ten Velde GPM, Schutte B, Vermeulen A, Volovics A, Reynders MMJ, Blijham GH: Flow cytometric analysis of DNA ploidy level in paraffin-embedded tissue of non–small-cell lung cancer. Eur J Cancer Clin Oncol 24:455–460, 1988.

285. Thorud E, Fossa SD, Vaage S, Kaalhus O, Knudsen OS, Bormer O, Shoaib MC: Primary breast cancer: Flow cytometric DNA pattern in relation to clinical and histopathological characteristics. Cancer 57:808–811, 1986.

286. Tirindelli-Danesi DF, Teodori L, Mauro F, Modini C, Botti C, Cicconetti F, Stipa S: Prognostic significance of flow cytometry in lung cancer. Cancer 60:844–851, 1987.

287. Toikkanen S, Eerola E, Ekfors TO: Pure and mixed mucinous breast carcinomas: DNA stemline and prognosis. J Clin Pathol 41:300–303, 1988.

288. Trask B, van den Engh G, Landegent J, Jansen in de Wal N, van der Ploeg M: Detection of DNA sequences in nuclei in suspension by in situ hybridization and dual beam flow cytometry. Science 20:1401–1403, 1985.

289. Trebeck CE, Friedlander ML, Russell P, Baird PJ: Brenner tumours of the ovary: A study of the histology, immunohistochemistry and cellular DNA content in benign, borderline and malignant ovarian tumours. Pathology 19:241–246, 1987.

290. Tribukait B, Hammarberg C, Rubio C: Ploidy and proliferation patterns in colorectal adenocarcinomas related to Dukes' classification and to histopathological differentiation. Acta Pathol Microbiol Immunol Scand 91:89–95, 1983.

291. Tribukait B, Rönström L, Esposti PL: Quantitative and qualitative aspects of flow DNA measurements related to the cytological grade in prostatic carcinoma. Anal Quant Cytol 5:107–111, 1983.

292. Tribukait B: Flow cytometry in assessing the clinical aggressiveness of genito-urinary neoplasms. World J Urol 5:108–122, 1987.

293. Tubiana M, Pejovic MJ, Ranaud A, Contesso G, Chavaudra N, Gioanni J, Malaise EP: Kinetic parameters and the course of disease in breast cancer. Cancer 47:937–943, 1981.

294. Ucelli R, Calugi A, Forte D, Mauro F, Polonio-Balbi P, Vecchioni A, Vizzone A, de Vita R: Flow cytometrically determined DNA content of breast carcinoma and benign lesions: Correlations with histopathological parameters. Tumori 72:171–177, 1986.

295. Uyterlinde AM, Schipper NW, Baak JPA, Petersen H, Matze E: Limited prognostic value of cellular DNA content to classical and morphometrical parameters in invasive ductal breast cancer. Am J Clin Pathol 89:301–307, 1988.

296. van Dilla MA, Trujillo TT, Mullaney PF, Coulter JR: Cell microfluorometry: A method for rapid fluorescence measurements. Science 163:1213–1214, 1969.

297. van Dilla MA, Dean PN, Laerum OD, Melamed MR: Flow cytometry: Instrumentation and data analysis. In Series on Analytical Cytology. Edited by JS Ploem. London, Academic Press, 1985.

298. van den Ingh HF, Griffioen G, Cornelisse CJ: Flow cytometric detection of aneuploidy in colorectal adenomas. Cancer Res 45:3392–3397, 1985.

299. Vindeløv LL, Hansen HH, Christensen IJ, Spang-Thomsen M, Hirsch FR, Hansen M, Nissen NI: Clonal heterogeneity of small-cell anaplastic carcinoma of the lung demonstrated by flow-cytometric analysis. Cancer Res 40:4295–4300, 1980.

300. Vindeløv LL, Christensen IJ, Jensen GJ, Nissen NI: Limits of detection of nuclear DNA abnormalities by flow cytometric DNA analysis. Cytometry 3:332–339, 1983.

301. Vindeløv LL, Christensen IJ, Keiding N, Spang-Thomsen M, Nissen NI: Long-term storage of samples for flow cytometric DNA analysis. Cytometry 3:317–322, 1983.

302. Vindeløv LL, Christensen IJ, Nissen NI: A detergent-trypsin method for the preparation of nuclei for flow cytometric DNA analysis. Cytometry 3:323–327, 1983.

303. Vindeløv LL, Christensen L, Nissen NI: Standardization of high-resolution flow cytometric DNA analysis by the simultaneous use of chicken and trout red blood cells as internal reference cells. Cytometry 3:328–331, 1983.

304. Vogelstein B, Fearon ER, Kern SE, Hamilton SR, Preisinger AC, Nakamura Y, White R: Allelotype of colorectal carcinomas. Science 244:207–211, 1989.

305. Volm M, Brüggemann A, Günther M, Kleine W, Pfleiderer A, Vogt-Schaden M: Prognostic relevance of ploidy, proliferation, and resistance-predictive tests in ovarian carcinoma. Cancer Res 45:5180–5185, 1985.

306. Volm M, Drings P, Mattern J, Sonka J, Vogt-Moykopf I, Wayss K: Prognostic significance of DNA patterns and resistance-predictive tests in non-small cell lung carcinoma. Cancer 56:1396–1403, 1985.

307. Volm M, Bak M, Hahn EW, Mattern J, Weber E: DNA and S-phase distribution and incidence of metastasis in human primary lung carcinoma. Cytometry 9:183–188, 1988.

308. Volpe JPG: Genetic instability of cancer. Cancer Genet Cytogenet 34:125–134, 1988.

309. von Roenn JH, Kheir SM, Wolter JM, Coon JS: Significance of DNA abnormalities in primary malignant melanoma and nevi: A retrospective flow cytometric study. Cancer Res 46:3192–3195, 1986.

310. Watson JV, Curling OM, Munn CF, Hudson CN: Oncogene expression in ovarian cancer: A pilot study of c-myc oncoprotein in serous papillary ovarian cancer. Gynecol Oncol 28:137–150, 1987.

311. Weiss H, Wildner GP, Jacobasch KH, Heinz U, Schaelicke W: Characterization of human adenomatous polyps of the colorectal bowel by means of DNA distribution patterns. Oncology 42:33–41, 1985.

312. Wiggers T, Arends JW, Schutte B, Volovics L, Bosman FT: A multivariate analysis of pathologic prognostic indicators in large bowel cancer. Cancer 61:386–395, 1988.

313. Williams NS, Durdey P, Quirke P, Robinson PJ, Dyson JED, Dixon MF, Bird CC: Pre-operative staging of rectal neoplasm and its impact on clinical management. Br J Surg 72:868–874, 1985.

314. Willen R, Trope C, Langström E, Ranstam J, Killander D, Clase L: Prospective malignancy grading and flow cytometry DNA distribution in biopsy specimens from invasive squamous cell carcinoma of the uterine cervix. Anticancer Res 7:235–242, 1987.

315. Winkler HZ, Rainwater LM, Myers RP, Farrow GM, Therneau TM, Zincke H, Lieber MM: Stage D1 prostatic adenocarcinoma: Significance of nuclear DNA ploidy patterns studied by flow cytometry. Mayo Clin Proc 63:103–112, 1988.

316. Wolley RC, Schreiber K, Koss LG, Karas M, Sherman A: DNA distribution in human colon carcinomas and its relationship to clinical behavior. J Natl Cancer Inst 69:15–22, 1982.

317. Xiang J, Spanier SS, Benson NA, Braylan R: Flow cytometric analysis of DNA in bone and soft-tissue tumors using nuclear suspensions. Cancer 59:1951–1958, 1987.

318. Zaloudik J, Moore M, Ghosh AK, Mechl Z, Rejthar A: DNA content and MHC class II antigen expression in malignant melanoma: Clinical course. J Clin Pathol 41:1078–1084, 1988.

319. Zimmerman PV, Hawson GAT, Bint MH, Parsons PG: Ploidy as a prognostic determinant in surgically treated lung cancer. Lancet i:530–533, 1987.

38

Immunocytochemistry

Mary Osborn
Wenancjusz Domagala

Immunocytochemistry (ICC) is an important adjunct method in cytologic diagnosis. Depending on the possible differential diagnosis and the markers employed, the information it yields can be critical in arriving at an unambiguous diagnosis. If markers are inappropriately chosen, ICC can have relatively little effect on the final diagnosis. The ICC data have to be considered together with the other information available to the cytopathologist, e.g., the clinical information and the morphologic features of cells in the smears. ICC should never be selected as the sole or only method of diagnosis but must be integrated into the cytologic decision-making process (Fig. 38–1).

The origin of ICC techniques lies in the pioneering work of Albert Coons, starting in 1941. He has described his first attempts to directly label antibodies with fluorescein isocyanate.[28] Fluorescein isothiocyanate was introduced as a label in 1958 and is still commonly employed as a label in fluorescence microscopy. Antigens today are usually detected by the indirect technique introduced in 1955, i.e., an unlabeled antibody is followed by a fluorescein- or enzyme-labeled second antibody. Contrary to the usual belief, fluorescein-labeled preparations that have been appropriately processed are quite stable. For certain applications in conventional cytology, fluorescein can still be the labeled reagent of choice, particularly when one desires to visualize subcellular details or to perform double labeling. However, evaluation of conventional morphologic features is difficult in such smears because they are usually not counterstained. Nuclei in smears can be stained with Hoechst dye, and morphology of cells and cell groups can be assessed in phase microscopy (Fig. 38–2).

Enzyme ICC methods in common use include those based on peroxidase, alkaline phosphatase, biotin-avidin and gold-silver techniques. They have a lower resolution but can have a higher sensitivity than fluorescence techniques. These methods can be utilized in a two- or three-step procedure. Antigens are revealed because they bind first the unlabeled antibody and then the labeled antibody, and after development a colored reaction product is visualized. These methods can be combined with a hematoxylin counterstain to show nuclei. They require only a simple light microscope, rather than the more expensive ultraviolet microscope necessary to visualize fluorescein-labeled compounds and have the further advantage that the cytologist does not need to examine the slides in the dark. In principle, however, if appropriate controls and antibody dilutions are employed, the different ICC methods should give the same results. (In this chapter most illustrations are

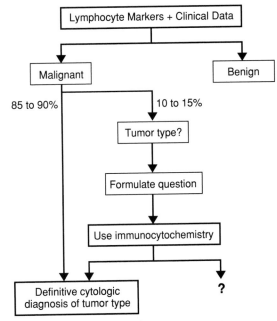

FIGURE 38–1. Integration of immunocytochemistry in the cytologic decision-making process.

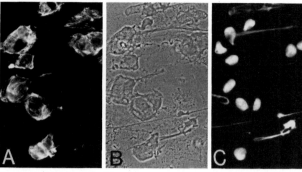

FIGURE 38–2. Fine needle aspiration, **breast carcinoma.** *A,* Morphology of tumor cells labeled with keratin mAb in indirect immunofluorescence. *B,* Morphology of cells in phase microscopy. *C,* Cell nuclei can be counterstained with Hoechst dye (×300).

from immunofluorescence studies because color reproduction was not possible.)

The immunologic techniques utilized are common to both histology and cytology. Although immunologic methods are relatively widely followed in routine histologic laboratories,[59, 63, 70, 116, 120, 140, 153] they are only beginning to be exploited in cytologic laboratories.[5, 23, 26, 41, 45, 55, 67, 86, 151] This occurrence is surprising because alcohol fixation, which is common in cytology, yields specimens that are usually optimal for immunologic procedures. In contrast, histology still relies largely on formaldehyde-fixed and paraffin-embedded material, a procedure that often results in the epitope no longer being recognized by the antibody.

Probably two advances are responsible for the increasing interest in immunologic markers for cell and tumor typing. First, protein chemical, DNA cloning and cell biologic studies have resulted in a clearer understanding of the number and cell type distribution of proteins that occur in multiple isoforms and multigene families. Those with expression rules that allow interesting histologic distinctions include intermediate filaments (IF),[139, 204] actins,[191] epithelial membrane antigen (EMA),[146] leukocyte common antigen (LCA)[96] and S-100 proteins.[92] Polyclonal and monoclonal antibodies have been raised that distinguish particular isoforms. Second, use of monoclonal antibody (mAb) technology means that antibodies can be isolated, by design or fortuitously, that distinguish antigens that are associated with particular cell types or mark various developmental stages along particular differentiation pathways, without the necessity of purifying each antigen to homogeneity. Because a monoclonal antibody sees usually only a single epitope, antibodies that can distinguish very similar molecules can be isolated. Once the mAb has been obtained, the molecular weight (Mr) of the antigen it recognizes can also be defined.

The choice of markers to be included in an immunologic panel of antibodies (Abs) is of course critical in fine needle aspirations (FNAs). It is usually simple to tell benign from malignant cells with only conventional cytology,[94] but a precise diagnosis of tumor type can be more difficult and may not be possible in 10 to 15% of cases by routine methods (see Fig. 38–1).

Differentiation, or cell- or tissue-specific markers that are located either in the cytoplasm or the membrane in normal cells, and are retained in tumor cells, seem to be helpful in the further differential diagnosis of such cases. In the first part of this chapter, these markers are divided according to the type of differentiation pathway in which they most often occur, e.g., epithelial, mesenchymal, glial, neural and neuroendocrine (NE). Certain melanoma and lymphoid markers are also included as are selected oncofetal markers. Markers discussed include the familiar, such as EMA, LCA, carcinoembryonic antigen (CEA), prostate-specific antigen (PSA) and S-100, and new promising markers, such as IF proteins,[140] individual keratins,[29, 120] synaptophysin and chromogranins.[207]

Our experience with ICC techniques is based in large part on aspiration cytology specimens, but we also discuss use on effusions, on cerebrospinal fluid (CSF) and on other cytologic preparations. Emphasis is placed on which markers may be helpful in solving diagnostic dilemmas that occur frequently in a cytologic laboratory. The utilization of ICC as a prognostic indicator is also considered. Figure 38–1 illustrates that although ICC allows a more definitive diagnosis in many cases it does not solve all of them. In particular there may be a small percentage of tumors that simultaneously express markers usually associated with two or more differentiation pathways. In addition, for a further small percentage, currently there may be no appropriate marker that allows a solution of the diagnostic question. The actual percentages in Figure 38–1 are rough estimates and obviously will vary depending on the cytologic material seen by a particular laboratory and on the expertise of the cytopathologist. Also, ICC as applied to routine cytologic specimens is still in its infancy. Indeed, up to 1986 by one count[86] there were only 42 primary reports, although this number is probably an underestimate. Here, we have tried to integrate information about the antigens with information about ICC in histology and cytology. More extensive overviews and additional references to ICC in tumor diagnosis can be found in other sources (see references 67, 141, 166 and 212). Methods are also discussed elsewhere (see references 149 and 186).

USEFUL MARKERS AND ANTIBODIES

The markers in current use in an immunologic laboratory represent a heterogeneous group of substances. Some, such as the different IF proteins[139, 204] (Table 38–1) and actins,[191] are cytoskeletal components and major proteins of the cell. Here, the particular isoform found by either ICC or biochemical techniques yields information on the differentiation pathway and hence the tumor type. Intermediate filaments and the actin-containing microfilaments are the major filamentous elements of the cytoplasm and can be visualized by ICC and electron microscopy. Alternatively, markers restricted to particular structures found only in a few differentiated cell types can be used, e.g., synaptophysin for neuroendocrine vesicles and titin for striated

TABLE 38–1. Complexity of Vertebrate Intermediate Filament Proteins

Source	Type	Molecular Weight	Number
Epithelia	Keratins	40–70 kD	19
appendages			8
Mesenchyme	Vimentin	54 kD	1
Myogenic	Desmin	53 kD	1
Glia	GFAP	51 kD	1
Neurons	NF-proteins		
	L	62 kD	1
	M	100 kD	1
	H	110 kD	1
	Peripherin	56 kD	1
Nuclear lamina	Lamins A, B, C	74, 64, 65 kD	3

GFAP = glial fibrillary acidic protein; NF = neurofilament; L = low; M = medium; H = high.

muscle. Membrane components, such as LCA or melanocyte surface antigens, can be found, which distinguish various stages in a given differentiation pathway. Oncofetal antigens, e.g., AFP and CEA, are also helpful, whereas antibodies to oncogene products are just beginning to be tested.

Epithelial Markers

Panepithelial Markers

Keratins. Epithelial cells share several common features that dictate their characteristic morphology. They contain the keratin type of IFs (see Table 38–1) often referred to as tonofilaments. These keratin filaments are anchored at special structures called desmosomes (macula-adherens type junctions). These structures link the keratin IFs in adjacent epithelial cells, thus giving the epithelium tensile strength. At least 27 human keratins exist, eight of which are associated with appendages such as hair and nails (Mr 40 to 68kD) (see Table 38–1).[29, 120] The different human keratins can be distinguished by their positions on two-dimensional gels, as estimated by their Mr and isoelectric points. Individual keratins are identified by numbers in the catalogue of Moll and coworkers.[120] Keratins are divided into two subfamilies: type II (keratins 1 to 8) and type I (keratins 10 to 19) (Fig. 38–3). At least one type I and one type II keratin are present in every epithelial cell, reflecting the fact that type I and type II keratins are obligatory heteropolymers. Carcinomas also express keratin IFs. Thus, pan or broad specificity keratin Abs, such as lu5[199] and KL1,[195] (which recognize most keratins, or a mixture of AE1 (several acidic keratins) and AE3 (keratins 1 to 8)[29] positively identify epithelial cells in complex tissues and tumors. Such Abs are of major use in distinguishing carcinomas from other tumors and are probably the best available reagents for this purpose. However, careful selection of a panepithelial mAb is essential, as exemplified by previous work in which with an Ab to stratum corneum keratins not all carcinomas were keratin positive.[200]

Desmosomes. These are characteristic of epithelia but are also present in certain nonepithelial cells, e.g.,

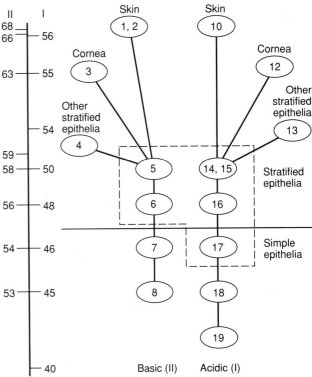

FIGURE 38–3. Members of the **two keratin subfamilies** arranged horizontally according to the "keratin pairs" found by coexpression and arranged vertically according to their molecular weights, which are given on the left of the figure. Keratins are designated by their number from the catalogue. (See Moll R, Franke WW, Schiller DL, Geiger B, Krepler R: Cell 31:11–24, 1982.) The horizontal line divides those keratins that are expressed by simple epithelia (below) from those expressed by stratified epithelia (above). The dashed box includes the keratins usually expressed by all stratified epithelia in neoplasms, hyperproliferative diseases and culture (Modified from Cooper D, Schermer A, Sun T-T: Lab Invest 82:243–256, 1985.)

in meningeal tissue, in intercalated discs in heart and between dendritic cells in lymph nodes. Desmosomes contain seven major polypeptides on sodium dodecyl sulfate (SDS) gels,[68] most of which have been given trivial names. Thus, Desmoplakins I and II (DPI and DPII) (Mr 250 and 215kD) are located on the cytoplasmic face of the desmosomal plaque. Desmoplakin I is common to all desmosomes, whereas DPII is restricted to stratified epithelia.[30] Desmoglein is a transmembrane glycoprotein (Mr ~ 165kD). Antibodies to DPI or selected Abs to desmoglein identify desmosomes in a wide variety of epithelial tissues and tumors.[119, 138] Desmosomes are visualized as dot-like structures—most dots represent single desmosomes—usually associated with the border between adjacent cells. Desmosomes provide a second specific marker for most types of carcinomas and allow a positive identification of meningiomas in which desmosomes are found associated, exceptionally, with vimentin IFs.[142]

Broad Specificity Epithelial Markers

Epithelial Membrane Antigen (EMA). This antigen is a high molecular weight glycoprotein (Mr 265 to 400kD) purified from the membranes of human milk fat globules.[80] It can be detected either with polyclonal Abs[80] or with mAbs, such as E29,[81] HMFG 2, 115 D8 and LICR LON M8. Epithelial membrane antigen belongs to the polymorphic epithelial mucin family.

Epithelial membrane antigen is a marker associated with most but not all normal and neoplastic epithelial cells.[81, 82, 93, 145, 146, 172] Usually, EMA positivity is visualized as membrane staining, but in occasional tumors additional cytoplasmic staining has also been reported. In breast the luminal cells show EMA positivity concentrated at the apical cell membranes but myoepithelial cells are negative. Endocrine glands such as pancreas, sweat and salivary glands show similar EMA distributions, whereas proximal tubules and hepatocytes appear negative. Squamous epithelia often either do not stain or show patchy expression. Non-epithelial cells are usually EMA negative, although positivity has been noted in occasional plasma cells.

In neoplasms, those that display glandular differentiation are EMA positive. Thus, adenocarcinomas of the breast, pancreas, lung, kidney, prostate and stomach are positive, as are squamous cell carcinomas (SCC) of the esophagus, cervix and skin. Undifferentiated carcinomas and mesotheliomas as well as epithelioid and synovial sarcomas, plasmacytomas and Kil-positive non-Hodgkin's lymphomas (NHLs) are usually EMA positive. Tumors negative for EMA include hepatocellular carcinomas (HCCs), neuroendocrine tumors, embryonal carcinomas and sarcomas excluding those already mentioned.

Restricted Specificity

Individual Keratin Polypeptides. Different epithelia are characterized by different but overlapping keratin subsets, with two to ten individual keratins being present in a particular epithelial cell. Complete listings of the keratin content of different epithelial cells and tumors can be found in other sources (see references 29, 118, 120 and 150). In general, expression of particular keratin polypeptides occurs in pairs (I and II) and is related to three factors.[29] First, simple epithelia display a different keratin subset than do stratified epithelia. Second, the particular differentiation program is important. Thus, for instance, skin, cornea and esophagus are characterized by different keratins (see Fig. 38–3). Third, the state of growth, e.g., whether normal or hyperproliferative, can affect the keratin complement. For diagnostic purposes, rather than employ two-dimensional gels, it is easier to employ mAbs to keratin that recognize only a single keratin polypeptide in ICC; selective single polypeptide–specific mAbs have been described for most human keratins.[36, 118, 189]

Simple epithelia express two to four of the lower molecular-weight keratins—keratins 7, 8, 18 and 19. Hepatocytes and pancreatic acini express only 8 and 18, and this keratin pair is expressed by all simple epithelia. Keratin 19 expression is characteristic of ductal and intestinal epithelia and can be detected with mAbs A531, B-A2, LP2K and CK19. Keratin 7 expression distinguishes a subpopulation of glandular cells. Usually, the same keratins that are present in simple epithelia are retained in adenocarcinomas. Thus, Abs to keratin 8 (e.g., CK8), 18 (e.g., CK1-CK4,[36] LE61 and RGE53[154]) or 8 and 18 (35 βH11[70]) can be helpful markers to distinguish adenocarcinoma from SCC.[36] Antibodies to keratin 7 (e.g., CK7 and RCK105) appear able to distinguish pancreatic carcinoma (positive) from gastrointestinal carcinoma (negative).[137] Interestingly, Tissue Polypeptide Antigen, which was originally thought to be a tumor marker and later a proliferation antigen, turns out to be obviously related to and almost certainly derived from keratins 8, 18 and 19.[205]

Stratified epithelia usually express higher molecular weight keratins (see Fig. 38–3).[29, 120, 150] Keratin 5 from the basic family is typically coexpressed with keratin 14 or 17 from the acidic family, and these keratins are typically present in most stratified squamous epithelia and in myoepithelial cells. Other "large" keratins are usually expressed in the suprabasal cells with the particular keratins dependent on the tissue (see Fig. 38–3). Thus, keratins 1, 2, 10 and 11 are typical of epidermis, 3 and 12 of corneal-type differentiation and 4 and 13 of esophageal-type differentiation. The presence or absence of particular keratins can be distinguished employing Abs specific for one or a few keratin polypeptides, e.g., keratin 14 (antibody CKB1,[3] LL002); keratins 1, 2 and 10 (AE2)[29]; keratin 3 (AE5)[29] or keratin 4 (6B10)[189] or keratin 13 (1C7, 1D7).[189] Squamous cell carcinomas often display large amounts of stratified epithelial–type keratins, e.g., SCC of skin display keratins 5 and 14 and, often, lesser amounts of keratins 1, 10 and 11. Squamous cell carcinomas of lung and cervix have complex patterns in which both stratified epithelial–type keratins and some simple epithelial–type keratins are present.

In complex epithelia, e.g., breast, luminal cells display simple epithelium–type keratins, whereas myoepithelial cells have keratins 5, 14 and 17 (for review, see reference 181). Keratin 17 can be recognized by mAb E3. Invasive ductal and lobular carcinomas of the breast usually express keratins 7, 8, 18 and 19. They thus appear to be derived from the luminal rather than the myoepithelial cells. Occasional tumors, however, express keratin 14, a typical keratin of myoepithelial cells, in the tumor cells.[3]

Although histologic data show that Abs to individual keratin polypeptides can be employed to further subdivide epithelial tissues and tumors,[36, 118, 137] little data exist from cytology. With FNAs, Abs CK2 and RGE53 have been utilized to distinguish adenocarcinomas from SCC.[45, 50]

However, other polypeptide-specific keratin Abs mentioned here should also prove to be suitable reagents for cytology.

Involucrin. Involucrin[157] (Mr 92kD) is a major component of the cornified envelope of keratinocytes. It is found in the upper half of the epidermis in cells of the intermediate and granular layers but not in the basal or immediately suprabasal cells. Other squamous epithelia, such as oral cavity, esophagus, anus, vagina and exocervix, show similar patterns of suprabasal staining. Transitional epithelia are less strongly stained. Normal glandular tissues are involucrin negative. In tumors,[157] the expression of involucrin in SCC of skin, tongue, esophagus, bronchus, lung and anus can be correlated with the amount of squamous differentiation. In many tumors, therefore, most tumor cells are negative for involucrin and show only focal staining of the squamous pearl formations, e.g., in lung tumors.[159] Mesotheliomas are negative for involucrin.

Prostate-specific Antigen (PSA) and Prostate-specific Acid Phosphatase (PSAP). The PSA is a glycoprotein (Mr ~ 33kD) restricted to prostate ductal epithelial cells. The PSAP, a glycoprotein (Mr ~ 100kD), is an acid phosphatase restricted primarily to the prostate gland. Both PSA and PSAP appear to be useful markers to confirm or exclude prostate cancer.[15, 89, 127] (See Prostatic Adenocarcinoma).

Thyroglobulin. Of thyroid tumors with follicular or papillary differentiation, 92 to 98% are positive when tested with Abs to thyroglobulin in ICC.[18, 60]

Mucins. Mucins are substances containing large amounts of carbohydrate attached in O-linkage to serine or threonine residues, or both, of the core proteins by the sugar N-acetylgalactosamine. Mucins are produced by epithelial cells lining the gastrointestinal tract and lungs and by many other glandular epithelia. The polymorphic epithelial mucins are the best defined human mucin family and are produced in large amounts by the lactating mammary gland and other glandular epithelia. They are characterized by a single core protein gene that shows tandem repeats.[180] Monoclonal antibodies to EMA, including HMFG-1 and HMFG-2, react with a synthetic peptide that contains the repeat sequence as well as with the fully glycosylated mucin. A further antibody, SM3,[17] which also reacts with the synthetic peptide, reacts with mucin produced by breast cancer cells but not with the fully glycosylated mucin. The SM3 reacts with 91% of breast carcinomas but does not stain benign mammary tumors, normal resting, pregnant or lactating breast. The SM3 is also positive on carcinomas of the lung, colon and ovary, but negative on intestine and most but not all normal tissues.

A second antibody to a mucin-like molecule, which seems to fall into a similar category as SM3 in its ability to distinguish malignant from benign epithelial cells, is B72.3.[85, 86] This antibody was generated against membrane-enriched extracts of liver metastases from two breast carcinomas and identifies a glycoprotein designated TAG-72 (Mr > 1000kD). The B72.3 recognizes more than 90% of adenocarcinomas of the ovary, colon and breast but does not react with melanomas, lymphomas, sarcomas and gliomas. A large series of benign FNAs and effusions studied in paraffin miniblocks do not stain with B72.3. However, note that mammary apocrine metaplasia and secretory and hyperplastic endometrium may be positive. This anti-

body appears able to discriminate between nonsmall-cell carcinoma of the lung (non-SCLC) (92% positive) and small-cell carcinoma of the lung (SCLC) (0% positive). A further interesting aspect is its ability to distinguish lung adenocarcinomas that are positive from malignant mesotheliomas that are negative.[176]

Mesenchymal Markers

Vimentin

Vimentin (54kD) is the most widely distributed of the intermediate filament proteins because it can be expressed alone or with any of the other IF types.[133, 140] Cells such as fibrocytes, osteocytes, osteoblasts, chondroblasts and chondrocytes are characterized by abundant vimentin IFs, and vimentin is the only IF type expressed in these cells. Most lymphatic cells seem to be vimentin positive, although reactive germinal center B cells may lack vimentin.[123] Vimentin is also the only IF type found in Langerhans's cells of the skin and in melanocytes. Vimentin-positive tumors include all nonmuscle soft tissue tumors (n. b., synovial sarcomas and epithelioid sarcomas coexpress vimentin and keratin), bone tumors (n. b., chordoma and adamantinoma are keratin positive), lymphomas, leukemias and melanomas. Some carcinomas coexpress vimentin (see subsequent discussion).

Markers of Muscle Differentiation

Muscle-specific markers discussed here include desmin, muscle-specific isoforms of actin and myosin, titin and myoglobin. The order of expression during embryonic development of these proteins, at least in the mouse,[58] is desmin, followed by muscle-specific actins and myosins, followed by titin.

Desmin. Desmin (53kD) is the IF protein associated with muscle differentiation.[37, 140] This protein is characteristic of skeletal, cardiac and visceral smooth muscle. Antibodies to desmin stain the Z disks of skeletal muscle; in heart muscle, they stain in addition intercalated discs. In mature skeletal muscle desmin is the only IF type present in muscle cells. Vascular smooth muscle cells may be vimentin positive and desmin negative or may coexpress vimentin and desmin (a small percentage express only desmin). The relative percentages of the first two types vary, depending on the blood vessel.[132]

Rhabdomyosarcomas,[7, 8, 114, 171] rhabdomyomas, leiomyosarcomas and leiomyomas react positively with desmin Abs. In histologic and cytologic specimens of rhabdomyosarcoma desmin Abs identify more than 95% of tumor cells, regardless of the state of differentiation. Vimentin can be coexpressed together with desmin in tumor cells. It is sometimes seen in all cells, sometimes in 5 to 50% of cells and sometimes not at all.[8]

Muscle-specific Actin Isoforms. Six different actins (Mr 45,000) are found in vertebrates, including humans, which are expressed in a tissue-specific manner.[191] The actins are classified according to the adult tissue in which they predominate. Thus, nonmuscle cells express β- and γ-cytoplasmic actins. Smooth muscle α actin predominates in visceral smooth muscle, and smooth muscle γ actin in vascular smooth muscle. The two sarcomeric muscle actins are referred to as cardiac and skeletal muscle α actins. However, tissues usually contain more than one actin form, e.g., the cardiac:skeletal α-actin ratio in adult human skeletal muscle is 0.05:1.0, as assayed by a sensitive amino terminal actin-typing procedure. Interestingly, when the same actin-typing procedure is used on rhabdomyosarcomas,[190] the ratio is ~4:1 and approaches the values inferred from animal studies for this ratio in fetal tissues.

Antibodies specific for different subsets of the actin isoforms are available.[35, 112, 171, 185] Of these, the most widely utilized is probably HHF35, which recognizes all four muscle actins but not β and γ cytoplasmic actins.[85] In formaldehyde-fixed histologic samples, it can distinguish muscle actin–positive tumors, e.g., rhabdomyosarcoma, leiomyosarcoma, leiomyoma, fibromatosis, nodular fascicles, glomus tumor and some gastrointestinal stromal tumors. Muscle actin–negative tumors include neuroblastoma, Ewing's sarcoma, malignant fibrous histiocytoma, glomus cell tumor and angiosarcoma. Other isotype-specific actin Abs that may be of use in pathology include anti-α sr[171] (both sarcomeric actins) anti-α sm, which sees smooth muscle α actin, and CGA-7,[185] which sees the smooth muscle α and γ actin forms.

Myosin. This occurs in nonmuscle- and muscle-specific isoforms (Mr 220kD). Antibodies specific for the muscle type of myosin heavy chain can identify rhabdomyosarcomas.[57]

Titin. Titin is restricted to skeletal muscle where it forms part of the elastic component (Mr 10^6kD). A single titin molecule spans the distance between the Z line and the M band. When employed in histology it specifically identifies rhabdomyosarcomas,[135] although in any given tumor fewer cells are stained than with the desmin antibody.

Myoglobin. Myoglobin antibodies stain only 40 to 80% of rhabdomyosarcomas, with the more differentiated tumors more likely to be positive. In many tumors only relatively few of the tumor cells are positive.[8]

Glial Markers

Glial fibrillary acidic protein (GFAP). This is the IF protein characteristic of glial cells and of tumors derived from them. Within the central nervous system (CNS), GFAP is characteristic of developing reactive and neoplastic astrocytes—processes of Bergmann's glial cells in tanycytes and in glial limitans.[11, 38, 140] It has also been reported in developing and neoplastic oligodendroglia. In the peripheral nervous system GFAP has been reported in human Schwann cells and in rat enteric glia. Reports of extraneural staining by GFAP are rare, but occasional unexpected reactivities may occur. In histologic sections most gliomas that are well differentiated are strongly GFAP positive.[105, 179] Anaplastic tumors suspected to be of glial origin sometimes do not stain. In glioblastoma multiforme the small round cells show little or no staining in contrast to the large multinucleated cells that are strongly positive. Unlike studies with antibodies to other IF proteins, studies with GFAP antibodies on histologic sections have mostly been performed retrospectively on formaldehyde-fixed paraffin-embedded material. Although GFAP can be readily identified on such material it may be that small amounts escape detection and that differences in fixation may account for some of the wide variations in the percentage of gliomas reported to be positive, e.g., for ependymomas. In this connection two studies of cytologic material are of particular interest. In one, a cocktail of three GFAP mAbs identified astrocytomas (3/3), anaplastic astrocytomas (3/3), glioblastomas 13/13) and oligodendrogliomas (2/2) but did not stain meningiomas and other nonglial tumors.[196] A second study of fewer specimens reached a similar conclusion, except that the single case of oligodendroglioma did not stain.[27] Clearly, therefore, oligodendrogliomas remain a problem area. In addition some cells in pleomorphic adenomas may coexpress GFAP, keratin and vimentin (Table 38–2).

Neural and Neuroendocrine Markers

Neuroendocrine (NE) Markers Associated with Vesicles and Secretory Granules

Synaptophysin. Synaptophysin was originally isolated from neuronal presynaptic vesicles. It is a glycoprotein with an apparent Mr of 38 to 42kD on SDS gels and after deglycosylation has an Mr of 34kD. This glycoprotein is found in the small transparent NE vesicles involved in the storage and release of classic

TABLE 38–2. Intermediate Filament Typing of Carcinomas

KER⁺		All
KER⁺, VIM⁺	MOST	Kidney
		Thyroid
		Papillary
		Follicular
		Large cell
		Endometrial
		Ovarian
	OFTEN	Lung*
		Breast
		Adenoid cystic
	RARE	GI tract
		Prostate
		Squamous cell other than lung
KER⁺, NF⁺, VIM⁻		Neuroendocrine (Merkel cell)
KER⁺, NF⁺, VIM⁺		Thyroid medullary

*Some cases KER and NF⁺.
KER = keratin; VIM = vimentin; NF = neurofilament.

neurotransmitters. These NE vesicles are characteristic of neuronal cells but are also found in some non-neuronal NE cells. Most immunologic studies to date have been performed with the mAb SY38, which recognizes the C terminal tail of the molecule located on the cytoplasmic side of the vesicles. In immunofluorescence, individual vesicles can be distinguished. Synaptophysin's distribution in human tissues and in tumors is reviewed in references 69 and 207. Synaptophysin positivity has been noted in neurons, in endocrine cells of the anterior pituitary, C cells of the thyroid, chromaffin cells of the adrenal medulla, NE cells of the bronchial and gastrointestinal tract and Merkel cells of the skin. Synaptophysin is present in a variety of neuronally derived tumors, including ganglioneuroblastomas, ganglioneuromas, medulloblastomas, neuroblastomas and paragangliomas. All such tumors checked with the SY38 antibody show strong staining. In addition, synaptophysin can also be employed to identify endocrine system–derived NE tumors. Pheochromocytomas, carcinoids and pancreatic NE tumors are positive in all cases. Other tumors, such as SCLC, are positive in only 50 to 70% of cases. Although many NE tumors stain positively for synaptophysin in all tumor cells, other NE tumors, e.g., Merkel cell carcinomas, appear only focally positive for synaptophysin and only some cases are positive. However, in general, synaptophysin appears to be an excellent marker for neural and NE tumors and should be more widely used.

Synapsins. Synapsins form a family of closely related synaptic vesicle membrane proteins.[175] They are involved in linking synaptic vesicles to other cellular elements and in the regulation of neurotransmitter release. Synapsins are usually considered to be neuron specific. When the distributions of synaptophysin and the four known synapsins are compared both stain vesicles.[175] Synapsin Ib shows a distribution very close to that of synaptophysin, whereas the other synapsins appear less widely distributed. These Abs have not yet been utilized in histology and cytology.

Chromogranins. These heat-stable proteins are associated with the matrix of the dense NE granules.[207] Chromogranins have a much wider distribution than the individual peptide hormones or neuropeptides with which such granules are filled. So far three members of the family have been identified: chromogranin A (Mr 48kD), chromogranin B (Mr 76kD) (also called secretogranin I) and chromogranin C (Mr 67kD) (also called secretogranin II). Their apparent molecular weights on SDS gels are much larger, probably because they undergo extensive post-translational modification and are sulfated on carbohydrates and on tyrosine residues. Studies of these proteins in human tissues show that they are distributed in a complementary and sometimes overlapping manner. The broadest specificity as an NE marker would therefore be obtained by mixing Abs to each of the three molecules, but only the mAb LK2H10 to chromogranin A is commercially available. All the normal cell types listed here as synaptophysin positive are also positive with chromogranin A Abs. Tumors derived from the nervous system may be either positive (most paragangliomas) for the chromogranins or negative (most neuroblastomas).[207] Neuroendocrine-derived tumors can express these proteins (e.g., pheochromocytomas and medullary thyroid carcinomas). Some NE tumors, such as gastrointestinal carcinoids and NE carcinomas, are strongly positive with chromogranin A Abs but are less strongly stained by Abs to the two other chromogranins. Small-cell carcinomas of the lung are chromogranin A positive only in a few cases, whereas other NE tumors (e.g., breast) show only focal immunoreactivity with chromogranin A Abs.

Leu 7 (HNK-1). This mAb was originally shown to "decorate" a T-cell leukemia cell line. Leu 7 (HNK-1) recognizes natural killer cells in blood and lymphoid tissues but in addition also recognizes a 75kD component of the NE granule matrix. Small-cell carcinomas of the lung, pheochromocytomas and other NE neoplasms are leu 7 positive.[16]

Gastrin-releasing Peptide. This is a 27 amino acid–long peptide from bovine intestine, which is thought to be the mammalian equivalent of bombesin. Abs to this peptide give a cytoplasmic staining pattern only in some neuroendocrine tumors, e.g., 5/8 carcinoids, 2/8 oat cell carcinomas, 0/20 nonoat cell carcinomas.[13]

Regulatory Peptides, Hormones and Amines. A great many hormones and amines associated with particular cells and neoplasms of the neuroendocrine system occurring in different but in part overlapping sets have been described. Unfortunately many neuroendocrine neoplasms produce such substances ectopically, and therefore their use in characterizing NE neoplasms of doubtful origin may be more limited than those markers previously described.

Intermediate Filament Proteins

The IF complement of NE cells is heterogeneous. Neurons and paraganglion cells express neurofilament proteins NF-L (62kD), NF-M (100kD) and NF-H (110kD) and are keratin negative. Most NE cells in contrast are keratin positive. A further indication of their epithelial nature is that they frequently express desmosomes. Neoplasms of the NE system will in general retain their IF complement but there are exceptions. Thus, paragangliomas, ganglioneuroblastomas, ganglioneuromas and almost all neuroblastomas are neurofilament positive[19, 125, 134, 184] and keratin negative.[69] Occasional neuroblastomas test negative for all three NF proteins. Pheochromocytoma is also NF positive, keratin negative. Most other NE tumors express keratin in all cases, but in a certain and usually minor fraction of cases NF proteins may be coexpressed. Medulloblastoma is unique in that it has vimentin as the only IF type. Other NE tumors with the exception of medullary thyroid carcinoma do not express vimentin (Table 38–2). Thus, NF and keratin antibodies can be employed to separate neural from NE tumors.

Peripherin (Mr 57kD) is an IF protein that is mostly

found in cells of the peripheral nervous system, although it is also expressed in select CNS populations. Peripherin or its message has been reported in sympathetic, parasympathetic and dorsal root ganglion neurons, in ventral horn motor neurons and in motor nuclei of cranial neurons in olfactory epithelium and in retinal ganglion cells.[72, 97, 101] Little information is currently available on its distribution in humans or in human tumors.

Neuron-specific Enolase

Enolases are glycolytic enzymes occurring as dimers composed of three subunits α, β and γ, which can be distinguished immunologically (Mr subunit 100kD). The γ subunit of enolase occurs at high concentrations in the central and peripheral nervous systems as αγ and γγ dimeric forms. The latter type is often called neuron-specific enolase (NSE), although this name also identifies the γ subunit. Both polyclonal and mAbs recognizing the γ subunit have been generated. Original claims that NSE was specific for NE cells have not been confirmed. Although CNS tissues display very high levels of this enzyme a wide variety of non-NE cells also display low levels of the γ subunit (see reference 77), but note that it includes certain smooth muscle cells, myoepithelial cells, the conducting system of the heart, epithelial cell loops of Henle, macula densa cells of kidney, T lymphocytes, plasma cells, platelets and so forth. Thus, diagnostically, Abs to the γ subunit may be of limited value, even if they are specific for γ enolase and do not stain the α and β forms. All NE neoplasms including those of neural and endocrine origin are NSE positive. It may be useful in typing lung carcinomas, in differentiating melanomas and neuroblastomas, in the differential diagnosis of neuroblastomas from Wilms' tumors and other small round cell tumors of children and in differentiating pheochromocytomas from adrenal cortical carcinomas (see reference 162). However, focal positivity of tumors other than those derived from the CNS system, such as schwannoma, carcinoma and fibroadenoma of the breast, renal cell carcinoma and chordoma have also been reported. Neuron-specific enolase should therefore be utilized in diagnosis only together with other NE markers and not alone.

Melanoma Markers

Melanomas have vimentin as their only IF protein[20] and are synaptophysin negative.[69] They therefore are placed in a separate category.

S-100 Proteins

S-100 (two subunits each 10.5kD) is a protein named because it is soluble in 100% ammonium sulfate. Characterization of certain other proteins selected by different criteria at the amino acid sequence or DNA levels has made it clear that there is a family of related

proteins that share sequence with S-100 proteins. The S-100 family[92] includes p11, the cystic fibrosis (CF) antigen and calcyclin for which the corresponding proteins have been isolated. However, four other members of the family—18A2, 42A, 42C and p9ka—are documented as homologous with S-100 by DNA sequence, whereas the corresponding proteins have not yet been isolated. This factor makes the interpretation of much of the existing literature on reactivity of S-100 Abs with different cell types very difficult, because it is not clear whether the Abs to S-100 that were used recognize only S-100 or whether they also recognize other members of the family as well. What is interesting, however, is that they display different specificities, suggesting that careful isolation and characterization of a set of Abs for each of these proteins might be helpful. Such arguments, for example, probably explain the different specificities of two mAbs to S-100 which, although blotting on both S-100 α and β, had different specificities when tested on normal and pathologic tissues.[192, 193]

Antibodies to CF antigen stain granulocytes, a subset of normal stratified epithelia, e.g., tongue, esophagus and buccal epithelium and also SCC derived from these tissues.[209] The p11 mAbs decorate a variety of tissues, including fibroblasts and certain epithelial cell types, but stain neither muscle nor neuronal cells. Because of the localization of at least some of these molecules under the cell membrane,[136] proper fixation prior to ICC may be especially important, and indeed a reduction of intensity in staining and number of positive cells has been noted on cytologic specimens if ethanol- rather than formaldehyde-fixed material is employed.[130]

S-100 was originally thought to be restricted to neural cells. Subsequently a much wider variety of cells in different tissues and tumors has been shown to contain material reactive with S-100 Abs. For the reasons previously given, rabbit Abs should be utilized with caution. However, in histologic sections,[206] S-100 reactive material is found in almost all benign nerve sheath tumors, with neurilemoma, neurofibroma and granular cell tumor showing strong staining of most cells. In malignant schwannoma 50 to 75% show rare-to-occasional positive cells. In some other soft tissue tumors S-100 staining of rare positive cells is noted. Carcinomas are generally S-100 negative but there are exceptions. In melanocytic tumors both cellular blue nevus and clear cell carcinoma of the tendon show occasional positive cells. In contrast most melanomas seem to be positive and to show moderate-to-strong staining of many cells (e.g., 9/9,[206] 62/62[71] and 21/23[130]).

Melanoma Surface Antigens

The mAbs generated against melanoma extracts have been isolated by several groups and may be useful in diagnostic pathology. The HMB-45[72] recognizes a 10kD polypeptide. Some 60/62 melanomas and 0/168 carcinomas, lymphomas and sarcomas were stained by HMB-45 in methacarn-fixed histologic material. Reactivity varied from <10% to >80% positive tumor cells.

The HMB-45 does not distinguish benign from malignant melanocytic growths and does not stain adult melanocytes. The HMB-45 can be utilized on cytologic specimens. A second antibody, HMB-50[197] recognizes a secreted 97kD polypeptide and displays a very similar specificity to HMB-45. Both the 97kD and the 10kD protein may be growth regulated. The mAb NK1/beteb,[194] which seems to recognize a different epitope on the 10kD molecule, has a reaction very similar to HMB-45 except that it recognizes adult melanocytes. It recognized 126/134 melanocytic tumors and other melanocytic lesions vs. 1/185 for other tumors. Other melanoma mAbs include NKC3, HMSA 1, HMSA 2, D6.1, melanoma-associated transferrin p97, anti GD3 and Abs to a 250 to 300,000 proteoglycan complex (see reference 197). Most have not yet been tested on cytologic specimens.

Lymphoid Markers

A huge variety of surface markers has been described for human leukocytes. Workshops on human leukocyte differentiation antigens were held in 1982, 1984, 1986 and 1988. Antigens were defined and assigned a cluster of differentiation (CD) number. This CD number is used to refer either to the antigen or sometimes also to the Abs that define an antigen. To be assigned a CD number putative antigens have to be recognized by at least two Abs, and the molecular weight of the antigen has to be known. Detailed lists of the 45 CD leukocyte antigens defined at the first three workshops, together with their Mr and the spectrum of cell types each recognizes, are beyond the scope of this chapter but can be found in McMichael and associates[108] or in commercial catalogues. Leukocyte common antigen (LCA) is a major membrane glycoprotein restricted to leukocytes.[96] Antigens that define pan B and pan T lymphocytes as well as others that recognize more restricted lymphocytic subsets are available.

Determination of the T- or B-cell phenotype, as well as the degree of maturation of lymphoid cells, can be important for treatment, particularly of lymphomas. Lymphocyte marker studies can alter the final cytologic diagnosis in up to 50% of selected cases.[158]

Some experiments allow a further identification of some of the CD antigens. Thus, specific Abs have been employed to clone and sequence the cDNA coding for some of these molecules. When the sequences were fed into the data banks several CD antigens were shown to correspond to surface peptidases,[90] e.g., CD10 and common acute lymphoblastic leukemia antigen (CALLA) are identical to endopeptidase 24.11, CD13 is identical to aminopeptidase N and CD 26 is identical to dipeptidyl peptidase.

Oncofetal Markers

The markers so far discussed distinguish particular differentiation pathways. They are not restricted to tumor cells but are found in both the tumor cell and the normal cell from which it is derived or with which it is related. The only exception so far covered that can help in distinguishing malignant from benign is SM-3[17] that recognizes an epitope on EMA, which is exposed in malignant but masked in certain benign tissues. Likewise, B72.3[85] also sees a mucin-like molecule in malignant but not in benign tissues.

However, another class of markers is known, i.e., proteins that are predominantly present in fetal tissues and in tumors but not in normal adult tissues. Two such oncofetal markers—CEA and AFP—are subsequently discussed. Attention is also drawn to the emergence of oncogene products as markers.

Carcinoembryonic Antigen

This antigen is a high molecular weight glycoprotein (Mr ~180,000, after deglycosylation ~85kD) originally described in 1965 in embryonic colon and in colon carcinomas. So far at least 13 CEA-related proteins[213] have been described by DNA cloning or by protein chemical techniques. These proteins can be divided into at least three families. Other related molecules in the CEA family include nonspecific cross-reacting proteins (NCA-95, 95kD and NCA 55, 55kD) and biliary glycoprotein (Mr 85kD). All three of these proteins are present in certain normal cell types and share up to 90% homology with CEA. All are made up of a repeating structure but differ in the number of repeats. These repeat domains have homology to the immunoglobulin constant region and to the neural cell adhesion molecule suggesting that these proteins may be evolutionarily related.

Considering the complexity of the CEA family it is not surprising that many of the mAbs and other Abs that have been isolated cross-react with other CEA-like molecules. Not all cases of a given tumor type are necessarily positive with CEA Abs. In one study of breast carcinomas 76% were CEA positive.[126] A good correlation was seen between results on FNAs and tissue sections, although some cases were CEA positive in the FNAs and negative in sections. Later, 82 mAbs were classified according to the epitope they recognize on CEA.[79] Interesting CEA-specific mAbs are contained in the GOLD 1 and GOLD 3 groups, which recognize two different peptide epitopes. It is probably from these groups that mAbs displaying a high degree of specificity for CEA in ICC should be selected. Other investigators have searched for CEA mAbs that are absolutely specific for colon carcinomas and that do not stain in normal colon. Thus, D14[87] reacts with all colon carcinomas (20/20) and some stomach carcinomas (4/9) on formaldehyde-fixed material but not with normal colon or stomach tissue. The mAb 7F reacted with all colorectal and stomach carcinomas, with adenocarcinomas of lung (2/5) and with ovary (1/3) and endometrium (1/3) but not with a wide variety of other tumors in frozen sections.[219] It was negative on most but not all other normal human tissues. Obviously, therefore, the exact spectrum seen with a CEA antibody will depend on which antibody is selected for the ICC studies of CEA.

Alpha₁-fetoprotein (AFP)

Alpha₁-fetoprotein is a glycoprotein (Mr 70kD) containing 3 to 5% carbohydrate and sharing sequence with albumin.[93] In the fetus, AFP is present in high concentration in blood and is synthesized in the liver, yolk sac and gastrointestinal tract.[93] After birth, AFP disappears from the blood but reappears in 80 to 90% of patients with HCC. However, it can be demonstrated by ICC in only 20 to 50% of HCC. An AFP staining is focal and most often found in the undifferentiated neoplasms. In some 66% of men with testicular teratomas, elevated levels of AFP are found and are usually associated with endodermal sinus tumor differentiation. Embryonal carcinomas can show AFP-positive cells, whereas pure seminomas, teratomas and choriocarcinomas are negative for AFP.

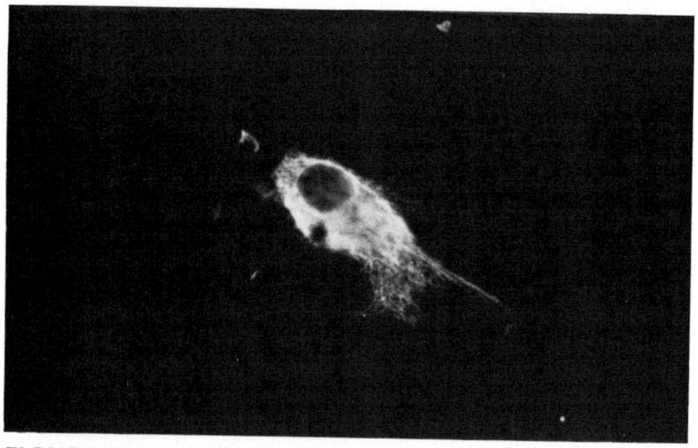

FIGURE 38–4. Fine needle aspiration, **kidney carcinoma,** stained with keratin mAb KL1. Note the filaments (indirect immunofluorescence; ×400).

Oncogenes[25]

Normal cellular genes that are involved in cell proliferation and differentiation and which when altered contribute to the development of a tumor are referred to as proto-oncogenes. The products of these genes can be secreted (e.g., c-sis), or they can be present on the cell surface (e.g., c-erb2), in the cytoplasm (e.g, c-ras) or in the nucleus (e.g., c-myc). Antibodies to a few normal and mutated proto-oncogenes are available. However, very careful characterization of such antibodies is required to make sure that they see only the proto-oncogene and not other cellular proteins.

DIAGNOSTIC SIGNIFICANCE OF IMMUNOCYTOCHEMISTRY IN CYTOLOGIC SPECIMENS

Fine Needle Aspirations—Tumor Typing

Carcinomas

The light microscopic and ICC features of tumor cells in aspirates depend on their site of origin, degree of differentiation and histologic make-up. As a rule, the better a carcinoma is differentiated the less difficult it is to diagnose its histologic type on a conventional smear. As a group, well-differentiated carcinomas share several distinctive morphologic features, which may permit their differentiation from other major tumor categories.[94] Hence, their diagnosis in FNAs is relatively simple in experienced hands in the majority of cases. The common diagnostic dilemmas in assessment of FNAs at the light microscopy level involve poorly differentiated (anaplastic) carcinomas. They include the differentiation of small-cell carcinomas from large-cell non-Hodgkin's malignant lymphomas or sometimes from small-cell sarcomas. Large-cell poorly differentiated (anaplastic, solid) carcinomas may be mistaken for malignant melanomas or a variety

of sarcomas. The ICC approach is therefore of most use in diagnosing poorly differentiated carcinomas composed of cells that cannot be readily classified by light microscopy.

As a group, carcinomas whether primary or metastatic are keratin positive regardless of the tumor site and of the degree of differentiation of the tumor cells. This finding is the same for both histologic[63, 70, 116, 140, 153] and cytologic[5, 55, 151] specimens. Thus, carcinomas can be detected by ICC techniques if appropriate broad specificity pan keratin antibodies, such as KL1[195] or Lu5,[199] are employed. Different carcinomas show varying amounts of keratin filaments. For example, squamous carcinomas always contain abundant keratin filaments, whereas SCLC may contain only delicate keratin networks. In some carcinoma cells individual keratin IFs can be resolved by immunofluorescence microscopy (Fig. 38–4). Although it is difficult to resolve individual filaments in many epithelial tumor cells, the pattern of keratin expression in the majority of carcinomas is clearly filamentous. In a very few tumor types keratin filaments aggregate into round bodies or "IF buttons." This fact can be exploited diagnostically as subsequently described.

Most carcinomas are negative for vimentin, although some carcinomas are keratin and vimentin positive. True coexpression of keratin and vimentin, i.e., simultaneous expression of both IF types in the same tumor cells, was first shown in salivary gland tumors.[21] It has since been shown in histologic sections and FNAs of the carcinomas listed in Table 38–2. Vimentin coexpression can be found in both primary and metastatic carcinomas.[10, 53, 109, 167] The frequency of coexpression differs with tumor type. For example, on histologic specimens the percentage of renal cell carcinomas in which vimentin and keratin coexpression was noted was variously reported as 47%, 57%, 80% and 100%.[48] On histologic specimens of thyroid carcinomas, all tumors expressed keratin and the majority showed coexpression of keratin and vimentin. In our material coexpression of keratin and vimetin was noted in FNAs

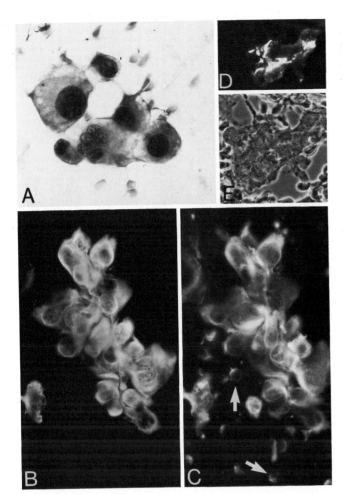

FIGURE 38–5. Fine needle aspiration, **metastatic kidney carcinoma.** *A,* Cytology showing anisocytosis, anisokaryosis and vacuolated cytoplasm of tumor cells (hematoxylin and eosin; ×600). *B* and *C,* Tumor cells labeled with both the keratin mAb Lu5 *(B)* and the guinea pig vimentin Ab *(C)* (double immunofluorescence on the same smear; ×600). Almost all tumor cells coexpress keratin and vimentin. Lymphocytes are vimentin positive (arrows in *C*) but keratin negative *(B).* *D,* Tumor cells labeled by epithelial membrane antigen mAb (Dako-EMA) in indirect immunofluorescence. Note granular membrane staining. *E,* Phase contrast of the cells shown in *D* (×380).

of all metastatic renal cell[48] (Fig. 38–5) and thyroid[4, 48] carcinomas (Figs. 38–6 and 38–7), in 23% of SCLC[45] and in 19% of breast carcinomas (Fig. 38–8).[42] In our FNAs series, single examples of adrenocortical, prostatic and squamous laryngeal carcinomas showing coexpression of keratin and vimentin were seen.[45] The percentage of tumor cells coexpressing keratin and vimentin varies, e.g., in breast carcinoma from <5% to >50%. Whatever the reasons for these differences, from the diagnostic viewpoint the cytopathologist has to be aware that while there are carcinoma types for which coexpression of keratin and vimentin is typical it may not occur in all cases or in all tumor cells of a positive case.

In summary, in some carcinomas coexpression of vimentin and keratin is very frequent (renal cell, thy-

roid, ovarian, endometrial), in some it is found in ~20% of cases (lung, breast) and in others it is rare or exceptional (gastrointestinal tract) (see Table 38–2). Therefore, a finding of coexpression of keratin and vimentin in a metastatic carcinoma can add important information relevant to the differential diagnosis in the search for the primary. That this can be of practical value is illustrated by two of our cases in which no significant clinical information was available when the FNA was taken from enlarged lymph nodes.[48] The IF typing showed a coexpression of keratin and vimentin, and on the basis of the combined morphologic and immunologic data a diagnosis of metastatic renal cell carcinoma was provided. Computed tomography and ultrasonography revealed kidney tumors, which were removed and shown by histology to be clear cell carcinomas. From the viewpoint of differential diagnosis it is important to note that keratin and vimentin can also be coexpressed in cells of mesotheliomas, synovial and epithelioid sarcomas and rare malignant rhabdoid tumors of soft parts (Table 38–3).[10, 53, 113]

Some carcinomas, i.e., neuroendocrine (Merkel cell) skin carcinomas (NSC), usually contain neurofilaments in addition to keratins.[122] Triple coexpression of keratin, vimentin and neurofilaments is characteristic of medullary thyroid carcinoma (see Table 38–2).[4, 48]

As a group, carcinomas are mostly EMA positive. In formalin-fixed, paraffin-embedded tissues adenocarcinomas from various primary sites, e.g., breast, lung, colon, stomach, pancreas, gallbladder, prostate, endometrium, ovary, kidney and thyroid, were immunoreactive for EMA.[146] Small-cell anaplastic carcinomas, transitional cell carcinomas and squamous carcinomas have also been shown to be EMA positive. The following carcinomas were shown to be EMA negative: adenocortical, medullary thyroid, embryonal and hepatocellular carcinomas. Some carcinoid tumors were also EMA negative. When utilized together with keratin, EMA seems to be a helpful diagnostic discrim-

TABLE 38–3. True Coexpression of Intermediate Filaments in Tumors Other than Carcinomas

Tumor Type	KER	VIM	NF	GFAP	DES
Carcinoid	+		(+)		
Pancreatic islet tumors	+		(+)		
Parathyroid adenoma	+		(+)		
Thyroid adenoma					
Hürthle cell	+	+			
Follicular	+	+			
Pleomorphic adenoma	+	+		+	
(parotid gland)					
Mesothelioma	+	(+)			
Leiomyosarcoma	f	(+)			+
Rhabdomyosarcoma	f	(+)			+
Papillary meningioma	+	+		+	
Ewing's tumor	(+)	+	f		
Synovial sarcoma	+	+			
Epithelioid sarcoma	+	+			
Malignant rhabdoid tumor of soft tissue	+	+			

(+) = Not all cases positive; f = focal positivity; KER = keratin; VIM = vimentin; NF = neurofilament; GFAP = glial fibrillary acidic protein; DES = desmin.

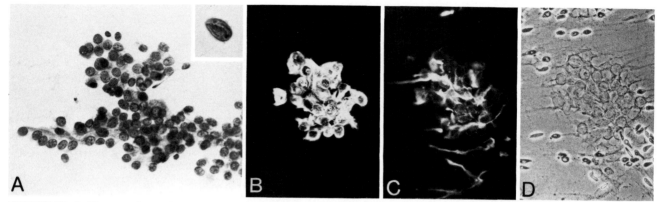

FIGURE 38–6. Fine needle aspiration, **metastatic papillary thyroid carcinoma.** *A,* Cytology (hematoxylin and eosin; ×250). *Inset,* "coffee-bean" nucleus of a tumor cell (hematoxylin and eosin; ×630). *B* and *C,* Cells stained with both the keratin mAb KL1*(B)* and the guinea pig vimentin Ab *(C)* (double immunofluorescence staining on the same smear; ×250). Note the different patterns of keratin and vimentin expression in tumor cells coexpressing both intermediate filament types. Elongated vimentin-positive, keratin-negative most likely endothelial cells are also visible in *C. D,* Phase contrast of cells in *B* and *C* (×250).

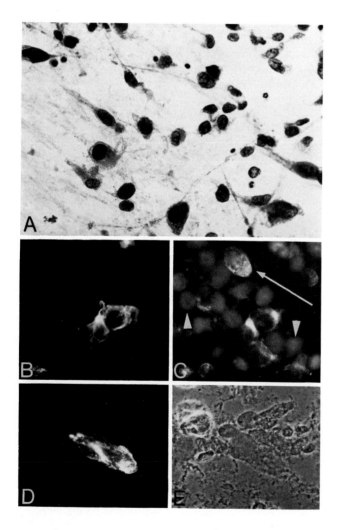

FIGURE 38–7. Fine needle aspiration, **large-cell anaplastic thyroid carcinoma.** *A,* Cytology showing dispersed tumor cells of variable size and shape (hematoxylin and eosin; ×400). *B* and *C,* Tumor cells labeled with both the keratin mAb KL1 *(B)* and the guinea pig vimentin Ab (double immunofluorescence staining on the same smear; ×400). Two tumor cells in the center coexpress keratin and vimentin. Some cells (macrophages?) express only vimentin (arrow in *C*). Many tumor cells are keratin and vimentin negative (arrowheads in *C*). *D,* Elongated tumor cell labeled by mAb to EMA (Dako-EMA; indirect immunofluorescence; ×400). *E,* Phase contrast of the cell in *D*.

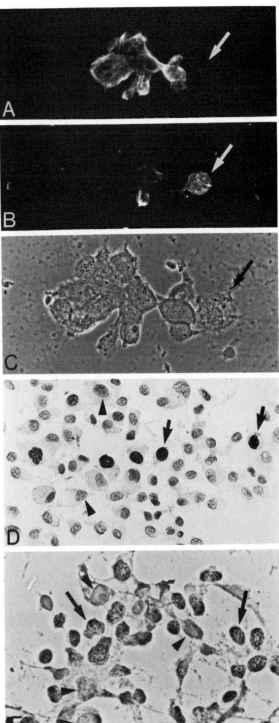

FIGURE 38–8. Fine needle aspiration, **breast carcinoma** (A and B). Cluster of tumor cells labeled by (A) keratin mAb KL1 and (B) the guinea pig vimentin Ab (double immunofluorescence on the same smear; ×380). Two tumor cells coexpress keratin and vimentin. Arrows in A, B and C show a vimentin-positive, keratin-negative macrophage. Compare the phase contrast appearance of the same cells in (C) (×600). Note the prominent nucleoli in tumor cells and distinctive morphology of the macrophage. D, Dispersed cancer cells labeled with Ki67 mAb to identify nuclei of proliferating cells (arrows) (immunoperoxidase; ×380). Positive nuclei (e.g., arrows) were brown, and negative nuclei (e.g., arrowheads) were blue due to hematoxylin counterstain in the original slide. E, Tumor cells labeled with mAb to estrogen receptor, which stains most (arrows) but not all nuclei (arrowheads, negative nuclei) (immunoperoxidase; ×940).

inant for carcinomas, especially those such as spindle cell carcinomas, which exhibit unusual morphology. However, some T-cell neoplasms, true histiocytic lymphomas, plasmacytomas, neuroblastomas as well as a few melanomas have been shown to be EMA positive,[2, 145, 146] although these tumors are keratin negative. In addition synovial and epithelial sarcomas are immunoreactive for EMA.

Relatively little experience has taken place with EMA on FNAs. In our FNA material, which was alcohol fixed, staining for EMA appeared less consistent and more variable in intensity than staining for keratin. Examples of granular membrane EMA expression in carcinomas are given in Fig. 38–5 D and Fig. 38–7 D. Carcinomas are nonreactive for LCA in FNAs.

Within the framework of appropriate clinical and morphologic information, several mAbs may be of use in the further subdivision of carcinomas.

Squamous Cell (Epidermoid) Carcinoma and Adenocarcinoma. Perusal of the two-dimensional catalogues of keratins of different adenocarcinomas shows that most adenocarcinomas are characterized by keratins 7, 8, 18 and 19.[118, 120, 150] Colon carcinomas have 8, 18 and 19. In contrast, many squamous cell carcinomas lack keratins 8 and 18. In general, they display a more complex keratin pattern often involving additional keratins, such as 4, 5, 14, 15 and 16, with the exact complement depending on the tumor type.

Studies on histologic sections with ICC have shown that discrimination can be obtained with antibodies specific for keratin 18.[36] Most adenocarcinomas originate from glandular (also called "simple" as opposed to stratified) epithelium. As previously mentioned, mAbs that recognize antigenic determinants appear only on particular keratin polypeptides associated with such epithelia, e.g., keratin 18 (CK2, RGE-53) stains simple epithelia but in general does not stain most stratified epithelia. Therefore, in general, adenocarcinomas arising from simple (glandular) epithelia are strongly keratin 18 positive in histologic[36] and cytologic[51, 55] specimens (Fig. 38–9), whereas SCC, such as those from skin, tongue and esophagus, are usually

negative. Likewise mAb 35βH11,[70] which recognizes keratins 8 and 18,[29] stains all adenocarcinomas positively irrespective of their origin and such tumors as renal cell carcinoma, hepatocellular carcinoma and carcinoid tumor, which are also known to contain these keratin polypeptides. However, Abs to keratin 18 do show occasional staining of SCC, e.g., of SCC of epiglottis and SCC of cervix uteri.[36] Such staining is nonuniform with areas of cornification remaining unstained.

Conversely, use of antibodies specific for keratin associated with squamous epithelia should allow a positive identification of SCC vs. adenocarcinomas. The antibody 34βE12[70] is often described as specific for large keratins and indeed does stain SCC positively. However, it also stains many adenocarcinomas and so should not be used for a distinction between SCC and adenocarcinoma by itself. The antibody 34βB4 stains only SCC, as do AE2,[29] RKSE 60[154] and CKS1.[3]

Although experience with chain-specific keratin Abs on FNAs is limited, we have employed CK2 and CKS1 to distinguish adenocarcinoma and SCC.[45, 50] Thus, keratin typing with several mAbs to different keratin polypeptides can be utilized to indicate whether a given carcinoma shows squamous or adenocarcinoma differentiation, especially when combined with the cytologic and clinical evidence.

Generally, EMA reactivity is found primarily in adenocarcinomas. However, some EMA-negative adenocarcinomas have been found, and SCCs can also be EMA positive. The mAb B72.3 reacts preferentially with adenocarcinomas from a variety of body sites and in particular with adenocarcinomas of the colon, breast and lung but clearly also reacts with some SCC.[86] Therefore, EMA and B72.3 are not reliable markers for discriminating between adenocarcinomas and SCC.

Neuroendocrine Carcinomas. Neuroendocrine carcinomas may arise at various sites in the body, particularly in the lung, thyroid and skin. They are characterized by the presence of NSE and cytoplasmic neurosecretory granules containing peptide hormones or substances such as serotonin. Some of these tumors can elaborate sufficient amounts of ACTH, gonadotrophins, parathyroid hormone and other hormones to induce clinical syndromes such as Cushing's. Neuroendocrine carcinoma comprises a spectrum that includes well-differentiated and intermediate types as well as small cell–type carcinomas. Consequently, some of them retain an organoid pattern and others display considerable pleomorphism. The precise diagnosis of NE carcinomas in FNAs only at the light microscopy level is difficult and often impossible. Fortunately, ICC has much to offer to help make this diagnosis more reliable. Synaptophysin,[69, 207, 208] chromogranin[203, 207] and keratins[69] are good markers in the search for NE differentiation of a tumor.

Neuroendocrine (Merkel Cell) Skin Carcinomas. Three histologic types have been identified: trabecular, intermediate cell and small cell. The term neuroendocrine skin carcinoma (NSC) was proposed to designate them. The cytologic differential diagnosis of NSC can be very difficult because this tumor must be distin-

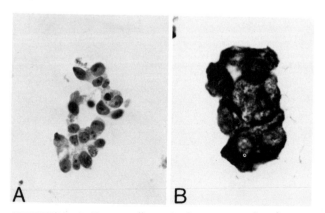

FIGURE 38–9. Fine needle aspiration, **metastatic adenocarcinoma of the breast.** *A,* Cytology of tumor cells (hematoxylin and eosin; ×260). *B,* Tumor cells labeled with keratin 18–specific mAb, CK2 (immunoperoxidase; ×630).

guished from metastatic undifferentiated small-cell carcinoma of the lung or other organs, metastatic carcinoid, malignant lymphoma, malignant melanoma, adult neuroblastoma, basal cell carcinoma of the skin and extraskeletal Ewing's sarcoma.

Only ten FNAs from NSCs have been described in the literature.[49, 144] We have seen six of these and five additional cases. The smears are usually highly cellular with numerous red blood cells present (Fig. 38–10 A and B). In some cases, tightly cohesive clusters of cells and rows with cellular and nuclear molding accompany dispersed cells (Fig. 38–10 C). The individual tumor cells are small, round or oval with slight anisocytosis.

The most characteristic light microscopy feature is the presence of pale, pink, homogeneous, relatively dense, well-circumscribed, round or oval buttons of cytoplasm that are found either in a perinuclear location still attached to the nucleus, often lying in an indentation of the nucleus, or detached from the nucleus freely dispersed in the smear (see Fig. 38–10 A and B).[49] They can be clearly distinguished from erythrocytes by their size, shape and color. We refer to them as IF buttons because they are button-like in morphology in FNAs and contain keratin and in the majority neurofilaments when studied with ICC techniques in smears[49, 144] or histologic sections.[122] In some tumor

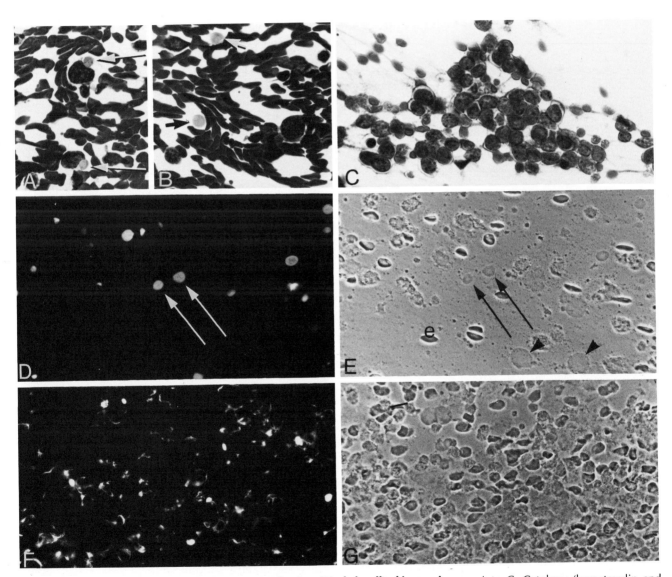

FIGURE 38–10. Fine needle aspiration, **neuroendocrine (Merkel cell) skin carcinoma.** A to C, Cytology (hematoxylin and eosin). A, Two intermediate filament (IF) buttons (arrows) in a perinuclear position. Note the invaginated nuclei (×400). B, Two "lost" IF buttons (arrows). Note the difference between IF buttons (arrows) and erythrocytes (×400). C, Tumor cell clusters showing nuclear molding (hematoxylin and eosin; ×250). D, "Lost" IF buttons stain positively with keratin mAb Lu5 (arrows) (indirect immunofluorescence; ×400). E, Phase contrast of the cells in D (×400). The "lost" IF buttons (arrows), nuclei of tumor cells (arrowheads) and erythrocytes (e). F, Cancer cells labeled by neurofilament mAb NR4. Note that both IF buttons and filaments are stained (indirect immunofluorescence; ×400). G, Phase contrast of cells in F. (Reproduced with permission from Domagala W, Lubinski J, Lasota J, et al.: Acta Cytol 31:267–275, 1987.)

TABLE 38–4. Differential Diagnosis of Neuroendocrine (Merkel Cell) Skin Carcinoma (NSC)

| | Intermediate Filaments (IF) | | | | | TEM | LM (FNA) | |
	KER	Type NF	VIM	Pattern Filamentous	IF Buttons	Neurosecretory Granules	If Buttons	Nuclear Molding
Malignant lymphoma	–	–	+	+	–	–	–	–
Malignant melanoma	–	–	+	+	–	–	–	–
Basal cell carcinoma	+	–	–	+	–	–‡	–	–
Neuroblastoma	–	+*	–	+	–	+	–	–
Carcinoid	+	–†	–	+	–†	+	–	–
Oat cell carcinoma	+	–†	–	+	–†	+	–	+
NSC	+	+*	–	+	+	+	+	+

*Majority positive, some cases negative.
†Majority negative, some cases positive.
‡Few cases positive.
(Reproduced with permission from Domagala W, Lubinski J, Lasota, J, Giryn I, Weber K, Osborn M: Acta Cytol 31:267–275, 1987.)
KER = keratin; NF = neurofilament; VIM = vimentin; TEM = transmission electron microscopy; LM (FNA) light microscopy (fine needle aspirate.

cells a filamentous network is revealed by antibodies against either keratins (Fig. 38–10 D) or neurofilaments (Fig. 38–10 F). The presence and number of cells containing IF buttons or fibrillar structures as well as their size and shape can differ in various smears. Thus far all our NSCs have been positive for keratin and neurofilaments, but by analogy with histologic specimens[122] one may expect the occasional NSC that will have only keratin filaments. The tumor cells are negative for vimentin; however, vimentin-positive macrophages can be found in the smears. Transmission electron microscopy reveals large aggregates of IFs (IF buttons) predominantly in the perinuclear region and round, membrane-bound, dense-core, neurosecretory type granules.[52, 122]

By immunohistochemistry, NSCs may contain calcitonin, bombesin, somatostatin, leuenkephalin and ACTH, but the expression of these neuropeptides in different cases is variable. Neuron-specific enolase is usually present, whereas synaptophysin seems to be focally present in some tumors.[207] These markers have not been tested yet on NSC aspirates.

The differential diagnosis of NSC can be aided by combining light microscopy, ICC and electron microscopy (Table 38–4). Intermediate filament typing can exclude malignant lymphoma and malignant melanoma without difficulty, because these tumors contain only vimentin, whereas NSC does not. The distinction of those NSCs that coexpress keratins and neurofilaments from oat cell carcinomas and carcinoids that contain only keratin is also relatively simple. However, a few oat cell carcinomas (variant type) express neurofilaments as may some carcinoids. These rare cases may be difficult to distinguish from NSC by microscopic techniques, especially as perinuclear aggregates of IFs have been revealed in some carcinoids of bronchial and intestinal origin as well as in a single instance of oat cell carcinoma.

In summary, NSCs are keratin and neurofilament positive, vimentin negative. They express both synaptophysin and NSE and contain IF buttons that can be revealed by light microscopy, ICC or electron microscopy.

Small-cell Carcinoma of the Lung (SCLC). Lung carcinomas, in general, and the small-cell type, in particular, manifest great heterogeneity both in morphology and in ICC.[14] According to a proposal, SCLC can be subdivided into the pure (classic) type, the small cell/large cell type (the variant type) and the combined type. The variant type of SCLC consists of a mixture of small cells and large cells with "open" nuclei and prominent eosinophilic nucleoli. This classification is supported by clinical studies, by tissue culture experiments in which three different types of cell lines growing from SCLC can be distinguished—classic, variant and multipotent—and by electron microscopy and ICC studies indicating that there might be a spectrum of characteristics of SCLC ranging from predominantly NE features of classic (oat) SCLC to minimal "epithelial" features of SCLC of the variant type. Small-cell lung carcinoma may occasionally produce multiple hormones (e.g., ADH and ACTH) and may be associated with paraneoplastic syndromes, such as Cushing's. The differential diagnosis, especially of metastatic SCLC, may be very difficult. Therefore, **a detailed clinical history is of the utmost importance for proper interpretation of light microscopy and ICC findings in FNAs.**

The majority of SCLC tumors seem to express **NE** features, such as neurosecretory granules detectable by transmission electron microscopy or by leu 7 or synaptic vesicles detectable by SY38. By ICC, NSE, bombesin, ACTH, serotonin, calcitonin, somatostatin and other hormones may be demonstrated in tumor cells. They may also be EMA and CEA positive. Occasional SCLC are positive for Leu-M1 Mab. The hemopoietic surface antigens, OKM1, OKM8, OKM9 and OKM10, may be found on SCLC cells. In contrast to other NE tumors SCLCs in cytologic specimens were chromogranin negative.[203] The nature of IFs in SCLC has been a matter of controversy. However, it now seems that (1) almost all SCLC contain keratin, whereas a few (probably a variant type) contain neurofilaments, and that (2) rarely, a coexpression of keratin and neurofilaments may be found in some tumor cells.[14] In the FNAs of all SCLCs in our series, sparse keratin filaments were present. In one case of SCLC globular keratin expression has been reported on tissue sections.

Differential Diagnosis. Primary SCLC has to be distinguished mainly from bronchial carcinoid and poorly differentiated epidermoid carcinomas and adenocarcinomas, as well as from large-cell carcinomas of the lung. Some tumors of this last type may coexpress keratin and neurofilaments. Differential diagnosis of metastatic SCLC includes poorly differentiated epidermoid carcinoma and adenocarcinoma, epidermoid carcinoma of the nasopharynx (lymphoepithelioma), NSC, metastatic carcinoid, malignant lymphoma, malignant melanoma, adult neuroblastoma, extraskeletal Ewing's sarcoma and occasionally seminoma. The clinical data and site of the metastasis, whether lymph node, skin or visceral organs, usually indicate some of these alternatives as more probable than others. Principal features that allow differentiation of SCLC from most of the tumors listed are given in Table 38–4.

In summary, SCLC may express keratin (majority), NF (occasional), NSE (majority), synaptophysin and chromogranin, neurosecretory granules (majority), EMA (some) and CEA (some). It does not express S-100 protein or LCA.

Medullary Thyroid Carcinoma. This carcinoma is thought to originate from calcitonin-producing parafollicular (C) cells of thyroid. Clinical paraneoplastic syndromes are frequently associated with this neoplasm—a fact to be reckoned with in the differential diagnosis. Some tumors can elaborate calcitonin and other hormones, such as ACTH, which can lead even to a Cushing-like syndrome in an occasional patient. Increased levels of circulating catecholamines can produce a carcinoid-like syndrome and sometimes prostaglandin-induced diarrhea occurs.

The most consistent morphologic features of medullary thyroid carcinoma in FNAs are elongated shape and a granular cytoplasm of tumor cells (Fig. 38–11). The majority of medullary thyroid carcinoma cells coexpress keratin and vimentin. In addition some cells—mostly triangular tumor cells—show positive staining with keratin, vimentin and neurofilament antibodies (see Fig. 38–11).[4, 48] This triple coexpression, i.e., the simultaneous expression of three classes of IF in one cell, is highly unusual. It has been shown both in smears of FNAs and on tissue sections from medullary thyroid carcinomas. Occasional carcinoids can also express keratin, vimentin and neurofilaments.

Calcitonin, which is regarded as a most constant and prominent product of medullary thyroid carcinoma, has been identified in tumor cells in FNAs.[127, 155] Some cases, however, show only a weak or borderline staining. Chromogranin has been demonstrated in cytologic specimens of medullary thyroid carcinoma.[203] Neuron-specific enolase represents a useful additional diagnostic marker, because it is positive in the majority of cases. A variety of regulatory peptide hormones, such as serotonin, somatostatin and ACTH, and a subunit of human chorionic gonadotropin can also be identified in tumor cells of some cases of medullary carcinoma. However, they are less reliable diagnostic markers.

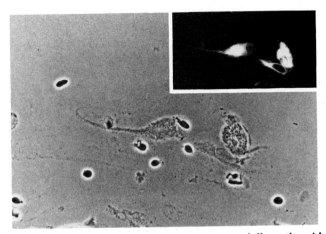

FIGURE 38–11. Fine needle aspiration, **medullary thyroid carcinoma.** Phase contrast of tumor cells. Note the tiny cytoplasmic granules (×380). *Inset,* The tumor cells and long cell processes are positively stained with the neurofilament mAb NR4 in indirect immunofluorescence (×600).

The few cases of medullary thyroid carcinoma studied to date in sections have been shown to be negative for EMA, LCA and S-100.[192, 193] S-100 may be helpful in differential diagnosis with other thyroid carcinomas, because the majority of papillary, follicular and anaplastic carcinomas were immunoreactive with polyclonal and mAbs to S-100. In contrast to follicular and papillary thyroid carcinomas, which are thyroglobulin positive, medullary carcinoma was negative for this marker on FNAs.[60]

Differential Diagnosis. Atypical variants of medullary thyroid carcinoma with follicular, papillary, glandular, pseudopapillary and anaplastic growth patterns, with production of mucus and with or without demonstrable amyloid have been described. Hence, the differential diagnosis of medullary thyroid carcinoma has to include, in addition to other types of thyroid carcinomas, adenocarcinomas, poorly differentiated carcinomas, sarcomas and occasionally carcinoids and plasmocytomas.

In summary, medullary thyroid carcinoma is characterized by (1) true coexpression of keratin, vimentin and neurofilaments in some cells, (2) calcitonin and (3) NSE. This triad is exceptionally specific and allows for precise diagnosis of this cancer in FNAs and its differentiation from all other malignant tumors.

Primary Hepatocellular Carcinoma. High serum levels of alpha$_1$-fetoprotein (AFP) and ferritin provide strong support for the diagnosis of HCC. Therefore, serologic tests and a detailed clinical history are important, especially in difficult cases. Only 20% of HCCs are positive for AFP in ICC. Thus, a positive ICC result strongly supports the diagnosis of HCC, but a negative result does not exclude HCC.

Tumor cells in the majority of HCCs contain only keratin,[10, 47, 137] although a few cases coexpress vimentin.[10] They were also mostly unreactive for EMA.[146] The diagnosis can further be aided by employing antibodies that detect endothelial cells,[47] because such cells, if present in large numbers in FNAs of a hepatic carcinoma and arranged in groups that envelope the clumps of tumor cells, are suggestive of primary HCC (Fig. 38–12). Their presence narrows the differential diagnosis with the most common metastatic cancers to renal cell carcinoma, where they have also been found, and perhaps to some endocrine carcinomas with high vascularity.

Some, mostly well-differentiated, primary HCC show positive staining for keratins 8 and 18 and are negative for keratins 7 and 19.[137] In contrast colorectal carcinomas are keratin-7 negative and keratin-19 positive, and pancreatic duct adenocarcinomas are keratin 7- and 19-positive. However, HCCs display great tumor cell heterogeneity, and at least half may have a keratin

composition identical with colorectal and pancreatic duct adenocarcinomas.[188] Therefore, ICC staining with mAbs to keratins 7, 8, 18, and 19 may not be reliable for distinction of primary and metastatic cancer of the liver.

Hepatocellular carcinomas and medullary thyroid carcinomas do not express S-100.[192, 193] However, cholangiocellular carcinoma as well as stomach and colon adenocarcinomas are positive for S-100 when tested with mAb S-2 but are negative with mAb S-1. In comparison, gallbladder carcinomas, pancreatic carcinomas and thyroid papillary, follicular and anaplastic carcinomas have been reported as S-100 positive with both mAbs. These differences in expression of S-100

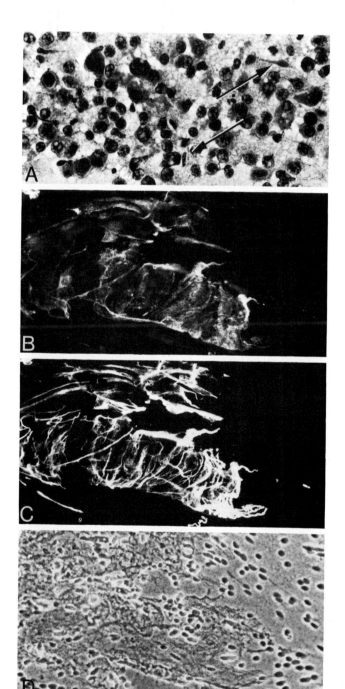

FIGURE 38–12. Fine needle aspiration, **hepatocellular carcinoma.** *A*, Cytology. Dispersed elongated cells (arrows) are intermingled with tumor cells (hematoxylin and eosin; ×250). *B* and *C*, A cluster of tumor cells is enveloped by endothelial cells. Elongated endothelial but not tumor cells are labeled by the mAb BMA 120 in *(B)* and in *(C)* by the guinea pig vimentin Ab (double immunofluorescence on same smear; ×400). *D*, Phase contrast of cells in *B* and *C* (×400). (*B* to *D* reproduced with permission from Domagala W, Lubinski J, Lasota J, et al.: Anal Quant Cytol Histol 11:8–14, 1989.)

as revealed by various mAbs may potentially be helpful in the differential diagnosis of primary and metastatic liver carcinoma and of hepatocarcinoma and cholangiocarcinoma. However, the aforementioned results refer to tissue sections and are based on a limited number of carcinomas.

Gastrointestinal Carcinomas. A gastrointestinal-specific mAb (mAb 29-10) has been isolated.[83] This mAb is sensitive to formaldehyde fixation because it recognizes 22 of 22 cytologic imprints but only two of 26 histologic sections of normal and neoplastic gastrointestinal tissues. On cytologic specimens this mAb appears to be more sensitive than a second widely utilized mAb 19.9. Interestingly, mAb 29-10 sees only 50% of colon polyps.

Thyroid Carcinomas. The presence of thyroglobulin has been found in primary and metastatic follicular and papillary carcinomas of the thyroid in tissue sections[16] and FNAs.[60] Most of them also coexpress keratin and vimentin. Thyroglobulin expression was not found in medullary thyroid carcinomas,[60] a fact that together with the characteristic immunophenotype of this tumor (see previous discussion) helps in differential diagnosis with other thyroid and extrathyroid carcinomas. Antiserum to parathyroid hormone was used in FNAs of parathyroid glands to confirm the parathyroid nature of cells and exclude a thyroid origin.[210] However, rare cases of thyroid carcinomas with features of both parafollicular and follicular differentiation do exist.

Prostatic Adenocarcinomas. Prostate-specific acid phosphatase (PSAP) and prostate-specific antigen (PSA) are helpful markers to determine or rule out the prostatic origin of a tumor in FNA.[89, 127] On tissue sections, in some cases, antisera to one marker may be more sensitive than antibodies to the other,[56] especially in poorly differentiated prostatic carcinomas. In 5 to 10% of such tumors, one of the markers may not be revealed and therefore use of both antisera is recommended.[89]

With regard to specificity, weak false-positive expression of PSAP may occur in some renal and breast carcinomas as well as in a variety of normal cells, e.g., islet cells, hepatocytes, parietal cells of stomach mucosa and granulocytes. Strong immunoreactivity with antisera to PSAP but not to PSA has been reported in some intestinal carcinoids, particularly rectal ones,[84] in some islet cell tumors[84] and in adenocarcinomas but not transitional cell carcinomas of the urinary bladder. A major challenge for differential diagnosis is carcinoid-like prostatic carcinoma. Absence of neurosecretory granules (by electron microscopy) in this tumor may help. Because demonstration of PSAP and PSA by ICC on FNAs is highly specific and sensitive, absence of both markers in a metastatic carcinoma is suggestive of a second tumor.[89]

Non-Hodgkin's Malignant Lymphoma (NHL)[100]

Fine needle aspiration cytology is frequently the first method employed to reveal the nature of enlarged lymph nodes or other lesions. The differential diagnosis between low-grade NHL and benign lymphoid hyperplasia or between high-grade NHL, anaplastic carcinoma and mesenchymal tumor may prove difficult in some cases.[45, 50, 61, 62] The first distinction is discussed later (see Effusions). Here we discuss the immunophenotype of NHLs and their distinction from anaplastic carcinomas.

Three markers are of particular interest: LCA, vimentin and keratin. In a series of 82 NHLs,[46] we found these markers to be sensitive, specific and reliable complementary diagnostic aids that were useful in the definitive diagnosis of NHL in alcohol-fixed FNAs. Tumor cells of all NHLs tested in this study were positive for vimentin and negative for keratin. In more than 85% of the cases, irrespective of their type, over 70% of the tumor cells were strongly vimentin positive (Fig. 38–13 B). Two dominant patterns of vimentin staining were seen in individual tumor cells: dispersed fine filaments and thick bundles of filaments in the form of a sickle, an ellipsoid or a round aggregate lying on one side of the nucleus. Similarly, tumor cells in other cases of NHL in FNA specimens were vimentin positive. In tissue sections differing results have been found. In some studies of frozen material the majority of tumor cells show vimentin,[59, 140, 154] whereas in other studies of formaldehyde-fixed material the majority of cases have been described as vimentin negative.[10, 65] These differences can be attributed to sensitivity of some vimentin antibodies to formaldehyde fixation. Although most lymphomas are vimentin positive, it has been suggested from results on frozen sections that Burkitt's lymphomas are vimentin negative.[123]

All NHLs except one tested for LCA on FNAs or Cytospins reported to date contained LCA-positive cells. The one LCA-negative NHL was a large cell T-cell lymphoma. Leukocyte common antigen positivity in FNAs was usually seen as membrane staining. In intact cells a prominent ring is seen at the periphery (Fig. 38–13 D), whereas membrane fragments stuck to the slide are also strongly stained. The intensity of staining and number of stained tumor cells varied from case to case. These findings are in agreement with the results obtained on cryostat sections, in which 100% of the NHLs, irrespective of their type and including large cell "histiocytic" lymphomas, were immunoreactive for LCA. A specificity of 100% and a sensitivity of 86% have been reported for LCA on paraffin sections,[110] and in another study, 93% of NHLs were positive.[96]

In general, from a practical point of view, vimentin and LCA can be regarded as sensitive, specific and reliable complementary diagnostic adjuncts in the definitive diagnosis of NHL on FNAs. When found together in the same keratin-negative population of tumor cells, they indicate NHL and make the differential diagnosis from other major tumor types possible in the majority of cases. In exceptional cases, when the ICC results with one or both of these markers are ambiguous or negative, one can look for specific gene rearrangements.

As described, the lymphoid nature of malignant tumor cells in FNA can be established by employing a

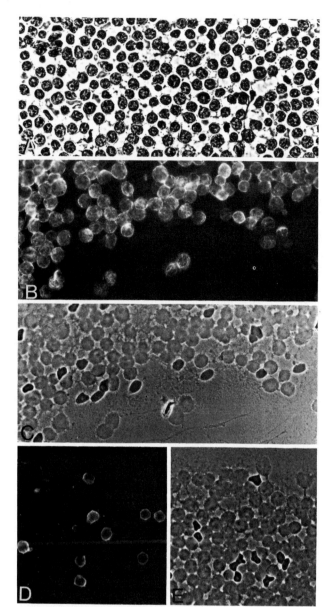

FIGURE 38–13. Fine needle aspiration, **lymphoblastic lymphoma.** *A,* Cytology (hematoxylin and eosin; ×600). *B,* Tumor cells stained with vimentin mAb V9. Note that almost all tumor cells are vimentin positive (indirect immunofluorescence; ×600). *C,* Phase contrast of cells in *B* (×600). *D,* Tumor cells from the same case stained with leukocyte common antigen (LCA) mAb (Dako-LCA; ×600). Less than 10% of the tumor cells are LCA positive (indirect immunofluorescence; ×600). *E,* Phase contrast of cells in *D* (×600). (Reproduced with permission from Domagala W, Lasota J, Chosia M, et al.: Anal Quant Cytol Histol 11:15–21, 1989.)

small panel of mAbs to LCA, keratin and vimentin. Epithelial membrane antigen can also be included. However, malignant lymphoid cells obtained by FNA can be analyzed further for both clonality and subtype utilizing antibodies to various lymphocyte surface markers expressed on B cells, T cells and monocytes.[9, 158, 177] Such an approach helped to confirm the original cytologic diagnosis in 46% of cases and modified it in

24%.[158] A successful subclassification was achieved on FNAs in high-grade NHLs that are diagnosed without difficulty on smears but usually subtyped on sections.[177] We share the opinion of Tani and associates[177] that ICC analysis of lymphoid cells obtained by FNA is comparable to analysis performed on excised lymph nodes. It is therefore helpful in the primary workup of patients with suspected NHLs, especially for diagnosis of rapidly growing tumors, in whom surgical access is difficult.

Epithelial membrane antigen, in principle an epithelial cell marker, is expressed on 100% of Ki-1 lymphomas and on some 12% of other NHLs. One third of T-cell NHLs were found to be EMA positive. Epithelial membrane antigen expression also was found on plasmacytomas and on Reed-Sternberg cells in the lymphocyte predominant type of Hodgkin's disease.[2] Despite this broad spectrum of reactivity the EMA antibody, when utilized with LCA, keratin and vimentin, may be useful in the differential diagnosis of anaplastic tumors and may help to recognize a subset of pleomorphic large-cell NHLs. An occasional Ki-1–positive tumor may be keratin positive. Some Ki-1–positive large-cell anaplastic NHLs, particularly those of T-cell origin, do not exhibit LCA reactivity.[178] Tumor cells of exceptional, large-cell NHLs may be nonreactive with LCA and keratin but stain positively for EMA.

A variable number of keratin-positive dendritic reticulum cells may be found in FNAs from both benign hyperplastic lymph nodes (Fig. 38–14 E) and from NHLs. Their characteristic morphology contrasts with that of NHL tumor cells.

Suggested panel consists of Abs to LCA, vimentin, keratin, κ, λ light chains and lymphocyte surface markers.

Malignant Melanoma

Tumor cells of both amelanotic and melanin-containing melanomas in FNAs express vimentin (Fig. 38–15) and are negative for keratin. In each case we have tested, over 90% of melanoma cells in aspirates were strongly positive for vimentin.[20, 45] Melanoma cells were also LCA negative. Non-Hodgkin's lymphomas and almost all nonmuscle sarcomas are also vimentin positive and keratin negative. Therefore, vimentin positivity supports the diagnosis of melanoma only when the clinical context and morphology of tumor cells are suggestive of this tumor type.

S-100 is helpful in the diagnosis of melanomas in FNAs (see S-100 Proteins).[130] All or almost all melanomas are S-100 positive.[71, 130, 206] Although S-100 is a sensitive marker in the diagnosis of melanomas, it is not a melanoma-specific marker. It can be expressed in a variety of tumors, e.g., occasional carcinomas (ovarian, breast, prostatic), sarcomas (neurogenic) gliomas and some histiocytic-derived tumors.[130]

Several mAbs that specifically react with melanoma cells have been developed (see Melanoma Surface Antigens). The mAb HMB45 gives finely granular

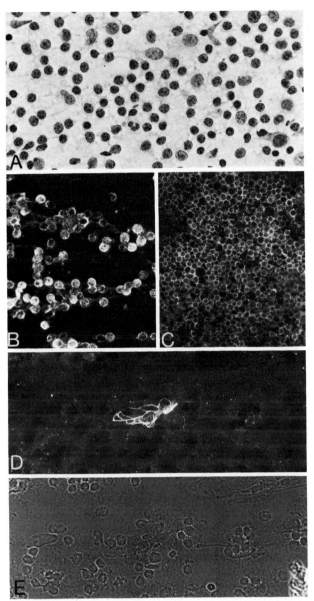

FIGURE 38–14. Fine needle aspiration, **reactive lymph node.** *A,* Cytology (hematoxylin and eosin; ×380). *B,* Dispersed lymphoid cells labeled with vimentin mAb V9. Almost all cells are positive (indirect immunofluorescence; ×380). *C,* Lymphoid cells labeled with leukocyte common antigen (LCA) mAb (Dako-LCA) (indirect immunofluorescence; ×290). *D,* Keratin-positive dendritic reticulum cell. Note the typical morphology that differs from that of lymphocytes. The lymphocytes are keratin negative (indirect immunofluorescence; ×380). *E,* Phase contrast of cells in *D* (×380).

cytoplasmic staining of melanoma cells in aspirates. This mAb has been reported to be highly specific (no false-positive results) but less sensitive (melanomas that are positive range from 70[130] to 92%[202]). However, these may be underestimates because the studies were retrospective on Papanicolaou-stained material (see Melanoma Markers). Therefore, when these or other melanoma-specific antibodies are employed to diagnose melanoma they should be employed preferably on freshly fixed material in a panel.

In summary, melanomas express S-100 and vimentin, are keratin and LCA negative and are positive with mAb HMB45 and other melanoma mAbs.

Suggested panel includes mAb HMB45, S-100, vimentin, keratin and LCA.

Sarcomas

Vimentin is a good general marker for nonmuscle sarcomas in FNAs. In our series of FNAs all nonmuscle sarcomas were vimentin positive (Fig. 38–16).[45] However, vimentin immunoreactivity needs careful interpretation. First, other tumors such as NHLs and malignant melanomas express vimentin. Second, a variety of carcinomas are keratin and vimentin positive (see Table 38–2). Third, a few sarcoma types can coexpress vimentin and keratin (see Table 38–3). They include synovial and epithelioid sarcomas and a rare malignant rhabdoid tumor of soft tissue.[45, 113, 117] In principle, these sarcomas have to be taken into account in differential diagnosis with those carcinomas that coexpress keratin and vimentin. However, these sarcomas are rare, and from a practical point of view only

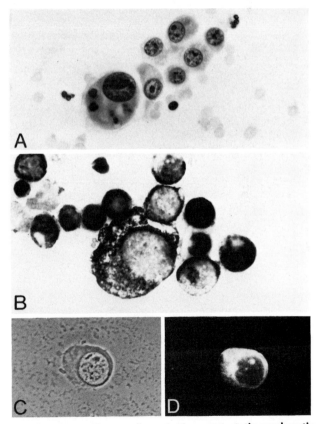

FIGURE 38–15. Fine needle aspiration, **metastatic amelanotic malignant melanoma.** *A,* Cytology (hematoxylin and eosin; ×500). Note anisocytosis, large nucleoli, abundant, sometimes cuboidal cytoplasm and lack of melanin pigment in tumor cells. *B,* Tumor cell cluster stained by mAb V9 to vimentin (immunoperoxidase; ×630). *C,* Phase contrast of a melanoma cell labeled in *(D)* by mAb V9 to vimentin in indirect immunofluorescence (×400).

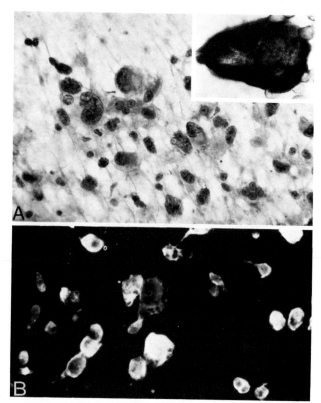

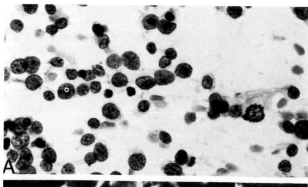

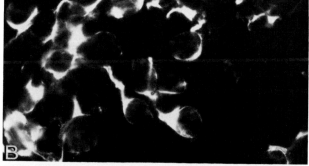

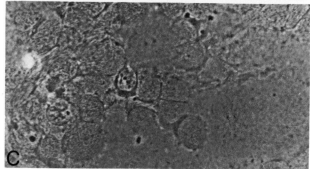

rescence microscopy abundant cytoplasm and long cytoplasmic processes are better revealed than in hematoxylin and eosin stained smears. On occasion, the cytopathologist is struck by the ample cytoplasm of the tumor cells evident in ICC that was thought to be rather scanty in light microscopy.

Poorly differentiated angiosarcomas express Factor VIII–related antigen and blood group antigens. Chordomas express S-100, keratin, EMA and CEA, whereas chondrosarcomas are also S-100 positive but keratin negative.

S-100, which is found in a variety of tumors, e.g., in tumors of glial and Schwann cell origin and in malignant melanomas, can also be found in certain sarcomas including some malignant schwannomas, chondrosarcomas, liposarcomas and clear cell sarcomas. This finding may prove helpful in the distinction of some

FIGURE 38–16. Fine needle aspiration, **osteogenic sarcoma.** A, Cytology (×400). Note pleomorphism of the tumor cells. Some cells with abundant cytoplasm resemble epithelial cells. Inset, A single tumor cell labeled in immunoperoxidase by vimentin mAb V9 (×630). Note that strong, intense staining obliterates the morphology of the nucleus. B, Dispersed sarcoma cells labeled in indirect immunofluorescence by vimentin mAb V9 (×400).

carcinomas metastatic to soft tissues would have to be considered. Clearly, vimentin coexpression in tumor cells in the smears, although helpful in the differential diagnosis of the tumor type, is informative only if specific differential diagnoses are formulated and a panel of several antibodies is used.

Markers of muscle origin have been considered. Desmin Abs distinguish sarcomas of muscle origin, e.g., rhabdomyosarcomas (Fig. 38–17) and leiomyosarcomas from other sarcomas, which contain only vimentin in both histologic and cytologic specimens. For use of desmin mAbs in the differential diagnosis of childhood tumors see the discussion that follows (Small Round Blue Cell Malignant Tumors of Childhood). Other muscle markers include the muscle-specific actin and myosin isoforms, titin and myoglobin, and some of these markers have been used to identify rhabdomyosarcomas in histologic sections.[4, 57, 114, 171, 185] Interestingly, titin is expressed in fewer tumor cells than is desmin,[135] whereas myoglobin is found only in relatively few cells in well-differentiated rhabdomyosarcomas.

The cytoplasm of tumor cells of the majority of sarcomas contains large amounts of intermediate filaments (see Fig. 38–16). Especially in immunofluo-

FIGURE 38–17. Fine needle aspiration, **embryonal rhabdomyosarcoma.** A, Cytology. Dispersed small tumor cells with scanty cytoplasm (hematoxylin and eosin; ×400). B, Elongated cytoplasm of tumor cells (mostly invisible in hematoxylin and eosin stained smears) is strongly labeled by desmin mAb DEB5 in indirect immunofluorescence (×630). C, Phase contrast of cells in B (×630).

malignant schwannomas (vimentin positive, S-100 positive) from conventional fibrosarcomas (vimentin positive, S-100 negative), S-100 positive malignant schwannomas, chondrosarcomas and liposarcomas can be distinguished from a variety of other sarcomas that seem to be nonimmunoreactive for S-100. With regard to the differential diagnosis, myxopapillary ependymoma, chordomas and extraskeletal myxoid chondrosarcoma are positive for S-100; LCA is not expressed in sarcomas.

In summary, nonmuscle sarcomas are vimentin positive; the majority are keratin and EMA negative; myosarcomas are desmin positive and synovial and epithelioid sarcomas and malignant rhabdoid tumor of soft tissues may express keratin, vimentin, EMA and CEA.

The suggested panel includes mAbs to vimentin, desmin, keratin, EMA and S-100.

Small Round Blue Cell Malignant Tumors of Childhood

Almost all neuroblastomas tested so far on tissue sections have been positive for neurofilaments (Fig. 38–18).[19, 91, 125, 134, 184] Although well-differentiated cases are strongly neurofilament positive and express all three NF proteins, in undifferentiated neuroblastomas heterogeneous staining is seen with NF-positive areas alternating with negative ones. In addition, occasional

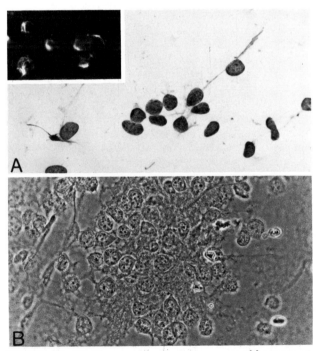

FIGURE 38–18. Fine needle aspiration, **neuroblastoma.** *A,* Cytology. Small round tumor cells in a rosette-like arrangement (hematoxylin and eosin; ×600). *Inset,* Tumor cells labeled by neurofilament mAb NR4 in indirect immunofluorescence; ×600). *B,* Phase contrast of cluster of tumor cells. Note the delicate meshwork of long, thin cell processes (×600).

NF negative (and indeed IF negative) neuroblastomas have been reported. In FNAs a variable number of tumor cells usually with a few delicate NFs in scanty cytoplasm are seen. Care must be taken in FNAs not to misdiagnose as NHL an NF-negative neuroblastoma containing a mixture of benign lymphoid cells (vimentin positive), especially in FNAs from lymph node metastases. All neuroblastomas are synaptophysin[69] and all[134] or almost all[19] are NSE positive. However, neuron-specific enolase does not seem to be a reliable marker because it has been found in some rhabdomyosarcomas and other tumors (see NE Markers Associated with Vesicles and Secretory Granules). Neuroblastomas were negative for keratin, vimentin, desmin and LCA. To distinguish neuroblastomas from primitive neuroectodermal tumors (PNETs) other markers have to be utilized.

The ICC marker profile of rhabdomyosarcomas is very helpful in the differential diagnosis of small round cell malignant tumors of childhood. Desmin has been found in all[8] or almost all[111, 171] rhabdomyosarcomas in tissue sections and in FNAs.[3, 34] Both the large rhabdomyoblasts and small poorly differentiated tumor cells were desmin positive and usually more than 95% of the tumor cells expressed the marker (see Fig. 38–17). Some tumor cells may coexpress vimentin with the percentage of cells that do so being higher in less differentiated tumors. Desmin is expressed in both rhabdomyosarcomas and leiomyosarcomas. However, if found in a small round cell tumor in a child it is more indicative of rhabdomyosarcoma because leiomyosarcomas are rare in a child. In adults, in whom pleomorphic leiomyosarcomas are more frequent than rhabdomyosarcomas, additional tests with mAbs specific for skeletal muscle actin, myosin and titin would be necessary to diagnose rhabdomyosarcoma.

Nephroblastomas (Wilms' tumors) are typically composed of three histologic components: tubuli or glomeruloid bodies, blastema cells and stromal cells. The stromal component can include various cell types, such as fibroblastic, smooth and skeletal muscle. However, Wilms' tumors with only two cell types or monomorphous tumors also occur. This histologic diversity is reflected in FNAs. Immunocytochemistry in FNAs and in tissue sections[6] has shown that the tubuli are keratin and desmoplakin positive and vimentin negative. The majority of stromal cells contain vimentin and in those tumors that show muscle differentiation desmin is found. The IF content of the blastema cells is tumor dependent. In well-differentiated tumors with tubule formation, blastema cells were keratin and vimentin positive. In poorly differentiated ones lacking tubuli, blastema cells were vimentin positive and keratin negative.

Ewing's tumors in FNAs and in tissue sections contain abundant vimentin filaments in almost all their cells.[115] In addition, on tissue sections desmoplakins[121] have been found in all tumors, less than 5% to more than 50% tumor cells. Keratin was coexpressed in scattered and clustered tumor cells in the majority of cases, and in three of 11 cases rare cells expressed neurofilaments.[121] Thus, cytoskeletal heterogeneity

TABLE 38–5. Immunocytochemistry in Malignant Small Round Cell Tumors of Childhood

Tumor Type	KER	VIM	DES	NF	NSE	SY	LCA	S-100
Neuroblastoma	−	−	−	+	+	+	−	+
Rhabdomyosarcoma	−	(+)	+	−	(+)		−	−*
Wilms' tumor								
Blastema	+†	+						
Stroma	−	+	(+)					
Epithelial part	+	−						
Ewing's tumor	F	+		f	f		−	−
Non-Hodgkin's lymphoma	−	+						

*Tumor cells in few cases positive.
†Tumor cells in few cases keratin negative, vimentin positive.
f = Focal positivity in few cases or F in almost all cases.
(+) Variable number of positive tumor cells in some cases.
KER = keratin; VIM = vimentin; DES = desmin; NF = neurofilament; NSE = neurospecific enolase; SY = synaptophysin; LCA = leukocyte common antigen.

(from case to case and among cells within a tumor) seems to be an important feature of Ewing's tumors as compared with other small round cell tumors of childhood. Abundant glycogen is a strong indicator in favor of Ewing's tumor, but it may also be found in neuroblastomas, rhabdomyosarcomas and even in about 10% of NHLs.[111]

Non-Hodgkin's lymphoma often has to be taken into account in the differential diagnosis of small round malignant tumors of childhood. For ICC characteristics see Non-Hodgkin's Malignant Lymphoma.

The salient ICC features that may be helpful in the differential diagnosis of small round blue cell tumors of childhood are listed in Table 38–5.

In summary, neuroblastomas express NF (all or almost all), synaptophysin (~all) and NSE (~all). Rhabdomyosarcomas express desmin (all). Wilms' tumor expresses vimentin or vimentin and keratin (blastema); keratin (tubuli) and vimentin and/or desmin (stroma). For Ewing's tumor, see text. Non-Hodgkin's lymphoma may express LCA (~all) and vimentin (~all) but do not express keratin, NF or desmin.

Suggested panel includes mAbs to keratin, vimentin, desmin, neurofilaments, LCA and synaptophysin.

Fine Needle Aspirations—Differential Diagnosis

Assessment of Need for Immunocytochemistry

With conventional light microscopy and clinical data we estimate that a definitive cytologic diagnosis of tumor type can be provided for 85 to 90% of our FNA material, leaving 10 to 15% of "difficult cases." Obviously, the exact percentages depend on the cytologic material seen in a particular laboratory. One way to try to assess the need for ICC in FNAs is to look at the FNAs in each of these categories employing ICC and compare the results obtained with this method with light microscopy and clinical data. As an example, we cite a study in which we have used IF proteins as markers of tumor type.[45]

Intermediate-filament typing of 271 consecutive cases in which a definitive diagnosis of tumor type had been made by conventional cytologic techniques provided an independent confirmation of tumor type in 262 cases (97%) and changed the diagnosis in nine cases (3%). In these nine cases, the IF content was inconsistent with the cytologic diagnosis. In eight cases diagnosed initially as anaplastic carcinoma only vimentin and no keratin was found. Of these, eight were reclassified as lymphoma and one as melanoma. All eight changes in diagnosis were confirmed by subsequent histology. One further case was reclassified as carotid body tumor rather than carcinoma (Table 38–6).

In the second group, 132 difficult cases were selected in which the tumor type could not be unambiguously diagnosed by conventional methods. In 7% of FNAs malignant cells were diagnosed but no further suggestion of tumor type was made. However, in 93% of FNAs one or two probable tumor types were suggested that greatly facilitated the subsequent use of ICC. Intermediate-filament typing of tumor cells confirmed the original cytologic suggestion of tumor type in 38%, changed it in 7% and could be employed to resolve ambiguities (two probable tumor types suggested) in 45% of cases. In 10% of these difficult cases ICC did not help in the diagnosis. The independent objective information provided by IF typing therefore seems to be of particular value in this second more difficult category of FNAs (see Table 38–5).

Differential Diagnosis of Major Tumor Categories: Carcinoma vs. NHL vs. Melanoma vs. Sarcoma

Immunocytochemistry in diagnostic cytology is perhaps most useful in assisting the differential diagnosis of major tumor categories. Careful interpretation of results of staining with a small panel of antibodies together with morphologic and clinical information can help in reaching the specific diagnosis. Accuracy of diagnosis of major tumor categories on FNAs depends not only on the morphologic features of cells but also

TABLE 38–6. Modification of Cytologic Diagnosis of Major Tumor Types as a Result of Intermediate Filament (IF) Typing of Tumor Cells in FNAs

Initial Diagnosis Based on Cytologic and Clinical Data	No. of Cases	Final Diagnosis Based on Cytologic and Clinical Data and IF Typing of Tumor Cells	
		No. of Cases Positive for Tumor Type Specified in Initial Cytologic Diagnosis	No. of Cases Other Tumor Type Diagnosed and New Diagnosis
1. Positive for Ca	198	189	9 (7 ML, 1 MM, 1 carotid body t)
m-suspicious for Ca	18	13	5 (4 ML, 1 MM)
m-suspicious for Ca or other tumor type	45	11	34 (22 ML, 4 MM, 7 Sa, 1 plasmacytoma)
			(48)
2. Positive for Sa	35	35	0
m-suspicious for Sa	14	14	0
m-suspicious for Sa or other tumor type	12	9	3 (2 Ca, 1 Wilms')
			(3)
3. Positive for ML	24	24	0
m-suspicious for ML	11	8	3 (3 Ca)
m-suspicious for ML or other tumor type	33	25	8 (6 Ca, 1 MM, 1 Sa)
			(11)
4. Positive for MM	10	10	0
m-suspicious for MM	9	9	0
m-suspicious for MM or other tumor type	5	3	2 (2 Ca)
			(2)
5. Positive for malignancy; no tumor type diagnosed or suggested	7		7 (1 Ca, 2 Sa, 3 Wilms, 1 neuroblastoma)

FNAs = fine needle aspirations; Ca = carcinoma; Sa = sarcoma; ML = malignant lymphoma; MM = malignant melanoma; m-suspicious = malignant.
(Reproduced with permission from Domagala W, Lasota J, Chosia M, Szadowska A, Weber K, Osborn M: Cancer 63:504–517, 1989.)

on the clinical, radiologic and other pertinent information available to the cytopathologist, which should be used to phrase the diagnostic question to be answered by ICC. Generally, the more specific the question asked, the less difficult it is to resolve by ICC.[45] Accurate classification of tumors is essential for selection of appropriate therapy.

One example may perhaps explain the importance of a comprehensive approach to the cytologic diagnosis of tumor type utilizing ICC. If malignant cells are present in FNA and the decision to be made is between carcinoma and NHL, use of only two antibodies, to keratin and vimentin, may point the decision in the right direction. If the tumor cells are keratin negative, vimentin positive, such a result is strongly against carcinoma and supports NHL. One may but does not have to (this depends on the degree of uncertainty of the initial cytologic diagnosis and the clinical context) pursue the matter further and confirm the diagnosis utilizing the antibodies to κ and γ chains in search for clonality and with LCA, pan B and pan T cell antibodies or CD markers to confirm and subdivide NHL. If, however, one is not sure whether the tumor is carcinoma, NHL or melanoma, expression of vimentin and lack of keratin merely excludes carcinoma but does not distinguish between NHL and melanoma, because both are vimentin positive. To arrive at a precise diagnosis in context, further tests with antibodies to LCA, pan B and pan T, κ and γ antibodies are required to confirm or exclude NHL. If NHL is excluded, S-100 and at least one melanoma-specific antibody (e.g., HMB45) should be employed to confirm or exclude melanoma.

Usually, from a practical viewpoint, a small panel of mAbs to markers is of great help in the differential diagnosis of major tumor types in FNAs such as carcinoma, NHL, melanoma and sarcoma. This panel may also help in establishing more specific diagnosis. For instance K+ V+ EMA+ S-100− LCA−phenotype in a sarcoma immediately draws attention to synovial or epithelial sarcomas. Alternatively, once a tumor is classified as a carcinoma, other markers with more restricted specificities (e.g., prostate-specific antigen) may be utilized to obtain more information. Table 38–7 may be used as a guideline with the clear understanding that there are exceptions to general rules as described elsewhere in this chapter and that ICC is still in an early stage of development. As larger numbers of tumors are studied the immunophenotypes of particular tumor types will become better defined.

Primary Hepatocellular Carcinoma vs. Metastatic Cancer

Metastases to the liver can be suspected from imaging techniques and abnormal liver test results. However, a definitive diagnosis requires confirmation by examining the morphology of cells in FNAs. The judicious use of ICC and electron microscopy may be of help in the differential diagnosis between HCC and metastases from other sites and in suggesting the primary origin of metastatic tumors. Thus, lengthy and expensive workups in the search for a primary in a patient with poor prognosis may be avoided.

TABLE 38–7. Immunocytochemistry in the Differential Diagnosis of Major Tumor Categories

Tumor	KER	VIM	EMA	LCA	S-100	CEA
Carcinoma	+	−/+	+/−	−	−/+	+/−
Lymphoma (NHL)	−*	+	−/+	+	−	
Melanoma	−	+	−	−	+/−	
Sarcoma	−†	+‡	−§	−	v‖	−§

−/+ Majority negative, some positive (see text); +/− Majority positive, a few negative (see text).
*Some Ki-1 NHL may express keratin.
†Synovial and epithelioid sarcomas and malignant rhabdoid tumor of soft tissue may coexpress keratin and vimentin. Occasional leiomyosarcomas may coexpress keratin and desmin.
‡ Some myosarcomas express only desmin.
§ Synovial and epithelioid sarcomas, positive.
‖ Variable reaction depending on sarcoma type. (KER = keratin; VIM = vimentin; EMA = epithelial membrane antigen; LCA = leukocyte common antigen; CEA = carcinoembryonic antigen.)

A *suggested panel* includes mAbs to AFP, vimentin, Factor VIII and to keratins nos. 7, 8, 18 and 19 and EMA and S-100.

Other Specific Problems of Differential Diagnosis

A parathyroid hormone antibody was utilized to confirm a parathyroid origin of cells in FNAs from patients with hyperparathyroidism.[210] This antibody and antibodies to calcitonin and thyroglobulin may help to distinguish cells of thyroid and parathyroid origin. Silver stains that demonstrate argyrophilic granules in the cytoplasm of parathyroid cells are not 100% specific, e.g., medullary thyroid carcinoma may also be argyrophilic.[155]

Immunocytochemistry may help to solve many other specific problems of differential cytologic diagnosis. For further details, see other discussions in this chapter, e.g., for differential diagnosis of mesothelioma versus adenocarcinoma see Mesothelioma vs. Adenocarcinoma, of NHLs and small-cell anaplastic carcinomas see Non-Hodgkin's Malignant Lymphoma and of small round cell tumors of childhood see Small Round Blue Cell Malignant Tumors of Childhood.

Effusions

In cytologic diagnosis of effusions five major practical areas of differential diagnosis have to be clarified: (1) reactive mesothelial cells vs. adenocarcinoma, (2) reactive mesothelial cells vs. mesothelioma, (3) mesothelioma vs. adenocarcinoma, (4) reactive lymphoid cells vs. NHL and (5) site of primary tumor.

Before discussing the immunologic markers attention is drawn to the claim that determination of the number of nuclear organizing regions can distinguish reactive mesothelial cells from mesothelioma from carcinoma see Benign vs. Malignant.[39]

Reactive Mesothelial Cells vs. Adenocarcinoma

The mAb B72.3, which is directed against a tumor-associated antigen—TAG-72—had a 95% overall recognition for adenocarcinomas on paraffin-embedded effusions,[85, 176] whereas reactive mesothelial cells were negative under the same conditions. Furthermore, no reactivity was demonstrated in any cell type in a series of 821 benign effusions.[86]

Adenocarcinoma cells in effusions are strongly positive for EMA and other epithelial membrane antigens (Fig. 38–19).[26, 37, 73, 75, 76, 183, 201] The percentage of positive cases is high, ranging from 54[183] to 100%.[75, 170, 201] Although immunoreactivity for EMA in mesothelial cells in effusions has been somewhat controversial,[64, 73, 75, 183, 187, 201] it seems that in most cases reactive mesothelial cells do not stain with mAb to EMA or show only weak reactivity.[73, 75, 170, 201]

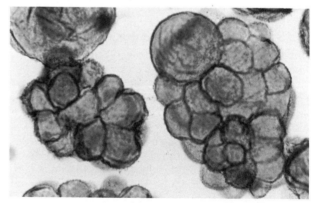

FIGURE 38–19. Ascites, **papillary serous adenocarcinoma of the ovary.** Surfaces of tumor cells forming clumps are labeled with mAb HEA-125 to epithelial membrane antigen (immunoperoxidase; ×450). (Reproduced with permission from Guzman J, Hilgarth M, Bross KJ, Costabel U, Yeck-Kapp G, Wiehle N, Huber A, Grunert F, v. Kleist S, Pfleiderer A: Gynäkol Prax 12:679–689, 1988.)

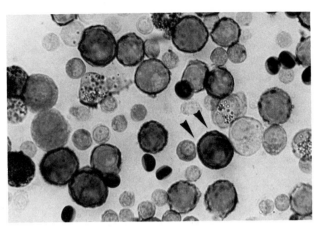

FIGURE 38–20. Pleural fluid, **metastatic breast carcinoma.** The surfaces of the tumor cells are labeled with mAb CEA3-13 (arrowheads) in immunoperoxidase. (CEA) Carcinoembryonic–antigen negative macrophages have phagocytosed latex particles. The CEA–negative small cells are lymphocytes. The small darkly stained small cells are erythrocytes with endogenous peroxidase staining (×520). (Reproduced with permission from Guzman J, Costabel U, Bross KJ, Wiehle U, Grunert F, Schaefer H-E: Acta Cytol 32:188–192, 1988.)

Adenocarcinomas also stain strongly for CEA (Fig. 38–20), however, with lower frequency. Tumor cells that are CEA positive support the diagnosis of adenocarcinoma, although it by no means excludes other histologic types and does not identify the origin of the tumor. A negative result does not exclude adenocarcinoma, because various percentages of carcinomas were negative for CEA in different series (e.g., as low as 37%[131]; as high as 70%, breast carcinomas[73]). Generally, mesothelial cells do not stain or stain only weakly for CEA, although strong positive staining for CEA in two benign effusions has been reported.[116]

In one study, a panel composed of CEA and EMA was positive in 91% of carcinomas.[170] When small-cell carcinomas of the lung were excluded, EMA identified 100% of carcinomatous effusions and CEA, 91%. Therefore, despite weak reactivity expressed by some reactive mesothelial cells and occasional rare cases of benign effusions with strong reactivity,[74, 170] it seems that EMA and CEA may be useful markers in the identification of adenocarcinoma cells in effusions.

Weak peripheral CEA staining of some reactive mesothelial cells or "spiky" or "hairy" EMA patterns on some mesothelial cells[74] may be explained in part by trapping of a reaction product among surface microvilli with which a subpopulation of such cells is endowed.[44] The morphologic pattern of EMA positivity may not be a reliable discriminator between mesothelial cells (spiky pattern) and adenocarcinoma cells ("linear" pattern) as suggested,[74] because cancer cells in effusions may also be covered by numerous microvilli. In addition, mAbs to Leu M1 (CD15 granulocyte antigen) and BMA/070 (CD 16 NK and cytotoxic cell antigen) did not react with mesothelial cells, although they stained carcinoma cells.[75]

Estrogen-receptor antibodies have been suggested as a tool to identify metastatic breast carcinoma in effusions from patients without solid tissue metastases.

Although reactive mesothelial cells were negative, in a larger series of cases ER-negative breast carcinomas would be misdiagnosed as false negative or as metastases from extramammary sites. In addition, ER has been reported in extramammary carcinomas (e.g., endometrial, endocervical, ovarian).

Adenocarcinomas are always keratin positive, if appropriately fixed material is used and if keratin antibodies, which have broad specificity or which recognize the simple epithelial keratins, e.g., keratins (7), 8, 18 and 19, are used. Fetal as well as normal diploid pleural and peritoneal mesothelial cells show keratins 8, 18 and 19 in two-dimensional gels. Thus, it is unlikely that antibodies specific for individual keratins will help in this differential diagnosis. Reactive and malignant mesothelial cells have been reported to contain a distinctive perinuclear pattern of keratin reactivity as opposed to the arborizing pattern typical of adenocarcinomas.[88] However, because of the overlap in patterns,[132, 170] this does not seem to be a reliable criterion. Vimentin is characteristic of mesothelial cells and of some, but not all, adenocarcinomas growing in effusions.

In summary, currently no reliable marker exists to distinguish exfoliated, reactive mesothelial cells from adenocarcinoma cells in effusions. However, a panel of four mAbs, to mAb B72.3, EMA, CEA and Leu M1 may help solve this problem. Strong reactivity with all four supports the diagnosis of adenocarcinoma or other carcinoma. A negative result with these mAbs favors reactive mesothelial cells over adenocarcinoma. Because not all adenocarcinomas show positivity for B72.3, EMA or CEA, a negative result must be interpreted with caution, although the probability of an adenocarcinoma being unreactive for these markers is low.

Suggested panel includes mAb B72.3 and mAbs to EMA, CEA and Leu M1.

Reactive Mesothelial Cells vs. Mesothelioma

Immunocytochemistry is of little help in distinguishing reactive from malignant mesothelial cells. As mentioned, mAb B72.3 and mAb to CEA are nonreactive with both types of cells. Variable numbers (3 to 99%) of moderately to intensely EMA-stained malignant cells were found in 100% or almost 100% of epithelial mesotheliomas.[73, 187, 201] Staining was diffuse and peripherally accentuated or confined mainly to the periphery of tumor cells owing to heavy stain of microvilli (Fig. 38–21). In most instances, mesothelial cells seem negative for EMA,[187, 201] although faint staining[201] as well as even strong staining in some cases[73, 183] has been reported. These results suggest that the interpretation of EMA staining in an effusion should be approached with the clear understanding that EMA-negative mesotheliomas do exist and that rare EMA-positive reactive mesothelial cells may occur.

Mesothelial cells and mesotheliomas are keratin positive and, in many instances, vimentin positive. Thus, neither the IF content nor the keratin patterns seem

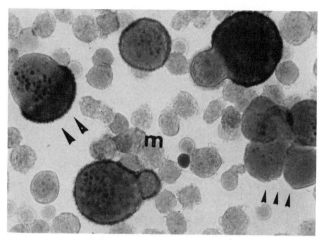

FIGURE 38–21. Pleural fluid, **mesothelioma.** Tumor cells are partially or totally positive with mAb to EMA (large arrowheads). Note the hairy reaction pattern at the surface indicating microvilli. Macrophages (m), lymphocytes and some tumor cells (small arrowheads) are negative (immunoperoxidase; ×580). (Reproduced with permission from Guzman J, Bross KJ, Würtemberg G, Costabel U: Chest 95:580–595, 1989.)

currently useful in this differential diagnosis (see also Reactive Mesothelial Cells vs. Adenocarcinoma and the following discussion).

Mesothelioma vs. Adenocarcinoma

The mAb B72.3 showed a highly selective reactivity for adenocarcinomas, particularly adenocarcinomas of the lung, vs. pleural malignant mesotheliomas in effusions.[86, 176]

Leu-M1 seems one of the more reliable markers in the differential diagnosis between malignant mesothelioma of epithelial type and adenocarcinoma, especially pulmonary adenocarcinoma. Although the majority of adenocarcinomas on tissue sections and in malignant effusions show cytoplasmic staining, mesotheliomas are Leu-M1 negative.[73, 75, 168]

Another useful marker may be CEA. In effusions, CEA in cell clusters seems to exclude a mesothelial origin.[73, 107, 131, 165] Adenocarcinomas are positive for CEA to different extents. However, different CEA mAbs can recognize different epitopes of the CEA molecule. These epitopes can have different patterns of cross-reaction with other glycoproteins, which may be present on mesotheliomas. Therefore, each mAb to CEA should be first tested carefully before it is selected for the differential diagnosis with mesothelioma. It seems that earlier reports claiming the presence of CEA in epithelial mesotheliomas could have been caused by the employment of antisera with contaminating antibodies to other antigens, such as to a nonspecific cross-reacting antigen (NCA), a glycoprotein that shares some antigenic sites with CEA. For instance, strong staining for CEA in myeloid or monocytic cells may be attributed to antibodies to NCA.

Regarding the expression of EMA on malignant mesothelial cells, conflicting results have been pub-

lished. In some reports, however,[73, 187] an EMA mAb (DAKO) has been utilized to show convincingly that effusions of almost all malignant mesotheliomas contained varying numbers of EMA-positive tumor cells (see Fig. 38–21). This finding is in agreement with some earlier reports.[183, 201] Thus, because many carcinomas stain with EMA, this marker seems not to be a reliable tool for differential diagnosis between malignant mesothelioma and carcinoma in effusions. Malignant mesotheliomas have also been reported as negative (0/7) for oncofetal antigens, such as AFP, SP1 and PLAP, whereas roughly half of carcinomas were positive with at least one of these markers.[131]

When one reviews the data on the IF content of mesotheliomas,[12] data from solid tumors show that in addition to keratins 8, 18 and 19, the epithelial and biphasic types can also coexpress keratin 7 (11/12 cases) and keratin 5 (11/12 cases), with different tumors showing very different amounts of keratins 7 and 5. Comparable data are not available for mesotheliomas growing in effusions. Perhaps it might be interesting to look with keratin 5 mAbs to see if they can discriminate mesothelioma from adenocarcinoma which does not express keratin 5. The keratin filament pattern again seems unreliable for this differential diagnosis. Interestingly, when vimentin was looked at in solid mesothelioma, tumor cells of the epithelial type of mesothelioma were vimentin negative or in one case focally positive. In the biphasic type only the spindle cells of the fibrous type expressed vimentin and keratin. In effusions most mesotheliomas are reported to be vimentin positive.[151] Thus, vimentin may not be able to discriminate between mesotheliomas and those adenocarcinomas that also express vimentin. In addition it is still not clear whether a higher percentage of carcinomas in effusions as opposed to FNAs coexpress both IF proteins.

Currently, no single reliable, mesothelial-cell specific antibody exists. Thus, the differential diagnosis of malignant mesothelioma and adenocarcinoma in effusions can be aided only by careful interpretation of negative results.

In summary, negative results with B72.3, Leu-M1 and CEA on tumor cells in effusions support mesothelioma over adenocarcinoma.

Suggested panel includes mAbs to B72.3, Leu-M1 and CEA.

Reactive Lymphoid Cells vs. NHL

The cytologic distinction of lymphocyte-rich effusions from NHL may be difficult purely on morphologic grounds. Inflammation (e.g., tuberculosis), nonspecific reaction due to other non-neoplastic diseases or chronic lymphocytic leukemia and lymphocytic or low-grade NHL have all to be considered. B- and T-cell enumeration using ICC may help obtain the proper diagnosis in some cases. Benign lymphocyte-rich effusions were characterized by a predominance of T cells (>80%),[43, 64, 67, 173] with an excess of helper to inducer cells (mean helper to suppressor ratio 3:0)[64, 173] and by a κ to λ chain ratio of 1:6 on B cells.[173] In B-cell NHLs, and in chronic lymphocytic leukemias, the percentage of T cells showed a decrease, whereas the percentage of B cells showed a dramatic increase.[43, 64, 95, 173] Monoclonal light chain immunoglobulin expression was reported in the majority but not in all B-cell NHLs. Use of mAbs to B and T cells, and to LCA,[106] allowed a definitive diagnosis of NHL or benign reactive effusion in every case studied. Immunocytochemistry results modified the morphologic diagnosis in over 50% of cases. However, the immunologic pattern of rare peripheral T-cell NHLs may not differ from that of benign lympho-cyte-rich fluids. Occasional equivocal results may be obtained in effusions that contain carcinoma cells and numerous lymphoid cells. Nevertheless, a panel of mAbs (to LCA, keratin, immunoglobulin κ and λ chains, "pan-B" mAbs) may help confirm a cytologic suggestion of NHL, especially in unusual locations that are difficult for surgical biopsy, e.g., in pericardial effusions due to primary cardiac NHL.

Some leukocyte differentiation antigens are expressed throughout most stages of lymphocyte maturation and differentiation, e.g., CD45 (leukocyte common antigen) or CD 19, CD 20 (known as "pan B") and CD3 (known as "pan T") antigens. Others are expressed only during a short phase of development. (For CD nomenclature for leukocyte antigens see reference 108.) Some monocyte/macrophage–specific antigens (e.g., CD 14 and CD 33) are known, but no pan monocyte/macrophage antigen has yet been found.

If lymphoma is to be distinguished from leukemia cells, CD 13 antigen (My 7, early myelomonocytic proliferations) and CD 15 (Leu-M1) or CD 33 (My 9, more mature proliferations) may be employed. B-cell NHLs may be defined by CD 19, 20 and 22 and T-cell NHLs by CD 2 and CD 3, although CD 2 and CD 3 are not expressed in immature T-cell cases. In interpreting negative results it is important to know that some antigens may be lost during malignant transformation. Kappa or λ light chain ICC may help distinguish NHL with intracytoplasmic immunoglobulin inclusions from adenocarcinoma with cytoplasmic mucin aggregates.

Site of Primary Tumor

Despite the overall poor prognosis in patients with disseminated cancer, a search for the primary seems to be justified because some patients with metastatic adenocarcinomas (e.g., of prostatic or breast origin) can still benefit from therapy.

Immunocytochemistry when utilized with clinical information and careful interpretation of morphology of the tumor cells may help to identify the site of origin of tumor cells in effusions in the patient with an unknown primary. Thus, a panel of six mAbs to tumor-associated glycoproteins and glycolipids helped to identify the site of the primary in 87% of effusions due to metastatic breast, ovarian and lung carcinomas.[124] These mAbs were not 100% specific for a given tumor type but when used together in a panel they yielded

fairly specific patterns. Some of these mAbs, e.g., OC125, react also with mesothelial cells. Further studies on a larger number of effusions are needed to evaluate the practical usefulness of these mAbs.

Expression of thyroglobulin indicates a thyroid origin of carcinoma cells in effusion.[143] Antibodies to PSAP or PSA can confirm or exclude the prostatic origin of a carcinoma in effusions.[15, 143] A positive result is important because hormonal therapy may be introduced. In patients with prostatic carcinomas, the majority of effusions are due to non-neoplastic processes, a few are due to metastases from prostatic cancer and some may be due to a second primary tumor.[15] For instance, ten of 33 effusions in patients with prostatic carcinoma with PSAP-negative tumor cells were found to be caused by a second primary tumor.[15] A panel of several Abs may help to find or exclude a second tumor metastasizing to serous cavities in patients with other malignancies.

Expression of CEA in carcinomas in effusions is variable but seems to show some preferences depending on the origin of the primary tumor.[131, 143] It is rare in serous ovarian carcinomas[143] but more frequent in gastrointestinal and bronchial carcinomas[131, 165] than in carcinomas of the breast.[143] Expression of CEA is absent[143] or very rare in prostatic carcinomas.[148] Elevated levels of CEA by an enzyme immunoassay in an effusion with an unknown primary seems to be a useful marker for the detection of gastrointestinal, pulmonary and breast carcinomas. Malignant ascites that is negative for CEA in a female suggests ovarian carcinoma.[148]

From a practical viewpoint a differential diagnosis between epithelial and nonepithelial tumor cells, excluding NHLs, is less important because the latter are rare in effusions. However, antibodies to S-100 may help to identify malignant melanoma in effusions. In one study,[99] four of seven melanomas were positive for S-100, whereas all benign effusions and other malignant effusions were negative.[147] Neuroendocrine origin of a metastatic tumor may be revealed by expression of synaptophysin (Fig. 38–22).

Cerebrospinal Fluid (CSF) and Other Cytologic Specimens from the Central Nervous System

Early diagnosis of disseminated cancer with meningeal involvement can be facilitated by a correct morphologic identification of tumor cells in CSF. However, especially in patients with no prior documentation of cancer even if the malignant nature of cells in CSF is recognized, it may be difficult to distinguish primary CNS tumors from metastatic carcinomas, lymphomas and leukemias or other malignant tumors. Furthermore, as in effusions, small lymphocytes have to be distinguished from well-differentiated NHL or leukemias. In principle, the ICC results on cells in effusions can also be applied to similar problems in CSF. However, because the amount of CSF for cytologic examination is usually small and the number of cells low, special preparative procedures may be required to

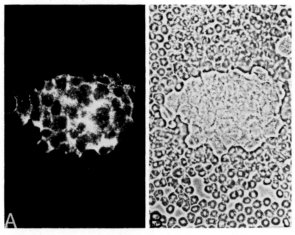

FIGURE 38–22. Ascites, **metastatic gastrointestinal carcinoid.** *A,* A cluster of tumor cells labeled with synaptophysin mAb SY 38 in indirect immunofluorescence (×320). Note the punctate pattern typical of synaptophysin reactivity. These cells were also keratin positive. *B,* Phase contrast of the cells in *A* (×320). (Reproduced with permission from Wiedenmann B, Kuhn C, Schwechheimer K, Waldherr R, Raue F, Brandeis WE, Kommerell B, Franke WW. Am J Clin Pathol 88:560–569, 1987.)

increase the cell yield.[174] (For a review of the various detection systems that can be used for ICC of CSF see reference 213). Immunocytochemistry analysis of CSF lymphoid cells with mAbs to lymphocyte/leucocyte markers seems to be a useful adjunct in CSF cytodiagnosis and may help to diagnose unequivocally NHL/leukemia of the CNS.[24, 106, 158, 214] Although no single antibody was diagnostic of any tumor type, a panel comprised of mAbs to GFAP, mAb B72.3 and a panleukocyte antibody helped to differentiate among primary brain tumors, metastases, NHLs and leukemias in a series of 53 specimens (CSF, brain cyst and ventricular fluids, needle washings and imprints).[196] The mAbs to GFAP have also been applied to cytologic diagnosis of brain tumors.[27]

Several difficult problems of CNS cytopathology cannot be resolved with the help of currently existing mAbs, e.g., the differential diagnosis between reactive gliosis and astrocytomas, the determination of the primary site of some metastases and the differential diagnosis between primitive tumors of CNS, such as retinoblastoma and medulloblastoma.

Benign vs. Malignant

Several instances occur in which ICC may help.

Non-Hodgkin's Lymphomas vs. Benign Lymphoproliferative Disorders. Analysis of clonality of the lymphoid cell population in FNA by monoclonal antibodies to immunoglobulin κ and λ light chains or to heavy chains (mu-chain) may help to distinguish between reactive lymphadenitis (polyclonal pattern) and NHLs (monoclonal staining pattern).[103, 177] This distinction is especially important in the diagnosis of low- and inter-

mediate-grade NHLs. However, some lymphomas do not show any clear-cut monoclonal pattern in FNAs or in surgical biopsy samples; therefore, ICC results may remain inconclusive. In such cases the detection of immunoglobulin gene, or T-cell receptor gene, rearrangements may help. Some cases with an early involvement of the lymph nodes may also present difficulties in both cytologic and ICC analyses. In lymphocyte-rich serous effusions, ICC studies of lymphoid cells may help to differentiate reactive from neoplastic lymphoproliferation (see Reactive Lymphoid Cells vs. Non-Hodgkin's Lymphoma).[215]

Carcinoma vs. Benign Lesions. In FNAs, positive staining with mAb B72.3 was observed in the great majority of "non-small cell" carcinomas of the lung, adenocarcinomas of the colon and breast and carcinomas from other body sites. In contrast benign lesions from the breast, lung, pancreas, parotid and thyroid showed no staining.[86] This antibody generally is unreactive with a variety of normal adult tissues including those of the colon, ovary and breast with the exception of mammary apocrine metaplasia and postovulatory endometrium. Phrases such as "great majority" or "most benign lesions" are not equivalent to "all" but imply the existence of exceptions in these studies.

Disseminated single carcinoma cells can be identified by mAbs in several anatomic sites against a contrasting background of benign cells of different histogenetic origin. For instance, in bone marrow, metastatic colorectal and breast carcinoma cells can be identified by employing a keratin antibody.[161] In patients with no distant metastases (Mo), ICC increased the percentage of cases in which such cells were found from 0 to 14%. In patients with metastasis (MI) such cells were found in 5 to 7% of cases with conventional cytology, but in 38% of cases with ICC.[161] The mAb to EMA has also been utilized to identify malignant cells in bone marrow, but because it cross-reacts with occasional plasma and lymphoid cells keratin is probably a better reagent for this purpose.

Demonstration of carcinocythemia in disseminated breast cancer has been facilitated by antibodies to CEA, EMA and LCA in mononuclear cell suspensions from blood. Carcinoma cells were CEA+, EMA+LCA− and OKMI−.[216]

In smears from FNAs of lymph nodes, a chance always exists that a few cancer cells might be overlooked. In comparison, enlarged histiocytes with prominent nucleoli can mimic cancer cells. Broadly reacting keratin antibodies can confirm a negative diagnosis of carcinoma if no positive cells are found. A positive reaction with antibody to keratin is a strong indication for the presence of metastatic carcinoma cells in FNA of the lymph node.[151] However, the cytopathologist must first exclude that they are benign keratin-positive cells, i.e., dendritic reticulum cells (see Fig. 38–14C), benign cells from rare glandular epithelial inclusions within the lymph nodes or epithelial cells from an epithelium through which the needle passed on its way to the lymph node.

Reactive Mesothelial Cells vs. Adenocarcinoma in Effusions. The use of mAb B72.3 is illustrated in Fig.

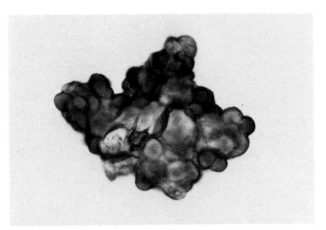

FIGURE 38–23. Malignant peritoneal effusion of **serous cystadenocarcinoma of the ovary** prepared by cytocentrifugation. Stained with mAb B72.3. Note staining at the membrane and in some cells in cytoplasm (×400). (Reproduced with permission from Johnston WW, Szpak CA, Thor A, Simpson JF, Schlom J: Cancer Invest 5:593–611, 1987.)

38–23. For further details on this mAb and mAbs to EMA, CEA and Leu-M1, see Reactive Mesothelial Cells vs. Adenocarcinoma.

Markers of Proliferative Activity. Classically, proliferative activity has been estimated by measuring the number of mitoses. However, this activity of a tumor can be determined with mAbs to the proliferation-associated nuclear antigen Ki67. The Ki67 growth fraction (GF) is four to five times higher in malignant breast tumors than in benign tumors. The Ki67 GF of benign tumors as assessed on cytologic specimens seems not to exceed 10%, whereas the range for malignant tumors is 0 to 70%.[99] A second antigen, PNCA/cyclin (Mr 36kD) is a nuclear protein found associated with DNA polymerase. Its expression peaks

in the late G1/S phase of the cell cycle. PNCA/cyclin can also be used to estimate the proliferative grade of tumors. Data on 41 methacarn-fixed tumors with antibody 19A2 in ICC showed a good correlation between the percentage of cells stained with cyclin antibodies and the percentage of cells in S phase calculated from flow cytometry.[61] The Ki67 GF seems also to correlate with the number of nuclear organizing regions (AgNORs) as measured by a silver colloid technique on NHLs.[31] In histologic sections it appears able to distinguish, for instance, malignant melanoma (mean 9.18 AgNORs) from melanotic nevi (mean 1.27 AgNORs).[102] On cytologic specimens, reactive mesothelial cells (mean 15.57 AgNORs) could be distinguished from mesothelioma (mean 30.08 AgNORs) from carcinoma (mean 43.45 AgNORs) (Fig. 38–24).[39] However, not all studies with this technique have been able to demonstrate such clear differences between benign and malignant cells (see reference 66).

Other Applications

Immunocytochemistry has been applied to the cytologic diagnosis of infections including the detection of human polyoma virus in urinary sediment,[1] human papilloma virus antigen in cervicovaginal smears, chlamydial antigen in both urethral scrapings and in prostatic aspirates,[128] in cytodiagnosis of herpes simplex keratosis and in a search for *Trichomonas vaginalis*.[129]

Nonsquamous cells (granulocytes, monocytes, lymphocytes, renal epithelial and urothelial cells) in urine, in acute tubular necrosis, in drug-related acute intestinal nephritis and in crescentic glomerulonephritis can be precisely identified employing mAbs in ICC.[164] In contrast by morphologic examination of the urine without such methods, it is impossible to determine from which part of the nephron epithelial cells are exfoliated.

Immunocytochemistry has also been utilized to demonstrate glial and neuronal cells in the amniotic fluid of anencephalic pregnancies.[198]

PROGNOSTIC SIGNIFICANCE OF IMMUNOCYTOCHEMISTRY IN CYTOLOGIC SPECIMENS

Immunocytochemistry staining on histologic specimens or on FNAs can yield information relevant to grading of particular tumor types and this information may be of relevance in planning primary treatment. We list several examples as follows.

Proliferation Markers. In FNAs of breast carcinomas high levels of Ki67 GF are associated with a poor prognosis.[99] Counts of AgNORs enabled discrimination between high-grade and low-grade NHLs in sections.[32]

Epidermal Growth Factor Receptor (EGFR). Epidermal growth factor acts by binding to EGFR on the cell surface. In early gastric carcinomas only 3.8% are EGFR positive, whereas in advanced ones 34.4% are

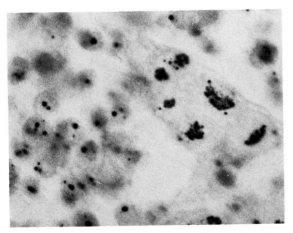

FIGURE 38–24. Adenocarcinomatous effusion. The six neoplastic cells on the right can be distinguished from the reactive non-neoplastic cells on the left on the basis of the silver staining for AgNOR proteins (×1250). (Reproduced with permission from Derenzini M, Nardi F, Farabegoli F, Ottinetti A, Roncaroli F, Bussolati G: Acta Cytol 33:491–500, 1989.)

EGFR positive.[217] In primary breast carcinoma relapse-free survival and overall survival were significantly worse in EGFR-positive than in EGFR-negative patients.[160]

ER Status. This is regarded as an important determinant of pathologic features and of clinical behavior of breast carcinomas and hence seems to have value in predicting recurrence-free survival and treatment planning. Estrogen receptors can be assayed on FNAs of breast carcinomas or on effusions by ICC methods (ER-ICA assay*) utilizing mAbs.[40, 104] The assay is simple and quick but requires formol and acetone and methanol fixation. The reliability of the ER-ICA assay on cytologic specimens is underscored by its 94% specificity and 100% sensitivity as compared with the dextran-coated charcoal assay performed on cytosols.[40] The ER-ICA assay on FNAs has several advantages. It facilitates preoperative evaluation. Estrogen receptors can be estimated at the time of recurrence or from a metastasis by less invasive procedures than a biopsy, and repetitive sampling can be applied in the therapeutic follow-up of breast cancers during hormone therapy.

Intermediate Filaments. We describe three examples. First, vimentin coexpression in breast carcinomas seems to be strongly associated with known poor prognostic indicators, such as high Ki67 GF, positive EGFR, negative ER and high histologic grade. Thus, vimentin has been shown to be preferentially expressed in ER-negative and low ER breast carcinomas.[22, 42] Vimentin expression is also associated with high Ki67 growth fraction,[42] with EGFR-positive breast carcinomas and with carcinomas of high histologic grade.[42, 156] In renal cell carcinomas, vimentin coexpression correlates well with high nuclear grade with vimentin-positive nuclear grade III tumors showing a particularly poor prognosis.[54] Second, breast carcinoma patients with keratin positive cells in the bone marrow relapse with a much higher rate than those without (81% vs. 11%).[141, 161] Third, mAb specific for keratin 18 stained only umbrella cells of transitional epithelium. In well-differentiated (grade I) transitional cell carcinoma, only the superficial layers of papillary structures were stained, whereas in high-grade invasive tumors almost all tumor cells were keratin 18 positive.[152]

S-100. This is present in Schwann cells in the well-developed stromal area of the more differentiated neuroblastic tumors, such as ganglioneuroblastoma and ganglioneuroma. The increased incidence of S-100 protein–positive cells found in the thin septal portion of the supportive stroma can indicate maturation and has been correlated with improved prognosis for neuroblastomas in general and undifferentiated neuroblastomas in particular.[169]

Oncogene Products. Some reports suggest that alterations in specific cellular proto-oncogenes may be associated with clinically aggressive tumors.[218] Amplification of *N-myc* in neuroblastomas[163] and of *c-erbB2* oncogene in breast carcinomas are perhaps the best

known examples. Strong membrane staining with antibody to the *c-erbB2* oncoprotein, which is known to correlate with gene amplification, was associated with earlier relapse, shorter post relapse and overall survival in breast cancer patients.[211]

Carbohydrates. Changes in carbohydrate expression have been correlated with the invasive and metastatic properties of tumor cells.[78] Binding of *Helix pomatia* agglutinin to *N*-acetyl-galactosaminyl oligosaccharide in ICC has been shown to be associated with a poor prognosis in a retrospective study of breast carcinoma.[98] (Other examples of lectins in ICC can be found in reference 33.)

TECHNIQUES

Common ICC techniques are presented in Figures 38–25 and 38–26. The decisions to be made by the cytologist before beginning with ICC include (1) how to fix, permeabilize and store cell smears, (2) which primary antibodies to purchase, (3) which method of detection should be used and (4) how to document the results.

Fixation. In general the methods employed to fix cell smears for routine light microscopy, i.e., immedi-

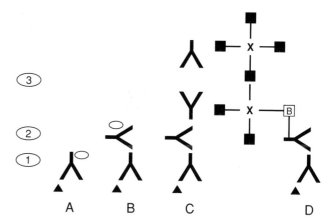

FIGURE 38–25. *A,* In a **one-step direct method** the labeled antibody reacts directly with the antigen. *B,* In a **two-step indirect method** the labeled second antibody is bound to the antigen via an unlabeled first antibody. *C,* In the **three-step method** a bridging antibody links the first antibody with a labeled antibody complex from the same species as the first antibody. *D,* Detection with a labeled avidin-biotin complex is shown (ABC method). Antigen is represented by triangles. Fluorochrome, peroxidase or gold label is represented by ovals with dots. Peroxidase or alkaline phosphatase is represented by the antibody used in step one, e.g., mouse mAb against, e.g., vimentin. Antibody in step two could then be a rabbit antimouse IgG. In *C,* step three, a preformed peroxidase antiperoxidase mouse mAb (PAP complex) or, alternatively, an alkaline phosphatase antialkaline phosphatase mouse mAb (APAAP complex) could be used. In *D* the unlabeled mouse mAb in step one is followed by a biotin-labeled rabbit antimouse IgG in step two. In step three an avidin-biotin complex is added. One site per avidin molecule is free to react with the biotinylated IgGs, while the other three sites are labeled with biotinylated peroxidase.

---

*Abbott Laboratories, Chicago.

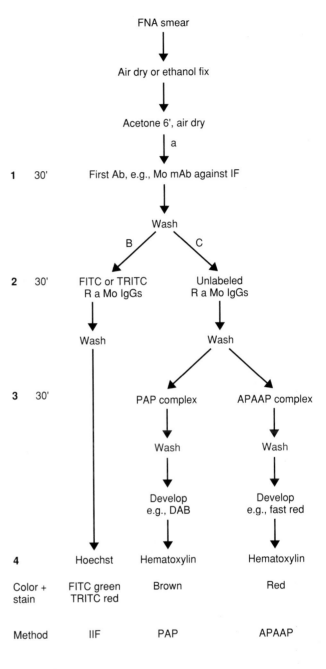

FIGURE 38–26. Protocols for method B (indirect immuno-fluorescence, IIF), C (peroxidase antiperoxidase, PAP) or D (alkaline phosphatase antialkaline phosphatase, APAAP). Endogenous peroxidase can be blocked at step a if necessary. (FNA = fine needle aspiration; Ab = antibody; Mo mAb = mouse monolonal antibody; FITC = fluorescein isothiocyanate; TRITC = rhodamine; R a Mo IgGs = rabbit anti-mouse IgGs; DAB = diaminobenzidine; and IIF = indirect immunofluorescence.)

ate fixation in 96% ethanol ("wet" cytology) or air drying ("dry" cytology), are adequate and are recommended for most ICC studies with cytoskeletal and membrane antigens. Fixation with glutaraldehyde (even low concentrations, e.g., 0.5%) or formaldehyde leads to inactivation of many epitopes (e.g., those containing a lysine) and often to higher backgrounds. In general, such steps are not recommended for most antigens, although for certain hormones and low molecular weight polypeptides it may be necessary to prefix prior to an organic solvent step so as to keep the antigen in the cell during the subsequent permeabilization with organic solvent. However, such steps if used should be kept short. Prior to immunostaining smears should be fixed with an organic solvent to make sure the cells are permeabilized and that the antibodies

have access (see Fig. 38–26). Because individual monoclonal antibodies can recognize many different epitopes on a single protein it is dangerous to generalize about appropriate fixation methods for a particular antigen. Reactivity is epitope dependent, not antigen dependent, provided the method of fixation keeps the antigen in the cell. For many antigens, e.g., IF, LCA, and EMA, it seems possible to prepare cell smears and store them for a considerable time (months) at $-70°C$ (or if $-70°C$ is not available then for shorter times at $-20°C$ to $-30°$) prior to immunostaining. However, with each new antigen and particularly for proteins that are present only in relatively small amounts in or on cells, it is important to check by using fresh smears as controls that the antigenicity is not reduced by the storage conditions.

Primary Antibodies. Most antibodies employed in routine cytologic diagnosis probably share the following characteristics: (1) they are available commercially, (2) they have been used previously on frozen histologic specimens and some of them may also work on paraffin-embedded, formaldehyde-fixed material and (3) they may or may not have been tested on cell smears.

In deciding which antibodies to purchase the following questions should be asked: (1) Is it monoclonal or polyclonal? (2) If monoclonal is it supplied as supernatant, as ascites fluid or as purified IgGs? (3) Has the manufacturer tested it on cell smears? and (4) Are working dilutions indicated for the method of detection used in the laboratory?

Monoclonal antibodies almost always come from mouse, whereas polyclonal antibodies come mostly from rabbits but may also come from other species. Each additional species necessitates purchase of appropriate second antibodies. Monoclonal antibodies in general recognize a single epitope on the molecule, whereas polyclonal antibodies usually are directed against several different epitopes. Different monoclonal antibodies, as well as a monoclonal vs. a polyclonal antibody, may display different specificities. Thus, it cannot *a priori* be assumed that, for instance, a CEA antibody sold by one manufacturer has the same spectrum of reactivities as that sold by a second. This is especially true for antigens that occur as multigene families. Conversely, it may be that the same monoclonal antibody is sold by different companies under different names or catalogue numbers. Monoclonal antibodies have the advantages that in principle they offer inexhaustible supplies of well-characterized reagents and that with carefully selected reagents it is often possible to distinguish very similar proteins, e.g., different IFs and different CEA molecules. In general, monoclonal antibodies appear to give staining patterns of the quality of affinity-purified polyclonal antibodies, i.e., of antibodies that have been purified by being bound on a column to which the original antigen has been coupled.

Monoclonal antibodies may be supplied as supernatants or as ascites. Supernatants are often used directly or can be diluted 1:40 or more, depending on the detection method. For ascites fluid dilutions of 1:300 to 1:3000 are commonly employed dependent on the original concentration of antibodies in the ascites fluid (usually 1-10 mg/ml). For purified IgGs usually a working dilution of 5 to 20 μg/ml is taken. The appropriate working concentration of each first antibody is established under the conditions of the routine cytologic laboratory. This saves not only in cost but the quality of the staining is often improved, and false-positive findings are avoided. This concentration should be redetermined if the method of detection is changed. Usually working dilutions of antibodies are stable for several months at 4°C if bovine serum albumin (BSA) is added to the diluent (0.5 mg/ml) and if azide is added (5×10^{-3} M) to prevent contamination. Sources of information that are often overlooked for methods are the manufacturers' catalogues. Perusal of these can often determine whether it has been

checked on cell smears, and some manufacturers, e.g., Dako, do this routinely. Antibodies that work on frozen sections from histologic specimens are a good choice for cytologic specimens. Often the method sheet accompanying the antibody will also give a rough indication of an appropriate dilution for a given detection method.

Detection Methods. An important decision is which detection method to employ, because this governs the choice of a second antibody. In immunofluorescence only a limited amount of detector antibody is bound, i.e., it is impossible to overdevelop. With the enzyme methods—peroxidase, alkaline phosphatase and biotin avidin—the time of development has to be carefully controlled to prevent underdevelopment or overdevelopment. Because of cost and time considerations, a laboratory usually chooses one method and stays with it, thus gaining experience in interpreting positive and negative reactions. High sensitivity methods are not always either necessary or desirable, particularly for major proteins, because they can introduce such problems as cross-reactivity between similar but not identical epitopes present, e.g., on different members of a multigene family. However, if minor proteins are not detected using a simple indirect method, one should consider trying to amplify the sensitivity by using a PAP or an APAAP method in which steps 2 and 3 can be repeated several times (see Fig. 38–25). Well-characterized antibodies and appropriate controls are again absolutely necessary.

Protocols. Space limitations prevent giving detailed protocols for each of the ICC methods in Figure 38–25. They can be found in histology laboratories, in reference sources[149, 186] or in the method sheets produced by some companies (e.g., Dako). Methods B and C of Figure 38–25 are further illustrated in the flow sheet given in Figure 38–26. After fixation with acetone to permeabilize the cells, areas of the smear where sufficient tumor cells are present are marked with a diamond pencil or with a special pen. Some protocols then employ a blocking step with undiluted sera. Supposedly, this step blocks unspecific binding of first and second antibodies. However, many sera contain autoantibodies and therefore either omission of this step or a careful selection of the blocking sera by testing several lots may help to reduce unwanted crossreactivities. About 5 to 10 μl of diluted antibody is usually sufficient for each antibody step if the slides are kept on damp paper in a closed container during the incubation steps. Multiple incubations can be performed on different areas of the same slide, but care must be taken so that the different antibodies do not mix. Alternatively, specially designed multihole slides can be utilized. After each antibody incubation, excess antibody is washed off in a sufficient volume of buffer (usually three changes of phosphate-buffered saline or Tris-NaCl). For further details of each protocol and for appropriate counterstains for nuclei see Figure 38–26. For all methods adequate positive and negative controls are necessary (see reference 82).

Double Staining. Sometimes it is advantageous to be able to visualize the distribution of two different antigens in the same smear (see Figs. 38–5 to 38–8). This step is relatively simple to do in immunofluorescence if antibodies to the two antigens made in two different species, e.g., mouse and rabbit, are available. In this case, for example, fluorescein-labeled goat anti rabbit (green) and rhodamine-labeled goat anti mouse (red) (or vice versa) can be employed provided the appropriate filters are available in the fluorescence microscope. It can be important to sieve each labeled antibody on purified IgGs from the other species, and controls utilizing each first antibody with both second antibodies are absolutely necessary. New labeled coumarin reagents have been introduced, which may allow triple labeling to be performed. Double labeling is also possible with the enzymatic methods provided a careful selection of labels is made and provided the antigens are present in different structures or, preferably, in different cellular compartments (see reference 149). Double labeling with different antibodies is of particular help in routine cytology to distinguish true coexpression of two antigens in tumor cells from normal cells of similar morphology (see Fig. 38–8) or to distinguish one particular cell type among many (see its use to "pick out" endothelial cells in Fig. 38–12). Other nonimmunologic methods can also sometimes be employed to distinguish a particular cell type (see the use of latex beads to distinguish macrophages in Fig. 38–20).

Paraffin Miniblocks. These may have some advantages over routinely prepared smears, as shown first with effusions. Often specific histologic patterns can be recognized in sections from miniblocks, which may not be identified without difficulty in smears from the same aspirate. Cellular morphology and nuclear detail are very well preserved. Multiple sections can be made from one block and stained either with conventional stains or with different antibodies. In one procedure that takes less than 4 hours, material from the FNA biopsy needle, which would normally be discarded, is concentrated in an Eppendorf centrifuge tube, fixed in ethanol and embedded in paraffin. Of 12 antibodies that worked well on conventional smears, 11 gave good results on the miniblock sections.

CONCLUSIONS

Immunocytochemistry with appropriate antibodies, such as some of those discussed in this chapter, can add independent objective information to the descriptive tumor typing currently used in diagnostic cytology. Immunocytochemistry is of most help in tumor typing. In the diagnosis of benign vs. malignant lesions and in prognosis ICC is much more restricted.

Success with ICC in diagnostic cytology depends on (1) using the light microscope and the clinical data to formulate a diagnostic question that can be answered by the employment of appropriate Abs in ICC, e.g., carcinoma vs. lymphoma; (2) using well-characterized Abs for which the specificity has been clearly defined both biochemically and by ICC on cytologic specimens of known origin and (3) evaluating the ICC data by a cytopathologist familiar with the light microscopy and clinical data (see Fig. 38–1). All three criteria should be taken into account in arriving at a final diagnosis. If the ICC results are inconclusive standard cytologic criteria should still be utilized to decide the final diagnosis.

Choice of antibodies to solve a particular problem should be governed by the following:
1. The realization that a panel of Abs may give more information than a single Ab.
2. If possible, markers that are present in all tumor cells rather than a minor population of tumor cells should be selected, e.g., desmin instead of myoglobin for rhabdomyosarcomas.
3. For antigens that occur as multigene families, it may be preferable to use mAbs, and mAbs in which the epitope is known may have advantages.

Thus, the approach to each diagnostic problem has to be individually designed in every case. Immunocytochemistry is currently certainly not a "magic bullet" approach in which, by adding antibodies, tumor cells turn red, brown or blue thus solving all diagnostic questions. However, the hope is that as more ICC data is accumulated algorithms can be constructed utilizing relatively few but well-characterized antibodies that allow a step-by-step approach to certain common diagnostic problems (see reference 166). In those algorithms constructed to date IF proteins, EMA and LCA seem to be the most general cell class-specific markers allowing fairly broad divisions according to tumor type with other markers allowing finer distributions.

Progress in applying ICC in diagnostic cytology will as in pathology depend on the continuing exchange of information between scientists interested in the antigens and those interested in using antibodies to these molecules in diagnosis. Only through understanding the complexities and limitations of ICC can its advantages be fully realized.

Complexities and Limitations

Immunocytochemistry will not solve all problems of differential diagnosis for a variety of reasons. These include the following:
1. No appropriate marker may exist to solve a particular problem, e.g., tumors with the same IF content cannot be separated if no additional markers are available.
2. Immunocytochemistry is in a stage of rapid development. Currently it is much simpler to make antibodies than to properly characterize them. The multitude of antigens and antibodies in present use makes it difficult sometimes to define "rules" let alone all exceptions to such rules. In this connection no substitute exists for more extensive testing of a few carefully selected antibodies on a large number of tumors of different types in several laboratories with well-defined protocols. Quality assurance programs for ICC are necessary for diagnostic cytology laboratories and for manufacturers.

3. For the increasing number of antigens that occur as members of multigene families, a better definition of reactivity profiles of mAbs on each individual member of a multigene family is required, e.g., for CEA and S-100 mAbs. Undoubtedly, the fact that some Abs recognize several and other Abs only one protein in a given family can account for some of the discrepancies in the literature. Additionally, certain currently used markers have to be moved from a specific to a less specific category, e.g., neuron-specific enolase should probably be replaced by neurofilaments and synaptophysin. Development of a standard nomenclature for mAbs would also help.

4. Technical problems occur for several reasons. ICC requires a good quality cellular smear, which has been appropriately fixed. Smears may contain a mixture of tumor cells from different parts of a tumor and may have a variable number of benign cells. Double immunostaining may be necessary to resolve these populations. Specificity of Abs has to be known under the conditions in which they are to be used. Appropriate Ab dilutions have to be utilized, and the method has to allow a cutoff between positive and negative cases.

5. No studies yet exist to show whether the immunologic phenotypes of particular tumors can be affected by treatment.

6. Expression of "ectopic" markers by minor subpopulations of tumor cells occurs in some tumors, e.g., keratin and neurofilaments in Ewing's tumor.

7. A minor percentage of tumors can probably never be classified by ICC because they exhibit signs of differentiation along more than one pathway. It would be interesting to know how large this category is.

Advantages

We believe the advantages of ICC include the following:

1. Immunocytochemistry provides independent objective differentiation or tissue-specific information that can confirm but also can contradict the initial cytologic diagnosis of tumor type (see Table 38–6). Its use can reveal features of the normal cytologic smear not previously recognized, e.g., IF buttons. It can strengthen the diagnosis reached on the basis of light microscopy and clinical data; it may help to resolve ambiguities in cytologic diagnosis and may help to prevent error.

2. A correct diagnosis of tumor type in a metastasis may either indicate the primary tumor or narrow the search for an unknown primary with obvious benefits for the patient and a reduction in cost for the hospital. Immunocytochemistry is of particular value when the differential diagnosis between major tumor types is in doubt.

3. Immunocytochemistry also provides the cytopathologist with the opportunity for a continuing education based on the most difficult and therefore the most informative cases.

For these reasons we believe that routine but judicious use of ICC in difficult cases in diagnostic cytology will benefit both the patient and the cytopathologist and that ICC should be more widely employed than it is at present.

References

1. Akura K, Hatakenaka M, Kawai K, Takenaka M, Kato K: Use of immunocytochemistry on urinary sediments for the rapid identification of human polyomavirus infection. A case report. Acta Cytol 32:247–251, 1988.
2. Al Saati T, Laveriviere P, Gorguet B, Delsol G, Gatter KC, Mason DY: Epithelial membrane antigen in hemopoietic neoplasms. Hum Pathol 17:533–534, 1986.
3. Altmannsberger M, Dirk T, Droese M, Weber K, Osborn M: Keratin polypeptide distribution in benign and malignant breast tumors—subdivision of ductal carcinomas using monoclonal antibodies. Virchows Arch B 51:265–275, 1986.
4. Altmannsberger M, Dralle M, Weber K, Osborn M, Droese M: Intermediate filaments in cytological specimens of thyroid tumors. Diagn Cytopathol 3:210–219, 1987.
5. Altmannsberger M, Osborn M, Droese M, Weber K, Schauer A: Diagnostic value of intermediate filament antibodies in clinical cytology. Klin Wochenschr 62:114–123, 1984.
6. Altmannsberger M, Osborn M, Schäfer H, Schauer A, Weber K: Distinction of nephroblastomas from other childhood tumors using antibodies to intermediate filaments. Virchows Arch B 45:113–124, 1984.
7. Altmannsberger M, Osborn M, Treuner J, Hölscher A, Weber K, Schauer A: Diagnosis of human childhood rhabdomyosarcoma by antibodies to desmin the structural protein of muscle specific intermediate antibodies. Virchows Arch B 39:203–215, 1982.
8. Altmannsberger M, Weber K, Droste B, Osborn M: Desmin is a specific marker for rhabdomyosarcoma of human and rat origin. Am J Pathol 118:85–95, 1985.
9. Aratake Y, Tamura K, Kotani T, Ohtaki S: Application of the avidin-biotin-complex method for the light microscope analysis of lymphocyte subsets with monoclonal antibodies on air-dried smears. Acta Cytol 32:117–122, 1988.
10. Azumi N, Battifora H: The distribution of vimentin and keratin in epithelial and nonepithelial neoplasms: A comprehensive immunohistochemical study on formalin- and alcohol-fixed tumors. Am J Clin Pathol 88:286–296, 1987.
11. Bignami A, Dahl D, Rueger DC: Glial fibrillary acidic protein (GFA) in normal neural cells and in pathological conditions. Adv Cell Neurobiol 1:285–310, 1980.
12. Blobel GA, Moll R, Franke WW, Kayser KW, Gould VE: The intermediate filament cytoskeleton of malignant mesotheliomas and its diagnostic significance. Am J Pathol 121:235–247, 1985.
13. Bostwick DG, Roth KA, Evans CJ, Barchas JD, Bensch KG: Gastrin-releasing peptide, a mammalian analog of bombesin, is present in human neuroendocrine lung tumors. Am J Pathol 117:195–200, 1984.
14. Broers JLV, Rot MK, Oostendorp T, Huysmans A, Wagenaar SS, Wiersman-van Tilburg AJM, Vooijs PG, Ramaekers FCS: Immunocytochemical detection of human lung cancer heterogeneity using antibodies to epithelial, neuronal, and neuroendocrine antigens. Cancer Res. 47:3225–3234, 1987.
15. Broghamer WL Jr, Richardson ME, Faurest WS, et al: Prostatic acid phosphatase immunoperoxidase staining cytologically positive effusions associated with adenocarcinoma of the prostate and neoplasms of undetermined origin. Acta Cytol 29:274–278, 1985.
16. Bunn PA, Linnoila I, Minna JD, Carney D, Gazdar AF: Small cell lung cancer endocrine cells of the fetal bronchus and other neuroendocrine cells express the Leu-7 antigenic determinant present on natural killer cells. Blood 65:764–768, 1985.
17. Burchell J, Gendler S, Taylor-Papadimitriou J, Girling A, Lewis A, Millis R, Lamport D: Development and characterization of breast cancer-reactive monoclonal antibodies directed

to the core protein of the human milk mucin. Cancer Res 47:5476–5482, 1987.

18. Burt A, Goudie RB: Diagnosis of primary thyroid carcinoma by immunohistochemical demonstration of thyroglobin. Histopathology 3:279–286, 1979.

19. Carlei F, Polak JM, Ceccamea A, Marangos PJ, Dahl D, Cocchia D, Michetti F, Lezoche E, Speranza V: Neuronal and glial markers in tumors of neuroblastic origin. Virchows Arch A 404:313–324, 1984.

20. Caselitz J, Jänner M, Breitbart E, Weber K, Osborn M: Malignant melanomas contain only the vimentin type IFs. Virchows Arch A 400:43–51, 1983.

21. Caselitz J, Osborn M, Wustrow J, Seifert G, Weber K: The expression of different intermediate-sized filaments in human salivary gland and their tumors. Pathol Res Pract 175:226–278, 1982.

22. Catoretti G, Andreola S, Clemente C, D'Amato L, Rilke F: Vimentin and p53 expression on epidermal growth factor-receptor-positive, oestrogen receptor-negative breast carcinomas. Br J Cancer 57:353–357, 1988.

23. Chess Q, Hajdu SI: The role of immunoperoxidase staining in diagnostic cytology. Acta Cytol 30:1–7, 1986.

24. Chin-Yang L, Witzig TE, Phyliky RL, Ziesmer SL, Yam LT: Diagnosis of B-cell non-Hodgkin's lymphoma of the central nervous system by immunocytochemical analysis of cerebrospinal fluid lymphocytes. Cancer 57:737–744, 1986.

25. Cline MJ: Molecular diagnosis of human cancer. Lab Invest 61:368–380, 1989.

26. Coleman DV, Ormerod MB: Tumor markers in cytology. *In* Advances in Clinical Cytology, vol 2. Edited by LG Kos and DV Coleman. New York, Masson Publing, 33–46, 1984.

27. Collins VP: Monoclonal antibodies to glial fibrillary acidic protein in the cytologic diagnosis of brain tumors. Acta Cytol 28:401–406, 1984.

28. Coons AH: The beginnings of immunofluorescence. J Immunl 87:499–503, 1961.

29. Cooper D, Schermer A, Sun T-T: Biology of disease: Classification of human epithelia and their neoplasms using monoclonal antibodies to keratins: strategies, applications and limitations. Lab Invest 52:243–256, 1985.

30. Cowin P, Kapprell H-P, Franke WW: The complement of desmosomal plaque proteins in different cell types. J Cell Biol 101:1442–1454, 1985.

31. Crocker J, Hull PA, Macartney AG, Stansfekld AG: A comparative study of nucleolar organizer regions (Ag-NORs), Ki-67 staining and DNA flow cytometry in non-Hodgkin's lymphomas. J Pathol 154:37a, 1988.

32. Crocker J, Nar P: Nucleolar organizer regions in lymphomas. J Pathol 151:111–118, 1987.

33. Damjanov I: Biology of disease: Lectin cytochemistry and histochemistry. Lab Invest 57:5–20, 1987.

34. de Jong ASH, van Kessel-van Vark M, van Heerde P: Fine needle aspiration biopsy diagnosis of rhabdomyosarcoma. An immunocytochemical study. Acta Cytol 31:573–577, 1987.

35. de Jong ASH, van Raamsdonk W, van Kessel-van Vark M, Albus-Lutter CE: Skeletal muscle actin as tumor marker in the diagnosis of rhabdomyosarcoma in childhood. Am J Surg Pathol 9:467–474, 1986.

36. Debus E, Moll R, Franke WW, Weber K, Osborn M: Immunohistochemical distinction of human carcinomas by cytokeratin typing with monoclonal antibodies. Am J Pathol 114:121–130, 1984.

37. Debus E, Weber K, Osborn M: Monoclonal antibodies to desmin, the muscle specific intermediate filament protein. EMBO J 2:2305–2312, 1983.

38. Debus E, Weber K, Osborn M: Monoclonal antibodies specific for glial fibrillary acidic protein (GFA) and for each of the individual neurofilament triplet proteins. Differentiation 25:193–199, 1983.

39. Derenzini M, Nardi F, Farabegoli F, Ottinetti A, Roncaroli F, Bussolati G: Distribution of silver-stained interphase nucleolar organizer regions as a parameter to distinguish neoplastic from nonneoplastic reactive cells in human effusions. Acta Cytol 33:491–498, 1989.

40. Devleeshouwer N, Faverly D, Kiss R, Legros N, de Launoit Y, Ryckaert, Andry M, Lenglet G, Paridaens R, Gomper M: Comparison of biochemical and immunoenzymatic macro-methods and a new immunocytochemical micromethod for assaying estrogen receptors in human breast carcinomas. Acta Cytol 32:816–824, 1988.

41. Dirk T, Droese M: Tumor typing in fine needle aspiration biopsies by immunocytochemistry. *In* New Frontiers in Cytology. Edited by K Goerttler, GE Feichter, S Witte. Berlin, Springer-Verlag, 1988, p199.

42. Domagala W, Lasota J, Bartkowiak J, Weber K, Osborn M: Vimentin is preferentially expressed in human breast carcinomas with low estrogen receptor and high Ki67 growth fraction. Am J Pathol 136:219–227, 1990.

43. Domagala W, Emeson EE, Koss LG: T and B lymphocyte enumeration in the diagnosis of lymphocyte-rich pleural fluids. Acta Cytol 25:108–110, 1981.

44. Domagala W, Koss LG: Surface configuration of mesothelial cells in effusions. A comparative light microscopic and scanning electron microscopic study. Virchows Arch B 30:231–243, 1979.

45. Domagala W, Lasota J, Chosia M, Szadowska A, Weber K, Osborn M: Diagnosis of major tumor categories in fine needle aspirates is more accurate when light microscopy is combined with intermediate filament typing: a study of 403 cases. Cancer 63:504–517, 1989.

46. Domagala W, Lasota J, Chosia M, Weber K, Osborn M: Leukocyte common antigen and vimentin are reliable adjuncts in the diagnosis of non-Hodgkin lymphoma in fine needle aspirates. Anal Quant Cytol Histol 11:15–21, 1989.

47. Domagala W, Lasota J, Weber K, Osborn M: Endothelial cells help in the diagnosis of primary versus metastatic carcinoma of the liver in fine needle aspirates: an immunofluorescence study with vimentin and endothelial cell–specific antibodies. Anal Quant Cytol Histol 11:8–14, 1989.

48. Domagala W, Lasota J, Wolska H, Lubinski J, Weber K, Osborn M: Diagnosis of metastatic renal cell and thyroid carcinoma by intermediate filament typing and cytology of tumor cells in fine needle aspirates. Acta Cytol 32:415–421, 1988.

49. Domagala W, Lubinski J, Lasota J, Giryn I, Weber K, Osborn M: Neuroendocrine (Merkel-cell) skin carcinoma: cytology, intermediate filament typing and ultrastructure of tumor cells in fine needle aspirates. Acta Cytol 31:267–275, 1987.

50. Domagala W, Lubinski J, Lasota J, Woyke S, Wozniak L, Szadowska A, Weber K, Osborn M: Decisive role of intermediate filament typing of tumor cells in differential diagnosis of difficult fine needle aspirates. Acta Cytol 31:253–266, 1987.

51. Domagala W, Lubinski J, Weber K, Osborn M: Intermediate filament typing of tumor cells in fine needle aspirates using monoclonal antibodies. Acta Cytol 30:214–224, 1986.

52. Domagala W, Lubinski J, Weber K, Osborn M: Intermediate filament typing vs. electron microscopy in the diagnosis of major tumor types in fine needle aspirates. *In* New Frontiers in Cytology. Edited by K Goerttler, F Feichter, S Witte. Berlin, Springer-Verlag, p 178, 1988.

53. Domagala W, Weber K, Osborn M: Diagnostic significance of coexpression of intermediate filaments in fine needle aspirates of human tumors. Acta Cytol 32:49–59, 1988.

54. Donhuijsen K, Schulz S: Prognostic significance of vimentin positivity in formalin-fixed renal cell carcinomas. Pathol Res Pract 184:287–291, 1989.

55. Droese M, Altmannsberger M, Kehl A, Lankisch PG, Weiss R, Weber K, Osborn M: Ultrasound-guided percutaneous fine needle aspiration biopsy of abdominal and retroperitoneal masses. Acta Cytol 28:368–384, 1984.

56. Ellis DW, Leffers S, Davies JS, Ng ABP: Multiple immunoperoxidase markers in benign hyperplasia and adenocarcinoma of the prostate. Am J Clin Pathol 81:279–284, 1984.

57. Eusebi V, Rilke F, Ceccarelli C, Fedeli F, Schiaffino S, Bussolati G: Fetal heavy chain skeletal myosin: an oncofetal antigen expressed by rhabdomyosarcoma. Am J Surg Pathol 10:384–389, 1986.

58. Fürst DO, Osborn M, Weber K: Myogenesis in the mouse embryo: differential onset of expression of myogenic proteins

and the involvement of titin in myofibril assembly. J Cell Biol 109:517–527, 1989.

59. Gabbiani G, Kapanci Y, Barazzone P, Franke WW: Immunochemical identification of intermediate-sized filaments in human neoplastic cells. Am J Pathol 104:206–216, 1981.

60. Gal R, Aronaf A, Gertzmann H, Kessler E: The potential value of the demonstration of thyroglobulin by immunoperoxidase techniques in fine needle aspiration cytology. Acta Cytol 31:713–716, 1987.

61. Garcia RL, Coltrera MD, Gown AM: Analysis of proliferative grade using anti-PCNA/cyclin monoclonal antibodies in fixed, embedded tissues: comparison with flow cytometric analysis. Am J Pathol 134:733–739, 1989.

62. Gatter KC, Alcock C, Heryet A, Mason DY: Clinical importance of analysing malignant tumors of uncertain origin with immunohistological techniques. Lancet 1:1302–1305, 1985.

63. Gatter KC, Alcock C, Heryet A, Pulford KA, Heyderman E, Taylor-Papadimitriou J, Stein H, Mason DY: The differential diagnosis of routinely processed anaplastic tumors using monoclonal antibodies. Am J Clin Pathol 82:33–43, 1984.

64. Ghosh AK, Spriggs AI, Taylor-Papadimitriou J, Mason DY: Immunocytochemical staining of cells in pleural and peritoneal effusions with a panel of monoclonal antibodies. J Clin Pathol 36:1154–1164, 1983.

65. Giorno R, Sciotto CG: Use of monoclonal antibodies for analyzing the distribution of the intermediate filament protein vimentin in human non-Hodgkin's lymphomas. Am J Pathol 120:351–355, 1985.

66. Giri DD, Dundas SAC, Sanderson PR, Howat AJ: Silver-binding nucleoli and nucleolar organizer regions in fine needle aspiration cytology of the breast. Acta Cytol 33:173–175, 1989.

67. Goerttler K, Feichter GE, Witte S (eds): New Frontiers in Cytology. Berlin, Springer Verlag, 1988.

68. Gorbsky G, Steinberg MS: Isolation of intracellular glycoproteins of desmosomes. J Cell Biol 90:243–248, 1981.

69. Gould VE, Wiedenmann B, Lee I, Schwechheimer K, Dockhorn-Dworniczak B, Radosevich JA, Moll R, Franke WW: Synaptophysin expression in neuroendocrine neoplasms as determined by immunocytochemistry. Am J Pathol 126:243–257, 1987.

70. Gown AM, Vogel AM: Monoclonal antibodies to human intermediate filament proteins. III. Analysis of tumors. Am J Clin Pathol 84:413–424, 1985.

71. Gown AM, Vogel AM, Hoak D, Gough F, McNutt MA: Monoclonal antibodies specific for melanocytic tumors distinguish subpopulations of melanocytes. Am J Pathol 126:243–257, 1987.

72. Greene LA: A new neuronal intermediate filament protein. Trends Neurosci 12:228–230, 1989.

73. Guzman J, Bross KJ, Würtemberger G, Costabel U: Immunocytology in malignant pleural mesothelioma. Expression of tumor markers and distribution of lymphocyte subsets. Chest 95:590–595, 1989.

74. Guzman J, Costabel U, Bross KJ, Wiehle U, Grunert F, Schaefer M-E: The value of the immunoperoxidase slide assay in the diagnosis of malignant pleural effusions in breast cancer. Acta Cytol 32:188–192, 1988.

75. Guzman J, Hilgarth M, Bross KJ, Costabel U, Yeck-Kapp G, Wiehle N, Huber A, Grunert F, von Kleist S, Pfleiderer A: Anwendung monoklonaler Antikörper in der Aszitesdiagnostik beim Ovarialkarzinom. Gynäkol Prax 12:679–689, 1988.

76. Guzman J, Hilgarth M, Bross KJ, Ross A, Wiehle U, Kresin V, Grunert F, von Kleist S: Malignant ascites of serous papillary ovarian adenocarcinoma. An immunocytochemical study of the tumor cells. Acta Cytol 32:519–522, 1988.

77. Haimoto H, Takahashi Y, Koshikawa T, Nagura H, Kato K: Immunohistochemical localization of γ-enolase in normal human tissues other than nervous and neuroendocrine tissues. Lab Invest 52:257–263, 1985.

78. Hakomori S, Kannagi R: Glycosphingolipids as tumor-associated and differentiation markers. J Natl Cancer Inst 71:231–251, 1983.

79. Hammarstrom S, Shively JE, Paxton RJ, Beatty BG, Larsson A, Ghosh R, Bormer O, Buchegger F, Mach J-P, Burtin P, Seguin P, Darbouret B, Degorce F, Sertour J, Jolu JP, Fuks A, Kalthoff H, Schmiegel W, Arndt R, Klöppel G, von Kleist S, Grunert F, Schwarz K, Matsuoka Y, Kuroki M, Wagener C, Weber T, Yachi A, Imai K, Hishikawa N, Tsujisaki M: Antigenic sites in carcinoembryonic antigen. Cancer Res 49:4852–4858, 1989.

80. Heyderman E, Steele K, Ormerod MG: A new antigen on the epithelial membrane: its immunoperoxidase localisation in normal and neoplastic tissues. J Clin Pathol 32:35–39, 1979.

81. Heyderman E, Strudley I, Powell G, Richardson TC, Cordell JL, Mason DY: A new monoclonal antibody to epithelial membrane antigen (EMA)-E29. A comparison of its immunocytochemical reactivity with polyclonal anti-EMA antibodies and with another monoclonal antibody, HMFG-2. Br J Cancer 52:355–361, 1985.

82. Heyderman E, Warren PJ, Haines AMR: Immunocytochemistry today—problems and practice. Histopathology, (in press).

83. Howell LP, Zipfel S, Steplewski Z, Koprowska I: A gastrointestinal specific monoclonal antibody that can be of clinical value in cytologic material. Acta Cytol 31:802–806, 1987.

84. Jobsis AC, De Vries GP, Meijer AEFH, Ploem JS: The immunohistochemical detection of prostatic acid phosphatase: its possibilities and limitations in tumor histochemistry. Histochem J 13:961–973, 1981.

85. Johnston WW, Szpak CA, Lottich SC, Thor A, Schlom J: Use of a monoclonal antibody (B72.3) as a novel immunocytochemical adjunct for the diagnosis of carcinomas in fine needle aspiration in biopsy specimens. Hum Pathol 17:501–513, 1986.

86. Johnston WW, Szpak CA, Thor A, Simpson JF, Schlom J: Applications of immunocytochemistry to clinical cytology. Cancer Invest 5:593–611, 1987.

87. Jothy S, Brazinsky SA, Chin-A-Loy MM, Haggarty A, Krantz MJ, Cheung M, Fuks A: Characterization of monoclonal antibodies to carcinoembryonic antigen with increased tumor specificity. Lab Invest 54:108–117, 1986.

88. Kahn HJ, Wedad H, Yeger H, Baumal R: Immunohistochemical localization of prekeratin filaments in benign and malignant cells in effusions—comparison with intermediate filament distribution by electron microscopy. Am J Pathol 109:206–214, 1982.

89. Katz RL, Ravel P, Brooks TE, Ordonez NG: The role of immunocytochemistry in the diagnosis of prostatic neoplasia by fine-needle aspiration biopsy. Diagn Cytopathol 1:28–32, 1985.

90. Kenny AJ, O'Hare MJ, Gusterson BA: Cell-surface peptidases as modulators of growth and differentiation. Lancet 2:785–787, 1989.

91. Kleihues P, Kiessling M, Janzer RC: Morphological markers in neuro-oncology. In Morphological Tumor Markers. Edited by G Seifert. Berlin, Springer-Verlag, p 307, 1987.

92. Kligman D, Hilt DC: The S-100 protein family. TIBS 13:437–443, 1988.

93. Klöppel G, Caselitz J: Epithelial tumor markers: oncofetal antigens (carcinoembryonic antigen, alpha-fetalprotein) and epithelial membrane antigen. In Morphological Tumor Markers. Edited by G Seifert. Berlin, Springer-Verlag, p 103, 1987.

94. Koss LG, Woyke S, Olszewski W: Aspiration Biopsy. Cytologic Interpretation and Histologic Bases. Tokyo, Igaku-Shoin, 1984.

95. Krajewski AS, Dewar AE, Ramage EF: T and B lymphocyte markers in effusions with non-Hodgkin's lymphoma. J Clin Pathol 35:1216–1219, 1982.

96. Kurtin PJ, Pinkus GS: Leukocyte common antigen—A diagnostic discriminant between hematopoietic and nonhematopoietic neoplasms in paraffin sections using monoclonal antibodies: Correlation with immunologic studies and ultrastructural localization. Hum Pathol 16:353–365, 1985.

97. Landon F, Lemonnier M, Benarous R, Huc C, Fiszman M, Gros F, Portier M-M: Multiple mRNAs encode peripherin, a neuronal intermediate filament protein. EMBO J 8:1719–1726, 1989.

98. Leathem AJ, Brooks SA: Predictive value of lectin binding on breast cancer recurrence and survival. Lancet 1:1054–1056, 1987.

99. Lellè RJ, Heidenreich W, Stauch G, Gerdes J: Growth fraction as determined in cytologic specimens of breast carcinomas: a study with the monoclonal antibody Ki67. In New Frontiers in Cytology. Edited by K Goerttler, GE Feichter, S Witte. Berlin, Springer-Verlag, p 212, 1988.

100. Lennert K: Classification of non-Hodgkin's lymphomas. In

Malignant Lymphomas Other Than Hodgkin's Disease. Edited by N Mohri, H Stein, E Kaiserling, E Müller-Hermelink. Berlin, Springer-Verlag, p 83, 1978.

101. Leonard DGB, Gorham JD, Cole P, Greene LA, Ziff EB: A nerve growth factor–regulated messenger RNA encodes a new intermediate filament protein. J Cell Biol 106:181–193, 1988.

102. Leong AS-Y, Gilham P: Silver staining of nucleolar organizer regions in malignant melanoma and melanotic nevi. Hum Pathol 20:257–262, 1989.

103. Levitt S, Cheng L, DuPuis MM, Layfield LJ: Fine needle aspiration diagnosis of malignant lymphoma with confirmation by immunoperoxidase staining. Acta Cytol 29:895–902, 1985.

104. Marchetti E, Bagni A, Querzoli P, Durante E, Marzola A, Fabris G, Nenci I: Immunocytochemical detection of estrogen receptors by staining with monoclonal antibodies on cytologic specimens of human breast cancer. Acta Cytol 32:829–834, 1988.

105. Marsden HB, Kumar S, Kahn J, Anderton BJ: A study of glial fibrillary acidic protein (GFAP) in childhood brain tumors. Int J Cancer 31:439–445, 1983.

106. Martin SE, Zhang HZ, Magyarosy E, Jaffe ES, Hsu SM, Chu EW: Immunologic methods in cytology: Definitive diagnosis of non-Hodgkin's lymphomas using immunologic markers for T and B cells. Am J Clin Pathol 82:666–673, 1984.

107. Mason MR, Bedrossian CWM, Fahey CA: Value of immuno-cytochemistry in the study of malignant effusions. Diagn Cytopathol 3:215–221, 1987.

108. McMichael AJ, et al (eds): Leucocyte Typing III. White Cell Differentiation Antigens. Oxford, Oxford University Press, 1987.

109. McNutt MA, Bolen JW, Gown AM, Hammar SP, Vogel AM: Coexpression of intermediate filaments in human epithelial neoplasms. Ultrastr Pathol 9:31–43, 1985.

110. Michels S, Swanson PE, Frizzera G, Wick MR: Immunostaining for leukocyte common antigen using an amplified avidin-biotin-peroxidase complex method and paraffin sections. A study of 735 hematopoietic and nonhematopoietic human neoplasms. Arch Pathol Lab Med 111:1035–1039, 1987.

111. Mierau GW, Berry PJ, Orsini EN: Small round cell neoplasms: Can electron microscopy and immunohistochemical studies accurately classify them? Ultrastr Pathol 9:99–111, 1985.

112. Miettinen M: Antibody specific to muscle actins in the diagnosis and classification of soft tissue tumors. Am J Pathol 130:205–215, 1988.

113. Miettinen M, Damjanov I: Coexpression of keratin in epithelioid sarcoma. Am J Surg Pathol 9:460–462, 1985.

114. Miettinen M, Lehto V-P, Badley RA, Virtanen I: Alveolar rhabdomyosarcoma: Demonstration of the muscle type of intermediate filament protein, desmin, as a diagnostic aid. Am J Pathol 108:246–251, 1982.

115. Miettinen M, Lehto V-P, Virtanen I: Histogenesis of Ewing's sarcoma: An evaluation on intermediate filaments and endothelial cell markers. Virchows Arch 41:277–284, 1982.

116. Miettinen M, Lehto V-P, Virtanen I: Antibodies to intermediate filament proteins in the diagnosis and classification of human tumors. Ultrastr Pathol 7:83–107, 1984.

117. Miettinen M, Virtanen I: Synovial sarcoma—A misnomer. Am J Pathol 11:18–25, 1984.

118. Moll R: Epithelial tumor markers: cytokeratins and tissue polypeptide antigen (TPA). In Morphological Tumor Markers. Edited by G Seifert. Berlin, Springer-Verlag, pp 71–101, 1987.

119. Moll R, Cowin P, Kapprell H-P, Franke WW: Desmosomal proteins—new markers for identification and classification of tumors. Lab Invest 54:4–25, 1986.

120. Moll R, Franke WW, Schiller DL, Geiger B, Krepler R: The catalog of human cytokeratins: patterns of expression in normal epithelia, tumors and cultured cells. Cell 31:11–24, 1982.

121. Moll R, Lee I, Gould VE, Berndt R, Roessner A, Franke WW: Immunocytochemical analysis of Ewing's tumors: Patterns of expression of intermediate filaments and desmosomal proteins indicate cell type heterogeneity and pluripotential differentiation. Am J Pathol 127:288–304, 1987.

122. Moll R, Osborn M, Hartschuh W, Moll I, Mahrle G, Weber K: Variability of expression and arrangement of cytokeratin and neurofilaments in cutaneous neuroendocrine carcinomas (Merkel cell tumors): Immunocytochemical and biochemical analysis of 12 cases. J Ultrastr Pathol 10:473–495, 1986.

123. Möller P, Momburg F, Hofmann WJ, Matthaei-Maurer DU: Lack of vimentin occurring during the follicular stages of B cell development characterizes follicular center cell lymphomas. Blood 1033–1038, 1988.

124. Mottolese M, Venturo I, Rinald M, Curcio CG, Donnorso RP, Natali PG: Immunocytochemical diagnosis of neoplastic effusions of unknown origin employing selected combinations of monoclonal antibodies to tumor-associated antigens. In New Frontiers in Cytology. Edited by K Goerttler, GE Feichter, S Witte. Berlin, Springer-Verlag, pp 237–240, 1988.

125. Mukai M, Torikata C, Iri H, Morikawa Y, Shimizu K, Shimoda T, Nukina N, Ihara Y, Kageyama K: Expression of neurofilament triplet proteins in human neuronal tumors. Am J Pathol 122:28–35, 1986.

126. Murthy L, Kapila K, Verma K: Immunoperoxidase detection of carcinoembryonic antigen in fine needle aspirates of breast carcinoma. Correlation with studies in tissue sections. Acta Cytol 32:60–62, 1988.

127. Nadji M: The potential value of immunoperoxidase techniques in diagnostic cytology. Acta Cytol 24:442–447, 1980.

128. Noble MA, Kwong A, Barteluk RL, Smith RP: Laboratory diagnosis of Chlamydia trachomatis using two immunodiagnostic methods. Am J Clin Pathol 89:205–210, 1988.

129. O'Hara CM, Gardner WA, Bennet BD: Immunoperoxidase staining of Trichomonas vaginalis in cytologic material. Acta Cytol 24:448–451, 1980.

130. Ordonez NG, Sneige N, Hickey RC, Brooks TE: Use of monoclonal antibody HMB-45 in the cytologic diagnosis of melanoma. Acta Cytol 32:684–688, 1988.

131. Orell SR, Dowling KD: Oncofetal antigens as tumor markers in the cytologic diagnosis of effusions. Acta Cytol 27:625–629, 1983.

132. Osborn M, Caselitz J, Weber K: Heterogeneity of intermediate filament expression in vascular smooth muscle: a gradient in desmin-positive cells from the rat aortic arch to the level of the arteria iliaca communis. Differentiation 20:196–202, 1981.

133. Osborn M, Debus E, Weber K: Monoclonal antibodies specific for vimentin. Eur J Cell Biol 34:137–143, 1984.

134. Osborn M, Dirk T, Käser H, Weber K, Altmannsberger M: Immunohistochemical localization of neurofilaments and neuron-specific enolase in 29 cases of neuroblastoma. Am J Pathol 122:433–442, 1986.

135. Osborn M, Hill C, Altmannsberger M, Weber K: Monoclonal antibodies to titin in conjunction with antibodies to desmin separate rhabdomyosarcomas from other tumor types. Lab Invest 55:101–108, 1986.

136. Osborn M, Johnsson N, Wehland J, Weber K: The submembranous location of p11 and its interaction with the p36 substrate of pp60 src kinase in situ. Exp Cell Res 175:81–96.

137. Osborn M, Van Lessen G, Weber K, Klöppel K, Altmannsberger M: Differential diagnosis of gastrointestinal carcinomas by using monoclonal antibodies specific for individual keratin polypeptides. Lab Invest 55:497–504, 1986.

138. Osborn M, Weber K: A monoclonal antibody recognizing desmosomes; use in human pathology. J Invest Dermatol 85:385–388, 1985.

139. Osborn M, Weber K: Intermediate filament proteins: a multigene family distinguishing major cell lineages. TIBS 2:461–472, 1986.

140. Osborn M, Weber K: Biology of disease: Tumor diagnosis by intermediate filament typing. A novel tool for surgical pathology. Lab Invest 48:372–394, 1983.

141. Osborn M, Weber K (eds): Cytoskeletal Proteins in Tumor Diagnosis. Current Communications in Molecular Biology. Cold Spring Harbor, Cold Spring Harbor Press, 1989.

142. Parrish EP, Garrod DR, Mattey DL, Hand L, Steart PV, Weller RO: Mouse antisera specific for desmosomal adhesion molecules of suprabasal skin cells, meninges and meningioma. Proc Natl Acad Sci 83:2657–2661, 1986.

143. Permanetter W, Wiesinger H: Immunohistochemical study of lysozyme, alpha₁-antichymotrypsin, tissue polypeptide antigen and carcinoembryonic antigen in effusion sediments. Acta Cytol 31:104–112, 1987.

144. Pettinato MD, De Chiava A, Insabato L: Diagnostic significance of intermediate filament buttons in fine needle aspirates of neuroendocrine (Merkel cell) carcinoma of the skin. Acta Cytol 33:420–421, 1989.

145. Pinkus GS, Etheridge CL, O'Conner EM: Are keratin proteins better tumor markers than epithelial membrane antigen? Am J Clin Pathol 85:269–277, 1986.

146. Pinkus GS, Kurtin PJ: Epithelial membrane antigen—a diagnostic discriminant in surgical pathology. Hum Pathol 16:929–940, 1985.

147. Pinto MM: An immunoperoxidase study of S-100 protein in neoplastic cells in serous effusions. Use as a marker for melanoma. Acta Cytol 30:240–244, 1986.

148. Pinto MM, Bernstein LH, Brogan DA, Criscuolo EM: Carcinoembryonic antigen in effusions. A diagnostic adjunct to cytology. Acta Cytol 31:113–118, 1987.

149. Polak JM, Van Noorden S (eds): Immunocytochemistry. Practical Applications in Pathology and Biology. London, Wright PSG, 1983.

150. Quinlan RA, Schiller DL, Hatzfeld M, Achtstatter T, Moll R, Jorcano J, Magin T, Franke WW: Patterns of expression and organization of cytokeratin intermediate filaments. Ann NY Acad Sci 455:282–306, 1985.

151. Ramaekers F, Haag D, Jap P, Vooijs PG: Immunochemical demonstration of keratin and vimentin in cytologic aspirates. Acta Cytol 28:385–392, 1984.

152. Ramaekers F, Huysmans A, Moesker O, Schaart G, Herman C, Vooijs P: Cytokeratin expression during neoplastic progression of human transitional cell carcinomas as detected by a monoclonal and a polyclonal antibody. Lab Invest 52:31–38, 1985.

153. Ramaekers F, Puts JJG, Moesker O, Kant A, Huysmans A, Haag D, Jap PHK, Herman CJ, Vooijs GP: Antibodies to intermediate filament proteins in the immunohistochemical identification of human tumours; an overview. Histochem J 15:691–713, 1983.

154. Ramaekers F, Vroom TM, Moesker D, Kant A, Scholte G, Vooijs GP: The use of antibodies to intermediate filament proteins in the differential diagnosis of lymphoma versus metastatic carcinoma. Histochem J 17:57–70, 1985.

155. Rastad J, Wilander E, Lindgren P-G, Ljnnghall S, Stenkvist BG, Akerström G: Cytologic diagnosis of a medullary carcinoma of the thyroid by Sevier-Munger silver staining and calcitonin immunocytochemistry. Acta Cytol 31:45–47, 1987.

156. Raymond WA, Leong A S-Y: Coexpression of cytokeratin and vimentin intermediate filament proteins in benign and neoplastic breast epithelium. J Pathol 157:299–306, 1989.

157. Rice RH, Pinkus GS, Warhol MJ, Antonioli DA: Involucrin: Biochemistry and immunohistochemistry. In Advances in Immunohistochemistry. Edited by S Sternber, R DeLellis. New York, Mason Publishing, p 111, 1984.

158. Robey SS, Cafferty LL, Beschorner WE, Gupta PK: Value of lymphocyte marker studies in diagnostic cytopathology. Acta Cytol 31:453–459, 1987.

159. Said JW, Nash G, Sassoon AF, Shintaku IP, Banks-Schlegel S: Involucrin in lung tumors: a specific marker for squamous differentiation. Lab Invest 49:563–568, 1983.

160. Sainsbury JR, Farndon JR, Needham GK, Malcolm AJ, Harris AL: Epidermal growth–factor receptor status as predictor of early recurrence of and death from breast cancer. Lancet 1:1398–1402, 1987.

161. Schlimok G, Funke I, Holzmann B, Göttlinger G, Schmidt G, Häuser H, Swierkot S, Warnecke HH, Schneider B, Koprowski H, Riethmüller G: Micrometastatic cancer cells in bone marrow: In vitro detection with anticytokeratin and in vivo labeling with anti-17-1A monoclonal antibodies. Proc Natl Acad Sci USA 84:8672–8676, 1987.

162. Schmechel DE: γ-Subunit of the glycolytic enzyme enolase: nonspecific or neuron specific? Lab Invest (Editorial) 52:239–242, 1985.

163. Seeger RC, Brodeur GM, Sather H, Dalton A, Siegel SE, Wong KY, Hammond D: Association of multiple copies of the N-myc oncogene with rapid progression of neuroblastomas. N Engl J Med 313:1111–1116, 1986.

164. Segasothy M, Lau TM, Birch DF, Fairley KF, Kincaid-Smith P: Immunologic dissection of the urine sediment using monoclonal antibodies. Am J Clin Pathol 90:691–699, 1988.

165. Sehested M, Ralfkjaer E, Rasmussen J: Immunoperoxidase demonstration of carcinoembryonic antigen in pleural and peritoneal effusions. Acta Cytol 27:124–127, 1983.

166. Seifert G (ed.): Morphological Tumor Markers. Berlin, Springer-Verlag, 1987.

167. Shah KD, Tabibzadeh SS, Gerber MA: Comparison of cytokeratin expression in primary and metastatic carcinomas: Diagnostic application in surgical pathology. Am J Clin Pathol 87:708–715, 1987.

168. Sheibani K, Battifora H, Burke JS, Rappaport H: Leu-M1 antigen in human neoplasms. An immunohistologic study of 400 cases. Am J Surg Pathol 10:227–236, 1986.

169. Shimada H, Aoyama C, Chiba T, Newton WA: Prognostic subgroups for undifferentiated neuroblastoma: immunohistochemical study with anti S-100 protein antibody. Hum Pathol 16:471–476, 1985.

170. Silverman JF, Nance K, Phillips B, Norris HT: The use of immunoperoxidase panels for the cytologic diagnosis of malignancy in serous effusions. Diagn Cytopathol 3:134–140, 1987.

171. Skalli O, Gabbiani G, Babai F, Seemayer TA, Pizzolato G, Schürch W: Intermediate filament proteins and actin isoforms as markers for soft tissue tumor differentiation and origin. II. Rhabdomyosarcomas. Am J Pathol 130:515–531, 1988.

172. Sloane JP, Ormerod MG: Distribution of epithelial membrane antigen in normal and neoplastic tissues and its value in diagnostic tumor pathology. Cancer 47:1786–1795, 1981.

173. Spieler P, Schmid U: Immunocytochemical differentiation of lymphocyte effusions. In New Frontiers in Cytology. Edited by K Goerttler, GE Feichter, S Witte. Berlin, Springer-Verlag, pp 223–225, 1988.

174. Stark E, Wurster U: Preparation procedure for cerebrospinal fluid that yields cytologic samples suitable for all types of staining, including immunologic and enzymatic methods. Acta Cytol 31:374–376, 1987.

175. Südhof TC, Czernik AJ, Kao H-T, Takei K, Johnston PA, Horiuchi A, Kanazir SD, Wagner MA, Perin MS, De Camilli P, Greengard P: Synapsins: mosaics of shared and individual domains in a family of synaptic vesicle phosphoproteins. Science 245:1474–1480, 1989.

176. Szpak CA, Johnston WW, Roggli V, Kolbeck J, Lottisch SC, Vollmer R, Thor A, Schlom J: The diagnostic distinction between malignant mesothelioma of the pleura and adenocarcinoma of the lung as defined by a monoclonal antibody (B72.3). Am J Pathol 122:252–260, 1986.

177. Tani EM, Christensson B, Porwit A, Skoog L: Immunocytochemical analysis and cytomorphologic diagnosis on fine needle aspirates of lymphoproliferative disease. Acta Cytol 32:209–215, 1988.

178. Tani E, Löwhagen T, Nasiell ST, Skoog L: Fine needle aspiration cytology and immunocytochemistry of large cell lymphomas expressing the Ki-1 antigen. Acta Cytol 33:359–362, 1989.

179. Tascos NA, Parr J, Gonatas NK: Immunocytochemical study of the glial fibrillary acidic protein in human neoplasms of the central nervous system. Hum Pathol 13:454–458, 1982.

180. Taylor-Papadimitriou J, Gendler SJ: Molecular aspects of mucins. Cancer Rev (in press).

181. Taylor-Papadimitriou J, Lane EB: Keratin expression in the mammary gland. In The Mammary Gland. Edited by MC Neville, CW Daniel. New York, Plenum Publishing Corp, pp 181–215, 1987.

182. Thomas ML: The leukocyte common antigen family. Ann Rev Immunol 7:339–369, 1989.

183. To A, Dearnaley DP, Ormerod G, Canti G, Coleman DV: Epithelial membrane antigen: its use in the cytodiagnosis of malignancy in serous effusions. Am J Clin Pathol 77:214–219, 1981.

184. Trojanowski JQ, Lee VM-Y, Schlaepfer WW: An immunohistochemical study of human central and peripheral nervous system tumors using monoclonal antibodies against neurofilaments and glial filaments. Hum Pathol 15:248–257, 1984.

185. Tsukada T, McNutt M, Ross R, Gown A: HHF35, a muscle actin-specific monoclonal antibody. II. Reactivity in normal, reactive, and neoplastic human tissue. Am J Pathol 127:389–402, 1987.

186. Tubbs RR, Gephardt GN, Petras RE: Atlas of Immunohistology. Chicago, American Society of Clinical Pathologists Press, 1986.

187. van der Kwast TH, Versnel MA, Delahaye M, de Jong A, Zondervan PE, Hoogsteden H: Expression of epithelial membrane antigen on malignant mesothelioma cells. An immunocytochemical and immunoelectron microscopic study. Acta Cytol 32:169–174, 1988.

188. Van Eyken P, Sciot R, Paterson A, Callea F, Kew MC, Desmet VJ: Cytokeratin expression in hepatocellular carcinoma. Hum Pathol 19:562–568, 1988.

189. Van Muijen GNP, Ruiter DJ, Franke WW, Achtstätter T, Haasnoot WHB, Ponec M, Warnaar SO: Cell type heterogeneity of cytokeratin expression in complex epithelia and carcinomas as demonstrated by monoclonal antibodies specific for cytokeratins nos. 4 and 13. Exp Cell Res 162:97–113, 1986.

190. Vandekerckhove J, Osborn M, Altmannsberger M, Weber K: Actin typing of rhabdomyosarcomas shows the presence of the foetal and adult forms of sarcomeric muscle actin. Differentiation 35:126–131, 1987.

191. Vandekerckhove J, Weber K: At least six different actins are expressed in a higher mammal: an analysis based on the amino acid sequence of the amino-terminal tryptic peptide. J Mol Biol 126:783–802, 1978.

192. Vanstapel M-J, Peeters B, Cordell J, Heyns W, De Wolf-Peeters C, Desmet V, Mason D: Methods in laboratory investigation: Production of monoclonal antibodies directed against antigenic determinants common to the α- and β-chain of bovine brain S-100 protein. Lab Invest 52:232–238, 1985.

193. Vanstapel M-J, Gatter KC, Wolf-Peeters C, Mason DY, Desmet VD: New sites of human S-100 immunoreactivity detected with monoclonal antibodies. Am J Clin Pathol 85:160–168, 1986.

194. Vennegoor C, Hageman P, Van Nouhuijs H, Ruiter DJ, Calafat J, Ringens PJ, Rümke P: A monoclonal antibody specific for cells of the melanocyte lineage. Am J Pathol 130:179–192, 1988.

195. Viac J, Reano A, Brochier J, Staquet M-J, Thivolet J: Reactivity pattern of a monoclonal antikeratin antibody (KL1). J Invest Dermatol 81:351–354, 1983.

196. Vick WW, Wikstrand CJ, Bullard DE, Kemshead J, Coakham HB, Schlom J, Johnston WW, Bigner DD, Bigner SH: The use of a panel of monoclonal antibodies in the evaluation of cytologic specimens from the central nervous system. Acta Cytol 31:815–824, 1987.

197. Vogel AM, Esclamado RM: Identification of a secreted Mr 95,000 glycoprotein in human melanocytes and melanomas by a melanocyte-specific monoclonal antibody. Cancer Res 48:1286–1294, 1988.

198. von Koskull H, Virtanen I, Lehto VI, Vartio T, Dahl D, Aula P: Glial and neuronal cells in amniotic fluid and anencephalic pregnancies. Pren Diagn 1:259–267, 1981.

199. Von Overbeck J, Staehli C, Gudat F, Carmann H, Lautenschlager C, Dorrmueller C, Tackacs B, Miggiani V, Staehlin T, Heitz P: Immunohistochemical characterization of an anti-epithelial monoclonal antibody (mab lu-5). Virchows Arch A 407:1–12, 1985.

200. Walts AE, Said JW, Banks-Schlegel S: Keratin and carcinoembryonic antigen in exfoliated mesothelial and malignant cells: an immunoperoxidase study. Am J Clin Pathol 80:671–676, 1983.

201. Walts AE, Said JW, Shintaku IP: Epithelial membrane antigen in the cytodiagnosis of effusions and aspirates: immunocytochemical and ultrastructural localization in benign and malignant cells. Diagn Cytopathol 3:41–49, 1987.

202. Walts A, Said J, Shintaku IP: Cytodiagnosis of malignant melanoma. Immunoperoxidase staining with HMB-45 antibody as an aid to diagnosis. Am J Clin Pathol 90:77–80, 1988.

203. Walts AE, Said JW, Shintaku IP, Lloyd R: Chromogranin as a marker of neuroendocrine cells in cytologic material. An immunocytochemical study. Am J Clin Pathol 84:273–277, 1985.

204. Wang E, Fischman D, Liem RKH, Sun TT: Intermediate filaments. Ann NY Acad Sci 455, 1985.

205. Weber K, Osborn M, Moll R, Wiklund B, Lüning B: Tissue polypeptide antigen (TPA) is related to the nonepidermal keratins 8, 18 and 19 typical of simple and nonsquamous epithelia: re-evaluation of a human tumor marker. EMBO J 3:2707–2714, 1984.

206. Weiss SW, Langloss JM, Enzinger FM: Value of S-100 protein in the diagnosis of soft tissue tumors with particular reference to benign and malignant Schwann cell tumors. Lab Invest 49:299–308, 1983.

207. Wiedenmann B, Huttner WB: Synaptophysin and chromogranins/secretogranins—widespread constituents of distinct types of neuroendocrine vesicles and new tools in tumor diagnosis. Virchows Arch B (in press).

208. Wiedenmann B, Kuhn C, Schwechheimer K, Waldherr R, Raue F, Brandeis WE, Kommerell B, Franke WW: Synaptophysin identified in metastases of neuroendocrine tumors by immunocytochemistry and immunoblotting. Am J Clin Pathol 88:560–569, 1987.

209. Wilkinson MM, Busuttil A, Hayward C, Brock DJH, Dorin JR, Van Heyningen V: Expression pattern of two related cystic fibrosis–associated calcium-binding proteins in normal and abnormal tissues. J Cell Sci 91:221–230, 1988.

210. Winkler B, Gooding GAW, Montgomery CK, Clark OH, Arnaud C: Immunoperoxidase confirmation of parathyroid origin of ultrasound-guided fine needle aspirates of the parathyroid glands. Acta Cytol 31:40–44, 1987.

211. Wright C, Angus B, Nicholson S, Sainsbury JRC, Cairns J, Gullick WJ, Kelly P, Harris AL, Horne CHW: Expression of c-erbB-2 oncoprotein: a prognostic indicator in human breast cancer. Cancer Res 49:2087–2090, 1989.

212. Wright GL: Monoclonal Antibodies and Cancer. New York, Marcel Dekker, 1984.

213. Yachi A, Shively JE (eds): The CEA Antigen Gene Family. New York, Elsevier, 1989.

214. Yam LT, English MC, Janckila AJ, Yiesmer S, Li CY: Immunocytochemistry of cerebrospinal fluid. Acta Cytol 31:825–833, 1987.

215. Yam LT, Lin DG, Janckila AJ, Li CY: Immunocytochemical diagnosis of lymphoma in serous effusions. Acta Cytol 29:833–841, 1985.

216. Yam LT, Janckila AJ: Immunocytodiagnosis of carcinocythemia in disseminated breast cancer. Acta Cytol 31:68–72, 1987.

217. Yasui W, Sumiyoshi H, Hata J, Kameda T, Ochiai A, Ito H, Tahara E: Expression of epidermal growth factor–receptor in human gastric and colonic carcinomas. Cancer Res 48:137–141, 1988.

218. Yokota J, Tsunetsugu-Yokota Y, Battifora H, Le Fevre C, Cline MJ: Alterations of myc, myb, and Harvey-ras protooncogenes in cancers are frequent and show clinical correlation. Science 231:261–265, 1986.

219. Zhang H-Z, Ordonez NG, Batsakis JG, Chan JC: Monoclonal antibody recognizing a carcinoembryonic antigen epitope differentially expressed in human colonic carcinoma vs. normal adult colon tissues. Cancer Res 49:5766–5773, 1989.

39

In Situ Hybridization

Christine Bergeron
Alex Ferenczy

Genetic information is carried by sequences of deoxyribonucleic acid (DNA), and DNA is a double helix made up of two polydeoxyribonucleotide strands. Each deoxyribonucleotide contains a nitrogen base, a five-carbon sugar (deoxyribose) and a phosphate group. Four kinds of nitrogen bases are found in a DNA molecule: two pyrimidines, which are thymine (T) and cytosine (C), and two purines, adenine (A) and guanine (G). The two polydeoxyribonucleotide chains are linked by hydrogen bonds between the nitrogen bases. The G hydrogen bonds specifically with C, whereas A bonds specifically with T. The genome is perpetuated by replication, a process involving duplication of the deoxyribonucleotide to give an identical copy. Ribonucleic acid (RNA) is made up of a single strand of ribonucleotides. Each ribonucleotide contains a nitrogen base, a five-carbon sugar (a ribose) and a phosphate group. The ribonucleotide contains guanine and cytosine (the same as in a DNA molecule), whereas uracil is bound to adenine instead of thymine. A single strand of the ribonucleotides is identical in sequence to one of the strands of the DNA and is generated by a *transcription* process.

Fragments of DNA from any source can be isolated and amplified by inserting them into a suitable replicon, such as a plasmid-vector, and subsequently transferred into bacteria cells, in a process called *DNA cloning*. Plasmids are small circular bacterial DNAs, which occur naturally and replicate freely in bacteria. As these transfected bacteria cells divide, the recombinant plasmid molecule carrying the DNA fragment of interest also replicates to produce a large copy number of the original DNA fragment. When the transfected cells are plated into a proper medium, the bacteria colony containing a recombinant plasmid can be identified by radioactive nucleic acid probes complementary to the cloned DNA fragment. How such probes are made is explained further.

Labeled cloned DNA or RNA probes are widely employed to identify specific nucleic acid sequences. The DNA fragment can be labeled radioactively by common, sensitive radioisotopes. These are phosphorus (^{32}P), sulfur (^{35}S) and tritium (^{3}H). These radioactive isotopes can be incorporated into DNA fragments by the *nick translation method*.[51] In nick translation, DNA is incubated with unlabeled and labeled nucleotides plus DNA nuclease (DNase I) and DNA polymerase enzyme. The DNase I introduces nicks into the DNA fragment while complementary radioactive nucleotides are incorporated by the DNA polymerase, which uses the original fragment DNA as the template. Labeled RNA probes can be generated from linear DNA recombinant SP6 vectors[13, 20, 30, 56] by using radioactive isotopes during the transcription process. The SP6 vector contains a promotor recognized specifically by an SP6 RNA polymerase. An SP6 RNA polymerase induces the transcription from SP6 promotor "upstream" of the inserted DNA. The transcript is either mRNA or "anti" mRNA depending on the orientation of the inserted DNA within the vector. The advantages of RNA probes over nick-translated DNA probes are a high specific activity, a noncompetitive hybridization to the complementary DNA strand and a low background with the use of RNase to digest unhybridized RNA probe. Radioactivity, however, in preparing DNA and RNA probes, has its disadvantages such as its high cost, radiation hazard and special disposal. The necessity to produce new labeled probes frequently because of rapid probe degradation by radiolysis is another disadvantage.

Nonisotopic markers have now been introduced that are easier to handle and offer more rapid signal detection. Nick-translated biotinylated DNA and biotinylated RNA probes are widely employed.[6, 9, 12, 48, 49, 54, 71, 85] Fluorochrome-[42, 69, 87] acetylaminofluorene-[47] and sulfonated-modified[80] DNA are other processes to label nonradioactive DNA probes.

The use of these probes is explained subsequently.

1052

For any single strand of DNA or RNA there is a predetermined complementary strand that will bind specifically to that single strand forming a *hybrid molecule* of double helix. This hybrid is stable under appropriate conditions of temperature, ionic strength and increased pH. The two strands can be dissociated into two single strands under high temperature or alkaline treatment. This process of strand separation is called *DNA denaturation* or *melting*. The average of the temperature range over which the strands of DNA separate is called the melting temperature, denoted Tm. When DNA is in solution under physiologic conditions, the Tm lies in a range of 85 to 95°C. The denaturation of DNA is reversible under appropriate conditions, in which the two separated complementary strands reform into a double helix. The reaction is called *renaturation* or *hybridization*. Hybridization conditions are commonly defined by the number of degrees below the Tm at which they are done. Hybridization under high stringency conditions corresponds to hybridization of perfectly or homologous complementary strands. These conditions are dependent on the ionic strength of the solution, the proportion of G-C base pairs, the presence of reagents such as formamide and the temperature that destabilizes hydrogen bonds. Alternatively, conditions in which hybridization of weakly homologous regions is possible are called low stringency conditions. They are much below the Tm, in comparison to high stringency conditions.

Single-stranded DNA probes can be produced simply from double-stranded DNA probes by denaturation. They can be mixed under hybridizing conditions with denatured viral and cellular DNA to detect the presence of a particular genome and its transcripts, respectively. RNA probes may be utilized to localize either DNA-RNA or mRNA-RNA hybrids depending on the denaturation conditions and the orientation of the transcription of DNA template.

Molecular probes may be employed effectively with a wide range of methods to detect specific nucleic acid sequences. The *Southern blot analysis* is a technique that localizes fragments of DNA in mixtures of DNA-restriction fragments obtained with restriction endonucleases and fractionated in bands by gel electrophoresis. The bands from the gel are transferred to a sheet of nitrocellulose paper, a process called blotting. The bands that hybridize to the radioactive DNA probe are identified by autoradiography. *Dot blot* is a simpler technique than is the Southern blot and utilizes total denatured cellular DNA, applied directly to nitrocellulose membrane in a small drop or dot. Hybridization with radioactive denatured DNA probes or RNA probes is performed and detected by autoradiography. The *polymerase chain reaction* (PCR) is a new technique of *in vitro* DNA amplification used in complement with Southern blot analysis. It is not a detection method per se, but rather it can enzymatically increase (amplify) the number of copies of a specific DNA sequence that otherwise could not be detected by the Southern blot method. The amplification is based upon the utilization of primers flanking both of the selected fragments of DNA. The DNA polymerase will extend

primers copying the DNA template with high fidelity in repeated amplification cycles up to 1 million-fold, providing ample DNA to be detected either by using restriction endonucleases in an acrylamide gel or by the Southern blot method. The *in situ hybridization* (ISH) technique is unique in that it localizes specific nucleic acid sequences *in situ* either in chromosomes or in particular types of cells in tissue sections or cell preparations. *In situ* hybridization was introduced in 1969 to localize DNA sequences.[8, 15, 41, 53, 68, 92] Since that time, ISH has been applied from localization of chromosomal mapping[42, 47, 69, 87] to neuroendocrine gene expression.[39] Application of ISH for the detection of oncogene expression in preneoplasia and early neoplasia is an interesting field of investigation for the experimental pathologist as well.

However, today the most widely used application of ISH in diagnostic pathology is viral detection,[37, 49, 53, 54, 78, 92] including human papillomaviruses (HPVs). These viruses are a heterogeneous group of small (55 μm) DNA viruses with a circular double-stranded genome of 8 kilobases (kb) and a nude capsid protein. They are well known to infect squamous and occasionally glandular epithelium.[29, 64] Currently, 63 different types of HPVs have been detected (S. Beaudenon, personal communication). Infection by certain HPV types has been shown to be clearly associated with an increased frequency of malignant progression of the infected epithelial cells.[29, 64] Epidermodysplasia verruciformis is the first human model in which infection with certain HPVs, such as types 5 and 8, has been shown to be associated with the development of squamous cell carcinoma of the skin.[64] A similar situation exists in the genital tract where 20 different HPV types have been detected (Table 39–1). Types 16, 18 and 33 and to a lesser degree 31, 35 and 39, and other newly characterized types, have been detected in a large proportion of invasive squamous cell carcinomas of the lower genital tract. These types are also associated with intraepithelial neoplasias of the lower female genital tract. Conversely, types 6 and 11, 42, 43 and 44 are found usually in benign acuminate and flat condylomata. It appears thus that although viruses such as 6 or 11 have negligible cancer risk potential, HPV 16, 18 and 33 are high risk viral types.

The techniques of molecular hybridization are powerful laboratory tools for investigating the prevalence of specific HPV types and defining high versus low risk populations (Table 39–2). Also, with their high sensitivity, clinically inapparent or latent infections, or both,

TABLE 39–1. Human Papillomaviruses Detected in Genital Lesions

Types	Associated Lesion
6,11	Condylomata acuminata
16,18,31,33,35,39	CIN + cervical carcinoma
42,43,44,54,55	Condylomata
45,51,52,56,58,63*	CIN + cervical carcinoma

*Beaudenon S, personal communication.
Adapted from Devilliers E: J Virol 63:4898–4903, 1989.
CIN = cervical intraepithelial neoplasia.

TABLE 39–2. Human Papillomavirus (HPV) Detection Methods by Molecular Biology

Methods	Characteristics
Southern blot	Sensitive
	HPV typing, integrated, episomal
	Detection of new HPVs
Dot blot	Sensitive
	False positives
	Typing limited to cloned HPVs
In situ hybridization	Sensitive
	(depending on probe type and detection system)
	Cellular localization
	Typing limited to cloned HPVs

and early precursor lesions may be detected, and data on mode or risk of transmission and progression to subclinical lesions may be obtained.[1, 29, 45, 64] Therefore, hybridization in all likelihood may lead to better detection rates, possibly more effective prevention and better understanding of the natural history of HPV infections of the lower genital tract.

The PCR is the most sensitive technique to assist the hybridization techniques to detect the presence of HPVs.[77] However, in routine practice, this technique remains limited because the choice of primers requires knowledge of DNA sequences and because possible external contamination can occur. Alternatively, Southern blot analysis is a highly sensitive and specific technique for detecting and typing HPV DNA. The specific DNA patterns of restriction fragments generated by using proper restriction endonuclease enzymes are hybridized under high and low stringency conditions with HPV probes to allow precise typing and detection of as yet uncharacterized HPV types. This technique also has the advantage of providing information on the physical status of the HPV DNA in the host cell, i.e., integrated into viral DNA or exists as free extrachromosomal episome. Dot blot hybridization, under high stringency conditions, indicates that the viral DNA to which the probe hybridizes is related to that probe type but is not necessarily identical. However, none of these techniques provides any information on the localization of the viral DNA or RNA in the specimen. This chapter focuses on the application of ISH to diagnosis of genital HPV infections in routine cytopathologic practice. The limitations of this technique as applied to cytology at present are also discussed.

METHODS OF HYBRIDIZATION

The purpose of ISH is to localize nucleic acid sequences in specific cells in either tissue sections or cell preparations. To maximize the sensitivity of ISH, several variables have to be taken into account: (1) preparation and appropriate fixation of tissue sections and cells, (2) preparation of probes and labeling, (3) hybridization conditions and (4) sensitivity of the detecting system.

Preparation and Fixation of Tissue Sections and Cells

The optimal preparation should keep the maximum number of sections or cells on the slide throughout the different steps of hybridization. For doing so, several approaches have been recommended: poly-L-lysine–coated slides, Elmer's glue diluted solution and gelatin-coated slides.[3, 18, 31, 79] The most simple procedure, however, is gelatin-coated slides.

The most appropriate method of fixation is the one that preserves the maximum amount of target DNA or RNA and provides optimal morphologic details. Cellular mRNAs are very unstable and to preserve and localize mRNAs, rapid fixation of biopsies or smears is necessary. The type of fixative must also be considered in individual situations, depending on the nature of the study. Recommended fixatives for fixed and embedded material are crosslinking agents, such as glutaraldehyde,[13, 15] 4% paraformaldehyde[39] and 4% buffered formalin,[59, 62, 63] and precipitants, such as ethanol-acetic acid[36] and Carnoy's.[14] For the study of DNA, Carnoy's fixative is superior with respect to the retention of morphologic detail;[14] however, for the study of RNA, buffered formalin is a better choice. Bouin's fixative should not be used for ISH, even if the morphology is very well preserved, as Bouin's fixation causes extensive degradation of DNA and RNA.[61] For a study at the ultrastructural level, glutaraldehyde is a good fixative.[15] Fixation of smears and cytocentrifuged cell suspensions can be done with routine ethanol, ethanol-acetic acid[36] or periodate lysine-paraformaldehyde-glutaraldehyde (PLPG).[31, 32]

Preparation of Probes and Labeling

All of the radioactive and nonradioactive probes described here are currently used for ISH. Single-stranded RNA probes labeled with ^{3}H, ^{35}S or biotin are increasingly employed because of their high specific activity and low background reaction.[13, 18, 19, 36, 79] The RNA probes of complete genomes have to be hydrolyzed to obtain a length not exceeding 400 base pairs—the optimal length for ISH.[13, 36] The DNA probes may be labeled with ^{3}H, ^{35}S or biotin by nick translation[4, 14, 15, 31] and have a small size (about 400 nucleotides) for diffusion into the cell. The positive signal by radioactively labeled probes can be detected by autoradiography[74] or by immunofluorescent and immunoenzymatic methods if nonradioactive probes are selected.[6, 54, 85]

Tritium remains the standard radioisotope in ISH for several reasons: localization of the signal by autoradiography is excellent at both the electron microscopic and light microscopic levels and high specific activities can be achieved when only a few copies of genomes are present.[13, 36] However, sections hybridized with ^{3}H-labeled probes require long exposure times (4 weeks) for signal detection.[74, 79] If more rapid detection is required, labeling with ^{35}S can yield results within 2 or 3 days, but the localization of the signal is more diffuse. High specific activity and efficient grain development can be achieved with ^{32}P-labeled probes, but localization is poor.[74] Nonradioactive biotinylated or sulfonated probes are detected in 1 day by the usual immunologic methods with antibodies to biotin or sulfonated agents. The enzymes, peroxidase and alkaline phosphatase, are revealed by H_2O_2 with diaminobenzidine and bromochloroindolyl phosphate with nitroblue tetrazolium, respectively. The sensitivity of these methods appears adequate, but none of the published work indicates that they are comparable in sensitivity to methods with radioactive probes.[19, 36, 59]

Hybridization Conditions

In the past few years, efforts have been made to simplify the initially complex methodology of ISH. For example, most investigators have eliminated HCL treatment believed to enhance probe penetration into cells and postfixation in paraformaldehyde,[14, 17–19, 76, 79] without loss of reaction signal. The protease treatment, however, remains an important step for enhancing diffusion in crosslinking fixed tissue, such as formalin. As a result, after deparaffinization of the tissue and rehydration through decreased concentrations of ethanol solutions, the tissue or cells are incubated for 15 minutes in proteinase K (2 μg/ml) at room temperature[13, 36] and washed in phosphate-buffered sodium containing 0.2% glycine. For Carnoy's fixed tissue or ethanol-fixed cells, this step may be omitted. Slides are then rinsed in 2XSSC (0.15 M NaCl; 0.015 sodium citrate) for 10 minutes.

Denaturation of cellular and viral DNA is done in a solution of 50% formamide and 2XSSC at 75°C for 10 minutes. The slides are then transferred quickly in ice cold 2XSSC for 5 minutes to stop denaturation and partial reannealing. In contrast, for localization of mRNA, hybridization should not include the denaturation process of the tissue or cells.

Hybridization conditions are similar for DNA or RNA, depending on the variables that influence the intensity of the signal. These variables are probe concentration, stringency of hybridization conditions and posthybridization washes. Final probe concentration of ^{3}H- or ^{35}S-labeled DNA or RNA probe is usually 1 μg/ml.[13, 31, 36, 79] If the DNA or RNA probes are not radioactively labeled, the concentration reaches a level between 2 μg/ml and 50 μg/ml.[4, 19] The aforementioned conditions approximately equal Tm −25°C for RNA or DNA-DNA hybridization and Tm −30°C for RNA-RNA hybridization. These provide optimal hybridization rates for HPV DNA and HPV RNA, respectively. The hybridization mixture contains 40% formamide, 10% dextran sulfate, 4XSSC, 100 μg/ml of yeast tRNA or 200 μg/ml salmon sperm DNA and the appropriate probe concentration. Approximately 20 μl and 60 μl of solutions are applied per histologic section and per smear, respectively, sealed with siliconized coverslips and incubated for 16 hours at 42°C in a humidified chamber (O. Croissant, personal communication).

They are washed under conditions of decreasing stringency using appropriate concentrations of formamide and SSC at different temperatures. If RNA probes are utilized, a step of RNase treatment should be included: incubation with a mixture of RNase A (20 μg/ml) and RNase T1 (5U/ml) in 2XSSC for 30 minutes at room temperature.

The slides are then processed for either autoradiographic exposure or immunoenzymologic analysis. They are dehydrated in graded ethanol and air dried for autoradiographic detection. Slides are dipped in Kodak emulsion at 38°C in a dark room, dried vertically in racks, transferred to containers with desiccant and exposed at 4°C for 4 days with ^{35}S and 30 days with ^{3}H probes. After developing, sections and smears are counterstained with hematoxylin and Papanicolaou, respectively, dehydrated and mounted. The distribution and density of silver grains are assessed microscopically with bright field illumination. For colorimetric detection, the usual immunologic procedures are employed (for details, see Chapter 38, Immunocytochemistry).

Controls of Specificity and Sensitivity

As for all histochemical procedures, controls have to be performed to prove specificity of ISH reactions. Several control reactions are available, depending on the probe and the target nucleic acid. Hybridization to positive or negative control cases confirmed by Southern blot analysis should reveal the expected distribution of reactivity or should be negative. Hybridization with nonspecific sequences and with probes prehybridized with specific DNA or RNA should yield negative results. For an exclusive DNA detection, pretreatment of the slides with RNase may be performed. When such sections are digested by DNase I prior to denaturation, the signal should be completely abolished. Alternatively, for RNA detection, the sections are pretreated with DNase I and are not denatured prior to hybridization. Nonspecific reactions in the detection system, such as chemography artifacts during autoradiography or nonspecific reactions in the immunohistochemistry procedure, are detected by omitting the labeled probe in the protocol.

The sensitivity of the method can be estimated by analyzing cultured cells from cervical cancers (CaSki, Hela) containing a define amount of HPV DNA. The amount of HPV DNA per cell can also be estimated by Southern blot analysis of cellular DNA extracted from a biopsy and histologic evaluation of the parenchyma stromal ratio. The lowest limit of HPV detection by ISH and ^{3}H-labeled antisense single-stranded RNA probes ranges between 20 and 50 integrated HPV genomes per cell[13, 19, 67, 76] and 25 copies of mRNA.[79] Dark field illumination increases the reaction contrast. The sensitivity of nonradioactive RNA and DNA probes depends on the hybridization conditions and the detection system.

APPLICATIONS

Histology and Cytology of HPV Infection

This section summarizes the main cytologic-histologic features that are helpful for diagnosing HPV infections. The reader may refer to Chapter 8 for more details.

Most HPV infections of the cervix are asymptomatic, grossly inapparent and detected by exfoliative cytology in about 3% of sexually active female patients.[45] Cytologic features of HPV infections are better understood when related to the biologic behavior of the virus. The first target cell of HPV is the basal cell of the squamous epithelium and probably the reserve cell of the endocervical glandular epithelium. Accessibility of HPV virions to these cells is enhanced by microfissures in the epithelium. These may occur after sexual contact or infection. The squamocolumnar junction of the transformation zone is also a site for direct virus-basal or -reserve cell contact.[27] Viral replication and full viral expression, including production of complete virions, are linked to the differentiation of the epithelium.[14] Full viral expression in genital HPV infections is manifested by koilocytosis and is considered to be a specific HPV-related cytopathic change.[5, 44, 55, 70] Cytologically, koilocytes are intermediate or superficial cells with an irregular cytoplasmic border, a distinct perinuclear zone of cytoplasmic clearing and a surrounding peripheral zone of dense cytoplasm. By definition, the nuclei of koilocytes are atypical. The atypical features include nuclear enlargement with irregular membrane, hyperchromasia and degenerative chromatin with margination and fragmentation. Binucleated and multinucleated cells, dyskeratocytes (individual cell keratinization) and hyperkeratosis or parakeratosis are also commonly found with HPV infections. However, they are not specific of HPV infections, rather they are related to increased growth (multinucleation) and disturbed keratin formation, which may be associated with either an HPV infection or a nonspecific regenerative process of the squamous epithelium. The number of koilocytes is proportional to cells in which HPV replicates, and when the lower parabasal cells are abnormal, koilocytes are associated with a neoplastic process.

The contrasting histologic features of cervical condyloma and cervical intraepithelial neoplasia (CIN) are summarized in Table 39–3. Condyloma is characterized by acanthosis, papillomatosis and well-oriented proliferation of basal or parabasal cells. Mitotic figures are confined to the lower part of the epithelium and are normal in configuration except for occasional tripolar and dispersed metaphases. Koilocytosis, dyskeratosis, hyperkeratosis and parakeratosis are found in intermediate and superficial layers of the epithelium. The overall morphologic alterations in condyloma are consistent with hyperplasia and degeneration of infected cells. In contrast to condyloma, CIN contains basal cellular disorientation with lack of basal polarity and a crowded, overlapping growth pattern. Cytologic ab-

TABLE 39–3. Morphologic Features of Cervical Condyloma and Cervical Intraepithelial Neoplasia (CIN)

	Condyloma	CIN
Koilocytosis	+ + +	±*
Chromatin clumping	−	+
Basal cell disorganization	−	+
Abnormal mitotic figures	−	+

*Depending on degree of differentiation.
Adapted from Fletcher S, Norval M: Lancet 1:546–549, 1983.

normalities include aberrant chromatin distribution, nuclear pleomorphism, increase in nucleocytoplasmic ratio and mitotic activity at all epithelial levels and morphologically aberrant mitotic figures.

Grading of intraepithelial neoplasia into I, II and III is classically based on the proportion of the epithelium occupied by basal, undifferentiated cells versus koilocytes.[57, 72] However, grading is subjective and difficult, if at all reproducible. This problem is particularly evident in low-grade squamous intraepithelial lesions, i.e., CIN grade I. A consensus panel has recommended to include condyloma in the group of CIN I lesions (see Chapters 4 and 9). Also, distinguishing grade I CIN from CIN II and HPV mimics may be a difficult task in routine pathologic practice. In such cases, tracing HPV DNA by the ISH method may be of great diagnostic help. Also, HPV typing of a given lesion is much more accurate with ISH than relying on the presence or absence of abnormal mitotic figures.[16, 72]

Detection of HPV in Tissue Sections by ISH

Prior to the development of the ISH method, HPV was detected in tissue sections or smears by transmission electron microscopy (TEM) and the immunologic peroxidase-antiperoxidase (PAP) technique. With TEM only fully formed virions can be detected in nuclei of differentiated cells, the material examined is of very limited volume and the technique is time-consuming.[10, 25, 38, 43, 91] As a result, TEM has no practical diagnostic value for HPV infections. Also, because any HPV type can be found in virions, TEM provides no information on HPV types. The PAP method utilizes rabbit antipapillomavirus antibody to react with the major capsid antigen of HPV, which is produced by the late gene of HPV (L1).[40] The gene L1 is predominantly expressed in nuclei of koilocytes for its expression is limited to differentiated cells.[25, 40, 46, 90] Such fully expressed virions are infectious in the susceptible host. The PAP method is thus useful if one is interested in a search for potentially infectious virions in a given tissue. Research is underway to develop antisera to type-specific epitopes.[7]

At present, ISH is the only technique that provides information on the localization and replication of a specific HPV genome in a cell type. Many more HPV-positive cells are detected by ISH than by the immu-

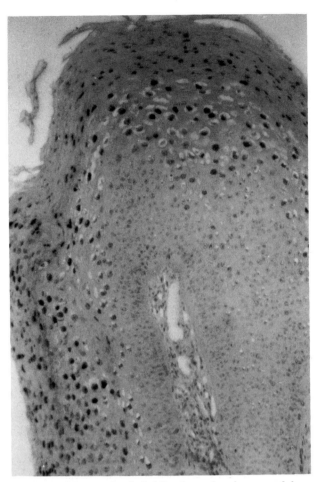

FIGURE 39–1. *In situ* **hybridization of vulvar condyloma acuminatum with ³H/HPV 6 probe.** Abundant grains in the nuclei of superficial cells indicate viral replication. Positive cells represent koilocytes or parakeratotic cells (hematoxylin stain; ×150). (Courtesy of O. Croissant, Unité des Papillomavirus Institut Pasteur.)

differentiation. Well-differentiated CIN lesions have larger amounts of HPV RNA than poorly differentiated lesions. Furthermore, RNA detection provides higher signals than DNA detection, reflecting the amplification of RNA copy number relative to DNA copy number.[79]

Attempts at correlating morphology of different genital lesional tissues of the female anogenital tract epithelium with HPV types using the ISH method have been reported.[3, 34, 35, 45, 66] Earlier studies found HPV types 6 and 11 in lesions diagnosed as condylomata and grade I intraepithelial neoplasias, whereas high-grade II and III intraepithelial neoplasias and invasive carcinomas contain oncogenic HPV types, namely, 16 and 18.[3, 35, 45, 66] However, in one study, low risk 6 and 11 type viruses were found in some CIN 2 and 3 lesions and high risk 16 and 18 and related viruses in condylomata.[81] More recent morphologic studies controlled by *in situ* DNA hybridization found that a majority of flat lesions of the cervix carry HPV type 16–related sequences.[28] Other potentially oncogenic types, such as 33, 35 and 39 and newly characterized types like S1, S2, S6 and S8, have been detected in half of low-grade CIN. Only acuminate condylomata of the cervix test positive for HPV type 6 and 11. Low risk HPV DNA types were found by ISH in juvenile laryngeal papillomatosis in children[84, 86] and in condylomata of the male urethra.[21] These results remain preliminary, however, because the probes were limited to types 6, 11, 16 and 18 and the plurality of HPVs that may infect the genital tract warrants that a larger scale of probes to obtain accurate correlation be used.[2, 22] Also, the morphologic criteria for low-grade genital lesions are

nohistochemical detection of antigen.[4, 32, 59, 90] *In situ* hybridization confirmed that HPV DNA is specifically localized in the nucleus of infected cells.[65] In many cases, HPV DNA sequences are present only focally in the epithelium. The amount of viral DNA detected increases towards terminally differentiated epithelial cells and koilocytes (Fig. 39–1).[4, 11, 79] In intraepithelial neoplasia, labeled cells are generally found in areas of cell differentiation;[17, 64, 65, 76] viral DNA rarely being detected in the parabasal cells (Fig. 39–2). In poorly differentiated, grade III intraepithelial neoplasia (without koilocytosis) and invasive carcinomas, it is often difficult to detect HPV DNA because it is often integrated into cellular target DNA.[11, 67, 76] *In situ* hybridization can also be used for localizing viral RNA transcription in individual cells or tissue sections.[19, 59, 79] In contrast to DNA detection, RNA detection is not confined to the nuclei but may also be present in the cytoplasm of infected cells.[19, 79] Early gene expression has been detected in basal epithelial cells in CIN and invasive carcinomas; however, the amount of HPV gene expression is inversely related to the degree of

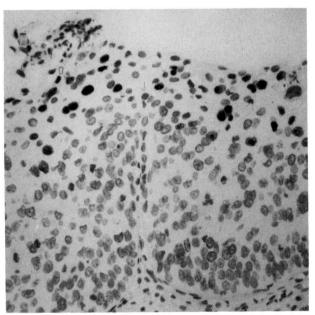

FIGURE 39–2. *In situ* **hybridization of cervical intraepithelial neoplasia 2 with a ³H/HPV 16 probe.** Numerous grains are found only in the superficial neoplastic cells' nuclei. The basal and parabasal layers are devoid of labeling (hematoxylin stain; ×350). (Courtesy of O. Croissant, Unité des Papillomavirus Institut Pasteur.)

still debated, a single biopsy may not have sampled the worst part of the lesion and ISH has significant false-negative rates. Also as mentioned previously, the limits of HPV DNA detection depend on conditions of hybridization and whether the viral genome is free or integrated in the host cell nuclei. The integrated genome gives a lower detection rate than the free viral genome.

In situ hybridization has also been employed to document the relative specificity of HPV type 18 in cervical glandular cells; HPV type 18 was found in most adenocarcinoma *in situ* (ACIS) and invasive carcinoma.[82, 83] *In situ* hybridization traced, furthermore, the same HPV type and HPV transcription level in intraepithelial squamous (CIN) or glandular (ACIS) and adjacent invasive squamous cell carcinoma and adenocarcinoma.[24, 89] The results support the concept of continuity between the aforementioned invasive carcinomas and their respective precursors.[24, 89] *In situ* hybridization is also helpful to document double or mixed infection for it can detect two HPV types in the same cell or different cells in serial sections.

HPV DNA has been reported in 10% of cases with histologically and cytologically normal squamous epithelium by Southern blot or dot blot hybridization.[23, 25] Detection of HPV DNA or mRNA in normal epithelium has never been reported with ISH. The discrepancy in these findings may reflect the limits of HPV DNA detection by ISH in situations of possible viral latency in which the copy number of viral DNA is very low and devoid of viral expression. Conversely, HPV DNA positivity by Southern blot may be a reflection of contaminated (viral shedding) normal epithelium from adjacent HPV lesion.[26] Perhaps searching for latent HPV DNA using PCR technology in sections adjacent to those tested by ISH may resolve the controversial latency issue.

Detection of HPV in Smears by ISH

In contrast to the biopsy, the Papanicolaou smear is a noninvasive technique. If taken appropriately,[58, 73] it samples extensively the cervix yet does not interfere with the biologic behavior of the lesion of interest. Therefore, it can be employed in prospective or retrospective studies for HPV cellular localization. In retrospective studies, it is particularly useful where usually no frozen tissue had been taken at the time of the original diagnosis, and biopsy specimens were fixed in Bouin's solution.

Genital HPVs have been first detected in smears by immunologic[33] and ultrastructural methods[38] in a small number of koilocytes. Most attempts at HPV typing in cervicovaginal smears have been performed by Southern or dot blot hybridizations.[50, 60, 75, 88] A few studies utilized radioactive ³H- or ³⁵S-labeled RNA or DNA probes.[31, 32, 52] Nonradiolabeled, biotinylated probes have as yet not been tried. Only one slide can be tested with ISH. As a result, individual slides have to be prepared according to the number of probes to be tested in the same cervical specimen. Cytospin prepa-

rations obtained from scraped cells collected in PBS and fixed in PLPG can be tested by ISH as well.

A good correlation exists between HPV DNA detection and presence of koilocytosis in a smear (Fig. 39–3). However, HPV infection is detected based on koilocytosis more frequently by routine cytologic screening than by ISH.[31, 32, 52] Hybridization signal is rarely positive in poorly differentiated neoplastic cells

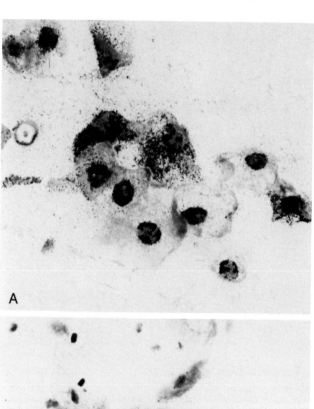

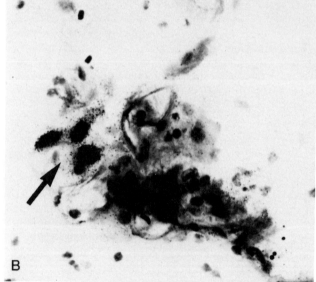

FIGURE 39–3. *A, **In situ** hybridization of a smear with ³H/HPV 39 probe.* Most of the intermediate and superficial koilocytotic cells' nuclei are labeled. Note the irregular clumping and nuclear margination of the grain distribution. The patient had a grade I cervical intraepithelial neoplasia in the cervical biopsy specimen (Papanicolaou stain; ×450). *B **In situ** hybridization of a smear with ³H/HPV 33 probe.* Only three koilocytotic cells' nuclei are heavily labeled (arrow) in this field. The adjacent morphologically similar nuclei are negative. The patient had cervical intraepithelial neoplasia grade II in the cervical biopsy specimen (Papanicolaou stain; ×450).

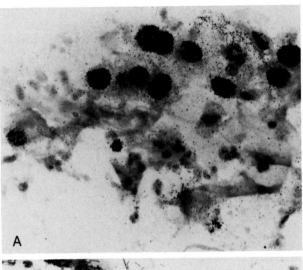

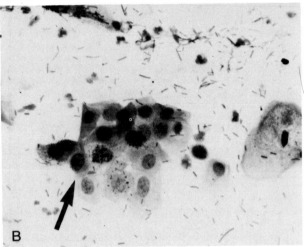

FIGURE 39–4. *A, In situ* **hybridization of a smear with ³H/HPV 35 probe.** Many nuclei of the neoplastic parabasal cells are strongly positive. The patient had grade III cervical intraepithelial neoplasia in the cervical biopsy specimen. (Papanicolaou stain; ×450). *B, In situ* **hybridization of a smear with ³H/HPV 16 probe.** Only three abnormal nuclei are labeled (arrow) in this group of parabasal cells. The patient had a grade III cervical intraepithelial neoplasia in the cervical biopsy specimen (Papanicolaou stain; ×450).

(Fig. 39–4), and HPV DNA is not detected by ISH in true negative smears. Because of the limited experience with ISH as applied to cytologic smears, the results should be considered preliminary at best. Also, the number of probes has been limited to 6, 11, 16 and 18. This may explain the higher yield of HPV detection by cytopathology than by ISH. At present, ISH in routine cytopathologic practice is not cost-effective.

Future Considerations for Using ISH

These, in routine practice, may include both cytology and histology. Technology should focus on reducing costs and improving the sensitivity of nonradioactive probes. Then the ISH method may be of great help in ascertaining cytologically and histologically equivocal HPV infections. These include questionable cytologic squamous atypia on routine smears and acetowhite lesions of the external anogenital epithelium, respectively. Ascertainment of their HPV relatedness has obvious clinical importance particularly as far as the management of HPV infections is concerned. Analysis of smears with ISH may also help to verify the light microscopic features considered to be specific for HPV

infections as well as the true significance of parakeratosis, hyperkeratosis and dyskeratosis of intermediate cells in relationship to HPV infections. As such, ISH may be of value for assessing the diagnostic expertise (quality control) of both the cytologic screener and the pathologist. *In situ* hybridization by virtue of its unique capability for tracing HPV DNA in routine histologic sections may contribute significantly to our insight into the cellular mechanisms of HPV infection and possibly lower genital carcinogenesis.

CONCLUSIONS

In situ hybridization is a method based on detecting nucleic acids in cells in either histologic tissue sections or smears. It is the method of choice to trace viral genome and its transcripts including HPV in possible target cells. *In situ* hybridization is also helpful to detect HPV nucleic acids in lesions in which only a very few cells harbor viral copies or when only alcohol-fixed Papanicolaou smears or formalin-fixed tissues are available, such as in retrospective studies. However, the relatively low sensitivity and high cost of ISH preclude its use in routine diagnostic practice for either cytologic screening or gynecologic pathology. Rather its primary role at present may be in resolving specific diagnostic problems involved with "equivocal" HPV infections and may serve as an adjunct for quality control of diagnostic expertise in cytologic and pathologic laboratories. Future considerations in the field of ISH should include DNA amplification with PCR in adjacent tissue sections, which may provide better insight into our understanding of HPV-related genital carcinogenesis.

Acknowledgments. The authors are grateful to O. Croissant, Unité des Papillomavirus, Institut Pasteur, for her advice in the preparation of the manuscript and for Figures 39–1 and 39–2. Brigitte Rubat du Mérac and Rosemary Rollet have also assisted in the preparation of the manuscript.

References

1. Barasso R, De Brux J, Croissant O, Orth G: High prevalence of papillomavirus-associated penile intraepithelial neoplasia in sexual partners of women with cervical intraepithelial neoplasia. N Engl J Med 317:916–923, 1987.
2. Beaudenon S, Kremsdorf D, Obalek S, Jablonska G, Pehan-Arnaudet G, Croissant O, Orth G: Plurality of genital human papillomaviruses: Characterization of two viral types with distinct biological projection. Virology 161:374–384, 1987.
3. Beckmann AM, Daling JR, Sherman KJ, Maden C, Miller BA, Coates RJ, Kiviat NB, Myerson D, Weiss NS, Hislop TG, Beagrie M, McDougall JK: Human papillomavirus infection and anal cancer. Int J Cancer 43:1042–1049, 1989.
4. Beckmann AM, Myerson D, Daling JR, Kiviat NB, Fenoglio CM, McDougall JK: Detection and localization of human papillomavirus DNA in human genital condylomas by in situ hybridization with biotinylated probes. J Med Virol 16:265–273, 1985.
5. Boon ME, Fox CH: Simultaneous condyloma acuminatum and dysplasia of the uterine cervix. Acta Cytol 25:393–399, 1981.
6. Brigati DJ, Myerson D, Leary JJ, Spalholz B, Travis SZ, Fong CKY, Hsung GD, Ward DC: Detection of viral genomes in cultured cells and paraffin-embedded tissue sections using biotin-labeled hybridization procedures. Virology 126:32–50, 1983.
7. Broker TR, Chow LT: Human papillomaviruses of the genital mucosa: electron microscopic analysis of DNA heteroduplexes formed with HPV types 6, 11 and 18. In Cancer Cell. Edited by M Botchan, T Grodzicker, PH Sharp. New York, Cold Spring Harbor Laboratory, 589–594, 1986.
8. Buongiorno-Nardelli N, Amaldi T: Autoradiographic detection of molecular hybrids between RNA and DNA in tissue sections. Nature 225:946–948, 1970.
9. Burns J, Chan VTW, Jonasson JA, Fleming KA, Taylor S, McGee JOD: Sensitive system for visualizing biotinylated DNA probes hybridized in situ: rapid sex determination of intact cells. J Clin Pathol 38:1085–1092, 1985.
10. Casas-Cordero M, Morin C, Roy M, Fortier M, Meisels A: Origin of the koilocyte in condyloma of the human cervix: ultrastructural study. Acta Cytol 25:383–392, 1981.
11. Caussy D, Orr W, Daya D, Roth P, Reeves W, Rawls W: Evaluation of methods for detecting human papillomavirus deoxyribonucleotide sequences in clinical specimens. J Clin Microbiol 26:236–243, 1988.
12. Chollet A, Kawashima EH: Biotin-labeled synthetic oligodeoxyribonucleotides: Chemical synthesis and uses as hybridization probes. Nucl Acid Res 13:1529–1541, 1985.
13. Cox KH, Delcon DV, Angerer LM, Angerer RC: Detection of mRNAs in sea urchin embryos by in situ hybridization using asymmetric RNA probes. Devel Biol 101:485–502, 1984.
14. Croissant O, Breitburd F, Orth G: Specificity of cytopathic effects of cutaneous papillomaviruses. In Clinical Dermatology. Edited by S Jablonska, G Orth. Philadelphia, JB Lippincott, 43–55, 1985.
15. Croissant O, Dauguet C, Jeanteur P: Application de la technique d'hybridation moléculaire in situ à la mise en évidence au microscope electronique de la replication végétative de l'ADN viral dans les papillomes provoqués par le virus de Shope chez le lapin cottontail. CR Acad Sci (Paris) 274:614–617, 1972.
16. Crum CP, Ikenberg H, Richart RM, Gissmann L: Human papillomavirus type 16 and early cervical neoplasia. N Engl J Med 310:880–883, 1984.
17. Crum CP, Mitao M, Levine RU, Silverstein S: Cervical papillomavirus segregate within morphologically distinct precancerous lesions. J Virol 54:675–681, 1985.
18. Crum CP, Nagai N, Levine RU, Silverstein S: In situ hybridization analysis of HPV 16 DNA sequences in early cervical neoplasia. Am J Pathol 123:174–182, 1986.
19. Crum CP, Nuovo G, Friedman P, Silverstein SJ: A comparison of biotin and isotope-labeled ribonucleic acid probes for in situ detection of HPV 16 ribonucleic acid in genital precancers. Lab Invest 58:354–359, 1988.
20. Davanloo P, Rosenberg AH, Dunn JJ, Studier FW: Cloning and expression of the gene for bacteriophage T7 RNA polymerase. Proc Natl Acad Sci USA 81:2035–2039, 1984.
21. Del Mistro A, Braunstein JP, Halwer M, Koss LG: Identification of human papillomavirus types in male urethral condylomata acuminata by in situ hybridization. Hum Pathol 18:936–940, 1987.
22. De Villiers E: Heterogeneity of the human papillomavirus group. J Virol 63:4898–4903, 1989.
23. De Villiers EM, Wagner D, Schneider A, Wesh H, Miklaw H, Walrendorf J, Papendick V, Zur Hausen H: Human papillomavirus infections in women with and without abnormal cervical cytology. Lancet 2:703–706, 1987.
24. Farnaworth A, Laverty C, Stoler MH: Human papillomavirus messenger RNA expression in adenocarcinoma in situ of the uterine cervix. Int J Gynecol Pathol 8:321–330, 1989.
25. Ferenczy A, Braun L, Shah KV: Human papillomavirus (HPV) in condylomatous lesions of cervix. A comparative ultrastructural and immunohistochemical study. Am J Surg Pathol 5:661–670, 1981.
26. Ferenczy A, Mitao M, Nagai N, Silverstein SJ, Crum CP: Latent papillomavirus and recurring genital warts. N Engl J Med 313:784–7, 1985.
27. Fletcher S, Norval M: On the nature of the deep cell disturbances in human papillomavirus infection of the squamous cervical epithelium. Lancet 1:546–549, 1983.
28. Franquemont DW, Ward BE, Andersen WA, Crum CP: Prediction of "high-risk" cervical papillomavirus infection by biopsy morphology. Am J Clin Pathol 92:577–582, 1989.
29. Gissmann L: Papillomaviruses and their association with cancer in animals and man. Cancer Surv 3:161–181, 1984.
30. Green MR, Maniatis T, Melton DA: Human betaglobin pre-mRNA synthesized in vitro is accurately spliced in Xenopus oocyte nuclei. Cell 32:681–694, 1983.
31. Gupta J, Gendelman HE, Naghashfar Z, Gupta P, Rosenshein N, Sawada E, Woodruff JD, Shah K: Specific identification of human papillomavirus type in cervical smears and paraffin sections by in situ hybridization with radioactive probes: A preliminary communication. Int J Gynecol Pathol 4:211–218, 1985.
32. Gupta J, Gupta PK, Rosenshein N, Shah KV: Detection of human papillomavirus in cervical smears: A comparison of in situ hybridization, immunocytochemistry and cytopathology. Acta Cytol 31:387–396, 1987.
33. Gupta JW, Gupta PK, Shah KV, Kelly DP: Distribution of human papillomavirus antigen in cervicovaginal smears and cervical tissues. Int J Gynecol Pathol 2:160–170, 1983.
34. Gupta J, Pilotti S, Rilke F, Shah K: Association of human papillomavirus type 16 with neoplastic lesions of the vulva and other genital sites by in situ hybridization. Am J Pathol 127:206–215, 1987.
35. Gupta J, Pilotti S, Shah KV, De Palo G, Rilke F: Human papillomavirus–associated early vulvar neoplasia investigated by in situ hybridization. Am J Surg Pathol 11:430–434, 1987.
36. Haase A, Brahic M, Stowring L, Blum H: Detection of viral nucleic acids by in situ hybridization. Methods Virol 7:189–227, 1985.

37. Harper ME, Marselle LM, Gallo RC, Wong-Stahl F: Detection of lymphocytes expressing human T-lymphotropic virus type III in lymph nodes and peripheral blood from infected individuals by *in situ* hybridization. Proc Natl Acad Sci USA 83:772–776, 1986.

38. Hills E, Laverty CR: Electron microscopic detection of papilloma virus particles in selected koilocytotic cells in a routine cervical smear. Acta Cytol 1:53–56, 1979.

39. Hofler H, Childers H, Montminy MR, Lechan RM, Goodman RH, Wolfe HJ: *In situ* hybridization methods for the detection of somatostatin mRNA in tissue sections using antisense RNA probes. Histochem J 18:597–604, 1986.

40. Jenson AB, Rosenthal JD, Olson C, Pass F, Lancaster WD, Shah K: Immunologic relatedness of papillomaviruses from different species. J Natl Cancer Inst 64:494–500, 1980.

41. John H, Birnstiel ML, Jones KW: RNA DNA hybrids at the cytological level. Nature 223:582–587, 1969.

42. Julien C, Bazin A, Guyot B, Forestier F, Daffas F: Rapid prenatal diagnosis of Down's syndrome with *in situ* hybridization of fluorescent DNA probes. Lancet 2:863–864, 1986.

43. Kadish AS, Burk RD, Kress Y, Calderin S, Romney SL: Human papillomavirus of different types in precancerous lesions of the uterine cervix. Histologic, immunocytochemical and ultrastructural studies. Human Pathol 17:384–392, 1986.

44. Koss LG, Durfee GR: Unusual patterns of squamous epithelium of the uterine cervix: Cytologic and pathologic study of koilocytotic atypia. Ann NY Acad Sci 63:1245–1261, 1956.

45. Koutsky LA, Galloway DA, Holmes KK: Epidemiology of genital human papillomavirus infection. Epidemiol Rev 10:122–163, 1988.

46. Kurman R, Shah KH, Lancaster WD: Immunoperoxidase localization of papillomavirus antigens in cervical dysplasias and vulvar condylomas. Am J Obstet Gynecol 140:931–935, 1981.

47. Landegent JE, Jansen in de Wal N, Van Ommen GJB, Baas F, de Vijlder JJM, Van Duijn P, Van der Ploeg M: Chromosomal localization of a unique gene by nonautoradiographic *in situ* hybridization. Nature 317:175–177, 1985.

48. Lawrence JB, Singer RH: Quantitative analysis of *in situ* hybridization methods for the detection of actin gene expression. Nucl Acid Res 13:1777–1799, 1985.

49. Loning T, Mildle K, Foss HD: *In situ* hybridization for the detection of cytomegalovirus (CMV) infections. Application of biotinylated CMV-DNA probes on paraffin embedded specimen. Virchows Arch 409:777–790, 1986.

50. Lorincz AT, Temple GF, Patterson JA, Jenson AB, Kurman RJ, Lancaster WD: Correlation of cellular atypia and human papillomavirus deoxyribonucleic acid sequence in exfoliated cells of the uterine cervix. Obstet Gynecol 68:508–512, 1986.

51. Maniatis T, Fritsch EF, Sanbrock J: Molecular cloning. A laboratory manual. New York, Cold Spring Harbor Laboratory, 1982.

52. Mayelo V: Detection de papillomavirus dans des frottis exocervicaux par hybridation *in situ*: correlations cytopathologiques et virologiques. Thèse DEA, Université Paris XI, France, 1986–87.

53. McDougall JK, Dunn AR, Jones KW: *In situ* hybridization of adenovirus RNA and DNA. Nature 236:346–348, 1972.

54. McDougall JK, Myerson D, Beckmann AM: Detection of viral DNA and RNA by *in situ* hybridization. J Histochem Cytochem 34:33–38, 1986.

55. Meisels A, Fortin R, Roy M: Condylomatous lesions of cervix and vagina. I. Cytologic patterns. Acta Cytol 20:505–509, 1976.

56. Melton DA, Krieg PA, Rebagliati MR, Maniatis T, Zinn K, Green MR: Efficient *in vitro* synthesis phage SP6 promoter. Nucl Acid Res 12:7035–7041, 1984.

57. Mitao M, Nagai N, Levine RU, Silverstein SJ, Crum CP: Human papillomavirus type 16 infection: A morphological spectrum with evidence for late gene expression. Int J Gynecol Pathol 5:287–296, 1987.

58. Morell ND, Taylor JR, Snyder RN, Ziel NK, Saltz A, Willie S: False-negative cytology rates in patients in whom invasive cervical cancer subsequently developed. Obstet Gynecol 60:41–45, 1982.

59. Nagai N, Nuovo G, Friedman D, Crum CP: Detection of papillomavirus nuclei acids in genital precancers with the *in situ* hybridization technique. Int J Gynecol Pathol 6:366–379, 1987.

60. Neumann R, Heiles B, Zippel C, Eggers HJ, Zippel HH, Holzmann L, Schulz KD: Use of biotinylated DNA probes in screening cells obtained from cervical swabs for human papillomavirus DNA sequences. Acta Cytol 30:603–606, 1986.

61. Nuovo GJ, Richart RM: Buffered formalin is the superior fixative for the detection of HPV DNA by *in situ* hybridization analysis. Am J Pathol 134:837–842, 1989.

62. Nuovo G, Silverstein SJ: Methods in laboratory investigation. Comparison of formalin, buffered formalin and Bouin's fixation on the detection of human papillomavirus deoxyribonucleic acid from genital lesions. Lab Invest 59:720–724, 1988.

63. Orth G, Breitburd F, Favre M: Evidence for antigen determinants shared by the structural polypeptides (Slope) rabbit papillomavirus and human papillomaviral type 1. Virology 91:213–255, 1978.

64. Orth G, Croissant O: Papillomavirus et cancer humain. Bull Inst Pasteur 86:297–315, 1988.

65. Orth G, Jeanteur P, Croissant O: Evidence for and localization of vegetative viral DNA replication by autoradiographic detection of RNA/DNA hybrids in sections of tumors induced by Shope papilloma virus. Proc Natl Acad Sci USA 68:1876–1880, 1971.

66. Ostrow RS, Manias DA, Clark BA, Fukushima M, Okagaki T, Twiggs LB, Faras AJ: The analysis of carcinomas of the vagina for human papillomavirus DNA. Int J Gynecol Pathol 7:308–314, 1988.

67. Ostrow R, Manias D, Clark B, Okagaki T, Twiggs L, Faras A: Detection of human papillomavirus DNA in invasive carcinomas of the cervix by *in situ* hybridization. Cancer Res 47:649–653, 1987.

68. Pardue ML, Gall JG: Molecular hybridization of radioactive DNA to the DNA of cytological preparations. Proc Natl Acad USA 64:600–604, 1969.

69. Pinkel D, Straume T, Gray JW: Cytogenetic analysis using quantitative, high-sensitivity, fluorescence hybridization. Proc Natl Acad Sci USA 86:2934–2938, 1986.

70. Purola E, Savia E: Cytology of gynecologic condyloma acuminatum. Acta Cytol 21:26–31, 1977.

71. Raap AK, Geelen JL, Van der Meer JWM, Van de Rijke FM, Van der Boogaard P, Van der Ploeg M: Nonradioactive *in situ* hybridization for the detection of cytomegalovirus infections. Histochemistry 88:367–374, 1988.

72. Richart RM: Causes and management of cervical intraepithelial neoplasia. Cancer 60:1951–1959, 1987.

73. Richart RM, Vaillant HW: Influence of cell collection techniques upon cytological diagnosis. Cancer 18:1474–1478, 1965.

74. Roger AW: Techniques of autoradiography. Amsterdam, Elsevier/North Holland Biomedical Press, 1979.

75. Schneider A, Meinhardt G, De Villiers EM, Gissmann L: Sensitivity of the cytologic diagnosis of cervical condyloma in comparison with HPV DNA hybridization studies. Diagnos Cytopathol 3:250–255, 1987.

76. Schneider A, Oltersdorf T, Schneider V, Gissmann L: Distribution pattern of human papilloma virus 16 genome in cervical neoplasia by molecular *in situ* hybridization of tissue sections. Int J Cancer 39:717–721, 1987.

77. Shibata D, Fu YS, Gupta JW, Shah KV, Arnheim N, Martin WJ: Detection of human papillomavirus in normal and dysplastic tissue by polymerase chain reaction. Lab Invest 59:555–559, 1988.

78. Siseberg JW, Nedrud JG, Raab-Traub N, Hanes RA, Pagano JS: Epstein-Barr virus replication in oropharyngeal epithelial cells. N Engl J Med 310:1225–1230, 1984.

79. Stoler MH, Broker TR: *In situ* hybridization detection of human papillomavirus DNAs and messenger RNAs in genital condylomas and cervical carcinoma. Hum Pathol 17:1250–1258, 1986.

80. Sverdlov ED, Monastyrskaya GS, Guskova LI, Levitan TL, Scheichenko VI, Budowsky EI: Modification of cytidine residues with a bisulfite-O-methylhydroxylamine mixture. Biochem Biophys Acta 340:153–165, 1974.

81. Syrjänen KJ, Mäntyjärvi R, Väyrynen M, Yliskoski M, Syrjänen SM, Saarikoski S, Nurmi T, Parkkinen S, Castren O: Cervical smears in assessment of the natural history of human papillomavirus infections in prospectively followed women. Acta Cytol 31:855–865, 1987.

82. Tase T, Okagaki T, Clark BA, Manias DA, Ostrow RS, Twiggs

LB, Faras AJ: Human papillomavirus types and localization in adenocarcinoma and adenosquamous carcinoma of the uterine cervix: A study by *in situ* DNA hybridization. Cancer Res 48:993–998, 1988.

83. Tase T, Okagaki T, Clark B, Twiggs LB, Ostrow RS, Faras AT: Human papillomavirus DNA in glandular dysplasia and microglandular hyperplasia: presumed precursors of adenocarcinoma of the uterine cervix. Obstet Gynecol 73:1005–1008, 1989.

84. Terry RM, Lewis FA, Griffiths S, Wells M, Bird CC: Demonstration of human papillomavirus types 6 and 11 in juvenile laryngeal papillomatosis by *in situ* DNA hybridization. J Pathol 153:245–248, 1987.

85. Unger E, Budgeon LR, Myerson D, Brigati DJ: Viral diagnosis by *in situ* hybridization. Description of a rapid simplified colorimetric method. Am J Surg Pathol 10:1–8, 1986.

86. Vallejo H, Del Mistro A, Kleinhaus S, Braustein JD, Halwer M, Koss LG: Characterization of human papilloma virus types in condylomata acuminata in children by *in situ* hybridization. Lab Invest 56:611–615, 1987.

87. Van Prooijen-Knegt AC, Van Hoek JFM, Bauman JGJ, Van Duijn P, Wool IG, Van der Ploeg M: *In situ* hybridization of DNA sequences in human metaphase chromosomes visualized by an indirect fluorescent immunocytochemical procedure. Exp Cell Res 141:397–407, 1982.

88. Vermund SH, Schiffman MH, Goldberg GL, Ritter DB, Weltman A, Burk RD: Molecular diagnosis of genital human papillomavirus infection: Comparison of two methods used to collect exfoliated cervical cells. Am J Obstet Gynecol 160:304–308, 1989.

89. Wilbur DC, Bonfiglio TA, Stoler MH: Continuity of human papillomavirus (HPV) type between neoplastic precursors and invasive cervical carcinoma. Am J Surg Pathol 12:182–186, 1988.

90. Wilbur DC, Reichman RC, Stoler MH: Detection of infection by human papillomavirus in genital condyloma. A comparison study using immunocytochemistry and *in situ* nucleic acid hybridization. Am J Clin Pathol 89:505–510, 1988.

91. Winkler BW, Crum CP, Fujii T: Koilocytotic lesions of the cervix: the relationship of mitotic abnormalities to the presence of papillomavirus antigens and nuclear DNA content. Cancer 53:1081–1087, 1984.

92. Wolf H, Zur Hausen H, Becker V: EB viral genomes in epithelial nasopharyngeal carcinoma cells. Nature New Biology 244:245–247, 1973.

Index

Note: Page numbers in *italics* indicate illustrations; those followed by t indicate tables.

A

G